PROVIDED
AS AN
EDUCATIONAL
SERVICE BY

Aventis

makers of

allegra®
fexofenadine HCl
180 mg tablets

ALG-SK-7734-1

© 2003 Aventis Pharmaceuticals Inc.

The
5-Minute
Pediatric
Consult

Third Edition

The
5-Minute
Pediatric
Consult

Third Edition

EDITOR

M. WILLIAM SCHWARTZ, M.D.

EMERITUS PROFESSOR OF PEDIATRICS

UNIVERSITY OF PENNSYLVANIA SCHOOL OF MEDICINE

AND SENIOR PHYSICIAN AT

CHILDREN'S HOSPITAL OF PHILADELPHIA

PHILADELPHIA, PENNSYLVANIA

LIPPINCOTT WILLIAMS & WILKINS

A **Wolters Kluwer** Company

Philadelphia · Baltimore · New York · London
Buenos Aires · Hong Kong · Sydney · Tokyo

Acquisitions Editor: Timothy Y. Hiscock
Developmental Editor: Joyce A. Murphy
Supervising Editor: Mary Ann McLaughlin
Manufacturing Manager: Benjamin Rivera
Compositor: TechBooks
Printer: World Color/Rand McNally

© 2003 by LIPPINCOTT WILLIAMS & WILKINS
530 Walnut Street
Philadelphia, PA 19106 USA
LWW.com

First edition, 1997
Second edition, 2000

The 5-Minute Logo ® is a registered trademark of Lippincott Williams & Wilkins. This mark may not be used without written permission from the publisher.

Printed in the USA

Library of Congress Cataloging-in-Publication Data

The 5-minute pediatric consult / editor, M. William Schwartz.—3rd ed.
    p. ; cm.
  Includes bibliographical references and index.
  ISBN 0-7817-3539-4
  1. Pediatrics—Handbooks, manuals, etc. I. Title: Five-minute pediatric consult. II.
Schwartz, M. William, 1935–
  [DNLM: 1. Pediatrics—Handbooks. WS 39 Z99 2002]
  RJ48 .A15 2002
  618.92—dc21   2002030013

10 9 8 7 6 5 4 3 2 1

TO

Mitchell, Anna Rose, Samuel, Eli, Perri and Chloe
Devin, Sarah, Sean, Chris, Michael, Amy and Sue
Dana
Marlene, Jordan and Jamie
Dr. Ed Baik and OkHung, Dennis, Marissa and Emma
Marisa, Elias, Henry and Isabel and Adele and Sidney
Elyse, Nathaniel, and memory of Nathan and Martin
Brandie, Mitchell, Chloe, my parents and GG

Preface

The publication of the third edition prompts reflection of the six-year history of this project. The book is a success in many ways, fulfilling its original mission to present succinct information that can be viewed efficiently. The easily recognized pink cover maintains its prominent position in offices, emergency rooms, and reference shelves. The editors and authors still think that the manuscript preparation is a fun job. It is a great satisfaction to see the book in use, at times worn out from frequent usage, a great tribute to the concept of a 5-Minute Consult.

In addition to a source of medical knowledge, *The 5-Minute Pediatric Consult* is a sociological study. The *5-Minute Pediatric Consult* serves as a metaphor for the effect of the past 6 years on our lives. In the aging process, the book has gained weight, has lost some color, and has become more organized. There is the constant hope of weight loss and resolutions to trim the midsection. The new topics reflect issues and problems of these times. We still included some childhood infections, such as rubella, even though that disease is joining the historical curiosities. On the other side, unfortunately, chapters on smallpox and anthrax reflect the updated knowledge required for 21st century world problems. Chapters on West Nile Fever and Prion Disease are included, as they span many differential diagnoses. A new chapter on heroin intoxication reflects the recurrence of the changing conditions in the drug culture. The list of authors, who formerly hailed mainly from the Children's Hospital of Philadelphia, now includes many medical centers and offices, as they move on to new positions of responsibility, another sign of the maturing process. The dedication list also reflects the life events of the editors. The list of dedicatees includes new children, memories of parents and friends and a blended family.

In an effort to keep the book current, the bibliography of most chapters includes recent articles and reviews. Many of the chapters were rewritten by new authors, keeping the information accurate and fresh, plus most of the surgical topics in this edition have new authors.

This venture involves the work of over 100 authors who kept to the schedule, although several required serious threats to return the manuscripts. The Associate Editors—Lou Bell, Peter Bingham, Esther Chung, Mitchell Cohen, David Friedman and Andy Mulberg—worked hard to recruit authors and to edit their work to bring the book to completion on time. Charlie Schwartz helped organize the tables and offered practical advice about the content. Their work and interest made the project move along with a minimum of problems. Special kudos to Cheryl Kosmowski, managing editor, who kept the project in order, finding lost letters and files. She is an exceptional person. She kept her pleasant façade while turning into a real pest at times to keep the project on schedule.

Likewise the professionals at Lippincott Williams & Wilkins did their jobs with a high degree of professionalism. Joyce Murphy, once again, did an admirable job, getting the material ready for production. She reminds me of a hockey goalie, tough under pressure, while nothing gets past her. My thanks to her for all her efforts. Tim Hiscock, acquisitions editor, took special interest in this project, organizing its start and overseeing the progress of the preparation. He seems *almost* as proud of the project as the editors. Thanks, too, to the many staff members of Lippincott Williams and Wilkins who worked on the marketing, production, and distribution of this book. They are important team players contributing to the success of this book. This exceptional team of editors, authors, and support staff has my sincere gratitude for their hard work and talented efforts in producing this third edition.

M. William Schwartz, M.D.
Philadelphia, 2002

Contributing Authors

Unless otherwise indicated, faculty appointments are at the University of Pennsylvania School of Medicine, and hospital appointments are at Children's Hospital of Philadelphia, Pennsylvania.

AKINYEMI O. AJAYI, M.D.
Fellow
Pulmonary Medicine

JULIAN L. ALLEN, M.D.
Chief, Division of Pulmonary Medicine

CRAIG A. ALTER, M.D.
Assistant Professor of Pediatrics
Division of Endocrinology

TIMOTHY ANDREWS, M.D.
Fellow
Immunology

RAANAN ARENS, M.D.
Assistant Professor
Department of Pediatrics
Director Sleep Disorders Center
Division of Pulmonary Medicine

LEE R. ATKINSON, M.D.
Staff Physician Pediatrics
Stanford University Medical Center
Palo Alto, California
Staff Physician Pediatrics
Lucille Packard Children's Hospital
Palo Alto, California

J. CHRISTOPHER AUSTIN, M.D.
Department of Urology

PHILIPPE F. BACKELJAUW, M.D.
Associate Professor of Pediatrics
Division of Endocrinology
Children's Medical Center
Cincinnati, Ohio

MARK L. BAGARAZZI, M.D.
Assistant Professor
Department of Pediatrics
MCP Hahnemann School of Medicine
Philadelphia, Pennsylvania
Attending Physician
Department of Pediatrics
St. Christopher's Hospital for Children
Philadelphia, Pennsylvania

ROBERT N. BALDASSANO, M.D.
Associate Professor of Pediatrics
Division of Gastroenterology and Nutrition

MEENA SCAVENA BALDI, M.D.
Division of Neurology

LOUIS M. BELL, JR., M.D.
Professor
Department of Pediatrics
Chief, Division of General Pediatrics
Department of Pediatrics

DEIRDRE BERNARD-PEARL, M.D.
Assistant Clinical Professor
General Pediatrics
University of California San Francisco

LISA BERNARD-PEARL, M.D.
Clinical Instructor
Obstetrics Gynecology and Reproductive Sciences
University of California
San Francisco, California

A.G. CHRISTINA BERGQVIST, M.D.
Assistant Professor of Neurology and Pediatrics
Division of Neurology

AMANDA K. BERRY, M.S.N, C.R.N.P
Pediatric Nurse Practitioner
Division of Urology

ANITA BHANDARI, M.D.
Attending Pulmonologist

SUMIT BHARGAVA, M.D.
Pulmonary Fellow

LISA M. BIGGS, M.D.
Medical Director
General Pediatrics

PETER M. BINGHAM, M.D.
Associate Professor
Department of Pediatric Neurology
University of Vermont
Burlington, Vermont

GEOFFREY L. BIRD, M.D.
Division of Cardiology,
Department of Pediatrics
Division of Critical Care Medicine,
Department of Anesthesiology and Critical Care Medicine

NATHAN J. BLUM, M.D.
Assistant Professor of Pediatrics
Division of Developmental and Behavioral Pediatrics
The Children's Seashore House

JULIE A. BOOM, M.D.
Assistant Professor
Department of Pediatrics
Baylor College of Medicine
Houston, Texas

AMY R. BROOKS-KAYAL, M.D.
Assistant Professor
Departments of Neurology and Pediatrics
Attending Physician
Department of Pediatrics
Division of Neurology

KURT A. BROWN, M.D.
Assistant Professor of Pediatrics
Department of Pediatrics
Attending Physician
Division of Gastroenterology and Nutrition

VALERIE BROWN, M.D., PH.D.
Fellow
Department of Oncology

LEAH BURKE, M.D.
University of Vermont
Burlington, Vermont

JAMES M. CALLAHAN, M.D.
Associate Professor
Department of Emergency Medicine
SUNY-Upstate Medical University Syracuse
Attending Physician
Pediatric Emergency Department
University Hospital
Syracuse, New York

CARLA CAMPBELL, M.D., M.S.
Clinical Assistant Professor of Pediatrics
Department of Pediatrics
CoMedical Director
Lead Poisoning and Toxicology Clinic

DOUGLAS CANNING, M.D.
Director, Division of Urology

WILLIAM B. CAREY, M.D.
Clinical Professor of Pediatrics
Senior Physician
Division of General Pediatrics

CHRISTINE A. CARMAN-DILLON, M.D.
Plastic Surgery Fellow

MICHAEL C. CARR, M.D., PH.D.
Attending Urologist
Department of Urology

AARON E. CARROLL, M.D.
RWJ Fellow
Department of Pediatrics
University of Washington
School of Medicine
Seattle, Washington

SUZETTE SURRATT CAUDLE, M.D.
Clinical Associate Professor of Pediatrics
University of North Carolina
Chapel Hill, North Carolina
Residency Program Director
Department of Pediatrics
Carolinas Medical Center
Charlotte, North Carolina

ELIZABETH CANDELL CHALOM, M.D.
Director
Pediatric Lyme Disease Program
Section Head
Pediatric Rheumatology
St. Barnabas Medical Center
Director
Pediatric Rheumatology
Children's Hospital of New Jersey
Livingston, New Jersey

LISA CHAMBERLAIN, M.D., M.P.H.
Department of Pediatrics
Stanford University
Palo Alto, California

CINDY W. CHRISTIAN, M.D.
Associate Professor of Pediatrics
Chair, Child Abuse and Neglect Prevention
Department of Pediatrics

EMIL CHUANG, M.D.
Attending Physician
Gastroenterology and Nutrition

THOMAS H. CHUN, M.D.
Assistant Professor of Pediatrics
Brown University School of Medicine
Providence, Rhode Island
Attending Physician
Emergency Department
Hasbro Children's Hospital
Providence, Rhode Island

ESTHER K. CHUNG, M.D., M.P.H.
Assistant Professor of Pediatrics
Thomas Jefferson University
Philadelphia, Pennsylvania

SUSAN SOHN CHUNG, M.D.
Department of Pediatrics
University of California San Francisco
San Francisco, California

RUSSELL G. CLAYTON, SR., D.O.
Assistant Professor of Pulmonology
Pulmonologist

MICHELE CLEMENT, M.D.
Urology

SUSAN E. COFFIN, M.D.
Assistant Professor of Pediatrics
Section of Infectious Diseases
Assistant Physician
Department of Pediatrics

MERYL S. COHEN, M.D.
Assistant Professor of Pediatrics
Department of Pediatric Cardiology

MITCHELL I. COHEN, M.D.
Arizona Pediatric Cardiology Consultant
Phoenix, Arizona

ROBERT M. COHN, M.D.
Deputy Director
Clinical Laboratories

PAULO F. COLLETT-SOLBERG, M.D.
Fellow
Division of Endocrinology

DANIEL H. CONWAY, M.D.
Assistant Professor of Pediatrics
St. Christopher's Hospital for Children
MCP/Hahnemann School of Medicine
Philadelphia, Pennsylvania

LUCY CRAIN, M.D.
Department of Pediatrics
University of San Francisco, California

PETER B. CRINO, M.D., PH.D.
Department of Neurology
University of Pennsylvania Medical Center
Philadelphia, Pennsylvania

RANDY Q. CRON, M.D., PH.D.
Assistant Professor of Pediatrics
Department of Rheumatology
Fellowship Director
Division of Rheumatology

MONICA DARBY, M.D.
Pharmacologist

RICHARD S. DAVIDSON, M.D.
Associate Professor of Orthopaedic Surgery
Department of Orthopaedic Surgery

MARK F. DITMAR, M.D.
Hospitalist
Atlantic City Hospital
Alfred I. Dupont Children's Hospital
Wilmington, Delaware

DENNIS J. DLUGOS, M.D.
Assistant Professor in Neurology
Departments of Neurology and Pediatrics

JOHN P. DORMANS, M.D.
Associate Professor of Orthopaedic Surgery
Chief of Orthopaedic Surgery

HENRY R. DROTT, PH.D.
Director
Clinical Chemistry Laboratory

DENNIS R. DURBIN, M.D.
Assistant Professor of Pediatrics and Epidemiology
Department of Pediatrics

NANCY DRUCKER, M.D.
Associate Professor
Department of Pediatrics
University of Vermont
Burlington, Vermont

JOEL A. FEIN, M.D.
Associate Professor of Pediatrics and Emergency Medicine
Attending Physician
Emergency Department

ROBERT J. FERRY, JR., M.D.
Assistant Professor-in-Residence
Department of Pediatrics
University of California Los Angeles School of Medicine
Attending Pediatric Endocrinologist
Division of Pediatric Endocrinology
Mattel Children's Hospital at UCLA
Los Angeles, California

RICHARD S. FINKEL, M.D.
Clinical Associate Professor
Department of Pediatrics and Neurology
Director, Neuromuscular Program
Department of Pediatrics

MICHAEL J. FISHER, M.D.
Department of Hematology and Oncology
University of Miami
Miami, Florida

JONATHAN FLEENOR, M.D.
Cardiology Fellow
Department of Cardiology

JOHN M. FLYNN, M.D.
Assistant Professor of Orthopedics
Associate Surgeon

BRIAN J.R. FORBES, M.D., PH.D.
Assistant Professor
Department of Ophthalmology
Pediatric Ophthalmologist
Department of Ophthalmology

JILL A. FOSTER, M.D.
Assistant Professor of Pediatrics
Allegheny University of the Health Sciences
Attending Physician
St. Christopher's Hospital for Children
Philadelphia, Pennsylvania

DAVID F. FRIEDMAN, M.D.
Clinical Assistant Professor
Division of Pediatric Hematology
Associate Director
Transfusion Services

DEBRA L. FRIEDMAN, M.D.
Assistant Clinical Professor
Department of Pediatrics
University of Washington School of Medicine
Children's Hospital and Regional Medical Center
Seattle, Washington

THEODORE J. GANLEY, M.D.
Assistant Professor of Orthopedics
Associate Surgeon of Pediatric Orthopedics

LYNETTE A. GILLIS, M.D.
Gastrointestinal Fellow

JILL P. GINSBERG, M.D.
Assistant Professor
Department of Pediatrics
Attending Physician
Division of Oncology

KENNETH R. GINSBURG, M.D., MS ED.
Assistant Professor of Pediatrics
Department of Pediatrics
Physician
Division of Adolescent Medicine

SCOTT M. GOLDSTEIN, D.O.
Ophthalmology Fellow

JOHN M. GOOD, M.D.
Department of Pediatrics
Lovelace Health Care Centers
Rio Rancho, New Maxico

MARC H. GORELICK, M.D.
Associate Professor of Pediatrics
Medical College of Wisconsin
Children's Hospital of Wisconsin
Milwaukee, Wisconsin

JANE M. GOULD, M.D.
Fellow
Department of Pediatric Infectious Diseases

WILLIAM R. GRAESSLE, M.D.
Assistant Professor
Department of Pediatrics
UMDNJ–Robert Wood Johnson Medical School–Camden
Camden, New Jersey
Director, Pediatric Medical Education
Department of Pediatrics
Cooper Hospital
Camden, New Jersey

ERNEST M. GRAHAM, M.D.
Assistant Professor
Department of Obstetrics and Gynecology
Johns Hopkins University School of Medicine
Baltimore, Maryland

JEANNE GREENBLATT, M.D.
Clinical Assistant Professor
Department of Psychiatry
University of Vermont

ADDA GRIMBERG, M.D.
Assistant Professor
Department of Pediatrics
Attending Physician
Division of Pediatric Endocrinology and Diabetes

BLAZE ROBERT GUSIC, M.D.
Instructor in Pediatrics
Department of Pediatrics
Attending Physician

BARBARA HABER, M.D.
Assistant Professor of Pediatrics
Department of Pediatrics

J. NATHAN HAGSTROM, M.D.
Assistant Professor
Department of Pediatrics
University of Connecticut
Farmington, Connecticut
Director
Hemostasis Program
Connecticut Children's Medical Center
Hartford, Connecticut

CHERYL L. HAUSMAN, M.D.
Medical Director
Primary Care Center of University City

MARK L. HELPIN, D.M.D.
Chief, Pediatric Dentistry

M. ELIZABETH HERNANDEZ, M.D.
Pulmonary Fellow

AMY HIRSHFELD, M.D.
Instructor
Department of Pediatrics
Fellow in Cardiology

TIMOTHY M. HOFFMAN, M.D.
Assistant Professor of Pediatrics
Division of Cardiology
Columbus Children's Hospital
The Ohio State University College of Medicine
Columbus, Ohio

MICHAEL D. HOGARTY, M.D.
Assistant Professor
Department of Pediatrics
Division of Oncology

SHELLY D. HOLSTRUM, M.D.
Department of Child Development

ZEV JACOBSON, M.D.
Cardiology Fellow

CYNTHIA R. JACOBSTEIN, M.D.
Instructor
Department of Pediatrics
Fellow
Division of Pediatric Emergency Medicine

STEPHANIE D. JAMES, M.D.
Primary Care and General Pediatrics

HELEN ANITA JOHN-KELLY, M.D.
Pediatric Gastroenterologist
Raymond Blank Children's Hospital
Des Moines, Iowa

ROBERT KAMEI, M.D.
Director
Pediatric Residency Training Program
Associate Professor of Clinical Pediatrics
University of California San Francisco
San Francisco, California

PETER B. KANG, M.D.
Fellow
Department of Neurology

TAMMY I. KANG, M.D.
Hematology Fellow
Department of Hematology

DOUGLAS KATZ, M.D.
St. Christopher's Hospital for Children
Philadelphia, Pennsylvania

LORRAINE KATZ, M.D.
Assistant Professor
Division of Endocrinology and Diabetes

ANDREA KELLY, M.D.
Assistant Professor
Department of Pediatrics

KARA M. KELLY, M.D.
Assistant Professor of Pediatrics
College of Physicians and Surgeons of Columbia University
Assistant Attending Physician
Division of Pediatric Oncology
The New York Presbyterian Hospital
New York, New York

THOMAS L. KENNEDY III, M.D.
Professor of Clinical Pediatrics
Department of Pediatrics
The Yale University School of Medicine
New Haven, Connecticut
Chairman
Department of Pediatrics
Bridgeport Hospital
Bridgeport, Connecticut

HO JIN KIM, M.D.
Clinical Assistant Professor of Dermatology
University of Virginia
McLean, Virginia

RICHARD E. KIRSCHNER, M.D.
Attending Surgeon
Director, Plastic Surgery Research

MICHELLE M. KLINEK, M.D.
Chief of Clinical Immunology and Asthma
Family Center for Allergy and Asthma
York, Pennsylvania

THOMAS F. KOLON, M.D.
Assistant Professor
Department of Urology
Assistant Professor
Department of Pediatric Urology

RICHARD MARK KRAVITZ, M.D.
Assistant Professor of Pediatrics
Department of Pediatrics
Division of Pediatric Pulmonary Diseases
Duke University Medical Center
Durham, North Carolina

REBECCA KRAYNAK, M.D.
Gastro-Intestinal

JANE M. LAVELLE, M.D.
Associate Professor
Department of Pediatrics
Attending Physician
Department of Emergency Medicine/Pediatrics

HAE-RHI LEE, M.D.
Clinical Assistant Professor
Department of Pediatric Cardiology
Clinical Associate
Department of Pediatric Cardiology

MARY B. LEONARD, M.D.
Assistant Professor of Pediatrics and Epidemiology

CHRIS A. LIACOURAS, M.D.
Associate Professor in Pediatrics
Director of Pediatric Endoscopy
Division of Gastroenterology and Nutrition

DANIEL J. LICHT, M.D.
Instructor in Neurology
Pediatrics Division
Child Neurology

JANET M. LI-TEMPEST, M.D.
Pediatrician
Gallup Indian Medical Center
Gallup, New Mexico

KAREN LIQUORNIK, M.D.
Fellow
Division of Gastroenterology

KATHLEEN M. LOOMES, M.D.
Fellow
Department of Gastroenterology and Nutrition

JEFFREY P. LOUIE, M.D.
Clinical Instructor
Childrens Hospital and Clinics
University of Minnesota
St. Paul, Minnesota

GRANT T. LIU, M.D.
Neuro-Ophthalmologist
Division of Ophthalmology

GORDANA LOVREKOVIC, M.D.
Pulmonary Fellow

DAVID W. LOW, M.D.
Associate Professor of Surgery
Hospital of the University of Pennsylvania
Division of Plastic Surgery
Philadelphia, Pennsylvania

ERIC S. MALLER, M.D.
Associate Director
GI Clinical Research
Merck Research Labs
Whitehouse Station, New Jersey

PETAR MAMULA, M.D.
Assistant Professor of Pediatrics
Division of Gastroenterology

BRADLEY S. MARINO, M.D., M.P.P.
Assistant Professor
Departments of Pediatric
Critical Care Medicine,
Pediatric Cardiology, Anesthesia and Critical Care Medicine, Pediatrics

MARIA R. MASCARENHAS, M.B.B.S.
Associate Professor of Pediatrics
Division of Gastroenterology and Nutrition
Department of Pediatrics
Director
Nutrition Support Services

JONATHAN E. MARKOWITZ, M.D.
Assistant Professor
Department of Pediatrics
Director, Inpatient Gastroenterology
Division of GI and Nutrition

TODD MAUGANS, M.D.
Assistant Professor
University of Vermont
Department of Neurosurgery

OSCAR HENRY MAYER, M.D.
Clinical Associate
Division of Pulmonary Medicine
Department of Pediatrics
Attending Physician
Division of Pulmonary Medicine
Department of Pediatrics

ANDREA McGEARY, M.D.
Attending Physician
Primary Care, Cobbs Creek

MARGARET McNAMARA, M.D.
Assistant Clinical Professor
Department of Pediatrics
University of California San Francisco
San Francisco, California

D. ELIZABETH McNEIL, M.D.
Division of Neurology

KEVIN E.C. MEYERS, M.D.
Pediatric Nephrologist
Department of Pediatrics

LISA MICHAELS, M.D.

MONTE D. MILLS, D.O.
Professor of Ophthalmology
Chief, Pediatric Ophthalmology

JANE E. MINTURN, M.D.
Hematology Fellow

ROBERT MARKHAM MITCHELL, M.D.
Private Practice
Loveladies, New Jersey

NAHUSH A. MOKADAM, M.D.

CYNTHIA J. MOLLEN, M.D.
Assistant Professor of Pediatrics
Division of Emergency Medicine

THOMAS J. MOLLEN, M.D.
Assistant Professor of Pediatrics
Division of Neonatology

ANDREW E. MULBERG, M.D.
Associate Professor of Pediatrics
Director, Pediatric Drug Development
Johnson and Johnson Pharmaceutical Research and Development
Titusville, New Jersey

LAURA T. MULREANY, M.D.
Pulmonary Fellow

MICHAEL P. MULREANY, M.D.
Children's Hospital of Philadelphia
Fellow-Cardiology

FRANCES M. NADEL, M.D.
Assistant Professor
Department of Pediatrics
Attending Physician, Emergency Medicine
Department of Pediatrics

KEITH NAGLE, M.D.
Assistant Professor of Neurology
University of Vermont
Burlington, Vermont

DIVA D. NG, M.D.

JULIEANA NICHOLS, M.D.
Baylor College of Medicine,
Academic Department of Pediatrics
Texas Children's Hospital
Houston, Texas

MICHAEL E. NORMAN, M.D.
Department of Pediatrics
Carolinas Medical Center
Charlotte, North Carolina

CYNTHIA F. NORRIS, M.D.
Clinical Associate in Pediatrics
Division of Hematology
Department of Pediatrics

KEVIN C. OSTERHOUDT, M.D.
Assistant Professor of Pediatrics
Attending Physician
Division of Pediatric Emergency Medicine

RITA PANOSCHA, M.D.
Clinical Assistant Professor
Department of Developmental Pediatrics
Children's Seashore House
Philadelphia, Pennsylvania

ELENA PEREZ, M.D., PH.D.
Fellow
Immunology

NADJA PETER, M.D.
Instructor
Department of Adolescent Medicine/Pediatrics
Co-Medical Director
Adolescent Care Center

SHANNON CONNOR PHILLIPS, M.D.
Clinical Assistant Professor
Department of Pediatrics
Indiana University School of Medicine
Indianapolis, Indiana

STEPHAN G. PILL, M.D.
Department of Orthopedics

JONATHAN R. PLETCHER, M.D.
Fellow
Division of Adolescent Medicine

ANN PODURI, M.D.
Fellow
Department of Neurology

BRENDA PORTER, M.D., Ph.D.
Post Doctoral Fellow
Division of Child Neurology

JILL C. POSNER, M.D., M.S.C.E.
Assistant Professor of Pediatrics
Department of Pediatrics
Attending Physician
Emergency Department

GRAHAM E. QUINN, M.D.
Professor of Ophthalmology
Attending Ophthalmologist
Division of Ophthalmology

LESLIE RAFFINI, M.D.
Fellow
Hematology

KRYSTAL REVAI, M.D.
University of Texas
Medical Branch
Division of General Academic Pediatrics
Galveston, Texas

SUSAN R. RHEINGOLD, M.D.
Assistant Professor
Department of Pediatrics
Director of Fellowship Education
Division of Oncology

PAMELA S. RO, M.D.
Cardiology Fellow
Pediatric Cardiology

HOWARD M. ROSENBERG, D.D.S., M.ED.
Department of Pediatric Dentistry

RICHARD M. RUTSTEIN, M.D.
Associate Professor of Pediatrics
Department of Pediatrics
Associate Division
Chief
Division of General Pediatrics

DENISE A. SALERNO, M.D.
Temple University
Children's Medical Center
Philadelphia, Pennsylvania

ZUHAIR SAYANY, D.M.D.
Pediatric Dentistry

THOMAS F. SCANLIN, M.D.
Professor of Pediatrics
Director, Cystic Fibrosis Center
Department of Pediatrics

SETH L. SCHULMAN, M.D.
Associate Professor
Department of Pediatrics and Surgery
Attending Physician
Divisions of Nephrology and Urology

CHARLES I. SCHWARTZ, M.D.
Assistant Clinical Professor
Department of Pediatrics
General Pediatrician
Department of Pediatrics
Phoenixville Hospital
Phoenixville, Pennsylvania

M. WILLIAM SCHWARTZ, M.D.
Emeritus Professor of Pediatrics
Senior Physician

MITCHELL SCHWARTZ, M.D.
Private Practice
Philadelphia, Pennsylvania

PHILIP V. SCRIBANO, D.O.
Assistant Professor
Department of Pediatrics
University of Connecticut School of Medicine
Farmington, Connecticut
Attending Physician
Division of Emergency Medicine
Connecticut Children's Medical Center
Hartford, Connecticut

STEVEN M. SELBST, M.D.
Professor and Vice Chairman
Director
Pediatric Residency Program
Jefferson Medical College of Thomas Jefferson University
Philadelphia, Pennsylvania
Attending Physician
Division of Emergency Medicine
A.I. Dupont Hospital for Children
Wilmington, Delaware

EDISIO SEMEAO, M.D.
Attending Physician
Department of Gastroenterology

TIMOTHY A.S. SENTONGO, M.D.
Assistant Professor
Division of Gastro-Enterology, Hepatology & Nutrition
Children's Memorial Hospital
Chicago, Illinois

SAMIR S. SHAH, M.D.
Instructor
Department of Pediatrics
Fellow
Divisions of General Pediatrics and Infectious Diseases

KATHY N. SHAW, M.D., M.S.C.E.
Associate Professor of Pediatrics
Director
Emergency Medical Services
Chief
Division of Emergency Medicine

ASEEM SHUKLA, M.D.
Fellow
Department of Urology

SUZANNE SHUSTERMAN, M.D.
Fellow
Department of Hematology and Oncology

EMILY L. SIEGE, M.D.
Fellow
Department of Urology

DEBORAH L. SILVER, M.D.
Clinical Assistant Professor
Department of Pediatrics
Medical Director
CHOP Connection at Abington Memorial Hospital
Abington, Pennsylvania

LAURA N. SINAI, M.D.
Pediatrician
Erdenheim Pediatrics
Abington Memorial Hospital
Abington, Pennsylvania

CHRISTOPHER A. SMITH, M.D.
Staff Physician
Department of Pediatrics
Cayuga Medical Center
Ithaca, New York

KIM SMITH-WHITLEY, M.D.
Assistant Professor of Pediatrics
Attending Physician
Division of Hematology

HOWARD M. SNYDER, M.D.
Associate Chief
Division of Urology

H. LYNN STARR, M.D.
Associate Director
Medical and Regulatory Science
McNeil Consumer and Specialty Pharmaceuticals

SCOTT STEM, M.D.
Fellow

JULIE W. STERN, M.D.
Fellow
Department of Hematology and Oncology

NICOLAS STETTLER, M.D., M.S.C.E.
Department of Gastroenterology and Nutrition

CATHERINE B. SULLIVAN, M.D.
Clinical Staff Associate
Department of Pediatrics

KATHLEEN E. SULLIVAN, M.D., PH.D.
Attending Physician
Department of Infectious Diseases

RONN E. TANEL, M.D.
Assistant Professor
Department of Pediatrics
Attending Cardiologist
Division of Cardiology

JOHN I. TAKAYAMA, M.D.
Associate Clinical Professor
Department of Pediatrics
University of California San Francisco
San Francisco, California

DANNA TAUBER, M.D., M.P.H.
Fellow
Division of Pulmonary Medicine

GREGORZ TELEGA, M.D.
Assistant Professor of Pediatrics
Medical Director of the Pediatric Liver Transplant Program
Medical Director of Pediatric Liver Disease Clinic
Division of Pediatric Gastroenterology
Department of Pediatrics
Gastroenterology Clinic
Children's Hospital of Wisconsin
Milwaukee, Wisconsin

BRUCE TEMPEST, M.D., M.A.C.P.
Consultant
Gallup Indian Medical Center
Indian Health Service (USPHS)
Gallup, New Mexico

OLAFUR THORARENSEN, M.D.
Department of Neurology

PAUL S. THORNTON, M.B.B.S.
Division of Pediatric Endocrinology

NICHOLAS TSAROUHAS, M.D.
Clinical Assistant Professor of Pediatrics
Department of Pediatrics
Attending Physician
Department of Pediatric Emergency Medicine

JOHN TUNG, M.D.
Pediatric Hepatologist
Department of Gastroenterology
Alfred I. Dupont Hospital for Children
Wilmington, Delaware

PAUL P. WANG, M.D.
Assistant Professor of Pediatrics
Divisions of Child Development and Neurology
Attending Physician

DROR WASSERMAN
Tel Aviv, Israel

BARBARA WATSON, M.D.
Director of Vaccine Evaluation
Department of Pediatrics
Albert Einstein Medical Center
Medical Immunization Specialist
Division of Disease Control
Philadelphia Department of Public Health
Philadelphia, Pennsylvania

STUART A. WEINZIMER, M.D.
Assistant Professor of Pediatrics
Division of Endocrinology and Diabetes

GEORGE ANTHONY WOODWARD, M.D., M.B.A.
Associate Professor
Department of Pediatrics
Medical Director, Section of Transport Medicine
Division of Emergency Medicine

HSI-YANG WU, M.D.
Assistant Professor
Department of Urology
University of Pittsburgh
Attending Physician
Department of Pediatric Urology
Children's Hospital of Pittsburgh
Pittsburgh, Pennsylvania

ALBERT C. YAN, M.D.
Pediatric Dermatology

THEOKLIS ZAOUTIS, M.D.
Instructor
Department of Pediatrics
Senior Fellow
Infectious Diseases

STEPHEN A. ZDERIC, M.D.
Assistant Professor of Pediatrics
Division of Urology

RAEZELLE ZINMAN, M.D.
Attending Pulmonologist

KATHY WHOLEY ZSOLWAY, D.O.
Assistant Professor of Pediatrics

Contents

SECTION III: SYNDROMES GLOSSARY / 893

SECTION IV: CARDIOLOGY LABORATORY / 899

Timothy M. Hoffman

SECTION V: SURGICAL GLOSSARY / 907

Aaron E. Carroll, Nahush A. Mokadam

SECTION VI: LABORATORY VALUES / 911

Henry R. Drott

SECTION VII: TABLES / 915

DEVELOPMENT

IMMUNIZATION

FEEDING AND NUTRITION

INFECTIOUS DISEASES

SECTION I
Chief Complaints

Abdominal Mass

 Database

DEFINITION

An abdominal mass is defined as either an unusually enlarged abdominal organ (i.e., hepatomegaly, splenomegaly, or an enlarged kidney) or a defined fullness in the abdominal cavity not directly associated with an abdominal organ.

 Differential Diagnosis

STOMACH

- Gastroparesis
- Duplication
- Foreign body/bezoar
- Gastric torsion

SPLEEN

- Infiltrative disease (Gaucher, Niemann-Pick)
- Histiocytosis X
- Leukemia
- Hematologic (hemolytic disease, sickle cell disease, hereditary spherocytosis/elliptocytosis)

INTESTINE

- Feces (constipation)
- Duplication
- Volvulus
- Intussusception
- Inflammatory bowel disease complications (abscess, phlegmon)
- Toxic megacolon
- Mesenteric/omental cyst
- Lymphoma
- Foreign body
- Appendiceal abscess

PANCREAS

- Pseudocyst (trauma)

LIVER

- Endocrinologic (glycogen storage disease)
- Infectious (hepatitis A, B, C)
- Congenital hepatic fibrosis
- Tumor (neuroblastoma, Wilms, leukemia)
- Vascular (hemangioma, hemangioendothelioma)

BLADDER

- Urethral valves
- Neurogenic bladder

OVARY

- Dermoid
- Follicular cyst
- Torsion
- Gonadal tumor

KIDNEY

- Hydronephrosis/ureteropelvic obstruction[1]
- Polycystic/multicystic disease[1]
- Wilms tumor
- Renal vein thrombosis
- Nephroblastomatosis

PERITONEAL

- Ascites
- Teratoma

UTERUS

- Pregnancy
- Hydrometrocolpos

ADRENAL

- Neuroblastoma
- Adrenal hemorrhage
- Pheochromocytoma

GALLBLADDER

- Choledochal cyst
- Hydrops
- Obstruction (stone, stricture, trauma)

ABDOMINAL WALL

- Umbilical/inguinal/ventral hernia
- Omphalocele/gastroschisis
- Trauma (rectus hematoma)
- Tumor (fibroma, lipoma, rhabdomyosarcoma)

OTHER

- Mesenteric cyst
- Omental cyst
- Lymphangioma

Approach to the Patient

GENERAL GOALS

Often, abdominal masses in children are found by an unsuspecting parent or by a physician during a routine physical examination. Most masses have no specific signs or symptoms. In children, abdominal masses require immediate attention. When evaluating a pediatric abdominal mass, an organized approach is paramount in determining its etiology.

Phase 1: Determine the location of the abdominal mass and its association with intraabdominal organs.

Phase 2: Perform diagnostic tests; the abdominal ultrasound is the most efficient way to start the evaluation.

Phase 3: Treatment (see Laboratory Aids)

[1] Most common in newborns

 Data Gathering

HISTORY

Question: Frequency and quality of bowel movements?
Significance: Constipation, intussusception

Question: History of abdominal trauma?
Significance: Pancreatic pseudocyst

Question: History of weight loss?
Significance: Tumor, posterior urethral valves, inflammatory bowel disease

Question: Presence of jaundice?
Significance: Liver/biliary disease

Question: Hematuria or dysuria?
Significance: Renal disease

Question: Sexual activity?
Significance: Pregnancy

Question: Fever?
Significance: Abscess

Question: What is the age of the patient?
Significance: The age of the patient is often a helpful clue in investigating the cause of the abdominal mass. The most common types of abdominal mass in newborns include renal disease (cystic kidney disease, renal vein thrombosis, hydronephrosis), adrenal hemorrhage, congenital anomalies, and teratoma. In preschool-aged children and adolescents, approximately 20% of abdominal masses arise from the gastrointestinal tract, while 5% have their origin in the liver or biliary tree. Wilms tumor typically occurs in preschool-aged children, while ovarian disorders present in adolescents.

Physical Examination

Finding: Location of the mass
Significance:

- Left upper quadrant mass typically involves the kidney or spleen
- Right upper quadrant mass involves the liver or gallbladder or indicates a choledochal cyst
- Right lower quadrant mass indicates an abscess (inflammatory bowel disease), intestinal phlegmon, intussusception, or ovarian process
- Left lower quadrant mass indicates constipation

Finding: Epigastric mass
Significance: Commonly arises from an abnormality of the stomach (bezoar, torsion) or the pancreas (pseudocyst)

Finding: Flank masses
Significance: Often represent renal disease

Finding: Hard and immobile
Significance: Palpable tumors

Finding: Large, extends across the midline
Significance: Teratomas

The abdomen of a normal infant and child should be completely soft and nontender. As a child ages, an increase in abdominal wall musculature may give greater resistance on examination, but the abdomen should continue to be soft to deep palpation.

 ## Laboratory Aids

Test: CBC
Significance: Anemia or hemolysis

Test: Chemistry panel
Significance: Renal disease (BUN, creatinine), liver disease (ALT, AST, alkaline phosphatase), gallbladder disease (bilirubin, GGTP), pancreatic disease (amylase), or intestinal disease (hypoalbuminemia)

Test: Abdominal ultrasound
Significance: Most useful pediatric diagnostic test for the evaluation of abdominal masses because the paucity of fat in children enhances its diagnostic detail; the disadvantage of ultrasound is its operator variability and its limitations when bowel gas obscures underlying abdominal tissues.

Test: Computed tomography scan
Significance: Can provide more detail when there is overlying gas or bone

Test: Plain abdominal x-ray studies
Significance: Presence of calcifications, extension into the chest

Test: Magnetic resonance imaging
Significance: Vascular lesions of liver, major vessels, and tumors

Test: Radioisotope HIDA scan
Significance: Liver, gallbladder, and intravenous urography (Wilms tumor, cystic kidney disease)

Test: Upper gastrointestinal, barium enema
Significance: Can be of benefit when the mass involves the intestine

Test: Laparoscopy
Significance: Can be useful for direct intraperitoneal visualization and biopsy of abdominal masses

Emergency Care

Of all the diseases listed in the differential diagnosis, patients who present with an abdominal mass and signs and/or symptoms of intestinal obstruction (intussusception, volvulus, gastric torsion, bezoar, foreign body), toxic megacolon, ovarian torsion, biliary obstruction (stone, hydrops), fever, or pancreatitis (pseudocyst) require immediate hospitalization. Initial diagnostic studies should include an abdominal ultrasound, plain abdominal x-ray studies, and a surgical consultation. The remaining causes of abdominal masses require urgent care and timely evaluation.

Issues for Referral

Except for the diagnosis of constipation, the presence of an abdominal mass requires immediate attention. For all masses in children, diagnostic studies should be performed expeditiously at a facility capable of diagnosing pediatric disorders. Once the abnormality is identified, the appropriate pediatric subspecialist should be consulted.

Clinical Pearls

In infants, a full bladder is often mistaken for an abdominal mass, while in neonates, a palpable liver edge can be normal and is often appreciated. Severe constipation in older children and adolescents can present as a large, hard mass extending from the pubis past the umbilicus. Finally, gastric distention should be considered in all children who present with a tympanitic epigastric mass.

BIBLIOGRAPHY

Mahaffey SM, Rychman RC, Martin LW. Clinical aspects of abdominal masses in children. *Semin Roentgenol* 1988;23:161–174.

Merten DF, Kirks DR. Diagnostic imaging of pediatric abdominal masses. *Pediatr Clin North Am* 1985;32:1397–1426.

Schwartz MW. Abdominal masses. In: Schwartz MW, Curry TA, Charney ED, et al., eds. *Principle and practice of clinical pediatrics*. Chicago: Yearbook, 1987:139–144.

Swischuk LE, Hayden CK Jr. Abdominal masses in children. *Pediatr Clin North Am* 1985;32:1281–1298.

Taylor LA, Ross AJ III. Abdominal masses. In: Walker WA, Durie PR, Hamilton JR, et al., eds. *Pediatric gastrointestinal disease*. Philadelphia: BC Decker, 1991:132–146.

Author: Chris A. Liacouras

Abdominal Pain

 Database

DEFINITION

Abdominal pain is a frequent complaint in the pediatric age group (see table More Common Causes of Abdominal Pain by Age, below). Pain may be acute or chronic, focal or nonspecific. A child's complaint of abdominal pain can originate from gastrointestinal and nongastrointestinal sources within the abdomen, or can be the manifestation of referred pain from extraabdominal sites.

 Differential Diagnosis

CONGENITAL/ANATOMIC

- Incarcerated hernia
- Intestinal adhesions
- Intussusception
- Malrotation with volvulus
- Ovarian torsion
- Testicular torsion
- Uteropelvic junction obstruction

INFECTIOUS

- Cystitis and urinary tract infections
- Fitz-Hugh-Curtis syndrome
- Gastroenteritis (bacterial, viral, or parasitic)
- *Helicobacter pylori* gastritis
- Mononucleosis with splenic enlargement/rupture
- Otitis media
- Pharyngitis
- Pelvic inflammatory disease
- Peritonitis
- Pneumonia
- Psoas abscess

- Sepsis
- Tubo-ovarian abscess
- Varicella

TOXIC, ENVIRONMENTAL, DRUGS

- Anticholinergic drugs
- Caustic ingestions
- Intestinal foreign body
- Heavy metal (i.e., lead) ingestion
- Mushroom poisoning
- Sympathomimetic drugs

TRAUMA

- Child abuse
- Duodenal hematoma
- Perforated viscus
- Splenic hematoma/rupture

TUMOR

- Any tumor, benign or malignant, leading to viscous obstruction
- Leukemia
- Lymphoma
- Nephroblastoma
- Wilms tumor

METABOLIC

- Diabetic ketoacidosis

ALLERGIC/INFLAMMATORY

- Appendicitis
- Cholecystitis
- Eosinophilic gastroenteritis
- Hemolytic-uremic syndrome
- Henoch-Schönlein purpura
- Hepatitis
- Inflammatory bowel disease
- Mesenteric adenitis
- Necrotizing enterocolitis
- Pancreatitis
- Peptic ulcer or gastritis
- Esophagitis or duodenitis

FUNCTIONAL

- Depression
- Functional abdominal pain
- Malingering
- Munchausen syndrome (± by proxy)

MISCELLANEOUS

- Abdominal migraine
- Cholelithiasis
- Colic
- Constipation
- Dysmenorrhea
- Ectopic pregnancy
- Endometriosis
- Ileus
- Intestinal pseudo-obstruction
- Irritable bowel syndrome
- Lactose intolerance
- Mittelschmerz
- Nephrolithiasis
- Ovarian cyst
- Pregnancy
- Porphyria
- Sickle-cell disease
- Typhlitis (in the presence of an immunocompromised host)

Approach to the Patient

GENERAL GOALS

Decide if abdominal pain complaints require emergent, urgent, or nonimmediate intervention.

Phase 1: Careful and complete history and physical examination to narrow this extensive differential diagnosis.

Phase 2: Directed laboratory evaluations should be made to support more likely portions of the differential diagnosis. If a narrowed differential is difficult to formulate, every effort should be made to ensure that the patient is clinically stable. A limited blood and/or radiographic evaluation screening with a CBC, ESR, comprehensive metabolic panel (i.e., Na^+, K^+, Cl^-, CO_2, BUN, creatinine, glucose, total protein, albumin, ALT, uric acid, LDH) and/or abdominal x-ray for significant abnormalities could be made to ensure there are no significant abnormalities above one's clinical suspicion.

Phase 3: Institute appropriate therapy related to diagnosis.

More Common Causes of Abdominal Pain by Age

INFANTS	TODDLERS TO PRETEENS	ADOLESCENTS
Colic	Appendicitis	Appendicitis
Child abuse	Child abuse	Constipation
Infectious gastroenteritis	Constipation	Dysmenorrhea
Intestinal obstruction	Infectious gastroenteritis	Infectious gastroenteritis
Intussusception	Ingestions	Inflammatory bowel disease
Incarcerated hernia	Otitis media	Irritable bowel disease
Necrotizing enterocolitis	Pancreatitis	Lactose intolerance
Pneumonia	Pharyngitis	Mittelschmerz
Pancreatitis	Pneumonia	Ovarian cyst
Sepsis	Trauma	Pancreatitis
Testicular torsion	Urinary tract infections	Pelvic inflammatory disease
Urinary tract infections		Sickle cell disease
		Trauma
		Urinary tract infections

Data Gathering

HISTORY

Question: Location of pain?
Significance: Pain etiology (see table below)

Question: Duration of pain?
Significance: Acute versus chronic illness

Question: Onset and progression of symptoms?
Significance: Evolution of painful process to help discriminate the exact pathological process

Question: Frank hematochezia?
Significance: Colonic bleeding or massive upper gastrointestinal bleeding

Question: Abdominal distention?
Significance: Distention of an abdominal viscus by air, stool, or fluid

Question: Radiation of pain?
Significance: Certain entities characteristically have radiation of pain (i.e., pancreatitis to the back, appendicitis to the right lower quadrant, gallstones to the shoulder).

Question: Pain relieved by bowel movements?
Significance: Etiology may be related to colonic distention (by air or stool) or inflammation (colitis).

Question: Bowel movement pattern?
Significance: Constipation

Question: Relationship to emesis?
Significance: Usually upper intestinal tract disorders

 ## Physical Examination

Finding: Location of pain
Significance: See table Etiology of Abdominal Pain Based on Most Common Symptom Location, below

Finding: Reexaminations by the same health care provider for changing characteristics
Significance: Evolution of abdominal process

Finding: Rebound tenderness
Significance: Peritonitis and the potential need for surgical intervention

Finding: Rectal examination
Significance: Peritoneal irritation, additional localization of pain, masses, presence and consistency of stool, and/or heme positive stools

 ## Laboratory Aids

Test: CBC with differential
Significance: Total white count is nonspecific and may be a poor indicator of intestinal inflammation.

Test: Erythrocyte sedimentation rate (ESR)
Significance: Nonspecific indicator of systemic inflammation

Test: Urinalysis
Significance: General screen for urinary tract abnormalities

Test: Two position abdominal x-ray
Significance: Possible clue to ileus, intussusception, intestinal obstruction, retained feces, or gas.

 ## Emergency Care

Every effort should be made to ensure that the patient is clinically stable. Frequent evaluation of vital signs and physical examination are a means of assessing evolving pain and ensure the patient is well enough for potential discharge.

Common Questions and Answers

Q: What is the most common cause of abdominal pain in children?
A: Constipation is probably still the most common presentation of abdominal pain. It can easily imitate the presentation of any organic disease, with localization of pain to any quadrant with any symptoms, including vomiting, diarrhea, or reflux.

Q: What are some of the physical findings associated with various abdominal pain syndromes?
A: In the presence of acute pancreatitis, there may be discoloration of the umbilicus (Cullen sign) and/or flank area (Grey Turner) sign. These are seen only in severe hemorrhagic pancreatitis. The presence of Murphy's sign is associated with gallbladder pathology. Tenderness over McBurney's point could suggest a process in the appendix.

Q: What is Rovsing sign?
A: This is tenderness over the left lower quadrant, which also causes pain in the right lower quadrant. This is highly suspicious for appendicitis.

Issues for Referral

Persistent abdominal pain without clear etiology or chronic gastrointestinal diseases should be referred to a pediatric gastroenterologist.

Clinical Pearls

• The farther the complaint of pain is away from the periumbilical region, the more likely the pain etiology represents organic disease.
• True nighttime waking with pain is more often correlated with organic disease than functional pain.

BIBLIOGRAPHY

Apley J. Psychosomatic aspects of gastrointestinal problems in children. *Clin Gastroenterol* 1977;6:311–320.

Hatch EI. The acute abdomen in children. *Pediatr Clin North Am* 1985;32:1151–1164.

Mason JD. The evaluation of acute abdominal pain in children. *Emerg Med Clin North Am* 1996;14:629–643.

Pearigen PD. Unusual causes of abdominal pain. *Emerg Med Clin North Am* 1996;14:593–613.

Author: Kurt A. Brown

Etiology of Abdominal Pain Based on Most Common Symptom Location*

LEFT UPPER QUADRANT	EPIGASTRIC	RIGHT UPPER QUADRANT
Splenic trauma	Esophagitis	Cholecystitis
	Gastritis	Cholelithiasis
	Gastroesophageal reflux disease	Fitz-Hugh-Curtis syndrome
	Pancreatitis	Pneumonia
	Peptic disease	

	SUPRAPUBIC	RIGHT LOWER QUADRANT
	Cystitis	Appendicitis
	Dysmenorrhea	Crohn disease
	Pelvic inflammatory disease	Mesenteric adenitis

*Nonlateralizing symptoms are not listed.

Abnormal Bleeding

 Database

DEFINITION
Abnormal bleeding may present as (1) an increase in severity or frequency of nose bleeds, bruising, or menstrual bleeding; (2) as bleeding in unusual sites such as joints or internal organs; or (3) as excessive bleeding for the degree of trauma experienced (see table Common Causes of Abnormal Bleeding).

 Differential Diagnosis

Abnormal bleeding can be the result of an acquired or congenital disorder of the procoagulant factors, platelets, or the vessel wall; disorders of procoagulant factors may be singular or multiple, disorders of platelets may be quantitative or qualitative, and disorders of the vessel wall may be inflammatory or structural. Consider child abuse in children with unusual bruising.

THROMBOCYTOPENIA: DEFECTIVE PRODUCTION
Congenital/Genetic
- Thrombocytopenia with absent radii (TAR) syndrome
- Amegakaryocytic thrombocytopenia
- Fanconi anemia
- Metabolic disorders
- Wiskott-Aldrich syndrome
- Bernard-Soulier syndrome
- Other rare familial syndromes (e.g. May-Hegglin anomaly)

Acquired
- Aplastic anemia
- Drug-associated marrow suppression
- Virus-associated marrow suppression (e.g., HIV)
- Chemotherapy
- Radiation injury
- Nutritional deficiencies (e.g., vitamin B_{12} and folate)

Marrow Infiltration
- Neoplasia (e.g., leukemia, neuroblastoma)
- Histiocytosis
- Osteopetrosis
- Myelofibrosis
- Hemophagocytic syndromes
- Storage diseases

THROMBOCYTOPENIA: INCREASED DESTRUCTION
- Idiopathic thrombocytopenic purpura (ITP)
- Neonatal alloimmune thrombocytopenia
- Maternal autoimmune thrombocytopenia
- Drug-induced (heparin, sulfonamides, digoxin, chloroquine)
- Sepsis/DIC
- Infection: viral, bacterial, fungal, rickettsial
- Microangiopathic process (e.g., TTP/HUS)
- Kasabach-Merritt syndrome
- Hypersplenism

PLATELET FUNCTION DISORDERS
- Storage pool disorders (e.g., dense granule deficiency, Hermansky-Pudlak syndrome)
- Platelet receptor abnormalities (e.g., Glanzmann's thrombasthenia, ADP receptor defect)
- Drugs (e.g., aspirin, NSAIDs, guaifenesin, antihistamines, phenothiazines, anticonvulsants
- Uremia
- Paraproteinemia

COAGULATION DISORDERS
Prolongation of aPTT
- Deficiency of factor VIII, IX, XI, or XII*
- Acquired inhibitor or lupus anticoagulant*
- von Willebrand disease (vWD) (often normal)

Prolongation of PT
- Mild vitamin K deficiency
- Liver disease, mild to moderate
- Deficiency of factor VII
- Factor VII inhibitor

Prolongation of PT and aPTT
- Liver disease, severe
- DIC
- Severe vitamin K deficiency
- Hemorrhagic disease of the newborn
- Deficiency of factors II, V, or X or fibrinogen
- Dysfibrinogenemia
- Hypoprothrombinemia associated with a lupus anticoagulant

Normal Screening Laboratory Tests
- vWD
- Factor XIII deficiency
- α_2 antiplasmin deficiency
- Plasminogen activator inhibitor-I deficiency

VESSEL WALL DISORDERS
Congenital
- Hereditary hemorrhagic telangiectasia
- Ehlers-Danlos syndrome
- Osteogenesis imperfecta
- Marfan syndrome

Acquired
- Vasculitis (SLE, HSP, etc.)
- Scurvy

*Factor XII deficiency and lupus anticoagulant not associated with abnormal bleeding.

Approach to the Patient
Phase 1: Includes a thorough history and physical examination as well as standard screening laboratory tests: PT/aPTT and platelet count. A familial history is an important component of this phase.

Phase 2: If a bleeding disorder is suspected but the initial screening tests are negative, then testing for vWD, factor XIII deficiency, and dysfibrinogenemia is warranted. A bleeding time should be performed at this phase if a platelet dysfunction is suspected.

Phase 3: Any abnormal screening tests need further evaluation with additional testing to define the specific disorder (e.g., factor assays, platelet aggregations).

 Data Gathering

HISTORY
Questions that help confirm presence of a bleeding disorder and assist in determining severity:
- Spontaneous bleeding?
- Bleeding in unusual places without significant trauma (intracranial, joints, etc.)?
- Bruising and bleeding disproportionate to injury? Large or palpable bruising?
- Poorly controlled epistaxis? [localized trauma (nose-picking) can exacerbate epistaxis, or be the sole cause of it; unilateral epistaxis may indicate local vascular problems, rather than bleeding disorder]
- Excessive bleeding with tooth extraction?
- Abnormal bleeding during or following circumcision or surgical procedure?
- Prolonged bleeding with minor cuts?
- Excessive bleeding following a fracture?
- Familial history of bleeding disorder?

Questions that help target the defective component of hemostasis:

Question: Mucosal bleeding (gum bleeding, epistaxis)?
Significance: Platelet disorder, vWD, hereditary hemorrhagic telangiectasia, dysfibrinogenemia

Question: Petechiae?
Significance: Platelet disorders, vWD

Question: Menorrhagia?
Significance: Common in vWD and platelet disorders

Question: Recent medications?
Significance: Aspirin and other drugs affect platelet function

Common Causes of Abnormal Bleeding

	COAGULATION FACTORS	PLATELET DISORDERS	VASCULAR DEFECTS
Congenital/Genetic	• Hemophilia (factors VIII, IX, or XI • Von Willebrand disease	• Neonatal alloimmune thrombocytopenia • Storage pool disease • ITP	• Hereditary hemorrhagic telangiectasias
Acquired	• Liver disease • DIC	• Leukemia	• Vasculitis: HSP

Question: Presence of renal or liver disease?
Significance: Azoturia contributes to bleeding. Liver disease reduces clotting factors.

Question: Severe malnutrition?
Significance: Scurvy, decreased hepatic synthesis

Physical Examination

Finding: Petechiae in skin and mucous membranes
Significance: Disorder of platelet number or function, vWD

Finding: Small bruises in unusual places
Significance: Possible platelet disorder, vWD

Finding: Large bruises or palpable bruises
Significance: Coagulation deficiencies, severe platelet disorders, or vWD

Finding: Delayed wound healing
Significance: Factor XIII deficiency and dysfibrinogenemia

Finding: Purpura localized to lower body (buttocks, legs, ankles)
Significance: Henoch-Schönlein purpura (HSP)

Laboratory Aids

Phase 1: Initial Laboratory Screening
• Platelet count
• PT and aPTT
• Bleeding time (may be delayed until phase 2)

Phase 2:
• Qualitative platelet defect suspected
—Bleeding time (may also help identify vWD)
—Platelet aggregation and ATP release studies with ristocetin, collagen, thrombin, arachidonic acid and ADP
• vWD suspected
—Factor VIII:C
—von Willebrand factor (vWF; VIIIR:Ag)
—Ristocetin cofactor activity
—Von Willebrand factor activity (new ELISA-based assay)
—vWF multimeric analysis
• Thrombin time or fibrinogen assay to screen for hypo- or dysfibrinogenemia

Phase 3: Discriminating Laboratory Studies for Abnormal Phase 1 Tests

When thrombocytopenia is present:
• Inspection of blood smear (screening for bone marrow diseases)
• Mean platelet volume (elevated in destructive causes, low in Wiskott-Aldrich)
• Bone marrow aspiration (rarely necessary)

When DIC is suspected (infection, liver disease, massive trauma, PT/aPTT prolonged):
• Fibrinogen
• D-dimer or fibrin split products
• Peripheral smear inspection for RBC fragments

Prolonged aPTT
• Inhibitor screen (50:50 mixing study of patient's and normal plasma)
• If aPTT fully corrects:
—Specific factor assays in the following order: VIII, IX, XI, X
• If partial or no correction after mixing study:
—Inhibitor present
—Confirmatory test for the presence of a lupus anticoagulant with a platelet neutralizing procedure

Prolonged PT
• Specific factor levels (II, VII, X)
• Inhibitor screen should also be considered for prolonged PT

Prolonged PT and aPTT
—Test for DIC, liver disease, and fibrinogen disorders, as described previously
—Vitamin K deficiency, moderate to severe
—Factor assays: V, X, II (prothrombin) and fibrinogen

PITFALLS OF TESTING
Bleeding Time
• Prolonged when platelets below 100,000/mm³
• Affected by medications such as aspirin, NSAIDs, antihistamines
• Does not correlate well with bleeding risk
• Accurate result depends on proper technique

PT and aPTT
• Normal ranges age dependent
• Polycythemia (Hct.65%) or too little blood collected may result in a spuriously high result
• Heparin contamination in samples from arterial or venous catheters

vWD Studies
• Normal ranges depend on patient's ABO blood group type
• Values fluctuate over time and may periodically be normal in affected individuals
• May require repeated testing to make diagnosis

Emergency Care

• Pressure, elevation, and ice are generally helpful for most bleeding disorders when active bleeding is present.
• Monitoring for complications of significant blood loss in the acute setting is important.
• More definitive care is dictated by the nature of the underlying hemostatic defect. Platelet transfusions are useful in disorders of thrombocytopenia due to decreased production and for intrinsic qualitative platelet disorders but not for immune platelet disorders. Frozen plasma should only be used in severe cases when the exact diagnosis is not readily available but a defect in coagulation is suspected.
• Head injuries in patients with thrombocytopenia or hemophilia require immediate medical attention.

Common Questions and Answers

Q: What are the proper preoperative screening tests for bleeding disorders prior to elective surgery such as tonsillectomy?
A: A thorough personal history, familial history, and physical examination are by far the most important screening tests. The bleeding time is not recommended. A CBC and PT/aPTT are often requested by the surgeon but normal results do not ensure that a bleeding complication will not occur. Overall the sensitivity and specificity of these screening tests is poor.

Q: Bruising is a normal part of childhood. How does one know when bruising is "too much"?
A: There is no proven set of clinical criteria that can reliably predict who should undergo an evaluation and who should not.

Issues for Referral
Indications
• If the history and physical examination strongly suggest the presence of a bleeding disorder or if the screening tests are abnormal, the patient should be referred to a pediatric hematologist.
• If von Willebrand disease is suspected, referral to a pediatric hematologist is usually necessary to determine the exact type and for testing that will assess the patient's response to ddAVP therapy.
• Patients with hemophilia should have regular visits to a hemophilia treatment center for follow-up and coordination of care.
• Consultation with a hematologist is recommended prior to invasive procedures, surgery, or dental work.

Screening Tests
Most clinical laboratories can do PT/aPTT and CBC, but may not be able to do bleeding times in young children.

Clinical Pearls
Children with bleeding disorders are more likely to have large bruises (greater than 5 cm), hematomas (palpable bruises), and bruises on more than one body part.

BIBLIOGRAPHY
Laposata M, Connor AM, Hicks DG, et al. *The clinical hemostasis handbook*. Chicago: Year Book, 1989.

Lusher JM. Approach to the bleeding patient. In: Nathan DG, Orkin SH, eds. *Nathan and Oski's hematology of infancy and childhood*. Philadelphia: WB Saunders, 1998:1574–1584.

Manno CS. Difficult pediatric diagnoses—bruising and bleeding. *Pediatr Clin North Am* 1991;38:637–655.

Pramanik AK. Bleeding disorders in neonates. *Pediatr Rev* 1992;13(5):163–173.

Author: J. Nathan Hagstrom

Allergic Child

Database

DEFINITION
The allergic child has the tendency toward IgE-mediated reactions in response to pollens, molds, environmental allergens, drugs, or foods. These reactions may manifest as any of the following: eczema, allergic rhinitis, asthma, angioedema, hives, or anaphylaxis.

Differential Diagnosis

EYES
- Physical and chemical irritants
- Viral or bacterial infection

NOSE
- Recurrent upper respiratory tract infections
- Rhinitis medicamentosum—reaction to nasal sprays
- Drugs that cause nasal congestion
—Oral contraceptives
—Reserpine
—Guanethidine
—Propranolol
—Thioridazine
—Tricyclic antidepressants
—Aspirin
- Airway irritants
—Smoke
—Environmental pollution
—Cold air
- Kartagener syndrome—sinusitis, bronchiectasis, immobile cilia
- Cystic fibrosis
- Sinusitis

LUNGS
- Intrinsic asthma
- Airway irritants
—Smoke
—Environmental pollution
—Cold air
- Gastroesophageal reflux
- Foreign body aspiration
- Anatomic defect in airway
- Cystic fibrosis
- Kartagener syndrome
- Immune deficiency

SKIN
- Viral exanthems
- Autoimmune disorders
- Physical and chemical irritants

Approach to the Patient

Phase 1: Characterize symptoms and identify target organ. Determine if symptoms are related to one season, which environment, medication. Which organ system(s) is involved?

Phase 2: Focused laboratory tests when in doubt of cause.

Phase 3: Treatment with antihistamines

Data Gathering

HISTORY
The history may reveal seasonal or year round symptoms.
Specific questions are best asked systematically in a review of systems format.

Ears
- Otitis
- Myringotomy tubes
- Hearing loss

Nasal
- Frequent URIs
- Sinusitis
- Polyps
- Epistaxis
- Snoring
- Sneezing
- Rhinitis
- Deviated septum
- Obstruction
- Itch
- Mouth breathing
- Nasal discharge

Throat
- Sore throat
- Throat clearing
- Postnasal drip
- Palate itch
- Tonsillitis
- Tonsillectomy
- Croup

Chest
- Day cough
- Night cough
- Sputum production
- Pain
- Wheeze
- Shortness of breath
- Cyanosis

Eyes
- Itching
- Tearing
- Discharge
- Swelling
- Redness
- Rubbing

Gastrointestinal
- Anorexia
- Nausea
- Vomiting
- Diarrhea
- Constipation
- Gas
- Belching
- Abdominal pain
- Fatty or foul-smelling stools

Skin
- Eczema
- Hives
- Angioedema
- Contact dermatitis
- Seborrheic dermatitis
- Skin infections
- Pruritus

Genitourinary
- Dysuria
- Burning
- Polyuria
- Hematuria
- Enuresis

Headache
- Location
- Character
- Frequency
- Duration
- Nausea
- Vomiting
- Scotomata

Other important questions include:

Question: Does your child have food or drug allergies?
Significance: Be sure to ask what type of reaction the child had (many types of intolerances are called allergies by parents). Generally, allergies are IgE-mediated reactions resulting in wheezing, allergic rhinitis, hives, angioedema, eczema, or anaphylaxis. Intolerances generally include a nonspecific rash, diarrhea, gas, headache, or hyperactivity. Specifically ask about peanut, nut, and shellfish allergy (allergy to any of these is an indication for an EpiPen (Center Labs, Port Washington, NY), and lifelong avoidance).

Question: Has your child ever been stung by a bee, and, if so, what was the reaction?
Significance: Systemic reactions are an indication for referral to an allergist for venom desensitization. Venom desensitization can be potentially lifesaving. Ask parents if they know the type of bee involved with the reaction. (Honeybees are the only bees that leave their stinger at the sting site.)

Question: Does anyone in your family have hayfever (allergic rhinitis), asthma, or eczema?
Significance: Familial history of atopy increases the likelihood of atopy in other family members.

Questions to ask regarding the environment:

Question: Do you have a basement?
Significance: Damp basements are a source of mold spores.

Question: Are there any damp areas in your home?
Significance: Damp areas serve to propagate mold growth in the home.

Question: Do you have forced air or radiator heat?
Significance: Forced air heat tends to blow allergen-laden dust around the home.

Question: How do you cool your home?
Significance: Opening outside windows lets the pollens from outside into the house.

Question: Do you have a humidifier?
Significance: Molds can grow in the water, and increased ambient humidity will raise the dust mite population in the home.

Question: Are there any smokers in the home?
Significance: Cigarette smoke is an airway irritant and can exacerbate respiratory difficulties.

Question: Are there any pets in the home, at school, or in day care?
Significance: Animal dander is a common aeroallergen. Pets should be excluded from the bedroom (a pet that sleeps on the patient's bed is a common problem).

Question: Are there many stuffed animals or books in the bedroom?
Significance: Dust mites love these dust collectors, and they should be removed from the bedroom. Environmental control efforts should be focused on the bedroom. Patients can have significant allergen exposure during sleep.

Question: Does the bedroom have carpeting?
Significance: Hardwood or tile floors are best to keep the dust mite population under control.

Question: How often do you wash the bedding, what type of pillow do you have, and is the mattress encased in plastic?
Significance: To keep the dust mite population under control the bedding should be washed in hot water at least once every 2 weeks (hot water kills dust mites), the pillow should be fiber filled, and the mattress should be encased in plastic.

Question: Where does the patient spend most of his time?
Significance: Allergenic exposure where most of the patient's time is spent is most important.

Question: Does the patient attend day care?
Significance: Day care is a major source of upper respiratory tract infections, which can mimic allergies and exacerbate reactive airway disease.

 ## Physical Examination

These children may have dark circles under their eyes (allergic shiners), a nasal crease, or the child may give you an allergic salute (upward rubbing of nose to relieve a nasal itch). A careful environmental history is essential. A complete physical examination is essential to rule out systemic disease that can mimic allergies (i.e., clubbing, anatomic obstruction, heart murmur, etc.)

Finding: Ocular allergic signs
Significance:
• Allergic shiners are due to passive congestion in the nose, which impedes the venous return to the vessels under the eyes.
• Cobblestoning of the conjunctiva is associated with allergic conjunctivitis.
• Dennie sign (Morgan line), infraorbital folds associated with suborbital edema secondary to atopy.
• Clear stringy discharge is the characteristic eye discharge seen in allergic conjunctivitis.

Finding: Nasal allergic signs
Significance:
• Pale edematous nasal mucosa is characteristic of allergic rhinitis.
• Nasal crease across the bridge of nose is secondary to repeated upward rubbing of the nose.
• Clear nasal discharge with or without occlusion is characteristic of allergic rhinitis.

Finding: Ears allergic signs
Significance: Fluid in the middle ear, or retracted tympanic membranes may be associated with eustachian tube dysfunction seen with allergic inflammation.

Finding: Throat allergic signs
Significance: Cobblestoning of posterior pharynx secondary to submucosal lymphoid hyperplasia can be seen in allergic patients.

Finding: Lungs allergic signs
Significance: Wheezes, rhonchi, decreased air entry, and chronic obstruction can be secondary to allergic responses.

Finding: Skin allergic signs
Significance: Eczema, hives, angioedema, and dermatographism are all characteristic of allergic skin.

 ## Laboratory Aids

Test: Immediate hypersensitivity
Significance:
• Skin prick tests to suspected allergens based on history. These are the study of choice because of their low cost, high sensitivity, rapid results, and documented excellent correlation with clinical sensitivity especially to pollens and animal dander.
• Intradermal skin tests are reserved for patients who have a negative prick test and a suspicious history. These studies are more sensitive than prick tests but less specific, and pose a greater risk of systemic reactions.
• RAST tests (radioallergosorbent tests) measures free serum IgE to a specific antigen to which a particular patient may be sensitized. These tests are primarily reserved for patients at risk for a severe systemic reaction from skin testing (i.e., Latex allergic patients), or in patients in whom skin testing is not feasible (i.e., patients with extensive skin disease). These tests are less sensitive than skin prick and intradermal tests.
• Serum IgE levels have a low sensitivity and, generally, are of little help.
• Presence of blood eosinophilia. Eosinophils in the blood or respiratory secretions may be indicative of an allergic diathesis.

Test: Baseline laboratory
Significance: Baseline pulmonary function studies should be obtained on asthmatic children.

 ## Emergency Care

ANAPHYLAXIS
• Subcutaneous epinephrine 1:1,000
• Diphenhydramine
• Ranitidine
• Methylprednisolone
• Volume expander to correct hypotension

ACUTE ASTHMA
• Oxygen
• Inhaled B-agonist
• Subcutaneous epinephrine 1:1,000
• Steroids

Common Questions and Answers

Q: Do children outgrow allergies?
A: No. Actually, once patients are sensitized, they are sensitized for life. In addition, the older the patient becomes, the greater the chance to develop other sensitivities.

Q: Can allergic children acquire more allergies?
A: Allergic children have the biologic potential to become sensitized to many environmental allergens. The goal should be to limit exposure to these antigens to prevent sensitization.

Q: If a parent is allergic to a specific allergen, can the child inherit this allergy?
A: Children inherit the tendency to be allergic, but they do not inherit specific allergies.

Q: What treatments are available?
A: Specific environmental control (as determined by skin testing), antihistamines, topical steroids, and immunotherapy.

Issues for Referral
• Patient failing medical management of upper respiratory or ocular allergies with routine antihistamine/decongestant medications. The allergist can help identify triggers contributing to the allergic symptomatology.
• Poorly controlled asthma not responding to intermittent inhaled B-agonists or an asthmatic who is symptomatic between exacerbations, or one that has an atypical pattern of exacerbations.
• Asthmatics with frequent hospitalizations or steroid-dependent asthmatics should also be referred.
• Patients who miss school frequently due to allergic or asthmatic symptoms.
• Patients with limited activities due to allergies or asthma.
• Strong seasonal history to respiratory complaints
• Systemic reaction to bee sting
• Difficult to manage eczema (atopic dermatitis)
• Recurrent croup
• Food allergy
• History of anaphylaxis
• Egg allergic patient who require influenza vaccine
• Drug allergy
• Latex allergy

BIBLIOGRAPHY
Fireman P. Diagnosis of allergic disorders. *Pediatr Rev* 1995;16(5):178–183.

Hopkin JM. Asthma and allergy-disorders of civilization? *Q J Med* 1998;91(3):169–170.

Middleton E, Reed CE, Adkinson NF, et al. *Allergic principles and practice*, 4th ed. Philadelphia: Mosby, 1993.

Sites DP, Terr AI, Parslow TG. *Basic and clinical immunology*, 8th ed. Englewood Cliffs, NJ: Prentice Hall, 1994.

Author: Christopher A. Smith

Alopecia (Hair Loss)

 ## Database

DEFINITION
Alopecia is defined as "partial or complete loss of hair" and is frequently seen in general pediatrics. Three leading causes—tinea capitis, alopecia areata, and traction alopecia—comprise 90% of all cases seen in pediatrics.

 ## Differential Diagnosis

There are four categories of alopecia:
- Acquired and circumscribed (95%)
- Acquired and diffuse
- Congenital and circumscribed
- Congenital and diffuse

PATHOPHYSIOLOGY
The pathophysiology of the three most common disorders that account for the majority of cases are described below:

Tinea capitis: *Trichophytan tonsurans* has replaced *Microsporum canis* as the most common dermatophyte infection. *T. tonsurans* grows within the endothrix (hair shaft), whereas *M. canis* attacks the ecothrix (external hair shaft). Due to the endothrix involvement, *T. tonsurans* does not fluoresce with a Wood's lamp, whereas the ecothrix involvement of *M. canis* does fluoresce.
Dematophyte infections have two stages:
- Noninflammatory stage lasts 2 to 8 weeks. The hair breaks off, leaving a "black dot" appearance in area of alopecia.
- Inflammatory stage is characterized by diffuse fine scaling without obvious broken-off hairs, scaly, pustular bald areas, and kerions. A kerion is believed to be a hypersensitivity reaction to dermatophytes, not an infection.

Alopecia areata: The exact etiology of alopecia areata is not understood, but many suspect dysregulation of the immune system. The theory of stress-inducing alopecia areata is controversial, and while it may be one contributing factor, it is not the sole cause. Alopecia that involves the entire scalp is called alopecia areata totalis, and when it involves the entire body it is referred to as alopecia areata universalis.

Traumatic alopecia: The pathogenesis of the third most common cause of alopecia depends on the type of trauma. Common causes include:
- Trichotillomania—pulling, twisting, or breaking of one's own hair; lifetime prevalence of 1%. In some cases, emotionally traumatic events precipitate hair pulling. Denial is a common feature. For confirmation, a biopsy shows traumatic avulsion of hair shafts.
- Traction—hair loss secondary to certain hairstyles, such as tight braids or ponytails, chemical treatments, and hot irons or combs.
- Rub or friction alopecia—the pruritus from atopic dermatitis causes infants to rub their heads on the bed sheets, resulting in hair loss.
- Pressure induced alopecia—the occipital alopecia seen in infants who spend extended periods of time lying supine.

Approach to the Patient

GENERAL GOALS
Keep in mind the four broad categories of differential diagnosis and the fact that the most common causes of alopecia are tinea capitis, alopecia areata, and traumatic alopecia.

 ## Data Gathering

HISTORY
Question: Is the hair loss recent or has it been there since birth? Is the hair loss localized or diffuse?
Significance: This aids in categorizing the differential diagnosis.

Question: Has the child been in contact with anyone else with similar hair loss patterns?
Significance: Tinea capitis can be transmitted from one person to another via caps, combs, and hair brushes.

Question: Who cares for the hair, and how is it cared for?
Significance: Traumatic alopecia is caused by certain types of hairstyling.

Question: Have there been any skin changes?
Significance: Vitiligo is associated with alopecia areata and SLE.

Question: Has there been any abdominal pain?
Significance: Bezoars form with trichotillomania and trichophagy, which is the chewing and swallowing of hair.

Question: Does the child have any significant medical history?
Significance: Alopecia can be seen with diseases, including: SLE, celiac disease, and myasthenia gravis.

Question: Does the child take any medications?
Significance: Alopecia can be seen with use of heparin, coumadin, and chemotherapy.

Question: Was the newborn screen negative?
Significance: Congenital hypothyroidism is associated with alopecia.

Question: Does the child have any dietary restrictions?
Significance: Hypervitaminosis A, zinc deficiency, and marasmus can cause alopecia.

Question: Have there been any recent family or social stressors?
Significance: Stress can induce alopecia areata and trichotillomania.

Question: Is there any concern for child abuse?
Significance: Traumatic alopecia is a manifestation of abuse.

Question: Any dogs or cats in the home?
Significance: Such pets can transmit *M. canis*.

 ## Physical Examination

Finding: Scalp with black dots (hairs broken off), scaling, pustules, or kerions (boggy, indurated, raised masses).
Significance: Seen with tinea capitis.

Finding: Frontal or parietal scalp with smooth and bald, oval, or round patches with no redness or scaling. Hairs may have an "exclamation point" appearance, which is a narrowed proximal diameter.
Significance: Seen with alopecia areata. In the ophiasis variant, there is occipital or frontal scalp involvement, with spread to the hair margins.

Finding: Frontoparietal or frontotemporal hair loss with irregular borders, hair of different lengths, occasional petechiae and excoriations.
Significance: Seen with trichotillomania.

Finding: Smooth occipital bald spot in young infants
Significance: Supine position.

Finding: Pigmentation changes and/or scars evident
Significance: May be seen in aplasia cutis congenital and/or other birthmarks listed in the differential diagnosis table.

Finding: Hair loss with greasy yellow scales in 2- to 10-week-old infant
Significance: Seborrheic dermatitis.

Finding: Suboccipital or posterior cervical lymphadenopathy
Significance: Associated with kerions and other inflammatory or infectious processes.

Finding: Abnormal teeth
Significance: Ectodermal dysplasia.

Finding: Evidence of lash/brow loss
Significance: Seen with trichotillomania and alopecia universalis.

Finding: Loss of pubic hair
Significance: Seen in alopecia universalis.

Finding: Pigmentary changes
Significance: Vitiligo is associated with alopecia areata.

Finding: Nail pitting
Significance: Seen with alopecia areata and other disorders.

 ## Laboratory Aids

Test: A fungal culture.
Significance: The gold standard test to diagnose tinea capitis. Scrapings for 10% KOH prep are less reliable and require experience to be done correctly but can be useful if culture is unavailable.

Test: A Wood's lamp exam.
Significance: Tinea capitis due to *M. canis* will result in a yellow-green fluorescence. *T. tonsurans* does not fluoresce.

Test: Further systemic workup.
Significance: This is indicated in the presence of diffuse alopecia, acquired or congenital, to evaluate endocrine, metabolic/biochemical, or nutritional abnormalities.

 ## Therapy

Tinea capitis: The standard treatment is oral griseofulvin for a minimum of 8 weeks, and it is absorbed best when taken with a fatty meal. Topical treatment is not effective because it does not reach the inside of the hair shaft where hyphae exist. Beyond griseofulvin, new antimycotic agents, including itraconazole, terbinafine, and fluconazole, are effective treatment alternatives. Further studies are needed to determine the optimal treatment with agents, including antifungal shampoos, topical

agents, and corticosteroids. If the culture reveals *M. canis* as the causative agent, the suspected infected dog or cat should be treated by a veterinarian.
Alopecia areata: For extensive lesions, treatment with intralesional corticosteroid injections and topical immunotherapy (e.g., superpotent topical steroids, anthralin, minoxidil, contact sensitizers) have been successful but are considered palliative. They do not change the prognosis of the disease. Since there is a high rate of hair regrowth, and there are side effects, reassurance is frequently all that is required. Support and information for families can be found through the National Alopecia Areata Foundation (*www.naaf.org*).
Traumatic alopecia: Identify and stop the activity that is causing the problem.
• Traction—Emphasis should be placed on wide-toothed combs, and gentle shampoos and shampooing. Inform patients that regrowth may take 6 to 12 months.

• Trichotillomania—The first step in management is convincing the parents of the cause. A short haircut or applying oil to hair makes hair pulling more difficult. Behavioral modification, hypnosis, psychotherapy, and family therapy are other treatment modalities that are available. Psychiatric referral may be necessary.

Other causes of alopecia: There are many treatments for the other causes of alopecia, most of which are managed by specialists. Treatment for acquired diffuse alopecia depends on the cause.

Follow-Up

Follow-up for tinea capitis should occur every 4 weeks. Some literature suggests a follow-up culture to document clearance.

Common Questions and Answers

Q: What is the most common cause of alopecia?
A: Tinea capitis is the most common cause, and *Trichophyton tonsurans* is the predominant agent.

Q: When should a patient with alopecia be referred to dermatology?
A: When the hair loss pattern falls into any category other than acquired circumscribed, or when there is recurrent alopecia areata.

Q: How long will it take the hair to grow back after a case of tinea capitis?
A: Some regrowth will be seen at 2 weeks, but full regrowth requires 3 to 6 months.

Q: How long will it take the hair to grow back after alopecia areata?
A: 95% of children will have hair grow back within a year.

Q: What is the recurrence rate of alopecia areata?
A: Approximately 30% of people will have recurrent alopecia areata. With subsequent bouts the prognosis worsens.

BIBLIOGRAPHY
Elewski BE. Tinea capitis: a current perspective. *J Am Acad Dermatol* 2000;42:1–20.

Madani S. Alopecia areata update. *J Am Acad Dermatol* 2000;42:549–566.

Messinger ML, Cheng TL. Trichotillomania. *Pediatr Rev* 1999;20:249–250.

Naveh Y. Celiac disease-associated alopecia in childhood. *J Pediatr* 1999;134:362–364.

Whiting DA. Chronic telogen effluvium. *Dermatol Clin* 1996;14:723–731.

Author: Lisa Chamberlain

Table of Etiologies by Pattern of Hair Loss

	ACQUIRED	*CONGENITAL*
Circumscribed	Tinea capitis	Birthmarks:
	Kerion	Sebaceous, epidermal nevi
	Alopecia areata	Melanocytic nevi
	Trauma	Hemangioma
	Traction	Lymphangioma
	Trichotillomania	Aplasia cutis congenita
	Chemical/thermal/radiation	Incontinentia pigmenti
	Rub alopecia (infants with	Hallermann-Streiff syndrome
	atopic dermatitis)	Goltz syndrome
	Pressure alopecia (infants)	Chondrodysplasia punctata
	Scaring from kerion, varicella	Intrauterine trauma (scalp
	trauma, burns.	electrodes)
	Less common:	
	Systemic lupus erythematosus	
	Lichen planus	
	Darier disease	
Diffuse	Telogen effluvium	Genetic syndromes
	Anagen effluvium	Ectodermal dysplasias
	Endocrine-associated	Congenital hypothyroidism
	Hypopituitarism	Atrichia congenita
	Hypothyroidism	Cartilage-hair hypoplasia
	Hyperthyroidism	Hair shaft abnormalities
	Hypoparathyroidism	Trichorrhexis nodosa
	Diabetes mellitus	(broomstick)
	Anogenic alopecia	Proximal, distal, familial
	Drug associated	Argininosuccinicaciduria
	Heparin	Pili torti (twisted)
	Coumadin	Proximal, distal, familial
	Diet associated	Monilethrix (beaded)
	Hypervitaminosis A	Congenital hypothyroidism
	Zinc deficiency	Progeria
	Marasmus	
	Lamellar ichthyosis	
	Proximal trichorrhexis nodosa	
	Multiple rare syndromes and disorders	

Back Pain

 Database

DEFINITION

• Back pain refers to any condition in which a patient has complaints of discomfort of the thoracic, lumbar, or sacral spine.
• Back pain can result from a variety of causes, involving the bony or muscular structures of the back, intervertebral discs, spinal cord, or peripheral nerves.
• Inheritance patterns for some of the congenital (e.g., scoliosis, Scheuermann kyphosis) and inflammatory/rheumatologic causes of back pain have been described.
• There is a 30–50% lifetime incidence of back pain in adolescents. Eight percent of adolescents report recurrent or chronic back pain. Discitis and osteomyelitis are most commonly seen in children under 10 years of age. Spondylolysis, spondylolisthesis, Scheuermann's kyphosis, herniated disc, tumors, and apophyseal ring fractures are usually seen in children over 10 years.

COMPLICATIONS

Depending on the underlying etiology, complications of missed diagnosis or improper management can include paralysis or other permanent neuromuscular injury, and neoplastic/paraneoplastic or infectious syndromes.

PROGNOSIS

• Prognosis is dependent on the underlying cause of back pain. The majority, if properly diagnosed and treated, do well, without significant sequelae.
• It is not possible to predict when spondylolysis will worsen or progress to spondylolisthesis, or the future course of Scheuermann's kyphosis.

 Differential Diagnosis

CONGENITAL

• Tethered cord
• Syringomyelia (may also be traumatic)

INFLAMMATORY

• Ankylosing spondylitis
• Enteropathic arthritis
• Intervertebral disc calcification

INFECTIOUS

• Tuberculosis
• Discitis
• Epidural abscess

TRAUMA

• "Musculotendinous" strain
• Spondylolysis (stress fracture of posterior vertebral elements, thought to be a repetitive stress injury)
• Spondylolisthesis (anterior displacement or "slip" of the vertebral body, associated with bilateral spondylolysis)
• Herniated disc
• Apophyseal ring fracture (fracture separating the vertebral body and cartilaginous ring apophysis)
• Epidural hematoma (traumatic or due to bleeding diathesis)

NEOPLASTIC

Bony

• Osteoid osteoma, osteoblastoma
• Osteosarcoma
• Ewing sarcoma
• Aneurysmal bone cyst

Metastatic/Other

• Leukemia, lymphoma
• Eosinophilic granuloma
• Glioma
• Neuroblastoma
• Rhabdomyosarcoma

DEVELOPMENTAL

• Scheuermann's kyphosis (excessive kyphosis/"hunchback" due to abnormal ossification causing "wedging" of the vertebral bodies)
• Painful scoliosis

REFERRED

• Pyelonephritis
• Pancreatitis

PSYCHOGENIC

 Data Gathering

Warning signs of potentially serious causes of back pain in children include:

• Young age (less than 4 years old)
• Chronic interference with normal activity (e.g., school, sports, play)
• Duration of pain longer than 4 weeks
• Associated fever, weight loss, or other systemic symptoms
• Postural shift of trunk
• Any neurologic abnormality
• Limitation of spinal motion (e.g., bending forward, straight leg raise)
• Painful or left thoracic scoliosis

HISTORY

Question: Onset, duration, and frequency of pain?
Significance: Fleeting or short duration of pain is rarely serious.

Question: Interference with activity?
Significance: Often a marker of severe disease.

Question: Physical activity and trauma history?
Significance: Spondylolysis and spondylolisthesis are more commonly seen in children who repeatedly twist, bend, or hyperextend their spine (e.g., participate in gymnastics, diving, tennis, contact sports, weightlifting, etc.). Heavy lifting may contribute to Scheuermann kyphosis. Trauma causes one third of herniated disc injuries.

Question: Pain aggravated by activity and/or relieved by rest?
Significance: Overuse conditions, spondylolysis, or spondylolisthesis is likely.

Question: Radiation of pain?
Significance: Pain that shoots down the legs is suggestive of a herniated disc, spondylolisthesis, epidural abscess, or osteoid osteoma.

Question: Motor, sensory, or bowel/bladder symptoms?
Significance: Consider syringomyelia or spinal cord abnormalities (e.g., congenital, tumors, or herniated disc).

Question: Growth history?
Significance: Adolescents during growth spurts are more prone to musculotendinous strain.

Question: Previous history of scoliosis?
Significance: Idiopathic scoliosis is rarely painful or functionally limiting.

SPECIAL QUESTIONS

Pain that awakes the child from sleep, and/or relief with NSAIDs. Osteoid osteoma and osteoblastoma often presents with nighttime back pain and/or recurrent back pain relieved by NSAIDs.
Pain aggravated by prone position is suggestive of an epidural abscess.

Physical Examination

Finding: Inspect for any occult abnormalities
Significance: Sacral dimples, hair tufts, vascular anomalies, café-au-lait spots, or discrepancies in limb length. If the head is not midline, consider syringomyelia, tumor, spondylolisthesis, or herniated disc. Shortened waistline and flattening or "heart shaped" buttocks are often seen in spondylolisthesis.

Finding: With the child's feet together and knees and hips straight, observe the child from the back and side, both standing and through full range of motion of the spine.
Significance: This evaluates the patient for scoliosis, kyphosis, and range of motion. Lumbar lordosis should "reverse" when the child bends over; if it does not, significant pathology should be suspected.

During forward flexion: if thoracic kyphosis is accentuated, suspect Scheuermann kyphosis; if stiffness is observed, consider inflammatory, infectious, or neoplastic causes. Stiffness during extension is typical of discitis.

Finding: Palpate for any point or focal tenderness.
Significance: Fractures often manifest with point tenderness.

Finding: Assess neurologic function.
Significance: In young children, this may be evaluated by observing gait, heel- and toe-walking, and rising from a squat. Complete examination of the lower body, including examination of sensation and rectal tone, should be performed. Any abnormal neurologic findings should be thoroughly investigated.

Finding: Abnormal gait.
Significance: Consider spondylolisthesis (short stride or "pelvic waddle") or herniated disc.

Finding: Hamstring tightness and/or decreased hip flexion.
Significance: May be seen in spondylolisthesis and discitis.

Finding: With the patient supine, examine the abdomen and have the patient perform a straight leg raise.
Significance: Limitation in leg raise or radiating pain is suggestive of neurologic abnormality. Lack of abdominal reflexes may suggest syringomyelia.

SPECIFIC TESTS

• Standing hyperextension (bending backward) often reproduces the lower lumbar pain of spondylolysis.
• A bony "ledge"/step-off on palpation of the lumbar spine or an anterior bony mass on rectal examination is sometimes appreciated with spondylolisthesis.

• Asymmetry of lower extremity muscle circumference may be a sign of nerve impingement due to a herniated disc.

 ## Laboratory Aids

Test: Plain radiographs (AP and lateral, and if warranted, oblique and flexion/extension views) of the spine are indicated if any worrisome signs or symptoms are present.
Significance: Spondylolysis has the appearance of a "collar" (lucent line) on the "Scottie dog's" neck.

Test: Bone or SPECT scan
Significance: More sensitive for occult or subtle lesions, and should be obtained if a serious etiology is clinically suspected.

Test: MRI
Significance: The preferred examination for suspected neurologic or disc injury.

Test: Blood tests (e.g., sed rate, HLA-B27, ANA, rheumatoid factor, blood culture)
Significance: Indicated only if infectious or rheumatologic etiologies are considered.

Test: Bacterial cultures (needle aspiration or open biopsy)
Significance: Positive in only 25% to 50% of discitis patients. Routine biopsy, therefore, is not recommended in cases of suspected discitis. Staphylococcal species are the most frequently recovered organism.

 ## Therapy

• If no warning signs are present, conservative management with rest, activity modification, ice or heat (whichever is appropriate), acetaminophen or ibuprofen, muscle relaxants, physical therapy, and close follow-up is reasonable. A back brace may also be helpful in spondylolisthesis and Scheuermann kyphosis.
• Conservative medical treatment is indicated for spondylolysis and spondylolisthesis of less than 50% slip. Surgical treatment is warranted for slip greater than 50% or persistent back pain.
• Antistaphylococcal medications are indicated in cases of discitis. The choice between oral or intravenous medications depends on the severity of the patient's symptoms.
• There is limited evidence in adults that lumbar supports are effective in treating low back pain.

 ## Follow-Up

• Patients managed conservatively should be reevaluated within 2 weeks.
• All patients should be instructed to follow-up immediately for any worsening symptoms.

PREVENTION

• When the child has recuperated, back muscle strengthening and hamstring stretching exercises may be helpful.
• When participating in sports, appropriate protective equipment should be used and proper technique should be emphasized.
• In gymnasts, training more than 15 hours per week has been associated with increased risk of injury.
• In adult studies, lumbar supports do not appear to be effective at preventing low back pain.

PITFALLS

• Missed diagnosis of a serious cause of back pain.
• Plain films are often normal, even in cases with serious causes.

 ## Common Questions and Answers

Q: Which children should have activity restrictions?
A: "High-risk" children (e.g., those with spinal or bony abnormalities, or familial histories of spondylolysis) should avoid hyperextension and contact sports.

Q: When can/should the child resume normal activities?
A: "Low-risk" children, with a normal neurologic exam, can resume activity or sports when they are pain free.

BIBLIOGRAPHY

Gerbino PG, Micheli LJ. Back injuries in the young athlete. *Clin Sports Med* 1995;14(3):571–590.

Ginsburg GM, Bassett GS. Back pain in children and adolescents: evaluation and differential diagnosis. *J Am Acad Orthop Surg* 1997 5(2):67–78.

Jellema P, van Tulder MW, van Poppel MNM, et al. Lumbar supports for prevention and treatment of low back pain. *Spine* 2001;26(4):377–386.

Mason DE. Back pain in children. *Pediatr Ann* 1999;28(12):727–738.

Payne WK, Ogilvie JW. Back pain in children and adolescents. *Pediatr Clin North Am* 1996;43(4):899–917.

Author: Thomas H. Chun

Behavioral or Psychiatric Problems

 Database

DEFINITION

Behavioral, developmental, or psychosocial problems that require medical or psychiatric treatment, or that cause the child significant impairment. Epidemiologic research indicates that between 14% and 20% of American children have moderate to severe psychiatric disorders. Unfortunately, research also shows that 30% of children with mental retardation and other developmental disabilities, and 50–80% of children with other mental health problems are not recognized by their primary care providers.

 Differential Diagnosis

ORGANIC CAUSES

- CNS infections or parainfectious syndromes
- Substance abuse, toxic ingestions, medication adverse effects
- Intracranial trauma or other injury
- CNS tumors
- Endocrine disorders

—Thyroid or adrenal dysfunction

- Metabolic disorders

—Abnormal glucose
—Sodium
—Potassium
—Calcium

- Migraines
- Seizure disorders
- Hematologic disorders

—Porphyria
—Severe anemia

- Hypoxia
- Other cardiopulmonary disturbances

Among psychobehavioral disorders, many disorders have similar symptoms. For example:

- Attention deficit/hyperactivity disorder (ADHD) may be difficult to distinguish from mood (depression or bipolar disorder), anxiety (including school phobia), posttraumatic stress, and tic disorders, substance abuse, hearing or vision impairment, and learning disabilities.
- Social withdrawal may be a sign of depression, neglect, pervasive developmental disorder (PDD), sensory impairment (e.g., deafness), or learning disability.
- Psychotic symptoms are seen not only in psychotic disorders, but also in mood disorders (depression, bipolar disorder), borderline personality disorder, and substance abuse.

Aggressive or violent behavior is not a diagnosis unto itself, but can represent a final common pathway of depression, psychosis, delirium, substance abuse, ADHD (uncommon), physical or sexual abuse, or family dysfunction.

Approach to the Patient

GENERAL GOALS

Phase 1: Assess the patient for safety (i.e., suicidality, homicidality, and adequate support and supervision at home)

Phase 2: Rule out organic causes.

Phase 3: As organic causes are being investigated, establish psychiatric/ psychological causes as a possible diagnosis.

Phase 4: Work with the family to accept possibility of psychiatric/psychological diagnosis and if necessary, facilitate referral to mental health services.

HINTS FOR SCREENING PROBLEMS

- Parents and children often are reluctant to discuss psychosocial issues. Standard developmental checklists in pediatric encounter forms often are inadequate for this purpose. Asking "Do you have any concerns about your child's behavior or emotional well-being?" has been suggested as a way to increase the likelihood of identifying such problems.
- There is strong evidence for a heritable/ genetic risk of bipolar disorder (manic-depression), schizophrenia, and depression. There is less strong but growing evidence that other conditions, e.g., anxiety, ADHD, PDD, and tic disorders, may be genetically transmissible. Twin studies (monozygotic versus dizygotic) suggest that personality disorders have a significant genetic component.
- Many disorders, e.g., ADHD (between 3:1 to 9:1), depression (1:2), etc., have distinct male/female preponderance.
- Suicide is epidemic. Eight percent of high school students attempt suicide, 25% of which require medical attention. Fifty percent of attempters seek medical care in the month preceding their attempt, 25% in the preceding week.
- Conservative estimates of the prevalence of depression in children and adolescents range from 5% to 10%.
- Eating disorders, while relatively uncommon (0.5% to 1% prevalence), have a 5% to 15% mortality rate.

 Data Gathering

HISTORY

- A psychobehavioral assessment should include a history of the presenting complaint, a past medical, developmental, and behavioral/psychiatric history, and a complete familial history and review of systems.
- The "SHADSSS" mnemonic is a useful inventory of psychosocial functioning. It is structured such that the least threatening topics are asked first, the most intimate last. All of these areas of psychosocial functioning should be assessed in all patients.

—School (in school? grades? relationships with peers and teachers?)
—Home (living situation? relationship with parents? siblings?)
—Activities (how do patients spend their free time?)
—Depression
—Substance abuse (including alcohol and tobacco)
—Sexuality (including abuse, STDs, and pregnancy)
—Safety (suicidality, homicidality, plans for revenge or violence)

Children do not exist in a vacuum. All families should receive a family assessment. Families/support systems are crucial for the ultimate success of any treatment plan. At a minimum, a family assessment should include a discussion of:

- Constitution of household, custody/ visitation arrangements
- Who supervises the child or provides child care
- Stressors on the family (emotional, financial, interpersonal, violence within the family, involvement with law enforcement or social services, etc.)
- Strategies used by the family in coping with conflicts, problems, stressors, etc.

Behavioral or Psychiatric Problems

 Physical Examination

A thorough physical examination should be performed on all patients. The goal is to detect any abnormalities suggestive of an organic cause for the patient's symptoms (*see* Differential Diagnosis).

 Laboratory Aids

There is no set of "routine" laboratory tests that should be ordered to rule out an organic etiology of the behavioral or psychiatric symptoms. Tests should be performed on the basis of clinical suspicion.

SPECIFIC RESOURCES

• The use of screening questionnaires (*see* Bibliography), parent monitoring forms/diaries, and direct observation of parent–child interactions can be used, depending on the practitioner's experience, familiarity, and confidence with these modalities, as well as the practice setting. Screening for maternal depression may also be important in detecting psychosocial dysfunction.
• The Pediatric Symptom Checklist (PSC) is a well-validated 35-item, easily scored, parent-report screen of emotional and behavioral problems. It can be completed in 5 minutes and is easily administered in an office waiting area. The Child Behavior Checklist (CBCL) provides more in-depth assessment, but is more difficult to administer and score. A multitude of other screening tools have been developed, which are of varying utility to the pediatric practitioner.
• Conners Rating Scales alone are not sufficient to diagnose ADHD. It is a clinical diagnosis, based on pervasive inattention, hyperactivity, or impulsivity across different settings.
• Published in 1996 by the American Academy of Pediatrics, the *Diagnostic and Statistical Manual for Primary Care* (DSM-PC), child and adolescent version, is the result of collaborative efforts by pediatricians (primary care, and behavioral and developmental specialists), and child psychiatrists, psychologists, and neurologists. It provides a concise, user-friendly guide for diagnosing mental disorders in children and adolescents.

Clinical Pearls

• Children on psychotropic medications should be monitored for adverse effects.
• Stimulants: frequent assessment of growth, heart rate, and blood pressure every 3 to 6 months. Those on pemoline (Cylert) should have LFTs checked every 6 to 12 months.
• Tricyclic antidepressants: baseline ECG (before starting medication), and ECGs 1 month after starting medications and every 6 months thereafter.
• Antipsychotics: reassessment at 2, 4, and 12 weeks after starting medication, and every 3 to 6 months thereafter for adverse effects (dystonia, anticholinergic symptoms, movement disorders).

Pitfalls

• Not asking about behavioral or psychiatric problems. Parents are often reluctant to talk about such problems, thinking such problems are stigmatizing.
• Missed psychiatric diagnosis, especially suicidality, homicidality, or plans for revenge or violence.
• Confusing the degree of medical severity of a suicide attempt with the degree of suicide intent, i.e., "(S)he isn't significantly injured, so (s)he isn't seriously suicidal." Children and adolescents often misjudge the lethality of their suicide methods. All attempts must be taken seriously.
• Deciding on a diagnosis and/or treatment without a complete evaluation. Many psychiatric disorders can present in similar fashion (*see* Differential Diagnosis). The success of any treatment plan, as well as avoidance of erroneously "labeling" a child (with an incorrect diagnosis), depends on an accurate diagnosis, based on a thorough biopsychosocial evaluation.
• Many patients with primary psychiatric disorders will present with vague physical complaints. All patients with such complaints should be screened for psychiatric problems.
• Delay in diagnosis or referral for treatment, e.g., prognosis for learning disabilities and hearing impairment, is associated with timely intervention.

 Common Questions and Answers

Q: When should a child be referred to a specialist?
A: Whenever there is uncertainty about diagnosis or management, or when the treatment needs of the patient exceed the practitioner's capacity to provide them.

Q: How do you get children and families to talk about their problems?
A: There is no "trick." Being a patient, empathetic, nonjudgmental listener is the best strategy.

Q: What constitutes a psychiatric emergency?
A: Any situation where the safety or functioning of the child, family, or another person is endangered.

BIBLIOGRAPHY

Achenbach TM, Ruffle TM. The child behavior checklist and related forms for assessing behavioral/emotional problems and competencies. *Pediatr Rev* 2000;21(8): 265–271.

American Academy of Pediatrics, ADHD subcommittee. Clinical practice guideline: diagnosis and evaluation of the child with ADHD. *Pediatrics* 2000;105(5):1158–1170.

Cantwell DP. Attention deficit disorder: a review of the past 10 years. *J Am Acad Child Adolesc Psychiatry* 1996;35(8):978–987.

Clark LR, Ginsburg KR. How to talk to your teenage patients. *Contemp Adolesc Gynecol* 1995;Winter:23–27.

Casidy LJ, Jellinek MS. Approaches to recognition and management of childhood psychiatric disorders in pediatric primary care. *Pediatr Clin North Am* 1998;45(5):1037–1052.

Glascoe FP. Early detection of developmental and behavioral problems. *Pediatr Rev* 2000;21(8):272–279.

Roberts RE, Attkisson C, Rosenblatt A. Prevalence of psychopathology among children and adolescents. *Am J Psych* 1998;155(6):715–725.

Spencer T, Wilens T, Biederman J. Psychotropic medications for children and adolescents. *Child Adolesc Psych Clin North Am* 1995;4(1):97–121.

Stancin T, Palermo TM. A review of behavioral screening practices in pediatric settings: do they pass the test? *J Dev Behav Pediatr* 1997;18(3):183–194.

Wolralch ML. Diagnostic and statistical manual for primary care (DSM-PC) child and adolescent version: design, intent, and hopes for the future. *J Dev Behav Pediatr* 1997;18(3):171–182.

Author: Thomas H. Chun

Bruising

 Database

DEFINITION

Bruises are the result of extravasation of blood into the skin. Conventional usage often groups petechiae and bruises (or ecchymoses) together as purpura and defines them as follows:

• Petechiae: flat, red, or reddish purple, 1 to 3 mm, nonblanching
• Ecchymoses: larger than petechiae, due to local extravasation, nonpulsatile, sometimes palpable, color depends on age of lesion

 Differential Diagnosis

CONGENITAL/ANATOMIC

• Coagulation factor abnormality: hemophilia, von Willebrand disease
• Platelet defect: Bernard-Soulier syndrome, Glanzmann thrombasthenia, and storage pool defects
• Congenital alloimmune or isoimmune thrombocytopenia
• Neonatal extramedullary hematopoiesis
• Hereditary hemorrhagic telangiectasia

INFECTIOUS

• Meningococcemia
• Viral infections (coxsackieviruses, echoviruses)
• Rocky Mountain spotted fever (RMSF)
• Syphilis
• Pertussis—secondary to severe cough
• Septic or fat emboli
• DIC—acquired factor deficiency

TOXIC, ENVIRONMENTAL, DRUGS

• Warfarin—acquired factor deficiency
• Corticosteroids—striae caused by increased capillary fragility
• Aspirin and ibuprofen—cause a qualitative platelet abnormality
• Sulfonamides
• Bismuth
• Chloramphenicol

TRAUMA

• Normal activity
• Child abuse
• Valsalva, crying, forceful coughing
• Cupping or coin rubbing
• Tight garments

TUMOR (QUANTITATIVE PLATELET ABNORMALITY)

• Bone marrow replacement–leukemia, myelofibrosis

GENETIC/METABOLIC

• Uremia
• Vitamin C deficiency
• Vitamin K deficiency—due to antibiotics, biliary atresia, malabsorption (acquired factor deficiency)

ALLERGIC/INFLAMMATORY/VASCULITIC

• Henoch-Schönlein purpura (HSP)
• Bone marrow failure—aplastic anemia (including Fanconi, PNH)
• Increased destruction—idiopathic thrombocytopenic purpura, Evan syndrome, lupus
• Nephrotic syndrome
• Collagen vascular disease
• Ehlers-Danlos syndrome
• Snake bite (copperhead)

MISCELLANEOUS (DISORDERS THAT SIMULATE BRUISES)

• Ataxia telangiectasia
• Cherry angiomata
• Kaposi sarcoma

Approach to the Patient

GENERAL GOAL

To determine if the etiology of the bruising is due to thrombocytopenia, a coagulation disorder, or an extrinsic factor (such as trauma, infection, etc.).

Phase 1: Determine if the history of bruising and/or petechiae is acute or chronic in onset and if there is known trauma versus spontaneous lesions (see tables Most Common Causes of Bruising and How to Estimate the Age of Bruises).
The acute onset of diffuse subcutaneous bleeding with bruises of different ages may indicate severe thrombocytopenia. Generally, children will not bruise or develop petechiae spontaneously until the platelet count is under 20,000/mm². ITP, leukemia, aplastic anemia, etc., can cause this bleeding. A hematologist should be consulted, because of the risk of potentially life-threatening bleeding.
Chronic history of recurrent bleeding, such as mucosal, deep muscle or joint bleeds, may indicate an inherited coagulation defect such as von Willebrand disease or hemophilia. The familial history may be positive, although von

Willebrand disease often goes undiagnosed into adulthood if there has been no challenge such as surgery.

Phase 2: Perform screening tests for bleeding disorders to categorize the abnormality.

• Platelet count to assess level of thrombocytopenia
• PT/PTT: Prolongation of either one or both of these may aid in the diagnosis of von Willebrand disease, coagulation factor deficiencies, liver disease, and vitamin K deficiency.
• Bleeding time: Prolongation may indicate the presence of a platelet aggregation disorder or von Willebrand disease.

 Data Gathering

HISTORY

Question: At what age was the bruising first noticed?
Significance: Significant bruising in the neonatal period may indicate neonatal thrombocytopenia, congenital infections, and sepsis with DIC. Hemophilia more typically presents with bleeding in the neonatal period, such as with circumcision. Other inherited disorders coagulation, such as von Willebrand disease, may not be diagnosed until a child is older, as these tend to be mild in nature and may be uncovered with preoperative testing or postoperative bleeding complications. ITP may occur at any age.

Question: What is the pattern or distribution of the bruises?
Significance: The pattern of bruising, especially in a younger child, may indicate normal toddler activity, child abuse, or religious practices such as coining (common among Southeast Asians) in which warm or hot coins are rubbed on the skin to help in the healing process.

Question: What medications is the child taking?
Significance: Use of aspirin, ibuprofen, cough syrups with guaifenesin, and some antihistamines cause platelet dysfunction by inhibiting cyclooxygenase and, therefore, interfering with the release of platelet granules. Use of these drugs may also unmask an otherwise mild inherited bleeding disorder.

Most Common Causes of Bruising

1. Trauma (either accidental or intentional)
2. Infectious (viral etiology more common than bacterial)
3. Thrombocytopenia
4. Henoch-Schönlein purpura
5. Inherited coagulation defects (hemophilia, von Willebrand disease)

Question: Are there any signs or symptoms of systemic illness or infection?
Significance: Infections such as meningococcemia or viruses and collagen vascular diseases may present with ecchymosis or petechiae.

Question: Is there any familial history of a bleeding diathesis, easy bruisability, or heavy menstrual bleeding?
Significance: A positive familial history of inherited disorders of coagulation factors or platelet aggregation may aid in directing the workup. A negative familial history does not rule out any of these disorders, however.

 ## Physical Examination

Question: Does the child appear well or systemically ill?
Significance: A well appearance is often found in those with ITP, though there is often a history of an antecedent viral illness. An ill appearance should raise concerns about malignancy, infection (especially meningococcemia), or other acquired coagulation factor deficiencies such as those seen with liver failure.

Question: What is the distribution of the bruises?
Significance: Bruising in unusual locations such as the back, genitalia, or thorax should raise suspicions of child abuse, especially if the lesions are in different stages of healing (see table How to Estimate the Age of Bruises) or suggest the pattern of a hand, belt, etc. Purpura confined mostly to the legs are typical of HSP. Most toddlers will have multiple ecchymoses in the pretibial regions that occur with normal activity. Petechiae entirely above the nipple line is consistent with Valsalva maneuver, severe cough, and viral infections.

Question: Is the bleeding confined to the skin surface or are deeper tissues such as muscles and joints involved?
Significance: Hemophilia generally causes deeper bleeding, although bruising is common in the infant and younger child.

Question: Are the mucous membranes involved?
Significance: Severe thrombocytopenia, streptococcal pharyngitis, varicella, measles, and other viral infections can cause this finding. Von Willebrand disease can also present with gingival bleeding.

How to Estimate the Age of Bruises

1. New	Purple, dark red
2. 1–4 days	Dark blue to brown
3. 5–7 days	Greenish to yellow
4. >7 days	Yellow

Question: Is there hepatosplenomegaly or lymphadenopathy?
Significance: Involvement of the reticuloendothelial system can be found with malignancies such as leukemia or with viral or bacterial infections.

Question: Are there other congenital abnormalities?
Significance: Syndromes such as Fanconi anemia and thrombocytopenia absent radii (TAR) may present with upper extremity limb malformations and bruising.

 ## Laboratory Aids

Test: CBC
Significance: Platelet count is the most important, however, abnormalities of WBC or Hgb may aid in the diagnosis bone marrow infiltration or failure.

Test: PT
Significance: Elevation may indicate warfarin ingestion or factor VII deficiency or vitamin K deficiency.

Test: aPTT
Significance: Prolongation is seen with hemophilia and may be seen in von Willebrand disease.

Test: Both PT and PTT
Significance: Both are prolonged in DIC, liver failure, and vitamin K deficiency.

Test: Bleeding time
Significance: Lengthened in platelet aggregation disorders and with drug effects.

Test: Fibrinogen
Significance: Decreased in liver failure, DIC

Test: Urinalysis
Significance: Hematuria and/or proteinuria may indicate HSP, nephrotic syndrome, or other vasculitis.

 ## Emergency Care

Factors that make this an emergency include:

- Severe thrombocytopenia below 10,000–20,000/mm^3 carries a higher risk of spontaneous internal bleeding including intracranial bleeding.
- Bleeding or bruising accompanied by evidence of leukemia or other malignancy.
- Evidence of sepsis (DIC) or meningococcemia.

 ## Common Questions and Answers

Q: Is hemophilia always diagnosed in the newborn period?
A: No. A familial history may provide clues, but a significant number of patients represent a spontaneous mutation. Additionally, not all boys with hemophilia will bleed with circumcision and the diagnosis may not be made until the infants become more active.

Q: What is a common cause of bruising among girls?
A: Girls may first come to attention at menarche and be diagnosed at that time with von Willebrand disease. Rarely, girls whose fathers have hemophilia may be unfavorably "lyonized" and, therefore, have decreased factor levels consistent with mild hemophilia.

Issues for Referral

- ITP should be referred to a hematologist especially if the child is older, because there is a higher risk of chronic ITP or an underlying disorder such as lupus.
- Prolonged PT/PTT/BT often require referral to work up an inherited or acquired coagulation defect.
- Any concern about a malignancy, liver failure, or child abuse.

Clinical Pearls

- The amount of bruising may or may not correlate with the amount of internal bleeding that has occurred. Hemophiliacs can significantly drop their hemoglobin during a thigh or psoas bleed without having much in the way of ecchymosis.
- A child presenting with ITP may have bruises and petechiae from head to toe without changing the hemoglobin much at all.

BIBLIOGRAPHY

Manno CS. Difficult pediatric diagnoses: bleeding and bruising. *Pediatr Clin North Am* 1991;38(3):637–655.

Author: Julie W. Stern and Lisa Michaels

Chest Pain

 Database

DEFINITION

Chest pain is a common pain syndrome in childhood (see table Most Common Causes of Pediatric Chest Pain). It is less common than abdominal pain and headache.

 Differential Diagnosis

MUSCULOSKELETAL DISORDERS
- Chest wall strain
- Costochondritis
- Direct chest trauma
- Slipping rib syndrome

CARDIAC PATHOLOGY
- Arrhythmia (supraventricular tachycardia, premature ventricular contractions)
- Coronary-artery anomalies
- Coronary-artery aneurysms (Kawasaki disease)
- Infections (myocarditis, pericarditis)
- Myocardial infarction/ischemia
- Structural abnormalities
—Aortic stenosis
—Hypertrophic cardiomyopathy
—Pulmonic stenosis
—Mitral valve prolapse
—Severe coarctation of the aorta

GASTROINTESTINAL DISORDERS
- Caustic ingestions
- Esophageal foreign bodies
- Esophagitis (sometimes tetracycline, "pill," induced)

PSYCHOGENIC CAUSES
- Anxiety
- Hyperventilation

RESPIRATORY DISORDERS
- Asthma
- Cough (prolonged)
- Pleural effusion
- Pneumonia
- Pneumothorax—spontaneous, trauma-related, drug-related (cocaine)
- Pneumomediastinum
- Pulmonary embolism

Most Common Causes of Pediatric Chest Pain

Idiopathic
Musculoskeletal
  Chest wall strain
  Costochondritis
  Direct trauma
Respiratory conditions
  Asthma, cough, pneumonia
Gastrointestinal problems
  Esophagitis, esophageal foreign body
  Psychogenic—stress related
Cardiac pathology

MISCELLANEOUS
- Breast mass
- Cigarette smoke
- Pleurodynia
- Precordial catch syndrome
- Shingles
- Sickle cell crises
- Thoracic tumor

Approach to the Patient

GENERAL GOAL
Identify the rare child with a serious etiology for chest pain (see tables Important Physical Findings on General Examination of Child with Chest Pain and Important Physical Findings on Chest Examination of Child with Chest Pain).

Phase 1: Is the patient in acute distress? If so, begin emergency management and proceed rapidly to find the cause of pain.

Phase 2: For the majority of stable children with chest pain, determine whether laboratory tests are needed to help identify the etiology.

Phase 3: Treat specific conditions as appropriate. Begin analgesics, reassure the family and arrange for follow-up care.

HINTS FOR SCREENING PROBLEM
Take a thorough history and perform a careful physical exam. Examine the chest last—do not focus only on this area. Use laboratory tests sparingly, only to confirm clinical suspicions.

 Data Gathering

HISTORY
Question: How severe, how often is the pain?
Significance: Constant, frequent severe pain is more likely to be distressing, interruptive of daily activity. Serious etiology is not well correlated with frequency, severity of pain.

Important Physical Findings on General Examination of Child with Chest Pain

Severe distress
Chronically ill appearance
Skin rash or bruising
Abdominal pathology
Arthritis present
Anxiety apparent

From: Selbst SM. Evaluation of chest pain in children. *Pediatr Rev* 1986;8:56–62.

Question: What is the type of pain? Its location?
Significance: Burning pain is associated with esophagitis. Sharp, stabbing pain relieved by sitting up or leaning forward is typical of pericarditis. Young children do not describe or localize chest pain well.

Question: When was the onset of pain?
Significance: Acute pain (<48 hours) is more likely to have an organic etiology. Chronic pain (>6 months) is more likely to be psychogenic, idiopathic. In an older child with sudden onset of pain consider an arrhythmia, pneumothorax, or musculoskeletal injury. In a young child with sudden onset of pain consider a foreign body (coin) in the esophagus, or injury.

Question: Is the pain induced by exercise?
Significance: Exercise-induced chest pain may be related to serious cardiac disease or asthma.

Question: Recent trauma or muscle overuse?
Significance: Musculoskeletal (chest wall) pain

Question: Eaten spicy foods? Taken tetracycline or other pills?
Significance: Esophagitis. Teens often take pills with little water and then lie down. The undissolved pill may lodge in the esophagus and cause pain.

Question: Recent use of cocaine?
Significance: Hypertension, tachycardia, myocardial ischemia, or pneumothorax.

Question: Use of oral contraceptives or recent leg trauma?
Significance: Pulmonary embolism. This is very rare in the pediatric age group.

Question: Recent significant stress (e.g., move, death of loved one, serious illness)?
Significance: Psychogenic pain. We know children have headaches and abdominal pain related to stress. Chest pain may also relate to unusual stress.

Question: Associated complaints?
Significance: Fever may imply pneumonia, myocarditis, pericarditis. Syncope, palpitations may imply cardiac arrhythmias or severe anemia. Joint pain, rash may relate chest pain to collagen vascular disease. Pain that resolves with parental attention may indicate an emotional etiology.

Important Physical Findings on Chest Examination of Child with Chest Pain

Inspection: trauma, asymmetry, abnormal breathing pattern
Auscultation: tachycardia, arrhythmia, murmur, rub, rales, wheezing
Palpation: tenderness, subcutaneous emphysema

From: Selbst SM. Evaluation of chest pain in children. *Pediatr Rev* 1986;8:56–62.

Question: Positive familial history?
Significance: Hypertrophic cardiomyopathy is often familial. Those with a familial history positive for heart disease and chest pain may be concerned about the symptom in a child. Chest pain in such children often has a nonorganic etiology.

Question: Past medical history?
Significance: Previous Kawasaki disease, long-standing insulin-dependent diabetes mellitus, and sickle cell disease may have serious cardiac or pulmonary complications leading to chest pain. Marfan syndrome has increased risk for aortic dissection, pneumothorax. Asthma has increased risk for pneumonia, pneumothorax. Collagen vascular disease has increased risk for pleural effusion, pericarditis. Most underlying structural cardiac lesions rarely produce chest pain.

 ## Physical Examination

Finding: Child is in significant distress.
Significance: Requires emergency care; stabilization. Consider pneumothorax, arrhythmia.

Finding: Child appears chronically ill.
Significance: Chest pain may be found in serious illness such as malignancy (Hodgkin's lymphoma).

Finding: Fever
Significance: Consider pneumonia, myocarditis.

Finding: Skin bruising present
Significance: Chest pain may be related to unrecognized trauma.

Finding: Abdominal pathology
Significance: Pain may be referred to the chest.

Finding: Arthritis present
Significance: Collagen vascular disease may manifest as pleural effusion, chest pain.

Finding: Unusually anxious child
Significance: Underlying stress may lead to pain.

Finding: Breast enlargement, asymmetry, tenderness
Significance: Physiologic breast changes in young teens may be painful. Consider pregnancy in teenage girls.

Finding: Rubs, decreased breath sounds, wheezing
Significance: May suggest pneumonia, asthma with overuse of chest wall muscles.

Finding: Subcutaneous emphysema palpable on chest or neck
Significance: Pneumothorax, pneumomediastinum

Finding: Heart murmur, rub, arrhythmia
Significance: Congenital heart disease, cardiac infection such as myocarditis, pericarditis, supraventricular tachycardia, ventricular tachycardia.

Finding: Tenderness of chest wall, costochondral junctions
Significance: Musculoskeletal pain

 ## Laboratory Aids

Test: Electrocardiogram
Significance: Obtain if history suggests cardiac pathology, for instance:
- Acute onset of pain
- Pain on exertion
- Pain associated with syncope, dizziness, palpitations
- History of congenital heart disease
- Serious associated medical problems (Kawasaki disease, diabetes mellitus)
- Use of cocaine
Obtain also if physical exam is abnormal. For instance:
- Respiratory distress
- Cardiac abnormality
- Fever
- Significant trauma

Test: Chest radiograph
Significance: Same as for electrocardiogram. Also, obtain if history suggests cardiac or pulmonary pathology, tumor, Marfan syndrome, or foreign body (coin ingestion).

Test: Holter monitor
Significance: Arrange for this study if cardiac arrhythmia suspected. Electrocardiogram may fail to detect intermittent arrhythmia.

Test: Exercise stress test, pulmonary function tests
Significance: Obtain if pain induced by exertion.

Test: Drug screen
Significance: Obtain if cocaine use suspected.

Emergency Care

Factors that make this an emergency include:
- Pneumothorax: may present with severe sudden chest pain, respiratory distress, cyanosis, hypotension.
- Cardiac arrhythmia: ventricular tachycardia or supraventricular tachycardia in an older child may progress to heart failure or a lethal rhythm.
- Cocaine intoxication: may present with pneumothorax, cardiac arrhythmia, hypertension.
- Direct chest trauma: may lead to cardiac contusion, and arrhythmia.
- Caustic ingestions or esophageal foreign bodies require prompt attention.

 ## Common Questions and Answers

Q: How common is chest pain in children?
A: Chest pain is a common pain syndrome reported in 6 of 1,000 children who present to an urban emergency department. The complaint is less common than abdominal pain or headache. Although children of all ages may complain of chest pain, the mean age is about 12 years.

Q: Is follow-up important?
A: Yes. Serious pathology is unlikely to be found if not diagnosed initially. However, watch for signs of exercise-induced asthma or for emotional problems that were not obvious initially. Ensure that the child returns to normal activity when appropriate.

Q: What is the prognosis for most children with chest pain?
A: Most children with chest pain have an excellent prognosis. About 40% of children with chest pain will have continued symptoms for 6 to 24 months.

Issues for Referral
- Acute distress
- Significant trauma
- History of heart disease or related serious medical problem
- Pain with exercise, syncope, palpitations, dizziness
- Serious emotional disturbance
- Esophageal foreign body, caustic ingestion
- Pneumothorax, pleural effusion

Clinical Pearls
- If the child is febrile, consider pneumonia, or viral myocarditis.
- Treat specific etiology when found.
- Over-the-counter analgesics (acetaminophen, ibuprofen) suffice for most pain.
- Antacids may be diagnostic and therapeutic for esophagitis pain.
- Rest, heat, relaxation techniques may be useful.
- Avoid expensive, invasive laboratory studies with chronic pain and normal physical examination, benign history.

BIBLIOGRAPHY
Kocis KC. Chest pain in pediatrics. *Pediatr Clin North Am* 1999;46:189–203.

Perry RF, Garlisi AP, Allison EJ, et al. Acute myocardial infarction in a 16-year-old boy with no predisposing risk factors. *Pediatr Emerg Care* 1997;13:413–416.

Selbst SM, Ruddy RM, Clark BJ, et al. Pediatric chest pain; a prospective study. *Pediatrics* 1988;82:319–323.

Selbst SM. Chest pain in children; consultation with the specialist. *Pediatr Rev* 1997;18:169–173.

Author: Steven M. Selbst

Coma

Database

DEFINITION

Coma is defined as an unresponsive state with eyes closed, usually lasting less than 24 hours. This condition signals a medical emergency, and immediate attention/intervention is required for abnormalities in breathing, circulation, glucose, or electrolytes.

- *Lethargy* indicates a patient who is incoherent but arousable and has a tendency to sleep.
- *Stupor* is used when the patient is responsive only to pain.
- *Vegetative state* suggests a chronic state in which sleep–wake cycles persist but there is no evidence of cognition.
- *Locked-in* must be distinguished from coma; that is, cognitive functions are intact, though the patient may appear unconscious.

CAUSES OF COMA

- Trauma: epidural, subdural, intracerebral hematoma, diffuse cerebral swelling
- Poisoning
- Hypoxia/ischemia
- Infection—meningitis, encephalitis, toxic shock, subdural empyema, hemorrhagic shock
- Metabolic disorders

—Hypoglycemia (salicylate or ethanol intoxication, hyperinsulinemia)
—Diabetic ketoacidosis (DKA): rare catastrophic neurologic deterioration seen on initiation of insulin and/or fluid therapy
—Reye syndrome
—Electrolyte abnormalities (Na, K, Ca, Mg)
—Hepatic/uremic encephalopathy
—Inborn errors of metabolism
—Hormonal abnormalities (thyroid, adrenal, pituitary)
—Hypothermia/hyperthermia

- Tumor
- Seizure
- Vascular: hemorrhage [from arteriovenous malformation (AVM), aneurysm, coagulopathy, infarction, cerebral venous thrombosis, hypertensive encephalopathy]
- Hydrocephalus: ventriculoperitoneal (VP) shunt obstruction, mass/bleed obstructing ventricular outflow

PATHOPHYSIOLOGY

Coma may be localized to the reticular activating system (RAS) in the brainstem or bilateral cerebral dysfunction. Abnormalities of the protective reflexes of the upper airway or abnormalities of the respiratory pattern may signal impending respiratory failure.

COMPLICATIONS OF ACUTE COMA

- Respiratory failure
- Deep venous thrombosis
- Pneumonia
- Aspiration

Differential Diagnosis

DISORDERS MIMICKING COMA

- Psychogenic coma: patient may resist passive eye opening, regards self in mirror, and avoids passive arm fall over face
- Locked-in state: complete paralysis with normal cerebral function may occur in severe neuromuscular disorders (acute polyneuropathy) or in ventral pontine lesions (hemorrhage, demyelination)

Data Gathering

HISTORY

- Head trauma
- Ingestion
- Drugs/toxins in home
- Fever
- Nausea
- Headache
- Preceding viral illness
- Seizures
- Diabetes
- Preexisting neurologic disease
- Previous episodes of coma

Physical Examination

- Vital signs
- Abnormal respiratory pattern
- Bradycardia
- Hypertension
- HEENT—look for signs of head trauma: raccoon eyes (Battle signs, ecchymosis at mastoid equals basilar skull fracture)
- Retinal hemorrhages
- Bulging fontanelle
- Neck: nuchal rigidity, Kernig and Brudzinski signs associated with meningitis
- Neurologic: verbal or motor response to voice, touch, pain; eye opening/fixation; spontaneous movements/posturing; pupil symmetry/reactivity, abnormal oculocephalic response (doll eyes); worsening signs in any of the above may indicate increased intracranial pressure (ICP)
- Reflexes specific to rostral brainstem function include pupillary light reflex, corneal reflex, jaw jerk
- Reflexes specific to caudal brainstem function include oculocephalic reflex (horizontal eye deviation with passive head rotation), gag, spontaneous respirations

Laboratory Aids

Initial blood studies obtained with placement of an IV line include:

- Glucose
- Electrolytes
- BUN/creatinine
- Calcium
- Arterial blood gas
- CBC
- Toxicology screen
- Ammonia
- Liver transaminases
- Radiology—noncontrast head CT scan first to look for hemorrhage, may be followed by contrasted images or MRI to look for infection/mass lesions
- Cervical spine series (CT or lateral and AP x-ray studies)—indicated if evidence of trauma by history or on examination
- Cervical spine must be stabilized until injury is ruled out
- Lumbar puncture, to rule out infection, bleed; defer until after CT if focal exam or signs of increased ICP
- Question of "traumatic tap" can often be settled by spinning out red cells promptly and examining fluid for xanthochromia
- EEG—helpful to rule out nonconvulsive status epilepticus

Emergency Care

- First priority is stabilization of respiratory and hemodynamic status.
- Endotracheal intubation—often required to ensure airway protection and adequate oxygenation.
- Large-bore IV lines should be placed and isotonic fluids administered as needed to replace intravascular volume and maintain adequate blood pressure.
- If finger-stick glucose determination is low, give 2 to 4 mL of 25% dextrose (D25) per kilogram intravenously (D10 if young infant).
- If ingestion is suspected, administer naloxone (0.01 mg/kg IV).

- When there is evidence of increased ICP:
—Hyperventilate to decrease blood CO_2 to 25 to 30 torr and give mannitol (0.5–1 g/kg IV).
—Dexamethasone, 1 to 2 mg/kg IV, can also be administered.
—All fluids given should be isotonic and the volume limited to that needed to maintain adequate perfusion.
—Head should be elevated 30 degrees above horizontal to maximize cerebral venous drainage.
—Hospitalization is usually in the intensive care unit for close monitoring for changes in respiratory status or signs of increased ICP.
—Drug indications depend on underlying etiology.
—IV antibiotics should be given if infection is suspected.

Therapy

As above

Follow-Up

PROGNOSIS

Prognosis depends on underlying etiology. Complete recovery is frequently seen after toxic-metabolic coma. In contrast, patients with coma resulting from severe head trauma or hypoxic injury often have significant neurologic sequelae and may require physical, occupational, and cognitive therapies.

PITFALLS

- Quadriparesis due to neuromuscular weakness may resemble coma; responsiveness is determined by patient questioning, using whatever movements may be preserved (often, eye movements).
- In psychogenic coma, defensive movements may be elicited (resistance to passive eye opening, arm falls away from face); presentation of a mirror may induce involuntary visual fixation.

Common Questions and Answers

Q: What is the role of EEG in the diagnosis of coma?
A: EEG is useful in diagnosis of psychogenic coma (should be normal) and in coma from brainstem lesions, in nonconvulsive status epilepticus (shows electrographic seizures), and in possible herpes encephalitis (temporal or frontal sharp activity).

Q: Should anticonvulsants be given to comatose victims of trauma?
A: While there is no clear evidence that anticonvulsants improve outcome or reduce incidence of posttraumatic seizures, they are often given when posttraumatic intracranial hypertension and/or edema is suspected because seizures are known to raise ICP.

Issues for Referral

Neurosurgical intervention may be required in cases of head trauma, hemorrhage, mass lesion, or hydrocephalus. Neurology consultation is usually indicated.

Clinical Pearls

Trauma and near-drowning are leading causes among children, and boys are more often victims of trauma/near-drowning than girls.

BIBLIOGRAPHY

Chiappa KH, Hill RA. Evaluation and prognostication in coma. *Electroencephalogr Clin Neurophysiol* 1998;106(2):149–155.

Feske SK. Coma and confusional states: emergency diagnosis and management. *Neurol Clin* 1998;16(2):237–256.

Jacizo SJ, Gieron-Korthals M, Ferreira JA. Predicting outcome in hypoxic-ischemic brain injury. *Pediatr Clin North Am* 2001;48(3):647–660.

Tasker RC. Neurological critical care. *Curr Opin Pediatr* 2000;12(3):222–226.

Author: Amy R. Brooks-Kayal

Cough

Database

DEFINITION

Cough is a symptom of a variety of underlying conditions, which results from a complex reflex phenomenon initiated by cough receptors and mediated in the brainstem's cough center. These receptors are located throughout the large- to medium-sized airways (and not the lower airways), pharynx, paranasal sinuses, external auditory canal, and stomach, and are triggered by thermal, chemical, mechanical, or inflammatory stimuli. The resultant high-velocity expiration, which removes airway secretions, is generally reflexive, but may sometimes be voluntarily initiated or suppressed.

Differential Diagnosis

Infection and reactive airway disease are the most common causes of cough in all age groups and should always be considered.

CAUSES OF ACUTE COUGH

- Infection
- Reactive airway disease (RAD)
- Sinusitis
- Irritative
- Allergic
- Foreign body

CAUSES OF CHRONIC COUGH

- Infection
- Asthma or asthmatic bronchitis
- Sinusitis
- Irritative/postinfectious
- Allergic
- Foreign body (FB)
- Gastroesophageal reflux (GER)
- Habitual or psychogenic
- Anatomic abnormalities

—Tracheoesophageal fistula
—Tracheobronchomalacia
—Laryngeal cleft
—Polyps
—Adductor vocal cord paralysis
—Pulmonary sequestration
—Bronchogenic cyst
—Cystic hygroma
—Vascular ring
—Tumor

- Cystic fibrosis (CF)
- Ciliary dyskinesia syndromes

- Immunodeficiency states

—Human immunodeficiency virus (HIV)
—Immunoglobulin deficiencies (IgA, IgG)
—Phagocytic defects
—Complement deficiency

- Pulmonary hemosiderosis
- Angiotensin-converting enzyme inhibitors
- External auditory canal irritation

Approach to the Patient

GENERAL GOAL

The presenting symptom of cough is a familiar one to most physicians and accounts for nearly 7% of chief complaints to pediatricians. Cough is an easily identifiable symptom that frequently provokes parental concern and can be troublesome to the physician. The possible etiologies of cough are diverse, and may range from a minor illness to a life-threatening condition. Therefore, a stepwise approach is required in an effort to prevent a costly and lengthy investigation. In particular, a thorough history and physical examination are of paramount importance in the evaluation.

Phase 1: Complete history and physical examination to determine time course and severity of cough and to ascertain whether it represents a significant problem of respiratory function or a serious underlying disease.

Phase 2: Initiate focused workup and treatment plan depending on differential diagnosis (see previous section).

Phase 3: Refer to pediatric pulmonologist if cough persists or if concerned about significant pathology (see following section).

Data Gathering

HISTORY

Question: Is the cough acute or chronic?
Significance: Generally considered to be chronic if present longer than 3 weeks. Although there is significant overlap, differential diagnosis varies depending on the time course.

Question: How is this problem different in children as compared with adults?
Significance: Differential diagnosis varies considerably based on the patient's age.

Question: Is there a recent history of upper respiratory infection (URI)?
Significance: Consider serial URIs (children have average of 6 to 8 per year with each lasting up to 2 weeks), postinfectious/irritative or sinusitis (which complicates up to 5% of URIs).

Question: What are the associated symptoms?
Significance:

- Fever, nasal discharge suggest infection.
- Fever with chills or night sweats suggests tuberculosis.
- Sputum production indicates bronchiectasis or other lower airway pathology.
- With headache or facial edema, consider sinusitis.
- With respiratory distress, suspect RAD.

Question: What is the quality of the cough?
Significance:

- Productive cough suggests lower airway infection, CF/bronchiectasis.
- Dry cough suggests RAD, fungal infection.
- Barking cough is usually associated with croup.
- Honking or brassy cough is typical in habitual or psychogenic cough.

Question: What is the pattern of the cough?
Significance:

- Nighttime cough suggests RAD.
- With nighttime/early morning cough, consider sinusitis.
- Seasonal cough suggests allergy.

Question: Are there any known triggers of cough (e.g., cold air, dust, smoke, URI)?
Significance: Consider irritant, allergic, or reactive airway disease.

Question: Is there any personal or familial history of atopy?
Significance: Consider RAD.

Question: Is there a history of recurrent infections?
Significance: Consider immunodeficiency, CF.

Question: Is there any relation of cough to feedings?
Significance: Consider aspiration, tracheoesophageal fistula.

Question: Is there a history of a choking episode?
Significance: Consider retained foreign body, although there may not be a history of a choking episode in this case and cough may be episodic as FB moves along respiratory tract.

Question: Is there failure to thrive?
Significance: Rule out CF, immunodeficiency.

Physical Examination

Finding: Patient's general appearance
Significance:

- Evidence of failure to thrive—consider CF, immunodeficiency.
- Cyanosis or pallor—rule out hypoxemia.
- Signs of respiratory distress such as tachypnea, accessory muscle use—most likely RAD or infection.

Finding: Barrel chest
Significance: Suggests air-trapping due to chronic disease.

Finding: Clubbing
Significance: May be seen with bronchiectasis.

Finding: Nasal polyps
Significance: May be associated with allergic conditions or CF.

Finding: Tracheal deviation
Significance: Suggests mediastinal mass or FB aspiration.

Finding: Signs of atopic disease
Significance: Eczema, allergic shiners, transverse nasal crease, rhinitis, mucosal cobblestoning, injected conjunctivae suggest allergy, RAD.

Finding: Periorbital edema, sinus tenderness, purulent posterior pharyngeal drainage, halitosis
Significance: Sinusitis

Finding: Wheezing
Significance: Polyphonic inspiratory or expiratory wheezes suggest RAD, while monophonic or fixed wheezes should make one consider FB or mass/congenital lesion.

Laboratory Aids

Laboratory investigation should reflect a rational, stepwise approach based on likely etiologies after a thorough history and physical examination.

Test: Chest radiograph
Significance:

- Infiltrates may suggest pneumonia, bronchiolitis, pneumonitis, TB, CF, bronchiectasis, FB.
- Volume loss may be seen with FB aspiration; sometimes need to obtain lateral decubitus views in young children who cannot cooperate with inspiratory/expiratory views.
- Hyperinflation suggests RAD or CF.
- Mediastinal nodes may indicate infection (especially TB, fungus) or malignancy.

Test: Mantoux test—purified protein derivative (PPD)
Significance: Rule out tuberculosis.

Test: Complete blood count
Significance: Eosinophilia suggests atopic disease or, rarely, parasitic infection; anemia should prompt one to consider chronic disease or, rarely, pulmonary hemosiderosis.

Test: Sputum sample must contain alveolar macrophages.
Significance:

- Eosinophils suggest asthmatic process or hypersensitivity reaction of lung.
- Polymorphonuclear cells suggest infection.
- Predominance of macrophages suggests postinfectious hyperresponsive cough receptors.
- Hemosiderin staining suggests pulmonary hemosiderosis.
- Lipid-laden macrophages suggest recurrent aspiration.
- Routine or special cultures based on likely pathogens.

Test: Serum IgE
Significance: Significant elevation indicates allergy or, rarely, parasites.

Test: Sweat chloride test
Significance: Cystic fibrosis. Need to be sure that laboratory has experience with this test.

Test: Wright peak flow rate
Significance:

- Easy to perform in the office with the proper flow meter.
- Helpful to get prebronchodilator and postbronchodilator rates if RAD suspected.
- Standardized tables available with values based on height and race.

Test: Immune workup
Significance: HIV; immunoglobulins

Test: Barium swallow or pH probe
Significance: Reflux

Test: Bronchoscopy
Significance: To remove FB or obtain tissue samples.

Emergency Care

- Cough should be considered an emergency if there are associated signs or symptoms of respiratory distress.
- Routine emergency airway assessment (i.e., ABCs) should be undertaken on presentation and appropriate supportive measures started in cases in which there is concern.
- Refer for additional treatment as outlined previously.

Common Questions and Answers

Q: Is whooping cough still a problem despite routine childhood immunization?
A: Yes. Pertussis often goes unrecognized as a cause of acute and chronic cough, particularly in infants who have not completed their immunization series and in adolescents (and adults) in whom immunity from vaccination will have waned.

Q: Is it possible for children to have asthma if they have never wheezed?
A: Yes, there is cough-variant reactive airway disease.

Issues for Referral

Factors that may alert you to make a referral include:

- The cough is unresponsive to treatment.
- The cause is likely to be an anatomic malformation or FB aspiration.
- There appears to be involvement of other organ systems (e.g., failure to thrive, GER, congestive heart failure, immunodeficiency, unusual infection).
- There is hemoptysis.

Clinical Pearls

- The goal is to treat the underlying cause of the cough, not the symptom.
- Educate parents about the beneficial function of cough to remove irritants and about the potential harm of suppressing a productive cough or cough secondary to RAD.
- Specific pharmacologic interventions:

—RAD: bronchodilators ± inhaled antiinflammatory agents (e.g., cromolyn sodium), oral or inhaled steroids, removal of irritants
—Infection: appropriate antibiotics
—Cough suppressants have not been shown to be efficacious in children under 5 years, and have been associated with significant toxicity in this age group.

BIBLIOGRAPHY

Committee on Drugs. Use of codeine and DM-containing cough remedies in children. *Pediatrics* 1997;99(6):918–920.

Kamei RK. Chronic cough in children. *Pediatr Clin North Am* 1991;38(3):593–605.

Katcher ML. Cold, cough and allergy medications: uses and abuses. *Pediatr Rev* 1996;17(1):12–17.

Kemper KJ. Chronic asthma: an update. *Pediatr Rev* 1996;17(4):111–117.

Taylor JA, Novack AH, Almquist JR, et al. Efficacy of cough suppressants in children. *J Pediatr* 1993;122(5):799–802.

Author: Margaret McNamara

Crying

 Database

DEFINITION

Crying is usually a normal physiologic response to distress, discomfort, or unfulfilled needs. Crying is felt to be potentially pathologic if it is interpreted by caregivers as differing in quality and duration without apparent explanation and/or persists without consolability beyond a reasonable time (generally 1 to 2 hours).

 Differential Diagnosis

CONGENITAL/ANATOMIC

- Intussusception
- Gastroesophageal reflux/esophagitis
- Volvulus
- Gaseous distention (2° to improper feeding or burping)
- Incarcerated hernia
- Peritonitis (acute abdomen)
- Testicular/ovarian torsion
- Constipation
- Anal fissure
- Meatal ulceration
- Glaucoma
- Urinary retention (secondary to posterior urethral valves)
- Cardiac—anomalous coronary artery, hypoxia

INFECTIOUS

- Otitis media/externa
- Urinary tract infection
- Stomatitis/gingivitis
- Meningitis
- Discitis
- Gastroenteritis
- Arthritis
- Osteomyelitis
- Perianal cellulitis
- Balanitis
- Dermatitis (especially pruritic as in scabies or painful as in staphylococcal scalded skin syndrome)

TOXIC, ENVIRONMENTAL, DRUGS

- Neonatal drug withdrawal
- Prenatal/perinatal cocaine exposure
- Immunization reactions (especially DTP)
- Cow's milk intolerance
- Isolated fructose intolerance
- Drug reactions (especially antihistamines, pseudoephedrine, phenylpropanolamine), including maternal medications in breast milk
- Vitamin A toxicity
- Emotional/physical neglect

TRAUMA

- Corneal abrasion
- Foreign body (hypopharynx, eye, ear)
- Skull fracture/subdural hematoma
- Intracranial hemorrhage
- Retinal hemorrhage
- Other fractures (especially extremities)
- Hair tourniquet syndrome (encircling finger, toe, penis, clitoris)
- Open diaper pin
- Bite (human, animal, insect)

GENETIC/METABOLIC

- Sickle cell crisis
- Phenylketonuria
- Hypothyroidism
- Electrolyte abnormalities (especially sodium)
- Hypoglycemia
- Hypocalcemia
- Inborn error of metabolism

ALLERGIC/INFLAMMATORY

- Cow's milk allergy
- Celiac disease (gluten enteropathy)

FUNCTIONAL

- Parental expectations/responses

MISCELLANEOUS

- Overstimulation
- Persistent night awakening
- Night terrors
- Congestive heart failure
- Caffey disease (infantile cortical hyperostosis)
- Dysrhythmia (especially supraventricular tachycardia)
- Autism
- Teething
- Headache/migraine
- Temperament
- Colic
- Discomfort (cold, heat, itching, hunger)

Approach to the Patient

GENERAL GOAL

Decide if the crying represents a normal physiologic response, a protracted multifactorial physiologic/developmental response (colic), or a potentially pathologic problem.

Phase 1: How urgent is the need for evaluation? A classic and difficult triage issue. One must identify the periodicity of the problem, associated symptoms, impression of wellness, and parental anxiety/reliability.

Phase 2: When in doubt, particularly if "colic" seems unlikely, see the patient as soon as possible.

 Data Gathering

HISTORY

Question: Onset after 1 month of age or persistent in infants older than 4 months?
Significance: Colic less likely as a cause.

Question: First episode?
Significance: Recurrent episodes, particularly with a diurnal pattern, are more likely due to colic.

Question: Fever?
Significance: Potential need for evaluation of meningitis, other infections.

Question: Do attempts at consolation make the crying worse?
Significance: Paradoxically increased crying (especially with lifting, rocking) can be seen in meningitis, peritonitis, long-bone fractures, arthritis.

Question: Stridor?
Significance: Implies possible upper airway obstruction (mechanical, functional).

Question: Expiratory grunting?
Significance: Higher likelihood of significant pathologic cause of crying (especially cardiac, respiratory, and/or infectious disease).

Question: Cold symptoms and/or day-care attendance?
Significance: Increased likelihood of otitis media.

Question: Vomiting?
Significance: Higher likelihood of pathologic gastrointestinal cause (e.g., obstruction, G-E reflux with possible esophagitis), particularly in infant <3 months, or CNS disease.

Question: What is the pattern of feeding?
Significance: Over/underfeeding, excessive air swallowing, inadequate burping, improper formula preparation may contribute to excessive crying.

Question: Recent fall or trauma?
Significance: Possible fracture, increased intracranial pressure, abuse.

 Physical Examination

Finding: Tympanic membrane with loss of landmarks, poor mobility.
Significance: Otitis media

Finding: Tenderness on palpation of extremities or clavicle.
Significance: Suggests fracture or osteomyelitis.

Finding: Conjunctival redness, eye tearing, scratches near the eye.
Significance: Suggests corneal abrasion (fluorescein testing of eye warranted) or foreign body in eye (eversion of lid recommended).

Finding: Impacted or bloody stool on rectal exam, abdominal mass
Significance: Constipation or intussusception

Finding: Geographic scars, frenulum tears, retinal hemorrhages, suspicious bruises, decreased weight/height ratio
Significance: Neglect/abuse (physical, emotional)

Finding: Bulging fontanel
Significance: Possible increased ICP (meningitis, subdural hematoma, vitamin A toxicity)

Finding: Edema of individual toes, fingers, or penis
Significance: Hair tourniquet syndrome

Finding: Tender swelling in inguinal or scrotal area
Significance: Incarcerated hernia, testicular torsion

Finding: Heart rate >200 with minimal variability
Significance: Possible supraventricular tachycardia

 Laboratory Aids

Test: Stool for occult blood
Significance: Possible intussusception, anal fissure

Test: Fluorescein testing of eye
Significance: Corneal abrasion (may occur without significant conjunctival redness)

Test: Urinalysis/urine culture
Significance: Urinary tract infection

Test: Urine toxicology screen
Significance: Drug withdrawal (neonatal), ingestions, passive exposures (e.g., cocaine)

Test: Pulse oximetry
Significance: Hypoxia (from cardiac causes) may cause increased irritability

 Emergency Care

Factors that make this an emergency include:

• Suspicion of meningitis: stiff neck, bulging fontanel, fever (especially infants <2 to 3 months)
• Suspicion of intestinal obstruction: vomiting (especially bilious or projectile), mass on abdominal palpation, and/or bloody stools
• Suspicion of incarcerated hernia or testicular/ovarian torsion
• Evidence of cardiac compromise (CHF, SVT): tachycardia, poor perfusion (capillary refill >3 seconds, poor distal pulses), rales
• Evidence of acute dehydration: weight loss, decreased urine output, orthostatic changes, poor perfusion
• Evidence of child abuse or neglect

Common Questions and Answers

Q: What is the most likely cause of inconsolable crying in the first few months of life?
A: Without question, infantile colic. A practitioner needs to be familiar with the clinical pattern of infantile colic, so that deviations from this most common pediatric syndrome are readily recognized.

Q: Is teething a common cause of excessive crying?
A: Grandparents everywhere insist that it is (as well as a common cause of fever, diarrhea, rashes, etc.). Objective data do not support a strong association. Be careful in ascribing symptoms and signs to teething. Trust the grandparents, but verify.

Issues for Referral

Factors that may help alert you to make a referral include: ill versus well-appearing. Although observation alone is less reliable in infants <3 months, judgment of an infant to be ill-appearing (e.g., pallor, grunting, poor arousability, poor response to social overtures) warrants more urgent and extensive evaluation. Weight loss or abnormal development implies a much higher likelihood of an organic cause of repetitive bouts of crying.

Clinical Pearls

• Quality of cry: Objective acoustic analyses of cries may become a common future modality to distinguish pathologic from physiologic crying. However, subjective interpretation can be helpful.

—High-pitched (shrill, piercing) crying in short bursts: associated with CNS pathology, especially with increased intracranial pressure
—High-pitched crying in longer bursts: seen in SGA infants, neonatal drug withdrawal
—Hoarse crying: seen in hypothyroidism, laryngeal diseases, hypocalcemic tetany
—Weak crying: may be seen in neuromuscular disorders, such as Hoffman-Werdnig syndrome, infant botulism, and/or the very ill infant
—Cat-like cry: as noted on every pediatric board exam for the last 35 years, a mewing cry can be associated with cri du chat syndrome (5p syndrome or absence of short arm of chromosome 5)

• Neonatal drug withdrawal has other characteristic findings in addition to excessive crying.

—Wakefulness
—Irritability
—Tremulousness, temperature variation, tachypnea
—Hyperactivity, high-pitched persistent cry, hyperacusis, hyperreflexia, hypertonia
—Diarrhea, diaphoresis, disorganized suck
—Rub marks, respiratory distress, rhinorrhea
—Apnea, autonomic dysfunction
—Weight loss or failure to gain weight
—Alkalosis (respiratory)
—Lacrimation

BIBLIOGRAPHY

Barr RG, Hopkins B, Green JA, eds. *Crying as a sign, a symptom and a signal.* London: Cambridge University Press, 2000.

Committee on Drugs. Neonatal drug withdrawal. *Pediatrics* 1998;101(6)72:1079–1088.

Corwin MJ, Lester BM, Golub HL. The infant cry: what can it tell us? *Curr Probl Pediatr* 1996;26(9):325–334.

Poole SR. The infant with acute, unexplained, excessive crying. *Pediatrics* 1991;88(3):450–455.

Author: Mark F. Ditmar

Diarrhea

 Database

DEFINITION

Diarrhea should be considered whenever there is an increase in frequency, volume, or liquidity of patients' stool as compared to their normal bowel movement pattern. While an adult excretes 100 to 200 g of stool each day, a child typically passes 10 g/kg in 24 hours. Diarrhea can also be characterized by duration. Chronic diarrhea is generally defined as the persistence of loose or more frequent stools for more than 2 weeks. Tenesmus, perianal discomfort, and incontinence may also occur. Diarrhea is caused whenever there is an alteration in the normal intestinal fluid-electrolyte balance. Malabsorption, maldigestion, cellular electrolyte pump dysfunction, and intestinal colonization or invasion by microorganisms can cause diarrhea.

 Differential Diagnosis

ACUTE DIARRHEA

- Dietary causes

—Sorbitol, fructose
—Intolerance to specific foods (beans, fruit, peppers, etc.)

- Infectious causes

—Bacterial (*Salmonella, Shigella, Campylobacter, Yersinia, Plesiomonas, Aeromonas, Escherichia coli*)
—Viral (rotavirus, Norwalk agent, adenovirus)

- Medication

—Antibiotics
—Laxatives: Magnesium-containing

CHRONIC DIARRHEA

- Allergic/autoimmune

—Milk/soy protein allergy
—Eosinophilic enteritis
—Henoch-Schönlein purpura
—AIDS
—IgA deficiency
—Combined immunodeficiency
—Vasculitis

- Anatomic abnormalities

—Short intestine
—Malrotation

- Bile salt malabsorption
- Celiac disease
- Congenital causes

—Cystic fibrosis
—Villous atrophy
—Holovisceral myopathy

- Hirschsprung enterocolitis
- Encopresis
- Endocrine disorders

—Hyperthyroidism
—Diabetes
—Congenital adrenal hyperplasia

- Infectious causes

—Bacterial
—Viral
—Parasites (*Giardia, Entamoeba, Cryptosporidium*)
—*Clostridium difficile*
—Bacterial overgrowth

- Inflammatory bowel disease

—Ulcerative colitis
—Crohn disease

- Intestinal lymphangiectasia: primary and secondary
- Irritable bowel syndrome
- Lactose intolerance (primary, secondary, congenital)
- Medication
- Necrotizing enterocolitis
- Pancreatic dysfunction

—Shwachman syndrome
—Chronic pancreatitis

- Postinfectious diarrhea
- Pseudo-obstruction
- Secretory tumors (VIPoma, somatostatinoma, gastrinoma)

—Hemolytic uremic syndrome

Approach to the Patient

GENERAL GOAL

Determine the type of diarrhea (osmotic versus secretory).

Phase 1: Secretory Diarrhea Absorption of intestinal fluid and electrolytes is accomplished through multiple cellular pumps transporting sodium, glucose, and amino acids. Factors that interrupt these pumps (cholera toxin, prostaglandin E, VIP, secretin) can cause a severe active isotonic secretory state manifested by profuse diarrhea, dehydration, and acidosis.

Phase 2: Osmotic Diarrhea In general, the solute composition of intestinal fluid is similar to plasma. Osmotic diarrhea occurs when poorly absorbed or nonabsorbable solute is present in the intestinal lumen. This can occur with the ingestion of nonabsorbable sugars or cathartics, with carbohydrate malabsorption secondary to mucosal damage, with maldigestion secondary to pancreatic or hepatic dysfunction, with rapid transit of intestinal fluid, or with a rare congenital transport defect.

 Data Gathering

HISTORY

Question: Has the diarrhea lasted less than 2 weeks?
Significance: A distinction should be made between acute and chronic diarrhea. The cause of acute diarrhea is almost always related to an infection, a medication, or the addition of a new food.

Question: Travel history?
Significance: Questions should be asked regarding travel to areas where drinking water is contaminated (e.g., Mexico—*Entamoeba*) or the ingestion of infected meat (*E. coli*) or fresh water (well water) infected with *Giardia*.

Question: Is the patient an adolescent who is concerned about his or her weight?
Significance: Laxative abuse causing an osmotic diarrhea is common among adolescents who have an eating disorder.

Question: Does the patient have other systemic symptoms?
Significance: Systemic symptoms such as fever, gastrointestinal bleeding, rash, or vomiting should be ascertained. Specific infections and inflammatory bowel disease have associated systemic symptoms.

Question: Hematochezia?
Significance: The occurrence of acute, bloody stools and fever generally indicates a bacterial infection or amebiasis; however, these same symptoms coupled with thrombocytopenia, anemia, and azotemia, or with a purpuric rash can indicate hemolytic uremic syndrome or Henoch-Schönlein purpura (HSP), respectively. Chronic bloody diarrhea, abdominal pain, and weight loss are characteristic of inflammatory bowel disease.

Question: What is the age of the child?
Significance: The age of the child is important because a number of diseases present between birth and 3 months of life including congenital villus/transport abnormalities, cystic fibrosis, or milk/soy allergy. In a previously well infant who had a recent viral illness with subsequent protracted diarrhea, the diagnosis of postviral enteritis should be suspected. This disorder is characterized by severe mucosal injury resulting in disaccharidase deficiency and prolonged malabsorption. Chronic nonspecific diarrhea should be considered in otherwise normal preschool-aged children who have 2 to 10 watery stools/day without other symptoms and/or etiology. Lactose intolerance commonly occurs in many older children and adults, with over a 95% occurrence rate in some ethnic groups.

Question: Chronic diarrhea with weight loss?
Significance: Inflammatory or immunologic disorders such as ulcerative colitis, Crohn disease, and celiac disease must be considered in older children with chronic diarrhea.

Question: Water supply?
Significance: Patients may acquire *Giardia* infection from well water or water from some rural areas.

 ## Physical Examination

Finding: What are the child's growth parameters?
Significance: An important part of the physical examination is height, weight, head circumference, and height/weight measurements. Previous measurements are necessary to make an accurate evaluation. Findings of a chronically malnourished child with years of unsuspected weight loss or poor growth velocity would indicate a divergent differential diagnosis from that of a healthy-appearing child with normal growth.

Finding: Does the child have arthritis?
Significance: Arthritis and diarrhea can occur in diseases such as inflammatory bowel disease, celiac disease, HSP, and in specific bacterial infections.

Finding: Is there nailbed clubbing?
Significance: Cystic fibrosis

Finding: Is there a right lower quadrant mass?
Significance: A right lower quadrant mass could suggest an abscess (Crohn disease, appendiceal abscess).

 ## Laboratory Aids

Test: Stool culture
Significance: Stool examination not only for blood/mucus/inflammatory cells but also for microorganisms is important in determining the etiology of the diarrhea. Stool cultures for parasites (*Giardia, Entamoeba*), bacterial pathogens (*Salmonella, Campylobacter, Shigella, Yersinia, Aeromonas, Plesiomonas*), and *C. difficile* toxin should be obtained in all children with unexplained diarrhea.

Test: Stool Gram stain
Significance: Useful in determining the presence of polymorphonuclear leukocytes suggesting a colitis.

Test: Stool pH
Significance: Useful in identifying carbohydrate malabsorption; normal stool pH is 5 to 6.

Test: Hemoccult
Significance: Documents blood

Test: 72-hour quantitative fecal fat evaluation
Significance: A sensitive test for steatorrhea. Patients need to be placed on a high-fat diet (3 g/kg) for 3 days. During this time, all stools are collected and frozen, and on completion the amount of ingested fat is compared to excreted fat. When malabsorption is present, disorders of pancreatic function (cystic fibrosis, Shwachman syndrome) or severe intestinal disease should be suspected.

Test: Lactose breath test
Significance: A noninvasive test that measures hydrogen levels in expired air and is based on the principle that hydrogen gas is produced by colonic bacterial fermentation of malabsorbed carbohydrates. When abnormal in older healthy-appearing children, primary lactose deficiency is suggested. However, in young children, secondary lactase deficiency should be considered and small-bowel disease should be suspected.

Test: D-xylose test
Significance: Based on the principle that D-xylose absorption occurs independently of bile salts, pancreatic secretions, and intestinal disaccharidases. A specific dose of D-xylose (0.5 gm/kg, maximum 25 g) is given orally after an 8 hour fast and the serum level of D-xylose is determined after 1 hour. Typically, disorders that alter or disrupt the intestinal mucosa produce abnormal results.

Test: Endoscopy and colonoscopy
Significance: These procedures have become extremely useful tests. These diagnostic tests not only allow direct visualization of the intestinal mucosa but also provide access for intestinal culture, disaccharidase and pancreatic enzyme evaluation, and intestinal biopsy.

 ## Emergency Care

Diarrhea can lead to dehydration. Any child suspected of clinical dehydration should be closely observed. If oral rehydration is ineffective, intravenous therapy is indicated. In addition, rarely acute right lower abdominal pain with diarrhea may indicate appendicitis. Culture-negative gastrointestinal bleeding associated with severe abdominal pain and diarrhea should always be treated urgently.

Issues for Referral

Because the occurrence of diarrhea in children is quite common, the decision to pursue an evaluation rests with the primary care physician. Children who present with growth failure, noninfectious heme-positive diarrhea, or unexplained chronic diarrhea should be considered for referral to a pediatric gastroenterologist.

BIBLIOGRAPHY

Ammon HV. Diarrhea. In: Haubrick WS, Schaffner F, Berk JE, eds. *Gastroenterology*, 5th ed. Philadelphia: WB Saunders, 1995:87–101.

Arnold L. Acute diarrhea. In: Schwartz MW, Curry TA, Sargent AJ, et al., eds. *Principles and practice of clinical pediatrics*. Chicago: Year Book, 1997:227–231.

Chronic diarrhea: a practical approach for the pediatrician. *Pediatr Clin North Am* 1991;38:667–685.

Fontaine O. Oral rehydration therapy: a critical component in integrated management of childhood illness. *J Pediatr Gastroenterol Nutr* 2000;30(5):490.

Rhoads JM, Powell DW. Diarrhea. In: Walker WA, Durie PR, Hamilton JR, et al., eds. *Pediatric gastrointestinal disease*. Philadelphia: BC Decker, 1990:62–78.

Vanderhoof JA. Diarrhea. In: Wyllie R, Hyams JS, eds. *Pediatric gastrointestinal disease*. Philadelphia: WB Saunders, 1993:187–197.

Waters V, Ford-Jones EL, Petric M, et al. Etiology of community-acquired pediatric viral diarrhea: a prospective longitudinal study in hospitals, emergency departments, pediatric practices and child care centers during the winter rotavirus outbreak, 1997 to 1998. The Pediatric Rotavirus Epidemiology Study for Immunization Study Group. *Pediatr Infect Dis J* 2000;19(9):843–848.

Author: Chris A. Liacouras

Dyspnea

 Database

DEFINITION

Shortness of breath, a subjective feeling of having difficulty breathing.

 Differential Diagnosis

CONGENITAL/ANATOMIC

- Subglottic stenosis
- Vocal cord paralysis
- Macroglossia
- Pierre Robin syndrome
- Laryngeal atresia
- Pulmonary sequestration
- Pulmonary hypoplasia

INFECTIOUS

- Lower airway

—Bronchiolitis
—Pertussis
—Pneumonia
—Tuberculosis

- Upper airway

—Croup
—Epiglottitis
—Tracheitis
—Peritonsillar abscess

TOXIC, ENVIRONMENTAL, DRUGS

- Aspiration

—Fluid
—Foreign body

- Carbon monoxide poisoning
- Methemoglobinemia
- Smoke inhalation

TUMORS/CYSTS

- Head/neck

—Dermoid cysts
—Branchial cleft cysts
—Lingual thyroid
—Hemangioma
—Teratoma
—Papilloma
—Brainstem tumor

- Thoracic

—Teratoma
—Cystic hygroma
—Bronchogenic cyst
—Pericardial cyst
—Neurogenic tumor
—Lymphoma
—Leukemia

- Abdominal mass

—Hepatic mass
—Hepatoblastoma
—Neuroblastoma

ALLERGY

- Anaphylaxis

PULMONARY

- Asthma
- Atelectasis
- Pneumothorax
- Pleural effusion
- Hemorrhage
- Embolism

CARDIAC

- Pulmonary edema

RENAL

- Renal failure causing fluid overload
- Metabolic acidosis

HEMATOLOGY

- Anemia
- Sickle cell crisis
- Acute chest syndrome

MUSCLE WEAKNESS

- Duchenne muscular dystrophy
- Spinal muscle atrophy

MISCELLANEOUS

- High altitude
- Exercise
- Psychogenic hyperventilation
- Anxiety
- Panic disorders

Approach to the Patient

GENERAL GOALS

To identify the organ system responsible for the dyspnea and to determine whether the process is acute or chronic.

Phase 1: Determine if the cause is respiratory or cardiac in nature. Are patients clinically stable and can they protect their airway? It is important to identify those who will need intensive/emergency care and those who can be worked up in the office.

Phase 2: Inquire about the duration of symptoms and the circumstances around the onset of the dyspnea. History and physical examination should focus on respiratory and cardiology. If these two have been ruled out, other etiologies must be evaluated.

Phase 3: Inquire about other medical problems of the patient.

 Data Gathering

HISTORY

Question: Onset of dyspnea? What was the patient doing at the time of onset (if acute)?
Significance: In a small child, acute onset may be related to aspiration of a foreign body or liquid. If the patient was unsupervised, foreign body is a high probability. If the dyspnea occurred over days, other respiratory, cardiac, or renal should be suspected.

Question: Any fever, cough, chest pain, runny nose?
Significance: This would suggest an infectious etiology. The chest pain could be related to a pneumothorax, which can occur spontaneously in some individuals.

Question: Anyone at home sick or have respiratory problems and/or illness?
Significance: Leading toward infection. However, in some cases of congenital heart disease a respiratory virus such as RSV can make an otherwise stable patient into a critically ill child.

Question: Is there history of wheezing or asthma?
Significance: Children who have a history of wheezing are likely to reexacerbate their lung disease.

Question: Has the child ever been hospitalized or had respiratory problem in the past?
Significance: Children who have been hospitalized for respiratory problems are likely to have subsequent difficulty with other respiratory problems.

Question: Any history of cardiac problems or ever been diagnosed with a murmur?
Significance: In the absence of an infectious type or wheezing type of history, a murmur can help the examiner focus on the cardiac examination.

Physical Examination

LUNG

Finding: Crackles or rhonchi auscultate
Significance: Lower lung disease such as pneumonia or bronchiolitis. Fluid overload can cause bilateral crackles.

Finding: Wheezing auscultated
Significance: Wheezing is usually heard on expiration. Suggests an obstructive lung disease such as asthma or reactive airways disease or anaphylaxis.

Finding: Distant or absent breath sounds
Significance: Foreign body aspiration blocking air movement. Pneumothorax should also be suspected.

Finding: Barking cough
Significance: Croup, which is usually caused by parainfluenza virus. It also could be foreign body.

Finding: Symptoms worse in supine position.
Significance: Could be secondary to pulmonary edema or compression by a mediastinal mass.

Finding: Egophony auscultate
Significance: Pleural effusion should be suspected.

HEART

Finding: Loud murmur or gallop auscultated
Significance: Cardiac disease in which pulmonary edema can be etiology of the dyspnea.

Finding: Cyanosis
Significance: Poor oxygen perfusion

Finding: Low blood pressure and poor skin perfusion
Significance: The patient can be in shock. Quick identification of the type of shock is needed to correct the underlying problem.

Finding: Clubbing of the digits
Significance: Suggests chronic disease such as cystic fibrosis or cardiac disease

Finding: Drooling, with mouth open in an ill-appearing child
Significance: Suggests epiglottitis and need for careful evaluation (see Epiglottitis)

Finding: Abdominal mass palpated
Significance: Could be causing compression of lungs

Finding: Ascites or edema
Significance: Fluid overload either from renal or cardiac etiology

Laboratory Aids

Test: Chest radiograph
Significance: Look for appearance of the lung fields for the different types of pneumonia. Evaluate the heart size and the pulmonary vascularity for fluid overload. Hyperinflation suggests an obstructive pulmonary disease such as asthma. A hyperinflated (usually right lobe) darkened lobe is suspicious of a foreign body present. Seeing a shift in the heart and seeing a lung edge is common in pneumothorax or effusion. Fluid in the costophrenic angle suggests an effusion.

Test: Pulse oximetry
Significance: A quick assessment of oxygen perfusion

Test: Arterial blood gas
Significance: A more detailed assessment of oxygenation and acidosis. A blood gas will also delineate metabolic versus respiratory acidosis and also can show if compensation has occurred.

Test: Complete blood count with differential
Significance: First, an elevated white blood count with a left shift differential can be a sign of infection. If the patient has pallor, the hemoglobin can be evaluated to see if the patient is anemic. A CBC also can be helpful in patients in whom leukemia or other oncologic diseases are suspected.

Test: Mantoux (PPD)
Significance: If there is a history of family members with tuberculosis or immigrants from a country where TB is prevalent, a PPD should be placed with anergy panel.

Common Questions and Answers

Q: Is dyspnea, in most cases, pulmonary in nature?
A: Yes, it is in most cases. However, if infectious, foreign body, and asthma etiologies are ruled out, a nonrespiratory cause must be investigated

Issues for Referral

• Any patient who has unstable vital signs, inability to oxygenate, and needs critical care services.
• Any patient with a suspected foreign body aspiration will need a bronchoscopy surgical consult.
• If asthma is suspected, use criteria as noted in asthma (see Asthma).
• Any patient with epiglottitis will need an otolaryngologist to evaluate the patient under general anesthesia (see Epiglottitis).
• Anaphylaxis is a medical emergency and mandates immediate action. Epinephrine, Benadryl, and possibly steroids are the drugs of choice for treatment.
• Any patient who has a pneumothorax. May need surgical aspiration or chest tube placement (see Pneumothorax).
• Any patient in whom an oncologic process is suspected. Referral to a tertiary care center with a critical care unit and with a pediatric oncologist (see Leukemia).

Clinical Pearls

• A child who presents with dyspnea, anxiety, or panic disorder should only be considered once the more serious etiologies have been ruled out.
• If hyperventilation is suspected, a brown paper bag can be useful to break the cycle of hypocarbia.

BIBLIOGRAPHY

Chang AB. Cough, cough receptors, and asthma in children *Pediatr Pulmonol* 1999;28(1):59–70.

Denny FW. Acute respiratory infections in children: etiology and epidemiology. *Pediatr Rev* 1987;9(5):135–146.

Dibs SD, Baker MD. Anaphylaxis in children: a 5-year experience. *Pediatrics* 1997;99(1):E7.

Holroyd HJ. Foreign body aspiration: potential cause of coughing and wheezing. *Pediatr Rev* 1988;10(2):59–63.

McIntosh K. Respiratory syncytial virus infections in infants and children: diagnosis and treatment. *Pediatr Rev* 1987;9(6): 191–196.

Schidlow DV, Callahan CW. Pneumonia. *Pediatr Rev* 1996;17(9):300–309.

Segel GB. Anemia. *Pediatr Rev* 1988;10(3): 77–88.

Author: Charles I. Schwartz

Dysuria

 Database

DEFINITION

Painful urination

 Differential Diagnosis

CONGENITAL/ANATOMIC

- Meatal stenosis
- Urethral stricture
- Posterior urethral diverticula
- Urethral stones
- Urethral valves
- Ureterocele
- Ectopic ureter
- Vesicovaginal fistula

INFECTIOUS

- Viral infection
- Gonorrhea
- Herpes simplex
- Tuberculosis
- Cystitis
- Urethritis
- Pinworms
- Prostatitis

TOXIC, ENVIRONMENTAL, DRUGS

- Bubble bath urethritis
- Cytoxan

TRAUMA

- Diaper dermatitis
- Foreign body
- Bicycle injury
- Masturbation
- Sexual abuse

TUMOR

- Sarcoma botryoides

GENETIC/METABOLIC

- Cystinuria

ALLERGIC INFLAMMATORY

- Food allergy
- Stevens-Johnson syndrome
- Contact dermatitis such as poison ivy

FUNCTIONAL

- Attention mechanism

MISCELLANEOUS

- Appendicitis

Approach to the Patient

GENERAL GOALS

Determine the cause and begin treatment.

Phase 1: Rule out common causes such as trauma, infection, chemical irritant, constipation, and masturbation. Consider attention-getting behavior.

Phase 2: Continue investigation–look for congential problems that cause infection, strictures. Metabolic disease and allergies.

Phase 3: Begin treatment.

HINTS FOR SCREENING PROBLEMS

Ask about medications and food allergens. Ask about special situations such as sand in bathing suit to cause irritation.

 Data Gathering

HISTORY

Question: Do the symptoms occur at any special time of day?
Significance: May indicate an attention mechanism if occurs before school.

Question: What kinds of medicine do you take?
Significance: Some medications such as cytoxin will cause irritation of the urethra.

Question: Have there been any new foods or known food allergens?
Significance: Milk and citrus fruits can cause dysuria in certain patients. Best determined if symptoms regress on elimination of possible offending food.

Question: Do you use bubble bath?
Significance: Bubble bath is fun but depletes the protective lipids in the urethra

Question: Any signs of bleeding?
Significance: Can indicate trauma, infection, or congenital anomalies. Calcium excretion can cause dysuria as well as hematuria.

Question: Fever
Significance: Common sign of urinary tract infection.

Question: Frequency
Significance: Both frequency and dysuria are common findings in urinary tract infections.

Question: Past history of urologic operations
Significance: Antireflux surgery may have a side effect of dysuria

Question: What have you taken for the discomfort?
Significance: Although cranberry juice is used for many urinary problems, the volume needed is usually more than what is ingested.

Question: Quality and strength of the urinary stream
Significance: Patients with posterior urethral valves have small, frequent voidings with low pressure because of the obstruction in the posterior urethra.

Physical Examination

Finding: Any signs of redness or ecchymoses?
Significance: May indicate trauma from masturbation or abuse

Finding: Any bleeding?
Significance: Seen in trauma, tumors, and infection.

Finding: Any change in behavior?
Significance: This symptom may be an attention-seeking device.

Finding: Abnormal swelling?
Significance: May occur in trauma or rare tumors.

Finding: Abnormal urethra?
Significance: Prolapsed urethra or diverticula

Finding: Grape-like structures in vagina?
Significance: Sarcoma botryoides

Finding: Abdominal pain?
Significance: Intraabdominal abscess or low-lying inflamed appendix can cause dysuria

Laboratory Aids

Test: Urinalysis
Significance: Most urinary tract infections will have white cells in the urine.

Test: Urine culture
Significance: Check for infection.

Test: Ultrasound
Significance: Not routinely requested unless a congenital anomaly is suspected.

Test: Metabolic screens
Significance: If sediment shows crystals; if familial history of metabolic disease.

Common Questions and Answers

Q: How does bubble bath cause dysuria?
A: The bubble bath depletes lipids that protect the urethra, causing the tissue to swell and become inflamed.

Q: Can allergies cause dysuria?
A: It is difficult to directly prove allergies as a cause of dysuria. However, in some cases, elimination of certain foods such as spices, citrus fruits, or known skin allergens have improved symptoms.

Q: How do children get infected with gonococcus?
A: This is a red flag of sexual abuse, which must be investigated.

Q: Which viruses cause dysuria?
A: Adenovirus has been identified.

Issues for Referral

- Evidence of congenital anomaly
- Increasing severity of symptoms
- Failure to respond to symptomatic or specific treatment

Clinical Pearls

- Sometimes difficult to differentiate dysuria from frequency, which may cause an uncomfortable feeling or pressure that is described by the child as "pain."
- Discharge with dysuria suggests gonococcal or chlamydia infection.
- Low lying inflamed appendix may cause bladder irritation and dysuria.
- Urethral prolapse may present as hematuria or frequency.

BIBLIOGRAPHY

Anonymous. 1998 guidelines for treatment of sexually transmitted diseases. Centers for Disease Control and Prevention. *MMWR* 1998;47(RR-1):1–111.

Lee HJ, Pyo JW, Choi EH, et al. Isolation of adenovirus type from the urine of children with acute hemorrhagic cystitis. *Pediatr Infect Dis J* 1996;15(7):633–634.

Rushton HG. Urinary tract infections in children. Epidemiology, evaluation, and management. *Pediatr Clin North Am* 1997;44(5):1133–1169.

Author: M. William Schwartz

Earache

Database

DEFINITION

Primary otalgia refers to pain originating from the ear structures. Secondary otalgia is the sensation of ear pain as a result of referred pain from other areas of the head and neck. Secondary pain is referred through cranial and cervical nerves that share distributions with the ear.

Differential Diagnosis

PRIMARY OTALGIA

Infectious

- Otitis media—most common cause of pediatric otalgia, acute onset.
- Otitis externa—more common in summer months; pain increases with traction on pinna.
- Varicella—chickenpox may involve the auricle and ear canal, as may herpes zoster.
- Herpes simplex—appears as grouped vesicles.
- Cellulitis
- Furunculosis—localized abscess of cartilaginous portion of ear canal (outer third)
- Mastoiditis—complication of otitis media; ear protrudes anteriorly.
- Myringitis-inflammation and blisters on the tympanic membrane.
- Perichondritis—inflammation of auricle without ear lobe involvement.

Trauma

- Foreign body—child may have an intense inflammatory reaction.
- Lacerations, abrasions—usually from putting objects in ear or cleaning.
- Blunt trauma—may be associated with tympanic membrane perforation, inner ear injury, or basilar skull fractures.
- Barotrauma—arising from abrupt changes in middle ear pressure (airplanes, scuba diving).

Tumor

- Rare in pediatric patients, but may involve any of the ear structures including skin, bone, vascular, and neural components: rhabdomyosarcoma, lymphoma, eosinophilic granuloma, Wegener granulomatosis pheochromocytoma.

Allergic/Inflammatory

- Serous otitis media—child may complain of pain, fullness, hearing loss, or "hearing things."
- Dermatologic conditions such as eczema and psoriasis.

- Allergy to topical antibiotic and cerumenolytic agents.

Functional

- Eustachian tube dysfunction

Miscellaneous

- Impacted cerumen
- Thermal injury to auricle
- Caustic burns from hearing aid batteries
- Aural neuralgia—brief sharp pain localized deep in ear without radiation; etiology unclear.

SECONDARY OTALGIA

Infectious

- Dental infections—abscess and gingivitis.
- Stomatitis—herpes simplex and Coxsackie
- Tonsillitis
- Peritonsillar abscess
- Retropharyngeal abscess—drooling, stridor, child usually appears ill
- Mumps
- Sinusitis
- Cervical adenitis
- Laryngitis
- Sialadenitis
- Ramsay Hunt syndrome (viral neuritis of facial nerve secondary to herpes zoster)

Trauma

- Dental trauma
- Penetrating injuries to the oropharynx
- Lacerations
- Posttonsillectomy/adenoidectomy—pain worsens with swallowing.
- Burns—caustic, thermal, or electrical
- Injuries to the neck and C-spine including fractures and muscle tension

Tumor

- Oropharyngeal/laryngeal tumors—may be cystic, benign, or malignant
- Rarely intracranial tumors will present with ear pain.

Allergic/Inflammatory

- Allergic rhinitis
- Cervical spine arthritis

Miscellaneous

- Aphthous ulcers (canker sores)
- Foreign body lodged in piriform sinus or esophagus.
- Esophagitis—usually secondary to severe gastroesophageal reflex (GER).
- Temporomandibular joint (TMJ) disease
- Migraine
- Thyroid inflammation of any etiology
- Psychogenic (rarely)

Approach to the Patient

GENERAL GOALS

As with the approach to any sick child, the primary determination is whether or not the child needs acute/emergent treatment for life-threatening disease. Ear pain can arise from disease involving almost any part of the head and neck; therefore, history taking and physical examination should be directed toward assessing symptoms from the entire region, not just the ear. Preceding symptoms and a history of events leading up to the onset of pain are of particular importance, as there are classic historic features to many of the diseases of the ear (e.g., URI symptoms with otitis media, wrestling history with auricle disease, swimming history with otitis externa).

Phase 1: Each encounter should begin with a careful history and physical examination. If the examination of the ear does not reveal the cause of pain, thoroughly examine the entire head and neck region.

Phase 2: An abnormal audiogram or tympanogram may help to determine if ear pathology is present in the face of a normal or difficult physical exam.

Phase 3: Referral to an otorhinolaryngologist and/or dentist is indicated in cases of ear pain with no identifiable cause.

Data Gathering

HISTORY

Question: Duration of symptoms?
Significance: Acute onset suggests recent trauma or infection.

Question: Severity of pain?
Significance: Severe pain is usually otogenic.

Question: Precipitating factors?
Significance: Pain increased with auricle movement—OE, furunculosis, perichondritis, cellulitis. Pain increased with jaw movement—TMJ disease, furunculosis.

Question: Associated symptoms?
Significance: Symptoms that point to primary otalgia include: aural discharge, deafness, tinnitus, and vertigo.

Question: Hoarseness?
Significance: Suggestive of oropharyngeal or laryngeal pathology including infections, foreign body, and GER.

Question: Choking/coughing?
Significance: Consider foreign body, mass, or GER.

Question: Location of additional pain or symptoms?
Significance: If referred pain, will likely have symptoms at primary site as well.

Question: Fever?
Significance: Suggestive of infectious etiology.

Question: Trauma and barotrauma?
Significance: Ask about recent ear cleaning, falls, accidents, air travel, diving.

Question: History of recurrent otitis media?
Significance: Consider serous otitis media, cholesteatoma.

 ## Physical Examination

Finding: Intense pain elicited by traction on pinna
Significance: Suggestive of otitis externa or furunculosis.

Finding: Areas of trauma
Significance: There may be an isolated abrasion or laceration; however, inspect carefully for hemotympanum and associated injuries and evidence of basilar skull fracture.

Finding: Foreign bodies
Significance: May be isolated, or associated with otitis externa; there are several case reports of foreign bodies behind the tympanic membranes.

Finding: Bulging, red, immobile tympanic membrane
Significance: Consistent with otitis media.

Finding: Retracted, immobile tympanic membrane
Significance: Suggests otitis media with effusion and eustachian tube dysfunction.

Finding: Redness, swelling, or tenderness of auricle
Significance: With lobe involvement—cellulitis; without lobe involvement—perichondritis.

Finding: Laterally displaced auricle
Significance: Highly suggestive finding in mastoiditis.

Finding: Normal ear exam
Significance: Suggests secondary otalgia. Be sure to examine head and neck carefully (see subsequent findings).

Finding: Dental caries
Significance: Multiple dental caries should raise the suspicion of a possible dental abscess.

Finding: Tonsillar asymmetry or uvular deviation from midline
Significance: May represent peritonsillar cellulitis/abscess or mass.

Finding: Assess facial-nerve function and other cranial nerves
Significance: Bell palsy may be a complication of otitis media. Other cranial nerve dysfunction suggests possible intracranial lesion.

 ## Laboratory Aids

The history and physical examination are usually sufficient to make the diagnosis.

Test: Audiometry
Significance: Assess for hearing loss suggestive of primary otalgia.

Test: Tympanometry
Significance: Useful in assessment of otitis media with effusion, eustachian-tube dysfunction, and tympanostomy tube obstruction.

Test: Culture of aural discharge
Significance: Indicated when otitis externa or otitis media with perforation of the tympanic membrane does not resolve as expected with routine antibiotic usage.

Test: CT scan
Significance: Important if symptoms suggest retropharyngeal mass/abscess (neck), to rule out sinusitis in complicated cases (sinus study), or to further evaluate for mastoiditis

Test: MRI or CT imaging of head
Significance: Rarely needed unless intracranial lesion suspected.

Test: Blood tests
Significance: Not routinely useful.

 ## Emergency Care

Disorders with potential to cause airway compromise (e.g., mass lesions, foreign bodies, abscess, penetrating injuries, posttonsillectomy complications):

- Establish "ABCs" as indicated.
- Consult otorhinolaryngologist (ORL).
- Hospitalize.

Trauma resulting in hearing loss, significant bleeding, or fractures:

- Establish "ABCs" as indicated.
- Promptly consult ORL.
- Do not attempt to remove debris from ear if suspected basilar skull fracture (can introduce bacteria).
- Hospitalize as indicated.

Infectious etiologies that cause toxic-appearing or "septic" child:

- Establish "ABCs" as indicated.
- Hospitalize and administer intravenous antibiotics.

Issues for Referral

Factors that may alert you to make a referral to ORL when otalgia is primary in origin include:

- Pain with unexplained hearing loss, vertigo, tinnitus
- Unexplained or persistent otorrhea

- Suspected neoplasm
- History suggestive of severe barotrauma
- Otitis media with complications
- Foreign bodies that cannot be removed easily from the ear
- Potential for auricle destruction (e.g., perichondritis can lead to permanent deformation, cauliflower ear)
- Ear pain without an identifiable source

Therapy

- Therapy is directed at the identified underlying cause.
- Pain medication such as topical benzocaine for otitis media, and acetaminophen or ibuprofen is always important, as many of the infectious etiologies are exquisitely painful.

Follow-Up

Varies depending on ultimate diagnosis.

 ## Common Questions and Answers

Question: Which nerves are involved in referred pain to the ear?
Answer: Sensory innervation of the ear arises from branches of the fifth (trigeminal), seventh (facial), ninth (glossopharyngeal), and tenth (vagus) cranial nerves as well as the second and third cervical nerves.

Question: What is the most common source of referred ear pain?
Answer: Dental disease.

Question: What are the most common organisms in otitis externa?
Answer: Pseudomonas aeruginosa, Staphylococcus aureus, Staphylococcus epidermidis, streptococci, *Enterobacter aerogenes, Proteus mirabilis, Klebsiella pneumoniae, Candida, Aspergillus.*

Question: What are the most common organisms in otitis media?
Answer: Streptococcus pneumoniae, Haemophilus influenzae, Moraxella catarrhalis, and viral agents.

BIBLIOGRAPHY

LeLiever W. *Nonotalgic otalgia. JAMA* 1990;264(17):2302.

Leung AK, Fong JH, Leong AG. Otalgia in children. *J Natl Med Assoc* 2000;92(5): 254–260.

Licameli GR. Diagnosis and management of otalgia in the pediatric patient. *Pediatr Ann* 1999;28(6):364–368.

Yellon R. The spectrum of reflux-associated otolaryngologic problems in infants and children. *Am J Med* 1997;103(3S):125S–129S.

Authors: Laura N. Sinai and Lisa M. Biggs

Edema

 Database

DEFINITION

Presence of abnormal amount of fluid in the extracellular spaces of the body. Edema is usually secondary to low albumin, obstruction of venous or lymphatic channels, or trauma.

CAUSES

- Excessive losses

—Renal loss of protein
—Gastrointestinal

- Inadequate production

—Liver disease
—Malnutrition

- Local trauma
- Increased hydrostatic pressure

—Congestive heart failure
—Pericardial effusion
—Venous obstruction
—Lymphatic obstruction

Differential Diagnosis

LOCALIZED

- Trauma—pressure or sun damage
- Infection
- Allergy
- Lymphatic obstruction (less common)
- Bee stings or insect bites

GENERALIZED

Congenital

- Lymphatic obstruction of legs or thoracic duct

Infection

- Hepatitis and liver failure
- Pericarditis

Toxic, Environmental, Drugs

- Sodium poisoning
- Toxic effect on liver and/or heart (chemotherapy)
- Cirrhosis

Tumor

- Obstruction of venous return from enlarged abdominal lymph nodes

Genetic/Metabolic

- Sickle cell renal failure

Allergic Inflammatory

- Protein losing enteropathy

Miscellaneous

- Nephrotic syndrome
- Renal failure
- Congestive heart failure
- Pericarditis
- Gastrointestinal protein loss
- Postpericardiotomy or congenital heart surgery
- Endocrine—sodium retention, hypothyroidism
- Hepatobiliary diseases

Approach to the Patient

GENERAL GOALS

Determine the cause of swelling. Is it localized, are there any losses of protein, or is there underproduction of protein? Determine the serum protein/albumin, which would make you consider increased losses or decreased production.

Phase 1: Is the swelling localized as seen in trauma, lymphatic, or venous obstruction?

Phase 2: Are there urinary or gastrointestinal losses? This will be associated with decreased serum albumin. Most likely the source of the loss is renal disease and less frequently gastrointestinal losses.

Phase 3: Search for other causes of edema such as insect bites, pericardial effusion, metabolic disease.

Data Gathering

HISTORY

Question: Is the edema localized or generalized?
Significance: See Differential Diagnosis section.

Question: Is the patient asymptomatic or in some distress specifically due to the edema?
Significance: Determines treatment urgency.

Question: Is there evidence of cardiac, renal, or gastrointestinal disease?
Significance: These are the major causes of edema.

Question: Has waist size become larger? Are shoes difficult to put on?
Significance: Evidence of edema in body.

Question: What is the salt intake in diet?
Significance: In some patients, excess salt contributes to edema.

Question: Is there shortness of breath?
Significance: There may be ascites, which compresses the diaphragm or causes pleural effusions.

Question: Is there chronic diarrhea?
Significance: Seen in protein-losing enteropathy or lymphatic obstruction.

Question: Have any urinalyses been performed in the past?
Significance: May help date the onset of the problem.

Question: History of allergies?
Significance: Allergies will commonly cause swelling around the eyes or face.

 ## Physical Examination

Finding: Dependent edema
Significance: Lumbosacral area pretibial pressure to detect edema scrotum/labia

Finding: Percussion of chest
Significance: Pleural effusion

Finding: Shifting dullness
Significance: Early signs of ascites

Finding: Soft ear cartilage
Significance: Common finding in nephrotic syndrome

Finding: Pitting edema
Significance: Pitting edema is seen in cases of protein loss and obstruction of venous/lymphatic flow, whereas nonpitting edema is seen in salt poisoning.

 ## Laboratory Aids

DISCRIMINATING LABORATORY TESTS

Test: Dipstick urinalysis
Significance: If there is generalized edema with heavy proteinuria and hypoalbuminemia, the presumptive diagnosis is always nephrotic syndrome until proven otherwise.

Test: Serum albumin
Significance: If there is generalized edema with no proteinuria but hypoalbuminemia, consider cardiac, gastrointestinal, or hepatobiliary disease and direct additional studies to evaluate these three organ systems specifically. If there is either localized edema or generalized edema but a normal urinalysis and a normal serum albumin, consider other unusual causes for edema such as mechanical or lymphatic obstruction, certain endocrine disorders, or the effects of drugs or toxins.

Test: Stool albumin
Significance: Seen in protein losing enteropathy.

Issues for Referral

Referral to a specialist for edema is indicated for the following reasons:

- Nephrotic edema with impaired glomerular function—pediatric nephrologist
- Protein-losing enteropathy or hepatobiliary disease—pediatric gastroenterologist
- Congestive heart failure secondary to occult cardiac disease—pediatric cardiologist
- Endocrine-mediated edema—pediatric endocrinologist
- Lymphatic or other mechanical obstructions—vascular surgeon or pediatric surgeon, if readily available

 ## Emergency Care

Any child or adolescent with an edema-forming state that compromises either cardiorespiratory function or the vascular integrity of a peripheral organ or limb should be referred immediately to an appropriate specialist for emergency care.

Clinical Pearls

- If edema is massive, the patient may awaken with swollen eyelids. Place blocks under the head of the bed to keep head elevated.
- If there is scrotal edema, jockey shorts will help support scrotum and protect the skin from breaking down.

Common Questions and Answers

Q: At what level of serum albumin will edema occur?
A: Edema is generally associated with serum albumin below 2.5 g/dL.

Q: Why does pericardial effusion cause edema?
A: The pericardial effusion is associated with decreased lymphatic flow and increased venous pressure.

Q: Is there a certain group of allergens that will cause edema?
A: No special allergens are associated with edema. The usual causes include such foods as peanuts and drugs such as penicillin.

BIBLIOGRAPHY

Bohn D. Problems associated with intravenous fluid administration in children: do we have the right solutions? *Curr Opin Pediatr* 2000;12(3):217–221.

Dudin A, Othman A. Acute periorbital swelling: evaluation of management protocol. *Pediatr Emerg Care* 1996;12(1):16–20.

Jacobs ML, Rychik J, Byrum CJ, et al. Protein-losing enteropathy after Fontan operation: resolution after baffle fenestration. *Ann Thorac Surg* 1996;61(1):206–208.

Kelsch RC, Sedman AB. Nephrotic syndrome. *Pediatr Rev* 1993;14:30–38.

Molina JF, Brown RF, Gedalia A, et al. Protein losing enteropathy as the initial manifestation of childhood systemic lupus erythematosus. *J Rheumatol* 1996;23(7): 1269–1271.

Rosen FS. Urticaria, angioedema, anaphylaxis. *Pediatr Rev* 1992;13:387–390.

Vande Walle JG, Donckerwolcke RA. Pathogenesis of edema formation in the nephrotic syndrome. *Pediatr Nephrol* 2001;16(3):283–293.

Author: Michael E. Norman

Failure to Thrive

 Database

DEFINITION

• *Failure to thrive* (FTT) is a term used to describe infants and children who fail to meet standards for appropriate growth. FTT is more a sign or symptom of an underlying problem than a final diagnosis or disease state.
• The different criteria for malnutrition are: mild, weight for age 75% to 90% of median; moderate, weight for age 60% to 74% of median; and severe, weight for age less than 60% of median.

 Differential Diagnosis

CONGENITAL/ANATOMIC

• Congenital syndromes
• Chromosomal abnormalities
• Congenital heart disease
• Hirschsprung disease
• Pyloric stenosis
• Malrotation
• Vascular slings

INFECTIOUS

• Hepatitis
• Tuberculosis
• Human immunodeficiency virus (HIV)
• Parasitic infection
• Urinary tract infection
• Chronic sinusitis

TOXIC, ENVIRONMENTAL, DRUGS

• Inadequate caloric intake due to emotional deprivation
• Maternal depression
• Poor feeding techniques
• Poor child–caregiver interactions
• Improper formula preparation
• Lack of proper environment for mealtimes
• Parental drug/alcohol abuse
• Child abuse/neglect
• Lead/mercury poisoning
• Hypervitaminosis
• Fetal exposure to alcohol/anticonvulsants

GENETIC/METABOLIC

• Malabsorption (lactase deficiency, celiac disease)
• Cystic fibrosis
• Renal tubular acidosis
• Diabetes mellitus
• Thyroid disease
• Pituitary disease
• Adrenal disease
• Parathyroid disease
• Galactosemia
• Aminoaciduria

• Organic acidurias
• Storage diseases
• Hypercalcemia

ALLERGIC/INFLAMMATORY

• Food allergies
• Inflammatory bowel disease
• Chronic lung disease, including aspiration

FUNCTIONAL

• Gastroesophageal reflux (GER)
• Chronic constipation

NEUROLOGIC

• Cerebral palsy
• Oral-motor dysfunction
• Structural abnormalities
• Degenerative diseases
• Diencephalic syndrome

RENAL

• Chronic renal insufficiency

HEMATOLOGIC

• Sickle cell disease
• Thalassemia
• Iron-deficiency anemia

ORTHOPEDIC

• Rickets
• Osteogenesis imperfecta
• Chondrodystrophies

MISCELLANEOUS

• Upper airway obstruction, including adenoidal hypertrophy
• Acquired heart disease
• Dental abnormalities (caries, infection)

Approach to the Patient

GENERAL GOALS

Determine whether the patient has growth failure by measuring the child's weight, height, and head circumference accurately, plotting them on standard growth curves, and comparing them to previous growth points.

Phase 1:

• Is the malnutrition acute or chronic, symmetric or asymmetric? With acute malnutrition, weight is the first parameter to be affected, leading to wasting. After weeks to months of malnutrition, stunted linear growth occurs. Finally, with long-standing and/or severe malnutrition, head circumference is affected. Symmetric FTT suggests long-standing malnutrition, chromosomal abnormalities, congenital infection, or teratogenic exposures as etiologies.

• When growth failure is recognized, the prenatal, developmental, and nutritional history must be complete. Search for indicators of diminished intake, excessive losses, and medical diseases. The physical examination should be thorough. The laboratory evaluation is guided by the results of the history and physical examination. Although some laboratory tests can be useful in the evaluation of FTT, random screening in search of a medical diagnosis is usually unrevealing, and is not recommended.

Phase 2: If the history and physical examination suggest a medical disease as a cause of the growth failure, appropriate diagnostic evaluation should be done. In the majority of cases, the cause of growth failure is environmental or psychosocial. Medical diseases are identified in fewer than 50% of children hospitalized for growth failure and even less frequently in children evaluated in the outpatient setting.

Phase 3: If organic disease is not a consideration, begin education and psychosocial interventions to improve nutrition.

HINTS FOR SCREENING PROBLEM

Always plot growth on the same standardized growth chart so that the child's percentiles are known and can be compared to percentiles at previous ages.

 Data Gathering

HISTORY

Question: When did the FTT begin?
Significance: Consideration of the age at which growth failure begins can be helpful in determining the cause of the failure.

Question: Does the child have a medical problem that explains the FTT?
Significance: Ask about symptoms that would lead you to believe the child has a medical illness, including vomiting, chronic diarrhea, abdominal distention, exercise intolerance, developmental problems, etc.

Question: What is the child's typical daily diet?
Significance: Because FTT is commonly an environmental problem, and represents undernutrition, the child's feeding history may yield clues to the problem. Have the parent describe in detail what the child eats and drinks each day, the daytime schedule, how formula is prepared. Determine who is responsible for meal preparation, when and where the child eats, and what problems the parent identifies related to mealtime.

Question: Are there indications of parental stress, drug abuse, or other family factors that may be contributing to the child's growth failure?
Significance: Children do not live in isolation, and growth failure may be a manifestation of family dysfunction.

 ## Physical Examination

Start with a complete physical examination.

Finding: Changing growth patterns on a plotted growth chart.
Significance: In practice, FTT is identified when a child's weight falls below the fifth percentile for age, when the weight falls more than two major percentile groups, or when the weight for height is below 80% of the median.

Finding: Look for wasted, thin extremities, with loose skin hanging from the buttocks; temporal wasting; thin, sparse hair or alopecia.
Significance: Signs of malnutrition.

Finding: Otitis media, respiratory infections
Significance: Children with FTT have more infections than age-matched controls.

Finding: Cheilosis, or cracking and irritation at the corners of the mouth.
Significance: Riboflavin and other vitamin B complex deficiencies.

Finding: Edema
Significance: Protein deficiency

Finding: Oropharyngeal abnormalities (dental caries, tonsillar hypertrophy, submucosal clefts, etc.).
Significance: These factors may interfere with eating.

Finding: Neurologic abnormalities
Significance: Cerebral palsy and other neurologic abnormalities may result in oral-motor dysfunction, swallowing incoordination, and difficulty eating.

Finding: Bruises, burns, patterned cutaneous injuries
Significance: These injuries suggest possible child abuse.

 ## Laboratory Aids

The laboratory evaluation of the child with growth failure should be guided by the history and physical examination findings. Avoid extensive random evaluations.

Test: A complete blood count (CBC)
Significance: Iron-deficiency anemia

Test: Lead level
Significance: Lead poisoning

Test: Urinalysis and urine culture
Significance: Screens for urinary tract infection and renal tubular acidosis.

Test: PPD
Significance: Tuberculosis.

Test: Chemical screening can assess underlying metabolic problems and renal insufficiency.
Significance: These tests are indicated to help prevent the refeeding syndrome. The refeeding syndrome includes potentially dangerous disorders in serum phosphorus, calcium, potassium, and other minerals and electrolytes at the time of reintroduction of nutrition, in severely malnourished children.

 ## Emergency Care

SEVERE MALNUTRITION

• Children meeting criteria for severe malnutrition are at risk for refeeding syndrome, and should be hospitalized.
• Early hospitalization of the severely malnourished child focuses on slowly reinstituting nutrition while avoiding potentially life-threatening changes in electrolytes. In the most severe cases, life support and hyperalimentation are needed. Hospitalization provides a controlled environment in which to assess the causes of growth failure, and determine the child's caloric needs for catch-up growth.
• Therapy aimed at improving and sustaining the child's nutrition, however, needs to continue well after the child is discharged from the hospital and requires frequent weight checks, careful monitoring, and support of the family.

 ## Common Questions and Answers

Q: How can you differentiate between FTT and alternative diagnoses related to growth?
A: Recognize that 3% to 5% of the population will naturally fall below the 3rd to 5th percentile using growth charts. These children usually are proportional (normal weight for height). Growth velocity and height for weight determinations may be helpful in identifying children with malnutrition.

Q: How quickly will a child respond to nutritional therapy?
A: Initiation of catch-up growth depends on the severity of the malnutrition. Initially, weight gains of 2 to 3 times the normal growth rate for age may be observed. Weight gain will precede improvements in height. Months of refeeding are required to restore the patient's weight for height, stature, and head circumference.

Issues for Referral

• Indications of child abuse or neglect: State laws in every state require that physicians report suspected child abuse and neglect to child welfare agencies for investigation.
• Multidisciplinary team referral: For children with moderate FTT, those who do not improve after therapy has been initiated, or families with psychosocial problems, nutritionists, nurses, social workers, feeding specialists, and psychologists can participate in providing continual assessment and care to the child and family.

Clinical Pearls

• Remember that medical and psychosocial causes of malnutrition often coexist and should be considered.
• Don't forget to ask about how much juice the infant or toddler drinks. This is a common cause of FTT.
• In cases of moderate-severe neglect, it may be necessary to increase the caloric density of the child's foods, as many malnourished children cannot increase the volume of food ingested to meet the requirement for catch-up growth. A diet with approximately 30% to 35% more energy and nearly twice the amount of protein is needed for catch-up growth.
• Provide a multivitamin.
• Continued, close follow-up of the malnourished child is essential to prevent recurrent growth failure and to monitor the child's development, which can be adversely affected in moderate and severe growth failure.

BIBLIOGRAPHY

Bithoney WG, Dubowitz H, Egan H. Failure to thrive/growth deficiency. *Pediatr Rev* 1992;13:453–460.

Gahagan S, Holmes R. A stepwise approach to evaluation of undernutrition and failure to thrive. *Pediatr Clin North Am* 1998;45(1): 169–187.

Maggioni A, Lifshitz F. Nutritional management of failure to thrive. *Pediatr Clin North Am* 1995;42;791–810.

Zenel JA. Failure to thrive: a general pediatrician's perspective. *J Pediatr Rev* 1997;18(11):371–378.

Author: Cindy W. Christian

Fever of Unknown Etiology

 Database

DEFINITION

Fever of unknown origin (FUO) is defined as a febrile illness (38.5°C on multiple occasions) that has been present for more than 10 days, with no apparent source despite careful history taking, physical examination, and preliminary laboratory studies.

 Differential Diagnosis

CAUSES

FUO is more often an unusual presentation of a common disease than a common presentation of an unusual disease. An underlying cause is never established in approximately 10% to 20% of cases. Possible etiologies include:

- Bacterial infections

—Sinusitis
—Urinary tract infection (UTI)
—Tuberculosis (TB)
—Liver or pelvic abscess
—Osteomyelitis
—Endocarditis
—Salmonellosis
—Cat-scratch disease

- Viral infections

—Cytomegalovirus
—Epstein-Barr virus (EBV)
—Viral hepatitis

- Other infections

—Rocky Mountain spotted fever (RMSF)
—Toxoplasmosis

- Collagen vascular disease

—Juvenile rheumatoid arthritis (JRA)
—Systemic lupus erythematosus
—Rheumatic fever
—Serum sickness

- Malignancy

—Leukemia/lymphoma
—Neuroblastoma
—Hodgkin disease

- Other

—Factitious fever
—Drug fever
—Inflammatory bowel disease (IBD)
—Kawasaki syndrome

Uncommon causes of FUO include:

- Bacterial infections

—Endocarditis
—Brucellosis
—Tularemia
—Leptospirosis
—Rat-bite fever

- Other infections

—Disseminated histoplasmosis
—Coccidioidomycosis
—Blastomycosis
—Malaria
—Babesiosis

- Collagen vascular disease

—Sarcoidosis
—Hypersensitivity vasculitis
—Polyarteritis nodosa

- Malignancy

—Atrial myxoma
—Brain tumors

- Other

—Diabetes insipidus
—Thyroiditis
—Familial Mediterranean fever
—Cyclic neutropenia

Approach to the Patient

GENERAL GOALS

Find the cause of the fever and begin treatment of the underlying illness.

Phase 1: Attempt to diagnose more common causes of fever. Observe the pattern of fever. Determine whether constitutional symptoms (growth failure, developmental arrest, etc) may suggest more serious underlying diseases are present.

Phase 2: Begin invasive studies to seek rarer forms of fever such as lymphoma, brucellosis, baseosis, subacute bacterial endocarditis (SBE).

Phase 3: Reexamine patient and repeat tests to reconsider etiologies such as JRA, sarcoidosis, factitious fever.

 Data Gathering

HISTORY

Question: Exposure to animals?
Significance: Cat-scratch disease, brucellosis, tularemia, leptospirosis

Question: Travel history?
Significance: Malaria, coccidioidomycosis, blastomycosis

Question: Ingestion of raw meat, fish, or unpasteurized milk??
Significance: Trichinosis, TB, hepatitis

Question: Pica?
Significance: Fungal infection

Question: Change in behavior or activity?
Significance: Brain tumor, TB, EBV, Rocky Mountain spotted fever

Question: Pattern of fever?
Significance: May correlate with underlying etiology, but unlikely.

Question: Medications (including over-the-counter medications and eye drops)?
Significance: Drug fever, atropine-induced fever

Question: Well-water ingestion?
Significance: Giardia infection

Question: Evidence of behavior problems?
Significance: Factitious fever

Physical Examination

Finding: Impaired weight gain or linear growth
Significance: Collagen disease, malignancy, IBD

Finding: Toxic appearance
Significance: Kawasaki syndrome

Finding: Rash, sparse hair
Significance: Systemic lupus erythematosus, JRA

Finding: Conjunctivitis
Significance: Kawasaki syndrome

Finding: Funduscopic lesions
Significance: Brain tumor, TB, systemic lupus erythematosus

Finding: Sinus tenderness
Significance: Sinusitis

Finding: Nasal discharge
Significance: Sinusitis

Finding: Pharyngitis
Significance: Kawasaki syndrome, EBV, SBE

Finding: Tachypnea
Significance: SBE

Finding: Rales
Significance: Histoplasmosis, sarcoidosis, coccidioidomycosis

Finding: Cardiac murmur
Significance: SBE

Finding: Hepatosplenomegaly
Significance: Hepatitis, EBV

Finding: Rectal abnormalities
Significance: Pelvic abscess, IBD

Finding: Arthritis
Significance: JRA, IBD

Finding: Bony tenderness
Significance: JRA, leukemia, osteomyelitis

 Laboratory Aids

The laboratory evaluation for a child with FUO should be directed toward the most likely diagnostic possibilities. All patients should have:

Test: CBC with differential and careful examination of WBC morphology
Significance: Kawasaki, cyclic neutropenia, malignancy

Test: Blood cultures
Significance: Endocarditis, salmonellosis

Test: Urinalysis and urine culture
Significance: UTI, Kawasaki

Test: ESR and/or C-reactive protein
Significance: Collagen-vascular disease, IBD

Test: PPD skin test
Significance: TB

Additional studies to be considered include:

Test: Chest and/or sinus x-ray studies
Significance: TB, sinusitis, histoplasmosis

Test: Stool bacterial culture and examination for ova and parasites
Significance: Salmonella, Giardia

Test: Bone marrow examination and culture
Significance: Salmonella, histoplasmosis

Test: Slit lamp examination
Significance: Kawasaki

Test: Chest and/or abdominal CT scan
Significance: TB, liver abscess

Test: Gallium or bone scan
Significance: Osteomyelitis

- Cardiac catheterization
- Lumbar puncture
- Hepatitis serologies

 Common Questions and Answers

Q: How do you explain factitious fever?
A: The patient may twirl the thermometer under the tongue. If left unattended, the child may place the thermometer under hot water or shake it to elevate temperature reading.

Q: When should antibiotics be used?
A: Empiric use of antibiotics should be avoided because of the risk of delaying the discovery of the appropriate underlying diagnosis. A trial of antipyretics or NSAIDs may be considered if collagen-vascular disease is likely.

BIBLIOGRAPHY

Baker MD. Evaluation and management of infants with fever. *Pediatr Clin North Am* 1999;46(6):1061–1072.

Hoberman A, Wald ER. Urinary tract infections in young febrile children. *Pediatr Infect Dis J* 1997;16(1):11–17.

Kramer MS, Shapiro ED. Management of the young febrile child: a commentary on recent practice guidelines *Pediatrics* 1997;100(1):128–134.

Lorin MI, Feigin RD. Fever without localizing signs and fever of unknown origin. In: Feigin RD, Cherry JD, eds. *Textbook of pediatric infectious diseases*, 3rd ed. Philadelphia: WB Saunders 1992:1012–1022.

McCarthy PL. The pediatric clinical evaluation and pneumonia. *Curr Opin Pediatr* 1996;8(5):427–429.

McCarthy PL, Klig JE, Shapiro ED, et al. Fever without apparent source on clinical examination, lower respiratory infections in children, and other infectious diseases, and acute gastroenteritis and diarrhea of infancy and early childhood. *Curr Opin Pediatr* 1996;8(1):75–93.

McClung HJ. Prolonged fever of unknown origin in children. *Am J Dis Child* 1972;124:544–550.

Miller LC, Sisson BA, Tucker LB, et al. Prolonged fevers of unknown origins in children, patterns of presentation and outcome. *J Pediatr* 1996;129(3):419–423.

Rehm KP. Fever in infants and children. *Curr Opin Pediatr* 2001;13(1):83–88.

Author: Susan E. Coffin

Hematuria

 Database

DEFINITION

Hematuria is defined as an abnormal number of red blood cells in the urine. This means >3 red blood cells per high-power field using a standard urinalysis technique on a centrifuged sample, which correlates with a peroxidase dipstick reaction of 1+ or greater (see table Central Aids in Distinguishing the Origin of Gross Hematuria).

 Differential Diagnosis

CAUSES

• Hematuria may originate at any site along the urinary tract.
• Factitious causes, urine appears bloody, but there is no hematuria.

ENDOGENOUS PIGMENTS

• Myoglobin
• Hemoglobin
• Bile pigments
• Urate crystals ("pink diaper" syndrome)
• Beeturia and iron deficiency anemia

EXOGENOUS PIGMENTS

• Food and beverage dyes
• Drugs that cause urinary discoloration

—Phenazopyridine (Pyridium)
—Deferoxamine
—Rifampin
—Sulfa

GLOMERULAR CAUSES

Common

• Strenuous exercise
• Acute postinfectious glomerulonephritides
• IGA nephropathy
• Thin basement membrane disease (benign familial hematuria)

Uncommon

• Membranoproliferative glomerulonephritis
• Nephritis of systemic disease (Henoch-Schönlein or systemic lupus)
• Alport syndrome, hereditary nephritis

NONGLOMERULAR RENAL CAUSES

Common

• Hypercalciuria/nephrolithiasis
• Renal trauma (contusion)
• Hemoglobinopathies [sickle cell (SC) disease, SC trait, SC disease]
• Ureteropelvic junction obstruction

Uncommon

• Drug-induced interstitial nephritis (penicillins, cephalosporins, NSAIDs, phenytoin)
• Cystic disease
• Neoplasm—Wilms tumor
• Coagulopathy
• Vascular thrombosis

NONRENAL CAUSES

Common

• Cystitis (bacterial, viral, occasionally chemical)
• Meatal stenosis in males
• "Terminal hematuria" syndrome (trigonitis)
• Perineal trauma or irritation

Uncommon

• Bladder tumor
• Polyp
• Foreign body in bladder or urethra

External causes of "hematuria"

• Menstrual contamination
• Diaper rash

Approach to the Patient

GENERAL GOALS

Determine the source of the bleeding and select problems that respond to treatment.

Phase 1: Determine if the pigment in urine is from blood or other source.

Phase 2: Determine the source of bleeding, i.e., kidney, bladder, urethra.

Phase 3: Select those who will need treatment versus those who will stop bleeding without treatment.

 Data Gathering

HISTORY

Question: Prior episodes of any gross hematuria, or abnormal urinalyses?
Significance: Chronic versus acute process

Question: Medications and diet?
Significance: Food or drug pigment, drug nephrotoxicity. Excessive calcium intake.

Question: Antecedent infection or concurrent infection?
Significance: Antecedent suggests postinfections glomerulonephritis (GN). Concurrent suggests IgA nephropathy, basement membrane disease.

Question: Any precipitating factors (trauma, exercise)?
Significance: Renal contusion, exercise hematuria, or myoglobinuria

Question: Voiding symptoms?
Significance: Suggests lower tract source.

Question: Renal colic or other pain?
Significance: Suggests stones.

Question: Fever, rash, arthritis?
Significance: Signs or symptoms of systemic illness

Question: Bleeding from any other source?
Significance: Suggests coagulopathy.

Question: Hematuria in family members?
Significance: Familial benign hematuria or Alport syndrome

Question: SC disease in family members?
Significance: Sickle nephropathy or hemoglobinuria

Question: Renal stone disease in family members?
Significance: Hypercalciuria or metabolic disease

Question: Cystic kidney disease in family members?
Significance: Autosomal-recessive or -dominant polycystic kidney disease

Question: Premature deafness in family members?
Significance: Suggests Alport syndrome.

Question: Anyone in family with kidney failure or identified kidney disease?
Significance: Suggests hereditary nephritis, cystic disease, or stones.

Clinical Aids in Distinguishing the Origin of Gross Hematuria

TEST FOR	GLOMERULAR OR RENAL	EXTRARENAL
Urine color	Brown, cloudy, red	Red
Clots	Usually absent	Frequently present
RBC casts	Frequently present	Never present
Red-cell morphology	Dysmorphic or distorted	Normal RBC shape
Urine stream	Constantly bloody	More bloody at initiation (suggesting distal urethral origin) or termination (suggesting trigonitis)

Physical Examination

Finding: Cardiovascular exam
Significance: Hypertension in glomerulonephritis, renal failure, tachycardia, murmur on gallop in volume overload

Finding: Abdominal exam
Significance: Volume overload ascites, organomegaly, tenderness, or masses

Finding: Genital exam
Significance: External source of bleeding or infection

Finding: Extremities
Significance: Edema or joint swelling

Finding: Skin and mucosal exam
Significance: Petechial, vasculitic rash, ulcerations

Laboratory Aids

Test: Gross and microscopic analyses of fresh urine specimen
Significance: Urinalysis should guide additional evaluation.

Test: Screening of the family members for occult hematuria
Significance: Baseline test for child with isolated asymptomatic hematuria

Test: Screening the child for hypercalciuria (random urine calcium:creatinine ratio, 0.2)
Significance: Hypercalcemia causes hematuria.

Test: Serum creatinine
Significance: Renal function

Test: Renal ultrasound
Significance: To rule out obvious structural etiology of the hematuria.

Test: SC preparation should be considered.
Significance:

Test: Evaluation for glomerulonephritis
Significance: Hematuria occurring in combination with proteinuria, edema, hypertension, or signs or symptoms suggestive of a systemic illness.

Test: CBC with platelets
Significance: May suggest clotting problem.

Test: Serum electrolytes, BUN and creatinine
Significance: Renal function

Test: Streptococcal serology
Significance: Acute GN

Test: Complement studies
Significance: Immune complex disease

Test: Antinuclear antibody titer
Significance: Collagen disease (lupus)

Test: Quantitation of proteinuria
Significance: A low C3 complement suggests postinfectious glomerulonephritis or the nephritis of systemic lupus.

Test: Urine culture
Significance: Voiding symptoms, fever, and concurrent pyuria

Test: Trauma to the perineum should be avoided and periodic reassessment.
Significance: Symptomless "terminal" hematuria, indicating trigonitis.

Test: Radiographic evaluation of lower urinary tract
Significance: Anatomic or trauma

ADDITIONAL INVESTIGATIONS

Rarely, additional studies such as cystourethrogram, renal angiography, cystoscopy, or renal biopsy will be required, in conjunction with an appropriate referral. Audiometry may be indicated if hereditary nephritis is suspected. Hematuria without proteinuria is less likely to be renal in origin.

Follow-Up

The well child with asymptomatic isolated hematuria and a negative workup should be reassessed annually with a complete physical examination and a urinalysis. If hematuria is persistent, periodic assessment of renal function and evaluation for proteinuria should also be performed.

PROGNOSIS

• The majority of children with asymptomatic isolated microscopic hematuria detected on a well-child examination will not be found to have serious underlying pathology and will simply require longitudinal follow-up.
• Children with asymptomatic microscopic or gross hematuria combined with proteinuria have a high likelihood of significant pathology.
• For children with either microscopic or gross hematuria associated with findings suggestive of glomerulonephritis (proteinuria, systemic symptoms), the prognosis will depend on the type of glomerulonephritis identified.

Issues for Referral

• Uncontrollable bleeding—can be seen in SC disease with papillary necrosis or unlocalized source.
• Bleeding after trauma may expose a congenital anomaly such as ureteropelvic obstruction.
• Bleeding secondary to coagulopathy
• Bleeding and proteinuria

Clinical Pearls

There is usually no treatment for hematuria per se, but in some children with an identified cause of hematuria, specific treatment measures may be indicated for control of the underlying process. In many cases, no specific treatment is indicated, only longitudinal follow-up.

Pitfalls

• Positive test for blood on urine dip sticks may be myoglobin or hemoglobin. If the urinary sediment does not show red cells, investigate for problems such as muscle breakdown or hemolysis.

Epidemiology

• Hematuria may be gross or microscopic, symptomless, or associated with a constellation of other complaints and physical findings.
• Asymptomatic microscopic hematuria may be found in 1% to 4% of all healthy school-aged children.
• The complaint of gross hematuria may account for 0.1% to 0.15% of pediatric acute care walk-in visits.
• The majority of children with asymptomatic hematuria will be healthy, and no serious underlying cause will be found.

BIBLIOGRAPHY

Ahn JH, Morey AF, McAninch JW. Workup and management of traumatic hematuria. *Emerg Med Clin North Am* 1998;16(1):145–164.

Feld LG, Meyers KE, Kaplan BS, et al. Limited evaluation of microscopic hematuria in pediatrics. *Pediatrics* 1998;102(4):E42.

Feld LG, Waz WR, Perez LM, et al. Hematuria. An integrated medical and surgical approach. *Pediatr Clin North Am* 1997;44(5):1191–1210.

Meglic A, Cavic M, Hren-Vencelj H, et al. Chlamydial infection of the urinary tract in children and adolescents with hematuria. *Pediatr Nephrol* 2000;15(1–2):132–3.

Piqueras AI, White RH, Raafat F, et al. Renal biopsy diagnosis in children presenting with haematuria. *Pediatr Nephrol* 1998;12(5): 386–391.

Roy S 3rd. Hematuria. *Pediatr Rev* 1998;19(6): 209–212; quiz 213.

Ward JF, Kaplan GW, Mevorach R, et al. Refined microscopic urinalysis for red blood cell morphology in the evaluation of asymptomatic microscopic hematuria in a pediatric population. *J Urol* 1998;160(4): 1492–1495.

Author: Mitchell Schwartz
Roberta S. Gray, 2nd edition

Hemolysis

Database

DEFINITION
The premature destruction of red blood cells either intravascularly or extravascularly leading to a shortened red cell survival time.

Differential Diagnosis

See table Common Mechanisms of Hemolysis.

CONGENITAL/ANATOMIC
- ABO and Rh incompatibility between infant and mother
- Cardiac lesions with turbulent flow, left-sided more common than right-sided
- Prosthetic heart valve (especially aortic)
- Kasabach-Merritt syndrome
- Hypersplenism

INFECTIOUS
- Congenital infections with syphilis, rubella, cytomegalovirus (CMV), and toxoplasmosis
- Malaria
- Bartonellosis
- *Clostridium perfringens* (via a toxin)
- *Mycoplasma pneumoniae*
- HIV
- Hemolytic uremic syndrome (HUS)

TOXIC, ENVIRONMENTAL, DRUGS
- Immune-complex "innocent bystander" mechanism
—Quinidine
—Acetaminophen
—Amoxicillin
—Cephalosporins
—Isoniazid
—Rifampin
- Immune-complex drug-adsorption mechanism
—Penicillin
—Cephalosporins
—Erythromycin
—Tetracycline
—Isoniazid
- Drug-induced autoimmune hemolytic anemia
—α-Methyldopa

Common Mechanisms of Hemolysis

ACQUIRED DISORDERS	HEREDITARY DISORDERS
Infectious	Hemoglobinopathies
Drug induced	RBC membrane defects
Immune mediated	RBC enzyme defects
Microangiopathic	

- Toxic drug-induced hemolysis
—Ribovirin (generally mild and not clinically significant)
- Snake and spider venoms
- Extensive burns

TRAUMA (MECHANICAL HEMOLYSIS)
- Cardiac hemolysis
- Abnormal microcirculation
—Thrombotic thrombocytopenic purpura (TTP)
—Disseminated intravascular coagulopathy (DIC)
—Malignant hypertension
—Eclampsia
—Hemangiomas
—Renal graft rejection
- "March" hemoglobinuria (due to prolonged physical activity)

TUMOR
- Lymphomas
- Thymoma
- Lymphoproliferative disorders

GENETIC/METABOLIC
- RBC membrane defects
—Hereditary spherocytosis (HS)
—Hereditary elliptocytosis (HE)
—Pyropoikilocytosis
—Paroxysmal nocturnal hemoglobinuria
- Enzyme defects
—Pyruvate kinase deficiency (PK)
—Glucose-6-phosphate dehydrogenase deficiency (G-6-PD)
- Thalassemias (β-thalassemia major is the most severe)
- Hemoglobinopathies
—Sickle cell anemia (Hgb SS and SC variants)
—Unstable hemoglobins

ALLERGIC/INFLAMMATORY/IMMUNE
- Autoimmune hemolytic anemia (AIHA)
—Warm antibody mediated
—Cold antibody mediated
—Hemolytic transfusion reaction

Approach to the Patient

GENERAL GOALS
Establish existence of hemolysis versus other causes of anemia such as blood loss, hypoproduction, etc.

Phase 1: Determine acuity and severity of the hemolysis. If the process has been acute in onset, there will be evidence of unstable vital signs and possibly heart failure. Parents may give a history of a rapid deterioration of the child's physical and/or mental state. Patients with a chronic hemolytic anemia that has progressed slowly over time may have a "critically low" hemoglobin yet be well compensated with fairly normal vital signs (except for tachycardia). A CBC with a corrected reticulocyte count will help determine if there is an appropriate bone marrow response to the level of anemia, and, therefore, whether the process is acute or chronic in onset.

Phase 2: Determine the cause of the hemolysis. Treatment approaches will vary depending on the underlying etiology.

Data Gathering

HISTORY

Question: Is the patient pale, fatigued, or jaundiced? Is there a history of tea colored urine?
Significance: The presence of hemoglobinuria is a sign of intravascular hemolysis, while pallor, fatigue, and jaundice may occur with either intravascular or extravascular hemolysis.

Question: Is there a history of anemia, splenectomy, or early cholecystectomy in multiple family members?
Significance: While hereditary membrane defects and enzyme deficiencies are autosomal-dominant and X-linked disorders, respectively, a negative familial history does not always rule out these diagnoses. In some cases, the diagnosis of HS has not been identified, yet multiple members of a family have had their gallbladders removed at an early age, which may indicate the presence of this defect. Thalassemia (especially β-thal) and sickle cell anemia may present in early childhood with chronic hemolysis with or without a familial history.

Question: Is there a history of travel?
Significance: Malaria is endemic to Africa, India, and parts of Central America.

Question: What drugs is the patient taking? What is the diet history? Specifically ask about exposure to fava beans, mothballs, and antibiotics.
Significance: Drugs can themselves cause hemolysis or can induce hemolysis if there is an underlying disorder such as G-6-PD deficiency.

Question: How old was the child at the first signs and symptoms of hemolysis (pallor or jaundice)?
Significance: Hereditary causes of hemolysis are most often chronic or recurrent, although the diagnosis may be delayed until the child is older if the process is mild. Acute, acquired hemolytic disorders may also recur (such as AIHA, Evan syndrome, lupus, etc.).

Physical Examination

Question: What is the general appearance of the child? Is there any vital sign instability?
Significance: Acute processes such as autoimmune hemolytic anemia (both warm and cold antibody mediated) may present with a child in extremis. Tachycardia is a common finding in nearly all cases of acute hemolysis. Blood pressure instability is a late finding. More chronic processes such as HS, G-6-PD and PK deficiencies, thalassemia, intermedia, or sickle cell disease may be picked up on routine physical or laboratory examination. These children often appear well (except for jaundice) but may become more anemic with an acute illness.

Question: Is there an underlying systemic illness?
Significance: Hemolysis that is a secondary problem (i.e., due to infection, tumors, etc.) may be found incidentally during evaluation of the primary process.

Question: Is there any hepatosplenomegaly or lymphadenopathy?
Significance: Splenomegaly, often impressive, as well as hepatomegaly are common findings in extravascular hemolysis. Hepatomegaly may be more pronounced if the child is in heart failure due to acute, severe anemia. Remember that splenomegaly may be either the cause of, or more frequently, a result of a hemolytic process. If significant lymphadenopathy is present, look for any underlying etiology like lymphoproliferative disorders or other tumors.

Question: What is the skin exam?
Significance: Pallor is nearly a universal finding in acute hemolysis and in exacerbations of chronic hemolysis. Jaundice is more common in intravascular hemolysis. The presence of ecchymoses or petechiae suggest DIC or thrombocytopenia.

Laboratory Aids

Test: CBC with differential and reticulocyte count
Significance: The level of anemia and the reticulocyte count must be interpreted together. Chronic hemolysis due to HS, for example, may have a nearly normal hemoglobin but usually has an increased reticulocyte count. With a rapid fall in Hgb, as in acute autoimmune hemolytic anemia, the reticulocyte count may be low at the start, rise in response to anemia, and fall during recovery. Thrombocytopenia should raise suspicions about TTP or HUS.

Test: Peripheral blood smear
Significance: Fragmented RBCs, schistocytes, and helmet cells are seen in DIC, TTP, HUS, and cardiac valve hemolysis. Other findings on the smear that may be helpful in the diagnosis are spherocytes (HS and warm AIHA), target cells (hemoglobin C and thalassemias), and acanthocytes (anorexia nervosa).

Test: Bilirubin
Significance: Total and unconjugated bilirubins are elevated in most cases.

Test: Urinalysis
Significance: Hemoglobinuria is present in intravascular hemolysis. This is established by a urine dipstick positive for heme with no intact red cells microscopically. Myoglobinuria can also give this picture.

Test: Coombs test
Significance: Direct Coombs test (direct antiglobulin test or DAT) detects antibodies or complement fragments present on the patient's RBCs, while the indirect antiglobulin test detects antibodies in the patient's serum that can bind normal RBCs. The DAT provides direct evidence of immune-mediated hemolysis. Warm antibody AIHA is caused by an IgG antibody that coats RBCs, which are subsequently removed by the spleen. Cold antibody AIHA is caused by an IgM antibody that binds RBCs, fixes complement, and can cause both extravascular as well as intravascular hemolysis.

Test: Haptoglobin, hemopexin, and LDH
Significance: In intravascular hemolysis, haptoglobin levels may be undetectable, hemopexin is reduced and LDH is significantly increased. In extravascular hemolysis, haptoglobin is decreased (but detectable) and LDH may be increased, but not to the level seen in intravascular hemolysis.

Test: Bone marrow aspiration
Significance: Rarely indicated, but if performed, erythroid hyperplasia should be present.

Emergency Care

Factors that constitute an emergency include:
• Hemoglobin under 5 g/dL, especially with signs of cardiovascular compromise, requires immediate attention. Attempts to stabilize cardiovascular compromise with volume should be undertaken with care, as hemodilution may occur. Transfusion may be difficult in autoimmune hemolysis because of potential problems with crossmatching.
• Renal failure may accompany severe hemolysis in TTP or HUS.
• Hemolysis in the neonatal period secondary to ABO or Rh incompatibility may require exchange transfusion either for anemia or for hyperbilirubinemia.

Common Questions and Answers

Q: When are blood transfusions indicated in patients with active hemolysis?
A: Patients with severe, acute hemolysis that is causing cardiovascular compromise may require a transfusion if the process cannot be stopped with standard therapy (steroids for warm AIHA, plasmapheresis for TTP, etc.). Transfusions must be given slowly if the hemolytic process has been chronic and the patient's blood volume is expanded.

Q: Can hemolysis always be identified on a peripheral blood smear?
A: No. Schistocytes, fragments, spherocytes, targets, or other morphology may provide clues to specific diagnoses but are not always present. The presence of a hemolytic process is inferred from a fall in hemoglobin, rise in the reticulocyte count and elevation of the bilirubin and LDH levels.

Issues for Referral
• Most patients with severe, acute hemolysis, either primary or due to an underlying chronic hemolytic disorder, will need to be evaluated by a hematologist.
• Suspected RBC membrane and enzyme defects, as well as hemoglobinopathies, should be referred at least for initial evaluation. Ongoing involvement of a hematologist will depend on the ultimate diagnosis.
• A CBC with a reticulocyte count is the most important screening test. Other tests depend on clinical suspicion of the underlying etiology but may include a direct and indirect Coombs test.

Clinical Pearls
• Hereditary RBC membrane defects may be mild and may be diagnosed at an older age. Although these disorders are autosomal dominant, 20% of these patients represent new spontaneous mutations and have no affected family members.
• Blood for diagnostic RBC enzyme studies must be drawn prior to transfusion.

BIBLIOGRAPHY
Berkowitz FE. Hemolysis and infection: categories and mechanisms of their interrelationship. *Rev Infect Dis* 1991;13(6):1151–1162.

Tabbara IA. Hemolytic anemias. Diagnosis and management. *Med Clin North Am* 1992;76(3):649–668.

Author: Julie W. Stern

Hepatomegaly

Database

DEFINITION

Liver enlargement beyond age-adjusted normal values. Can be a common component of many diverse disease processes seen in infants and children.

Differential Diagnosis

CONGENITAL/ANATOMIC

- Alagille syndrome
- Biliary atresia
- Choledochal cyst
- Congenital hepatic fibrosis
- Obstruction of the common bile duct due to stones, strictures, or tumors

INFECTIONS

- Viral infections

—Hepatitis types A—E
—Cytomegalovirus (CMV)
—Epstein-Barr virus (EBV)
—Coxsackievirus

- Congenital infections

—Toxoplasmosis
—Rubella
—CMV
—Herpes
—Human immunodeficiency virus (HIV)

- Parasitic infections

—Amebiasis
—Flukes
—Schistosomiasis
—Malaria

- Fungal disease

—Candidiasis
—Histoplasmosis

- Sexually transmitted disease

—Gonococcal perihepatitis
—Syphilis
—HIV

- Zoonotic diseases

—Brucellosis

- Leptospirosis
- Hepatic abscess
- *Bartonella henselae*
- *Pasteurella multocida*
- Tuberculosis
- Septicemia

TOXIC, METABOLIC, DRUGS

- Drug-induced hepatitis

—Acetaminophen

—Alcohol
—Corticosteroids
—Erythromycin
—Hypervitaminosis A
—Iron
—Isoniazid
—Nitrofurantoin
—Oral contraceptives
—Phenobarbital
—Valproate

TRAUMA

- Hemorrhage
- Subcapsular hematoma
- Traumatic cyst

TUMOR

- Benign tumors

—Hemangioma
—Hemangioendothelioma
—Mesenchymal hamartoma
—Focal nodular hyperplasia
—Adenoma

- Malignant tumors

—Hepatoblastoma
—Hepatocellular carcinoma

- Metastatic tumors
- Histiocytic disease

GENETIC/METABOLIC

- α_1-Antitrypsin deficiency
- Amyloidosis
- Beckwith-Wiedemann syndrome
- Chédiak-Higashi syndrome
- Crigler-Najjar syndrome
- Cystic fibrosis
- Diabetes mellitus
- Galactosemia
- GM_1 gangliosidoses
- Glycogen storage diseases
- Hematochromatosis
- Hereditary fructose intolerance
- Homocystinuria
- Lipidoses
- Mucopolysaccharidoses
- Urea cycle defects
- Wilson disease
- Zellweger syndrome

ALLERGIC/INFLAMMATORY

- Chronic active hepatitis
- Sclerosing cholangitis
- Sarcoidosis
- Systemic inflammatory disease

—Juvenile rheumatoid arthritis
—Systemic lupus erythematosus
—Inflammatory bowel disease

MISCELLANEOUS

- Congestive heart failure
- Extramedullary hematopoiesis
- Pulmonary hyperinflation
- Restrictive pericarditis

- Veno-occlusive disease
- Malnutrition
- Reye syndrome
- Total parenteral nutrition

Approach to the Patient

- All patients with hepatomegaly should have a laboratory evaluation including complete blood count with differential, comprehensive metabolic panel (including liver function tests, total protein and albumin, total and direct bilirubin, basic electrolytes and glucose), a prothrombin time, and a partial prothrombin time.
- A detailed history and physical will direct the practitioner to any additional laboratory testing or appropriate radiologic evaluation.

Data Gathering

HISTORY

Question: Any prenatal history suggesting possible TORCH infection or HIV infection?
Significance: TORCH infections and HIV may cause hepatomegaly, although the liver involvement with HIV is usually secondary to disseminated opportunistic infections or neoplastic processes, rather than from the primary infection itself.

Question: Any history of blood product transfusions?
Significance: Hepatitis C is the most common cause of transfusion-associated hepatitis and the diagnosis should be considered in any child who had received transfusions prior to 1990.

Question: Any history of sexual activity or intravenous drug use?
Significance: Consider not only hepatitis B and HIV, but also gonococcal perihepatitis (Fitz-Hugh—Curtis syndrome), and syphilis.

Question: Any foreign travel?
Significance: Increased risk for parasitic infections or liver abscess.

Question: Any shellfish ingestion?
Significance: Contaminated shellfish has been the source of several large outbreaks of hepatitis A.

Question: What medications is the patient taking?
Significance: Many pharmaceuticals have hepatotoxic side effects. Remember to ask about nonprescription and recreational drug use, as vitamin A, alcohol, and certain mushroom species (*Amanita phalloides*) can be hepatotoxic.

Question: Any other chronic illnesses present?
Significance: Patients with heart disease may have liver enlargement due to congestive heart failure. Patients with cystic fibrosis can have focal biliary cirrhosis. Patients with

diabetes mellitus often have hepatomegaly secondary to increased glycogen secretion. Severely anemic patients have hepatomegaly because of extramedullary hematopoiesis.

Question: Has the patient received total parenteral nutrition (TPN)?
Significance: Cholestasis, bile duct proliferation, fatty infiltration, and early cirrhosis are all well-described complications of TPN.

Question: Any itching?
Significance: Pruritus can be a subtle sign of cholestasis.

 ## Physical Examination

Finding: Where is the liver edge?
Significance: In children younger than 2 years of age, the liver edge can extend from 1 to 3 cm below the right costal margin in the midclavicular line. In older children, the liver edge rarely extends beyond 2 cm. Verify all suspected cases of hepatomegaly by checking the liver span.

Finding: What are signs of chronic liver disease?
Significance: The liver is usually firm and enlarged, though actually may decrease in size eventually with advanced disease. Splenomegaly, caput medusae, spider angiomas, esophageal varices, and hemorrhoids suggest portal hypertension. Ascites may develop due to elevated hydrostatic pressures and decreased oncotic pressures secondary to hypoalbuminemia. Also look for signs of occult bleeding or bruising due to impaired vitamin K production.

Finding: Is splenomegaly present?
Significance: Splenic enlargement in the context of chronic liver disease implies portal hypertension. Splenomegaly in the context of other signs of viral illness like adenopathy, fever, malaise, and pharyngitis suggests acute viral hepatitis. Splenomegaly in the absence of these signs suggests storage disease or hematologic malignancy.

Finding: Are there conditions present that may be mimicking hepatomegaly?
Significance: Pulmonary hyperinflation, subdiaphragmatic abscesses, retroperitoneal mass lesions, or rib cage anomalies may all downwardly displace a normal-sized liver mimicking hepatomegaly.

 ## Laboratory Aids

Complete blood count with differential (CBC)

Test: Aminotransferase and alanine aminotransferase (AST and ALT).
Significance: Elevations reflect the amount of damage to hepatocytes. Elevations >1,000 indicate severe damage.

Test: Prothrombin time and partial prothrombin time (PT and PTT)
Significance: Good indicators of the liver's synthetic function. Elevations can occur with an acute injury or illness. Combined with albumin level, this test can be a sensitive indicator of chronic liver disease as well.

Test: γ-Glutamyltransferase (GGT) and alkaline phosphatase
Significance: Elevations of GGT out of proportion to elevations in AST and ALT can indicate an obstructive or infiltrative abnormality. If an elevated GGT is associated with elevations in bilirubin, cholesterol, and alkaline phosphatase, an obstructive process is more likely.

Test: Ammonia level
Significance: Rising ammonia levels with a prolongation of the PT and PTT suggests liver failure.

Test: Hepatitis profile
Significance: Should be obtained in all patients with appropriate prodromal illness.

Test: Mono spot
Significance: While this is a nonspecific heterophile antibody test for EBV infection, it can be predictive in association with an elevation of the atypical lymphocyte count. There is a high false-negative rate as well in children less than 4 years of age. EBV titer is the only confirmatory test.

Test: Alpha-fetoprotein (AFP) and carcinoembryonic antigen (CEA)
Significance: Tumor markers for hepatoblastoma and hepatocellular carcinoma, respectively.

Test: TORCH titers
Significance: Consider in newborns with hepatomegaly.

Test: Serum immunoglobulins, antinuclear antibody (ANA), smooth muscle antibody (SMA), antimicrosomal antibody, etc.
Significance: Additional autoimmune evaluation is indicated for those patients with chronic active hepatitis.

Test: Abdominal ultrasound
Significance: Should be performed on all patients with acholic stools, asymmetric liver enlargement, or abdominal mass.

Test: Serum ceruloplasmin level and urinary excretion of copper
Significance: Decreased ceruloplasmin levels and increased urinary excretion of copper characterize Wilson disease, especially after the administration of oral D-penicillamine. Consider the diagnosis for patients with unexplained liver disease.

 ## Emergency Care

Indications for immediate hospitalization include:

- Persistent anorexia and vomiting
- Mental status changes
- Worsening jaundice
- Relapse of symptoms after initial improvement
- Known exposure to a liver toxin
- Rising PT
- Rising ammonia level
- Bilirubin >20 mg/dL
- AST >2,000
- Development of new ascites
- Hypoglycemia
- Leukocytosis and thrombocytopenia

Common Questions and Answers

Q: Why does cholestasis cause pruritus?
A: This probably reflects an abnormal accumulation of bile acids in the skin.

Q: When following patients with chronic liver disease, are there any differences in their nutritional needs?
A: Patients may have impaired fat absorption, and therefore may have deficiencies of fat soluble vitamins A, D, E, and K, which may become evident as anemia, neuropathy, rickets, pathologic fractures, visual disturbances, or skin changes. Also consider supplementing the diet with medium-chain triglycerides, which are more easily absorbed. There may also be higher than normal requirements of trace minerals as well.

Q: What is the etiology of TPN cholestasis?
A: Certain amino acids present in TPN have been shown to increase the serum levels of bile acids, which may in turn affect peristalsis in the gallbladder. Fasting may also decrease the normal hormonal stimulation of bile secretion.

Clinical Pearls

- Until age 2, girls have a slightly larger liver span than boys.
- A Reidel lobe is a normal variant in which the right lobe of the liver appears elongated due to its adhesion to the mesocolon.
- The majority of cases of hepatic failure in children are due to acute viral hepatitis. Toxic exposure accounts for 25% of cases, with the most common drug being acetaminophen.
- Administration of vitamin K in an attempt to correct PT can be a valuable assessment of the liver's synthetic function.
- Fetor hepaticus is a sweetish odor that can be detected on the breath and urine of patients with liver failure.
- Asterixis or liver flap is rare in children.

BIBLIOGRAPHY

Roy C, Silverman A, Alagille D. *Pediatric clinical gastroenterology*. St. Louis: Mosby, 1995.

Author: John M. Good

Hypogammaglobulinemia

 Database

DEFINITION

Hypogammaglobulinemia is a humoral immunodeficiency signified by low or absent immunoglobulin levels, as compared with age-matched controls, and defective specific antibody production.

 Differential Diagnosis

- Selective IgA deficiency

—For details, refer to the topics Immune Deficiency, Common Variable Immunodeficiency (CVID), and Immune A Deficiency.

- X-linked agammaglobulinemia (XLA) (Bruton agammaglobulinemia)

—Intrinsic defect in B-cell maturation due to mutations in the gene on the X chromosome encoding a B-cell—associated tyrosine kinase. The protein is involved in cytoplasmic signal transduction.
—All immunoglobulin isotypes are significantly decreased or absent.
—Significant reduction or absence of B cells
—Bacterial infections with pyogenic encapsulated organisms due to *Staphylococcus aureus*, *Streptococcus Pneumoniae*, *Haemophilus influenzae*, and *Pseudomonas* species
—Recurrent respiratory tract infections including otitis, sinusitis, bronchitis, and pneumonia
—Associated complications include arthritis of the large joints, chronic meningoencephalitis due to echoviruses, chronic diarrhea due to *Giardia lamblia*, neutropenia, autoimmune hemolytic anemia, dermatomyositis, and an increased incidence of lymphoreticular malignancies.
—Patients are also susceptible to viral infections, particularly enteroviruses. Live viral vaccines are contraindicated in these patients because some patients have vaccine-associated poliomyelitis.

- Hyper-IgM syndrome

—Predominantly an X-linked inheritance pattern. Affected females have been described.
—Defect is caused by mutations in the gene encoding the CD40 ligand surface molecule on T cells. This leads to defective T-cell signaling for B-cell immunoglobulin class switching.
—Normal to elevated IgM levels with low to absent IgG, IgA, and IgE
—Recurrent upper respiratory tract infections, otitis, pneumonia, sinusitis

—Associated complications include autoimmune hemolytic anemia/thrombocytopenia/neutropenia, opportunistic infections with *Pneumocystis carinii*, and lymphoproliferative disease.

- Transient hypogammaglobulinemia of infancy

—It is difficult to differentiate this from the normal physiologic nadir of IgG that occurs between 3 and 6 months of age due to the loss of maternally derived immunoglobulin. This nadir is normally short lived.
—Affected infants have abnormally prolonged delay in the onset of their own immunoglobulin production to compensate for this nadir.
—The cause is unknown.
—Self-limited, most infants recover by 18 to 36 months.
—Clinical course is typically benign. Therapy with intravenous immunoglobulin (IVIG) should be considered only in infants with severe recurrent infections.
—This syndrome is frequently seen in infants with a familial history of SCID or other immunodeficiencies.

- Selective IgG subclass deficiency (the four subclasses of IgG, in decreasing order of serum levels: IgG1, IgG2, IgG3, and IgG4)

—Total serum IgG levels can be normal even when one subclass is low or absent.
—Deficiency of IgG3 is most common in adults while deficiency of IgG2 is seen more frequently in children.
—IgG2 deficiency has been associated with an inability to respond to polysaccharide antigens.
—The clinical significance of IgG subclass deficiency has not been fully defined. Many patients have been described as having an increased frequency of upper and lower respiratory tract infections while others are asymptomatic.
—There is no consensus on standard therapy for these patients in regard to replacement IVIG.

- Kappa-chain deficiency

—Absence of the kappa subtype of light chains in immunoglobulin molecules
—Described in two families
—Associated with variable defects in specific antibody formation

- Immunodeficiency with thymoma

—Seen in adults, typically between 40 and 70 years old
—Associated with significantly decreased to absent IgG, IgA, and IgM

- Secondary causes of hypogammaglobulinemia

—Viruses: Epstein-Barr virus (EBV), cytomegalovirus (CMV), congenital rubella

—The mechanism by which antibody responses and immunoglobulin production are altered in infected patients is not clearly defined.
—Infectious mononucleosis has been associated with defective specific antibody responses to neoantigens and impaired *in vitro* B-cell function in normal individuals. These defects are transient and resolve within 6 to 8 weeks after the onset of the disease. A disastrous response to EBV infection is seen in X-linked lymphoproliferative syndrome. These patients develop fatal infectious mononucleosis, marrow aplasia, B-cell lymphoma, and agammaglobulinemia.
—HIV, CMV, and rubella infections have been associated with abnormal specific antibody responses.

DRUGS

- Immunosuppressive/chemotherapeutic agents, phenytoin
- The associated defects in immune function and antibody production usually resolve after the therapy is discontinued.

OTHER

- Protein-losing enteropathy
- Intestinal lymphangiectasia
- Nephrotic syndrome
- The hypogammaglobulinemia is due to direct loss through the gastrointestinal (GI) tract or kidneys.
- Lymphoreticular malignancies have been associated with various immune defects and decreased immunoglobulin production.

 Data Gathering

HISTORY

A detailed history for recurrent infection is key to evaluating suspected humoral immunodeficiency.

- Patients with humoral immunodeficiencies usually present with recurrent infections due to encapsulated bacteria, such as *Haemophilus influenzae* type B and *Streptococcus pneumoniae*.
- It is important to rule out hypogammaglobulinemia in patients with recurrent infections because replacement therapy with intravenous IgG is readily available.

Question: At what age did the recurrent infections start?
Significance: Patients with hypogammaglobulinemia usually present after 3 to 6 months of age. Late onset of infections may be more consistent with CVID.

Question: What type of infections have been diagnosed?
Significance: Hypogammaglobulinemia typically results in bacterial infections with encapsulated organisms.

Question: Have there been recurrent severe infections such as meningitis, sepsis, and osteomyelitis?
Significance: Some of the congenital immunodeficiency syndromes are signified by specific infections such as chronic meningoencephalitis with echoviruses, vaccine-associated poliomyelitis, and *Pneumocystis carinii* pneumonia.

Question: Is there a familial history of immunodeficiencies?
Significance: Previously affected males suggests an X-linked inheritance pattern.

Question: Early infant deaths?
Significance: Early infant deaths due to overwhelming infection may indicate a previously undiagnosed congenital immunodeficiency.

Question: Any other associated signs or symptoms?
Significance: Many of the congenital immunodeficiencies have associated arthritis, autoimmune disease, chronic lung disease, and GI manifestations.

 ## Physical Examination

In general, patients should be examined for signs of acute and chronic infections.

Finding: Growth parameters
Significance: Children with significant, recurrent infections and GI disease related to immunodeficiency may present with failure to thrive.

Finding: Signs of chronic otitis media or conjunctival recurrent disease
Significance: Patients with XLA frequently have signs of chronic conjunctivitis.

Finding: Gingivitis and stomatitis
Significance: May occur with the neutropenia-associated hypogammaglobulinemia syndromes.

Finding: Lymphoid tissue
Significance: Absence of tonsillar tissue and palpable lymph nodes is suggestive of X-linked agammaglobulinemia.

Finding: Lymphadenopathy and tonsillar hypertrophy
Significance: Can be seen in hyper-IgM syndrome and CVID. Persistently enlarged nodes should be investigated.

Finding: Wheezes, rales
Significance: Acute pneumonia or chronic lung disease

Finding: Hepatosplenomegaly or masses
Significance: May be seen in hyper-IgM syndrome and CVID. Abdominal masses should be investigated promptly to rule out malignancy.

Finding: Arthritis, clubbing
Significance: Arthritis can be seen in patients with XLA and CVID. Clubbing can be seen in the presence of chronic lung disease/bronchiectasis.

 ## Laboratory Aids

Test: Complete blood count with differential
Significance: Autoimmune hemolytic anemia, neutropenia, and thrombocytopenia can be seen in XLA, hyper-IgM, and CVID.

Test: Quantitative immunoglobulin levels
Significance: Each isotype should be measured (IgG, IgA, IgM, IgE). A normal or elevated IgM level in face of low to absent IgG, IgA, is characteristic of hyper-IgM syndrome.

Test: Serial testing of immunoglobulins
Significance: Should be done in infants suspected of transient hypogammaglobulinemia to document subsequent normalization of immunoglobulin levels.

Test: Qualitative antibody levels
Significance: Isohemagglutinins are primarily IgM antibodies to the main blood groups. They should be present in normal patients. However, they will be absent in patients with AB blood type. In addition, their presence is inconstant in children under 1 year of age.

Test: Antibody titers to tetanus, diphtheria, *Streptococcus pneumoniae*, and *Haemophilus influenzae* type B measured postvaccination.
Significance: The ability to mount a protective antibody response to childhood vaccinations may indicate a less severe clinical course in hypogammaglobulinemia.

Test: B-cell enumeration
Significance: Numbers of peripheral B-cell will be decreased to absent in XLA and rare in CVID. They are usually normal in other hypogammaglobulinemia syndromes.

Test: Total lymphocyte count (derived from the CBC with differential)
Significance: Lymphocyte enumeration is done using monoclonal antibodies to cell-specific CD surface markers measured by flow cytometry.

Test: Chest and sinus radiography and CT scans
Significance: May be helpful in evaluating for acute and chronic disease. Bronchiectasis can be a long-term sequela of chronic pulmonary infection.

• Prompt and appropriate antibiotic therapy is an important part of routine treatment.
• There may be a role for prophylactic antibiotics in patients with persistent recurrent infections.
• Replacement therapy with IVIG is the primary therapeutic modality for XLA, hyper-IgM syndrome, and CVID. Usual initiating doses are 200 to 400 mg/kg every 3 to 4 weeks. Nadir IgG levels should be greater than 300 mg/dL.
• Patients receiving IVIG therapy should not receive routine vaccinations; they are passively immunized with the therapy.
• Therapy is usually lifelong in patients with documented humoral immunodeficiency.

 ## Common Questions and Answers

Q: When should I make a referral?
A: Refer any patient suspected of having a primary humoral immunodeficiency to a specialist in allergy and immunology. These are patients with chronic disease who require prolonged follow-up and good communication between the referring physician and specialist.

BIBLIOGRAPHY

Huston DP, Kavanaugh AF, Rohane PW, et al. Immunoglobulin deficiency syndromes and therapy. *J Allergy Clin Immunol* 1991;87:1–17.

Ochs HD, Smith CI. X-linked agammaglobinemia: a clinical and molecular analysis. *Medicine* 1996;75(6):287–299.

Ochs HD, Winkelstein JA. Disorders of the B-cell system. In: Stiehm ER, ed. *Immunologic disorders in infants and children*, 4th ed. Philadelphia: WB Saunders. 1996:296–338.

Rosen FS, Cooper MD, Wedgwood RJP. The primary immunodeficiencies. *N Engl J Med* 1995;333:431–440.

Schaffer FM, Ballow M. Immunodeficiency: the office work-up. *J Respir Dis* 1995;16:523–541.

Skull S, Kemp A. Treatment of hypogammaglobulinaemia with intravenous immunoglobulin, 1973–1993. *Arch Dis Child* 1996;74(6):527–530.

Woroniecka M. Ballow M. Office evaluation of children with recurrent infection. *Pediatr Clin North Am* 2000;47(6):1211–1224.

Author: Timothy Andrews
Alex G. Yip, 2nd edition

Immune Deficiency

 Database

DEFINITION
- Immunodeficiencies represent a defect in host defense.
- Immunodeficiencies can be either congenital or acquired.
- Certain immunodeficiencies lead to specific types of infections, while others are associated with a more global predisposition to infection.

PATHOPHYSIOLOGY
- B-cell dysfunction: leads to antibody deficiency; poor opsonization of bacteria, loss of immunologic memory. The hallmark of B-cell disorders is recurrent infections with organisms typical for that age group.
- T-cell dysfunction: loss of cytolytic activity against viruses, loss of cytokines required for regulation of the immune response. Patients are vulnerable to viral infections, chronic indolent infections such as fungi, and opportunistic infections. Autoimmune disease due to impaired regulation is also common.
- Complement deficiency: complement serves as a major opsonin to tag pathogens for removal. Complement deficiencies are associated with systemic lupus erythematosus, infections with encapsulated organisms, or infections with neisserial species.
- Neutrophil disorders: either due to qualitative or quantitative dysfunction; impaired phagocytosis of bacteria.

GENETICS
There are six important immunodeficiencies
- X-linked (properdin deficiency, X-linked agammaglobulinemia, X-linked hyper-IgM, X-linked severe combined immunodeficiency, X-linked chronic granulomatous disease, X-linked lymphoproliferative syndrome).
- Most other inherited immunodeficiencies are autosomal recessive.
- hyper-IgE syndrome, which is typically autosomal dominant.
- IgA deficiency and common variable immunodeficiency which are polygenic in origin.

EPIDEMIOLOGY
The most common immunodeficiency is IgA deficiency with an estimated prevalence of 1:500 people. Other immunodeficiencies range in prevalence from 1:3,000 for chromosome 22q11.2 deletion syndrome (DiGeorge syndrome) to 1:200,000 for chronic granulomatous disease.

COMPLICATIONS
- Damage to end organs that occurs as a result of chronic or severe infections.
- Bronchiectasis.
- Deafness.
- Amyloidosis.
- Lymphoreticular malignancies occur in patients with T-cell disorders.
- Live viral vaccines administered to patients with T-cell dysfunction can result in unchecked viremia.

- Oral polio vaccine administered to patients with agammaglobulinemia can cause meningoencephalitis

PROGNOSIS
- Most antibody deficiencies have an excellent prognosis. Transient or developmental deficiencies of IgG or IgG subclasses typically resolve by 2 years of age.
- Antibody deficiencies such as X-linked agammaglobulinemia or common variable immunodeficiency have a good prognosis with IVIG treatment.
- The treatment of neutrophil disorders remains problematic and most children with chronic granulomatous disease will not have a full life expectancy
- Patients with T-cell disorders for whom bone marrow transplantation is not performed can do well if the defect is mild or suffer from autoimmune disease, malignancy, and recurrent infections.

 Differential Diagnosis

- Chronic inflammation of mucous membranes such as that due to reflux or allergies can lead to recurrent infections.
- Secondary immunodeficiency.
—Immunocompromise due to chemotherapy and immunosuppressive drugs
- Malnutrition, intercurrent viral infections such as EBV and CMV, toxin exposure, and medications such as Dilantin and gold.
—Many of the inborn errors of metabolism.
—Many chromosomal syndromes.
- HIV infection.

BRIEF DESCRIPTIONS OF CONGENITAL OR PRIMARY IMMUNODEFICIENCIES
Defects in Antibody Production
- X-linked agammaglobulinemia. Onset of symptoms after 6 months; sinopulmonary infections with typical bacterial pathogens. Markedly decreased immunoglobulins and B cells are characteristic.
- Hyper-IgM syndrome. Usually presents with recurrent bacterial infections; Pneumocystis carinii is seen in some infants; intermittent neutropenia is common. Decreased IgG, IgE, IgA with normal or increased IgM.
- Common variable immunodeficiency. Usually presents with recurrent bacterial infections; most commonly arises in the second or third decade of life (but is seen in all ages). Immunoglobulin levels and function gradually decline; often an associated mild T-cell defect.
- IgG subclass deficiency. IgG2 subclass deficiency is seen as a transient developmental delay in the acquisition of humoral immunity. May also precede the development of common variable immunodeficiency and can rarely be seen as an isolated defect.
- IgA deficiency. This is the most common congenital immunodeficiency (1:500); most are asymptomatic. Symptoms can be seen at any age; typically sinopulmonary infections; increased risk of allergy, autoimmune disease, and anaphylaxis from blood products.

- Transient hypogammaglobulinemia of infancy. A developmental delay of immunoglobulin production; function is intact; typically resolves between 9 and 15 months.

T-Cell Defects
- Severe combined immunodeficiency. Most common presentation is a respiratory virus that fails to clear or chronic diarrhea. Failure to thrive, thrush, and Pneumocystis carinii pneumonia are also common; presents before 6 months of age; early diagnosis is essential.
- Chromosome 22q11.2 deletion syndrome (DiGeorge syndrome/velocardiofacial syndrome). Classic constellation: cardiac anomaly, hypocalcemia, and hypoplastic thymus. Most patients have a partial phenotype; T-cell immunodeficiency is common and variable in severity. Few patients have an absent thymus and no T cells.
- Chronic mucocutaneous candidiasis. There are multiple forms of this disorder. One form is also called autoimmune polyendocrino-pathy—candidiasis—ectodermal dystrophy (APECED) and has a very strong association with polyendocrinopathies and ectodermal dysplasia. The other types are more likely to have an associated T-cell defect. Infants have extensive or recurrent Candida; predisposition to other infections is modest.

Neutrophil Defects
- Autoimmune neutropenia of infancy. Most common neutrophil defect of childhood; usually detected at about 6–12 months of age; often resolves by 2 years of age.
- Congenital neutropenia. Infections may be skin infections or sinopulmonary; patients have either absent or markedly low neutrophil counts, which are consistent.
- Leukocyte adhesion deficiency. Approximately 10% have delayed separation of the umbilical cord; most common presentations are recurrent skin ulcers and periodontitis.
- Chronic granulomatous disease. Recurrent skin abscesses common, deep hepatic abscesses, and pulmonary abscesses are also seen. Typical organisms are Staphylococcus aureus and Pseudomonas; Aspergillus and Candida are also seen; age of onset is usually 1–3 years.

Immunodeficiency Syndromes
- Ataxia telangiectasia. Progressive cerebellar ataxia beginning at about 12 months; ocular telangiectasias beginning at about 5 to 15 years; recurrent sinopulmonary infections; alpha-fetoprotein is elevated, IgA and IgG2 are diminished.
- Wiskott-Aldrich syndrome. Clinical triad of eczema, thrombocytopenia, and recurrent infections. IgM low; IgG normal or slightly low; IgA and IgE elevated; platelets range from 20–90K and are small.
- Hyper-IgE syndrome. Recurrent infections of the skin, lungs, middle ears, and sinuses; S. aureus is a major cause of infection and pulmonary infections typically heal with blebs.

• *X-linked lymphoproliferative syndrome.* Four main types of presentation: acute EBV infection with hemophagocytosis, lymphoma, hypogammaglobulinemia, and aplastic anemia. Family history is key to diagnosis.
• *Chédiak-Higashi syndrome.* Pigmentary dilution, progressive neuropathy, and frequent infections; associated with a hemophagocytic process. Neutrophil counts are low and neutrophils have giant inclusions.

Miscellaneous
Complement deficiency. Deficiencies of C5–C9 are associated with *Neisseria* infections; deficiencies of C1, C2, C4 are associated with lupus and recurrent bacterial infections. C3 deficiency is associated with glomerulonephritis and severe recurrent infections.
Familial hemophagocytic lymphohistiocytosis. A defect in natural killer cell function; presents with fever, pancytopenia and hepatosplenomegaly; usually before 5 years of age.

SECONDARY IMMUNODEFICIENCIES
• HIV infection
• Malignancy
• Viral suppression
• Nephrotic syndrome
• Malnutrition
• Medications
• Splenectomy

Approach to the Patient

GENERAL GOALS
• Immunologic laboratory evaluations are performed according to the suspected type of immunodeficiency. A patient with recurrent sinopulmonary infections with typical organisms could have a defect in antibody production. Therefore, laboratory evaluations should focus on the quantity and function of antibodies.
• Patients with chronic viral infections or opportunistic infections might have a T-cell defect. These patients would benefit from an evaluation of T-cell production and function.
• Neutrophil disorders typically present with skin abscesses or ulcers or deep infections with *Staphylococcus* or *Pseudomonas*. Patients with these problems would benefit from an evaluation of neutrophil numbers and function.
• In certain patients it may be difficult to differentiate between viral processes and bacterial processes. In these cases, a CBC and differential, IgG, IgA, IgM levels, and diphtheria and tetanus titers are a useful screen to evaluate for the most common immunodeficiencies.

 ## Data Gathering

HISTORY
• Family history (primarily inquiring about the possibility of maternally inherited disorders)
• Number and duration of infections (to determine whether the problem is one of

clearance, which implies a T-cell defect, or frequency, which implies a B-cell defect)
• Types of infections (infections of skin are frequently due to neutrophil problems, whereas recurrent infections of a single site implies an anatomic problem with clearance of organisms. Opportunistic infections are associated with both neutrophil defects and T-cell defects.
• HIV risk factors
• Associated health problems (syndromic features, medications)

PHYSICAL EXAMINATION
• The physical examination should be directed at defining organ damage as a result of infection, the presence of any current infections, the presence of any syndromic features, the presence of signs of autoimmune disease, and the characterization of accessible lymphoid organs. Examination of lymph nodes, tonsils, liver, and spleen will reveal hypoplasia or expansion.

 ## Laboratory Aids

Tests
• Complete blood count with differential
• Quantitative immunoglobulins
• Antibody responses to immunizations (must be certain that the child has been immunized)
• T-cell enumeration
• T-cell function measured as proliferation in response to maximal stimuli (PHA, PWM, ConA) or physiologic stimuli (recall antigens)
• Neutrophil respiratory burst assay (nitroblue tetrazolium, dichlorofluorescein, rhodamine)
• CH50: total hemolytic complement
• HIV ELISA and Western blot: If positive in children under 15 months of age, HIV infection should be confirmed with HIV PCR.

 ## Emergency Care

Suspected severe combined immunodeficiency requires isolation, CMV negative/irradiated blood products, and a prompt evaluation.

 ## Therapy

Bone Marrow Transplantation
• Severe combined immunodeficiency (SCID)
• Wiskott-Aldrich syndrome
• X-linked lymphoproliferative syndrome
• Chédiak-Higashi syndrome
• Familial hemophagocytic lymphohistiocytosis

Thymus Transplantation
Severe chromosome 22q11.2 deletion syndrome (DiGeorge syndrome)

Intravenous Immunoglobulin Replacement
• X-linked agammaglobulinemia
• Hyper-IgM
• Common variable immunodeficiency
• IgG subclass deficiency (infrequently)

Prophylactic Antibiotics/Antifungals
• IgG subclass deficiency
• Chronic mucocutaneous candidiasis
• Ataxia telangiectasia
• Hyper-IgE syndrome
• Chronic granulomatous disease

 ## Follow-Up

Patients with congenital immunodeficiencies usually require lifelong ongoing management.

 ## Common Questions and Answers

Q: I have many patients with recurrent episodes of green rhinorrhea. Do these episodes all need to be treated with antibiotics and should the child have an immunologic evaluation?
A: Many viral infections cause green rhinorrhea and thus do not require antibiotics. Children with no other infections may be safely observed, but children who have recurrent sinus disease and any other significant infections should be evaluated for the possibility of an immunodeficiency.

Q: Does a child with thrush require evaluation?
A: A child with severe thrush in the absence of risk factors should have an evaluation for T-cell dysfunction, HIV, and the possibility of chronic mucocutaneous candidiasis of childhood. Moderate thrush or recurrent simple thrush does not require evaluation unless it is occurring in an older child.

Q: A newborn in my practice still has his umbilical cord attached at 6 weeks. Is that abnormal and does it require an evaluation for leukocyte adhesion deficiency?
A: A completely healthy appearing cord at 6 weeks does not require any evaluation.

Clinical Pearls
• Boys with X-linked agammaglobulinemia and X-linked hyper-IgM do not have tonsils and adenoids
• Children and adults with hyper-IgE syndrome develop abscesses that aren't painful.

BIBLIOGRAPHY
Conley ME, Notarangelo L, Etzioni A. Diagnostic criteria for primary immunodeficiencies. *Clin Immunol* 1999;93:190–197.

Noroski L, Shearer WT. Screening for primary immunodeficiencies in the clinical immunology laboratory. *Clin Immunol Immunopathol* 1998;86:237–245.

Author: Kathleen E. Sullivan

Jaundice

Database

DEFINITION
- Jaundice—a yellow or green/yellow hue to the skin, sclerae, and mucous membranes—becomes recognizable at serum total bilirubin levels of approximately 5 mg/dL (see table Common Causes of Pathologic Jaundice).
- Conjugated hyperbilirubinemia is defined as a direct-reacting fraction of serum bilirubin exceeding 30% to 40% of the total serum bilirubin.
- Unconjugated hyperbilirubinemia, the direct-reacting fraction is <15% of the total serum bilirubin. Patients with direct-reacting bilirubin between 15% and 30% are, therefore, indeterminate.

Differential Diagnosis

UNCONJUGATED HYPERBILIRUBINEMIA
Congenital/Anatomic
- Placental dysfunction
- Upper gastrointestinal (GI) tract obstruction (e.g., pyloric stenosis, duodenal web, stenosis, or atresia)
- Congenital hypothyroidism
- Infants of diabetic mothers

Infectious
- Sepsis

Trauma
- Cephalohematoma; bruising

Genetic/Metabolic
- Inherited red cell enzyme or membrane structural defects (e.g., G-6-PD deficiency, phosphokinase deficiency, spherocytosis)
- Defect in hepatic bilirubin conjugation (Crigler-Najjar syndrome, types I and II)

ALLERGIC/INFLAMMATORY/IMMUNOLOGIC
- Rh or ABO incompatibility

Functional
- Physiologic jaundice (almost always less than 14 days of age)
- Breast-feeding—associated jaundice
- Swallowed maternal blood; infant bleeding from clotting disorder (increased bilirubin load; see Trauma)
- Familial benign unconjugated hyperbilirubinemia (Lucey-Driscoll syndrome)

CONJUGATED HYPERBILIRUBINEMIA
Congenital/Anatomic
- Biliary atresia
- Biliary hypoplasia
- Congenital or acquired bile duct stenosis
- Choledochal cyst and other anomalies of the choledochopancreatic ductal junction
- Spontaneous perforation of the bile duct
- Bile or mucus plug or "biliary sludge"
- Gallstone
- Cystic dilatation of intrahepatic bile ducts ("Caroli disease")
- Congenital hepatic fibrosis/polycystic kidney and liver disease

Infectious Etiologies
- Bacterial
—Gram-negative sepsis
—Urinary tract infection/pyelonephritis
- Viral
—Cytomegalovirus (CMV)
—Echovirus
—HIV
—Hepatitis B, C
- Toxoplasmosis
- *Pneumocystis carinii*
- *Entamoeba histolytica*
- *Mycobacterium tuberculosis*
- *M. avium-intracellulare*
- Syphilis

Toxic/Environmental/Drugs
- Postnecrotizing enterocolitis
- Postshock or postasphyxia
- Medications
- Hyperalimentation

Tumor
- Neuroblastoma
- Porta hepatis nodes

Genetic/Metabolic
- Arteriohepatic dysplasia (Alagille syndrome)
- Progressive familial intrahepatic cholestasis (several types including Byler disease, MDR3 deficiency)
- Defects in bile acid metabolism
- Defects in amino acid metabolism
- Defects in lipid metabolism
—Wolman disease (cholesterol ester storage disease)
—Niemann-Pick disease
—Gaucher disease
- Defects in carbohydrate metabolism
—Galactosemia
—Hereditary fructose intolerance
—Glycogenosis type IV
—Zellweger syndrome (cerebrohepatorenal)
- Defects in mitochondrial DNA and respiratory chain enzyme deficiencies
- α_1-Antitrypsin deficiency
- Cystic fibrosis
- Multiple acyl coenzyme A dehydrogenase deficiency
- Wilson disease (older child only)
- Inherited noncholestatic conjugated jaundice syndromes (e.g., Dubin-Johnson and Rotor syndromes)
- Familial benign recurrent cholestasis—inborn errors of bile acid synthesis
- Hereditary cholestasis with lymphedema (Aegenaes syndrome)

Allergic/Inflammatory/Immunologic
- Sclerosing cholangitis

Miscellaneous
- Idiopathic neonatal hepatitis
- Neonatal iron storage disease
- Idiopathic hypopituitarism

Approach to the Patient

GENERAL GOAL
Decide if disorder threatens acute or subacute hepatic failure (conjugated hyperbilirubinemia). Decide if disorder threatens neurologic injury (kernicterus).

Phase 1: Is the jaundice due entirely to unconjugated hyperbilirubinemia?

Phase 2: Is the jaundice due to conjugated hyperbilirubinemia? Obtain values for total, direct, and indirect serum bilirubin); serum aminotransferases (ALT and AST), γ-glutamyltransferase (GGT), prothrombin time (PT), and partial thromboplastin time (PTT).

Phase 3: Rule out those causes of direct hyperbilirubinemia for which delay in diagnosis and treatment may adversely affect outcome, i.e., biliary atresia, tyrosinemia, galactosemia, inborn error of bile acid synthesis, hereditary fructose intolerance, neonatal iron storage disease.

Data Gathering

HISTORY
Question: Does the patient have unexplained itching?
Significance: Suggests cholestatic liver disease (conjugated hyperbilirubinemia).

Question: Does the patient have a change in mental status, handwriting, or school performance?
Significance: Consider Wilson disease (generally children over 4 years of age).

Question: Is there a history of intravenous drug abuse or exposure to blood or blood products, especially prior to 1992?
Significance: The patient may have transfusion-associated hepatitis, most likely hepatitis C.

Common Causes of Pathologic Jaundice

NEWBORN AND EARLY INFANCY PERIOD	*OLDER CHILD*
Biliary atresia	Autoimmune hepatitis
Idiopathic neonatal hepatitis	Viral hepatitis
Alpha-1-Antitrypsin deficiency	Wilson disease
Infection	Biliary obstruction (e.g., gallstone or choledochal cyst)

Question: Is there a history of a sibling with prolonged jaundice or hepatic failure in infancy?
Significance: Because many of the causes of neonatal conjugated hyperbilirubinemia are due to recessive disorders, a sibling with prolonged neonatal jaundice, particularly if fatal and left undiagnosed, suggests an inborn error such as tyrosinemia, α_1-antitrypsin deficiency, etc., as the cause for the newborn patient's jaundice.

 Physical Examination

Finding: Scratch marks
Significance: Possibly attributable to pruritus, suggesting cholestasis.

Finding: Spider angiomata, palmar erythema
Significance: Evidence of chronic liver disease.

Finding: Petechiae, purpura, microcephaly
Significance: Evidence of thrombocytopenia, possibly due to congenital TORCH infection.

Finding: Severe bruising, cephalohematoma
Significance: Increased bilirubin load.

Finding: Pallor
Significance: Indicative of severe anemia, possibly due to ongoing hemolysis as a cause of indirect hyperbilirubinemia.

Finding: Heart murmur
Significance: Alagille syndrome (classically peripheral pulmonic stenosis).

Finding: Hepatosplenomegaly
Significance: Congenital TORCH infection or of significant liver scarring and portal hypertension

Finding: Ascites
Significance: Hypoalbuminemia, generally implying significant chronic liver disease and synthetic dysfunction

Finding: Acholic stool
Significance: Severe cholestasis; in the newborn, suggestive but not pathognomonic of biliary atresia; in the older child, may also suggest biliary obstruction due to a gallstone, mass, or other lesion obstructing the flow of bile.

 Laboratory Aids

Test: Total bilirubin with fractionation, preferably by HPLC into conjugated, unconjugated, and delta fractions (newborn or young infant).
Significance: If unconjugated hyperbilirubinemia, initiate workup with:
• Blood type and Rh factor of mother and infant—hemolysis due to blood group or Rh incompatibility

• Hemoglobin, hematocrit, reticulocyte count, peripheral smear for red cell morphology—rule out microspherocytes indicating hemolysis, or evidence of hereditary spherocytosis or elliptocytosis
• Coombs test—assess for autoimmune hemolytic anemia
• PT, PTT, platelet count—assess coagulopathy that may explain lost blood and increased bilirubin load causing unconjugated hyperbilirubinemia
• Sepsis evaluation (blood, urine, and spinal fluid cultures)
• T_4, T_3, TSH—screen for neonatal thyroid disease

Test: Serum aminotransferases (ALT, AST); GGT
Significance: Measures degree of liver inflammation and cholestasis

Test: Serum albumin, PT, PTT, fibrinogen, cholesterol
Significance: Measures degree of liver synthetic function; decrease in albumin, fibrinogen, or very low cholesterol and increases in PT, PTT implies significant liver disease.

Test: Stool color
Significance: Acholic (white) or very pale stools imply possibly obstructive lesion (such as biliary atresia).

• Sepsis evaluation (cultures of blood, urine, and spinal fluid).
• Hepatitis B surface antigen and hepatitis C antibody and RNA by polymerase chain reaction (PCR)

Test: TORCH titers and VDRL
Significance: Congenital infection

Test: α_1-Antitrypsin and Pi (protease inhibitor) type
Significance: Inherited homozygous deficient alleles

Test: Urine and plasma amino acids and urine organic acids
Significance: Screens for inherited amino and organic acidopathies.

Test: Urine dipstick for glucose and Clinitest for reducing substances
Significance: Implies the presence of another sugar such as galactose.

Test: Urine for bile acid analysis
Significance: Assesses for inborn error of bile acid synthesis.

Test: Ultrasonography
Significance: Dilated hepatic ducts implying an obstructive lesion; presence of gallstones or a choledochal cyst.

Test: Hepatobiliary scintigraphy (DISIDA scan)
Significance: The presence of excretion of labeled tracer from the liver into the bowel effectively rules out biliary atresia; the absence of excretion does not necessarily rule in an obstructive disorder.

Test: Percutaneous liver biopsy
Significance: Allows with greater than 90% to 95% certainty the assessment of findings that may suggest extrahepatic obstruction, such as biliary atresia, which merits surgical exploration and intraoperative cholangiogram.

 Common Questions and Answers

Q: Because biliary atresia is an obstructive lesion, are the intrahepatic bile ducts dilated?
A: Never!

Q: What disorders are life-threatening?
A: Biliary atresia, galactosemia, hereditary fructose intolerance, tyrosinemia, sepsis, hypopituitarism, inborn error of bile acid metabolism, neonatal iron storage disease. In the infant with unconjugated hyperbilirubinemia, sepsis, and hypothyroidism together with Crigler-Najar syndrome types I and II such as brisk hemolysis that causes a rapid rise of unconjugated bilirubin above 20 mg/dL. In the older child, suspected Wilson disease.

Issues for Referral
• Lack of excretion on hepatobiliary scintigraphy scan.
• Presence of choledochal cyst or dilated biliary ducts seen on ultrasound.
• Abnormal metabolic screen (urine and plasma, amino, or organic acids).
• Evidence of decompensated liver disease, e.g., PT >20 seconds; albumin <3.0, ascites, encephalopathy, bilirubin >20 mg/dL; ALT/AST >300, especially if associated with one or more of the previous criteria.

Clinical Pearls
• Crigler-Najar type II syndrome must be treated promptly with phototherapy and phenobarbital to prevent kernicterus.
• Older children presenting with Wilson disease may present with significant hemolysis, and therefore with a predominantly unconjugated hyperbilirubinemia but with significant parenchymal liver disease and even liver failure. Do not be fooled!

BIBLIOGRAPHY
Lasker MR, Holzman R. Neonatal jaundice: when to treat, when to watch and wait. *Postgrad Med* 1996;99(3):187–193.

Mews C, Sinatra FR. Chronic liver disease in children. *Pediatr Rev* 1993;14(11):436–444.

Author: Eric S. Maller

Learning Problems

 Database

DEFINITION

Learning disorders, or *learning disabilities*, are defined in the *Diagnostic and Statistical Manual of Mental Disorders*, 4th edition (DSM-IV) as academic achievement that is substantially below the level expected for age, schooling, and general intellectual ability, and that cannot be accounted for by psychosocial factors. The term *specific learning disability* is sometimes used with the same meaning. A learning disability may affect reading, writing, spelling, or math, and any given child may have more than one learning disability. Learning disabilities are neurobiologically based, and are believed to have a genetic etiology.

EPIDEMIOLOGY

Learning disorders have an estimated incidence of up to 10% in school-aged children. Learning disorders typically are not evident until academic demands are placed on the affected children. Psychiatric comorbidity is frequent, either as a complication of learning problems or as an etiologic factor in their development.

 Differential Diagnosis

Children's school problems may result from a specific learning disorder, or may be the secondary effect of some other medical or psychosocial problem.

- Attention deficit/hyperactivity disorder (ADHD) may present as a learning problem, especially when the inattentive and distractible symptoms of the diagnosis are greater than the hyperactive symptoms. ADHD may be difficult to distinguish from a learning disorder, and the two also may be found comorbidly. Careful psychoeducational assessment often may be needed to clarify these diagnoses.
- Sensory impairments: Hearing or vision impairments may cause learning problems. School screening results should be confirmed in children with learning problems.
- Neurologic: Absence seizures and other nonconvulsive epileptic disorders are much less common than ADHD but may mimic its symptoms. Narcolepsy also is associated with learning problems. Neurodegenerative disorders such as Niemann-Pick disease, adrenoleukodystrophy, ceroid lipofuscinosis, and subacute sclerosing panencephalitis may rarely present as school-age learning problems.
- Mental retardation: Borderline or mild mental retardation may not be recognized until school entrance.

- Genetics: Some genetic syndromes may show subtle dysmorphology that is not noted until learning problems arise. Examples are sex chromosome aneuploidies, fragile X syndrome in both boys and girls, neurofibromatosis, tuberous sclerosis, and velocardiofacial/DiGeorge syndrome.
- Nutritional, toxicologic, infections: Lead intoxication, chronic malnutrition, iron-deficiency, hypothyroidism, and HIV infection may have insidious effects on cognitive function.
- Iatrogenic interventions: Medical therapies may compromise learning abilities; for example, cranial irradiation for malignancies, and treatment with antiepileptic drugs or theophylline.
- Psychosocial: Issues related to family stress, peer relationships, illness, or adolescence may present as academic difficulty. Conversely, behavior problems at home or at school always should prompt evaluation of school functioning.
- Psychiatric comorbidity occurs commonly. Adjustment disorders, mood disorders, oppositional defiant disorder, conduct disorder, tic disorders, substance abuse, and other behavior problems may precede or follow the presentation of learning problems. Less commonly, psychotic disorders, personality disorders, and obsessive-compulsive disorder may underlie learning problems.
- Speculative etiologies: Food allergies, "developmental optometric" disorders, and exposure to food preservatives or sugar are widely discussed but are essentially unproven causes of learning problems.

Approach to the Patient

GENERAL GOAL

Determine whether the learning problems result from a primary medical or psychosocial condition. If no such condition is identified, then the patient may have a specific learning disability. The pediatrician also is in a good position to identify social and environmental factors that may be associated with learning problems, and can coordinate the appropriate medical, psychiatric, and/or psychoeducational evaluation, with consultation as indicated. Early identification of learning problems helps to prevent the cascade of negative consequences triggered by poor academic achievement.

Phase 1a: Identify and address medical factors that may affect learning (e.g., sensory impairments, lead intoxication, absence seizures, iatrogenic interventions). Consider subtle genetic syndromes (e.g., fragile X syndrome in girls) that may cause learning problems without causing other major medical abnormalities.

Phase 1b: Screen for psychiatric conditions, and for social and environmental factors that may be associated with learning problems. Psychosocial stresses may exacerbate learning difficulties, or be a primary etiologic factor. If indicated, refer to appropriate consultants.

Phase 2: For patients with learning problems that are suspected to be primary (i.e., specific learning disabilities), a complete psychoeducational evaluation is indicated. If ADHD is present, treatment may be directed by the primary care physician or by a subspecialist.

 Data Gathering

HISTORY

Question: When and how does the child fail in his daily academic pursuits?
Significance: For specific learning disabilities, problems may occur in only one class. For attention deficit, problems may be broad-based and may emerge as children move into more formal didactic settings. With borderline mental retardation or other chronic problems, there may be a long history of developmental concerns.

Question: Recent or new decline in school performance?
Significance: Consider new pathophysiologic processes, such as psychosocial issues, new vision or hearing impairment, side effect from new medication, or neurodegenerative disorder (rare).

Question: Reaction to the learning problem (mood, anxiety)?
Significance: Poor school performance commonly leads to depression, poor self-esteem, and possible behavior problems.

Question: Past medical history? Medications? Review of systems? Psychosocial stresses?
Significance: Identify factors that may affect learning. Early language delays are common among children with learning disorders.

Question: Family history?
Significance: May be positive for learning or attention problems that are similar to the child's.

Physical Examination

Finding: Subtle dysmorphology
Significance: May suggest the presence of a genetic syndrome or a pattern of malformation resulting from teratogenic fetal exposures (e.g., alcohol, hydantoin, etc.).

Finding: Abnormal neurological examination
Significance: Any focal signs demand additional evaluation. Soft signs (neuromaturational signs) are often present in children with learning problems, but are nonspecific.

Finding: Abnormal audiology or vision screening
Significance: May be direct cause of learning problem.

Laboratory Aids

No laboratory studies are routinely indicated. The history and physical examination may provide specific indications for further testing.

Test: Standardized behavior questionnaires
Significance: Diagnosis of attention deficit disorder is critically dependent on input from teachers and parents. Psychiatric complications, such as depression, should also be considered.

Test: Lead level, thyroid functions, karyotype, HIV testing, hearing and vision testing, EEG, neuroimaging
Significance: Each of these can be considered if the history and physical exam provide specific indications.

Test: Psychoeducational evaluation
Significance: A comprehensive psychoeducational evaluation serves as the cornerstone of diagnosis and educational intervention. This testing must be performed individually, and should include general intelligence and academic achievement testing. Federal law requires schools to provide comprehensive evaluations on written request by the parents to the school principal. (Specific information for each state can be obtained from the National Information Center for Children and Youth with Disabilities (800-695-0285; *www.nichcy.org*). Many centers outside the school system (e.g., hospital-based centers) also conduct evaluations of children with learning problems.

Test: Neuropsychological evaluation
Significance: For children who do not respond to first-line educational interventions, more extensive neuropsychological testing may elucidate specific cognitive strengths and weaknesses that may be helpful in developing an effective educational plan.

Issues for Referral

Referrals to medical and psychological professionals may be helpful for both diagnostic and therapeutic purposes. When a specific medical etiology is suspected, the choice of subspecialist for referral will be clear. When no specific etiology is apparent, consider referral to a clinician experienced with learning disabilities. This consultant may assist in comprehensive diagnostic formulation, pharmacologic treatment when indicated, developmental follow-up, and advocacy.

Therapy

- For children with specific learning disabilities (i.e., learning problems not caused by an identifiable medical factor), educational interventions are the centerpiece of treatment. Depending of the nature of the problem, possible classroom accommodations include preferential seating, extra time for test-taking, use of electronic word processors, provision of written rather than verbal instructions, tutoring, resource room assistance, and alternative classroom placement. For children with ADHD, behavioral therapy and pharmacologic therapy may also be required to optimize their potential for learning.
- Treatment is most effective when it employs a team approach, inclusive of parents, teachers, and other therapists.

Follow-Up

Children with learning disabilities require continued monitoring of academic progress. Even when the initial learning problems are resolved, later difficulties may arise in writing, note-taking, composition, organization, and with more abstract academic topics.

Clinical Pearls

- Comorbidity and symptomatic overlap are common among ADHD, specific learning disabilities, and other psychiatric disorders. Students who have a learning disability or are depressed may show symptoms of inattention. Academic or attention difficulties may lead to spiraling psychological problems, from depression or damaged self-esteem to conduct disorder and school dropout.

- Normal attention and activity in the physician's office do not rule out ADHD. Many children with ADHD show significant difficulties with inattention and distractibility, but little hyperactivity. Even children with severe ADHD may appear attentive in the intimidating and artificial milieu of the doctor's office, or when engaged in highly motivating and highly reinforcing computer games.

BIBLIOGRAPHY

Beitchman JH, Young AR. Learning disorders with a special emphasis on reading disorders: a review of the past 10 years. *J Am Acad Child Adolesc Psychiatry* 1997;36(8):1020–1032.

Buttross S. Attention deficit-hyperactivity disorder and its deceivers. *Curr Probl Pediatr* 2000;30(2):37–50.

Hechtman L. Assessment and diagnosis of attention-deficit/hyperactivity disorder. *Child Adolesc Psychiatr Clin North Am* 2000;9(3): 481–498.

Levy SE. Pediatric evaluation of the child with developmental delay. *Child Adolesc Psychiatr Clin North Am* 1996;5(4):809–826.

Mannuzza S, Klein RG. Long-term prognosis in attention-deficit/hyperactivity disorder. *Child Adolesc Psychiatr Clin North Am* 2000;9(3): 711–726.

Reiff MI. Adolescent school failure: failure to thrive in adolescence. *Pediatr Rev* 1998;19(6): 199–207.

Resnick MB, Gomatam SV, Carter RL, et al. Educational disabilities of neonatal intensive care graduates. *Pediatrics* 1998;102(2 pt 1): 308–314.

Shaywitz SE. Dyslexia. *N Engl J Med* 1998;338(5):307–312.

Author: Paul P. Wang

Leukocytosis

 Database

DEFINITION
An increase in white blood cell count above normal for age. The most frequent cause is an increase in the total neutrophil count but leukocytosis may result from an increase in any type of white blood cell, such as lymphocytosis, monocytosis, eosinophilia, basophilia, or atypical monocytosis.

 Differential Diagnosis

INFECTIOUS
- Bacterial
—*Streptococcus* (especially *pneumoniae*)
—*Staphylococcus aureus*
—*Haemophilus*
—*Neisseria*
—*Brucella*
—*Bartonella* (cat-scratch disease)
—Pertussis
- Viral
—Infectious mononucleosis
—Cytomegalovirus (CMV)
—Rubella
—Mumps
—Hepatitis
- Fungal
—*Aspergillus*
- Parasitic
—*Toxocara*
—*Toxoplasma*
—*Trichinella*
—Tapeworms
—*Strongyloides*
—*Coccidioidomycosis*
- Tuberculosis
- Syphilis
- Acute infectious lymphocytosis
—Benign viral mediated lymphocytosis (often >25,000/mm^3)
- Kawasaki disease

CONGENITAL/ANATOMIC
- Down syndrome
- Sickle cell disease
- Fanconi anemia

Causes of Neutrophilia

Bacterial infections
Inflammatory states
Acute hemorrhage
Stress
Drugs
  Corticosteroids, Epinephrine
Metabolic disorders
  Uremia
  Acidosis
Myeloproliferative disorders
  Myelofibrosis, Polycythemia vera, CML
Sickle cell disease

- Thrombocytopenia with absent radii
- Leukocyte adhesion factor deficiency

DRUGS
- Corticosteroids
- Epinephrine
- Lithium
- Granulocyte colony-stimulating factor (GCSF)
- Granulocyte-macrophage colony-stimulating factor (GM-CSF)

TRAUMA
- Acute hemorrhage
- Severe burns
- Inflammation

TUMOR
- Leukemia
- Lymphoma
- Myeloproliferative disorders

GENETIC/METABOLIC
- Hyperthyroidism
- Acidosis

INFLAMMATORY
- Juvenile rheumatoid arthritis (JRA)
- Rheumatoid arthritis (RA)
- Inflammatory bowel disease
- Chronic granulomatous disease (CGD)
- Pulmonary eosinophilic syndromes
—Transient infiltrates associated with a peripheral eosinophilia

ALLERGIC
- Asthma
- Seasonal or drug allergies
- Eczema
- Psoriasis

HEMATOLOGIC
- Severe hemolysis

ARTIFACTUAL
- Nucleated RBCs
- Clumped platelets on a mechanical differential

Approach to the Patient

Phase 1: Is the WBC count dangerously elevated? If the WBC count is greater than 50,000/mm^3, consult a pediatric hematologist/oncologist. WBC of 100,000/mm^3 can increase blood viscosity causing stroke or infarct of end-organs.

Causes of Lymphocytosis

Viral infections
Bordetella pertussis
Tuberculosis
Syphilis
Acute infectious lymphocytosis
Malignancy
  Acute lymphocytic leukemia, Lymphoma

Phase 2: Which white blood cell line is elevated?
- An elevated granulocyte count is more likely with bacterial infections and a lymphocytosis is usually associated with viral infections. Pitfall: Many laboratories provide only machine-generated differentials. If there are any abnormalities, a manual differential must be obtained. It may be necessary to review the smear with a hematologist or pathologist.

Phase 3: Lastly, the degree of elevation can be indicative of the diagnosis.
- Most elevations of WBC count are in the 10,000 to 20,000/mm^3 range. A WBC count in the 30,000/mm^3 range is more consistent with pertussis, pneumococcal infection, or acute infectious lymphocytosis. Higher counts are worrisome for malignant processes or leukemoid reactions.

 Data Gathering

HISTORY
Question: Is there any evidence for infection, such as fever, rash, or swelling?
Significance: Infection is the most common etiology for leukocytosis. A thorough history should be taken for apparent or occult infections. Fever can also be a symptom of inflammatory diseases such as JRA or CGD.

Question: What other complaints has the patient had over the preceding weeks to months?
Significance: Infectious etiologies tend to present acutely. If a patient has long-term complaints, one should broaden the differential or focus it based on specific complaints. A chronic cough may point to tuberculosis, whereas a whooping cough may indicate pertussis.

Causes of Eosinophilia

Allergic disorders
  Asthma
  Urticaria
  Drug hypersensitivity
Skin disorders
  Eczema, Psoriasis, Pemphigus
Parasitic infections
Fungal infections
Hypereosinophilic syndromes
Hereditary eosinophilia
Hematologic disorders
  Fanconi anemia
  Thrombocytopenia with absent radii
  Congenital neutropenias
Inflammatory disorders
  Gastrointestinal
  Sarcoid
  Polyarteritis nodosa

Question: Does the patient have any other medical problems?
Significance: Patients with sickle cell disease have an elevated WBC count probably secondary to chronic inflammation or marrow expansion. Children with Down syndrome can have a benign leukemoid reaction, especially in the first few months of life, that resolves spontaneously.

Question: Is the patient on any medications?
Significance: Corticosteroids will increase the neutrophil precursors. Epinephrine can cause a transitory increase in neutrophil count.

Question: Is there a familial history of any inflammatory diseases?
Significance: For example, collagen vascular disease such as RA, thyroid, Crohn disease.

Question: Has the patient lost weight, been fatigued, had night sweats, or been pale?
Significance: Malignancy (leukemia) must be ruled out.

 ## Physical Examination

Finding: Are there any foci of infection?
Significance: Look for cellulitis, otitis, pharyngitis, or abscesses on examination. A careful lung examination is necessary as pneumonia can cause a WBC count as high as 30,000 to 40,000/mm^3. A murmur or gallop may be a sign of bacterial endocarditis.

Finding: Lymphadenopathy or hepatosplenomegaly?
Significance: Points toward a possible viral etiology but is also of concern for malignancy.

Finding: Are joints tender or swollen?
Significance: JRA, septic arthritis, SLE

Finding: Mongoloid features?
Significance: Down syndrome.

Causes of Monocytosis

Infection
   Tuberculosis
   Malaria
   Brucellosis
   Bacterial endocarditis
Inflammatory disease
   Collagen vascular disease
   Sarcoid
   RA
   Crohn's, ulcerative colitis
   SLE
Malignancy
   Hodgkin disease
   Acute myelocytic leukemia
   Myelodysplastic syndromes

 ## Laboratory Aids

Test: WBC count including differential.
Significance: If neutrophilia is present, think of bacterial infections. One may also see Döhle bodies, toxic granulations, or vacuolization in bacteremia. A recovering or stressed marrow may have an increase in monocytes or eosinophils. Look for leukemic blasts.

Test: Hemoglobin/platelet count
Significance: If either is low, consider a marrow infiltrative process or a marrow that is hyperstimulated to compensate for a low hemoglobin or platelet count.

Test: Chemistry panel
Significance: Evaluate LFTs for possible viral etiology. Uric acid and LDH are elevated in leukemia and lymphoma.

Test: Cultures
Significance: Blood, urine, stool, throat, etc.

Test: Monospot, heterophil Ab, EBV titers
Significance: Screen for infectious mononucleosis. Monospot can be falsely negative in younger children.

Test: Leukocyte alkaline phosphatase
Significance: Elevated in infection but not in leukemia. Helps to differentiate CML from a leukemoid reaction.

Test: ANA
Significance: Screen for rheumatologic etiology.

Test: Bone marrow biopsy and aspirate
Significance: Necessary if any other blood cell line is abnormally low or if the WBCs appear dysmorphic. Need to rule out malignancy, myelodysplasia, or other marrow processes. Send cytogenetics when possible.

Test: Chest x-ray
Significance: Pneumonia, tuberculosis.

Issues for Referral
- WBC counts greater than 50,000/mm^3
- Any indication of malignancy
- Any indication of a rheumatologic etiology
- Inability to find an etiology with a persistent leukocytosis

 ## Emergency Care

- Antibiotics if a child appears septic.
- Fluids containing bicarbonate and allopurinol if leukemia is suspected.
- If the leukocytosis is >100,000/mm^3 and the patient has symptoms of end-organ failure, emergent leukapheresis should be performed. If the patient's condition is hemodynamically stable, avoid red cell transfusions, which will increase the blood viscosity.

Clinical Pearls
Beware of any differential that has a high percentage of monocytes or atypical lymphocytes whether machine generated or manual. These are the cell types most commonly mistaken for leukemic blasts.

Common Questions and Answers

Q: What does "left-shifted" mean?
A: There are early granulocyte precursors (metamyelocytes, myelocytes) seen in the peripheral smear with a bandemia and neutrophilia. Often seen with bacteremia or marrow recovery from a suppressing drug/virus.

Q: Infectious mononucleosis (IM) and acute lymphocytic leukemia have many similar signs and symptoms. How can I differentiate them?
A: Both can present with fever, malaise, headache, prominent lymphadenopathy, organomegaly, and suppressed hemoglobin and platelet counts. IM tends to be associated with a sore throat and children with ALL are more likely to complain of bony pain. The easiest way to differentiate the two is a careful exam of the peripheral smear. A heterophil AB or monospot can be sent and, if positive, help with the diagnosis.

Q: What are the signs and symptoms of acute infectious lymphocytosis (AIL)?
A: AIL is probably caused by several viruses from which the child can be totally asymptomatic except for a significant lymphocytosis (40,000–80,000/mm^3). On review of the peripheral smear there is a prevalence of small, mature lymphocytes. There can also be an eosinophilia. As a rule there is no anemia or thrombocytopenia. The lymphocytosis resolves spontaneously.

BIBLIOGRAPHY
Gin-Shaw S, Moore GP. Selected white cell disorders. *Emerg Med Clin North Am* 1993;11(2):495–516.

Hoffbrand AV, Pettit JE, eds. *Color atlas of clinical hematology*, 2nd ed. St. Louis: Mosby-Wolfe, 1994.

Peterson L, Hrisinko MA. Benign lymphocytosis and reactive neutrophilia. *Clin Lab Med* 1993;13(4):863–877.

Author: Susan R. Rheingold

Lower GI Bleeding

 Database

DEFINITION

Lower gastrointestinal (GI) bleeding refers to bleeding from the lower GI tract. It can be hematochezia (passage of bright red or dark blood per rectum) or melena (passage of dark, black, or tarry stools).

 Differential Diagnosis

- The majority of patients with lower GI bleeding have a fissure or infection.
- Mucosal lesions are more likely to be associated with antecedent occult bleeding.
- In most patients the bleeding stops spontaneously.

REASONS FOR LOWER GI BLEEDING AT DIFFERENT AGES

Neonatal Period

- Anal fissure
- Necrotizing enterocolitis
- Enteric infections
- Allergic colitis
- Lymphonodular hyperplasia (LNH)
- Upper GI source
- Duplication cyst
- Enterocolitis with Hirschsprung disease
- Meckel diverticulum
- Vascular malformations
- Shock with ischemic bowel
- Hemorrhagic disease of the newborn

Infancy

- Anal fissure
- Enteric infections
- Allergic colitis
- Intussusception
- Meckel diverticulum
- LNH
- Upper GI source
- Duplication cyst
- Enterocolitis with Hirschsprung disease
- Vascular malformation
- Shock with ischemic bowel
- Gangrenous bowel

Preschool Age

- Anal fissure
- Enteric infections
- Polyps
- Parasites
- Meckel diverticulum
- Intussusception
- LNH
- Inflammatory bowel disease (IBD)
- Enterocolitis with Hirschsprung disease
- Hemolytic uremic syndrome
- Shock with ischemic bowel

- Gangrenous bowel
- Vascular malformation
- Child abuse

School Age

- Anal fissure
- Enteric infections
- IBD
- Intussusception
- Meckel diverticulum
- Polyps
- Henoch Schönlein purpura (HSP)
- Hemolytic uremic syndrome (HUS)
- Parasites
- Child abuse
- Vascular malformations

Adolescent

- Anal fissure
- Enteric infections
- IBD
- HUS
- Intussusception
- Midgut volvulus
- Vascular malformations
- LNH
- Parasites

Approach to the Patient

GENERAL GOALS

Determine location of bleeding, the cause, and begin stabilization and treatment

Phase 1: Determine if there is blood or other cause of red or black stools. Hematest the stool.

Phase 2: Assess patient to determine etiology; follow history, physical, and laboratory.

Phase 3: Stabilize patient, decide if emergency treatment is needed or if referral is appropriate. (See Emergency Care.)

HINTS FOR SCREENING PROBLEM

- The rate of bleeding will determine the clinical presentation.
- The more rapid the rate, the larger the volume of lower GI bleeding, and greater the drop in hemoglobin and change in pulse and blood pressure.
- Any significant blood loss will lead to pallor, tachycardia, orthostasis, poor capillary refill, CNS changes (restlessness, confusion), and hypotension.
- Hypotension may not be seen even in the face of significant blood loss, because vasoconstriction will occur to maintain blood pressure until decompensation.
- Initial hemoglobin values may be unreliable since a delay in hemodilution may falsely result in near-normal values.
- In newborn, determine if this is swallowed maternal blood.

 Data Gathering

HISTORY

Question: Is this really blood?
Significance: Get a history and check if any recently ingested foods resemble blood, e.g., red dye, beets, Jell-O, Kool-Aid.

Question: Color of blood?
Significance: If bright red, then site of bleeding is probably in left colon, rectosigmoid, or anal canal; if darker red, then from right colon; if melena or tarry, then bleeding is proximal to ileocecal valve.

Question: Location of blood in relation to the stool?
Significance: In colitis the blood will be mixed with the stool, with a fissure it will be in streaks on the outer aspect of the stool.

Question: Consistency of the stool?
Significance: If diarrhea, more likely to be colitis; if hard, then more likely to be a fissure.

Question: Painful stools?
Significance: Suggest anal fissure or local proctitis.

Question: Painless rectal bleeding?
Significance: Associated with polyps and Meckel diverticulum.

Question: Abdominal pain?
Significance: Can be seen with colitis, IBD, or surgical abdomen.

Question: Any underlying known GI disease, previous GI surgery?
Significance: Past history of colitis, Hirschsprung disease, necrotizing enterocolitis.

Question: Any history of jaundice, hepatitis, liver disease, neonatal history?
Significance: Suggestive of portal vein thrombosis (sepsis, shock, exchange transfusion, omphalitis, IV catheters), portal hypertension, and variceal bleeding.

Question: Any familial history of bleeding diathesis?
Significance: von Willebrand disease, hemophilia

Question: Any medications that can cause bleeding—heparin, warfarin?
Question: Any associated symptoms?
Significance:

—Mouth ulcers
—Weight loss
—Joint pains as in IBD
—Petechiae
—Renal insufficiency
—History of ingestion of uncooked meat as in HUS
—Purpuric rash as in HSP
—Severe abdominal pain and vomiting as in a surgical abdomen

Physical Examination

Finding: Skin
Significance:

- Petechiae
- Ecchymosis
- Purpura
- Hemangiomas
- Evidence of chronic liver disease

—Spider angiomata
—Palmar erythema

- Jaundice

Finding: HEENT: freckles on buccal mucosa
Significance: Peutz-Jeghers syndrome

Finding: Mouth ulcers
Significance: Crohn disease

Finding: Abdomen: hepatosplenomegaly, ascites
Significance: Portal hypertension

Finding: Isolated splenomegaly
Significance: Cavernous transformation of the portal vein

Finding: Rectal examination: evidence of any perianal disease
Significance: Source of bleeding

- IBD, bright red blood in the perianal area or on the examining glove
- Polyps bright red blood in stool

Laboratory Aids

Test: CBC
Significance: Iron-deficiency anemia. If there is leukopenia, anemia, and thrombocytopenia, think chronic liver disease and portal hypertension. If there is anemia with normal RBC indices, then there is truly an acute cause for bleeding. If RBC indices indicate iron-deficiency anemia, think of varices or a mucosal lesion, i.e., chronic blood loss. If thrombocytopenia, think Hemolytic uremic syndrome (HUS).

Test: Coagulation profile
Significance: If PT and PTT are abnormal, then think of liver disease or disseminated intravascular coagulation (DIC) with sepsis. If DIC screen is negative, think liver disease.

Test: Renal function tests (BUN, creatinine, urine analysis)
Significance: Abnormal in HUS, HSP

Test: Liver function tests
Significance: Abnormal in chronic liver disease

Test: Stool tests
Significance: Stool culture (*Salmonella, Shigella, Campylobacter, Yersinia, Aeromonas, Escherichia coli*), stool for *Clostridium difficile* toxin A and B, three stool samples for ova

and parasites (amoeba). Stool smears for white blood cells (not always positive in colitis) and eosinophils (not always positive in allergic colitis).

Test: Abdominal x-ray
Significance: Helpful in surgical abdomen (dilated bowel, air-fluid levels, perforation), constipation (presence of excessive stool), or colitis (edematous bowel, thumb-printing) and toxic megacolon.

Test: Lower and upper endoscopy
Significance: Full colonoscopy to the terminal ileum helpful in diagnosing IBD. Upper endoscopy diagnostic in massive upper GI bleeds presenting with hematochezia.

Test: Barium tests
Significance: Barium enema is diagnostic and therapeutic in intussusception. Contraindicated in moderate and severe colitis. Air contrast barium enema is helpful in diagnosing mucosal lesions (polyps). Upper GI series with small bowel follow through is helpful in evaluating anatomy and Crohn's disease and its complications (fistula, sometimes ulcer may be identified). Enteroclysis or small bowel enema provides good mucosal detail.

Test: Meckel scan
Significance: Diagnostic for Meckel diverticulum that secrete acid. There may be false negatives if the Meckel diverticulum has different tissue expression.

Test: Bleeding scan
Significance: Useful in the patient in whom endoscopy was not diagnostic. Technetium sulfur colloids versus tagged RBC scan. The former detects rapid bleeding but can miss small bleeds, especially if patient is not bleeding during the scan. The latter can detect small bleeds, especially if intermittent.

Test: Angiography
Significance: Useful in detecting vascular causes for GI bleeding. Can also be therapeutic.

Emergency Care

- If patient critical, stabilize the patient with intravenous fluids and blood products.
- Order laboratory tests: CBC, PT/PTT, DIC screen, liver function tests, blood type, and crossmatch.
- Insert an NG tube and lavage with saline if it is unclear whether the patient is having hematochezia due to massive bleeding from the upper GI tract.
- Monitor patient's vital signs and hemoglobin as necessary.
- Make appropriate diagnosis and institute appropriate therapy, i.e., abdominal x-ray, colonoscopy, bleeding scans.

PITFALLS

- Make sure red substance in stool is really blood and not food coloring.

- Initial hemoglobin if normal may be misleading.

Common Questions and Answers

Q: What is the most common cause of lower GI bleeding?
A: Throughout all age groups fissures are the leading cause followed by infections. However, in infancy, the most common cause is a fissure, in toddlers and young children—polyps, and in older children—IBD.

Q: What common foods cause stools to be red? black?
A: Red: Raspberries, cranberries, artificial coloring in cereal. Black: Bismuth, licorice.

Issues for Referral

The following patients should be referred to a specialist:

- Any patient with significant acute lower GI bleeding after initial stabilization.
- Patients with less acute bleeding for whom an easily identifiable cause has not been found (e.g., fissures, infection, intussusception, Meckel diverticulum); patients with chronic or recurrent lower GI bleeding.

Clinical Pearls

- Anal fissure: Treat the underlying constipation (mineral oil, lactulose, high-fiber diet). Local therapy consists of sitz baths, local emollient cremes, and steroid suppositories.
- Polyp: Colonoscopy and polypectomy.
- Intussusception: Barium enema is both diagnostic and permits hydrostatic reduction.
- Parasites. Anti-parasitic drugs.
- Surgery: In cases of massive or persistent bleeding with no identifiable site, exploratory laparotomy may be required.

BIBLIOGRAPHY

Chaibou M, Tucci M, Dugas MA, et al. Clinically significant upper gastrointestinal bleeding acquired in a pediatric intensive care unit. *Pediatrics* 1998;102(4 pt 1):933–938.

Guritzky RP, Rudnitsky G. Bloody neonatal diaper. *Ann Emerg Med* 1996;27:662–664.

Irish MS, Pearl RH, Caty MG, et al. The approach to common abdominal diagnosis in infants and children. *Pediatr Clin North Am* 1998;45(4):729–772.

Silber G. Lower gastrointestinal bleeding. *Pediatr Rev* 1990;12:85–93.

Teach SJ, Fleisher GR. Rectal bleeding in the pediatric emergency department. *Ann Emerg Med* 1994;23:1252–1258.

Author: Maria R. Mascarenhas

Mediastinal Mass

 Database

DEFINITION

Any mass in the anterior, posterior, or middle mediastinum. The anterior mediastinum includes the thymus and other structures anterior to the pericardium. The middle mediastinum is a vascular space that contains the pericardium, heart, great vessels, ascending aorta, and the aortic arch. The posterior mediastinum contains the tracheobronchial tree, esophagus, descending aorta, and neural structures.

 Differential Diagnosis

CONGENITAL/ANATOMIC

- Thoracic meningocele
- Large normal thymus in neonate
- Bronchogenic cyst
- Pericardial cyst
- Aortic aneurysm

INFECTIOUS

May cause mediastinal adenopathy and/or pulmonary nodules.

- Tuberculosis
- Histoplasmosis
- Aspergillosis
- Coccidioidomycosis
- Blastomycosis

TOXIC, ENVIRONMENTAL, DRUGS

- Foreign body in the trachea or esophagus

TUMOR

- Benign

—Thymoma
—Teratoma/dermoid cyst
—Lymphangioma/cystic hygroma
—Hemangioma
—Pheochromocytoma
—Ganglioneuroma
—Neurofibroma

- Malignant

—Hodgkin's lymphoma
—Non-Hodgkin's lymphoma
—Leukemia
—Neuroblastoma
—Rhabdomyosarcoma
—Ganglioneuroblastoma
—Neurofibrosarcoma
—Ewing sarcoma
—Malignant germ cell tumor

ALLERGIC, INFLAMMATORY

- Sarcoid

Approach to the Patient

GENERAL GOAL

Promptly establish diagnosis and begin treatment as indicated. Leukemia and lymphoma may progress rapidly and become life-threatening. If you suspect a malignancy, the child should be immediately referred to an oncologist.

Phase 1: Identify and treat life-threatening complications promptly.

- Superior vena cava (SVC) syndrome—mass compression of the SVC resulting in decreased blood flow to the heart.
- Tracheal compression
- Spinal cord compression
- pleural and/or pericardial effusion
- Tumor lysis syndrome—metabolic triad of hyperkalemia, hyperuricemia, and hyperphosphatemia

Phase 2:

- If mass appears solid, attempt to obtain a tissue diagnosis via biopsy or excision of mass
- If mass appears cystic, a surgical consult may be indicated
- If patient exhibits signs of infection (fever, cough, etc.), obtain appropriate cultures, place PPD and anergy panel and begin broad-spectrum antibiotics

COMPLICATIONS

- Superior vena cava (SVC) syndrome: mass compressing the SVC resulting in decreased blood flow to the heart. Signs and symptoms include edema and cyanosis of the face, neck, and upper extremities, plethora, distended neck veins, cough, dyspnea, orthopnea, headache, anxiety, and confusion. Symptoms are exacerbated when child is recumbent.
- Tracheal compression: mass compression of the trachea resulting in respiratory compromise. Signs and symptoms include stridor, cough, dyspnea, orthopnea.
- Spinal cord compression: symptoms vary depending on the level of the lesion.
- Pleural and pericardial effusions: resulting in respiratory distress or cardiac tamponade.
- Infection: may be the primary mass (tuberculosis) or a complication of the mass (infected cyst, infected nodes).
- Horner syndrome: ptosis, miosis, and anhydrosis resulting from compression of the cervical sympathetic nerve trunk.
- Esophageal narrowing or erosion: may result in feeding difficulty or bleeding.

 Data Gathering

HISTORY

Question: Symptoms of respiratory distress: stridor cough, dyspnea, orthopnea, wheezing?
Significance: May indicate tracheal compression.

Question: Headache, syncope, dyspnea, orthopnea, anxiety, facial swelling, eye edema?
Significance: Seen in SVC syndrome.

Question: Systemic symptoms: fever, weight loss, night sweats, fatigue?
Significance: Associated with infection and malignancies.

 Physical Examination

Finding: Decreased breath sounds, wheezing, stridor
Significance: Mass may be impinging on trachea or bronchi.

Finding: Edema and cyanosis of face, neck, and upper extremities
Significance: Seen in SVC syndrome.

Finding: Venous distention (jugular and superficial chest veins)
Significance: Seen in SVC syndrome.

Finding: Conjunctival edema, retinal vessel engorgement
Significance: Seen in SVC syndrome.

Finding: Lymphadenopathy and/or hepatosplenomegaly
Significance: Suggests lymphoma/leukemia.

Finding: Generalized bruises, petechiae, mucosal bleeding
Significance: Suggests thrombocytopenia, which can be seen in leukemia.

Finding: Horner syndrome
Significance: Can be seen in neuroblastoma.

Laboratory Aids

Test: Chest x-ray (lateral film required)
Significance: Establish size and location of mass.

Test: CBC with differential
Significance: Anemia, thrombocytopenia, or leukocytosis frequently noted in leukemia or lymphoma syndromes.

Test: LDH, uric acid, electrolytes, BUN, Cr
Significance: Frequently abnormal in leukemia or lymphoma syndromes.

Test: Pulse oximetry
Significance: Helpful to assess tissue oxygenation.

Test: Computed tomography (CT) of the chest (if patient can tolerate recumbency)
Significance: Define size, location, and consistency of mass.

Test: Diagnostic:

- Lymph node aspiration/biopsy
- Bone marrow aspiration/biopsy
- PPD skin test for tuberculosis

Test: Diagnostic and therapeutic: pleurocentesis or pericardiocentesis, biopsy or excision of mass
Significance: Establish tissue diagnosis and relieve symptoms.

PROCEDURE

- Avoid supine position in suspected SVC syndrome.

Clinical Pearls

Do not treat a patient who has no history of asthma with steroids without a chest x-ray to confirm that there is no mediastinal mass.

General Therapy

Therapy will be based on the diagnosis and may include:

- Chemotherapy and/or radiation therapy for malignant tumors
- Surgical excision alone for benign tumors.
- Antibiotics for infectious processes

Emergency Care

If symptoms are progressing rapidly or there is evidence of SVC syndrome, tracheal compression, or spinal cord compression, steroids or radiation may be required.

Pitfalls

Circulatory collapse or respiratory failure can occur in children with SVC syndrome and/or tracheal compression. Avoid:

- General anesthesia: try to make the diagnosis with local or no anesthesia.
- Sedation: may cause irreversible respiratory depression.
- Supine position: keep head elevated to increase venous return.
- Placing intravenous line in the upper extremities due to poor venous return: try to use lower extremities.
- Long delays in establishing diagnosis: leukemia and lymphomas grow quickly and can rapidly impinge on vital structures.

Common Questions and Answers

Q: What should be done if the child is asymptomatic and mediastinal mass is an incidental finding on CXR?
A:

- Careful history and physical with specific attention to pulmonary, cardiac, and hematologic systems
- Vital signs to include temperature and pulse OX
- CBC, differential, ESR, tumor lysis labs
- PPD, anergy panel
- CT of chest
- Referral to oncologist, surgeon, or infectious disease specialist, pending above results

Q: When should an oncologist be consulted?
A: With any of the following:

- Rapidly enlarging mass
- Signs and symptoms of tracheal compression, SVC syndrome, or spinal cord compression
- Hepatosplenomegaly, lymphadenopathy, bruises, or petechiae on physical examination
- Anemia, thrombocytopenia, or leukocytosis suggesting bone marrow involvement
- Malignant histology is demonstrated with biopsy
- When help is needed in establishing the diagnosis

BIBLIOGRAPHY

Bower RJ, Kiesewetter WB. Mediastinal masses in infants and children. *Arch Surg* 1977;112: 1003–1009.

Buckley JA, et al. CT evaluation of mediastinal masses in children: spectrum of disease with pathologic correlation. *Clin Rev Diagn Imaging* 1998;39(5):365–392.

Hudson MM, Donaldson SS. Hodgkin's disease. *Pediatr Clin North Am* 1997;44:891–906.

Kelly KM, Lange B. Oncologic emergencies. *Pediatr Clin North Am* 1997;44:809–829.

Maity A, Goldweins JW, Lange BW, et al. Mediastinal masses in children with Hodgkin's disease. *Cancer* 1992;69(11):2755–2760.

Shad A, Magrath I. Non-Hodgkin's lymphoma. *Pediatr Clin North Am* 1997;44:863–890.

Shamberger RC, Holzman RS, Griscom NJ, et al. Prospective evaluation by computed tomography and pulmonary function tests of children with mediastinal masses. *Surgery* 1995;118(3):468–473.

Author: Leslie Raffini
Cynthia Norris, 2nd edition

Microcytic Anemia

 ## Database

DEFINITION

Inadequate hemoglobin synthesis leading to a decrease in hemoglobin concentration and red cell size. Caused by either iron deficiency or the inability to utilize iron. Hemoglobin (Hgb) and mean red cell volume (MCV) are below normal for age (see the table Hematologic Values in Children).

 ## Differential Diagnosis

METABOLIC

• Iron deficiency (most common)

ENVIRONMENTAL

• Chronic lead poisoning

CONGENITAL

• Thalassemia syndromes
• Selected congenital hemolytic anemias with unstable hemoglobin

INFLAMMATORY

• Recent or chronic inflammation or infection

MISCELLANEOUS

• Sideroblastic anemia (rare in children)

Approach to the Patient

Microcytic anemia in children is most commonly identified through routine screening and is usually the result of a chronic condition that does not require immediate intervention. Review of the child's history, red cell indices, and peripheral blood smear should guide further laboratory evaluation. General guidelines for evaluating a patient with microcytic anemia include:

• Initially identify severe anemia that requires inpatient observation and possible blood transfusion.
• Consider chronic lead intoxication early. If history is suspicious (e.g., peeling paint, pica, etc.), draw lead level to make diagnosis.
• Iron deficiency is the most common cause of microcytic anemia. Screen by history as described below. If history is suspicious, consider therapeutic iron trial prior to additional workup.
• If suspicious of thalassemia, send hemoglobin electrophoresis and complete blood counts from parents.

 ## Data Gathering

HISTORY

Question: What is the child's age?
Significance: Microcytic anemia in children age 9 months to 3 years and in adolescence is most commonly due to iron deficiency. Term infants are born with adequate iron stores for 6 months and therefore should not have nutritional iron deficiency causing anemia.

Question: What does the child's diet include?
Significance:

• Evaluate dietary iron intake as appropriate for age. Iron in breast milk is more bioavailable (50% vs. 10%) than iron in formula. However, infants who are exclusively breast-fed after 6 months are at an increased risk for iron deficiency if they do not receive supplements. Infant formulas and cereals should be iron-fortified. In preschool children and adolescents assess intake of high iron-containing foods including red meats, fish, poultry, beans, and peanut butter. Bran, vegetable fiber, and tannins found in tea can decrease iron absorption.
• Introduction of whole cow's milk before the age of 1 provides little dietary iron and can cause occult intestinal bleeding leading to iron loss. High intake of milk also causes a decreased appetite for other foods with a higher iron content.
• History of pica suggests iron deficiency and/or lead intoxication.

Question: Is there any history of blood loss?
Significance: Blood loss decreases iron stores. Ask about loss from stool, urine, chronic nosebleeds, and menorrhagia.

Question: Was the child born prematurely or was there a history of blood loss at birth?
Significance: Premature infants have lower total body iron stores and an increased growth rate that leads to increased iron requirements. Significant blood loss at birth can deplete iron stores.

Hematologic Values in Children

AGE	HEMOGLOBIN (G/DL)		HEMATOCRIT (%)		COUNT (10^{12}/L)		MCV (L)		MCH (PG)		MCHC (G/DL)	
	MEAN	−2 SD	MEAN	−2 SD	MEAN	−2 SD	MEAN	−2 SD	MEAN	−2 SD	MEAN	−2 SD
Birth (cord blood)	16.5	13.5	51	42	4.7	3.9	108	98	34	31	33	30
1 to 3 days (capillary)	18.5	14.5	56	45	5.3	4.0	108	95	34	31	33	29
1 week	17.5	13.5	54	42	5.1	3.9	107	88	34	28	33	28
~2 weeks	16.5	12.5	51	39	4.9	3.6	105	86	34	28	33	28
1 month	14.0	10.0	43	31	4.2	3.0	104	85	34	28	33	29
~2 months	11.5	9.0	35	28	3.8	2.7	96	77	30	26	33	29
~3 to 6 months	11.5	9.5	35	29	3.8	3.1	91	74	30	25	33	30
0.5 to 2 years	12.0	10.5	36	33	4.5	3.7	78	70	27	23	33	30
2 to 6 years	12.5	11.5	37	34	4.6	3.9	81	75	27	24	34	31
5 to 12 years	13.5	11.5	40	35	4.6	4.0	86	77	29	25	34	31
12 to 18 years												
Female	14.0	12.0	41	36	4.6	4.1	90	78	30	25	34	31
Male	14.5	13.0	43	37	4.9	4.5	88	78	30	25	34	31
18 to 49 years												
Female	14.0	12.0	41	36	4.6	4.0	90	80	30	26	34	31
Male	15.5	13.5	47	41	5.2	4.5	90	80	30	26	34	31

These data have been compiled from several sources. Emphasis is given to studies employing electronic counters and to the selection of populations that are likely to exclude individuals with iron deficiency. The mean ± 2 SD can be expected to include 95% of the observations in a normal population.

(From *Nathan and Oski's hematology of infancy and childhood*, 5th ed. Philadelphia: WB Saunders, 1998.)

Question: What is the child's ethnic background? Is there any familial history of anemia?
Significance: α-Thalassemia is most common among children of African or Asian descent. β-Thalassemia is most common in children of Asian or Mediterranean descent.

 ## Physical Examination

Finding: Child's general appearance
Significance: Most children with mild to moderate microcytic anemia are well appearing with a normal physical examination.

Finding: Irritability or pallor
Significance: Anemia is likely more severe than usual.

Finding: Cardiovascular examination
Significance: Check for instability including tachycardia, hypotension, and presence of a gallop. Flow murmurs are common with chronic anemia.

Finding: Abnormal sclerae
Significance: Blue sclera is associated with iron deficiency (very rare). Icterus is seen with severe thalassemia syndromes.

Finding: Mouth lesions
Significance: Glossitis and stomatitis are signs of iron deficiency.

Finding: Splenic enlargement
Significance: Splenic enlargement may be seen with thalassemia syndromes depending on the severity. The spleen is a site of extramedullary hematopoiesis and clears abnormal red cells.

 ## Laboratory Aids

PATIENT

Test: Complete blood count (CBC)
Significance: Low hemoglobin and low MCV.

Test: Red cell distribution width (RDW)
Significance: Measures the variation in red cell size. High in iron deficiency. Normal in thalassemia trait, infection, and lead poisoning.

Test: Ferritin
Significance: Serum ferritin reflects tissue iron stores. Low in iron deficiency. Acute phase reactant. Normal or increased in thalassemia and infection.

Test: Serum iron
Significance: Low in iron deficiency. Normal in thalassemia (unless chronically transfused). Normal or increased in infection or inflammatory states.

Test: Transferrin
Significance: Transferrin measures the total iron binding capacity. Increased in iron deficiency. Normal in thalassemia. Normal or increased in infection or inflammatory states.

Test: Transferrin saturation
Significance: Transferrin saturation measures the iron available for hemoglobin synthesis. Low in iron deficiency and chronic infection. Normal in thalassemia.

Test: Lead level
Significance: Increase in lead intoxication.

Test: Hemoglobin electrophoresis
Significance: Increased hemoglobin A2 in β-thalassemia trait. Normal in α-thalassemia trait and other microcytic anemias.

Test: Peripheral blood smear
Significance: Microcytosis and hypochromia. Marked poikilocytosis and anisocytosis with iron deficiency and thalassemia syndromes. Basophilic stippling with lead poisoning.

Test: Bone marrow aspirate
Significance: Bone marrow aspirate is rarely needed to establish diagnosis. Can assess iron stores by hemosiderin staining. In sideroblastic anemias, greater than 10% of the nucleated red cell precursors are ringed sideroblasts.

FAMILY STUDIES

- **Test:** CBC
- **Test:** Peripheral blood smear.
- **Test:** Hemoglobin electrophoresis

 ## Therapy

- Consider therapeutic trial of iron supplementation if history is suspicious.
- May require initial inpatient observation in cases of severe anemia.
- Red cell transfusion only if evidence of cardiovascular compromise (rarely indicated).
- Removal of environmental exposure and possible chelation for lead poisoning to prevent central nervous system toxicity.

 ## Follow-Up

In iron deficiency, the reticulocyte count should double in 1–2 weeks and the hemoglobin concentration should be increased at least 1.0 g/dL in 2–4 weeks following iron supplementation.
Children with thalassemia trait have a persistent mild, microcytic anemia that is not clinically significant, but require genetic counseling as they become older. Refer children with other thalassemia syndromes to a hematologist.

Pitfalls

Lead poisoning and iron deficiency can occur concurrently because iron deficiency causes increased lead absorption. If history is concerning for increased lead exposure in cases of documented iron deficiency, send lead levels.

 ## Common Questions and Answers

Q: What is a therapeutic iron trial and when is it indicated?
A: A therapeutic iron trial is a trial of oral iron therapy without additional laboratory testing in a patient with a microcytic anemia and a history of dietary deficiency or known history of blood loss. An increase in the hemoglobin concentration of 1 g/dL or greater after 2–4 weeks of therapy confirms the diagnosis of iron deficiency. If the hemoglobin does not increase, additional laboratory testing is necessary and other diagnoses should be considered.

Q: How does infection affect the diagnosis of anemia?
A: Common childhood infections can be associated with a mild microcytic anemia. Acute infection also affects some of the laboratory tests used to diagnose the cause of microcytic anemia. With infection there is a shift of iron from serum to storage sites causing a decrease in serum iron and an increase in ferritin and there is an increase in the FEP level. It is, therefore, preferable to evaluate a microcytic anemia 3–4 weeks after an infection resolves.

BIBLIOGRAPHY

Grantham-McGregor S, Ani C. A review of studies on the effect of iron deficiency on cognitive development in children. *J Nutr* 2001;131(2S-2):649S–666S; discussion 666S–668S.

Hoffbrand AV, Herbert V. Nutritional anemias. *Semin Hematol* 1999;36(4 suppl 7):13–23.

Nathan DG, Orkin SH, eds. *Nathan and Oski's hematology of infancy and childhood,* 5th ed. Philadelphia: WB Saunders, 1998.

Pappas DE. Iron deficiency anemia. *Pediatr Rev* 1998;19:321–322.

Segel GB. Anemia. *Pediatr Rev* 1988;10:77–88.

Walters MC, Abelson HT. Interpretation of the complete blood count. *Pediatr Clin North Am* 1996;43:599–622.

Author: Suzanne Shusterman

Pallor

 Database

DEFINITION

Pallor is defined as paleness of the skin and may be related either to reduced hemoglobin and/or decreased blood flow to the skin.

 Differential Diagnosis

CONGENITAL

• Diamond-Blackfan anemia

—Congenital pure red-cell aplasia (rare)

• Fanconi anemia

—Constellation of varied cytopenias
—Multiple congenital anomalies
—Abnormal bone marrow chromosomal fragility

• Thalassemia syndromes

—Defective globin synthesis

• Erythrocyte membrane defects

—Hereditary spherocytosis
—Elliptocytosis
—Stomatocytosis
—Pyropoikilocytosis
—Infantile pyknocytosis

• Erythrocyte enzyme defects

—Glucose-6-phosphate dehydrogenase (G-6-PD) deficiency
—Pyruvate kinase deficiency

• Hemoglobinopathies

—Sickle cell syndromes
—Other unstable hemoglobins

INFECTIOUS

• Septic shock
• Infection-related bone marrow suppression

—Parvovirus B19 infection

• Infection-related hemolytic anemias

—Epstein-Barr virus
—Influenza
—Coxsackievirus
—Varicella
—Cytomegalovirus
— *Escherichia coli*
— Pneumococcus
— Streptococcus
— Salmonella typhi
— Mycoplasma

TOXIC/ENVIRONMENTAL/DRUGS

• Iron-deficiency anemia

—Common cause of anemia in children, especially under the age of 3 years and in female adolescents

• Atropine ingestion
• Plumbism

—Anemia usually due to coexisting iron deficiency. Very high lead levels associated with altered heme synthesis

• Vitamin B_{12} and/or folate deficiency

—Results in a megaloblastic anemia

• Medication-induced bone marrow suppression

—Many chemotherapeutic agents for malignancy, antibiotics, especially trimethoprim-sulfamethoxazole

• Drug-related hemolytic anemia

—Antibiotics
—Antiepileptics
—Nonsteroidal antiinflammatory drugs
— Azathioprine
— Isoniazid

TRAUMA

• Acute blood loss

—Chronic blood loss often presents as iron deficiency

TUMOR

• Malignancies include leukemia, a primary bone marrow malignancy as well as any malignancy that metastasizes to the bone marrow, displacing normal marrow cells
• Histiocytosis syndromes

—Disseminated forms, marrow replacement

• Anemia of cancer even without bone marrow invasion

GENETIC/METABOLIC

• Metabolic derangements

—Severe electrolyte disturbance
—pH disturbance
—Inborn errors

• Shwachman-Diamond syndrome

—Marrow hypoplasia with associated pancreatic insufficiency and associated failure to thrive

• Systemic diseases

—Anemia of chronic disease
—Chronic renal disease
—Uremia

• Hypothyroidism

ALLERGIC/INFLAMMATORY

• Anaphylaxis
• Disseminated intravascular coagulation

OTHER

• Transient erythroblastopenia of childhood

—Acquired pure red blood cell aplasia

• Aplastic anemia

—Bone marrow failure syndrome with at least 2 of the 3 blood cell lines eventually affected

• Sideroblastic anemia

—Defective iron utilization within the developing erythrocytes

• Autoimmune and isoimmune hemolytic anemias
• Microangiopathic hemolytic anemias

—Thrombotic thrombocytopenic purpura (TTP)
—Hemolytic uremic syndrome (HUS)
—Disseminated intravascular coagulation (DIC)

• Mechanical destruction

—Vascular malformation
—Shunts
—Abnormal valves
—Prosthetic valves

Approach to the Patient

Determine first that the child appears pale, not simply fair-skinned. Decide if there is a medical emergency associated with circulatory failure. If not, the goal is to investigate the etiology and then intervene appropriately.

Phase 1: Quickly assess for signs of shock, indicating circulatory as opposed to hematologic etiology for pallor. If circulatory, initiate emergency procedures as required to support basic vital functions, such as airway, breathing, and circulation.

Phase 2: If patient is stable, perform history, physical examination, and CBC with reticulocyte count to establish time of onset of pallor and associated symptoms, and level of anemia.

Phase 3: Specific diagnostic workup based on findings in phase 2.

 Data Gathering

HISTORY

Question: Rapid onset? (Hours to few days)
Significance: Suggests acute blood loss, autoimmune hemolytic anemia, and/or circulatory compromise.

Question: Weight loss, fever, night sweats, cough, and/or bone pain?
Significance: Suggest an underlying systemic illness, such as leukemia, infection, collagen vascular disease.

Question: Jaundice, dark urine?
Significance: Suggests hemolysis

Question: Age between 6 months and 3 years, or adolescent females?
Significance: Peak age ranges for iron deficiency.

Question: Age less than 6 months?
Significance: May represent a congenital anemia or isoimmunization.

Question: Male?
Significance: Some red-cell enzyme X-linked defects, such as G-6-PD and phosphoglycerate kinase deficiencies are sex linked.

Question: African-American?
Significance: Hemoglobins S and C, α- and β-thalassemia trait, G-6-PD deficiency.

Question: Southeast Asian?
Significance: Hemoglobin E and α-thalassemia

Question: Mediterranean descent?
Significance: β-Thalassemia and G-6-PD deficiency

Question: Premature infant?
Significance: Increased risk of both iron and vitamin E deficiency. Exaggerated hyperbilirubinemia can be the presenting symptom of isoimmune hemolytic or other congenital hemolytic anemia.

Question: Pica?
Significance: Pica is often associated with both plumbism and iron and vitamin deficiency.

Question: Medications?
Significance: Can cause bone marrow suppression and/or hemolysis.

Question: Recent trauma and/or surgery?
Significance: Blood loss can result in iron deficiency.

Question: Recent infection?
Significance: Can be associated with hemolysis or bone marrow suppression.

Question: Familial history?
Significance: Some of the congenital hemolytic anemias are autosomal dominant. Familial history of splenectomy and/or early cholecystectomy can be a clue for a previously undiagnosed hemolytic anemia.

Physical Examination

Finding: Rapid respiratory rate, decreased blood pressure, weak pulses, slow capillary refill
Significance: Vital signs indicate pallor due to acute severe blood loss, shock, or other emergencies.

Finding: Frontal bossing and prominence of the malar and maxillary bones
Significance: Thalassemia, due to extramedullary erythropoiesis

Finding: Icterus of sclerae and mucous membranes
Significance: May indicate hemolysis

Finding: Systolic flow murmur
Significance: Chronic anemia

Finding: Bruits
Significance: May indicate vascular malformations

Finding: Enlarged spleen
Significance: Hemolytic anemias, malignancy, infection

Finding: Petechiae and bruising
Significance: May indicate an associated thrombocytopenia, coagulopathy, or vasculitis

Finding: Dysmorphic features
Significance: Both Diamond-Blackfan and Fanconi anemias are associated with other congenital defects, including thumb abnormalities, short stature, congenital heart disease.

Laboratory Aids

Test: Hemoglobin or hematocrit
Significance: Establishes the presence of anemia as the etiology for pallor

Test: Mean corpuscular volume (MCV)
Significance: Divides anemias into microcytic, normocytic, and macrocytic.

Test: Reticulocyte count
Significance: Distinguishes between decreased production and increased destruction of red cells.

Test: Coombs test and antibody screen
Significance: Identifies immune-mediated red-cell destruction.

Test: Peripheral blood smear
Significance: Specific morphologic findings can be diagnostic.

Test: Iron studies: iron-binding capacity, serum Fe, ferritin, transferrin
Significance: Diagnosis of iron deficiency anemia or anemia of chronic disease

Test: Hgb electrophoresis, quantitative Hgb A_2 or F
Significance: Diagnosis of hemoglobinopathy

Test: Lead studies: serum lead, free erythrocyte protoporphyrin
Significance: Diagnosis of plumbism

Test: Osmotic fragility
Significance: Diagnosis of red cell membrane defects

Test: Quantitative red-cell enzyme assays
Significance: Diagnosis of inherited RBC enzyme deficiencies

Test: Serum folate, RBC folate, and serum vitamin B_{12} levels
Significance: Diagnosis of deficiency of these vitamins

Test: Bone marrow aspiration and biopsy
Significance: Diagnosis of malignancy or bone marrow failure syndrome

Issues for Referral

- Hemodynamic compromise
- Severe anemia
- Anemias other than dietary iron deficiency or anemia of chronic disease
- All bone marrow failure or infiltrative processes

Tests to prepare for consult

- Complete blood count, reticulocyte count, past blood counts if available

Emergency Care

- If there is circulatory failure without anemia, treatment requires intensive monitoring and access to critical care in an emergency room or ICU. Fluid resuscitation and/or inotropic pressor support as needed.
- Acute blood loss: treat circulatory failure as described. Transfuse with packed red blood cells, platelets, and fresh frozen plasma as needed.
- Severe anemia of unclear etiology with hemodynamic instability: transfuse with packed red blood cells cautiously. In an autoimmune hemolytic process, the child is at significant risk of a hemolytic transfusion reaction. Obtain blood for diagnostic studies before transfusion.

Clinical Pearls

- Parents often fail to notice pallor of gradual onset. Grandparents or others who see child less often may be the first to suspect pallor.
- Hematologic pallor: Often well-appearing pale child with anemia. Pallor is clinically apparent when the hemoglobin is less than 9 g/dL.
- Nonhematologic pallor: Generally ill-appearing child. Any condition with peripheral vasoconstriction that alters the distribution of blood flow away from the skin surface.

BIBLIOGRAPHY

Glader BE. Hemolytic anemia in children *Clin Lab Med* 1999;19(1):87–111.

Graham EA. The changing face of anemia in infancy. *Pediatr Rev* 1995;15:175–183.

Monzon CM, Beaver D, Dillon TD. Evaluation of erythrocyte disorders with mean corpuscular volume (MCV) and red cell distribution width (RDW). *Clin Pediatr* 1987;26:632–638.

Segal GB. Anemia. *Pediatr Rev* 1988;10:77–98.

Sills RH. Indications for bone marrow examination. *Pediatr Rev* 1995;16:226–228.

Author: Debra L. Friedman

Proteinuria

 Database

DEFINITION
Presence of protein in urine. Usually greater than 0.3 g of protein in a 24-hour collection and/or 1 g/L (1+ or greater) on two random urine samples at least 6 hours apart on a midstream urine.

 Differential Diagnosis

CONGENITAL
- Congenital nephrotic syndrome
- Faconi syndrome
- Congenital syphilis
- Cystinosis

INFECTIOUS
- Viral
—Hepatitis B, Epstein-Barr virus, cytomegalovirus, HIV
- Bacterial
—Acute poststreptococcal glomerulonephritis
—Subacute bacterial endocarditis
—Urinary tract infections
- Parasitic
—Malaria
—Schistosomiasis

TOXIC, ENVIRONMENTAL, DRUGS
- Allergens
—Pollens, inhalants
- Venoms
—Bees and snakes
- Immunizations
- Heavy metals
- Heroin
- Medicines
—Captopril
—Penicillamine, nonsteroidal antiinflammatory drugs, aminoglycosides

INFLAMMATORY
Renal
Glomerular Disease
- Minimal change nephrotic syndrome
- Hereditary nephritis
- Membranoproliferative glomerulonephritis
- Membranous glomerulonephritis
- Mesangial proliferative glomerulonephritis
- Focal segmental glomerulosclerosis
- Henoch-Schönlein syndrome
- IGA nephropathy
- Systemic lupus erythematosus nephritis
- Systemic vasculitides
- Shunt nephritis
- Subacute bacterial endocarditis

METABOLIC
- Hypokalemic nephropathy
- Diabetic nephropathy
- Hypothyroidism

TUMOR
- Wilms tumor
- Carcinomas
- Lymphoma
- Leukemia

ISOLATED PROTEINURIA
- Orthostatic proteinuria
- Persistent asymptomatic proteinuria

HEMATOLOGY
- Sickle cell disease
- Renal vein thrombosis
- Hemolytic uremic syndrome (HUS)

MISCELLANEOUS
- Orthostatic proteinuria
- Strenuous exercise
- Fever
- Emotional stress
- Cold exposure
- Congestive heart failure
- Seizure

Tubulointerstitial Disease
- Ischemic tubular injury
- Reflux nephropathy
- Interstitial nephritis

Approach to the Patient

GENERAL GOAL
Determine the etiology of the proteinuria and determine what therapy there is to possibly treat the problem.

Phase 1: In most healthy patients proteinuria is a isolated finding that is usually benign; it is important based on the history, physical examination, and laboratory test to determine the severity of the proteinuria in order to determine which can safely be evaluated without referral.

Phase 2: If the finding is severe (e.g., in the nephrotic range proteinuria) it must be decided what should be done for the patient acutely to stabilize, and then whether or not to transfer to nephrologist care for additional evaluation.

Phase 3: If the patient is clinically stable, it is up to the primary care physician to do screening tests to help additionally delineate the etiology of the proteinuria. Phone consultation with a pediatric nephrologist may be helpful in this task of initial labs.

Phase 4: Inquire about other medical problems of the patient.

 Data Gathering

HISTORY
Question: Is there a preexisting history of renal disease?
Significance: In cases of proteinuria a prior history of renal disease will allow the physician to take a more aggressive approach to the patient. Even a history of nephritis can be an important finding in the evaluation.

Question: Is there a history of abnormal screening urinalyses?
Significance: It is common for primary care physicians to use a colorimetric urine dipstick at well-child checkups. In the case of proteinuria (1+ or greater), it is important to see if there is a previous history of protein in the urine.

Question: Is there a history of previous or multiple urinary tract infections?
Significance: Urinary tract infection can be associated with other renal/urinary tract problems, such as vesicoureteral reflux, which leads to damage of the kidneys and thus proteinuria.

Question: Is there history of a preceding illness?
Significance: Occasionally, a disease can precede the onset of nephrosis.

Question: Familial history of renal disease, metabolic disease, or mental retardation?
Significance: Some renal diseases are inherited or associated with genetic diseases, which cause mental retardation.

Question: Recent heavy exercise?
Significance: Strenuous exercise can cause a transient proteinuria trace to 1+ on urine dipstick. Follow-up urinalysis without exercise in previous 24 hours or test for orthostatic proteinuria should be done.

Question: Does the child have an unremarkable previous medical history?
Significance: A majority of children will have no significant past medical history for renal disease. Based on data a small percentage of patients will have persistent proteinuria on follow-up testing.

 Physical Examination

Finding: Hypertension
Significance: Hypertension greater than the 95 percentile for gender and age is important to evaluate for renal disease. Proteinuria and hypertension should quickly alert the primary care physician to focus on a renal etiology.

Finding: Edema (usually dependent and pitting)
Significance: In severe proteinuria, edema may be present in the patient. Edema is the result of third spacing of fluid into the interstitial tissues. In general, the appearance of edema can have intravascular hypovolemic dehydration. Potassium sparing diuretics are usually chosen in hypoproteinemic edema. Loop and thiazide diuretics can exacerbate a patient in the intravascular hypovolemic state (*see* Nephrotic Syndrome).

Finding: Ascites/pleural effusion
Significance: The spacing of fluid usually results of fluid in the peritoneal cavity (ascites). The fluid may move into the pleural cavity from the abdominal cavity. This fluid is at risk for secondary infection.

Finding: Shifting dullness in abdomen
Significance: As the patient is rolled from side to side, percussion of the abdomen will show dullness following the shifting of the ascitic fluid.

Finding: Purpura
Significance: Henoch-Schönlein purpura (HSP) can be a reason for renal disease. Purpura is usually on the buttocks, lower extremities, and dependent areas.

Finding: Suprapubic and costovertebral tenderness
Significance: Urinary tract infections or pyelonephritis can be a cause of isolated proteinuria. White blood cells, nitrites, and blood are also present with infection.

 Laboratory Aids

Test: Urine colorimetric dipstick
Significance: A quick and reliable method to evaluate proteinuria; 1+ or greater should lead a physician to evaluate a patient for etiology of the finding. This test also allows a family member to follow proteinuria at home and notify the physician of changes in a patient's physiology. If follow-up urines are 100% positive (1+ or greater), the physician should conduct a test 24-hour collection and then consider referral to a nephrologist. See table Relationship Between Urine Protein and Dipstick Results.

Test: 24-Hour collection of urine
Significance: After the collection, an analysis of total protein, creatinine, and electrolytes can be studied. In the evaluation of orthostatic proteinuria, the 24-hour collection can be split into standing and recumbent collections. In this case, the overnight

Relationship Between Urine Protein and Dipstick Results

GRADE	PROTEIN MEASUREMENTS (MG/DL)
Trace	10–20
1+	30
2+	100
3+	300
4+	1000–2000

24-Hour Urine Collection Values

Normal values: <4 mg/m^2/hr
Abnormal: 4–40/m^2/hr
Nephrotic range: >40 mg/m^2/hour

recumbent sample should be less than 100 mg and the rest of the collection should have protein. However, the standing protein can be 2 to 3 times the level of the recumbent. Normal result is less than 4 mg/m^2 per hour. A pediatric phone consult may necessary to help with the workup. If the results are greater than 2 g, *see* Nephrotic Syndrome. See table 24-Hour Urine Collection Values.

Test: Metabolic serum chemistry including blood urea nitrogen (BUN), creatinine, total protein, albumin, and cholesterol
Significance: Renal failure can be identified with a rise in BUN and creatinine as well as hyperkalemia. Hypoproteinemia, hypoalbuminemia, and hypercholesteremia are seen in nephrotic syndrome (*see* Nephrotic Syndrome).

Test: Urine culture
Significance: In a majority of cases of urinary tract infection, proteinuria can be present. Appropriate antibiotic therapy can treat the infection and in most cases the proteinuria will discontinue. Follow-up urinalysis as well as additional tests should be done if the proteinuria persists.

Test: Additional renal/immunology tests
Significance: Not all the tests are need to evaluate proteinuria, every patient history and physical examination will help determine which tests are needed. They may include an ASO titer, creatinine clearance, urine sediment evaluation by urinalysis, C3, and/or CTXT0 complement level, circulating immune complexes, antinuclear antibody (ANA), hepatitis B surface antigen.

 Common Questions and Answers

Q: Is proteinuria serious?
A: In most cases proteinuria is a benign condition usually related to strenuous exercise, orthostatic proteinuria. Most children will need serial physical examinations as well as checking the urine.

Q: Are most forms of proteinuria treatable?
A: In the case of orthostatic and transient proteinuria require no treatment. In some cases, autoimmune may be treated with immunosuppressives. Minimal change nephrotic syndrome can be treated (*see* Nephrotic Syndrome).

Issues for Referral
• The patient who has unstable vital signs or appears to be septic may need referral. Children with ascites are at risk of peritonitis and can develop complications from spreading of the bacteria. Correction of blood pressure should be done after close evaluation of fluid intravascular status. Children can have total body fluid overload and have decreased intracellular fluid. In these cases aggressive diuretic therapy can worsen the patient's condition.

• Children with signs of kidney failure, electrolyte abnormalities, nonorthostatic persistent proteinuria, hematuria, hypertension, edema, and or purpura/vasculitis.
• The child with positive familial history of severe renal disease and has developed similar symptoms. Renal biopsy may be needed to be performed by a nephrologist.
• Orthostatic, transient, persistent asymptomatic proteinurias are all diseases that should be followed with serial urine dipstick analysis and blood pressure measurement. Persistent asymptomatic proteinuria should be followed but many patients will persist without any additional progression.

Clinical Pearls
• In the routine screening of urine colorimetric dipsticks, first morning urine is preferable. Because orthostatic proteinuria's outlook is common, this is the first test that should be done.
• False-positive proteinuria exists and the usual causes can result from alkaline urine (pH >8), overlong emersions in urine, placing in the direct stream of urine, or pyuria; false negatives can exist also in cases when the urine is too dilute or a different protein is being excreted other than albumin.
• The urine dipstick should be read within 1 minute. After that, the color will become darker and give a false-positive test.
• Trace protein is normal.

BIBLIOGRAPHY
Ettenger RB. The evaluation of the child with proteinuria. *Pediatr Ann* 1994;(23)1:486–494.

Hodson EM, Knight JF, Willis NS, et al. Corticosteroid therapy for nephrotic syndrome in children. *Cochrane Database of Systematic Reviews* [computer file] 2000;4:CD001533.

Hogg RJ, Portman RJ, Milliner D, et al. Evaluation and management of proteinuria and nephrotic syndrome in children: recommendations from a pediatric nephrology panel established at the National Kidney Foundation conference on proteinuria, albuminuria, risk, assessment, detection, and elimination *Pediatrics* 2000;105(6): 1242–1249.

Norman ME. An office approach to hematuria and proteinuria. *Pediatr Clin North Am* 1987;34(30):545–560.

Author: Charles I. Schwartz

Pruritus

Database

DEFINITION
Itching, an unpleasant cutaneous sensation that provokes the desire to rub or scratch the skin to obtain relief.

Differential Diagnosis

CONGENITAL/ANATOMIC
- Cholestasis secondary to biliary obstruction

INFECTIOUS
- Pinworm (*Enterobius vermicularis*)
- Swimmer's itch: due to fresh water mammalian or avian schistosomes
- Herpes viruses: primary varicella infection or zoster, Herpes simplex
- *Borrelia burgdorferi*: erythema chronicum migrans lesion of Lyme disease
- Tinea
- *Toxocara canis*

TOXIC
- Contact dermatitis
- —Allergens
- —Plants (Rhus dermatitis—poison ivy/oak)
- —Cosmetics
- —Dyes
- —Medications
- —Irritants
- —Soaps
- —Detergents and other chemicals
- —Excrement
- —Wool
- —Fiberglass

ENVIRONMENTAL
- Papular urticaria: bites of fleas, mosquitoes
- Pediculosis (lice)
- Mites: scabies (*Sarcoptes scabei*), chiggers (*Enterobicula alfreddugesi*), etc.
- Subcutaneous foreign body
- Phytophotodermatitis occurs when skin is exposed to sunlight after contact with an offending plant

DRUGS
- Systemic use of medications such as aminophylline, aspirin, barbiturates, erythromycin, gold, griseofulvin, iodine contrast dyes, isoniazid, opiates, phenothiazines, vitamin A

ALLERGIC, INFLAMMATORY
- Atopic dermatitis (eczema)
- Psoriasis
- Seborrheic dermatitis

MISCELLANEOUS
- Nonspecific urticaria
- Pityriasis rosea
- Asteatotic eczema—"winter itch"
- Xerosis (dry skin)—from excess bathing with or without strong detergents or low humidity, idiopathic

Approach to the Patient

GENERAL GOALS
Determine severity and if pruritus is isolated or due to an underlying systemic illness primarily by assessing the presence or absence of associated signs and symptoms, especially rash.

Phase 1: Assess the severity of illness. Pruritus will rarely be an element of a medical emergency except in cases of anaphylaxis or erythema multiforme-major.

Phase 2: Determine if the itch is isolated or if there are any associated signs or symptoms. Pruritus is most frequently associated with rash. Pruritus with or without rash may be a manifestation of systemic illness.

Phase 3: A thorough history and examination should narrow the differential diagnosis considerably, enabling the clinician to determine the underlying cause of the complaint in the majority of causes. Laboratory tests may be indicated in cases where the diagnosis is unclear.

HINTS FOR SCREENING PROBLEM
One may want to ask if this is a new or recurrent problem. If it is new, one should ask if there is anything new in the child's life that may be associated with the onset of the pruritus (with or without rash). This is often the most revealing question, as one may find that the child recently came in contact with a new item, which is known to be a contact irritant (see table below).

Data Gathering

HISTORY
Question: How severe is the pruritus? On a scale of 1 to 10? Compared to a mosquito bite? Is it severe enough to interfere with the daily routine of the child (e.g., wakes the child from sleep)?
Significance: Waking from sleep may point to a more severe form resulting from systemic disease.

Question: Has anything new or different been introduced to the child, especially anything that comes in contact with his/her skin?
Significance: See table Potential Contact Irritants.

Question: How often is the child bathed and with what?

Significance: Different soaps or detergents contain additives that may be allergenic. Changes in soaps may be important. Some soaps cause excessive dryness or have heavy fragrances. Children who are bathed frequently with anything more than water may develop dry and irritated (pruritic) skin.

Question: Has the child been hiking or camping in a wooded area?
Significance: May be a clue to common skin irritation such as rhus dermatitis from poison ivy.

Question: Are there any underlying illness(es) or associated symptoms?
Significance: For example, pruritus associated with night sweats and fever may point to hematopoietic malignancy. There is a long list of illnesses that are associated with pruritus (see table Causes of Pruritus in Children).

Question: Is anyone who comes in frequent contact with the child also itching?
Significance: This may identify a common source of a contact irritant. Scabies or lice.

Question: Accompanied by rash or other signs and symptoms?
Significance: Elicits additional signs and symptoms of any of the systemic diseases listed in the table. For instance, arthritis and arthralgias in SLE or JRA, jaundice in the cholestatic disorders.

Physical Examination

Finding: If rash is present, what is the appearance?
Significance:
- Lesions appear in crops with varicella zoster, scabies, insect bites.
- Lesions are in groups of 3 or 4 with a central punctum in scabies.
- Papular lesions occur with insect bites, chiggers, pediculosis, contact dermatitis, pityriasis rosea, urticaria (wheal), and atopic dermatitis.
- Lichenification (plaque and scale formation) occur with psoriasis, xerosis, tinea, atopic dermatitis.
- Serpiginous lesions occur with cutaneous larva migrans and myiasis (or maggots).
- Vesicular lesions occur with varicella (generalized), scabies, poison ivy (linear), and atopic dermatitis.
- Dry skin (xerosis) occurs with atopic dermatitis.

Potential Contact Irritants

Shoes	Clothing	Diapers	Cosmetics
Dyes (for hair, etc.)	Detergents	Excrement	Plants (e.g., cacti)
Jewelry (nickel)	Systemic medications	Topical medications	Foods
Wool	Fiberglass	Animals	Capsaicin in hot peppers[a]

[a]Acts as an irritant when first applied but actually decreases pruritus if applied repeatedly over weeks

- Christmas tree pattern occurs with pityriasis rosea.

Finding: What is the location of the itch and/or rash?
Significance:
- Generalized distribution occurs with varicella.
- Anus: consider pinworms.
- Back: consider pityriasis rosea.
- Axillae and/or genital/diaper area: consider seborrheic dermatitis and scabies.
- Dorsal foot: consider shoe dermatitis from rubber or tanning agents.
- Exposed surfaces: consider swimmer's itch and poison ivy.
- Finger, ear lobe, wrist, or necklace distribution: consider irritant contact dermatitis (e.g., nickel).
- Nipples: consider scabies (burrows).
- Interdigital areas and ulnar borders: consider tinea pedis, scabies (burrows).
- Palms and/or soles: consider biliary cirrhosis.
- Plantar foot: consider cutaneous larva migrans.
- Scalp: consider pediculosis (nits found cemented to hair shaft) and tinea capitis.

Finding: Abnormal affect or mood?
Significance: One must consider whether the complaint is psychosomatic or due to neurotic excoriation, especially in cases of abnormal affect or mood.

 Laboratory Aids

Test: Complete blood count including differential

Significance: Presence of eosinophilia suggests atopy or parasitic infections.

Test: Wood light examination, KOH preparation
Significance: Screen for tinea infections.

Test: Skin scraping in oil under cover slip
Significance: Mites in scabies.

Test: Perianal adhesive tape slide (preferably early morning)
Significance: Verify pinworm.

Test: Serum for hepatic and renal function
Significance: Screen for underlying disease.

Test: Urine β-HCG
Significance: Cholestasis associated with pregnancy.

Test: Skin biopsy
Significance: Usually not of value since histologic changes are due to scratching.

Issues for Referral
- Identification of an underlying state, such as neoplasia, pregnancy, or hepatic, renal, or psychiatric disease.
- Some severe cases of atopic dermatitis or psoriasis (may require dermatologic referral).
- Identification of pubic pediculosis (may require investigation into abuse).

 Emergency Care

- Pruritus due to anaphylaxis will require initial management of airway, breathing, and circulation (ABCs) followed by sympathomimetics (such as epinephrine), antihistamines (such as diphenhydramine), corticosteroids, and possibly fluid resuscitation.

Clinical Pearls
- Pruritus that is worse at night is seen with scabies or pinworm.
- If the child was recently swimming in fresh water, one should consider swimmer's itch, caused by fresh water mammalian or avian schistosomes.

 Common Questions and Answers

Q: Does the time course of a pruritic rash give any clue in identifying the offending agent?
A: Yes, certain plants will cause an immediate welt on the skin but the urticaria will be short-lived (immediate contact dermatitis). Skin that is traumatized mechanically (e.g., cactus spine) or chemically (e.g., capsaicin in hot peppers) produces more persistent skin reactions.

Q: Are some antihistamines better than others for pruritus?
A: Possibly. There is conflicting evidence but several studies have shown that older systemic antihistamines that cause more somnolence are actually more effective at alleviating pruritus than newer, longer-acting antihistamines (e.g., astemizole, loratadine, terfenadine, cetirizine).

Q: Is there any symptomatic treatment for pruritus other than antihistamines?
A: Yes, systemic and topical corticosteroids and topical pramoxine and doxepin have been shown to be effective in placebo-controlled trials.

Q: Do topical antihistamines alleviate pruritus?
A: Not usually, except for pruritus seen with insect bites and urticaria.

Q: Does scratching make the pruritus better or worse?
A: Worse, scratching leads to the release of the mediators of inflammation including histamine that in turn leads to more pruritus, thus creating a vicious cycle.

Q: Are there any useful adjuncts to reduce pruritus?
A: Yes, keeping skin moist with moisturizers and avoiding dry environments. Avoid overwashing especially with hot water and/or alkaline soaps.

BIBLIOGRAPHY

Greaves MW. Anti-itch treatments: do they work? *Skin Pharmacol* 1997;10:225–229.

Greaves MW, Wall PD. Pathophysiology of itching. *Lancet* 1996;348:938–940.

Millikan LE. Pruritus: unapproved treatments or indications. *Clin Dermatol* 2000;18:149–152.

Rees JL. Laidlaw A. Pruritus: more scratch than itch. *Clin Exp Dermatol* 1999 24:490–493.

Wahlgren CF. Itch and atopic dermatitis: an overview. *J Dermatol* 1999;26:770–779.

Author: Mark L. Bagarazzi

Causes of Pruritus in Children

MOST COMMON	LESS COMMON	RARE
Atopic dermatitis (eczema)	Anaphylaxis	*Collagen—vascular disorders:*
Contact dermatitis	*Cholestasis:* Drug-induced	JRA, systemic lupus
Allergens: plants (poison ivy), cosmetics, dyes, medications	(e.g., total parenteral nutrition, estrogens,	erythematosus, Sjögren syndrome, dermatomyositis
Irritants: soaps, detergents and other chemicals, excrement, wool, fiberglass	phenothiazine, allopurinol), extrahepatic biliary obstruction, biliary cirrhosis	Congenital ectodermal disorders
Cutaneous infections:	*Cutaneous infections:*	*Systemic infections:* HIV/AIDS, parvovirus B19, giardiasis, ascariasis
Varicella-zoster virus (chicken pox), tinea infections, Pinworm	Cutaneous larva migrans— "creeping eruption," hookworm, cercariasis	*Endocrinological disorders:* diabetes mellitus,
Papular urticaria—bites of fleas, mosquitoes, etc.	(onchocercaria volvulus), trichinosis	hyper/hypothyroidism, hypoparathyroidism
Pediculosis (lice)	Myiasis (maggots)	*Neurologic syndromes:*
Mites—scabies (*Sarcoptes scabei*), chiggers (*Enterobicula alfreddugesi*), etc.	Neurotic excoriation Chronic renal failure—with or without "uremic frost"	cerebral abscess or tumor, multiple sclerosis Erythropoietic protoporphyria
Seborrheic dermatitis	*Hematopoietic neoplasms:*	Psychosomatic disorders
Xerosis (dry skin) Excess bathing, strong detergents, low humidity	Hodgkin disease, lymphoma, leukemia Iron deficiency anemia	Hematopoietic neoplasms Polycythemia vera Mastocytosis
Nonspecific urticaria		Paraneoplastic syndromes secondary to solid organ neoplasms

Short Stature

Database

DEFINITION

Short stature is defined as height below the 3rd percentile, but many pediatricians use the 5th percentile as the cutoff.

- Growth failure refers to downward crossing of the height percentile over the normal curves and eventually leads to short stature. With evidence of growth failure, diagnostic evaluation is required, even if short stature is not yet present.
- Failure to thrive refers to infants and children who fail to gain weight and often lose weight. They may or may not be short and are underweight for height.

Differential Diagnosis

EXTREMES OF NORMAL GROWTH

- Familial short stature

—Short parent(s)
—Normal height velocity
—Normal age of onset of puberty
—Normal bone age
—Short stature throughout childhood
—Final adult height close to the mid-parental height and around the 3rd or 5th percentile

- Constitutional short stature/delay of growth

—Height percentile below the target range defined by parental heights
—Delayed bone age
—Reduced height velocity (especially in late childhood—below 25th percentile)
—Associated with delay of puberty
—Positive family history, usually boys
—Final adult height in the normal range and commensurate with target height

- Idiopathic short stature

—Used to categorize patients otherwise normal, who cannot be diagnosed with a variant of normal growth or any of the causes of short stature. May not always turn out to be a true normal variant.
—This is a diagnosis of exclusion and groups patients whose calculated predicted height is more than 2 SD below the mid-parental height, whose height is below the 5th percentile, with or without delay of skeletal maturation, and without identifiable diagnosis after appropriate evaluation.

PRIMARY SHORT STATURE

- Usually the consequence of an abnormality of the skeletal system. Bone age often not delayed or only delayed mildly.
- Skeletal defect can be primary or secondary (to a metabolic abnormality). In either case this may lead to disproportionate short stature and/or significant dysmorphism. Occasionally, the skeletal abnormalities are subtle and do not lead to disproportionate short stature.
- Skeletal dysplasia

—Osteochondrodysplasia
—Genetic transmission—many cases represent new mutation
—Defects in growth of tubular bones and/or axial skeleton
—Typical radiologic findings on skeletal survey x-ray
—More common forms include: achondroplasia, hypochondroplasia

- Short stature due to congenital error of metabolism

—Diffuse skeletal involvement
—Mostly autosomal recessive inheritance
—Dysmorphic features
—Typical biochemical abnormalities
—More common type: mucopolysaccharidosis

- Chromosomal abnormalities

—Autosomes or sex chromosomes
—Usually associated with other somatic abnormalities or mental retardation
—Clinical findings may be subtle (mosaicism)
—More common forms: Trisomy 21, -18, -13, and Turner syndrome

- Intrauterine growth retardation (IUGR)

—Often with poor postnatal growth
—Cause for IUGR may come from mother, fetus, or placenta
—Primordial dwarfism: due to intrinsic fetal defect leading to both pre- and postnatal growth failure (may be associated with specific genetic anomaly)
—IUGR is seen in congenital infection, fetal exposure to toxin, placental abnormalities, maternal disease, Russell-Silver syndrome and other congenital anomalies.

SECONDARY SHORT STATURE

- Malnutrition

—Especially under 2 years of age (most common in first 6 months of life)
—Caloric—malnutrition and/or protein—malnutrition
—Vitamin and mineral deficiencies (vitamin D, iron, zinc deficiency)

- Chronic illness

—Many chronic diseases present first with poor growth
—Cardiovascular: VSD, PDA, TOF, TGV, AS, PS, aortic coarctation, AV canal
—Pulmonary: asthma, CF, BPD
—GI/liver: inflammatory bowel disease, celiac disease, malabsorption, short bowel syndrome, chronic gastroenteritis, CF
—Renal: NS, CGN, RTA, CRF, nephrogenic DI, uropathy, congenital anomalies
—Metabolic: poorly controlled diabetes mellitus, storage disorders
—Chronic infections (HIV) and immune deficiencies
—Hematopoietic: anemia, leukemia, SCD

- Drugs

—Corticosteroids
—Sex steroids
—Methylphenidate, dextroamphetamine

- Psychosocial growth retardation
- Endocrine short stature

—Among secondary short stature, endocrine causes are least frequent

Approach to the Patient

GENERAL GOAL

Determine if the patient has short stature and/or growth failure. Determine if height alone is affected, or if growth problem includes weight and head circumference.

Phase 1: Determine if patient's profile fits normal variant of growth.

Phase 2: Determine if patient's profile fits with pathologic short stature.

Phase 3: Screening evaluation, referral to pediatric endocrinologist or observation.

Data Gathering

HISTORY

Question: Is the child short for his/her parents?
Significance: Mid-parental height is calculated to estimate the expected target height. To calculate mid-parental height for a boy, add his father's height to his mother's height plus 13 cm, and divide by 2. To calculate mid-parental height for a girl, add her mother's height to her father's height minus 13 cm, and divide by 2. If the child's height percentile is out of keeping with the calculated target height, this is likely significant.

Question: What is the child's growth (or height) velocity?
Significance: Height velocity for a specific interval can be annualized and plotted on a height velocity curve. This becomes an important criterion in a patient's growth and is different from height at any point in time, which, for a major part, is a representation of the influence of things past.

Question: What is the weight-to-height?
Significance: Usually increased in hypothyroidism, Cushing syndrome, pseudohypoparathyroidism, and growth hormone deficiency. Normal or decreased in emotional deprivation, anorexia, chronic renal failure, renal tubular acidosis, inflammatory bowel disease, malabsorption, malnutrition, lung and heart disease.

Question: Were there any complications during pregnancy, labor, and delivery?
Significance: Clues from the pregnancy can provide information about possible maternal disorders, intrauterine drug exposure, or placental abnormalities that lead to IUGR. Birth trauma can be associated with hypopituitarism. An inquiry about the perinatal and neonatal history is also necessary.

Question: Familial history. What are the heights of the parents and grandparents? What are the heights of the siblings? Was puberty on time in both parents? Any history of endocrine disorder or chronic illness affecting a major organ system?
Significance: Calculate mid-parental height. If short stature is running in the family, this could point toward familial or genetic short stature, isolated growth hormone deficiency, or skeletal dysplasia. Delayed pubertal maturation in the parents is important for a diagnosis of constitutional growth delay. Disorders such as diabetes mellitus and insipidus, thyroiditis, hypophosphatemic rickets, arthritis, and inflammatory bowel disease can affect different family members.

Question: What is the social situation?
Significance: Emotional stresses affect growth and development, either directly (abnormal growth hormone production), or indirectly (inadequate nutrition).

Question: What are current eating habits and how is the past dietary history? Any evidence of underutilization of calories ingested?
Significance: Estimate approximate total daily caloric intake. Detect deficiencies in certain nutrients, or the existence of abnormal eating habits (malabsorption, rickets, anorexia, inadequate parenting).

Question: Any chronic illness? Any hospitalization, surgery, or trauma to the head?
Significance: Chronic disorders can present with growth failure first, without specific symptoms (rheumatoid arthritis, celiac disease), and a previous hospitalization or surgery could be a clue for an underlying pathology (jaundice and hepatitis—chronic liver disease, asthma exacerbation and high-dose corticosteroids, head trauma and pituitary insufficiency).

The history should be completed by obtaining a detailed review of systems, with specific questions inquiring about the occurrence of headache, vomiting, visual disturbance (brain tumor), anorexia, diarrhea, or constipation (bowel disease, hypothyroidism), polyuria and polydypsia (diabetes mellitus, diabetes insipidus, and renal problems), and medication as well as activity pattern, sleep hygiene, and general development.

 ## Physical Examination

Finding: Abnormal upper/lower segment ratio
Significance: Primary short stature

Finding: Low weight/height ratio
Significance: Points toward malnutrition

Finding: Edema
Significance: Chronic renal failure

Finding: Frontal bossing, flat nasal bridge, and truncal fat deposition
Significance: Growth hormone deficiency

Finding: Abdominal distention and gluteal wasting
Significance: Malabsorption and celiac disease

Finding: Webbed neck, increased carrying angle, shield chest
Significance: Turner syndrome

Finding: Smooth tongue
Significance: Iron deficiency

Finding: Round face, ear lobe abnormality, and mental retardation
Significance: Pseudohypoparathyroidism

Finding: Temporal thinning of the hair, sparse hair, dry hair
Significance: Hypothyroidism, growth hormone deficiency, hypopituitarism

Finding: Delayed pubertal maturation
Significance: Turner syndrome, constitutional delay, hypopituitarism, hypothyroidism, inflammatory bowel disease, chronic renal disease

Finding: Leg bowing, rachitic rosary, widening of wrists
Significance: Rickets, malabsorption

 ## Laboratory Aids

If no specific cause found, screening tests are indicated.

Test: Complete blood count and differential
Significance: Anemia, infection, leukemia

Test: Sedimentation rate
Significance: Infection, inflammation.

Test: Electrolyte panel, glucose
Significance: Renal disorders, diabetes mellitus, and -insipidus

Test: Metabolic panel
Significance: Malnutrition, liver problem, bone disorder, pseudohypoparathyroidism

Test: Urinalysis
Significance: Urinary tract infection, diabetes, renal disorder, metabolic problem

Test: Thyroxine and thyroid-stimulating hormone
Significance: Hypothyroidism, hypopituitarism

Test: X-ray study of the left hand and wrist
Significance: Bone age determination

Test: Karyotype
Significance: Turner syndrome in short girls, chromosomal disorders

Test: IGF-I and IGFBP-3 concentrations
Significance: Shows little fluctuation over 24 hours, but interpretation of values needs to take age-related norms into account. IGF-I and IGFBP-3 are low in GH-deficiency, but can also be low due to hypothyroidism, chronic illness, or poor nutrition. Normal IGF-I and IGFBP-3 concentrations make growth hormone deficiency less likely.

Additional workup may be necessary, as determined by history and physical examination (transglutaminase antibodies, sweat chloride test, urine metabolic screening, skeletal survey, etc.).

Issues for Referral

- Flat growth curve, delayed bone age, abnormal thyroid test, poorly controlled diabetes, physical findings consistent with growth hormone deficiency, hypothyroidism, rickets—pediatric endocrinologist
- Protein-losing enteropathy, malabsorption, hepatic disorder—gastroenterologist
- Chronic lung disease, abnormal sweat chloride test—pulmonologist
- Congenital heart disease, occult cardiac disease—cardiologist
- Elevated creatinine, low serum bicarbonate, abnormal urinalysis—nephrologist

Growth failure is usually a relatively slow or subacute process and, therefore, does not require emergency workup. It is of basic importance, however, to pay special attention to correct measurements of height, weight, and head circumference, to evaluate the abnormally growing child adequately.

BIBLIOGRAPHY

Blizzard RM, Johanson A. Disorders of growth. In: Kappy MS, Blizzard RM, Migeon CJ, eds. *Wilkins' the diagnosis and treatment of endocrine disorders in childhood and adolescence*, Charles C Thomas, 1994;9: 383–456.

Rosenfield RL. Essentials of growth diagnosis. *Endocr Metab Clin North Am* 1996;25(3): 743–758.

Author: Philippe F. Backeljauw

Sore Throat

 Database

DEFINITION

Sore throat or pain with swallowing is a common presenting complaint in the pediatric population. The majority of cases have an infectious etiology, with viral causes being the most common.

 Differential Diagnosis

INFECTIOUS

• Pharyngitis/Tonsillitis

—Respiratory viruses: adenovirus/influenza/ parainfluenza; Epstein-Barr virus (EBV)
—Bacterial: Group A β-hemolytic streptococcus (*Streptococcus pyogenes*); group C streptococcus; diphtheria; *Neisseria gonorrhoeae;* anaerobic bacteria; tularemia; *Chlamydia*; *Mycoplasma*; *Arcanobacterium haemolyticum*
—Stomatitis: Herpes simplex virus, coxsackievirus
—Peritonsillar cellulitis/abscess
—Retropharyngeal abscess
—Epiglottitis/supraglottitis

ENVIRONMENTAL

• Irritative pharyngitis: exposure to smoke or dry air

TRAUMA

• Foreign body: either retained or causing laceration to posterior pharynx
• Burns: hot liquids/foods
• Voice overuse

TUMOR

• Rare in pediatric population

ALLERGIC/INFLAMMATORY

• Allergens causing chronic postnasal drip that leads to irritant pharyngitis

MISCELLANEOUS

• Kawasaki disease
• Psychogenic pain
• Referred pain

Approach to the Patient

GENERAL GOAL

The majority of cases of sore throat have an infectious cause, with most (~70–80%) of these having a viral etiology. Once the life-threatening and/or noninfectious causes have been excluded, the goal is to determine if the pharyngitis is caused by group A β-hemolytic streptococci (GABS), which should be treated with antibiotics, or one of the many other infectious etiologies.

Phase 1: Use history and physical exam to separate infectious from noninfectious causes. If etiology seems infectious, consider throat culture for group A streptococci infection.

 Data Gathering

HISTORY

Question: Sore throat in association with fever, headache, and/or abdominal pain?
Significance: Common association of symptoms present in group A streptococci pharyngitis.

Question: Sore throat in association with fever, URI symptoms (cough, rhinorrhea, conjunctivitis)?
Significance: More suggestive of viral pharyngitis.

Question: Presence of drooling, voice changes?
Significance: Possibility of more severe infectious etiology, including retropharyngeal or peritonsillar abscess, epiglottitis.

Question: Foreign body exposure?
Significance: Retained foreign body (e.g., fishbone) or laceration/irritation from foreign body.

Question: Irritant exposure (e.g., dry air from heating or cooling system)?
Significance: Pharyngeal mucosal drying.

Question: Immunization status and travel history?
Significance: Possibility of diphtheria in the non- or incompletely immunized patient, especially if recent travel to countries of the former Soviet Union.

Question: Sexual activity (including oral sex and possibility of abuse)?
Significance: Gonococcal pharyngitis.

Physical Examination

Finding: Pharyngeal erythema with or without exudate
Significance: Suggestive of infectious etiology, though does not reliably differentiate viral from bacterial causes.

Finding: Tender cervical adenopathy
Significance: Suggestive of infectious etiology; anterior cervical nodes described in classic GABS infection; posterior cervical nodes ± hepatosplenomegaly suggest possibility of EBV.

Finding: Stridor/drooling
Significance: Raises concern for etiologies that may cause airway obstruction

Finding: Asymmetric enlargement of tonsillar pillar with deviation of uvula away from enlarged side
Significance: Peritonsillar abscess

Finding: Mild erythema with cobblestoning of posterior pharyngeal mucosa
Significance: Suggests allergic or irritant etiology

Finding: Vesicular or ulcerative lesions in oropharynx
Significance: Suggestive of viral etiologies including herpes simplex (lesions commonly in anterior oropharynx) or coxsackievirus (lesions commonly in posterior oropharynx)

 ## Laboratory Aids

Test: Throat swab for strep antigen test with subsequent culture if antigen test is negative.
Significance: Useful for definitive diagnosis of group A streptococci infection. A negative antigen test should be followed by throat culture to improve sensitivity.

Test: Lateral neck x-ray
Significance: Enlarged epiglottis suggests epiglottitis; widened prevertebral soft tissue space suggestive of retropharyngeal abscess.

Test: Complete blood count and Monospot if indicated
Significance: Atypical lymphocytosis/presence of heterophil antibodies suggestive of EBV infection. EBV titers (if indicated) should be sent in those less than 4 years of age because of low sensitivity (~50%) of Monospot in this age group.

 ## Emergency Care

Factors that make sore throat an emergency include:

- Airway compromise

—Epiglottitis
—Retropharyngeal abscess
—Peritonsillar abscess
—Significant tonsillar hypertrophy
—Diphtheria

The patient may present with toxic appearance, fever, drooling, voice change, and sitting in the sniffing position (to optimize airway). Make NPO, supplemental oxygen; consider airway adjuncts (e.g., NP airway), intravenous access to facilitate airway management (if patient able to tolerate). Consider anesthesia consult for endotracheal intubation in most controlled setting.

 ## Common Questions and Answers

Q: What is the incidence of group A streptococci disease as the cause of pharyngitis?
A: Group A streptococci is the most common bacterial etiology of infectious pharyngitis. The incidence of this disease is approximately 15% to 30% of all cases of infectious pharyngitis.

Q: When must antibiotic therapy begin in group A streptococci pharyngitis in order to prevent rheumatic fever?
A: Antibiotics should be started within 9 days from the onset of symptoms in order to prevent this nonsuppurative complication of group A streptococci pharyngitis.

Issues for Referral

- Signs/symptoms of airway compromise—general toxicity, stridor, drooling. Patient may need emergent airway protection/stabilization.
- Fluctuant peritonsillar abscess—drainage may be done by otolaryngologist.
- Presence of foreign body—may need removal by otolaryngologist or x-ray to look for air in retropharyngeal soft tissue

Clinical Pearls

The clinical appearance of a GABS pharyngitis may be indistinguishable from pharyngitis of viral etiologies. The therapy for these illnesses is different: antibiotics for group A streptococci versus symptomatic care for viral pharyngitis. The practitioner should perform diagnostic testing (i.e., rapid strep antigen and/or culture) when GABS pharyngitis is considered. In general, it is not recommended to treat pending the culture results; rather, wait until the GABS pharyngitis is confirmed with a positive antigen or culture before starting antibiotics.

BIBLIOGRAPHY

Bisno AL. Acute pharyngitis. *N Engl J Med* 2001:344(3):205–211.

Bisno AL. Acute pharyngitis: etiology and diagnosis. *Pediatrics* 1996;97(6 pt 2): 949–954.

Fleisher GR. Sore throat. In: Fleisher GR, Ludwig S, eds. *Textbook of pediatric emergency medicine*. Philadelphia: Lippincott Williams & Wilkins, 2000:581–585.

Schwartz B, et al. Pharyngitis-principles of judicious use of antimicrobial agents. *Pediatrics* 1998;101(1 pt 2):171–174.

Author: Cynthia R. Jacobstein

Speech Delay

 Database

DEFINITION

Speech development significantly below the norm for children of the same age

 Differential Diagnosis

See table Most Common Causes of Speech Delay.

CONGENITAL/ANATOMIC

- Cerebral palsy
- Cleft palate
- Congenital infections (e.g., cytomegalovirus, syphilis, herpes, HIV)
- Lateralized (left-sided) brain lesion
- Mental retardation
- Microcephaly
- Sensorineural impairment (hearing or vision disorder)
- Sturge-Weber syndrome

INFECTIOUS

- Bacterial meningitis
- Human immunodeficiency virus (HIV)
- Recurrent otitis media

TOXIC

- Fetal alcohol syndrome/effects
- Kernicterus

TRAUMA

- Head injury
- Intracranial hemorrhage
- Stroke

GENETIC/METABOLIC

- Autism
- Pervasive developmental disorder (PDD)
- Developmental language disorder (DLD)
- Fragile X syndrome
- Neuromuscular disease
- Neurodegenerative disorder
- Tuberous sclerosis
- Velocardiofacial syndrome
- Williams syndrome

Most Common Causes of Speech Delay

Mental retardation
Hearing loss
Developmental language disorder
Autistic spectrum disorder (pervasive developmental disorder/autism)

MISCELLANEOUS

- Environmental deprivation
- Iatrogenic causes: endotracheal tube placement, tracheostomy
- Prematurity

Approach to the Patient

GENERAL GOALS

Determine if true delay in acquisition of speech. Determine if treatable etiology.

Phase 1: Determine if delays in attainment of other skills. Assess for impaired hearing.

Phase 2: Evaluate for presence of genetic, neuromuscular, or metabolic disorder.

Phase 3: Refer for treatment or additional evaluation.

HINTS FOR SCREENING PROBLEM

Screening tools (appropriate milestones, see the table Patterns of Emerging Speech Development)

- Denver Developmental Screening Test II: agent most commonly used for screening language; less sensitive for identifying delays in expressive language than delays in other areas of development.
- Early Language Milestone Scale (ELM) and Clinical Linguistic and Auditory Milestone Scale (CLAMS): more sensitive measures for children from birth to 36 months of age.
- Other useful screening measures: Peabody Picture Vocabulary Test-III (PPVT-III) and the Receptive-Expressive Emergent Language Screen (REEL). All can be used to assess language in children from 1 to 36 months old.

 Data Gathering

HISTORY

Question: At what age did the child demonstrate a social smile? Have first word? Use meaningful words? Demonstrate intelligible speech?
Significance: Knowledge of developmental speech milestones will enable the physician to determine if skills are delayed.

Question: Does the child have normal hearing and vision?
Significance: Children with impaired hearing (and vision to a lesser degree) often suffer from delayed language despite normal oral skills and an otherwise normal neurologic status.

Question: Does the child appear to be developmentally normal in other skills?
Significance: Mental retardation and other developmental disabilities (e.g., cerebral palsy) often present with delayed or aberrant language skills. Some neuromuscular disorders also present with delayed onset of speech with gross motor delay.

Question: Does the child appear medically ill?
Significance: Failure to thrive can signify a multitude of underlying problems (e.g., encephalopathy, chronic neglect), which can cause speech delay.

Question: Does the child exhibit appropriate social relatedness?
Significance: Deviant or delayed speech is a cardinal feature of autism. Children with autism (or pervasive developmental disorder) exhibit a restricted repertoire of activities and interests as well as impairment in social interactions.

Patterns of Emerging Speech Development

AGE	SPEECH
2 months (8 weeks)	Coos, social smile, attends to voice
3 months (12 weeks)	Some vocal sounds; "aah, ooh"
4 months (16 weeks)	Laughs
6 months (28 weeks)	Repetitive vowel sounds (e.g., babbling)
9 months (40 weeks)	Waves bye-bye, repetitive consonant sounds (e.g., "dadada")
12 months (52 weeks)	One or more words (e.g., "mama," "dada")
15 months	Points, single words besides "mama/dada"
18 months	Up to 10 words, jargoning; names pictures, identifies 1 or more body parts
21 months	Two-word phrases
24 months	30–50 words, 3-word sentences
30 months	Refers to self as "I," knows name
36 months	Counts to 3, knows age and sex
	Speech intelligible
48 months	Counts four objects, tells story
60 months	Counts ten objects correctly, asks meanings of words

Question: Is the child's home environment adequately stimulating?
Significance: Environmental deprivation and neglect are well-documented causes of delayed speech.

Question: Is there evidence of a familial or hereditary condition?
Significance: Hearing impairment, stuttering, and autism are found in higher numbers among first-degree relatives. The effects of fragile X syndrome are also well documented.

Question: Is there any history of seizure activity?
Significance: Seizures may indicate an underlying neurologic impairment (e.g., Landau-Kleffner syndrome) or, if severe and poorly controlled, can themselves directly interfere with achieving milestones.

 ## Physical Examination

Finding: Macrocephaly, microcephaly, hypertelorism, or hair whorls?
Significance: May indicate an underlying brain defect or *in utero* exposure.

Finding: Unusual facies or other dysmorphisms?
Significance: Suggest genetic problem or syndromes, some of which are associated with speech problems and/or mental retardation (e.g., Down syndrome, fetal alcohol syndrome, fragile X syndrome, Williams syndrome, velocardiofacial syndrome).

Finding: Abnormal (misshapen), low set, or small ears or eyes?
Significance: May point to a sensorineural impairment and/or a syndrome including mental retardation (e.g., Treacher Collins syndrome, trisomies).

Finding: Scarred tympanic membranes?
Significance: May represent chronic otitis media with resultant prolonged (transient) hearing impairment.

Finding: Tracheostomy or suprasternal scar?
Significance: Raises the question of damage to the vocal cords.

Finding: Skin abnormalities?
Significance: May represent (e.g., café-au-lait spots, hypopigmented macules, port-wine stains) syndrome associated with hearing impairment or mental retardation.

Finding: Malnutrition and social withdrawal?
Significance: May point to environmental deprivation or chronic disease.

Finding: Abnormal or impaired muscle control?
Significance: May indicate an underlying neurologic process (e.g., facial diplegia in Mobius syndrome, brisk tendon reflexes with clonus in cerebral palsy).

 ## Laboratory Aids

Test: Behavioral audiometry or brainstem auditory evoked response testing
Significance: Children with severe hearing loss will demonstrate speech delay.

Test: Computed tomography (CT) or magnetic resonance imaging (MRI) of the head
Significance: Indicated when speech delay is accompanied by focal neurologic abnormalities, moderate to profound mental retardation, or dysmorphic features.

Test: Karyotype and fragile X screen
Significance: Indicated in the presence of stereotyped or unusual behaviors, dysmorphic features, and developmental delay.

Test: Metabolic screens
Significance: Liver function tests, serum for amino acids, and urine for organic acids are suggested only in the presence of changes in skin or hair, growth failure, lethargy, loss of milestones, organomegaly, or severe developmental delay.

Test: Electroencephalogram (EEG)
Significance: An EEG should be performed if there is a concern or history of seizure activity or regression in or loss of language skills.

Test to Prepare for Consult

• Audiometry
• Office language screen (Denver II, ELM, CLAMS)

 ## Emergency Care

Urgent evaluation is indicated with the presence of seizures, and regression in developmental milestones.

 ## Common Questions and Answers

Q: Do later-born children speak later than first-born children do?
A: No. Parents and siblings often speak for the child in question, but this is a result of, not a cause of, the child's delay.

Q: Is the child being "lazy"?
A: Children who are lazy usually demonstrate normal language skills.

Q: Do bilingual children speak later than children in single-language homes do?
A: No. Developmental constants are normal, and by 36 months of age these children are often fluent in both languages.

Q: Do deaf infants show absence of vocalizations?
A: No. Deaf infants may coo and babble in a normal pattern until 6 months of age.

Q: Should a child demonstrating speech delay who has normal results on an office hearing screen be referred for further evaluation?
A: Yes. Hearing screens in the office setting may miss a mild, high-frequency sensorineural hearing loss.

Special Insight

The initial complaint of parents of preschool-aged children with an autistic disorder is almost always inadequate language. All children with mental retardation exhibit language delay, but not all children with language delay have mental retardation.

Issues for Referral

• Children requiring referral include those without meaningful words by 18 months of age, meaningful phrases by 2 years of age, or those with unintelligible speech at age 3 years.
• Professionals to make referrals to include:

—Speech-language pathologists: they evaluate the oral-peripheral mechanism, and provide additional information about communication skills.
—Developmental pediatricians: they identify whether there is a discrepancy between communication skills and other developmental skill areas, and evaluate the possible etiologies for the speech problems. This referral is indicated when speech delay is accompanied by other developmental delays.
—Child psychologists or neuropsychologists: they evaluate abnormal behaviors and provide information regarding cognitive skills.
—Pediatric neurologists: they evaluate seizures, motor abnormalities, and/or neurodegenerative features, and assist in the evaluation and management of unusual behaviors.

BIBLIOGRAPHY

Coplan J. Normal speech and language development: an overview. *Pediatr Rev* 1995;16(3):91–100.

Leung A. Evaluation and management of the child with speech delay. *Am Fam Physician* 1999;59:3121–3128.

Shonkoff JP. Language delay: late talking to communication disorder. In: Rudolph AM, Hoffman JI, Rudolph CD, eds. *Rudolph's pediatrics*, 20th ed. London: Prentice-Hall, 1996:124–128.

Tanguay P. Pervasive developmental disorders: a 10-year review. *J Am Acad Child Adolesc Psychiatry* 2000;39(9):1079–1095.

Author: H. Lynn Starr

Speech Problems

Database

DEFINITION
Disorders of word production and language expression. They can be found as isolated difficulties or in conjunction with more complex disorders. See tables below.

Differential Diagnosis

CONGENITAL/ANATOMIC
- Cerebral palsy
- Cleft lip/palate
- Hearing impairment
- Intracranial hemorrhage
- Isolated language disorder
- Laryngeal abnormalities
- Mid-facial defects
- Mobius syndrome
- Stroke

INFECTIOUS
- Human immunodeficiency virus (HIV)

TOXIC
- Fetal alcohol syndrome/effects

TRAUMA
- Traumatic brain and/or laryngeal injuries

GENETIC/METABOLIC
- Autism and pervasive developmental disorders
- Mental retardation
- Neuromuscular disease
- Velocardiofacial syndrome
- Williams syndrome

MISCELLANEOUS
- Acquired aphasias (e.g., Landau-Kleffner syndrome, related language-epilepsy syndromes)
- Acquired deafness
- Iatrogenic causes: endotracheal tube placement, tracheostomy
- Prematurity
- Severe environmental deprivation

Approach to the Patient

GENERAL GOAL
Determine if speech is abnormal, or if the problem is transient, progressive, or static.
Phase 1: Determine if the patient has a hearing impairment or delays in other areas of development.
Phase 2: Determine if problem is an articulation or experience language disorder (see table directly below).

Most Common Causes of Speech Problems

Developmental language disorder
Hearing loss
Mental retardation

Phase 3: Refer for additional evaluation and treatment if warranted.

Data Gathering

HISTORY
Question: Does the child have normal hearing and vision?
Significance: Children with sensorineural hearing impairments often have disrupted speech (e.g., articulation disorders) and/or language skills (e.g., semantic-pragmatic disorders).
Question: Is there evidence of developmental delay in other areas of skills?
Significance: Mental retardation and other developmental disabilities (e.g., cerebral palsy) often present with delayed or aberrant skills (dysarthric or dyspraxic speech, lexical-syntactic disorder, and nonverbal and verbal communication impairment).
Question: Does the child have dysmorphic features or other medical conditions?
Significance: Speech problems are manifested in several genetic syndromes such as:
- Williams syndrome
- Fragile X syndrome
- Velocardiofacial syndrome
Question: Does the child exhibit unusual behaviors?
Significance: Children with autism/pervasive developmental disorder may exhibit stereotyped behaviors, with impaired social interactions, as well as deviant speech patterns (delayed language development, nonverbal and verbal communication impairment, semantic-pragmatic disorder).
Question: When was the child noted to have a speech problem?
Significance: Abrupt onset is seen with head trauma, encephalitis, and other acute illnesses.

Question: Has there been any change in the child's speech, especially loss of milestones?
Significance: Progressive loss of speech may be seen in Landau-Kleffner syndrome and neurodegenerative disorders. Classic features of Landau-Kleffner syndrome include: normal early language, acquired aphasia, clinical seizures, or a frankly paroxysmal electroencephalogram (EEG).
Question: Is there evidence of a familial or hereditary condition?
Significance: Hearing impairment, stuttering, and autism are found in higher numbers among first-degree relatives.
Question: Is there a history of seizure activity?
Significance: Seizures may be indicative of Landau-Kleffner syndrome, a seizure disorder, or of an underlying neurologic impairment.

HINTS FOR SCREENING FOR THE PROBLEM
Children with speech problems may be identified by signs of inadequate language and/or vocabulary, and by evaluation of the conversation skills, comprehension, and syntax in comparison to other children of the same age.

Physical Examination

Finding: Macrocephaly, microcephaly, hypertelorism, or hair whorls?
Significance: May indicate an underlying brain defect, *in utero* exposure to medication (e.g., hydantoin) or infection (e.g., CMV).
Finding: Abnormal (misshapen) or small ears?
Significance: May point to a sensorineural impairment.
Finding: Scarred tympanic membranes?
Significance: May represent chronic otitis media and the resultant prolonged (although temporary) hearing impairment.

Speech Disorders

ARTICULATION DISORDERS	
Dysarthria	Articulation impaired by poor oral muscle control
Dyspraxia	Difficulty with the production of speech despite normal oral musculature
Language disorders	An impaired ability to use meaningful words, phrases, or gestures. They include two major types: expressive and receptive language disorders.
Resonance disorders	Difficulty in the volume or tone of speech, often due to abnormalities of the nasal and/or oral airways
Stuttering	Difficulty with the rhythm or fluency of speech, accompanied by signs of distress (e.g., facial grimacing)
Voice disorders	Production of speech impaired by an abnormal larynx
EXPRESSIVE LANGUAGE DISORDERS	
Lexical-syntactic disorders	Difficulties with word-finding and sentence structure
Semantic-pragmatic disorders	Impairment in production and understanding of conversation, including echolalia
Nonverbal and verbal communication impairments	Limited comprehension of language with or without speech
Speech programming deficit	Fluency with interspersed jargon

Finding: Cleft lip or palate?
Significance: May cause resonance abnormalities in the production of speech (hyponasal speech).

Finding: Unusual facies or other dysmorphic features?
Significance: Suggest genetic or hereditary syndromes, some of which are associated with speech problems and/or mental retardation (e.g., fetal alcohol syndrome, fragile X syndrome, Williams syndrome, velocardiofacial syndrome).

Finding: Tracheostomy or suprasternal scar?
Significance: May indicate a history of damage to the vocal cords.

Finding: Malnutrition and social withdrawal?
Significance: May point to environmental deprivation or chronic disease.

Finding: Abnormal or impaired muscle control?
Significance: May be significant for an underlying neurologic process (e.g., facial diplegia in Mobius syndrome, brisk tendon reflexes with clonus in cerebral palsy).

Finding: Behavioral problems?
Significance: Children with stereotyped behavior, avoidance of eye contact, and poor social skills may have autism/pervasive developmental disorder.

Finding: Shortened frenulum?
Significance: Probably an incidental finding, as this does not result in deviant speech in most instances.

 ## Laboratory Aids

Test: Behavioral audiometry or brainstem auditory evoked response testing
Significance: Hearing loss may impair a child's ability to discriminate between certain speech sounds. This may result in abnormalities of articulation and resonance.

Test: Computed tomography (CT) or magnetic resonance imaging (MRI) of the head
Significance: One of these studies is indicated when speech problems are accompanied by focal neurologic abnormalities (such as hearing loss, abnormal muscle tone, etc.), moderate to profound mental retardation, skin abnormalities or dysmorphic features. MRI is the procedure of choice; however, CT scans are superior in imaging cranial bones, and when making the determination of intracranial calcifications.

Test: Karyotype and fragile X screen
Significance: These studies are indicated in the presence of stereotyped or unusual behaviors, dysmorphic features, and developmental delay. No more than 2–5% of persons with autism have a fragile X mutation.

Test: Metabolic screen
Significance: Liver function tests, serum for amino acids, and urine for organic acids are suggested only in the presence of changes in or abnormal skin or hair, growth failure, lethargy, loss of milestones, organomegaly, or severe developmental delay.

Test: Electroencephalogram
Significance: An EEG should be performed if there is a concern or history of seizure activity or regression in or loss of language skills. Autism and atypical autism have been reported in approximately 40% of persons with tuberous sclerosis.

Tests to Prepare for Consult
• Audiometry
• Office language screens:
—Denver Developmental Screening Test II: most commonly used for screening language; is most sensitive for detecting severe speech delay.
—The Early Language Milestone Scale (ELM) and the Clinical Linguistic and Auditory Milestone Scale (CLAMS) the preferred measures in screening speech problems.
—The Peabody Picture Vocabulary Test-III is a better measure of receptive than expressive language skills.

Clinical Pearls
• Dysfluency, or transient loss of normal speech rate and rhythm, is frequently seen in children $2\frac{1}{2}$ to 4 years of age. Dysfluency involves repetition of whole words, without signs of distress, should not be confused with stuttering, which involves repetition of shorter speech segments or difficulty initiating a word, accompanied by signs of distress.
• Males are more likely to exhibit speech problems.

 ## Therapy

In many cases, the mainstay of management of children with speech problems is education.

SPECIFIC
• Auditory feedback has been used with some success for stutterers (e.g., delayed auditory feedback) and selective mutism (e.g., auditory feed forward).
• Auditory integration and facilitated communication are two techniques demonstrating little improvement in patient status.

DRUGS
• Haloperidol, although not routinely used, has been successful in the management of stuttering.
• Fluoxetine has demonstrated limited effect in selective mutism.
• Antiepileptic medications have been used with success when EEGs demonstrate spike forms.

 ## Follow-Up

• Coordination and periodic follow-up of services are crucial to treatment success.
• As the child grows, the need for specific services may change, requiring the primary physician to be vigilant to ensure that treatment goals are being met.

 ## Common Questions and Answers

Q: When should children with stuttering be referred to a speech-language therapist?
A: A child should be referred when dysfluency persists for more than 6 months, has an onset or persistence after 5 years of age, when there are five or more breaks per 100 words, or when stuttering is accompanied by significant distress.

Q: What are some ways parents can help their child who stutters?
A: A parent should be encouraged to avoid criticizing the child, reminding the child to speak more slowly and/or to repeat words.

Q: When a child exhibits selective mutism, is a referral to a speech therapist indicated?
A: Initial referral to a behavioral specialist.

Issues for Referral
• A speech-language pathologist is needed to evaluate the oral-peripheral mechanism, and to provide additional information about communication skills.
• Developmental pediatricians are able to identify whether there is a discrepancy between communication skills and other developmental skill areas, evaluate the possible etiologies for the speech problems, and to act as coordinators for needed therapies.
• Child psychologists or neuropsychologists are able to evaluate abnormal behaviors and to provide information regarding cognitive skills.
• School systems may serve as a center for the provision of evaluations and services for children over 3 years of age, and for children with disabilities under the age of 3.

BIBLIOGRAPHY
Blum NJ, et al. Case study: auditory feedforward treatment of selective mutism. *J Am Acad Child Adolesc Psychiatry* 1998;37(1):40–43.

Coplan J. Normal speech and language development: an overview. *Pediatr Rev* 1995;16(3):91–100.

Lawrence M, Barclay DM. Stuttering: a brief review. *Am Fam Physician* 1998;57(9):2175–2178.

Rapin I. Practitioner review: developmental language disorders: a clinical update. *J Child Psychiatry* 1996;37:643—655.

Author: H. Lynn Starr

Splenomegaly

 Database

DEFINITION

A palpable spleen is found in most premature infants and in 30% of term infants. A spleen tip is still palpable in 10% of infants at 1 year of age and in 1% of children 10 years of age. Normal spleens are soft, at the midclavicular line, and often palpable only on deep inspiration. Dullness on percussion beyond the 11th intercostal space suggests splenomegaly. Splenic tenderness is abnormal.

 Differential Diagnosis

INFECTION

- Bacterial
- Bacteremia
- Pneumonia
- Sepsis
- Subacute bacterial endocarditis
- *Salmonella*
- Tuberculosis
- Brucellosis
- Staphylococcal shunt infections
- Tularemia
- Syphilis
- Leptospirosis

VIRAL

- Epstein-Barr virus (mononucleosis)
- Cytomegalovirus
- HIV
- Rubella
- Herpes
- Hepatitis A, B
- Rickettsial/protozoan
- Rocky Mountain spotted fever
- Malaria
- Toxoplasmosis
- Trypanosomiasis
- Babesiosis
- Schistosomiasis
- Visceral larval migrans
- Kala-azar

FUNGAL

- Histoplasmosis
- Coccidioidomycosis

BLOOD DISEASE: HEMOLYTIC DISEASES

- Hereditary spherocytosis
- Sickle cell disease
- Thalassemia major autoimmune hemolytic anemia
- Hemoglobin C disease
- Pyruvate kinase deficiency
- Glucose-6-phosphate dehydrogenase deficiency
- Isoimmunization disorders
- Infantile pyknocytosis
- Iron-deficiency anemia (rare)
- Thrombocytopenic purpura

VASCULAR CONGESTIVE DISORDERS

- Cavernous transformation of the portal vein
- Congenital hepatic fibrosis

CIRRHOSIS SECONDARY TO:

- Hepatitis
- Biliary atresia
- Wilson disease
- Cystic fibrosis
- α_1-Antitrypsin deficiency
- Tyrosinemia
- Hereditary fructose intolerance
- Hemosiderosis
- Thrombosis of the hepatic vein
- Budd-Chiari syndrome
- Congestive heart failure
- Constrictive pericarditis
- Galactosemia
- Congenital portal vein stenosis or atresia
- Splenic artery aneurysm
- Splenic hematoma
- Splenic hemangioma

METABOLIC DISEASES

- Gangliosidoses
- Mucolipidoses
- Metachromatic leukodystrophy
- Wolman disease
- Gaucher disease
- Niemann-Pick disease
- Amyloidosis
- Hyperlipoproteinemia
- Familial hemophagocytic reticulosis
- Porphyria
- Lysinuric protein intolerance
- Dibasic aminoaciduria
- Cystinosis

NEOPLASTIC DISEASES

- Leukemia
- Lymphoma
- Lymphosarcoma
- Neuroblastoma
- Histiocytosis X

MISCELLANEOUS

- Serum sickness
- Connective-tissue disorders
- Juvenile rheumatoid arthritis
- Systemic lupus erythematosus
- Sarcoidosis
- Beckwith-Wiedemann syndrome
- Infant of a diabetic mother
- Splenic hamartoma
- Cysts: congenital and posttraumatic
- Hyperparathyroidism
- Gingival fibromatosis and digital anomalies

NONSPLENIC LEFT ABDOMINAL MASSES

- Large kidney
- Retroperitoneal tumor
- Adrenal neoplasm
- Ovarian cyst
- Pancreatic cyst
- Mesenteric cyst

Approach to the Patient

GENERAL GOALS

Determine the etiology of the large spleen.

Phase 1: Establish the presence of enlarged spleen, not a palpable spleen that is pushed down by inflated lungs.

Phase 2: Rule out common causes as a viral infection, bacterial infection, or anemia.

Phase 3: Rule out malignancy or storage disease or other rare causes of large spleen.

Data Gathering

HISTORY

Question: History of acute illness?
Significance: Suggests infection.

Question: History of GI bleeding?
Significance: With splenomegaly, suggests increased portal venous pressure.

Question: Familial history of hematologic or immune disease?
Significance: Suggests bleeding disorder or genetic disorder.

Question: Systemic symptoms: fever, jaundice, pallor, bleeding, hematuria, anorexia, abdominal distention?
Significance: Suggests infectious disease.

Question: Are there signs of cardiac distress?
Significance: Congenital heart disease or failure.

Physical Examination

Begin the abdominal examination in the lower quadrant, as an enlarged spleen may be missed in the upper quadrant exam.

Finding: Auscultate for rub or bruit
Significance: Look for signs of storage disease: retina, facies, etc.

Finding: Complete evaluation of lymph nodes
Significance: Look for ascites.

Finding: Pain
Significance: Suggests capsular distention due to infiltration, trauma, or infection.

Finding: Prominent abdominal veins or hemorrhoids
Significance: Suggest increased portal venous pressure.

Laboratory Aids

Test: Complete blood count with differential and platelets
Significance: Sickle cell, hemolytic anemia, leukemia

Test: Reticulocyte count
Significance: Hemolytic anemia

Test: Liver tests: transaminases: AST, ALT, albumin, bilirubin, PT/PTT, glucose
Significance: Cirrhosis, hepatic obstruction

DISCRIMINATING LABORATORY TESTS

If no hemolytic disease, with signs of infection:

* Blood culture
* Thick smear of blood for malaria
* Viral testing

If no hemolytic disease, no sign of infection, no sign of congestion:

* Ultrasound
* Liver spleen scan
* Biopsy: bone, lymph node, liver

If no hemolytic disease, no sign of infection, but sign of congestion:

* Ultrasound
* Computed tomography
* Magnetic resonance imaging

Emergency Care

* Life-threatening etiologies: sepsis, severe hemolytic anemia, trauma, hypersplenism
* Rapid placement of a large-bore intravenous access route should occur when a life-threatening etiology is suspected.

Common Questions and Answers

Q: How long will the enlarged spleen secondary to a viral infection be present?
A: The enlarged spleen may persist for several months.

SPECIAL INSIGHTS OR CUES

Asthmatic patients may have palpable spleen secondary to overinflation of lungs and depressed diaphragm.

Issues For Referral

* Disproportionate size of spleen
* Increasing size over serial examinations
* Unexplained lymphadenopathy
* Liver dysfunction
* Ascites
* Signs of storage or metabolic disease
* Howell-Jolly bodies on peripheral smear, suggesting splenic dysfunction

BIBLIOGRAPHY

Bale JF Jr, Blackman JA, Sato Y. Outcome in children with symptomatic congenital cytomegalovirus infection. *J Child Neurol* 1990;5(2):131–136.

Donnelly LF, Foss JN, Frush DP, et al. Heterogeneous splenic enhancement patterns on spiral CT images in children: minimizing misinterpretation. *Radiology* 1999;210(2): 493–497.

Imrie J, Wraith JE. Isolated splenomegaly as the presenting feature of Niemann-Pick disease type C. *Arch Dis Child* 2001;84(5): 427–429.

Sheth S, Ruzal-Shapiro C, Piomelli S, et al. CT imaging of splenic sequestration in sickle cell disease. *Pediatr Radiol* 2000;30(12):830–833.

Zimmerman SA, Ware RE. Palpable splenomegaly in children with haemoglobin SC disease: haematological and clinical manifestations. *Clin Lab Haematol* 2000;22(3):145–150.

Author: Andrew E. Mulberg

Teething

Database

DEFINITION

• Teething is the normal developmental process of primary tooth eruption (see table, Guidelines for the Time of Tooth Eruption), often characterized by parental reports of fever, fussiness, increased drooling, increased finger sucking, alterations in bowel pattern, and/or decreased appetite.
• Of note, fever >102°F, irritability, or diarrhea should not be attributed to teething and other etiologies should be considered such as otitis media, urinary tract infection, septicemia, meningitis, septic arthritis, or viral infection.

Differential Diagnosis

CONGENITAL/ANATOMIC

• Natal teeth, neonatal teeth
• Gastroesophageal reflux resulting in esophagitis with decreased appetite

INFECTIOUS

• Primary herpes gingivostomatitis causing pain or drooling
• Human herpesvirus 6 causing fever
• Coxsackievirus oral infection causing fever or drooling
• Epiglottitis causing severe drooling with fever
• Viral illness causing fever >101°F, diarrhea, or upper respiratory symptoms

TOXIC

• Toxic ingestion causing drooling

TRAUMA

• "Lancing" of gums (i.e., incising the gum to expose the erupting tooth) causing pain
• Hair tourniquet syndrome causing pain and irritability
• Corneal abrasion causing pain

MISCELLANEOUS

• Drooling, gum rubbing, and finger sucking may be normal developmental behaviors

Approach to the Patient

GENERAL GOAL

Determine if the infant has any other signs or symptoms of another illness that would require additional investigation (e.g., fever >102°F, diarrhea, or irritability); avoid over diagnosing teething, which might delay diagnosis of a more serious illness.

Phase 1: Careful history and physical.

Phase 2: Workup of specific signs or symptoms that are not consistent with teething.

Phase 3: Provide relief of discomfort for the child who is teething.

Data Gathering

Question: How old is the child?
Significance: The average age for the eruption of the first tooth is approximately 6 months. One percent of infants acquire the first tooth before 4 months, and 1% after 12 months. Rule of thumb: age (months) − 6 = average number of teeth (up to 2 years of age). Eruption usually begins with the lower central incisors.

Question: Has the parent noted any swelling or bluish discoloration of the gums?
Significance: Primary tooth eruption is frequently associated with swelling of the gums. A bluish area of gum swelling may represent an eruption cyst secondary to a hematoma. This condition requires parental reassurance only.

Question: Is the infant consolable?
Significance: Infants who are teething may be fussy but should be consolable. An infant who is irritable and not consolable should be evaluated for serious systemic illness such as septicemia, meningitis, septic arthritis, or urinary tract infection.

Question: Have the parents documented any fever?
Significance: Several studies suggest that mild temperature elevation can occur 1 to 3 days prior to tooth eruption. Fevers >102°F cannot be attributed to teething and require workup for other causes of illness such as upper respiratory infection, otitis media, urinary tract infection, meningitis, septic arthritis, or other viral infection.

Question: What other symptoms is the child experiencing?
Significance: One recent study found that the following symptoms may be seen during the 4 days before and the 3 days after tooth eruption: increased biting, drooling, gum-rubbing, sucking, irritability, wakefulness, ear-rubbing, facial rash, decreased appetite for solid foods, and mild temperature elevation. In this study, congestion, sleep disturbance, stool looseness, increased stool number, decreased interest in drinking, cough, nonfacial rashes, vomiting, and fever >102°F were not associated with the teething period. Another recent study did not validate these findings.

Question: How is the child sleeping?
Significance: A teething child should be able to sleep with minimal disturbance. Changes in sleeping habits, such as frequent nighttime awakening, should suggest common problems with sleep associations often seen in young children 6 to 12 months of age.

Question: Are other contacts in the home ill?
Significance: An acute illness should be investigated as the cause of the child's symptoms.

Question: What home remedies or treatments have the parents tried?
Significance: Most over-the-counter preparations marketed for the relief of teething symptoms contain 7.5% to 10% benzocaine as the active ingredient. Excessive use of benzocaine preparations has been associated with methemoglobinemia. Homeopathic remedies may contain a variety of ingredients including belladonna alkaloids, chamomile, and ground coffee. Depending on the size of the child and the amount of medication or herb ingested, toxicity is possible. Excessive use of topical 2% lidocaine may cause seizures. Other remedies have been associated with salicylate toxicity and lead poisoning. If toxicity is suspected, the local poison control center should be consulted.

Question: Have the parents tried applying cold/frozen objects locally onto the gums?
Significance: Though many find that cold objects work well, care must be taken because direct contact with a frozen object may, on occasion, result in local irritation.

Question: What objects have the parents offered the child to chew or bite?
Significance: Choking hazards, such as raw carrots, must be avoided. Teething rings should not be placed around the child's neck as they represent a strangulation hazard.

Guidelines for the Time of Tooth Eruption

TEETH	MAXILLARY ERUPTION	MANDIBULAR ERUPTION
Central incisors	6–8 months	5–7 months
Lateral incisors	8–11 months	7–10 months
Cuspids	16–20 months	16–20 months
First molars	10–16 months	10–16 months
Second molars	20–30 months	20–30 months

Teething

Physical Examination

Question: Is there swelling with slight pallor over the gum where the tooth will erupt?
Significance: This is a normal finding.

Question: Is there bluish discoloration overlying the gum where a tooth is expected?
Significance: This represents a hematoma, known as an "eruption cyst," which is a normal finding.

Question: Is the child irritable?
Significance: Irritability on physical examination suggests a more serious illness other than teething. In addition to the infectious etiologies noted, the child should be evaluated for hair tourniquet syndrome and/or corneal abrasion.

Question: Are there oral ulcers?
Significance: Viral enanthems, such as herpes or Coxsackie, should be considered.

Question: Is cervical lymphadenopathy present?
Significance: Oral, dental, or pharyngeal infections should be considered.

Question: Are there signs of dehydration, such as dry mucous membranes, absent tears, sunken fontanel, or tenting of the skin?
Significance: Infectious etiologies that result in poor oral intake or diarrhea should be considered.

Question: Is there oral erythema, and abrasions with excessive drooling?
Significance: The possibility of caustic ingestion should be explored.

Laboratory Aids

No laboratory tests are indicated in the otherwise healthy child with teething.

Common Questions and Answers

Q: What are some common remedies for relieving the pain caused by teething?
A: Children with teething should find temporary relief from biting or chewing on hard or cold items, such as refrigerated plastic teething rings, a cold wet washcloth, or teething biscuits. Gum massage with a clean finger may also provide relief.
Over-the-counter products containing benzocaine should be used with caution. Acetaminophen (15 mg/kg by mouth every 4 hours) or ibuprofen (10 mg/kg by mouth every 6 hours) may be used for pain relief as needed, but should not be given to mask fever. Remedies that have been used in the past and are no longer recommended include: alcoholic liquors, paregoric, 2% lidocaine solution, lancing the gums, and rubbing the gums with a thimble until the tooth breaks through the gum.

Q: What is the difference between natal teeth and neonatal teeth?
A: Natal teeth are present at birth, whereas neonatal teeth erupt during the first month of life. The incidence of natal teeth is 1:2,000 to 1:6,000 live births and usually involves the lower central incisor. Natal teeth can be associated with various conditions including Pierre Robin sequence, cleft lip, or cleft palate. There is often a familial history of natal or neonatal teeth. Ninety-five percent of natal teeth are normal primary incisors that may have formed superficially and erupted early. Only 5% of natal teeth are supernumerary (extra) teeth. Therefore, if a natal tooth is removed, a primary tooth will not erupt in its place in most cases. Because primary teeth act as space holders for the secondary teeth, early loss of a primary tooth may result in significant crowding of the permanent successors.

Q: Does primary tooth eruption in preterm infants occur at the same time as in full-term infants?
A: In healthy preterm infants who had relative uneventful neonatal courses, the first primary tooth erupts at the usual chronological age. In premature infants who required prolonged oral intubation and or who experienced inadequate nutrition due to the severity of neonatal disease may have delayed eruption. The initial eruption sequence remains the same (lower central incisors first).

Issues for Referral

• Children who have delayed eruption of their first primary tooth beyond 12 months require additional investigation for the following: adontia, osteodystrophies, hypothyroidism, hypopituitarism, Down syndrome, rickets, Gardner syndrome. Most of these conditions require referral to a specialist for management.
• Children with premature eruption may have a familial cause, however, referral for evaluation of hyperpituitarism should be considered.
• Referral to a dentist should be considered for children with significant variation in eruption caused by dental infections, additional teeth in the path of eruption, insufficient space in the dental arch, and/or ectopic placement of teeth.
• Natal teeth that are stable and do not interfere with breast-feeding may remain. Loose natal teeth may need to be removed to prevent choking and aspiration. Natal teeth can interfere with breast-feeding and cause ulceration, which is another indication for removal.

BIBLIOGRAPHY

Jaber L, Cohen IJ, Mor A. Fever associated with teething. *Arch Dis Child* 1992;67:233–234.

Kates GA, Needleman HL, Holmes LB. Natal and neonatal teeth: a clinical study. *J Am Dent Assoc* 1984;109:441–443.

Macknin ML, Piedmonte M, Jacobs J, et al. Symptoms associated with infant teething: a prospective study. *Pediatrics* 2000;105:747–752.

Mofenson HC, Caraccio TR, Miller H, et al. Lidocaine toxicity from topical mucosal application. *Clin Pediatr* 1983;22:190–192.

Paynter AS, Alexander FW. Salicilate intoxication caused by teething ointment. *Lancet* 1979;2:1132.

Townes PL, Geertsma MA, White MR. Benzocaine induced methemoglobinemia. *Am J Dis Child* 1977;13:697–698.

Viscardi RM, Romberg E, Abrams RG. Delayed primary tooth eruption in premature infants: relationship to neonatal factors. *Pediatr Dent* 1994;16:23–28.

Wake M, Hesketh K, Lucas J. Teething and tooth eruption in infants: a cohort study. *Pediatrics* 2000;106:1374–1379.

Author: Julie A. Boom

Thrombosis

 Database

DEFINITION

Pathologic arterial or venous intravascular occlusion by thrombus, which interferes with normal blood flow. Arterial events are often embolic. The following are common thrombotic events:
- Deep venous thrombosis (DVT): involves large systemic veins outside the CNS.
- Dural sinus thrombosis: involves the intracranial venous sinuses often with extension into the cerebral veins.
- Superficial thrombophlebitis.
- Ischemic stroke: arterial occlusion or insufficiency with infarction of brain tissue.
- Hemorrhagic stroke: follows an ischemic event with reperfusion.
- Intracardiac thrombosis: mural, valvular, or hardware associated.
- Neonatal aortic thrombosis: can be spontaneous or catheter associated.
- Renal vein thrombosis: in the neonatal period or in children with nephrotic syndrome.
- Myocardial infarction: Kawasaki disease or with severe familial hypercholesterolemia.
- Budd-Chiari syndrome: thrombosis of the hepatic vein.
- Portal vein thrombosis.

EPIDEMIOLOGY
- The incidence of venous thrombosis in children is estimated at 0.7 per 100,000 per year. It is likely that the actual incidence is higher.
- Two-thirds of children with thromboembolic disease have a predisposing underlying condition, the most common being an indwelling catheter.

COMPLICATIONS
- Complications vary depending on the location and severity of the thrombosis.
- For deep venous thrombosis, pulmonary embolism is the most significant acute complication with recurrent thrombosis and postphlebitic syndrome common chronic complications.
- For arterial thromboembolic disease the ischemic injury to the involved organ determines the acute and long-term complications.

 Differential Diagnosis

PRIMARY PROTHROMBOTIC STATES
Inherited
- Factor V Leiden
- Protein C deficiency
- Protein S deficiency
- Antithrombin (formerly antithrombin III) deficiency
- Plasminogen deficiency
- Dysfibrinogenemia
- Heparin cofactor II deficiency
- Plasminogen activator inhibitor type 1 excess
- Homocystinemia (mild to moderate) from minor defects in enzymes such as methylenetetrahydrofolate reductase (MTHFR)

- Prothrombin excess (e.g., prothrombin 20210A allele)
- Factor VIII excess
- Factor IX excess
- Factor XII deficiency
- Lipoprotein (a) excess
- Activated protein C resistance other than factor V Leiden (factor V Cambridge, factor V Hong Kong)

Acquired
- Antiphospholipid antibody syndrome
- Postinfectious protein C or S deficiency
- Severe neonatal acquired protein C or S deficiency

RISK FACTORS FOR THROMBOSIS
Neonatal
- Birth trauma
- Prematurity
- Maternal diabetes
- Severe RDS
- Hypernatremic dehydration
- Umbilical catheters
- Sepsis
- Polycythemia
- Perinatal asphyxia

Malignancy/Bone Marrow Disorders
- Leukemia (hyperleukocytosis, APML)
- Myeloproliferative disorders
- Paroxysmal nocturnal hemoglobinuria

Medications
- L-Asparaginase
- Oral contraceptives

Anatomic
- Indwelling catheters
- Cardiac catheterization
- Congenital heart disease
- Prosthetic heart valves
- Intracardiac baffles
- Tumor compression

Disorders Associated with Thrombosis
- Nephrotic syndrome
- Inflammatory disorders (e.g., IBD, SLE)
- Liver disease
- Heart failure/increased venous pressure
- Sickle cell disease
- Behçet disease
- Homocystinuria
- Diabetes mellitus

Miscellaneous Risk Factors
- Infection
- Trauma
- Orthopedic surgery (Hip)
- Strenuous exercise
- Prolonged immobilization or paralysis
- Prolonged sitting

Risk Factors/Conditions Specific for Arterial Disease
- Kawasaki disease
- Takayasu arteritis
- Other vasculitides
- Hyperlipidemia
- Blalock-Taussig shunts
- Organ transplantation

 Data Gathering

HISTORY
- Thromboembolic disease is commonly overlooked.
- A familial and/or personal history of thrombosis is an important risk factor for thrombosis.
- Neonatal seizure is a common and often sole presenting sign for dural sinus thrombosis.
- Presenting signs and symptoms of pulmonary embolism can be subtle and include dyspnea and chest pain.

 Physical Examination

- Pain, decreased perfusion/pulses, color change.
- Superficial dilated cutaneous veins distal to the site of venous occlusion.
- Unilateral swelling/edema of a limb (may be bilateral if the IVC or SVC is extensively involved).
- Chronic discoloration (darkening) of the skin, ulcerations, pain, intermittent swelling.
- Unexplained hepatosplenomegaly may be the only sign of hepatic or portal vein thrombosis.
- Abdominal pain and ileus may be present with involvement of mesenteric, portal, or hepatic vessels.

Approach to the Patient

Phase 1:

- D-dimer may be useful as a screening test in certain situations.
- Rapid evaluation of the hemostatic system prior to initiating therapy (CBC, PT/aPTT, fibrinogen).
- Therapy for thromboembolic disease should not be delayed.
- Whenever possible an antithrombin III level, a thrombin time, and a screen for the lupus anticoagulant should be drawn before starting heparin. Protein C and S levels should be drawn before starting warfarin and plasminogen levels prior to any thrombolytic therapy.

Phase 2:

- Serial imaging to assess response to treatment may be necessary.
- Search for an etiology of the thrombosis and evaluate risk factors.
- Test for factor V Leiden and anticardiolipin antibodies if not done with initial blood work.

Phase 3:

- Additional testing if a primary prothrombotic condition is strongly suspected.

Laboratory Aids

General evaluation of the hemostatic system:
- PT/PTT/fibrinogen
- CBC with platelet count
- FSP/d-dimer
- Thrombin time

The following tests are used to investigate for a prothrombotic state:

Phase 1:

- Factor V Leiden mutation analysis by PCR
- Prothrombin 20210A allele by PCR
- Lupus anticoagulant screen (dRVVT, TTI, dilute PTT)
- Anticardiolipin antibodies (IgG, IgM, IgA)
- Protein C activity
- Protein S activity
- Antithrombin activity
- Lipid profile for arterial disease

Phase 2:

- MTHFR-T by PCR
- Factor VIII activity
- Lipoprotein a
- Plasminogen
- Thrombin time or dysfibrinogenemia screen
- Activated protein C resistance clotting assay
- Plasma homocysteine levels

Phase 3:

- Heparin cofactor II
- Tissue plasminogen activator (post-veno-occlusion)
- Plasminogen activator inhibitor type 1
- Factor XII activity
- Factor IX activity

IMAGING

- Ultrasound—least invasive but sensitivity for DVT in upper extremities variable.
- Magnetic resonance imaging with contrast (MRA/MRV)—expensive, time-consuming, and not adequately studied in children against the gold standard.
- Contrast angiography—is the gold standard but invasive and sometimes technically difficult to perform in small children.

PITFALLS

- Normal ranges for coagulation tests are age dependent: diagnosing an inherited deficiency in any of the anticoagulants can be difficult in the neonatal period. Repeat testing at 6 to 12 months of age is necessary.
- Consumption can occur during acute thrombosis, therefore, low levels must be repeated.
- Warfarin will decrease the levels of protein C and protein S.

Therapy

- Therapy for acute thrombosis and long-term management is individualized.
- Consult a pediatric hematologist or someone with expertise in pediatric anticoagulant therapy.

DRUGS

- Standard heparin (SH): Given as a bolus followed by an infusion, adjusted to maintain the aPTT at about two times baseline. The younger the child the more heparin per weight is required to achieve a therapeutic level.
- Low molecular weight heparin (LMWH): More predictable dose response. Given subcutaneously twice a day. Equivalent in efficacy to SH in the acute management of uncomplicated DVT.
- Urokinase: Agent with most experience in pediatric patients. Given as a bolus followed by an infusion for 12 to 24 hours.
- Recombinant tissue plasminogen activator (tPA): a recombinant thrombolytic agent with theoretical advantages over urokinase.
- Warfarin: an oral anticoagulant given as a loading dose, adjusted to maintain the INR at 2.0–3.0.
- Aspirin

Follow-Up

- Growth of involved limbs, especially following an arterial event.
- Avoid acquired risk factors for vascular disease.
- Medical risk factors should be controlled.

PITFALLS

Central venous catheter related thrombosis may be completely asymptomatic despite extensive damage to the venous system. The long-term consequences of this are not known, but recurrent thrombosis years after the line has been removed, when the patient is older, is a possibility.

Common Questions and Answers

Q: What is the optimal strategy for preventing thrombosis associated with indwelling catheters?
A: Low-dose warfarin holds some promise in that the rate of thrombosis is decreased with minimal adverse effects. Using urokinase instead of heparin to flush the lines is an option; however, there is no strong evidence to suggest it is better than heparin.

Q: If an inherited prothrombotic condition is identified, should family members be tested?
A: If they have other risk factors for thrombosis such as malignancy, major surgery, oral contraceptives, obesity, etc.

Q: When is it appropriate to use LMWH rather than standard heparin?
A: There are several potential advantages to LMWH. The pharmacokinetics are much more predictable and frequent monitoring is not necessary. It is administered subcutaneously, not intravenous. The risk of bleeding may be slightly lower.

Q: When is it appropriate to use thrombolytic therapy?
A: Studies do not clearly demonstrate a role for thrombolytic therapy in DVT. However, if a thrombus extends on heparin therapy, a pulmonary embolus is suspected, or if the disturbance in blood flow causes ischemia, thrombolytic therapy can be used. Intracranial bleeding is a contraindication. For arterial thrombotic events, thrombolytic therapy is often the treatment of choice because of the rapid resolution of the clot and restoration of blood flow.

Q: What precautions should be taken for invasive procedures and for athletics when a patient is on anticoagulant therapy?
A: Lumbar punctures, arterial punctures, and surgical procedures should be avoided. If they are necessary, then the child should have the anticoagulant partially or fully reversed prior to the procedure. The child should not participate in contact sports such as football, karate, and boxing. For baseball, a helmet should be worn at all times.

Issues for Referral

- Pediatric hematologists should be consulted to assist in evaluating for primary hypercoagulable states and assisting in the management of anticoagulant therapy. The management of these children can be problematic and the advice of a specialist is recommended.
- Interventional radiologists should be consulted for choosing the best imaging study for diagnosis and follow-up.
- Surgical thrombectomy or vascular reconstruction is rarely necessary and carries considerable risk.

BIBLIOGRAPHY

Andrew M, Michelson AD, Bovill E, et al. Guidelines for antithrombotic therapy in pediatric patients. *J Pediatr* 1998;132: 575–588.

Andrew M, Monagle PT, Brooker L. *Thromboembolic complications during infancy and childhood*. Hamilton, Ont: BC Decker, 2000.

Author: J. Nathan Hagstrom

Upper GI Bleeding

 Database

DEFINITION

Vomiting of blood whether bright red or dark constitutes upper gastrointestinal (GI) bleeding or hematemesis. This usually represents bleeding from the GI tract proximal to the ligament of Treitz. One has to differentiate from hemoptysis (coughing up of blood), nose bleeds, and bleeding from the mouth and pharynx. Sometimes upper GI bleeding can present with melena or the passage of tarry stools.

 Differential Diagnosis

- 95% of the causes of UGI bleeding are due to mucosal abnormalities or esophageal varices.
- Mucosal lesions are more likely to be associated with antecedent occult bleeding.
- In about 80% to 95% of patients the bleeding stops spontaneously.
- Age of the patient is important.

NEONATAL PERIOD

- Swallowed maternal blood
- Hemorrhagic disease of the newborn
- Esophagitis/gastritis
- Stress ulcer
- Foreign body irritation
- Vascular malformation

INFANCY

- Esophagitis/gastritis
- Stress ulcer
- Mallory-Weiss tear
- Pyloric stenosis
- Vascular malformation
- Duplication cysts

PRESCHOOL AGED

- Esophageal varices
- Esophagitis/gastritis/ulcer
- Foreign body/bezoar
- Mallory-Weiss tear
- Vascular malformation

SCHOOL AGED

- Esophageal varices
- Esophagitis/gastritis/ulcer
- Mallory-Weiss tear
- Inflammatory bowel disease

Approach to the Patient

GENERAL GOALS

Determine the cause of the bleeding and begin treatment.

Phase 1: Determine if blood or food coloring, beets. Hematest material.

Phase 2: Assess severity of bleeding. Is there a change in vital signs, hematocrit, blood pressures, capillary filling, pulse?

Phase 3: Determine the site of bleeding and begin treatment. Examine airway for bleeding—epistaxis may contaminate vomitus to appear as upper GI bleeding. Usually will require imaging or endoscopy.

HINTS FOR SCREENING PROBLEM

- Bright red blood signifies active bleeding.
- Darker blood or "coffee grounds" usually means that the blood has had some time to be denatured by gastric acid.
- The rate of bleeding will determine the clinical presentation. The more rapid the rate, the larger the volume of upper GI bleeding and the greater the drop in hemoglobin and change in pulse and blood pressure. Slower bleeding usually presents with anemia and heme positive stools.
- Any significant blood loss will lead to pallor, tachycardia, orthostasis, poor capillary refill, CNS changes (restlessness, confusion), and hypotension. Hypotension may not be seen even in the face of significant blood loss because vasoconstriction will occur to maintain blood pressure until decompensation.
- Initial hemoglobin values may be unreliable because a delay in hemodilution may falsely result in near normal values.
- Absence of blood in the emesis or in nasogastric lavage fluid does not rule out the upper GI tract as the site of bleeding, because a competent pylorus may mask bleeding from a duodenal site. In fact, in some cases of massive UGI bleeding, the patient may not vomit blood but may pass large, black, tarry, or sticky stools, called melena.

 Data Gathering

HISTORY

Question: Amount of blood, i.e., drops versus 1 teaspoon versus 1 tablespoon? Any clots?
Significance: Indicates severity of bleeding.

Question: Vomitus contains blood?
Significance: Indicates bleeding from upper GI tract or swallowed blood.

Question: Any recently ingested foods resemble blood, e.g., red food dye, beets, Jell-o, Kool-Aid, antibiotic syrups, food fibers?
Significance: Vomitus may not have blood.

Question: Can one determine the source of bleeding?
Significance: Hematemesis from the esophagus, stomach, or duodenum versus hemoptysis versus swallowed blood from the nose, mouth, or pharynx.

Question: Was the blood coughed or vomited?
Significance: Indicative of hemoptysis.

Question: Was it from the nose—swallowed and then vomited?
Significance: Not bleeding from the upper GI tract.

Question: Was there prolonged vomiting preceding the bleeding?
Significance: Prolonged retching prior to hematemesis suggests a Mallory-Weiss tear.

Question: History of recent stress (burns, head trauma, surgery)?
Significance: Suggests an ulcer or gastritis.

Question: History of toxic ingestion?
Significance: May result in an ulcerated esophagus, which can bleed.

Question: Ingestion of certain medications?
Significance: Aspirin, steroids can lead to gastritis and ulcers. Ingestion of drugs (nonsteroidal antiinflammatory drugs) and alcohol can lead to gastritis.

Question: Abdominal pain and vomiting blood?
Significance: Suggests esophagitis, gastritis, and peptic ulcers

Question: Is there breast-feeding?
Significance: Cracked nipples in the mother can lead to the infant swallowing maternal blood and then having hematemesis.

Question: Is there history of gastroesophageal reflux?
Significance: Suggests esophagitis.

Question: Is there past history of GI disease?
Significance: Gastroesophageal reflux, peptic ulcer disease, or previous GI surgery may suggest that the current symptoms may be due to recurrence of disease.

Question: Is there history of jaundice, hepatitis, or liver disease?
Significance: Suggests portal hypertension and variceal bleeding.

Question: Was there any neonatal history of umbilical vein catheterization or infection?
Significance: Portal vein thrombosis (sepsis, shock, exchange transfusion, omphalitis, IV catheters) suggests portal hypertension and bleeding varices due to cavernous transformation of the portal vein.

Question: Familial history of bleeding?
Significance: Familial history of bleeding diathesis, e.g., von Willebrand disease, hemophilia.

Physical Examination

Finding: Are there any skin petechiae, ecchymosis, hemangiomas?
Significance: Evidence of chronic liver disease (spider angiomata, palmar erythema, jaundice). Look for evidence of chronic liver disease and bleeding diathesis.

Finding: HEENT: Nasopharyngeal source of bleeding
Significance: Swallowed blood

Finding: Freckles on buccal mucosa
Significance: Osler-Weber-Rendu syndrome; Peutz-Jeghers syndrome

Finding: Oral thrush
Significance: *Candida* esophagitis

Finding: Oral mucosal lesions
Significance: Corrosive ingestions

Finding: Abdomen

- Hepatosplenomegaly
- Ascites

Significance: Portal hypertension

Finding: Isolated splenomegaly
Significance: Cavernous transformation of the portal vein; portal hypertension

Finding: Rectal examination
Significance: Heme-positive stool may or may not be present. If positive, confirms the presence of UGI bleeding.

 ## Laboratory Aids

Test: Guaiac or Hematest
Significance: If possible check the red substance for blood. In neonates, may need to check for fetal hemoglobin with the Apt test.

Test: CBC
Significance: If there is leukopenia, anemia, and thrombocytopenia, think chronic liver disease and portal hypertension. If there is anemia with normal RBC indices, then there is truly an acute cause for bleeding. If RBC indices indicate iron-deficiency anemia, think of varices or a mucosal lesion, i.e., chronic blood loss.

Test: Coagulation profile
Significance: If PT/PTT are abnormal, then think of liver disease or disseminated intravascular coagulation (DIC) with sepsis. If DIC screen is negative, think liver disease. Make sure, however, that blood sample was not contaminated with heparin.

Test: Bleeding time
Significance: Abnormal in patients with previous history (or family history) of bleeding disorders.

Test: Liver function tests
Significance: Abnormal in chronic liver disease

Test: Upper endoscopy
Significance: Useful, as diagnosis can be made in 75% to 90% of patients.

Test: Barium tests
Significance: Not as useful as esophagogastroduodenoscopy (EGD) but can identify a large ulcer. Air-contrast UGI better than regular UGI test.

Test: Bleeding scan
Significance: Useful in the patient with significant bleeding in whom endoscopy was not diagnostic. Can get two types of scans: technetium sulfur colloid or tagged RBC scan. The former detects very rapid bleeding but can miss small bleeds, especially if patient is not bleeding during the scan. The latter can detect small bleeds, especially if intermittent.

Test: Angiography
Significance: Useful in detecting vascular causes for UGI bleeding. Can also be therapeutic, i.e., injection of coils into a vascular malformation to occlude it. Invasiveness and need for specialized training are limitations.

 ## Therapy

Initial management of the emergency depends on diagnosis and clinical condition of the patient.

- Stabilize the patient with intravenous fluids and blood products if necessary.
- Order laboratory tests: CBC, PT/PTT, DIC screen, liver function tests, blood type, and crossmatch.
- Insert an NG tube and lavage with saline to determine site as well as rate of ongoing bleeding. No need for cold saline.
- Monitor patient's vital signs and hemoglobin as necessary.
- Make appropriate diagnosis and institute appropriate therapy, i.e., EGD, bleeding scans.

DISEASE-SPECIFIC THERAPY

- Peptic ulcer disease

—Proton pump inhibitors
—H_2 blockers
—Sucralfate
—Prokinetic agents

- Esophageal varices

—Vasopressin or somatostatin infusion
—Sclerotherapy or banding
—Sengstaken-Blakemore tube

If bleeding stops quickly, then workup is less emergent.

 ## Follow-Up

- Monitor hemoglobin in the hospital until stable
- Once patient is discharged, monitor hemoglobin weekly as well as Hemoccult cards until stable.
- More specific follow-up depends on the underlying condition.

PREVENTION

- Avoid drugs that are likely to cause bleeding or gastritis especially in a susceptible patient.
- In patients with chronic GI conditions, optimize therapy and monitoring.
- Correct coagulopathy
- Prophylactic sclerotherapy or banding for patients with known variceal bleeds

PITFALLS

- Make sure the vomited material is really blood.
- A negative nasogastric aspirate for blood does not indicate the absence of upper GI bleeding.
- Initial hemoglobin may not be accurate and serial hemoglobins should be obtained.

 ## Common Questions and Answers

Q: When do you refer a patient?
A: Any bleed—immediate referral if bleed is large, the patient is hemodynamically unstable, and bleeding will not stop. Patient with evidence of chronic iron deficiency anemia and heme-positive stools.

Q: What makes upper GI bleeding an emergency?
A: Any persistent bleed with change in vital signs. Significant drop in hemoglobin.

BIBLIOGRAPHY

Ament M. Diagnosis and management of upper gastrointestinal bleeding in the pediatric patient. *Pediatr Rev* 1990;12:107–116.

Hassal E. Sclerotherapy for extrahepatic nonvariceal upper GI bleeding. *Med Clin North Am* 1993;77:973–992.

Sherman PM. Peptic ulcer disease in children—diagnosis, treatment and the implication of *Helicobater pylor*. *Gastroenterol Clin North Am* 1994;23(4):707–725.

Vinton NE. Gastrointestinal bleeding in infancy and childhood. *Gastroenterol Clin North Am* 1994;23(1):93–122.

Author: Maria R. Mascarenhas

Vomiting

Database

DEFINITION

The expulsion of gastric contents through the mouth in varying degrees. Regurgitation is defined as small, effortless mouthfuls of food or stomach contents. Vomiting is usually associated with large, forceful amounts of stomach contents.

Differential Diagnosis

DISORDERS OF GASTROINTESTINAL TRACT

• Anatomic

—Esophageal: stricture, web, ring, atresia
—Stomach: pyloric stenosis, web, duplication
—Intestine: duodenal atresia, malrotation, duplication
—Colon: Hirschsprung disease, imperforate anus

• Motility

—Achalasia
—Gastroesophageal reflux
—Intestinal pseudo-obstruction

• Foreign body/bezoar
• Obstruction

—Intussusception
—Volvulus
—Incarcerated hernia

• Cholecystitis or cholelithiasis
• Eosinophilic enteritis
• Appendicitis
• Necrotizing enterocolitis
• Peritonitis
• Celiac disease
• Peptic ulcer
• Trauma

—Duodenal hematoma
—Pancreatitis (pseudocyst)

NEUROLOGIC

• Intracranial mass lesions

—Tumor
—Cyst
—Subdural hematoma

• Cerebral edema
• Hydrocephalus
• Pseudotumor cerebri
• Migraine (head, abdominal)
• Seizures

RENAL

• Obstructive uropathy

—Ureteropelvic junction obstruction
—Hydronephrosis
—Nephrolithiasis

• Renal insufficiency
• Glomerulonephritis
• Renal tubular acidosis

METABOLIC

• Inborn errors of metabolism

—Galactosemia
—Fructose intolerance
—Hereditary fructose intolerance
—Amino acid or organic acid metabolism
—Urea cycle defects
—Fatty acid oxidation disorders
—Lactic acidosis

INFECTION

• Sepsis
• Meningitis
• Urinary tract infection
• Parasites
• *Giardia*
• Ascaris
• *Helicobacter pylori*
• Otitis media
• Viral/bacterial

—Gastroenteritis
—Viral hepatitis (A, B, C)
—*Bordetella* pertussis

ENDOCRINE

• Diabetes

—Diabetic ketoacidosis (DKA)
—Gastroparesis

• Adrenal insufficiency

RESPIRATORY

• Pneumonia
• Sinusitis
• Laryngitis

IMMUNOLOGIC

• Milk/soy protein allergy
• *Cryptosporidium* (AIDS)
• Graft-versus-host disease
• Chronic granulomatous disease

OTHER

• Pregnancy
• Rumination
• Bulimia
• Psychogenic
• Cyclic emesis syndrome
• Overfeeding
• Medications

—Drugs
—Vitamin toxicity

• Vascular (superior mesenteric artery syndrome)

Approach to the Patient

Vomiting is a prominent feature of many disorders of infancy and childhood and is often the only presenting symptom of many diseases. Vomiting can occur as a defense mechanism to expel ingested toxins, as an abnormality of the vomiting center related to increased intracranial pressure, as a result of intestinal obstruction or anatomic/mucosal abnormalities, or as the result of a generalized metabolic disease. A full history should include medication and drug use, trauma, and, in adolescents, questions regarding feeding disorders (bulimia) and intercourse (pregnancy).

Data Gathering

History

Question: Fever?
Significance: Infectious causes of vomiting are common.

Question: Abdominal pain and frequent, forceful or bilious emesis?
Significance: Often associated with anatomic or obstructive intestinal disorder.

Question: Age of patient?
Significance: Pyloric stenosis and inborn errors of metabolism almost always present in infancy with vomiting, dehydration, and biochemical abnormalities.

Question: Mental retardation, pica, and patchy baldness?
Significance: Foreign body or hair ingestion and the development of a gastric bezoar.

Question: Nausea and epigastric pain related to meals?
Significance: Often indicates gastritis, gastric emptying delay, or gallbladder disease.

Question: Alleviated by meals?
Significance: Gastroesophageal reflux and gastric ulcer disease

Question: Alternating vomiting and lethargy?
Significance: Intussusception

Question: Chronic headaches, fatigue, weakness, weight loss, and early morning vomiting?
Significance: Neurologic causes of vomiting secondary to increased intracranial pressure

Question: Right- or left-sided abdominal pain?
Significance: Renal disease, inflammatory bowel disease

Physical Examination

A careful and complete physical examination can often provide excellent clues as to the cause of vomiting in children.

Finding: Visible bowel loops
Significance: Obstruction

Finding: Palpation for a mass effect and tenderness, and auscultation for evidence of absent bowel sounds or borborygmi (rumbling bowel sounds)
Significance: Intestinal obstruction

Finding: Rectal examination
Significance: Testing the stool for occult blood

Finding: Discoloration of skin and sclera
Significance: Jaundice (liver/gallbladder or metabolic disease)

Finding: Orange tint of sclera or skin
Significance: Hypervitaminosis A

Finding: Unusual odor
Significance: Metabolic disease

Finding: Chronic vomiting
Significance: Evidence of neurologic dysfunction, including nystagmus, head tilt, papilledema, abnormal reflexes, and weakness

Finding: Tense anterior fontanelle
Significance: May indicate meningitis, hydrocephalus, or vitamin A toxicity

Finding: Enlarged parotid glands and hypersalivation
Significance: Bulimia and other feeding disorders

Finding: Pelvic examination
Significance: Pregnancy, pelvic inflammatory disease, or ovarian disease

 ## Laboratory Aids

Test: CBC
Significance: Anemia and iron deficiency can occur with intestinal duplication and obstruction, gastritis/esophagitis, and ulcer disease.

Test: Blood chemistry
Significance: Electrolyte abnormalities are found in pyloric stenosis, metabolic abnormalities, while an elevated ALT, total bilirubin, and GGT can indicate liver, gallbladder, or metabolic disease.

Test: Urinalysis
Significance: Pyelonephritis

Test: Amylase
Significance: Pancreatitis

Test: BUN/creatinine
Significance: If elevated—renal disease

Test: Urine culture
Significance: UTI

Test: Plain abdominal x-ray study
Significance: Obstruction

Test: Abdominal ultrasound
Significance: Liver, gallbladder, renal, pancreatic, ovarian, or uterine disease. In infants, abdominal ultrasound is the test of choice for pyloric stenosis. Useful when considering abdominal abscess and appendicitis.

Test: Contrast radiography
Significance: Intestinal anatomic abnormalities (malrotation, intussusception, volvulus)

Test: Computed tomography
Significance: Not generally indicated for evaluation of vomiting, although it is an effective tool when more anatomic abdominal detail is required (abscess, tumor).

Test: Endoscopy
Significance: Esophageal, gastric, and duodenal inflammation (esophagitis, gastritis, ulcer disease, celiac disease, eosinophilic enteritis) as well as for obtaining cultures for unusual infections (duodenal *Giardia*, *Helicobacter pylori*/cytomegalovirus gastritis).

Issues for Referral

- Chronic vomiting (2–3 weeks)
- Weight loss
- Severe abdominal pain or irritability
- Gastrointestinal bleeding
- Evidence of intestinal obstruction
- Serum electrolyte abnormalities
- Abnormal neurologic examination
- Dehydration
- Signs of an acute abdomen
- Lethargy

 ## Emergency Care

Evidence of hematemesis, intestinal obstruction (bilious vomiting), dehydration, neurologic dysfunction, or an acute abdomen should be treated as a medical emergency, and hospitalization should be considered.

BIBLIOGRAPHY

Silverman A, Roy CC, eds. *Pediatric clinical gastroenterology*, 3rd ed. St. Louis: CV Mosby, 1983.

Sondheimer J. Vomiting and regurgitation. In: Walker WA, Durie PR, Hamilton JR, et al., eds. *Pediatric gastrointestinal disease*. St. Louis: Mosby, 1996:19.

Author: Chris A. Liacouras

Weight Loss

 Database

DEFINITION

Weight loss is a documented decrease in weight from a previous measurement. Outside of the newborn period (weight loss in the first 2 weeks is common), acute illnesses resulting in fluid loss, and obese adolescents voluntarily on a designed weight reduction program, weight loss is an unusual and worrisome symptom, regardless of the percentage decline.

 Differential Diagnosis

CONGENITAL/ANATOMIC

- Congenital heart disease
- Pyloric stenosis
- Gastrointestinal malformation (duodenal atresia, annular pancreas, volvulus)
- Short bowel syndrome
- Lymphangiectasia
- Superior mesenteric artery syndrome
- Gastroesophageal reflux
- Immunodeficiency disorders
- Hirschsprung disease

INFECTIOUS

- Urinary tract infection
- Tuberculosis
- Stomatitis
- Osteomyelitis
- Human immunodeficiency virus
- Hepatitis
- Parasitic disease
- Abscess, intraabdominal
- Gastroenteritis
- Pericarditis
- Histoplasmosis
- Acute severe febrile illness (pyelonephritis, pneumonia, septic arthritis)

TOXIC, ENVIRONMENTAL, DRUGS

- Lead poisoning
- Mercury poisoning
- Vitamin A poisoning
- Chronic methylphenidate, dextroamphetamine, or valproic acid use
- Substance abuse, especially amphetamines and crack cocaine

TRAUMA

- Chronic subdural hematomas

TUMOR

- Diencephalic syndrome
- Leukemia
- Lymphoma
- Pheochromocytoma
- Other neoplasms

GENETIC/METABOLIC

- Diabetes mellitus
- Diabetes insipidus
- Hyperthyroidism
- Cystic fibrosis
- Schwachman syndrome
- Addison disease
- Hypercalcemia
- Congenital adrenal hyperplasia
- Lactose intolerance
- Renal tubular acidosis
- Chronic renal failure
- Hypopituitarism
- Inborn errors of metabolism
- Storage diseases
- Muscular dystrophy
- Lipodystrophy

ALLERGIC/INFLAMMATORY

- Inflammatory bowel disease
- Juvenile rheumatoid arthritis
- Systemic lupus erythematosus
- Sarcoidosis
- Pancreatitis
- Hepatitis
- Celiac disease (gluten enteropathy)

FUNCTIONAL/MISCELLANEOUS

- Malnutrition
- Child abuse
- Postoperative
- Dieting
- Rumination syndrome
- Depression/affective disorders
- Anorexia nervosa
- Chronic congestive heart failure
- Chronic pulmonary disease
- Chronic renal disease
- Iron deficiency
- Zinc deficiency
- Cerebral palsy
- Postinfectious malabsorption
- Factitious (e.g., scale error)

Approach to the Patient

GENERAL GOAL

Determine the acuity or chronicity and severity of weight loss, and the need for hospitalization.

Phase 1: Attempt to narrow the diagnostic possibilities by history and examination, particularly by assessing if the loss might be attributable to diminished intake, diminished absorption, or increased requirements.

 Data Gathering

HISTORY

Question: Is the weight loss real?
Significance: Scale error, different scales, different technique (e.g., clothed versus unclothed)

Question: What is the child's diet?
Significance: A prospective 3-day dietary record can be very useful for demonstrating insufficient caloric intake.

Question: Less than 2 weeks of age?
Significance: Physiologic weight loss, underfeeding, inappropriate feeding, inborn errors of metabolism, congenital heart disease, gastroesophageal reflux

Question: Less than 4 months?
Significance: Malnutrition, improper formula preparation, cystic fibrosis, gastroesophageal reflux, pyloric stenosis, congenital heart disease, congenital adrenal hyperplasia, inborn errors of metabolism

Question: 4 months to 8 years?
Significance: Chronic infection, cystic fibrosis, malabsorption, neglect/abuse, renal disease, liver disease, diabetes mellitus

Question: Older than 8 years?
Significance: Eating disorder, chronic infection, neoplasm, renal disease, liver disease, substance abuse, diabetes mellitus, inflammatory bowel disease, collagen vascular disease

Question: Cramping, bloating or abnormally greasy, voluminous stools?
Significance: Possible malabsorption

Question: Vomiting, especially projectile?
Significance: Suggestive of intestinal obstruction, G-E reflux, inborn errors of metabolism

Question: Polyuria, polydipsia, and polyphagia?
Significance: Possible diabetes mellitus

Question: Headaches, especially early morning?
Significance: Possible increased intracranial pressure, CNS malignancy

Question: Maternal history of multiple miscarriages, neonatal deaths, or consanguinity?
Significance: Possible inborn error of metabolism

Question: History of severe infections, persistent candidal infections?
Significance: Immunodeficiency, congenital or acquired

Question: Fear of fatness, preoccupation with food, distorted body image, and/or amenorrhea?
Significance: Possible eating disorder

Question: Delayed puberty?
Significance: Suggests chronic severe weight loss, pituitary abnormalities, anorexia nervosa

Question: Foreign travel?
Significance: Possible chronic infection (e.g., tuberculosis, parasitic disease)

Question: Tiring during feeding or difficulty feeding due to cough and dyspnea?

Significance: Suggests CHF in newborn/infant, hypothyroidism

Question: Increased appetite with weight loss?
Significance: Suggests hyperthyroidism, cystic fibrosis, pheochromocytoma

Question: Altered mental status, seizures, unusual body/fluid odors
Significance: Inborn error of metabolism

Physical Examination

Finding: Clubbing
Significance: Suggests chronic cardiac, pulmonary, or intestinal disease

Finding: Significant abdominal distension
Significance: Suggests celiac disease

Finding: Hypothermia, bradycardia
Significance: Suggests anorexia nervosa, hypothyroidism

Finding: Tachycardia, resting
Significance: Hyperthyroidism, pheochromocytoma, anemia, acute weight loss

Finding: Orthostatic changes
Significance: Significant weight loss, possibly acute

Finding: Hypotension, resting
Significance: Addison disease, anorexia nervosa, significant acute dehydration

Finding: Visual field abnormalities
Significance: Suggests possible CNS malignancy

Finding: Swollen joint
Significance: Juvenile rheumatoid arthritis, inflammatory bowel disease

Finding: Muscle weakness
Significance: Connective tissue disorder, electrolyte abnormality, muscular dystrophy

Finding: Enlarged liver and/or spleen
Significance: Suggests malignancy, chronic infection, storage disease, inborn error of metabolism

Laboratory Aids

Test: Complete blood count
Significance:

• Evidence of

—Anemia—macrocytic associated with folate/B_{12} deficiency, microcytic with iron deficiency or chronic infection
—Polycythemia—suggestive of chronic pulmonary or cardiac disease
—Neutropenia—suggestive of hematologic malignancy, Schwachman syndrome, immunodeficiency

—Lymphopenia—suggestive of immunodeficiency
—Eosinophilia—suggestive of parasitic disease
—Leukocytosis—suggestive of infection
—Thrombocytosis—suggestive of chronic infection, malignancy
—Lymphoblasts—suggestive of leukemia

Test: ESR
Significance: May be elevated in inflammatory bowel disease, chronic infections, rheumatoid diseases

Test: Serum electrolytes
Significance: Abnormalities in dehydration, adrenal insufficiency (low Na, high K), renal disease, anorexia nervosa

Test: BUN, creatinine
Significance: Abnormal in renal disease, dehydration

Test: Stool for occult blood and pH, reducing substances (Clinitest)
Significance: Occult blood suggests inflammatory bowel disease; low pH and positive reducing substances suggest malabsorption

Test: Urinalysis
Significance: Hematuria and/or proteinuria suggest renal disease; glycosuria suggests diabetes mellitus; very low specific gravity suggests diabetes insipidus, chronic renal failure, hypercalcemia; pyuria suggests UTI; pH >6 suggests RTA (type I)

Test: Urine culture
Significance: Evaluation for UTI

Test: Serum protein levels
Significance: Very low levels imply impaired liver function, severe chronic weight loss or protein malabsorption

Test: Tuberculosis skin test
Significance: Possible chronic infection

Test: Liver function tests
Significance: Evaluation for hepatitis, chronic liver disease

Depending on age and clinical findings, other tests to consider include thyroid function tests, sweat test, tests for malabsorption (e.g., lactose breath test, stool fat, stool for trypsin), tests for metabolic disease (e.g., plasma ammonia, lactate, serum/urine amino acids, urine organic acids), imaging studies (e.g., CT, MRI, bone scan), immunologic studies.

Emergency Care

• Significant dehydration: abnormal vital signs with orthostasis, decreased urine output, decreased skin turgor, delayed capillary refill (>3 seconds). Mandates cardiovascular support (intravenous hydration) and a more urgent diagnosis (e.g., inborn error of metabolism, obstructive GI disease, congenital adrenal hyperplasia, diabetic ketoacidosis).

• Abnormal mental status, significant lethargy: May be seen in severe dehydration, hypoadrenalism, hypoxic states, toxic ingestions, renal or respiratory failure, increased intracranial pressure, severe electrolyte abnormalities.
• Increasing vomiting in the setting of known weight loss in infants: high risk for dehydration, hypoglycemia, and electrolyte abnormalities. Need to evaluate for treatable conditions (e.g., obstructive GI disease, inborn errors of metabolism, congenital adrenal hyperplasia, congenital heart disease) in which a delay is life-threatening.
• Severe malnutrition (weight loss >20% of ideal body weight): high risk for metabolic derangements, including dysrhythmias secondary to electrolyte abnormalities. Aggressive evaluation is warranted.

Common Questions and Answers

Q: How common is weight loss in the first 2 weeks of life?
A: Formula-fed babies may lose up to 7% of birth weight and breast-fed newborns up to 10% before regaining their birth weight by 2 weeks of age.

Issues for Referral

Weight loss is a diagnostic exigency—a cause must be found or the loss self-resolved. If a diagnosis is not uncovered in the setting of continued weight loss, referral to a pediatric diagnostic center is indicated.

Clinical Pearls

• Be certain that the weight loss is real. In some studies, up to 25% of weight loss is artifactual as a result of measurement errors (e.g., excessive movement of scale, dressed versus undressed patient).
• Newborns with weight loss, especially at the 2-week visit, may manifest passivity and paradoxical lack of interest in breast-feeding, although the reason for their problem is malnourishment due to inadequate intake (often from improper positioning or too infrequent feedings). They may not act "hungry." Observation of the feeding technique (by a practitioner with expertise or a lactation consultant) is vital.

BIBLIOGRAPHY

Kleinman RE, ed. *Pediatric nutrition handbook*, 4th ed. Elk Grove Village, IL: American Academy of Pediatrics, 1998.

Maisels MJ, Gifford K. Breast-feeding, weight loss, and jaundice. *J Pediatr* 1983;102:117–118.

Schechter M. Weight loss/failure to thrive. *Pediatr Rev* 2000;21:238–239.

Author: Mark F. Ditmar

Wheezing

 Database

DEFINITION

Wheezing is a continuous sound that occurs primarily during expiration due to airway narrowing anywhere along the respiratory tract. The sound is due to the turbulent flow of air through the obstructed region. It is often described as musical in nature and with a variable pitch.

 Differential Diagnosis

CONGENITAL/ANATOMIC

Anterior Mediastinum

- Thymic mass, teratoma, angioma, lymphoma

Middle Mediastinum

- Vascular anomalies
- Double aortic arch, vascular ring, pulmonary sling
- Left atrial enlargement
- Lymphoma
- Lymphadenopathy
- Bronchogenic cyst

Posterior Mediastinum

- Neurogenic tumor
- Duplication/bronchogenic cyst
- Intrinsic to airway

Airway Wall

- Tracheomalacia
- Bronchomalacia
- Laryngotracheal stenosis

Intraluminal

- Foreign body
- Neoplasia
- Hemangioma, endobronchial tumor
- Paralyzed vocal cord

Peripheral

- Asthma
- Bronchopulmonary dysplasia
- Pulmonary edema

INFLAMMATORY/INFECTIOUS

- Bronchiolitis/viral pneumonia/laryngotracheitis
- Pneumonia

—Streptococcus, Staphylococcus, Haemophilus, Moraxella, Mycoplasma, Chlamydia

- Recurrent aspiration
- Pneumonitis
- Bronchiectasis
- Bronchial papilloma
- Pulmonary hemosiderosis

GENETIC/METABOLIC

- Cystic fibrosis
- Immotile cilia syndrome (Kartagener syndrome)

ALLERGIC

- Asthma
- Allergic bronchopulmonary aspergillosis

PSYCHOSOMATIC

- Vocal cord dysfunction
- Psychogenic wheezing

Approach to the Patient

GENERAL GOALS

Phase 1: Quickly determine the severity of the patient's general status and degree of respiratory distress and triage accordingly.

Phase 2: Determine the most likely causes of wheezing.

Phase 3: Initiate appropriate therapies.

 Data Gathering

HISTORY

Question: What is/has been the pattern of the wheezing?
Significance: A rapid onset is suggestive of a foreign body or a postexposure exacerbation, while a slow onset may suggest an infectious etiology. Periods of recurrent wheezing are suggestive of asthma. Nocturnal and early morning wheezing can go along with gastroesophageal reflux, sinusitis, and dust mite or mold sensitivity. Wheezing in association with or soon after a meal can be seen in swallowing dysfunction and gastroesophageal reflux. Wheezing that worsens with crying is suggestive of tracheomalacia and/or bronchomalacia or a fixed intraluminal or extraluminal obstruction.

Question: Timing to exertion?
Significance: Onset after stopping exercise—

—Exercise induced asthma.

Question: Multiple exacerbations with clearing or persistent symptoms?
Significance: Multiple cycles of exacerbations with clearing in between suggests a chronic process such as asthma, cystic fibrosis, and bronchopulmonary dysplasia, while persistent wheezing is more common with fixed anatomic abnormalities.

Question: What are the triggers?
Significance: Common triggers include smoke, dust, animal dander, change in humidity or temperature, change in seasons (pollens, grasses, molds), and exercise.

Question: Is there a family history?
Significance: A positive family history of wheezing, asthma, or atopy—asthma.

Question: Did an episode of choking precede the onset of wheezing?
Significance: A history of choking mandates consideration of foreign body aspiration.

 Physical Examination

- Observe: assess the patient's degree of respiratory difficulty.

—Tachypnea—The body's compensation to maintain minute ventilation after loss of ventilatory capacity due to airway obstruction.
—Accessory muscle usage—
—use of intercostal and sternocleidomastoid muscles and abdominal musculature, and indicates increased expiratory effort to overcome airway obstruction.

- Subcostal retractions—With air-trapping and hyperinflation, the diaphragm is in a more horizontal position and its contraction causes inward motion of the ribs.
- Nasal flaring—With increasing respiratory difficulty the nares will be dilated to decrease the resistance to air flow of the nares.
- Palpate: Assess symmetry of chest motion.

—Thoracoabdominal asynchrony
—Asymmetric inflation

- Auscultate: Assess airflow, symmetry of breath sounds, and for adventitious sounds.

Significance: Aeration—Decreased aeration is much worse prognostically than wheezing since it is directly related to the amount of aeration and, therefore, ventilation and gas exchange. With decreased aeration wheezing may not be audible.

Timing in respiratory cycle—Inspiratory continuous sounds (stridor) typically indicate an extrathoracic obstruction except in situations with a *fixed* intrathoracic obstruction. Continuous expiratory sounds (wheezing) typically indicate intrathoracic obstruction.
Ratio of inspiration to exhalation—With increased intrathoracic airways obstruction the time needed to exhale will become greater because of a greater decrease in airway caliber during exhalation.

Other Findings

• Clubbing

—congenital heart diseases chronic bronchopneumonia (cystic fibrosis, ciliary dyskinesia).

• Presence of allergic shiners, Dennie lines, nasal crease, the "allergic salute" (i.e., rubbing the nose with the palm of the hand), atopic dermatitis, boggy nasal turbinates, and clear postnasal drainage.

Significance: These are all suggestive of coincident allergic/atopic disease, which increases the likelihood of coexisting asthma.

Diagnostic Aids

• Bronchodilator responsiveness.
Significance: A postbronchodilator *improvement* in wheezing indicates a reversible process such as asthma. *Worsening* can be seen in disorders of airway wall rigidity such as bronchomalacia or tracheomalacia. No change can be seen in situations with foreign bodies, fixed airway obstruction, due to significant inflammation, or due to airway remodeling.
• Pulmonary function testing (spirometry)
Significance: Spirometry remains the standard and most helpful measure of pulmonary function, and normative data have been described in children >3 years of age.
• Pulse oximetry measurement of oxygen saturation (Sao_2).
Significance: Pulse oximetry is an insensitive measure of mild to moderate respiratory difficulty during wheezing, but oxyhemoglobin saturation below 92% may be seen in severe compromise.
• Arterial blood gas (ABG)
Significance: ABGs provide a direct measure of oxygenation (Pao_2) and ventilation ($Paco_2$).
• Chest radiography (anteroposterior and lateral)
Significance: It should be strongly considered in all patients with new-onset wheezing or an asymmetric lung exam.

—Can show findings suggestive of airway obstruction (hyperinflation, hyperlucency, flattening of the diaphragms)

Asymmetry in aeration on right and left lateral decubitus films suggests foreign body on the side having the greatest air trapping.
• Microbiologic studies.
• Tuberculosis skin test—Mantoux purified protein derivative (PPD)
• Complete blood count including eosinophil count, quantitative immunoglobulins, IgE, complement, HIV testing, allergy skin testing

 ## Emergency Care

Factors that may indicate a respiratory emergency:

• Signs of mild to moderate respiratory difficulty—tachypnea, intercostal and suprasternal retractions, nasal flaring, head bobbing and exaggerated shoulder movement during breathing, abdominal breathing and subcostal retractions, relative difficulty speaking in complete sentences, significant wheezing, prolonged exhalation, and low $Paco_2$ in the face of tachypnea.
• Signs of impending respiratory failure—cyanosis, fatigue, inability to speak in greater than 1- to 2-word phrases, altered mental status (e.g., confusion, agitation), decreased respiratory drive, inadequate ventilation (poor air flow), no audible wheezing, normal or rising $Paco_2$ in the face of respiratory distress.
• Determine which patients require assisted ventilation (e.g., bag-mask ventilation, noninvasive (nasal) ventilation or endotracheal intubation).
• Lack of response to aggressive albuterol therapy (continuous over 1 hour) and/or the presence of stridor (biphasic adventitious sounds) should immediately raise the suspicion of a fixed lesion.

 ## Therapy

• A trial of bronchodilator therapy (e.g., albuterol) may be both therapeutic and diagnostic of the reversible airway obstruction characteristic of asthma.
• For acute asthma exacerbation—corticosteroids
• In the acute setting ipratropium bromide may be helpful in reducing airway secretions and reduce airway obstruction of little value out of the acute setting.
• Antibiotics should be used in patients with suspected pneumonia.
• Antiviral agents.

 ## Common Questions and Answers

Q: How common is wheezing in childhood?
A: Wheezing is common in childhood. By 1 year of age, 25% to 30% of infants will have an episode of wheezing. This percentage may increase to 40% by 3 years of age, and nearly 50% by 6 years.

Q: What percent of recurrent wheezing resolves by school age?
A: In one prospective study up to 6 years of age, roughly 40% of children with one or more episodes of wheezing by 3 years of age no longer wheezed by 6 years of age.

Q: Should chest x-rays be routinely obtained in children experiencing their first episodes of wheezing?
A: Though the likelihood of discovering an abnormal finding may be minimal (reported to be 5–6%), the potential risk of not diagnosing an abnormality with the potential for worsening if therapy is delayed should greatly outweigh the risk of and the difficulty in obtaining a chest x-ray.

Issues for Referral

Factors that may help alert you to make a referral include:

• Foreign body aspiration requires *immediate* referral.
• Patients with specific congenital/anatomic malformations and genetic syndromes.
• Patients with asthma who experience a life-threatening episode or poor control.

Clinical Pearls

• "All that wheezes is not asthma." While most episodes of wheezing will represent viral infections or asthma, clinicians need to be mindful of alternative diagnoses. This is especially true in patients with first-time, persistent, or atypical episodes of wheezing.
• Toy safety: Toys that fit inside toilet paper roll (1.75 inches) are too small for child <3 years.

BIBLIOGRAPHY

Expert Panel Report 2. *Guidelines for the diagnosis and management of asthma: National Heart, Lung, and Blood Institute.* National Asthma Education Program Expert Panel report. NIH Publication No. 97-4051. April 1997.

Martinez FD, Wright AL, Taussig LM, et al. Asthma and wheezing in the first six years of life. The Group Health Medical Associates. *N Engl J Med* 1995;332(3):133–138.

Panitch HB. Bronchiolitis in infants. *Curr Opin Pediatr* 2001;13(3):256–260.

Author: Hank Mayer
Alan Uba and Gerd Cropp 2nd edition

SECTION II
Specific Diseases

Abdominal Migraine (Epilepsy)

 Database

DEFINITION

• Recurrent identical attacks of periumbilical pain, which can include nausea, vomiting, headache, pallor, perspiration, slowing of pulse rate, fever, occasional diarrhea, limb pains
• Synonyms include: periodic syndrome, cyclical vomiting, growing pains

PATHOLOGY

• Controversy exists between the migraine hypothesis and the epileptic root. Although nonspecific EEG changes are seen more commonly among these children, very few go on to develop signs of epilepsy. On the other hand, children with abdominal migraine are more likely than controls to go on to develop more typical migraine headaches later in life; 10% of children who have migraine headaches are found in retrospect to have suffered from unexplained abdominal pain prior to the onset of headache. Adult migraine headache sufferers experience abdominal pain more frequently than tension headache sufferers.
• May involve neuronal activity originating in the hypothalamus with involvement of the cortex and autonomic nervous system. Serotonin is implicated, and blockade of serotonin receptors has been shown to act prophylactically in abdominal migraine.
• May involve some as yet ill-defined local intestinal vasomotor factor.

EPIDEMIOLOGY

• Mostly occurs in children between the ages of 3 and 10, peaking at about age 9
• More common in girls
• May affect as many as 1–2% of children at some point in their lives
• Declining frequency toward adulthood

GENETICS

• Parents of affected children often have history of migraine headaches

 Differential Diagnosis

INFECTION

• *Giardia*
• Environmental: lead intoxication
• Tumors
• Metabolic: porphyria, lactose intolerance
• Psychosocial: functional abdominal pain/irritable bowel syndrome
• Surgical: appendicitis, intussusception, biliary colic
• Inflammation: inflammatory bowel disease, peptic ulcer disease, mesenteric adenitis
• Gastrointestinal: irritable bowel, GE reflux, wandering spleen.
• Anatomic: Meckel diverticulum, ureteropelvic junction (UPJ) obstruction
• Miscellaneous: constipation, abdominal epilepsy—but has a shorter duration of pain (minutes), altered consciousness during event, abrupt onset, abnormal discharges in EEG in 80%

 Data Gathering

HISTORY

• Pain usually lasts less than 6 hours.
• Pain can be located anywhere in abdomen, but more often in upper quadrants.
• No abdominal pain in between attacks
• Repetition of identical abdominal crises, anywhere from one per week to several times a year
• Migraine in the history of patient or relatives
• Occasionally, presence of other migrainous syndromes such as nausea, vomiting, perspiration, body temperature changes, focal paresthesias, radiation of pain to a limb, general malaise
• Absence of impaired consciousness

 Physical Examination

The physical examination is unremarkable, with a benign abdomen.

SPECIAL QUESTIONS

Ask about a family history of migraine headache or unexplained bouts of abdominal pain as children.

Laboratory Aids

Test: Normal CBC, differential, sedimentation rate, urinalysis
Significance: R/O infection, i.e., UTI

Test: Stool heme test, and stool for cultures
Significance: IBD, GI causes of pain

Test: Lactose breath test
Significance: Lactose intolerance

Test: Lead test, porphyria workup (depending on situation)
Significance: Porphyria

Test: Urine organic acids, ammonia level
Significance: Underlying metabolic disorders may cause episodic vomiting.

Test: EEG
Significance: May help differentiate between abdominal migraine and abdominal epilepsy.

Test: Visual evoked response (VER) to red and white flash light
Significance: Has been shown to be helpful in diagnosing abdominal migraine, as children with clinically diagnosed abdominal migraine display a specific fast-wave activity response compared to normal controls, or children with migraine headaches alone.

Test: Obstruction series
Significance: Intermittent or partial bowel obstruction

Test: Upper GI
Significance: To rule out anatomic abnormalities

Test: Ultrasound
Significance: To rule out tumor, chronic appendicitis, etc.

Test: Renal ultrasound
Significance: To rule out UPJ obstruction

Test: Barium enema
Significance: During painful crisis to rule out intussusception

PITFALLS

Because it is usually a diagnosis of exclusion, many patients go through a large workup to rule out other causes of pain, sometimes including laparotomy.

Therapy

DRUGS

• Ergotamine, used for treatment of migraine headaches
• Serotonin receptor antagonists
• If EEG or other data point to possible epilepsy, empiric treatment with anticonvulsants may be considered and weighed against possible side effects of these agents.

PITFALLS

The medications must be given on a daily basis, as they are used in a prophylactic fashion. For the majority of patients, the side effects and complications from the use of these medications may outweigh the relief of pain, especially in children who are experiencing infrequent episodes.

Follow-Up

Most children outgrow abdominal migraines by early adolescence. However, a substantial percentage of them may then develop more typical migraine headaches.

PITFALLS

Even if a patient meets most criteria for abdominal migraine, various studies as outlined above should be done to ensure that a more serious disorder does not exist. Thus, the labeling of a child with abdominal migraine is a diagnosis of exclusion.

Common Questions and Answers

Q: Does this mean my child will develop migraine headaches?
A: There is an association between abdominal migraines in childhood and migraine headaches in later life. There is no good way to predict for sure whether your child will be a sufferer.

Q: I have two other younger children. What chance do they have of developing abdominal migraines?
A: Although there is a genetic tendency—i.e. abdominal migraines do tend to run in families—there is no known mendelian inheritance pattern. This is as opposed to a disease that is known to be recessive or dominant, such as cystic fibrosis, for which a probability can be given.

Q: What can I do to help my child during bouts of pain?
A: The parent should allow the child to do whatever makes him or her comfortable. This may mean rest, positioning, quiet, etc. Acetaminophen and other pain relievers may help to a certain degree. Whether the patient should be excused from school depends on various factors, such as the frequency, severity, and duration of the pain, as well as the age, maturity, and coping skills of the child.

ICD-9-CM 346.2

BIBLIOGRAPHY

Barlow, CF. The periodic syndrome—cyclic vomiting and abdominal migraine. *Clin Dev Med* 1984;91:83–84.

Bruyn GW. Migraine equivalents. *Handbook Clin Neurol* 1986;4(48):155–171.

Mortimer MJ, Good PA. The VER as a diagnostic marker for childhood abdominal migraine. *Headache* 1990;30:642–645.

Mortimer MJ, Kay J, Janon A. Clinical epidemiology of childhood migraine in an urban general pediatric practice. *Dev Med Child Neurol* 1993;35:243–248.

Symon DY. Abdominal migraine: a childhood syndrome defined. *Cephalalgia* 1986;6:223–228.

Author: Karen Liquornik

Acne

 Database

DEFINITION

• Acne vulgaris, or acne, is a common disorder of the pilosebaceous units (pilosebaceous follicles and sebaceous glands), initially characterized by microcomedo.
• The classification includes acne vulgaris, neonatal acne, and cosmetic or "pomade" acne. Rare, highly inflammatory types include acne fulminans (associated with fever, arthralgias, leukocytosis, and inflammatory bone lesions) and pyoderma faciale (numerous large pustules and nodular furuncles). Acne conglobata (numerous deep, coalescing inflammatory nodules, often with sinus tracks on face and trunk) is the most common type of intense inflammatory acne.

The manifestations of acne range from mild to severe:

• Mild: noninflammatory, focal comedonal lesions
• Moderate: inflammatory lesions: comedonal, papules, and possible pustules
• Moderate-severe: more severe localized inflammatory acne with comedones, papules, and pustules
• Severe: generalized inflammatory acne with nodules, pustules, and cysts

PATHOPHYSIOLOGY

Primary Cause

• Excessive sebum production by increasingly active sebaceous gland activity caused by androgen production initially by adrenal glands (prepubertal adrenarche) and then by gonads (pubertal)

Other Contributing Causes

• *Propionibacterium acnes* (common skin anaerobe) proliferates in excess sebum and follicular cell mixture.
• Linoleic acid deficiency (present in patients with acne) increases surface epithelial desquamation.
• Stress appears to exacerbate acne, as do hormonal factors associated with normal menstrual cycles.
• Higher levels of dehydroepiandrosterone sulfate (DHEAS), as with polycystic ovary disease, or testosterone.
• Cosmetics, creams, elevated androgen levels, certain drugs (topical or systemic corticosteroids, androgenic oral contraceptives, isoniazid, phenytoin, rifampin, and lithium) can worsen acne.
• Diet does not cause acne. Topical application of cocoa butter and other fatty acid based cosmetics to skin is comedogenic, as is working over a deep fat fryer for prolonged time.

Progression of Pathology

• Follicular obstruction leads to formation of microcomedo, which can progress to a comedo (i.e., blackhead = open comedone, and whitehead = closed comedone).
• Bacterial colonization (most commonly *P. acnes*) fosters the development of inflammatory papules, pustules, and nodules or cysts.
• Initial noninflammatory comedonal acne presents most commonly on the face and/or trunk and may progress to increasing numbers of inflammatory facial lesions, before becoming more generalized on face and trunk.

GENETICS

• Familial or possible genetic predisposition to severe acne seems likely (including expression of systemic linoleic acid deficiency); mechanisms have not yet been determined.
• Infants with severe neonatal acne appear to be at increased risk for more severe acne in their pubertal years, suggesting genetic predisposition.

COMPLICATIONS

• Comorbid conditions include: loss of self-esteem, embarrassment, and overt behavioral and psychiatric pathology, including depression.
• Keloid formation and permanent scarring are potential complications of nodular, cystic acne.

PROGNOSIS

• Less serious acne bumps ("zits" or papules) may resolve in 5–7 days.
• Major improvement usually noted 2–4 weeks after initiating an effective new treatment.
• Acne improves or resolves in >90% of individuals with proper care and treatment.

 Differential Diagnosis

• Steroid folliculitis
• Periorificial dermatitis
• Rosacea

 Data Gathering

HISTORY

Question: Age of onset?
Significance: Average age of onset is 11 years (or Tanner stage II) in both sexes.

Question: Location?
Significance: Most commonly on face, next on trunk, then upper arms, thighs, and buttocks.

Question: Current skin care?
Significance: Comedogenic cosmetics, moisturizers, sunscreens, soaps, and abrasive cleansers may worsen acne.

Question: Noted provocative factors?
Significance: Provocative factors include stress, menstrual cycle, occupational exposures, head or facial gear (including ball caps, 'do rags, helmets), allergies, contact irritants.

Question: Past or current use of nonprescriptive (OTC) or prescriptive medications for acne?
Significance: Assesses efficacy of current therapy.

Question: Any other medications or drugs, prescriptive and nonprescriptive?
Significance: Steroids, phenytoin, other medications with androgenic side effects may contribute.

Question: Any evidence for androgenic/hormonal disorder (amenorrhea, hirsutism, obesity)
Significance: Endocrine/metabolic evaluation indicated.

Question: Extent of concern with appearance?
Significance: Potential damage to self-esteem, mental health, depression.

 Physical Examination

• Determine types, location, and numbers of lesions present, classify as to severity. Document evidence of inflammation, any scarring (describe as hypertrophic or atrophic), or hypo- or hyperpigmentation.
• Note any signs of hirsutism, striae, obesity.

 Laboratory Aids

Females with severe acne (especially those with oligomenorrhea or hirsutism); check FSH, LH, free testosterone, DHEAS levels.

 Therapy

Patient education: Dispel common myths about acne:

• Not caused by dirt or lack of scrubbing the skin, lack of sexual activity, too much chocolate, fried foods, too much or too little sex or masturbation.
• Carefully prescribed antibiotics should not be harmful, including long-term tetracycline.
• Accutane (isotretinoin) is not warranted for every teenager with acne, does not work miracles overnight, and can have major side effects.

Acne

Mild acne (comedones without inflammation)

- General skin care: Wash gently with nonabrasive, noncomedogenic soap 1–2 times per day. Harsh scrubbing is contraindicated (may increase inflammation). Occasional (not more than once daily) astringent or alcohol pads may help remove excess oil or makeup without necessity of repeated washing. If makeup is used, be sure it is noncomedogenic or nonacneogenic.
- Add benzoyl peroxide gel 0.025% or wash (5%) **or** tretinoin (Retin-A) 0.025–0.05% cream at bedtime, at least 20 minutes after washing.

Moderate acne (comedones and papules, ± local inflammation)

- General skin care
- Benzoyl peroxide 5% wash **or** 0.025% tretinoin (Retin-A) gel at bedtime
- Add topical antibiotics 1–2× daily if any inflammation present.

Moderate-severe acne (comedones, papules, and pustules)

- General skin care
- Benzoyl peroxide 2.5–5.0% gel or 5.0% wash in the morning
- Tretinoin (Retin-A) 0.025–0.05% cream or 0.025% gel at bedtime
- Topical antibiotics twice daily
- Add systemic antibiotics (e.g., tetracycline 500–750 mg twice daily, adult dose)
- Consider azeleic acid (Azelex) 20% cream b.i.d. instead of benzoyl peroxide and tretinoin, if scars or pustules appear hyperpigmented.

Severe acne (cystic, nodular lesions)

- General skin care.
- Benzoyl peroxide 2.5–5.0% gel in the morning
- Tretinoin (Retin-A) 0.025–0.05% cream or 0.025% gel at bedtime
- Systemic antibiotics (e.g., tetracycline 500–1,000 mg b.i.d. or minocycline HCl, doxycycline, or erythromycin of recommended equivalent dose)
- Surgery or isotretinoin (Accutane): Refer to a dermatologist

MEDICATIONS

- Tretinoin, a vitamin A derivative and photosensitizer, increases the risk of sunburn. Benzoyl peroxide is synergistic with tretinoin, but both tend to dry the skin. Alert patients to risks of sun exposure and drying effects of most acne medications.
- Topical antibiotics have limited efficacy in papular and pustular acne. Clindamycin and erythromycin topical preparations are equally effective. Lotions are less drying than gel formulas.
- Tetracycline should not be used in children until the permanent teeth have erupted, due to risk of permanent discoloration of enamel.

- Isotretinoin (Accutane) is a remarkably effective drug for severe cystic acne that has been unresponsive to conventional therapy. Accutane stops sebum production during the recommended 4- to 5-month course of therapy, and this effect usually persists for lengthy periods after cessation of treatment. It is expensive ($500 to $700 or more for a treatment course) and has significant side effects, necessitating routine 2- to 4-week blood counts, liver function tests, cholesterol and triglyceride determination. Accutane has serious teratogenic capability (affecting more than 60% of infants with gestational exposure and resulting in incurable and usually fatal birth defects). This necessitates a negative pretreatment pregnancy test and effective birth control methods for female patients of childbearing age, who should not become pregnant for at least 1 month following cessation of Accutane therapy. Common side effects include significant dryness of mucous membranes, lips, face, and conjunctivae. Bone pain and arthralgias are also relatively common.

OTHER, NEW, AND FUTURE TREATMENT CONSIDERATIONS

"Emergency" Treatment Modalities

- Intralesional corticosteroids (injection of 0.5 to 2.5 mL of triamcinolone acetate into a severely inflamed acne cyst or papule, usually by a dermatologist.)
- Incision and drainage of an inflamed comedone, preferably using a comedone extractor to drain the contents of cystic lesions.

Newer and Future Acne Medications

- **Azaleic acid** 20% cream (Azelex), a dicarboxylic acid, FDA approved in 1996 as a topical treatment for acne, has antikeratinizing and antimicrobial properties and fewer side effects than other topicals. Recommended for twice daily application, it is an effective comedolytic.
- **Adapalene** gel 0.1% (Differin), a synthetic derivative of naphthoic acid with retinoid-like activity. Has comedolytic and antiinflammatory effects and reportedly better efficacy than Retin-A gel 0.025%. Inconsistent results reported and not used as commonly as more familiar retinoids.
- **Spironolactone**, an effective oral treatment of inflammatory acne lesions, blocking androgen receptors and inhibiting androgen synthesis. Has common side effects of breast tenderness, menstrual irregularities, and hyperkalemia.

 Follow-Up

- Patients with moderate acne requiring antibiotic treatment should initially be seen in 2–4 weeks, then at least every 3–4 months.
- Patients receiving Accutane therapy should be seen at least monthly.
- Patients with keloids or scarring acne should be referred for dermatologic consultation.
- Accutane not warranted for every teen with acne, does not work miracles overnight, and can have major side effects.
- Use good general skin care daily, washing face and other acne-involved skin with mild noncomedogenic soap (Cetaphil, Neutrogena, Lever 2000, Dial) 1–2 times per day.
- Avoid harsh scrubbing of skin and frequent application of alcohol or astringents.
- Avoid comedogenic cosmetics, moisturizers, sun lotions, cocoa butter, oily hair and skin products.
- Avoid wearing hair on face, sweat bands, hats, or caps with forehead contact.
- Avoid picking or squeezing lesions (may encourage scarring.

 Common Questions and Answers

Q: What's the best medication to use for mild acne?
A: Topical tretinoin is one of the best for mild acne and should be used nightly or on alternate nights, if the skin is especially dry.

Q: Does chocolate cause acne?
A: Only if you rub cocoa butter on your skin.

Q: Does diet affect acne?
A: No, but food preparation over hot grease can be comedogenic.

BIBLIOGRAPHY

Brown SK, Shalita AR. Acne vulgaris. *Lancet* 1998;351:1871–1876.

Krowchuk DP. Managing acne in adolescents. *Pediatr Clin North Am* 2000;47(4):841–857.

Krowchuk DP, Lucky AW. Managing adolescent acne. *Adolesc Med* 2001;12(2):vii,355–374.

Leyden JJ. Therapy for acne vulgaris. *N Engl J Med* 1997;336:1156–1162.

Strasburger VC. Acne: what every pediatrician should know about treatment. *Pediatr Clin North Am* 1997;44(6):1505–1523.

Author: Lucy S. Crain

Acquired Hypothyroidism

 Database

DEFINITION

Hypothyroidism that occurs after the neonatal period.

PATHOPHYSIOLOGY

- There are myriad causes (*see* Differential Diagnosis).
- Decreased synthesis or release of thyroid hormone can result from thyroid gland dysfunction (primary hypothyroidism) or from pituitary/hypothalamic dysfunction leading to understimulation of the thyroid gland (secondary and tertiary hypothyroidism).

GENETICS

- A genetic predisposition exists in patients with chronic lymphocytic thyroiditis (CLT), the most common cause of acquired thyroiditis in nonendemic areas; 30% to 40% of patients have a familial history of thyroid disease, and up to 50% of their first-degree relatives have thyroid antibodies.
- Associations of CLT with certain human leukocyte antigen (HLA) haplotypes are weak and not consistently reproducible.
- Autoimmune thyroid disease may be part of Schmidt syndrome (type II polyglandular autoimmune disease), which also involves Addison disease and type 1 diabetes mellitus. This incompletely penetrant autosomal-dominant disorder demonstrates stronger HLA linkage.
- Genetic syndromes associated with higher incidence of autoimmune thyroiditis:

—Down syndrome
—Turner syndrome (especially those with isochromosome Xq)

EPIDEMIOLOGY

- May develop at any age.
- CLT prevalence correlates with iodine intake, such that countries as the United States and Japan with the highest dietary iodine also have the highest CLT prevalence. Experiments with T cells from CLT patients and with NOD-H_2(h4) mice, a model for autoimmune thyroiditis, suggest that iodine increases the autoantigenicity of thyroglobulin.
- Autoimmune thyroid disorders occur more frequently in children and adolescents with type 1 diabetes mellitus.

COMPLICATIONS

- The most significant complication during childhood is impaired linear growth.
- Myxedema coma may occur.
- Encephalopathy of varied clinical presentation has been associated with high titers of thyroid antibodies, especially antimicrosomal, and responds well to corticosteroid treatment.

 Differential Diagnosis

IMMUNOLOGIC

- Chronic lymphocytic thyroiditis (often referred to as Hashimoto thyroiditis)
- Autoimmune polyendocrine syndrome (Schmidt syndrome)

INFECTIOUS

- Postviral subacute thyroiditis
- Associated with congenital infections

—Rubella
—Toxoplasmosis

ENVIRONMENTAL

- Goitrogen ingestion

—Iodides
—Expectorants
—Thioureas

IATROGENIC

- Following surgical thyroidectomy for thyroid cancer, hyperthyroidism, or extensive neck tumors.
- Following radioiodine ablative therapy for hyperthyroidism or thyroid cancer.
- Following irradiation to the head or neck for cancer treatment.
- Medications: lithium, amiodarone, iodine contrast dyes.

METABOLIC

- Cystinosis
- Histiocytosis X

CONGENITAL

- Late-onset congenital-large ectopic gland

GENETIC SYNDROMES

- Down syndrome
- Turner syndrome

SECONDARY OR TERTIARY HYPOTHYROIDISM

- Hypothalamic or pituitary disease

 Data Gathering

HISTORY

Question: Growth pattern?
Significance: Linear growth failure can be the first sign of thyroid dysfunction.

Question: Declining school performance?
Significance: Sensitive marker for lethargy and reduced focusing.

SYMPTOMS

Question: Any symptoms of hypothyroidism and their duration?
Significance: Early primary hypothyroidism can be asymptomatic. The presence of hypothyroid-related symptoms indicates progression from compensated to uncompensated hypothyroidism.

Question: Notice any thyroid gland enlargement? Its duration? Tenderness?
Significance: Goiter may be the presenting sign of acquired hypothyroidism. Tenderness suggests an infectious process.

Question: Any past medical history factors associated with hypothyroidism? (e.g., genetic syndromes, radiation exposure, medications, history of diabetes).
Significance: Any of these factors should raise the concern for possible acquired hypothyroidism.

Question: Familial history of thyroid disease (hyper or hypo) or other autoimmune endocrinopathies
Significance: Family history of thyroid disease or other autoimmune endocrinopathies increases the risk of developing autoimmune thyroid disease.

 Physical Examination

Finding: Bradycardia
Significance: Thyroid hormone has cardiac effects.

Finding: Short stature (or fall-off on growth curve), and increased upper/lower segment ratio
Significance: Euthyroidism is required to maintain normal growth.

Finding: Goiter: note consistency, symmetry, nodularity, signs of inflammation
Significance: Goiter characteristics may give a clue regarding the cause of the hypothyroidism and provide a clinical marker to follow during therapy.

Finding: Myxedema (water retention)
Significance: Myxedema is not limited to the subcutaneous tissue. It may also lead to cardiac failure, pleural effusions, and coma.

Finding: Muscle hypertrophy, yet muscle weakness most obvious in arms, legs, and tongue.
Significance: Hypothyroidism causes disordered muscle function.

Finding: Delayed relaxation phase of deep tendon reflexes
Significance: Due to slowed muscle contraction, not a change in the transmission rate of the nervous impulse.

Finding: Pale, cool, dry, carotenemic skin
Significance: Due to decreased cell turnover.

Finding: Increase in lanugo hair
Significance: Can be seen in children with hypothyroidism and reversed with treatment.

SPECIAL QUESTIONS

Sexual development is an important factor because hypothyroidism can be associated with both delayed puberty (due to low thyroid hormone level) as well as precocious puberty and galactorrhea (due to elevated TSH).

 ## Laboratory Aids

TESTS

Test: T_4 (low) and TSH (elevated)
Significance: Elevated TSH with normal T_4 represents a state of compensated primary hypothyroidism.

Test: Free T_4
Significance: The most sensitive marker for secondary/tertiary hypothyroidism (in which case, TSH elevation is lost and total T_4 may still be in the low end of the normal range).

Test: Antithyroglobulin and antimicrosomal (antiperoxidase) antibodies
Significance: Markers for CLT.

IMAGING

Test: Head MRI
Significance: Suspected secondary/tertiary hypothyroidism; pituitary or hypothalamic lesion

The following conditions may test false-positive for acquired hypothyroidism:

Test: Thyroid-binding globulin deficiency
Significance: Low total T_4, but normal free T_4 and TSH

Test: Peripheral resistance to thyroid hormone
Significance: Normal/high total T_4

Test: "Euthyroid sick" syndrome
Significance: Low T_4 and T_3; normal/low TSH; increased shunting to reverse T_3

 ## Therapy

L-THYROXINE (SYNTHETIC THYROID HORMONE) REPLACEMENT

- Indicated for the treatment of overt or compensated hypothyroidism.
- 2 to 5 μg/kg/d po, once daily
- Monitor T_4 and TSH and titrate dose to maintain normalized TFTs.
- Duration of therapy

—Lifetime
—30% of children with CLT will undergo spontaneous remission, and reassessment of need for treatment can be done after growth is completed.

 ## Follow-Up

CHANGES IN TFTS

- Whenever starting medication or adjusting dose, check T_4 and TSH 4 to 6 weeks later, to assess adequacy of the new dose.

WHEN TO EXPECT IMPROVEMENT

- Treated patients often resume growth at a rate greater than normal (catch-up growth).
- Other signs and symptoms resolve at a variable rate.
- Goiters in CLT may not completely regress with treatment (enlargement due to persistent inflammation does not correct, though TSH-mediated hypertrophy will).

SIGNS TO WATCH FOR TO INDICATE PROBLEMS

- Monitor response to treatment by measuring T_4 and TSH levels to ensure compliance.

PROGNOSIS

- If patients are compliant, prognosis is excellent.
- In children in whom treatment has been delayed, catch-up growth may not fully normalize height to predicted values.

 ## Common Questions and Answers

Q: What happens if my child forgets a dose?
A: Give the dose as soon as you remember. If it is the next day, give two doses.

Q: How long will my child have to take these pills?
A: Probably for life.

Q: Are there any side effects from the medication?
A: No. The medication contains only the hormone that your child's thyroid gland is not making. The hormone is made synthetically, so there is also no infectious risk.

Q: If my child takes twice the dose, will his or her growth catch up faster?
A: Your child may grow a little faster but will also have adverse effects from having too much thyroid hormone.

Q: Does the medication have to be taken at any particular time of day?
A: No, but consistently choosing the same time of day helps to remember taking it.

ICD-9-CM 244.9

BIBLIOGRAPHY

Barbesino G, Chiovato L. The genetics of Hashimoto's disease. *Endocrinol Metab Clin North Am* 2000;29:357–374.

Betterle C, Volpato M, Greggio AN, et al. Type 2 polyglandular autoimmune disease (Schmidt syndrome). J Pediatr Endocrinol Metab 1996;(9 suppl 1):113–123.

Dayan CM, Daniels GH. Chronic autoimmune thyroiditis. *N Engl J Med* 1996;335:99–107.

Hunter I, Greene SA, MacDonald TM, et al. Prevalence and aetiology of hypothyroidism in the young. *Arch Dis Child* 2000;83:207–210.

Rickees SA, Bode HH, Crawford JD. Long-term growth in juvenile acquired hypothyroidism: the failure to achieve normal adult stature. *N Engl J Med* 1988;318:599–602.

Roldan MB, Alonso M, Barrio R. Thyroid autoimmunity in children and adolescents with Type 1 diabetes mellitus. *Diabetes Nutr Metab Clin Exp* 1999;12:27–31.

Rose NR, Rasooly L, Saboori AM, et al. Linking iodine with autoimmune thyroiditis. *Environ Health Perspect* 1999;107(suppl 5):749–752.

Vasconcellos E, Pina-Garza JE, Fakhoury T, et al. Pediatric manifestations of Hashimoto's encephalopathy. *Pediatr Neurol* 1999;20(5):394–398.

Watemberg N, Willis D, Pellock JM. Encephalopathy as the presenting symptom of Hashimoto's thyroiditis. *J Child Neurol* 2000;15(1):66–69.

Author: Adda Grimberg
Marta Satin-Smith, 2nd edition

Acute Lymphoblastic Leukemia

 Database

DEFINITION

Acute lymphoblastic leukemia (ALL) is a malignant disorder of lymphoblasts occurring as a result of indefinite clonal proliferation of a single lymphoblast that has undergone malignant transformation. This lymphoblastic clonal proliferation leads to overgrowth and the crowding out of normal bone marrow precursors, invasion of nonhematopoietic tissues, and suppression of differentiation of normal cells causing ineffective hematopoiesis.

CAUSES

• Unknown

Following factors have been associated:

• Genetic predisposition: 25% risk of ALL in monozygotic twin if one twin develops ALL before 5 years of age
• Trisomy 21 (Down syndrome)
• Immunodeficiencies

—Prolonged immunosuppressive therapy
—Congenital hypogammaglobulinemia
—Ataxia telangiectasia
—Wiskott-Aldrich syndrome
—Bloom syndrome

• Exposure to ionizing radiation (not diagnostic x-rays)

PATHOLOGY

• Bone marrow aspirate shows >25% leukemic lymphoblasts

French American British (FAB) Classification: based on morphology:

• L1: size <2 RBC; scant, subtle nucleoli; <10% cytoplasm; round or oval nucleus
• L2: size >2 RBC; prominent nucleoli; >20% cytoplasm; folded nuclei
• L3: big, blue vacuolated cells ("Burkitt cell")

Immunologic classification:

• B cell lineage

—80% to 85% of childhood cases
—Early pre-B and pre-B cell most common
—ALL antigen (CALLA) positive and TdT positive

• T-cell lineage

—15% to 20% of all cases
—10% of these are CALLA positive

Cytogenetics:

• Hyperdiploid state (>50 chromosomes or DI >1.16) associated with good prognosis
• Hypodiploid state (<46 chromosomes or DI <1.16) associated with poor prognosis
• Karyotype of malignant cells is reported normal in up to 50% of cases

EPIDEMIOLOGY

• most common leukemia of childhood
• Incidence of ALL is 1/1700 in children under the age of 15 years; 75–80% of acute leukemia in childhood is ALL
• Peak incidence at 4 years of age; more common in whites and boys
• Higher incidence in industrialized countries

COMPLICATIONS

Due to disease:

• Hyperleukocytosis (WBC >400,000)—can lead to stroke
• Mediastinal mass (usually T-cell lineage)—can lead to cardiorespiratory arrest
• Tumor lysis syndrome—can lead to renal failure, cardiac arrhythmias
• Coagulopathy—can lead to stroke and hemorrhage
• Severe anemia—can lead to CHF
• Hypercalcemia—can lead to renal failure, cardiorespiratory arrest
• Febrile neutropenia—can lead to infections, shock, sepsis

Due to therapy:

• Cranial radiation (XRT)

—Brain tumors
—Leukoencephalopathy and deterioration of intellectual functions/learning deficits
—Growth retardation
—Decreased bone density

• Glucocorticoid steroids (prednisone/dexamethasone)

—Avascular necrosis of bones
—Cushingoid habitus (reversible)
—Hypertension (reversible)
—Hyperglycemia (reversible)
—Decreased bone density

• Vincristine (VCR)

—Syndrome of inappropriate antidiuretic hormone
—Footdrop (reversible)
—Hair loss (reversible)

• L-asparaginase

—Pancreatitis
—Coagulopathy leading to cerebral infarcts or thrombosis

• Adriamycin/doxorubicin/daunorubicin

—Cardiac toxicity

• Cyclophosphamide

—Hemorrhagic cystitis
—Sterility

• Methotrexate (MTX)

—Hepatotoxicity

PROGNOSIS

• Remission induction in all risk categories with presently available therapy is 95%.

• Long-term survival in standard risk group is about 85% (>5 years after completion of therapy) and slightly higher for girls than for boys.
• Long-term survival is about 60% to 65% for high-risk group.

 Differential Diagnosis

NONMALIGNANT CONDITIONS

• Juvenile rheumatoid arthritis
• Infectious mononucleosis
• Idiopathic thrombocytopenic purpura
• Pertussis and parapertussis
• Aplastic anemia

MALIGNANT CONDITIONS

• Neuroblastoma with bone marrow involvement
• Lymphoma with bone marrow involvement
• Rhabdomyosarcoma
• Retinoblastoma
• Acute myeloid leukemia

 Data Gathering

HISTORY

• Common findings: Fatigue; feeling the "blahs" and not recovering quickly after a recent viral illness
• Fever
• Bleeding (cutaneous and mucosal); easy bruising; petechiae
• Bone pains; arthralgia, limp
• Fatigue and pallor
• Lymph node enlargement
• Stridor, orthopnea, shortness of breath, any respiratory distress
• Ocular pain; blurred vision; photophobia
• Headache, vomiting, seizures

 Physical Examination

• Pallor, Congestive heart failure
• Lymphadenopathy (generalized)
• Hepatosplenomegaly
• Sternal tenderness/bone tenderness
• Petechiae and purpura
• Subconjunctival and retinal hemorrhages
• Hypopyon (layering of leukemia cells in anterior chamber of eye)
• Painless testicular enlargement in boys
• Papilledema in CNS leukemia
• Swelling of the face, orthopnea
• Subcutaneous nodules (leukemia cutis)
• Extremity weakness; numbness or tingling (Spinal cord compression)

Laboratory Aids

Test: CBC
Significance: Increased white blood count >10,000/mm^3 (50% cases); >50,000/mm^3 (20%)

Neutropenia (<500/mm^3) common; Hb <10 g/dL (80%); Thrombocytopenia (<100,000/mm^3) (75%)
Peripheral smear may show characteristic leukemic lymphoblasts

Test: Bone marrow aspirate
Significance: >25% Lymphoblasts is diagnostic

Test: Immunophenotyping and cytogenetic studies on bone marrow aspirate
Significance: Diagnostic and prognostic

Biochemical tests

• Increased uric acid
• Slight abnormality of liver function tests due to leukemic infiltrate

Test: Chest x-ray
Significance: 5% to 10% cases have mediastinal mass

Test: CSF examination with lymphoblasts
Significance: CNS leukemia (5% at diagnosis)

PROGNOSTIC FACTORS

• Patients with any of the following criteria belong to high-risk group.

—Age <1 year or >10 years of age
—WBC count >50,000/mm^3
—Translocations—t(9;22), t(4;11), t(1;19)
—Hypodiploidy (<46 chromosomes or DI >1.16 by karyotype)

Emergency Care

• Hyperleukocytosis
• Spinal cord compression
• Mediastinal mass

Therapy

Stratified according to risk groups

• Standard risk—age 1 to 10 years; WBC <50,000 at diagnosis; karyotype does not have t(9;22), t(4;11)
• High risk—age 1 to 10 years with WBC ≥50,000; age <1 or >10 years regardless of WBC or karyotype; karyotype t(9;22), t(4;11)

FOUR PHASES OF THERAPY

• Induction to achieve remission (>5% blasts in bone marrow). Usually with four drugs

—Vincristine
—Glucocorticoid steroids (prednisone or dexamethasone)
—L-asparaginase
—Doxorubicin or daunorubicin
—Intrathecal methotrexate to prevent CNS disease
—Consolidation

• Delayed intensification (one or two): To further decrease leukemic burden

—Vincristine
—Glucocorticoid steroids (prednisone or dexamethasone)
—L-asparaginase
—Doxorubicin
—Cyclophosphamide
—Cytosine arabinoside (ARA-C)
—6 thioguanine (6TG)
—Intrathecal MTX

• Maintenance

—2.5 years for girls and 3 years for boys
—Daily oral 6MP
—Weekly MTX and monthly pulses of VCR and glucocorticoid steroids
—Intrathecal MTX every 3 months

• CNS leukemia at diagnosis

—Cranial radiation (2400 cGy)
—Triple intrathecal (MTX, ARA-C, Hydrocortisone), in addition to therapy above.

RELAPSE

Reappearance of leukemia cells at any site in the body

• Responsiveness of recurrent ALL to therapy depends on duration of first remission (prognosis for early bone marrow relapse and for late bone marrow relapse is 10–20% and 30–40% respectively).
• Most relapses occur during treatment or within the first 2 years after completion of therapy, but some initial relapses can occur >10 years after diagnosis.
• Most common sites of relapse are bone marrow, CNS, testis.
• Bone marrow relapse

—May present with anemia, leukocytosis, leukopenia, thrombocytopenia, hepatosplenomegaly, bone pain, fever, or sudden decrease in tolerance to chemotherapy.
—Bone marrow relapse with or without extramedullary involvement usually points to poor clinical outcome.
—Treat with allogeneic hematopoietic stem cell transplant.

• Extramedullary relapse (CNS, testis)

—Patients who initially present with high WBC, t(9;22) karyotype, or CNS leukemia have a increased risk of CNS relapse.

Common Questions and Answers

Q: Can the child on treatment for ALL go to school?
A: Yes.

Q: Will the hair fall out and the child be sick for all 3 years on chemotherapy?
A: The hair usually falls out within a few weeks of initiating therapy and the child remains with alopecia for first 6 to 8 months. The hair grows back once maintenance therapy begins. Most children feel well during the maintenance chemotherapy.

Q: Does the child need to be isolated from other children?
A: The child should be isolated from any child who has varicella or is obviously sick due to any other infection.

ICD-9-CM 204.0

BIBLIOGRAPHY

Brenner MK, Pinkel D. Cure of leukemia. *Semin Hematol* 1999;36(4, suppl 7):73–83.

Pui CH. Acute lymphoblastic leukemia. *Pediatr Clin North Am* 1997;44(4):831–846.

Pui CH. Acute lymphoblastic leukemia in children. *Curr Opin Oncol* 2000;12:3–12.

Author: Valerie I. Brown

Acute Myeloid Leukemia

 ## Database

DEFINITION

Acute myeloid leukemia (AML) is a block in differentiation and an unregulated proliferation of myeloid progenitor cells.

PATHOPHYSIOLOGY

- Principal defect is a block in the differentiation of primitive myeloid precursor cells.
- Two predominant mechanisms have been identified:

—Defect at the level of transcriptional activation.
—Defects in the signaling pathway of hematopoietic growth factors. In particular the proto-oncogene Ras is mutated in up to one third of patients with AML.

ETIOLOGY

- Exact cause unknown.
- Acquired risk factors

—Exposure to benzene
—Exposure to ionizing radiation
—Therapy induced from chemotherapy for a prior malignancy
—Alkylating agents such as cyclophosphamide, nitrogen mustard, chlorambucil, melphalan. Typically presents several years after therapy.
—Epi-podophyllotoxins such as VP16, VM26. Typically occurs within 2 years after therapy and are characterized by rearrangements involving 11q23.

- Associated congenital syndromes carry an increased risk of AML

—Fanconi anemia
—Bloom syndrome
—Neurofibromatosis type I
—Down syndrome
—Severe congenital anemia, i.e., Kostmann disease with exposure to granulocyte colony-stimulating factor
—Diamond Blackfan anemia
—Paroxysmal nocturnal hemoglobinemia
—Li-Fraumeni syndrome

PATHOLOGY

- Bone marrow aspirate must contain >30% myeloblasts.
- Classified according to the French-American-British Classification (FAB)

—Divides AML into 7 subtypes—M1-M7

- Immunophenotyping

—Blasts positive for myeloid associated surface antigens (CD11b, CD13, CD14, CD15, CD33, or CD36) in 90% of cases
—Lymphoid markers, both T and B cell may be present in 30–60% of pediatric patients
—CD41 and CD42 (megakaryocytic)

- Morphology

—Large blasts with low nuclear/cytoplasmic ratio
—Multiple nucleoli and cytoplasmic granules

- Cytochemistry

—Blasts are positive for myeloperoxidase and Sudan black and usually negative for periodic acid-Schiff (PAS) and terminal deoxynucleotide transferase (TdT)

CYTOGENETICS

- Only 20–30% of pediatric blasts have a normal karyotype vs. 40–50% in adults
- 60% of abnormal karyotypes fall into known subgroups
- Translocations of duplications of the MLL gene at 11q23 are found in many cases of therapy-induced AML as well as in infants
- Techniques such as fluorescence *in situ* hybridization, Southern blotting, and reverse transcriptase–polymerase chain reactions are becoming necessary diagnostic tools for AML

EPIDEMIOLOGY

- Seventh most common pediatric malignancy
- 500 children/year in the U.S.
- Incidence peaks at 2 years and again at 16 years
- Leukemia in first 4 weeks of life is usually AML
- Ratio of AML to ALL throughout childhood is 1:4
- Boys and girls equally affected

COMPLICATIONS AT DIAGNOSIS

- Bleeding—usually secondary to thrombocytopenia
- Disseminated intravascular coagulation (DIC) occurs in some types of AML including APML (M3).

—Should be aggressively treated with fresh frozen plasma and platelet transfusions.

- Infection

—40% of patients are febrile at diagnosis.
—Empiric antibiotic therapy must be started after blood cultures are obtained.

- Leukostasis

—Intravascular clumping of blasts causing hypoxia, infarction, and hemorrhage.
—Usually with white blood count (WBC) >200,000/mm^3.
—Brain and lung are commonly affected organs.
—Leukopheresis or exchange transfusion may be indicated with patients who are symptomatic with extremely high blast counts.

- Tumor lysis syndrome

—Refers to the metabolic consequences from the release of cellular contents of dying leukemic cells.

—Hyperuricemia can lead to renal failure.
—Hyperkalemia, hyperphosphatemia, and secondary hypocalcemia can be life threatening.
—Patients should be hydrated with fluid containing bicarbonate and given allopurinol.

PROGNOSIS

- 85% achieve remission with intensive chemotherapy.
- About 30% to 40% achieve long-term survival (more than 5 years after diagnosis).

 ## Differential Diagnosis

- Myeloid blast crisis of chronic myeloid leukemia (Philadelphia chromosome positive)
- Acute lymphoblastic leukemia
- Leukemoid reaction
- Exaggerated leukocytosis

 ## Data Gathering

HISTORY

- Children with AML can present with very few symptoms or with life-threatening sepsis or hemorrhage.

Common symptoms include

—Fever: 30–40%
—Pallor: 25%
—Weight loss/anorexia: 22%
—Fatigue: 19%
—Bleeding, i.e., cutaneous, mucosal, menorrhagia: 33%
—Bone or joint pain: 18%

 ## Physical Examination

- Signs of anemia

—Pallor, fatigue, headache, dyspnea, systolic flow murmur
—Signs of thrombocytopenia
—Petechiae, bruising, epistaxis, gingival bleeding

- Signs of infection

—Fever
—Lingering bacterial infections of lung, sinuses, gingiva, perirectal area, skin

- Other exam findings

—Hepatomegaly
—Splenomegaly
—Lymphadenopathy
—Gingival hyperplasia
—Papilledema, cranial nerve palsies (rare)
—Colorless or slightly purple subcutaneous nodules—"blueberry muffin" lesions of leukemia cutis (more commonly seen in neonates)

Laboratory Findings

- CBC

—Anemia, thrombocytopenia, elevated or low total WBC count

- Peripheral smear

—Myeloblasts may be seen

- Bone marrow aspirate

—>30% myeloblasts is diagnostic
—Confirm with immunophenotyping and cytochemistry

- PT/PTT fibrin spit products

—Can be elevated with some cases especially with acute promyelocytic leukemia (M3)
—Can have severe, life-threatening DIC

- Electrolytes—abnormalities associated with tumor lysis syndrome

—Hyperkalemia
—Hypocalcemia
—Hyperphosphatemia
—Hyperuricemia

- CSF for cell count and cytology

—>5 WBC/mm^3 is suggestive of CNS disease.
—5–15% of cases have CNS involvement at diagnosis.

PROGNOSTIC FACTORS

Factors associated with low remission induction rate:

- WBC count >100,000/mm^3
- Monosomy 7
- Secondary AML or prior myelodysplastic syndrome

 ## Emergency Care

- Children with suspected AML should have immediate evaluation with physical exam, history, and laboratory data including CBC, PT/PTT, electrolytes, calcium, phosphorus, uric acid, creatinine.

 ## Therapy

INDUCTION

- Most effective drugs for remission induction in AML are anthracyclines, e.g., doxorubicin, daunomycin, mitoxantrone, and cytarabine
- 6-thioguanine (6TG), VP-16, and dexamethasone are added in some regimens
- Remission rate is approximately 70–85%
- High rate of remission induction with all trans retinoic acid in acute promyelocytic leukemia
- Consolidation therapy usually with ARA-C and L-asparaginase
- Intrathecal ARA-C for CNS prophylaxis
- Maintenance with VP16, ARA-C, 6TG, daunomycin, dexamethasone
- Duration of therapy is usually 6–9 months
- Allogeneic bone marrow transplant may be the best treatment for AML in first remission

SUPPORTIVE CARE

- Hydration, alkalization, and allopurinol during induction
- Blood product support

—Avoid products from family members due to the possibility of allogeneic bone marrow transplant

- Broad-spectrum antibiotics and antifungal therapy for fever and neutropenia
- Prophylactic trimethoprim/sulfamethoxazole for *Pneumocystis*
- Nystatin/fluconazole for fungal prophylaxis
- Heparin may be needed for treatment of DIC.

 ## Follow-Up

Blood counts monthly for first year, then every 3 months for the second year and then every 6 months. Liver and kidney function tests are done every 3 months. Cardiac function should be checked every 6 to 12 months. Endocrine function should be tested in pubertal children.

 ## Common Questions and Answers

Q: Is an indwelling line required for therapy?
A: Always.

Q: Are repeated hospitalizations likely?
A: Repeated hospitalizations are needed for chemotherapy and infectious complications.

Q: Can the child go to school?
A: May be able to go intermittently during therapy.

ICD-9-CM 205.0

BIBLIOGRAPHY

Ebb DH, Weinstein HJ. Diagnosis and treatment of childhood AML. *Pediatr Clin North Am* 1997;44(4):847–862.

Golub, TR, Weinstein HJ, Grier HE. Acute myelogenous leukemia. In: Pizzo PA, Poplack DG, eds. *Principles and practices of pediatric oncology*, 3rd ed. Philadelphia: Lippincott-Raven, 1997.

Hurwitz CA, Mounce KG, Grier HE. Treatment of patients with AML: review of clinical trials of past decade. *J Pediatr Hematol Oncol* 1995;17(3):185–197.

Kersey JH. Fifty years of studies of biology and therapy of childhood leukemia. *Blood* 1997;90(11):4243–4251.

Langmuir P, Aplenc R, Lange B. Acute myeloid leukemia in children. *Best Pract Res Clin Haematol* 2001;14(1):77–93.

Author: Tammy Kang
Sadhna M. Shankar, 2nd edition

Adenovirus Infection

 Database

DEFINITION

Adenoviruses are ubiquitous double-stranded DNA viruses. There are 47 human serotypes.

PATHOPHYSIOLOGY

Adenoviruses may cause a lytic or chronic/latent infection. They have also been shown to be capable of inducing oncogenic transformation of cells, although the clinical significance of this observation remains unclear.

EPIDEMIOLOGY

• Primary infection usually occurs early in life (by age 10 years) and is most often characterized by upper respiratory symptoms.
• Military trainees are especially susceptible to infection, probably due to crowded living conditions.
• Respiratory and enteric infections may occur at any time of year. Epidemics of respiratory disease occur in winter and spring.
• Transmission of respiratory disease occurs via contact with infected secretions. Transmission of enteric adenoviruses is via the fecal–oral route.
• Outbreaks of pharyngoconjunctival fever have been associated with inadequately chlorinated swimming pools.

COMPLICATIONS

• Bronchiolitis obliterans (rare), corneal opacities with visual disturbance (usually resolves spontaneously)

PROGNOSIS

Most syndromes are self-limited.

ASSOCIATED ILLNESSES

• Respiratory infection responsible for 10% of all pediatric respiratory illnesses; may cause upper respiratory symptoms, whooping cough syndrome; pneumonitis; lower respiratory tract disease associated with adenovirus types 4 and 7.
• Pharyngoconjunctival fever: low-grade fever associated with conjunctivitis, pharyngitis, rhinitis, and cervical adenitis; 15% of patients may have meningismus; increased incidence in summer months; common-source outbreaks most often associated with type 3.
• Epidemic keratoconjunctivitis: bilateral conjunctivitis with preauricular adenopathy; may persist for up to 4 weeks; corneal opacities may persist for several months; associated with types 8, 19, and 37.
• Hemorrhagic cystitis may cause microscopic or gross hematuria; if present, gross hematuria persists on average for 3 days; often associated with dysuria and urinary frequency; more common in males than females; associated with types 11 and 21.
• Infantile diarrhea: watery diarrhea associated with fever; symptoms may persist for 1 to 2 weeks; associated with types 40 and 41.
• Central nervous system (CNS) infection epidemics (associated with outbreaks of respiratory disease) and sporadic cases of encephalitis and meningitis have been observed; often associated with pneumonia.
• Miscellaneous adenoviruses have been associated with intussusception (isolated in up to 40% of cases), fatal congenital infection, disseminated disease in immunocompromised patients.

 Differential Diagnosis

• Respiratory infection

—Influenza
—Parainfluenza
—Pertussis
—Mycoplasma
—Bacterial pneumonia

• Pharyngoconjunctival fever group A streptococcus

—Epstein-Barr virus
—Parainfluenza
—Enterovirus
—Measles

• Epidemic keratoconjunctivitis herpes simplex

—Chlamydia
—Enterovirus

• Hemorrhagic cystitis glomerulonephritis

—Vasculitis
—Renal tuberculosis

• Infantile diarrhea rotavirus

—Norwalk agent
—Astrovirus
—Salmonella
—Shigella
—Campylobacter

• CNS infection herpes simplex virus

—Enterovirus
—Mycoplasma
—Bacterial meningitis

Data Gathering

HISTORY

Question: Fever
Significance: Nonspecific

Question: Rhinitis
Significance: URI

Question: Laryngitis, sore throat
Significance: URI

Question: Nonproductive or croupy cough
Significance: Respiratory infection

Question: Headache, myalgias
Significance: CNS infection

Question: Hematuria (gross or microscopic), dysuria, urinary frequency
Significance: Hemorrhagic cystitis

Question: Watery diarrhea
Significance: Enteric adenovirus

Physical Examination

Finding: Head and neck conjunctivitis, rhinitis, exudative pharyngitis, meningismus
Significance: Typical findings of adenovirus

Finding: Pulmonary tachypnea, wheezing, rales
Significance: Pneumonia

Finding: Abdomen tenderness, distention
Significance: Gastroenteritis

Laboratory Aids

Test: CBC
Significance: Leukocytosis or leukopenia, often with left shift in the differential count.

Test: Erythrocyte sedimentation rate
Significance: Often elevated

Test: Chest radiograph
Significance: Bilateral patchy interstitial infiltrates (lower lobes).

Test: Serology
Significance: Diagnosis may be made by a documented 4-fold rise in serum antibody.

Test: Viral isolation
Significance: From nasopharyngeal secretions, urine, conjuctivae, or stool.

Test: Viral identification
Significance: Either visualization of virion by electron microscopy or demonstration of viral antigen in infected cells by immunofluorescence; highest yield from nasopharyngeal swab or stool.

Therapy

PREVENTION

Precautions that Should Be Used for Hospitalized Patients

SYMPTOMS	TYPE OF PRECAUTIONS
Respiratory disease	Contact
Gastrointestinal	Enteric disease
Conjunctivitis	Drainage and secretion

Oral vaccines have been used by the military.

ICD-9-CM 079.0

Diarrhea secondary to adenoviral infection 008.62
Conjunctivitis-pharyngoconjuctival fever 007.2
Conjunctivitis 077.3

BIBLIOGRAPHY

Baum SG. Adenovirus. In: Mandell GL, Douglas RG, Bennett JE, eds. *Principles and practice of infectious diseases*, 4th ed. New York: Churchill Livingstone 1995:1382–1387.

Claesson BA, Trollfors B, Brolin I, et al. Etiology of community-acquired pneumonia in children based on antibody responses to bacterial and viral antigens. *Pediatr Infect Dis J* 1989;8(12):856–862.

Krajden M, Brown M, Petrasek A, et al. Clinical features of adenovirus enteritis: a review of 127 cases. *Pediatr Infect Dis J* 1990;9:636–641.

Wirsing von Konig CH, Rott H, Bogaerts H, et al. A serologic study of organisms possibly associated with pertussis-like coughing. *Pediatr Infect Dis J* 1998;17(7):645–649.

Author: Susan E. Coffin

Alcohol (Ethanol) Intoxication

 Database

DEFINITION

• Alcohol intoxication is the ingestion of toxic quantities of ethanol (ethyl alcohol), which results in common signs, including lack of coordination, slurred speech, ataxia, nausea, vomiting, increased urination, vasodilatation, coma, shock, hypoglycemia, and seizures.
• Ingestion of 1 g/kg yields peak blood level 100 mg/dL (legal limit defining intoxication).
• Blood level of 50 mg/dL can cause intoxication in children.

ETIOLOGY

• Alcoholic beverages contain 20% to 50% alcohol (hard liquor), 10% to 14% (wine), and 3% to 8% (beer); 1% = 1 mg/dL.
• Ethanol is also in liquid cold remedies, mouthwashes, after-shave lotion, liniments, tinctures, some rubbing alcohols, perfumes, colognes, glass cleaners, and paint removers.
• When ingestion is intentional, it often occurs concurrent with multiple drug ingestions and trauma from risk-taking behaviors.

PATHOPHYSIOLOGY

• Ethanol is rapidly absorbed (20% in stomach, 80% in small intestine)
• Blood levels peak 30 to 60 minutes after ingestion
• It is metabolized primarily in the liver utilizing alcohol dehydrogenase
• 2% to 10% of ethanol is excreted unchanged by the kidneys
• Ethanol depresses the central nervous system (CNS) via the reticular activating system by interfering with ion transport at the cell membrane and interacting with γ-aminobutyric acid receptors.
• Hypoglycemia is caused by impaired gluconeogenesis and lactic acidosis or ketoacidosis may develop. Seizures are a frequent manifestation of hypoglycemia in children.

EPIDEMIOLOGY

• Intentional intoxication is most common in adolescents.
• Accidental intoxication occurs most frequently in toddlers.

COMPLICATIONS

• Death: associated with ingestion of >3 g/kg (which corresponds to an approximate serum level of 300 mg/dL)
• CNS depression: apnea, hypoxia, poor judgment, and risk taking
• Vomiting and aspiration
• Vasodilatation and hypotension
• Increased urinary losses and dehydration
• Hypoglycemia and seizures and coma

PROGNOSIS

• Blood levels >300 mg/dL: survival expected if treated.
• Blood levels >500 mg/dL: high risk of death despite therapy.

 Differential Diagnosis

INFECTION

• Meningitis
• Encephalitis
• Overwhelming infection

ENVIRONMENTAL

• Inhalations and toxic exposures (e.g., carbon monoxide poisoning)
• Other ingestions

TUMOR

• Brain tumor and sudden increase in intracranial pressure secondary to obstruction by mass

TRAUMA

• Head trauma

METABOLIC

• Other causes of hypoglycemia
• Ketoacidosis
• Hyperammonemic states

Data Gathering

HISTORY

Question: Quantity and time of ingestion?
Significance: May help in determining expected blood level and the development of additional symptoms.

Question: Other possible ingestions?
Significance: Concurrent ingestions are common and effects can vary as well as treatment.

Question: Did the ingestion occur as an intentional or unintentional act?
Significance: Assess risk of suicidal ideation.

Question: Past medical problems?
Significance: Because alcohol may exacerbate underlying conditions (e.g., diabetes, liver disease, renal failure), it is important to obtain a history on past medical problems.

Question: When did the patient last eat?
Significance: Determines the risk for aspiration.

Physical Examination

Finding: Complete neurologic examination
Significance: Assesses level of consciousness, ability to protect airway.

Finding: Signs of trauma
Significance: Head trauma can occur concurrently or mimic symptoms of ethanol intoxication. Falls and motor vehicle accidents are also common secondary problems.

Laboratory Aids

Test: Estimated peak ethanol level
Significance: Calculated as mg ingested/ (volume of distribution × body weight), where volume of distribution is 0.6 L/kg in adults and 0.7 L/kg in children

Test: Drug screen
Significance: Usually includes drugs of abuse, antidepressants, benzodiazepines, and others.

Test: Electrolytes, glucose, renal function (BUN, creatinine), liver enzymes, arterial blood gas
Significance: Dehydration, hypoglycemia, renal impairment, liver toxicity, metabolic and respiratory acidosis can occur.

RADIOGRAPHIC IMAGING

Computed tomography of head: if head trauma suspected.

Therapy

- ABCs (airway, breathing, circulation); life support measures including mechanical ventilation may be required.
- Gastric lavage if within 30 to 60 minutes of ingestion (do not induce emesis because of CNS depression).
- Activated charcoal if ingestion of other substances suspected; not useful in alcohol intoxication alone.
- Treat hypoglycemia with IV dextrose. Treat until clinically stable and blood ethanol level is <50 mg/dL.
- Treat dehydration and hypotension with intravenous fluids.
- Monitor for hypothermia.
- Hemodialysis may be required if levels exceed 300 to 350 mg/dL.
- No specific antidote exists

Follow-Up

- If ingestion was intentional, psychiatric evaluation is highly recommended.
- Accidental ingestions require parental education about child safety.

PREVENTION

- Child safety caps on medicine bottles
- Locks on medicine and liquor cabinets
- Avoid purchasing medicines containing alcohol for use by children.

PITFALLS

Ingestion of other toxic substances may be missed.
Failure to assess neurologic morbidity from trauma.

BIBLIOGRAPHY

Ernst AA, Jones K, Nick TG, et al. Ethanol ingestion and related hypoglycemia in a pediatric and adolescent emergency department population. *Acad Emerg Med* 1996;3(1):46–49.

Hagymasi K, Blazovics A, Lengyel G, et al. Oxidative damage in alcoholic liver disease. *Eur J Gastroenterol Hepatol* 2001;13(1):49–53.

Leung AK. Ethyl alcohol ingestion in children. *Clin Pediatr* 1986;25(12):617–619.

Raroque SSU, Weibe, RA. Household products and environmental toxins. In: Levin DL, Morriss, FC, eds. *Essentials of pediatric intensive care*, 2nd ed. New York: Quality Medical Publishing and Churchill Livingstone, 1997:922–923.

Rodgers GC, Matyunas NJ. *Handbook of common poisonings in children*, 3rd ed. Committee on Injury and Poison Prevention. Evanston, IL: American Academy of Pediatrics, 1994:149–152.

Author: Deborah L. Silver

Alpha-1 Antitrypsin Deficiency

 Database

DEFINITION

Alpha-1 antitrypsin deficiency is a disease characterized by the deficiency of the serum protease inhibitor, α-1 antitrypsin, leading to premature development of lung emphysema and chronic liver disease.

CAUSES

• Deficiency of α-1 antitrypsin, a serum protease inhibitor, a glycoprotein of approximately 52 kd, which inhibits the activity of elastase, an enzyme involved in the remodeling of connective tissue.
• In the absence of regulated protease activity, alteration in the structure of end organs, lung, and liver can develop and cause disease.

EPIDEMIOLOGY

• Most common metabolic cause of emphysema in adults and liver disease in children, for which they receive orthotopic liver transplantation.
• Incidence and prevalence change with the population studied, ranging from 1:1,639 live births in Sweden to 1:2,000 individuals in the United States.

GENETICS

• Autosomal-recessive inheritance
• Multiple structural forms of the α-1 antitrypsin protein are encoded on chromosome 14.
• 75 different alleles with the most common phenotypes are characterized as Pi, protease inhibitors, by gel electrophoresis.
• The most common normal variant is referred to as M.
• Individuals with the most severe deficiency have an α-1 antitrypsin allele variant, referred to as Z.

COMPLICATIONS

• Cirrhosis and emphysema are common.
• Individuals expressing the homozygous ZZ alleles.
• Infants are often diagnosed with neonatal hepatitis and jaundice and may develop one of three patterns of disease in the future: death, continuing evidence of liver damage, possibly necessitating liver transplantation for development of normal liver function.
• In adults with cirrhosis and chronic active hepatitis, the heterozygous allele variant, MZ, may be detected.

 Differential Diagnosis

Alpha-1 antitrypsin deficiency in infancy and childhood may have diverse presentations, including jaundice and hepatosplenomegaly or ascites and cirrhosis in the neonatal period to asymptomatic hepatosplenomegaly in adulthood. Differential diagnosis of idiopathic neonatal hepatitis, cholestasis, and cirrhosis should be considered for the varying presentation of α-1 antitrypsin deficiency

 Data Gathering

HISTORY

Question: Was there jaundice in the newborn?
Significance: Neonatal hepatitis and jaundice may be the first signs of α-1 antitrypsin deficiency.

Question: Was there prolonged jaundice?
Significance: Common to see persistent elevation of neonatal bilirubin level, often within the first 4 months of life.

Question: What is the significance of resolved cholestasis in infants?
Significance: May then have long asymptomatic periods with persistence of hepatocellular injury.

Question: What is the usual adult presentation?
Significance: Adults present with cirrhosis and ascites.

 Physical Examination

Finding: Jaundice and hepatosplenomegaly
Significance: Evidence of chronic liver disease in older children and adults.

 Laboratory Aids

Test: The diagnosis of the allele variants is made by serum protein electrophoresis, which characterizes the most common of the protein forms.
Significance: The most common variants are the normal allele variant, M; deficient variant, Z and S, the latter leading to lung disease and the former leading to both liver and lung disease; and the null and dysfunctional variants.

Test: *MM*
Significance: Gives a serum α-1 antitrypsin level of 20 to 53 mmol/L, the normal state.

Test: *PiZZ*
Significance: Gives a low concentration of 2.5 to 7 mmol/L.

Test: *Pinull/nul*
Significance: Gives zero levels.

Test: *PiSZ*
Significance: Gives a mildly increased risk.

IMAGING TECHNIQUES

Testing for diagnosis for complications of α-1 antitrypsin deficiency may include ultrasonography with Doppler study to evaluate a candidate for transplantation or the presence of portal hypertension.

Therapy

DRUGS

• No appropriate drug therapy currently exists for the deficient state.
• Ursodeoxycholic acid, a choleretic agent, is used in doses of 20 to 30 mg/kg/day in one or divided doses for management of cholestasis and pruritus.
• Other medications for treatment of complications of chronic liver disease may be necessary.
• Future treatment options will include definitive gene therapy for ZZ and possibly other genotypes.

DURATION

• Lifelong expectant management and treatment of complications

SURGICAL

• Only definitive therapy is orthotopic liver transplantation

 ## Follow-Up

PROGNOSIS

• One fourth of children will need a future liver transplantation as a result of worsening liver function and evidence of cirrhosis and portal hypertension.
• One fourth will stabilize and liver function will normalize.
• One fourth will slowly develop chronic liver disease and cirrhosis.
• One fourth will have less severe liver function and live into adulthood.

 ## Common Questions and Answers

Q: What is the usual medical course for my child with this problem?
A: In general, one fourth of children will need future liver transplantation as a result of worsening liver function and evidence of cirrhosis and portal hypertension; one fourth will stabilize and liver function will normalize; one fourth will slowly develop chronic liver disease and cirrhosis; and one fourth will have less severe liver function and live into adulthood.

Q: Is there a cure for my daughter at present?
A: Yes; at present treatment options range from treating for complications and definitively performing a liver transplantation to remove the affected organ. Since prognosis can change for children, we wait until the liver is no longer functioning before it is replaced. Eventually, it is possible to consider gene therapy for this disorder since there are investigations in this area but these are years away from fulfillment.

ICD-9-CM 277.6

BIBLIOGRAPHY

α-1-Antitrypsin deficiency. In: Sherlock S, Dooley J, eds. *Diseases of the liver and biliary system*. London: Blackwell Scientific, 1992:425–427.

Balistreri W. Neonatal cholestasis. *J Pediatr* 1987;106:171.

Balistreri W. Liver disease associated with a α-antitrypsin deficiency. In: Balistreri W, Stocker J, eds. *Pediatric hepatology*. New York: Hemisphere, 1990:159–175.

Marcus N, Teckman JH, Perlmutter DH. α-Antitrypsin deficiency in childhood disease. *J Pediatr Gastroenterol Nutr* 1998;27(1):65–74.

Perlmutter DH. a-Antitrypsin deficiency. In: Walker WA, Durie PR, Hamilton JR, et al., eds. *Pediatric gastrointestinal disease*. Philadelphia: BC Decker, 1991:976–991.

Author: Andrew E. Mulberg

Altitude Illness

 Database

DEFINITION

- Acute mountain sickness (AMS): Failure to adapt to the hypoxic demands of altitude. Includes a group of clinical signs and symptoms seen in travelers to altitudes greater than 2,500 meters.
- Mild mountain sickness: Headache in morning and on exertion, anorexia, nausea, dizziness, vomiting, shortness of breath on exertion, insomnia, irritability, periodic breathing (Cheyne-Stokes respiration), poor performance
- Moderate mountain sickness: Severe headache, lassitude (weariness, indifference, antisocial), weakness, anorexia, nausea, ataxia, decreased urine output, diminished judgment and coordination. Capable of activities with difficulty
- Severe mountain sickness: Insidious or acute onset, usually 2 to 4 days after ascent. Can progress to life-threatening within hours. Can include pulmonary and cerebral edema
- High-altitude cerebral edema (HACE): Develops over 1–3 days after ascent. Headache, vomiting, lassitude, irritability, drowsiness, ataxia, slurred speech, cranial nerve paralysis, hypo- or hyperreflexia, hemiparesis, hemiplegia, mental status changes (confusion, unreasonableness, depression, disorientation, amnesia, hallucinations, severe nightmares), decreased urine output, seizures, papilledema, coma, death.
- High-altitude pulmonary edema (HAPE): Often develops over several days. Initially with dyspnea on exertion, then at rest, decreased exercise capability, dry cough, fatigue, tachypnea, low-grade temperature (<38.5°C). Develop pink frothy sputum, cyanosis, wheezing, rales, tachycardia, low-grade fever, orthopnea.
- Other altitude related issues: High-altitude syncope, amnesia, edema (facial and extremity), retinopathy (hemorrhages), pharyngitis and bronchitis, flatus, immune suppression, thrombosis, coagulation abnormalities (thrombolic events), platelet changes, chronic mountain illness (Monge disease).

PROGNOSIS AND COMPLICATIONS

- Excellent if recognized quickly, ascent stopped, and/or descent and treatment begun
- Can be poor if symptoms not recognized or appreciated and appropriate descent and therapy not initiated
- Symptoms insidious or acute onset, usually 2 to 4 days after ascent
—Can progress to life-threatening within hours

ASSOCIATED ILLNESSES

- Ophthalmologic

—Retinal vessel engorgement
—Retinal hemorrhages: Usually resolves in 7 to 10 days without symptoms. 100% of people at 6,500 m (21,450 ft)
—Macular hemorrhages: More severe, associated with visual changes. Ultraviolet keratitis.

 Differential Diagnosis

ENVIRONMENTAL

- Alcohol toxicity
- Hangover
- Drug effects
- Hypothermia
- Carbon monoxide poisoning

MEDICAL/METABOLIC

- Dehydration
- Viral illness

PSYCHOSOCIAL

- Exhaustion, sleep deprivation
- Personality traits (irritability)
- Insomnia

 Data Gathering

HISTORY

Question: Previous altitude illness?
Significance: Suggests symptoms in future with ascent to similar altitude.

Question: Location (altitude) where symptoms occurred, how did the patient arrive at that altitude, and what was the rate of ascent?
Significance: Rapid ascent minimizes time for natural acclimatization and increases risk of developing altitude illness.

Question: Exertion level?
Significance: Increased exertion on ascent may increase speed of symptom development.

Question: Medication, drug or alcohol use, predisposing medical illness (asthma, restrictive lung disease)?
Significance: Underlying medical conditions, such as sickle cell disease, hypertension, sleep apnea, obstructive lung disease, cerebrovascular disease or concurrent infections, may predispose one to development of altitude illness. Medication use or presumed medical illness may mask or mimic signs and symptoms of altitude illness.

Question: Symptom complex (variable)?

Question: Morning headache, progressive with ascent?
Significance: Suggests HACE.

Question: Insomnia, difficulty falling asleep, frequent waking?

Significance: Suggests hypoxia and development of altitude illness.

Question: Periodic breathing (hyperpnea to apnea)?
Significance: Suggests moderate to more advanced altitude illness.

Question: Gastrointestinal: anorexia, nausea, vomiting, abdominal cramps, flatus?
Significance: Potentially related to ascent.

Question: Pulmonary: dry cough, shortness of breath, sore throat, dyspnea on exertion and at rest, decreased exercise capability?
Significance: Potential progression to HAPE.

Question: Neurologic: lassitude, weariness, indifference, fatigue, irritability, dizziness, ataxia, weakness?
Significance: Progression to HACE.

Question: Decreased urine output edema, fluid retention?
Significance: Indicative of fluid shifts, fluid losses, inadequate replacement, or dehydration.

 Physical Examination

Finding: Normal in early AMS
Significance: Physical examinations are nondescript early in development.

Abnormalities usually occur after 12 to 24 hours at altitude (range 2 to 96 hours).

 Laboratory Aids

Test: Chest x-ray study (CXR)
Significance: Vasocongestion, patchy or diffuse infiltrates; often worse than physical examination would suggest.

Test: ECG
Significance: Rule out myocardial etiology of symptomatology or consequence of ascent.

Test: Toxicologic screen
Significance: Rule out medication effect for presenting symptomatology.

Test: Electrolytes
Significance: Assess hydration status, fluid shifts, glucose.

Test: Arterial blood gas
Significance: Assess oxygenation, ventilation, and acid–base status.

Test: Carbon monoxide level
Significance: Ensure carbon monoxide poisoning not a factor in presentation.

Test: CBC
Significance: Assess oxygen carrying capacity of blood. Look for anemia, polycythemia, and platelet abnormalities.

Test: Ventilation and perfusion scan
Significance: Structural pulmonary assessment.

Test: Brain CT
Significance: Assess for structural abnormalities and cerebral edema.

Therapy

GENERAL

- Suspect AMS
- Stop ascent
- Partial or full descent
- Oxygen if available
- Fluids
- Consider acetazolamide to hasten acclimatization
- Avoid alcohol, codeine, sedative-hypnotics
- Avoid respiratory depressants

SPECIFIC

- Mild AMS: Treatment may not be needed. Symptomatic headache relief with ibuprofen, acetaminophen, aspirin, prochlorperazine (Compazine). Temporal artery massage. Halt descent until symptoms improve.
- Moderate to severe AMS

—Descent
—Oxygen (relieves hypoxia, reduces pulmonary hypertension)
—Furosemide (be careful of volume depletion)
—Acetazolamide
—Consider dexamethasone (if allergic to sulfa or cannot take acetazolamide)
—Vasodilators (nifedipine, morphine)

- HACE: Descend immediately. Oxygen, furosemide, dexamethasone. Consider intubation and hyperventilation.
- HAPE

—Descend immediately
—Oxygen
—Furosemide
—Acetazolamide
—Vasodilators (nifedipine, morphine) may be useful
—Consider antibiotics
—Positive-pressure breathing
—Pursed-lip breathing, mask, intubation
—Knee-chest position with abdominal squeeze
—Portable hyperbaric chamber
—Symptoms may recur when positive pressure removed.

MEDICATIONS

- Acetazolamide (Diamox, a carbonic anhydrase inhibitor)

—Hastens natural respiratory changes that occur during acclimatization
—Can help prevent AMS. Effectiveness in treating established AMS not clear.
—General guidelines for use

—Use in conjunction with (not in place of) gradual ascent, with passive transport to 3,000 m (9,850 ft) and rapid active transport
—Prophylaxis if previous history of AMS, history of periodic breathing, insomnia
—Treatment of early AMS
—May be useful if sulfa allergy is present
—Dosage: 5 to 10 mg/kg/day divided b.i.d. (125–500 mg b.i.d. or t.i.d. in adults), 24 hours prior to ascent and 1 to 2 days at altitude
—Side effects: mild diureses, paresthesias, nausea, drowsiness, taste changes, anorexia, blurred vision

- Dexamethasone (Decadron): Helpful for AMS treatment and early cerebral edema. Dosage: 4 mg b.i.d. to q.i.d.
- Oxygen: Helpful at low flow at night (for headache, insomnia, cyanosis). Increases Pao_2
- Nifedipine: Dosage: 20 mg sustained release q8 hours may be useful for treatment and prevention of HAPE, 24 hours prior to ascent and for 2 to 3 days at altitude
- Diet: Increase fluid and calorie consumption with altitude and exertion. Increased carbohydrate diet. Avoid alcohol, tobacco, sedatives, recreational drugs.

Follow-Up

- Expect improvement with mild mountain sickness in 1 to 2 days.
- Moderate mountain sickness clears with descent and acclimation.
- Severe mountain sickness clears with descent and therapy.

PROGNOSIS

Good if recognized and treated appropriately. Poor if not recognized or treated appropriately

PREVENTION

- Avoid rapid ascent: Do not go too high too fast. Do not fly or drive to heights >3,000 m (>10,000 ft).
- Gradual acclimatization: Limit ascents to 300 m (1,000 ft) per day above 3,000 m (10,000 ft). Allow at least 24 hours for each 1,000 m (3,300 ft) gained. Exercise is not a substitute for acclimatization (or protection against AMS).
- Be aware and respectful of symptoms (even if minor): Assume symptoms secondary to AMS unless proven otherwise. Go no higher until symptoms resolve. Descend if worsening.
- Climb high, sleep low.
- Avoid alcohol, codeine, sedative-hypnotics, respiratory depressants.
- Exercise within individual capacity; avoid heavy exercise after passive ascent for at least 24 hours.

Common Questions and Answers

Q: Can one develop AMS at moderate altitudes, such as during a ski vacation?
A: Yes, although the altitudes encountered rarely lead to the development of severe symptoms in this population.

Q: Will physical conditioning prior to ascent decrease the risk of developing altitude illness?
A: No, in fact better conditioning may inadvertently increase the risk of developing altitude illness as one may achieve higher altitudes more quickly.

Q: Should everyone in whom a headache develops when at a higher than usual altitude be treated (pretreated) with acetazolamide?
A: No. One must weigh other options and severity of illness prior to decision to treat or provide prophylaxis for AMS.

BIBLIOGRAPHY

Carpenter TC, Niermeyer S, Durmowicz AG. Altitude-related illness in children. *Curr Probl Pediatr* 1998;28(6):177–198.

Dumont L, Mardirosoff C, Tramer MR. Efficacy and harm of pharmacological prevention of acute mountain sickness: quantitative systematic review. *Br Med J* 2000;321(7256): 267–272

Woodward GA. Altitude Illness. Clinical pediatric emergency medicine: Environmental Emergencies 2001;(3):168–178

Author: George Anthony Woodward

Amblyopia

Database

DEFINITION

Amblyopia is poor vision, usually just in one eye, resulting from poor visual input during early childhood (the critical period for visual development).

- Although the cause of amblyopia may be correctable (refractive blur, strabismus, cataract), vision is not restored immediately due to poor neurovisual development.

PATHOPHYSIOLOGY

Normally, equal and clear visual input from both eyes is necessary for the visual system to develop. Any condition that prevents a clear, fusible (capable of being integrated into a single binocular image in the brain) image during the first 8–10 years of life is capable of causing amblyopia.

- In general, the earlier the abnormal input, the greater the likelihood and severity of amblyopia. In an infant, amblyopia can result from as little as 1 week of abnormal visual input.
- Asymmetrical input between the two eyes (unilateral cataract, anisometropia, etc.) is more likely to cause amblyopia than symmetrically poor images, due to competitive influences between the two eyes. As a result, amblyopia is almost always unilateral.
- Bilateral amblyopia may result from severe, symmetrical bilateral image degradation such as bilateral cataract, bilateral high ametropia (high refractive error), etc.
- Visual acuity in amblyopic eyes varies from minimal impairment (20/25) to legal blindness (<20/200). Other significant impairments may include reduced contrast sensitivity, reduced or absent binocularity and depth perception, and impaired or distorted spatial perception. Peripheral visual fields are preserved, and vision is never completely lost (no light perception) from amblyopia alone.

CLASSIFICATION

Amblyopia is generally classified by cause, with three primary types:

- Anisometropic amblyopia—resulting from asymmetrical refractive error and resultant unilateral blurring. This is the most common cause of amblyopia.
- Strabismic amblyopia—resulting from misalignment of the eyes, and subsequent lack of an image that can be "fused" or integrated into a single image in the brain. This is most likely with early onset, constant strabismus. Up to 60% of patients with strabismus will also have amblyopia.
- Deprivation amblyopia—resulting from optical imperfection (cataract, ptosis, corneal opacity, prolonged patching or bandage), which prevents the formation of a clear image in one or both eyes.

GENETICS

Amblyopia is thought to be primarily environmental, although some of the conditions leading to amblyopia, including strabismus, cataracts, ptosis, and anisometropia, have a genetic basis. For this reason, the family history is frequently positive for amblyopia.

EPIDEMIOLOGY

- Large population-based studies suggest that 2–5% of the adult population has amblyopia.
- Amblyopia is the most common cause of unilateral vision loss in children and young adults.

Differential Diagnosis

Amblyopia is diagnosed by exclusion: residual vision loss after correction or elimination of all other optical and anatomic factors is defined as amblyopia. Conditions that cause vision loss without easily recognized pathology might be mistaken for amblyopia. In children, the differential diagnosis of vision loss in normal-appearing eyes includes:

- Uncorrected refractive error (hyperopia, myopia, astigmatism)
- Congenital optic nerve hypoplasia
- Optic atrophy
- Compressive, toxic, or hereditary optic neuropathies
- Retinopathies, including Leber congenital amaurosis, Stargardt disease, retinitis pigmentosa, and others
- Central visual impairment (cortical blindness)
- Glaucoma
- Factitious or functional causes (hysterical blindness)

Vision loss from amblyopia will persist even after the condition that originally caused the amblyopia has resolved. In some cases, when there is no obvious cause, a history of past episodes of anisometropia, occlusion, or strabismus must be considered.

Data Gathering

HISTORY

- Age of onset of vision loss
- History of eye trauma, injury, or surgery
- History of refractive error or glasses
- History of ptosis or ocular occlusion
- Family history of strabismus, anisometropia, or amblyopia

Physical Examination

Visual acuity is the single most significant sign in detection of amblyopia. Vision must be tested with each eye separately, with reliable occlusion (adhesive patch, opaque card, or plastic occluder). Since most amblyopia is monocular, testing vision with both eyes open is inadequate as a screening tool.

- In older children (>4 years) capable of reliable testing, monocular recognition visual acuity is tested by reading standard charts. Interocular difference of >1 line, or vision in either eye <20/30 that is not corrected with glasses should be investigated with full ophthalmologic examination. Charts may use illiterate symbols (pictures, numbers, E's) or letters.
- Younger children or children not capable of recognition visual acuity testing with charts can be tested by fixation preference, by induced tropia test (using vertical prism to induce diplopia and observing fixation preference).
- Binocularity tests such as Titmus stereopsis (3-D fly) will detect suppression, which is frequently associated with amblyopia.
- Other tests for amblyopic factors, while not directly measuring reduced vision, are useful for screening purposes, including:

—Cover test, Hirschberg corneal light reflex test, and Bruchner tests for strabismus (see Strabismus)
—Photoscreening, which uses the characteristics of the red reflex to detect amblyogenic factors such as optical aberrations and strabismus
—Inspection of the red reflex for cataract, optical opacities, and high refractive errors

Because the outcome of amblyopia depends entirely on early detection and treatment within the first few years of life, all children should be screened by monocular recognition visual acuity as early as possible (at the 3- or 4-year well-child visit) and testing should be repeated annually until 8 years of age. Children with interocular difference of >1 line, or acuity in one or both eyes <20/30, should be referred for complete ophthalmologic evaluation and treatment. Children who are not capable of accurate visual acuity testing by 4 years should also be referred for complete evaluation.

Laboratory Aids

TESTS

Electrophysiologic testing using visual evoked cortical potential (VEP) is capable of detecting amblyopia. As typically performed, using very bright diffuse flashes, however, VEP is not sensitive enough to accurately detect amblyopia. Special VEP techniques using patterns (SVEP), however, show promise as a useful technique to measure resolution visual acuity in very young and nonverbal children. Psychophysical tests such as Teller preferential visual acuity testing have been used clinically to detect amblyopia and quantify visual acuity in young children, but are less useful for population-based screening because of the time and skill required to administer the tests.

Imaging studies of the optic nerves and posterior visual pathways may be useful to exclude other causes of vision loss.

Therapy

Treatment for children with unilateral amblyopia consists of treating the underling cause of vision loss (strabismus, anisometropia, optical opacity, etc.) and forced preferential use of the amblyopic eye. The classic and most common treatment is occlusion with an adhesive patch worn over the opposite eye for several hours per day. The amount of time of occlusion necessary to reverse amblyopia depends on variables including the density of amblyopia, cause of amblyopia, age, and other ocular conditions. Typically patches are worn from hours to full time, from a few weeks to months. Infants and very young children will require closer observation to prevent reversing the amblyopia to the previously preferred eye (occlusion amblyopia) from excessive patching. Other techniques include:

- Occlusion of the opposite eye with opaque or translucent lens in glasses or opaque contact lens
- Optical penalization of the opposite eye with intentional overcorrection of refractive error (usually +3.00 diopters or more overcorrection)
- Cycloplegia for penalization, using atropine or other long-acting cycloplegic in the opposite eye

Treatment should be attempted in amblyopic children within the "sensitive period" of birth to 8 years of age. Improvement of vision with treatment of older children has been reported, but is much less likely.

In strabismic amblyopia, initiation of treatment for amblyopia need not wait for correction of the strabismus. In fact, the stability of the surgical strabismus correction is improved if amblyopia therapy is initiated prior to surgery. Treatment is usually continued until visual acuity in both eyes is equal, or until vision in the amblyopic eye shows no further improvement after several examinations over a period of time.
For bilateral amblyopia, correction of the underlying cause is the only treatment available.

Follow-Up

- In general, the younger the patient, the more intensive the patching therapy, and the milder the amblyopia, the more frequent vision testing is necessary to ensure that vision in the opposite, occluded eye is not harmed. For full-time patching, testing is generally done at intervals of about 1 week per year of age, e.g., 2 weeks for a 2-year-old, etc.
- In younger children, amblyopia may recur after successful treatment. Children should be retested frequently, and re-treated if vision drops after finishing successful initial treatment. Testing should continue at least annually until the child is at least 8 years old.

PITFALLS

- Vision testing in young children is difficult and sometimes unreliable. Children must be tested with each eye separately. Repeating the tests and adjunctive tests including the Titmus test (-D fly), cover testing, photoscreening, and Bruchner red reflex test will increase the sensitivity of screening.
- Prompt referral of failures and children suspected of poor vision for complete ophthalmic examination is essential for successful amblyopia screening programs.
- Once treated, amblyopia may recur and vision should be retested regularly.
- Patients with strabismus, even if previously treated with glasses or surgery, must be followed for amblyopia. Amblyopia is found in 40–60% of patients with strabismus, and is not reversed by strabismus surgery.

Common Questions and Answers

Q: How long will patching be necessary?
A: It is not possible to predict exactly how long treatment will be necessary to restore vision. In general, the younger the patient, the milder the impairment, and the more intensive the patching, the more quickly vision is restored. In general, patching is usually continued for 1–4 months in most cases of anisometropic or strabismic amblyopia.

Q: Will vision be normal after treatment?
A: The degree of recovery with amblyopia therapy depends on the density of the amblyopia, the cause, and the age at which treatment is initiated. In almost all children under 6–8 years of age, some visual improvement can be expected with amblyopia treatment, although not all patients will improve to 20/20 vision.

Q: Will patching eliminate the need for glasses?
A: No

Q: Will patching for amblyopia improve the strabismus?
A: No

Q: Is "vision therapy" without patching an effective treatment for strabismus?
A: Although eye exercises, pleoptics, and other vision therapies have been used to treat amblyopia, none is as effective as patching or other occlusive therapy. Current vision therapy techniques have not been proven to improve amblyopia.

Q: My child refuses to wear a patch. Are there alternatives to patching?
A: Yes, optical penalization with glasses, atropine cycloplegic penalization, and even contact lens occlusion can be effective.

BIBLIOGRAPHY

Ching FC, Parks NMN, Friendly DS. Practical management of amblyopia. *J Pediatr Ophthalmol Strabismus* 1986;23:12–17.

Lam GC, Repka MX, Guyton DL. Timing of amblyopia therapy relative to strabismus surgery. *Ophthalmology* 1993;100:1751–1756.

The Pediatric Eye Disease Investigator Group. A randomized trial of atropine vs. patching for treatment of moderate amblyopia in children. *Archives of Ophthalmology* 2002; 120:268–278.

The Pediatric Eye Disease Investigator Group. The clinical profile of moderate amblyopia in children younger than 7 years. *Archives of Ophthalmology* 2002;120:281–287.

Sengpien F, Blakemore C. The neural basis of suppression and amblyopia in strabismus. *Eye* 1996;10:250–258.

Weakley DR, Holland DR. Effect of ongoing treatment of amblyopia on surgical outcome in esotropia. *J Pediatr Ophthalmol Strabismus* 1997;4:275–278.

Author: Monte D. Mills

Amebiasis

 Database

DEFINITION

• Clinical syndromes associated with *Entamoeba histolytica* infection.
• Most common clinical manifestation is intestinal amebiasis.
• Intestinal disease may be asymptomatic or have mild symptoms such as abdominal discomfort, flatulence, constipation, and occasionally diarrhea.
• Nondysenteric colitis is characterized by intermittent diarrhea and abdominal pain.
• Acute amebic colitis (dysenteric) is associated with grossly bloody stools with mucus, abdominal pain, and tenesmus.

CAUSES

• *Entamoeba histolytica* is nonflagellated protozoan parasite.
• Other species of the *Entamoeba* family are nonpathogenic including the morphologically identical *E. dispar*.

PATHOPHYSIOLOGY

• Fecal-oral transmission
• *E. histolytica* is excreted as cysts or trophozoites in the stool of infected patients.
• Ingested cysts are unaffected by gastric acid and produce trophozoites that colonize and invade the colon. The parasite has the ability to lyse human cells including colonic epithelium and immune effector cells such as neutrophils, macrophages, and lymphocytes. The host immune response contributes significantly to the destruction of host tissues.
• Amebas disseminate directly from the intestine to the liver in up to 10% of patients. Dissemination from the liver to the lung, heart, brain, and spleen has been described.
• The incubation period is typically 1–3 weeks but can range from a few days to months or years.

EPIDEMIOLOGY

• Spreads person to person via fecal-oral transmission.
• Less common modes of transmission include food and water. Sexual transmission can occur among homosexual males.
• Worldwide distribution involving an estimated to 10% or more of the world's population. Most common in tropical areas with infection rates as high as 20–50%. The highest morbidity and mortality is seen in developing countries in Central America, South America, Africa, and Asia.
• Amebiasis accounts for 40–50 million cases of colitis worldwide and leads to 40,000–110,000 deaths annually.
• The estimated prevalence in the United States is 4%.
• The very young, the elderly, and patients with underlying immunosuppression or malnutrition are at highest risk for severe disease.

COMPLICATIONS

• Amebic liver abscess—second most common presentation of amebiasis, often not associated with amebic dysentery
• Ameboma—abdominal mass representing granulation tissue in the colon
• Extraintestinal manifestations of amebiasis are presumed to be a result of direct extension from liver abscesses. These include:
• Pericarditis
• Pleuropulmonary abscess or empyema
• Bronchohepatic fistula
• Genitourinary tract abscess
• Cerebral abscess
• Cutaneous amebiasis

 Differential Diagnosis

INFECTION

• *Salmonella*
• *Shigella*
• *Campylobacter*
• *Yersinia*
• *Clostridium difficile*
• *Escherichia coli* (enteroinvasive and enterohemorrhagic)
• Pyogenic abscess
• Echinococcal cyst

INFLAMMATORY BOWEL DISEASE

• Crohn disease
• Ulcerative colitis

MISCELLANEOUS

• Ischemic colitis
• Diverticulitis
• Arteriovenous malformations
• Hepatoma

 Data Gathering

The diagnosis is often missed in children because the disease is not included in the differential. Patients in whom the diagnosis should be considered include:

• Immigrants from or travelers to endemic areas
• Children with bloody stools or mucus in stools
• Children with hepatic abscess
• The febrile child with right upper quadrant pain and tenderness, abdominal pain, or discomfort
• The child with hepatomegaly, typically without jaundice.

Laboratory Aids

The diagnosis of amebiasis depends on the recognition of typical symptoms and:

ROUTINE LABORATORY TESTS

- Complete blood count typically reveals a leukocytosis.
- Transaminases are often not elevated.
- Occult blood is detected in stool.

MICROSCOPIC DIAGNOSIS

Identification of trophozoites or cysts in the stool.

- Serial stool samples, usually three, are recommended.
- Samples obtained within 1–2 hours of passage should be examined by wet mount and fixed in formalin and polyvinyl alcohol.
- Serial stool samples are necessary since cysts may be shed intermittently. Three serial stool samples will detect up to 70% of patients with amebic colitis and 50% of patients with hepatic abscess.
- Stool samples should not be contaminated by urine, water, barium, enema substances, laxatives, or antibiotics since these substances may destroy or interfere with identification of the trophozoites.

SEROLOGY

- Serum antiamebic antibodies are considered an adjunct to diagnosis. Approximately 85% of patients with amebic dysentery and 99% of patients with liver amebiasis will have positive serology.

RADIOGRAPHIC STUDIES

- Ultrasound, CT, or MRI of the liver.
- Chest radiographs in patients with hepatic amebiasis may reveal elevation of the right hemidiaphragm.

BIOPSY STUDIES

- Amebae are difficult to visualize in abscess aspirates and substantial risk is associated with CT or ultrasound-guided procedures including bleeding, peritonitis secondary to spillage of amebae or rupture of echinococcal cysts.
- Colonic or rectal mucosa visualized by colonoscopy reveals ulcerations and amebae can often be found around these lesions.

 Therapy

SPECIFIC

- The goal of treatment is the elimination of tissue-invading trophozoites and intestinal cysts.
- The choice of treatment regimens depends on the clinical presentation. Agents that are active against *E. histolytica* are divided into two categories: drugs with activity against intraluminal amebae and drugs with activity against extraintestinal and invasive amebiasis.

—Asymptomatic intestinal amebiasis—intraluminal agents
—Iodoquinol is the drug of choice. The recommended dosage is 30–40 mg/kg/day (max. 1,950 mg) given orally in three divided doses for 20 days.
—Alternative agents include diloxanide furoate (Furamide) at doses of 20 mg/kg/day (max. 1,500 mg/day) given orally in three divided doses **OR** paromomycin, 25–35 mg/kg/day given orally in three divided doses for 7 days.
—Acute amebic colitis or extraintestinal amebiasis
—Metronidazole (a tissue active agent) 35–50 mg/kg/day given orally in three divided doses for 10 days (max. 2,250 mg/day) PLUS a course of treatment with an intraluminal active agent (as above). Approximately one third of patients treated with metronidazole alone will relapse.

- Patients with large liver abscesses or who have failed medical therapy should be considered candidates for surgical or percutaneous drainage.

PREVENTION

- Treatment of drinking water
- Hand washing
- Appropriate disposal of human fecal waste
- Use of condoms

INFECTION CONTROL MEASURES

- Standard precautions are recommended for the hospitalized patient.

 Follow-Up

- Clinical improvement is expected within 72 hours of initiation of therapy
- Follow-up stool examination is always necessary to insure eradication of intestinal amebae
- For amebic abscesses, drainage should be considered if response to medical therapy has not occurred in 4 to 5 days

PITFALLS

Misdiagnosis is a common problem with amebiasis. Since it is not common in the United States, amebiasis may initially be misdiagnosed as bacterial dysentery.

BIBLIOGRAPHY

American Academy of Pediatrics. Amebiasis. In: Pickering LK, ed. *2000 Red book: report of the Committee on Infectious Diseases* , 25th ed. Elk Grove, IL: American Academy of Pediatrics, 2000:164–166.

Hotez PJ, Strickland AD. Amebiasis. In: Feigin RD, Cherry JD, eds. *Textbook of pediatric infectious diseases*, 4th ed, vol 2. Philadelphia: WB Saunders, 1998:208:2389–2397.

Purdy JE, Petri WA Jr. *Entamoeba histolytica* (amebiasis). In: Long SS, Pickering LK, Pober CG, eds. *Principles and practice of pediatric infectious diseases*, 1st ed. New York: Churchill Livingstone, 1997;275:1380–1386.

Ravdin JI. *Entamoeba histolytica* (amebiasis). In: Mandell GL, Bennett JE, Dolin R, eds. *Principles and practice of infectious diseases*, 5th ed, vol 2. Philadelphia: Churchill Livingstone, 2000:2798–2810.

Author: Theoklis Zaoutis

Anaerobic Infections

 Database

DEFINITION

Anaerobes are organisms capable of growing in a reduced oxygen tension, either exclusively (obligate anaerobes) or in addition to growing in air (facultative anaerobes). They are the predominant organisms in normal bacterial flora.

PATHOPHYSIOLOGY

- Usually caused by endogenous organisms.
- Occurs when there is a break in a mucocutaneous barrier.
- Infections are often polymicrobial and include aerobic organisms.
- Increased risk associated with impaired host immunity or presence of devitalized tissue (due to surgery, trauma, vascular insufficiency).
- Numerous virulence factors including exotoxins (e.g., *Clostridia* spp.), antiphagocytic capsule (e.g., *Bacteroides* spp.), endotoxin (gram-negative anaerobes).
- Infections may be characterized by suppuration, abscess formation, or tissue destruction.

EPIDEMIOLOGY

- Less frequent in children than in adults.
- Responsible for up to 10% of significant bacteremic episodes in infants and children.

COMPLICATIONS

- Vary with nature of infection.

PROGNOSIS

- Determined by speed with which infection is appropriately treated with surgery and antibiotics.
- Up to 40% mortality associated with clinically apparent anaerobic bacteremia.
- Soft tissue infections caused by *Clostridial* spp. may cause up to 20% mortality despite aggressive therapy.

ASSOCIATED ILLNESSES

- Central nervous system (CNS) infections

—Brain abscess
—Subdural empyema
—Epidural abscess

- Head and neck infections

—Sinusitis
—Chronic otitis media
—Ludwig angina
—Cervical adenitis
—Peritonsillar abscess
—Dental abscess
—Gingivitis

- Pleuropulmonary infections

—Aspiration of oral and/or gastrointestinal fluids
—Secondary to aspirated foreign bodies
—Actinomycosis

- Peritonitis/peritoneal abscess

—Appendiceal abscess
—Perforated viscus
—Postoperative complication
—Trauma related

- Cholangitis

—Ascending infection may occur following Kasai procedure.
—Infection is often polymicrobial.

- Bacteremia

—Often associated with underlying GI disease.

- Soft tissue infection

—Paronychia
—Crepitant cellulitis
—Necrotizing fasciitis
—Gas gangrene

- Infected bite wounds

—Anaerobes isolated from 50% of human or animal bites.

 Differential Diagnosis

- Likely pathogens not recovered from aerobic cultures.
- Failure of empiric antibiotic coverage that is not active against anaerobes.

 Data Gathering

HISTORY

Question: Impaired mental status?
Significance: Increased risk of aspiration.

Question: History of thumb-sucking?
Significance: Anaerobes frequently isolated from paronychia.

Question: Recent surgery or trauma?
Significance: Poor drainage or devitalized tissue associated with anaerobic infection.

Question: Underlying immunodeficiency or chronic illness?
Significance: Impaired phagocytic function.

Question: Discharge with foul odor?
Significance: Characteristic of anaerobic infection.

Physical Examination

Finding: Location of infection
Significance: Increased incidence of anaerobic infections associated with oropharyngeal, abdominal, and female genital tract.

Finding: Poor dentition
Significance: Increased colonization of oropharynx with anaerobic organisms.

Finding: Gas in tissue, crepitus
Significance: Infection with gas-forming organism

Finding: "Dishwater" pus
Significance: Characteristic of anaerobic infections

 ## Laboratory Aids

Test: Gram stain
Significance: Small, pleomorphic gram-negative bacilli (*Bacteroides* spp.); large gram-positive organisms with "box-car" morphology (*Clostridia* spp.).

Test: Anaerobic cultures
Significance: Should be performed on tissue or aspirated fluid obtained in a sterile fashion from the infected site. Avoid sending a swab for culture. Specimens need to be transported promptly to the microbiology laboratory.

Test: Antibacterial susceptibility testing
Significance: Due to usual efficacy of empiric regimens, susceptibility studies should be limited to organisms involved in potentially life-threatening or difficult-to-treat infections.

Test: X-ray studies
Significance: Air-fluid level, cavity formation, gas in tissue.

Test: Special imaging studies
Significance: CT and/or MRI scans often important to define anatomic location and extent of disease.

 ## Therapy

EMPIRIC DRUG THERAPY

• CNS infections

—Cefotaxime/metronidazole or oxacillin/chloramphenicol

• Head and neck infections

—Penicillin or clindamycin

• Pleuropulmonary infections

—Penicillin or clindamycin or ampicillin/sulbactam

• Peritonitis/peritoneal abscess

—Ampicillin/sulbactam or cefoxitin

• Cholangitis

—Ampicillin/sulbactam and gentamicin

• Bacteremia

—Isolate-dependent

• Soft tissue infection

—Site dependent

• Infected bite wounds

—Amoxicillin/clavulinic acid

ADJUNCTIVE THERAPY

• Surgery

—Effective drainage of abscesses and debridement of devitalized tissue essential.

• Hyperbaric oxygen

—Especially for extensive *Clostridial* infections.

ICD-9-CM 041.84

BIBLIOGRAPHY

Dunkle LM. Anaerobic infections. In: Feigin RD, Cherry JD, eds. *Textbook of pediatric infectious diseases*, 3rd ed. Philadelphia: WB Saunders, 1992:1044–1052.

Finegold SM. Anaerobic bacteria: general concepts. In: Mandell GL, Douglas RG, Bennett JE, eds. *Principles and practice of infectious diseases*, 4th ed. New York: Churchill Livingstone, 1995:2156–2173.

Goldstein EJ. Selective nonsurgical anaerobic infections: therapeutic choices and the effective armamentarium. *Clin Infect Dis* 1994;18:S273–S279.

Gorbach SL. Antibiotic treatment of anaerobic infections. *Clin Infect Dis* 1994;18:S305–S310.

Nichols RL, Smith JW. Anaerobes from a surgical perspective. *Clin Infect Dis* 1994;18: S280–S286.

Author: Susan E. Coffin

Anaphylaxis

 Database

DEFINITION

Anaphylaxis is an explosive antigen specific IgE-mediated response resulting in the release of potent biologically active mediators from mast cells and other inflammatory cells. However, non–IgE-mediated direct mast cell degranulation can result in the same response. Patients may develop any combination of the following symptoms: cutaneous (urticaria/angioedema), respiratory (bronchospasm/laryngeal edema), cardiovascular (hypotension, arrhythmias, myocardial ischemia), and gastrointestinal (nausea, vomiting, pain, diarrhea).

PATHOPHYSIOLOGY

Inducing agents stimulate mast cells to release inflammatory mediators either via an antigen-specific or antigen-nonspecific manner. These mediators may then act either locally or systemically. Mediator release results in the table Pathophysiology of Anaphylaxis.

GENETICS

Atopy can be familial and atopics are at more risk for anaphylaxis.

EPIDEMIOLOGY

- Incidence 0.4 cases per million individuals annually
- Increased hospital incidence of 0.6 cases per 1,000 patients
- 400 to 800 deaths annually in the United States

COMPLICATIONS

- Pulmonary edema, pulmonary hemorrhage, and pneumothorax
- Laryngeal edema with or without airway obstruction
- Myocardial ischemia and infarction
- Death may result from asphyxiation from upper airway obstruction or profound shock or both.

PROGNOSIS

Excellent provided the trigger can be avoided.

 Differential Diagnosis

GENETIC/METABOLIC

- Hereditary angioedema
- Systemic mastocytosis
- Pheochromocytoma
- Carcinoid

ALLERGIC/IMMUNOLOGIC

- Idiopathic
- IgE-mediated
- Nonimmunologic mast-cell degranulation
- Exercise-related
- Sulfiting agents
- Nonsteroidal antiinflammatory drug reaction
- Serum sickness

MISCELLANEOUS

- Vasovagal collapse

COMMON CAUSES

- IgE mediated
—Antibiotics (penicillin and others)
—Foreign protein agents (bee-sting venom, latex antigens, fire ant venom, and others)
—Therapeutic agents (allergen extracts, vaccines, and others)
—Foods (peanuts, nuts, shellfish, and others)
- Non–IgE-mediated (activates histamine release from mast cells without IgE)
—Radiocontrast media
—Opiates
—Dextran
—Vancomycin
—Polymyxin B
—Quaternary ammonium muscle relaxants (i.e., methyl scopolamine bromide, homatropine methylbromide, methantheline bromide, and ProBanthine bromide)

Approach to the Patient

GENERAL GOAL

Rapidly decide whether the symptoms the patient is experiencing are consistent with anaphylaxis (profuse rhinorrhea, urticaria, wheezing, throat tightness, tachycardia, and hypotension).

Phase 1: Initiate therapy for anaphylaxis. This generally includes: epinephrine 1:1000 administered subcutaneously, 1H antihistamines, and H1 antihistamines (refractory cases).

Phase 2: Attempt to identify the agent that induced the anaphylactic reaction.

Data Gathering

HISTORY

Question: How long does it take for a patient to react to an offending allergen?
Significance: Anaphylactic reactions usually begin within seconds to minutes after contact with offending antigen. This can help the physician identify the responsible antigen.

Question: Can a patient have an anaphylactic reaction on their first exposure to an allergen?
Significance: A patient must have had a previous exposure to the offending allergen for sensitization to occur. Therefore, anaphylactic reactions should not occur on first exposure.

Question: What does the patient sense during an anaphylactic reaction?
Significance: Patients commonly describe an impending doom. This may be the first sign of an impending anaphylactic reaction.

Question: What organ systems are affected in an anaphylactic reaction?
Significance: The target organs may include: the heart, the lungs, the skin, and the gastrointestinal tract. Any or all of these target organs may be affected.

Question: What is the mechanism of fatal anaphylaxis?
Significance: Death may occur from upper airway obstruction and/or shock. When treating a patient with anaphylaxis upper airway obstruction, and hypotension should be taken very seriously.

Question: Has the patient had anaphylaxis in the past?
Significance: The patient likely knows the responsible allergen. Efforts should be directed toward allergen avoidance.

Question: Does the patient have autoinjectable epinephrine?
Significance: Most deaths from anaphylaxis are associated with delayed administration of epinephrine. Most patients with a history of anaphylaxis are candidates for autoinjectable epinephrine.

Question: Did the patient experience a bee sting, or is the patient allergic to any foods?
Significance: Bee venom allergy can result in anaphylaxis. It is important to identify the bee (remember honey bees leave their stinger at the sting site). Immunotherapy is indicated and effective for bee venom–allergic patients. Any food can cause anaphylaxis, but peanuts, nuts, and shellfish are notorious.

Pathophysiology of Anaphylaxis

PATHOLOGIC PROCESS	SIGN OR SYMPTOM	PUTATIVE MEDIATOR RESPONSIBLE
Vascular permeability	Urticaria, angioedema, laryngeal edema, abdominal swelling, cramps	Histamine (H_1) leukotrienes, prostaglandins
Vasodilation	Flushing, headache	Histamine (H_1 and H_2), leukotrienes, prostaglandins
Smooth-muscle contraction	Wheezing, gastrointestinal cramps, diarrhea	Histamine (H_1), leukotrienes, prostaglandins
Congestion	Rhinorrhea, bronchorrhea	Histamine (H_2), prostaglandins, leukotrienes

Source: From Atkinson et al., with permission.

Question: Does the patient have asthma or heart disease?
Significance: Asthma and cardiovascular disease are risk factors for death during anaphylaxis.

Question: Does the patient take any medications?
Significance: Beta-blockers make treatment of anaphylaxis more difficult. Alternative medications should be sought in patients with a history of anaphylaxis.

 ## Physical Examination

Finding: Angioedema
Significance: May be noted anywhere during a systemic allergic reaction, but it is much more significant if it involves the lips, tongue, mouth, or larynx (can result in airway obstruction).

Finding: Urticaria
Significance: Cutaneous manifestation of a systemic allergic reaction.

Finding: Profuse rhinorrhea
Significance: May signal upper respiratory tract involvement in a systemic allergic reaction.

Finding: Wheezing
Significance: May signal lower respiratory tract involvement in a systemic allergic reaction.

Finding: Tachycardia and hypotension
Significance: May signal cardiovascular involvement in a systemic allergic reaction. Tachycardia usually represents a compensatory mechanism in order to maintain the patient's blood pressure.

 ## Laboratory Aids

The treatment of anaphylaxis should never be withheld while awaiting laboratory confirmation.

Test: Plasma histamine
Significance: Plasma histamine is elevated during anaphylaxis.

Test: Serum tryptase
Significance: Serum tryptase becomes elevated during anaphylaxis.

Test: Complete blood count
Significance: Hemoconcentration (as judged by an increased hematocrit or hemoglobin) is common as fluid exits the intravascular space during an anaphylactic reaction.

Test: Chest x-ray
Significance: The bronchospasm associated with anaphylaxis may result in air trapping and hyperinflated lung fields on chest x-ray.

Test: ECG
Significance: Anaphylaxis may show rhythm abnormalities, ischemic changes or infarction on an ECG.

Test: Cardiac enzymes
Significance: Myocardial ischemia during anaphylaxis may result in a myocardial infarction, and elevated cardiac enzymes.

REFERRAL
Factors that may help alert you to make a referral include:
• History of idiopathic anaphylaxis. The allergist can help by testing to likely triggers.
• History of anaphylaxis to bees. Anaphylaxis to bees is an indication for venom desensitization.
• History of food anaphylaxis. The allergist can assist with an appropriate avoidance diet and support resources.
• History of latex anaphylaxis. The allergist can assist with strict latex avoidance precautions, and latex testing if the history is unclear.

 ## Therapy

• Subcutaneous epinephrine 1:1000 concentration. Early administration of epinephrine is very important.
• Maintain airway. Laryngeal edema can be managed with racemic epinephrine from a meter dose inhaler or nebulizer.
• A tourniquet may be applied (above the injection or sting site) to decrease venous blood return from the site of antigen entry.
• Supplement with oxygen, place in recumbent position and elevate legs. Patients during anaphylaxis have an increased oxygen consumption.
• Diphenhydramine IV. H1 blockade is very important in the control of an anaphylactic reaction.
• Cimetidine IV or ranitidine IV. H1 blockade may be helpful in refractory anaphylaxis.
• Maintain blood pressure with volume expanders or pressors. Hypotension is a serious manifestation of anaphylaxis.
• Aminophylline may be added for wheezing.
• Hydrocortisone or another systemic steroid should be started. These are most helpful to prevent a late-phase reaction, and they are of little help during an immediate anaphylactic reaction.

 ## Follow-Up

• All patients who have had anaphylaxis should be discharged with epinephrine in an autoinjecting apparatus.
• Patients with a known trigger should be counseled on strict avoidance.
• All patients should follow up with an allergist.
• Patients not admitted to the hospital should be observed for several hours because late reactions can begin as late as 12 hours after the initial anaphylaxis. These patients are at risk for a second episode of anaphylaxis. These patients, therefore, should be bolused with steroids during the acute treatment, and they should be given a short course of oral corticosteroids to finish at home. In addition, these patients must be discharge with autoinjecting epinephrine (this will provide temporary relief so the patient will have time to seek medical assistance). Patients must know to seek immediate medical help if symptoms return.

 ## Common Questions and Answers

Q: When should the autoinjectable epinephrine be used?
A: It is intended for severe allergic reactions as manifested by any of the following: bronchospasm, angioedema of the lips or tongue, or hypotension (dizziness). The patient must seek immediate medical help if the autoinjectable epinephrine is required.

Q: Do patient's outgrow this condition?
A: No. Subsequent reactions tend to have a more rapid onset, and tend to be more severe.

Q: Who should be referred to an allergist?
A: All patients who have experienced anaphylaxis would benefit from consultation with an allergist. Patients with anaphylaxis from bee stings, and certain antibiotics can be desensitized. In addition, the allergist can be helpful in identifying obscure triggers of anaphylaxis.

BIBLIOGRAPHY
Atkinson TP, Kaliner MA. Anaphylaxis. *Med Clin North Am* 1992;76:841–853.

Bochner BS, Lichtenstein LM. Anaphylaxis. *N Engl J Med* 1991;324:1785–1790.

Cahaly RJ, Slater JE. Latex hypersensitivity in children. *Curr Opin Pediatr* 1995;7(6): 671–675.

Kaliner MA. Anaphylaxis. In: Lockey RF, Bukantz SC, eds. *Fundamentals of immunology and allergy*. Philadelphia: WB Saunders, 1987:203.

Middleton E, Reed CE, Ellis EF, et al. *Allergy principles and practice*, 4th ed. Philadelphia: Mosby, 1993.

Stites DP, Terr AI, Parslow TG. *Basic and clinical immunology*, 8th ed. Englewood Cliffs, NJ: Prentice Hall, 1994.

Author: Christopher A. Smith

Anemia of Chronic Disease

 Database

DEFINITION

Anemia that accompanies a variety of systemic diseases with the common features of chronicity and inflammation

PATHOPHYSIOLOGY

- Associated with collagen vascular disease, inflammatory bowel disease, malignancy, severe tissue injury, renal failure, and infections.
- Three common pathophysiologic factors

—Shortened red-cell survival—not seen in the anemia of all chronic disorders. The mechanism has not yet been defined.
—Impaired bone marrow erythropoietic response to the anemia with a blunted increase in red-cell production. Decreased marrow response to erythropoietin.
—Impaired iron utilization. Poor iron release from the reticuloendothelial system. This leads to a fall in plasma iron levels, a decrease in marrow sideroblasts, and a rise in red cell protoporphyrin concentration.

- Impaired erythroid progenitor response.
- Iron absorption may be normal or decreased.
- Cytokines such as interleukin-1 and interleukin-6 can activate ferritin synthesis. The ferritin can lead to sequester iron, which eventually is converted into hemosiderin.

EPIDEMIOLOGY

May be associated with chronic infectious, collagen vascular disorders, other chronic inflammatory diseases, and cancer.

COMPLICATIONS

If severe, patients may be transfusion dependent and thus be at risk for complications associated with packed red blood cell transfusions.

 Differential Diagnosis

- Often confused with iron deficiency anemia.
- In both iron deficiency and anemia of chronic disease

—Decreased plasma iron
—Decreased transferrin saturation
—Decreased marrow sideroblasts
—Elevated free erythrocyte protoporphyrin (FEP)
—Decreased reticulocyte count

- In anemia of chronic disease

—Mild to moderate anemia
—Mild anisocytosis
—Usually normochromic normocytic but can be hypochromic with microcytosis
—Decreased plasma iron
—Decreased iron-binding capacity
—Normal or slightly low transferrin saturation
—Decreased marrow sideroblasts
—Normal or elevated reticuloendothelial iron
—Elevated free erythrocyte protoporphyrin
—Normal or elevated ferritin

- In iron deficiency

—Decreased plasma iron
—Increased iron-binding capacity
—Decreased transferrin saturation
—Decreased marrow sideroblasts
—Decreased reticuloendothelial iron
—Increased free erythrocyte protoporphyrin
—Decreased serum ferritin

 Data Gathering

HISTORY

- Underlying disease process exists. Disease entities often associated with anemia of chronic disease include infections, both acute and chronic; inflammatory disease; collagen vascular diseases; malignancies, and renal failure.
- The anemia develops over the first month of the disease process and then remains fairly stable over time.

 Physical Examination

Various abnormal physical findings may be present depending on the underlying chronic disease process.
May have mild pallor but will not have signs of circulatory collapse.

Laboratory Aids

- Complete blood count with indices: normocytic, normochromic (can be microcytic, hypochromic) anemia with hematocrit rarely less than 20%
- Reticulocyte count: Usually in the normal range, but low for the level of anemia.
- Iron studies: Low plasma iron, with low total iron-binding capacity, low transferrin saturation by iron, normal or high ferritin, elevated FEP.
- Hemosiderin in bone marrow macrophages is increased if bone marrow aspiration is done and the aspirate is viewed with iron stains. This is generally not indicated.
- Albumin and transferrin: Both low.
- Acute-phase reactants like C-reactive protein may be elevated.

PITFALLS

- If only the serum iron is obtained without the remainder of iron studies, the child may be inappropriately diagnosed with iron deficiency.
- Anemia of chronic disease often coexists with other causes of anemia, including: occult blood loss, hemolysis, dietary iron deficiency, and drug-related marrow suppression.

 ## Therapy

DRUGS

- Iron: There is no role for iron therapy unless there is coexisting iron-deficiency anemia.
- Recombinant human erythropoietin: Effective, but indications for use are still not universally accepted. Often utilized in chronic renal failure. Has been used in inflammatory bowel diseases with good results. Should be used for more severe and symptomatic anemia where the underlying disease is likely to be prolonged and difficult to treat. May be used in childhood cancer to decrease the exposure to blood products.

OTHER THERAPIES

- Treatment should be directed at the underlying disease process.
- Transfusion of packed red blood cells is sometimes indicated intermittently in severe anemia with hemodynamic compromise.

 ## Follow-Up

- Treatment of underlying disease process may promote slow resolution of associated anemia.
- Hematocrit increases about 6–8 weeks after start of recombinant human erythropoietin therapy. Continues to rise over 6 months.

 ## Common Questions and Answers

Q: Does anemia that is associated with a chronic disease require further evaluation?
A: If the anemia fits within the general guidelines of diagnosis as outlined above, there is no need to pursue further investigation, except in specific cases. If there is an associated malignancy where marrow metastasis is possible, a bone marrow aspirate and biopsy should be done. In conditions with malabsorption, nutritional deficiencies and blood loss should be ruled out.

ICD-9-CM 281.9

BIBLIOGRAPHY

Andrews NB, Bridges KC. Disorders of iron metabolism and sideroblastic anemia. In: Nathan DG, Oski FA, eds. *Hematology of infancy and childhood*, 5th ed. Philadelphia: WB Saunders, 1998:450–451.

Means RT. Erythropoietin in the treatment of anemia in chronic infectious, inflammatory, and malignant disease. *Curr Opin Hematol* 1995;2:210–213.

Means RT. Clinical application of recombinant erythropoietin in the anemia of chronic disease. *Hematol Oncol Clin North Am* 1994;8:933–944.

Stockman JA III, Ezekowitz, AB. Hematologic manifestations of systemic diseases. In: Nathan DG, Oski FA, eds. *Hematology of infancy and childhood*, 5th ed. Philadelphia: WB Saunders, 1998:1841–1879.

Author: Tammy I. Kang

Angioedema

 Database

DEFINITION

Angioedema is an autosomal-dominant disorder in which mutations in the C1-INH (C1 esterase inhibitor) gene results in a deficiency (or an inactive form) of plasma C1-INH. This permits unregulated activation of the complement and plasma kinin-forming pathways leading to angioedema.

COMMON CAUSES

Classic Hereditary Form

• Defect in one of the two genes coding for C1-INH on chromosome 11.

Acquired Forms

• In one form, normal amount and functionally normal C1-INH is secreted into the plasma, but it is bound to circulating antibodies that inactivate it (associated with benign and malignant monoclonal B-cell lymphoproliferative disorders)
• In the other form, an autoantibody not associated with lymphoproliferative disorders binds to C1-INH, which makes the C1-INH-C1s complex unstable, resulting in increased degradation of C1-INH.

PATHOPHYSIOLOGY

• Deficiency of C1-INH leads to unopposed activation of the first complement component, resulting in the formation of bradykinin, which produces angioedema.
• Angioedema may occur in the upper airway, gastrointestinal tract, and extremities.
• Life-threatening upper airway obstruction may develop.

GENETICS

• Autosomal dominant
• Mutations may be in either of two genes for C1-INH located on chromosome 11.
• Acquired forms lack a genetic predisposition (there is no mutation in the C1-INH gene).

COMPLICATIONS

• Life-threatening upper airway obstruction.
• Severe abdominal pain often mistaken for a surgical abdomen.

PROGNOSIS

Good with prophylactic and recombinant C1-INH therapies.

 Differential Diagnosis

TOXIC, ENVIRONMENTAL, DRUGS

Patients on angiotensin-converting enzyme (ACE) inhibitors

ALLERGIC INFLAMMATORY

• IgE-mediated allergic reactions

—Drug allergy
—Food allergy
—Contact allergy

• Transfusion reaction

TUMOR

Associated with neoplasms via unknown mechanism

GENETIC/METABOLIC

• Urticaria pigmentosa/mastocytosis
• Familial cold urticaria
• C3b inactivator deficiency
• Amyloidosis with deafness and urticaria
• Hereditary vibratory angioedema

PHYSICAL

• Physical urticarias

—Cold urticaria
—Cholinergic urticaria
—Pressure urticaria (angioedema)
—Vibratory angioedema
—Solar urticaria
—Aquagenic urticaria

• Exercise-induced anaphylaxis

RHEUMATOLOGIC

Collagen vascular disease

PSYCHOLOGICAL

• Panic attacks
• Globus hystericus
• Vocal cord dysfunction

MISCELLANEOUS

Idiopathic angioedema

 Data Gathering

HISTORY

Question: At what age did the recurrent episodes of subcutaneous and submucosal edema begin?
Significance: Recurrent episodes of angioedema usually begin at puberty.

Question: How are the episodes of angioedema characterized?
Significance: Angioedema episodes are characterized by edema of the upper airway, extremities, or bowels (can cause severe abdominal pain).

Question: Are the angioedema episodes associated with hives?
Significance: Episodes of angioedema are not associated with hives.

Question: How long do the episodes of angioedema last?
Significance: The duration of an angioedema episode usually last 1 to 4 days.

Question: What triggers the angioedema episode?
Significance: Episodes of angioedema can be triggered by emotional stress and physical trauma.

Question: Do other family members have similar episodes of angioedema?
Significance: Angioedema can be inherited in an autosomal-dominant fashion. There may be other affected family members.

Question: Do the episodes of angioedema respond to epinephrine, antihistamines, or corticosteroids?
Significance: Angioedema related to angioedema responds poorly to epinephrine, antihistamines, and corticosteroids.

 Physical Examination

Aside from angioedema, the physical examination is normal.

Laboratory Aids

GENERAL GOAL

Decide if the patient's symptoms are consistent with angioedema (recurrent angioedema after minor trauma, family history, onset at puberty, lack of hives, poor response to epinephrine).

- Measure C1 esterase inhibitor level.
- If C1 esterase inhibitor level is normal, and an acquired deficiency is suspected, order a functional assay of C1 esterase inhibitor. Samples for complement assays must be placed on ice immediately, otherwise the results may be falsely low.

Test: Direct measurement of C1-INH (study of choice to identify the hereditary form of C1-INH deficiency).
Significance: This is an antigenic assay. Affected patients have a minimal quantity of C1-INH detected, and heterozygotes (carriers) have approximately one-half normal levels detected.

Test: Direct measurement of C4 and C2 during attacks.
Significance: In acquired C1-INH deficiency the direct measurement of C1-INH is normal, but the C2 and C4 levels are decreased during attacks.

Test: CH50
Significance: The CH50 is a general screen of the complement system, and if abnormal can indicate a deficiency of any of the complement components.

REFERRAL

Factors that may help alert you to make a referral include:

- Any patient diagnosed with angioedema. An allergist can help evaluate these patients for possible androgen prophylaxis therapy. In addition, they can assist in the creation of an emergency plan for recombinant C1 esterase infusion.
- Patients with difficult-to-control angioedema without an identified trigger. An allergist/immunologist can assist with the appropriate evaluation.

Therapy

PROPHYLAXIS

- Anabolic steroids (Danazol or Stanozolol) cause increased production of C1-INH resulting in near-normal C2 and C4 levels (decreased degradation by activated C1), and a significantly decreased episode frequency. This therapy is indicated in patients with frequent or life-threatening episodes.
- Plasmin inhibitors (ϵ-aminocaproic acid or tranexamic acid) do not correct C2 and C4 levels, but are clinically effective.
- Recombinant C1-INH concentrate recently available.

ACUTE ATTACKS

- Recombinant C1-INH concentrate
- Intermittent administration of subcutaneous epinephrine (this type of angioedema is usually poorly responsive, but in an emergent situation this may be considered).

MEDICAL MANAGEMENT

Treatment of the underlying condition often results in resolution of the angioedema.

Follow-Up

- Patients should be seen at least annually.
- Follow-up should include:

—Review of triggers
—Prospective genetic counseling
—Reinforcement of the need for prophylaxis
—Review of attacks during the previous year
—Creation of an emergency plan for the administration of recombinant C1 esterase inhibitor during severe attacks

- Regular follow-up with an endocrinologist is indicated for patients requiring androgen steroid therapy

Common Questions and Answers

Q: What is a good screening test for angioedema?
A: The CH50 is a good screening test. Patients with angioedema have a low CH50. Remember that the specimen must be placed on ice immediately. Failure to ice the specimen will result in a falsely low CH50.

Q: What are the side effects of the prophylactic androgen therapy?
A: The side effects include: masculinization, menstrual irregularities, enhanced epiphyseal growth plate closure, water retention, hypertension, cholestatic hepatitis, hepatic carcinoma, decreased spermatogenesis, and gynecomastia.

BIBLIOGRAPHY

Agostoni A, Cicardi M. Hereditary and acquired C1-inhibitor deficiency: biological and clinical characteristics in 235 patients. *Medicine* 1992;71:206–215.

Borum ML, Howard DE. Hereditary angioedema. Complex symptoms can make diagnosis difficult. *Postgrad Med* 1998;103(4):251–256.

Frank MM, Gelfand JA, Atkinson JP. Hereditary angioedema: the clinical syndrome and its management. *Ann Intern Med* 1976;84: 580–593.

Gratten C, Powell S, Humphreys F. Management and diagnostic guidelines for urticaria and angio-edema. *Br J Dermatol* 2001;144(4):708–714.

Middleton E, Reed CE, Ellis EF, et al. *Allergy principles and practice*, 4th ed. Philadelphia: Mosby, 1993.

Sim TC, Grant JA. Hereditary angioedema: its diagnostic and management perspectives. *Am J Med* 1990;88:656–664.

Stites DP, Terr AI, Parslow TG. *Basic and clinical immunology*, 8th ed. Englewood Cliffs, NJ: Prentice Hall, 1994.

Author: Christopher A. Smith

Ankylosing Spondylitis

 Database

DEFINITION

Ankylosing spondylitis is an inflammatory arthritis that tends to be asymmetric peripherally and to involve the insertion of tendons, ligaments, as well as the sacroiliac joints and spine.

CAUSES

- Idiopathic

PATHOLOGY

- Inflammatory synovitis of joints and calcification of the anterior and posterior longitudinal ligaments of the spine

EPIDEMIOLOGY

- Typically affects adolescent males
- About 1 per 1,000 white boys
- Much less common in blacks

GENETICS

- HLA-B27 associated

COMPLICATIONS

- Acute anterior uveitis
- Aortic insufficiency

 Differential Diagnosis

INFECTION

- Reiter syndrome caused by enteric pathogens or *Chlamydia*
- Whipple disease
- Intestinal-bypass–associated arthritis
- Discitis
- Pott disease

TUMORS

- Osteoid osteoma

TRAUMA

- Traumatic injury causing low back pain/spasm
- Herniated disc

METABOLIC

- Ochronosis

CONGENITAL

- Kyphosis

IMMUNOLOGIC

- Inflammatory bowel disease–associated arthropathy
- Pauciarticular juvenile rheumatoid arthritis

PSYCHOLOGICAL

- Feigning low back pain/stiffness

MISCELLANEOUS

- Psoriasis-associated arthritis
- SEA (seronegative enthesopathy and arthropathy) syndrome

 Data Gathering

HISTORY

Question: Ankylosing spondylitis
Significance: Signified by back pain of insidious onset that has been present for at least 3 months. There is usually a family history of a male relative with disease and inactivity stiffness resulting in gelling of peripheral joints and back.

 Physical Examination

Finding: Sacroiliac tenderness
Significance: Indicates site of inflammation

Finding: Pain on direct palpation at insertion of Achilles tendon and plantar fascia at calcaneal insertion
Significance: Indicates site of inflammation

Finding: Schober test of lumbar spine flexibility
Significance: Mark 15-cm span at mid-low back at level of iliac crest while patient is standing. Have patient flex back as far as possible. Remeasure span. Abnormal if less than 5 cm increase in span.

Laboratory Aids

Test: CBC, ESR, HLA-B27, rheumatoid factor (RF), and antinuclear antibody (ANA) tests should be done.
Significance: Note that ESR is occasionally not elevated. RF and ANA are typically negative.

Test: Imaging
Significance: Sacroiliac views should be obtained to demonstrate evidence of pseudo-widening and/or sclerosis.

Test: False positives
Significance: HLA-B27 occurs in 8% of whites and 6% of blacks.

 ## Therapy

DRUGS

- NSAIDs: naproxen, indomethacin, meclofenamate
- Disease-modifying drugs: sulfasalazine, methotrexate, and tumor necrosis factor inhibitors.

PHYSICAL THERAPY

Physical therapy is an essential component of treatment. Must encourage range-of-motion exercises and avoid prolonged neck flexion.

DURATION OF THERAPY

- May be lifelong

DIET

- Food intake should be good with NSAIDs
- Ensure folate intake with methotrexate

 ## Follow-Up

WHEN TO EXPECT IMPROVEMENT

Over weeks to several months should see some improvement in stiffness, synovitis, and range of motion.

SIGNS TO WATCH FOR TO INDICATE PROBLEMS

- Worsening stiffness
- Acute or chronic eye pain
- Chest pain or shortness of breath

PROGNOSIS

- Poor if disease remains active for 10 years or more

PITFALLS

Overdiagnosis in HLA-B27–positive individuals in whom other causes for joint swelling should be considered.

 ## Common Questions and Answers

Q: Should HLA-B27 be checked routinely in boys with back pain?
A: Detection of HLA-B27 alone should not precipitate an extensive workup because it is so common in the normal healthy population. However, the risk for developing a spondyloarthropathy is 16 times greater than in the HLA-B27–negative individual.

Q: Can affected individuals play contact sports?
A: This is probably not a good idea because as the spine fuses, the risk for fracture of the spine (especially the C-spine) increases.

ICD-9-CM 720.0

BIBLIOGRAPHY

Burgos-Vargas R, Pacheco-Tena C, Vazquez-Mellado J. Juvenile-onset spondyloarthropathies. *Rheum Dis North Am* 1997;23:569–585.

Flato B, Aasland A, Vinje O, et al. Outcome and predictive factors in juvenile rheumatoid arthritis and juvenile spondyloarthropathy. *J Rheumatol* 1998;25(2):366–375.

Pepmueller PH, Moore TL. Juvenile spondyloarthropathies. *Curr Opin Rheumatol* 2000;12:269–273.

Prieur AM. Spondyloarthropathies in childhood. *Baillieres Clin Rheumatol* 1998;12:287–307.

Rosenberg AM. Juvenile onset spondyloarthropathies. *Curr Opin Rheumatol* 2000;12:425–429.

Authors: Randy Q. Cron
Gregory F. Keenan, 2nd edition

Anomalous Coronary Artery

 Database

DEFINITION

In this disorder, the left coronary artery arises from the pulmonary trunk rather than the aorta.

CAUSES

- Abnormal septation of the conotruncus into aorta and pulmonary artery.
- Persistence of the pulmonary buds and involution of the aortic buds that will eventually form the coronary arteries.

PATHOPHYSIOLOGY

- Left ventricle is perfused with desaturated blood.
- Collateral flow tends to steal blood from the myocardial blood vessels into the pulmonary artery, resulting in myocardial ischemia.

EPIDEMIOLOGY

- Rare anomaly
- 87% of patients with this anomaly present in infancy.

 Differential Diagnosis

- Cardiomyopathy
- Mitral-valve incompetence
- Left ventricular failure from other causes
- Colic
- Bronchiolitis

 Data Gathering

HISTORY

- Paroxysms of poor feeding, pallor, and sweats
- Irritability (crying), especially after meals
- May have intractable congestive heart failure
- Sometimes asymptomatic
- Occasionally may be symptomatic in infancy and then gradually improve (with adequate coronary collateralization)
- Older children and adults may have dyspnea, syncope, or angina pectoris on effort
- Sudden death

 Physical Examination

- Signs of congestive heart failure
- Loud P_2 component of S_2
- Gallop rhythm
- Murmur: mitral incompetence or a continuous murmur reminiscent of a coronary arteriovenous fistula
- Diagnosis should be entertained in any infant presenting with cardiomegaly or perplexing cardiorespiratory symptoms.

Laboratory Aids

Test: Chest x-ray study
Significance: Cardiomegaly, pulmonary edema

Test: Nuclear imaging
Significance: Thallium myocardial perfusion imaging shows reduced uptake in ischemic regions.

Test: Electrocardiography
Significance: Anterolateral infarct pattern in an infant (Q in I, aVL, V4–V6), abnormal R wave progression in precordial leads

Test: Echocardiogram
Significance: Attachment of coronary artery to pulmonary artery by two-dimensional Doppler interrogation shows flow passing from coronary artery to great artery rather than vice versa.

- Large right coronary artery
- Function and wall-motion abnormalities of left ventricle
- Echogenic papillary muscles
- Mitral regurgitation
- Cardiac catheterization
- Low cardiac output
- High filling pressures
- Pulmonary hypertension
- Aortic root angiography shows passage of contrast medium from left coronary to pulmonary artery

Test: Pulmonary artery angiogram
Significance: Shows reflux of contrast medium into the left coronary artery.

Emergency Care

Referral to cardiac center

Therapy

The first priority is stabilization of the patient.

SURGERY

- Ligation of origin of left coronary artery and reconstitution of flow with saphenous or internal mammary graft.
- Direct reimplantation of the left coronary (with a button of pulmonary artery around the origin) into the aorta.
- Creation of an aortopulmonary window and tunnel that directs blood from aorta to the left coronary ostium (Takeuchi procedure).
- Ligation of the origin of the left coronary artery to prevent steal in very sick infants

PROGNOSIS

- Untreated, 65% to 85% die before the age of 1 year, usually after 2 months of age (when pulmonary vascular resistance falls).
- Few improve spontaneously.
- Late results after surgery are fairly good.
- Mitral-valve incompetence may progress in spite of surgery and its repair may be required later.

Common Questions and Answers

Q: How do you differentiate the crying from colic?
A: This is not easy but the crying in patients with this lesion classically occurs after meals as blood is shunted to liver and intestines. This is not a highly sensitive finding.

Q: How does one proceed with the evaluation?
A: An ECG may show the classic pattern of an infarct or ischemia

ICD-9-CM 746.85

BIBLIOGRAPHY

Davis JA, Cecchin F, Jones TK, et al. Major coronary artery anomalies in a pediatric population: incidence and clinical importance. *J Am Coll Cardiol* 2001;37(2):593–597.

Emmanouilides GC, Riemenschneider TA, Allen HD, et al., eds. *Moss and Adams' heart disease in infants, children and adolescents including the fetus and young adult*, 5th ed. Baltimore: Williams & Wilkins, 1995:776–780.

Fyler C. *Nadas' pediatric cardiology.* Philadelphia: Henley & Belfins; St. Louis: Mosby, 1992:51:715–718.

Pelliccia A. Congenital coronary artery anomalies in young patients: new perspectives for timely identification. *J Am Coll Cardiol* 2001;37(2):598–600.

Author: Geoffrey Bird
Maully Shah, 2nd edition

Anorexia Nervosa

 Database

DEFINITION

Anorexia nervosa (AN) is a potentially life-threatening psychopathologic disorder of eating, involving profound weight loss, and abnormal body image. The impact on overall nutritional status and multisystem involvement of the individual's health can be significant and potentially life-threatening. Diagnostic criteria:

• Weight loss or failure to attain expected weight gain leading to body weight less than 85% of normal weight for height
• Disordered perception of experience of personal body weight or shape, undue influence of body image on self-assessment, and/or denial of seriousness and abnormality of current low body weight
• Intense, abnormal fear of becoming fat or of weight gain, although significantly underweight for height
• In females, the absence of at least three consecutive menstrual periods (i.e., amenorrhea)

DSM-IV specifies two types of AN:
• Restricting type: Absence of regular binge eating or purging (i.e., misuse of laxatives, enemas, or diuretics or self-induced vomiting) during the current episode of anorexia nervosa
• Binge eating/purging type: Presence of regular purging or binge eating behaviors during the current episode of anorexia nervosa

A third category, eating disorder not otherwise specified (EDNOS), describes patients who present with emotional concerns similar to those with AN or bulimia, and are considered pre-anorexic, at risk, or subthreshold anorexia

SPECTRUM OF SEVERITY

Mild: Weight proportionate (at or >90%) for height
• More exaggerated concern about body image and thinness than among normal adolescent and young adult population in the U.S.
• Mild distortion of body image (self-perception as overweight)
• No symptoms or signs of excess weight loss are noted.
• Daily diet contains 1,000 calories or more
• No purging
• Exercise moderate, not excessive

Moderate: Increasing distortion of body image (escalating self-perception of being overweight)
• Weight <90% of average weight for height
• Symptoms and signs of weight loss
• Constant dieting
• Abnormal concern with weight (either avoiding being weighed or weighing him/herself frequently, sometimes several times daily)
• Excessive exercise
• Diet contains <1,000 calories per day
• Withdrawal from family and friends
• Denial of weight loss, thinness, or the existence of any problem with weight loss or thinness

Severe: Pathologic and dramatic distortion of body image plus ongoing weight loss
• Weight only 85% (or less) of height
• Ongoing determination to lose additional weight
• Signs and symptoms of malnutrition (may include bradycardia and/or hypotension)
• Denial regarding thinness
• Pathologic or unhealthy means of weight loss (consuming <1,000 calories/day, purging, enemas, laxatives, anorexic drugs)
• Markedly excessive exercise

Profound: Body weight 75% or less than expected for height, as well as continuing rapid weight loss
• Increasingly disordered perception of body image and denial of thinness
• Electrolyte imbalances
• Associated cardiac abnormalities (e.g., arrhythmias, prolonged QT interval, bradycardia)
• Hypotension, with potential cardiovascular collapse

GENETICS
• Familial and genetic predisposition likely, but not yet clearly defined

EPIDEMIOLOGY
• More common in adolescents and young adults
• Much more prevalent in industrialized societies
• 85–95% female, but increasing evidence of AN in teenage males
• Age of presentation: 9 to 25 years; most common ages of onset: 14 and 18 years, with occasional onset after age 40

COMPLICATIONS
• Cardiac failure, dysrhythmia, hypotension, syncope
• Cardiac ventricular enlargement, cardiovascular collapse, shock, and potential death
• Esophagitis, hematemesis (including Mallory-Weiss syndrome)
• Constipation, decreased intestinal motility, rectal prolapse
• Delayed gastric emptying
• Gastric dilatation and even rupture
• Pancreatitis
• Renal calculi
• Delayed onset of puberty, amenorrhea, infertility
• Convulsive seizures (due to hypophosphatemia, hypocalcemia, other severe electrolyte/metabolic abnormalities)
• Peripheral neuropathies
• Severe bone loss, potential persistent osteopenia, and related fracture risk growth arrest
• Depression, anxiety, obsessive-compulsive disorder, potential suicide risk
• Euthyroid sick syndrome
• Malnutrition and/or acute and chronic malnutrition states
• Anemia, leukopenia, thrombocytopenia

PROGNOSIS
• Mortality rate of AN is 0.56% per year (>12 times the mortality rate among young females in general population)
• Most common causes of death: cardiac dysfunction or suicide
• 50% fully recover; 30% have partial recovery, including recurrences; 20% may have no substantial improvement in symptoms

 Differential Diagnosis

TUMORS
• Malignancy, including CNS malignancy

GASTROINTESTINAL
• Inflammatory bowel disease

METABOLIC
• Diabetes mellitus
• Addison disease
• Estrogen deficiency

 Data Gathering

HISTORY
• Weight changes (duration, extent, exact or estimated weight loss, including clothing sizes, past history)
• Diet patterns
• Menstruation history
• Exercise
• Energy level
• Sleep
• Emesis, other purging, including laxatives, diuretics, enemas
• Other drugs, including anorexic drugs, caffeine, other stimulants
• Other concomitant illnesses or family history of illnesses, including thyroid disorders, malignancies, diabetes mellitus, inflammatory bowel disease, psychiatric disorders

QUESTIONS TO ASK PATIENT
Question: How do you feel about your body size. Do you consider your weight too thin, too heavy, or just right for your height? How much would you like to weigh?

Question: When did you last weigh yourself? How often do you weigh yourself?

Question: What foods do you not eat? What foods make you feel anxious/guilty to eat? *Significance:* Fatty or high calorie foods may be specifically avoided by those with AN.

Other questions to include:
• When did you last eat something? Drink something? What? How much?
• How did you feel after you last ate (or drank) something?
• Do you feel sick (nauseated, bloated, etc.) after you eat (and how often)?
• When did you last vomit after eating (and was it spontaneous or provoked)?

Physical Examination

Finding: Flat affect, despondent
Significance: Depression, potential suicidal risk, poor self-image

Finding: Bradycardia, hypothermia, orthostasis, and/or hypotension
Significance: Volume depletion, dehydration, potential for cardiovascular collapse and shock

Finding: Dry skin, lanugo hair, carotinemic skin coloration
Significance: Chronic malnutrition and vitamin deficiency

Finding: Peripheral edema, acrocyanosis, diminished capillary refill
Significance: Increased severity of malnutrition and possible cardiovascular, electrolyte, and/or renal pathology

Finding: Bladder distention
Significance: Water loading to falsely increase weight for exam

Finding: Scars on knuckles, eroded dental enamel, parotid enlargement
Significance: Suggestive of self-induced vomiting, bulimia

Finding: Scars, old cuts, evidence of self-inflicted burns
Significance: Risk-taking behaviors

Laboratory Aids

- Complete blood count
- Sedimentation rate
- Serum electrolytes, including magnesium, calcium, phosphate, random glucose
- Electrocardiogram
- Thyroid function studies (TSH, free T_3), FSH/LH, and pregnancy test
- Bone density (if patient amenorrheic for >6 months)

Therapy

Inpatient hospitalization indicated for:
- Very low weight (75% or less of expected body weight)
- Excessive and rapid weight loss
- Acute electrolyte imbalance
- Cardiac disturbance
- Determination of need for parenteral or enteral rehydration and nutrition
- High suicide risk or psychosis
- Symptoms not responding to outpatient treatment
- Note: Specialized eating disorder centers are not readily available in all locations, often necessitating local hospitalization and stabilization with telephone subspecialty consultation.

Outpatient: The majority of mild and moderate eating disorders are amenable to care in ambulatory settings.

Components of intervention may include any of the following:
- Patient and parent education
- Collaboration with experienced and knowledgeable treatment team (including primary care physician, dietitian/nutritionist, psychotherapist, or psychiatric social worker)
- Stabilize nutritional status and medical concerns
- Individual and family therapy
- Assessment of suicide risk and extent of any concomitant psychiatric pathology
- Appropriate limitations on exercise, as indicated
- Calcium (1,000–1,500 mg/day) and multivitamin supplementation (assuring adequate vitamin D 400 IU/day)
- Psychiatric consultation and treatment for concomitant psychiatric illness
- Consider fluoxetine, desipramine, or imipramine for stabilization of recovery (with psychiatric/psychopharmacologic consultation), when weight at or <85% appropriate for height. (Note: Obtain baseline ECG to rule out prolonged QT interval before considering tricyclic antidepressants.)

Follow-Up

- Must be coordinated with patient, parents, primary health providers and psychiatric consultant for moderate and severe AN.
- Should involve at least one key contact at school and/or work: teacher, coach, counselor.
- At least weekly follow up appointments for 2 months or longer are warranted for patients with moderate or severe AN until weight gain and full activities resumed.
- Resumption of weight gain should occur gradually over weeks.
- Resumption of academic and extracurricular activities, sports participation, and exercise must be monitored in view of general health, nutritional status.

SIGNS TO WATCH FOR TO INDICATE PROBLEMS
- Failure to regain weight or weight loss
- Noncompliance with scheduled follow-up appointments
- Unexcused or unwarranted school absenteeism
- Deterioration in academic performance, impaired cognitive abilities, distractibility
- Sleep disturbance, excessive fatigue
- Behavioral problems, acting out, risk-taking behaviors
- Depression, other symptoms or signs of psychopathology
- Electrolyte abnormalities, or other signs of recurrent AN or bulimia

PITFALLS
- Excessively rapid refeeding (may produce gastric bloating, edema, or congestive heart failure)
- Potential electrolyte imbalances during refeeding
- Premature hospital discharge

Common Questions and Answers

Q: When can the patient resume regular school attendance?
A: As soon as possible, or when weight is at >85% of ideal body weight.

Q: When can the patient resume sports participation?
A: Exercise restrictions apply until there is no evidence of cardiac or electrolyte abnormalities.

Q: When can the patient safely be discharged from close monitoring and frequent follow-up medical care?
A: Individually determined, with consideration given to the severity of the eating disorder, duration of symptoms, and compliance with treatment plan, as well as consistency of weight gain. At least annual physical examinations with detailed nutritional assessment are advised for the lifetime of individuals with significant eating disorders.

ICD-9-CM 307.1

BIBLIOGRAPHY

American Psychiatric Association. *Diagnostic and statistical manual of mental disorders*, 4th ed, text revision. Washington, DC: American Psychiatric Association, 2000.

Becker AE, Grinspoon SK, Klibanski A, et al. Eating disorders. *N Engl J Med* 1999;340(14): 1092–1098.

Author: Lucy S. Crain

Anthrax

 Database

DEFINITION

Bacillus anthracis is a spore-forming, gram-positive rod that can cause acute infection (anthrax) in both animals and humans.

PATHOPHYSIOLOGY

- After inhalation, wound inoculation, or ingestion, *B. anthracis* spores infect macrophages, germinate, and proliferate. Proliferation occurs at the site of infection and in regional lymph nodes. Replicating bacteria release toxins leading to edema, hemorrhage, and necrosis.
- The incubation period of anthrax depends on the route of transmission.

—Inhalational anthrax: Infection requires inhalation of >8,000 spores. Incubation period is 2–60 days.
—Cutaneous anthrax: Spores enter a cut or abrasion in the skin. Incubation period is 1–12 days.
—Gastrointestinal anthrax: Spores are ingested in undercooked, infected meat. Incubation period is 1–7 days. Infection occurs in the upper (oral-pharyngeal lesions) or lower (intestinal lesions) GI tract.

- Hematogenous spread of the bacteria causes infection at other sites including the CNS, liver, spleen, and kidney.

ASSOCIATED DISEASES

- If anthrax is intentionally released, physicians must be alert for diseases caused by other potential biologic warfare agents. These include plague, tularemia, Q fever, smallpox, and botulism.

EPIDEMIOLOGY

- Anthrax is primarily zoonotic. Most naturally acquired anthrax infections are cutaneous (95%). Inhalational (5%) and GI (<1%) forms are particularly rare.

—Only 18 cases of inhalational anthrax were reported in the U.S. during the 20th century.
—No human-to-human spread of inhalational anthrax has been reported.
—Rare cases of human-to-human transmission via direct contact with cutaneous lesions have occurred.

- Anthrax has also been developed as a biologic warfare agent.

COMPLICATIONS

- Antibiotic therapy does not change the course of the eschar formation and healing in cutaneous anthrax, but it does decrease the likelihood of systemic disease.

- Systemic dissemination of inhalational, cutaneous, or GI anthrax leads to sepsis, meningitis, and death.

PROGNOSIS

- Inhalational anthrax

—Case fatality rates are >85% once symptoms develop.
—50% of patients develop hemorrhagic meningitis.
—Survival rate is higher if symptoms develop >30 days after exposure.

- Cutaneous anthrax

—Case-fatality rate is 20% without antibiotic treatment and <1% with antibiotic treatment.

- GI anthrax

—Case-fatality rate is 25–60%.

 Differential Diagnosis

- Many viral respiratory illnesses resemble the prodrome of inhalational anthrax.
- CXR findings in patients with inhalational anthrax may resemble those with aortic aneurysm and bacterial mediastinitis.
- Skin lesions: staphylococcal disease, plague, tularemia, ecthyma gangrenosum, and brown recluse spider bite.
- Bloody diarrhea: other infectious causes (*Shigella, Salmonella, Yersinia, Campylobacter,* enterohemorrhagic *Escherichia coli, C. difficile* colitis), intussusception, Meckel diverticulum, and inflammatory bowel disease.

 Data Gathering

HISTORY

- Inhalational anthrax

—Clinical presentation is a two-stage illness.
—Initial symptoms are nonspecific and last 1–3 days. They include low-grade fever, dry cough, headache, vomiting, chills, weakness, abdominal pain, and substernal discomfort. This stage is followed by a brief period of apparent recovery.
—Second-stage symptoms develop abruptly and include fever, hemoptysis, dyspnea, chest pain, and profuse diaphoresis. Death usually occurs within 1–2 days.

- Cutaneous anthrax

—Lesions develop on affected areas soon after exposure.
—Systemic symptoms of fever, malaise, and headache may occur.

- GI anthrax

—Oral-pharyngeal form causes sore throat, dysphagia, and fever.

—Intestinal form also causes nausea, vomiting, anorexia, severe abdominal pain, and bloody diarrhea.

 Physical Examination

- Inhalational anthrax
  - Tachypnea, hypoxia, cyanosis
  - Stridor, rales, signs of pleural effusion
  - Hemoptysis, hematemesis, melena
  - Cutaneous anthrax
  - Initial painless, pruritic macule or papule enlarges into a 1- to 3-cm round ulcer by the 2nd day
  - 1- to 3-mm vesicles with clear or serosanguinous fluid surround the ulcer
  - A painless, depressed, black eschar follows, often with extensive local edema
  - Over 1 to 2 weeks, the eschar dries, loosens, and falls off, occasionally with scarring.
  - Painful, regional lymphadenopathy may occur.

- GI anthrax
  - Oral or esophageal ulcers, cervical lymphadenopathy
  - Cecal or terminal ileal ulcers
  - Massive ascites
  - Acute abdomen

- Disseminated anthrax (potential complication of any of the above forms of anthrax)

—Sepsis syndrome: tachycardia, hypotension, septic shock
—Meningitis: meningismus, delirium, obtundation

 Laboratory Aids

Test: Chest X-ray (or chest CT scan)
Significance: Inhalational anthrax causes a hemorrhagic mediastinitis. CXR shows a widened mediastinum and pleural effusions. No infiltrates are present.

Test: Gram stain smear and culture from vesicular fluid
Significance: Diagnose cutaneous anthrax. Gram stain reveals large, gram-positive, boxcar-shaped bacilli. Capsule is visible on polychrome methylene blue stain. *B. anthracis* grows readily on blood agar.

Test: Anthraxin skin test
Significance: Measures anthrax cell-mediated immunity. It is positive in 80% of patients within 72 hours of infection and >95% of cases within 3 weeks. The test was positive in 72% of patients >16 years after recovery.

Test: Serologic enzyme-linked immunosorbent assay (ELISA)
Significance: Measures antibodies to the lethal and edema toxins of *B. anthracis*. Positive if a single acute-phase titer is >1:32 or if there is

a fourfold or greater rise between acute and convalescent titers collected 4 weeks apart.

Test: PCR, immunohistochemical staining

Test: Nasopharyngeal swab or induced respiratory secretion culture
Significance: Used for epidemiologic investigation to determine who was at the highest risk of exposure in the setting of a confirmed case. The sensitivity, specificity, and predictive value of nasal swab testing are unknown. It should not be used to diagnose anthrax or to guide prophylaxis or treatment.

Test: Blood culture (or lumbar puncture)
Significance: Patient with cutaneous anthrax may have bacteremia with *B. anthracis* even without significant signs of systemic disease.

Test: Complete blood count

Test: Serum electrolytes, glucose, and calcium
Significance: Hypokalemia, acidosis, hypoglycemia, and hypocalcemia occurred during experimental anthrax infection in animals.

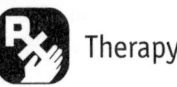 ## Emergency Care

• When a person has had direct physical contact with a substance alleged to be anthrax, the following measures should be taken:

—Wash exposed skin and articles of clothing with soap and water.
—Administer postexposure prophylaxis until the substance is proved not to be anthrax.
—Contact the public health department or the Centers for Disease Control and Prevention.

Therapy

• Postexposure prophylaxis

—Ciprofloxacin 15 mg/kg (up to 500 mg) OR doxycycline 2 mg/kg (up to 100 mg) po b.i.d. for 60 days.
—In children, use ciprofloxacin for initial prophylaxis. Switch to amoxicillin or penicillin if susceptibility testing permits.

• Treatment

—For all forms of anthrax, begin with IV therapy and switch to oral therapy when clinically appropriate. Treat for 60 days (IV and po combined).
—Inhalational or GI anthrax: Ciprofloxacin 15 mg/kg (up to 400 mg) or doxycycline 2 mg/kg (up to 100 mg) IV every 12 h PLUS clindamycin or rifampin.
—Cutaneous anthrax: Ciprofloxacin or doxycycline IV.
—In children, begin therapy with ciprofloxacin (plus clindamycin or rifampin for inhalational/GI anthrax) and convert to penicillin G IV if susceptibility testing permits and when clinical improvement is documented.

 ## Follow-Up

INFECTION CONTROL

• Immediately notify the hospital epidemiologist, infection control department, or local health department of suspected cases.
• No data suggest that patient-to-patient transmission of inhalational anthrax occurs. Standard barrier isolation precautions are recommended for all hospitalized patients with all forms of anthrax infection. High-efficiency particulate air filter masks or other measures for airborne precautions are not indicated.
• These is no need to immunize or provide prophylaxis to patient contacts unless they, like the patient, were exposed to the aerosol.
• If anthrax is used as a bio-weapon, spores may be detected on environmental surfaces. Inhalational anthrax is unlikely to be caused by secondary aerosolization of these spores.

PREVENTION

• Antibiotics are effective against germinating *B. anthracis* but not against the spores. Therefore, if prophylactic antibiotics are stopped prematurely, remaining spores can cause disease when they germinate. This phenomenon of delayed onset disease does not occur with cutaneous or GI exposures.
• In situations where the threat of transmission of *B. anthracis* spores is deemed credible, decontamination of skin and potential fomites (e.g., clothing) may be considered to reduce the risk for cutaneous and GI forms of the disease.
• AVA (anthrax vaccine adsorbed) is the only licensed human anthrax vaccine in the U.S. Primary vaccination consists of subcutaneous injections at 0, 2, and 4 weeks, and three booster vaccinations at 6, 12, and 18 months. Annual booster injections are required to maintain immunity. Most common adverse event is injection-site discomfort (e.g., edema, pain, local hypersensitivity).

PITFALLS

• Failure to remember that the pulmonary disease caused by anthrax is a hemorrhagic mediastinitis with pleural effusions and NOT a bronchopneumonia.

 ## Common Questions and Answers

Q: Does the government have a plan in place if there were mass exposure to anthrax?
A: Yes. Under emergency plans, the federal government would ship appropriate antibiotics from its stockpile to wherever they are needed.

Q: Should individuals ask their physicians to write a prescription for ciprofloxacin (or other antibiotics) so they have prophylaxis available?
A: No. Ciprofloxacin and other antibiotics should not be prescribed unless there is a clearly indicated need. Additionally, indiscriminate prescribing and widespread use of ciprofloxacin could hasten the development of drug-resistant organisms.

Q: Can a person get screened or tested for anthrax?
A: No screening test is available to determine whether anthrax exposure has occurred. The only way exposure can be determined is through a public health investigation.

ICD-9-CM

Anthrax 022.9;
Cutaneous 022.0;
Pulmonary 022.1

BIBLIOGRAPHY

CDC. Use of anthrax vaccine in the United States: recommendations of the Advisory Committee on Immunization Practices (ACIP). *MMWR* 2000;49(RR-15):1–20.

CDC. Update: investigation of bioterrorism-related anthrax and interim guidelines for exposure management and antimicrobial therapy, October 2001. *MMWR* 2001;50:909–919.

Sellman Br, Mourez M, Collier RJ. Dominant-negative mutants of a toxin subunit: an approach to therapy of anthrax. *Science* 2001;292:695–697.

Weber DJ, Rutala WA. Risks and prevention of nosocomial transmission of rare zoonotic diseases. *Clin Infect Dis* 2001;32:446–456.

Author: Samir S. Shah

Aplastic Anemia

 Database

DEFINITION

Aplastic anemia is a heterogeneous disorder within the bone marrow failure syndromes. It is characterized by a marked decrease or absence of blood forming elements in the bone marrow and peripheral pancytopenia. The disorder exists in both acquired and congenital forms.

CAUSES

Acquired

- Idiopathic (70% of cases)
- Drugs (idiosyncratic)—e.g., chloramphenicol, oxyphenylbutazone, quinacrine, cimetidine, carbamazepine
- Hepatitis (A, B, C and seronegative)
- HIV, EBV, influenza, parainfluenza, parvovirus B19, CMV
- Chemicals/toxins—e.g., insecticides (DDT, parathion); benzene, carbon tetrachloride, toluene, glues
- Irradiation
- Malnutrition
- Kwashiorkor, marasmus, anorexia nervosa
- Paroxysmal nocturnal hemoglobinuria (PNH)
- Pregnancy
- Autoimmune mechanisms
- Preleukemia, myelodysplastic syndrome (MDS)

Congenital

- Fanconi anemia
- Dyskeratosis congenita
- Shwachman-Diamond syndrome
- Reticular dysgenesis

PATHOLOGY/PATHOPHYSIOLOGY

- Intrinsic proliferative defect and reduction in number of hematopoietic stem cells
- Autoimmune-mediated destruction of hematopoietic stem cell
- Abnormal stromal cells within the bone marrow microenvironment (minority of cases)
- Aberrant cytokine production by host T-lymphocytes suppressing hematopoietic cell proliferation and triggering apoptosis of CD34 progenitor cells
- Genetic predisposition

GENETICS

- Most cases are sporadic
- Moderately correlated with specific histocompatibility antigen frequency (HLA-DR2 antigen is twice as frequent in aplastic anemia patients as in the unaffected population)

- Familial aplastic anemia is associated with congenital syndromes, with heterogeneous hematologic manifestations, and usually recognized congenital physical anomalies. This diagnosis should always be considered even without a positive family history or obvious syndromic features. Testing for Fanconi anemia is considered mandatory in all new AA patients.

EPIDEMIOLOGY

- Annual incidence of 2 new cases per 1 million population in U.S. and Europe
- Incidence in Asia is about threefold higher than in West; likely related to environmental/infectious exposures.
- Two major age peaks: 15 to 25 years and over 60 years
- Males and females equally affected.

COMPLICATIONS

- Infection: overwhelming bacterial sepsis and fungal (Aspergillus) infections are most frequent cause of death.
- Hemorrhage: intracranial, especially if refractory to platelet transfusions
- Iron overload secondary to long-term red blood cell transfusions, with subsequent organ dysfunction if untreated.

PROGNOSIS

- In patients with severe aplastic anemia, 80% to 90% mortality at 1 year if untreated.
- **Bone marrow transplant from HLA-identical sibling donor**

—77% overall survival in patients ≤20 years of age
—80% to 90% survival for the young, uninfected, and minimally transfused patient

- **Bone marrow transplant from HLA-identical unrelated donor**

—30–55% survival (due to older population, frequent graft rejection, infection from delayed engraftment with prolonged neutropenia)

- **Immunosuppressive therapy**

—75% response rate (initial treatment)
—90% 5-year survival among responders

- Factors associated with poor outcome:

—Bleeding at presentation
—Severe pancytopenia (ANC $<200/mm^3$, platelet $<20,000/mm^3$)
—Bone marrow cellularity <20%
—Prolonged pancytopenia (>1 month)
—Male gender
—Posthepatitis
—Active infection at diagnosis

 Differential Diagnosis

- Acute leukemia
- Myelodysplastic syndrome
- Paroxysmal nocturnal hemoglobinuria
- Folate or B_{12} deficiency (macrocytic anemia)
- Acute drug reaction with bone marrow suppression
- Acute infection (viral) with bone marrow suppression, e.g., HIV-1, CMV, parvovirus B19, EBV, seronegative hepatitis
- Marrow infiltration by malignant tumors, e.g., non-Hodgkin lymphoma, neuroblastoma
- Hemophagocytic lymphohistiocytosis (aka: familial erythrophagocytic lymphohistiocytosis)

 Data Gathering

HISTORY

Evidence of Bone Marrow Failure

- Pallor, lethargy, easy fatigue, weakness, and loss of appetite are signs of anemia. These may not be noticed by patient/parent due to slow onset of anemia (with compensation).
- Petechiae, easy and excessive bruising, prolonged epistaxis, gingival bleeding, hematuria and bloody stools are signs/symptoms of thrombocytopenia.
- Infections that don't respond to antibiotics, oral ulcers, and gingival hyperplasia may be signs of neutropenia.

EVIDENCE OF CAUSE

- Drug or toxin exposure (although usually not identified)
- History of hepatitis, jaundice, or other viral infections

 Physical Examination

- Tachycardia from severe anemia
- Excessive bruising, petechiae, and pallor as signs of severe anemia and thrombocytopenia
- Oral mucosal ulcerations and bleeding, thrush, palatal petechiae, and gingival hypertrophy as signs of neutropenia, and thrombocytopenia
- Systolic ejection murmur from anemia
- Lymphadenopathy and hepatosplenomegaly suggest acute leukemia/malignant process, and are not associated with aplastic anemia.
- Perianal ulcerations/infection from neutropenia
- Skeletal anomalies, dysmorphic features may be signs of Fanconi anemia

Laboratory Aids

TO CONFIRM THE DIAGNOSIS

Test: CBC with differential and reticulocyte count
Significance:

• Severe aplastic anemia (at least 2 of the following):

—Granulocyte count <500/mm^3
—Platelet count <20,000/mm^3
—Reticulocyte count (corrected for hematocrit) <1%

• Mild or moderate aplastic anemia (hypoplastic anemia)

—Less severe cytopenias

Test: Bone marrow aspirate and biopsy
Significance:

• Severe aplastic anemia:

—Hypocellular with fatty infiltration
—Less than 25% cellularity on biopsy

• Mild or moderate aplastic anemia

—Normal or increased cellularity

Supplemental Laboratory Studies

• LFTs, clotting profile, hepatitis A, B, and C antibody panel
• Viral serologies: EBV, parvovirus B19 (IgG and IgM), VZV, CMV, HIV, HHV-6

TO EXCLUDE OTHER CAUSES

• Bone marrow aspirate for chromosomal analysis to rule out Fanconi anemia, myelodysplastic syndromes, acute leukemia
• Diepoxybutane (on peripheral blood) to test for Fanconi anemia
• Ham test, sucrose hemolysis, and flow cytometry to exclude paroxysmal nocturnal hemoglobinuria
• Red cell folate and B$_{12}$ levels to rule out vitamin deficient macrocytic anemia with neutropenia

Emergency Care

• Broad-spectrum antibiotics for febrile neutropenic patients. Consider antifungal therapy for patients with prolonged fevers.
• Platelet transfusions for bleeding. Maintain platelet count >15,000/mm^3 in nonbleeding adolescent/adult patients (single donor units, irradiated, leukocyte depleted)
• Red cell transfusions in severely anemic patients should occur slowly to prevent congestive heart failure (unless anemia is acute and due to blood loss rather than lack of production). Use irradiated, leukocyte-depleted, CMV safe red cell product from unrelated donors.

 ## Therapy

• Bone marrow transplantation

—Treatment of choice for patients <50 years with severe aplastic anemia and HLA-identical sibling.
—Transplant early, minimize supportive transfusions.
—Alternative donor BMT should be used only for patients who have failed immunosuppressive therapy (>1 course of immunosuppressive treatment reduces success with BMT).
—Peripheral blood stem cell and umbilical cord blood regimens currently being tested.

• Immunosuppressive therapy

—Antithymocyte globulin (ATG), cyclosporin A, methylprednisolone, and growth factors (G-CSF or GM-CSF)
—High-dose cyclophosphamide and cyclosporin A without BMT (if failure to respond/relapse using ATG regimen)

• Androgens

—Used for the treatment of aplastic anemia associated with Fanconi anemia
—Effective in moderate and mild aplastic anemia

• Supportive therapy

—Transfusion support: family donors should not be used (to avoid alloimmunization), use CMV negative, irradiated, leuko-reduced product; minimize number of transfusions.
—Infectious disease support: pan culture and institute broad-spectrum parenteral antibiotics for fever/neutropenia; antifungal therapy for persistent fevers. Maintain good hand washing and oral hygiene. Avoid raw fish, fruits, and vegetables. No rectal temperatures.

 ## Follow-Up

TIME TO RECOVERY

Most responders to medical therapy will recover (normal ANC and transfusion independent) within 70 to 100 days (90% by 3 months); some patients may remain cyclosporine dependent

SIGNS OF RECOVERY

Signs of recovery include normalization of mean corpuscular volume (MCV), increasing reticulocyte, neutrophil and monocyte count. Full platelet recovery may take months. Partial recovery is possible.

RELAPSE

• Risk of relapse is 30–40% at 5 years; many are salvageable.
• Salvage therapy: second course of immunosuppressive therapy (50% salvage); matched-unrelated donor BMT (30–55% overall survival).

OTHER

• 8–10% risk of MDS and/or myeloid leukemia at 10 years
• 15% risk of PNH at 5 years

 ## Common Questions and Answers

Q: Can family members donate blood for a child with aplastic anemia?
A: This is not recommended, as transfusion with blood products from parents or siblings increases the risk of graft rejection of bone marrow in the setting of a related-donor bone marrow transplant.

Q: What activities should a child with aplastic anemia avoid?
A: Patients with low red blood cell counts should avoid excessive exercise or high-altitude exposure. Patients with low white blood cell counts are more susceptible to bacterial infections. Patients should avoid dental work, as this may introduce bacteria into the bloodstream through the mouth. Patients with low platelet counts should avoid contact sports, including football, hockey, lacrosse, skiing, etc.

Q: How does one learn more about experimental therapies for the treatment of aplastic anemia?
A: Inquiries to the National Institutes of Health (NIH) in Bethesda, Maryland, or to the hematology division of the nearest medical school or NIH-designated cancer center should result in information about the availability of experimental therapies.

ICD-9-CM 284.9

BIBLIOGRAPHY

Ball, SE. The modern management of severe aplastic anaemia. *Br J Haematol* 2000;110: 41–53.

Frickhofen N, Rosenfeld, SJ. Immunosuppressive treatment of aplastic anemia with antithymocyte globulin and cyclosporine. *Semin Hematol* 2000;37:56–68.

Horowitz, MM. Current status of allogeneic bone marrow transplantation in acquired aplastic anemia. *Semin Hematol* 2000;37:30–42.

Young NS. Acquired aplastic anemia. *JAMA* 1999;281:271–278.

Author: Jane E. Minturn
Kara M. Kelly, 2nd edition

Appendicitis

 Database

DEFINITION

Acute inflammation of the appendix

CAUSES

• Obstruction of appendiceal lumen by fecalith, calculi, or hyperplastic lymphoid tissue

PATHOLOGY

• Acute obstruction raises intraluminal pressure, leading to ischemia.
• Bacteria invade the appendiceal wall at sites of ulceration producing inflammation.
• Necrosis of appendiceal wall results in perforation with fecal contamination of the peritoneum.

EPIDEMIOLOGY

• Usually occurs in children over 2 years of age.
• Peak incidence in teens and young adults aged 15 to 25.
• Affects 1 in 500 people each year worldwide.

 Differential Diagnosis

INFECTION

• Gastroenteritis (e.g., *Yersinia, Campylobacter*)
• Constipation
• Right lower lobe pneumonia
• Mesenteric adenitis
• Typhlitis
• Urinary tract infection
• Pelvic inflammatory disease, tubo-ovarian abscess, or ectopic pregnancy

INFLAMMATORY

• Inflammatory bowel disease exacerbation
• Anaphylactic purpura
• Hemolytic uremic anemia
• Cholecystitis
• Pancreatitis
• Diverticulitis

GENETIC/METABOLIC

• Diabetes
• Sickle and sickle cell disease
• Renal stones
• Hypernatremia
• Crohn disease

MISCELLANEOUS

• Function abdominal pain
• Fecalith
• Torsion of testes or ovaries
• Ovarian cyst
• Endometriosis
• Small bowel obstruction
• Rupture of rectus abdominis

 Data Gathering

HISTORY

Question: Is there constipation and inability to pass gas?
Significance: These are considered traditional cardinal signs for irritation associated with peritoneal or abdominal mesentery.

Question: Is there nausea or vomiting?
Significance: Many surgeons feel that vomiting is the cardinal symptom associated with appendicitis.

Question: Is there fever?
Significance: Low-grade fever is common in appendicitis; higher fever can be an abscess or other infectious disease.

Question: Does the pain move or is there point tenderness associated in the right lower quadrant (RLQ)?
Significance: Typically, there is poorly localized, cramp-like midabdominal pain that migrates to the RLQ.

Question: Other classic features?

• Rectal tenderness
• Nausea, anorexia
• Patient prefers to lie still
• Rarely secretory diarrhea
• Change in bowel habits, especially diarrhea
• Guarding, i.e., voluntary contraction of the abdominal muscle

Significance: Appendicitis may be presenting with unusual features.

Physical Examination

Finding: Focal peritoneal signs
Significance: Peritoneal irritation

Finding: Pain at McBurney point
Significance: Peritoneal irritation

Finding: Psoas sign
Significance: Peritoneal irritation

Finding: Abdominal rebound tenderness
Significance: Peritoneal irritation

Finding: Focal tenderness on rectal examination
Significance: Appendicitis or abscess

Finding: Following perforation, abdomen becomes rigid and tender with absent bowel sounds; patients often febrile, tachypneic, and tachycardic
Significance: Peritonitis

SPECIAL QUESTION

Question: Was the car ride painful, e.g., going over bumps?
Significance: Another way to elicit peritoneal irritation.

SPECIAL EXAMINATION TRICKS

- Palpation with stethoscope
  Jiggling bed should produce RLQ pain.
- Pain may be elicited by asking patient to cough or hop on right foot (psoas sign).

Laboratory Aids

TESTS

Test: CBC
Significance: Elevated white blood cell (WBC) count with left shift

IMAGING

Test: Abdominal x-ray
Significance:

- often normal
- 8% to 10% show calcified fecalith
  Cecal-wall thickening
- Air-fluid levels
- Indistinct psoas margins

Test: Barium enema—not routine
Significance: May show evidence of RLQ mass or partial or complete nonfilling of appendix.

Test: Ultrasound
Significance: Edema, inflammation, and/or abscess formation

Test: CT abdomen
Significance: Gaining popularity for diagnostic problems.

Therapy

- IV fluids to correct hypovolemia, electrolyte abnormalities
- Exploratory laparotomy
- Emergency appendectomy
- Broad-spectrum antibiotics should be used if perforation is suspected.
- Nasogastric tube and pain medications may provide comfort preoperatively.
- Abscess may require external drainage.

Follow-Up

- Recovery rapid
- Prognosis excellent without perforation, good with perforation (mortality, 1%)

PITFALLS

- Position of appendix may vary, i.e., location of pain may vary
- Retroiliac appendix, poorly localized pain
- Retrocecal appendix, right upper quadrant (RUQ) pain
- Appendix in gutter, flank pain
- Pelvic appendix, pain on rectal examination, or diarrhea caused by direct irritation of sigmoid colon.
- Appendicitis progresses rapidly in children; perforation often occurs due to delayed diagnosis
- Pain may resolve briefly following perforation.

DIETARY GUIDELINES

Postoperative

- Patient diet should consist of clear liquids, i.e., broth, juices, and herbal teas.
- Introduce foods high in beta-carotene.

Significance: beta-carotene soothes injured mucous membrane and heals tissue.

- Avoid gas-producing foods i.e., nuts, legumes broccoli.
- Introduce nutritional supplements or foods high in vitamin B-complex for strength, vitamin C for tissue repair, vitamin E for antioxidant and zinc to aid healing tissue.

Common Questions and Answers

Q: Why is perforation more commonly observed in children with appendicitis?
A: There is more rapid progression of symptoms that may not follow the classic pattern of RLQ pain. Young children may not be capable of describing their pain. The mesentery in children is thin walled and less effective at walling off an infection.

Q: Is appendicitis genetically inherited?
A: Appendicitis does show a tendency to occur in families.

Q: How long is the typical postoperative recovery period?
A: Traditional recovery period rule of thumb is 6 weeks.

ICD-9-CM 541

BIBLIOGRAPHY

Andersen BR, Kallehave FL, Andersen HK. Antibiotics versus placebo for prevention of postoperative infection after appendicectomy (Cochrane Review). Cochrane Database Syst Rev 2001;2.

Brender JD, Marcuse EK, Koepsell T, et al. Childhood appendicitis: factors associated with perforation. *Pediatrics* 1985;76:301–306.

Kokoska, ER, Minkes RK, Silen ML, et al. Effect of pediatric surgical practice on the treatment of children with appendicitis. *Pediatrics* 2001;107(6):1298–1301.

Lawrence J. Computed tomography in diagnosing suspected appendicitis. *Pediatrics* 2001;107(5):1231.

Authors: Scott Stem and Andrew E. Mulberg

Arthritis—Juvenile Rheumatoid

 Database

DEFINITION

• Juvenile rheumatoid arthritis (JRA) is chronic synovial inflammation of unknown etiology in at least one joint, for at least 6 weeks. Age of onset must be less than 16 years old. It can be subdivided into three major types.
• Pauciarticular JRA is JRA affecting less than 5 joints.

—Type I usually affects young girls. Peak age of onset is 1–6 years; 80% are antinuclear antibody (ANA)-positive.
—Type II (spondyloarthropathies) generally affects boys, many of whom are human leukocyte antigen (HLA)-B27 positive, in late childhood or adolescence.

• Polyarticular JRA affects 5 or more joints and can occur at any age, but peak ages of onset are 1–4 and 7–10 years.
• Rheumatoid factor positive (RF+) polyarticular JRA is like adult onset RA that occurs in a child.
• Rheumatoid factor negative (RF−) polyarticular JRA is usually less aggressive and easier to control.
• Systemic-onset JRA is characterized by high, spiking quotidian or diquotidian fevers and an evanescent pink/salmon-colored macular rash. Affected children may also have lymphadenopathy, hepatosplenomegaly, pericarditis, or pleuritis. The arthritis may not appear until weeks to months after the onset of the systemic symptoms. Systemic-onset JRA can occur at any age.

CAUSES

The etiology of JRA is unknown, but genetic predisposition, autoimmunity, infection, and trauma may all play a role.

PATHOLOGY

• Chronic synovial inflammation

EPIDEMIOLOGY

• JRA affects approximately 70,000–100,000 children in the United States.
• Affects girls twice as often as it affects boys, but pauciarticular type II usually affects boys (male/female ratio, 10:1).
• Approximately 50% of children with JRA have the pauciarticular type.
• 40% have the polyarticular type.
• 10% have systemic-onset JRA.

GENETICS

Some studies have indicated that various HLA markers may be associated with different subtypes of JRA. For example, HLA-DR4 seems to be associated with rheumatoid factor-positive (RF1) polyarticular JRA, HLA-DR1 is associated with pauciarticular disease without uveitis, and HLA-DR5 is associated with pauciarticular JRA with uveitis.

COMPLICATIONS

• Joint degeneration with loss of articular cartilage
• Soft tissue contractures
• Leg-length discrepancies
• Micrognathia
• Cervical spine dislocations
• Rheumatoid nodules
• Growth retardation

Pauciarticular JRA, especially with a positive ANA, is also associated with a chronic uveitis, which can lead to loss of vision if not detected early with routine slit-lamp eye examinations. Pericarditis and pleuritis, as well as severe anemia, may develop in patients with systemic-onset JRA.

 Differential Diagnosis

• Monoarticular JRA

—Septic joint
—Trauma
—Hemarthrosis
—Villonodular synovitis

• Monoarticular or pauciarticular JRA

—Lyme disease
—Acute rheumatic fever
—Malignancies
—Sarcoidosis
—Inflammatory bowel disease

• Polyarticular JRA

—Viral or postviral illness (especially parvovirus)
—Lyme disease
—Lupus

• Systemic-onset JRA

—Infection
—Oncologic process (leukemia)
—Inflammatory bowel disease
—Lupus

 Data Gathering

HISTORY

• Morning stiffness that improves after a warm shower/bath or with stretching and mild exercise is common in JRA.
• The joints often become sore/painful again in the late afternoon or evening.
• Patients with JRA generally do not complain of severe pain, but rather they avoid using joints that are particularly affected. If a child has severe pain in a joint, especially pain that seems out of proportion to the physical findings, diagnoses other than JRA should be entertained.
• In systemic JRA the fever curve is important to document. Between fever spikes the child is often completely afebrile. The rash is evanescent and the patients often have a history of fatigue, malaise, and weight loss.

 Physical Examination

• Arthritis must be present in at least one joint. There may be restricted range of motion in the affected joints and soft tissue contractures as well.

—Enthesitis and sacroiliac tenderness are often seen in spondyloarthropathies.

• In systemic JRA the rash, if present, is almost pathognomonic for this disease.
• Lymphadenopathy and hepatosplenomegaly may be seen.
• A careful cardiac and pulmonary examination must be done to look for pericarditis and pleuritis.

Laboratory Aids

- No laboratory finding is diagnostic for JRA.
- Many patients with JRA, especially the polyarticular and systemic types, have elevated sedimentation rates and anemia.
- Patients with systemic JRA often have a leukocytosis, predominantly neutrophils, a thrombocytosis as well.
- ANA is a useful test in classifying patients with JRA.

—Positive in 80% of pauciarticular type I
—40% to 60% polyarticular
—15% normal population

- RF will be positive in 15% to 20% of patients with polyarticular arthritis and usually indicates a more aggressive form of arthritis.

IMAGING

- Radiography is often normal early in JRA.
- Later, if arthritis persists, bone demineralization, loss of articular cartilage, erosions, and joint fusion may be seen.

Therapy

DRUGS

- Nonsteroidal antiinflammatory drugs (NSAIDs)

—First-line therapy for JRA
—If there is no response to the initial NSAID after 4 to 6 weeks of an adequate dose, a different one should be tried. Patients will often respond differently to the various nonsteroidal drugs.

- If NSAIDs are ineffective in controlling the disease, a second-line agent should be added, such as methotrexate, hydroxychloroquine, or sulfasalazine.
- Methotrexate: If the arthritis is relatively severe, methotrexate is often started. Laboratory values must be monitored closely in these patients, looking for bone marrow suppression or elevation of transaminase levels.
- Antitumor necrosis factor therapy (etanercept) is often added in patients not responding adequately to methotrexate plus NSAIDs.
- Glucocorticoids

—In systemic JRA with high fevers, systemic glucocorticoids are often necessary, either as oral (daily or every other day) doses or as intravenous pulses, every 2 to 8 weeks. Steroids are also used for patients with polyarticular JRA whose arthritis is unresponsive to other medications. Because of the many side effects of systemic steroids, patients should be weaned off steroids as soon as possible.

- Intraarticular steroids are often used in patients with only one or two active joints.

PHYSICAL AND OCCUPATIONAL THERAPY

Physical and occupational therapy are important in the management of JRA. The goal is to maintain range of motion, muscle strength, and function.

DIET

Patients with systemic or polyarticular JRA, especially those on steroids, should maintain adequate calcium intake to minimize osteoporosis. Patients on methotrexate should take folate supplements daily, except on the days that the methotrexate is given.

WHEN TO EXPECT IMPROVEMENT

- Responses to treatments for JRA vary tremendously.

—Some patients may respond to NSAIDs within a week or two.
—Others take 4 to 6 weeks to improve, or they may not respond at all.
—Steroids usually start to relieve symptoms within a few days.
—Methotrexate usually takes 4–8 weeks until a benefit is seen.
—Anti-TNF therapy can start decreasing symptoms in as little as 1–2 weeks, or it may take up to 3 months.
—Other second-line agents can take up to 16 weeks until the maximum benefit is seen.

- The waxing and waning nature of JRA itself adds to the variability of patient responses to treatments.

PROGNOSIS

- Varies considerably
- Children with pauciarticular JRA usually do well and often go into remission within a year or two of starting treatment. They may have flares, however, even up to 10 years after being symptom-free and off all medications.
- Patients with polyarticular JRA who are RF+ often develop a severe arthritis that may persist into adulthood.
- RF− polyarticular patients generally do better and many outgrow their disease.
- 50% of patients with systemic-onset JRA will develop chronic polyarticular arthritis.

PITFALLS

Overdiagnosis: arthritis must be present for at least 6 weeks before a patient can be diagnosed with JRA. Many viral illnesses can give joint pain and swelling that mimics JRA, but resolves within 4 to 6 weeks.

Common Questions and Answers

Q: Will the patient outgrow JRA?
A: Prognosis depends of the type of JRA. In some studies, up to 50% of patients with JRA still had active disease 10 years after diagnosis. Only 15%, however, had any loss of function.

Q: Will siblings of patients with JRA develop the disease?
A: Rarely, but it can occur.

ICD-9-CM 714.30

BIBLIOGRAPHY

Aaron S, Fraser PA, Jackson JM, et al. Sex ratio and sibship size in juvenile arthritis kindreds. *Arthritis Rheum* 1985;28:753.

Singsen BH. Epidemiology of rheumatic diseases of childhood. *Rheum Dis Clin North Am* 1990;16:581–599.

Towner SR, Michet CJ Jr, O'Fallon WM, et al. The epidemiology of juvenile arthritis in Rochester, Minnesota. *Arthritis Rheum* 1983;26:1208.

Wallace CA, Levinson JE. Juvenile rheumatoid arthritis: outcome and treatment for the 1990s. *Pediatr Rheum* 1991;17:891–905.

Author: Elizabeth Candell Chalom

Ascaris Lumbricoides

 Database

DEFINITION

Ascaris lumbricoides is a large roundworm, 15 to 40 cm in length, which infects humans via eggs found in soil. Animals are not affected. Approximately one fourth of the world's population is infested with this worm.

PATHOPHYSIOLOGY

- The life cycle begins when eggs are ingested from soil contaminated with human feces.
- Subsequently, the larvae are liberated in the small intestine.
- The rhabdoid larvae invade the venous system and travel to the portal circulation, inferior vena cava, and finally, pulmonary capillaries.
- They penetrate the alveoli, and are subsequently expelled by coughing across the epiglottis and swallowed. During the migration of the parasite through the pulmonary vessels, an eosinophilic response is evoked.
- The larvae become adult worms in the small intestine.
- The cycle takes 2 months.
- In the intestinal stage, mechanical obstruction from the mass of worms in the gut may be observed in children.

EPIDEMIOLOGY

- One female worm produces 200,000 eggs per day.
- Fertilized eggs must incubate in the soil for 2 to 3 weeks.
- The eggs are viable for up to 6 years in temperate climates; they survive freezing but not direct sunlight.
- All ages may be affected; however, children are more frequent hosts due to oral behavior.
- Ascariasis is more common where sanitation is poor and population dense.

COMPLICATIONS

- Bronchopneumonia may be seen during the migrational stage, producing fever, cough, dyspnea, wheeze, eosinophilia, and pulmonary infiltrates.
- Heavy infestations may cause abdominal pain, malabsorption, and growth failure.
- Children may experience obstruction (ileocecal), malabsorption, or intussusception.
- Perforation of a viscus, or migration into the appendix, biliary, or pancreatic ducts may rarely occur.

PROGNOSIS

- Once intestinal infection is detected and treated, the prognosis is excellent. If obstructive or respiratory complications have occurred, the prognosis is less favorable.
- The case fatality rate in the United States is 3%.

 Differential Diagnosis

- Ascariasis should be considered in the differential diagnosis when a patient presents with pneumonia and peripheral eosinophilia.
- The diagnosis of *Ascaris* infection should be considered whenever intestinal obstruction is seen in an endemic area.
- This infection may be associated with other parasites acquired from contaminated soil.

 Data Gathering

HISTORY

Question: Do patients infected with *Ascaris* always have symptoms?
Significance: The majority of patients with moderate infections are asymptomatic.

Question: Do patients actually see worms in their stool?
Significance: History or passage of large worms in the stool or vomitus is suggestive.

Question: What are pulmonary symptoms?
Significance: During the pulmonary stage, cough, dyspnea, fever, and pulmonary infiltrates in the presence of eosinophilia suggest the diagnosis.

Question: Are there symptoms of obstruction?
Significance: Rarely, the infection presents as intestinal obstruction, with an incidence of approximately 2 children per 1,000 infected.

Laboratory Aids

LABORATORY TESTS

- Complete white blood cell count
- Electrolytes
- Liver-function tests: transaminases, PT/PTT
- Amylase and lipase (to exclude pancreatitis)
- Creatinine and blood urea nitrogen
- Blood cultures
- Urine for specific gravity
- Viral serologies, including hepatitis B and C viruses, coxsackievirus, enteroviruses

IMAGING

- Abdominal radiography
- Ultrasound of the abdomen to differentiate between free and loculated fluid collection and the presence of intraabdominal masses
- Abdominal computed axial tomography

ABDOMINAL PARACENTESIS

Abdominal paracentesis is a safe procedure in the evaluation of etiologies of ascites. The two complications are perforation of the bowel and hemorrhage. With sterile conditions, a narrow-bore angiocatheter, usually 23-gauge, is inserted through the linea alba 2 cm below the umbilicus, using the Z-technique. Paracentesis is done for routine studies, including white blood cell count, culture, LDH, total protein, albumin, glucose, Gram stain, amylase, cholesterol with triglycerides, and cytology. These tests require approximately 10 to 20 mL of fluid. Interpretation of these data is reflected in the table below.

- When glucose in the ascitic fluid is below 30 mg/dL, tuberculous peritonitis must be excluded.
- When ascitic amylase is greater than the normal serum amylase, pancreatitis is suggested.

 ## Therapy

The management of the ascites should be directed toward the underlying etiology. In a patient with cirrhosis, accumulation of ascites should be avoided by preventing complications such as esophageal hemorrhage, spontaneous bacterial peritonitis, hepatorenal syndrome, inferior vena cava obstruction, and renal and cardiac circulatory disturbances.

- Sodium intake should be restricted to 1 to 2 mEq/kg/d (low-salt diet).
- Water should be restricted to 75% of maintenance requirements.
- Diuretics may be used to promote negative sodium and water balance. When diuretics are used, urine output and serum electrolytes should be monitored to prevent prerenal azotemia and decrease effective blood flow to the kidneys.
- Therapeutic abdominal paracentesis should be used only in resistant cases, because ascitic fluid tends to reaccumulate. Paracentesis of volumes greater than 1 L should be accompanied by the IV infusion of salt-poor albumin during the procedure.
- LeVeen shunt (peritoneal venous shunting) is rarely used as a therapeutic option because of the high frequency of infection, obstruction, and other complications.
- Portosystemic shunting may be valuable in cases where portal hypertension is felt to be the underlying etiology of ascitic accumulation.

 ## Follow-Up

Weight and effects of diuretics should be assessed closely with attention to preservation of renal function. Urine and serum electrolytes should be monitored. Abdominal girth should be measured frequently. In cases of infection or peritonitis, a repeat paracentesis should be performed approximately 48 hours after the initiation of antibiotics for culture and white blood cell count.

PITFALLS

- With congenital ascites, evaluate for lysosomal storage diseases.
- When performing paracentesis, make certain that the fluid is ascitic and not intraluminal.
- Ultrasonography may be helpful to determine the location of this fluid.
- With new onset of ascites, make certain to evaluate for abdominal neoplasia.
- With marginally compensated liver disease, attempt to identify the source of the patient's acute decompensation.

 ## Common Questions and Answers

Q: What is the common thought regarding neonatal ascites?
A: Exclude lysosomal storage and/or other metabolic diseases.

Q: What is the best test to discriminate the type of ascites?
A: Analysis of the peritoneal fluid collected by abdominal paracentesis is required for this purpose. Differentiation of a serous effusion versus exudate is thus achieved.

ICD-9-CM 789.5

BIBLIOGRAPHY

Clark JH, Fitzgerald JF, Kleinman MB. Spontaneous bacterial peritonitis. *J Pediatr* 1984;104(4):495–500.

Fitzgerald JF. Ascites. In: Wyllie R, Hyams J, eds. *Pediatric gastrointestinal diseases*. Philadelphia: WB Saunders, 1993:151–160.

Gillan JE, Lowden JA, Gaskin K, et al. Congenital ascites as a presenting sign of lysosomal storage disease. *J Pediatr* 1984;104:225–231.

Hoefs JC, Runyon BA. Spontaneous bacterial peritonitis. *Dis Mon* 1985;31(9):1–48.

Machin GA. Diseases causing fetal and neonatal ascites. *Pediatr Pathol* 1985;4(3–4):195–211.

Wasserman D. Ascites. In: Altschuler S, Liacouras C, eds. *Clinical pediatric gastroenterology*. Philadelphia: Churchill Livingstone, 1997:323–325.

Author: Dror Wasserman

Aspergillosis

Database

DEFINITION

Aspergillosis is infection caused by the fungus *Aspergillus*. The two most common etiologic agents are *Aspergillus fumigatus* and *Aspergillus flavus*.

PATHOPHYSIOLOGY

- Macrophage phagocytic response is the first and main line of defense against infection with *Aspergillus*.
- Relative lack of importance of cell-mediated immunity in host defense for this infection (therefore, not a common infection in patients with acquired immunodeficiency syndrome).
- The lung is the most common site of both noninvasive and invasive *Aspergillus* infection.

ASSOCIATED ILLNESSES

- *Allergic bronchopulmonary aspergillosis* is characterized by periodic episodes of wheezing, low-grade fever, eosinophilia on peripheral smear, transient infiltrates on chest x-ray film, and a cough productive of brown mucus plugs. It occurs when patients with chronic respiratory disease, (i.e., in children with cystic fibrosis) trap *Aspergillus* spores in mucus, which leads to an immune response and a worsening of respiratory symptoms.
- *Paranasal sinusitis* and *otomycosis* in healthy hosts in warm, wet climates.
- *Aspergillomas* are noninvasive pulmonary fungus balls that grow in bronchogenic cysts or other lung cavities. They are the most frequent form of pulmonary aspergillosis.
- *Invasive aspergillosis* occurs in the immunocompromised host, most commonly in patients treated with long-term broad-spectrum antibiotics, cytotoxic chemotherapy, or immunosuppressive therapy, or in patients with an underlying disease that causes neutrophil or macrophage dysfunction (i.e., acute leukemia or chronic granulomatous disease). In the immunocompromised host, invasion of blood vessels by *Aspergillus* leads to infarction, necrosis, and hematogenous dissemination.

EPIDEMIOLOGY

- *Aspergillus* species are saprophytic molds that are ubiquitous and worldwide, growing in soil, grain, dung, bird droppings, and decaying plant matter.
- Spores are resistant to desiccation, lightweight, and easily dispersed in air currents.
- Main route of transmission is via inhalation of airborne spores; person-to-person spread does not occur.
- Other than those with otomycosis or allergic bronchopulmonary disease, most patients infected with *Aspergillus* are immunocompromised in some way (see above).
- Nosocomial outbreaks have occurred when ventilation or heating systems become contaminated, or when large numbers of spores become airborne during building construction or renovation.
- The incubation period in the human host has not been defined.

COMPLICATIONS

- Disseminated infection: defined as infection of two or more organs, can involve any of the previously discussed sites, as well as the CNS, heart, bones, or skin. Invasiveness depends on the immune state of the host, as well as the period of time and number of spores in the exposure.
- Patients with underlying diseases that predispose them to pulmonary cavitations, blebs, or cysts (such as asthma, chronic bronchitis, TB, sarcoid, histoplasmosis, and bronchiectasis) may develop an aspergilloma (fungus ball) after seeding their pulmonary secretions with *Aspergillus*. When the mass is large enough to be demonstrated on chest x-ray study, serum levels of IgG antibody to *Aspergillus* are characteristically high. Patients may present with hemoptysis, exacerbation of their underlying disease, or rarely, invasion or dissemination.

PROGNOSIS

- Good in noninvasive disease, such as simple otomycosis or paranasal sinusitis
- Immunosuppressed or severely neutropenic patients can have rapid extension or dissemination of disease; prognosis is often very poor. Early recognition and aggressive treatment and debridement are necessary.

Differential Diagnosis

- Other overwhelming systemic infections, both bacterial and fungal
- Allergic pneumonitis (other causes)
- Neoplasm

Data Gathering

HISTORY

Question: Is there a history of the chronic otitis externa?
Significance: Associated with otomycosis

Question: Is there history of sinusitis that does not clear?
Significance: Indolent or noninvasive paranasal sinusitis presents with signs and symptoms of chronic sinusitis that is unresponsive to antibiotic therapy.

Question: Does an asthmatic patient cough up large, dark mucus plugs?
Significance: Allergic bronchopulmonary aspergillosis should be considered in the asthmatic patient with a history of expectorating dark mucus plugs, or a history of fleeting pulmonary infiltrates on chest x-ray (due to bronchial plugging).

Question: Is the patient immunocompromised?
Significance: Immunocompromised patients, especially those with prolonged neutropenia, are at highest risk for invasive aspergillosis. Neutropenic patients who are profoundly neutropenic and febrile for 1 week despite broad-spectrum antibiotics are likely to have invasive fungal disease.

Physical Examination

- Otomycosis is characterized by a mass of black spores (*A. niger*) that start close to the eardrum and eventually fill the external canal, pain on tragal movement, and occasionally a purulent discharge. It is only rarely an invasive disease.
- Invasive sinus aspergillosis may present with severe pain, proptosis, monocular blindness, and bony destruction on x-ray films, with evidence of direct extension to the anterior fossa or orbit, or with widespread dissemination.
- Invasive pulmonary aspergillosis may be indistinguishable from other causes of pneumonia on physical examination. Findings may include fever, tachypnea, rales, hypoxemia, and hemoptysis (secondary to the angioinvasive potential of the organism).

Laboratory Aids

- Isolation of *Aspergillus* species by culture is required for definitive diagnosis.
- *Aspergillus* can be recovered from samples of blood, CSF, sputum, urine, BAL sample, or tissue biopsy. Types of specimens collected are guided by history and physical examination.
- *Aspergillus* species recovered from cultures of the respiratory tract (e.g., sputum and nasal cultures) are usually a result of colonization in the immunocompetent host but may indicate invasive disease in the immunocompromised host. The positive predictive value may be as high as 80–90% in patients with leukemia or bone marrow transplants.
- Microscopic examination of specially stained tissue samples, or of 10% potassium hydroxide wet preparation samples, that are positive for branching, septate hyphae are suggestive of *Aspergillus* or other fungal invaders.
- Elevated serum IgE eosinophilia, serum antibody for *Aspergillus* and an immediate-type skin test response to *Aspergillus* antigen are often present in patients with allergic aspergillosis and are helpful in establishing the diagnosis.
- Radiographic studies may include characteristic findings such as wedge-shaped pleural-based densities or cavities on plain radiographs. Findings on CT scans include the "halo sign" (an area of low attenuation surrounding a nodular lung lesion) initially (caused by edema or bleeding surrounding an ischemic area) and later the "crescent sign" (an air crescent near the periphery of a lung nodule, caused by contraction of infarcted tissue).
- Recent developments in early diagnosis include the use of: high-resolution chest CT, new rapid stain techniques and monoclonal antibodies for BAL samples, and serum ELISA for *Aspergillus galactomannan*.

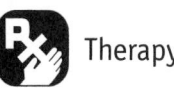

Therapy

- Allergic bronchopulmonary aspergillosis is frequently managed with oral or inhaled corticosteroids. In patients with corticosteroid-dependent allergic bronchopulmonary aspergillosis, the addition of itraconazole has been shown to be an effective adjunctive agent.
- If paranasal sinusitis is noninvasive, surgical drainage or debridement usually results in clearance of the infection.
- Otomycosis (most commonly secondary to *A. niger*) is often found in association with a bacterial external otitis. Debridement of the external canal and treatment of underlying bacterial external otitis usually produces a good therapeutic response.

- Invasive or systemic disease is treated with amphotericin B, with recommended doses ranging from 0.8 to 1.5 mg/kg/d.
- The lipid-based amphotericin preparations are indicated for patients with invasive aspergillosis who develop nephrotoxicity while receiving conventional amphotericin. The lipid-based formulations may be preferred as initial therapy in patients with marginal renal function or in patients receiving other nephrotoxic drugs.
- Itraconazole has been shown to be efficacious in the treatment of invasive aspergillosis. The oral form of itraconazole may be considered as an alternative to amphotericin for prolonged treatment once disease progression has been halted with IV amphotericin therapy.
- Surgical excision, in addition to amphotericin B, is sometimes required for localized debridement in invasive disease.

Follow-Up

The course of illness is variable, depending on host immune function and location and invasiveness of disease.

PITFALLS

- Any immunocompromised patient with persistent fevers or signs of invasive infection not improving on treatment with broad-spectrum antibiotics must be evaluated for fungal infection and the empiric use of antifungal medications considered.
- The rare finding of diffuse nodular pneumonia in children may be indicative of an underlying diagnosis of chronic granulomatous disease and aspergillosis.

PREVENTION

Infection Control

- Hospitalized, immunosuppressed patients are at risk for invasive aspergillosis.
- Environmental measures to control airborne spread of conidiospores in hospitals during construction are indicated.
- Laminar-flow rooms with appropriate filters will significantly decrease contact with airborne conidiospores.

Common Questions and Answers

Q: What are rare complications of aspergillosis?
A: Endocarditis, osteomyelitis, and cutaneous disease.

Q: Does person-to-person spread occur?
A: No. The principal route of transmission is inhalation of airborne spores.

ICD-9-CM 117.3

BIBLIOGRAPHY

American Academy of Pediatrics. Aspergillosis. In: Pickering L, ed. *2000 red book: report of the Committee on Infectious Diseases* , 25th ed. Elk Grove Village, IL: American Academy of Pediatrics, 2000:178–179.

Denning DW. Aspergillus species. In: Mandell GL, et al., eds. *Principles and practice of infectious diseases*, 5th ed. New York: Churchill Livingstone, 2000:2674–2684.

Blum MD, Wiederman BL. Aspergillus. In: Feigen RD, Cherry JD, eds. *Textbook of pediatric infectious diseases*, 4th ed. Philadelphia: WB Saunders, 1998:2288–2296.

Stevens DA, Kan VL, Judson MA, et al. Practice guidelines for diseases caused by Aspergillus. *Clin Infect Dis* 2000;30:696–709.

Author: Theoklis Zaoutis
Molly (Martha) W. Stevens, 2nd edition

Asplenia/Hyposplenia

 Database

DEFINITION

Hyposplenia and asplenia are defined by the functional capacity of the spleen to filter blood and perform immunogenic functions.

CAUSES

Hyposplenia/asplenia occurs in association with a number of illnesses and after splenectomy. A complete listing of causes is given below (see Differential Diagnosis).

PATHOLOGY

• Most patients with hyposplenism have no problems handling antigens. However, if the spleen is minimally functional, problems develop. The major consequence is an inability to handle infections.
• The spleen is a major component of reticuloendothelial system; it is important both for antibody synthesis and removal of opsonized organisms. The encapsulated microbes such as pneumococcus, meningococcus and *Haemophilus* are usually handled by this mechanism.
• Under the age of 4 years where few alternate routes of bacterial clearance exist, significant pathology can result for the patient with impaired splenic function.
• Asplenia syndrome should be viewed separately as its morbidity is distinctly unfavorable. Asplenia syndrome is characterized by complex congenital heart defects, asplenia, and abdominal heterotaxy.

—The common associated anomalies include: atrioventricular canal defects, conotruncal anomalies, anomalous systemic pulmonary venous connections, and abnormalities of visceroatrial situs.
—The embryologic basis is thought to be a disturbance in embryogenesis in the fifth week of development that results in bilateral right-sidedness with abnormal pulmonary lobation in 80% of patients and abdominal heterotaxy in 72%. The mouse model and family history are suggestive of an autosomal-recessive inheritance pattern. A review of 519 autopsy cases calculated survival to be 2.6 months with death typically resulting from cardiorespiratory failure or infection.

 Differential Diagnosis

Diminished splenic function is found in:

• Normal infants
• Congenital asplenia
• Asplenia syndrome
• Old age
• Sequestration rises (sickle hemoglobinopathies, essential thrombocytosis, malaria, thrombosis of the splenic vessels)
• Autoimmune disorders (glomerulonephritis, SLE, rheumatoid arthritis, GVHD, sarcoid)
• Gastrointestinal disorders (celiac disease—30–50% are hyposplenic, Crohn disease, ulcerative colitis, dermatitis herpetiformis)
• Space-occupying lesions (tumors, amyloid, cysts)
• Splenic irradiation
• Postsplenectomy

 Data Gathering

HISTORY

The history taking should be directed toward the differential diagnosis given above. However, in the apparently healthy child with no identified risk factors who presents with an overwhelming infection with an encapsulated organism, the hematologic smear should be examined.

 Physical Examination

On physical exam the spleen may be normal, large, or atretic. Therefore, the size of the spleen cannot be used as an index of splenic function. The size is most closely linked to the underlying etiology. Complete splenic replacement by cysts, neoplasm, or amyloid is an example of hyposplenic splenomegaly. Similarly, sequestration crises such as that associated with sickle cell and malaria clog the spleen with cellular debris, which results in increased spleen size and decreased function.

Laboratory Aids

- The reduction or absence of splenic function can be determined by specific hematologic changes.
- Nonspecific changes include a modest increase in WBC and platelet count.
- More specific changes include target cells, Howell-Jolly bodies (nuclear fragments that normally are removed in the spleen) and pitted erythrocytes.
- Pits or pox on the red cell surface are the most sensitive indicator of hyposplenism. These are submembranous vacuoles that can be seen only in wet preparations of red cells using direct interference-contrast microscopy.
- ^{51}Cr-labeled heat damaged red cells can be used as a measure of the capacity of the spleen to clear particulate matter from the bloodstream.
- Size of the spleen can be determined by either ultrasound or CT scan.

 ## Therapy

- Immunization with a polyvalent pneumococcal vaccine should be carried out in all patients with hyposplenism. In those patients who will be undergoing splenectomy, the vaccine should be given prior to the operation.
- No revaccination is needed according to the present recommendations.
- Children should also receive HiB vaccine.

PITFALLS

Under the age of 4 years, splenectomy is contraindicated because of the risk of developing bacterial infection.

 ## Common Questions and Answers

Q: What should I do if my child has a fever?
A: In hyposplenic patients, especially those under the age of 4 years, all fevers should be taken seriously. If the child is not on prophylactic penicillin, he/she should be treated for all symptomatic infections.

Q: Are there any special times I need to worry about infections?
A: In these patients dental work, especially tooth extraction, should always be covered with antibiotics.

ICD-9-CM 459.0

BIBLIOGRAPHY

Phoon CK, Neill CA. Asplenia syndrome—risk factors for early unfavorable outcome. *Am J Cardiol* 1994;73:1235–1237.

Phoon CK, Neill CA. Asplenia syndrome: insight into embryology through an analysis of cardiac and extracardiac anomalies. *Am J Cardiol* 1994;73:581–587.

Suchy F. *Liver disease in children*. Philadelphia: Mosby, 1994.

Author: Barbara Haber

Asthma

 Database

DEFINITION

- Characterized by three components:

—Reversible airway obstruction
—Airway inflammation
—Airway hyperresponsiveness to a variety of stimuli

DIAGNOSIS—THE THREE R'S

- Recurrence—symptoms are recurrent
- Reactivity—symptoms brought on by specific occurrence or exposure (trigger)
- Responsive—symptoms diminish in response to bronchodilator or antiinflammatory agent

PATHOPHYSIOLOGY AND CAUSES

- Immune and inflammatory responses in the airways triggered by an array of environmental antigens, irritants, or infectious organisms
- Atopy and asthma are related

—Eosinophilia and the ability to make excess IgE in response to antigen is associated with increased airway reactivity.
—Asthma is more common in children who have allergic rhinitis and eczema.

- Viral infections, particularly respiratory syncytial virus (RSV), during infancy may play a role in the development of asthma or may modify the severity of asthma.
- Exposure to cigarette smoke and other airway irritants influences the development and severity of asthma.
- Airway stimulated and primary inflammatory mediators released.
- Airway is invaded by inflammatory cells (mast cells, basophils, eosinophils, macrophages, neutrophils, B and T lymphocytes).
- Inflammatory cells respond to and produce various mediators (cytokines, leukotrienes, lymphokines), augmenting the inflammatory response.
- Airway epithelium is inflamed and becomes disrupted, and basal membrane is thickened.
- Airway smooth muscle is hyperresponsive, and bronchoconstriction ensues.
- Airway smooth muscle hypertrophy and airway epithelial hyperplasia are characteristic chronic changes resulting from poorly controlled asthma.

GENETICS

- Children of asthmatics have higher incidence of asthma:

—6% to 7% risk if neither parent has asthma
—20% risk if one parent has asthma
—60% risk if both parents have asthma

- Several genes are known to be associated with the development of atopy and bronchial muscle responsiveness.

EPIDEMIOLOGY

- Most common chronic illness in children
- Death from asthma in children nearly tripled form 1980 to 1995, and incidence of death from asthma does not seem to correlate with severity.
- Wheezing in children is extremely common in the industrialized world (cumulative prevalence, 30–60%).
- In younger children, most episodes occur following viral infections.
- Over 50% of children who wheeze in early childhood stop wheezing by age 6 years.
- 14% of all young children (40% of those who wheeze during infancy) continue to wheeze.

COMPLICATIONS

- Morbidity

—Frequent hospitalizations and absence from school
—Psychologic impact of having a chronic illness
—Decline in lung function over time

PROGNOSIS

- With proper therapy and good adherence with treatment regimen: excellent

 Differential Diagnosis

INFECTIOUS

- Pneumonia
- Bronchiolitis
- *Chlamydia* infection
- Laryngotracheobronchitis
- Sinusitis

MECHANICAL

- Extrinsic airway compression
- Vascular ring
- Foreign body
- Vocal cord dysfunction
- Tracheobronchomalacia

MISCELLANEOUS

- Cystic fibrosis
- Bronchopulmonary dysplasia
- Pulmonary edema
- Gastroesophageal reflux (GER)
- Recurrent aspiration
- Bronchiolitis obliterans

 Data Gathering

HISTORY

Inquire about these symptoms: coughing, wheezing, shortness of breath, chest tightness

- Frequency of symptoms defines severity
- Precipitating factor (trigger)
- Response to bronchodilator or antiinflammatory medication

PATTERN OF SYMPTOMS

- Perennial versus seasonal
- Continuous versus acute
- Duration and frequency of episodes
- Diurnal variation/nocturnal symptoms

Do any of the following set off the breathing difficulty?

- Infections (upper respiratory, sinusitis)
- Exposure to:

—Dust (mites)
—Animal dander
—Pollen
—Mold

- Cold air or weather changes
- Exercise or play
- Environmental stimulants

—Cigarette smoke
—Strong odors
—Pollutants

- Emotional factors

—Laughing
—Crying
—Fear

- Drug intake

—Aspirin
—NSAIDs
—β-blockers

- Food additives
- Endocrine factors

—Menses
—Pregnancy
—Thyroid dysfunction

- Family history of asthma or atopy

REVIEW OF SYSTEMS

- Symptoms of complicating factors (gastroesophageal reflux, sinusitis, allergies)

—Dyspepsia, sour taste (GE reflux)
—Throat clearing, purulent nasal discharge, halitosis, cephalgia, or facial pain (sinusitis)
—Nasal itching, ("allergic salute"), eye rubbing, sneezing, watery nasal discharge (allergies)

IMPACT OF ASTHMA

- Number of hospitalizations/ICU admissions
- Number of ER visits/doctor's office visits
- Asthma attack frequency
- Number of missed school days/parent workdays
- Limitation on activity
- Number of courses of systemic steroids needed

ENVIRONMENTAL HISTORY

- Type of home
- Location of home (urban, suburban, rural)
- Heating system/air conditioning
- Use of humidifier
- Presence of molds, cockroaches, rodents
- Fireplace
- Carpeting
- Stuffed animals
- Pets
- Exposure to cigarette smoke

 ## Physical Examination

- Pulmonary examination may be normal when asymptomatic.
- Assess work of breathing

—Level of distress
—Intercostal/supraclavicular muscle retractions

- Chest shape (i.e., normal vs. barrel-shaped)
- Lung auscultation

—Wheezing
—End-expiratory involuntary cough
—Prolonged expiratory phase
—Crackles or coarse breath sounds
—Stridor (indicates extrathoracic airway obstruction)

- HEENT examination: signs of allergies or sinusitis

—Watery or itchy eyes
—Allergic shiners
—Dennie lines
—Nasal congestion
—Boggy nasal turbinates
—Nasal polyps
—Postnasal drip

- General examination: vital signs

—Blood pressure (pulsus paradoxus)
—Respiratory rate (tachypnea)

- Skin: evidence of eczema
- Extremities: digital clubbing (suggests alternative diagnosis)

PHYSICAL EXAMINATION TRICK

Forced exhalation maneuver to observe for wheezes or for precipitating coughing

 ## Laboratory Aids

TESTS

- Pulmonary function tests

—Essential for the assessment and ongoing care of children with asthma.
—Spirometry measures the degree of airway obstruction and the response to bronchodilators.
—Values obtained can measure absolute degree of airway obstruction.
—Serial values can follow progress of disease and response to treatment.
—Children as young as 3 years old can usually perform spirometry with practice.

- Provocational testing

—Exercise challenge: determines effect of exercise on triggering airway obstruction
—Cold air challenge: indirect test of airway hyperresponsiveness
—Methacholine challenge: a positive test supports the diagnosis of asthma; useful in cases where history is equivocal and pulmonary function test is normal; measures the degree of airway hyperreactivity

- Allergy evaluation

—Blood tests (eosinophilic count, IgE level)
—Skin testing (best test for assessing allergen sensitivity)
—RAST testing (not as accurate as skin testing)
—Sputum/nasal examination for presence of eosinophilia

- Other studies

—GER evaluation
—pH probe
—Milk scan
—Barium swallow (confirms normal anatomy)

- Bronchoscopy to rule out:

—Anatomic malformations
—Foreign bodies
—Mucus plugging
—Vocal cord function

- Assess for aspiration (lipid-laden macrophages)

IMAGING

- Chest radiograph should usually be obtained at least once for all children to rule out congenital lung malformations or obvious vascular malformations. Findings can be normal. Common findings are peribronchial thickening, subsegmental atelectasis, and hyperinflation.
- Sinus CT is useful if symptoms suggest sinusitis.
- Chest CT should be performed if bronchiectasis or anatomic abnormality is suspected.

HOME TESTING

- Peak flow meter

—Measures peak flow rate (PEFR)
—Used with patients who have poor symptom recognition or labile asthma
—Dips in PEFR precede onset of clinical asthmatic symptoms.
—PEFR should be performed at least once a day

PEFR values are divided into three zones:

—Green: 80% of baseline or higher
—Yellow: 50% to 80% of baseline
—Red: 50% of baseline
—Specific PEFR guidelines should be individualized for each patient based on the best measurement obtained during a 14-day period when the child is well.

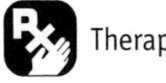 ## Therapy

DRUGS

Antiinflammatory Agents

- Indicated for all patients with asthma except for those with very infrequent and mild symptoms.
- Three classes described below

Corticosteroids

- Most effective antiinflammatory agent
- Preparations
- Inhaled
  —Reduce airway inflammation and hyperresponsiveness more than any other inhaled agent
  —Inhibit production and release of cytokines and arachidonic acid–associated metabolites
  —Enhance β-adrenoceptor responsiveness
  —Side effects: oral thrush; may minimally affect growth velocity at moderate or high doses

- Dosage individualized to each patient
  —Agents vary in topical potency and systemic bioavailability
  —Available as pressurized metered dose inhaler (pMDI), dry powder inhaler (DPI), or nebulized as indicated below
  —Fluticazone (44, 110, 220 μg/puff pMDI) (Flovent)
  —Budesonide (200 μg/puff DPI; 250 and 500 μg vials for nebulizer) (Pulmicort)
  —Beclomethasone (42, 84 μg /puff) (Beclovent, Vanceril)
  —Triamcinolone (100 μg /puff) (Azmacort)
  —Flunisolide (250 μg /puff) (Aerobid)

- Oral—used for asthma exacerbations or for severe asthma that cannot be otherwise controlled

—Exacerbations—prednisone 1–2 mg/kg/d 3 to 7 days or longer; usually tapered if more

Asthma

than 7 days of therapy required or if systemic steroids are used frequently

—Ongoing therapy—0.5 to 1 mg/kg/day daily or every other day for patients with severe asthma
—Undesirable side-effect profile
—When used daily, assess bone density and for cataract formation at least yearly

• Intravenous

—Methylprednisolone (Solumedrol) 1 mg/kg IV q6–12h until able to take oral medication

Leukotriene Modifiers

• Block the synthesis and/or action of leukotrienes
• 5-Lipoxygenase inhibitors; zileuton. May cause hepatic dysfunction.
• Leukotriene receptor antagonists; zafirlukast (10 mg; Accolate) and montelukast (4, 5, and 10 mg; Singulair)
• Indicated as monotherapy for mild or exercise induced asthma and in combination with an inhaled corticosteroid for more effective symptom control or using a lower dose of inhaled corticosteroid

Mast-Cell Stabilizers

• Weak antiinflammatory agents
• Preparations

—Cromolyn sodium (Intal)
—Nedocromil sodium (Tilade)

• Decrease bronchial hyperresponsiveness
• Can be used prior to exercise for exercise-induced symptoms
• No significant side effects
• Inhaled

—Nebulizer
—MDI

Bronchodilators

• Relaxes airway smooth muscle
• Three classes described below

β_2-Agonists

• Indication is for relief of acute bronchoconstriction (quick relief medicine)
• Used as needed in people with asthma who have breakthrough symptoms
• Used prior to exercise in exercise-induced bronchospasm
• Regular use or overuse associated with worsened control of asthma
• Routes

—Inhaled (most effective): metered dose inhaler or nebulizer
—Oral (least effective; most side effects)

• Preparations: Short-acting (effect lasts 4–6 hours):

—Albuterol (Ventolin, Proventil)
—Terbutaline (Brethaire, Brethine)
—Metoproterenol (Alupent)

• Preparation: Long-acting (lasts up to 12 hours)

—Salmeterol (Serevent)—available as pMDI and DPI
—Can be used daily in conjunction with antiinflammatory agent for improved symptom control

Theophylline

• Second line agent used when more conventional therapies are unsuccessful
• Indications

—Chronic, poorly controlled asthma
—Nocturnal asthma (if no GER)
—Adjunctive therapy with β_2 drugs and steroids in hospitalized patients in selected cases

• Route: oral or IV
• Serum levels must be routinely monitored

—Therapeutic levels: 5 to 15 mg/mL
—Side effects are seen with increased levels.
—Many factors affect theophylline levels.
—Increased levels seen with:
—Erythromycin
—Ciprofloxacin
—Cimetidine
—Viral illnesses
—Fever
—Decreased levels seen with:

—Phenobarbital
—Phenytoin
—Rifampin

Anticholinergic Agents

• Adjunctive bronchodilator, may be useful in patients who only partially respond to β-agonists
• Preparations

—Ipratropium bromide MDI or ampule for nebulization (Atrovent)

MISCELLANEOUS DRUGS USED IN SEVERE CASES

Steroid-Sparing Agents

Troleandomycin (Tao)

• Macrolide antibiotic
• Decreases clearance of corticosteroids, thus prolonging the effects of corticosteroids on the lung
• Lower corticosteroid dosing required

Methotrexate

• Potent immunosuppressive drug
• Needs further investigation in children

Cyclosporine

• Has been shown to have steroid-sparing effect in adult population with asthma
• Side effects are significant and may limit use.

IVIG

• High-dose therapy under investigation

$MgSO_4$

• Used intravenously as smooth muscle relaxer in severe acute asthma exacerbation

HELIUM

• May improve airflow in severe asthma
• Can improve ventilation and potentially oxygenation

IMMUNOTHERAPY

• Efficacy in asthma is controversial.
• Use only in selected cases if medical management and environmental control measures are ineffective.

Duration of Therapy

• Antiinflammatory agents

—Use every day.
—May be decreased in patients as asthma comes under long-standing control.

• Bronchodilators

—Should be used as needed

EDUCATION/ENVIRONMENTAL CONTROL

• Patient and caregiver education is mandatory to establish provider/caregiver partnership and ensure adherence with treatment plan.
• Every patient/caregiver should be taught that asthma is a chronic, inflammatory condition that can be controlled with proper therapy.
• All medications should be explained and potential risks (side effects) and benefits reviewed.
• A written asthma management plan should be provided, outlining daily therapy and an "action plan" for managing exacerbations of asthma.
• Environmental counseling

—Avoid airborne irritants (tobacco smoke, wood stoves, noxious fumes).
—Minimize dust-mite exposure.
—Avoid using in room humidifier or vaporizer.
—Minimize stuffed animals, quilts, books, and clutter.
—Use dust mite–proof coverings on mattresses, pillows, and box springs.
—Wash pillows, blankets, and sheets in hot water.
—Avoid molds by decreasing relative humidity to 50%.
—Remove pets from child's bedroom, and from house if patient is allergic to animal.

DIET

• Avoid foods or food additives (if truly allergic).
• Food-induced asthma is uncommon.

Follow-Up

WHEN TO EXPECT IMPROVEMENT

- In acute asthma attacks, with appropriate therapy, improvement is usually seen within 24 to 48 hours.
- Long-term control of symptoms can usually be obtained within 2 to 4 weeks

SIGNS THAT MAY INDICATE PROBLEMS

- Increased symptoms (cough day or night, wheeze)
- Exercise limitations or symptoms during exercise
- Decrease in PEFR
- Increasing use of inhaled bronchodilators
- Subject not improving on enhanced home therapy

PITFALLS

- Not recognizing that asthma can manifest as chronic cough
- Reluctance to "label" child with having asthma (uses terms like *reactive airways disease* or *bronchitis*)
- Frequent antibiotic or cough medicine use to treat asthma symptoms
- "Recurrent pneumonias" many times are actually asthma exacerbations; subsegmental atelectasis on chest radiography misdiagnosed as infiltrate
- Underreporting of asthma symptoms
- Poor adherence with therapy once symptoms are controlled
- Failure to properly use inhaled medications

—Inhaled medication use must be taught and reviewed at each visit.
—A fixed volume holding chamber should always be used with a pMDI, regardless of patient age.
—PMDIs should be refilled based on the number of doses used, not by estimating contents by shaking or spraying.

Common Questions and Answers

Q: Will my child outgrow his or her asthma?
A: Family history and allergies affect the ultimate outcome. Wheezing during the first 3 years of life is extremely common, with 40% to 50% of all children wheezing at some time. Many of these children do not develop asthma and "outgrow" their illness by school age. Some patients develop asthma again as young adults.

Q: Can my child become dependent on asthma medications?
A: Children do not become "dependent" on these medications as they would with narcotic agents. Daily asthma medications are required to maintain airway patency and to control airway inflammation.

Q: Will my child be on medications for the rest of his or her life?
A: This depends on the severity of the asthma. The types, doses, and frequency of asthma medications will change over a patient's lifetime.

Q: Do inhaled steroids affect patient growth?
A: There is some transient and slight decrease in growth velocity seen in children who receive moderate-dose inhaled corticosteroids (approximately 0.5 mg/day). Ultimate height does not seem to be affected.

ICD-9-CM 493.01

BIBLIOGRAPHY

Crater SE, Platts-Mills TA. Searching for the cause of the increase in asthma. *Curr Opin Pediatr* 1998;10(6):594–599.

Hakonarson H, Grunstein MM. Management of childhood asthma. In: Barnes P, Grunstein MM, Leff A, et al., eds. *Asthma*, vol 2. New York: Raven Press, 1997:1847–1868.

Hill M, Szefler SJ. Asthma pathogenesis and the implications for therapy in children. *Pediatr Clin North Am* 1992;39:1205–1224.

National Asthma Education and Prevention Program. *Expert Panel Report 2: Guidelines for the diagnosis and management of asthma.* NIH-NHLBI publication, Washington, DC: US Government Printing Office, February 1997.

Reid MJ. Complicating features of asthma. *Pediatr Clin North Am* 1992;39:1327–1341.

Silverstein MD, Mair JE, Katusic SK, et al. School attendance and school performance: a population-based study of children with asthma. *J Pediatr* 2001;139(2):278–83.

Turktas I, Ozkaya O, Bostanci I, et al. Safety of inhaled corticosteroid therapy in young children with asthma. *Ann Allergy Asthma Immunol* 2001;86(6):649–654.

Author: Russell G. Clayton Sr.
Hakon Hakonaarson, 2nd edition

Ataxia

 ## Database

DEFINITION

Ataxia is defined as a problem with orientation of movement due to abnormal coordination of agonist-antagonist muscle groups. Though cerebellar dysfunction is the most common cause of ataxia in children, other localizations should also be considered—peripheral nerve, dorsal-root ganglion, brainstem, and inner ear (labyrinth).

- Appendicular ataxia affects limb movement.
- Truncal ataxia, gait ataxia, dysarthria, and nystagmus often occur together in cerebellar ataxia.

CLINICAL PRESENTATION

- Acute cerebellar ataxia following a benign viral infection is common in children.
- Chronic ataxia usually signals serious underlying pathology (tumor, hereditary, or metabolic disorder).

PATHOPHYSIOLOGY

The cerebellum "fine-tunes" coordination of agonist-antagonist muscle groups and is sensitive to any structural (e.g., tumor, stroke) or metabolic (e.g., intoxication) injury. Disturbance of pathways to (e.g., vestibular nerve, proprioceptive sensory nerves, dorsal-root ganglion cells) or from (e.g., superior cerebellar peduncles, brainstem) the cerebellum.

EPIDEMIOLOGY

Metabolic/heredodegenerative causes are rare. Ataxia telangiectasia incidence is near 1/100,000.

GENETICS

Hereditary causes of chronic ataxia include Friedreich ataxia, ataxia telangiectasia, mitochondrial disease, and aminoacidopathies.

ASSOCIATED CONDITIONS

- Acute ataxia, most often due to intoxication; in association with opsoclonus-myoclonus syndrome, may be symptomatic of underlying neuroblastoma/ ganglioneuroma, though more often isolated, transient "cerebellitis" associated with EBV, varicella, and other viruses.
- Friedreich ataxia is associated with cardiomyopathy, diabetes, and peripheral neuropathy.
- Mitochondrial disorders—short stature, seizures, retinopathy, heart block, myopathy

 ## Data Gathering

HISTORY

Establish acute vs. chronic onset of ataxia to narrow the differential diagnosis.

- In acute ataxia, history should be directed to possible intoxication, head trauma, or migraine.
- History of episodic change in consciousness or convulsions point to seizure disorder (postictal ataxia).
- Recent varicella or other infection suggests postviral cerebellar ataxia, labyrinthitis, or Guillain-Barré syndrome (GBS) (see Guillain-Barré Syndrome)
- Congenital heart disease or other known circulatory disorder raises the possibility of cerebellar stroke.
- History of extreme irritability or progressive macrocrania (from well-care records) in an infant or toddler suggest brain tumor.
- History of recurrent vomiting (metabolic disorders), psychiatric disturbance (conversion disorders), or other family members with neurologic disease (hereditary neuropathies, familial periodic ataxia) may lead to specific diagnoses.

 ## Physical Examination

The neuroanatomic localization of the ataxia must be determined.

- Cerebellar ataxia often interferes with speech; unless the brainstem is affected, consciousness is normal, despite "drunken" movements and gait. Signs include:

—Intention tremor—oscillations seen (e.g., on finger nose testing) when agonists and antagonists co-contract to orient limb movement
—Disdiadochokinesia—impairment of rapid alternating movements
—Titubation, truncal ataxia, and pathologic nystagmus point to cerebellar or vestibular disease.
—Cranial nerve findings, especially third, sixth, or lower cranial nerves, point to possible brain tumor; hyperreflexia or up-going toes may be present.
—Asymmetric ataxia or weakness may signify tumor, stroke, or demyelinating disease.

- Sensory ataxia also spares consciousness; other signs include:

—Romberg fall—ataxia worsened by eye closure. Indicates sensory dysfunction, either proprioceptive (peripheral nerves, dorsal-root ganglia), or vestibular (inner ear, vestibular nerve).
—Areflexia—not seen in central causes of ataxia; key sign in distinguishing sensory ataxia (as in GBS) from cerebellar ataxia.

- Toxic/metabolic causes—intoxications, postictal ataxia, and sleep drunkenness usually alter consciousness.

 ## Differential Diagnosis

Chorea, tremor, or athetosis may be mistakenly diagnosed as ataxia.

ACUTE ATAXIA

- Intoxication: depressed mental status; toxicologic screen; medications at home
- Posttraumatic: history/physical findings
- Postinfectious: acute cerebellar ataxia (dysarthria, mild hypotonia)
- Paraneoplastic: more indolent/subacute onset; ataxia may precede opsoclonus/ myoclonus; neuroblastoma/ganglioneuroma
- Migraine: resolves in hours; headache may precede ataxia
- Labyrinthitis: fast phase of nystagmus is unidirectional
- Acute disseminated encephalomyelitis (ADEM) white matter changes on MRI, variable on CT
- Acute polyneuropathy: GBS (areflexia, signs of sensory ataxia)
- Stroke: focal deficits; abnormal imaging studies
- Postictal: rapidly resolving ataxia with negative studies, slowing on EEG; history of convulsion
- Familial periodic ataxia: (family history)
- Acute ataxia: can be a rare presentation of meningitis/encephalitis
- Psychogenic: "astasia abasia" (variable effort; no pathologic nystagmus, characteristic gait)

CHRONIC ATAXIA

- Brain tumor (esp. under 10 years): associated cranial neuropathies, papilledema, headache, pyramidal tract signs
- Friedreich ataxia: onset 5–15 years; family history, associated cardiomyopathy, polyneuropathy, diabetes
- Leukodystrophy: adrenoleukodystrophy, metachromatic leukodystrophy, Pelizaeus-Merzbacher disease (abnormal MRI signal in white matter)
- Other metabolic diseases: Niemann-Pick, maple syrup urine disease (MSUD), Hartnup disease (amino acid screen)
- Abetalipoproteinemia: onset in second decade; hypocholesterolemia/decreased LDL
- Hereditary neuropathy: decreased reflexes, weakness usually more prominent, family history, molecular diagnosis
- Thiamine deficiency (Wernicke encephalopathy) associated with malnutrition, TPN
- Celiac disease
- Hereditary ataxia: autosomal dominant, molecular diagnosis
- Long-term phenytoin: primarily adults
- Metabolic: variable onset; may be episodic, with other systemic symptoms; Hartnup disease, MSUD, organic acidemias, Niemann-Pick C (visceromegaly?, foam cells in marrow)
- Intermittent or chronic ataxia may be a feature of mitochondrial disease, usually in association with other systemic signs/symptoms—retinopathy, sensorineural hearing loss, diabetes, growth delay, seizures, myopathy.
- Rare: ataxic cerebral palsy, brain dysgenesis, Joubert syndrome, multiple sclerosis, Gerstmann-Straussler (familial; prion disease)

Laboratory Aids

- Toxicologic screen is usually a good initial screen in acute ataxia.
- Radiologic studies are necessary when intoxication has been ruled out (rule out tumor, stroke, demyelination); MRI is superior to CT for imaging the cerebellum, though contrast CT is adequate to rule out posterior fossa tumor.
- Spinal tap may reveal a few cells/mild increase in protein in benign acute cerebellar ataxia of childhood or in acute demyelinating encephalomyelitis.
- EEG if postictal ataxia is a possibility.
- Full workup for neuroblastoma in ataxia opsoclonus/myoclonus includes body CT, serum ferritin, urine homovanillic/vanillylmandelic acid (HVA/VMA).
- Low cholesterol in chronic ataxia suggests abetalipoproteinemia.
- Genetic test for Friedreich (chronic) ataxia may soon become available.
- Laboratory testing for mitochondrial ataxia, that may produce intermittent or chronic ataxia, usually with other systemic abnormalities (see above) includes urine organic acids, plasma lactate/pyruvate, genetic testing on blood, muscle biopsy.

Therapy

- As indicated for any underlying condition; precautions and limitation of activity to decrease the chance of injury/aspiration
- Steroids (2 mg/kg IV prednisolone) and IVIG (400 mg/kg/day for 5 days) have been used for ADEM, though there is no proven benefit.
- Immunomodulatory therapies have been tried (plasmapheresis, IVIG) for paraneoplastic ataxia-opsoclonus/myoclonus, since the movement disorder may persist long after therapy for the tumor.
- Acetazolamide may be helpful for familial periodic ataxia.

Follow-Up

- Acute postinfectious cerebellar ataxia usually resolves over days to weeks; if imaging studies show demyelination, recovery may take longer and the chance of recurrence may be higher.
- If initial studies in opsoclonus/myoclonus do not reveal a neoplasm, follow-up studies should be repeated.

PITFALLS

- Children with acute recurrent ataxia should be evaluated for metabolic disease, even if examination is normal between attacks. Possibilities include ornithine transcarbamoylase deficiency, mitochondrial disorders, or one of the paroxysmal dyskinesias (ion channelopathies)
- Inadvertent intoxication with anticonvulsants in the household may not be detected on routine toxin screen. Ask about carbamazepine, phenytoin.
- Symptoms of progressive herniation of the cerebellar tonsils in a child or adolescent with Arnold-Chiari type 1 malformation may mimic migraine. A head scan should be done on a child with ataxia and a headache.

Common Questions and Answers

Q: What intoxications are most likely to cause ataxia?
A: Benzodiazepines, the major anticonvulsants (except valproate), ethanol, tricyclics, antihistamines, others.

Q: How long can postinfectious cerebellar ataxia last?
A: Rarely, it may last for months, but should be improving during that time.

Q: What is the role of physical therapy for cerebellar ataxia?
A: Physical therapy for ataxia is of limited value.

ICD-9-CM 334.3

BIBLIOGRAPHY

Connolly AM, Dodson WE, Prensky AL, et al. Course and outcome of acute cerebellar ataxia. *Ann Neurol* 1994;35(6):673–679.

Bushara K, Goebel SU, Shill H, et al. Gluten sensitivity in sporadic and hereditary cerebellar ataxia. *Ann Neurol* 2001;49:540–543.

Gieron-Korthals MA, Westberry KR, Emmanuel PJ. Acute childhood ataxia: 10-year experience. *J Child Neurol* 1994;9(4):381–384.

Snodgrass SR. Syndromic diagnosis in para-infectious neurologic disease: varicella ataxic syndrome. *J Child Neurol* 1998;2:83–85.

Author: Peter M. Bingham

Atelectasis

 Database

DEFINITION

- State of collapsed and airless alveoli
- May be subsegmental, segmental, or lobar, or may involve the entire lung
- A radiographic sign of an underlying disease and not a diagnosis unto itself

CAUSES

- Airway obstruction (resorption atelectasis)
  —Most common cause for atelectasis in children
  —Obstructed communication between alveoli and trachea

  - Large airway obstruction:
    —Intrinsic: i.e., foreign-body aspiration, mucus plug, inflammatory tumor
    —Extrinsic: i.e., hilar adenopathy, mediastinal mass, congenital lung malformations

  - Small airway obstruction:
    —Altered mucociliary clearance: i.e., CNS depression, smoke inhalation, pain
    —Acute infection: i.e., bronchiolitis, pneumonia (respiratory infections are the most common cause of acute atelectasis)

- Mechanical compression of the pulmonary parenchyma or pleural space (compressive atelectasis)
  - Intrathoracic compression: i.e., pneumothorax, pleural effusion, lobar emphysema, intrathoracic tumors, cardiomegaly, diaphragmatic hernias
  - Abdominal distention: i.e., large intraabdominal tumors, hepatosplenomegaly, massive ascites, morbid obesity

- Decreased surface tension in the small airways and alveoli (adhesive atelectasis)
  —Stems from surfactant deficiency
  —Diffuse surfactant deficiency: e.g., hyaline membrane disease, ARDS, smoke inhalation
  —Localized surfactant deficiency: e.g., acute radiation pneumonitis, pulmonary embolism

- Neuromuscular weakness (hypoventilation)
  —Inherent weakness: e.g., muscular dystrophy, spinal muscle atrophy, paralysis
  —Acquired weakness: e.g., postanesthesia (hypoventilation)

PATHOPHYSIOLOGY

- Reduced lung compliance
- Loss of alveoli (if extensive) may lead to hypoxia.
- Intrapulmonary shunting develops from hypoxia-induced pulmonary arterial vasoconstriction, which may lead to areas of ventilation/perfusion (V/Q) mismatch and further hypoxia.
- If atelectasis is extensive, pulmonary hypertension may develop.
- Atelectatic areas are prone to bacterial overgrowth.

GENETICS

- Depends on the underlying disease causing atelectasis

EPIDEMIOLOGY

- Depends on the underlying disease causing atelectasis
- Resorption atelectasis the most common form

COMPLICATIONS

- Recurrent infections
- Bronchiectasis
- Hemoptysis
- Abscess formation
- Fibrosis of the pulmonary parenchyma

PROGNOSIS

- Dependent on the underlying disease process

—In otherwise healthy individuals: excellent

 Differential Diagnosis

- Pneumonia

—Viral pneumonia versus subsegmental atelectasis
—Bacterial pneumonia versus segmental or lobar atelectasis

- Thymus (may be mistaken for atelectasis in an upper lobe)
- Congenital malformations (i.e., sequestration, bronchogenic cyst)
- Pleural effusion

 Data Gathering

HISTORY

- Dependent on the underlying disease process
- May be asymptomatic
- Cough and/or wheeze can be present
- Dyspnea
- Chest pain

Special Questions

- Is the atelectasis acute, recurrent, or chronic in terms of its duration?
- Is there a history of asthma, chronic lung disease, or exposure to smoke or toxic fumes that would increase the risk for atelectasis?

 Physical Examination

- May be normal
- Tachypnea
- Rales or rhonchi
- The most specific sign is localized decrease or loss of breath sounds.
- Dullness to percussion if large area involved
- Tracheal deviation and shift of heart sounds toward atelectatic side
- Localized wheezes in cases of partial obstruction
- Cyanosis (seen when extensive atelectasis is present causing impairment of oxygenation and areas of V/Q mismatch)

Laboratory Aids

TESTS

Appropriate test is dependent on the underlying etiology

- Asthma
  —Spirometry
  —Sweat test (if CF suspected)
- Infection
  —Cultures (sputum, blood, bronchoalveolar lavage fluid)
  —Nasal washing (especially for viruses)
  —PPD (when tuberculosis is suspected)
- Foreign body aspiration
  —Bronchoscopy (to remove the obstructing agent)
- Immunodeficiency
  —CBC with differential
  —Immunoglobulins (IgG, IgA, IgM)
  —HIV testing
- Congenital malformations
  —CT scan of the chest (for lung malformation)
  —bronchoscopy [for H-type tracheoesophageal fistula (TEF) or bronchial stenosis]

Imaging

Chest Radiography

- Most important diagnostic tool
- Radiographic signs of atelectasis:
  —Loss of lung volume from the affected lobe
  —Compensatory hyperexpansion of the remaining lobes on the affected side
  —Shift of interlobar fissures
  —Elevation of diaphragm
  —Mediastinal shift toward the affected side
  —Approximation of ribs on the affected side

CT of Chest

- Confluence of bronchi and blood vessels converge toward the affected side
- Provides information in regard to precise location and extent of any obstructing process

 Therapy

- Treat underlying disease (i.e., removal of aspirated foreign body)
- Chest physical therapy with bronchodilators—usually for at least 1 month
- If no improvement with conservative therapy, a bronchoscopy with lavage to remove possible mucus plug is indicated (lavage may be with saline or in select cases, with recombinant human DNase)
- Surgery to remove the affected region should be considered when the atelectasis:

—is chronic or recurrent
—is unresponsive to therapy
—Focal bronchiectasis has developed
—When significant morbidity is seen

- Prevention of recurrent or future atelectasis: directed toward underlying cause, when applicable

 Follow-Up

WHEN TO EXPECT IMPROVEMENT

- 1 to 3 months in typical, uncomplicated cases

 Common Questions and Answers

Q: When is the optimal time for bronchoscopy?
A: There are no established criteria for when a bronchoscopy should be performed. A bronchoscopy should be done early in the course of illness when there is a high suspicion of a foreign body, significant respiratory distress is present, or if the atelectasis is extensive and conservative treatment is ineffective.

ICD-9-CM 518.0

BIBLIOGRAPHY

Karlson KH. *Pediatric respiratory disease: diagnosis and treatment.* Philadelphia: WB Saunders, 1993:436–440.

Oermann CM, Moore RH. Foolers: things that look like pneumonia in children. *Semin Respir Infect* 1996;11:204–213.

Redding GJ. Atelectasis in childhood. *Pediatr Clin North Am* 1984;31:891–905.

Slattery DM, Waltz DA, Denham B, O'Mahony M, Greally P. Bronchoscopically administered recombinant human dnase for lobar atelectasis in cystic fibrosis. *Pediatr Pulmonol* 2001;31:383–388.

Woodring JH, Reed JC. Types and mechanisms of pulmonary atelectasis. *Thorac Imaging* 1996;11:92–108.

Author: Richard M. Kravitz

Atopic Dermatitis

 Database

DEFINITION

Atopic dermatitis or eczema is a chronic, recurrent, pruritic skin eruption seen in individuals with associated personal or family history of atopy—asthma, allergies, hay fever, or rhinitis. The disease is characterized by intermittent acute flares. It most commonly begins in infancy or early childhood.

CAUSES

- Etiology of atopic dermatitis is multifactorial, with genetic, environmental, physiologic, and immunologic factors.
- Decreased resistance to sensitization and increased viral and dermatophyte infections seen in these patients suggest decreased cell-mediated immunity.
- Patients often have elevated IgE levels and decreased chemotaxis of neutrophils.
- Up to 70% of patients have a family history, but the mode of inheritance is not well defined.

PATHOLOGY

- Histologic findings are dependent on the stage of atopic dermatitis—acute or chronic.
- Lymphocytes can be seen infiltrating the epidermis.
- The acute form shows spongiosis and intercellular edema that can lead to vesicle formation.
- The chronic form is characterized by epidermal psoriasiform hyperplasia and hyperkeratosis.

GENETICS

- There is a genetic trait seen in atopic dermatitis, with 30% to 70% of family members having atopy—allergies, asthma, eczema, or hay fever.
- The exact mode of inheritance is not well defined and appears to be multifactorial.

EPIDEMIOLOGY

- Atopic dermatitis is a common disease, occurring in up to 18% of children.
- Approximately 60% of patients with atopic dermatitis will develop it in the first year of life, and 30% between the ages of 1 and 5 years.
- A family history of atopy—allergies, asthma, eczema, or hay fever—is present in 30% to 70% of patients.
- Atopic dermatitis is usually worse in the winter.

COMPLICATIONS

- Decreased cell-mediated immunity and decreased chemotaxis can result in increased infection—viral, dermatophyte, and bacterial. Patients with atopic dermatitis have a high density of *Staphylococcus aureus* on their skin, and given the fissures and open excoriations, there is a risk of superinfection of these lesions.
- The decreased integrity of the skin can result in widely spread cutaneous infections such as herpes simplex infection, known as Kaposi varicelliform eruption or eczema herpeticum. Similar problems can also be seen with coxsackievirus or molluscum contagiosum and used to occur with vaccinia.
- Cataracts can be found in patients with atopic dermatitis.
- Overuse of potent topical steroids can result in hypopigmentation, telangiectasias, atrophy, and striae, as well as excess systemic absorption leading to hypothalamic-pituitary axis suppression and growth retardation.
- Early growth delay is not uncommon among children with atopic dermatitis, although later catch-up growth is generally seen. This may be related to various mechanisms including impaired growth hormone release. This growth delay can occur independent of topical steroid exposure.

 Differential Diagnosis

Diagnostic criteria have been established for atopic dermatitis. The differential diagnosis of atopic dermatitis includes:

- Severe seborrheic dermatitis
- Contact dermatitis
- Allergic or irritant, psoriasis
- Wiskott-Aldrich syndrome
- Histiocytosis X
- Acrodermatitis enteropathica
- Scabies
- Xerosis
- Hyper-IgE syndrome
- Metabolic deficiencies

—Carboxylase
—Prolidase deficiencies

 Data Gathering

HISTORY

- Age of onset
- Location
- Prior treatment
- Bathing habits
- Family history of atopy—allergies
- Asthma
- Eczema
- Hay fever

 Physical Examination

- Acute flares reveal weeping and crusted erythema.
- Chronic disease is characterized by hyperpigmentation or hypopigmentation, lichenification, and scaling.
- The distribution of the disease is dependent on age.

—During infancy to approximately 2 years of age, the disease is widespread and includes cheeks, forehead, scalp, and extensor surfaces.
—In children from approximately 3 to 11 years, the disease involves the more characteristic flexural sites with lichenification.
—The hands and face can also be involved.
—From adolescence to adulthood, the flexures, neck, hands, and feet are frequently involved, with the face and neck flaring occasionally.

- When the disease is severe, it can present as exfoliative erythroderma with diffuse scaling and erythema.
- Other associated findings include geographic tongue, Dennie-Morgan folds (infraorbital folds), pityriasis alba, (dry white patches), hyperlinear palms, facial pallor, infraorbital darkening, follicular accentuation, keratosis pilaris (dry, rough hair follicles on extensor surfaces of upper arms and thighs), and ichthyosis.

Special Questions

Excessive dryness exacerbates this disease; therefore, inquiry about bathing habits, frequency, and emollients is helpful.

 Laboratory Aids

- No tests are diagnostic of atopic dermatitis.
- Biopsy can be helpful to rule out papulosquamous disease, such as psoriasis.
- IgE levels are often elevated. Cultures can help identify superinfection during acute flares and viral cultures, and Tzanck smear can identify complications of eczema herpeticum.
- Patch testing can help differentiate atopic dermatitis from contact dermatitis.

Atopic Dermatitis

 Therapy

- There is no cure for atopic dermatitis.
- Parents must understand that this is a chronic disease with intermittent flares and that control is the aim of treatment.
- Good skin care is critical to maintenance and includes use of mild soaps, frequent use of emollients, and avoidance of excessive bathing.
- Avoidance of irritants from the environment, such as wool sweaters or blankets, is recommended. Protective clothing at night to avoid scratching while sleeping is also helpful, as is trimming the nails.
- Antihistamines such as hydroxyzine or diphenhydramine may help to decrease itching.
- Topical steroids control inflammation and mid- to high-potency steroids can be used during acute flares, with tapering of steroids to milder potency when control is achieved. Once cleared, topical steroids can be held and substituted with emollients. Long-term use of steroids can lead to atrophy, telangiectasias, tachyphylaxis, and occasionally, stunting of growth.
- Oral antibiotics are indicated when there is superinfection of lesions.
- Tacrolimus ointment and pimecrolimus cream are topical therapies recently approved for use in children 2 years of age and older. It is a calcineurin phosphatase inhibitor that acts to suppress T-cell function. Since tacrolimus ointment is not a steroid, it is not atrophogenic and does not appear to alter hypothalamic-pituitary axis function. However, little is known regarding its long-term effects in children. Children who receive this medication should receive instructions for diligent sun protection and sunscreen use to minimize potentiation for sun damage.
- Antivirals are needed for cases of eczema herpeticum. During acute flares with oozing and crusting and when there is superinfection with bacteria or herpes simplex virus, compresses can be helpful.
- Systemic steroids are generally not used because of the chronicity of atopic dermatitis, and are reserved for when control of the eruption is very difficult, and then use should be of short duration.
- Phototherapy with ultraviolet B can be used in patients with extensive disease resistant to other therapy.

 Follow-Up

It should be emphasized to the parents that atopic dermatitis is a chronic disease and that good skin care is necessary to control disease activity. Up to 40% to 50% of children will outgrow their atopic dermatitis after the age of 5 years.

 Common Questions and Answers

Q: Will the child outgrow this?
A: Up to 40% to 50% of children will outgrow their atopic dermatitis after the age of 5 years. In some patients, however, the disease will persist to variable extents throughout adulthood.

Q: When atopic dermatitis is controlled, is any treatment necessary?
A: Excessive dryness can exacerbate or flare disease; therefore, less use of soaps and frequent use of emollients are recommended.

Q: Do food hypersensitivities play a role in atopic dermatitis?
A: This is a debated issue. In general, the majority of patients are probably not adversely affected by foods. However, some individuals, particularly those unresponsive to routine therapy, may benefit from screening for food hypersensitivity and a trial of avoidance to any foods that test positive. The most common foods associated with exacerbation when an association can be made are eggs, milk, wheat, soy, peanuts, and fish.

ICD-9-CM 691.8

BIBLIOGRAPHY

Boguniewicz M. Advances in the understanding and treatment of atopic dermatitis. *Curr Opin Pediatr* 1997;9(6):577–581.

Bondi EE, Jegasothy BV, Lazarus GS. *Dermatology diagnosis and therapy*. Norwalk, CT: Appleton & Lange, 1991.

Burks AW, James JM, Hiegel A, et al. Atopic dermatitis and food hypersensitivity reactions. *J Pediatr* 1998;132(1):132–136.

Fitzpatrick TB, Eisen AZ, Wolfe K, et al. *Dermatology in general medicine*, 4th ed. New York: McGraw-Hill, 1993:1543–1564.

Hill DJ, Hosking CS. Emerging disease profiles in infants and young children with food allergy. *Pediatr Allergy Immunol* 1997; 8(10 suppl):21–26.

Lever WF, Schaumberg-Lever G. *Histopathology of the skin*, 7th ed. Philadelphia: Lippincott, 1990.

Oakes RC, Cox AD, Burgdorf WH. Atopic dermatitis: a review of diagnosis, pathogenesis, and management. *Clin Pediatr* 1983;22(7):467–475.

Author: Albert C. Yan
Christen Mowad, 2nd edition

Atrial Septal Defect

 Database

DEFINITION

An opening in the atrial septum, other than a patent foramen ovale (PFO).

- Four major types of atrial septal defects (ASDs):

—Secundum ASD
—Primum ASD
—Sinus venosus ASD.
—Coronary sinus ASD

- A PFO usually does not cause a significant intracardiac shunt. A probe patent PFO can be found in up to 25% of normal hearts at pathologic examination.
- Secundum defects make up 60–70% of all ASDs; usually there is a shunt from the left atrium to the right atrium.
- Primum defects occur in about 30% of all ASDs. They are usually associated with a cleft mitral valve. This defect is the result of an abnormality of the endocardial cushions, and therefore is also referred to as an incomplete AV canal defect.
- Sinus venosus defects can be of the superior or inferior venal caval type and occur in about 5–10% of all ASDs. In ASDs of the superior venal caval type, the right pulmonary veins (usually right upper lobe) may drain anomalously.
- Coronary sinus ASDs are rare and occur in <1% of all ASDs. They are often associated with absence of the coronary sinus and a persistent left SVC that joins the roof of the left atrium (also known as an "unroofed coronary sinus").

PREVALENCE

The incidence of ASD is difficult to determine. It occurs in 6–10% of all cardiac anomalies encountered and is seen more frequently in females than males (2:1).

ASSOCIATED LESIONS

An ASD may be associated with partial or total anomalous pulmonary venous drainage, mitral valve anomalies, transposition of the great arteries or tricuspid atresia. Although usually spontaneous, ASDs may occur as part of a syndrome [Holt-Oram (autosomal dominant)].

PATHOPHYSIOLOGY

A left-to-right shunt occurs through the ASD. For large defects this results in right atrial and right ventricular (RV) volume overload. There is usually increased pulmonary blood flow. The left-to-right shunt generally increases with time as pulmonary resistance drops and RV compliance normalizes. Moderate and large defects are associated with a Qp/Qs ratio of more than 2:1. The direction of atrial shunting is determined by the relative compliance of the RV and LV.

PROGNOSIS

- The prognosis of small ASDs seems excellent without specific therapy.
- Spontaneous closure of some small secundum ASDs can occur in up to 80% of infants in the first year of life. Isolated secundum ASDs of moderate and large size do not typically cause symptoms in most infants and children.
- Pulmonary hypertension is rare in childhood.
- Atrial flutter and fibrillation present in up to 13% of unoperated patients over 40 years of age.
- Bacterial endocarditis is rare in children with isolated ASD.
- Paradoxical emboli may occur, and should be considered in patients with cerebral or systemic emboli.

 Differential Diagnosis

- Ventricular septal defect
- Patent ductus arteriosus
- AV canal defect
- Valvar pulmonary stenosis

 Data Gathering

HISTORY

- Most infants are asymptomatic.
- Older children with moderate left-to-right shunts are often asymptomatic, but may have mild fatigue or dyspnea.
- Children with large left-to-right shunts may complain of fatigue and dyspnea, which may become noticeable when the child gets older.
- Growth failure is uncommon. Older patients with large atrial shunts may develop atrial arrhythmias.

 Physical Examination

- Inspection and palpation of the precordium are usually normal.
- Older children with a large shunt may have a hyperdynamic precordium and RV heave.
- Auscultation reveals three important features:

—Wide and "fixed" splitting of S_2; splitting of S_2 (A_2 and P_2 components) is caused by delay in emptying of a volume loaded right ventricle.
—A systolic ejection murmur at the upper left sternal border; murmur is caused by increase in blood flow across a normal pulmonary valve. It may be differentiated from the murmur of pulmonary stenosis because there is no click.
—A diastolic murmur at the lower sternal border, indicating a Qp/Qs ratio of at least 2:1. This murmur is caused by increased flow across the tricuspid valve.

Laboratory Aids

ECG

Usually normal sinus rhythm with an rSR' (incomplete right bundle branch block pattern) in lead V1, indicating RV volume overload. First-degree AV block may be present. For larger shunts ECG may have evidence of right atrial enlargement. A late finding suggestive of pulmonary hypertension is right ventricular hypertrophy.

CXR

Cardiomegaly, increased pulmonary vascular markings, and a dilated pulmonary trunk are seen in patients with significant left-to-right shunts.

ECHO

A two-dimensional echo study is diagnostic; it reveals the location, size, and associated defect, if any. It may demonstrate dilated right-heart structures. Color Doppler generally permits visualization of the direction of shunt flow. Older children and adolescents may require transesophageal echo to best define the ASD.

CARDIAC CATHETERIZATION

Generally unnecessary; it is indicated when pulmonary vascular disease is suspected (determination of pulmonary vascular resistance) or for associated cardiac defects.

 ## Therapy

Infants with congestive heart failure should be treated with digoxin and diuretics. Elective surgical repair is indicated for ASDs associated with large left-to-right shunts, cardiomegaly, or symptoms. Other indications may include: prevention of paradoxical emboli and cerebrovascular accidents or refractory supraventricular arrhythmias. High PVR (i.e., >8 Wu/M^2) increases the morbidity and may worsen the prognosis. Sinus venosus and ostium primum defects require elective surgery regardless of the defect size. The timing of the repair is usually deferred until 3 to 4 years of age. The mortality of surgical repair for an uncomplicated ASD approaches 0%. For some secundum ASDs, device closure of the defect can be done in the cardiac catheterization laboratory.

 ## Follow-Up

• Children with typical auscultation and ECG findings should undergo an echocardiographic evaluation to determine the location and size of the ASD.
• Children with ASDs should have regular follow-up to assess for signs of congestive heart failure or RV volume overload. Restriction on activity is unnecessary. SBE prophylaxis is not indicated in isolated secundum ASDs. Residual ASD after surgery is rare.
• SBE prophylaxis is indicated for the first 6 months (assuming no residual defect) after closure of a secundum defect.
• Complications related to surgery include:

—Sinus node dysfunction
—Venous obstruction (facial or pulmonary edema) may occur after a sinus venous ASD repair.
—Postpericardiotomy syndrome, which manifests with nausea, vomiting, abdominal pain or fever, may occur a few weeks after surgical repair. Although a friction rub may not be present, CXR may demonstrate cardiomegaly, and echo may reveal a pericardial effusion.

 ## Common Questions and Answers

Q: When should a moderate secundum ASD be closed?
A: This can generally be performed in children prior to their starting grade school.

Q: What is the significance of a patient having gastrointestinal complaints (nausea and vomiting) 2–3 weeks after surgical closure of an ASD?
A: This may represent a pericardial effusion (postpericardotomy syndrome).

ICD-9-CM 745.61

BIBLIOGRAPHY

Chang AC, Hanley FL, Wernovsky G, et al. *Pediatric cardiac intensive care.* Baltimore: Williams & Wilkins, 1998:207–211.

Emanouilides G, Allen H, Reimenschneider T, et al. *Heart disease in infants, children and adolescents,* 5th ed. Baltimore: Williams & Wilkins, 1995:687–703.

Garson A, Bricker J, McNamara D. *The science and practice of pediatric cardiology.* Philadelphia: Lea & Febiger, 1990:1023–1036.

Radzik D, Davignon A, van Doesburg N, et al. Predictive factors for spontaneous closure of atrial septal defect diagnosed in the first 3 months of life. *J Am Coll Cardiol* 1993;22:851–853.

Author: Jonathan Fleenor
Song-Gui Yang, 2nd edition

Attention-Deficit Hyperactivity Disorder

 Database

DEFINITION

Attention-deficit hyperactivity disorder (ADHD) is a syndrome characterized by persistent and developmentally inappropriate levels of inattention and/or hyperactivity and impulsivity. It can be classified into three subtypes—hyperactive/impulsive, inattentive, or combined.

GENETICS

- Risk of ADHD in first-degree relatives is approximately 25%.
- Concordance in monozygotic twins: 59% to 81%; dizygotic twins: 33%

EPIDEMIOLOGY

- Affects 3% to 10% of school-aged children
- Male/female ratio of 4:1. Females are more likely to have inattentive type.
- Prevalence in adults is less well studied, but estimated at 1% to 2%.

COMPLICATIONS

- School failure (33% kept back a grade before reaching high school)
- Learning disabilities (30%)
- Poor peer relationships
- Sleep problems (over 50%)
- Poor fine-motor skills
- Increased risk of accidental injury and motor vehicle accidents
- Adolescent risk-taking behavior (sexual promiscuity, tobacco, and illicit drug use)
- Additional psychiatric diagnosis (over 50%, depression, anxiety, other)

PROGNOSIS

- Many individuals with ADHD are quite successful. As a group, however, individuals with ADHD tend to complete fewer years of school and have lower occupational status.
- Children with ADHD and aggressive or antisocial behaviors are at relatively high risk for continuing to demonstrate these behaviors as adults. Thus, these children will usually need to be referred for intensive treatment, including pharmacotherapy, counseling, academic interventions, and family therapy.
- Good prognostic factors include positive parental and peer relationships, higher IQ and socioeconomic status, and possibly early multimodal treatment.

 Differential Diagnosis

- Medical: seizures (absence), sleep disorder, sensory impairment (vision, hearing), thyroid disorder, medication side effects, nutritional disorders, neurodegenerative disorders (early in course)
- Developmental: mental retardation, pervasive developmental disorders (autism)
- Educational: learning disabilities, inappropriate school environment
- Psychiatric: depression, mania, anxiety disorders, obsessive-compulsive disorder, oppositional defiant disorder, conduct disorder
- Family: disorganized/chaotic family environment, psychosocial stressors

 Data Gathering

HISTORY

- A detailed history of the child's behavior at home, school, and with peers is needed. Inquire about frequency, duration, and intensity of the behaviors.
- Symptoms of ADHD usually present prior to age 7 years.
- Obtain medical, developmental, academic, family, and social history, focusing on the complications and differential diagnosis. Behavior that changes with the environment suggests that other diagnoses should be considered. Multiple visits and/or a multidisciplinary team approach are often necessary.
- Specific questions include: see also DSM-IV (APA, 1994)
—Does the child fail to pay close attention to detail or make careless mistakes?
—Does the child have difficulty finishing work or chores?
—Does the child squirm, fidget, or act excessively active?
—Does the child lose or forget things needed for homework or other tasks?
—Does the child interrupt work, games, or conversations?
—Does the child have difficulty waiting his/her turn?

 Physical Examination

- Children with ADHD have "soft" neurologic signs such as overflow movements, choreiform movements and finger gnosis. However, these signs are not specific.
- The remainder of physical and neurologic examination is usually normal.
- To rule out other diagnoses the following should be conducted: mental status examination, hearing and vision tests, examination of the skin for neurocutaneous syndromes and developmental testing with IQ and academic screening.

 Laboratory Aids

RATING SCALES

- There are many rating scales to assess ADHD (see Mercugliano et al., 1998).
- Parent and teacher ratings are routine components of the assessment.
- Significant discrepancy between parent and teacher ratings suggests more information is needed.
- Scales designed specifically to assess attention, activity, and impulsivity, tend to be the most sensitive in detecting ADHD.
- Scales designed to assess more than just ADHD symptoms may be helpful in detecting co-occurring conditions.

OTHER TESTS

- Laboratory tests are usually not needed. Psychoeducational testing can be very helpful in identifying learning difficulties. Computerized continuous performance tasks are sometimes used, but scores on these tests are not sensitive in detecting ADHD.

 Therapy

NONPHARMACOLOGIC

- See Mercugliano et al., 1998, for an in-depth discussion.
- Behavioral counseling and educational interventions are important components of treatment.
- Information on resources and support groups for parents should be provided.
- Alternative therapies such as diet modifications may have a beneficial effect in a small percentage of children.

MEDICAL MANAGEMENT

- Results from a national multisite study showed medication management is the most effective intervention for controlling core ADHD symptoms of inattention, hyperactivity, and impulsivity.
- Treatment with medication should be considered when target symptoms are severe enough to impair function.
- Stimulant medications (methylphenidate, dextroamphetamine) are first-line treatment for ADHD symptoms.
- A trial of multiple doses is helpful to determine the optimum dose for an individual.
- Somatic complaints are common in children with ADHD and should be inquired about before medication is started.

Methylphenidate (Ritalin, Metadate, Concerta)

• Efficacy: Eighty percent of children with ADHD improve significantly. Individual response is highly variable. Teacher rating scales are helpful in documenting positive response to the medication.
• Pharmacokinetics: Onset, 20 to 30 minutes. Duration, 3 to 4 hours. Three times per day (TID) dosing is often superior to two times per day (BID) dosing. Longer acting forms (Metadate, Concerta) are available and helpful for children who dislike taking medication in school.
• Dose: 0.3 to 0.6 mg/kg per dose titrated for effect. Higher doses may be needed in some patients.
• Common side effects: appetite suppression, insomnia, stomachaches, headaches
• Less common side effects: rebound (increased activity or moodiness as medication wears off), dizziness, growth suppression (at high doses), dysphoria , tics (5–10%), Tourette syndrome (1%; medication may unmask underlying disorder); excessive dose may result in tired or withdrawn appearance.
• Rare side effects: thrombocytopenia, neutropenia, eosinophilia
• Interactions: may inhibit metabolism of anticonvulsants, coumadin, tricyclic antidepressants.
• Should not be used with MAO inhibitors. Other sympathomimetic medications (e.g., ephedrine, pseudoephedrine) may increase side effects. Antihistamines may decrease efficacy.

Dextroamphetamine (Dexedrine, Adderall)

Effects and side effects are similar to those of methylphenidate. Start at 2.5–5.0 mg/d. Usual dose range, 0.15 to 0.3 mg/kg per dose. Unusual to exceed 30 mg/d. Adderall and Dexedrine spansule capsules are long acting (5 to 8 hours).

Pemoline (Cylert)

Onset, 1 to 2 hours. Plasma half-life, 5 to 6 hours. Usual dose, 1 to 3 mg/kg/d. Liver function tests need to be monitored. Liver failure resulting in death or liver transplantation has occurred.

α-Adrenergic Agonists

• Clonidine (Catapress), Guanfacine (Tenex)
• Indications
—Nonresponders to stimulants: ADHD with significant hyperactivity or aggression. ADHD with tics or Tourette syndrome.
• Side effects: sedation (very common), rebound hypertension if medications are stopped suddenly, decreased blood pressure (dizziness), depression

Tricyclic Antidepressants

• Imipramine (Tofranil), nortriptyline (Pamelor), desipramine (Norpramin)
• Indications
—Nonresponders to stimulants: ADHD with tics or Tourette syndrome; ADHD with anxiety or mood disorders
• Side effects: anticholinergic effects, cardiac arrhythmias (must monitor ECGs), fatigue
• Warn families that overdoses can be fatal.

Atypical Antidepressants

• Bupropion (Wellbutrin)
• Indications
—Nonresponders to stimulants: ADHD with anxiety or mood disorders
• Side effects: irritability, insomnia; limited experience in children, but in adults drug-induced seizures can occur, especially at high doses.
• Venlafaxine (Effexor)
• Indications
—Nonresponders to stimulants: ADHD with coexisting anxiety, mood or obsessive-compulsive disorders
• Side effects: irritability/insomnia, nausea/weight loss, sexual dysfunction

 ## Follow-Up

• Evidence for improved efficacy with close follow-up.
• Assess family and peer relationships.
• Assess school performance.
• Check for associated behavioral and psychiatric problems.
• Check for medication side effects.
• Assess continuing need for medication yearly.

PITFALLS
• Insufficient time for thorough evaluation
• Lack of information on symptoms from both school and home
• Missing associated learning problems and/or psychiatric disorders
• Not using high enough or frequent enough a dose, especially for shorter acting medications
• Individual response to stimulant medication is idiosyncratic. Higher doses do not always result in improvement in symptoms.

 ## Common Questions and Answers

Q: At what age can you begin to make the diagnosis of ADHD?
A: No lower limit has been identified. There is a wide range of normal activity levels and attention spans in preschool-aged children that may improve with time. Be cautious about making the diagnosis in children under the age of 4 years. Developmental disorders such as developmental delays and autistic spectrum disorders need to be ruled out.

Q: Should stimulant medication be prescribed on weekends and over the summer?
A: Evaluate the risk vs. benefit. Children engaged in school-like or school-related tasks during the summer or on weekends may need to be on medication for these activities. Family and peer relationships of some children with ADHD benefit from medication use during these times. However, periods off medication may minimize the long-term effects on weight and growth.

Q: Can methylphenidate be used to treat ADHD in children with tics or Tourette syndrome?
A: Methylphenidate will cause an exacerbation of tics in some children with chronic tic disorder or Tourette syndrome. However, many children will not experience any significant change in tic frequency on methylphenidate.

Q: Can methylphenidate be used to treat ADHD in children with seizures?
A: Although the *Physicians' Desk Reference* states that methylphenidate lowers the seizure threshold, the medication can be used in children with well-controlled seizure disorders.

Q: Why is my child's medication no longer working?
A: If a recent growth spurt or change in metabolism is suspected, consider a trial of varying medication dosages. After initial success in controlling symptoms with behavioral management, it is common to slowly revert to old negative patterns of behavior. Change in environment, new psychosocial stressors, change in health, and emerging learning disabilities with increasing academic demands can all play a role.

ICD-9-CM 314.01

BIBLIOGRAPHY

American Academy of Pediatrics. Clinical practice guideline: diagnosis and evaluation of the child with attention-deficit/hyperactivity disorder. *Pediatrics* 2000;105(5):1158–1170.

Barkley RA. *Taking charge of ADHD: the complete authoritative guide for parents*, revised ed. New York: Guilford, 2000.

Jensen PS, Hinshaw SP, Swanson JM, et al. Findings from the NIMH multimodal treatment study of ADHD (MTA): implications and applications for primary care providers. *Dev Behav Pediatr* 2001;2(1):60–73.

Mercugliano M, Power TJ, Blum NJ. *The clinician's practical guide to attention-deficit/hyperactivity disorder*. Baltimore: Brookes, 1998.

Miller KJ, Castellanos FX. Attention deficit/hyperactivity disorders. *Pediatr Rev* 1998;19(11):373–384.

Authors: Shelly D. Holstrum and Nathan J. Blum

Atypical Mycobacterial Infections

 ## Database

DEFINITION

Atypical mycobacterial (ATM) infection refers to disease caused by *Mycobacterium* other than *tuberculosis, bovis,* and *leprae,* and usually involves *Mycobacterium avium-intracellulare* or *M. scrofulaceum.* These diseases are also referred to as nontuberculous mycobacterial infections, environmental mycobacterial infections, and mycobacteria other than tuberculosis (MOTT) infections.

CAUSES

- The most common associated illness is unilateral chronic cervical adenopathy/adenitis in preschool-aged children.
- In adults, ATM infection may cause a chronic single pulmonary nodule or more extensive chronic lung disease.
- In children and adults infected with HIV, disseminated disease is common, yet it is not common in other acquired or congenital immunodeficiencies that affect T-cell function.
- Rarely, it may cause otitis/mastoiditis in immunocompetent children.
- Chronic skin, bone, or soft tissue infections may develop after trauma/surgery, usually with *M. chelonei* or *M. fortuitum* as the etiologic agents.
- Infections of indwelling central venous catheters appear to be on the increase.

PATHOPHYSIOLOGY

- Organisms are ubiquitous in the environment: soil, fresh water, ocean water, home and hospital water, dust, and food (eggs, dairy products, meat).
- It is spread by aerosol inhalation or ingestion of contaminated food, dust, or water.
- Person-to-person spread has never been documented and is not a concern.

EPIDEMIOLOGY

- 80% to 90% of cases of adenitis caused by ATM infection occur in preschool-aged children (ages 1–5 years).
- Early in the HIV epidemic, the incidence rate of disseminated disease in HIV-infected adults was approximately 40%; in HIV-infected children, 10% to 20%. This rate has decreased markedly in recent years through the routine use of prophylaxis and because of the improved immunologic function in HIV-infected individuals on newer antiretroviral agents.

COMPLICATIONS

- Chronic draining of infected cervical nodes
- Rarely, pulmonary disease or dissemination
- Chronic skin/bone infections
- Disseminated disease

PROGNOSIS

- For localized adenopathy: excellent
- For disseminated disease, generally treatable in the rare immunocompetent individual
- In patients with AIDS, treatable in terms of symptom relief, but requires lifelong therapy

 ## Differential Diagnosis

- For unilateral adenopathy/adenitis:

—Viral/bacterial adenitis-affected nodes are tender, warm, and erythematous; usually associated with upper respiratory symptoms and/or fever.
—Cat-scratch disease (contact with cat, usually kitten). Frequently, child will have scratch/puncture mark on arm. There are rarely any systemic signs/symptoms.

- Neoplastic disease

 ## Data Gathering

HISTORY

- Region of residence
- Recent travel
- Length of time of adenopathy, associated systemic symptoms
- Contact with cats (for differential of cat-scratch disease or toxoplasmosis)
- Systemic symptoms, such as fever and weight loss, make neoplastic disease more likely.
- Chronic cough would suggest *M. tuberculosis.*
- Recent upper respiratory symptoms/fever suggest viral or bacterial cause.

Physical Examination

- Most common: single or regional cervical adenopathy, 90% of the time, is unilateral, firm, not fixed, and not especially tender nor warm; occasionally, there is spontaneous drainage.
- Generalized adenopathy makes ATM disease unlikely.
- Systemic signs of infection are absent.
- Hepatosplenomegaly indicates other diagnosis, especially neoplastic disease or HIV-related illness.
- Normal nutritional status

Laboratory Aids

- Specific PPD tests are not readily available at this time. Many children with ATM adenitis will have 5- to 10-mm reactions to standard PPD.
- Definitive diagnosis is made by isolation and identification of organism. The most frequently identified strains are: *M. avium-intracellulare, M. kansasii, M. chelonei, M. fortuitum,* and *M. scrofulaceum.*
- Normal chest radiograph
- In disseminated disease, cultures are positive from blood and bone marrow aspirates.

Therapy

- Complete surgical excision for isolated adenopathy secondary to ATM; chemotherapy unnecessary in most cases.
- For disseminated or pulmonary disease, or when complete surgical excision of an infected node is not possible, three- or four-drug treatment regimens based on sensitivity. Combinations generally include several of the following antibiotics: rifabutin, clarithromycin or azithromycin, ethambutol, ciprofloxacin, and amikacin.

PREVENTION

For HIV-infected children with severe immunodeficiency, prophylaxis with daily clarithromycin or rifabutin, or once-weekly azithromycin, decreases the risk of development of disseminated disease.

Follow-Up

Routine follow-up should be done for 1 year after excision to monitor for possible local/contralateral recurrence.

PITFALLS

Use of incision and drainage/aspiration for treatment of adenitis, which can lead to chronically draining node. Aspiration may be needed to make the original diagnosis, but total excision results in almost 100% cure rates.

Common Questions and Answers

Q: Should all cases of cervical adenitis be tested for ATM?
A: The typical case of cervical adenitis, presenting with the usual prodrome, responds rapidly to appropriate oral or parenteral antibiotics, which would not be the case if ATM were the culprit. Certainly, a PPD test should be done on all children with cervical adenitis. If the node is aspirated, in addition to routine bacterial cultures, fluid should be sent for mycobacterial culture. In addition, testing for cat-scratch disease should be part of the evaluation of all cases of cervical adenitis.

Q: Should patients with disease secondary to ATM undergo a chest x-ray study?
A: Yes. Though uncommon, ATM-related pulmonary disease can be seen in children.

Q: If the node is excised, should oral therapy be instituted?
A: Most studies suggest that oral therapy is unnecessary following total excision.

ICD-9-CM 031.9

BIBLIOGRAPHY

Hazra R, Robsin CD, Perez-Atayde AR, et al. Lymphadenitis due to nontuberculous mycobacteria in children: presentation and response to therapy. *Clin Infect Dis* 1999;28:123–129.

Schaad UB, Votteler TP, McCracken GH, et al. Management of atypical mycobacterial lymphadenitis in childhood: a review based on 380 cases. *J Pediatr* 1979;95:356–360.

Smith MHD, Starke JR, Marquis JR. Tuberculosis and opportunistic mycobacterial infections. In: Feigin R, Cherry J, eds. *Pediatric infectious diseases*, 3rd ed. Philadelphia: WB Saunders, 1992:1354–1356.

Starke JR. Management of nontuberculous mycobacterial cervical adenitis. *Pediatr Infect Dis J* 2000;19:674–675.

Taha AM, Davidson PT, Bailey WC. Surgical treatment of atypical mycobacterial lymphadenitis in children. *Pediatr Infect Dis J* 1985;4:664–667.

Author: Richard M. Rutstein

Autism/Pervasive Developmental Disorder Spectrum

 Database

DEFINITION

Autism and pervasive developmental disorders (PDD) are neuropsychiatric syndromes characterized by:

- Delays and impairments in development of social, communicative, and play/behavioral skills.
- Onset in the first years of life.
- Frequent association with mental retardation.
- Increased risk of seizure disorder.

Autism and PDD are a spectrum of related disorders. Pervasive developmental disorders include: PDD–NOS (subthreshold autism), Asperger disorder (restricted range of interest/activities, normal language and cognitive abilities), childhood disintegrative disorder (developmental deterioration after 24 months), and Rett syndrome (females, hand-washing/hand-wringing movements, head growth deceleration before 48 months). Autistic disorder implies onset of symptoms prior to age 3, with impairments seen in social relatedness, communication, and play and restricted interests/activities.

EPIDEMIOLOGY

PDD-NOS: 5 cases per 1000 children. Prevalence of autism is 1 per 1000 children.

- 3–4 times more common in males than females.
- Females with autism tend to be more severely mental retarded than males.
- In population-based samples of autistic disorder:

—50% of cases exhibit severe to profound mental retardation.
—30% of cases have mild to moderate mental retardation.
—20% of cases have normal cognitive abilities.

Asperger Disorder

- Much more common in boys than girls.
- Estimates for prevalence range from 2–4 cases per 1000

Rett Disorder

- Prevalence estimated as 0.83 per 1000 female births

Childhood Disintegrative Disorder

- Occurs predominately in males.
- As of 1999 there were 106 cases reported.
- Prevalence of this disorder is 0.011 per 1000.

ETIOLOGY

No single cause for autism identified. May be multiple etiologies leading to expression of the same syndrome. Twin genetic studies strongly implicated role of genetic factors in pathogenesis of autism. Siblings of proband at higher risk. Monozygotic twins consistently have higher concordance rate than dizygotic twins. Approximately 1 in 100 persons with autism exhibits fragile X anomaly. Rate of autism in tuberous sclerosis is also elevated.

Disorders found in association with PDD spectrum disorders include:

- Prenatal: toxemia, rubella, cytomegalovirus, toxoplasmosis
- Perinatal: anoxia, trauma, hyperbilirubinemia
- Chromosomal: Angelman syndrome, Prader-Willi syndrome, fragile X syndrome, trisomy 21, XYY syndrome, tuberous sclerosis
- Metabolic: phenylketonuria, hyperthyroidism, lead ingestion, histidinemia, lipidosis
- Congenital: microcephaly, hydrocephalus, Dandy-Walker syndrome
- Acquired: infantile spasms, meningitis, encephalitis

CLINICAL PRESENTING SIGNS AND SYMPTOMS

- Delays or impairments in development of language
- Marked inability to initiate and sustain conversation with others (when speech is present)
- Cognitive delays
- Impairment in eye contact, facial expression and other nonverbal social behaviors
- Lack of interest in or impairments in social interactions
- Failure to develop developmentally appropriate peer relationships
- Stereotypies (e.g., rocking, hand flapping)
- Preoccupation with a restricted range of interests
- Attachment to unusual objects and fascination with parts of objects
- Rigid adherence to routine and distress with changes in routine
- Lack of spontaneous imaginary play appropriate to developmental level

Rett Disorder features severe mental retardation, scoliosis, breathing problems, seizures, and motor problems.

 Differential Diagnosis

Differential diagnoses of autistic symptoms include:

- **Mental retardation**—Differs from PDD spectrum disorders in that communication, behavior, play, and social skills are appropriate for developmental age.
- **Deafness**—May present with delayed or absent oral language acquisition. Behavioral difficulties and social skill deficits related to delays in language acquisition
- **Mixed Receptive-Expressive Language Disorder**—Language impairment is not associated with qualitative deficits in social interactions or with restrictive, repetitive, patterns of interests and activities.
- **Selective mutism**—The child has developmentally appropriate communication in some social situations and does not exhibit qualitative impairments in social interactions or restrictive, repetitive, patterns of interests and activities.

 Data Gathering

HISTORY

- Complete developmental history including: prenatal, neonatal, medical, family and childhood history essential in accurate diagnosis.
- Diagnosis based on a history of impaired verbal/nonverbal communication, impaired/delayed social skills, and restrictive/repetitive range of behaviors.
- History may indicate presence of stereotyped behavior, behavioral rigidity, and tactile defensiveness.
- History of incoordination, symptoms suggesting epilepsy and poor appetite and sleep frequently present
- Gather history regarding possible comorbid symptoms of: attention problems, OCD traits, tics, anxiety symptoms, mood instability, sleep problems, aggression, and self-injury.

 Physical Examination

- Examine growth curves for possible secondary growth disturbance due to rigid/restrictive eating behavior.
- Evaluate for signs of self-injurious behavior
- Physical findings may suggest alternate (metabolic) disorders or the underlying basis of autism:

—Long, thin face and prominent ears are characteristic of fragile X, and macroorchidism may not be present until after puberty.

—Pigmented lesions may suggest neurocutaneous syndromes, especially hypopigmented macules or fibromas indicating tuberous sclerosis.
—Microcephaly suggests TORCH infection (toxoplasmosis, rubella, cytomegalovirus, herpes infection), Angelman syndrome or Rett syndrome.
—Macrocephaly suggests neurocutaneous disorder, storage disease, or hydrocephalus, or may have no clear underlying cause.
—Presence of spasticity, visual loss, or ataxia suggests leukodystrophy.
—Neurologic examination necessary for assessment of stereotypic behavior, involuntary movements, abnormalities in motor coordination and mirror or other overflow movements.
—Ophthalmologic and audiologic evaluations necessary to rule out visual and hearing deficits.

 Laboratory Aids

Neurodiagnostic tests may not be useful unless specific neurologic disorders are suspected. Routine neuroimaging is of limited diagnostic or practical value.

TESTS

• EEG

—Significance: 20% to 40% of autistic patients develop seizures.

• Chromosomes/fragile X studies

—Significance: appropriate for all autistic patients; helpful for genetic counseling.

• Inborn error screen

—Significance: to detect PKU, other amino acid disorders.

• Head MRI/CT

—Significance: evaluation of structural CNS if focal neurologic deficit or microcephaly/macrocephaly is present.

• TORCH (toxoplasmosis, rubella, cytomegalovirus, herpes virus) titers

—Significance: evaluation of microcephaly

• Complete blood count

—Significance: evaluation of growth delay and/or pica

• Blood lead level

—Significance: R/O lead intoxication.

• Thyroid function tests

—Significance: R/O hyper/hypothyroidism.

• Audiogram/BAER

—Significance: evaluation of speech and language delay, R/O hearing loss.

 Therapy

MEDICAL MANAGEMENT

Pharmacotherapy does not treat core symptoms of autism. Medication can help in treating comorbid symptoms that interfere with the patient's ability to function at his/her highest potential in educational/social activities:

• Self-injurious behavior: typical and atypical antipsychotics, naltrexone, clomipramine
• Sleep disturbances: melatonin, clonidine, Benadryl
• Seizures: barbiturates (may worsen hyperactivity), carbamazepine, phenytoin, valproate, others
• Hyperactivity /attention difficulties: psychostimulants, bupropion, venlafaxine, clonidine
• OCD symptoms/perseveration: SSRIs, clomipramine
• Tic disorders: guanfacine, clonidine, typical and atypical antipsychotics
• Depression: SSRIs, bupropion, venlafaxine
• Anxiety: SSRIs, buspirone, venlafaxine, benzodiazepines (may increase disorganization)
• Aggression: typical and atypical antipsychotics, SSRIs

EDUCATIONAL/PSYCHOSOCIAL/MEDICAL MANAGEMENT

• A complete psychoeducational assessment and treatment plan for intellectual, developmental, adaptive, functional, communication, and social skills is warranted.
• Early and sustained structured behavioral intervention using applied behavior analysis and behavior modification appears to be highly beneficial in many children with PDD and autism.
• Intensive educational and behavioral interventions should target acquisition of communicative, social, and cognitive skills.
• Vocational training important for some adolescents and adults with PDD and autism.
• Consider social skills training for higher functioning patients.
• Education and support for parents and siblings is integral to treatment.
• Psychotherapy not indicated to address core features of autism and PDD.

PITFALLS

• Autism and the PDD spectrum disorders vary greatly in symptom presentation.
• Symptom presentation often differs at different stages of development.
• Patient's with PDD and autism may be more likely to develop side effects to medication.
• Subclinical seizure types, including absence spells, may be detected only on EEG.

 Follow-Up

• Prognosis is closely linked to cognitive ability and acquisition of social and communication skills.
• If no language acquired by 6 years, language development is unlikely and probable outcome is poor.
• Children with autism or PDD often require lifelong treatment and support.

 Common Questions and Answers

Q: What are the chances of having a second child with autism?
A: In families with one child with autism the recurrence risk for subsequent children is 4.5%. This is in contrast to the risk in the general population, which is 0.1%.

Q: What is the value of brain imaging in autism?
A: MRI may help diagnose a heritable syndrome with genetic counseling implications (e.g., leukodystrophy, tuberous sclerosis), but is not recommended in all cases.

ICD-9-CM 299.0

BIBLIOGRAPHY

Cook EH. Genetics of autism. Child Adolesc Psychiatr Clin North Am 2001;10(2)333–350.

Edwards DR, Bristol MM. Autism: early identification and management in family practice. Am Fam Pract 1991;44(5): 1755–1764.

Filipek PA, et al. The screening and diagnosis of autistic spectrum disorders. J Autism Dev Disord 1999;29:439–484.

Piven J. The biological basis of autism. Curr Opin Neurobiol 1997;7(5):708–712.

Volkmar F., Cook EH Jr, Pomeroy J, Realmuto G, Tanguay P. Practice parameters—autism and pervasive developmental disorders. J Am Acad Child Adolesc Psychiatry 1999;38(12):32S–54S.

Wing L. The autism spectrum. Lancet 1997;350(9093):1761–1766.

Author: Jeanne Greenblatt

Autoimmune Hemolytic Anemia

 Database

DEFINITION

Autoimmune hemolytic anemia (AIHA) is characterized by shortened red-cell survival that is caused by autoantibodies directed against red blood cells, with or without the participation of complement on the red-cell membrane.

CAUSES
- Idiopathic
- Passive transfer of maternal antibodies
- Secondary to an underlying disorder
—Infection: viral [e.g., *Mycoplasma,* Epstein-Barr virus (EBV), cytomegalovirus (CMV), hepatitis, HIV] or bacterial (e.g., *Streptococcus,* typhoid fever, *Escherichia coli* septicemia)
—Drugs: antimalarials, antipyretics, sulfonamides, penicillin, rifampin
—Hematologic disorders: leukemia, lymphoma
—Immunopathic/autoimmune disorders: lupus, mixed connective tissue disorders, Wiskott-Aldrich syndrome, ulcerative colitis, rheumatoid arthritis, scleroderma
—Tumors: ovarian, carcinomas, thymomas, dermoid cysts

PATHOPHYSIOLOGY
- Warm autoantibodies
—Maximal activity of *in vitro* red-cell binding at 37°C
—IgG-class antibody sometimes with relative specificity for Rh erythrocyte antigens
—IgG-coated RBCs cleared—predominantly in the spleen by macrophages
—Complement not required for clearance, although complement fixation may contribute to clearance
- Cold autoantibodies (cold agglutinins)
—Maximal activity of *in vitro* red-cell binding at temperatures between 0°C and 30°C
—Almost always caused by IgM antibody with specificity for antigens of the I/T system on RBCs
—Anti-I antibodies characteristic of *Mycoplasma pneumoniae*-associated hemolysis
—Anti-I antibodies usually found in infectious mononucleosis
—IgM-coated RBCs are cleared primarily in the liver by hepatic macrophage C3b receptors.
—Hemolysis is complement-dependent.
- Paroxysmal cold hemoglobinuria (PCH)
—IgG autoantibody binds RBC at cooler areas of the body (i.e., extremities), causing irreversible binding of complement components (C3 and C4). When coated RBCs enter warmer areas of the body, IgG falls off and complement causes hemolysis (Donath-Landsteiner biphasic hemolysin).
—Unusual IgG antibody with anti-P specificity
—Most frequently found in children with viral infections (30%)

EPIDEMIOLOGY
- Occurs at an incidence of about 1:50,000 to 80,000 persons per year
- Less common in children and adolescents than in adults
- No apparent racial or sexual preponderance (in childhood)
- Peak incidence in childhood is in first 4 years of life with warm AIHA.
- Mortality in pediatric series ranged from 9% to 19%.

COMPLICATIONS
- Heart failure may be seen in severe anemia; requires aggressive supportive care.
- Morbidity is usually secondary to treatment (see Therapy section).

 Differential Diagnosis

- Defects intrinsic to RBC
—Membrane defects
—Enzyme defects
—Hemoglobin defects
—Congenital dyserythropoietic anemias
—Paroxysmal nocturnal hemoglobinuria
- Defects extrinsic to RBC
—Immune-mediated
—Isoimmune: hemolytic disease of the newborn, blood-group incompatibility
—Autoimmune: see in Database section, Causes
—Drug-dependent red-cell antibodies
—Nonimmune mediated
—Idiopathic
—Secondary to an underlying disorder [i.e., hemolytic uremic syndrome (HUS), thrombotic thrombocytopenic purpura (TTP)]
—Mechanical: march hemoglobinuria, heart valves

 Data Gathering

NATURAL HISTORY
- Acute disease
—Onset with rapid fall in hemoglobin level over hours to days
—Usual course: complete resolution of disease within 3 to 6 months
—Resolution more likely in children who present between 2 and 12 years of age
- Chronic disease
—Slower onset of anemia over weeks to months, with some having persistence of hemolysis or intermittent relapses
—More likely to be associated with underlying disorder
—More common in adults and children <2 years or >12 years of age

HISTORY
- Pallor
- Jaundice
- Dark urine
- Fever
- Weakness
- Dizziness
- Syncope
- Exercise intolerance

 Physical Examination

- Pallor
- Jaundice
- Splenomegaly
- Hepatomegaly
- Tachycardia, systolic flow murmur
- Orthostasis in acute onset

 Laboratory Aids

- CBC: Hb level decreased (occasionally, thrombocytopenia seen in Evans's syndrome); MCV may be normal
- Reticulocyte count increased
- Peripheral smear: spherocytes, polychromasia, macrocytes, rouleaux formation
- Direct antiglobulin test (Coombs): positive
—Single most important test
—Warm AIHA will have IgG ± C3 positive
—Cold AIHA and PCH will have C3 positive
- Haptoglobin level decreased
- Indirect hyperbilirubinemia
- Elevated LDH
- Urinalysis: hemoglobinuria, increased urobilinogen
- Bone marrow aspiration—erythroid hyperplasia (to rule out leukemia or lymphoma associated with AIHA)
- Cold agglutinin titer: positive (usually 1:64)
- Donath-Landsteiner test should be performed in cases of suspected PCH.

PITFALLS
A negative Coombs test can occur when small numbers of IgG or C3 molecules are present on the red-cell membrane (i.e., in cases of less severe hemolysis). Radiolabeled Coombs test or enzyme immunoassays are more sensitive diagnostic tests in these circumstances. Reticulocytopenia may occur in most severe cases where the antibody coats and removes reticulocytes.

Therapy

PATIENT MONITORING
- Hemoglobin level q4h to q12h (depending on severity)
- Reticulocyte count: daily
- Spleen size: daily
- Hemoglobinuria: daily
- Coombs test: weekly

BLOOD TRANSFUSION
- Indication
—Blood transfusion is indicated in cases of physiologic compromise from the anemia (usually only in severe acute onset) or with continued blood loss.
- Complications
—The blood bank may be unable to find compatible blood. In IgG-mediated disease, autoantibody is usually panreactive; therefore, you must use the least incompatible unit of blood. In cold agglutinin disease, you must prewarm all infusions to decrease IgM binding and must monitor for acute hemolysis during transfusion.
- Dose
—Use only a volume of blood sufficient to relieve compromise from anemia.

CORTICOSTEROIDS
- Indication
—In IgG-mediated disease, steroids have been shown to interfere with macrophage Fc and C3b receptors responsible for RBC destruction. They also have been shown to elute IgG Ab from the RBC surface (improving survival).
—In chronic warm AIHA, pulsed high-dose dexamethasone has been shown to be effective in some cases.
- Complications
—There are both short- and long-term side effects of steroids. Corticosteroids are generally not effective in cold agglutinin disease.
- Dose
—Start prednisone po/methylprednisolone IV at 2 mg/kg/d in divided doses. Tapering of steroids should begin once a therapeutic response is achieved (may take several weeks to months). Alternative treatments should be considered for patients unresponsive to steroids or who require high doses for maintenance of hemoglobin level.
- Goal
—The goal is initially to return to normal hemoglobin level with nontoxic levels of steroid, or no steroids. However, in some patients, the goal may be achieving decreased hemolysis and a clinically asymptomatic state with minimal steroid side effects.

INTRAVENOUS IMMUNE GLOBULIN (IVIG)
- Indication
—IVIG may be useful in selected cases of immune hemolytic anemia unresponsive to steroids. The mechanism of action is not entirely clear.
- Complications
—The effect is usually temporary; re-treatment may be required q3 to q4 weeks. There may be a risk of hepatitis C. IVIG is expensive.
- Dose
—Up to 1 g/kg/d for 5 days has been required to achieve a beneficial effect.

PLASMAPHERESIS/EXCHANGE TRANSFUSION
- Indication
—This treatment will slow the rate of hemolysis in severe disease.
—Indicated for AIHA associated with TTP
- Complications
—It is only of short-term benefit and is expensive.
- Dose
—The frequency and duration depend on response.

SPLENECTOMY
- Indication
—Patients unresponsive to medical management, who require moderate to high maintenance doses of steroids or who develop steroid intolerance may be candidates for splenectomy. It is not effective in cold agglutinin disease.
- The response rate is about 50% to 70%, with the majority only partial remissions.
- Complications
—There is a high morbidity rate for the surgical procedure and during the postoperative period.
—There is an increased risk of sepsis.

IMMUNOSUPPRESSIVE AGENTS (ANTIMETABOLITES & ALKYLATING AGENTS)
- Indication
—When there is a clinically unacceptable degree of hemolysis that is refractory to steroids and splenectomy, immunosuppressive agents are indicated. Some have been effective in cold agglutinin disease.
- Complications
—There are varying side effects dependent on the agent used. Therefore, clinical indications must be strong and exposure to drug should be limited.
- Dose
—Adjusted to maintain WBC >2,000, ANC >1,000, and platelet count at 50,000 to 100,000 cells/mm^3

PROGNOSIS
Dependent on age, underlying disorder (if any), and response to therapy. See also in Data Gathering section, Natural History.

Common Questions and Answers

Q: Will the anemia go away?
A: Children with cold autoantibodies tend to have short-lived illness, whereas children with warm antibodies often have a chronic clinical course characterized by periods of remissions and relapses.

Q: Is this contagious?
A: No. Another child may acquire the same viral illness; however, the body's response to produce an autoantibody is dependent on the individual patient.

ICD-9-CM 283.0

BIBLIOGRAPHY
Domen RE. An overview of immune hemolytic anemia. *Cleve Clin J Med* 1998;65(2):89–99.

Engelfriet CP, Overbeeke MAM, Kr. von dem Borne AEG. Autoimmune hemolytic anemia. *Semin Hematol* 1992;29(1):3–12.

Lanzkowsky P. Hemolytic anemia. In: Lanzkowsky P, ed. *Manual of pediatric hematology and oncology*. New York: Churchill Livingstone, 2000:137–199.

Meyer O, Stahl D, Beckhove P, et al. Pulsed high-dose dexamethasone in chronic autoimmune hemolytic anemia. *Br J Haematol* 1997;98(4):860–862.

Ware RE, Rosse WF. Autoimmune hemolytic anemia. In: Nathan DG, Oski FA, eds. *Hematology of infancy and childhood*, 5th ed. Philadelphia: WB Saunders, 1998:499–522.

Ware RE. Autoimmune hemolytic and thrombocytopenic disease in the adolescent patient. *Adolesc Med* 1999;10(3):377–384.

Author: Tammy I. Kang
Deborah L. Kramer, 2nd edition

Avascular (Aseptic) Necrosis of the Femoral Head (Hip)

 Database

DEFINITION

Avascular (aseptic) necrosis (AVN) results from the interruption of the blood supply of bone (either traumatic or nontraumatic occlusion). The femoral head is the most common site of AVN. When idiopathic AVN of the hip occurs in children, this is known as Perthes disease (See Perthes Disease)

CAUSES

- Traumatic

—After fracture
—After hip dislocation
—After slipped capital femoral epiphysis
—After casting, bracing, surgery

- Nontraumatic

—Idiopathic (older, after physeal closure); similar to adult AVN
—Idiopathic (younger, before physeal closure, Perthes disease)
—Caisson disease
—With sickle cell disease
—After septic arthritis
—With steroids or chemotherapy

PATHOPHYSIOLOGY

- Death and necrosis of bone with gradual return of blood supply
- Necrotic bone gradually resorbed and replaced by new bone

EPIDEMIOLOGY

- Variable, depending on cause

GENETICS

- Variable, depending on cause

COMPLICATIONS

- Decreased range of motion, pain, limping
- Osteoarthritis
- Physeal arrest with growth disturbance

PROGNOSIS

- Variable, depending on cause

 Differential Diagnosis

- Trauma

—Osteochondral fracture
—Impaction fracture
—Epiphyseal/physeal fracture

- Infection

—Osteomyelitis
—Septic arthritis

- Neoplastic process

—Epiphyseal tumors (chondroblastoma, Trevor disease, etc.)

- Rheumatologic processes

 Data Gathering

HISTORY

- Onset (gradual or after traumatic event)
- Association with:

—Trauma
—Medications (steroids or chemotherapy)
—Casting, splinting, surgery (iatrogenic)
—Pain, limping?
—Stiffness (decreased range of motion)

 Physical Examination

- Gait

—Limping
—Antalgic gait (decreased)
—Trendelenburg gait

- Range of motion

—Flexion and extension
—Abduction and adduction
—Internal and external rotation

- Hip joint irritability (short arc rotation)
- Sign of other disease process (e.g., sickle cell disease)
- Physical examination trick

—Loss of internal rotation is usually the first and most affected loss of motion seen.

Laboratory Aids

TESTS

Laboratory examinations should be normal in most forms of AVN of the femoral head. Exceptions:

–Sickle cell disease
–Septic arthritis
–Chemotherapy

IMAGING

Usual

–Sclerosis
–Subchondral fracture
–Collapse
–Reossification
–Repair

Variable

–Cysts
–Physeal growth arrest (young)
–Early osteoarthritis
–Subluxation

Therapy

DRUGS

• NSAIDs may be effective in decreasing associated inflammation.
• If associated with steroid use, discontinuation or elimination if appropriate

TREATMENT PRINCIPLES

• Maintain range of motion (physical therapy, traction, continuous passive motion).
• Contain the femoral head in the acetabulum (see Perthes Disease principles).
• Surgery

—Redirectional osteotomy
—Femoral or acetabular (see containment operations of Perthes)
—Core decompression to introduce new blood supply (older patient)

DURATION OF THERAPY

• Variable, depending on cause

DIET

• Thought not to alter disease process; recommend general balanced diet

Follow-Up

WHEN TO EXPECT IMPROVEMENT

• Variable, depending on cause

SIGNS TO WATCH FOR

• Subluxation
• Early osteoarthritis
• Growth arrest

PROGNOSIS

• Overall, good if mild involvement (usual) and patient is young
• See Prevention, below

PREVENTION

• Traumatic

—After fracture: early anatomic reduction is key.
—After hip dislocation: early reduction is key.
—After slipped capital femoral epiphysis: associated with unstable grade 3 slips.
—After casting, bracing, surgery: prevention is key.

• Nontraumatic

—Idiopathic (older, after physeal closure); similar to adult AVN
—Idiopathic Perthes (younger, before physeal closure); see Perthes Disease
—Caisson disease: rare now
—With sickle cell disease: good medical management key
—After septic arthritis: early surgical drainage of hip key to prevention
—With steroids or chemotherapy: do not use unless no other alternatives

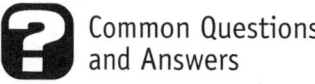

Common Questions and Answers

Q: What type of medication is associated with AVN of the hip?
A: Steroids

Q: For AVN in children (Perthes disease of the hip, for example), is younger or older age associated with a better prognosis?
A: Younger age

ICD-9-CM

Legg Perthe 731.1
Avascular Necrosis 733.40

BIBLIOGRAPHY

Lahdes-Vasama T, Lamminen A, Merikanto J, et al. The value of MRI in early Perthes disease: an MRI study with a 2 year follow up. *Pediatr Radiol* 1997;27(6):517–522.

Sanders JO, Browne RH, Mooney JF, et al. Treatment of femoral fractures in children by pediatric orthopedists: results of a 1998 survey. *J Pediatr Orthop* 2001;21(4):436–441.

Author: John P. Dormans

Babesiosis

Database

DEFINITION

Human babesiosis is a tick-borne malaria-like illness characterized by fever, malaise, and hemolytic anemia. However, most infected individuals are asymptomatic.

CAUSES

• Human babesiosis is caused by the intraerythrocytic parasite of the *Babesia* genus.
• In the northeast United States, *Babesia microti* is transmitted by *Ixodes dammini*, the same tick responsible for Lyme disease.
• A babesiosis-like syndrome caused by the WA1 protozoan is found in the western part of the United States.
• Rarely, the disease has been acquired through transfusion of contaminated blood products or vertical transmission from mother to fetus.

PATHOPHYSIOLOGY

• A bite from an infected tick transmits the protozoa.
• The incubation period is usually 1 to 4 weeks but can be as long as 9 weeks.
• Infection of the erythrocyte causes membrane damage and lysis, which promotes adherence to the endothelium and microvascular stasis.
• The spleen plays an important role in decreasing the protozoal load through antibody production and filtering abnormally shaped infected red blood cells (RBCs).

EPIDEMIOLOGY

• The first case in the United States was reported from California in 1966.
• The most severely affected are those who are at the extremes of age, functionally or anatomically asplenic, or otherwise immunocompromised.
• Transmission usually occurs in the summer and early fall.
• Most cases have been reported from the northeast United States and the West Coast. Endemic areas include Rhode Island, Massachusetts, and New York. There also have been cases from Maryland, Virginia, Georgia, Wisconsin, and Minnesota.

COMPLICATIONS

• Rarely fatal in the United States.
• Pancytopenia and overwhelming secondary bacterial sepsis may occur.
• Other unusual complications in adults include:

—Pulmonary edema and adult respiratory distress syndrome, often happening after treatment has begun.
—Renal failure
—Hemophagocytic syndrome
—Seizures

• Those co-infected with Lyme disease are susceptible to more severe disease and complications.

ASSOCIATED ILLNESSES

It is estimated that 23% of patients have concurrent Lyme disease.

Differential Diagnosis

• Infection
• Nonspecific viral syndrome
• Malaria

Data Gathering

• Few patients recall a tick bite.
• Patients live in or have had recent travel to an endemic region.
• Initial symptoms are vague and may include progressive fatigue, malaise, and anorexia, accompanied by intermittent fevers as high as 40°C.
• Chills, myalgias, and arthralgias may follow these symptoms.
• Less common complaints include headache, cough, sore throat, abdominal pain, and emotional lability.

Physical Examination

• Fever is often the only finding.
• Some may have a mildly enlarged liver and/or splenomegaly.
• Jaundice or hematuria may also be seen.
• Petechiae and ecchymosis are rare.

Laboratory Aids

SPECIFIC TESTS

• Giemsa- or Wright-stained thick and thin blood smears may demonstrate the intraerythrocytic ring form.
• Indirect immunofluorescent assay (IFA) is antigen-specific for *B. microti* and can be used when blood smears are negative. In general, a titer = 1:64 indicates exposure, and titers = 1:256 suggest acute infection. In endemic areas, the IFA test has a sensitivity of 91% and a specificity of 99%.
• Polymerase chain reaction (PCR) is highly specific.
• Isolation of the parasite can be done by intraperitoneal injection of a patient's blood into a golden hamster, but this takes weeks to perform.

OTHER TESTS

Most of the abnormal routine tests are the result of hemolysis.

• Urinalysis: proteinuria, hemoglobinuria
• Complete blood count: normocytic/normochromic anemia, thrombocytopenia, and atypical lymphocytosis
• Possible positive Coombs test
• Elevated erythrocyte sedimentation rate
• Liver function tests: elevated bilirubin, lactate dehydrogenase, and liver transaminases

In asymptomatic patients, these tests are often normal.

FALSE NEGATIVES

• The blood smears may not demonstrate the protozoan at low levels of parasitemia.
• Serologic false positives for *B. micoti* include cross-reactivity with other *Babesia* species or malarial organisms.
• Theoretical serologic false positives for WA1: rheumatoid factor, antinuclear antibody and antibody to *Toxoplasma gondii*.

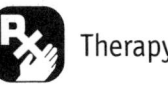 Therapy

- Those with mild clinical disease usually recover without treatment.
- Asplenic, immunodeficient, or symptomatic patients should be treated with clindamycin and quinine.

—The dose of clindamycin is 20 to 40 mg/kg/day divided into three doses for 7 days.
—Quinine is dosed 10 to 25 mg/kg/day divided into three doses for 7 days.
—Atovaquone and azithromycin together and in combination with the above drugs have also been used successfully.

- For life-threatening infections, exchange transfusion has been successful. Progressive respiratory distress may require mechanical ventilation.

 Follow-Up

WHEN TO EXPECT IMPROVEMENT

- Those who are only mildly affected usually have resolution of their symptoms over a few weeks.
- For the severely affected and immunodeficient patients, the convalescent period may be as long as 18 months.

SIGNS TO WATCH FOR

- Respiratory distress, especially after treatment has begun
- Pancytopenia and lymphadenopathy: may indicate the development of hemophagocytic syndrome

PITFALLS

- Children who are from endemic areas and have an acute febrile illness may be misdiagnosed with a nonspecific viral illness.
- One should be suspicious for a co-infection with Lyme disease in those who are not responding to standard therapy.
- Delayed recognition of this uncommon disease may be life threatening in the immunocompromised patient.

PREVENTION

- Prevention begins with avoidance of tick bites.
- For most individuals, simple measures include wearing long-sleeved shirts and long pants, with pants tucked into the socks in tick-infested areas.
- Light clothing will make ticks easier to see.
- Spraying the bottoms of one's pants with a tick repellent may also be helpful.
- Children and dogs should be inspected for ticks after being outside.
- High-risk individuals may want to avoid endemic areas from May to September.
- Currently, there is no universal laboratory screening of blood products.
- No prophylaxis treatment after a tick bite is recommended.

 Common Questions and Answers

Q: How long does a tick have to be attached for infection to occur?
A: In general, successful transmission requires at least 24 hours of attachment.

Q: How should a tick be removed?
A: The tick should be grasped with forceps as close to its head as possible and pulled straight up. If possible, it should be saved for identification.

Q: Does infection confer lifetime immunity?
A: Reinfection is possible.

ICD-9-CM 088.82

BIBLIOGRAPHY

American Academy of Pediatrics. Babesiosis. *Red book: report of the Committee of Infectious Diseases* .Washington, DC: American Academy of Pediatrics, 2000:181–182.

Bonoan JT, Johnson DH, Cunha BA. Life-threatening babesiosis in an asplenic patient treated with exchange transfusion, azithromycin, and atovaquone. *Heart Lung* 1998;27:424–428.

Boustani MR, Gelfand JA. Babesiosis. *Clin Infect Dis* 1996;22:611–615.

Krause PJ, Telford SR, Spielman A, et al. Comparison of PCR with blood smear and inoculation of small animals for diagnosis of Babesia microti parasitemia. *J Clin Microbiol* 1996;34:2791–2794.

Krause PJ, Telford SR, Spielman A, et al. Concurrent Lyme disease and babesiosis. Evidence for increased severity and duration of illness. *JAMA* 1996;275:1657–1660.

Krause PJ, Telford SR 3d, Pollack RJ, et al. Babesiosis: an underdiagnosed disease of children. *Pediatrics* 1992;89:1045–1048.

New DL, Quinn JB, Qureshi MZ, et al. Vertically transmitted babesiosis. *J Pediatr* 1997;131:163–164.

Author: Frances M. Nadel

Barotitis

 Database

DEFINITION

Barotrauma of the middle or inner ear, most often caused by scuba diving or flying.

PATHOPHYSIOLOGY

• The eustachian tube is responsible for equalizing pressure of the middle ear to external ear/environment. Differences in the atmospheric pressure between the inner ear, middle ear, and the environment result in injury to the middle and/or inner ear. When ambient pressure decreases (e.g., airplane ascent) the tympanic membrane bulges outward and the eustachian tube vents the excess middle ear pressure. With a functioning eustachian tube, barotitis does not develop; the pressure is easily equalized. When ambient pressure increases (e.g., scuba diving, airplane descent) the tympanic membrane bulges inward and the eustachian tube resists inward flow of air to the middle ear. Even with a normally functioning eustachian tube, pressure equalization is difficult.
• Middle ear barotitis results in vascular engorgement, bleeding, and exudate formation.
• Inner ear barotrauma can cause labyrinthine window rupture.
• At a pressure differential of 60 mm Hg (greater ambient to middle ear pressure), subjective discomfort is reported. At a pressure differential of 90 mm Hg, the eustachian tube becomes "locked," because the palatal musculature is not strong enough to open the tube and air will not be able to enter the middle ear to equalize the pressure. The tympanic membrane can rupture at pressure differentials over 100 to 500 mm Hg.
• Barotitis is sometimes classified using Teed's classification of disease severity (see Physical Examination section).
• Nasal congestion has been shown to increase the likelihood of developing barotitis.

EPIDEMIOLOGY

• Significant disease is uncommon in commercial (pressurized) aircraft, although mild negative pressure of the middle ear is common after flying.
• Significant symptoms or injury can occur in scuba divers, and those who fly military aircraft and experience rapid altitude changes during tactical maneuvers.

COMPLICATIONS

• Vertigo
• Hearing loss
• Tympanic membrane rupture
• Oval or round window rupture
• Hemorrhage

PROGNOSIS

• Complete spontaneous resolution in mild cases
• Rarely, tympanotomy or tympanostomy is required to relieve pressure and pain, as well as prevent complications.
• Variable outcome for auditory and vestibular symptoms and injuries to the inner ear

 Differential Diagnosis

INFECTION

Otitis media with effusion can cause decreased hearing, sensation of fullness, tympanic membrane hyperemia, and pain.

TRAUMA

• Blunt trauma to the tympanic membrane (e.g., cotton swabs) can cause rupture and bleeding.
• Exposure to extremely loud noise can result in pain and hearing loss.

HISTORY

• Questions regarding exposure to pressure change (e.g., diving or flying) or trauma (e.g., ear clapping, "heavy metal" concert) are critical to making the proper diagnosis.
• Ear pain, sensation of pressure, and decreased hearing are the most common symptoms.
• Symptoms of inner ear damage may include vestibular and/or auditory complaints.

 Physical Examination

Teed's Classification:

Grade 0: Normal

Grade 1: Retraction, redness in Shrapnell membrane and along manubrium

Grade 2: Retraction, with redness of entire ear drum

Grade 3: Grade 2 plus hemotympanum or clear exudate

Grade 4: Perforation of tympanic membrane

• Nystagmus
• Hearing loss

 Laboratory Aids

TESTS

Hearing Tests

• Should be performed on all patients who have signs of barotrauma, and on patients with normal physical examinations but who are symptomatic.

Radiographic Studies

• MRI: may be indicated in patients with vestibular symptoms or hearing loss to rule out inner ear damage.

Therapy

- When diving or descending in an airplane, performing a Valsalva maneuver (blowing the nose while pinching the nostrils closed) will force air into the middle ear via the eustachian tube, thereby equalizing the pressure between the middle ear and the environment.
- Swallowing, yawning, and chewing can aid release of pressure through the eustachian tube when ascending in an airplane or when returning to the surface when scuba diving.
- A Politzer bag is an instrument used for clearing pressure disequilibrium that has not improved with Valsalva maneuvers and a trial of decongestants. (See Brown, 1994, for a description of the device and its use.)
- Otovent is another instrument that can be used for treatment or prevention. Usage can be taught to children as young as 2 to 6 years of age.
- Severe disease may require tympanotomy or tympanostomy to relieve pressure.
- For the patient with excruciating pain or unrelenting eustachian tube dysfunction, myringotomy is effective. It is best performed by an otorhinolaryngologist.

DRUGS

- Nasal decongestant sprays may be helpful by constricting mucosal arterioles and enhancing eustachian tube function. Topical decongestants are used 1 hour prior to plane travel/diving and one-half hour prior to plane descent.
- Oral decongestants may be helpful through the same physiologic pathway as topical agents. They should be initiated 1 to 2 days prior to the expected pressure change.
- Antihistamines may also be helpful by reducing mucosal edema and enhancing the eustachian tube orifice. They can be used on the day of the expected pressure change.

 Follow-Up

- Pressure differential without damage to the middle or inner ear usually resolves within a few days of returning to normal atmospheric pressure.
- Barotitis that resulted in injury to the middle or inner ear has a variable rate of improvement; some damage is permanent (e.g., organ of Corti), while other injury is reversible (e.g., tympanic membrane).

PREVENTION

- Travel in commercial aircraft will generally not result in severe barotitis.
- Most items in the Therapy section can be used as prevention: antihistamines, decongestants, avoidance of dehydration, frequent Valsalva maneuver, and Otovent use.
- Ascend and descend carefully when scuba diving.

 Common Questions and Answers

Q: Is the Valsalva maneuver also effective on plane ascent?
A: Yes, creating even greater pressure in the middle ear by performing the Valsalva maneuver can overcome a resistant eustachian tube and result in sudden venting of increased middle ear pressure.

Q: Can children with otitis media travel in airplanes?
A: Yes, Weiss and Frost (1987) have shown that commercial air travel did not result in worsening of symptoms, and, in fact, the presence of otitis media with effusion seemed protective against barotitis.

Q: How can I help my baby not have ear pain when traveling in an airplane?
A: Have the child nurse, take a bottle, or eat during ascent and descent. This will result in pharyngeal movements that will repeatedly open the eustachian tube and equalize middle ear pressure to environmental pressure. Also, if the child is currently experiencing an upper respiratory infection, use of decongestants prior to flight may be helpful.

ICD-9-CM 993.0

BIBLIOGRAPHY

Brown TP. Middle ear symptoms while flying: ways to prevent a severe outcome. *Postgrad Med* 1994;96:135–142.

Nakashima T, Itoh M, Sato M, et al. Auditory and vestibular disorders due to barotrauma. *Ann Otol Rhinol Laryngol* 1988;97:146–152.

Stangerup SE, Tjernstrom O, Harcourt J, et al. Barotitis in children after aviation: prevalence and treatment with Otovent. *J Laryngol Otol* 1996;110:625–628.

Stangerup SE, Tjernstrom O, Klokker M, et al. Point prevalence of barotitis in children and adults after flight, and effect of autoinflation. *Aviat Space Environ Med* 1998;69(1):45–49.

Weiss MH, Frost O. May children with otitis media with effusion safely fly? *Clin Pediatr* 1987;26:567–568.

Author: Laura N. Sinai

Bell Palsy

Database

DEFINITION

Bell palsy is an acute facial paralysis due to extracranial or peripheral involvement of the seventh cranial nerve. The facial nerve innervates muscles of facial expression, and its branches include the stapedius nerve, chorda tympani nerve (taste in anterior two thirds of tongue), greater petrosal nerve (lacrimal and nasal glands), and the nervus intermedius (cutaneous sensory fibers). Although facial nerve dysfunction manifests primarily as facial paralysis, varying degrees of the following symptoms may occur: dysgeusia, decreased salivation/lacrimation, epiphora, hyperacusis, facial numbness, and pain.

PATHOPHYSIOLOGY

• The facial nerve travels through a tortuous and narrow path from the brainstem to the peripheral face. As it courses through the temporal bone, it reaches the narrowest portion in the labyrinthine segment of the internal auditory canal, measuring only 0.68 mm in diameter. This segment is also a watershed zone between the blood supply from the vertebral and carotid artery systems. It is here that the nerve is exquisitely vulnerable to edema, inflammation, and ischemia.

EPIDEMIOLOGY

• Most common cause of facial paralysis worldwide
• Annual incidence: approximately 3/100,000 in the first decade, 10/100,000 in the second decade, and 25/100,000 in adults
• 1% of cases have bilateral involvement
• 10% recurrence rate

COMPLICATIONS

Seen in 10% to 15% of all cases:

• Corneal abrasions
• Keratitis
• Incomplete recovery
• Aberrant reinnervation of the facial nerve resulting in facial tics, synkinesis, or "crocodile tears" (lacrimation after exposure to smell or taste of food)
• Facial contractures
• Facial hyperkinesis: blepharospasm, hemifacial spasm

PROGNOSIS

• More than 60–70% will have complete recovery without treatment
• Signs of recovery should be evident within 1 month. Greatest degree of recovery is seen within first 4 months
• Continued recovery may occur for up to 12 months

• Paralysis is progressive for 7 to 10 days from onset of symptoms
• Younger patients have a better prognosis.
• Patients with complete paralysis have worse prognosis.

Differential Diagnosis

IDIOPATHIC

• Melkersson-Rosenthal syndrome (recurrent alternating facial palsy, furrowed tongue, faciolabial edema)

TRAUMA

• Intrauterine birth trauma (e.g., skull and facial molding)
• Forceps-assisted delivery
• Temporal bone fractures from blunt trauma
• Skull/facial puncture wounds or lacerations
• Iatrogenic from otologic surgery

INFECTIOUS

• Mastoiditis
• Acute otitis media
• Sinusitis
• Meningitis
• Osteomyelitis of skull base
• Ramsay Hunt syndrome/herpes zoster oticus (facial paralysis, vesicular eruption, vestibulocochlear dysfunction, pain)
• Lyme disease
• EBV
• CMV
• HIV
• Syphilis

CONGENITAL

Usually associated with craniofacial or bony anomalies

• Mobius syndrome
• Goldenhar syndrome
• McCune-Albright syndrome
• Osteopetrosis

NEOPLASTIC

Central tumors affecting structures in the brainstem/cerebellopontine angle or peripheral tumors following the course of the facial nerve

NEUROLOGIC

• Stroke
• Guillain-Barré syndrome
• Multiple sclerosis
• Aneurysm of vertebral, basilar, or carotid arteries

IMMUNOLOGIC/INFLAMMATORY

• Sarcoidosis

TOXIC

• Thalidomide embryopathy
• Alcoholism

METABOLIC

• Diabetes mellitus
• Hypothyroidism

Data Gathering

HISTORY

• Viral prodrome or pain/tingling around the ear of the affected side 1 to 2 days before onset of facial weakness is seen in the majority patients with Bell palsy.
• Onset of facial weakness is usually acute (several hours) but can be subacute (1 to 2 days).
• Tick bites may be suggestive of Lyme disease.
• Rule out trauma, focus on birth history in neonates.
• Rule out toxin exposure.
• Ask about symptoms suggestive of an underlying medical disorder or systemic illness, including infections.

Physical Examination

• Neurologic exam: facial nerve palsy will manifest as upper and lower unilateral facial weakness with abnormalities of taste, fungiform papillae on the anterior tongue, hyperacusis with decreased or absent stapedial reflex, decreased lacrimation and salivation, and possibly numbness with postauricular pain. Rule out upper motor neuron facial paralysis. Use tuning fork to assess hearing. The Schirmer test can be used to assess lacrimation by measuring the degree of moisture absorbed on a strip of filter paper when placed over the conjunctival sac of the lower lid. Neurologic abnormalities in addition to a seventh nerve palsy are suggestive of another diagnosis.
• Face and neck exam: rule out parotid gland swelling or mass. Rule out infectious etiology such as otitis media, mastoiditis, Lyme disease, meningitis, osteomyelitis of the skull base. Look for tick bites, erythema chronicum migrans. Examine ipsilateral ear for herpetic lesions seen in Ramsay Hunt syndrome. Observe for any craniofacial anomalies.
• Signs of trauma: Battle sign, hemotympanum, skull deformity. Trauma patients with nerve injury may be candidates for emergent surgical decompression with nerve repair.

Laboratory Aids

TESTS

- Serology for Lyme, EBV, mumps, rubella, HIV, RPR if history or presentation suggestive (e.g., tick bite, hepatosplenomegaly, lack of proper vaccination, recurrent infections, history of chancre)
- Thyroid function tests if signs or symptoms suggest hypothyroidism
- Chemistry panel if history of ingestion or toxin exposure
- ESR if signs of autoimmune disease (e.g., sarcoidosis)
- CBC may show leukocytosis if bacterial etiology, such as osteomyelitis, meningitis, or suppurative otitis media is present.
- Lumbar puncture if meningitis or HSV encephalitis is suspected as the underlying cause

RADIOGRAPHIC AND OTHER STUDIES

- MRI—mass lesions should be considered in cases with an atypical course, persistent symptoms, recurrence, exam concerning for intracranial process (e.g., bilateral nerve involvement, multiple cranial nerve deficits, upper motor neuron weakness, etc). In Bell palsy, gadolinium-enhanced MRI will show increased uptake in the labyrinthine segment of the facial nerve due to inflammation/ neuritis.
- CT—high-resolution CT can be used to rule out temporal bone fractures as well as intracranial bleeds or hemorrhagic stroke.
- EMG/nerve conduction studies—may be helpful in determining the extent of nerve damage and prognosis. Use in pediatric Bell palsy is not well studied.
- Audiology—absence of stapedial reflex indicates poorer prognosis. Conductive hearing loss may suggest middle ear disease or cholesteatoma. Sensorineural hearing loss indicates eighth nerve dysfunction as seen in Ramsay Hunt syndrome or acoustic neuromas.

Therapy

- Eye protection—artificial tears 3 to 4 times during the day, glasses or goggles to protect from light, wind, foreign body, and Lacri-Lube applied at night, serve to prevent corneal abrasions and keratitis. Very active children may benefit from eye patching while playing outside to avoid foreign body exposure.
- Prednisone—must be started within 72 hours of onset of symptoms to be effective. May be contraindicated in certain patients with hypertension, diabetes, pregnancy, and granulomatous disease. Recommended dose: 1 mg/kg/day for 5 days, tapered over the next 5 days for a total of 10 days; adult dose: 30 mg bid for 5 days, tapered over the next 5 days.

- Acyclovir—double therapy of acyclovir combined with prednisone has been advocated based on hypothesis of HSV-induced neuritis. Single therapy with acyclovir may be considered when patient is unable to take prednisone. Dosage for children >2 years: 20 mg/kg/day for 10 days; adult dose: 200–400 mg 5 times/day for 10 days. Most common side effect is GI upset.
- Surgical decompression—indicated in cases of trauma or iatrogenic injury during otologic surgery. In Bell palsy patients, surgical treatment is reserved for severe cases after 1 year of observation.

Follow-Up

- Close follow-up every 2 weeks during the first month of symptoms is essential.
- After the first month, follow monthly until full recovery, usually achieved by 4 months

PITFALLS

Misdiagnosis can lead to delayed treatment and poor outcome. The following red flags should prompt the clinician to investigate other causes of facial nerve palsy:

- Slowly progressive facial paralysis for more than 3 weeks or lack of function after 6 months suggests neoplasm.
- Simultaneous bilateral nerve paralysis commonly seen with Lyme disease, leukemia, sarcoidosis, multiple sclerosis or other systemic conditions.
- Intact forehead movement suggests upper motor neuron disease but can be seen in up to 5% Bell palsy patients.
- Recurrent unilateral paralysis seen in 30% of tumor patients compared to 1% of Bell palsy patients.
- Facial hyperkinesis seen in vascular compression syndromes and neoplasms.
- Multiple cranial nerve involvement suggests systemic disease or tumor.

Common Questions and Answers

Q: What is the recommendation for prednisone and/or acyclovir treatment in pediatric patients?
A: The decision to treat with prednisone and acyclovir remains controversial. A 1999 randomized control trial of 42 pediatric patients did not show a statistically significant difference in degree of recovery or risk of complications between those treated with prednisone versus those treated with placebo. In adult studies, patients treated with prednisone tended to have better outcomes than patients who were not treated. However, there are not enough clinical studies in the pediatric

population to say definitively whether steroids and/or acyclovir improve outcomes.
Q: When is it appropriate to consult a neurologist?
A: Red flags at the time of presentation may be signs of an intracranial or underlying neurologic disease. Multiple cranial neuropathies, associated headache, intact forehead innervation, hearing loss, bilateral facial involvement, focal neurologic findings in the extremities (e.g., spasticity or weakness) are more suggestive of an intracranial or upper motor neuron process than an isolated peripheral facial nerve palsy, and patients with these conditions should be referred to a neurologist.

If a patient has progressive symptoms, lack of clinical improvement after 1 month, or recurrence of symptoms, s/he may have an underlying disease or may go on to have complications requiring more aggressive management and should be referred to a neurologist.

ICD-9-CM 351.0

BIBLIOGRAPHY

Adour K. Bell's palsy treatment with acyclovir and prednisone compared with prednisone alone: a double-blind, randomized, controlled trial. *Ann Otol Rhinol Laryngol* 1996;105: 371–378.

Bauer C, Coker N. Update on facial nerve disorders. *Otolaryngol Clin North Am* 1996;29(3):445–454.

De Diego J. Idiopathic facial paralysis: a randomized, prospective, and controlled study using single-dose prednisone versus acyclovir three times daily. *Laryngoscope* 1998;108:575–575.

Morgan M. Facial palsy and infection: the unfolding story. *Clin Infect Dis* 1992;14: 263–271.

Unuvar E. Corticosteroid treatment of childhood Bell's palsy. *Pediatr Neurol* 1999; 21: 814–816.

Author: Susan Sohn Chung

Bezoars

 Database

DEFINITION

Bezoars are accumulation of foreign material in the gastrointestinal tract.

- The peak age of onset reported in the literature is 10 to 19 years.
- Ninety percent of patients reportedly are female.
- Have been documented over two millennia and served some medical value in some cultures.

CAUSES

The classification of bezoars is dependent on the most prominent substance from which they are formed. This includes:

- Trichobezoars: hair
- Phytobezoars: indigestible fruit and vegetable matter
- Lactobezoars: milk
- Foreign bodies
- Fungal
- Less common materials include vitamins, antacids, psyllium, sucralfate, cimetidine, and nifedipine.

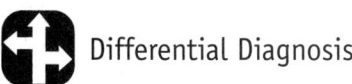 Differential Diagnosis

Any gastric foreign body can mimic a gastric mass and may present on palpation.

 Data Gathering

TRICHOBEZOARS

- Associated with trichotillomania and trichophagia
- Retention of hair strands in the gastric folds
- Bezoars may become large and form a cast of the stomach.
- The bezoar may extend through the pylorus into the small bowel. This "tail" may obstruct the papilla of Vater, leading to jaundice and pancreatitis.
- Presents with abdominal mass, crepitation over the stomach, iron-deficiency anemia.
- Most trichophagia does not result in bezoar formation.
- History of trichophagia is obtained in only 50% of cases.

PHYTOBEZOARS

- Most common form among adults
- Associated with gastric dysmotility and poor gastric emptying (either primary or following gastric surgery) and hypochlorhydria
- Composed primarily of cellulose, hemicellulose, lignins, and tannins

LACTOBEZOARS (MILK)

Most often reported in premature, low-birth-weight infants (although there are reports in full-term infants and exclusively breast-fed infants)

- Factors contributing to lactobezoar formation include:

—Formulas with a high casein content
—Early and rapid feeding advancement in small infants
—High-caloric-density formulas
—Formulas with high calcium/phosphate content
—Continuous tube feedings
—Altered gastric motility in low-birth-weight infants

 Physical Examination

HISTORY

Symptoms and signs of bezoar formation include:

- Pain
- Halitosis
- Nausea
- Vomiting
- Diarrhea
- Gastric ulceration
- Upper gastrointestinal bleeding and perforation
- Left upper quadrant (LUQ) mass

TRICHOBEZOARS

- Unusual patterns of balding
- Palpable LUQ mass in the abdomen is often detected.

PHYTOBEZOARS

Abdominal mass is palpable in less than half of patients.

Laboratory Aids

- Iron-deficiency anemia, steatorrhea, or protein-losing enteropathy
- Plain abdominal radiography of the abdomen
- Upper gastrointestinal studies may outline the mass.
- Endoscopy may provide the diagnosis of the specific type of bezoar.

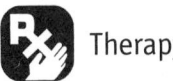 ## Therapy

TRICHOBEZOARS

Surgical: they are normally too large, and hair is not dissolvable. Any trial to break the hairball may lead to metastatic migration and need of small intestinal surgery.

PHYTOBEZOARS

- Diet alteration
- Medications such as prokinetic agents to stimulate gastric motility
- Enzyme therapy to help dissolve the material
- Acetylcysteine treatment via nasogastric tube has been documented in one case report.
- Papain has shown to be approximately 87% effective. [Papain tablets are not currently available in the United States, so monosodium glutamate (MSG) dissolved in clear liquids has been used.] Complications of this therapy include the development of gastric ulceration and hypernatremia secondary to the high sodium content of MSG.
- Endoscopic fragmentation or extraction
- Surgical extraction

LACTOBEZOARS

- Withholding feedings for approximately 48 hours while the patient is sustained on IV fluids

 ## Common Questions and Answers

Q: What are some commonly used medications that can lead to bezoar formation?
A: Vitamins, antacids, psyllium, sucralfate, cimetidine, and nifedipine.

Q: What may place an infant at risk for formation of a bezoar?
A: The literature suggests that formulas with a high casein contact may be linked with lactobezoar formation. Other possible contributing factors include early and rapid feeding advancement in small infants, high-density formulas; formulas with high calcium/phosphate content, continuous tube feedings, and altered gastric motility in low-birth-weight infants.

ICD-9-CM 938

BIBLIOGRAPHY

Walker-Renard P. Update on the medicinal management of phytobezoars. *Am J Gastroenterol* 1993;88(10):1663–1666.

Wyllie R, Hyams J. *Pediatric gastrointestinal disease: pathophysiology, diagnosis, and management*. Philadelphia: WB Saunders, 1993.

Author: Dror Wasserman
Donna Zeiter, 2nd edition

Biliary Atresia

 Database

DEFINITION

Biliary atresia is a progressive obliteration of the lumen of the extrahepatic (EHBA) and intrahepatic biliary duct systems of the liver.

PATHOPHYSIOLOGY

The etiology is unclear. Each of the following etiologies has been suggested but has never been substantiated:

- Infection [reovirus 3, rotavirus, cytomegalovirus (CMV)]
- Vascular insufficiency
- Autoimmune obliteration of the bile ducts
- Pancreatic reflux leading to destruction of the biliary duct system
- Developmental anomaly such as ductal plate malformation

PATHOLOGY

Gross Anatomy

EHBA can affect all or any part of the extrahepatic biliary tree. When the affected portion is limited to the distal common bile duct, cystic duct, or gallbladder, the form is considered correctable because biliary drainage may be established. This situation occurs in less than 10% of patients. Coexisting anomalies are found in approximately 20% of patients. Some of the reported associations include:

- Absence of the inferior vena cava with azygous continuation
- Preduodenal portal vein and symmetric liver
- Malrotation
- Situs inversus
- Bronchial anomalies
- Multiple spleens

HISTOLOGY

Because this is a progressive disease, the pathologic findings vary with stage. Extrahepatic biliary obstruction begins near the time of birth and progresses. Early in the course of the disease (approximately the first year), the liver biopsy shows cholestasis, interlobular bile duct proliferation, and a mononuclear infiltrate invading the periductal tissue. Later biopsies show degeneration and loss of bile ducts. If the biopsy is performed prior to 4 weeks of age, the pathology may be confused with other causes of neonatal cholestasis, such as giant-cell hepatitis.

GENETICS

- No clear genetic inheritance can be demonstrated, as indicated by discordance for both monozygotic and dizygotic twins.
- However, HLA-B12, HLA-A9-B5, and HLA-A28-B35 are found with a higher frequency in affected individuals.

EPIDEMIOLOGY

EHBA accounts for 25% to 30% of the cases of neonatal cholestasis and occurs with a frequency of 1 per 8,000 to 15,000 live births. It is the most common cause of neonatal jaundice for which surgery is indicated.

 Differential Diagnosis

The differential diagnosis includes all causes of neonatal cholestasis (NC).

EXTRAHEPATIC CAUSES OF NEONATAL CHOLESTASIS

- Biliary atresia
- Choledochal cyst
- Sclerosing cholangitis
- Bile duct stenosis
- Anomalies of the choledochopancreatico-ductal junction
- Spontaneous perforation of the common bile duct
- Obstructing neoplasia or stone
- Inspissated bile or mucus plug

INTRAHEPATIC DISORDERS OF NEONATAL CHOLESTASIS

Infection

- Sepsis
- Urinary tract infection (UTI)
- TORCH
- Coxsackie B virus, echovirus

Metabolic Abnormalities

- Tyrosinemia
- Galactosemia
- Hereditary fructose intolerance
- Inborn errors of bile acid metabolism
- Zellweger syndrome
- Benign familial recurrent cholestasis
- α_1-Antitrypsin deficiency
- Neonatal iron-storage disease
- Cystic fibrosis
- Hypopituitarism
- Bile duct paucity (Alagille syndrome and nonsyndromic paucity)
- Trisomy 17, 18, 21 and Turner syndrome

Drugs/Toxins

- Medications
- Total parenteral nutrition (TPN)

Systemic Disease

- Post-shock
- Post-asphyxia
- Congestive heart failure

Inherited Jaundice Syndromes

- Dubin-Johnson syndrome
- Rotor syndrome
- Idiopathic neonatal giant-cell hepatitis

 Data Gathering

HISTORY

Typically, the patient is an otherwise healthy infant who develops jaundice within the first 90 days of life, and laboratory data demonstrate a conjugated hyperbilirubinemia.

 Physical Examination

- Jaundice is best visualized by examination of the hard palate, buccal mucosa, or sclera and may not be present until the bilirubin exceeds 5 to 7 dL in the newborn period and 2 dL in the older child.
- Acholic stools, hepatomegaly, and abnormal liver consistency are variable findings and do not need to be present to establish the diagnosis of biliary atresia.

 Laboratory Aids

- Conjugated hyperbilirubin is defined as a conjugated fraction greater than 2.0 dL or a conjugated/total greater than 15%.
- Any child with a conjugated hyperbilirubinemia should undergo the following examinations:

—Fractionated bilirubin
—AST, ALT, PT/PTT, total protein, albumin, CBC
—Bacterial cultures (blood, urine, stool)
—Viral studies [hepatitis B, hepatitis C, Epstein-Barr virus (EBV), TORCH, HIV, adenovirus, enterovirus]
—α_1-Antitrypsin with Pi typing
—Urine and serum amino acids
—Urine organic acids
—Urine for reducing substance while the child is taking lactose-containing formula; if positive, assay of galactose-1-phosphate uridyl transferase
—X-ray studies to exclude evidence of congenital infections and Alagille syndrome (i.e., calcifications of brain and butterfly vertebrae)
—Eye examination for congenital infections
—Sweat test

—HIV serology
—Thyroid-function tests
—Abdominal ultrasound
—Hepatobiliary scintigraphy
—Liver biopsy
—Operative cholangiogram, if nonexcreting scintigraphy

 Therapy

• General approach

—Once the diagnosis of EHBA is established, a surgical drainage procedure is performed.
—Subsequent management is directed at providing nutrition and monitoring for common problems.
—Although surgical intervention is helpful, liver disease progresses and the majority of patients will ultimately require liver transplantation.

• Surgical drainage

—Correctable biliary atresia occurs in up to 10% of patients and is defined as obstruction limited to the distal common bile duct, cystic duct, and/or gallbladder. These patients may undergo a more limited operation linking the patent distal portion of the tree to the intestine, bypassing the obstruction.
—Noncorrectable biliary atresia occurs most frequently and is manifested as an absent extrahepatic biliary tree. The standard surgical procedure is the hepatoportoenterostomy (Kasai procedure).

• Nutrition

—Malabsorption due to decreased concentration of bile acids within the duodenal lumen is common and leads to fat-soluble vitamin deficiency and malnutrition. Patients receive routine supplementation with vitamins A, D, E, and K. The diet should be enriched with medium-chain triglycerides to ensure adequate fat ingestion. Nasogastric tube feedings should be implemented.

• Prevention of cholangitis—During the first year of life most children are maintained on daily oral antibiotics to prevent infections from ascending into the liver.
• Pruritus is common and develops when there is increased serum bile acid concentration. Many approaches to treatment with only limited success have included ursodeoxycholic acid, antihistamines, cholestyramine, improved nutrition (e.g., nasogastric supplements), rifampin, phenobarbital, naloxone, and biliary diversion.

• Hyperlipidemia/xanthomas: Hyperlipidemia develops as a complication of chronic liver disease and can be treated with choleretic agents such as ursodeoxycholic acid as well as with improved nutrition.
• Ascites

—Spironolactone, chlorothiazide, and furosemide are commonly used diuretics. Acute changes in fluid balance or a rapid diuresis can be achieved by the use of furosemide in conjunction with albumin replacement

• Liver transplantation: indications for transplantation include life-threatening hemorrhage from portal hypertension, failure to thrive, intractable pruritus, and liver failure.

 Follow-Up

COMMON LONG-TERM PROBLEMS

• Poor growth
• Fat-soluble vitamin deficiency
• Cholangitis
• Portal hypertension
• Pruritus
• Progression of liver damage despite a surgical drainage procedure

The clinician should:

• Keep notes in a flow chart.
• Monitor growth parameters and fat-soluble vitamins.
• Monitor liver span, liver texture, and spleen size to follow progress of disease.
• Follow liver-function tests and CBC.
• Watch closely for cholangitis: the most important findings suggestive of cholangitis are fever and elevated transaminases and GGT levels.

PITFALLS

Because age at the time of surgical intervention is the most important determinant of outcome, a delay in diagnosis can be tragic. Surgery is successful in 86% of infants prior to 8 weeks, 36% of infants between 8 and 12 weeks, and only 20% for those over 12 weeks.

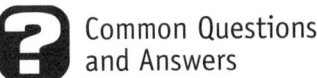 Common Questions and Answers

Q: When should a patient with neonatal jaundice have a fractionated bilirubin test?
A: If hyperbilirubinemia has not resolved by 6 weeks, fractionation should be performed to allow ample time for evaluation of neonatal cholestasis and the possible need for surgical intervention.

Q: Can the physician prioritize the diagnostic evaluation?
A: In general, the answer is no. Because the diagnosis must be made as early as possible and because many tests are performed only in special laboratories, the full workup should be complete within a few days to 2 weeks, depending on the age of the child.

Q: Will a Kasai operation hurt the chances of successful liver transplantation?
A: No. A review of children who underwent transplantation at Boston Children's Hospital reported an 89% 10-year survival for patients who had the Kasai procedure.

ICD-9-CM 751.61

BIBLIOGRAPHY

Gitnick G, LaBrecque DR, Moody FG. *Diseases of the liver and biliary tract*. Philadelphia: Mosby-Year Book, 1992.

Haber BA, Lake A. Neonatal cholestatis. *Clin Perinatol* 1990;17:483–506.

Karrer FM, Bensard DDM. Neonatal cholestasis. *Semin Pediatr Surg* 2000;Nov(4):166–169.

Loomes K, Mulberg AE. The infant with cholestasis: diagnosis and management. In: Brandt LJ, Daum F, eds. *Clinical practice of gastroenterology*. Philadelphia: Churchill Livingstone, 1999.

Mowat AP. *Liver disorders in childhood*. Boston: Butterworth-Heinemann, 1987.

Ohi R. Biliary atresia: a surgical perspective. *Clin Liver Dis* 2000;4:779–804.

Suchy F. *Liver disease in children*. Philadelphia: Mosby-Year Book, 1994.

Author: Barbara Haber

Blastomycosis

 Database

DEFINITION

Blastomycosis is infection caused by the dimorphic soil fungus *Blastomyces dermatitidis*.

PATHOPHYSIOLOGY

• Blastomycosis is a chronic disease characterized by granulomatous and suppurative lesions.
• It may cause asymptomatic infection or be associated with acute, chronic, or rapidly progressive systemic disease.
• It causes a large number of different presenting symptoms and different radiographic appearances.

EPIDEMIOLOGY

• Infection occurs after inhalation of conidia (spores of mycelial form).
• No person-to-person transmission
• Human infection is not uncommon. It is endemic in the United States in the southeast and central states and in the towns bordering the Great Lakes, with the highest incidence in Arkansas, Kentucky, Louisiana, Mississippi, North Carolina, Tennessee, and Wisconsin. Other reported areas of infection include parts of Canada (Ontario, Manitoba), Africa, India, and South America.
• Natural infection occurs only in two mammalian species: humans and dogs.
• It may be associated with immune compromise, but is not common in patients with HIV.
• Uncommon in the pediatric age group (<4% of cases in the most extensive patient review)
• Incubation period estimated at 30 to 45 days

COMPLICATIONS

• Dissemination is the main complication of the infection.
• Systemic infection may be well advanced before symptoms are noted, making eradication more difficult. Long-term therapy and follow-up may be necessary.

PROGNOSIS

• Self-limited pulmonary infection is often undiagnosed and resolves without dissemination (almost 50% of those infected may be asymptomatic).
• Early treatment with amphotericin B in progressive, severe, or disseminated disease is effective, with excellent rates of cure.
• The prognosis for chronic cutaneous disease is better than that for systemic disease.
• The number of deaths from blastomycosis is decreasing with the use of antifungal agents. Prevalence of blastomycosis remains high, however, in endemic areas.

ASSOCIATED ILLNESSES

• *Pulmonary blastomycosis:* most common form of infection by *Blastomyces* in children; can be acute, subacute, or chronic. Illness severity can vary greatly, from asymptomatic to presentations of URI, bronchitis, pleuritis, pneumonia, or severe respiratory distress.
• *Cutaneous blastomycosis:* skin manifestations are variable and include nodules, verrucous lesions, subcutaneous abscesses, or ulcerations. Cutaneous disease occurs following pulmonary inoculation in most cases, but can be inoculated primarily to skin.
• *Disseminated blastomycosis:* usually begins as pulmonary infection, with subsequent spread to involve skin (most commonly), bone, GU tract, and CNS.

 Differential Diagnosis

• Tuberculosis
• Neoplasm
• Sarcoidosis
• Other bacterial, viral, and fungal infections causing URI, bronchitis, pleuritis, and pneumonia

 Data Gathering

HISTORY

• Symptoms of common respiratory infections (nonproductive cough, pleuritic chest pain, poor appetite) that last more than 2 weeks. There may also be a history of fever, chills, weight loss, fatigue, night sweats, or, rarely, hemoptysis.
• History of residence or travel to an endemic area

Physical Examination

• Initial pulmonary infection may present as a mild respiratory infection. Respiratory signs and symptoms often have resolved by the time cutaneous manifestations are apparent.
• Skin involvement appears as nodules, nodules with ulceration, and, finally, granulomatous lesions with advancing borders.
• Sites in disseminated disease include lung, skin, bone, GU tract, CNS, and, infrequently, liver and spleen, lymph nodes, thyroid, heart, adrenals, omentum, GI tract, muscles, and pancreas.
• CXR indicated by physical examination or history may show localized consolidation in acute disease, and cavitations or pulmonary nodules with a more chronic course.

 ## Laboratory Aids

• Direct visualization of the yeast form may be performed on samples of sputum, urine, CSF, BAL sample, or tissue biopsy after 10% potassium hydroxide preparation.
• Culture of the organism from samples can be performed and a DNA probe used to identify *B. dermatitidis*.
• Serologic testing may be helpful in disseminated disease.
• Immunodiffusion testing is reliable for indication of infection, but a negative test does not rule out infection with *Blastomyces*.
• Severe pulmonary infection may develop with cavitation, pneumonia, or pulmonary nodules apparent on chest x-ray films.

 ## Therapy

• Mild or moderate disease is treated with oral itraconazole or ketoconazole, with or without an initial short course of amphotericin B.
• Severe or CNS or other severe infection should be treated with intravenous amphotericin B. Therapy for some patients may be switched to oral itraconazole after clinical stabilization with amphotericin B.
• The use of lipid formulations of amphotericin B has not been reported for CNS blastomycosis, but this treatment may be an alternative for patients unable to tolerate amphotericin B.
• Length of therapy is site-dependent: at least 6 months for pulmonary disease and at least 12 months for bone disease.

PREVENTION

• Infection control
• No special precautions for hospitalized patients are indicated.
• Outbreaks have occurred, with clustering of cases occurring at the same place and time.
• A natural reservoir is undetermined.

ICD-9-CM 116.0

BIBLIOGRAPHY

American Academy of Pediatrics. Blastomycosis. In: Pickering L, ed. *2000 red book: report of the Committee on Infectious Diseases* , 25th ed. Elk Grove Village, IL: American Academy of Pediatrics, 2000:189–190.

Chapman SW. Blastomyces dermatitis. In: Mondell GL, et al., eds. *Principles and practice of infectious diseases*, 5th ed. New York: Churchill Livingstone, 2000:2733–2746.

Chapman SW, Bradsher RW, Campbell GD Jr, et al. Practice guidelines for the management of patients with blastomycosis. *Clin Infect Dis* 2000;30:679–683.

Maxon S, Jacobs RF. Community-acquired fungal pneumonia in children. *Semin Respir Infect* 1996;11(3):196–203.

Schutze G. Blastomycosis. In: Feigin RD, Cherry JD, eds. *Textbook of pediatric infectious diseases*, 3rd ed. Philadelphia: WB Saunders, 1998:2297–2303.

Varkey B. Blastomycosis in children. *Semin Respir Infect* 1997;12(3):235–242.

Author: Theoklis Zaoutis
Molly (Martha) W. Stevens, 2nd edition

Blepharitis

 Database

DEFINITION

Blepharitis is inflammation or infection of the margins of the eyelid. The hallmark clinical features include redness, itching or burning, and crusting or scaling of the lid margins.

Various types:

- Seborrheic blepharitis—notable for easy-to-remove, yellow, greasy scales along the eyelashes; occurs in conjunction with similar seborrheic scales of the eyebrow, scalp and external ears.
- Staphylococcal blepharitis—localized infection of the eyelid margin caused by *Staphylococcus aureus* or *S. epidermidis*. The hallmark features of staphylococcal-induced blepharitis are fibrinous, difficult-to-remove scales at the eyelash bases with concomitant inflammation of the lid margin, and occasionally loss of eyelashes.
- Mixed blepharitis—presence of a staphylococcal infection complicating seborrhea of the eyelids.
- Parasitic blepharitis—inflammation of the eyelids due to infestation by crab lice (*Pediculus pubis*) or head lice (*Pediculus capitis*).

PATHOPHYSIOLOGY

- There are several glands (meibomian glands, pilosebaceous glands of Zeiss, and the apocrine glands of Moll) that exit along the eyelid margin. These glands produce the lipid component of tears.
- When these glands become infected or dysfunctional, the clinical features notable for blepharitis may occur.
- Spread of bacteria to the glands of Zeiss or the meibomian glands can lead to development of a hordeolum or stye.
- Staphylococcal exotoxins can lead to conjunctivitis or keratitis.

EPIDEMIOLOGY

Atopic or allergic contact dermatitis as a cause of blepharitis occurs in up to 65% of patients.

COMPLICATIONS

- Loss of eyelashes (madarosis) from traction of hair due to rubbing
- Hordeolum (stye)
- Conjunctivitis
- Keratitis
- Chalazion

PROGNOSIS

- Blepharitis is frequently a chronic and relapsing process.
- With appropriate treatment, symptoms may resolve within a week.

 Differential Diagnosis

- Atopic or contact dermatitis
- Psoriasis
- Rosacea (usually accompanied by dilated telangiectasia of the blood vessels in the lid margins, cheeks, nose, and chin)
- Dacryostenosis
- Acute conjunctivitis (bacteria, viral, or allergic)

 Data Gathering

HISTORY

Ask about:

- History of previous inflammation of eyelid margins, or presence of symptoms for a prolonged period of time
- Pruritus
- Use of any medications or products (i.e., contacts lens, soaps, or makeup) used on or around the eye
- Frequent rubbing of the eye or contact with eyelids by hands
- Hand-washing practices
- Cleansing of eyelids
- Past medical and family histories of atopy
- Seasonal variation of symptoms (suggests allergic etiology)
- History of lice

 Physical Examination

- Evaluate eyelid margins and eyelashes for crust, erythema, loss of hair, and ulceration. With chronic infection, you may see thickening of the eyelid margin. With herpes simplex viral infection, you may see grouped vesicles along the eyelid.
- Evaluate remainder of eye, particularly the conjunctiva and sclera, for evidence of inflammation or infection.
- Examine the scalp and skin of the head for evidence of seborrhea, atopic dermatitis, contact dermatitis, louse infestation, or rosacea.

 Laboratory Aids

- Laboratory testing is only indicated in cases that do not respond to treatment.
- Bacterial or viral culture of the lid margins
- Giemsa staining of conjunctival scrapings—may show the presence of neutrophils, which is useful in cases where cultures do not conclusively show signs of infection.

Therapy

- Eyelid margin cleansing twice daily is considered first-line therapy.

—First a warm compress should be placed over closed eyelids for 5 to 10 minutes to loosen debris.
—Next the eyelid margins should be cleansed with a dilute mixture of baby shampoo (brands that do not irritate the eyes) and water.
—Commercial eyelid cleansers are also available.

- In cases associated with seborrhea, treatment of the accompanying scalp and eyebrow involvement should be initiated with selenium sulfide shampoo once to twice a week, with manual removal of the crusting in those areas with a fine-toothed comb or soft bristle brush.
- More resistant cases, or those that fail the above treatments, can be treated with application of a topical antibiotic ointment with efficacy against staphylococcal species (e.g., bacitracin or erythromycin ophthalmic ointment) for 1 to 2 weeks.
- The most severe cases, particularly those associated with rosacea, may need to be treated with an oral antibiotic.

Follow-Up

- Once symptoms have resolved, there is no need for routine follow-up of blepharitis.
- If symptoms begin to recur, encourage early initiation of eyelid hygiene with the soap and water wash.

PREVENTION

- Treat seborrheic dermatitis of scalp early.
- Discourage eye rubbing in patients.
- Encourage frequent hand washing for children.
- For children with allergic symptoms, oral antihistamines can decrease rubbing of their eyes.

Common Questions and Answers

Q: Is blepharitis contagious?
A: Blepharitis is not spread to other family members. However, the bacteria that can cause the infection are frequently transmitted by hand contact, so frequent hand washing is recommended.

Q: Will this problem happen again?
A: Blepharitis may recur. In cases of children with seborrhea and atopic dermatitis, treatment of these conditions can limit the frequency of flare-ups. Early eyelid hygiene can limit the severity of future recurrences.

ICD-9-CM 373.00

BIBLIOGRAPHY

Baum J. Infections of the eye. *Clin Infect Dis* 1995;21:479–488.

Beltrani VS. Dermatologic disorders of the eyelids. *Immunol Allergy Clin North Am* 1997;17(1):103–129.

Carter SR. Eyelid disorders: diagnosis and management. *Am Fam Physician* 1998; 57(11):2695–2702.

Denton P, Barequet IS, O'Brien TP. Ocular infections: update on therapy. Therapy of infectious blepharitis. *Ophthalmol Clin North Am* 1999;12(1):9–14.

Hara JH. The red eye: diagnosis and treatment. *Am Fam Physician* 1996;54(8): 2423–2430.

Shields SR. Managing eye disease in primary care: part 2. How to recognize and treat common eye problems. *Postgrad Med* 2000;108(5):83–96.

Author: Lee R. Atkinson

Bone Marrow/Stem Cell Transplantation

 Database

DEFINITION

Reconstitution of damaged, defective, or infiltrated bone marrow with IV infusion of hematopoietic progenitor (stem) cells from:

- The patient (autologous)
- An identical twin (syngeneic)
- A histocompatible donor (allogeneic)

INDICATIONS

Accepted indications if a human leukocyte antigen (HLA) identical sibling is available:

- Acute lymphoblastic leukemia (ALL) in second complete remission (CR) and in certain patients in first CR (Philadelphia chromosome positive ALL)
- Acute myelogenous leukemia in first CR
- Chédiak-Higashi and other severe neutrophil defects
- Chronic myelogenous leukemia (CML) when in the chronic phase and within a year from time of diagnosis
- Congenital bone marrow failure syndromes
- Diamond-Blackfan anemia (resistant to medical therapy)
- Schwachman-Diamond syndrome (resistant to therapy)
- Fanconi anemia
- Juvenile myelomonocytic leukemia (formerly called JCML)
- Lymphoma after second CR
- Myelodysplastic syndromes
- Myelofibrosis
- Osteopetrosis
- Severe aplastic anemia
- SLE especially if unresponsive or intolerant to conventional medical therapy
- Severe combined immunodeficiency and other congenital immunodeficiencies
- Thalassemia major (treatment of choice in Italy)
- Wiskott-Aldrich syndrome

Autologous transplantation is an accepted treatment for lymphoma in second CR and for high-risk or stage IV solid tumors in CR or very good partial response.
Tandem autologous peripheral stem cell transplants also are under investigation for treatment of high-risk neuroblastoma, PNET, brain tumors.
Also under investigation:

- Sickle cell disease: A national trial is studying bone marrow transplant (BMT) in patients who have developed significant sequelae, such as stroke, severe, multiple pain episodes or acute chest syndrome. European investigators have successfully performed BMT on asymptomatic patients, but the risk/benefit ratio is unknown.
- Mucopolysaccharidoses, lipidoses, and mucolipidoses

BMT can lead to restoration of enzymatic activity in white cells and removal of accumulated substrate in affected tissues. In some diseases, such as adrenoleukodystrophy (childhood onset), it has been successful. In others, such Krabbe disease (infantile form), it has been a failure. Of concern is that improvement in organ function has not always led to improvement in intellectual function.

DONOR SELECTION (IN ORDER OF PREFERENCE)

- Identical twin: The increased risk of relapse of leukemia is offset by decreased treatment-related mortality.
- HLA identical sibling
- Other family members
- Rarely (i.e., in 5% of families), a nonsibling relative who is phenotypically mismatched for one antigen will be found. Such transplantations have comparable results to HLA-identical sibling BMT.
- Haploidentical transplantations (2 or 3 HLA-antigen mismatch) have been performed but require depletion of T cells from the graft to avoid fatal graft-versus-host disease (GVHD). T-cell depletion can help prevent or ameliorate GVHD, but T-cell depletion can cause graft failure, delay in immunologic recovery, and/or loss of graft versus leukemia (GVL) effect. Haploidentical transplantations are associated with a lower survival than conventional BMT.
- Unrelated donors

- Autologous (either peripheral stem cells or bone marrow)—Peripheral blood or bone marrow stem cells are provided by the patient in remission.
- Gene-marking studies have shown that infused marrow containing tumor can contribute to relapse. To ensure that the graft stem cells do not contain viable tumor cells, the stem cells undergo purging or positive selection prior to infusion into the recipient. However, these methods still need to be improved.

NONMYELOABLATIVE TRANSPLANTS

- Use less cytotoxic preparative regimens
- Require immunosuppression of host and a generous infusion of hematopoietic stem cells
- Leads to mixed chimerism

PREPARATIVE REGIMENS (CONDITIONING)

- The purpose of conditioning (either chemoradiotherapy or chemotherapy alone) is threefold:

—To provide immune suppression in order to avoid destruction of the allograft by residual, immunologically active cells in the host
—To destroy any residual cancer cells
—To provide space for the new bone marrow to grow

- Agents used primarily for immunosuppression:

—Cyclophosphamide
—Antithymocyte globulin (ATG)

- Agents used primarily for antineoplastic effects or bone marrow ablation:

—Busulfan
—Cytarabine (ARA-C)
—Etoposide (VP-16)
—Carmustine (BCNU)
—Carboplatin
—Melphalan
—Agents used for both purposes:
—Total-body irradiation (TBI)
—Thiotepa

Note: Few randomized trials have compared one regimen to another. Choice depends on the disease being treated, the type of donor available, and previous treatment received.

STEM-CELL COLLECTION METHODS

- Conventional bone marrow

—Harvested from the posterior iliac crests under general anesthesia (alternative sites include anterior iliac crests, sternum).
—100–300 million stem cells per kilogram of the recipient's weight are harvested.
—T-cell depletion is performed on allografts to reduce risk of GVHD, but it increases risk of graft failure/rejection and of relapse in the patient with leukemia.
—Average time to engraftment is 12–28 days for allograft and 14–21 days for autograft.
—Peripheral blood stem-cell (PBSC) collections via apheresis
—Hematopoietic stem cells normally circulate in the peripheral blood in small numbers but can be mobilized by chemotherapy and/or growth factors (e.g., GM-CSF or G-CSF) and then collected by apheresis and cryopreserved.
—Autologous and allogeneic PBSC transplants have shorter time to engraftment than allogeneic bone marrow transplants, but have increased risk for more severe acute GVHD and chronic GVHD (but may have better GVL).
—Convincing survival advantage overall has not been demonstrated yet.
—Average time to engraftment is 14–15 days.

- Umbilical cord blood (UCB)

—A rich source of hematopoietic stem cells; 45 mL of cord blood can reconstitute the hematopoietic system of a child.
—Decreased incidence and severity of acute GVHD and chronic GVHD, but has longer engraftment time.
—Advantages: abundant source of stem cells is harvested at no risk to the mother or fetus; UCB is cryopreserved and banked, so it is available on demand; can target minority populations; do not "lose" donors because of increased donor age, the donor's developing a new medical conditional or donor geographic relocation.

—Disadvantages: limited number of hematopoietic stem cells in collected UCB may contribute to delay or failure of engraftment; newborn donor may have a medical condition affecting stem cells that has not been diagnosed; cannot collect additional donor stem cells for recipient experiencing graft failure; cannot collect donor lymphocytes for recipient who has relapsed.

TOXICITIES

Chemoradiotherapy

- Universal: nausea/vomiting/diarrhea, alopecia, pancytopenia
- Possible and agent-specific:
- TBI: skin erythema, parotitis
- Cyclophosphamide: hemorrhagic cystitis, SIADH, cardiomyopathy
- ATG: allergy, serum sickness
- Busulfan: seizures, pulmonary fibrosis, bronzing of the skin
- ARA-C: fever, neurologic symptoms, acute respiratory distress syndrome (ARDS)
- VP-16: allergic reactions
- BCNU: pulmonary fibrosis
- Graft failure

—Usually due to destruction of the graft by the immunologically active cells in the host
—Predisposing factors:
—Previous blood transfusions
—Less intensive high-dose preparative regimens
—Use of methotrexate rather than cyclosporine to prevent GVHD
—T-cell depletion of donor cells
—Can occur early (failure to engraft) or even after successful engraftment
—Rare in HLA-identical sibling transplantations
—Risk increases with unrelated donors (6%) or T-cell depletion (approximately 14% but depends on the degree of T-cell depletion and the use of ATG seems to decrease incidence of graft rejection markedly)
—Usually fatal

- Graft-versus-host disease (see chapter on GHVD)
- Infection: the major cause of nonrelapse mortality
- Immune dysfunction is caused by the period of severe myelosuppression immediately following stem cell transplant, lack of sustained transfer of clinically significant donor-derived B- and T-cell immunity, the recapitulation of normal lymphoid ontogeny, and the effects of GVHD and its treatment.

—In the first month posttransplantation, bacterial and fungal infections predominate. Use of prophylactic broad-spectrum antibiotics and fluconazole during the time of severe myelosuppression has helped considerably.

—In the second and third months, viral infections predominate, which include cytomegalovirus (CMV), adenovirus, herpesvirus, varicella virus, and polyomaviruses as well as PCP.
—After 3 months: herpes zoster and bacterial infections in patients with chronic GVHD
—Acyclovir is used prophylactically in patients who are HSV or VZV positive. Gancyclovir is used prophylactically in CMV seropositive donors or recipients, and is started 100 days after transplant because of drug-related neutropenia.

Note: After T-depleted transplantations, the risk of fatal Epstein-Barr virus infection is significant.

- Hepatic veno-occlusive disease

—Clinical criteria met when two of the following are present:
—Hepatomegaly and/or right upper quadrant pain
—Hyperbilirubinemia (>2.0 mg/dL)
—Greater than 5% weight gain and/or ascites
—Incidence of approximately 25% (range, 1–54%) and mortality of 30% (range, 3–67%) have been reported.
—Progressive hepatic failure and often renal failure develop in severely affected patients.
—Therapy is largely supportive. Currently, there is no definitive therapy.

- Interstitial pneumonitis

—Typically appears 40 to 80 days post-BMT as rapid-onset tachypnea, fever, and hypoxia associated with bilateral interstitial infiltrates
—Common etiologies include:

　—CMV
　—*Pneumocystis carinii*
　—Idiopathic: when no bacterial, viral, fungal, or protozoan cause is identified. Radiation to the lungs probably also plays a role.

LATE COMPLICATIONS

- Endocrine

—Hypothyroidism: seen in approximately 20% of patients after TBI; rare after chemotherapy alone
—Growth hormone deficiency: seen in over half of patients receiving TBI
—Primary gonadal failure and absence of development of secondary sexual characteristics are common, especially if the recipient was prepubertal at the time of transplantation or received TBI.

- Infertility: Sterility is expected after TBI; fertility may be preserved after cyclophosphamide alone.
- Ophthalmologic: Cataracts are seen in 40% of patients after TBI and in 20% after chemotherapy alone. A higher incidence is seen in those who also receive steroids.

- Dental: Poor calcification of teeth and root blunting have been seen. The defects are more severe in children younger than age 7 at transplantation.
- Renal

—Radiation nephritis
—Hemolytic uremic syndrome and thrombocytopenic purpura occur, especially during treatment with cyclosporine

- Secondary malignancies: Fifteen-year cumulative incidence rates are 20% and 6% after regimens with and without TBI, respectively.
- Recurrent leukemia—current treatment options include donor leukocyte infusions to induce GVL effect, nonmyeloablative "mini"-transplants, or full allogeneic bone marrow transplant.
- Intellectual function: Few prospective studies published

 ## Common Questions and Answers

Q: When should I immunize a patient after transplantation?
A: At 1 year post-BMT, patients free of chronic GVHD should begin a primary immunization schedule with DPT and Salk polio; at 1–2 years, HiB, hepatitis B, pneumovax, and prevnar. MMR is usually given at 2 years post-BMT. Influenza vaccine should be given after 1 year and then annually.

Q: If my patient relapses after BMT, can a second BMT be done?
A: Previously, there were few therapeutic options for patients who relapsed less than 1 year post-BMT. Remissions after an infusion of buffy coat (containing T cells) from the patient's donor, called donor leukocyte infusion, have been achieved. Although the majority of successful infusions have been in patients with CML, success has also been seen in acute leukemia. Chronic GVHD will often result.

ICD-9-CM 996.85

BIBLIOGRAPHY

Cutler C, Antin JH. Peripheral blood stem cells for allogeneic transplantation: a review. *Stem Cells* 2001;19:108–117.

Laughlin MJ. Umbilical cord blood for allogeneic transplantation in children and adults. *Bone Marrow Transplant* 2001;27:1–6.

Sanders JE. Bone marrow transplantation for pediatric malignancies. *Pediatr Clin North Am* 1997;44(4):1005–1020.

Author: Valerie I. Brown

Botulism

 Database

DEFINITION

An illness produced by neurotoxins elaborated by *Clostridium botulinum,* which causes an acute, descending, flaccid paralysis. The neurotoxin may be ingested or absorbed from infected wounds, or ingested spores germinate, producing toxin. There are three types of illness:

- In infant botulism, ingested spores germinate and colonize the infant's colon and elaborate toxin.
- In adults, the patient ingests preformed toxin while eating improperly prepared or stored foodstuffs.
- In wound botulism, spores germinate in an infected wound and toxin is absorbed.

CAUSES

C. botulinum, the etiologic agent, is a gram-positive, spore-forming, obligate anaerobic bacteria that is found in soil throughout the world.

PATHOPHYSIOLOGY

- Neurotoxin is taken up by nerve endings and irreversibly blocks acetylcholine release in peripheral cholinergic synapses.
- Cranial nerves are usually affected first and most severely, leading to difficulty swallowing and loss of airway protective reflexes. Respiratory failure develops.
- Botulinum toxin does not cross the blood–brain barrier; therefore, the sensorium remains clear.
- Recovery occurs with the regeneration of terminal motor neurons and the formation of new motor end plates.
- Infants are particularly prone to colonic colonization with *C. botulinum.* When foods other than breast milk are introduced in breast-fed infants, changes in flora may be especially important.

EPIDEMIOLOGY

- *Infant botulism* occurs in the first year of life, with more than 95% of cases reported in the first 6 months.
- Infants are usually white, breast-fed, and from middle-class families. Infants who have less than one bowel movement per day may be at increased risk. Cases are seen more frequently in rural and suburban areas.
- Most cases have been reported in California, Utah, and Pennsylvania.
- There often is a history of a recent change in feeding practice (addition of formula or solids or changing from breast- to bottle-feeding).
- Honey seems to be a particularly contaminated food and has been implicated in California. Corn syrup has also been reported to contain botulinum spores but much less frequently than honey and has been associated with significantly fewer cases of infant botulism.
- Breast-fed infants get ill at an older age than do bottle-fed infants; all cases of sudden infant death syndrome (SIDS) associated with infant botulism have been in bottle-fed infants.
- *Food-borne* cases are usually associated with the use of home-processed foods—especially vegetables, fruits, and condiments.
- *Wound botulism* is very rare.

COMPLICATIONS

- The most serious and fatal complication is respiratory failure due to paralysis of the respiratory muscles.
- Bulbar dysfunction in infant botulism may lead to dehydration before presentation.
- The loss of airway protective reflexes can lead to aspiration and pneumonia.
- Constipation and urinary retention may precede the onset of paralysis and may complicate later management as well. Cases of severe *Clostridium difficile* enterocolitis with hypovolemia, hypotension and prolonged ICU stays have been reported in infants with botulism.
- The earliest symptoms in adults and older children may be visual changes, including blurred vision, loss of accommodation, and diplopia.
- SIADH and urinary tract infections have been reported in infants with infant botulism.

PROGNOSIS

- *Food-borne* botulism carries a mortality rate of 20% to 25%. This rate is lower in patients younger than 20 years old (about 10%).
- Patients with a shorter incubation period usually have more severe involvement and a worse prognosis, probably related to an increased amount of toxin ingested.
- If recognized early and treated aggressively, botulism carries a good prognosis, and complete recovery can be expected. Fatigability may persist for up to 1 year.
- *Infant botulism* has an estimated mortality rate of less than 5% in hospitalized patients. Complete recovery can be expected when disease is recognized early and treated appropriately.

 Differential Diagnosis

INFECTIONS

- In noninfants, bacterial sepsis, meningitis, poliomyelitis, tick paralysis, and diphtheric polyneuritis.
- In infants, sepsis and meningitis may present in a similar way.

—Absence of fever and a clear sensorium make sepsis and meningitis less likely.

NEUROLOGIC

- Myasthenia gravis usually spares the pupillary response, while it is fatigable in botulism, if not absent.
- In Werdnig-Hoffman disease (type I spinal muscle atrophy), facial muscles are spared.

TOXINS

Drug ingestions may lead to weakness and lethargy.

 Data Gathering

HISTORY

- Usually constipation. With a progressive course of lethargy, weakness, and poor feeding.

—Occasionally, the progression may be quite rapid, and the abrupt onset of lethargy and weakness may suggest the diagnosis of bacterial sepsis or meningitis.

- *Food-borne* cases result in complaints of emesis in about 50% of patients.

—There may initially be complaints of diarrhea followed by constipation.
—The incubation period from ingestion to the onset of symptoms is usually 18 to 36 hours (range, a few hours to several days).
—Patients complain of weakness and dry mouth.
—Visual complaints include blurry vision, loss of accommodation, and diplopia.
—Patients may complain of dysphagia or dysarthria.
—Patients may have urinary retention.
—Fever is absent.
—Within 3 days, there is the onset of the characteristic descending, symmetrical paralysis. The cranial nerves are usually affected first.
—Mentation is clear, except for understandable anxiety and agitation.

- *Wound botulism* has an incubation period of 4 to 14 days.

—Fever may or may not be present.
—Patients often report constipation but rarely nausea or vomiting.
—They may complain of unilateral sensory changes and of purulent discharge from the wound.

Physical Examination

- Older children and adults often appear alert and are afebrile.
- Ptosis, extraocular palsies, and fixed and dilated pupils are often the first signs of descending paralysis. Loss of airway protective reflexes and respiratory muscle weakness lead to respiratory failure.

- The triad of bulbar palsies, a lucid sensorium, and the absence of fever should prompt one to strongly consider the diagnosis of botulism.
- Infant botulism presents in a similar way. Patients are usually afebrile. They are usually weak, with decreased spontaneous activity at presentation. They have an expressionless (masklike) face, ptosis, a weak cry, poor head control, and generalized weakness and hypotonia.
- Pupils are often midposition initially and may be at least weakly reactive. The pupillary response is fatigable. The pupils become fixed and dilated for a period in many cases. Except for the symmetric, descending paralysis, the remainder of the physical examination is normal.
- Signs of autonomic instability include unexpected fluctuations in skin color, blood pressure, and heart rate.

PHYSICAL EXAMINATION TRICK

In infants, early in the course of the disease, pupillary and corneal reflexes may fatigue easily.

Laboratory Aids

TESTS

- Tests for the presence of toxin or the organism can be conducted on patient samples (serum, gastric aspirates, feces, or wound exudate) or suspected foodstuffs.
- Anaerobic cultures of a wound or the GI tract may yield the organism.
- Electromyography (EMG) shows a characteristic pattern of brief duration, sharp amplitude, overly abundant motor unit action potentials (brief short-acting potentials, BSAPs).
- EEG, MRI, and CT are nonspecific and usually normal in the absence of any complications.

Requirements for Testing

- Most tests for toxin and cultures are conducted by state health departments.
- The most common test performed is an assay for botulinum toxin in stool.
- Specimens must be shipped in sealed, break-proof, and leak-proof containers. Even small amounts of toxin, if inhaled or ingested, can lead to disease.
- Suspect foods should be shipped refrigerated and in their original containers if possible.

Emergency Care

- Good supportive care with emphasis on respiratory support, including intubation and mechanical ventilation when needed, is the most important consideration in emergency therapy.
- In suspected infant botulism, aminoglycoside antibiotics (e.g., gentamicin) should be avoided as they may produce an abrupt worsening of the weakness and ensuing respiratory failure.

Therapy

- All patients with suspected botulism should be admitted to the hospital and have continuous monitoring of their heart rate, respiratory rate, and oxygenation, as well as frequent assessment of their respiratory effort and airway protective reflexes.
- The mainstay of therapy is meticulous supportive care. Particular attention is paid to respiratory and nutritional needs.
- Endotracheal intubation may be necessary both for patients with frank respiratory failure and when airway protective reflexes are lost.
- Wounds should be explored and debrided, and anaerobic cultures should be obtained.
- Cases of suspected toxin ingestion should be treated early with induced emesis and/or gastric lavage in an attempt to decrease toxin exposure.
- All cases should be reported to the state health department and the CDC.

DRUGS

- Antibiotics are not helpful in infant botulism.
- Equine antitoxin is not recommended for infant botulism.
- Antibiotics are indicated only for documented complications such as pneumonia.
- Cathartics are not beneficial, and enemas may cause colonic distention and increased toxin absorption.
- Cases of botulism resulting from *ingested toxin* or *wound infection* should be treated with botulism equine trivalent antitoxin (ABE), available from the CDC. Antitoxin should not be administered to asymptomatic individuals who have only eaten suspect foods.
- Wound botulism should be treated with IV penicillin G 250,000 units/kg/d.

DURATION

- In wound botulism, antibiotics should be continued for 10 to 14 days.
- Supportive care should be continued until the patient is able to be weaned from respiratory support and begin PO feedings.

Follow-Up

The nadir of the paresis in infants is usually 1 to 2 weeks after presentation. Infants remain at their nadir for 1 to 3 weeks. Infants are ready for discharge when gag, suck, and swallow reflexes are adequate to protect against aspiration. In food-borne and wound botulism, recovery may be prolonged, with symptoms of fatigability persisting for up to 1 year.

PREVENTION

- Botulinum toxin is heat-labile; 5 minutes of boiling will destroy the toxin.
- Home-canned foods should be boiled for at least 10 minutes before serving.
- Spores are more resistant to heat. Home canners must use temperatures well above boiling to destroy spores effectively (120°C for 30 minutes). Pressure cookers are needed to achieve these conditions.

Common Questions and Answers

Q: Can infant botulism recur?
A: True recurrence in infant botulism has not been documented.

Q: Should antitoxin be given to persons who have ingested food that they think might be contaminated with botulinum toxin?
A: Since the antitoxin carries a significant risk of serum sickness, it should be given only to persons with neurologic symptoms.

Q: Where is antitoxin obtained?
A: Antitoxin may be obtained from the Centers for Disease Control and Prevention, Atlanta, Georgia; 404-639-3753 (days), 404-639-2888 (nights).

ICD-9-CM 005.1

BIBLIOGRAPHY

Muensterer OJ. Infant botulism. *Pediatr Rev* 2000;21(12):427.

Passaro DJ, Werner SB, Mcgee J, et al. Wound botulism associated with black tar heroin among injecting drug users. *JAMA* 1998;279:859–863.

Shapiro RL, Hatheway C, Swerdlow DL. Botulism in the United States: a clinical and Epidemiologic review. *Ann Intern Med* 1998;129:221–228.

Author: James M. Callahan

Brachial Plexus Palsy

 Database

DEFINITION

Weakness or paralysis of muscles of shoulder girdle, arms, or hand. The brachial plexus is a network of peripheral nerves derived usually from the ventral rami of the fifth cervical through the first thoracic nerve roots, forming three trunks from the five roots.

CLINICAL-ANATOMIC RELATIONSHIPS

• 5th and 6th cervical (C5, C6) nerve roots fuse to form the upper trunk of the plexus.

—C5 impairment causes arm abduction (deltoid and supraspinatus) weakness, while C6 causes elbow flexion (mainly biceps) and partial supination (supinator) weakness.
—If the lesion is at the C5, C6 root level or very proximal upper trunk, then winging of the scapula (serratus anterior) occurs. The biceps and brachioradialis deep tendon reflexes (DTRs) are depressed or absent.

• 7th cervical (C7) nerve root alone forms the middle trunk of the plexus and is largely responsible for elbow extension (triceps), wrist extension and flexion (extensor carpi ulnaris and flexor carpi radialis), and finger extension (extensor digitorum).
• 8th cervical (C8) and 1st thoracic (T1) nerve roots fuse to form the lower trunk of the plexus and innervate the intrinsic hand muscles responsible for grip and thumb opposition/abduction. The triceps DTR reflects the C7, C8 roots, but is difficult to obtain in newborns. The pectoralis DTR has the same distribution and is easier to elicit.

CAUSES

Traumatic

• The most common etiology which occurs in infancy and childhood.

Neonatal Brachial Plexus Injury

• Erbs palsy is the most commonly encountered partial lesion of the plexus seen in children, accounting for approximately 73–90% of all newborn cases, and occurs in approximately 1 in 1,000 live births.

—Risk factors: mainly large for gestational age and shoulder dystocia.
—Not all cases are due to a traumatic delivery; antepartum compressive causes are well described in a minority of cases.

1) Mild Approximately half of patients have a mild injury, with mild to moderate weakness, but usually not full flaccidity after birth.

—All have at least antigravity strength in the affected muscles by age 2 weeks.
—Full recovery between 2 weeks and 2 months of age.

2) Moderate Another third of babies with a moderate injury are very weak to fully flaccid at birth, and have less than antigravity strength at 2 weeks of age, but do develop at least antigravity strength in shoulder abduction and elbow flexion/extension within 4.5 months (50% at 2.3 months and 79% by 3 months).

—Will eventually recover full functional strength, although this may take up to 15 months (mean age 7.5 months).

3) Severe Remaining 10% to 15% is the most severely affected group, with a full flaccid paralysis at birth and less than antigravity deltoid and biceps strength elicited at 2 weeks.

—By 6 months antigravity strength may have evolved in elbow flexion and extension but not in the deltoid.
—Ipsilateral diaphragm weakness is seen in about 5%, due to phrenic nerve (C4, C5) compromise. Bilateral arm weakness, typically asymmetric in degree, is noted in about 10%. Associated subluxation of the cervical spine and related spinal cord injury is identified in about 5%. Torticollis and facial palsy are seen in about 10%.
—Ultimately, there is very poor arm abduction and weak elbow flexion/extension.
—If severe wrist and finger extensor weakness is present at 6 months, there is little chance that a good functional recovery will occur spontaneously.

• Rarely, the lower trunk (C8 and T1 roots) portion of the plexus is solely involved (Klumpkes palsy), resulting in a weak hand grip and absent palmar grasp reflex, with preserved shoulder and arm strength.

—It occurs more in breech and face presentation deliveries.

• Inherited

—Neuralgic amyotrophy with predilection for the brachial plexus

—Autosomal-dominant inherited condition that maps to a chromosome 17q25.1 locus.
—Episodes of recurrent unilateral or bilateral brachial neuritis begin in childhood and are characterized by recurrent pain followed by weakness, with sensory impairment and absent reflexes.
—There may be mild lumbar involvement or dysmorphic features.
—Attacks are often triggered by recent infection or immunization. It remits spontaneously over weeks to months.
—Hereditary neuropathy with liability to pressure palsy is an autosomal-dominant inherited disorder

—Deletion of the peripheral myelin protein 22 gene. The myelin sheath is particularly sensitive to sustained pressure, resulting in painless weakness that slowly recovers.

Inflammatory

—Postinfectious brachial neuritis:
—Reported following EBV, CMV, and herpes zoster infection.
—Spontaneous recovery with supportive care is the rule.
—Postimmunization brachial neuritis: Only the tetanus toxoid component of the DPT immunization has been clearly associated with brachial neuropathy in infants. It resolves fully, but may recur with future such immunizations.

 Differential Diagnosis

• Lesions of the brain and spinal cord can produce focal weakness in mainly one limb. Usually the ipsilateral leg will have at least mild findings to indicate a hemiparesis.
• The pattern of weakness and hyperreflexia distinguish a central brain or spinal cord lesion from a peripheral nerve, root or plexus lesion.
• Congential malformations and contractures may mimic a BPP.

 Data Gathering

HISTORY

• Birth history, birth weight
• Recent viral infection
• Recent tetanus injection

PHYSICAL EVALUATION

• Testing of tone, strength, muscle bulk, joint range of motion, sensation, muscle stretch reflexes (DTRs), diaphragm excursion, pupil size, pulses, and perfusion of the affected limb.
• Sensory loss is difficult to assess when only part of the plexus is impaired, because of overlap of dermatomes.
• **Erbs palsy**
—Upper trunk of the plexus is typically traumatized, sometimes also with C5, C6 root avulsion.
—Arm hangs limply at the shoulder, adducted and internally rotated, the elbow extended and the forearm pronated.
—Hand grip is preserved.
—Sensory impairment is often present over the lateral deltoid.
—The biceps and brachioradialis muscle stretch reflexes are unelicitable.
—The triceps reflex is preserved (difficult to elicit in normal neonates). Testing the pectoralis reflex is preferred. The Moro reflex is asymmetric.

Klumpkes palsy
- Lower trunk of the plexus is traumatized, often with C8, T1 root avulsion
- Elbow flexion, supination of the forearm, wrist and finger extension, and an odd cupped-hand position.

—Triceps jerk is often absent.
—Sensation may be impaired in the C8-T1 dermatomes.
—An ipsilateral Horner sign (ptosis and miosis) indicates T1 involvement.
—With **a complete lesion of the plexus,** the entire upper limb and shoulder girdle is flaccid, anesthetic, and areflexic

Laboratory Tests

For complicated cases

- Chest and arm radiograph

—Identifies subluxation of the spine, fracture of the humerus or clavicle, and diaphragmatic palsy
—Imaging of the cervical spinal cord, nerve roots, and plexus
—Often valuable in identifying the nature and extent of injury and is useful in the more severely affected patient when surgery is being planned.
—High-resolution MRI has now largely replaced the CT-myelogram.

- There are occasional false positive and negative findings for root avulsion on MRI
- Electromyography (EMG) and nerve conduction velocity studies (NCV) can confirm the localization of the lesion.

—Sometimes the timing of the lesion can be estimated.
—Acute denervation is usually not evident on EMG until 10 to 21 days after the injury and reinnervation often takes 3 months to evolve.
—Less useful early after a traumatic insult in determining the prognosis, but can be helpful after 3 months or postoperatively.

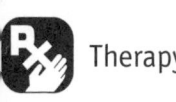 ## Therapy

For severe injury
Mild weakness will recover in most cases without special treatment

- Flaccid shoulder girdle
- *Immobilization:* babies should have the limb partly immobilized for 2 weeks, to prevent further traction injury on the plexus.
- Cuff can be pinned to the midline of the jersey at the umbilicus level.
- Caregivers should be instructed in proper lifting and positioning techniques to avoid pressure at the axilla.

- *Passive range of motion stretching:* After 3 weeks, physiotherapy should be initiated with gentle passive range of motion.
- Fracture needs to be excluded on x-ray.
- Regular visits to a pediatric occupational or physiotherapist are necessary.
- *Electrical muscle stimulation:* External and implantable devices that directly stimulate muscle can prevent atrophy while awaiting nerve healing and reinnervation. This may hasten recovery of strength and function, although the data are limited and there is no consensus at present regarding selection of patients for this treatment.
- *Surgical issues:* Important to identify as early as possible those babies who are not likely to spontaneously recover normal strength and function, so that a surgical referral can be considered. Serial exams between 1 and 6 months of age and sometimes EMG testing at 3 to 6 months can estimate prognosis.
- When there is no movement in the deltoid and biceps muscles at 3 months and the EMG shows ongoing active denervation without reinnervation features, the prospect of spontaneous recovery to a functional level is poor.
- Early surgical intervention at that time may be warranted in this setting, particularly if there is full plexus involvement.
- When there is some movement at 3 months and slow but steady improvement is seen, then defer the decision about referral to surgeon until 6 months of age.
- Good functional recovery is unlikely to then occur spontaneously if strength is still less than antigravity in the deltoid-biceps, progress has plateaued, and there is little reinnervation on EMG.
- Critical window of time to consider surgical intervention is at 3 months when the deltoid-biceps remain flaccid and between 6 and 12 months when at least some early recovery of strength is seen.

 ## Follow-Up

- The newborn with BPP should be reevaluated at 2 weeks and if not nearly back to normal, then referred for occupational or physical therapy and seen again at 3 months.
- When steady improvement is noted between 2 weeks and 3 months, the patient is monitored closely with the following prognostic guidelines kept in mind as to whether full functional recovery is likely to occur spontaneously or whether an operation may be indicated between 6 and 18 months of age.

PROGNOSIS

- Peripheral nerve stretch injury has the most favorable prognosis.
- Axonal disruption with preserved continuity of the nerve sheath (axonotmesis), can recover fully, but is more variable and tends to take longer as axonal regrowth is about 1 mm/day. If the nerve is ruptured and not in continuity (neurotmesis), the prognosis is very poor. Lesions of mixed and partial types can result in recovery occurring in phases.
- Nerve root avulsion from the spinal cord harbors the worst prognosis.
- Full recovery to normal reported has been reported in 69% to 95% of patients, and up to 90% of these babies do so by 4 months of age.
- Pure C5, C6 Erbs palsy patients do the best as a group.
- Prognosis is more guarded when C7 is involved.
- Involvement of the whole plexus or C8, T1 (Klumpkes palsy) distribution fares least well.

—Significant permanent weakness occurs in 3% to 16%.

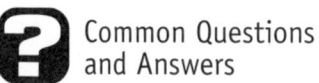 ## Common Questions and Answers

Q: Will my baby get better?
A: The majority of babies gain full recovery, but this may take several weeks or months. S/he will need to be followed closely to monitor the progress and determine if any therapy or future testing will be necessary.

Q: What if my baby does not get better?
A: About one in seven babies have poor or limited recovery within the first few months, in which case we would consider seeing if a surgeon can try to fix the nerves or improve function by tendon transfers.

ICD-9-CM 767.6, ERB'S PALSY

BIBLIOGRAPHY

Useful Web sites for Erb's and brachial plexus lesions include *www.ubpn.org, www.ninds.gov* (see NINDS Brachial Plexus Information Page) and *www.injurednewborn.com.*

Semin Pediatr Neurol 2000;7(1). This entire issue is devoted to the evaluation and management of brachial plexus injuries in the newborn and child.

Author: Richard S. Finkel

Brain Abscess

Database

DEFINITION

A suppurative infection involving the brain parenchyma; it may be a single (or multiple) lesion.

CAUSES

- Bacteria are the most common causes of brain abscesses.
- *Streptococcus* sp. and *Staphylococcus* sp. are the two most common cultured microorganisms.
- Neonates may develop abscesses after a gram-negative meningitis (*Proteus* and *Citrobacter*).
- A single organism is found in about 70% of patients.
- Anaerobic organisms are being found with increasing incidence with improved laboratory and culture techniques.
- Parasitic infections are often caused by *Taenia solium* (neurocysticercosis).
- Fungi and protozoa are common with immunocompromised patients.

PATHOPHYSIOLOGY

- Microorganisms enter the brain parenchyma by contiguous or hematogenous (metastasis) pathways.

LOCATION OF BRAIN ABSCESSES

- Cyanotic congenital heart disease patients tend to have abscesses within the middle meningeal artery distribution: frontal, parietal, and temporal lobes.
- Frontal abscesses are commonly seen with frontal sinusitis.
- Temporal, parietal, or cerebellar abscesses tend to occur with mastoiditis or otitis media infections.
- Brain abscesses can occur anywhere in the brain parenchyma regardless of a predisposing risk factor secondary to hematogenous metastasis.

PREDISPOSING RISK FACTORS

- Cyanotic congenital heart disease (CCHD)
- Otorhinolaryngologic infections such as sinusitis, mastoiditis, chronic otitis media, or cholesteatomas
- Meningitis (especially with neonates)
- Penetrating head trauma
- Surgical manipulation of the brain (ventriculoperitoneal shunts, tumor removal, etc.)
- Esophageal manipulation (sclerotherapy or dilation)
- Cystic fibrosis
- Dental infections
- Lung infections
- Any site of infection (osteomyelitis, orbital, cellulitis, urinary tract infections, etc.)

- Patients who have traveled to endemic areas with neurocysticercosis (Latin America, parts of Africa, Asia, and the Indian subcontinent)
- Immunocompromised patients
- Unknown etiology is found in about 30% of patients

EPIDEMIOLOGY

- Incidence is about 2 to 3 per 10,000 general hospital admissions.
- A majority of children are male (2:1 male to female predominance).
- Average age of presentation is about 7 years of age.
- About 2–4% of children with CCHD will develop a brain abscess (tetralogy of Fallot is the most common CCHD).

COMPLICATIONS

- These arise from the location, size, and number of intracranial abscesses and can vary from SIADH, seizures, to focal neurologic deficits.

PROGNOSIS

- A high index of suspicion is required to diagnose a brain abscess. A delay in diagnosis or performing a lumbar puncture (LP) for suspected meningitis increases mortality and morbidity.
- With the advent of computed tomography (CT) and magnetic resonance imaging (MRI) scans, the mortality rate has dropped from 30% to <14%.
- Multiple abscesses, coma on presentation, less than 2 years of age, performance of an LP and rupture of abscess into the ventricle carries a higher mortality rate. About 30% to 40% of patients will have some morbidity. This ranges from seizures, hemiparesis, focal neurologic deficits, hydrocephalus to cognitive/behavior problems.

Differential Diagnosis

- Infectious: meningitis, encephalitis, subdural empyema, epidural abscess
- Vascular: Venous sinus thrombosis, migraine, cerebral infarct, cerebral hemorrhage
- Miscellaneous: Primary or secondary tumor, pseudotumor cerebri, hydrocephalus

Data Gathering

HISTORY

- It should be noted that the location of the brain abscess or abscesses will often influence the history of presentation and physical exam.
- Classic triad of fever, headache, and focal neurologic findings occurs in less than 30% of cases.
- Headache is the most common complaint.
- The average duration of symptoms prior to diagnosis is about 4 weeks.
- Vomiting and mental status changes can often be the presenting chief complaints.
- Neonates will often have a history of meningitis before developing a brain abscess.
- Questions should focus on acute or chronic otolaryngologic infections such as sinusitis, chronic otitis media and mastoiditis, as well as a history of cholesteatomas.
- Cyanotic congenital heart disease (CCHD) should be determined, as well as a partially repaired CCHD.

Physical Examination

- Neonates may present with a full fontanel, increasing head circumference, seizures, or vomiting.
- Older children may have signs of a focal neurologic deficit, hemiparesis, or even found to have papilledema.
- Meningeal signs may be diagnosed in about 30% of patients.
- Ataxia is seen with cerebellar lesions.

Brain Abscess

 ## Laboratory Aids

- CBC may be mildly elevated and less than 10% will show a left shift.
- Erythrocyte sedimentation rate (ESR) is a poor indicator of brain abscesses.
- Electrolytes may show low sodium, indicating SIADH.
- LP is contraindicated if any mass lesion is suspected, but if CSF is obtained, it may show a mild to moderate pleocytosis (20% of patients may have normal values); the opening pressure is always elevated; glucose may be decreased in 30% of patients; the protein is elevated in 70% of cases; and only 10% of cultures are positive, unless the abscess ruptures into the ventricles.

STUDIES

- CT and MRI scans are the studies of choice in diagnosing brain abscesses.

 ## Therapy

- Broad-spectrum antibiotics should be started at the time of diagnosis until identification of the microorganism is determined. At that time, the antibiotics can be tailored to the offending microorganism.
- Most brain abscesses are surgically removed. A few may require CT-guided aspiration.
- When multiple abscesses are found on CT scan, one lesion should be aspirated to determine the identification of the microorganism.
- There are patients successfully managed with antibiotics alone.
- Antiparasitic medications are controversial in the treatment of neurocysticercosis.
- Antifungals should be considered with immunocompromised patients.
- The use of steroids is controversial.
- If a patient is manifesting signs and symptoms of increased intracranial pressure (Cushing triad: bradycardia, hypertension, and abnormal respirations) or if the patient is comatose and is unable to protect his/her airway, the patient should be intubated, hyperventilated, and given mannitol.
- Those patients with unknown predisposing factors should be evaluated by cardiology, dental, and otorhinolaryngology.

 ## Follow-Up

- Neonates and older patients may be discharged with home physical therapy and home nursing for intravenous antibiotics.
- Patients will need intravenous antibiotics for a total of 3 to 4 weeks. Some may require longer courses of antibiotics.
- Some children will need follow-up CT scans.
- Follow-up with neurosurgical, rehabilitation, and neurology clinics are usually required.
- Some children may need in-patient rehabilitation services.

PREVENTION

- During recreational activities, wearing helmets may prevent penetrating head trauma.
- Preventive medicine: dentistry and otorhinolaryngology

PITFALLS

- About 40% of children will not have fevers.
- Failing to consider a brain abscess in a child with altered mental status, fevers, and meningismus
- LP is contraindicated with mass lesions.

 ## Common Questions and Answers

Q: Do all brain abscesses require surgery?
A: No. Some will regress with antibiotics and follow-up with MRI.

Q: What is the best way to diagnose brain abscess?
A: MRI.

ICD-9-CM 324.0

BIBLIOGRAPHY

Carmel PW. Purulent focal infections. In: Rudolph AM, ed. *Rudolph's pediatrics*, 19th ed. Stamford: Appleton and Lange, 1991: 1845–1849.

Cochrane DD. Brain abscess. *Pediatr Rev* 1999;20:209–214.

Jadavji T, Humphreys RP, Prober CG. Brain abscesses in infants and children. *Pediatr Infect Dis J* 1985;4:394–398.

Kaplan K. Brain abscess. In: Symposium on infections of the central nervous system. *Med Clin North Am* 1985;69:345–360.

Mitchell WG. Neurocysticercosis and acquired cerebral toxoplasmosis in children. *Semin Pediatr Neurol* 1999;6:267–277.

Patrick CC, Kaplan SL. Current concept in the pathogenesis and management of brain abscesses in children. In: New concepts in pediatric infectious disease. *Pediatr Clin North Am* 1988;35:625–636.

Renier D, Flandin C, Hirsch E, et al. Brain abscesses in neonates. *J Neurosurg* 1988;69:877–882.

Rennels MB, Woodward CL, Robinson WL, et al. Medical cure of apparent brain abscesses. *Pediatrics* 1983;72:220–224.

Saez-Llorens XJ, Umana MA, Odio CM, et al. Brain abscess in infants and children. *Pediatr Infect Dis J* 1989;8:449–458.

Yogev R. Focal suppurative infections of the central nervous system. In: Long SS, Pickering LK, Prober CG, eds. *Principles and practice of pediatric infectious diseases*, 1st ed. New York: Churchill Livingstone, 1997:349–358.

Author: Jeffrey P. Louie

Brain Injury—Traumatic

 Database

DEFINITION

Traumatic brain injury (TBI) is damage to the brain sustained as a result of accidental or nonaccidental trauma. Manifestations may include loss of consciousness, seizures, posturing, hemiparesis. Concussion implies a transient alteration in neural functioning, which frequently—but not necessarily—involves a loss of consciousness. Head injury frequently is associated with trauma to the face, neck, or spine without permanent brain injury.

PATHOPHYSIOLOGY

Rapid acceleration/deceleration injuries, causing cerebral contusions, skull fractures, diffuse axonal injury (DAI), and intracranial hematomas; cervical spine injuries; penetration injuries, causing brain lacerations; intracerebral hemorrhage. Secondary phenomena produced by alterations in cerebral perfusion, oxygenation, edema formation, etc.

Age-Specific Pathophysiology

Infants

- A large head causes vulnerability to injury (head size is 64% adult size at birth, 83% by 1 year, and 92% by 2 years).
- A deformable, expansile skull usually protects from herniation due to cerebral edema or hematoma.
- The most commonly seen injuries are shear injuries, contusions, and subdural hematomas (SDHs) secondary to venous sinus tears in nonaccidental trauma.
- The most common cause of head injury in infants (before capacity to ambulate is achieved) is nonaccidental trauma.
- Diffuse injuries secondary to shaken impact syndrome can lead to cerebral swelling with secondary infarction and/or decreased central respiratory control, leading to apnea, hypoxia, and cerebral edema.
- Birth trauma commonly results in subgaleal hematoma, cephalohematoma (below the periosteum), and caput succedaneum (confined to the superficial scalp).
- More severe birth trauma can result in SDH due to tearing of the dura of falx.

Children/Adolescents

- Usually due to falls and motor vehicle accidents
- Projectile injuries in adolescent population
- Can result from nonaccidental trauma (usually correlated with other stigmata of assault)

EPIDEMIOLOGY

- Incidence of general trauma is approximately 86 per 1,000, of which 50% is head trauma.
- In children, 2 years of age, falls are the most common cause of trauma.

ASSOCIATED CONDITIONS

- Intoxications (of child, caregiver, others in the environment)
- Physical abuse/neglect
- Epilepsy

 Differential Diagnosis

- Neurologic presentation varies in severity from a normal examination through coma similar to that of other hypoxic-ischemic brain injuries (e.g., near-drowning), other causes of stupor/coma, seizure activity (postictal encephalopathy).
- Distinction between simple concussion, DAI, and hypoxic-ischemic injury may be difficult at initial presentation but will clear as clinical picture/neuroimaging evolves.

 Data Gathering

HISTORY

- Eyewitness accounts are invaluable.
- A history of previous concussions or seizures
- Details of who was caring for the child
- Try to determine if the patient fell and injured the head or collapsed from a neurologic problem and fell with no additional injury.
- Although mild head injury [Glasgow coma score (GCS) of 13–15] was found to have no long-term effects on cognition in a large British study ($n = 513{,}000$), recent studies have found measurable impairments on detailed neuropsychiatric testing.
- Patients who have sustained moderate-to-severe head injury (GCS of 13) often have academic difficulties, memory abnormalities, disinhibition, and other complications as described above.
- Static encephalopathy after head injury can be manifested as any combination of learning disabilities, seizure disorder, speech disorder, memory disturbance, and visual/hearing loss.

 Physical Examination

- Stabilization of neck to avoid exacerbation of potential spine injury is an immediate concern once airway, breathing, and circulation are ensured.
- Elevation of the head to 30 degrees may help to alleviate intracranial hypertension.
- Vital sign changes indicative of Cushing reflex (bradycardia, hypertension, irregular respirations) suggest intracranial pressure/impending brain herniation; these signs warrant prompt intubation and IV access.
- A C-spine collar should be worn until x-ray studies are done and found to be negative.
- HEENT examination for ecchymoses, retinal hemorrhages, bullet holes, penetrating bone fragments, herniating brain, hemotympanum, CSF leak (nasal or otic)
- The postresuscitation GCS score should be recorded in all trauma patients.
- Neurologic examination should document responsiveness (to voice, touch, pain), resting posture (flaccid, extensor, flexor), spontaneous movements (convulsions, writhing/agitated movements, purposeful), and oculomotor findings (see below).
- When carefully documented over time, these observations provide far more useful information to other caregivers than do coma scores.
- Papilledema is a late finding with intracranial hypertension
- Pupils: Marked asymmetry suggests brain herniation causing third-nerve palsy (see Follow-Up section, Pitfalls). Reactivity of pupils is best examined through an otoscope.
- Eye movements: Dysconjugate gaze is common in the unconscious patient and may not indicate a focal structural problem or elevated ICP. Absence of contraversive, lateral movement of eyes with passive head-turning (doll's-eyes maneuver—if cervical spine has been cleared) suggests midbrain damage due to hemorrhage or axonal shear.
- Heart: Narrow pulse pressure or hypotension may be due to shock or pericardial tamponade. Bradycardia or irregular respirations may be due to intracranial hypertension.
- Careful examination for trauma or other clues: ecchymoses, open fractures, hematuria
- Remember to examine a patient after sufficient clearance times for chemical paralytics, sedatives, and narcotics.

Laboratory Aids

- An unenhanced CT scan of the brain is the imaging study of choice for initial evaluation of a patient with suspected traumatic brain injury.
- Three-view (AP, lateral, odontoid) C-spine plain films in any case of altered mental status or with a mechanism of injury that could produce cervical spine injury; any patient with cervical pain after trauma
- Many trauma centers now obtain fine-cut CT scans with 3-D reconstructions of the cervical spine in patients rather than plain films since the later may be difficult to accomplish (e.g., in a large patient with high shoulders).
- Long-bone films if degree of injury is not consistent with history or history of fall from unclear height
- With CT scan showing normal brain/ventricular spaces: consider EEG and lumbar puncture if a nontraumatic etiology for altered mental status is suspected.
- In all patients with suspected traumatic brain injury, one should obtain:

—CBC (infants can have a large amount of intracranial blood loss)
—PT/PTT (to evaluate a possible bleeding disorder as a possible preoperative laboratory test)
—Electrolytes

HINTS

- Unenhanced CT: first-line study in all patients with LOC or focal neurologic findings
- MRI: useful for DAI (with a negative head CT) as well as showing small lesions (e.g., punctate contusions)
- EEG: to evaluate suspected seizures
- Audiometry: especially with speech delay after head trauma
- CSF tracer study: CSF leaks, not responding to head elevation, lumbar drainage

Therapy

- Studies in adults showed no prophylactic benefit to phenytoin beyond 1 week postinjury.
- Once laboratory values are obtained, appropriate corrective measures should be undertaken as needed (e.g., packed RBC or platelet transfusion, fluid restriction).
- Anticonvulsants may be used in those with persistent coma and elevated intracranial pressure (ICP), and in those with intracranial hemorrhage, since seizures cause ICP spikes. Otherwise, anticonvulsant therapy is reserved for children with documented seizure(s).
- Consultations.

Emergency Care

- Immobilize C-spine in a firm (e.g., Philadelphia or Aspen) collar until radiographic and clinical clearance of fracture/dislocations/soft tissue injuries can be accomplished.
- Radiologic findings may prompt specific interventions, including:

—Normal CT scan: consider a neurosurgery consultation, close monitoring overnight with frequent neurologic checks, seizure precautions
—Abnormal CT scan showing structural injury, including cerebral edema, hemorrhage, hypodense white matter: mandatory neurosurgical consultation; consider transport to ICU for medical management of elevated ICP; measures should include maintaining a euvolemic state, heart monitoring, urine output measurements, elevation of head of bed; airway protection/mechanical ventilation if necessary. Possible ICP monitoring with mannitol, and hyperventilation as needed

- Normal neuroimaging in coma due to trauma may still be present in the setting of major CNS injury and attendant complications; alternate diagnoses (meningitis, epilepsy) and other laboratory investigation (spinal tap, EEG) should be considered if the traumatic basis of stupor/coma remains in doubt.

Follow-Up

- Monitoring for cognitive difficulties, hyperactivity, seizures, hydrocephalus, movement disorders, paralysis, visual/hearing disturbance, headache; psychologists, neurologists, neurosurgeon, ophthalmologists, audiologists, and physical therapists may be helpful.
- Children <3 years old can sustain growing fractures due to prolapse of meninges into the skull fracture, leading to formation of a leptomeningeal cyst. Almost always develops within 6 months of injury.
- The pediatrician should refer any patient with a known skull fracture who manifests a new swelling in area of old fracture to neurosurgery for 3-D CT imaging of the head.
- Approximately 10% of patients with severe head injury will develop epilepsy.

PITFALLS

- Pupil asymmetry may be due to pharmacologic treatment (i.e., mydriatic agents for examination).
- Bacterial meningitis in a child who has had TBI may be indicative of a CSF leak.
- Basilar skull fracture may be missed on routine CT scan—review bone windows or skull films frequently a diagnosis can be made on the findings of raccoon eyes, Battle sign (retromastoid discoloration), hemotympanum, or CSF rhinorrhea/otorrhea.
- Witnesses and or primary caregivers may have personal reasons to conceal part or all of the circumstances regarding the child's injury. Speak to as many people as possible who can provide historically relevant information.

Common Question and Answers

Q: What are the specific signs of increased intracranial pressure (ICP)?
A: Cushing's reflex in association with deterioration in mental status. A change in pupils or ocular motility, or onset of posturing may also indicate increased ICP.

Q: When is mannitol used?
A: In patients with increased ICP in the absence of intracranial hemorrhage, mannitol may exacerbate elevated ICP if extravascular blood is present.

ICD-9-CM 854.0

BIBLIOGRAPHY

Bijur PE, Haslum M, Golding J. Cognitive and behavioral sequelae of mild head injury in children. *Pediatrics* 1990;86:337–344.

Duhaime A-C, Gennarelli TA, Thibault LE, et al. The shaken baby syndrome. *J Neurosurg* 1987;66:409–415.

Lee MS, Rinne JO, Ceballos-Baumann A, et al. Dystonia after head trauma. *Neurology* 1994; 44:1374–1378.

Luke A, Micheli L. Sports injuries: emergency assessment and field-side care. *Pediatr Rev* 1999;20(9):291–301.

Zimmerman RA, Bilaniuk LT. Pediatric head trauma. *Neuroimaging Clin North Am* 1994;4: 349–366.

Author: Todd Maugans
D. Elizabeth McNeil, 2nd edition

Brain Tumor

 Database

DEFINITION

A brain tumor is a primary neoplasm arising in the central nervous system (CNS).

PATHOPHYSIOLOGY

- No specific causative agents are known, but there is an association with radiation, chemical exposure, other malignancies, familial/heritable diseases, immunosuppression (lymphoma).
- The majority of tumors are classified based on their histology. The most common:
- Glioma

—Arises from astrocytes (supportive tissue)
—>50% of childhood CNS tumors
—Ranges from benign or low grade (often in the cerebellum or optic pathway) to malignant or grade III to IV (in the cerebrum or brainstem)
—Locally recurrent and invasive when malignant

- Primitive neuroectodermal tumor (PNET)/medulloblastoma

—Malignant embryonal tumor arising from unknown cell type
—Comprises about 20% of childhood CNS tumors
—Most common malignant brain tumor in children
—Majority arise in the midline of the cerebellum (referred to as medulloblastoma)
—Predisposition for leptomeningeal dissemination

- Ependymoma

—Arises from ependymal cells that line the ventricular system
—Comprises about 5% to 10% of childhood CNS tumors
—Most commonly occurs in the fourth ventricle; may arise in the spinal cord
—Locally recurrent and invasive; spinal metastases rare at initial diagnosis

- Germ cell tumor

—Derived from totipotent germ cells
—3–5% of childhood CNS tumors
—Majority are located in the pineal or suprasellar region

- Rhabdoid or atypical teratoid tumor

—Rare embryonal tumor arising from unknown cell type; often misdiagnosed as PNET
—Comprises less than 3% of childhood CNS tumors
—Majority arise in children younger than 5 years of age
—Propensity to arise in the posterior fossa with frequent leptomeningeal dissemination; reported in association with malignant rhabdoid tumors of the kidney

- Craniopharyngioma

—6–9% of childhood CNS tumors

- Tumors of the choroid plexus
- Ganglioglioma
- Meningioma and hemangioblastoma, rare in children

GENETICS

- Not a heritable condition
- Primary CNS tumors are associated with several familial syndromes:

—Neurofibromatosis (NF) with optic pathway gliomas (NF1) and meningiomas (NF2)
—Tuberous sclerosis with gliomas and rarely ependymomas
—Li-Fraumeni syndrome with astrocytomas
—Von Hippel–Lindau with cerebellar hemangioblastoma
—Turcot syndrome with PNET

EPIDEMIOLOGY

- Most common solid neoplasm of childhood (second to leukemia in overall incidence)
- Incidence rising (about 2,000 new cases/yr)
- 2.5–4 cases/100,000 children/year
- Peak incidence in children 7 years of age and younger
- Slight male predominance
- Majority arise infratentorially (within cerebellum or brainstem) in children 1–11 years of age
- Majority arise supratentorially in children <1 year of age

COMPLICATIONS

- Secondary to disease

—Increased intracranial pressure (ICP)
—Obstruction of cerebrospinal fluid (CSF) flow
—Requires immediate neurosurgical evaluation

- Secondary to therapy
- Radiation

—Neurocognitive sequelae (age- and dose-related)
—Endocrinopathy (growth hormone deficiency, hypothyroidism, gonadal dysfunction)
—Risk of second malignancies (meningioma, glioma, sarcoma)

- Chemotherapy

—Risks associated with bone marrow suppression (infection, bleeding, anemia)
—Hearing loss
—Risk of secondary leukemia

PROGNOSIS

Dependent on histology of tumor, location, and extent of initial resection.

- Glioma

—Low grade: 70–90% 5-year event-free survival (EFS)

—High grade: 16–46% 5-year EFS

- Intrinsic pontine: median overall survival of 9–13 months from diagnosis
- Medulloblastoma

—60–90% survival at 5 years if localized, gross totally resected, and >3 years old at diagnosis
—30–40% survival if disseminated

- Ependymoma

—50–70% survival at 5 years with total resection
—Less than 30% survival with subtotal resection

- Infants overall have a worse prognosis, possibly due to the limitations of therapy and/or the aggressiveness of the tumor.

 Differential Diagnosis

- Infection

—Cerebral abscess

- Tumors

—Metastatic tumor to brain uncommon with childhood solid tumors

- Trauma

—Hemorrhage unlikely to be confused with tumor

- Congenital

—Arteriovenous malformation
—Hamartoma
—Dysplastic brain

- Psychosocial

—Some patients with nausea, vomiting, or behavior changes are first diagnosed with psychiatric disorders, gastrointestinal disorders, failure to thrive, or anorexia nervosa prior to discovery of a brain tumor.

 Data Gathering

- Tumor location dictates symptoms and signs

HISTORY

Question: Headache and vomiting (particularly in the morning), irritable, lethargy?
Significance: Associated with increased intracranial pressure (ICP)

Question: Difficulty swallowing, slurred speech, and diplopia?
Significance: Brainstem tumor

Question: Visual field deficits (bumps into things)?
Significance: Optic tract lesion

Question: Focal weakness?
Significance: Pyramidal tract lesion

Question: Ataxia?
Significance: Cerebellar lesion

Question: Changes in behavior or school performance, new-onset seizures, weakness?
Significance: Supratentorial lesion

Question: Polyuria/polydipsia?
Significance: Hypothalamic/pituitary lesion

Question: Failure to thrive, emaciation, euphoria, and increased appetite in an infant?
Significance: Hypothalamic lesion (diencephalic syndrome)

Question: Back pain, extremity weakness, bowel/bladder dysfunction?
Significance: Spinal cord metastases (often seen with PNET/Medulloblastoma and germ cell tumors)

 ## Physical Examination

Finding: Macrocephaly, bulging fontanelle, papilledema, impaired upgaze
Significance: Increased ICP

Finding: Focal deficit on neurologic examination
Significance: Localizes mass lesion

Finding: Isolated cranial nerve VI and VII palsies
Significance: Brainstem tumor

Finding: Ataxia, dysmetria
Significance: Cerebellar mass

Finding: Decrease visual acuity, visual field deficit, absent pupillary light response, strabismus
Significance: Optic tract tumor

Finding: Changes in cognitive function, mood, and affect
Significance: Supratentorial lesion

Finding: Impaired upgaze, convergence nystagmus, pupils respond to accommodation but poorly to light
Significance: Pineal lesion (Parinaud's syndrome)

Finding: Signs of neurocutaneous disease (e.g., café-au-lait spots, Lisch nodules)
Significance: Syndrome like neurofibromatosis

 ## Laboratory Aids

IMAGING

Test: MRI with and without gadolinium enhancement
Significance: Gold standard for identification, localization, and characterization of tumor

Test: CT
Significance: Can be used as an initial study, but if negative with a high index of suspicion, follow with MRI. Useful to evaluate for hydrocephalus and hemorrhage.

STAGING OF TUMOR

Test: Postoperative head MRI within 24 to 48 hours
Significance: To determine residual disease before postoperative inflammatory changes are prominent

Test: Spine MRI; CSF cytology
Significance: Neuraxis staging for tumors with high risk of leptomeningeal dissemination

Test: α-Fetoprotein (AFP), quantitative B-HCG
Significance: Serum and CSF markers for germ cell tumors

 ## Therapy

SURGERY

• Both for histology and to attempt maximal tumor debulking; should be performed by experienced pediatric neurosurgeon
• Rarely indicated in intrinsic pontine (brainstem) glioma
• Ventriculoperitoneal (VP) shunt when needed for obstructive hydrocephalus (risk of peritoneal seeding minimal)

DRUGS

• Dexamethasone to control increased intracranial pressure (0.5 mg/kg divided q6h)
• Chemotherapy

—Drugs are most often used in combination
—CCNU, vincristine, procarbazine for high-grade glioma
—Cisplatin, CCNU, vincristine for PNET/medulloblastoma
—Carboplatin, vincristine or 6-thioguanine, procarbazine, CCNU, vincristine for low-grade glioma

• New protocols currently under development
• High-dose chemotherapy with stem cell rescue for high-risk PNET/medulloblastoma
• Targeted therapies, angiogenesis inhibitors

RADIATION THERAPY (XRT)

• Volume and dose vary depending on histology.
• XRT to the tumor bed is used for most patients with brain tumors.
• Medulloblastoma/PNET patients need craniospinal XRT. The one exception is in infants and young children (<3 years of age) in whom cognitive deficits from XRT can be devastating.

DURATION OF THERAPY

• Radiation therapy: 6 weeks
• Chemotherapy: 1 to 2 years

POSSIBLE CONFLICTS WITH OTHER TREATMENTS

Chemotherapy can alter anticonvulsant levels.

 ## Follow-Up

• Neurologic deficits can take months to improve or stabilize with permanent deficit.
• Any relapse or worsening of symptoms must be evaluated for tumor recurrence.
• MRI every 3 months the first year, every 6 months for the next 2 years, and annually thereafter. Benefit of routine surveillance imaging is controversial.

PITFALLS

• New onset of psychoses should prompt imaging to rule out tumor.
• Even benign tumors may be life-threatening if their location precludes resection.
• Not referring the patient to a pediatric brain tumor/oncology center at diagnosis (preoperatively). This requires an experienced (pediatric) neurosurgeon.

 ## Common Questions and Answers

Q: Are my other children at risk for getting a brain tumor?
A: No (except in rare cases of certain familial syndromes).

Q: Did something I do cause this?
A: No. In addition, the claims made about high-power lines and cellular phones causing brain tumors or cancer are unproven.

ICD-9-CM 191.9

BIBLIOGRAPHY

Packer RJ. Brain tumors in children. *Arch Neurol* 1999;56:421–425.

Valentino TL, Conway EE Jr, Shiminski-Maher T, et al. Pediatric brain tumors. *Pediatr Ann* 1997;26(10):579–587.

Author: Michael J. Fisher
Deborah L. Kramer, 2ⁿᵈ edition

Branchial Cleft Malformations

 Database

DEFINITION

• The fetal branchial apparatus is a foregut derivative and develops in the second fetal week.
• Five paired pharyngeal arches are separated by four endodermal pouches internally and four ectodermal clefts externally.
• Overgrowth of the second through fourth cleft creates the cervical sinus and occurs during weeks 4 and 5.
• Persistence of the cervical sinus produces a spectrum of cysts, sinus tracts, and fistulas.

CLASSIFICATION

• First branchial cleft anomalies

—Site: anywhere from external auditory canal to angle of mandible, usually superior to or within parotid
—Fistula tract: external auditory canal

• Second branchial cleft anomalies

—Site: ventral to anterior border of sternocleidomastoid muscle, lateral to carotid sheath, and dorsal to submandibular gland
—Fistula tract: palatine tonsil

• Third branchial cleft anomalies

—Site: posterior triangle in middle to lower left side of the neck near level of upper thyroid lobe
—Fistula: upper lateral piriform sinus wall to lower lateral neck posterior to sternocleidomastoid muscle

• Fourth branchial cleft anomalies

—Site: close association to thyroid gland associated with clinical thyroiditis if cyst infected
—Fistula: apex of piriform sinus to base of neck anterior to sternocleidomastoid muscle

GENETICS

• Familial history of branchial defects occasionally noted

EPIDEMIOLOGY

• Overwhelming majority of cysts in newborns and infants are developmental, whereas in children and adults they are inflammatory or neoplastic.
• Midline malformations are most often thyroglossal duct cysts or dermoids.
• Cysts occurring in the laterocervical region are usually branchial cleft malformations, the most common of these are derivatives of the second cleft, followed by those of the first cleft, of the fourth pouch and thymic cysts.
• Third and fourth branchial cleft anomalies are rare, with most presenting as sinus tracts rather than cysts.
• Suspect congenital anomaly in the clinical setting of recurrent infection.

COMPLICATIONS

• Cysts, sinus tracts, and fistulas can become recurrently infected (especially with abscess formation).
• Surgery is more difficult if there has been previous infections or previous surgery.
• Damage to facial, hypoglossal, and glossopharyngeal nerves or carotid artery can occur during surgical repair.
• Recurrence of the lesion seen if not fully removed.
• Thyroiditis
• Parotiditis (more common in first branchial arch malformation)

PROGNOSIS

• If lesion completely excised: excellent. Many patients require multiple procedures.

 Differential Diagnosis

CONGENITAL

Anterior Triangle of Neck

• Thymic cyst

Midline and Anterior Triangle of Neck

• Ranula
• Laryngocele
• Sialocele
• Thyroglossal cyst
• Dermoid/teratomatous cyst
• Bronchogenic cyst

Posterior Triangle of Neck

• Lymphangioma
• Hemangioma

INFLAMMATORY

• Adenitis
• Granulomatous disease (sarcoidosis, tuberculosis)
• Lymphoepithelial cysts (HIV)
• Otorrhea
• Parotiditis
• Retropharyngeal abscess
• Thyroiditis

TUMORS

• Lymphoma
• Rhabdomyosarcoma
• Cystic schwannoma (anterior triangle of neck)

 Data Gathering

HISTORY

• Present since birth
• Recurrent neck infections
• Intermittent discharge from neck
• Fever
• Tenderness

Physical Examination

- Mass usually mobile
- Usually a single lesion
- Nonpulsatile
- Lesion usually nontender (unless actively infected)
- Assess for sites of drainage:

—At the anterior or posterior border of the sternocleidomastoid muscle
—In the posterior pharynx at the tonsillar fossa or piriform sinus

 ## Laboratory Aids

Test: CBC with differential
Significance: Increased WBC with left shift seen with infection.

Test: Tuberculin test
Significance: to rule out tuberculosis

IMAGING

Test: Chest radiography
Significance: Assess for hilar adenopathy, suggesting a systemic process (such as tuberculosis or malignancy)

Test: Lateral neck radiography
Significance: Assess for airway compromise (not usually seen)

Test: Ultrasound
Significance: Help differentiate solid masses from cystic masses

Test: Fistulogram
Significance: Inject contrast into the fistula to delineate its course

Test: CT scan of neck
Significance: Superior spatial delineation and definition of anatomic compartment of the lesion

Test: MRI
Significance: More detailed soft tissue characterization and recognition of solid components within cystic masses

 ## Therapy

DRUGS

- Antibiotics are indicated if the defect is infected.

SURGERY

- Excision of the entire lesion
- Surgery should be delayed if infection present.

 ## Follow-Up

- Postoperative follow-up as outpatient for wound inspection
- Observation for recurrence or reinfection

PITFALLS

- Lesion may recur if not completely excised.
- High incidence of reinfection if not properly treated.

 ## Common Questions and Answers

Q: Can the cyst, fistula, or sinus recur?
A: Only a 3% recurrence rate is seen if the lesion is completely excised. A higher rate of recurrence is seen in cases of incomplete excision or with previous surgeries.

Q: Should the lesion be removed as soon as it is discovered?
A: The lesion should not be removed if there is an active infection present; treat the infection first and then schedule elective surgery.

ICD-9-CM 744.41

BIBLIOGRAPHY

Karmody CS. Developmental anomalies of the neck. In: Bluestone CD, Stool S, Kenna M, eds. *Pediatric otolaryngology*, 3rd ed. Philadelphia: WB Saunders, 1996:1497–1511.

Langman's medical embryology, 6th ed. Baltimore: Williams & Wilkins, 1990:298–327.

Lev S, Lev MH. Imaging of cystic lesions. *Radiol Clin North Am* 2000;38:1013–1027.

Lusk RP. Neck masses. In: Bluestone CD, Stool S, Kenna M, eds. *Pediatric otolaryngology*, 3rd ed. Philadelphia: WB Saunders, 1996:1488–1496.

McGuirt WF. The neck mass. *Med Clin North Am* 1999;83:219–234

Nicollas R, Guelfucci B, Roman S, et al. Congenital cysts and fistulas of the neck. *Int J Pediatr Otorhinolaryngol* 2000;55:117–124.

Nusbaum AO, Som P, Rothschild MA, et al. Recurrence of deep neck infection: a clinical indication of an underlying congenital lesion. *Arch Otolaryngol Head Neck Surg* 1999;125: 1379–1382.

Authors: Anita Bhandari and Raezelle Zinman

Breast Abscess

 Database

DEFINITION

Breast abscess is breast inflammation with pus localized in the breast bud or breast tissue.

CAUSES

- In newborns, infection is most often due to *Staphylococcus aureus*. Gram-negative enteric organisms should be considered (e.g., *Escherichia coli, Pseudomonas aeruginosa,* group B streptococcus can be causative).
- In adolescents, most often due to *S. aureus*; other organisms to consider include *Pseudomonas, E. coli,* tuberculosis, *Neisseria gonorrhea,* and syphilis.

ASSOCIATED ILLNESSES

- Mammary duct ectasia characterized by dilatation of subareolar ducts with fibrosis and chronic inflammation
- Epidermal cysts
- Skin infection or acne

PATHOPHYSIOLOGY

- Newborn—breast hypertrophy secondary to maternal hormones appears to increase the risk of breast abscess formation. Potentially pathogenic bacteria may colonize the skin and move retrograde into the ducts and deeper tissues.
- Adolescents—breast infection usually occurs during lactation, other causes include trauma (e.g., sexual manipulation, nipple rings), mammary duct ectasia, and local skin infections (e.g., acne).

EPIDEMIOLOGY

- Most often neonates age 1 to 5 weeks
- Neonatal M:F ratio 1:2
- Bilateral abscesses are rare, and may occur in neonates.
- Breast-feeding is the most common cause of mastitis in adolescents (2% of all postpartum women develop breast abscesses)

COMPLICATIONS

- In newborns, septicemia may occur.
- Extending cellulitis or necrotizing fasciitis has been described.
- Long-term destruction of mammary glands with scar formation

 Differential Diagnosis

INFECTION

- Cellulitis

TRAUMA

- Fat necrosis from trauma with painless firm, circumscribed, mobile mass
- Contusion with firm, tender, poorly defined mass
- Hematoma—sharply defined mass with ecchymosis

MISCELLANEOUS

- Mondor disease is a superficial phlebitis in the skin, often due to trauma (i.e., postbiopsy). Resolves spontaneously.
- Carcinoma

 Data Gathering

HISTORY

- Evaluate for history of manipulation of breast, trauma, sudden onset of swelling, warmth, tenderness, or erythema.
- Ask about fever, irritability, nipple discharge.

 Physical Examination

- Warmth, erythema, tenderness of breast tissue, may have fluctuance
- Fever
- Purulent nipple discharge
- Regional adenopathy

 Laboratory Aids

TESTS

- Culture nipple discharge from aspirated or incisional specimens
- Culture blood in neonates to rule out bacteremia (consider full sepsis workup).
- Consider culturing the throat and nose of neonate for colonization of *S. aureus*.

RADIOGRAPHIC STUDIES

- Ultrasound as needed

Therapy

DRUGS

- Neonates: IV oxacillin or other β-lactamase–resistant penicillin, with or without an aminoglycoside
- Adolescents: IV β-lactamase–resistant penicillin (e.g., oxacillin, methicillin)

OTHER TREATMENTS

- Incision and drainage when fluctuance present
- Warm compresses
- If adolescent is breast-feeding, continued expression of milk is necessary to avoid engorgement and areas of milk stasis

DURATION

- Neonates: 10 to 14 days; may give at home by mouth
- Adolescents: 14 days or longer, initially IV, then by mouth

PREVENTION

- Avoid manipulation of breast tissue

 Follow-Up

- Expect improvement within 48 hours of initiating IV antibiotics
- Need to follow both neonatal and adolescent patients closely for the risk of recurrence

 Common Questions and Answers

Q: Is fluctuance always found on examination?
A: No, yet breast swelling and/or warmth and erythema are nearly universally present.

Q: Is fever necessary for the diagnosis?
A: No, fever is not always present at time of presentation.

Q: Should a mother discontinue breast-feeding if she has a breast abscess?
A: The *2000 Red Book* recommendations are to discontinue breast-feeding from the affected breast, but the unaffected breast can be used for breast-feeding. After treatment is complete, the affected breast can be utilized in breast-feeding again.

ICD-9-CM

BIBLIOGRAPHY

American Academy of Pediatrics, Pickering LK, ed. *2000 red book: report of the Committee on Infectious Diseases* , 25th ed. Elk Grove, IL: American Academy of Pediatrics; 2000:99.

Bailey LA, Waecker NJ Jr. *Pseudomonas aeruginosa* mastitis in a neonate. *Pediatric Infect Dis J* 1993;12(1):104.

Bodemer C, Panhans A, Chretien-Marquet B, et al. Staphylococcal necrotizing fasciitis in the mammary region in childhood: a report of five cases. *J Pediatr* 1997;131(3):466–469.

Bodsworth NH, Price R, Nelson MJ. A case of gonococcal mastitis in a male. *Genitourinary Med* 1993;69:222–223.

Greydanus DE, Parks DS, Farrell EG. Breast disorders in children and adolescents. *Pediatr Clin North Am* 1989;36(3):601–638.

Walsh M, McIntosh K. Neonatal mastitis. *Clin Pediatr* 1986;25:395–399.

Author: Andrea McGeary

Breast-Feeding

 Database

DEFINITION

Human lactation produces breast milk, a species-specific nutrient for infants, term and preterm. The composition of breast milk changes during the establishment of milk production, from colostrum to transitional milk to mature milk within 2 weeks of delivery. **Colostrum**, a thick yellowish fluid is produced in the first 24 hours of delivery. Colostrum's higher protein content partially reflects increased delivery of immunoglobulins, especially secretory IgA. Colostrum also provides a high level of immunologically competent mononuclear cells along with other antiinfective agents. It also has a cathartic effect, promoting the passage of meconium. Colostrum provides from 5 to 20 mL of fluid per feeding.

Transitional milk represents the gradual change, beginning at about the 3rd to 5th day of life, from colostrum to mature milk. Transitional milk provides a gradually increased volume of fluid as well as a higher caloric content associated with the increased fat and carbohydrate content.

Mature milk is established at about 2 weeks postpartum. Each feeding session of mature milk is composed of **fore-milk** and **hind-milk**. At the initiation of nursing, the milk has a relatively higher protein and carbohydrate content; the hind-milk produced in the last 2 to 5 minutes of nursing has a higher fat content. It has been postulated that the increased fat content leads to satiation in the infant, promoting adequate rest until the next meal. Components unique to breast milk include:
- Antibodies
- Interferon
- Growth factors that confer maturational factors to gut
- Live cells, including polymorphonuclear neutrophils, lymphocytes, and macrophages

See table Comparison of Nutrients.
Benefits of breast-feeding in the first 6 to 12 months of life:
- Reduced incidence of diarrheal illnesses
- Reduced incidence of otitis media
- Potential protective effect against atopic disease

Positions in which a mother may nurse her infant: the classic "cradle" hold involves the mother supporting the infant with his/her trunk positioned across the mother's chest and upper abdomen. The "football" or "clutch" hold is ideal for the first several days following a cesarean section. In this position, the newborn is supported under the mother's arm and along her side, with the head of the baby in front of the mother's body. The "side-lying position" allows the mother to nurse her infant while both mother and baby lie on their sides.

PATHOPHYSIOLOGY

- In pregnancy: maternal prolactin is elevated and leads to an increase in secretory cells plus prolactin receptors in the breast; and significantly elevated progesterone levels inhibit prolactin action (production of breast milk). After birth, placenta delivery leads to a prolactin surge while progesterone and estrogen levels decrease. Prolactin stimulates secretory cells that result in milk production.
- With each nursing session, there is a prolactin burst. Prolactin remains elevated for the duration the infant breast-feeds.
- Oxytocin, whose elevated levels lead to the uterine contractions that result in the delivery of the fetus, also is released upon infant suckling at the breast. Oxytocin then goes on to cause contraction and involution of the uterus to the nonpregnant dimensions.

EPIDEMIOLOGY

- 60% of mothers initiate breast-feeding at birth; by 6 months only 18% are still nursing.
- Factors associated with higher prevalence and longer duration breast-feeding include higher level of maternal education and greater maternal age.
- Factors negatively associated with breast-feeding include:
—Single motherhood, whether widowed, divorced, or never married
—Maternal employment outside of home

COMPLICATIONS

- Engorgement: breasts are firm, hard, hot, painful. They may be so firm that the infant cannot latch on.
- Sore and/or cracked nipples: nipples erythematous, with or without fissures, sometimes scabs may form; pain may be mild to pronounced.
- Candidiasis of maternal nipples: nipples may be erythematous, have deep burning or soreness.
- Inadequate milk supply.

- Poor weight gain in the infant may result from inadequate supply or poor feeding technique.

PROGNOSIS

- Breast-fed infants in first 3 months have similar increase in weight, length, and head circumference, compared to formula-fed infants but proportionately slower weight gain for the next 9 months, resulting in a leaner infant with height and head circumference being maintained.

 Data Gathering

HISTORY

Consider the following decision factors that contribute to feeding practices:
- Maternal preference, knowledge base
- Paternal preference, knowledge base
- Cultural/societal supports including mother's mother
- Parity: feeding method of mother's previous infants

For the mother uncertain about how much milk infant is getting:

Question: How long does the infant nurse on each side?
Significance: Infants should nurse for 10 to 15 minutes on each side.
Question: Do her breasts feel softer after each feeding?
Significance: Breasts should feel softer if milk has been removed adequately by the infant.
Question: Does the infant seem satisfied?
Significance: To ensure that a baby has received enough, the baby should seem satisfied after a feeding.
Question: How many wet diapers a day is the infant making?
Significance: Infants receiving adequate hydration should void 6 to 8 times per day. Since it is difficult to change diapers after each voiding, several voidings may occur, so this number is an estimate.
Question: Mother complaining of sore or cracked nipples?
Significance: Determine frequency of feeds, varied positions when feeding, and the nature of any home therapy attempted. Also, ask about concomitant infant oral thrush or infant diaper rash consistent with candidal dermatitis.
Question: Mother concerned about the quantity of milk being provided to the baby?
Significance: Confirm she is taking a vitamin supplement, offering breast at least q2h initially, drinking enough fluids herself, eating a balanced diet, and getting adequate rest.

 Physical Examination

Finding: Ensure that the neonate has not lost more than 10% of the birth weight in the first couple of weeks, and that he/she has regained the birth weight by the end of the second week.

Comparison of Nutrients

	PROTEIN	FAT	CHO	CA	FE
Per 100 mL	Total (whey/casein)		(Lactose)		
Colostrum	2.3 g (total)	2.9 g	5.3 g	39 mg	70 μg
Term	1.1 g (20%/80%)	3.8 g	7.0 g	35 mg	100 μg
Preterm	1.81 g	4.0 g	6.95 g	22 mg	100 μg
Cow milk	3.3 g (80%/20%)	3.3 g	4.8 g	130 mg	70 μg

Adapted from Lawrence RA, with permission.

Significance: Minimal criteria for adequate breast milk supply.
Finding: Assess for jaundice.
Significance: Infants who breast-feed are at risk for breast-feeding jaundice.
• Observe the infant's feeding, positioning, adequacy of latch-on, and suck.

Laboratory Aids

Test: Electrolytes
Significance: Infant appears dehydrated.
Test: Bilirubin
Significance: Infant jaundice is present.

Therapy

• Engorgement (due to production of milk, and increased circulation of blood and lymph in breasts)
—Feed infant often, avoid supplements (e.g., formula, sugar water), express milk if infant must skip feeding.
—When time to wean, do so gradually.
—Use warm, moist compresses just before nursing, gently massage breasts during feeding. After nursing, reduce swelling with ice packs.
• Sore and/or cracked nipples
—Prevent by changing nursing positions often (various nursing styles should be demonstrated by lactation consultant before mother and baby are discharged from hospital).
—Ensure that the baby has much of the areola in his/her mouth when nursing, allow nipples to air dry completely between feedings, and always break suction seal before removing infant from breast.
—If pain occurs with nursing, change positioning (e.g., cradle position to football position). The infant's suck in one position may irritate a region of the nipple, which is uninvolved when the suck is from a different angle.
—Clean nipples with clear water, dry completely, and apply expressed breast milk to nipple. Pure lanolin cream may be helpful.
—If mother has fever, malaise, and/or discharge from affected area, she may have mastitis and should seek care from her health care provider.
• Nipple candidiasis or "thrush nipples"— after each feed massage nystatin cream into nipple(s); concurrently treat infant with nystatin suspension for 10 days.
• Inadequate milk supply, poor feeding, and weight gain: mother should drink 32 to 40 oz of fluids daily, preferably water; eat balanced diet (500 kcal/day). Offer breast q1–2h to increase milk supply; wake infant at least once between 12 A.M. and 6 A.M. to nurse; sleep when baby sleeps to maximize mother's rest necessary for milk production.
• For the sleepy infant: change diaper, undress to diaper only, increase mother–baby skin-to-skin contact. Rule out infant illness.

Follow-Up

• Aggressive follow-up by primary care provider is ideal. In addition, if mother does not have adequate sources for a lactation consultant from nursery, local directories are available. Women, Infants, and Children (WIC) programs in many regions have developed strong lactation support staff.
• Monitor weight on a weekly basis, if necessary, until milk supply is well established and infant is nursing successfully.
• Women who return to work may continue exclusively breast-feeding their infants. Support of her employer including a time and place to express milk is paramount for successful breast-feeding. For milk expression, an electric double pump is ideal for time considerations and for maintaining milk supply.
• Weaning: nutritional and developmental studies suggest exclusive breast-feeding for up to 6 months. Weaning should be done gradually both for mother's physical comfort and her infant's psychological acceptance.

PREVENTION
Contraindications to breast-feeding include:
• Galactosemia
• Maternal neoplasm, life-threatening or debilitating illness
• Maternal medications: recreational drugs, chemotherapeutic drugs, bromocriptine, ergotamine, lithium, pheanindione
• Maternal infection: HIV–absolute contraindication in developed world

PITFALLS
• Inadequate support of nursing mother who may give up and have a sense of failure.
• Dispensing of formula samples on hospital discharge to breast-feeding mothers promotes acceptance of formula feeding as cultural norm.

Common Questions and Answers

Q: How frequently should I feed the baby? What does "on-demand" mean?
A: At first, newborn infants should be offered the breast at least every 1.5 to 2 hours as the milk supply is established. In the first 2 weeks, newborns should nurse 8 to 12 times/day and should be awakened to nurse if the baby sleeps more than 4 hours.

Q: How much is too much? Can I overfeed the baby?
A: An infant will usually stop eating if full but may continue to suck with less vigor for comfort. This less vigorous sucking is called "grazing." The mother will soon notice the difference and should cease nursing and choose to cuddle and rock the infant at that time. Allowing grazing at the nipple can lead to obesity or even nursing caries; by the end of the first month the infant should take most of the feed in 10 to 15 minutes.

Q: Does my baby need vitamins?
A: If the mother continues her prenatal vitamins and eats a well-balanced diet, vitamin supplementation for the infant may not be necessary. Vitamin D is not in sufficient amounts in breast milk; however, its precursor is in the infant's skin and is converted to the active metabolite if the infant is exposed to sunlight at least 15 minutes/day. For a dark-skinned infant in winter, it is recommended to give liquid vitamin drops with 5 to 7.5 μg vitamin D daily. Vitamin drops are safe for all babies when used at the recommended dosage. Fluoride is recommended for the breast-fed infant greater than 6 months of age if the baby is not receiving any fluoridated water. The recommended dosage in this setting is 0.25 mg fluoride daily.

Q: Is it not just easier to bottle-feed?
A: Breast-feeding is convenient, always available, sterile, at the proper temperature, and mother may modestly nurse in most settings. It is also inexpensive. Compare the nominal increase of maternal nutrition costs to more than $1,000/year of infancy spent on proprietary formula.

BIBLIOGRAPHY

Banta-Wright SA. Minimizing infant exposure to and risks from medications while breast-feeding. *J Perinat Neonat Nurs* 1997;11(5):71–84.

Briggs GG, Freeman RK, Yaffe SJ. *Drugs in pregnancy and lactation: a reference guide to fetal and neonatal risk*. Baltimore: Williams & Wilkins, 1998

Campbell C. Breast-feeding and health in the western world. *Br J Gen Pract* 1996;46: 613–617.

Dewey KG. Cross-cultural patterns of growth and nutritional status of breast-fed infants. *Am J Clin Nutr* 1998;67:10–17.

Dillon AE, Wagner CL, Wiest D, et al. Drug therapy in the nursing mother. *Clin Obstet Gynecol* 1997;24(3):675–696.

Golding J, Rogers I, Emmett P. Association between breast feeding, child development and behavior. *Early Hum Dev* 1997;49(suppl): S175–S184.

Jacobsen SW, Jacobsen JL. Breast feeding and intelligence. *Lancet* 1992;339:926.

Krishna RV, Plichta SB. The role of social support in breast-feeding promotion: a literature review. *J Hum Lact* 1998;14:41–45.

Lawrence RA. *Breast-feeding: a guide for the medical profession*. St. Louis: Mosby-Year Book, 1999:Appendix A.

Vandenplas Y. Myths and facts about breast-feeding: does it prevent later atopic disease? *Acta Pediatr* 1997;86:1283–1287.

Xanthou M. Human milk cells. *Acta Pediatr* 1997;86:1288–1290.

Author: Stephanie D. James

Breast-Feeding Jaundice and Breast-Milk Jaundice

 Database

DEFINITION

Early-onset breast-feeding jaundice (BFJ) and late-onset breast-milk jaundice (BMJ) are the two major overlapping causes of jaundice in otherwise healthy breast-fed infants.
• BFJ: associated with inadequate breast-feeding; exaggerated early-onset (3–5 days) physiologic unconjugated hyperbilirubinemia (>12 mg/dL)
• BMJ: associated with being fed breast milk; late-onset (1–6 weeks) unconjugated hyperbilirubinemia (>10 mg/dL)

PATHOPHYSIOLOGY

Bilirubin is a breakdown product of hemoglobin and other heme-containing proteins.
In newborns, the shorter life span of a larger number of erythrocytes, the immaturity of the bilirubin uptake and conjugation system in the liver, and the increased enterohepatic circulation (initiated by a more rapid hydrolysis of the conjugated bilirubin to the unconjugated form) contribute to hyperbilirubinemia and physiologic jaundice.
• BFJ: inadequate intake of milk and calories with or without relative dehydration leading to increased intestinal bilirubin absorption and enterohepatic circulation
• BMJ: several hypotheses proposed but remain unproven:
—Pregnanediol isomer (steroid metabolite of progesterone, competitive inhibitor of hepatic glucuronyl transferase) present in milk of mothers of infants with BMJ
—Increased concentrations of nonesterified (free) fatty acids (inhibitor of hepatic glucuronyl transferase) in milk of mothers of infants with BMJ
—Factors present in human breast milk of mothers of infants with BMJ that increases enterohepatic circulation of bilirubin, e.g., β-glucuronidase, which can hydrolyze conjugated to unconjugated bilirubin (this has been disproven since newborns already have much higher endogenous concentration of intestinal beta glucuronidase)
—Defects in bilirubin uridine diphosphate-glucuronosyltransferase gene (UGT1A1) associated with breast-milk–related unconjugated hyperbilirubinemia

EPIDEMIOLOGY

• BFJ likely to be the predominant cause of early-onset jaundice; however, often difficult to distinguish from jaundice related to other causes because of considerable overlap.
• Jaundice occurs in 3% to 23% of breast-fed infants compared to 2% to 8% of formula-fed infants.
• BMJ affects 10% to 30% of breast-fed newborns during the second to sixth weeks of life.

GENETICS

• BFJ: subsequent siblings of infants with jaundice are more likely to develop jaundice.

• BMJ: mutations in the bilirubin uridine diphosphate-glucuronosyltransferase gene have been identified in a Japanese population and were felt to be associated with breast-milk jaundice.

COMPLICATIONS

• BFJ and BMJ: kernicterus (bilirubin encephalopathy; extremely rare), characterized acutely by opisthotonus and seizures & on a more chronic basis by hearing loss, upward gaze palsy, & cerebral palsy
• Cessation of breast-feeding
• Parental and health care provider anxiety

PROGNOSIS

• BFJ and BMJ: excellent if hyper-bilirubinemia identified and treated appropriately; however, both evaluation and treatment may contribute to interruption of breast-feeding and increased parental anxiety, leading to cessation of breast-feeding.

 Differential Diagnosis

INFECTIOUS
• Sepsis (jaundice is usually not the sole presenting sign)

HEMATOLOGIC
• Blood group incompatibility
• Rh incompatibility
• Erythrocyte enzyme defects (e.g., glucose-6-phosphate dehydrogenase deficiency)
• Erythrocyte membrane defects (e.g., hereditary spherocytosis)
• Polycythemia

GASTROINTESTINAL
• Intestinal obstruction (e.g., meconium ileus, Hirschsprung disease, pyloric stenosis)

CONGENITAL
• Transient familial neonatal hyperbilirubinemia

METABOLIC
• Hypothyroidism
• Galactosemia
• Gilbert syndrome
• Crigler-Najjar syndrome

MISCELLANEOUS
• Dehydration
• Cephalohematoma
• Maternal oxytocin use

 Data Gathering

HISTORY
Question: Is there a family history of jaundice in a sibling?
Significance: Prior history may indicate similar risk factors and genetic propensities for developing jaundice. Severe neonatal jaundice suggests familial or inherited hemolytic disease.
Question: Are there relatives with a history of anemia, gallbladder disease, or splenectomy?

Significance: Hemolytic anemias constitute an inheritable cause of severe and prolonged jaundice.
Question: Are there maternal risk factors?
Significance: Maternal illness (e.g., diabetes) and medication use (e.g., oxytocin) are associated with jaundice. Infants born to mothers positive for group B streptococcus are at increased risk for neonatal sepsis.
Question: Are there birth-related risk factors?
Significance: Sepsis will be included in the differential diagnosis for presence of fever, prolonged rupture of amniotic membranes, or cloudy or odorous amniotic fluid. Traumatic delivery, including the use of instruments such as forceps or vacuum, may contribute to significant bruising and cephalohematoma formation.
Question: How is early infant feeding?
Significance: Infrequent and difficult breast-feeding are predictors of breast-feeding jaundice. Many such infants have increased enterohepatic circulation and dehydration reflected by delayed passage of meconium and significant weight loss.
Question: When did jaundice become noticeable?
Significance: Jaundice before 24 hours of age suggests a hemolytic process. Early jaundice beyond 24 hours is associated with BFJ while prolonged jaundice beyond 1–2 weeks suggests BMJ.
Question: How is the infant doing?
Significance: Infants with breast-milk jaundice are in good health, vigorous, eating well, and gaining weight.

 Physical Examination

• Onset of jaundice before 24 hours of age suggests a pathologic process.
• Jaundice generally progresses from the face to the lower extremities in proportion to rising serum bilirubin concentrations, which can be estimated by degree of skin involvement: jaundice on face and neck (6 mg/dL); down to trunk and umbilicus (9 mg/dL); groin and upper thighs (12 mg/dL); knees and ankles (15 mg/dL); feet (>15 mg/dL); however, this method of assessment is not accurate.

Finding: Cephalohematoma, facial bruising
Significance: May contribute to hyperbilirubinemia
Finding: Increased respirations, cyanosis, grunting, nasal flaring, intercostal retractions
Significance: May suggest infection
Finding: Hepatosplenomegaly
Significance: Suggests infectious, metabolic or severe hemolytic causes of hyperbilirubinemia
Finding: Abdominal distention
Significance: Suggests intestinal obstruction
Finding: Dry mucous membranes and skin tenting
Significance: Consistent with dehydration and may contribute to BFJ

Finding: Well-appearing older infant who is gaining weight
Significance: Consistent with BMJ

Laboratory Aids

Generally, no tests are needed in a healthy breast-fed infant with mild to moderate jaundice in the absence of risk factors for other causes of jaundice. However, BFJ and BMJ are diagnoses of exclusion. The following tests should be considered depending on the clinical presentation:

Test: Total serum bilirubin
Significance: Quantification of bilirubin levels can assist in diagnosis and choice of therapy (e.g., phototherapy); bilirubin must be measured in all infants with very early jaundice <24 hours of age
Test: Maternal blood type and Rh status; and infant blood type and Coombs test from cord blood if indicated (mother's blood type is O and/or Rh is negative)
Significance: Identification of risk for hemolytic anemia from blood type and/or Rh incompatibility, with considerations for treatment at lower levels of total serum bilirubin.
Test: Conjugated serum bilirubin
Significance: Elevated conjugated bilirubin (>1 mg/dL or 10% of total serum bilirubin) may indicate infection, biliary obstructive disease, cholestasis, metabolic disease, or severe hemolysis.
Test: Complete blood count and smear
Significance: Abnormal red cell count can indicate polycythemia or anemia; in an infant with anemia, blood smear can demonstrate erythrocyte morphology suggestive of hemolysis and hereditary spherocytosis; abnormal white cell count may indicate infection, although unlikely in an otherwise healthy infant; decreases in red cell count over time may reflect ongoing hemorrhage or hemolysis.
Test: G6PD activity
Significance: G6PD deficiency is common worldwide and a rapid increase in bilirubin may occur later than in other types of hemolytic disease; risk of kernicterus seems to be higher in infants with G6PD deficiency, indicating consideration of treatment at lower levels of total serum bilirubin.

Therapy

Goal of therapy is to maintain the total serum bilirubin concentration at a level to minimize the risk of encephalopathy.

BFJ
• Increase frequency of breast-feeding to 10–12 times per day during the first 3 days of life.
• Supplement with formula if significant feeding problems or poor milk production.
• Phototherapy if serum bilirubin levels exceed the American Academy of Pediatrics recommended threshold levels for phototherapy for full-term infants based on infant's age in hours (i.e., implement phototherapy for infants 25–48 hours old if total serum bilirubin ≥15 mg/dL; 49–72 hours old if bilirubin ≥18 mg/dL; >72 hours old if bilirubin ≥20 mg/dL); for infants <24 hours, phototherapy is recommended if bilirubin is greater than half of the infant's age (in hours).
• Consider exchange blood transfusion for infants 25–48 hours old and total serum bilirubin above 25 mg/dL and for infants ≥48 hours old and total serum bilirubin above 30 mg/dL

BMJ
• Continue observation.
• Refrain from complete or partial interruption of nursing and the feeding of formula.
• If bilirubin >20 mg/dL and/or evidence of significant starvation or dehydration, consider supplementation with formula or interruption of breast-feeding temporarily and substitution with formula; and/or administration of phototherapy.

SUPPORTIVE CARE
• BFJ and BMJ: monitor serum bilirubin levels
• BFJ: lactation consultation
• BMJ: close observation

DURATION OF THERAPY
• BFJ and BMJ: continue treatment until serum bilirubin levels consistently within acceptable levels

POSSIBLE CONFLICTS WITH OTHER TREATMENTS
• Home phototherapy poses less of an obstruction to effective breast-feeding than hospitalization
• Phototherapy may contribute to dehydration
• Exchange transfusion should be considered in conjunction with phototherapy

Follow-Up

WHEN TO EXPECT IMPROVEMENT
• BFJ: if phototherapy instituted, significant improvement in jaundice expected within 24 hours
• BMJ: after temporary interruption of breast-feeding for 24 to 48 hours

PROGNOSIS
• Increased risk for hyperbilirubinemia in subsequent siblings

PITFALLS
• Visual assessment of jaundice may be inaccurate.
• Thresholds for starting phototherapy are lower for infants with hemolytic diseases including G6PD deficiency and Rh incompatibility; and for premature infants and infants who are ill.
• Discharge follow-up at 48 to 72 hours of age important to identify significant hyperbilirubinemia given decreasing duration of postpartum hospital stay.

Common Questions and Answers

Q: Will my baby have developmental or neurologic problems afterward?
A: Not from jaundice as long as the hyperbilirubinemia is appropriately monitored and treated.
Q: Will exposure to sunlight decrease the level of jaundice?
A: Yes. However, avoid prolonged exposure and direct sunlight to avoid sunburn. Periodic indirect sunlight (e.g., exposure in a warm sunlit room) is sufficient.
Q: Should I stop breast-feeding?
A: The frequency of breast-feeding should be increased and appropriate lactation consultation obtained for BFJ. Early frequent breast-feeding can decrease the risk. For BMJ, temporary cessation of breast-feeding will lower the total serum bilirubin; however, this recommendation should be considered along with supplementation with formula and phototherapy only if total serum bilirubin ≥20 mg/dL.
Q: Should all babies be screened for hyperbilirubinemia?
A: Some researchers suggest universal bilirubin screening of infants at 1 day of life because of the inaccuracy of visual assessment of infants for jaundice. Poor room lighting, skin color, and other factors contribute to such difficulties. A bilirubin of 5 mg/dL at 1 day of life has been shown to be associated with a higher rate of hyperbilirubinemia; however, it remains unclear whether targeted screening using appropriate context (e.g., family history of neonatal jaundice, hemolytic disease, cephalohematoma) might minimize the potential financial and nonfinancial cost of universal screening. With development of new technology, including transcutaneous bilirubin and expiratory CO (carbon monoxide) measurements, the current serum bilirubin screening may be supplanted.

ICD-9-CM
Breast-Feeding Jaundice 774.39
Breast-Milk Jaundice 776.0;774.6

BIBLIOGRAPHY
American Academy of Pediatrics. Provisional Committee for Quality Improvement and Subcommittee on Hyperbilirubinemia. Practice parameter: management of hyperbilirubinemia in the healthy term newborn [published erratum appears in *Pediatrics* 1995;95: 458–461]. *Pediatrics* 1994;94:558–565.

Gartner LM, Lee K. Jaundice in the breast-fed infant. *Clin Perinatol* 1999;26:431–445.

Koh AY, Bernstein HH. Neonatal jaundice, animal-induced injuries and immunizations. *Curr Opin Pediatr* 2000;12:413–425.

Maisels MJ, Newman TB. Jaundice in full-term and near-term babies who leave the hospital within 36 hours: the pediatrician's nemesis. *Clin Perinatol* 1998;25:295–302.

Author: John I. Takayama

Breath-Holding Spells

 Database

DEFINITION

• Simple breath-holding spells (BHSs) are involuntary (reflexive), nonepileptic, paroxysmal events in which the child becomes apneic and often bradycardic at end expiration.
• BHSs are classified as severe when they are prolonged and associated with loss of consciousness and/or seizure activity.
• Often divided into cyanotic spells or pallid spells, based on child's coloration during episodes.

ETIOLOGY

• Usually brought on by anger, frustration, fear, or minor injury.
• Cyanotic spells thought to be related to an autonomic dysregulation leading to prolonged expiratory apnea.
• Pallid spells thought to be related to an overactive vagal response resulting in bradycardia or asystole.
• Anemia has been reported to worsen the severity and frequency of BHSs.
• Family history of BHSs identified in one third of families, with equal frequency between maternal and paternal sides.

EPIDEMIOLOGY

• Lifetime prevalence of up to 25% during childhood.
• Severe BHSs occur in less than 1% of the population.
• Onset is typically between 6 months and 2 years of age, with some presenting younger than 6 months.
• Peak frequency of spells occurs between 12 and 18 months.
• Mean age at termination 36–42 months; rare after age 6 years.
• Cyanotic spells more common than pallid spells.
• Some children have both types of BHSs, with one type predominating.
• Within families, multiple children may have different types of BHSs.

COMPLICATIONS

• No clear evidence of long-term sequelae.
• Reports of neurodevelopmental abnormalities, and rarely, death in children with severe BHSs do exist, but the association of these outcomes with the BHS is very controversial.

 Differential Diagnosis

Look for alternative diagnoses in children whose course differs from the expected natural history.

• Seizures: the presence of a precipitating event and the occurrence of cyanosis or pallor prior to the tonic-clonic movements usually allows BHSs to be distinguished from seizures by history.
• Familial dysautonomia
• Long QT syndrome
• Brainstem lesions: tumor, Arnold-Chiari malformation
• Munchausen Syndrome by proxy

 Data Gathering

HISTORY

Focus on preceding circumstances and parents' reaction to the event(s).

Question: Was there an injury, anger, frustration?
Significance: Helps identify situations likely to precede the spells.

 Physical Examination

Finding: Results of the general physical examination are normal. To rule out other disorders, brainstem and spinal cord function should be evaluated on neurologic examination.
Significance: Familial dysautonomia is a rare disorder that causes symptoms from infancy. Symptoms include failure to thrive, chronic aspiration, insensitivity to pain, and crying without tears.

 Laboratory Aids

Test: CBC
Significance: Check for anemia and iron deficiency

Test: EEG
Significance: Helpful in distinguishing BHSs from seizure disorder when history unclear

Test: ECG
Significance: Indicated to rule out long QT syndrome when there is syncope and history is atypical for BHS.

Therapy

- Reassure parents that these spells will not harm the child.
- Parental education for severe BHSs. Normal breathing resumes after loss of consciousness.
- Calm parental reaction is associated with a reduced frequency.
- Place child on the floor to prevent falling.
- Clear the mouth of food/foreign bodies during episode to prevent aspiration.
- Activate the emergency medical system if the loss of consciousness is longer than 1 minute.

DRUGS

- Iron: Treatment with ferrous sulfate (5 mg/kg/day) for 16 weeks resulted in a cessation of BHSs in over 50% of cases. Not all responders were iron deficient on laboratory evaluation, but children with iron deficiency were more likely to benefit from this treatment. Mechanism of action was unknown. Consider treatment with iron in children with severe BHSs.
- Atropine: Has been used in severe pallid BHSs to prevent bradycardia and loss of consciousness, but is not currently available as a single agent oral drug in the United States.

 ## Follow-Up

- Based on the amount of support the parents need in learning to manage these spells
- Referral to a mental health professional if parents unable to discipline child for fear of inducing BHSs

PITFALLS

- Child may learn to trigger spells if they result in the child getting what he or she wants.
- Attempts to give mouth-to-mouth resuscitation to children with BHSs are unnecessary and may result in aspiration.

 ## Common Questions and Answers

Q: Are children with BHSs more stubborn or disobedient than other children?
A: No. Recent studies found no difference in the behavioral profiles of children with BHSs and controls.

Q: Will BHSs occur in other children in the family?
A: There does seem to be a tendency toward having BHSs that can be inherited. Twenty to thirty percent of first-degree relatives of probands with severe BHSs will have a current or past history of severe BHSs. In severe BHSs, this is most consistent with an underlying genetic inheritance pattern of autosomal dominance with reduced penetrance.

Q: Should all children with BHSs have an EEG and ECG?
A: No, in most cases, history is sufficient to distinguish BHSs from other problems. See Laboratory Aids, above.

Q: Are BHSs more common in boys?
A: No, they are found equally in both sexes.

ICD-9-CM 786.9

BIBLIOGRAPHY

Daoud AS, Batieha A, Al-Sheyyab M, et al. Effectiveness of iron therapy on breath-holding spells. *J Pediatr* 1997;130: 547–550.

DiMario FJ. Breath-holding spells in childhood. *Am J Dis Child* 1992;146:125–131.

DiMario FJ. Prospective study of children with cyanotic and pallid breath-holding spells. *Pediatrics* 2001;107:265–269.

DiMario FJ, Sarfarazi M. Family pedigree analysis of children with severe breath-holding spells. *J Pediatr* 1997;130(4): 647–651.

Evans OB. Breath-holding spells. *Pediatr Ann* 1997;26:410–414.

McWilliam RC, Stephenson JBP. Atropine treatment of reflex anoxic seizures. *Arch Dis Child* 1974;59:473–475.

Schmitt BD. *Instructions for pediatric patients.* Philadelphia: WB Saunders, 1992:172.

Authors: Emily L. Siege and Nathan J. Blum

Bronchiolitis

Also see Respiratory Syncytial Virus

 Database

DEFINITION

Acute lower respiratory illness causing obstruction of the small conducting airways of the lung.

PATHOPHYSIOLOGY AND CAUSES

- Respiratory syncytial virus (RSV) is the most common cause of this illness (40–90%).
- Other agents associated:
—Human parainfluenza viruses (type 3 is second most common cause)
—Influenza A
—Adenovirus
—Rhinovirus
—*Mycoplasma pneumoniae*
- RSV is transmitted by:
—Direct contact with nasal secretions from an infected individual (secretions remain infectious on countertops and stethoscopes for more than 6 hours and on hands or tissue for about 30 minutes)
—Aerosol spread (less common)
- Viral shedding: 3 to 8 days (in some infants: 3 to 4 weeks)
- Leukocytes (predominantly lymphocytes) infiltrate the peribronchial epithelial tissue, leading to airway wall edema. In addition, inflammation causes necrosis of the bronchiolar epithelium, loss of cilia, and sloughing of dead cells causing mucus plugging, which may result in partial airway obstruction, increased airways resistance, hypoxemia, and cyanosis.
- RSV-induced changes in the bronchiolar epithelium can last beyond the acute infection. Regeneration of bronchiolar epithelium may take months and lags behind clinical signs of recovery.

EPIDEMIOLOGY

- Seen in all geographic areas
- Peaks during the winter and early spring
- Most children infected are within the first 2 years of life; 57% of those hospitalized were younger than 6 months.
- Infection rate peak in infants aged 6 weeks to 6 months, highest rates occurring under 3 months of age.
- Mortality associated with primary RSV infection in otherwise healthy children is 0.005% to 0.02%, and is approximately 1% to 3% among hospitalized children.
- Risk factors for acquisition of RSV infection: Birth during the months of April through September; day-care attendance or older siblings in day care; crowded living condition; lower socioeconomic class; exposure to cigarette smoke; lower cord serum RSV antibodies; delayed immunizations; multiple births
—Approximately 30% to 40% of infants with bronchiolitis develop subsequent wheezing, specifically those with eosinophilia during RSV bronchiolitis.

GENETICS

- Genetic background is unclear.

COMPLICATIONS

- Common complications
—Pneumonia
—Aspiration syndrome
—Respiratory failure requiring mechanical ventilation
—Apnea
—Syndrome of inappropriate ADH (risk for overhydration)
- Patient groups at high risk of severe RSV disease:
- Premature infants (<35 weeks' gestation)
- Congenital heart disease
- Chronic lung disease [including bronchopulmonary dysplasia (BPD)]
- Cystic fibrosis
- Compromised immune function (from chemotherapy, transplant, congenital or acquired immunodeficiencies)

PROGNOSIS

- For most infants, prognosis is good.
- Mortality associated with primary RSV infection in otherwise healthy infants is 0.005% to 0.02% (usually as a result of unrecognized apnea, respiratory failure, or untreated bacterial superinfection).
- Morbidity and mortality is considerable in patients with an underlying chronic disease.
- Approximately 30% to 40% of infants with bronchiolitis develop subsequent wheezing until 7 years of age, specifically those with eosinophilia during RSV bronchiolitis.
- Bronchiolitis obliterans may be a sequela in a few patients infected with *Mycoplasma pneumoniae* or adenovirus.

 Differential Diagnosis

- Pneumonia (viral or bacterial)
- Asthma
- Gastroesophageal reflux (GER)
- Foreign body aspiration
- Exposure to noxious agents (chemicals, fumes, toxins)
- Congestive heart failure
- Cystic fibrosis

INDICATIONS FOR HOSPITALIZATION

- <3 months of age (has increased risk for apnea and severe illness)
- Gestational age younger than 34 weeks
- Presence of risk factors
- Presence of apnea, tachypnea, retractions, poor feeding, and agitation (signs of impending respiratory failure)
- Pulse oximetry <95% on room air
- Atelectasis on chest x-ray
- High-risk group for developing severe RSV disease

 Data Gathering

HISTORY

Question: Rhinorrhea with thick nasal secretions?
Significance: Characteristic of disease

Question: Coughing?
Significance: Initially hoarse cough for 3–5 days; Progresses to deep wet cough of increased frequency

Question: Poor feeding?
Significance: Early sign of respiratory fatigue; may lead to dehydration

Question: Low-grade fever?
Significance: Characteristic of disease; not a reliable marker of severity of disease

Question: Restlessness or lethargy?
Significance: May indicate impending respiratory failure (hypoxemia and/or CO_2 retention)

Question: Apnea (seen in younger infants)?
Significance: Impending respiratory failure

Question: Cyanosis/color change or increased work of breathing?
Significance: Impending respiratory failure

 Physical Examination

GENERAL APPEARANCE

- Interactive vs. ill-appearing
- Paroxysmal cough (most common sign), not associated with "whoop"
- ± Poor oral intake

HEENT EXAMINATION

- Nasal flaring
- Nasal congestion with thick, purulent secretion

PULMONARY EXAMINATION

- Pattern of breathing: presence or absence of apnea or periodic breathing
- Tachypnea

Significance: >70/min is associated with severe illness
- Nasal flaring and accessory muscle retractions
- Thoracoabdominal asynchrony
- Hyperresonance to percussion
- Diffuse, high-pitched heterophonous wheezing
- Prolonged expiratory phase
- Fine inspiratory crackles (may be heard in both bronchiolitis and pneumonia)
- ± Diffuse rhonchi

OTHER FINDINGS

- Signs of dehydration
- Low-grade fever
- Tachycardia
- Bradycardia associated with apnea
- Possible cyanosis of nailbeds and oral mucosa

- Liver and spleen typically pushed down by hyperinflated lungs
- Digital clubbing (may alert the presence of underlying chronic lung disease)

 ## Laboratory Aids

BLOOD TESTS
Test: Pulse oximetry
Significance: To assess oxygenation

Test: arterial blood gas
Significance: Useful in assessment
- Degree of hypoxemia (determine A-a gradient)
- Evidence of respiratory failure and respiratory acidosis with CO_2 retention

Test: Serum electrolytes (Chem 7)
Significance: Useful in hospitalized patients to assess adequacy of hydration; infer chronic CO_2 retention if serum bicarbonate is elevated

Test: RSV serology (acute and convalescent serum samples)
Significance: No practical application for clinical use

RAPID VIRAL IDENTIFICATION
- Immunofluorescence (direct or indirect IFA)
- Enzyme immunoassay (EIA): Advantage: rapid results (15 to 30 minutes), does not require the presence of a viable virus. Sensitivity ranges from 57% to 97%; specificity: 69% to 100%

VIRAL CULTURE
Test: Culture of nasopharynx
Significance: Should be done for all patients with negative rapid respiratory studies

IMAGING
Chest radiography: findings include
- Hyperinflation, flattened diaphragms
- Peribronchial thickening
- Patchy or more extensive atelectasis
- Possible collapse of a segment or a lobe
- Diffuse interstitial infiltrates commonly seen

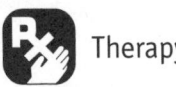 ## Therapy

GENERAL MANAGEMENT
- Most cases are mild and may be treated at home.

SUPPORTIVE OUTPATIENT MANAGEMENT
- Adequate fluid intake
- Maintenance of nasal airway patency:
—Short-term nasal decongestant
—Suction secretions with suction bulb

SUPPORTIVE INPATIENT MANAGEMENT
- Careful fluid hydration

Supplemental Oxygen
- Given to any patient with hypoxemia
- Preferably warmed, humidified, by head box or tent

Bronchodilators
- All infants with bronchiolitis with significant wheezing should receive a trial of at least one aerosolized β-adrenergic treatment to see if there is any relief of symptoms.
- Infants with history of prior wheezing or familial history of asthma or atopy are more likely to respond to bronchodilators.
- Theophylline is not usually useful as a bronchodilator, and may potentially worsen GE reflux, if present. This may be considered if apnea is present (keep level 5–10 mg/mL).

Nebulized Epinephrine
- Potentially beneficial in the early stage of bronchiolitis. It has combined α- and β-receptor agonists.
- Both racemic epinephrine (0.1 mL/kg of 2.25% solution) and L-epinephrine have been studied separately and showed beneficial results compared with β-agonists. To date, there is no specific guideline regarding the optimal dose and frequency for the treatment of bronchiolitis.

Corticosteroids
- Use of oral or inhaled steroid in children with bronchiolitis has not been evaluated adequately and current investigations have conflicting results. In previously healthy infants, corticosteroids are not routinely recommended.

Antibiotics
- Not usually indicated
- Superimposed bacterial infection is rare

Antiviral Agents (Ribavirin)
See Respiratory Syncytial Virus
- The major means of preventing RSV disease is strict observance of infection control.
- Comprehensive RSV-prevention programs should be implemented on all high-risk infants.

 ## Follow-Up

WHEN TO EXPECT IMPROVEMENT
- Most infants improve within 3 to 5 days. In some, nasal congestion and cough may continue for 1 to 3 weeks.
- Those who need mechanical ventilation may have difficulties with extubation due to excessive secretions and atelectasis.
- Approximately 30% to 40% of infants may have recurrent wheezing until 7 years of age.

SIGNS TO WATCH FOR
- Impending respiratory failure (increased work of breathing, retractions, hypoxemia, CO_2 retention, lethargy).
- Sudden deterioration suggesting atelectasis due to mucous plugging.
- Fatigue may occur in infants who have prolonged and extensive disease.
- Fatigue will manifest with increased pco_2 and worsening hypoxemia.

PITFALLS
- Hypoxia is common, so always follow oxygen saturation.
- Be aware of apnea.
- Respiratory failure may have a sudden presentation.
- In cases of clinical bronchiolitis, causes of false-negative ELISA tests:
—Poor quality of sample
—Sample contamination
—Insufficient sample
—Non-RSV bronchiolitis

 ## Common Questions and Answers

Q: How did my child get bronchiolitis?
A: RSV bronchiolitis is a common, seasonal, lower respiratory tract infection that is easily transmissible.

Q: Can my child become reinfected?
A: Children can become reinfected with RSV bronchiolitis, and infection can occur more than once during the same respiratory season.

Q: Do patients with bronchiolitis need to be isolated?
A: RSV-positive patients need to be isolated with other RSV-positive patients and from uninfected patients. Patients receiving ribavirin should be kept in isolation.

Q : Will my child develop asthma?
A : Recurrent wheezing has been described in about 30% to 40% of infants with RSV bronchiolitis. However, most data are retrospective and observational. Whether RSV per se can contribute to the development of asthma and allergic sensitization remains unclear.

ICD-9-CM 466.1

BIBLIOGRAPHY
American Academy of Pediatric. Respiratory syncytial virus. In: Pickering LK, ed. *2000 red book: report of the Committee on Infectious Diseases*, 25th ed. Elk Grove Village, IL: American Academy of Pediatrics, 2000:483–487.

Ehlenfield DR, Cameron K, Welliver RC. Eosinophilia at the time of respiratory syncytial virus bronchiolitis predicts childhood reactive airways disease. *Pediatrics* 2000;105:79–83.

Holberg CJ, Wright AL, Martinez FD, et al. Risk factors for respiratory syncytial virus- associated lower respiratory illness in the first year of life. *Am J Epidemiol* 1991;133:1135–1151.

Menon K, Sutcliffe T, Klassen TP. A randomized trial comparing the efficacy of epinephrine with salbutamol in the treatment of acute bronchiolitis. *J Pediatr* 1995;126:1004–1007.

Sigurs N, Bjarnason R, Sigurbergsson F, et al. Respiratory syncytial virus bronchiolitis in infancy is an important risk factor for asthma and allergy at age 7. *Am J Respir Crit Care Med* 2000;161:1501–1507.

Author: M. Elizabeth Hernandez

Bronchopulmonary Dysplasia

 Database

DEFINITION

Subsequent improvements in the care of premature neonates have decreased incidence of severe bronchopulmonary dysplasia (BPD), as described by Northway, and many authors have proposed refinement in the original definition, making the precise definition of BPD somewhat controversial.

PATHOPHYSIOLOGY

- Barotrauma is the result of positive-pressure applied to a surfactant-deficient lung, causing unequal pressures and thus unequal aeration of the tracheobronchial tree.
- Terminal bronchioles and alveolar ducts are prone to damage and rupture when subjected to higher than normal pressures.
- Ruptured bronchioles can lead to pulmonary interstitial emphysema (PIE), which increases the risk of BPD sixfold.
- Free radical damage is increased in premature lung, from hyperoxia and impaired antioxidant activity.

GENETICS

- Premature infants with a strong familial history of asthma and eczema are more likely to develop BPD.
- There is an association with HLA-A2.

EPIDEMIOLOGY

- Risk is inversely proportional to birth weight.
- Rare in infants weighing more than 1,500 g; common in infants weighing less than 1,000 g.
- Most common form of chronic lung disease in infancy.

COMPLICATIONS

- Prolonged intubation may cause subglottic stenosis and tracheomalacia.
- Pulmonary hypertension may occur as a result of vasculature damage and subsequent intimal proliferation, which may, in turn, produce right ventricular hypertrophy and, if severe enough, cor pulmonale.
- Pulmonary edema often occurs secondary to increased pulmonary capillary permeability and increased pulmonary pressures.
- Reactive airways, bronchospasm, and altered pulmonary mechanics due to a poorly compliant lung may result in abnormal pulmonary function testing and increased work of breathing.
- Malnutrition and growth failure may occur as a result of increased work of breathing and a subsequently high caloric expenditure.
- Impaired lung defenses result in an increased susceptibility to infection, especially respiratory syncytial virus (RSV).

PROGNOSIS

- Majority of survivors demonstrate slow, steady improvement.

- High death rate (17–47%) for patients with severe disease requiring prolonged mechanical ventilation.
- Despite multiple and varied treatment modalities, none has shown significant impact on the long-term outcome of chronic BPD.
- BPD survivors often have long-term pulmonary sequelae including hyperinflation, reactive airways, and exercise intolerance.
- Even older children and young adults who were felt to be asymptomatic have been shown to have abnormal responsiveness to exercise.
- Newer technologies, in particular the use of high-frequency ventilation and the widespread use of exogenous surfactant, have definitely improved survival rates for premature infants; however, concomitant reduction in the incidence and severity of BPD has been difficult to demonstrate.

 Differential Diagnosis

- Asthma
- Bronchiolitis obliterans
- Congenital heart disease
- Cystic adenomatoid malformation
- Cystic fibrosis
- Idiopathic pulmonary fibrosis
- Infections
- Meconium aspiration syndrome
- Recurrent aspiration

 Data Gathering

HISTORY

- Maternal use of antenatal steroids?
- Gestational age, birth weight, APGAR score?
- Initial resuscitative efforts, need for intubation, use of surfactant, duration in intubation, type of ventilation, duration of supplemental oxygen therapy, and other factors? These may have influenced the type and degree of lung injury.
- Familial history of asthma, atopy, or other children with BPD?
- Social support structure?
- Any potentially exacerbating factors such as exposure to smoking?

 Physical Examination

- Review of systems to include careful assessment of work of breathing both at rest and during activity.
- Feeding and sleeping history, and a review of growth charts.
- Vitals to include respiratory rate and pulse oxymetry both at rest and with activity.
- Signs of pulmonary hypertension, including peripheral edema, hepatomegaly, and venous distention.

 Laboratory Aids

Test: Changes on chest radiography
Significance: Include hyperinflation, emphysema, cyst formation, pulmonary edema, fibrosis, and cardiovascular changes. The severity of these changes may help predict the severity of the disease.

Test: Electrocardiogram
Significance: Often followed serially to assess for right ventricular hypertrophy (RVH).

Test: Echocardiogram
Significance: Often a useful adjunct to follow those patients with RVH.

Test: Cardiac catheterization
Significance: Reserved for those patients with evidence of pulmonary hypertension and cardiac dysfunction.

Test: Pulmonary function testing
Significance: Often used to follow patients and evaluate responsiveness to interventions.

Test: Blood gases
Significance: Useful both in the acute and chronic management of BPD to follow the degree of hypoxia and hypercapnia.

Test: Bronchoscopy, barium swallow, PH probe, and sleep studies
Significance: May reveal other underlying conditions possibly contributing to pulmonary dysfunction.

 Therapy

DIURETICS

- Diuretics are used for treating pulmonary edema, often improving lung mechanics and gas exchange.
- Furosemide may have other nondiuretic benefits, including effects on prostaglandin synthesis, direct vasodilatation, and improved surfactant production.
- There are many side effects from long-term furosemide therapy including azotemia, ototoxicity, electrolyte abnormalities, excessive urinary calcium loss, osteopenia, and nephrocalcinosis.
- Thiazide diuretics, usually used in conjunction with a potassium-sparing diuretic such as spironolactone, are generally considered to be not as effective as furosemide.
- Routine monitoring of electrolytes recommended for patients on long-term diuretic therapy.
- Electrolyte supplementation often required with long-term diuretic usage.

BRONCHODILATORS

Inhaled β-agonists are effective treatment for reversible bronchospasm, though the safety and efficacy of long-term usage of these agents has yet to be established.

Albuterol is often the drug of choice, though longer acting agents often used as well.

Muscarinic antagonists, such as ipratropium, may be useful adjuncts, especially in patients who are not significantly responsive to albuterol. Felt to work on large- and medium-sized airways.

- Cromolyn, though not a bronchodilator, is often used for its antiinflammatory effects and has a low side-effect profile.
- Methylxanthines, such as caffeine and theophylline, are often used in the treatment of apnea because of their effects on respiratory drive, also have a mild diuretic effect and help improve diaphragmatic contractility, making them a potentially useful adjunct in BPD as well.

PULMONARY VASODILATORS

Supplemental oxygen is an effective vasodilator and remains a mainstay of treatment for infants with either chronic or intermittent hypoxia.

STEROIDS

- Steroid usage in BPD is controversial.
- Increased risk for sepsis has probably been overstated.
- Often used successfully in short regimens to wean ventilatory support and hasten extubation.
- No long-term benefits of steroid therapy have been demonstrated, including reduced hospitalization, improved survival, or reduced incidence of BPD.
- Inhaled steroids may provide the desired antiinflammatory effects, without systemic side effects, making them attractive as both prevention and treatment, although their routine use in premature infants is an active area of investigation. Linear growth retardation has been a concern. Newer agents that can be nebulized are now available, improving drug delivery in small infants.

NUTRITION

- Infants with BPD may have increased caloric needs as much as 150 kcal/kg/d.
- Premature and critically ill infants may be deficient in antioxidants such as vitamin A, vitamin E, and superoxide dismutase (SOD).
- Supplementation of vitamin A, vitamin E, and SOD at therapeutic and supratherapeutic levels have not yet shown to affect outcomes in BPD, though antioxidant supplementation remains an area of ongoing research.

 Follow-Up

- A multidisciplinary approach is recommended for all patients with moderate and severe BPD.

- Team may include primary care physician, pediatric pulmonologist, pediatric cardiologist, nutritionist, speech, respiratory, occupational, and physical therapists.
- Monitor growth and nutritional status.
- Monitor neurodevelopmental status, including NICU "high-risk" follow-up.

PREVENTION

- Antenatal steroids for all mothers with irreversible preterm labor, less than 35 weeks' gestation.
- Surfactant administration clearly improves mortality, though a reduction in the incidence or severity of BPD has been difficult to demonstrate.
- A change in ventilatory strategy toward "permissive hypercapnia," which favors the acceptance of lower pH and higher Pco_2 in exchange for lower peak inspiratory pressures and less barotrauma, has been widely adopted.
- High-frequency ventilation, with either oscillatory or jet technology, may prevent barotrauma, though has yet to be shown to affect the incidence or severity of BPD.
- Avoidance of pulmonary edema, including the prophylactic and early treatment of patent ductus arteriosis may be of benefit.
- Early nutritional support, including the supplementation of antioxidant vitamins and minerals at therapeutic and supratherapeutic levels, may be of benefit.

PITFALLS

- Ensure adequate calcium and phosphorus intake in patients at risk for hyperparathyroidism and rickets.
- Patients less than 2 years old are candidates for RSV immune globulin prophylaxis, if not contraindicated.
- Patients older than 6 months are candidates for influenza vaccine, if not contraindicated.
- Chest physiotherapy may cause pathologic fractures in patients with osteopenia.

 Common Questions and Answers

Q: Will antibiotics help my child?
A: While some evidence suggests that infection with ureaplasm may be important in the pathogenesis of BPD, it remains to be seen whether or not treatment of this particular organism affects outcome. Excessive usage of antibiotics increases occurrence of antibiotic resistance.

Q: Which babies should get RSV immune globulin (Respigam or Synagis)?
A: Immunoprophylaxis has been recommended by the AAP Committee on Infectious Diseases for infants with BPD who are less than 2 years old at the onset of RSV season. Other premature infants may be candidates as well, regardless of their BPD status, according to their gestational age at birth and their age at the onset of RSV season. Those infants who were born at 28 weeks or less at the onset of RSV season

and who are 12 months or less should receive immunoprophylaxis monthly for the entire RSV season. Those infants who were born between 29 and 32 weeks' gestation and who are 6 months old or younger at the beginning of RSV season should also receive immunoprophylaxis. Those in between 32 and 35 weeks may or may not be candidates depending on other risk factors, such as day-care attendance, exposure to tobacco smoke, and the number of other small children in the home.

Q: Will anti-RSV immunoprophylaxis prevent my baby from getting RSV?
A: It won't prevent RSV, but it will help your child's own immune system attack the virus.

Q: Will my child have asthma when he grows up?
A: Asthma occurs in over 50% of older children who survived BPD.

Q: What types of additional therapies can help my child?
A: Chest physiotherapy may be of benefit in infants with both early and late BPD, helping to mobilize secretions and to prevent atelectasis. Speech and occupational therapy may be of benefit as infants who have had prolonged intubation or other interventions that may have interfered with oral functioning may have some degree of oral-motor dysfunction and oral aversion. Other infants simply with increased work of breathing may have discoordinated suck and swallow, making oral feedings difficult. Physical therapy may be of benefit to help infants with gross and fine motor delays, poor tone, and abnormal posture. Parents can learn many of the therapies in order to incorporate therapeutic exercises and positioning into their daily routines.

ICD-9-CM 770.7

BIBLIOGRAPHY

Bader D, Ramos AD, Lew CD, et al. Childhood sequelae of infant lung disease exercise and pulmonary function abnormalities after bronchopulmonary dysplasia. *J Pediatr* 1987;10:693–699.

Hageman JR, ed. *The pediatric clinics of North America: neonatology update*. Philadelphia: WB Saunders, 1998.

Jobe AH, Ikegami M. Prevention of bronchopulmonary dysplasia. *Curr Opin Pediatr* 2001;13(2):124–129.

Northway WH Jr, Rosan RC, Porter DY. Pulmonary disease following respiratory therapy of hyaline membrane disease. *N Engl J Med* 1967;276:357–368.

Author: John M. Good

Bruxism

 Database

DEFINITION

Bruxism is a nonfunctional grinding of the teeth. It is a poorly understood phenomenon with many suggested etiologies. It is usually a subconscious activity that can occur during the day or night. Clenching is a related condition that also is considered to be a nonfunctional habit. Nonfunctional (or "parafunctional") habits include mandibular movements not involved with normal chewing, swallowing, or speaking. Some examples of these include chewing pencils, nail, cheek, or lip biting.

INCIDENCE

• Bruxism may occur throughout life. Its frequency tends to peak up to the ages of 7 to 10 and then decreases with age.
• Infants have been known to brux with the eruption of the first primary tooth. Bruxism may sometimes be temporarily or intermittently present, making diagnosis difficult.
• Incidence of bruxism in children has been reported to be from 5% to 88% (with most reports indicating an average of 15% to 30%)

ETIOLOGY

The exact cause of bruxism is not known, but several factors have been implicated:

• Dental (local) factors

—Occlusal interferences, including malocclusions, where teeth do not interdigitate smoothly
—"High" dental restorations (e.g., fillings or crowns)
—Intraoral irritation (e.g., sharp tooth cusp)
—Teething

• Psychological factors

—Nervous tension (related to stress, anger, and aggression)
—Personality disorders
—Mental retardation

• Systemic factors: common

—Neuromuscular disorders (e.g., cerebral palsy)
—Brain injury
—Burn injuries

• Uncommon or rare

—Asthma
—Genetics
—Allergies
—Nutritional and vitamin deficiencies
—Intestinal parasites
—Endocrine disorders
—Restricted mobility of the cervical spine
—Mouth breathing

SIGNS/SYMPTOMS AND ASSOCIATED PROBLEMS

• Teeth

—Wear facets; abraded areas on teeth
—Extreme wear of the primary teeth is occasionally observed, but it is extremely rare that the pulp becomes exposed or nerve damage occurs
—Broken dental restorations
—Loosening of the teeth
—Exacerbation of preexisting periodontal disturbances (gingival inflammation and recession, alveolar bone loss)
—Tooth pain or sensitivity

• Muscular symptoms in any of the head and neck muscles- -Most often seen in the lateral pterygoids, followed by the medial pterygoids and masseters

—Pain
—Trismus
—Spasm

• Headache (especially in the morning)
• Temporomandibular joint (TMJ) disorders

—Pain in the TMJ area
—Symptoms (pain, trismus, spasm) in the masticatory muscles
—Limited mandibular range of motion
—Degenerative changes in the TMJ (very rare, especially in children)

(The evidence equating bruxism as an etiologic factor in temporomandibular joint disorders is contradictory and insufficient to support active therapy on this basis)

• Grinding sounds, nocturnal and/or diurnal, which can be extremely distressing for parents and caregivers.

 Differential Diagnosis

• Dental problems
• Seizures
• Drug reaction
• Stress

 Therapy

• Treatment for bruxism is **rarely** indicated in children. Practical considerations include:
• Therapy is justified if damage to the *permanent* dentition or periodontal structures is observed (occasionally in adolescents)

Treatment should be limited to the most simple and reversible measures. There are inadequate data to support the efficacy of irreversible treatment in children. (Irreversible approaches include selective tooth grinding and orthodontics.)

COMMONLY UTILIZED MODES OF TREATMENT

• Patient and family education

—Ensure that the bruxism itself does not become an issue generating stress for the child

• Behavior (habit) therapy
• Stress counseling

—Identify and address sources of stress
—Biofeedback exercises
—Counseling/psychotherapy
—Hypnosis

UNCOMMONLY UTILIZED MODES OF TREATMENT

• Plastic or vinyl bite guard
• Occlusal adjustment (selective tooth grinding to balance the bite)
• Dental restorations

—Treat and restore carious lesions
—Stainless steel crowns for extreme wear in primary teeth in order to stop tooth sensitivity and/or prevent pulpal exposure

RARELY UTILIZED MODES OF TREATMENT

• Physical therapy

—Warm compresses for muscle or TMJ symptoms
—Limit affected muscle activity (e.g., "do not open wide," "take very small bites," "do not chew gum")
—Ultrasound
—TENS
—Acupressure and/or acupuncture
—Correct cervical spine dysfunction (particularly head position)

• Medications

—Analgesic for symptoms
—Antiinflammatory (e.g., ibuprofen) for symptoms
—Muscle relaxants for symptoms
—Mild tranquilizers if anxiety plays an etiologic role

• Orthodontics

PROGNOSIS

Although the associated problems are well documented, there are no data that establish cause-and-effect relationships for bruxism in childhood continuing on in adulthood.

- Preschool children

—Bruxism typically ceases without therapeutic interventions.
—Associated problems are rare.

- School-age children

—Bruxism typically ceases without therapeutic interventions.
—Monitor for associated conditions without treatment.

- Adolescents

—More commonly benefit from therapeutic intervention.
—Associated problems may also require therapy (e.g., abrasion of teeth, muscular, TMJ symptoms).

- Special needs children

—The long-term prognosis for bruxism in special needs children is poor.
—Acute situations in children who are comatose or those who have suffered traumatic brain injuries or severe burns can be managed by the use of prefabricated bite blocks, or in rare cases, by the fabrication of custom-fitted mouth guards. These appliances are primarily used to prevent soft tissue damage from parafunctional habits such as lip, cheek, and tongue biting.

 Follow-Up

- Continue to monitor for significant associated problems.
- Intercede if damage to permanent dentition and/or periodontal structures is observed

 Common Questions and Answers

Q: How should bruxism in a preschool child be treated?
A: The great majority of bruxism in children stops without any therapy.

Considering the controversial nature of treatment modalities, it is prudent to advise no treatment for childhood bruxism and to advise the parents that the condition is common and is usually outgrown.

Q: What about treating bruxism in adolescence?
A: Because damage to the permanent teeth or periodontal structures may have long-term consequences, bruxism in adolescence can be a concern. Still, treatment should be limited to the most simple and reversible approaches. Careful dental evaluation would be an important first step.

Q: Does damage to the primary teeth result in problems with the permanent teeth or with the TMJ?
A: There is no evidence that bruxism in children leads to problems during adolescence or later.

Q: Should custom-fitted mouth guards be fabricated for children with traumatic brain or burn injuries, who engage in lip or tongue biting?
A: The long-term prognosis for bruxism is often poor in these patients. For patients with transitory soft tissue injuries, conservative measures such as prefabricated bite-blocks to get through the acute stage should be tried first. Patients who exhibit chronic chewing may require the fabrication of custom-fitted mouth guards, which may require the use of deep sedation or general anesthesia procedures in order to construct the appliance. The risk of these procedures would need to be weighed against the benefit of the bite guard.

ICD-9-CM 306.8

BIBLIOGRAPHY

Ahmad R. Bruxism in children. *J Pedodont* 1986;10:105–126.

Ash M, Ramfjord S. Concepts of dysfunction. In: *Occlusion*, 4th ed. Philadelphia: WB Saunders, 1995:144–146.

Cash R. Bruxism in children: review of the literature. *J Pedodont* 1988;12:107–125.

Faulkner D. Bruxism: a review of the literature. *Aust Dent J* 1990;35(4):355–361.

American Academy of Pediatric Dentistry. Guidelines for temporomandibular disorders in children and adolescents. In: *Reference manual 1999-00: pediatric dentistry*. 1999;21(5):66–67.

Okeson J. Etiology of functional disturbances in the masticatory system. In: *Management of temporomandibular disorders and occlusion*, 4th ed. St. Louis: Mosby, 1998:149–173.

Authors: Zuhair Sayany, Howard M. Rosenberg, and Mark L. Helpin

Bulimia

Database

DEFINITION
Bulimia nervosa is an eating disorder characterized by:
- Recurrent episodes of binge eating characterized by rapid consumption of large amounts of food in discrete periods of time, usually less than 2 hours.
- Accompanied by compensatory behavior such as self-induced vomiting, laxative or diuretic use, strict dieting or vigorous exercise to induce weight loss.
- Minimum average of two binge-eating episodes per week for at least 3 months
- Feeling of lack of control over eating behavior during eating binges.
- Frenzied quality, often occurring alone and secretively.
- Associated feelings of guilt, anxiety, low self-esteem, and depression.
- Persistent overconcern with body shape and weight

PATHOPHYSIOLOGY
- Personality traits of low self-esteem, self-regulatory difficulties, frustration intolerance, and impaired ability to recognize and directly express feelings have been described in patients with bulimia nervosa.
- May be two subtypes
—Multi-impulsive: rely on binging and purging as a way of regulating intolerable states of tension, anger, and fragmentation.
—Post-dieting: binge eating precipitated by dietary restraint with compensatory behaviors maintained by reduction of guilty feelings associated with fears of weight gain.
- Neuroendocrine abnormalities may also play a role:
—Abnormalities in serotonergic function have been demonstrated in patients with bulimia nervosa. Serotonin is thought to be involved in development of satiety.
- Cholecystokinin response to a meal is decreased in patients with bulimia nervosa, which also may indicate abnormal satiety signaling.
- May be abnormalities in other hormones or neurotransmitters such as leptin, dopamine, and endorphins, but unclear if these are cause or effect.

GENETICS
Recent studies, including twin studies suggest that bulimia nervosa and binge-eating is familial.

EPIDEMIOLOGY
- Onset in late adolescence to early adulthood (range: 13–28 years of age)
- Females account for 85% to 90% of cases
- Affects 1% to 3% of young females in Western countries
- Affects 4% to 10% of adolescent and college-age females
- Ten times more common than anorexia nervosa

- 83% have lifetime history of an anxiety disorder and 63% have a lifetime history of depression

COMPLICATIONS
Pulmonary
- Aspiration pneumonia
- Pneumomediastinum

Gastrointestinal
- Pancreatitis
- Parotid-gland enlargement
- Gastric and esophageal irritation
- Mallory-Weiss tears
- Paralytic ileus (due to laxative abuse and hypokalemia)
- Cathartic colon (due to laxative abuse)

Metabolic
- Hypokalemia (due to laxative abuse or vomiting)
- Secondary cardiac dysrhythmias, myopathy, ileus
- Electrolyte imbalances, including hypomagnesemia
- Fluid imbalances
- Hyperamylasemia
- Edema (secondary to hypoproteinemia or renal sodium and water retention secondary to hypovolemia)
- Bone loss (if amenorrhea; significantly more common in anorexia nervosa)

Dental
- Enamel erosion
- Caries and periodontal disease

PROGNOSIS
- Very low mortality: 0.3% (but may be underestimation secondary to poor follow-up in studies)
- Most have episodic course with trend toward improvement
- No studies of long-term prognosis in adolescents
- Adult studies: 5- to 10-year follow-up
—50% made full recovery
—30% relapsed
—20% still met full criteria for bulimia nervosa
- Poor prognostic indicators:
—Concomitant depression, personality disorder, or substance abuse
—Frequent vomiting
—History of substance abuse
- Good prognostic indicators:
—High motivation for treatment
—No concurrent disruptive psychopathology
—Good self-esteem

Differential Diagnosis

Psychosocial
- Psychogenic vomiting
- Drug abuse

MISCELLANEOUS
- Gastrointestinal obstruction
- Hiatal hernia

Data Gathering

HISTORY
Eating-Disorder Specific
- Eating habits
- Rituals, behaviors
- Body image
- Actual and desired weights, minimum and maximum weights
- Use of laxatives, diuretics, diet pills, emetics
- Presence of binge or purge behavior
- Menstrual history
- History of exercise

General
- Weakness or fatigue or hyperactivity
- Thirst, frequent urination
- Headaches
- Abdominal pain, fullness, bloating, or nausea
- Constipation or diarrhea

Psychiatric
- Mood disorder
- Substance abuse
- Anxiety
- Personality disorders
- Suicidal tendencies
- Low self-esteem
- Feelings of ineffectiveness

Family
- Medical and psychiatric histories

Physical Examination

Finding: Vital signs
Significance: Check for hypotension

Finding: Weight
Significance: May be normal, overweight, or underweight

Finding: Edema of hands and feet
Significance: Evidence of low albumin or compensatory renal sodium and water retention

Finding: Calluses on knuckles or hands
Significance: Russell sign secondary to inducing vomiting

Finding: Erosion of dental enamel
Significance: Exposure to gastric juices secondary to frequent vomiting

Finding: Muscle cramps or weakness
Significance: Hypokalemia

SPECIAL QUESTIONS
- How much do you want to weigh?
- How do you control your weight?
- How do you feel about yourself?
- How often do you vomit, use diuretics or laxatives?

Laboratory Aids

Perform a laboratory evaluation as part of the diagnostic workup. Laboratory evaluation is most useful for assessing complications. There is no diagnostic or confirmatory laboratory test for bulimia nervosa. Many patients have normal laboratory studies.

Test: CBC
Significance: Iron-deficiency anemia

Test: Electrolytes, including calcium, magnesium, and phosphate
Significance: Abnormalities may occur as a result of prolonged vomiting or use of laxatives

Test: BUN and creatinine
Significance: Renal function usually normal but BUN may be elevated secondary to dehydration or low secondary to protein loss.

Test: Glucose
Significance: Patient may be hypoglycemic

Test: Cholesterol, lipids
Significance: May be elevated in starvation states.

Test: Amylase
Significance: Pancreatitis

Test: Total protein, albumin, prealbumin
Significance: Usually normal but may be low as evidence of malnutrition

Test: Liver function tests
Significance: Transaminases may be mildly elevated (up to twice normal)

Test: ESR
Significance: Almost invariably normal. If elevated consider occult organic process.

Test: HCO_3^-
Significance: Metabolic alkalosis from vomiting or metabolic acidosis if using laxatives

Test: Urine toxicology screen, optional
Significance: May be positive, as this disorder often is associated with substance abuse

Test: ECG with rhythm strip
Significance: May reveal U waves associated with hypokalemia

RADIOGRAPHIC STUDIES
• Consider upper GI series with small-bowel follow-through
• Consider DEXA scan if prolonged amenorrhea to evaluate bone density

Therapy

• Hospitalize in cases of:
—Hypovolemia
—Severe electrolyte disturbances
—Intractable vomiting
—Acute psychiatric emergencies (e.g., suicidal ideation, acute psychosis)

—Medical complication of malnutrition (e.g., aspiration pneumonia, cardiac failure, pancreatitis, Mallory-Weiss syndrome, etc.)
—Comorbid diagnoses that interfere with the treatment of the eating disorder (e.g., severe depression, obsessive-compulsive disorder, severe family dysfunction)
—Failure of outpatient therapy

PSYCHOTHERAPY
• Outpatient therapy
• Cognitive behavioral therapy:
—More effective than interpersonal psychotherapy or behavioral therapy alone
—Focuses on patient's preoccupation with weight and body shape, persistent dieting, and binging and purging cycles
—Patients are directed to monitor the thoughts, feelings, and circumstances surrounding binge-purge episodes, cease dieting, begin regular eating, and challenge their assumptions that their weight is linked to self-esteem.
• Individual psychotherapy
• Family treatment (to help with dysfunctional family dynamics)
• Group therapy

DRUGS
• Antidepressants
—Decrease the binge-purge behavior
—Improve attitudes about eating
—Lessen preoccupation with food and weight
—Fluoxetine (Prozac), sertraline (Zoloft), desipramine, and fluvoxamine (Luvox) have been used with good results in patients with bulimia nervosa.
—One study showed fluoxetine to be helpful in patients with a poor response to psychotherapy.
—Effect of antidepressant may diminish over time and patients may relapse when stopped.
• Stool softeners may be used for constipation, but avoid laxatives.
• Ondansetron shown in one study to decrease vomiting frequency. It may help normalize the physiologic mechanism controlling satiation.

Follow-Up

• Reduction in binge and purge episodes may take months or years.
• Behavioral and thought disorders associated with bulimia nervosa may be of long duration.

SIGNS TO WATCH FOR
• Weight loss or major weight fluctuations
• Electrolyte abnormalities
• Muscle cramps
• Fatigue
• Depression or mood disturbance
• Willful behavior or acting out

PREVENTION
• Emphasize healthy self-esteem and body image during visits with preadolescents and adolescents.

PITFALLS
• During treatment, patients and their families may cause "splitting" of the hospital staff. To avoid this, always be supportive and maintain consistency in stating goals.

Common Questions and Answers

Q: How do I determine if a patient has anorexia with vomiting or bulimia?
A: The key feature of bulimia nervosa is the binge episode, which distinguishes it from anorexia nervosa. If there are not at least two binge eating episodes per week for at least 3 months, the diagnosis is not bulimia.

Q: What laboratory abnormalities should I look for in my patients with bulimia?
A: Electrolyte abnormalities, particularly hypokalemia. Patients may develop a hypochloremic metabolic alkalosis. If electrolytes are significantly abnormal, the patient should be hospitalized until they have normalized.

ICD-9-CM 133.6

BIBLIOGRAPHY
Agras WS, Walsh BT, Fairburn CG, et al. A multicenter comparison of cognitive-behavioral therapy and interpersonal psychotherapy for bulimia nervosa. *Arch Gen Psychiatry* 2000;57:459–466.

Bulik CM, Sullivan PF, Kendler KS. Heritability of binge-eating and broadly defined bulimia nervosa. *Biol Psychiatry* 1998;44:1210–1218.

Comerci GD. Medical complications of anorexia and bulimia nervosa. *Med Clin North Am* 1990;74:1293–1310.

Faris PL, Kim SW, Meller WH, et al. Effect of decreasing afferent vagal activity with odansetron on symptoms of bulimia nervosa: a randomized, double-blind trial. *Lancet* 2000;355:792–797.

Haller E. Eating disorders. A review and update. *West J Med* 1992;157:658–662.

Herzog DB, Keller MB, Sacks NR, et al. Psychiatric comorbidity in treatment-seeking anorexics and bulimics. *J Am Acad Child Adolesc Psychiatry* 1992;31:810–818.

Kaye WH, Klump KL, Frank GKW, et al. Anorexia and bulimia nervosa. *Annu Rev Med* 2000;51.

Keel PK, Mitchell JE. Outcome in bulimia nervosa. *Am J Psychiatry* 1997;154:131–321.

Kreipe RE, Birndorf SA. Eating disorders in adolescent and young adults. *Med Clin North Am* 2000;84:1027–1049.

Walsh BT, Agras WS, Devlin MJ, et al. Fluoxetine for bulimia nervosa following poor response to psychotherapy. *Am J Psychiatry* 2000;157:1332–1334.

Author: Nadja Peter
Liana R. Clark, 2nd edition

C1 Esterase Inhibitor Deficiency

 Database

DEFINITION

• C1 esterase inhibitor deficiency is a hereditary and acquired form of recurrent angioedema. The attacks are usually without urticaria.
• C1 esterase inhibitor deficiency has now been classified into a number of types including:

—Hereditary angioedema (HAE) type I (transmitted as autosomal dominant)
—HAE type II (transmitted as autosomal dominant)
—Acquired angioedema (AAE) type I
—AAE type II

• HAE type I accounts for approximately 85% of the C1 esterase deficiencies and is a genetic alteration that leads to impairment of mRNA transcription or translation and, therefore, decreased enzyme synthesis.
• HAE type II is a genetic alteration that leads to production of an inactive protein.
• In acquired deficiency of C1 esterase inhibitor, there appears to be a normal ability to synthesize the enzyme; however, the enzyme is metabolized at an increased rate. This syndrome may be seen in patients with autoimmune diseases or malignancy and usually occurs after the fourth decade of life.
• AAE type I is a very rare syndrome usually associated with lymphoproliferative (usually B cell), carcinomas, autoimmune diseases, and paraproteinemias. Because of the other disease processes, complement-activating factors and idiotype-antiidiotype complexes act to increase consumption of C1 esterase inhibitor.
• AAE type II develops when an auto antibody is produced against the C1 esterase inhibitor protein. When these antibodies adhere to the C1 esterase molecule and conformational change occurs leading to decreased function or enhanced metabolism.
• AAE forms may be differentiated from HAE by genetic studies and serologically by significantly decreased C1q, C1r, C1s levels and decreased functional activity of the enzyme in AAE.

PATHOPHYSIOLOGY

• C1 esterase inhibitor is a single chain polypeptide with a molecular weight of 108 kd. The gene has been identified on chromosome 11 (11q12-q13.1)
• This protein inhibits the classic complement pathway by inhibiting activation of C2 and C4. In the fibrinolytic system, C1 esterase inhibitor inhibits formation of plasmin, the activation of C1r and C1s, and the formation of bradykinin from kininogen.
• With a deficiency of this enzyme, the classic complement system becomes activated along with fibrinolysis and kinin formation, which is felt to participate in the production of angioedema.
• Kinin is known to cause similar histologic lesions to histamine but without pruritus.
• The complement activation leads to production of C2b, a product that also has kinin-like activity, and bradykinin, a vasoactive peptide that may also participate in the formation of angioedema.

GENETICS

HAE type I and II are transmitted as autosomal dominant.

 Differential Diagnosis

• IgE mediated

—Episodic angioedema
—Allergic reactions to food and drugs
—Physically induced angioedema

• Hypocomplementemic (hereditary angioedema)
• Idiosyncratic

—Nonsteroidal antiinflammatory drugs
—Other drugs

• Lupus erythematosus
• Idiopathic

 Data Gathering

HISTORY

Question: What is the presentation?
Significance: Patients with HAE usually present in the second decade of life with angioedema involving the subcutaneous tissues (mostly involving the extremities).

Question: What gastrointestinal effects are present?
Significance: Angioedema involving the gastrointestinal tract may lead to severe pain, vomiting, and diarrhea.

Question: Are there respiratory complications?
Significance: Two out of three patients will have orofacial or laryngeal swelling.

Question: Can there be hives?
Significance: The edema usually occurs without evidence of inflammation; however, episodes of urticaria have also been documented.

• The variability of clinical manifestations, even among individuals with the same genetic mutation, is striking, implicating nongenetic factors or other genes as possible mediators of clinical presentation.
• Emesis?
• Diarrhea?
• Hypotension from extravasation of plasma into the skin?
• Hemoconcentration?
• Azotemia?
• Central nervous system complaints including headache, hemiparesis, and seizures, may be triggered by trauma or stress.
• AAE presents in the same way but usually in the fourth decade of life, not associated with a familial history.

Physical Examination

Depending on the clinical features, angioedema causes pale, well-demarcated, tense, brawny, nonpruritic and nonpitting single or multiple localized swellings. These may involve the periorbital tissues, genitalia, face, tongue, lips, larynx, extremities, and gastrointestinal tract.

Laboratory Aids

- C1 esterase inhibitor concentration
- C1 esterase inhibitor activity
- C4 concentration
- C1q concentration (usually lower in patients with AAE)

Therapy

- For these entities, therapy is divided into management of the acute attack, maintenance therapy for HAE, and more specific interventions for those with AAE.
- During an acute episode, management focuses on adequate respiratory and fluid resuscitation, and the treatment of pain.
- In HAE, acute attacks are treated with replacement of the C1 esterase inhibitor with IV concentrates. Fresh frozen plasma may also be used.
- For prophylaxis, androgens (such as danazol and stanozolol) are used in postpubertal patients with HAE of both types.
- These androgens stimulate the synthesis of C1-INH, and, while the level of activity is not normalized, it is increased sufficiently to be clinically efficacious.
- In prepubertal children, androgens are used only in those with severe attacks or purified C1-INH if available.
- For those patients who do not tolerate androgens, tranexamic acid and ϵ-aminocaproic acid (antifibrinolytic inhibitors or plasmin activity) may be used, although they carry the risk of significant side effects.
- AAE type I requires an intensive search for malignancy, although this form of AAE occasionally appears before the development of clinical signs of the malignancy.
- Androgens are also effective in preventing attacks in individuals with this syndrome.
- AAE type II requires immunosuppression to decrease formation of the autoantibody.
- Androgen treatment has not led to good clinical response.

Common Questions and Answers

Q: What are other causes of angioedema?
A: There are classic allergic reactions to food and drugs, physically induced angioedema, IgE-mediated episodic angioedema, idiosyncratic reactions to NSAIDs and other drugs, lupus erythematosus, and idiopathic causes.

Q: What are the usual precipitating factors in causing reactions?
A: Recurrent episodes of angioedema, abdominal pain, nausea, vomiting occur wither spontaneously or after local trauma, especially of the upper respiratory tract. Other causes include vigorous exercise, emotional stress, and with menstrual periods.

ICD-9-CM

Hereditary angioedema 277.6
Angioedema 955.1

BIBLIOGRAPHY

Buckley RH, Mathews KP. Common allergic skin diseases. *JAMA* 1982;248:2611.

Csepregi A, Nemesanszky E. Acquired C1 esterase inhibitor deficiency. *Ann Intern Med* 2000;133(10):838–839.

Green M. *Pediatric diagnosis*. Philadelphia: WB Saunders, 1986.

Heymann WR. Acquired angioedema. *J Am Acad Dermatol* 1997;36:611–615.

Huston DP, Bressler RB. Urticaria and angioedema. *Med Clin North Am* 1992;76(4):805–840.

Kaplan AP. The pathogenic basis of angioedema and urticaria, recent advances. *Am J Med* 1981;70:755.

Oski FA, DeAngelis CD, Feign RD, et al. *Principles and practice of pediatrics*. Philadelphia: JB Lippincott, 1990.

Winnewisser J, Rossi M, Spath P, et al. Type I hereditary angio-oedema. Variability of clinical presentation and course within two large kindreds. *J Intern Med* 1997;241:39–46.

Zuraw BL. Urticaria, angioedema, and autoimmunity. *Clin Lab Med* 1997;17(3):559–569.

Author: Andrew E. Mulberg

Campylobacter Infections

 Database

DEFINITION

- *Campylobacter* species involved in human infections include *C. jejuni* (which causes enteritis), and *C. fetus* (implicated in systemic illness).
- *Campylobacter* is a motile, curved, microaerophilic, non–lactose-fermenting, gram-negative rod that requires oxygen and carbon dioxide for optimal growth.

PATHOPHYSIOLOGY

- *C. jejuni* adheres to epithelial cells and mucus, secretes cytotoxins (which play a role in the development of watery diarrhea), and induces an inflammatory ileocolitis.
- Enteritis, the best-known disease of *C. jejuni,* has been isolated more often than *Salmonella* or *Shigella,* with an incidence of 4% to 12% of diarrheal illness.
- Bacteremia, although uncommon, can occur, especially in the neonate and immunocompromised host; *C. fetus* is the species most likely to be isolated.
- *C. upsaliensis* has been identified in immunocompromised individuals and is usually associated with a self-limiting enteritis.

EPIDEMIOLOGY

- *Campylobacter* infections equal and perhaps exceed the number of cases of inflammatory enteritis due to other causes, with the highest attack rates observed in young children.
- 30% to 100% of chickens, turkeys, and water fowl are infected asymptomatically in addition to swine, cattle, sheep, horses, rodents, and household pets (especially young). Contaminated water and milk sources also act as reservoirs for infections.
- Transmission of disease is by the fecal-oral route from contaminated food and water or by direct contact with fecal material from animals or persons infected with the organism.
- Person-to-person transmission of *C. jejuni* has been reported when the index cases were young children who were incontinent of feces; vertical transmission from mother to neonate has also been reported.
- Asymptomatic hospital personnel or food handlers have not been implicated as sources.
- The peak rate of isolation occurs in the warmer months of the year (late summer, early fall).

COMPLICATIONS

- Postinfectious immunologic complications include reactive arthritis, Guillain-Barré syndrome (GBS), Reiter syndrome, and erythema nodosum.
- *C. jejuni* is the most frequently identified cause of GBS with serotypes 0:19 and 0:41, and is responsible for up to 40% of GBS cases.
- HLA-B27 antigen is associated with reactive arthropathy.
- Seizures may develop in young children with enteritis and high fevers.
- A typhoid-like syndrome and meningitis have also been reported in patients with *Campylobacter* infection.
- Spontaneous abortion, and hemolytic-uremic syndrome have been described with *C. upsaliensis.*

PROGNOSIS

- For patients with enteritis, the prognosis is very good, regardless of whether antibiotic treatment is given.

 Differential Diagnosis

Campylobacter infection should be considered in all patients with a diarrheal illness, especially those with a history of bloody or mucous stools, recurrent gastritis or in immunocompromised hosts.

 Data Gathering

HISTORY

Question: Exposure to unpasteurized milk products?
Significance: Source of *Campylobacter* infection.

Question: Well water used?
Significance: Contaminated water serves as a reservoir.

Question: Inadequately cooked poultry?
Significance: Chickens are asymptomatic carriers.

Question: Fever, abdominal pain, bloody diarrhea?
Significance: Illness is characterized by fever, abdominal pain, and bloody diarrhea. Symptoms can last for 24 hours and be indistinguishable from a viral gastroenteritis, or can be relapsing, thus mimicking inflammatory bowel disease.

Question: Inflammatory ileocolitis?
Significance: The most common manifestation in children.

Question: Duration of symptoms?
Significance: Incubation period is 1 to 7 days and is usually self-limited by 5 to 7 days.

Physical Examination

Finding: Abdominal pain, diarrhea, malaise, and fever.
Significance: Signs and symptoms of *C. jejuni* infection. If the infection establishes a chronic phase (20% of infected patients), symptoms may mimic inflammatory bowel disease and other immunoreactive complications such as reactive arthropathy, GBS, Reiter syndrome, and erythema nodosum may occur.

Laboratory Aids

Test: Examination of fecal specimen for darting motility of *C. jejuni* by darkfield or phase-contrast microscopy
Significance: If examined within 2 hours of passage, it can permit presumptive diagnosis.

Test: Stool culture
Significance: Can be used, but selective media (Skirrow, Butzler, or campy-BAP) must be used to isolate *Campylobacter* species.

Test: DNA-based testing
Significance: Development of this diagnostic tool will improve the ability to detect and differentiate *Campylobacter* species much faster than the gold standard of stool culture.

Therapy

• If treated early in the course of disease (less than 4 days), erythromycin or azithromycin for 5 to 7 days appears to be effective in eradicating the organism from the stool within 2 to 3 days.
• Ciprofloxacin, tetracycline, aminoglycosides, and imipenem are alternative antimicrobials if resistant or bacteremic strains are present.

Follow-Up

• Once treated, symptoms should improve in 2 to 3 days.
• In the untreated patient, the median excretion of organism is up to 2 to 3 weeks, and it was 3 months before all patients in one study were free of the organism. Asymptomatic carriage is uncommon.
• The expected course of treatment of *C. pylori* infection is variable since *in vitro* sensitivities are not reliable predictors of the response to treatment.

PREVENTION

• The importance of hand washing after contact with animals or animal products, proper cooling and storage of foods, pasteurization of milk, and chlorination of water supplies will decrease the overall risk for infection.
• In the hospital setting, enteric precautions are recommended for infected infants and children who are incontinent of stool and should be maintained until the patient receives at least 48 hours of antibiotic treatment.

PITFALLS

Not all bacterial colitis presents with blood- or mucus-appearing diarrhea. Therefore, suspicion should exist if the diarrhea is prolonged or environmental exposures pose a risk for developing infection.

Common Questions and Answers

Q: Is treatment necessary if the child is asymptomatic by the time the *Campylobacter* is isolated as the pathogen causing the enteritis?
A: No treatment is needed in this situation. Therapy for symptomatic patients, although it may be of benefit, has not been proven efficacious.

Q: Are there any risks of *Campylobacter* infection to the pregnant patient?
A: Women infected symptomatically or asymptomatically may experience recurrent abortions or preterm deliveries. Life-threatening infections to the fetus or newborn are also possible.

Q: Can you develop immunity to *Campylobacter* infections?
A: Immunity to *C. jejuni* is acquired after one or more infections. For children living in endemic areas, effective natural immunity is due to significant repeated early exposure with a progressive decrease in the illness/infection ratio as age increases.

Q: What is the relationship between GBS and *C. jejuni* infection?
A: Many strains of *C. jejuni* have surface glycolipids that are similar to gangliosides, which are abundant in the central and peripheral nervous systems. Antibody formation from this infection binds to the gangliosides causing the demyelinating process characteristic of GBS.

ICD-9 CM 559.008.43

BIBLIOGRAPHY

Blaser MJ, Reller LB. Campylobacter enteritis. *N Engl J Med* 1981;305:1444–1452.

Bourke B, Chan VL, Sherman P. Campylobacter upsaliensis: waiting in the wings. *Clin Microbiol Rev* 1998;11:440–449.

Fields PI, Swerdlow DL. Campylobacter jejuni. *Clin Lab Med* 1999;19:489–504.

McCarthy N, Giesecke J. Incidence of Guillain-Barre syndrome following infection with Campylobacter jejuni. *Am J Epidemiol* 2001;153(6):610–614.

Peter G, Halsey NA, Marcuse EK, et al. Campylobacter infections. In: *2000 red book: report of the Committee on Infectious Diseases*, 25th ed. Elk Grove Village, IL: American Academy of Pediatrics, 2000:196–198.

Ruiz-Palacios G, Pickering LK. Campylobacter infections. In: Feigin RD, Cherry JD, eds. *Pediatric infectious diseases*, 3rd ed. Philadelphia: WB Saunders, 1992:1073–1081.

Tauxe RV, Hargrett-Bean N, Patton CM, et al. Campylobacter isolates in the United States, 1982–1986. *MMWR* 1987;37:10–25.

Thorson SM, Lohr JA, Dudley S, et al. Value of methylene blue examination, dark-field microscopy, and carbol-fuchsin Gram stain in the detection of Campylobacter enteritis. *J Pediatr* 1985;106:941–943.

Author: Philip V. Scribano

Candidiasis

Database

DEFINITION

Candida albicans remains the most common pathogen in oropharyngeal and cutaneous candidiasis, but non-*albicans* species of *Candida* are increasingly frequent problems in both invasive and vaginal candidiasis.

PATHOPHYSIOLOGY

- Colonizes the mouth, gastrointestinal (GI) tract, respiratory tract, and vagina.
- Neonatal infection acquired from infected vaginal mucosa during birth. Transmission also occurs during nursing from the mother's breast or from imperfect sterilization of bottle nipples.
- Serious candidal disease in the immunocompetent host is rare but may occur when changes in host defense (locally or systemically) allow for overgrowth of the organism.
- Systemic infection results from subsequent hematogenous spread.

ASSOCIATED DISEASES

Candida spp. may cause disease at any site.

Mucosal Candidiasis

- Oropharyngeal candidiasis (thrush) occurs in up to 40% of healthy newborns. Patches of white, curdish material are visible on the buccal and gingival mucosa. It may cause mouth pain and poor nursing. In older children, it is associated with the use of antibiotics or immunosuppressive drugs, conditions of endocrine or immune dysfunction, and malignancy.
- Candidal glossitis occurs secondarily to antibiotic therapy. The tongue is smooth and erythematous, and patients complain of glossodynia (painful tongue). Perlèche (angular cheilosis) results from chronic licking of the corners of the mouth and is characterized by fissuring, erythema, and pain.
- Esophageal candidiasis occurs in HIV-infected patients and those on immunosuppressive therapy; 30% have associated thrush.

Cutaneous Candidiasis

- Diaper dermatitis is most common during infancy due to predisposing factors found with diaper use.
- Intertriginous candidiasis is characterized by a confluent, erythematous, weeping rash with a scaling edge found at skin folds: axillae, groin, gluteal folds, intramammary region, interdigital spaces, and umbilicus. Predisposing factors in healthy patients include chronic moisture, recent antibiotic use, and obesity.

Vaginal Candidiasis

Characterized by vaginal discharge (curdlike or mucoid), pruritus, vulvar burning, and dysuria. Oral contraceptives, antibiotics, pregnancy, corticosteroids, and immunodeficiency are predisposing conditions. Classified as uncomplicated or complicated.

- Uncomplicated
—90% of patients
—Condition is mild to moderate; frequency is sporadic; organism is *C. albicans;* and the host is immunocompetent.
- Complicated
—10% of patients
—Presence of any one of the following factors defines a complicated infection: severe, recurrent infection by non-*albicans Candida* species; or predisposing host factor.
- The reliability of self-diagnosis is poor (<50% correct); therefore, KOH/pH testing is suggested for diagnosis.

Disseminated or Systemic Candidiasis

- Occurs in the immunocompromised host. Risk factors include:
—Malignancy, immunodeficiency syndromes, and diabetes mellitus.
—Broad-spectrum antibiotic therapy, corticosteroids, chemotherapy, and hyperalimentation.
—Indwelling catheters, recent complex surgery, and organ transplantation.
- The most frequent sites of involvement are the GI tract, lungs, kidneys, liver, spleen, eyes, and brain. Fungal sepsis may occur. Peritoneal, urinary tract, and cardiac valve candidal infections are most often related to instrumentation or catheterization in the immunocompromised host.

EPIDEMIOLOGY

- Colonization of the oral mucosa, GI tract, respiratory tract, and vaginal mucosa is common in healthy children. Rates of colonization are substantially higher in hospitalized or chronically ill children.
- 80% of vaginal candidiases are due to *C. albicans,* the remainder are due to other *Candida* species, including *C. glabrata* and *C. tropicalis* .

COMPLICATIONS

- Persistent oropharyngeal candidiasis, especially in immunocompromised patients.
- Systemic dissemination (see above).

Differential Diagnosis

- Oral lesions: aphthous stomatitis, acute necrotizing gingivitis, herpes gingivostomatitis or other viral causes of stomatitis (e.g., coxsackievirus).
- Diaper dermatitis: atopic, seborrheic, bacterial, or occlusional.
- Intertriginous infections: seborrheic and atopic dermatitides
- Vaginitis: *Neisseria gonorrheae, Trichomonas vaginalis, Chlamydia trachomatis, Gardnerella vaginalis, Bacteroides* spp., *Mycoplasma hominis, Peptostreptococcus,* and chemical or mechanical irritants
- Systemic disease: bacterial infection or sepsis

Data Gathering

HISTORY

Question: Is the infection recurrent?
Significance: In oral thrush, reinfection can occur from nipples, pacifiers, or toys (see Prevention and Pitfalls, below). In recurrent vaginitis, bacterial or non-*albicans Candida* species infections are possible.

Question: Recent antibiotic use?
Significance: Oral thrush often occurs in infants, but can occur in normal older children after treatment with systemic antibiotics.

Question: Are there predisposing conditions?
Significance: Oropharyngeal candidiasis in an immunocompromised host often requires oral azole therapy. Systemic dissemination of infection is more likely with impaired immunity.

Question: Visual changes or discomfort?
Significance: Features of endophthalmitis include eye pain, blurred vision, scotomata, and photophobia.

Physical Examination

Finding: Oral lesions
Significance: Buccal or lingual mucosa, gingiva, and tongue lesions have a characteristic white, friable pseudomembrane that when scraped away reveals reddened, denuded, and sometimes ulcerated mucosa.

Finding: Rash
Significance: The rash of monilial diaper dermatitis is initially scattered. Erythematous papules progress and coalesce into a deeply erythematous, weeping, confluent rash with a scaling border and satellite lesions.

Laboratory Aids

LABORATORY STUDIES

Test: Direct light microscopic examination of specimen
Significance: Clinical diagnosis of mucosal, cutaneous, and vaginal candidiasis can be confirmed by microscopic examination of material scraped gently from lesions. KOH preparation (10% or 20% potassium hydroxide) allows visualization of the long, branching, hyphae of *C. albicans.* Vaginal pH remains normal (<4.5) with vaginal candidiasis.

Test: Fungal culture
Significance: *Candida* species can be isolated from culture of mucosal or cutaneous scrapings, blood, urine, CSF, bone marrow, tissue biopsy, abscess aspirate, and bronchoalveolar lavage fluid. Isolation of the organism permits susceptibility testing, which is important for patients with disseminated infection or impaired immunity.

OTHER STUDIES

Test: Dilated retinal examination (by an ophthalmologist)
Significance: Endophthalmitis, a sight-threatening complication, should be excluded in all patients with candidemia.

Test: CT scan and echocardiogram
Significance: Important to identify deep organ lesions (liver, spleen, brain, kidney, or heart) associated with disseminated infection.

 Therapy

Treatment of candidiasis is dependent on the site of infection, immune status of the host, and the risk of systemic dissemination.

OROPHARYNGEAL CANDIDIASIS
Oral Candidiasis
• Treat with nystatin suspension until 2 days after the lesions have cleared. Miconazole oral gel, while more effective, is not yet available in the U.S.
• In older patients, nystatin as a swish-swallow suspension or in oral tablet form for >7 days is effective. Clotrimazole lozenges are also effective; 10 mg dissolved in mouth 5 times daily for 7 days.
• Gentian violet is no longer recommended for the treatment of oral candidiasis.
• Fluconazole and ketoconazole are effective for infections that are persistent or occur in immunocompromised hosts. Azole-resistant *C. albicans* has been described in HIV-infected individuals with recurrent infection.

Esophageal Candidiasis
• A therapeutic trial with fluconazole for patients with presumed esophageal candidiasis is a cost-effective alternative to endoscopy; symptoms should resolve within 7 days after the start of therapy. A 14- to 21-day course is recommended. Itraconazole solution and IV amphotericin B are acceptable alternatives.
• Patients with advanced AIDS commonly have recurrent infections and may benefit from chronic suppressive fluconazole therapy.

Cutaneous or Intertriginous Candidiasis and Candidal Diaper Dermatitis
Both are treated by keeping the area dry and using nystatin cream (100,000 units/g qid) until the rash has cleared. Topical regimens of clotrimazole 1%, miconazole 2%, ketoconazole 2%, and econazole 1% are also effective.

Vaginal Candidiasis
Uncomplicated
• Topical agents are highly effective in uncomplicated infections (cure rates >80%): clotrimazole, miconazole, butoconazole, and terconazole (dose varies with 1-, 3-, or 7-day treatment).
• Oral agents are also effective: fluconazole (10 mg/kg up to 150 mg as a single-dose), ketoconazole (400 mg qd for 5 days), and itraconazole (200 mg bid for 1 day or 200 mg qd for 3 days).

Complicated
• Extend antimycotic therapy to 7–14 days.
• Non-*albicans* species of *Candida* usually respond to topical boric acid (600 mg/day for 14 days). Azole-resistant *C. albicans* infections are extremely rare in the immunocompetent host.

Recurrent (>4 episodes of proven infection during a 12-month period)
• Recurrent vaginitis is usually due to azole-susceptible *C. albicans*. Induction therapy with 2 weeks of a topical or oral azole is followed by a maintenance regimen for 6 months. Suitable maintenance regimens include fluconazole (150 mg weekly), ketoconazole (100 mg daily), itraconazole (100 mg qod), or daily therapy with a topical azole.

Systemic or Disseminated Candidiasis
• Begin treatment in hospital due to severity of illness, underlying disease process, and need for the intravenous route of drug administration.
• Address predisposing factors (e.g., removal of indwelling catheters).
• Antifungal agents commonly used:
—Amphotericin B: 0.5 to 1.0 mg/kg/d qd, or 1.5 mg/kg qod IV. Preferred for initial therapy because of its broader spectrum. Duration of treatment for candidemia is 14 days from first negative blood culture and when signs and symptoms of infection have resolved. Flucytosine may provide synergy.
—Fluconazole: 12 mg/kg/d up to 600 mg/d, oral or IV. May be used in those with a fluconazole-susceptible organism (check susceptibility testing before changing from amphotericin B).
—Lipid-based amphotericin B: 3–6 mg/kg/d IV. Appropriate for patients who are refractory to, intolerant of, or at high-risk of being intolerant of conventional amphotericin B preparations.
• Intolerance to conventional amphotericin B is usually defined as initial renal insufficiency (CrCl <25 mL/min), significant rise in creatinine during therapy (to 2.5 mg/dL in adults or 1.5 mg/dL in children), or severe acute administration-related toxicity. The toxicity of amphotericin (rigors, anemia, thrombocytopenia, and renal failure) requires close monitoring and may limit its use.
• Duration of therapy is longer for candidal meningitis (4 weeks), endophthalmitis (6–12 weeks), endocarditis (>6 weeks following surgical therapy), and osteomyelitis (6–12 months).

PREVENTION
• Sterilize bottle nipples and toys to prevent reinoculation of oral candidiasis.
• Avoid unnecessarily long courses of broad-spectrum antibiotics.
• Maintain intravenous catheters and catheter-skin insertion sites appropriately.

 Follow-Up

Follow-up is required only for disseminated/systemic candidiasis.

PITFALLS
• Failure to eliminate source of re-infection. Recurrent thrush in a breast-fed infant may indicate *C. albicans* colonization of the mother's nipples; this can be eliminated by treatment of the nipples with nystatin cream.
• Failure to consider that symptoms of persistent vaginitis may be caused by non-*albicans Candida* species or by bacteria (see Vaginitis).
• Failure to maintain a high index of suspicion for disseminated disease in an immunocompromised patient. Persistent fevers despite antibiotic therapy, diffuse rash, and visual complaints are important clues.

 Common Questions and Answers

Q: When should an older child with thrush be worked up for possible immunodeficiency?
A: Thrush in the older child is usually caused by recent antibiotic or steroid treatment. If no apparent cause is found, an immunologic evaluation that includes HIV testing, should be considered.

ICD-9-CM 112.9

BIBLIOGRAPHY
Hoppe JE. Treatment of oropharyngeal candidiasis and candidal diaper dermatitis in neonates and infants: review and reappraisal. *Pediatr Infect Dis J* 1997;16:885–894.

Hughes WT, Flynn PM. Candidiasis. In: Feigin RD, Cherry JD, eds. *Textbook of pediatric infectious diseases*, 4th ed. Philadelphia: WB Saunders, 1998:2303–2313.

Mermel LA, Farr BM, Sheretz RJ, et al. Guidelines for the management of intravascular catheter-related infections. *Clin Infect Dis* 2001;32:1249–1272.

Rex JH, Walsh TJ, Sobel JD, et al. Practice guidelines for the treatment of candidiasis. *Clin Infect Dis* 2000;30:662–678.

Sobel JD, Faro S, Force RW, et al. Vulvovaginal candidiasis: epidemiologic, diagnostic, and therapeutic considerations. *Am J Obstet Gynecol* 1998;178:203–211.

Authors: Samir S. Shah
Molly (Martha) W. Stevens, 2nd edition

Cardiomyopathy

 Database

DEFINITION

Cardiomyopathy is defined as a disease of the myocardium, which can be either a primary process or secondary to an associated disorder.
• Dilated cardiomyopathy (DCM): Impairment of biventricular systolic function with predominant involvement of the left ventricle eliciting congestive heart failure.
• Hypertrophic cardiomyopathy (HCM): Characterized with an asymmetric hypertrophy of the left ventricle with 20% to 25% of the patients exhibiting left ventricular outflow tract obstruction.
• Restrictive cardiomyopathy (RCM): Cardiac muscle disease that impairs ventricular filling (normal or decreased diastolic volume of the ventricles), yet systolic function generally remains normal.

PATHOPHYSIOLOGY

• DCM: There are many associated diseases that cause DCM, which are grouped as inborn errors of fatty-acid oxidation, disorders of mitochondrial oxidative phosphorylation, X-linked muscular dystrophies, toxin-induced cardiomyopathy (i.e., anthracycline), postinfectious (viral myocarditis associated with coxsackievirus B or echovirus), nutritional deficiencies, primary and secondary carnitine deficiency, and chronic tachyarrhythmias. Similarly, idiopathic DCM is manifested by abnormally dilated ventricular chambers with frequently noted mural thrombi and atrioventricular valve leaflet scarring with secondary annulus dilatation, and hypertrophy and degeneration of myocytes.
• HCM: This disease is manifested by ventricular hypertrophy, which is often asymmetrical and involves the interventricular septum most commonly but may also affect the free walls. Dynamic obstruction of the left ventricular outflow tract can occur and anatomically relates to the presence of mitral valve systolic anterior motion causing subaortic obstruction.
• RCM: Causes of RCM include amyloidosis, infiltrative and storage diseases (Gaucher disease, Hurler syndrome, Fabry disease), carcinoid syndrome, and radiation-induced fibrosis. Idiopathic RCM can also be familial. The disease is manifested by increased stiffness of the myocardium; therefore, small increases in volume will cause a disproportionately greater increase in ventricular pressure.

GENETICS

• DCM: A portion of cases of idiopathic DCM may have a genetic cause with approximately 20% of patients with the disease having a first-degree relative with abnormalities of myocardial function.
• HCM: A familial hypertrophic cardiomyopathy is known and is an autosomal-dominant disease with variable penetrance. Other studies have noted areas of chromosome 1, 14, and 15 to be involved, and can document 60% of patients who have a first-degree relative with morphologic evidence of HCM.
• RCM: Idiopathic cases may have a familial occurrence and may be associated with a skeletal myopathy. Also, an autosomal-dominant form of the disease with variable penetrance has been associated with Noonan syndrome.

EPIDEMIOLOGY

• DCM: Idiopathic DCM has a prevalence of 36/100,000. Overall survival of 50% to 60% at 2 years.
• HCM: Prevalence of 1/500 with a heterogeneous natural history of the disease.
• RCM: Least common of the cardiomyopathic disorders.

COMPLICATIONS

• In some studies, the overall actuarial survival of those with DCM is 63% to 90% at 1 year with a 5-year survival of 20% to 80%.
• Arrhythmias may be seen and are most often ventricular in origin.
• Thrombus formation can be seen in DCM due to the stasis of blood in a hypocontractile state and, therefore, systemic or pulmonary emboli are possible.

PROGNOSIS

• A general rule for idiopathic DCM is that one third exhibit improved cardiac function, one third have stable cardiac dysfunction, and one third progress to significant cardiac dysfunction.
• Overall rate of sudden death is 2% to 4% in HCM with deaths occurring most commonly in children and young adults.
• The reported median survival in RCM is 1.4 years in children.

 Differential Diagnosis

• DCM: Children and young adults often present with symptoms that mimic other disease states. For example, abdominal distention, right upper quadrant pain, nausea, and anorexia that indicates right heart failure could be mistaken for hepatic or gallbladder disease. Dyspnea on exertion may mimic exercise-induced asthma. The cardiomegaly on chest radiograph may be mistaken for a large pericardial effusion.
• HCM: This disease must be differentiated from the left ventricular hypertrophy that is seen in an athlete.
• RCM: Must be distinguished from constrictive pericarditis (a history of tuberculosis, trauma, or cardiac surgery may suggest constrictive pericarditis).

 Data Gathering

HISTORY

Question: Respiratory distress?
Significance: A manifestation of congestive heart failure.

Question: Irritability?
Significance: A manifestation of congestive heart failure or a pericardial effusion.
Question: Diaphoresis?
Significance: A manifestation of congestive heart failure.
Question: Gastrointestinal complaints (nausea, emesis)?
Significance: Right-sided congestive heart failure, pericardial effusion, or decreased systemic output.
Question: Tachypnea with feeding, pallor, and poor weight gain?
Significance: A manifestation of congestive heart failure.
Question: Chest pain?
Significance: Carditis, pericardial effusion, or arrhythmia.
Question: Syncope?
Significance: Low cardiac output or arrhythmia.
Question: Palpitations?
Significance: Arrhythmia.
Question: Orthopnea, paroxysmal nocturnal dyspnea?
Significance: A manifestation of congestive heart failure.
Question: Peripheral edema?
Significance: Right-sided heart failure.
Question: Reduced exercise capacity?
Significance: Congestive heart failure or low cardiac output.
Question: Neurologic changes (delayed development)?
Significance: Systemic emboli in DCM.
Question: Recent febrile illness?
Significance: In DCM, 50% of cases have a history of fever within 3 months of the diagnosis.

 Physical Examination

CARDIAC

Finding: DCM: tachycardia, cardiomegaly, hepatomegaly, S3 or S4 gallop
Significance: Evidence of heart failure and decreased cardiac output.
Finding: HCM: Can be normal.
Significance: The presence of outflow tract obstruction produces a systolic ejection murmur of variable intensity related to the degree of obstruction, the murmur increases in intensity with Valsalva and decreases in magnitude with squatting. A parasternal or carotid thrill may be present
Finding: RCM: Jugular venous pulse either fails to fall or rises in inspiration (Kussmaul sign), S3 or S4
Significance: Advanced cases may exhibit weak peripheral pulses as evidence of low cardiac output.

RESPIRATORY

Finding: Tachypnea, rales, or cardiac wheezing
Significance: Signs of congestive heart failure

ABDOMINAL
Finding: Hepatomegaly, ascites, tenderness to palpation
Significance: Right-sided congestive heart failure.

EXTREMITIES
Finding: Peripheral edema in advanced cases
Significance: Congestive heart failure.

Laboratory Aids

NONSPECIFIC TESTS

Test: Chest radiograph
Significance: Cardiomegaly, pulmonary edema, Kerley B lines, and pleural effusions
Test: Electrocardiogram
Significance: Nonspecific ST-T wave changes, hypertrophy or enlargement of chambers (although generalized low voltages may be seen), ventricular and supraventricular tachyarrhythmias, atrioventricular block, localized Q waves

SPECIFIC TESTS
Laboratory tests aimed at a specific etiology or an associated disease state should be accomplished in certain cases. For example, carnitine levels may prove helpful as well as polymerase chain reaction assay testing (evidence for an enteroviral infection) on endomyocardial biopsies performed on selected cases of DCM. Storage and metabolic disease states should be investigated if there is clinical suspicion.

Test: Echocardiography
Significance: Allows for measurement of systolic function, ventricular dimensions, outflow tract obstruction, and diastolic filling properties.
Test: Cardiac catheterization
Significance: DCM: Low cardiac output with possible alterations in pulmonary vascular resistance, performance of endomyocardial biopsies, aortography to assure usual coronary anatomy (rule out anomalous coronary origin) HCM: Determination of the presence or absence of left ventricular outflow tract obstruction, hypertrophy, "spike and dome" arterial pulse tracing, Brockenbrough phenomenon (a beat following a premature ventricular contraction exhibits an arterial pulse pressure less than that of the control beat). RCM: Atrial pressures are elevated and equal, the ventricular pressure exhibits a rapid and deep early decline at the onset of diastole followed by a rapid rise to a plateau in early diastole (so-called square-root sign).

Therapy

• DCM: Afterload reduction (enalapril, captopril), inotropic agents (milrinone, dobutamine, digoxin), aldactone [improves New York Heart Association (NYHA) functional class], anticoagulation to avoid embolic complications, antiarrhythmics as needed, β-adrenergic blockers (metoprolol, carvedilol),

and at the time of diagnosis, a trial of intravenous gamma globulin and/or other immunomodulators (prednisone, azathioprine). Ventricular assist devices have been used in those with end-stage heart failure either as a bridge to recovery or to transplantation.
• HCM: β-Adrenergic blockers, verapamil, nifedipine, diltiazem, antiarrhythmics as needed. If medical therapy is not effective, other options may include myotomy-myectomy, atrioventricular sequential pacing, or intracoronary ethanol injection to decrease the extent of outflow tract obstruction.
• RCM: Diuretics can be used with caution to treat venous congestion, antiarrhythmics as needed, anticoagulation to avoid embolic complications, regulated physical activity, and supportive care.
• Transplantation: Heart or heart-lung (if the pulmonary vascular resistance is elevated) transplantation may be necessary if all therapeutic endeavors prove to be futile.

Follow-Up

All of these patients require careful follow-up by a cardiologist in addition to their primary care physician to note any adverse alterations in their cardiac status including arrhythmia control and surveillance. Patients should be referred for a transplant evaluation if deemed necessary by their clinical status.

PREVENTION
There is no specific prevention; however, a physician should evaluate individuals with a familial history of cardiomyopathy even if they are asymptomatic.

PITFALLS
In cases of HCM, the cardiac examination can be completely normal; therefore, those patients that raise suspicion for the disease either by family or clinical history should be carefully evaluated.

Common Questions and Answers

Q: Should family members be evaluated once a cardiomyopathy is diagnosed in a first-degree relative?
A: Yes. In some types of cardiomyopathy, there is a strong genetic component and family members should be evaluated. Certainly the diagnosis of certain subtypes of cardiomyopathy (i.e., postinfectious DCM, toxin-induced DCM) do not require evaluation of relatives.
Q: Does the cardiomyopathy of infants of diabetic mothers carry the same clinical course and outcome as that of patients with HCM?
A: No. The pathophysiology initially is similar in that asymmetric hypertrophy of the ventricular septum is often seen in the cardiomyopathy in infants of diabetic mothers and can be obstructive to left ventricular outflow. However, the clinical course of the cardiomyopathy in infants born to diabetic

mothers is usually benign and resolves within the first 6 months of life.
Q: What are the differentiating features of HCM and the benign physiologic hypertrophy of an athlete's heart?
A: Several criteria are used to make this distinction. For example, a familial history of HCM leads one to be suspicious of this entity. Studies have suggested specific left ventricular dimensions by echocardiography to differentiate benign hypertrophy and HCM (i.e., a wall thickness of 15 mm or left ventricle cavity dimensions of <45 mm are more consistent with HCM). Also, echocardiographic evidence of abnormal mitral valve inflow is suggestive of HCM.

ICD-9-CM 425.4

BIBLIOGRAPHY
Akagi T, Benson LN, Lightfoot NE, et al. Natural history of dilated cardiomyopathy in children. *Am Heart J* 1991;121:1502–1506.

Chan DP, Allen HD. Dilated congestive cardiomyopathy. In: Emmanouilides GC, ed. *Moss and Adams heart disease in infants, children, and adolescents including the fetus and young adult,* 5th ed. Baltimore: Williams & Wilkins, 1995:1365–1381.

Dec GW, Fuster V. Idiopathic dilated cardiomyopathy. Medical progress: idiopathic dilated cardiomyopathy. *N Engl J Med* 1994;330(13).

Kelly DP, Strauss AW. Mechanisms of disease: inherited cardiomyopathies. *N Engl J Med* 1994;330(13):913–919.

Kappenberger LJ, Linde C, Jeanrenaud X, et al. Clinical progress after randomized on/off pacemaker treatment for hypertrophic obstructive cardiomyopathy. Pacing in cardiomyopathy study group. *Europace* 1999;1(2)77–84.

Kushwaha SS, Fallon JT, Fuster V. Restrictive cardiomyopathy. *N Engl J Med* 1997;336(4):267–276.

Lewis AB, Chabot M. Outcome of infants and children with dilated cardiomyopathy. *Am J Cardiol* 1991;68:365–369.

Maron BJ. Hypertrophic cardiomyopathy. In: Emmanouilides GC, ed. *Moss and Adams heart disease in infants, children, and adolescents including the fetus and young adult,* 5th ed. Baltimore: Williams & Wilkins, 1995:1337–1365.

Mazur W, Nagueh SF, Lakkis NM, et al. Regression of left ventricular hypertrophy after nonsurgical septal reduction therapy for hypertrophic obstructive cardiomyopathy. *Circulation* 2001;103(11):1492–1496.

Pelliccia A, Maron BJ, Spataro A, et al. The upper limit of physiologic cardiac hypertrophy in highly trained elite athletes. *N Engl J Med* 1991;324:295–301.

Spirito P, Seidman CE, McKenna WJ, et al. Medical progress: The management of hypertrophic cardiomyopathy. *N Engl J Med* 1997;336(11):775–785.

Author: Timothy M. Hoffman

Cataract

Database

DEFINITION
A cataract is any opacification of the normally clear, crystalline lens of the eye. Some are small and nonprogressive and do not cause visual symptoms. Cataracts that are clinically significant and decrease visual acuity in children represent a major challenge.

CAUSES
• Of congenital cataracts, about one third are inherited; one third are associated with systemic genetic, metabolic, or maternal infectious disorders; and about one third are idiopathic, referring to being of a cause of unknown etiology.
• A small number of cataracts are associated with other primary ocular abnormalities that are inherited.
• Developmental cataracts can result from some metabolic disorders, toxic agents (steroids, radiation), and localized trauma.

PATHOPHYSIOLOGY
• Cataracts represent a derangement of the normal developmental growth of the crystalline fibers of the central lens nucleus or peripheral cortex and are frequently classified according to their morphology or etiology.
• The age at which they occurred is often determined by the location of the opacity within the lens.
• Dense central opacities of 3 mm or more usually produce substantial visual disability.

GENETICS
• Estimated that some 8% to 33% of congenital cataracts are inherited. Primary inherited congenital cataracts usually follow an autosomal-dominant mode of inheritance, though there are also autosomal-recessive and X-linked–recessive varieties.

EPIDEMIOLOGY
• Cataracts occur in about 0.4% of children, and it has been variously estimated that between 10% and 40% of all blindness in children throughout the world are secondary to cataracts.

COMPLICATIONS
• Lack of removal of a visually significant cataract at the appropriate early time will lead to irreversible deprivation amblyopia in which case no amount of surgery, optical correction, and amblyopia therapy is of any benefit.
• Surgical removal of a cataract in children previously left the eye without a lens (aphakic) and unable to focus without some type of optical correction (spectacles, contacts, or intraocular lenses). Unless rapid restoration of optical correction occurs, irreversible deprivation amblyopia may still occur after the cataract is removed. This is especially true when cataracts are unilateral.
• The aphakic pediatric eye is more prone to elevated intraocular pressures (glaucoma) and early retinal detachments, either of which can cause permanent visual loss, than an anatomically normal eye. More recently, intraocular lenses have become commonly accepted as a means of optical rehabilitation in pediatric patients requiring cataract extraction primarily in children older than two years of age. Investigational studies have been implemented to evaluate the use of intraocular lenses in children younger than 2 years of age.

PROGNOSIS
• Prior to 1980, the majority of children treated for monocular cataracts had their best corrected vision only in the 20/200 to 20/800 range (legal blindness—best corrected visual acuity of 20/200 or worse); and bilateral cataracts usually obtained only best corrected visual acuity's in the 20/80 to 20/200 range.
• Early surgery, better surgical techniques, and rapid optical correction now affords frequent corrected visual acuities in the 20/40 or better range for bilateral cataracts, and in the 20/40 to 20/200 range for monocular cataracts.
• In all cases, the onset or presence of nystagmus, a to and fro motion of the eyes, before the cataract is removed is an ominous sign of poor outcome.
• In general, successful treatment of cataracts in a child can be extremely difficult and must be accomplished very early in life in the case of congenital cataracts.
• Useful vision in children with unilateral cataracts in the newborn period can be restored/obtained if the surgery is completed within the first 8 to 12 weeks of life.
• After 8 to 12 weeks, because of irreversible deprivation amblyopia, visual restoration becomes progressively more difficult.
• With bilateral congenital cataracts, the prognosis for visual rehabilitation is slightly better providing surgical removal and optical correction is also accomplished early, preferably by 3 months of age.
• Later onset cataracts have a better prognosis because the visual system is maturer.

Differential Diagnosis

The differential diagnosis of cataracts in children is more concerned with the underlying cause of the leukokoria itself rather than the presence of some other entity, as the cataract is readily defined by the ophthalmologist.

• Retinoblastoma, retinopathy of prematurity, juvenile retinoschisis, persistent hyperplastic primary vitreous, severe uveitis, and retinal detachment can all cause primary leukokoria or result in a cataract.
• In addition, the cataract may be an expression of some more severe underlying, previously undiagnosed systemic disease that must be defined to benefit the child's overall health.

ASSOCIATED DISEASES
• Systemic disorders include the TORCH syndromes, including congenital rubella.
• Fetal alcohol syndrome
• Chromosomal disorders such as Down syndrome, trisomy 13–15, Turner syndrome
• Many craniofacial and mandibulofacial syndromes
• Dermatologic syndromes such as congenital ichthyosis, hereditary ectodermal dysplasia, infantile poikiloderma
• Skeletal syndromes such as Marfan and Conradi syndromes
• Renal disorders such as Lowe or Alport syndrome
• Neurofibromatosis
• Myotonic dystrophy
• Metabolic and endocrine disorders such as galactosemia, hypoglycemia, diabetes mellitus
• Fabry disease and hypoparathyroidism
• Local ocular disorders with cataracts include aniridia; many of the anterior chamber dysgenesis syndromes, trauma, and those associated with ocular inflammatory processes (chronic iritis, uveitis) such as juvenile rheumatoid arthritis.

Data Gathering

HISTORY
Question: Decreased visual responses?
Significance: Cataracts may decrease vision.

Question: Sun sensitivity (squinting in bright light)?
Significance: Cataracts may increase light sensitivity.

Question: Strabismus?
Significance: Strabismus may indicate loss of vision in one eye.

Question: White pupil?
Significance: White pupil cataracts appear as white object in or under pupil.

Question: Unequal or abnormal pupillary reflections in photographs?
Significance: Cataract will block the standard red reflex.

Question: Nystagmus?
Significance: Nystagmus can be an ominous sign for degree of vision loss.

Question: Careful family and prenatal history?
Significance: Some 8% to 33% of congenital cataracts are inherited.

Question: Positive family history or known history of disorder associated with cataracts?
Significance: See associated disease section.

Physical Examination

Finding: Decreased vision
Significance: Cataracts may decrease visual acuity.

Finding: Strabismus
Significance: May indicate loss of vision in one eye.

Finding: White pupil (leukokoria) on flashlight examination
Significance: Cataracts appear as white pupil.

Finding: Unequal or poor red fundus reflections by direct ophthalmoscopy
Significance: Cataract will interfere with seeing red reflex.

Finding: Visual acuity assessment
Significance: Determine if cataracts caused visual loss.

Finding: Presence or absence of nystagmus
Significance: Nystagmus is poor prognostic sign.

Finding: Bilaterality of disease
Significance: Bilateral cataracts are primarily idiopathic, hereditary, or secondary to systemic disease.

Finding: Size of globe
Significance: Microphthalmia suggests congenital cataracts.

Finding: Thorough physical examination for systemic syndrome
Significance: Many diseases are associated with cataracts. See associated disease sections.

Laboratory Aids

- Complete ophthalmic examination.
- Biomicroscopy
- Ultrasonography if unable to visualize media behind opacity
- Electrophysiologic analysis of visual system
- Selective workup
- TORCH titers, including syphilis
- Urine for reducing substance (galactosemia), protein, and pH (Lowe syndrome)
- Blood glucose, calcium, phosphate
- Quantitative amino acids, RBC enzyme levels (galactokinase, gal-1-uridyltransferase)
- Genetic consultation; chromosome analysis

Therapy

- With monocular, small cataracts, sometimes simple dilatation of the pupil of the cataractous eye and occlusion of the normal eye help overcome mild amblyopia and preserve acceptable vision without surgical removal of the cataract. Glasses may or may not be of additional help.
- With visually significant cataracts, surgical removal is the therapy. However, without optical correction of the operated, aphakic eye, visual rehabilitation is impossible.
- Prior to age 2, optical correction of aphakia is most frequently accomplished with contact lenses or spectacles when the cataracts are bilateral. In unilateral cases, successful visual rehabilitation always requires extensive occlusion therapy to the normal eye for years. In this instance, optical correction of the unilateral aphakia is best obtained with a contact lens. Even when visual rehabilitation of the monocular aphakia is successful, normal binocular vision with three-dimensional and perfect depth perception is rarely possible.
- Refractive corneal surgery for optical correction of the aphakic is not at this time indicated in children.
- In children older than 2 years, especially those with unilateral cataracts, intraocular lenses (IOLs) have proved successful in appropriate cases, and are now used frequently. They can afford faster visual rehabilitation and excellent chances of normal binocular vision.

PREVENTION
There is currently no known way to prevent congenital cataracts other than correcting any underlying metabolic abnormality.

Follow-Up

- Without treatment, progressive visual loss is the course of a visually significant cataract. When the opacity is present at birth or very early in life, the visual loss quickly becomes irreversible.
- Once surgical removal and optical correction is started, the child, parents, and physician enter into an intensive and long rehabilitation period, lasting until visual maturity and stability is reached (usually, around 9 years old). Following this, yearly eye examinations are the minimum requirement.
- Parental and educational support services may be needed for those with residual visual handicap.
- Special local, state, and federal services for the visually handicapped and/or blind may be required, as not all children who have successful surgical results will have good vision.

Common Questions and Answers

Q: Is surgical removal the same as visual cure?
A: No. This is the beginning of treatment that includes optical correction and amblyopia therapy.

Q: Once the cataract is removed, is intensive, extensive follow-up needed?
A: Yes. The visual prognosis is directly related to postsurgical treatment compliance.

Q: Is the cataract easier to treat when the child is older?
A: No. Irreversible deprivation amblyopia develops when the child is older, which precludes the chance for normal vision.

ICD-9-CM 366.9

BIBLIOGRAPHY
Childhood cataracts and other lens disorders. In: Del Monte MA, eds. *Pediatric ophthalmology and strabismus: basic and clinical science course*, section 6. San Francisco: American Academy of Ophthalmology, 1994–95:93–95.

Gimbel HV, Basti S, Ferensowicz M, et al. Results of bilateral cataract extraction with posterior chamber intraocular lens implantation in children. *Ophthalmology* 1997;104:1737–1743.

Hiles DA, Hered RW. Disorders of the lens. In: Isenberg SJ, ed. *The eye in infancy*. Chicago: Year Book, 1989:284–319.

Nelson LB, Ullman S. Congenital and developmental cataracts. In: Tasman W, Jaeger EA, eds. *Duane's clinical ophthalmology*. Philadelphia: JB Lippincott, 1994:1–10.

Zwann J, Mullaney PB, Awad, AA, et al. Pediatric intraocular lens implantation: surgical results and complications in more than 300 cases. *Ophthalmology* 1198;105:112–119.

Author: Brian J. R. Forbes

Cat-Scratch Disease

 Database

DEFINITION

Cat-scratch disease (CSD) is a subacute, regional lymphadenitis syndrome that occurs following cutaneous inoculation. The majority of patients have had an identifiable contact with a cat, most notably in the form of a scratch or bite.

CAUSES

The etiologic agent for CSD is now referred to as *Bartonella henselae* (previously, *Rochalimaea henselae*), a pleomorphic gram-negative rod. Skin inoculation with the organism through cat contact is the typical mechanism of infection.

PATHOPHYSIOLOGY

Following infection, both the primary inoculation site and the affected lymph nodes show a characteristic central avascular necrotic area surrounded by lymphocytes with some giant cells and histiocytes. Involved nodes develop generalized enlargement, cortex thickening, and germinal-center hypertrophy. Progression leads to pus-filled sinuses within the affected nodes.

EPIDEMIOLOGY

- Occurs in patients of all ages, with 80% of cases being in those less than 21 years old
- Approximately 24,000 cases each year and likely represents the most common cause of chronic benign regional adenopathy
- More common when scratched by a cat less than 12 months of age

COMPLICATIONS

- Unilateral subacute or chronic tender nodes of the axillary, epitrochlear, and preauricular area support a diagnosis of CSD, especially in the face of a consistent cat contact.
- Regional lymphadenitis
- Parinaud oculoglandular syndrome. This occurs when the site of primary inoculation is the conjunctiva or eyelid. A mild to moderate conjunctivitis develops along with preauricular lymph nodes.
- Encephalopathy/encephalitis: may occur suddenly 2 to 6 weeks after the initial symptoms of CSD, and seizures may be the heralding symptom. Patients may become delirious and then comatose for several days before recovering. Spinal fluid is typically normal or shows minimal WBC and protein elevation. Recovery is generally complete.
- Erythema nodosum: likely represents a delayed hypersensitivity reaction to the infection. Most often involves the subcutaneous fat of the legs and, at times, dorsum of arms, hands, and feet.
- Osteolytic bone lesions occur as a rare complication.
- Other rare complications include thrombotic thrombocytopenic purpura, erythema marginatum, mesenteric lymphadenitis, pneumonia, arthralgias, subacute iriditis, urethritis, lymphedema, thyroiditis, and anicteric hepatitis.

PROGNOSIS

Most patients with CSD have a benign course. Patients with significant complications such as encephalopathy, thrombocytopenic purpura, or bone lesions usually have a more prolonged course, but also have a good long-term prognosis.

 Differential Diagnosis

Most known causes of lymphadenopathy (*see* neck masses). Location of the abnormal lymph nodes may supply a strong clue.

 Data Gathering

HISTORY

Question: Cat contact?
Significance: The majority of patients have an antecedent cat contact.

Question: A skin rash?
Significance: May describe the appearance of a papule on the skin at the site of inoculation 3 to 5 days after the initial injury.

Question: Changes in rash?
Significance: This papule generally progresses through a vesicular and crusty stage.

Question: When did large lymph nodes appear?
Significance: Within 1 to 2 weeks, lymphadenopathy in the region of drainage may be noted.

Question: Other symptoms?
Significance: Mild associated symptoms of generalized achiness, malaise, anorexia may also be present. Fever is present in less than 10%.

Physical Examination

- One or more red papules at the inoculation site may be detectable.
- The true sign of CSD (present in 10% of cases) is chronic or subacute lymphadenitis involving the first or second set of nodes draining the inoculation site.
- The groups affected, in decreasing order of frequency, are the axillary, cervical, submandibular, periauricular, epitrochlear, femoral, and inguinal lymph nodes.
- Usually tender with overlying erythema, warmth, and induration.
- Less than half become suppurative or form a sinus tract to the skin.

Laboratory Aids

Test: Direct fluorescence antibody testing
Significance: For detection of antibodies to *B. henselae,* conducted on serum samples at the Centers for Disease Control and Prevention. This test should be used to confirm a CSD diagnosis.

Test: Enzyme immunoassay
Significance: For detection of IgG antibodies to *B. henselae,* also commercially available (Specialty Laboratories, Santa Monica, CA).

Test: Blood cultures
Significance: Using lysed or centrifuged blood may at times yield *B. henselae* growth from infected individuals in whom bacteremia is suspected.

Isolation of organism from skin lesions and nodal aspirates may be possible.

Therapy

- Antibiotic therapy for CSD is somewhat controversial.
- Some experts still suggest the use of an oral antibiotic such as trimethoprim-sulfamethoxazole (TMP-SMX), 6 to 8 mg/kg of TMP b.i.d. to t.i.d. for 7 days.
- Alternatively, azithromycin 500 mg initially then 250 mg for a total of 5 days in patients more than 45.5 kg and 10 mg/kg on the first day and 5 mg/kg for the subsequent 4 days in children for uncomplicated CSD may be used. Many experts suggest conservative, symptomatic treatment only.
- Percutaneous drainage of tender, fluctuant adenitis can provide relief of pain.
- For immunocompromised patients and those with severe disease (including encephalitis) gentamicin sulfate, 5 mg/kg/d divided q8h intramuscularly or intravenously, is recommended. The duration of treatment should be based on response.

PREVENTION

Measures to prevent CSD should be directed toward minimizing contact between infected cats and people. Keeping kittens and older cats indoors and avoiding rough play may decrease the likelihood of infection. Avoidance of stray animals and good local care of any sustained bite or scratch is essential.

Follow-Up

Most patients will have a benign course and can expect resolution of systemic symptoms in less than 2 weeks. Slow resolution of enlarged or painful lymph nodes will occur over weeks to months. As mentioned, percutaneous drainage of tender, fluctuant lymph nodes may be required to relieve pain. As stated previously, the course for patients with severe complications, including encephalitis, will be more prolonged, but without lasting sequelae.

Common Questions and Answers

Q: Can a sibling develop CSD from an infected patient?
A: No. Person-to-person transmission is not reported.

Q: Should the parents of a child with cat-scratch disease get rid of the cat?
A: In general, this is not recommended. These animals are not ill. The capacity to transmit disease appears to be transient, and recurrent disease is rare.

ICD-9-CM 078.3

BIBLIOGRAPHY

Adal KA, Cockerell CJ, Petri WA. Cat-scratch disease, bacillary angiomatosis, and other infections due to Rochalimaea. *N Engl J Med* 1994;330:1509–1515.

Bass JW, Freitas, BC, Freitas AD, et al. Prospective randomized double blend placebo-controlled evaluation of azithromycin for treatment of cat-scratch disease. *Pediatr Infect Dis J* 1998;17:447–452.

Boyer KM, Cherry JD. Cat-scratch disease. In: Feigin RD, Cherry JD, eds. *Textbook of pediatric infectious diseases*, 3rd ed. Philadelphia: WB Saunders, 1992:1084–1088.

Carithers HA. Cat-scratch disease: acute encephalopathy and other neurologic manifestations. *Am J Dis Child* 1991;145: 48–101.

Carithers HA. Cat-scratch disease: an overview based on a study of 1,200 patients. *Am J Dis Child* 1985;139:1124–1133.

Case records of the Massachusetts General Hospital. Weekly clinicopathological exercises. Case 1-1998. An 11-year-old boy with a seizure [clinical conference] [published erratum appears in *N Engl J Med* 1998;338(7):483]. *N Engl J Med* 1998;338(2): 112–119.

Kelly CS, Kelly RE Jr. Lymphadenopathy in children. *Pediatr Clin North Am* 1998;45(4): 875–888.

Margileth AM. Antibiotic therapy for cat-scratch disease: clinical study of therapeutic outcome in 268 patients and a review of the literature. *Pediatr Infect Dis J* 1992;11:474–478.

Schutze GE. Diagnosis and treatment of *Bortonella henselae* infections. *Pediatr Infect Dis J* 2000;19(12):185–187.

Stone JE. Encephalitis associated with cat-scratch disease—Broward and Palm Beach Counties, Florida, 1994. *JAMA* 1995;273:614.

Author: Louis M. Bell
Susan Dibs, 2nd edition

Cavernous Sinus Syndrome

 Database

DEFINITION

• The cavernous sinus syndrome (CSS) includes a variety of disease processes localized to the cavernous sinus—a venous plexus that drains the face, mouth, tonsils, pharynx, nasal cavity, paranasal sinuses, orbit, middle ear, and parts of the cerebral cortex.
• Small lesions in this region may produce dramatic neurologic signs.

CAUSES

• Infectious agents include *Staphylococcus aureus, Streptococcus pneumoniae*, gram-negative rods, and anaerobes.
• Mucormycosis and *Aspergillus* may be found in immunocompromised patients.
• Aseptic venous thrombosis has been associated with sickle cell anemia, trauma, dehydration, vasculitis, pregnancy, oral contraceptive use, congenital heart disease, inflammatory bowel disease, and hypercoagulable states.
• Neoplasms involving the cavernous sinus include pituitary adenomas, meningiomas, trigeminal schwannomas, craniopharyn-giomas, lymphomas, neuromas, chordomas, chondrosarcomas, nasopharyngeal carcinomas, and very rarely teratomas. Neoplasms may present with diplopia, visual-effect deficits, headache, or isolated cranial nerve deficits. The lateral extension of pituitary neoplasms into the cavernous sinus usually affects the third cranial nerve, with the fourth and sixth nerves less commonly involved. Rupture of a cystic craniopharyngioma may appear as acute CSS.
• Carotid-cavernous fistulas, which often have a more chronic course, are direct high-flow shunts between the internal carotid artery and the cavernous sinus. Almost always sequelae of trauma, they may present with a history of ocular motility deficits, arterialization of conjunctival vessels, and a bruit usually heard best over the orbit.
• Nonspecific and idiopathic inflammation of the cavernous sinus, also called idiopathic cavernous sinusitis or Tolosa-Hunt syndrome, has been reported in patients as young as $3\frac{1}{2}$ years. This is a diagnosis of exclusion.

PATHOPHYSIOLOGY

• The cavernous sinus is located lateral to the pituitary gland and sella turcica, superior to the sphenoid sinus, and inferior to the optic chiasm. Within the cavernous sinus are the carotid artery, the pericarotid sympathetic fibers, and the abducens nerve (VI); within its lateral wall are the oculomotor nerve (III), the trochlear nerve (IV), and the ophthalmic and maxillary divisions of the trigeminal nerve (V1, V2).

• CSS is typically caused by septic or aseptic sinus thrombosis, neoplasm or trauma, or idiopathic inflammation. Acute obstruction by mass or thrombosis may progress rapidly if not diagnosed and treated quickly.

COMPLICATIONS

Complications are dependent on the etiology of CSS.

• Septic CSS thrombosis and fungal infections may rapidly evolve to life-threatening sepsis and meningitis.
• Mucormycosis, usually seen in patients with diabetic ketoacidosis, is especially devastating.
• Aseptic CSS thrombosis may evolve to more extensive intracranial venous sinus thrombosis.
• Local spread of neoplasms will continue if not treated appropriately.

PROGNOSIS

Prognosis depends on the underlying etiology. Bacterial infections usually respond if diagnosed and treated promptly.

 Differential Diagnosis

Other disorders that may resemble CSS include:

• Orbital cellulitis, sphenoid sinusitis, thyroid eye disease, cavernous carotid aneurysm, orbital apex tumor, orbital pseudotumor, ocular migraine, and ocular trauma.

First priority is to rule out septic cavernous sinus thrombosis, a life-threatening complication of infections of the face, sinuses, middle ear, teeth, and orbit.

 Data Gathering

HISTORY

Question: Is there a history of a recent local infection?
Significance: Facial furuncle or cellulitis, sinusitis, dental infection, otitis, or orbital cellulitis may predispose to CSS.

Question: Are local or systemic symptoms present?
Significance: Fever, headache, eye pain, diplopia, and facial paresthesias may be present.

 Physical Examination

Finding: Conjunctival injection with lid swelling and proptosis
Significance: Signs of cavernous sinus venous congestion.

Finding: Ptosis, anisocoria, ophthalmo-paresis, and facial sensory changes
Significance: Signs of cranial nerve involvement.

Finding: Horner syndrome
Significance: Sympathetic nerve fibers traveling with V1 may be affected. This usually occurs in conjunction with an abducens nerve (CN VI) palsy with an inability to abduct the eye.

Finding: Signs and symptoms begin unilaterally.
Significance: But may rapidly spread bilaterally.

Finding: The optic nerve and visual acuity are spared early in CSS.
Significance: But can be affected as it progresses.

Finding: Funduscopic findings include venous dilatation and hemorrhages.
Significance: Papilledema is rare in acute cavernous sinus disease.

Finding: Resistance to retropulsion
Significance: May be very painful to elicit, but is a helpful sign.

Finding: Ocular bruit
Significance: May be heard in any acute CSS, but especially in carotid-cavernous fistula.

Finding: Signs of meningitis and systemic toxicity
Significance: These rapidly evolve if infections are untreated.

 Laboratory Aids

Test: CBC, ESR, PT/PTT, blood culture
Significance: Basic studies in any child with suspected acute CSS. Blood cultures are positive in 70% of cases of septic venous sinus thrombosis.

Test: MRI or CT
Significance: Any child with proptosis, cranial-nerve findings, or an ocular bruit should have an urgent MRI or CT. MRI, with and without gadolinium, with special attention to the cavernous sinus and parasellar region, is the imaging study of choice. Magnetic resonance venography (MRV) may be helpful.

Test: Lumbar puncture (LP)
Significance: LP should be performed if there is no contraindication and infection is suspected. About 35% of patients with septic cavernous sinus thrombosis have CSF findings consistent with bacterial meningitis—excess neutrophils, increased protein, and/or decreased glucose.

Test: Angiography
Significance: Suspected carotid-cavernous fistulas require angiography.

Test: Nasopharyngeal biopsy and culture
Significance: Helpful if mucormycosis or *Aspergillus* is suspected.

Test: ANA panel, HIV test
Significance: Obtain before a diagnosis of Tolosa-Hunt syndrome (diagnosis of exclusion) is made.

 ## Emergency Care

Depending on the clinical condition of the patient and suspected etiology, emergency imaging, lumbar puncture, antibiotics and/or anticoagulation may be indicated.

 ## Therapy

- For septic cavernous sinus thrombosis, broad-spectrum antibiotics (including coverage of penicillinase-resistant staphylococci and anaerobes) are begun immediately. Duration of therapy is usually 2 to 4 weeks beyond the resolution of symptoms.
- Amphotericin B is given if mucormycosis or *Aspergillus* is suspected.
- Surgical drainage of the primary infection (i.e., sinusitis) may be indicated (avoiding surgical manipulation of the cavernous sinus itself).
- Anticoagulation is controversial, but one study in adults found heparin reduced morbidity from septic cavernous sinus thrombosis.
- Posttraumatic carotid-cavernous fistulas rarely close spontaneously and have been treated with endoarterial balloon embolization.
- Consultation with a neuro-oncologist and a neurosurgeon are important for suspected neoplasms or surgical lesions.
- Idiopathic cavernous sinusitus, a diagnosis of exclusion, responds to corticosteroids. Treatment should not be started until neoplasm and infection have been ruled out.

 ## Follow-Up

- Septic cavernous sinus thrombosis may relapse, or embolic abscesses may develop, 2 to 6 weeks after therapy has been stopped. Mortality remains 13% to 30%, and less than 40% of patients recover fully from cranial-nerve deficits.
- Patients with carotid-cavernous fistulas frequently have persistent cranial-nerve deficits even after embolization.
- Idiopathic cavernous sinusitis responds to steroids, but relapses can be problematic. Clinical follow-up and serial MRI scans are indicated to rule out a low-grade neoplasm or fungal infection.

PREVENTION

- Local bacterial infections—sinusitis, facial cellulitis, dental abscesses, otitis, preseptal cellulitis and orbital cellulitis—should be treated promptly.
- Patients with suspected hypercoagulable states should be evaluated fully; dehydration must be avoided in such patients and anticoagulation may be necessary.

PITFALLS

- Ophthalmoplegic migraine must be distinguished from CSS by neuroimaging studies and history.
- Proptosis does not occur in migraine. This is a diagnosis of exclusion, especially on first presentation.
- Acute infection and hemorrhage of the pituitary gland—pituitary apoplexy—may present with acute bilateral ophthalmoplegia and signs of acute pituitary insufficiency. This most commonly occurs with pituitary neoplasms, but may also occur in pregnant women at the time of delivery.
- Chronic granulomatous disorders and tuberculosis may underlie CSS.

 ## Common Questions and Answers

Q: Will my child's eye movements return to normal?
A: In most cases, oculomotor nerves regain function as other signs improve, though they may take the longest to recover.

Q: Can more pain medicine be given?
A: There is often an attempt to balance side effects of sedation and hypoventilation against the need for pain control, especially when intracranial pressure is a concern.

ICD-9-CM

325 Thrombophlebitis of intracranial venous sinuses
437.6 Nonpyogenic Thrombosis of intracranial venous sinuses

BIBLIOGRAPHY

Berge J, Louail C, Caille JM. Cavernous sinus thrombosis diagnostic approach. *J Neuroradiol* 1994;21:101–117.

Doyle KJ, Jackler RK. Otogenic cavernous sinus thrombosis. *Otolaryngol Head Neck Surg* 1991;104:873–877.

Eisenberg MB, Al-Mefty O, DeMonte F, et al. Benign nonmeningeal tumors of the cavernous sinus. *Neurosurgery* 1999;44:949–955.

Gallagher RM, Gross CW, Phillips CD. Suppurative intracranial complications of sinusitis. *Laryngoscope* 1998;108:1635–1642.

Keane JR. Cavernous sinus syndrome— analysis of 151 cases. *Arch Neurol* 1996;53:967–971.

Liu GT, Volpe NJ, Galetta SL. *Neuro-ophthalmology: diagnosis and management.* Philadelphia: WB Saunders, 2001:550–561.

Author: Dennis J. Dlugos

Cavernous Transformation and Portal Vein Obstruction

 Database

DEFINITION

Cavernous transformation is defined as the collection of collaterals that develop around an obstructed vessel. In pediatrics, the obstruction is most typically of the portal vein. In portal vein obstruction the main portal vein or splenic vein is obstructed somewhere along its course, between the hilum of the spleen and the porta hepatis.

PATHOPHYSIOLOGY

Patients present with asymptomatic splenomegaly or upper gastrointestinal hemorrhage, resulting from portal hypertension. Less commonly, the patient presents with ascites or failure to thrive. And 50% of portal vein obstructions are idiopathic. Identified etiologies include:

- Congenital lesions
- Web
- Vascular anomaly
- Clot that develops as a result of hypercoagulable states
- Malignancy
- Protein C deficiency
- Protein S deficiency
- Antithrombin III deficiency
- Clot from other etiologies
- Omphalitis
- Umbilical-vein catheterization
- Portal pyelophlebitis
- Intraabdominal sepsis
- Surgery near the porta hepatis
- Sepsis
- Cholangitis
- Dehydration
- Trauma

GENETICS

A genetic basis of this problem has not been identified. Congenital abnormalities of the heart, major blood vessels, biliary tree, and renal system are found in 40% of cases.

EPIDEMIOLOGY

Even if the lesion developed in infancy, patients present at any age. Patients in the 7th decade have been reported, but most patients present between birth and 15 years of age. Bleeding is more typical of patients presenting before 7 years of age; splenomegaly in the absence of symptoms is more typical for patients between ages 5 and 15.

COMPLICATIONS

Most of the complications are secondary to portal hypertension, such as variceal hemorrhage and splenomegaly with hypersplenism. In some cases, steatorrhea and protein-losing enteropathy occur secondary to venous congestion of the intestinal mucosa. Ascites may also develop around the time of the onset of portal hypertension. Often, it develops in the period immediately following an upper gastrointestinal (GI) hemorrhage due to acute hepatic decompensation and decreasing albumin. Both the albumin and the ascites resolve in several weeks.

 Differential Diagnosis

The differential diagnosis must exclude other causes of splenomegaly and portal hypertension. Once portal vein obstruction has been identified, a search for the underlying etiology must be pursued.

 Data Gathering

Clinical examination reveals no jaundice or other evidence of chronic liver disease. Splenomegaly is the only intraabdominal abnormality that can be identified. Ascites is rarely present.

HISTORY

Question: Other causes of splenomegaly?
Significance: Exposure to infectious mononucleosis, metabolic storage disease, and malignancy.

 Physical Examination

Finding: Splenomegaly and possible hemorrhoids
Significance: The spleen is measured from the left anterior axillary line at the costal margin diagonally toward the umbilicus.

Laboratory Aids

Test: CBC
Significance: Leukopenia and thrombo-cytopenia will be present if there is hypersplenism.

Test: AST/ALT/GGT
Significance: Should be normal

Test: PT/PTT
Significance: May be abnormal if malabsorption is present.

Test: Protein C, protein S, antithrombin III
Significance: Associated with hypercoagulable states.

Test: Ultrasound with Doppler
Significance: To examine portal vein flow and to identify collateral veins if there is cavernous transformation of the portal vein. The liver may be slightly small, but may be normal in texture.

Test: Liver biopsy
Significance: Exclude other etiologies.

Test: Upper endoscopy
Significance: To define extent of varices.

Test: Bone marrow examination
Significance: To determine if there is an underlying myeloproliferative disease.

 Therapy

Therapy is designed to manage variceal hemorrhage and to identify an underlying etiology to determine if the patient is at risk for additional venous thrombosis or malignancy. The therapy for GI hemorrhage is:

- Prophylactic sclerotherapy
- β-blocker therapy
- Shunt in order to decompress varices

 Follow-Up

Follow-up by the pediatrician should focus on growth parameters and early detection of malabsorption. The gastroenterologist will manage GI hemorrhage and supplemental nutrition, if needed.

PITFALLS

The patient should be advised about activity restrictions due to splenomegaly and should be told to avoid medicines that interfere with platelet function.

 Common Questions and Answers

Q: What is the long-term prognosis?
A: Good. Upper GI hemorrhage becomes less problematic as the child becomes older. Shunting is rarely recommended. Most patients undergo prophylactic sclerotherapy. As liver function is normal, it is rare for encephalopathy to develop.

Q: Should I restrict my child's activities?
A: Contact sports should be limited or a spleen guard used. NSAIDs, including aspirin, should be avoided because of the risk of hemorrhage.

ICD-9-CM 747.49

BIBLIOGRAPHY

Gitnick G, LaBrecque DR, Moody FG. *Diseases of the liver and biliary tract.* Philadelphia: Mosby-Year Book, 1992.

Mowat AP. *Liver disorders in childhood.* Boston: Butterworths, 1987.

Suchy F. *Liver disease in children.* Philadelphia: CV Mosby, 1994.

Author: Barbara Haber

Celiac Disease

 Database

DEFINITION

This is defined as a lifetime sensitivity to gluten, a protein fraction that is present in wheat, barley, rye, and possibly in oats.

CLINICAL PRESENTATION

• Typical presentation is in the toddler under the age of 2 years who presents with failure to thrive, malabsorption, wasting of muscles, bloated abdomen, fractious and unhappy behavior. The stools are explosive and foul, and vomiting is common. About 80% of all children with celiac disease present with this picture.
• Atypical forms are:

—Late presentation in schoolchildren with recurrent abdominal pain
—Recurrent aphthous stomatitis
—Cryptogenic hepatitis
—Dental defects

• Disease also causes:

—Iron-deficiency anemia resistant to iron therapy
—Gastrointestinal bleeding
—Short stature
—Joint problems
—Dermatitis herpetiformis without obvious symptoms of malabsorption

• With increasingly sensitive methods for detection more cases of celiac disease have been found where the disease is clinically silent when the enteropathy is found incidentally in a healthy child. With detailed studies of these patients, there is a higher prevalence of these patients with vague symptoms such as behavioral problems, anemia, fatigue, and osteopenia.
• In latent celiac disease, patients have mild symptoms of celiac disease but on endoscopy there is no evidence of enteropathy, but once challenged with 20 g of gluten there is obvious enteropathy. These patients probably present with a milder form of the disease.
• Finally, some toddlers present with classic celiac disease on endoscopy and gluten challenge but after a few years they tolerate a gluten-containing diet with no endoscopic evidence of enteropathy. This is probably a form of transient protein intolerance, such as with milk protein intolerance.

PATHOPHYSIOLOGY

Small bowel biopsy is done by direct endoscopy with forceps or with the Crosby capsule. The Crosby capsule takes better aligned biopsies to demonstrate the entire crypt-villus architecture, but using a dissecting microscope it is quite easy to align the biopsy for the pathologist. The aligning is crucial since the diagnosis is made based on visualizing flattening of the villus, which can be easily mimicked by a poorly aligned biopsy from a healthy patient.
Features that characterize celiac disease are:

• Total villus atrophy
• Crypt hyperplasia
• Increased crypt cell mitosis
• Infiltration of lamina propria with excess lymphocytes (CD4 T cells mainly)

EPIDEMIOLOGY

• Prevalence of 90 per 100,000
• Women more affected than men
• Uncommon in the United States but more common in Europe
• Including asymptomatic patients may affect as many as 1 in 300 people based on blood donor studies.

GENETICS

• There is 5% to 15% of first-degree concordance in first-degree relatives with celiac disease and 75% concordance in twins demonstrating the genetic causality.
• In addition 90% of patients have the HLA-DQ2 molecule coded by the alleles DQA1*0501 and DQB1*0201 and 5% carry the HLA-DR4, DQ8 haplotype.

OTHER ASSOCIATED DISEASES

• Ankylosing spondylitis, scleroderma systemic lupus erythematosus (SLE), Sjögren syndrome
• Chromosomal anomalies such as Down and Turner syndrome
• Addison disease, autoimmune thyroiditis, Graves disease, parathyroid adenoma, diabetes mellitus
• Alopecia, atopic eczema, dermatitis herpetiformis, psoriasis
• Mouth diseases such as cancer, lichen planus, and recurrent stomatitis
• Inflammatory bowel disease and oropharyngeal cancers
• Chronic active hepatitis, primary biliary cirrhosis, primary sclerosing cholangitis
• Neurologic and behavioral disorders
• IgA deficiency
• Asthma, alveolitis, sarcoidosis

 Differential Diagnosis

• Milk protein intolerance
• Toddler's diarrhea
• Giardiasis
• Gastritis
• Gastroenteritis
• Eosinophilic gastroenteritis
• Autoimmune enteropathy
• Immunodeficiency
• Cystic fibrosis
• Inflammatory bowel disease
• Celiac disease has been associated with other diseases including:

—Diabetes mellitus
—Thyrotoxicosis
—Hypothyroidism
—IgA deficiency
—Sarcoidosis
—Vasculitis
—Dermatitis herpetiformis
—Pernicious anemia

Celiac Disease

Data Gathering

HISTORY

Question: Diet?
Significance: Determine the relationship between intake of gluten and symptoms. Find out the amount of wheat, rye, and barley.

Question: Growth pattern?
Significance: Most patients have short stature.

Question: Description of stools?
Significance: Stools tend to be explosive and foul smelling.

Question: Description of behavior?
Significance: Patients tend to be irritable.

Physical Examination

Finding: Growth pattern
Significance: Often have short stature

Finding: Classic presentation is large abdomen with wasted buttocks.
Significance: Many patients do not have that appearance.

Laboratory Aids

Test: IgG and IgA quantification
Significance: 2% of patients with celiac disease are IgA deficient; it is best to check both IgG and IgA antigliadin antibodies concurrently. If patients are IgA-deficient, then IgA antibody tests are unreliable.

Test: Antigliadin antibody (AGA) IgA and IgG
Significance: 50–90% with active celiac disease are positive

Test: Antireticulin antibody (AR) IgA
Significance: More specific but less sensitive than antigliadin Ab

Test: Antiendomysial antibody (AEA) IgA
Significance: More specific than AGA but in treated patients titers fall more than AGA (90–100% sensitive and specific).

Test: Antitransglutaminase (AtTG) IgA
Significance: The autoantigen responsible for the endomysial pattern is tissue transglutaminase (90–100% sensitive and specific).

BIOPSY

- Before a biopsy is done it is usual to check all the celiac antibodies as a screening test. With diagnosed patients AGA and AEA titers are useful monitoring tools for compliance and recovery.
- Should be performed on a regular diet.
- Reveals flattened villi with plasma cell infiltrate.

CBC

- Microcytic anemia is common.

DIAGNOSIS

- Because AEA and AtTG are so specific for celiac disease, some people have advocated treatment based on these antibodies alone. However the current standard is still to obtain a small bowel biopsy on a gluten-containing diet. Symptoms should resolve on a gluten-free diet with reversal of enteropathy on subsequent biopsy.
- Additional monitoring is done with symptoms and antibody testing.
- Finally, to diagnose transient gluten intolerance, a gluten challenge is carried out after an interval. There is no consensus as to when this should be performed.

TREATMENT

Gluten-free diet with normalization of symptoms and enteropathy, which can take up to 6 months.

PROGNOSIS

On patients with strict diet there is very little risk of malignant lymphoma and other malignancies. Therefore, in patients with proven celiac disease it is advisable to remain on gluten-free diet for life.

Follow-Up

Compliance of patients can be monitored by the fall of AEA or AtTG antibodies with a gluten-free diet. This should be accompanied by improvement of presenting symptoms such as failure to thrive, diarrhea, and anemia.

Common Questions and Answers

Q: Why do you do a gluten challenge when celiac disease is a lifelong disease?
A: This is to exclude the diagnosis of transient gluten intolerance, which is more like a milk protein intolerance and disappears when the gut heals. In such patients, a gluten challenge is normal.

Q: Are oats included in the gluten containing cereal?
A: Strictly speaking, wheat, rye, barley, and oats are more closely related in their development from the primitive grains such as rice, corn, sorghum, and millets, which do not activate celiac disease. Gluten-free means a diet devoid of all wheat, rye, barley, and oats but some adult studies have shown that ingestion of even up to 50 g of oats did not cause clear-cut histologic or clinical deterioration in celiac patients. It appears that of the four grains, oats is the least "toxic" to celiac patients.

Q: Can patients with celiac disease drink beer?
A: Not if the beer is derived from barley, rye, wheat, or oats.

ICD-9-CM 579.0

BIBLIOGRAPHY

Catassi C, Fabiani E. The spectrum of coeliac disease in children. In: Walker-Smith JA, ed. *Paediatric gastroenterology, Bailliere's clinical gastroenterology international practice and research.* Bailliere Tindall, 1997:485–507.

Kagnoff MF. Genetic basis of celiac disease: role of HLA genes. In: Marsh M, ed. *Coeliac disease.* Boston: Blackwell Scientific Publications, 1992:215–238.

McPherson RA. Advances in the laboratory diagnosis of celiac disease. *J Clin Lab Anal* 2001;15(3):105–107.

Author: John Tung

Cellulitis

 Database

DEFINITION

- Inflammation/infection of the skin/subcutaneous tissues
- Often classified by body area involved:

—Periorbital
—Orbital
—Buccal
—Peritonsillar
—Extremity
—Breast
—Perianal
—Cellulitis-adenitis

CAUSES

- *Staphylococcus aureus*
- Group A *β*-hemolytic streptococci (*Streptococcus pyogenes*)
- *Streptococcus pneumoniae*
- Group B streptococci, gram-negative bacilli (neonates)
- *Haemophilus influenzae* type b (very rare since advent of childhood immunization)
- *Pseudomonas aeruginosa*, anaerobic bacteria (immunocompromised children)

PATHOPHYSIOLOGY

- Most commonly secondary to local trauma

—Abrasions
—Lacerations
—Bites
—Excoriated dermatitis
—Other breaches in the integument

- May develop secondary to local invasion or infection (e.g., sinusitis leading to orbital cellulitis).
- Hematogenous dissemination

EPIDEMIOLOGY

- The most common cause of cellulitis in children is *Staphylococcus aureus* or *Streptococcus pyogenes* infection, which develops secondary to local trauma of the integument.
- Bacteremic disease, previously seen commonly when *H. influenzae* type b was prevalent, has now been surpassed by *S. pneumoniae*.
- Clinical failures with penicillin-resistant *S. pneumoniae* have not yet become a significant problem in cases of uncomplicated cellulitis.

ASSOCIATED ILLNESSES

- Periorbital

—Usually secondary to local trauma
—Impetigo
—Varicella
—Eczema
—Much less common, hematogenous
—Rarely associated with infectious conjunctivitis

- Orbital

—Most commonly associated with severe sinusitis
—Less common, dental abscess

- Buccal

—Same pathophysiology and epidemiology as periorbital cellulitis (not including conjunctivitis)

- Peritonsillar

—Commonly secondary to severe group A *β*-hemolytic streptococcal pharyngitis
—Often progresses or associated with a peritonsillar abscess

- Extremity

—Almost always secondary to local trauma

- Breast

—Usually with mastitis (most often in neonates)

- Perianal

—Seen in infants and young children
—Etiology: Group A *Streptococcus*
—Perianal pain, pruritus, and erythema; sometimes associated with bloody stools.

- Cellulitis-Adenitis Syndrome

—Uncommon infection seen in neonates and young infants
—Etiology: Group B Streptococcus, *Staphylococcus aureus*, gram-negative bacilli
—Bacteremia almost always documented
—Meningitis also common

COMPLICATIONS

- Local as well as distant spread of infection is possible.
- Suppuration and abscess formation may occur (e.g., peritonsillar abscess).
- Extremity cellulitis may extend into the deep tissues to produce an arthritis or osteomyelitis, or it may extend proximally as a lymphangitis.
- Orbital cellulitis may be complicated by visual loss and/or cavernous sinus thrombosis.
- Prior to widespread immunization against *H. influenzae* type b, the bacteremia associated with facial cellulitis was not uncommonly associated with pneumonia, meningitis, pericarditis, epiglottitis, as well as arthritis and osteomyelitis.

PROGNOSIS

- The prognosis for complete recovery is good as long as appropriate antimicrobials are administered in a timely fashion.

 Differential Diagnosis

- Allergic angioedema is the most common entity; it can usually be excluded by its lack of tenderness and the absence of fever.
- Contact dermatitis, similarly, is distinguished by its painlessness, pruritus, and the Koebner phenomenon (appearance of isomorphic lesions in the lines of scratching).
- A traumatic contusion may be mistaken for cellulitis, but the history should be confirmatory.
- Severe conjunctivitis may mimic periorbital cellulitis; conjunctival injection, chemosis, and discharge usually implicate a conjunctivitis.
- "Popsicle panniculitis," a cold-induced fat injury to the cheeks of infants, may be almost indistinguishable from buccal cellulitis; a history of cold weather exposure, or ice or popsicle sucking should be sought.
- A primary eye malignancy (retinoblastoma), locally invasive tumor (rhabdomyosarcoma), or metastatic disease (neuroblastoma, leukemia, lymphoma), may simulate periorbital or orbital cellulitis.

 Data Gathering

HISTORY

Question: Is there an expanding, red, painful area of swelling?
Significance: This is the most common presentation.

Question: Are there associated, mild constitutional symptoms (with or without fever)?
Significance: Commonly associated with cellulitis.

Question: Is there a history of local trauma to the integument?
Significance: This is the clue to the portal of bacterial entry.

Cellulitis

Physical Examination

Finding: Erythema, edema, tenderness, and warmth
Significance: The classic clinical findings of cellulitis.

Finding: Distinct demarcation of raised erythema
Significance: The classic description of erysipelas, a superficial cellulitis usually associated with *S. pyogenes*.

Finding: A red streak extending proximally from the extremity
Significance: Lymphangitis, which usually implies more serious involvement.

Finding: Regional adenopathy
Significance: Commonly associated with minor cellulitis. Occasionally complicated by lymphadenitis.

Laboratory Aids

Test: CBC
Significance: May be normal or show leukocytosis in more severe cases.

Test: Blood cultures
Significance: As invasive *H. influenzae* type b disease has virtually disappeared, obtaining blood cultures has become less mandatory with cellulitis. Blood cultures are now rarely positive in most routine cases of cellulitis. Ill-appearing children, however, should have a culture obtained. Additionally, some experts still recommend blood cultures in facial and other serious cases of cellulitis.

Test: Needle aspiration and culture
Significance: "Leading edge" cultures, etc., are generally not indicated.

Test: Lumbar puncture
Significance: Indicated only in ill-appearing children and young infants (to rule out sepsis).

Test: X-ray studies
Significance: Sometimes helpful to rule out complications such as arthritis or osteomyelitis. Also useful in cases of suspected foreign bodies.

Test: Head CT scan
Significance: Important in orbital cellulitis to delineate extent of disease, and also in some cases when distinction from periorbital cellulitis is clinically difficult.

Test: Bone marrow aspirate and biopsy (as well as CT scan)
Significance: To rule out malignancies.

Therapy

- Most cases of uncomplicated cellulitis can be treated with oral antibiotics active against *Staphylococcus* and *Streptococcus* (e.g., amoxicillin-clavulanate, cephalexin, and erythromycin).
- Ill-appearing children or extensive cellulitic lesions require intravenous antibiotics.
- Initial intravenous therapy should be directed against *S. aureus* and *Streptococcus* (e.g., oxacillin, nafcillin, cefazolin, or ampicillin/sulbactam).
- When hematogenous dissemination is a strong possibility, an agent active against *H. influenzae* type b also should be added (e.g., ceftriaxone, cefotaxime, cefuroxime, or chloramphenicol).
- Neonates (<7 weeks of age) should have gram-positive and gram-negative coverage (e.g., oxacillin/nafcillin and gentamicin, or oxacillin/nafcillin and cefotaxime) to cover the enterics as well.
- The duration of antibiotics (intravenous and oral) should generally be 7 to 10 days.
- Abscesses should be surgically drained.

Follow-Up

- Rapid, steady improvement should be expected.
- If daily improvement is not noted, inappropriate antimicrobial therapy, a deeper infection or abscess, or some other complication should be suspected (e.g., foreign body).

PREVENTION

- Good wound care can prevent most cases of cellulitis.
- Parents should be instructed to cleanse all wounds thoroughly with soap and water, then cover with a clean, dry cloth.
- Topical antibiotic ointment is optional.
- The heptavalent-conjugated pneumococcal vaccine will likely dramatically decrease the occurrence of bacteremic *S. pneumoniae* cellulitis.

PITFALLS

- Avoid trying to make distinction between staphylococcal and streptococcal by clinical presentation—it is always safest to cover cellulitis patients with an agent active against both (i.e., penicillin and amoxicillin are *not* good empiric choices).
- The "violaceous hue" touted as an indicator of *H. influenzae* type b cellulitis is neither sensitive nor specific.

Common Questions and Answers

Q: Is ophthalmology consultation necessary in all cases of periorbital cellulitis?
A: Ophthalmology consultation is not necessary in simple, uncomplicated cases of periorbital cellulitis that clearly have no associated proptosis, limitation in extraocular eye movement, or visual impairment that would suggest a more serious orbital cellulitis; if, however, the diagnosis is in question, consultation is indicated.

Q: Is cefuroxime adequate coverage in cases of facial cellulitis?
A: If meningitis is suspected, cefuroxime should not be used, as its CSF penetration is suboptimal.

ICD-9-CM 682.9

BIBLIOGRAPHY

Albanyan EA, Baker CJ. Is lumbar puncture necessary to exclude meningitis in neonates and young infants: lessons from the group B streptococcus cellulitis-adenitis syndrome. *Pediatrics* 1998;102(4 pt 1):984–986.

Barone SR, Aiuto LT. Periorbital and orbital cellulitis in the Haemophilus influenza vaccine era. *J Pediatr Ophthalmol Strabismus* 1997;34(5):293–296.

Barzilai A, Choen HA. Isolation of Group A streptococci from children with perianal cellulitis. *Pediatr Infect Dis J* 1998;17(4):358–360.

Berger-Sadow K, Chamberlain JM. Blood cultures in the evaluation of children with cellulitis. *Pediatrics* 1998;101(3). URL: http://www.pediatrics.org/cgi/content/full/101/3/e4.

Ciarallo LR, Rowe PC. Lumbar puncture in children with periorbital and orbital cellulitis. *J Pediatr* 1993;122(3):355–359.

Danik SB, Schwartz RA, Oleske JM. Cellulitis. *Cutis* 1999;64:157–164.

Donahue SP, Schwartz G. Preseptal and orbital cellulitis in childhood: a changing microbiologic spectrum. *Ophthalmology* 1998;105(10):1902–1906.

Givner LB, et al. Pneumococcal facial cellulitis in children. *Pediatrics* 2000;106(5). URL: http://www.pediatrics.org/cgi/content/full/106/5/e61.

Lessner A, Stern GA. Preseptal and orbital cellulitis. *Infect Dis Clin North Am* 1992;6(4):933–952.

Powell KR. Periorbital and orbital cellulitis. *Pediatr Rev* 1995;16(5):163–167.

Zenel JA. A febrile infant who has hand edema and erythema. *Pediatr Rev* 2000;21(9):321–323.

Author: Nicholas Tsarouhas

229

Cerebral Palsy

Database

DEFINITION AND CLASSIFICATION
- Cerebral palsy (CP) is a nonprogressive motor impairment condition that result from damage to or dysfunction of the brain.
- Subtypes are defined by type of neurologic impairment and anatomic distribution:
—Spastic CP (pyramidal CP) (40%): increased deep tendon reflexes, sustained clonus, hypertonia, and the clasp-knife response
—Spastic diplegia—lower extremity involvement
—Spastic hemiplegia—one side of the body involved
—Spastic quadriplegia—total-body involvement.
—Dyskinetic CP (30%): fluctuating tone, rigidity total-body involvement by definition. Persistent primitive reflex patterns [e.g., asymmetric tonic neck reflex (ATNR), labyrinthine] often seen. Subtypes:
—Athetoid CP: slow writhing movements (or chorea: rapid, random, jerky movements),
—Dystonic CP: posturing of the head, trunk, and extremities.
—Ataxic CP (10%): characterized by cerebellar signs (ataxia, dysmetria, past-pointing, tremor, nystagmus) and abnormalities of voluntary movement
—Mixed CP (10%): two or more types codominant, most often spastic and dyskinetic
- Other CP (10%): criteria for CP met but specific subtype cannot be defined
- Extrapyramidal CP: sometimes applied to nonspastic types of CP as a group

EPIDEMIOLOGY
- Prevalence approximately 2 per 1,000
- Approximately 50% of cases are associated with prematurity.
- Increased incidence with multiple gestation (10% were twins in one study)
- Increased concordance among monozygotic versus dizygotic twins in some studies (not in others)
- Intrauterine growth retardation (IUGR) more common in CP than controls, especially for full-term infants in whom CP develops.
- Male/female ratio, 1.3:1
- Inconsistent correlation to maternal age, socioeconomic status, and parity
- Epidemiologic studies suggest that prenatal factors are more strongly associated with subsequent CP than perinatal or postnatal factors; however, individual risk factors are poorly predictive of subsequent CP in the individual child.
- Diagnosis of perinatal asphyxia requires evidence of multiorgan system hypoxic-ischemic insult and severe encephalopathy (e.g., neonatal seizures, severe hypotonia), and accounts for only about 9% of cases of CP.

ETIOLOGY
- In the majority of cases, etiology is not apparent.

- Epidemiologic studies indicate two types of vulnerability to CP: prematurity-related and IUGR-related.
—Prematurity-related: unique vulnerability of the periventricular white matter between 28 and 32 weeks of gestation results in periventricular leukomalacia.
—IUGR-related: in full-term infants, fetal abnormalities associated with CNS dysgenesis, non-CNS malformation, teratogens, growth retardation, evidence of hypoxic-ischemic encephalopathy more often seen.

ASSOCIATED IMPAIRMENTS
- Sensory
—Sensorineural and conductive hearing loss
—Impairments of visual acuity
—Oculomotor dysfunction
—Strabismus
—Somatosensory impairments
- Cognitive
—Mental retardation (MR) in about 50%, especially in spastic quadriparesis
—High incidence of learning disabilities
—Attention deficit/hyperactivity disorder
—Sleep and behavioral disturbances
- Neurologic
—Seizures
—Hydrocephalus
- Musculoskeletal
—Contractures
—Hip subluxation/dislocation
—Scoliosis
- Cardiorespiratory
—Upper airway obstruction
—Aspiration pneumonitis
—Restrictive lung disease
—Secondary to thoracic deformity
—Reactive airway disease
- Gastrointestinal tract/nutrition
—Failure to thrive
—Gastroesophageal reflux
—Constipation
—Oral motor dysfunction/dysphagia
- Gastrourinary tract
- Neurogenic bladder
- Skin
—Decubitus ulcers
- Dental
—Caries
—Gingival hyperplasia
—Abnormalities of enamel (congenital)

Differential Diagnosis

- Motor impairment syndromes related to spinal cord, lower motor neuron, peripheral nerve, or primary muscular disease
- Connective-tissue disorders (primary and secondary) resulting in musculoskeletal abnormalities (e.g., arthrogryposis multiplex, skeletal dysplasias)
- Inborn errors of metabolism and CP: protean manifestations, dyskinesia, ataxia, postnatal growth failure, neurologic deterioration (especially associated with recurrent vomiting) are clues, but presentation can be insidious.

Data Gathering

HISTORY
Question: Prenatal history?
Significance: Exposure to toxins/drugs, infections or fever, HIV/STD risk, vaginal bleeding, abnormal fetal movement, preeclampsia (especially proteinuria), breech position, poor maternal weight gain, premature labor, fetal distress, IUGR, prenatal testing, placental disorders.
Question: Perinatal history?
Significance: Premature delivery, neonatal resuscitation, low Apgar scores (7 at 5 and 10 minutes), birth trauma, evidence of neonatal encephalopathy (seizures, severe hypotonia), complicated neonatal course (intraventricular hemorrhage, prolonged respiratory support, meningitis, sepsis, hyperbilirubinemia).
Question: Postnatal history?
Significance: Hospitalization for severe infection or trauma, periodic or persistent deterioration in function (suggests neurodegenerative/metabolic disease).
Question: Development?
Significance: Severe delay in motor milestones (e.g., not rolling at 7 months, not sitting at 8 months, not walking at 15 months) associated with persistent primitive reflexes (e.g., prominent tonic neck and labyrinthine responses at 1 year of age) and delayed or absent development of protective reactions (e.g., lateral prop at 7 months, parachute at 13 months). Associated delays in language, play, social, and adaptive behavior.

Physical Examination

GENERAL
Finding: Respiratory pattern
Significance: Obstruction, aspiration risk, evidence of dysmorphism/pigmentary skin changes and growth abnormalities contribute to assessment of etiology.
Finding: Head circumference
Significance: To evaluate for microcephaly/macrocephaly/hydrocephaly.
Finding: Strabismus/cataracts/iris or retinal abnormalities
Significance: Either cranial nerve damage, muscle imbalance, metabolic disease, or congenital infection.

MUSCULOSKELETAL
Finding: Range of motion
Significance: Decreased with contractures
Finding: Leg-length discrepancy
Significance: Hip dislocation
Finding: Spinal curvature
Significance: Neuromuscular imbalance

NEUROLOGIC

Finding: In addition to formal examination, documentation of best level of visual motor/manipulative skills (e.g., able to run, transfer, hold a cup, etc.)
Significance: Helpful in following the course of the motor impairment.
Finding: Cranial nerves
Significance: Especially strabismus, speech and swallowing, vision and hearing.
Finding: Tone
Significance: Spasticity versus rigidity versus hypotonia
Finding: Strength
Significance: Often decreased
Finding: Clasp-knife response
Significance: Hyperactive deep tendon reflexes, and clonus in spasticity; Babinski reflex (extensor response to plantar stimulation)
Finding: Persistent primitive reflexes
Significance: CNS damage
Finding: Protective reactions
Significance: Head and trunk righting, prop reactions, parachute; cerebellar signs
Finding: Postural stability
Significance: Neuromuscular imbalance
Finding: Gait abnormalities, subtle seizures
Significance: Motor or CNS damage

Laboratory Aids

Test: Hearing and vision
Significance: All in first year with regular follow-up examinations (identification of sensory deficits and clues to etiology)
Test: Brain imaging
Significance: Should be performed when hydrocephalus is suspected; frequently useful in determining etiology
Test: Genetic and metabolic studies
Significance: Indicated when the history and physical examination suggest a progressive or hereditary disorder.
Test: X-ray studies
Significance: Should be done routinely in spastic diparesis for hip dislocation; usefulness of scoliosis films depends on physical findings.
Test: Audiologic evaluation
Significance: Required for those with language delay or those who manifest hearing impairment.
Test: Radionucleotide studies or pH probe
Significance: "Milk scan"; evaluate gastroesophageal reflux (GER), gastric emptying, aspiration
Test: Blood tests—chemistries, liver-function studies, cell counts
Significance: Evaluate nutritional/metabolic status, anticonvulsant levels
Test: Urodynamic studies
Significance: Spastic bladder, indicated in those with recurrent urinary tract infections or voiding dysfunction.

Test: Sleep study
Significance: May disclose treatable obstructive sleep apnea in those with excessive somnolence or abnormal sleep-wake cycles.
Test: Pulmonary-function studies
Significance: Helpful in documenting progressive restrictive pulmonary dysfunction (e.g., in severe scoliosis).
Test: EEG
Significance: Seizure disorder is suspected

Therapy

- Family-centered care is directed toward optimizing function/minimizing handicap (habilitation).
- Interdisciplinary clinics: to provide multiple services (medical, surgical, therapy, etc.) coordinated with primary care physician.
- Education services: recent emphasis on inclusion/mainstreaming; for many children, special education services are still required and appropriate.
- Physical, occupational, speech/language therapy, other allied health professionals: therapy provided in home, school, and hospital settings, directed primarily at improved functioning in the areas of mobility, self-care, and communication; orthodontists for braces.
- Social services: provided in a variety of contexts to aid in the coordination of care

Follow-Up

- Requirements for follow-up vary greatly with the degree of disability and the scope of impairments. An interdisciplinary clinic setting may be more appropriate for a child with severe CP.
- Early referral to a pediatric orthopedist is indicated, especially for monitoring of early hip subluxation, which is best managed before progression to frank dislocation.
- Early referral for developmental assessment to establish need for early intervention, to optimize development, and to promote family coping

PITFALLS

- Overdiagnosis of CP in infants with spastic hypertonia (especially those born prematurely); normalization of tone/function may take up to 2 years.
- Slowly progressive neurogenerative disease may masquerade as CP.
- Cervical cord lesions may masquerade as quadriparetic spastic CP. Swallowing reflexes may be preserved; cognitive development is normal.
- Determination of ideal body weight may be complex in CP; growth standards according to CP type are under development.

Common Questions and Answers

Q: Is severe clumsiness a form of CP?
A: Mild spastic diplegia or hemiplegia may present this way, but spasticity and contractures distinguish these from developmental coordination disorders.
Q: Do children with CP also have mental retardation?
A: Not necessarily; although 50% have mental retardation, it is not a part of the definition of CP.
Q: What about surgery for CP?
A: Spasticity in the lower extremities may be addressed directly with selective dorsal rhizotomy (interruption of afferent limb of stretch reflex arch). Otherwise, surgical therapy in CP is directed at associated conditions; many children with CP undergo orthopedic procedures for hip dislocation, release of contractures, and scoliosis. Surgery for correction of strabismus or placement of a gastrostomy tube is commonly performed.

ICD-9-CM 343.9

BIBLIOGRAPHY

Badawi N, Watson L, Petterson B, et al. What constitutes cerebral palsy? *Dev Med Child Neurol* 1998;40(8):520–527.

Fennell EB, Dikel TN. Cognitive and neuropsychological functioning in children with cerebral palsy. [erratum appears in *J Child Neurol* 2001;16(3):225]. *J Child Neurol* 2001;16(1):58–63.

Freeman JM, Nelson KB. Intrapartum asphyxia and cerebral palsy. *Pediatrics* 1988;82:240–249.

Golden CG. Apgar scores as predictors of chronic neurologic disability, by Karin B. Nelson, MD, and Jonas H. Ellenberg, PhD. *Pediatrics* 1981;68:36–44. *Pediatrics* 1998;102(1 pt 2):262–264.

Goldstein EM. Spasticity management: an overview. *J Child Neurol* 2001;16(1):16–23.

Kirschner J, Berweck S, Mall V, et al. Botulinum toxin treatment in cerebral palsy: evidence for a new treatment option. *J Neurol* 2001;248(suppl 1):28–30.

Nelson KB, Ellenberg JH. Antecedents of cerebral palsy: multivariate analysis of risk. *N Engl J Med* 1986;315:81–86.

Patrick JH, Roberts AP, Cole GF. Therapeutic choices in the locomotor management of the child with cerebral palsy—more luck than judgment *Arch Dis Child* 2001;85(4):275–279.

Petersen MC, Palmer FB. Advances in prevention and treatment of cerebral palsy. *Mental Retardation Dev Disabil Res Rev* 2001; 7(1):30–37.

Author: Robert Markham Mitchell
Louis Pelligrino, 2nd edition

Cervicitis

Database

DEFINITION

Cervicitis is infection of the endocervix resulting in inflammation leading to mucopurulent cervical discharge, edema, erythema, and friability of the cervix and endocervical canal.

CAUSES

In the majority of young women, no pathogen is isolated. Common identifiable causes include:

- *Chlamydia trachomatis*
- *Neisseria gonorrhoeae*
- Herpesvirus hominis
- *Trichomonas vaginalis*
- *Candida albicans*

ASSOCIATED DISEASES

The presence of other sexually transmitted diseases must be considered including:

- *T. vaginalis*
- Syphilis
- Hepatitis B
- HIV
- Bacterial vaginosis

EPIDEMIOLOGY

The true incidence of mucopurulent cervicitis is unknown; however, it is quite common. As many patients are asymptomatic and the interpretation and presence of the clinical signs is quite variable, many cases go undiagnosed.

COMPLICATIONS

The patient with endocervical infection is at risk for:

- Reinfection
- Sexually transmitted diseases
- pregnancy
- Symptomatic or asymptomatic upper genital tract disease with all its sequelae

—Infertility
—Ectopic pregnancy
—Chronic pelvic pain

PROGNOSIS

If treated appropriately, these patients are cured and have no sequelae from the infection.

Differential Diagnosis

- Inflammation of the vulva, the urethra and/or bladder, the vagina, and the endocervical canal
- In patients presenting with abnormal menstrual bleeding, these infectious causes are common.

Data Gathering

HISTORY

Symptoms Consistent with But Not Diagnostic of Cervicitis

Question: Abnormal vaginal bleeding and/or discharge?
Significance: Inflamed cervix may bleed; may indicate vaginal infection.

Question: Dysuria?
Significance: May indicate urethritis or bladder infection.

Question: Vulvar itching?
Significance: May indicate extension of infection to vagina.

Question: Dyspareunia?
Significance: Common finding of sensitive cervix.

Medical History

Important questions of women's health assessment but not diagnostic of cervicitis:

Question: Previous sexually transmitted disease (STD)?
Significance: Common association

Question: Last menstrual period?
Significance: May lead to ectopic pregnancy.

Question: Birth control method?
Significance: Condoms are protective.

Question: Exposure to infected partner?
Significance : Important to treat both partners.

Question: Gravity?

Question: Parity?

Physical Examination

ABDOMEN

Finding: No tenderness on palpation of the abdomen
Significance: Infection is limited to the cervix.

PELVIC

Finding: Mucopurulent discharge from the cervical os or yellow exudative discharge present on a cotton-tipped swab from the endocervical canal
Significance: Evidence of cervical infection

Finding: No cervical motion or adnexal tenderness or masses
Significance: Pathology has not extended beyond the cervix.

Finding: Friability of the exocervix.
Significance: Easily induced bleeding from the cervical canal, not to be confused with normal cervical ectopy (area of columnar epithelium around the cervical os presenting as a discrete, nonfriable pinkish circle)

Etiology of Infection

VULVITIS	VAGINITIS	CERVICITIS	URETHRITIS	CYSTITIS
Herpes simplex	Gardnerella	C. trachomatis	C. trachomatis	Coliforms
C. albicans	C. albicans	N. gonorrhoeae	N. gonorrhoeae	S. sapprophyticus
HPV	T. vaginalis	T. vaginalis	HSV	
C. albicans	C. trachomatis	HSV	U. urealyticum	
	Foreign body			
	N. gonorrhoeae			

Laboratory Aids

Test: Cervical Gram stain from cervical discharge (uncontaminated by vaginal secretions)
Significance: Positive findings: >10 polymorphonuclear leukocytes per high-power field and/or gram-negative intracellular diplococci

Test: Cervical gonococcal culture or LCR (cannot be used if there is any amount of bleeding)

Test: Cervical chlamydia culture, fluorescence antibody test or LCR
Significance: Common association cause

Test: HSV culture
Significance: Common association cause

Test: Wet preparation or culture for *T. vaginalis*
Significance: Common association

Test: Potassium hydroxide preparation for budding hyphae
Significance: Test for *Candida*

Therapy

• Patients should receive therapy for *N. gonorrhoeae* and *C. trachomatis*. Treat other pathogens if clinically indicated or if documented by laboratory studies.
• Gonorrhea

—Cefixime, 400 mg PO, single dose
—Ceftriaxone, 125 mg IM, single dose
—Ciprofloxacin, 500 mg PO, single dose

• *C. trachomatis*

—Azithromycin, 1 g PO, single dose
—Doxycycline, 100 mg PO b.i.d. for 7 days
—Erythromycin base, 500 mg PO q.i.d. for 7 days

• *T. vaginalis*

—Metronidazole, 2 g PO single dose
—Metronidazole, 500 mg PO b.i.d. for 7 days

• *H. hominis*

—Acyclovir, 200 mg PO five times daily for 7 to 10 days, or until resolution

• *C. albicans*

—Butoconazole 2% cream 5 g intravaginally for 3 days
—Clotrimazole 1% cream, 5 g intravaginally for 7–14 days
—Clotrimazole 100 mg vaginal tablet, for 7 days
—Clotrimazole 500 mg vaginal tablet, single application
—Miconazole 2% cream, 5 g intravaginal for 7 days
—Fluconazole 150 mg PO single dose

Follow-Up

The recommended treatment regimens have an excellent cure rate. The patient should have resolution of symptoms 3 to 5 days after starting therapy. Routine follow-up cultures are not necessary unless the patient remains symptomatic. Reculturing may be considered 2 to 3 months following therapy to identify reinfection.

PITFALLS

Failure to recognize the importance of evaluating the internal pelvic organs by physical examination with the presenting symptoms of dysuria, vaginal discharge, or abnormal menstrual bleeding in the postpubertal female.

Common Questions and Answers

Q: How much cervical motion tenderness is present in patients with cervicitis?
A: None. Patients with cervicitis have inflammation and infection of the cervix only. They do not have any evidence of peritoneal inflammation on physical examination. Therefore, patients with tenderness should be treated with the protocols set forth by the CDC for pelvic inflammatory disease. This does not include the use of a single dose of azithromycin.

Q : Which partners should be referred for treatment?
A : Sex partners from the preceding 60 days should be referred for evaluation and treatment. Treatment is based on documented or presumptive etiologies.

ICD-9-CM 616.0

BIBLIOGRAPHY

American Academy of Pediatrics. Sexually transmitted diseases. In: Pickering LK, ed. *2000 red book: report of the Committee on Infectious Diseases*, 25th ed. Elk Grove Village, IL: American Academy of Pediatrics, 2000.

Holmes KK. Lower genital tract infections in women: cystitis, urethritis, vulvovaginitis, and cervicitis. In: Holmes KK, Mardh P, Sparling PF, et al., eds. *Sexually transmitted diseases*, 2nd ed. New York: McGraw-Hill, 1990:527–545.

Neinstein LS. *Adolescent health care: a practical guide*, 4th ed. Baltimore: Urban and Schwarzenberg, 2002.

U.S. Department of Health and Human Services. 1998 Guidelines for treatment of sexually transmitted diseases. *MMWR* 1998;47(RR-1).

Author: Jane Lavelle

Chancroid

 Database

DEFINITION/CAUSES

Infection with the gram-negative rod *Haemophilus ducreyi* resulting in painful genital ulcers.

PATHOPHYSIOLOGY

Trauma and abrasion allow the organism to penetrate the epidermis, leading to infection, ulcer formation, and lymphadenitis with a pyogenic inflammatory response.

ASSOCIATED DISEASES

• Associated with HIV transmission and infection
• Co-infection with syphilis and human herpesvirus can occur (10%).

EPIDEMIOLOGY

Initially considered a rare disease in developed countries, but over the past decade there has been a dramatic rise in the number of cases in the United States. It is transmitted via sexual contact with an individual with an ulcer. It is seen more commonly in males.

COMPLICATIONS

• Draining bubo

 Differential Diagnosis

• Common causes of genital ulcers include infection with *Treponema pallidum* or herpes simplex.
• Uncommon etiologies include:

—Trauma
—Fixed drug eruptions
—Lymphogranuloma venereum
—Inflammatory bowel disease
—Behçet syndrome

 Data Gathering

HISTORY

• Males usually present with symptoms referable to an ulcer.
• Females present with nonspecific symptoms such as dysuria, dyspareunia, vaginal discharge or rectal pain, or bleeding.

 Physical Examination

Classic findings include:

• Presence of an extremely painful ulcer with an irregular border and a gray, necrotic center.
• Males: Found on prepuce and coronal sulcus
• Females: Often found at the entrance to the vagina
• Inguinal lymphadenopathy, present in 50%, may spontaneously drain (bubo)
• Extragenital sites very rare

 Laboratory Aids

Diagnosis is made by clinical findings and exclusion of other causes of genital ulcers. The following can be considered:

Test: Gram stain from the base of the ulcer
Significance: May show short gram-negative bacilli in parallel "school of fish" arrangement. This is nonspecific.

Test: Cultures from the ulcer
Significance: H. ducreyi can be isolated from the ulcer, but special culture media and conditions are required for its isolation. This is the gold standard, but it is difficult to perform, not widely available and insensitive.

• Specimens are taken from the base of the ulcer using a cotton or calcium alginate swab.
• A culture for herpes should be done.
• An RPR should be done.

Chancroid

 Therapy

- Azithromycin, 1 g PO
- Ceftriaxone, 250 mg IM
- Ciprofloxacin, 500 mg b.i.d. for 3 days (patients >18 years)
- Erythromycin base, 500 mg q.i.d. for 7 days

PREVENTION

- Condom use, consider HIV testing.
- Partners should be treated whether or not symptoms are present.
- Patients should be evaluated for the presence of other sexually transmitted diseases.

 Follow-Up

- Patients are symptomatically improved within 48 to 72 hours.
- Ulcers themselves heal between 1 and 4 weeks.
- Lymphadenopathy may take longer to regress and may progress to fluctuance in spite of adequate therapy.
- Patients should be followed weekly until symptoms resolve.
- For patients who do not follow the typical course, consider other causes of genital ulcers, noncompliance, presence of a coexisting STD, especially HIV infection, and, rarely, presence of a resistant organism.
- Recent sexual partners (within the preceding 10 days), should be treated.

 Common Questions and Answers

Q: How do the ulcers of chancroid differ from those caused by herpes simplex and *T. pallidum*?
A: The ulcers caused by chancroid have irregular margins and deep undermined edges. They are very painful and occur singularly or in small numbers. Herpes simplex lesions occur as grouped vesicles that when ruptured leave behind painful shallow ulcers. The ulcers of syphilis are painless and solitary and have smooth margins surrounding a clean indurated base.

ICD-9-CM 099.0

BIBLIOGRAPHY

Pickering LK, ed. *2000 red book: report of the Committee on Infectious Diseases*, 25th ed. Elk Grove Village, IL: American Academy of Pediatrics, 2000.

Piot P, Plummer FA. Genital ulcer adenopathy syndrome. In: Holmes KK, Mardh P, Sparling PF, et al., eds. *Sexually transmitted diseases*, 2nd ed. New York: McGraw-Hill, 1990.

U.S. Department of Health and Human Services. 1998 Guidelines for treatment of sexually transmitted diseases. *MMWR* 1998;47(RR-1).

Author: Jane Lavelle

Chickenpox (Varicella, Herpes Zoster)

 Database

DEFINITION

Varicella-zoster virus (VZV) is a herpesvirus. Only one strain is recognized. Humans are the only source of infection.

PATHOPHYSIOLOGY

• The virus can be demonstrated in the vesicular lesions by immunofluorescence, viral culture, and polymerase chain reaction (PCR) in specimens obtained from skin lesions, organs such as brain, lung, and placenta, or cerebrospinal fluid.
• Humoral immunity is sometimes insufficient to provide protection. Severe varicella is due more to impairment of the cell-mediated immune response than to a defect in humoral immunity.
• Healthy children in whom a cell-mediated immune response develops after the varicella exanthem have mild primary VZV infection, whereas in immunodeficient children in whom VZV-specific lymphocytes fail to proliferate progressive disseminated varicella develops.
• Adults have impaired cell-mediated responses and, consequently, are 35 times more likely to die of varicella than healthy children who contract chickenpox.
• Elderly adults and patients on immunosuppressive therapy have lower VZV-specific lymphocyte proliferation and are more likely to reactivate VZV, resulting in herpes zoster. A decrease in cell-mediated immunity is a necessary but not a sufficient setting for the development of zoster.

ASSOCIATED DISEASES/COMPLICATIONS OF VARICELLA INFECTION

• Secondary bacterial infection—especially virulent group A streptococcal infections and staphylococcal (drug resistance, an increasing problem)
• *Varicella pneumonitis* (more common in adults and infants)
• Gastrointestinal complications associated with viscous involvement, such as pancreatitis, appendicitis and hepatitis, idiopathic thrombocytopenia (ITP), and bleeding diathesis
• Nephritis
• Transverse myelitis
• Encephalitis, 60 cases per year
• Disseminated intravascular coagulation (hemorrhagic VZV)
• Individuals with AIDS may have chronic VZV
• Arthritis, which can become superinfected usually with *Staphylococcus aureus*
• Congenital varicella syndrome that occurs in the first or second trimester of pregnancy, characterized by limb atrophy and scarring of the extremity. Central nervous system and eye manifestations also occur.
• Death—1 to 2 deaths per week in the United States; varicella is the most common vaccine preventable cause of death.

• These complications are associated with significant morbidity and may occur irrespective of the use of acyclovir.

EPIDEMIOLOGY

• Person-to-person transmission occurs by direct contact with varicella or zoster and respiratory secretions.
• Varicella is most common during late winter and early spring, although in cases of high vaccine coverage this seasonality is now less pronounced.
• The introduction of an index case of varicella into a home results in transmission of the virus to susceptible persons and secondary cases of disease in 98% of susceptible persons.
• Secondary cases in this situation usually have more severe disease.
• Most reported cases occur between the ages of 5 and 9 years, although in areas of the United States, where many 1 to 4 year olds are in child care, this age group predominates with an increase in complications.
• Immunity from natural disease is usually lifelong, but symptomatic reinfections do occur; more common are asymptomatic reinfections, with a fourfold boost in antibody level.
• Immunocompromised individuals with either primary varicella or zoster are at risk for severe disease.
• Disease is also more severe in infants older than 3 months of age, adolescents, adults, those on oral and/or intravenous steroids or long-term aspirin therapy, or those with pulmonary disorders including asthma.
• Congenital varicella syndrome risk is about 2%, and is greatest from the 12th to 20th week.
• Incubation 10 to 21 days after contact; cases most contagious 2 days before the rash appears and until 5 days after lesions stop cropping (longer in immunocompromised patients).
• In varicella active surveillance sites, breakthrough varicella now represents 25% of all varicella cases. Breakthrough disease needs to be verified and the question of whether significant transmission of disease occurs from this state needs to be answered.

 Differential Diagnosis

• With limited or mild rash, the differential diagnosis includes other causes of vesiculation such as:
• Coxsackie virus infection with hand, foot, and mouth disease
• Rickettsial pox
• *Mycoplasma*
• *Pseudomonas* (in immunocompromised individuals)
• Eczema herpeticum
• Herpes zoster with dissemination
• Toxic epidermal necrosis, and various noninfectious vesicular conditions of the skin
• Scabies

 Data Gathering

HISTORY

Question: Time of year?
Significance: More common in winter and spring

Question: Typical rash that has multiple stages identified?
Significance: Classic finding

Question: Does a history of not previously having had varicella usually make the diagnosis?
Significance: Varicella infection provides immunity, although recent studies have implicated 10% who may have had a previous history.

 Physical Examination

• The appearance of a typical rash that occurs in successive crops of macules, papules, and vesicles is distinctive; crops usually appear every 3 days.
• Vesicles may appear in the mouth, conjunctiva, vagina, urethra.
• Some lesions may be secondarily infected.

 Laboratory Aids

• Immunofluorescence of the vesicular fluid
• Culture of the vesicular fluid
• PCR of any tissue of vesicular fluid (reference labs include Dr. Philip LaRussa, NY, and Dr. Scott Schinid, CDC National Viral Hepatitis, *dssi@cdc.gov*).
• The complement-fixation test is not reliable in determining immunity, and has been abandoned.

Test: Acute and convalescent sera for antibody testing by a number of assays, including enzyme immunoassay (EIA), immunofluorescence assay (IFA), latex agglutination (LA), fluorescent antibody to membrane antigen (FAMA), and, through the CDC laboratory group, ELISA, which is important in determining vaccine immunity.
Significance: These tests can also be used to determine immunity.

The whole-cell EIA is better for immunity from "wild/national" diseases.
The latex agglutination in commercial laboratories is not recommended for screening health care workers.

 Therapy

• Acyclovir, vidarabine, Famvir, foscarnet, and a number of antiviral agents—pending licensure—have been shown in clinical trials to be effective against VZV.
• Acyclovir is the drug of choice in children.

• Who benefits? Any child who is ill enough to warrant hospitalization and whose rash demonstrates new vesicle formation should be treated with acyclovir (IV dose is 1,500 mg/m² divided into three doses q8h).
• Consider oral acyclovir (80 mg/kg divided in four doses q6h) for children over 12 years of age, those with chronic cutaneous or pulmonary disorders, persons on short or intermittent corticosteroids or aerosolized corticosteroids, newborn infants, and selected immunocompromised persons at risk for severe varicella.
• Children with varicella should not receive salicylates because of the association with Reye syndrome. Acetaminophen may be used to control the fever. NSAIDs may increase complications from bacterial superinfection.
• In the era of a preventable disease, acyclovir should be considered before complications of varicella warrant hospitalization.

ISOLATION OF HOSPITALIZED PATIENTS
• Strict isolation for the duration of vesicular eruption (usually 5 days, longer in immunocompromised patients)
• Patients should be in negative-pressure rooms if possible.
• Exposed susceptible persons should be in strict isolation for 8 to 21 days after the onset of the rash in the index patient.
• Those who received varicella zoster immune globulin (VZIG) should be kept in isolation for 28 days after exposure.
• Immunocompromised patients who have zoster (localized or generalized) and normal patients with disseminated zoster should remain in strict isolation for the duration of the illness. For normal patients with localized zoster drainage and secretion, precautions are recommended until all lesions are crusted.

PREVENTION
• This is now a vaccine-preventable disease and is incorporated in the harmonized immunization schedule recommended by the AAP and ACIP since 1995, and is covered by the vaccine for children's program
• Extensive clinical trials conducted in Japan, Belgium, and the United States evaluating the safety, immunogenicity, and transmissibility of vaccine virus, including comparative studies of various vaccine preparations, dose titration, efficacy (of which there is only one placebo-controlled study), consistency, and persistency of the immune response resulted in licensure of the varicella vaccine in March 1995.
• The vaccine is recommended for routine immunization of all healthy susceptible children, adolescents, and adults.
• One dose (0.5 mL subcutaneously) is required for children 12 months to 13 years of age.
• Individuals over 13 years of age require 2 doses, 1 to 2 months apart.
• The vaccine is safe, with a <4% rash rate from immunization. Postlicensure surveillance has documented three incidences of transmission in 25 million doses.

• The vaccine is 93% efficacious against natural disease in clinical trials, and field experience using the secondary family attack rate methodology has shown 84% efficacy.
• Duration of immunity from individuals followed in the clinical trials has shown that both humoral and cell-mediated immune responses persist for at least 10 years (U.S. data) and 20 years (Japanese data).
• The vaccine is not currently recommended for immunocompromised individuals, but there are studies in process. HIV positive children whose CD4 is 25% of normal value should get 2 doses of vaccine 1–3 months apart.
• Vaccine is available by protocol for acute lymphatic leukemia in remission (Tel: 215-283-0897).
• For those individuals who cannot receive VZV vaccine because of an immunocompromised state, varicella-susceptible pregnant women (until the VZV vaccine registry has data to make alternate recommendations), and newborns, VZIG would continue to be recommended.
• Varicella vaccine is recommended for postexposure prophylaxis within 5 days of a household exposure, or if an outbreak in a school is identified as soon as the local health authorities notify the parents.

 Follow-Up

• In the postvaccine era, accurate diagnosis of "breakthrough varicella" chickenpox varicella occurring more than 42 days after vaccine is crucial as it may point to *lowered efficacy* of improperly stored and administered VZV vaccine. Accurate diagnosis of VZV vaccine strain would be made by sending a PCR specimen to the CDC. Email *dssi@cdc.gov* for instruction or telephone 404-639-0066.

For normal healthy individuals follow-up is not necessary.

PROGNOSIS
• 50 to 100 previously healthy children die each year (1–2 each week) from varicella. This rate is about 35 times higher in the immunocompromised and adult populations.
• For most children, this childhood exanthem is a benign disease that lasts 6 to 8 days.
• With the advent of universal immunization, complications of varicella will become historical, as with those associated with measles, as we reach for the goal of measles eradication.

 Common Questions and Answers

Q: What do you do for a patient on corticosteroids who has not had VZV and is exposed to VZV?
A: These patients are immunosuppressed (if the dose of steroids is >0.2 mg/kg/d) and would require VZIG or treatment with acyclovir within 72 hours of developing VZV, if VZIG had not been administered.

Q: What about asthmatics on inhaled steroids? Can they be immunized safely and are they at risk of more severe varicella if not immunized?
A: Asthmatics on inhaled steroids can be immunized as the dose of inhaled steroids is not immunosuppressive. Recent data show that asthmatic children who are unimmunized do get more severe varicella.

Q: Is there any patient who should not receive VZV vaccine?
A: Yes. Immunosuppressed individuals, pregnant patients, and infants <1 year.

Q: How contagious is breakthrough varicella disease?
A: There are no good prelicensure data to answer this question; surveillance studies are in process. Breakthrough varicella is expected to be less contagious because of its mildness; however, a definitive answer is needed because of exposure to high-risk susceptible patients in health care settings.

Q: Will a booster dose of VZV vaccine be necessary?
A: Surveillance procedures must be put into place to track the baseline incidence of varicella prior to licensure of the varicella vaccine and follow the patterns of disease postlicensure. Current data do not support the need for a "booster" dose because seroconversion following one dose in children and 2 doses in those individuals over 13 occurs in 98% of vaccinees. However, trials with two dose series demonstrate higher titers and lower breakthrough rates. In the near future a combination measles-mumps-rubella vaccine may be available, making this question moot. Current epidemiologic data demonstrate the head immunity from the vaccine; unvaccinated susceptible older children are less likely to be exposed, thus causing a susceptible cohort of adolescents and adults. Catch-up VZV vaccination of all susceptible patients needs to be aggressively practiced.

ICD-9-CM 052.9

BIBLIOGRAPHY
Arvin AM. Cell-mediated immunity to varicella-zoster virus. *J Infect Dis* 1992;166(suppl 1):S35–S41.

Meyer P, Seward J, Jumaan A, et al. Varicella mortality: trends before vaccine licensure in USA 1970–1994. *J Infect Dis* 2000;182: 383–390.

Seward JF, Watson B, Petersen C, et al. Varicella disease after introduction of varicella vaccination in the United States, 1995–2000. *JAMA* 2002;287:606–611.

Author: Barbara Watson

Child Abuse-Physical

 Database

DEFINITION

Injuries or illnesses that occur to children as a result of family dysfunction. In practice, child abuse is considered nonaccidental injury of children at the hands of their caregivers. Physical abuse is legally defined by state laws.

• Multifactorial etiology:

—Include societal, familial, and individual factors
—Associated with poverty, family stress, family isolation

• Associated problems:

—Domestic violence
—Sexual abuse
—Neglect
—Emotional abuse
—Juvenile delinquency
—Poverty
—Parental substance abuse, including alcohol

EPIDEMIOLOGY

• Approximately 250,000 substantiated cases identified in the U.S. each year
• Almost 2,000 deaths/year, by conservative estimates
• Parents who were abused as children are at much greater risk for abusing their own children. It is estimated that 30% of abused children become abusive parents.
• Domestic violence and child abuse have a 50% concurrence.

COMPLICATIONS

• Death
• Mental retardation
• Cerebral palsy
• Seizures
• Learning disabilities
• Emotional problems

PROGNOSIS

Varies greatly depending on injuries sustained, family problems, available support systems.

 Differential Diagnosis

Varies depending on injury sustained.

INFECTION

• Sepsis
• Meningitis
• Congenital syphilis
• Osteomyelitis
• Impetigo
• Staphylococcal scalded-skin syndrome
• Purpura fulminans

ENVIRONMENTAL

• Phytophotodermatitis
• Coining: rubbing oiled coin over the child's body as part of a medicinal ritual. Seen in some Asian cultures.
• Cupping: a cup with a small amount of alcohol is ignited and inverted over the skin. As the heated air cools, a vacuum is produced. It is believed that this suction from the cup will draw out illness. This is a folk remedy used by Mexican-American, Southeast Asian, and other cultures.
• Moxibustion: Chinese folk remedy in which cones or balls of the moxa herb are burned on the skin.

TRAUMA

• Accidental injury

METABOLIC

• Copper deficiency
• Rickets
• Scurvy
• Vitamin K deficiency
• Glutaric aciduria type 1

CONGENITAL

• Osteogenesis imperfecta
• Ehlers-Danlos syndrome
• Familial dysautonomia, with congenital indifference to pain
• Mongolian spots
• Minor skeletal anomalies

IMMUNOLOGIC

• Henoch-Schönlein purpura
• Immune thrombocytopenic purpura

MISCELLANEOUS

• Apparent life-threatening event (ALTE)
• Epidermolysis bullosa
• Erythema multiforme

HEMATOLOGIC

• Leukemia
• Hemophilia
• von Willebrand disease
• Disseminated intravascular coagulation (DIC)

 Data Gathering

HISTORY

The following should raise the question of child abuse:

Question: History provided does not correlate with findings
Significance: Makes one suspect the truthfulness of the historian

Question: Denial of trauma to child
Significance: Typical response of child abuse

• Child's development not compatible with mechanism described
• History of events changes with time
• Unexpected delay in seeking care
• A detailed history of injury is essential for comparing the mechanism provided by the historian to the injuries sustained
• If no history of trauma is provided, ask when the child was last well, and who the caregivers were around that time. This may be helpful in identifying when the child was injured, and by whom.
• Search for indications of family stress, isolation, substance abuse, and violence, including domestic violence.

 Physical Examination

Always perform a complete examination in a well-lit room. Assess child for:

• Growth failure
• Bruises
• Burns
• Retinal hemorrhages
• Oral injuries
• Palpable rib fractures
• Abdominal injuries
• Genital injuries
• Are the findings explained by any medical condition?

 Laboratory Aids

For children with bruising and/or bleeding:

Test: CBC, including a platelet count
Significance: Evaluate for anemia and thrombocytopenia.

Test: PT/PTT
Significance: Evaluate for hemophilia and other bleeding disorders.

Test: Bleeding time/von Willebrand panel
Significance: Screen for von Willebrand disease.

Test: Liver function tests
Significance: Evaluate for possible liver injury.

Test: Amylase, lipase
Significance: Evaluate for pancreas injury.

Test: Urinalysis
Significance: Screen for genitourinary injury, abdominal trauma, or myoglobinuria.

Test: Creatine kinase (if muscle injury)
Significance: Evaluate for muscle injury; possible myoglobinuria.

Test: Lumbar puncture
Significance: Evaluate for meningitis; identify bloody CSF.

Test: Toxicology screens
Significance: Child may have been poisoned.

RADIOGRAPHIC STUDIES

• Skeletal survey: useful for all children <2 years old, for some children 2 to 5 years old. Not generally used for children older than 5 years. Bony injuries highly suggestive of abuse include rib, metaphyseal, scapular, sternal, and spinous process fractures.
• Clavicle, long bone shaft, and linear skull fractures are common fractures and are sometimes related to abuse, but have low specificity for abuse.
• Radionuclide bone scan: serves as an adjunct to skeletal survey
• CT and MRI: for suspected head, thoracic, or abdominal trauma. Subdural hemorrhage is a hallmark of inflicted head injury. Subdural hemorrhages associated with abuse can be located anywhere around the brain, but are often found in the posterior interhemispheric fissure.

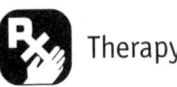

Therapy

• Report all suspected abuse to local child welfare agency.
• Report abuse to law enforcement when injuries warrant police investigation.
• Consult social worker.
• Children with head injury should be examined by an ophthalmologist.
• Subdural hemorrhages do not usually require surgical evacuation.

DRUGS

• Dependent on injury sustained
• Pain medication

Follow-Up

• Cases will be investigated by child welfare agents and/or the police.
• Need for foster care placement and/or ongoing supervision decided by investigators.
• Changes in family functioning often require intensive, long-term intervention.
• Improvement of individual injuries varies according to the injury; family functioning may improve with intervention for some families, but may never improve for others.
• Noncompliance with medical follow-up or additional injuries to child may indicate ongoing abuse, parental substance abuse, etc.

PREVENTION

• Much of what is considered prevention is actually early intervention in high-risk families.
• Primary prevention would include universal parenting education and home visitation for all families. Currently, families thought to be at risk for abuse are identified and offered services.
• Home visitation by nurses for first-time, low-income women is shown to decrease child abuse.

PITFALLS

• Failing to consider abuse in the differential diagnosis of all pediatric trauma.
• Failing to consider abuse in the differential diagnosis of all infants and toddlers with mental status changes (especially ALTEs), even in the absence of bruising.
• Failing to consider alternative medical diagnoses in children who are thought to be abused.
• Acute (<10 days) rib fractures are easily missed on plain films.

 Common Questions and Answers

Q: What are the signs of abusive head trauma (also known as shaken-baby syndrome)?
A: Abusive head trauma is a clinical diagnosis based on history, physical examination findings, and radiologic data. The hallmark of abusive head trauma is subdural hemorrhage, which is often a marker for diffuse, acceleration-deceleration brain injury. The majority of victims have retinal hemorrhages, which tend to be bilateral and are sometimes severe. Some, but not all, children have old and/or new skeletal or skin injuries, although these are not needed to make the diagnosis. The symptoms of head trauma in young children are nonspecific, and include mental status changes, ALTEs, vomiting, lethargy, irritability, seizures, etc. Abusive head injury in infants is often missed by physicians who fail to consider the diagnosis in babies with the above-mentioned symptoms, leading to further injury or death of abused infants.

Q: Are retinal hemorrhages pathognomonic for physical abuse?
A: No, retinal hemorrhages may be seen in a variety of diseases and in some normal newborns. They occur in approximately 30% of newborns delivered vaginally. In these children they usually resolve in a few days, but may rarely last for 5–6 weeks. Outside of the newborn period, severe inflicted injury is the leading cause of retinal hemorrhages in children. Retinal hemorrhages may also result from increased intracranial pressure, severe hypertension, carbon monoxide poisoning, meningitis, vasculitis, endocarditis, and

coagulopathy, but severe, bilateral hemorrhages are almost always due to abuse.

Q: What is the differential diagnosis for subdural hemorrhages?
A: It includes birth injury, accidental trauma, coagulopathy, hemorrhagic disease of the newborn, and vascular malformations. Trauma remains the leading cause of subdural hemorrhages in children.

Q: When is a child-abuse report filed?
A: Whenever there is a suspicion, based on the history, physical examination, laboratory data, and/or psychosocial assessment, that a child's injuries or illnesses were a result of abuse or neglect. Certainty regarding the diagnosis is not needed.

Q: Can I be held liable for reports that are made that are not substantiated?
A: No. Health care workers who report suspected abuse "in good faith" are protected from civil and criminal litigation arising from allegations of false reports.

ICD-9-CM 995.81

BIBLIOGRAPHY

Block RW. Child abuse-controversies and impostors. *Curr Probl Pediatr* 1999;29:249–272.

Duhaime AC, Christian CW, Rorke LB, et al. Nonaccidental head injury in infants—the "shaken-baby syndrome." *N Engl J Med* 1998;338:1822–1829.

Helfer ME, Kempe RS. *The battered child*, 5th ed. Chicago: University of Chicago Press, 1997.

Jenny C, Hymel KP, Ritzen A, et al. Analysis of missed cases of abusive head trauma. *JAMA* 1999;282:29.

Kleinman PK. *Diagnostic imaging of child abuse*. St. Louis: Mosby Yearbook, 1998.

Olds D, Eckenrode J., Henderson CR, Kitzman H, Powers J, Cole R, Sidora K, Morris P, Pettitt LM, Luckey D. Long-term effects of homevisitation on maternal life conrse and child abuse, and neglect. Fifteen-year follow-up of a randomized trial. *JAMA* 1997;278:637–43.

Reece R, Ludwig S, eds. *Child abuse medical diagnosis and management*. Philadelphia: Lippincott Williams & Wilkins, 2001.

Sugar NF, Taylor JA, Feldman KW. Bruises in infants and toddlers: those who don't cruise rarely bruise. *Arch Pediatr Adolesc Med* 1999;153:399–403.

Author: Cindy W. Christian

Chlamydial Infections

 Database

DEFINITION

Chlamydiae are obligate intracellular bacteria responsible for pulmonary infections, ocular trachoma, sexually transmitted disease, and infections of the genital tract in the pediatric and adult population.

- The genus *Chlamydia* has three species known to affect humans:
  —*C. trachomatis* (CT)
  —*C. psittaci*
  —*C. pneumoniae* (CP).
- All three species can produce the clinical manifestations of the so-called atypical or interstitial pneumonia.
- CT can cause afebrile pneumonia in 10–20% of infants born to infected mothers. Infected infants usually present prior to 2 months of age. Up to 50% of patients have a history of inclusion conjunctivitis.
- *C. psittaci* is mainly pathogenic for birds and occasionally affects humans, typically causing interstitial pneumonitis with associated fever, headache, malaise, and nausea.
- CP causes pneumonia, pharyngitis, sinusitis, and bronchitis in humans. Along with *Mycoplasma pneumoniae,* CP probably accounts for most of the community-acquired pneumonias (CAPs) in school-age children and adolescents.

EPIDEMIOLOGY
Chlamydia Trachomatis

There are at least 15 serologically distinct variants (serovars).
- This is the most common reportable sexually transmitted infection in the United States.
- CT pneumonia usually develops in infected infants under 2 months of age (2 weeks to 5 months). The contagiousness of pulmonary disease is unknown, but is considered low.
- Half of the neonates born to infected mothers via vaginal delivery will acquire CT.
  —Conjunctivitis may develop in 25% to 50%.
  —Pneumonia may develop in 5% to 20%.
- Ocular trachoma caused by serovars A, B, Ba, and C is the most common cause of preventable blindness in the world, but is rare in the United States.
- Incubation period: at least 1 week

Chlamydia Psittaci
(Psittacosis/Ornithosis)

- Both healthy and sick birds can transmit the bacteria via the airborne route by their excrement or secretions.
- Workers in poultry slaughter plants, poultry farms, pet shops, laboratory workers, and pet owners are at high risk.
- Though usually rare in children, it should be considered in any child with environmental exposure who develops an atypical pneumonia. The incubation period is 7–14 days.

Chlamydia Pneumoniae

- *C. pneumoniae* is antigenically, morphologically, and genetically distinct from other chlamydiae.
- It is assumed to be transmitted from person to person through aerosolized respiratory secretions.
- Increased prevalence rates of CP specific antibody have been documented in school-age children, reaching 30–45% in adolescents.
- Studies of community acquired pneumonias in children, have found *C. pneumoniae* in 6–19% of cases. Evidence of lower respiratory tract infection has been found in 0–18% of the pediatric population.
- CP has recently been associated with atherosclerotic cardiovascular disease. Limited evidence associates CP with asthma and bronchospasm, Alzheimer disease, multiple sclerosis, Kawasaki disease, HIV and other immune disorders, malignancy, otitis media, and episodes of acute chest syndrome in patients with sickle cell disease.
- The majority of infections are mild or asymptomatic. Acute infection does not appear to vary by season. A carriage state has been detected in 2–5% of patients. Recurrent infection is common, especially in adults.
- Co-infection with other respiratory pathogens, especially *M. pneumoniae* and *Streptococcus pneumoniae,* is frequent.
- Incubation period: about 21 days.

COMPLICATIONS

- In very young infants, chlamydial pneumonia can lead to apnea or respiratory failure. Untreated infection can persist for weeks to months.
- Complications of psittacosis include myocarditis, hepatitis, pancreatitis, and secondary bacterial pneumonia.

PROGNOSIS

- In general, good
- Infection with CT has been associated with long-term respiratory sequelae, such as an increased incidence of reactive airway disease and abnormal pulmonary function tests.

 Differential Diagnosis

CHLAMYDIA TRACHOMATIS

- Viral respiratory pathogens:
  —Respiratory syncytial virus (RSV)
  —Adenovirus
  —Influenza A and B
  —Parainfluenza
- Other agents that can cause pneumonitis:
  —Cytomegalovirus
  —*Pneumocystis carinii*
  —*Ureaplasma urealyticum*
  —*Bordetella pertussis*

CHLAMYDIA PNEUMONIAE

- *Mycoplasma pneumoniae*
- Influenza A and B
- Parainfluenza
- Adenovirus
- RSV

- Can resemble typical bacterial pneumonia
- Less frequently: *C. psittaci, Coxiella burnetii,* or *Legionella pneumophila*

 Data Gathering

HISTORY
Chlamydia Trachomatis

- Presents between 4 and 12 weeks of age
- Insidious onset
- Afebrile illness
- Rhinorrhea
- Repetitive cough
  —Staccato type in more than 50% of infants
  —Sometimes pertussis-like coughing spells
- Conjunctivitis in up to 50% of infants
- Mild-to-moderate respiratory distress

Chlamydia Pneumoniae

- Often insidious onset
- May manifest as pharyngitis, sinusitis, bronchitis, or pneumonia
- Fever
- Hoarseness
- Prolonged cough; can be productive
- Biphasic course

 Physical Examination

CHLAMYDIA TRACHOMATIS

- Afebrile
- 50% of patients will have conjunctivitis with discharge (can be seen up to several weeks after birth)
- Rhinitis with mucoid discharge or nasal stuffiness, sometimes causing significant airway obstruction.
- Hypoxia frequently present
- Moderate tachypnea (50–60 breaths/min)
- Frequent cough during examination
- Scattered rales on chest auscultation
- Wheezing is an uncommon finding.

CHLAMYDIA PNEUMONIAE

- Patients may be asymptomatic or mildly to moderately ill.
- Cervical lymphadenopathy
- Postnasal discharge
- Nonexudative pharyngitis
- Wheezing, frequently without rales on chest auscultation

 Laboratory Aids

TESTS
Chlamydia Trachomatis

- Definitive diagnosis is by isolation of the organism in tissue culture. Confirmation is by microscopy of the characteristic inclusions by fluorescent antibody staining. Specimens are obtained from the nasopharynx, conjunctiva, vagina, or rectum. Dacron polyester–tipped swabs should be used for collection.

- Nucleic acid amplification methods such as polymerase chain reaction (PCR) and ligase chain reaction (LCR) are more sensitive than cell culture and more specific and sensitive than DNA probe, direct fluorescent antibody (DFA), or enzyme immunoassay (EIA).
- DNA probe, DFA, and EIA are the most common nonculture direct antigen-detection tests approved by the FDA. These are most sensitive (90%) and specific (95%) in conjunctival specimens. These methods can have false-positive results when used for vaginal or rectal specimens.
- Serum antibody detection can be performed by microimmunofluorescence (MIF). These are difficult to perform and are not widely available.
—*Chlamydia*-specific IgM titer of 1:32 or greater is diagnostic for CT pneumonia.
- Eosinophilia of 300 to 400/mm^3, hyperinflation, and bilateral diffuse infiltrates on chest radiograph and elevation of IgM (>110 mg/dL) and IgG (>500 mg/dL) are indirect evidence that suggest CT pneumonia.

Chlamydia Pneumoniae
- No reliable test is available commercially.
- The nasopharynx is the optimal site for recovery of CP. It has also been isolated from sputum and pleural fluid.
- The organism can be grown in tissue culture. Its presence can be detected by using PCR and a fluorescent antibody test.
- Serologic diagnosis by MIF is the most sensitive and specific test. Evidence of acute infection:
—Fourfold elevation of IgG titers
—Specific IgM titer of 1:16 or greater
—Specific IgG titer of 1:512 or greater
- WBC count is usually normal.

Imaging
- Chest radiography
—*C. trachomatis*: the most consistent finding is hyperinflation with bilateral diffuse infiltrates
—*C. pneumoniae*: presents with focal to bilateral infiltrates; pleural effusions have been reported.

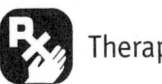

Therapy

DRUGS
Chlamydia Trachomatis
- Erythromycin, 50 mg/kg/d divided q.i.d. for 14 days (therapy is effective in 80% of cases). Additional topical therapy is unnecessary. An association between oral erythromycin and infantile hypertrophic pyloric stenosis (IHPS) has been reported, in infants younger than 6 weeks of age. Parents should be informed of the possible risk of IHPS and its signs.
- If the patient does not tolerate erythromycin, oral sulfonamides may be used after the immediate neonatal period. Children older than 8 years can be treated with tetracycline, 25–50 mg/kg/d divided q.i.d. for 7 days.

Chlamydia Pneumoniae
- Erythromycin, 50 mg/kg/d divided q.i.d. for 14 days. For adolescent patients, erythromycin 500 mg q.i.d. for 14 days or 250 mg q.i.d. for 21 days.
- An alternative for children over 9 years of age is doxycycline 100 mg b.i.d. for 14 days.
- Clarithromycin 15 mg/kg/d divided b.i.d. for 10 days was proven as effective as erythromycin.
- Azithromycin 10 mg/kg on day 1 (maximum, 500 mg) followed by 5 mg/kg days 2 to 5 (maximum, 250 mg) has been shown as efficacious as erythromycin in pediatric studies.

Follow-Up

- Slow recovery
- Cough and malaise may persist for several weeks.

PREVENTION
Adequate surveillance and treatment of CT colonizing the genital tract of pregnant women is the best way of preventing disease in the infant.

PITFALLS
Chlamydia Trachomatis
- Infection can occur in infants delivered by cesarean section, even without rupture of amniotic membranes.
- Ocular prophylaxis at birth does not reliably prevent *Chlamydia* conjunctivitis or extraocular infection, even if erythromycin ointment is used. Topical treatment alone is not recommended because it does not eradicate the nasopharyngeal colonization.
- Antibiotic treatment failure rate is about 20%. A second course of therapy is sometimes needed.

Chlamydia Pneumoniae
- Lack of commercially reliable test for diagnosis. MIF is proven diagnostic in less than 50% of infected children. An increase in antibody titer may be delayed for several weeks after onset of symptoms. Early antimicrobial therapy may interfere with the development of detectable antibodies.
- Sometimes it is difficult to differentiate between infection and carrier state, and recent and past infection.
- Recurrent infections are common. Prolonged nasopharyngeal shedding can occur for months after acute disease.
- Isolation: standard precautions for both CP and CT
- Control measures: In infants infected with CT, the mother and her sexual partner should be treated. None for CP pneumonia.

Common Questions and Answers

CHLAMYDIA TRACHOMATIS
Q: If the mother has an untreated genital infection, should we treat the asymptomatic newborn?
A: Yes. The child should receive oral erythromycin for 14 days.

Q: Do we need to pursue the diagnosis of other sexually transmitted diseases?
A: Yes. Gonorrhea, syphilis, hepatitis B, and HIV infection need to be ruled out. If conjunctivitis is present, an ocular swab to exclude *Neisseria gonorrhoeae* infection must be included.

Q: When do we need to suspect CT pneumonia?
A: In any infant younger than 4 months of age who presents with cough, tachypnea, and rales on examination, when the chest x-ray shows bilateral infiltrates with hyperinflation.

ICD-9-CM 483.1
BIBLIOGRAPHY
American Academy of Pediatrics. *2000 red book: report of the Committee on Infectious Diseases* .Elk Grove Village, IL: American Academy of Pediatrics, 2000:205–212.

Darville T. Chlamydia. *Pediatr Rev* 1998;19(3).

Hamerschlag MR. *Chlamydia trachomatis* and *Chlamydia pneumoniae* infections. In: Taussig LM, Landau LI, LeSouef PN, et al., eds. *Textbook of pediatric respiratory medicine*, 1st ed. St. Louis: Mosby, 1999.

Hammerschlag MR. Atypical pneumonias in children. *Adv Pediatr Infect Dis* 1995;10:1–39.

Hammerschlag MR. *Chlamydia* infections. In: Feigin RD, Cherry JD, eds. *Textbook of pediatric infectious diseases*, 3rd ed. Philadelphia: WB Saunders, 1998.

Schidlow DV, Callahan CW. Pneumonia. *Pediatr Rev* 1996;17(9).

Author: Sumit Bhargava
Roberto Nachajon, 2nd edition

Cholelithiasis

 Database

DEFINITION

Cholelithiasis, defined as cholesterol and/or pigment stones in the gallbladder, is primarily a disease of adulthood. Since the introduction of ultrasonography in the late 1970s, incidental or silent gallstones are detected more often in children. In addition, gallstones can be found in high-risk populations in pediatrics (sickle cell disease, newborns) and should always be evaluated as a potential cause of colicky abdominal pain.

CAUSES

- Hemolytic disease (17–29% of children with sickle cell disease)
- Total parenteral nutrition
- Prematurity
- Necrotizing enterocolitis
- Cystic fibrosis
- Obesity
- Pregnancy
- Oral contraceptives
- Down syndrome

PATHOLOGY

- Bile is composed of five major components: water, bilirubin, cholesterol, pigments, and phospholipids and calcium salts. Stones are of two types: pigment and cholesterol stones. The formation of cholesterol stones is associated with sludge and cholesterol supersaturation. Other important factors include:

—Gallbladder stasis
—Excess lecithin
—Increased biliary mucus secretion
—Rapidity of nucleation time

- Total parenteral alimentation is associated with decrease in bile flow, stasis, sludge, and stone formation.
- The formation of gallstones secondary to ileal disease or resection has been reported in children and adults because of a decreased bile acid pool and cholesterol supersaturation of the bile.

EPIDEMIOLOGY

- Cholelithiasis is relatively uncommon in childhood; however, gallstones have even been detected *in utero*.
- Pigment stones are more prevalent in prepubertal children, whereas cholesterol stones are predominant in adolescence and adulthood.
- The incidence of gallstones remains negligible in males throughout childhood and adolescence to adulthood.
- In females, the incidence is 0.27% during ages 6 to 19 years and increases to 2.7% between the ages of 18 and 29; gallstones predominate in females.
- Canadian Eskimos and native Africans have the lowest risk of cholelithiasis.
- Native Americans, Swedes, and Czechs have the highest risk.

SYMPTOMS

- Silent gallstones present coincidentally in infancy and preschool-age children.
- The classic symptoms of right-upper-quadrant (RUQ) pain and vomiting exist in older children and adolescents.
- Younger children present with nonspecific symptoms, including obstructive jaundice.
- Fever is unusual in all age groups and often indicates the development of complications such as cholecystitis, choledocholithiasis, cholangitis, or gallbladder perforation, all of which are rare in children.
- Pancreatitis develops in 8% of patients with gallstones and is the most common complication. Pancreatitis is more common in obese adolescents who have undergone rapid weight reduction, as reported in the adult population.

 Data Gathering

HISTORY

- Most gallstones are incidental findings on abdominal ultrasound and are clinically silent.
- Biliary colic, pancreatitis, obstructive jaundice, cholangitis, or other complications should be excluded.
- Intolerance to fatty food rarely exists in children.

The history should always include questions concerning:

- Previous episodes of RUQ abdominal pain
- Any risk factors for hemolysis
- History of prematurity and necrotizing enterocolitis
- Total parenteral nutrition
- Diuretic use
- Short gut syndrome
- History of resection of the terminal ileum.

Physical Examination

- The physical examination may be completely normal or may uncover the acute abdomen of pancreatitis.
- In adolescents, the Murphy sign (tenderness on palpation of the RUQ of the abdomen associated with inspiration) may be elicited.

Laboratory Aids

TESTS

- Blood testing is usually unrewarding.
- Occasionally, a leukocytosis, elevation in liver enzymes, or elevated amylase/lipase may be detected.
- Abdominal radiography may show the presence of a gallstone; 50% of these are radiopaque.
- Ultrasound is the diagnostic procedure of choice—noninvasive, sensitive, and specific.
- Endoscopic retrograde cholangiopancreatography (ERCP) is especially good for evaluation of choledocholithiasis and removal of common bile duct stones.

Therapy

- In children with asymptomatic gallstones, observation is the best therapy.
- In infants, there is a chance for spontaneous stone dissolution, especially in cholelithiasis linked to total parenteral nutrition (TPN). In children who are dependent on TPN, such as patients with short-bowel syndrome, pseudo-obstruction, and inflammatory bowel disease, gallstones should be removed.
- Cholecystectomy remains the procedure of choice in children with symptoms or in the presence of silent gallstones.
- Laparoscopic cholecystectomy may decrease the length of the hospital stay and the extent of the required abdominal incision.
- Medical treatment for cholesterol gallstones in children may include chenodeoxycholic acid and ursodeoxycholic acid. This treatment is not recommended in the pediatric age group because of low success rate.
- Prevention of gallstone formation is done by treating underlying risk factors (small enteral feeds in addition to TPN, early pancreatic enzyme supplements in patients with cystic fibrosis, using alternative forms of contraception in high-risk populations, and weight control in obese infants and children with known hemolytic disease).
- Pigment stone formation increases with age. Cholecystectomy, even for the asymptomatic patient, is warranted. Sickle cell patients should have the gallbladder removed once stones are identified. This will decrease the risk of cholecystitis and other complications, and will also help to differentiate between biliary colic and sickle cell crisis.
- Patients with a history of cholecystitis are at increased risk for further episodes (69% will have biliary colic within 2 years, and 6% will require cholecystectomy).

Follow-Up

- Asymptomatic patients: Follow up every year with ultrasound; monitor for onset of symptoms.
- Symptomatic patients: Consider cholecystectomy.

Common Questions and Answers

Q: Does my child with cystic fibrosis (CF) have a greater problem with gallstones?
A: Yes, children with CF may have more frequent development of gallstones than will normal children. Reports of gallstones while on ursodeoxycholic acid therapy have also been noted.

Q: Why does my child with sickle cell disease have gallstones?
A: Because the process involves breakdown of hemoglobin, which is then derived into bilirubin, this process may accelerate the formation of pigmented gallstones.

Q: If my child has repeated attacks of abdominal pain and there are gallstones in the gallbladder, should he have surgery? What kind?
A: Yes; in older adolescents, laparoscopic cholecystectomy is recommended. For younger children or infants, open cholecystectomy is the preferred choice of treatment. There is no role for Actigall in their therapy.

ICD-9-CM 574.20

BIBLIOGRAPHY

Gilger MA. Cholelithiasis and cholecystitis. In: Wyllie R, Hyams J, eds. *Pediatric gastrointestinal diseases*. Philadelphia: WB Saunders, 1993:931–944.

Haller JO. Sonography of the biliary tract in infants and children. *AJR* 1991;157(5):1051–1058.

Heubi JE, Lewis LG. Diseases of the gallbladder in infancy, childhood, and adolescence. In: Suchy F, ed. *Liver diseases in children*. Chicago: Mosby-Year Book, 1994:609–621.

Irish MS, Pearl RH, Caty MG, et al. The approach to common abdominal diagnosis in infants and children. *Pediatr Clin North Am* 1998;45(4):729–772.

Kasirajan K, Obermeyer RJ, Kehris J, et al. Microinvasive laparoscopic cholecystectomy in pediatric patients. *J Laparoendosc Adv Surg Techniques Part A* 1998;8(3):131–135.

Rescorla FJ. Cholelithiasis, cholecystitis, and common bile duct stones. *Curr Opin Pediatr* 1997;9(3):276–282.

Rescorla FJ, Grosfeld JL. Cholecystitis and cholelithiasis in children. *Semin Pediatr Surg* 1992;1(2):98–106.

Author: Dror Wasserman

Chronic Active Hepatitis

 Database

DEFINITION

Chronic active hepatitis is a continuing inflammation of the liver that may become cirrhotic. Features include inflammation not due to acute self-limiting infection or past drug exposure with raised transaminases and histologic evidence of hepatitis.

CAUSES

- Autoimmune liver disease
- Chronic viral hepatitis
- Bile acid synthetic defects
- Progressive familial intrahepatic cholestasis (PFIC) syndromes
- Wilson disease
- Tyrosinemia
- Persistent biliary disease: post-Kasai, choledochal cyst
- Sclerosing cholangitis
- Immunodeficiency
- Glycogen storage disease
- Cystic fibrosis
- Iron storage disorders/chronic transfusion
- Mitochondrial respiratory chain defects
- Peroxisomal defects

PATHOPHYSIOLOGY

Pathology has been traditionally classified as chronic persistent hepatitis, chronic aggressive hepatitis, and chronic lobular hepatitis. The hepatocytes are damaged, with inflammatory cellular infiltration accompanied by liver regeneration.

Chronic Persistent Hepatitis

Minimal portal tract fibrosis, slightly widened portal tracts. The limiting plate is intact and inflammation does not extend beyond this. There is no bridging fibrosis between portal tracts.

Chronic Aggressive Hepatitis

Perilobular hepatitis, with inflammatory cells extending from portal tracts into parenchyma with fibrosis. Piecemeal necrosis is necrotic hepatocytes surrounded by lymphocytes and fibroblasts. In advanced disease, fibrosis bridges the portal tracts (bridging fibrosis). Cirrhosis occurs when there is loss of architecture due to fibrosis.

Chronic Lobular Hepatitis

Liver architecture is preserved with scattered changes of acute hepatitis with hepatocyte necrosis in the lobules (perivenular regions). These changes are most often associated with hepatitis B and non-A, non-B (NANB) hepatitis.

EPIDEMIOLOGY

- More common in females

 Differential Diagnosis

INDICATED FURTHER INVESTIGATIONS

- Congenital hepatic fibrosis, Niemann-Pick type C, or other storage disorders
- Lysosomal storage disease, glycogen storage disease
- Congenital or acquired venous or arterial malformations
- Wilson disease
- Cystic fibrosis
- Byler disease (PFIC-1)
- Alagille syndrome

 Data Gathering

HISTORY

- Symptoms of chronic illness, poor growth, intermittent jaundice, abdominal pain, bleeding, malabsorption, fever, amenorrhea, poor school achievement, and itching
- Variceal bleeding can be a presenting syndrome in patients with portal hypertension.
- A history of jaundice in infancy, family history of liver disease or autoimmune liver disease, blood transfusions, intravenous drug abuse, or multiple sexual partners can suggest an etiology of hepatitis.
- Chronicity is often defined by the persistence of hepatitis for at least 6 months.

 Physical Examination

Stigmata of chronic liver disease are:

- Spider nevi
- Cutaneous shunts
- Palmar erythema
- Cyanosis (hepatopulmonary syndrome)
- Jaundice
- Itching
- Enlarged liver or small, shrunken liver
- Splenomegaly
- Ascites
- Rickets

Laboratory Aids

TESTS

Laboratory Tests

- Albumin, creatinine, GGT, AST, ALT, bilirubin, PT, FBC, blood group, Coombs test
- Serum ceruloplasmin, serum copper, 24-hour urine copper (penicillamine challenge), liver copper
- Cholesterol, triglycerides
- Immunoglobulins
- Complement levels (C3, C4)
- Tissue autoantibodies
- Virology: Hep A, Hep B, Hep C, Hep D
- α_1-Antitrypsin phenotype
- Urinary succinylacetone
- Urinary bile acids
- Sweat test
- AFP

Imaging

- CXR
- Ultrasound scan of abdomen, focusing on liver, spleen, and kidney
- Echocardiogram
- Liver biopsy

INDICATED FURTHER INVESTIGATIONS

- PTC or ERCP (or MRCP): congenital hepatic fibrosis, sclerosing cholangitis
- Colonoscopy: sclerosing cholangitis associated with inflammatory bowel disease
- Bone marrow aspirate: exclude Niemann-Pick type C or other storage disorders
- Enzyme from white cells or cultured fibroblasts (skin biopsy): to exclude lysosomal storage disease, glycogen storage disease
- Angiography: congenital or acquired venous or arterial malformations, assessment of portosystemic shunt
- Cardiac catheterization: to assess pulmonary hypertension and cardiac status
- Microaggregate albumin scan: to assess hepatopulmonary syndrome and hepatic encephalopathy
- Muscle biopsy: to assay respiratory chain enzymes in mitochondrial disorders
- Genotyping: Wilson disease, cystic fibrosis, Byler disease (PFIC-1), Alagille syndrome
- Liver biopsy can be postponed until coagulopathy improves.
- Repeat biopsies have shown histologic relapse rates to be very high—87% to 100%. Forty percent of treated patients develop cirrhosis after 10 years.
- Malignancies developed in 5%, with the mean time of onset 9.7 years after diagnosis. In rare instances, in which the autoimmune process cannot be controlled by steroids and azathioprine, cyclosporine or tacrolimus may be used.

- ERCP is done routinely in some centers on all patients with active hepatitis, and when changes of sclerosing cholangitis are detected, patients are started on ursodeoxycholic acid. The success of liver transplantation is the same as for other causes, but the disease occasionally recurs.

Therapy

The management of patients is that of any chronic liver disease and treatment specific to a diagnosis.

GENERAL MANAGEMENT

- Maintaining growth and development is of paramount importance to optimize the physical and mental well-being of the patient. Fat-soluble vitamins given orally are poorly absorbed and levels must be monitored. Anthropometric parameters must be recorded, including skinfold thickness. The use of medium-chain triglycerides for fat malabsorption and branched-chain amino acids in hepatic encephalopathy are useful nutritional maneuvers.
- Proactive involvement of the clinical psychologist and play therapist can help alleviate some of the problems, such as depression and fear. Chronic debilitating pruritus is an indication for liver transplantation after failure of medical therapy, which may include antihistamines, cholestyramine, naltrexone, rifampicin, and ursodeoxycholic acid.
- Monitoring portal hypertension by assessment of portal flow on ultrasound and splenic size may provide some indication of disease progression. Airplane cabin pressures are maintained at levels lower than atmospheric, and this can predispose to variceal bleeding.
- The physician must be vigilant in monitoring for spontaneous bacterial peritonitis in patients with ascites; it carries a mortality rate between 55% and 78% and a recurrence rate of 69% after 1 year.

SPECIFIC MANAGEMENT

- Chronic viral hepatitis B and C: Hepatitis B that causes chronic active hepatitis is currently treated with interferon-α for at least 6 months. The success rate based on adult studies is 33% and 37% for the loss of HBeAg and HBV DNA, respectively. In patients with cirrhosis, the use of interferon is risky, because it can cause liver disease decompensation, and should be given only in centers that are familiar with and have access to liver transplantation.
- There may be a role for Lamivudine, an oral nucleoside analogue that inhibits viral DNA replication; it has been shown to markedly reduce HBV DNA levels in 98% of patients during therapy, but there is a high recurrence rate after the drug is discontinued.

- Treatment of hepatitis C with interferon in children is not established. In adults, it is licensed for use, with good response in the region of 41% improvement in ALT; 70% of patients show improved histology, but with a 50% to 70% relapse rate.
- The treatment for end-stage liver failure is liver transplantation.
- Patients may deteriorate rapidly if not treated aggressively, and in some cases develop fulminant liver failure. Corticosteroids are started, and the dose slowly weaned over 4 to 6 weeks to maintain normal transaminases up to 6 months.
- Remission is induced in 70% of patients within 24 months of therapy, but relapses occur in 50% in 6 months and in 70% in 36 months.
- Azathioprine is used when corticosteroid doses cannot be weaned. Liver function tests, immunoglobulin levels, and autoantibody titers are monitored closely. In one report, discontinuation of treatment occurred in 20% of type 1 active hepatitis but not in type 2.

DRUGS

- Azathioprine: 1 to 2 mg/kg/d
- Cholestyramine: 240 mg/kg/d in three divided doses; avoid giving with other medications because it can bind and reduce absorption. Give other medications 1 hour before or 4 hours after cholestyramine.
- Cyclosporine: 1 to 2 mg/kg/d orally (bd)
- Interferon-α (dose from published pediatric trials):

—Chronic HBV: 5 to 10 μg/m^2 given three times a week for 6 to 12 months
—Chronic HCV: 3 μg/m^2 given three times a week for 6 to 12 months

- Interferon is not licensed for use in children. Very common side effects are hematologic, infectious, autoimmune, neuropsychiatric, and systemic with myelosuppression. If platelets fall below 50,000/mm^3 and neutrophils below 1,500/mm^3, then interferon dose is lowered or temporarily discontinued.
- Lamivudine (trial basis): 25 to 100 mg/d in adult for 1 year
- Naltrexone: 25 to 50 mg/d in adults (tablets, 50 mg)
- Tacrolimus: 0.15 mg/kg/d orally (bd)
- Ursodeoxycholic acid: 20 mg/kg/d (bd)

Common Questions and Answers

Q: Can patients with autoimmune liver disease be transplanted? Will the disease not recur?
A: Patients who end up with end-stage liver failure should be transplanted. It is not common to see the recurrence of the original autoimmune liver disease after transplant, but it occurs.

Q: What are the risks of providing very young patients with a liver transplant?
A: There is a theoretical advantage in transplanting the very young, in that less rejection occurs and immunosuppression requirements are less. Using split liver techniques, outcomes of orthoptic liver transplantation (OLT) in infants have improved.

Q: Why should we be aggressive with vitamin supplementation?
A: There is significant malabsorption of vitamins A, D, E, and K. Vitamin D and E deficiencies are the most significant causing rickets and neuropathy.

Q: Oral supplements of vitamins are sometimes very difficult to administer in the very young. How can I overcome this problem?
A: It is common practice in some centers to give vitamins D and E as an intramuscular injection on a monthly basis, with levels done in between.

Q: Why do jaundiced children scratch?
A: It is the accumulation of bile salts that causes pruritus.

Q: Are the stigmata of chronic liver disease also seen in children?
A: It is very common to find spider nevi, liver palms, splenomegaly, cutaneous shunts, and clubbing.

ICD-9-CD 571.40

BIBLIOGRAPHY

Hyams KC. Risks of chronicity following acute hepatitis B virus infection: a review. *Clin Infect Dis* 1995;20(4):992–1000.

Johnson PJ, McFarland IG, et al. Meeting report: International Autoimmune Hepatitis. *Hepatology* 1993;18:998–1005.

Lai, CL, Chien RN, Leung NW, et al. One year trial of lamivudine for chronic hepatitis B. *N Engl J Med* 1998;339(2):61–68.

Ruiz-Moreno M, Rua MJ, Castillo I, et al. Treatment of children with chronic hepatitis. *Hepatology* 1992;16:882–885.

Trivedi P, Mowat AP. Chronic hepatitis. In: Suchy FJ, ed. *Liver disease in children*, 1st ed. St. Louis: Mosby, 1994:510–523.

Vergani GM, Vergani D. Immune mechanisms in pediatric liver disease. In: Suchy FJ, ed. *Liver disease in children*, 1st ed. St. Louis: Mosby, 1994:173–180.

Authors: Andrew E. Mulberg and John Tung

Chronic Diarrhea

 Database

DEFINITION

Chronic diarrhea is arbitrarily defined as diarrhea lasting more than 3 weeks, whereas acute diarrhea, generally caused by enteric pathogens, is self-limiting and duration of symptoms is less than 2 weeks. Stool output in excess of 200 g per day in children and adults, or 10 g per kg per day in infants is considered diarrhea.

PATHOPHYSIOLOGY

The major categories are osmotic and secretory. Inflammatory and motility disorders are smaller but important subcategories to consider. In many conditions, more that one process may be present.

- *Osmotic diarrhea* occurs when unabsorbable solute accumulates in the lumen of the distal small intestine and colon. This increases the intraluminal osmotic pressure and results in excessive fluid and electrolyte losses in stool. Osmotic diarrhea will improve with fasting.
- *Secretory diarrhea* occurs when the net secretion of fluid and electrolyte is in excess of absorption in the intestine. The intestinal mucosa is normally very active in both of these processes. The diarrhea occurs independently of the osmotic load in the intestinal lumen and does not improve with fasting.
- *Inflammation* in the intestine causes a disruption of the epithelial lining, resulting in exudative loss of mucus, blood, and/or protein. Increased permeability of the mucosal lining may affect absorption and result in secondary secretory diarrhea.
- *Motility* disorders will affect the intestinal transit time. Hypermotility will cause rapid transit through the intestine and hence, shorten the effective absorptive capacity of the bowel. This can be a primary cause of diarrhea, but is more commonly associated with another pathologic process.

EPIDEMIOLOGY

Chronic diarrhea is a common childhood ailment that results in significant morbidity and mortality worldwide. The etiology varies according to age and geographic location. Chronic diarrhea seen in the tropics and developing countries is more likely infectious in nature than in the United States. Gender and genetic factors do not play a significant role in most cases of chronic diarrhea.

COMPLICATIONS

The most common complications include:

- Dehydration
- Failure to thrive
- Electrolyte abnormalities

 Differential Diagnosis

The causes of chronic diarrhea differ markedly depending on the age of the child.

- Infants younger than 1 year of age:

—Intractable diarrhea of infancy is associated with diffuse mucosal injury beginning prior to 6 months of age resulting in malabsorption and malnutrition.
—The two most commonly identified etiologies are cow's-milk and/or soy protein intolerance
—Protracted postinfectious diarrhea
—Microvillus inclusions disease
—Autoimmune enteropathy
—Hirschsprung disease with enterocolitis
—Transport defects (e.g., congenital chloridorrhea)
—Nutrient malabsorption (e.g., congenital glucose-galactose malabsorption and congenital lactase deficiency, sucrase-isomaltase deficiency)
—Munchausen syndrome by proxy

- Children between 1 and 5 years of age:

—Chronic nonspecific diarrhea of infancy (toddler's diarrhea)
—Postinfectious enteritis
—Giardiasis
—Eosinophilic gastroenteritis
—Sucrase-isomaltase deficiency
—Tumors (neuroblastoma, VIPoma with secretory diarrhea)
—Inflammatory bowel disease
—Celiac disease
—Cystic fibrosis
—Small bowel bacterial overgrowth
—AIDS enteropathy

- Children older than 5 years of age:

—Acquired lactose deficiency
—Inflammatory bowel disease
—Constipation with (overflow) encopresis
—Appendiceal abscess
—Laxative abuse (adolescents)

 Data Gathering

HISTORY

- Dietary intake. The occurrence of diarrhea in close relationship to specific food intake (e.g., dairy products) may be diagnostic.
- Evaluation of the stool pattern, including consistency, frequency, and appearance. The history of blood and mucus in stool is strongly suggestive of an inflammatory process.
- Nutritional status and growth parameters need to be assessed. The presence of growth failure or malnutrition has considerable implications compared with a child with normal growth and no history of weight loss.

 Physical Examination

- Nutritional status of the patient by initially comparing height, weight, and head circumference with normal standards and old measurements.
- Anthropometric measurements are important in assessing loss of body fat and muscle mass.
- Peripheral edema, ascites, rash, dystrophic nails, alopecia, chronic chest findings, and pallor.
- A rectal examination may reveal stool impaction with overflow as the apparent cause of "uncontrolled diarrhea."
- Evidence of infection should be considered, such as fever and vital sign instability.

 Laboratory Aids

- Stool samples:

—Stool should be tested for occult blood and for the presence of fecal leukocytes, which indicate the presence of inflammation (usually colonic).
—Stools pH and reducing substances can be done in the office setting or sent to a laboratory. If stool is positive for reducing substances and/or the pH <5.5, carbohydrate malabsorption with or without proximal small-bowel injury is likely. (Note: Sucrose is not a reducing substance. If sucrose malabsorption is suspected, stool sample has to be hydrolyzed with hydrochloric acid and heat before analysis.)

—A positive Sudan stain of the stool is indicative of fat malabsorption. However, a 72-hour fecal fat collection remains the gold standard to diagnose fat malabsorption.
—Stool should be cultured for bacteria, ova and parasites, and viral organisms. *Clostridium difficile* toxins A and B are heat labile and stool must be kept cool during transport.

• Blood samples have an important role for both screening and diagnostic purposes.

—Hemoglobin and RBC indices may show evidence of deficiencies in iron, vitamins, or other micronutrients.
—Prealbumin and albumin are good parameters of protein and overall nutritional status.
—Electrolytes may be helpful in the diagnostic process if significant changes exist in the Na^+, Cl^-, HCO_3^-.

• Several other tests are available that look at more specific causes of chronic diarrhea:

—In the evaluation for celiac disease, serum antitissue transglutaminase antibody has now replaced antigliadin and antiendomysial antibodies as the screening antibody test of choice, so long as the serum IgA is normal.
—A D-xylose absorption test is helpful in screening for small bowel injury. Timed serum D-xylose following oral ingestion is significantly lower in diseases causing diffuse mucosal damage to the small bowel, i.e., postviral enteropathy, celiac disease.
—A hydrogen breath test may be helpful in evaluating for the possibility of small bowel bacterial overgrowth. Lactose or sucrose hydrogen breath tests are done if lactose or sucrase-isomaltase is suspected respectively.
—Viral serologies such as HIV and cytomegalovirus need to be considered in the immunocompromised host with diarrhea.
—Plain x-ray studies are not usually helpful in the evaluation of chronic diarrhea. Upper gastrointestinal series may show partial small bowel obstruction, strictures, or evidence of inflammatory bowel disease.

• If the less invasive studies are unhelpful, esophagogastroduodenoscopy (EGD) and colonoscopy may be necessary.

—Endoscopy with small-bowel biopsy and small-bowel aspirate for culture can be helpful in diagnosing certain congenital, immunologic, or infective causes of diarrhea.
—Colonoscopy will diagnose colitis related to inflammatory bowel disease or infection.

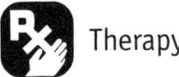 Therapy

• In cases in which infection is detected, appropriate antibiotic therapy should be initiated.
• In infants in whom the infection is severe or protracted in its course, a predigested (elemental or semi-elemental) formula may be necessary early in the recovery phase of the illness. These formulas tend to be much better tolerated and absorbed by the injured small bowel. Once the infant has shown good improvement, transition to a regular diet can be attempted. If the diarrhea is severe and oral nutrition appears inadequate, the formula can be given in a slow, continuous fashion via a nasogastric/nasojejunal tube. This again allows for better absorption of nutrients by the injured bowel.
• When the offending agent is identified as the cause of the diarrhea, e.g., cow's-milk protein, soy protein, lactose, or gluten, these agents should be promptly removed.
• Many causes of congenital diarrhea do not have specific therapy available and treatment is supportive.
• Congenital microvillus atrophy leads to an intractable diarrhea, and the patient is supported with the use of hyperalimentation (HAL). No current treatment has been found to correct this entity. Patients eventually die from complications of long-term HAL. Small bowel transplant remains experimental and should be offered only in select cases.
• In cases in which there is increased motility and thus rapid transit time, such as in chronic nonspecific diarrhea, alterations in the diet can be very helpful.
• Elimination of sorbitol-containing juices, which increases the osmotic load, and low-carbohydrate diet will help to lower the osmotic load delivered to the intestine. Furthermore, a high-fat diet will slow the intestinal transit time and increase the time available to absorb fluid, electrolytes, and nutrients from the intestinal tract.
• Certain causes of chronic diarrhea require specific therapy. Tumors, inflammatory bowel disease, or cystic fibrosis requires chronic and multifactorial treatment regimen to manage the underlying disease.
• The use of antimotility agents such as loperamide or antisecretory agents, such as octreotide, have a role in noninfective causes of diarrhea. However, identification and treatment of the underlying cause of diarrhea is always preferable.

 Follow-Up

With many of the chronic and complicated causes of chronic diarrhea, the best markers to follow as indicators of disease activity tend to be growth and nutritional status. If the patient is able to thrive and grow, the disease is being well controlled.

PITFALLS

• In certain cases in which the diet is altered as a therapeutic intervention, the physician must ensure that the patient is still absorbing adequate calories and micronutrients so that the nutritional status of the patient is not further compromised.
• Avoid the reinstitution of a regular diet too quickly following a severe and/or protracted insult to the gut since this may further exacerbate the diarrhea.
• The use of antimotility and antisecretory agents should be judicious and as an adjunct to other therapy, but not as the mainstay in the treatment regimen.
• In patients with cow's-milk and/or soy allergy, rechallenge should be after 12 months of age and should be in a controlled environment in case anaphylaxis occurs.

ICD-9-CM 558.9

BIBLIOGRAPHY

Baldassano RN, Liacouras CA. Chronic diarrhea, a practical approach for the pediatrician. *Pediatr Clin North Am* 1991;38(3):667–686.

Guerrant RL, Bobak DA. Bacterial and protozoal gastroenteritis. *N Engl J Med* 1991;325:327–340.

Hyams JS, Stafford RJ, Grand RJ, et al. Correlation of the lactose breath test, intestinal morphology and lactase activity in young children. *J Pediatr* 1980;97:609–612.

Lentze MJ. Persistent diarrhea. In: Walker WA, Durie PR, Hamilton JR, et al., eds. *Pediatric gastrointestinal disease*, 3rd ed. St. Louis: Mosby, 2000.

Salvilahti E. Food-induced malabsorption syndromes. *J Pediatr Gastroenterol Nutr* 2000;30(suppl):S61–66.

Smith MM, Lifshitz F. Excess fruit juice consumption as a contributing factor in nonorganic failure to thrive. *Pediatrics* 1994;93(3):438–443.

Vanderhoof JA. Chronic diarrhea. *Pediatr Rev* 1998;19(12):418–422.

Author: Emil Chuang

Chronic Granulomatous Disease

 Database

DEFINITION

Chronic granulomatous disease is a rare inherited defect involving phagocytes. The defective phagocytes (neutrophils and monocytes) have a decreased or absent ability to generate reactive oxygen intermediates, leaving the host susceptible to recurrent bacterial and fungal infections.

PATHOPHYSIOLOGY

The associated defects involve the NADPH oxidase complex of the neutrophil. Neutrophils in chronic granulomatous disease have an impaired ability to combat infection via an impaired respiratory burst. The NADPH oxidase complex is composed of four subunits, any of which may be defective in chronic granulomatous disease. Sixty percent of patients with chronic granulomatous disease have a defect in the gp91-*phox* subunit, which is inherited in an X-linked manner. Thirty-three percent of patients have a defect in the p47-*phox* subunit, which is inherited in an autosomal-recessive manner. Defects occur less frequently in the p22-*phox* and p67-*phox* subunits.

GENETICS

• Gene mutations may occur spontaneously and are inherited as an X-linked variant, or autosomal-recessive variant.
• Mutations may occur in any one of the four subunits of the neutrophil NADPH oxidase complex:

—gp91-*phox:* X chromosome
—p22-*phox:* chromosome 16
—p47-*phox:* chromosome 7
—p67-*phox:* chromosome 1

EPIDEMIOLOGY

• Prevalence: approximately 1 in 500,000 individuals

COMPLICATIONS

These patients have an increased susceptibility to bacterial and fungal infections that usually are not pathogenic in normal hosts

• Recurrent skin infections
• Sepsis
• Chronic lung disease (secondary to recurrent infections)
• Chronic liver disease (secondary to recurrent infections)
• Chronic osteomyelitis of large and small bones
• Malabsorption
• Systemic and discoid lupus erythematosus: increased incidence in female Carriers

The diagnosis of chronic granulomatous disease should be considered in patients with:

• Recurrent lymphadenitis
• Staphylococcal hepatic abscess
• *Aspergillus* or *Nocardia* pneumonia
• *Serratia marcescens* osteomyelitis
• Infections with *Pseudomonas cepacia*
• *Salmonella* sepsis
• Perirectal abscesses
• Brain abscesses

PROGNOSIS

Survival beyond the fourth decade is common. Bone marrow transplantation is curative.

 Differential Diagnosis

INFECTIOUS

Infections are related to the immune deficiency.

GENETIC/METABOLIC

• Leukocyte glucose-6-phosphate dehydrogenase deficiency
• Myeloperoxidase deficiency
• Humoral immune deficiencies
• Complement deficiencies

COMMON CAUSES

• Chronic granulomatous disease is not acquired; it is inherited as an X-linked variant or as an autosomal variant.

 Data Gathering

HISTORY

Question: At what age did the patient present?
Significance: Patients with chronic granulomatous disease usually present before 2 years of age with marked lymphadenopathy, hepatosplenomegaly, draining lymph nodes, and pneumonias.

Question: What is the infecting organism?
Significance: Patients with chronic granulomatous disease tend to develop infections with unusual organisms, such as *S. aureus, S. epidermidis, S. marcescens, Pseudomonas, Escherichia coli, Candida, Aspergillus, Nocardia,* and *Salmonella.*

Question: Are there other affected family members?
Significance: Chronic granulomatous disease is inherited in an X-linked and autosomal-recessive pattern. Therefore, there may be other affected family members.

Question: Does the mother have lupus?
Significance: There is a higher incidence of lupus in females who are carriers for chronic granulomatous disease.

 Physical Examination

Finding: Skin abscess or boils
Significance: Patients with chronic granulomatous disease develop frequent skin infections.

Finding: Mucous membrane and perirectal infections
Significance: Patients with chronic granulomatous disease commonly develop infections at mucous membrane and epidermal junctions, especially in the perirectal area.

Finding: Lymphadenopathy
Significance: Patients with chronic granulomatous disease commonly develop lymphadenopathy and draining lymph nodes.

Finding: Hepatosplenomegaly
Significance: Hepatosplenomegaly is a common finding in patients with chronic granulomatous disease.

Finding: Abnormal lung examination
Significance: Pulmonary disease is common in patients with chronic granulomatous disease.

Chronic Granulomatous Disease

 Laboratory Aids

APPROACH TO THE PATIENT

• General goal: Decide whether the patient's type of infections (osteomyelitis, perirectal abscess, etc.) and infecting organisms are consistent with the diagnosis of chronic granulomatous disease.
• Order a nitroblue tetrazolium (NBT) test.
• If abnormal, initiate sulfamethoxazole/trimethoprim prophylaxis.

Test: The NBT
Significance: The NBT is the most widely available test for chronic granulomatous disease. Neutrophils from normal individuals can reduce the dye, resulting in a color change. Neutrophils from patients with chronic granulomatous disease cannot reduce the dye, and it remains colorless. Neutrophils and monocytes from patients with chronic granulomatous disease have an impaired hexose monophosphate shunt. Therefore, they have a decreased conversion of NADP to NADPH, and a decreased oxidative burst, which results in an inability to reduce the NBT in this study.

Test: The 2,7-dichlorofluorescin (DCF)
Significance: DCF can directly measure the production of hydrogen peroxide utilizing a fluorescent label and flow cytometry. Patients with chronic granulomatous disease have decreased hydrogen peroxide production.

Test: Immunoblotting
Significance: Immunoblotting can be used to quantify the amount of each NADPH subunit present.

ISSUES FOR REFERRAL

Factors that may help alert you to make a referral include:

• A new diagnosis of chronic granulomatous disease: Immunologists can assist with antibiotic prophylaxis and with parameters for when to seek medical attention, and they can help identify which genetic variant is responsible for the patient's disease.
• Pregnant carrier for chronic granulomatous disease: Immunologists can help with prenatal diagnosis. Furthermore, some centers may consider *in utero* bone marrow transplantation for an affected fetus.
• Fever or suspected infection: Patients with chronic granulomatous disease tend to develop infections in unusual sites with unusual organisms. An immunologist can help with the evaluation and appropriate antibiotic coverage.

 Therapy

• *Antibiotic prophylaxis:* Trimethoprim-sulfamethoxazole is the antibiotic of choice, because both components are concentrated in the neutrophil, and for its bacterial spectrum.
• *Recombinant interferon-γ:* This is reserved for patients with severe disease. This therapy may decrease the incidence of infection.
• *Bone marrow transplant:* Chronic granulomatous disease has been cured in patients with matched transplants.
• *Acute infections:*

—*Broad-spectrum intravenous antibiotics:* There should be a low threshold to start this therapy. Severe infections should be treated with broad-spectrum intravenous antibiotics until an organism is identified. Good initial antibiotics include intravenous penicillins, aminoglycosides, and antipseudomonal antibiotics.
—*Amphotericin B:* This should not be withheld if a fungal infection is suspected, or if the patient's clinical status is deteriorating despite broad-spectrum antibiotics.
—*Leukocyte transfusions:* These are reserved for severe infections, and efficacy is controversial.

 Follow-Up

Chronic granulomatous disease is a lifelong disease. These patients tend to develop chronic lung disease; therefore, pulmonary function studies should be followed at least annually. Liver disease is also common; therefore, liver function studies should also be followed at least annually. Female carriers should be observed for signs of lupus erythematosus.

 Common Questions and Answers

Q: How do you interpret an NBT test reported as 50% of normal?
A: This is generally consistent with a carrier state. The carrier is not at increased risk for infection. However, carrier females have an increased risk of developing lupus.

Q: What do the infecting organisms have in common?
A: Patients with chronic granulomatous disease are most susceptible to catalase-positive organisms.

Q: Are all chronic granulomatous disease patients with fever admitted automatically?
A: No. It is true that these patients are more prone to invasive and systemic infections, but these patients are not admitted with every febrile episode (especially if there is evidence of a minor bacterial or viral infection). However, subtle signs of an invasive infection must be taken very seriously, and these patients are certainly admitted.

Q: Can a prenatal diagnosis be made?
A: Yes. However, currently this can only be done in a limited number of research laboratories, and the testing is not commercially available. Testing involves chorionic villus sampling, and it can be done only on families in which the specific mutation has been mapped.

ICD-9-CM 288.1

BIBLIOGRAPHY

Curnutte JT. Chronic granulomatous disease: the solving of a clinical riddle at the molecular level. *Clin Immunol Immunopathol* 1993;67(3 pt 2):S2–S15.

Heyworth PG, Curnutte JT, Noack D, et al. Hematologic important mutations: X-linked chronic granulomatous disease—an update. *Blood Cells Mol Dis* 1997;23(3):443–450.

Horwitz ME, Barrett AJ, Brown MR, et al. Treatment of chronic granulomatous disease with nonmyeloablative conditioning and a T-cell-depleted hematopoietic allograft. *N Engl J Med* 2001;344(12):881–888.

Kamani N, Douglas SD. Natural history of chronic granulomatous disease. *Diagn Clin Immunol* 1988;5:314–317.

Sites DP, Terr AI, Parslow TG. *Basic and clinical immunology*, 8th ed. Englewood Cliffs, NJ: Prentice Hall, 1994.

Author: Christopher A. Smith

Cirrhosis

 ## Database

DEFINITION

Cirrhosis is a diffuse, dynamic liver process reflecting the competing processes of hepatocyte injury (necrosis), response to injury (fibrosis), and regeneration (nodule formation). Cirrhosis may occur as a result of any progressive liver disease. As cirrhosis advances, there is distortion of liver architecture with altered hepatic blood flow, and development of portal hypertension and shunting of blood from the liver. This results in irregular delivery of oxygen and nutrients to the liver and may perpetuate cirrhosis even after original insult has ceased.

CAUSES

In children, a wide range of causes of hepatocellular injury may result in cirrhosis.

- Biliary

—Extrahepatic biliary atresia
—Choledochal cyst
—Tumors
—Common bile duct and biliary lithiasis
—Alagille syndrome
—Biliary hypoplasia
—Primary familial intrahepatic cholestasis (PFIC)
—Sclerosing cholangitis
—Graft-vs-host disease
—Drugs (e.g., trimethoprim-sulfamethoxazole)
—Histiocytosis X (Langerhans cell histiocytosis)

- Hepatic

—Neonatal hepatitis, including TORCH infections
—Viral—hepatitis B, C, D, EBV, CMV
—Autoimmune hepatitis
—Drugs/toxins and alcohol

- Genetic/metabolic

—Cystic fibrosis
—α_1-Antitrypsin deficiency
—Metal storage defects—Wilson's disease, neonatal hemochromatosis
—Carbohydrate defects—galactosemia, hereditary fructose intolerance, glycogen storage III and IV
—Amino acid defects—tyrosinemia, urea cycle disorders
—Lipid storage diseases—Gaucher's disease, Niemann-Pick type C
—Mitochondrial disorders—fatty acid β-oxidation defects, respiratory chain defects
—Peroxisomal disorders—Zellweger's syndrome

- Vascular

—Budd-Chiari syndrome
—Veno-occlusive disease
—Cardiac

GENETICS

In several disorders, including sclerosing cholangitis and hemochromatosis, there have been identified HLA markers. However, no specific markers correlate with cirrhosis.

EPIDEMIOLOGY

Based on the varying etiologies, no specific epidemiologic pattern can be identified.

COMPLICATIONS

- Malnutrition and growth failure
- Malabsorption (steatorrhea, fat-soluble vitamin deficiencies)
- Portal hypertension and variceal bleeding
- Hypersplenism (associated with anemia, thrombocytopenia, and neutropenia)
- Ascites
- Encephalopathy
- Coagulopathy
- Hepatopulmonary syndrome
- Hepatorenal syndrome
- Bacterial infections, spontaneous bacterial peritonitis
- Hepatocellular carcinoma

PROGNOSIS

The prognosis for cirrhosis leading to decompensation depends on the etiologic agent. Knowledge of the natural history of particular disease states is of value (i.e., tyrosinemia and biliary atresia). Most available liver tests have poor predictive value until liver decompensation has occurred. Poor prognostic features in children include prolonged prothrombin time unresponsive to vitamin K, ascites, malnutrition, low plasma cholesterol, elevated bilirubin level, and partial thromboplastin time prolonged more than 20 seconds.

 ## Data Gathering

CLINICAL PRESENTATION

- Compensated cirrhosis—asymptomatic, with no signs or symptoms of liver disease. Discovered incidentally either during routine physical examinations with an enlarged liver and/or palpable spleen, or as a result of an investigation for an unrelated condition.
- Decompensated cirrhosis—acute, precipitous presentation of liver failure with a life-threatening complication of cirrhosis, such as an esophageal variceal hemorrhage.

HISTORY

Based on the varying etiologic agents, one should elicit pertinent historical features characteristic of each specific problem as detailed:

- Exposure to hepatitis, antecedent viral illnesses
- Exposure to hepatotoxins
- Family history of genetic, metabolic, or autoimmune diseases
- Neurologic problems (Wilson disease)

 ## Physical Examination

- General—poor growth, malnutrition, fever, cachexia
- Skin—jaundice, flushing or pallor, palmar erythema, spider angiomata, easy bruising
- Abdomen—ascites (distention, fluid wave, shifting dullness), caput medusa, splenomegaly, rectal varices, hepatomegaly or a shrunken liver
- Extremities—digital clubbing, hypertrophic osteoarthropathy
- Endocrine—gynecomastia, testicular atrophy, delayed puberty
- CNS—asterixis, positive Babinski sign, mental status changes, hyperreflexia, muscle wasting

Laboratory Aids

TESTS

These tests focus on determining the etiology and the severity of liver disease prior to a liver biopsy.

- Tests of liver cell injury—alanine aminotransferase, aspartate aminotransferase, lactic dehydrogenase
- Tests of synthetic function—albumin and other serum proteins, prothrombin time, ammonia, plasma and urine amino acids, serum lipids and lipoproteins, cholesterol and triglycerides
- Tests of cholestasis—fractionated bilirubin, alkaline phosphatase, γ-glutamyltransferase, 5'-nucleotidase, serum and urine bile acids
- Miscellaneous disease-specific serum tests

—Viral serologies—TORCH, hepatitis B, C, EBV, CMV
—Wilson disease—ceruloplasmin, serum and urine cooper, hemolytic anemia, and slit-lamp exam for Kaiser-Fleischer rings
—α_1-Antitrypsin deficiency—α_1-antitrypsin serum level and protease inhibitor (Pi) phenotype
—Autoimmune hepatitis—sedimentation rate, autoantibodies, immunoglobulins
—Metabolic/genetic—fasting blood sugar, lactate, pyruvate, uric acid, sweat test, carnitine, CPK, iron ferritin, porphyrins, serum amino acids, urine organic acids, fatty acid degeneration products

IMAGING

- Ultrasound with Doppler images—evaluates for anatomic variation or obstruction of the biliary tree. Doppler images evaluate for portal hypertension and venous outflow obstruction.
- Hepatobiliary radioisotope scanning—assess for biliary excretion in neonatal cholestasis.
- Cholangiography (ERCP, MRCP, intraoperative)—assess for extrahepatic biliary disease (stones, choledochal cyst, sclerosing cholangitis).

LIVER BIOPSY

- Percutaneous needle biopsy, intraoperative wedge biopsy, transjugular liver biopsy
- Confirm the presence, type, and degree of activity of cirrhosis
- Various hepatic diseases that progress to cirrhosis have characteristic histologic findings. The process of cirrhosis in chronic liver disease may obscure the nature of the original insult, rendering morphologic and histologic classifications unhelpful.

 ## Therapy

DRUGS

- Fat-soluble vitamins—vitamins A, D, E, and K.
- Diuretic therapy (furosemide, spironolactone, chlorothiazide) for patients with ascites.
- Albumin infusions for patients with refractory ascites.
- Beta-blockers shown to decrease portal pressure and reduce the risk of variceal bleeding in adults.
- Lactulose and neomycin are used for patients with hepatic encephalopathy.
- Antibiotics if suspicious of spontaneous bacterial peritonitis.

NUTRITION

Malnutrition is common in chronic liver diseases because of metabolic derangements, fat malabsorption, anorexia, and increased energy requirements. It is important to achieve adequate caloric intake, often with nocturnal nutritional supplementation. Fluid and electrolyte homeostasis (e.g., salt and water retention with ascites) is also a vital part of management. Can optimize fat absorption with medium- and long-chain triglycerides, and supplement with fat-soluble vitamins.

SURGERY AND PROCEDURES

- Endoscopic variceal band ligation or sclerotherapy for GI bleeding
- Paracentesis for refractory ascites or diagnosis of spontaneous bacterial peritonitis
- Porta-systemic shunt placement (surgical or radiologic TIPS procedure) for uncontrolled portal hypertension
- Liver transplantation for decompensated cirrhosis

 ## Follow-Up

Close monitoring and management of any complications of chronic liver disease.

 ## Common Questions and Answers

Q: Will my child with cystic fibrosis develop cirrhosis?
A: The medical literature cites a 5% to 20% incidence of cirrhosis in children with cystic fibrosis. Many factors seem to relate to the development of cirrhosis in these children, but the genetic type of cystic fibrosis does not seem to be a cause only.

Q: Will every child with cirrhosis need a liver transplant?
A: Most children who develop cirrhosis from causes such as biliary atresia or metabolic disease will ultimately require a liver transplant.

ICD-9-CD 571.0

BIBLIOGRAPHY

Hardy S, Kleinman RE. Cirrhosis and chronic liver failure. In: Suchy FJ, Sokol RJ, Balistreri WF, eds. *Liver disease in children*. Philadelphia: Lippincott Williams & Wilkins, 2001:89–127.

Kelly DA. Current results and evolving indications for liver transplantation in children. *J Pediatr Gastroenterol Nutr* 1998;27(2):214.

Poupon R, Chazouilleres O, Poupon RE. Chronic cholestatic diseases. *J Hepatol* 2000;32(1 suppl):129.

Shepherd R. Complications and management of chronic liver disease. In: Kelly DA, ed. *Diseases of the liver and biliary system in children*. London: Blackwell Science, 1999:189–210.

Author: Lynette A. Gillis

Cleft Lip and Palate

 Database

DEFINITION

A cleft lip (CL) is a deformity of the upper lip that may include a discontinuity of vermilion, skin, muscle, and mucosa, as well as the underlying gingiva and bone. It can be unilateral or bilateral. A complete cleft extends into the nose, while an incomplete cleft has at least some bridge of intact tissue separating the oral and nasal cavities. A cleft palate (CP) usually represents a visible separation between the two halves of the roof of the mouth, involving mucosa, muscle, and often the bones of the hard palate. A submucous CP has intact mucosa, but the underlying muscle and bone are at least partially divided.

ETIOLOGY

- Cleft lip may result from failure of the medial nasal and maxillary processes to join *in utero*, or possibly from lack of adequate mesenchymal reinforcement, leading to subsequent breakdown and separation. CP results from failure of the palatal shelves to fuse.
- Lower-than-expected incidence of CL and CP has been noted with prenatal dietary supplementation with folic acid and vitamin B_6. Folic acid supplementation has also been clearly associated with a decreased incidence of neural tube defects.

PATHOPHYSIOLOGY

Muscle fibers are atrophic and disorganized in the region of the cleft, and mitochondrial abnormalities are noted at the cleft margins by histochemical and electromyographic studies.

ETIOLOGY AND GENETICS

- One-third of patients with CL and/or CP have a positive family history; positive family history is noted twice as often in CL with or without CP as in CP alone.
- Although a number of recognized patterns of malformation that include CL and/or CP may be caused by exposure to teratogens such as alcohol, anticonvulsants, and isotretinoin, there is little evidence linking isolated clefts to exposure to any single teratogenic agent. One notable exception is the anticonvulsant phenytoin, the use of which during pregnancy has been associated with a tenfold increase in the incidence of CL.
- The incidence of CL in infants born to mothers who smoke during pregnancy is twice that of those born to nonsmoking mothers.

- Among patients with clefts of the secondary palate alone, those syndromes associated with microdeletions of chromosome 22q11.2 (velocardiofacial syndrome, DiGeorge syndrome, and conotruncal anomaly face syndrome) are currently the most common syndromic diagnoses. Inheritance is autosomal dominant with considerable variability in phenotypic expression, which may include facial dysmorphism, developmental delay, cardiovascular anomalies, immunologic abnormalities, CP, and velopharyngeal dysfunction.
- The next most common syndrome associated with palatal clefts is Stickler syndrome, characterized by autosomal dominance, CP, epicanthal folds, flat facies, severe myopia, retinal detachment, and glaucoma, caused by a mutation of the gene for type 2 collagen (chromosome 12q).
- Other syndromes linked to specific chromosomal abnormalities include Van der Woude (autosomal dominant, CP and/or CL, lower lip pits, 1q32), and Smith-Lemli-Opitz (defect in cholesterol synthesis, 7q34).
- The majority of clefts are nonsyndromic and may be either multifactorial in origin or the result of changes at a major single-gene locus.

EPIDEMIOLOGY

- Incidence of CL with or without CP is 1 in 700 births.
- Racial heterogeneity noted in CL and CP (Asians, 2.1 in 1,000 births; whites, 1 in 1,000; blacks, 0.41 in 1,000)
- Isolated CP is in 1 in 2,000 births across races.
- Bilateral CL is associated with CP in 86% of cases, and unilateral CL is associated with CP in 68% of cases.
- CL/CP is more common on the left side, particularly in boys.
- Incidence of CL with or without CP increases with parental (especially paternal) age greater than 30 years. Some association with low socioeconomic class may be nutrition-related.

COMPLICATIONS

- Airway obstruction and feeding disorders, particularly with Pierre Robin sequence (micrognathia, glossoptosis, airway obstruction, with or without CP)
- Chronic otitis media
- Speech problems, including hypernasality and articulation errors
- Associated malformations
- About one third of patients with CP have associated anomalies, with isolated having the highest. CNS, cardiac, and urinary tract malformations and clubfoot are commonly associated with clefting.

 Data Gathering

HISTORY

Prenatal exposure to alcohol, cigarettes, phenytoin, isotretinoin; family history of CL or CP, or speech problems in first-degree relative

 Physical Examination

- Incomplete or complete cleft of lip, alveolus, hard and soft palate, or uvula. Soft palate and uvula clefts are always midline, while lip, alveolar, and hard palatal clefts can be unilateral or bilateral.
- A bifid uvula may indicate a submucous cleft.
- A small mandible and retropositioned tongue may indicate a risk for airway obstruction (Pierre Robin sequence).
- Look for associated anomalies of the face, heart, and extremities that may indicate a clefting syndrome.

TRICKS

Examine the palate from the top of the patient, with the head in your lap, using a tongue depressor and flashlight. Palpate the posterior hard palate for a possible notch in the bone. Palpate the gums and maxilla for a possible notch in the floor of the nose.

 Laboratory Aids

The following tests should be performed if indicated by history and physical examination:

- Complete ophthalmologic examination to check for myopia, glaucoma, retinal detachment
- Pulse oximetry to check for desaturation while feeding or while supine
- Polysomnography to distinguish central from obstructive apnea
- Increased serum 7-dehydrocholesterol and decreased serum cholesterol to rule out Smith-Lemli-Opitz syndrome
- Karyotype to rule out specific genetic abnormalities
- Fluorescence *in situ* hybridization (FISH) to rule out a chromosome 22q11.2 deletion
- Echocardiography, renal ultrasound, IV pyelography if indicated

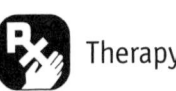

Therapy

NEONATAL

Airway management, prone positioning if tongue is causing airway obstruction. Cleft patients may have significant feeding problems because of inability to generate negative intraoral pressure necessary to feed efficiently. Premie nipples with enlarged or cross-cut openings, or soft plastic squeezable bottles, can facilitate milk flow. Poor weight gain may necessitate NG tube feedings.

SURGICAL

• Significant airway obstruction and desaturation in the neonatal period refractory to prone positioning may indicate the need for a tongue-lip adhesion, release of the floor of the mouth musculature, mandibular distraction, or tracheostomy.
• Wide clefts of the lip may benefit from preliminary lip adhesion at 2–3 months of age. Timing of definitive lip repair varies from 2 to 6 months of age.
• Palate repair is generally done prior to 1 year of age to decrease speech and language difficulties.
• Otitis media is more common with CP, and bilateral myringotomy tubes can be inserted at the time of cleft repair.
• Correction of secondary deformities may include lip scar revision, cleft nasal deformity correction (infancy to adulthood), alveolar bone grafts (usually when permanent canines are erupting), pharyngoplasty for soft palate–velopharyngeal incompetence, closure of palatal fistulas, and orthognathic surgery for severe jaw deformities.

ORTHODONTICS

May include obturators to facilitate feeding and speech, nasal molding and palatal repositioning prior to lip and palate repair, palatal expansion prior to bone grafting, conventional orthodontics (appliances, prosthetic teeth, bridgework), and preorthognathic surgery manipulation of the dentition.

Follow-Up

MULTIDISCIPLINARY TEAM

• Pediatrician
• Plastic surgeon
• Speech pathologist
• Orthodontist
• Pediatric dentist
• Psychologist
• Social worker
• Nurse practitioner
• Anthropologist (facial growth specialist)
• Geneticist
• Support groups

POTENTIAL PROBLEMS

• Hypernasal resonance and nasal air emission during speech may indicate velopharyngeal incompetence or palatal fistula. Up to 30% of patients may require additional palatal or pharyngeal surgery following initial palate repair.
• Multiple ear infections may require prolonged use of myringotomy tubes to prevent hearing impairment. Audiograms should be obtained regularly.
• Delays in speech and language development may require detailed evaluation, early intervention programs, and speech therapy.
• Poor dentition, occlusal problems (crossbite), gingivitis, and crowding have been noted. Behavior disorders and psychosocial adjustment disorders may require attention.

PROGNOSIS

Good, for normal growth and development with long-term follow-up by a multidisciplinary team and with good parental support

PITFALLS

• Failure to diagnose airway obstruction in infants with Pierre Robin sequence may lead to failure to thrive or, in severe cases, in death.
• Failure to diagnose associated anomalies may lead to missed syndromes and inaccurate genetic counseling.
• A submucous CP can be easily missed until hypernasal speech is noted later in life.

Common Questions and Answers

FOR NONSYNDROMIC CL WITH OR WITHOUT CP

Q: What is our risk of having a second child with a cleft, if neither of us has a cleft?
A: Two percent.

Q: What is my child's risk of later having a child with a cleft?
A: Four percent.

Q: What is our risk of having a third child with a cleft, if we have two affected children, but neither of us is affected?
A: Nine percent.

Q: What is our risk of having a second child with a cleft, if one of us also has a cleft?
A: Seventeen percent.

FOR NONSYNDROMIC ISOLATED CP

Q: What is our risk of having a second child with a cleft, if neither of us has a cleft?
A: Two percent.

Q: What is my child's risk of later having a child with a cleft?
A: Six percent.

Q: What is our risk of having a third child with a cleft, if we have two affected children, but neither of us is affected?
A: One percent.

Q: What is our risk of having a second child with a cleft, if one of us also has a cleft?
A: Fifteen percent.

Q: Will my child look normal?
A: All CL repairs will leave some type of permanent scar, with potential asymmetry that may benefit from later additional lip scar revision. The goal is to create a lip that does not attract undue attention. The nose is often the most difficult to correct, because of asymmetry in cartilage and skin contour.

Q: Will my child speak normally?
A: Most children will achieve velopharyngeal competence and normal speech, but may require additional speech therapy to achieve this goal.

ICD-9-CM 749.10, 749.20

BIBLIOGRAPHY

Byrd HS. Cleft lip I: primary deformity. *Select Read Plast Surg* 1994;7(21):1–34.

Hardesty RA, ed. Advances in the management of cleft lip and palate. *Clin Plast Surg* 1993;20(4):597–821.

Hobar PC. Cleft lip II: secondary deformities. *Select Read Plast Surg* 1994;7(22):1–28.

Hodges PL, Pownell PH. Cleft surgery and velopharyngeal function. *Select Read Plast Surg* 1994;7(23):1–36.

Kaufman FL. Managing the cleft lip and palate patient. *Pediatr Clin North Am* 1991;38(5): 1127–1147.

Witt PD, Marsh JL. Advances in assessing outcome of surgical repair of cleft lip and cleft palate. *Plast Reconstr Surg* 1997;100(7):1907–1917.

Authors: Richard E. Kirschner, Christine A. Carman-Dillon, and David W. Low

Clubfoot

 Database

DEFINITION

Clubfoot is a congenital or neuromuscular deformity in which the hindfoot is fixed in equinus and varus and the forefoot is fixed in varus and often cavus.

CAUSES

• Most cases are idiopathic (multifactorial inheritance pattern with significant environmental influence).
• Infrequently, neuromuscular imbalance may underlie the deformity (cerebral palsy, myelo-meningocele, lipomas of the cord, caudal or sacral agenesis, polio, arthrogryposis, fetal alcohol syndrome).

PATHOPHYSIOLOGY

• Many anatomic abnormalities have been postulated as causing clubfoot: anomalous or deficient muscles, myoblasts, mast cells, abnormal primary bone formation, joint and muscle contractures, vascular anomalies (absent dorsalis pedis artery), nerve anomalies, and abnormalities of the fibrous connective tissue.
• Interruption of the development of the embryonic foot has also been suggested.

EPIDEMIOLOGY

• Prevalence is 1 to 1.4 per 1,000 live births, but can vary among different ethnic groups.
• The risk of deformity increases by 20 to 30 times where there is an affected first-degree relative. Male/female ratio is 2:1.

 Differential Diagnosis

• Distinguish other deformities of the foot:

—Metatarsus adductus or varus (heel is in neutral position)
—Calcaneovalgus (foot is in valgus)
—Vertical talus (foot is in valgus, heel in equinovalgus)
—Many children with clubfoot also have tibial torsion.

 Data Gathering

HISTORY

• Family history of clubfoot (3%)
• Onset of deformity (congenital or developmental)

 Physical Examination

Careful examination is called for, especially of the following:

• The neuromuscular system for neuromuscular etiologies such as lumbosacral sinuses, dimples, and lipomas
• The hips for hip dysplasia
• The neck for torticollis

PHYSICAL EXAMINATION TRICKS

Push the foot into a corrected position. Is the deformity fully correctable? Overcorrectable?

 Laboratory Aids

• X-ray studies (after 3 months of age)
• Tarsal bones are poorly ossified in the newborn. Diagnosis is clinical.
• At 3 to 6 months of age, anteroposterior (AP) and lateral x-ray films in dorsiflexion (maximal correction) may help in defining residual deformity. The beam should be focused on the hindfoot for both the AP and lateral x-rays, as the measured angles will be hindfoot angles.
• Decreased talocalcaneal angle on the AP and lateral views (25 degrees or less) confirm persistent deformity.
• Medial displacement of the cuboid on the calcaneus and persistent plantar flexion of the forefoot on the hindfoot (talar to first metatarsal angle) indicate more complex deformities.

Emergency Care

• Care can begin in the first week after birth.

Clubfoot

Therapy

- Initial treatment is serial (weekly) manipulation and casting.
- Taping may be useful for treatment of the infant requiring ICU care; access to the feet should be maintained for blood tests.
- Failure to correct the deformity completely by manipulation within 3 to 9 months should lead to surgical treatment.
- Long-leg serial casting by the Ponseti technique has improved the nonoperative results.

Follow-Up

- Realignment of the deformity is the goal and should be achieved at surgery or by casting.
- Most surgeons cast the feet for 3 months postoperatively.
- Some brace the feet for 6 months.
- Remember, the cause of the deformity is not corrected. Only the alignment of the bones and lengthening of the soft tissues are corrected.
- Depending on the severity of the deformity, calf narrowing and weakness, and ankle and subtalar stiffness, a difference between the feet of one to two shoe sizes and even a leg-length discrepancy will be present in all corrected clubfeet.
- There will also be decreased ankle and subtalar motion as compared to the normal.
- Adolescent children with clubfeet often will get leg cramps and will tire easily while doing normally strenuous activities in sports.
- All true recurrences should lead to further evaluation for neuromuscular or syndrome causes that might have been missed in the infant.

Common Questions and Answers

Q: How can a rigid clubfoot be distinguished from a positional clubfoot?
A: During initial evaluation of the child, it is important to assess the amount of flexibility in a clubfoot. This can be most easily done by flexing the hip to 90 degrees, flexing the knee to 90 degrees, and then gently trying to turn the forefoot into a straight position lined up with the thigh. If the foot easily spins around into a normal position, it can be assumed that this is a flexible or positional clubfoot. If deformity persists, this is a rigid deformity. If possible, the examining physician should palpate the heel to see if the os calcis comes out of its equinus position filling the heel pad. In some children, particularly with a rocker bottom sole, the heel pad looks as if it is in the correct position, but the os calcis remains in equinus with the posterior aspect of the os calcis proximal to the heel pad.

Q: What percentage of clubfeet are successfully treated by casting?
A: To some extent, the amount of success depends on how much correction is desired. Occasionally, cast correction will provide a partial correction. Some feet, after casting, can be held in the corrected position, only to spin back to the clubfoot deformity when released. Positional clubfeet are likely to improve with casting in perhaps 80% of cases. Rigid clubfeet are much less likely to be corrected by casting. The success rate in the rigid feet is likely to be about 10% to 20%.

Q: What will be the permanent disability of a congenital clubfoot deformity?
A: While casting and surgical correction of a congenital clubfoot can realign the bones, the surgery does little to correct the underlying neuromuscular problems. As a result, all children with rigid clubfeet are likely to have a leg-length inequality (usually less than 1.5 inches), a smaller foot (usually one to two sizes), calf narrowing that cannot be significantly improved with exercise, and joint stiffness (ankle, subtalar, and midfoot). Even children with optimal realignment of the deformity will notice their inability to perform gymnastic activities or running activities requiring normal range of motion of the ankle and foot. Many will complain of the inability to keep up with their peer group during adolescent and young-adult sports activities.

Q: How soon should an infant with congenital clubfoot be referred to an orthopedic surgeon?
A: If casting is to be even partially successful, cast treatment should begin within the first week or two of life. Clearly, medical and life-threatening conditions will take precedence over the treatment of the clubfoot. Access to the feet for IV or blood studies will interfere with a casting regimen. Casting should begin as soon as is practical. It may even be possible to begin taping of the foot as an alternative to casting, which will still allow IV access to the feet. Referral to an orthopedic surgeon should therefore follow as soon as is practical.

ICD-9-CM 754.70

BIBLIOGRAPHY

Hamel J, Becker W. Sonographic assessment of clubfoot deformity in young children. *J Pediatr Orthop B* 1996;5(4):279–286.

Johnston CE II, Hobatho MC, Baker KJ, et al. Three-dimensional analysis of clubfoot deformity by computed tomography. *J Pediatr Orthop B* 1995;4(1):39–48.

Napiontek M. Clinical and radiographic appearance of congenital talipes equinovarus after successful nonoperative treatment. *J Pediatr Orthop* 1996;16(1):67–72.

Yamamoto H, Muneta T, Morita S. Nonsurgical treatment of congenital clubfoot with manipulation, cast, and modified Denis Browne splint. *J Pediatr Orthop* 1998;18(4):538–542.

Ponseti I. Treatment of congenital clubfoot. *J Bone Joint Surg* 1992;74(3):448–454.

Author: Richard S. Davidson

Coarctation of Aorta

 Database

DEFINITION

Discrete stenosis of the upper thoracic aorta, usually just opposite the site of insertion of the ductus arteriosus (juxtaductal). A defect in the vessel media giving rise to a prominent posterior infolding ("the posterior shelf"). The lesion is most often discrete, but may be long-segment or torturous in nature. It is usually juxtaductal but may occur in other sites (ascending or abdominal aorta).

PATHOPHYSIOLOGY

• Decreased systemic blood flow to lower extremities after ductal closure
• Increased resistance to left ventricular outflow causes systolic hypertension and LV hypertrophy.
• If the coarctation of the aorta (CoA) is severe, left ventricular dysfunction and congestive heart failure result, with low cardiac output and increased left ventricular end-diastolic pressure.
• Decreased myocardial perfusion may be present in cases of very low output.

GENETICS

• Multifactorial; occurs in 35% of patients with Turner syndrome (XO)
• Has been described in cases of monozygotic twins

EPIDEMIOLOGY

Approximately 6% to 8% of patients with congenital heart disease have CoA. Male/female ratio is 1.2 to 2.0:1.

COMPLICATIONS

• Systemic hypertension
• Shock
• Mesenteric ischemia
• Congestive heart failure
• Cerebrovascular accident

PROGNOSIS

Untreated CoA has a poor natural history, with the onset of congestive heart failure. Claudication is common in older children with previously undiscovered CoA. Generally, the prognosis following successful repair in infancy or childhood is excellent. Clinical conditions that may affect long-term prognosis after repair of CoA include:

• Residual or recurrent coarctation
• Hypertension (rest and exercise)
• Aortic aneurysm
• Associated intracardiac lesions

ASSOCIATED LESIONS

• Bicuspid aortic valve occurs in 85% of patients with CoA.
• Patent ductus arteriosus
• Ventricular septal defect
• Valvar or subvalvar aortic stenosis
• Mitral stenosis: often associated with structural mitral valve abnormalities (i.e., supravalvar mitral ring, thickening of mitral leaflet, single papillary muscle with parachute deformity, or short dysplastic chordae tendinae)
• Shone syndrome: multiple left-sided obstructive lesions, including mitral stenosis, subaortic membrane, aortic valve stenosis, and coarctation
• Berry aneurysm of the circle of Willis
• Renal artery stenosis associated with abdominal coarctation

 Differential Diagnosis

• Other left-sided heart obstructive lesions
• Hypoplastic left-heart syndrome
• Critical aortic stenosis

 Data Gathering

HISTORY

There are two typical patterns of the clinical presentation of CoA:

• An infant with congestive heart failure or shock—a small, pale, irritable child in respiratory distress. This is caused by closure of ductus and is more common in infants with complex CoA (20–30%).

—Poor feeding
—Dyspnea
—Diaphoresis
—Poor weight gain
—Oliguria

• An otherwise asymptomatic child with systolic hypertension and/or a heart murmur (70–80%)

—Lower extremity claudication
—Headaches

 Physical Examination

• Tachypnea and tachycardia
• Discrepant arterial pulses and systolic blood pressure in the upper and lower extremities
• Weak "thready" pulses
• Grades 2 to 3/6 systolic ejection murmur
• Gallop rhythm in an infant with congestive heart failure
• Ejection click from bicuspid aortic valve

—The most important finding: decreased or absent lower extremity pulses. Are pulses present? Is there a delay between the brachial and femoral pulses?
—Heart murmur: best heard at the upper left sternal border (LSB), at the base and radiating to the left interscapular area posteriorly
—An infant with critical CoA with patent ductus arteriosis (PDA) "differential cyanosis." The lower part of the body appears cyanotic because the descending aortic flow is provided by the right ventricle through PDA (check postductal saturation).

 Laboratory Aids

• ECG: Right ventricular hypertrophy is usually present in symptomatic infants. ECG is often normal in children. Left ventricular hypertrophy is apparent with more severe coarctation or coarctation of longer standing.
• Chest x-ray: in the infant, moderate-to-severe cardiomegaly with increased pulmonary vascular markings (PVM). In an asymptomatic child, the heart size is often normal with normal PVM. Rib notching may be seen in older children secondary to erosion of the ribs by dilated intercostal collateral vessels.
• Echocardiography: localization and degree of CoA and associated findings; PDA, isthmus hypoplasia. Assessment of associated left-sided obstruction (severity of which may be underestimated in patients with congestive heart failure, low cardiac output, or the presence of a PDA): mitral valve abnormality, left ventricular outflow obstruction, and aortic stenosis (bicuspid aortic valve)
• MRI: clearly defines the location and severity of CoA. Is useful for serial follow-up postoperatively (especially aortic aneurysms)
• Cardiac catheterization and angiography: usually not indicated unless there are further questions to be answered and/or a planned intervention.

Coarctation of Aorta

 Therapy

MEDICAL

For the sick neonate who presents with severe congestive heart failure or shock (ductal-dependent left-sided obstructive lesion):

- Prostaglandin infusion: 0.05 μg/kg/min
- Inotropic support
- Diuretics for pulmonary venous hypertension or pulmonary edema
- Correction of metabolic disturbances caused by systemic hypoperfusion
- Surgical intervention should follow as soon as possible.

For the asymptomatic child, elective repair and medical management of hypertension are appropriate.

SURGICAL

Infancy

- Surgical repair of CoA and associated intracardiac anomalies
- The surgical mortality rate for infants with CoA and a large VSD ranges from 5% to 15% and is higher for children with more complex intracardiac anomalies.

Childhood

- Elective CoA repair between ages 3 and 5 years in asymptomatic children without severe upper extremity hypertension. Later repair is associated with increased risk of sustained hypertension and atherosclerosis.

Types of Surgical Repair

- End-to-end anastomosis
- Subclavian flap aortoplasty
- Prosthetic patch aortoplasty
- Bypass graft

Nonsurgical Option

- Percutaneous balloon angioplasty of native CoA is still controversial because of concern about recurrent stenosis and aneurysm formation.

POSTOPERATIVE COMPLICATIONS

- Bleeding
- Postcoarctectomy syndrome/mesenteric arteritis
- Paradoxical hypertension
- Spinal cord ischemia (0.4%)
- Residual coarctation
- Chylothorax
- Stridor
- Diaphragm paralysis
- Subclavian steal
- Aortic aneurysm or dissection

 Follow-Up

- Reexamine every 12 months.
- Residual or recurrent CoA (25–60%); occurs most commonly after repair in infancy; percutaneous balloon angioplasty can be performed as early as 2 months postoperatively.
- Residual systemic hypertension; most commonly in patients whose CoA repair is delayed beyond late childhood
- Aneurysm formation
- Cerebrovascular accidents
- Monitor four-extremity blood pressure for recoarctation or residual hypertension.
- Antibiotic prophylaxis to prevent endocarditis or endarteritis
- May have hypertension with exercise, even if normotensive at rest
- Exercise-induced hypertension without anatomic stenosis may respond to beta-blocker therapy.

PITFALLS

- The most reliable clinical findings to diagnose CoA are the presence of pressure differences in upper and lower extremities and decreased or absent femoral pulses. Palpable pulses do not exclude coarctation. What one palpates is pulse pressure, not absolute systolic pressure.
- Four-extremity blood pressure measurement is very important in assessing infants and children with possible congenital heart disease. Proper cuff size must be used.

 Common Questions and Answers

Q: When is the most appropriate time to perform surgical repair of simple CoA?
A: Currently, it is recommended that elective CoA repair be performed between 3 and 5 years of age in asymptomatic children without severe upper extremity hypertension, based on the risk of recoarctation (higher incidence under 3 years, especially under 1 year, of age) and residual hypertension and subsequent atherosclerotic cardiovascular disease.

Q: What is the incidence of residual hypertension after surgical repair of CoA?
A: The incidence of late residual hypertension may be reduced to approximately 6% if CoA repair is performed under 5 years of age, as opposed to 30% to 50% in patients whose CoA is repaired at an older age.

ICD-9-CM 747.10

BIBLIOGRAPHY

Beekman RH. Coarctation of aorta. In: Moss AJ, Adams FH, *Heart disease in infants, children, and adolescents*, 5th ed. Philadelphia: Lippincott, 1977:1111–1113.

Brickner ME, Hillis LD, Lange RA. Congenital heart disease in adults. First of two parts. *N Engl J Med* 2000;342(4):256–263.

Chang AC, Hanley FL, Wernovsky G, et al. *Pediatric cardiac intensive care*. Baltimore: Williams & Wilkins, 1998:247–254.

Fyler DC. *Nadas' pediatric cardiology*. Philadelphia: Hanley and Belfur, 1992:535–556.

Jenkins NP, Ward C. Coarctation of the aorta: natural history and outcome after surgical treatment. *Q J Med* 1999;92(7):365–371.

Liberthson RR. Coarctation of the aorta: review of 234 patients and clarification of management problems. *Am J Cardiol* 1979;43:835–840.

McCrindle BW. Coarctation of the aorta. *Curr Opin Cardiol* 1999;14(5):448–452.

Morriss MJH, McNamara DG. Coarctation of the aorta and interrupted aortic arch. In: Gasson A Jr, Bricker JT, Fisher DJ, et al., eds. *The science and practice of pediatric cardiology*. Philadelphia: Lea & Febiger, 1990:1353–1381.

Author: Geoffrey Bird

Coccidioidomycosis

 Database

DEFINITION

Coccidioidomycosis is an infection caused by the dimorphic fungus *Coccidioides immitis*.

PATHOPHYSIOLOGY

- Inhalation of arthrospores from disturbed, arid soil is the major route of infection.
- Sixty percent of acute infections are subclinical (asymptomatic).
- Most patients have infection limited to a localized area of lung and hilar nodes after mounting an intense inflammatory response with granuloma formation.
- Dissemination occurs in a minority of patients (<1%) via lymphatic or hematologic spread.
- The course of illness is highly variable and dependent on host immune response and amount of exposure. HIV-infected patients and other patients with immunosuppression due to T-lymphocyte dysfunction (lymphoma, organ transplantation) are particularly susceptible to severe forms of pulmonary and extrapulmonary coccidioidomycosis.

EPIDEMIOLOGY

- *C. immitis* is found in the soil and is endemic in the southwestern United States (west Texas, New Mexico, Arizona, California), northern Mexico, and parts of South and Central America. Up to one third of the population in endemic areas has been infected.
- There is no person-to-person spread.
- The average incubation period is 10 to 16 days (range 1 to 4 weeks).
- Primary infection is most commonly seen in the summer and fall months.

COMPLICATIONS

- Localized complications of primary pulmonary infection are infrequent and include pleural effusions and pericarditis.
- Approximately 5% of lung infections result in residual pulmonary sequelae, usually nodules or abscess cavities. One third of these cavities spontaneously resolve within 2 years. Hemoptysis and rupture of the abscess, with formation of an empyema, are potential complications in patients with unresolved cavities.
- Risk factors for disseminated coccidioidomycosis include immunosuppression, male gender, extremes of age (neonates and elderly), African or Filipino descent, and pregnancy.

- Extrapulmonary dissemination usually develops within a year after the initial infection, but may appear much later if immunity is impaired (e.g., HIV infection, malignancy, immunosuppressive therapy).
- Hydrocephalus may occur with CNS involvement.

PROGNOSIS

- Most infections are asymptomatic (60%) or mild (35%) and self-limited.
- Primary infection of the lungs is usually self-limited, with a course of illness lasting 1 to 3 weeks; complications (see above) may prolong the course.
- Dissemination is infrequent (see above for risk factors). Morbidity and mortality have improved with use of antifungal therapy, but immunocompromised patients still have a poor prognosis after the development of disseminated infection. The mortality rate is 70% in HIV-infected patients with diffuse pulmonary coccidioidomycosis.
- Meningitis, untreated, is nearly always fatal within 2 years of diagnosis.

ASSOCIATED DISEASES

- *Primary pulmonary* infection is usually asymptomatic.
- *Symptomatic pulmonary infection* is characterized by cough, chest pain, and fever. Rash, myalgias, and arthralgias may be present. Chronic pulmonary lesions are rare in children (see Complications).
- Extrapulmonary dissemination is rare (<1%) and usually involves the skin, skeletal system, and CNS.
- Primary cutaneous coccidioidomycosis occurs by direct inoculation of the skin (trauma). A relatively painless, indurated nodule with occasional central ulceration develops at the site of injury. Regional lymphadenopathy is often present.
- Secondary cutaneous coccidioidomycosis occurs by hematogenous spread to the skin. Lesions range from superficial maculopapular lesions to verrucous ulcers. Lesions can occur anywhere but are most common along the nasolabial fold.
- Osteomyelitis is subacute or chronic and frequently involves more than one bone (40%). Common sites are the hands, feet, ribs, and vertebrae.
- Meningitis develops within 6 months of initial infection. Hydrocephalus is a common complication. CNS vasculitis and intracerebral abscesses are rare.

 Differential Diagnosis

- Other pulmonary mycoses (e.g., *Histoplasma capsulatum, Aspergillus fumigatus,* and *Blastomyces dermatitidis*)
- *Mycobacterium tuberculosis* (lung or CSF)
- *Mycoplasma pneumoniae*
- Influenza and other viral infections that present as bronchopneumonia

 Data Gathering

HISTORY

- Travel or residence in an endemic area is typical. Risk factors for disseminated infection should be sought.
- Fever, dry or productive cough, and pleuritic chest pain suggest pulmonary infection.
- Hemoptysis, although rare in children, is reported in 15% of adults with symptomatic pulmonary infection.
- Trauma precedes primary cutaneous disease.
- Myalgias, arthralgias, chills, night sweats, and anorexia suggest systemic dissemination.
- Headache, vomiting, and altered mental status suggest meningitis.

 Physical Examination

- Most infections (60%) are asymptomatic.
- Signs of pneumonia and pleural effusions are often present with symptomatic pulmonary infection.
- Indurated nodules and regional lymphadenopathy are seen with primary cutaneous infection.
- Erythematous maculopapular rash suggests secondary cutaneous involvement and is seen in 50% of symptomatic children. It is usually limited to the lower trunk and thighs, but may be diffuse.
- Erythema nodosum occurs later in the course of infection. Erythema nodosum correlates with the development of cell-mediated immunity and is associated with a low incidence of dissemination.
- Chorioretinal lesions are present in up to 40% of patients with disseminated disease.
- Stridor is present with infection of the subglottic tissues.
- Signs of increased intracranial pressure are seen with CNS infection. Classic signs of meningeal irritation are usually absent.

Coccidioidomycosis

Laboratory Aids

DIRECT EXAMINATION AND CULTURE

• Cytologic examination of bronchoalveolar fluid is diagnostic in only about one third of persons and is less sensitive than culture. Visualization of large spherules is possible in stained specimens of sputum, tracheal aspirates, urine, or tissue biopsy. They are rarely seen in CSF.
• The organisms can be detected by culture in experienced laboratories. The yield is highest from purulent material. The yield from other sources, such as pleural fluid, blood, and gastric aspirates is lower.

SKIN TESTING

• Coccidioidin or spherulin intradermal skin test is positive (delayed type hypersensitivity; >5 mm induration) within 2 weeks of symptom onset (range 2 days to 4 weeks). Recent conversion is diagnostic; reactivity persists after infection, thereby limiting its usefulness as a diagnostic test for acute infections.
• Skin tests are often negative in progressive or disseminated disease and in immunocompromised patients.

SEROLOGIC STUDIES

• *C. immitis*–specific IgM antibody is detectable in 75% of patients 1 to 3 weeks after symptom onset and usually is absent after 6 months. False-positive results are seen in 15% of patients with cystic fibrosis.
• IgG is detected by the complement fixation (CF) assay from serum or CSF. It is positive in 50% of patients at 4 weeks and 83% at 3 months following symptomatic primary infection. In general, higher titers reflect more extensive infection and rising CF antibody concentrations are associated with worsening disease.
• Hematologic findings include elevated ESR, leukocytosis, and, eosinophilia (in 10%).

OTHER STUDIES

• CSF findings in meningitis include hypoglycorrhachia and pleocytosis with mononuclear cell predominance.

RADIOLOGIC STUDIES

• Chest x-ray may reveal well-circumscribed nodules, lobar or patchy pulmonary infiltrates, pleural effusions, cavitary lesions, and hilar adenopathy.
• X-rays of involved bones may reveal lytic lesions. Scintigraphy of bone is more sensitive for the diagnosis of osteomyelitis.

Therapy

• Uncomplicated or minor disease is self-limited and should not be treated with antifungal therapy (>95% of cases).
• Treatment of uncomplicated respiratory infection is recommended for infants, pregnant women, and patients with continuous fever for >1 month, >10% weight loss, extensive or progressive pulmonary disease, negative skin test results, or immunodeficiency (either from HIV or as a result of immunosuppressive medications). Use either oral fluconazole or itraconazole for 3 to 6 months.
• Surgical debridement is used for localized and persistent lesions in bone and lung.
• Diffuse pneumonia: Start therapy with amphotericin B and replace with oral fluconazole or itraconazole when clinical improvement is demonstrated. The total length of therapy should be at least 1 year, and for patients with severe immunodeficiency, oral azole therapy should be continued as secondary prophylaxis.
• Disseminated infection, nonmeningeal: Treat with oral fluconazole or itraconazole. Amphotericin B is alternative therapy, especially if lesions worsen or are at critical locations, such as the vertebral column. The duration of therapy may be longer than for those with pneumonia only.
• Meningitis: Oral fluconazole is preferred (800–1,000 mg/day). Itraconazole (400–600 mg/day) is also effective. Therapy should be continued indefinitely.
• Intrathecal amphotericin B may be useful in CNS infections.

PREVENTION

Infection Control

• No special isolation or precautions for the hospitalized patient.
• Contaminated dressings from skin lesions should be handled and discarded with care.
• Preventive efforts are aimed at dust control and trials to eliminate organisms from soil.
• Avoidance of field activities or travel in highly endemic areas is recommended for children with a negative skin test.

PITFALLS

• Skin test in disseminated disease may be negative.
• Clinicians in endemic areas should maintain a high level of clinical suspicion.
• Diagnosis in nonendemic areas may be missed due to low clinical suspicion or missed travel history.

Common Questions and Answers

Q: Do all patients with symptomatic primary respiratory infection due to *C. immitis* require treatment?
A: No, since >95% of initial pulmonary infections are self-limited, treatment is not always required. Patients with concurrent risk factors (e.g., HIV infection, organ transplant, or high doses of corticosteroids) or evidence of unusually severe infections should always be treated. Factors suggesting increased severity of infection include weight loss of >10%, night sweats, infiltrates involving more than half of one lung or portions of both lungs, complement fixation antibody to *C. immitis* >1:16, and failure to develop dermal hypersensitivity of coccidioidal antigens.

Q: How should pregnant women with coccidioidomycosis be managed?
A: Diagnosis of primary infection during the third trimester of pregnancy or immediately in the postpartum period should raise consideration for treatment. During pregnancy, amphotericin B is the treatment of choice because fluconazole and other azole antifungals are likely teratogenic.

ICD-9-CM 114.9

BIBLIOGRAPHY

Dosanjh A, Theodore J, Pappagianis D. Probable false positive coccidioidal serologic results in patients with cystic fibrosis. *Pediatr Transplant* 1998;2:313–317.

Galgiani JN. *Coccidioides immitis*. In: Mandell GL, Bennett JE, Dolin R, eds. *Principles and practice of infectious diseases*, 5th ed. New York: Churchill Livingstone, 2000: 2746–2757.

Galgiani JN, Ampel NM, Catanzaro A, et al. Practice guidelines for the treatment of coccidioidomycosis. *Clin Infect Dis* 2000;30:658–661.

Galgiani JN, Catanzaro A, Cloud GA, et al. Comparison of oral fluconazole and itraconazole for progressive, nonmeningeal coccidioidomycosis: a randomized, double-blind trial. *Ann Intern Med* 2000;133: 676–686.

Shehab ZM. Coccidioidomycosis. In: Feigin RD, Cherry JD, eds. *Textbook of pediatric infectious diseases*, 4th ed. Philadelphia: WB Saunders, 1998:2314–2325.

Stevens DA. Coccidioidomycosis. *N Engl J Med* 1995;332:1077–1082.

Authors: Samir S. Shah
Molly (Martha) W. Stevens, 2nd edition

Colic

Database

DEFINITION

A poorly defined and incompletely understood state of prolonged or excessive crying in young infants who are otherwise well

- No standard definition of this phenomenon
- Best definition available: more than 3 hours a day of irritability, fussing, or crying on more than 3 days in any 1 week during the first 3 to 4 months of life in an infant who is otherwise healthy and well fed. Some add the criterion of a duration of 3 weeks or more.
- Crying is not qualitatively different, but quantitatively. It is considerably more than the average.

PATHOPHYSIOLOGY

- No single cause is always found.
- Typically, the problem lies in the interaction between factors in the infant and the environment.

—In the infant there is a normal physiologic or temperamental predisposition to be more sensitive, irritable, intense, or harder to soothe than average for the age.
—Parents generally have not yet learned how to read the infant's needs correctly and respond appropriately. They may be manipulating the infant in ways that increase rather than decrease the amount of crying.

- Colic generally occurs in the absence of any abnormality in the infant or the parents, but rather when the parents have not yet learned to interact harmoniously with the infant.
- There is no evidence that the bowel is at fault; flatus is more likely to be the result of the crying than the cause.
- Psychosocial risk factors, such as poor support for the mother and various stressors, are probably more common than in noncolicky infants, but they are not necessary.

—When such external factors present, they seem to exert their effects by reducing the parent's ability to respond appropriately to the infant.

- In the case of a physical problem in the infant, such as milk allergy, the prolonged crying is, by definition, not colic.

GENETICS

No genetic influence has been discovered, but it has not been investigated. Temperamental traits are known to be largely inherited, however.

EPIDEMIOLOGY

- Colic typically begins shortly after a baby comes home from a newborn nursery.
- It can last until 3 to 4 months of age if not successfully managed.
- If excessive crying lasts after 4 months, other diagnoses should be considered.

COMPLICATIONS

- Excessive crying does not turn into any other condition, but the factors that caused it may contribute to sleep problems and other behavioral concerns in the infant after the colic has gone.
- Parents are usually exasperated by it.
- The most serious outcome is that, due to parental exasperation, the infant may be physically abused.
- The infant is likely to be overfed.

PROGNOSIS

The long-term outcome of these infants has not been studied adequately. Predictions are hazardous. Temperamental predispositions may continue. The parents' perceptions of themselves and of the infant may be altered unfavorably.

Differential Diagnosis

- Normal crying. Average, normal infants cry about 2 hours a day at 2 weeks of age, just under 3 hours at 6 weeks, and then decrease to about 1 hour by 12 weeks. Normal crying, like colic, tends to occur predominantly in the evening.
- Prolonged or excessive crying from physical causes:

—Faulty feeding techniques: overfeeding or underfeeding and inadequate burping or sucking
—Physical problems in the infant: acute disorders such as otitis media, intestinal cramping with diarrhea, corneal abrasion, and incarcerated hernia; or chronic ones such as gastroesophageal reflux
—Cow's-milk allergy, lactose intolerance, or transmission of irritating substances such as caffeine via breast milk

Data Gathering

HISTORY

- Define symptoms: intensity, duration, and frequency of crying. Some parents complain more than others about the crying.
- Ask parents to describe a typical day.

—Description of a typical day or keeping a crying diary is helpful.
—This will give insights into the daily routine, feeding, rest, and interpretive skills of parents.

- Ask parents to describe and demonstrate their soothing techniques.
- Information on the baby's temperament can be obtained by asking the parents to describe the baby's typical reaction patterns.
- Medical history should include concerns about the pregnancy and the newborn period, anxieties related to parents' own experiences as children or with previous children, and the quality of family supports and other stressors.

Physical Examination

- No findings are expected if the child has colic. However, examination should always be performed to reassure both parents and physician.
- Attempts at management over the telephone without a physical examination are likely to be unsuccessful.

Laboratory Aids

No tests are indicated unless specifically suggested by history and physical examination.

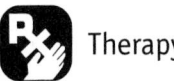

Therapy

• The most effective form of treatment is counseling, which should consist of these main points:

—*The infant is not sick.* Crying may be persistent, but there is no evidence of a physical problem. There is no proof the infant is having pain, just distress. Avoid iatrogenic problems caused by suggesting that something is wrong with the infant. The infant is probably just overaroused and tired.

—*Education about infant crying.* Parents need to know how much normal infants cry and how they vary in sensitivity, irritability, and soothability. The way parents react to their infants can affect the amount of crying. Parents often do not understand that a common reason for infant crying is fatigue and a need to be left alone.

—*The excessive crying can be reduced.* Parents have to learn to tune in more sensitively to infants' needs and to be more effectively responsive to them.

• Basic strategy: Soothe more, as by a pacifier, repetitive sound, or a hot water bottle, and stimulate less by decreasing the picking up, holding, and feeding the infant when it is not appropriate.

—A quiet environment, correction of any faulty feeding techniques, and a minimum of unnecessary handling without changing the composition of the feedings. Pertinent psychosocial issues should be dealt with.

• Expression of optimism by the pediatrician about the immediate outcome is justified and in itself improves chances of success. Simply saying that the colic will be gone by 3 to 4 months of age is not comforting and may be quite the opposite.
• Extra carrying does not help.
• Drugs, such as phenobarbital or diphenhydramine, are seldom necessary. Some observers have reported beneficial effects, when used for a week or two in conjunction with counseling, but these results have not as yet been subjected to double-blind studies. Simethicone has not been shown to be helpful.
• Formula changes are frequently attempted by physicians hoping for a simple solution, but they rarely are effective. Sometimes they seem to be helpful for a few days, only to cease being so a day or two later.
• Almost any procedure done with conviction is likely to be followed by a temporary reduction in crying because of the placebo effect.

Follow-Up

• It is important to keep in close touch with parents of an excessively fussy baby. Telephone contact every 2 to 3 days is essential until improvement. Reexamination is rarely needed.
• Standard pediatric textbooks state that colic usually goes away by itself by 3 to 4 months of age and that little can be done to change that pattern. However, several studies report that colic can be sharply reduced within 2 to 3 days if management such as that described above is used. Some infants take longer, but virtually all respond to suitable management.

PREVENTION

No study has yet demonstrated any certain way of preventing this prolonged or excessive crying. Two methods that are likely to be helpful are education of all parents about infant crying and soothing, and dealing with parental anxieties when they occur.

PITFALLS

Numerous pitfalls await the unprepared physician:

• Overdiagnosing the condition of the infant or caregiving inadequacies of parents
• Overtreatment of the infant with changes of feedings, medications, and various inappropriate procedures such as enemas and rectal manipulations. Despite the widely held, popular view that cow's-milk allergy is a principal reason for excessive crying, no study of acceptable double-blind design has demonstrated its occurrence in infants who are free of respiratory, gastrointestinal, or cutaneous manifestations of allergy.
• Unnecessary laboratory tests
• Colic is defined as a pattern of recurring episodes of crying. Other explanations should be carefully considered first for an acute bout of crying.

Common Questions and Answers

Q: What is wrong with my baby? What can we do to relieve the pain? Why is he/she so gassy? How do you know that it is not due to an allergy? Shouldn't we strengthen the formula? You mean it's all my fault? Will this ever stop? What will he/she be like later?
A: All the answers are to be found above.

ICD-9-CM 789.0

BIBLIOGRAPHY

Barr RG, Hopkins B, Green JA, eds. *Crying as a sign, a symptom and a signal*. London: MacKeith Press, 2000.

Carey WB. "Colic": prolonged or excessive crying in young infants. In: Levine MD, Carey WB, Crocker AC, eds. *Developmental-behavioral pediatrics*, 3rd ed. Philadelphia: WB Saunders, 1999.

Carey WB. The effectiveness of parent counseling in managing colic. *Pediatrics* 1994;94:333–334.

Lester BM, Barr RG, eds. *Colic and excessive crying*. 105th Ross Conference on Pediatric Research. Columbus, OH: Ross Products Division, Abbott Laboratories, 1997.

Wessel MA, Cobb JC, Jackson EB, et al. Paroxysmal fussing in infants, sometimes called "colic." *Pediatrics* 1954;14:421–434.

Author: William B. Carey

Common Variable Immunodeficiency

 Database

DEFINITION

Common variable immunodeficiency (CVID) is a heterogeneous immunodeficiency syndrome characterized by hypogammaglobulinemia, recurrent infections, and a wide spectrum of immunologic abnormalities, including autoimmune disease, inflammatory conditions, and the development of lymphomas.
It is a common primary immunodeficiency.
Other terminology for this disease includes:

- Acquired hypogammaglobulinemia
- Adult-onset hypogammaglobulinemia
- Dysgammaglobulinemia
- Common variable hypogammaglobulinemia

ETIOLOGY

- The primary immunologic defect(s) leading to this syndrome is (are) unknown, but B-cell defect is likely.
- Hypogammaglobulinemia is the main characteristic.
- Most patients have impaired immunoglobulin and specific antibody production despite normal B-lymphocyte numbers. An increased proportion of immature B cells is often present.
- Functional defects of both B and T lymphocytes occur.

GENETICS

- Some evidence for potential susceptibility locus on 6p21 (proximal part of MHC locus).
- Some families have a pattern consistent with autosomal-recessive inheritance.
- IgA deficiency more likely in offspring of parents with CVID (mothers more likely to transmit).

EPIDEMIOLOGY

- Incidence is estimated to be 1 in 25,000 to 1 in 66,000 in the general population.
- Can present at any age, but usually seen in the second to third decade of life. CVID has been described in patients as young as 6 months.
- Diagnosis is usually made several years after the onset of recurrent infections (pneumonia, sinusitis, otitis).
- A subgroup of children has been described in which the onset of disease was most often before 5 years of age. This group was characterized by a relapsing and remitting course in which autoimmune disease predominated.
- About 20–25% of patients with CVID have one or more autoimmune conditions at the time of diagnosis.

COMPLICATIONS

- Autoimmune disease in 20% of CVID patients. Most common are autoimmune hemolytic anemia (AHA) and idiopathic thrombocytopenia purpura (ITP).
- GI complications include chronic diarrhea, malabsorption, and weight loss. Inflammatory bowel disease and *Helicobacter pylori* infection have also been observed.
- Granulomatous infiltrations may mimic sarcoidosis.
- Lymphoproliferative disease: overall risk is 8% to 10%. The most common are lymphomas, usually non-Hodgkin lymphoma, well differentiated, mostly Epstein-Barr virus (EBV) negative.
- Chronic sinusitis and lung disease with abnormal pulmonary function tests (PFTs).
- Progressive decline in T-lymphocyte function

 Differential Diagnosis

- Other primary antibody-deficiency disorders: X-linked agammaglobulinemia and transient hypogammaglobulinemia of infancy
- Severe malabsorption with protein-losing enteropathy
- HIV infection
- Chronic lung disease: cystic fibrosis, immotile cilia syndrome, and α_1-antitrypsin deficiency
- Primary autoimmune diseases: immune thrombocytopenic purpura (ITP), autoimmune hemolytic anemia (AIHA), systemic lupus erythematosus (SLE), and thyroiditis

 Data Gathering

HISTORY

- Recurrent sinopulmonary infections, especially sinusitis and pneumonias, with encapsulated bacteria
- Autoimmune diseases such as AIHA, ITP, thyroid disease, and chronic active hepatitis
- Persistent diarrhea of infectious (e.g., *Giardia lamblia*) or noninfectious etiologies
- Severe or unusual viral infections with herpes simplex, cytomegalovirus (CMV), and varicella, such as pneumonitis, hepatitis, or encephalitis. Chronic meningoencephalitis can be seen with enteroviral infection.

 Physical Examination

- Evaluation should focus on the presence of infection.
- Thirty percent of patients will have lymphadenopathy and/or splenomegaly.

 Laboratory Aids

TESTS

- IgG, IgA, IgM, and IgE below age-appropriate norms
- CBC with differential: examine smear for evidence of hemolysis in AIHA.
- Autoimmune antibody screen: ANA, autoantibody panel
- Stool culture for bacteria and ova/parasites to evaluate chronic diarrhea
- Isohemagglutinins as well as functional antibody titers to bacterial antigens such as tetanus, diphtheria, and pneumococcus are usually low to absent.
- Spirometry may be helpful in following chronic lung disease.
- Mitogen/antigen stimulation studies will help assess lymphocyte function.
- T- and B-lymphocyte enumeration by flow cytometry
- Absent B lymphocytes suggests X-linked agammaglobulinemia (XLA) rather than CVID.
- Appropriate cultures based on site of infection

IMAGING

Chest and sinus x-ray studies/CT scans may be warranted for evaluation of chronic disease.

DIAGNOSTIC PROCEDURES

- GI endoscopy with biopsies for cases of idiopathic persistent diarrhea
- Lymph node biopsy in suspected malignancy

Therapy

- Appropriate antibiotics for acute infections. Prophylactic antibiotics may be helpful in chronic/recurrent infections.
- Monthly IV immunoglobulin (IVIG) replacement: nadir IgG levels should be greater than 300 mg/dL.
- Cautious use of corticosteroids may be necessary in the treatment of GI and autoimmune manifestations.

Follow-Up

- Close and frequent follow-up is warranted for patients with severe, recurrent symptoms. It may be as frequent as monthly, depending on symptoms.
- Signs and symptoms suggesting malignancy (e.g., persistent adenopathy in absence of infection, significant weight loss, or abdominal mass) should be evaluated expeditiously.

Common Questions and Answers

Q: What is the life expectancy of patients with the diagnosis of CVID?
A: Since the clinical presentations and symptoms are variable, it is difficult to predict the life expectancy in individual patients. The availability of IVIG, in addition to antibiotic therapy, has greatly improved the outlook for these patients. However, despite adequate therapy, a large percentage of patients with CVID have a progressive decline in immune function. Major morbidity and mortality usually result from the associated complications of malignancy, chronic lung disease, and severe autoimmune disease. Lymphoma is the major single cause of death. In one study, the mortality is estimated between 23% and 27% over a median follow-up of 7 years (0–25 years).

Q: Do children differ in their presentation compared with adults?
A: In a subgroup of children with CVID, autoimmune disease may be the major clinical problem rather than infections.

Q: Should patients with CVID receive live viral vaccines?
A: In general, patients receiving IVIG therapy do not require any vaccinations. Live viral vaccines should be avoided in these patients, especially if they have deteriorating immune function.

Q: Can CVID be diagnosed prenatally?
A: Since there are no clear genetic inheritance patterns, prenatal diagnosis is unavailable.

ICD-9-CM 279.06

BIBLIOGRAPHY

de Asis ML, Iqbal S, Sicklick M. Analysis of a family obtaining three members with common variable immunodeficiency. *Ann Allergy Asthma Immunol* 1996;76(6):527–529.

Conley ME, Park CL, Douglas SD. Childhood common variable immunodeficiency with autoimmune disease. *J Pediatr* 1986;916:915–922.

Cunningham-Rundles C. Common variable immunodeficiency. *Curr Allergy Asthma Rep* 2001;1:421–429.

Eisenstein EM, Sneller MC. Common variable immunodeficiency: diagnosis and management. *Ann Allergy* 1994;73:285–294.

Hausser C, et al. Common variable hypogammaglobulinemia in children. *Am J Dis Child* 1983;137:833–837.

Sneller MC, et al. New insights in common variable immunodeficiency. *Ann Intern Med* 1993;118:720–730.

Winkelstein JA, et al., eds. *Patient and family handbook for the primary immune deficiency diseases*, 2nd ed. Immune Deficiency Foundation, 1993.

Yocum MW, Kelso JM. Common variable immunodeficiency: the disorder and treatment. *Mayo Clin Proc* 1991;66:83–96.

Author: Elena Perez
Alex Yip, 2^(nd) edition

Complement Deficiency

 Database

DEFINITION

Complement consists of plasma and cell membrane proteins that function as cofactors in defense against pathogenic microbes and in the generation of many immunopathogenic disorders. Biologic actions include:

- Cytolysis: destruction of cells by disrupting cell membrane
- Opsonization of organisms, which facilitates phagocytosis
- Inflammation by generation of peptides, which can upregulate chemotaxis and can cause vasodilatation
- Clearance of immune complexes

PATHOPHYSIOLOGY

- Two pathways, the classic and the alternate, that converge on same terminal pathway—the membrane attack complex
- Primary or congenital deficiencies of complement
- Secondary deficiencies of complement
- Usually secondary to a consumptive or decreased productive state:

—Newborn state
—Malnutrition, anorexia nervosa
—Liver cirrhosis
—Reye syndrome
—Nephrotic syndrome

See the table Complement Deficiency and Related Clinical Problems.

GENETICS

- Deficiencies of either pathway are usually autosomal-recessive traits.
- Properdin deficiency is X-linked.
- Heterozygotes are usually phenotypically normal.

EPIDEMIOLOGY

Prevalence of known primary immunodeficiency is 1 per 100,000. Complement accounts for approximately 2% of all primary immunodeficiencies.

SYMPTOMS/COMPLICATIONS

Deficiencies can lead to:

- Recurrent infection
- Immune complex disease
- Autoimmunity

 Differential Diagnosis

Humoral deficits such as immunoglobulin deficiency or dysfunction; consumptive process such as sepsis

 Data Gathering

HISTORY

Indications for Evaluating Complement System

- SLE, juvenile rheumatoid arthritis (JRA), or other immune complex disease
- Recurrent pyogenic infections
- Second episode of bacteremia at any age
- Second episode of meningococcal meningitis or gonococcal arthritis
- Recurrent angioedema
- Pneumococcal bacteremia after infancy

Complement Deficiency and Related Clinical Problems

DEFICIENCY	CLINICAL MANIFESTATIONS
C2	Systemic lupus erythematosus (SLE), vasculitis, glomerulonephritis
C4	SLE, glomerulonephritis
C3	Glomerulonephritis, pyogenic infection, immune complex disease
C1(qrs)	SLE, pyogenic infections, hereditary angioedema
Properdin	Neisserial infections
Factor D	Neisserial infections
C5, C6, C7, C8	Disseminated neisserial infections

 Physical Examination

- Failure to thrive
- Scars from various infections
- Joint destruction

Laboratory Aids

- CH50: to assess integrity of classical pathway. It is the quantity of serum required to lyse 50% of an aliquot of antibody-sensitized sheep RBC. Handling of the specimen is paramount because complement components are thermolabile, and a common cause of an abnormal value is improper handling. Procedure may require use of dry ice.
- APH50: to assess integrity of alternate pathway
- C3, C4, and other individual components

Therapy

- Fresh-frozen plasma for acute severe infections
- Aggressive workup and management of infections
- Prophylactic antibiotics may be useful for recurrent infections.
- Immunization for pneumococci, *Haemophilus influenzae,* and *Neisseria meningitidis* for patient and household members
- Close monitoring for onset of autoimmune disease
- Study other family members for genetic counseling.

PITFALLS

- Special care is required for the proper handling of blood test to prevent falsely low values.
- Sometimes the complement cascade can be activated and consume the complement factor, leading to the improper diagnosis of a complement deficiency.

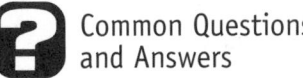

Common Questions and Answers

Q: How common are complement deficiencies?
A: Very uncommon. They account for 2% of all immunodeficiencies.

Q: When should I evaluate for a complement deficiency?
A: Any child with recurrent sinopulmonary infections or more than one episode of a Neisserial infection.

ICD-9-CM 279.3

BIBLIOGRAPHY

Berger M, Frank MM. The serum complement system. In: Stiehm ER, ed. *Immunologic disorders in infants and children*, 3rd ed. Philadelphia: WB Saunders, 1989:97–115.

Colten HR. Complement deficiences. *Annu Rev Immunol* 1992;10:809–834.

Ernst T, Spath PJ, Aebi C, et al. Screening for complement deficiency in bacterial meningitis. *Acta Paediatr* 1997;86(9):1009–1010.

Frank MM. Complement deficiencies. In: Stites DP, Terr AI, eds. *Basic and clinical immunology*. Norwalk, CT: Appleton & Lange, 1991:36–366.

Frank MM. Detection of complement in relation to disease. *J Allergy Clin Immunol* 1992;89:641–648.

Author: Michelle M. Klinek

Concussion

 Database

DEFINITION

Concussion is an alteration of consciousness secondary to head trauma, which may or may not involve a loss of consciousness. Symptoms of concussion can be categorized into early and late symptoms.

• Early symptoms most commonly include confusion and amnesia but also include headache, dizziness/vertigo, and nausea/vomiting, and are expected to resolve in minutes to hours.
• Late symptoms evolve over days to weeks after the injury and include persistent low-grade headache, poor attention, memory difficulties, easy fatigability, photo-/phonophobia, anxiety, and sleep disturbance. Late symptoms are most prominent after repeated concussive injury.

A grading scale has been established in sports medicine to determine the severity of injury:

• Grade 1: (a) transient confusion, (b) no loss of consciousness, (c) mental status changes resolve in less than 15 minutes.
• Grade 2: (a) transient confusion, (b) no loss of consciousness, (c) mental status changes longer than 15 minutes.
• Grade 3: any loss of consciousness, either brief or prolonged.

PATHOPHYSIOLOGY

The brain is buoyed in the cranium by cerebrospinal fluid (CSF), which surrounds it and acts as protective insulation from the hard bone. In acceleration-deceleration accidents the brain continues to experience forward momentum and slams against hard bone. The temporal and frontal lobes of the brain are particularly prone to injury by this mechanism because of their location inside the skull.
Depressed level of consciousness is thought to be the result of rotational stretch injury to the dorsal aspect of the brain stem where the reticular activating system lies. The injuries are usually mild and rarely visible on MRI scans.

EPIDEMIOLOGY

Concussions per 1,000 athlete exposures:

• Sports played with helmets

—Ice hockey 0.27
—Football 0.25
—Men's lacrosse 0.19
—Women's softball 0.11

• Sports played without helmets

—Men's soccer 0.25
—Women's soccer 0.24
—Field hockey 0.20
—Wrestling 0.20

COMPLICATIONS

• Concussion

—Confusion
—Alteration of consciousness
—Headaches and vomiting
—May also be symptoms of more serious complications of head injury.

• Serious head injury

—Contusion (brain bruise)
—Epidural bleed (from tearing of arteries that feed the membranous covering of the brain)
—Subdural bleed (tearing of the veins that drain blood from the brain)
—Intraparenchymal bleeds (bleeds in the brain tissue itself)

These may occur with or without fracturing the skull.

PROGNOSIS

• In general the prognosis is excellent but depends on the severity of the injury.
• The typical adult patient with a concussion will recover to baseline function in 6 to 12 weeks.
• Athletes and children usually recover in 48 hours. However, children with previous head injury, learning difficulties, or neurologic, psychiatric, or family problems may continue to show significant ongoing problems at 3 months.
• Chronic headaches, persistent difficulty with short- and long-term memory and episodic confusion are common sequelae of the cumulative damage that occurs with repeated concussive injuries.

 Data Gathering

HISTORY

Sideline Evaluation: Mental Status

Question: What happened?
Significance: Insight into injury

Question: Orientation?
Significance: Person, place, and time should be known if mental status is normal

Question: Concentration (backward digits/months)
Significance: A higher level test of brain function

Question: Memory?
Significance: If patient can recall five objects at 5 minutes, recent events, and the president's name, then memory is fine.

 Physical Examination

NEUROLOGIC EXAMINATION

• Cranial nerves: equally reactive pupils, conjugate eye movements, full visual fields, symmetric grimace, normal speech.
• Motor: moves all 4 extremities, normal and symmetric strength
• Sensory: intact and symmetric light touch, no paresthesias
• Coordination, agility: finger-to-nose-to-finger, rapid alternating movements (finger tapping, toe tapping), heel/toe/tandem gait
• Exertional provocative tests: 5 push-ups, 5 sit-ups, 5 knee bends, 40 yard sprint; look for change in exam

 Laboratory Aids

BLOOD

Blood tests are not useful for diagnosing concussion.

IMAGING

• Computed tomogram of the head (HCT) is essential to rule out intracranial bleeding in grade 3 concussions.
• Magnetic resonance imaging (MRI) may be necessary in patients experiencing long-term effects of repeated head injury.

Therapy

MEDICAL

Medical intervention is dependent on the grade of concussion. In athletic competition the following guidelines apply:

• Grade 1

—Remove from contest.
—Examine the patient immediately and at 5 minutes postinjury.
—The patient may return to the contest if all postconcussive symptoms clear within 15 minutes.
—A second grade 1 concussion in the same contest eliminates the player from competition that day. If asymptomatic for 1 week, the player may return to competition.

• Grade 2

—Remove from contest and disallow return to competition that day.
—Examine patient frequently for signs of evolving intracranial pathology (e.g., intracranial hemorrhage).
—Follow-up examination by a trained physician on the day after injury.
—Head CT or MRI should be performed in instances where the postconcussive symptoms persist or worsen after injury.
—The patient may return to competition if asymptomatic for 1 week and a physician has performed a neurologic examination.
—Following a second grade 2 concussion players should not return to play until they have been asymptomatic for at least 2 weeks.

• Grade 3

—Transport the injured player to the nearest emergency room by ambulance with cervical spine immobilization.
—A thorough neurologic examination should be performed with the appropriate neuroimaging (HCT or MRI).
—Hospitalization is indicated if any signs of pathology are detected on physical exam, on neuroimaging, or if the mental status remains abnormal.
—If the findings are normal at the time of initial medical evaluation, the patient may return home with explicit written instructions on observation.
—Neurologic status should be assessed daily until all symptoms have stabilized or resolved.
—Prolonged unconsciousness, persistent mental status alterations, worsening postconcussive symptoms, or abnormalities on neurologic examination require urgent neurosurgical evaluation or transfer to a trauma center.
—After brief (seconds) grade 3 concussions the patient may return to competition only after being asymptomatic for 1 week. After prolonged (minutes) grade 3 concussions the patient should be withheld from play for at least 2 asymptomatic weeks.

—Following a second grade 3 concussion, the patient should be withheld from play for at least 1 asymptomatic month.
—Neuroimaging is recommended for any postconcussive symptoms that persist or worsen for over 1 week.
—Any abnormality of neuroimaging consistent with brain swelling, contusion, or other intracranial pathology should result in termination of the athletic season and return to play in the future should be seriously discouraged.

SURGICAL

• Neurosurgical evaluation or transfer to a trauma center should be considered for symptoms of prolonged unconsciousness, persistent mental status alterations, worsening postconcussive symptoms, or abnormalities on neurologic examination.

Follow-Up

• Grade 1

—Examinations are required at 0 and 5 minutes after injury

• Grade 2

—Frequent examinations are required immediately after injury to assess for signs of evolving intracranial pathology (e.g., intracranial hemorrhages).
—Follow-up examination by a trained physician on the day following the injury.

• Grade 3

—A trained physician should see the patient on a daily basis until all symptoms have stabilized or resolved.
—Neuroimaging is recommended for any postconcussive symptoms that persist or worsen for over 1 week.

Signs to watch for:

• First 24 hours: worsening of headache, depression of mental status, increased confusion, photophobia, or blurred or double vision.
• First week: insidious worsening of symptoms (continued nausea and vomiting past first 24 hours, dizziness, photophobia, or blurred or double vision); emotional liability or mental status changes.

Prevention: Rest and fluids for the first 24 hours after injury. Avoid exertion and reinjury.

Common Questions and Answers

Q: Should athletes with two or more grade 3 concussions be allowed to resume team play?
A: Brain injury from concussions is cumulative; even with normal neuroimaging results the athlete should be discouraged from returning to the sport.

Q: What is second-impact syndrome?
A: Second-impact syndrome is the result of second concussion injury while an individual is still symptomatic from a first concussion. In this syndrome the athlete suffers malignant brain swelling as a result of vascular engorgement.

Q: What are some symptoms of postconcussion syndrome in children?
A: Hyperactivity, impulsivity, and aggressive behaviors were once thought to be the pediatric manifestations of postconcussive syndrome, but these were most likely premorbid conditions. In reality, children experience the same constellation of symptoms as adults, with depression, dizziness, headaches, and memory problems being the most common.

ICD-9-CM

850.1 Brief
850.2 Moderate
850.3 Prolonged

BIBLIOGRAPHY

Bijur P, Haslum M, et al. Cognitive outcomes of multiple mild head injuries in children. *J Dev Behav Pediatr* 1996;17(3):183–185.

Kelly JP, Rosenberg JH. Diagnosis and management of concussion in sports. *Neurology* 1997;48:575–580.

Kushner D. Mild traumatic brain injury: toward understanding manifestations and treatment. *Arch Intern Med* 1998;158(15):1617–1624.

McCrea M, Kelly JP, et al. Standardized assessment of concussion in football players. *Neurology* 1997;48:586–588.

Ponsford J, Willmott C, et al. Cognitive and behavioral outcome following mild traumatic head injury in children. *J Head Trauma Rehabil* 1999;14(4):360–372.

Report of the Quality Standards Subcommittee. Practice parameter: the management of concussion in sports. *Neurology* 1997;48:581–585.

Author: Daniel Licht

Condyloma (Condyloma Acuminata)

 Database

DEFINITION

Members of the Papovaviridae family, the human papillomaviruses cause warts of the skin and mucous membranes. Exophytic venereal warts or condylomata acuminata are caused by human papillomavirus (HPV) types 6 and 11. Virus types 16, 18, 31, 33, and 35 cause subclinical infection in the anogenital region and have been associated with genital carcinomas.

PATHOPHYSIOLOGY

- Transmission is primarily through sexual contact.
- It can also be acquired during the birth process.
- Transmission from nongenital sites occurs rarely.
- The incubation period ranges from 3 months to several years.
- The virus is trophic for epithelial cells and infects the basal layer of actively dividing cells.
- Infection results in koilocytosis, nuclear atypia, and so forth. These changes may progress to severe dysplasia and CIS (carcinoma in situ).

EPIDEMIOLOGY

- HPV infection is not a reportable disease.
- It is the most common viral STD.
- A minimum of 10% to 20% of sexually active women are infected with HPV.
- Genital warts and HPV infection are diseases of young adults 16 to 25 years of age.

PROGNOSIS

Therapy will not eradicate the virus; thus, HPV causes recurrent disease.

ASSOCIATED DISEASES

- Laryngeal papillomas
- Other sexually transmitted diseases

 Differential Diagnosis

- Condyloma lata
- Molluscum contagiosum
- Pink pearly papules or hypertrophic papillae of the penis
- Lipomas
- Fibromas
- Adenomas

 Data Gathering

HISTORY

- Most patients have no symptoms.
- Presence of warts
- Vaginal or urethral discharge, bleeding, local pain
- Dysuria
- Pruritus

 Physical Examination

- Warts appear as soft, sessile tumors with surfaces ranging from smooth to rough with many finger-like projections.
- HPV may also cause flat keratotic plaques that project only slightly with a hyperpigmented surface and are difficult to identify without the addition of acetic acid.
- Subclinical infection is common, causing many foci of epithelial hyperplasia invisible to the examiner.
- In males, infection is found on the penis, urethra, scrotum, perianal, and rectal area.
- In females, infection involves the vulva, vagina, cervix, perianal area, and rectum.
- Diagnosis is made by visual inspection of the anogenital region and/or Pap smear.

 Laboratory Aids

- Application of 3% to 5% acetic acid for 5 minutes causes lesions to appear white and thus more readily apparent and can help with the detection of cervical disease.
- Tissue specimens may show koilocytosis typical for HPV infection.
- Colposcopy aids the diagnosis of cervical lesions.
- No cultures are available currently, but PCR is commercially available.

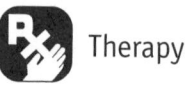 Therapy

- To date, no therapy exists that eradicates the virus. Recurrences are likely due to reinfection.
- All available therapies have equal efficacy in eradicating warts, ranging from 22% to 94%, with the significant rate of relapse of 25% within 3 months (see table Specific Therapies).

—Consider size, location, number of warts, previous treatment, and patient preference.
—Also consider patient preference, expense, and side effects.
—Patients with extensive lesions should be referred to physicians who routinely treat these lesions.

SURGICAL EXCISION

- External: see table
- Meatal: cryotherapy or podophyllin
- Anal: cryotherapy or TCA
- Vaginal: TCA
- Cervical: Refer to an expert.

PREVENTION

- Condom use may diminish transmission.
- Examine partners; treat those infected.

Specific Therapies

MEDICATION	PROCEDURE	SIDE EFFECT
Podofilox 0.5%	Apply with cotton swab b.i.d. for 3 days. After 4 days, repeat as necessary for four cycles total; should not exceed 0.5 mL/d.	Local
Imiquimod 5% cream	Patients apply at bedtime 3 times per week for up to 16 weeks. Wash off after 6–10 hours.	Local
Podophyllin 10%–25%	Applied by practitioner and then washed off 1–4 hours later. Dose is limited, 0.5 mL per treatment, to avoid systemic toxicity.	Local
Trichloroacetic acid (TCA) 80%–90%	Applied to warts directly, then talc is applied to remove unreacted acid. Washed off after 4 hours	Local
Laser surgical excision	Requires special equipment and training; often requires general anesthesia; controlled tissue destruction	Local

Condyloma (Condyloma Acuminata)

Follow-Up

- Follow up for expected course of disease.
- Scheduled follow-up is not necessary.
- Latent infection and recurrent disease are common.

Common Questions and Answers

Q: What treatment is indicated during pregnancy?
A: Most experts recommend surgical removal if necessary. Podophyllin is absolutely contraindicated.

Q: Should partners of patients with genital warts be referred for examination?
A: Recurrence is due to reactivation of the virus; reinfection plays no role. Therefore, partner examination is not necessary. However, the partner may benefit from treatment and counseling. The majority of partners have subclinical infection. It is important that female partners have routine Pap smears.

Q: Are genital warts in children always indicative of sexual abuse?
A: No. The HPV virus has an incubation period of many months. Thus, warts transmitted to infants at the time of birth may not become clinically apparent for 1 to 2 years. Whether the incubation period can be longer than this remains unknown. Thus, maternal history and, potentially, examination are both important factors. Children older than 2 years with anogenital warts should be carefully evaluated by experienced clinicians for child abuse. It is possible that caregivers may transmit the virus to children through close but nonsexual contact; thus, this history is also important in older children.

ICD-9-CM 078.0

BIBLIOGRAPHY

1998 guidelines for treatment of sexually transmitted disease. *MMWR* 1998;47(RR-1).

American Academy of Pediatrics. Papillomavirus. In: Pickering LK, ed. *2000 red book: report of the Committee on Infectious Diseases* , 25th ed. Elk Grove Village, IL: AAP, 2000.

Emans SJ, Goldstein DP. Human papillomavirus (HPV) and human immunodeficiency virus (HIV). In: Emans SJ, Goldstein DP, eds. *Pediatric and adolescent gynecology*, 3rd ed. Boston: Little, Brown, 1990:385–410.

Nienstein LS. *Adolescent health care, a practical guide*, 4th ed. Baltimore: Urban & Schwarzenberg, 2002.

Oriel D. Genital human papillomavirus infection. In: Holmes KK, Mardh P, Sparling PF, et al., eds. *Sexually transmitted diseases*, 2nd ed. New York: McGraw-Hill, 1990:433–441.

Author: Jane Lavelle

Congenital Hepatic Fibrosis

 Database

DEFINITION

Congenital hepatic fibrosis (CHF) is an inherited, noncirrhotic liver disease associated with cystic disease of the kidneys. Prominent clinical features include portal hypertension and an increased risk of ascending cholangitis. Liver biopsy shows the classic lesion of ductal plate malformation. Patients are typically divided into two groups: those presenting in infancy with severe renal disease (autosomal-recessive polycystic kidney disease, ARPKD) and those presenting later in childhood with symptoms of liver disease predominating. Mortality is high in the group presenting early, but if these patients survive, they later demonstrate hepatic lesions identical to those seen in CHF. The patients presenting in later childhood typically have more mild renal disease. The relationship of ARPKD to CHF is controversial, but many believe that these two developmental disorders of the liver and kidneys represent a single disease entity.

PATHOPHYSIOLOGY

- Ductal plate malformation is a characteristic histologic lesion of the liver, implying a disturbance of the normal formation of the bile ducts. Hallmarks on pathology include persistence of the ductal plate, or increased numbers of large and abnormally shaped duct elements, and increased amounts of noninflammatory fibrosis in the portal tracts. Hepatocytes and lobular architecture appear normal.
- Genetic etiology is currently unknown, but the gene locus has been identified. The developmental abnormalities involve the liver and kidneys, as well as, less commonly, the vasculature and the heart.
- Portal hypertension is thought to result from the fibrosis in the portal tracts, as well as, in some patients, from portal vein abnormalities.

 GENETICS

- Inheritance is autosomal recessive in most families.
- The gene causing ARPKD/CHF has not yet been identified, but the locus has been mapped to chromosome 6p21-p12.

EPIDEMIOLOGY

The incidence of ARPKD is 1 per 4,000 to 1 per 8,000 live births.

COMPLICATIONS

- Portal hypertension with hypersplenism and variceal bleeding
- Cholangitis
- Renal and/or hepatic failure
- Associated vascular anomalies in the liver and brain
- Increased risk of hepatocellular or cholangiocarcinoma
- May be associated with congenital heart disease
- Systemic hypertension due to renal involvement

 Differential Diagnosis

- Varies with presentation. Usually differential diagnosis is that of cirrhosis.
- Liver histology is highly characteristic.

Data Gathering

HISTORY

- CHF most commonly presents with hematemesis or melena, generally between the ages of 5 and 13 years.
- Patients may present with fever and jaundice (cholangitis) or, rarely, with signs of liver failure.
- The majority have hepatosplenomegaly or GI bleeding within the first decade.

Physical Examination

- Firm, enlarged liver with a prominent left lobe
- Splenomegaly
- Kidneys may be palpable.

Laboratory Aids

TESTS

Blood Tests

- Thrombocytopenia and leukopenia associated with hypersplenism
- Liver enzymes and bilirubin are typically normal, although transaminases may be mildly elevated in some patients.
- Usually hepatic synthetic functions (albumin, PT) are normal.
- May see elevated BUN and creatinine with renal involvement.

IMAGING

- Ultrasound with Doppler: increased echogenicity, splenomegaly, and evidence of portal hypertension
- Angiography: may show duplication of intrahepatic branches of the portal vein
- Renal ultrasound and IVP: minor abnormalities in up to 70% of Patients

LIVER BIOPSY

- Characteristic histology of ductal plate malformation
- Send specimen for bacterial culture.

Therapy

- Suspected cholangitis should be managed with liver biopsy, culture, and appropriate antibiotics. Some patients with chronic cholangitis may require antibiotic prophylaxis.
- Choleretic agents, including ursodeoxycholic acid, are used in bile stasis and refractory cholangitis.
- Prophylactic sclerotherapy provides relief from variceal hemorrhage in many cases.
- Portosystemic shunting may be required.
- Liver transplant may be indicated for chronic cholangitis, recurrent bleeding, or progressive hepatic disease.

Follow-Up

- Watch for recurrent upper gastrointestinal tract bleeding.
- Morbidity occurs mainly from portal hypertension and cholangitis.
- Mortality often results from ascending cholangitis associated with sepsis and hepatic failure.
- Those presenting in infancy may develop chronic renal failure.
- The prognosis is good when the disease presents in older children.

Common Questions and Answers

Q: Will other children of mine be affected?
A: Maybe. The inheritance pattern is autosomal recessive, with the possibility of an affected sibling being 1:4.

Q: Is my child at increased risk if he contracts viral hepatitis?
A: Yes, the underlying liver disease places these patients at increased risk. They should be immunized against hepatitis A and B.

Q: If my child has a fever, does she need to be seen by her doctor?
A: Yes. Patients with CHF who have fever without an obvious source should be evaluated for possible cholangitis, at least by obtaining a blood culture and liver enzymes.

ICD-9-CM 571.5

BIBLIOGRAPHY

Desmet VJ. Congenital diseases of the intrahepatic bile ducts: variations on the theme "ductal plate malformation." *Hepatology* 1992;16(4):1069–1083.

Mucher G, Becker J, Knapp M, et al. Fine mapping of the autosomal recessive polycystic kidney disease locus (PKHD1) and the genes MUT, RDS, CSNK2b, and GSTA1 at 6p21.1-p12. *Genomics* 1998;48(1):40–45.

Perisic VN. Long-term studies on congenital hepatic fibrosis in children. *Acta Paediatr* 1995;84:695–696.

Author: Andrew E. Mulberg

Congenital Hypothyroidism

 Database

DEFINITION

- Primary thyroid failure that is present at birth

PATHOPHYSIOLOGY

- Thyroid gland malformation

—Agenesis: absent thyroid gland
—Dysgenesis: ectopic (e.g., sublingual) or incorrectly formed (e.g., hemigland) thyroid

- Dyshormonogenesis

—Fifteen known defects of thyroxine (T_4) synthesis, including those in iodide transport and iodide organification

- Transient hypothyroidism

—Maternal ingestion of antithyroid drugs
—Transplacental transfer of maternal antithyroid antibodies (can be transient or permanent damage)
—Exposure to high levels of iodine (povidone) in neonatal period

GENETICS

- Dysgenesis is usually sporadic.

—Familial occurrence in 1%.
—Mutations have been found in the TSH-receptor gene and in the transcription factors PAX-8 and TTF-2.

- Dyshormonogenesis is inherited in an autosomal-recessive pattern. Most commonly:

—Chromosome 2p: Mutations in the thyroid peroxidase gene result in partial or complete loss of iodide organification function.
—Chromosome 19p: Mutations in the sodium-iodide symporter gene result in an inability to maintain the normal thyroid-to-plasma iodine concentration difference.

EPIDEMIOLOGY

- Worldwide, the incidence of congenital hypothyroidism is 1 in 3,000 to 4,000 births; in North America, it is 1 in 3,700.
- Male/female ratio is 1:2 to 3.
- Eighty percent dysgenesis or agenesis; 20% dyshormonogenesis
- Racial differences: prevalence in black infants about one-third that in whites.
- Higher prevalence of congenital hypo-thyroidism in low birth weight (<2,000 g) and macrosomic (≥4,500 g) babies.

COMPLICATIONS

- If untreated:

—Severe mental retardation (cretinism)
—Poor motor development
—Poor growth

- Children with hypothyroidism as part of hypopituitarism do not seem to be as significantly affected by their low thyroid hormone levels as do those with primary hypothyroidism.

PROGNOSIS

Excellent, if treatment is started within the first 4 weeks of life. Level of T_4 at birth is an important indicator of long-term sequelae.

 Differential Diagnosis

- Developmental

—Transient hypothyroxinemia in the first weeks of life in premature babies

- Metabolic

—Sick euthyroid syndrome in severely ill neonates

- Secondary or tertiary hypothyroidism

—Panhypopituitarism

- Genetic

—Thyroid-binding globulin (TBG) deficiency (X-linked recessive)

- Environmental

—Iodine exposure (e.g., delivery by cesarean section, surgery in the neonatal period)
—Maternal ingestion of antithyroid drugs

- Immunologic

—Transfer of maternal antithyroid and TSH-receptor blocking antibodies

 Data Gathering

Most children are diagnosed by the neonatal screening program.

- Five percent to 10% false-negative rate
- Neonatal screening protocols differ state to state (i.e., whether they screen T_4 levels, TSH levels, or both).
- Beware in severely ill neonates who are transferred from one unit or hospital to another that sending off the state screen is not overlooked! If missed by the state screening procedure, the findings below are seen within the first 2 months of life.

HISTORY

- Symptoms that may relate to hypothyroidism:

—Prolonged jaundice
—Poor feeding
—Constipation
—Sedate or placid child
—Poor linear growth

- Family history of thyroid disorders:

—Autoimmune thyroid disease
—Vague histories of "mild hypothyroidism" not requiring treatment are often found in families with TBG deficiency.

- Maternal medications
- Birth history
- Results of the newborn screen

 Physical Examination

- Signs that may relate to hypothyroidism:

—Hypothermia
—Large fontanelles (especially posterior) with wide cranial sutures
—Coarse facial features, including macroglossia
—Hoarse cry
—Hypotonia
—Delayed deep tendon reflex release
—Distended abdomen
—Umbilical hernia

- Examine for possible goiter; helpful tricks:

—Inspect the base of the tongue for an ectopic gland.
—While supporting the posterior neck and occiput, allow the infant's head to hang back over a parent's arm or examination table. This will extend the neck and allow better visualization of the anterior region.

 Laboratory Aids

TESTS

Neonatal Screening Program (Filter Card)

- Although methods vary from state to state, most screen for T_4 and then run TSH levels on the lowest tenth percentile of that day's T_4 values.
- Abnormal results on state screen should prompt *immediate* examination and confirmatory tests.

Confirmatory Tests

- Serum T_4 and TSH are preferable to a repeated filter screen, which may result in delayed diagnosis and treatment.
- If abnormalities in binding are suspected, also check TBG level and free T_4 level or triiodothyronine (T_3) resin uptake.
- Free T_4 level is the most sensitive indicator of secondary or tertiary hypothyroidism (hypopituitarism).

IMAGING

- ^{123}I or technetium thyroid scan will define gland anatomy (agenesis, dysgenesis, or ectopic gland).
- ^{123}I scan with perchlorate washout may also help to identify dyshormonogenesis (especially organification defects).
- ^{123}I scan must be obtained prior to the initiation of thyroxine replacement therapy. If this significantly delays the commencement of treatment, defer scanning until brain growth is complete (2 years of age), when a period off medication can be more safely pursued.

FALSE POSITIVES

- Blood specimens obtained before 48 hours of life may have "elevated" TSH as a result of the normal postnatal surge.
- TBG deficiency: total T_4 is low, but TSH is normal. Especially consider in males (X-linked).

 ## Therapy

DRUGS

- L-thyroxine

—10 to 15 μg/kg/d once a day. Titrate dose to keep T_4 in the upper range of normal.
—TSH levels may not come into the normal range for several weeks, even with good T_4 values.
—A minority of infants have variable pituitary-thyroid hormone resistance, with relatively elevated serum levels of TSH for their free T_4, that improves with age.

Duration

- Lifelong
- If medication is started without imaging studies and diagnosis is not clear-cut, can stop L-thyroxine following completion of brain growth (2–3 years of age). Reevaluate need for continued supplementation after a 6-week trial off.

DIET

- No restrictions
- Soy formulas may interfere with absorption of L-thyroxine.

 ## Follow-Up

WHEN TO EXPECT IMPROVEMENT

- Most children are asymptomatic at diagnosis.
- Parents may note an increase in activity, improvement in feeding, and increase in urination and bowel movements soon after starting treatment.

SIGNS TO WATCH FOR

Poor growth and low T_4 and elevated TSH values suggest poor compliance or undertreatment.

NEUROPSYCHOLOGICAL SEQUELAE

Although IQ scores are predominantly in the normal range, subtle impairments in language and motor skills and specific learning disabilities may occur despite early treatment. Neurocognitive evaluation and rehabilitation should be provided.

PITFALLS

- X-linked TBG deficiency: low total T_4, normal TSH, and normal free T_4. Diagnose with low TBG level or high T_3 resin uptake. No treatment is necessary!
- Panhypopituitarism: low T_4 and low or low-normal TSH (i.e., loss of the negative feedback loop). Screen with free T_4. Treat with L-thyroxine as would primary hypothyroidism, and investigate for other pituitary hormone deficiencies.

 ## Common Questions and Answers

Q: Will my child be retarded?
A: It depends on when the diagnosis was made and how quickly treatment was started. Some long-term studies have suggested an increase in learning disabilities when compared with siblings, even in patients treated within the first 4 weeks of life.

Q: What if I forget a dose?
A: Give it as soon as you remember. If it is the next day, give two doses.

Q: How do I give this medicine to my baby?
A: L-thyroxine is only available in tablet form. Crush the tablet between two spoons and dissolve the powder in a small amount of formula or breast milk, which you offer to the baby at the *start* of a feeding to ensure complete ingestion.

Q: Are there side effects from the medication?
A: None. The tablet contains only the hormone that your child's thyroid is not making. It is synthetically produced, so there are no infectious risks.

Q: Should the transient hypothyroxinemia of prematurity be treated with L-thyroxine?
A: Severe hypothyroxinemia in preterm infants has been associated with increased problems in neurologic and mental development later in childhood, but causality has not been established. A randomized, placebo-controlled, double-blind trial of thyroxine supplementation in 200 infants born before 30 weeks' gestation, revealed no improvement in mental, motor, or neurologic outcome at 2 years of age, though higher developmental testing was seen for those born before 27 weeks' gestation.

ICD-9-CM 243

BIBLIOGRAPHY

American Academy of Pediatrics AAP Section on Endocrinology and Committee on Genetics, and American Thyroid Association Committee on Public Health. Newborn screening for congenital hypothyroidism: recommended guidelines. *Pediatrics* 1993;91(6):1203–1210.

Bargagna S, Canepa G, Costagli C, et al. Neuropsychological follow-up in early-treated congenital hypothyroidism: a problem-oriented approach. *Thyroid* 2000;10:243–249.

Fisher DA. Hypothyroxinemia in premature infants: is thyroxine treatment necessary? *Thyroid* 1999;9:715–720.

Fisher DA, Schoen EJ, La Franchi S, et al. The hypothalamic-pituitary-thyroid negative feedback control axis in children with treated congenital hypothyroidism. *J Clin Endocrinol Metab* 2000;85:2722–2727.

Krude H, Biebermann H, Schnabel D, et al. Molecular pathogenesis of neonatal hypothyroidism. *Horm Res* 2000;53 (suppl 1):12–18.

LaFranchi S. Congenital hypothyroidism: etiologies, diagnosis, and management. *Thyroid* 1999;9:735–740.

Macchia PE, Felice MD, Lauro RD. Molecular genetics of congenital hypothyroidism. *Curr Opin Genet Dev* 1999;9:289–294.

Reuss ML, Paneth N, Pinto-Martin JA, et al. The relation of transient hypothyroxinemia in preterm infants to neurologic development at two years of age [editorial]. *N Engl J Med* 1996;334:821–827,857–858.

Rovet JF, Ehrlich R. Psychoeducational outcome in children with early-treated congenital hypothyroidism. *Pediatrics* 2000;105:515–522.

Van Vliet G. Neonatal hypothyroidism: treatment and outcome. *Thyroid* 1999;9:79–84.

Van Wassenaer AG, Kok JH, deVijlder JJM, et al. Effects of thyroxine supplementation on neurologic development in infants born at less than 30 weeks' gestation. *N Engl J Med* 1997;336:21–26.

Waller DK, Anderson JL, Lorey F, et al. Risk factors for congenital hypothyroidism: an investigation of infant's birth weight, ethnicity, and gender in California, 1990–1998. *Teratology* 2000;62:36–41.

Author: Adda Grimberg
Marta Satin-Smith, 2nd edition

Congestive Heart Failure

 Database

DEFINITION

Congestive heart failure (CHF) is the pathophysiologic state in which the heart is unable to pump sufficient blood to meet the metabolic demands of the body.

ETIOLOGY

- Excessive workload (volume and/or pressure) secondary to congenital heart disease (CHD) or acquired heart disease in the presence of normal myocardial function
- Normal workload in the presence of myocardial dysfunction

CAUSES

In Utero

- Arrhythmias: supraventricular or ventricular tachycardia, complete heart block (CHB)
- Volume overload: atrioventricular (AV) valve regurgitation or arteriovenous malformations (AVM)
- Primary myocardial disease: cardiomyopathy, myocarditis
- Anemia: Rh isoimmune disease, thalassemia, and twin-twin transfusion
- Premature closure of foramen ovale or ductus arteriosus

In Neonates

- Myocardial dysfunction: asphyxia, sepsis, myocarditis, hypoglycemia
- Pressure overload: left-sided obstructive lesions (e.g., aortic stenosis, coarctation of the aorta, hypoplastic left-heart syndrome)
- Volume overload: patent ductus arteriosus, truncus arteriosus, aortopulmonary window, total anomalous pulmonary venous return, AVM
- Arrhythmias: supraventricular or ventricular arrhythmias, CHB

In Infants

- Volume overload: left-to-right shunt physiology (e.g., patent ductus arteriosus, truncus arteriosus, aortopulmonary window, ventricular septal defect, common AV canal defect, total anomalous pulmonary venous return)
- Myocardial dysfunction: endocardial fibroelastosis, glycogen storage disease, myocarditis, Kawasaki syndrome, anomalous left coronary artery from pulmonary artery
- Secondary causes: renal disease, hypertension, hypothyroidism, sepsis
- Arrhythmias: supraventricular

—Ventricular tachycardia, complete heart block

- Pressure overload: coarctation of the aorta, residual aortic stenosis, subaortic membrane

In Childhood and Adolescence

- Unrepaired CHD with volume and/or pressure overload
- Repaired CHD with residual defects that result in volume and/or pressure overload
- Acquired heart disease: pericarditis, myocarditis, endocarditis, acute rheumatic fever
- Secondary causes: hypertension, thyrotoxicosis, chemotherapy (doxorubicin, radiation), sickle cell anemia, cor pulmonale, neuromuscular disease (e.g., Duchenne muscular dystrophy)

 Differential Diagnosis

- Respiratory disease
- Hypoalbuminemia
- Anemia
- Hypothyroidism
- Poisoning: parathion, salicylates
- Arrhythmias
- Viral myocarditis
- Syndromes: Marfan, Hurler, Noonan
- Sepsis

 Data Gathering

HISTORY

Infants and Neonates

- Prolonged feedings associated with tachypnea, retractions, and excessive perspiration
- Emesis, inadequate caloric intake, and failure to thrive
- Irritability with feeding and frequent respiratory infections

Childhood and Adolescence

- Exercise intolerance with exertional dyspnea
- Chronic cough, wheezing, orthopnea, fatigue, weakness, anorexia, nausea, and edema
- Weight loss secondary to anorexia and nausea
- Weight gain secondary to fluid retention

 Physical Examination

INFANTS AND NEONATES

- Tachycardia
- Gallop
- Tachypnea
- Wheezing
- Crackles
- Retractions
- Nasal flaring
- Grunting
- Hepatomegaly
- Splenomegaly
- Edema (periorbital)
- Cool and/or mottled extremities
- Poor capillary refill
- Weak pulses

CHILDHOOD AND ADOLESCENCE

- Tachycardia
- Gallop
- Tachypnea
- Cool and pale extremities, with cyanosis and poor capillary refill
- Jugular venous distension
- Wheezing ("cardiac asthma")
- Hepatomegaly
- Splenomegaly
- Edema (periorbital or peripheral)
- Pulsus alternans
- Pulsus paradoxus

Laboratory Aids

TESTS

CHEST X-RAY

Cardiomegaly, increased pulmonary vascular markings, hyperinflation, pleural effusion

Electrocardiography

- Abnormal P-waves and nonspecific ST-T wave changes
- May help in the diagnosis of a cardiac anomaly (e.g., anomalous left coronary, pericarditis, arrhythmia)

Echocardiography

- Rule out CHD
- Assessment of cardiac function

Cardiac Catheterization

- Delineation of cardiac hemodynamics and anatomy (used only in selected cases)
- Cardiac biopsy may be helpful in the diagnosis of myocarditis or cardiomyopathy
- Electrophysiologic study to delineate arrhythmia

Other Laboratory Findings

- Abnormalities in the pH, Pa_{O_2}, and Pa_{CO_2} may be seen.
- Hyponatremia, hypokalemia, and/or hypochloremia (secondary to chronic diuretic therapy)
- Anemia, leukocytosis, or leukopenia (e.g., viral myocarditis)
- Elevation of ESR (e.g., rheumatic fever or Kawasaki syndrome)
- Proteinuria, high urine specific gravity, microscopic hematuria

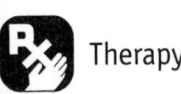

Therapy

TREATMENT OF UNDERLYING CAUSE

- Surgical palliation or correction of structural abnormality
- Medical therapy or radiofrequency ablation of arrhythmia
- Interventional cardiac catheterization (e.g., balloon dilation of aortic or pulmonary stenosis, coil embolization of patent ductus arteriosus, device closure of atrial septal defect)
- Medical treatment of endocarditis, myocarditis, anemia, or hypertension
- Administration of antiarrhythmic agents to the mother has been used to control congestive heart failure in the fetus secondary to an arrhythmia

MANAGEMENT

- General measures: restriction of physical activity, oxygen, tube feedings, increase in caloric content of feedings, limit of salt intake
- Pharmaceutical management

—Inotropic agents (digoxin, dopamine, dobutamine)
—Diuretics (loop diuretics: e.g., furosemide)
—Afterload reducing agents (angiotensin-converting enzyme inhibitors: e.g., captopril and enalapril)

- Heart and heart/lung transplantation in select cases

Follow-Up

Depends on the etiology and degree of CHF

PREVENTION

- Intravenous immunoglobulin (IVIG) for myocarditis
- Limited use of cardiac anthracycline drugs
- SBE prophylaxis to prevent infective endocarditis
- Controlling arrhythmias with pharmacotherapy, or
- Treatment of tachyarrhythmias with radiofrequency ablation and bradyarrhythmias (CHB) with pacing

PITFALLS

- In patients with CHF, on the basis of left-to-right shunting, spontaneous clinical improvement of CHF may indicate the development of pulmonary vascular disease.
- Patients with a VSD can develop a right ventricular muscle bundle even if the VSD spontaneously closes. Some patients may also develop a subaortic membrane or prolapse of a coronary cusp with subsequent aortic insufficiency.
- In ductal dependent lesions, an increase in Pa_{O_2} with metabolic acidosis may be secondary to increased pulmonary blood flow with decreased systemic blood flow.

Common Questions and Answers

Q: My child has a large ventricular septal defect and is on digoxin and Lasix. Should I take salt out of his diet?
A: No. Excessive salt restriction is not necessary. A no-added-salt diet is sufficient.

Q: What is the importance of tachycardia and bradycardia in heart failure?
A: Tachycardia limits diastolic filling time and may result in a decreased output. However, bradycardia may be poorly tolerated in patients with heart failure and a relatively fixed stroke volume who are dependent on heart rate to maintain an appropriate output.

ICD-9-CM 437.8

BIBLIOGRAPHY

Emmanoulides GC, Riemenscheider TA, Allen HD, et al., eds. In: Moss AJ, Adams FH, eds. *Heart disease in infants, children, and adolescents, including the fetus and the young adult,* 5th ed. Baltimore: Williams & Wilkins, 1995.

Fyler DC, ed. *Nadas' pediatric cardiology.* Philadelphia: Hanley & Belfus, 1992.

Garson A Jr, Bricker JT, Fisher DJ, et al., eds. In: *The science and practice of pediatric cardiology,* 2nd ed. Baltimore: Williams & Wilkins, 1998.

Moller JH, Hoffman JIE, eds. In: *Pediatric cardiovascular medicine,* 1st ed. New York: Churchill Livingstone, 2000.

Author: Hae-Rhi Lee

Conjunctivitis

 Database

DEFINITION

Conjunctivitis is an inflammatory process involving the mucous membrane of the eye or the conjunctiva that is manifested by redness and edema of the conjunctiva, frequently with associated discharge.

PATHOPHYSIOLOGY

Bacterial, viral, allergic, or toxic activation of the inflammatory response that causes dilation and exudation from conjunctival blood vessels or conjunctivitis.

PATHOLOGY

- Dilated conjunctival capillaries with leukocytic infiltration and edema of conjunctiva and substantia propria.
- In children with competent lymphocyte function (>3 months of age), visible conjunctival lymphoid follicles may develop.

GENETICS

There is no clear genetic profile.

EPIDEMIOLOGY

- Viral conjunctivitis is extremely common and highly contagious. Adenovirus is the common cause of viral conjunctivitis.
- Conjunctivitis is also caused by bacteria (staphylococci, streptococci, and *Haemophilus*) and serious complications of these are rare.
- Ophthalmia neonatorum or neonatal conjunctivitis remains a significant cause of blindness worldwide.
- *Chlamydia,* herpes simplex, and chemicals such as silver nitrate are other causes of conjunctivitis.

COMPLICATIONS

- Significant complications are extremely rare for common bacterial, viral, or allergic conjunctivitis.
- Blindness may result from untreated neonatal conjunctivitis.

 Differential Diagnosis

FOR NEONATAL CONJUNCTIVITIS

- Chemical conjunctivitis

—Noninfectious, mild, self-limited
—Result of silver nitrate or povidone iodine administration

- Birth trauma

—Unilateral, often with associated eyelid contusion
—History of forceps use or difficult delivery

- Congenital glaucoma

—Mild conjunctival redness, minimal discharge
—Look for enlarged eye, cloudy cornea, tearing, and photophobia

- Nasolacrimal duct obstruction

—Unilateral or bilateral discharge
—May be clear to mucopurulent with reflux from nasolacrimal sac
—The conjunctiva is usually white and nonerythematous

FOR ALL CONJUNCTIVITIS

- Preseptal cellulitis

—Early eyelid edema/erythema
—Looks like conjunctivitis, especially in young children, with the difficulty of examination
—Motility deficit, proptosis, decreased vision, afferent pupillary defect are consistent with orbital cellulitis.

- Keratitis

—Keratitis signifies corneal infection and may have associated conjunctivitis.
—Primary herpes keratitis is associated with vesicular eyelid rash and pain.
—Consult an ophthalmologist for specific treatment. Bacterial keratitis may be caused by staphylococci, streptococci, and *Pseudomonas*; Lyme spirochete; or vitamin A deficiency.

- Iritis

—Frequently unilateral, with or without a history of trauma
—Photophobia, decreased vision, and constant pain (except associated with juvenile rheumatoid arthritis)
—A contagious history is rare.
—Consult an ophthalmologist for full evaluation, including pupillary dilation.

 Data Gathering

HISTORY

- Type I ophthalmia neonatorum (<40–60 days of age)

—Acute perinatal conjunctivitis with purulent discharge.

- Type 2 ophthalmia neonatorum

—"Pink eye"
—Red, watery eyes with acute onset, with or without upper respiratory tract infection
—Often, history of similar infection in siblings or contacts
—Usually viral, occasionally bacterial, commonly self-limited

 Physical Examination

- Discharge ranges from clear, watery (often viral) to mucopurulent (often bacterial).
- Conjunctiva is inflamed and edematous.
- May have eyelid swelling or submandibular or preauricular lymphadenopathy.
- Cornea is clear.
- Vision, pupils, and motility are normal.
- Refer to an ophthalmologist if vesicular rash is present on eyelids and corneal changes are present, as the condition may be caused by herpes simplex.

 Laboratory Aids

TESTS

- Gram stain of discharge (always in ophthalmia neonatorum):

—Gonococcus (GC): gram-negative intracellular diplococcus
—Polymorphonuclear leukocytes without bacteria likely chemical (neonatal) or viral conjunctivitis
—*Chlamydia*: intracytoplasmic, paranuclear inclusion bodies on Gram stain and basophilic intracytoplasmic inclusion bodies, PMLs, and lymphocytes on Giemsa stain

- Culture

—Thayer-Martin test for GC
—Blood agar, chocolate agar for bacterial
—Viral cultures for herpesvirus and adenovirus are not clinically useful.
—*Chlamydia* culture techniques are not widely available.

- Immunofluorescence staining

—May be useful in identifying *Chlamydia* infection.

Therapy

- GC: Ceftriaxone, 28 to 50 mg/kg/d IV q8–12h and ocular irrigation followed by topical 0.5% erythromycin or 1.0% tetracycline ophthalmic ointments q.i.d. for 14 days. Also treat for *Chlamydia* as below.
- *Chlamydia*: Oral erythromycin syrup, 12.5 mg/kg/d in four doses for 14 days. Topical 0.5% erythromycin or 1.0% tetracycline ophthalmic ointment q.i.d. both eyes for 14 days above.
- Bacterial: Empiric antibiotic treatment if bacterial infection is suspected, including erythromycin 0.5%, tetracycline 1% ointment, or polymyxin B solution four times a day.
- Herpes simplex: Topical trifluorothymidine (viroptic solution), nine times a day for at least 14 days with or without systemic acyclovir (IV solution)
- Chemical

—Close observation only
—Self-limited

- Viral or epidemic keratoconjunctivitis

—Cool compresses
—No specific antiadenovirus treatment is available.

 Follow-Up

- Daily follow-up is necessary for GC, *Chlamydia*, and herpes simplex virus.
- For epidemic viral conjunctivitis, frequency is dictated by severity (daily to weekly).

NATURAL HISTORY

- GC conjunctivitis is benign if recognized early, and devastating if misdiagnosed or delayed.
- *Chlamydia* chronic infection leads to scarring and corneal opacity; chlamydial pneumonia develops in 20% of these patients.
- Viral: usually benign course, but may rarely lead to conjunctival scarring.
- HSV may lead to significant visual loss from recurrence and corneal scarring, even with proper therapy.

PITFALLS

- Failure to diagnose GC conjunctivitis may lead to corneal perforation.
- Recommending no follow-up routinely

—Follow atypical conjunctivitis closely until a more serious disease can be excluded.
—A nonresponsive or worsening condition needs ophthalmic consultation.

- Treating any red eye with steroids

—Activates or accelerates unrecognized HSV infection
—Chronic administration may raise intraocular pressure or cause cataracts.

- Chronic use of empiric broad-spectrum antibiotics for self-limited conjunctivitis promotes bacterial resistance.
- It is critical to rule out GC infection because of the destructive nature of eye disease and associated systemic infection.

 Common Questions and Answers

Q: Is conjunctivitis contagious?
A: All infectious conjunctivitis is contagious, but to varying degrees. Viral or epidemic keratoconjunctivitis (EKC) is the most contagious. Careful handling of secretions, tissues, towels, bed linens, and strict hand washing usually prevent spread. Wipe surfaces with isopropyl alcohol or dilute bleach to prevent recontamination. GC, *Chlamydia*, and HSV can be transmitted through infected discharge or secretions, but this is less common. The most common source is the infected birth canal.

Q: Should the patient with "pink eye" (non-GC, non-*Chlamydia*, non-HSV conjunctivitis) be treated with empiric antibiotics?
A: Empiric treatment with topical antibiotics does little harm except for sulfa-containing compounds. Antibiotic toxicity, including Stevens-Johnson reactions, can occur from sulfa antibiotics, and use of antibiotics long term promotes selection of resistant strains of bacteria. Empiric treatment also increases manipulation of the infected eye and thus increases the risk of spread.

Q: How long is the patient with "pink eye" (non-GC, non-*Chlamydia*, non-HSV conjunctivitis) contagious and when can the patient return to school?
A: The organism can be recovered from the eye for up 2 weeks after onset of symptoms, demonstrating that patients are infectious during this time. Practically, children should probably be kept out of school for at least 1 week.

ICD-9-CM 372.30

BIBLIOGRAPHY

Bell TA, Grayston JT, Krohn MA, et al., Eye Prophylaxis Study Group. Randomized trial of silver nitrate, erythromycin and no prophylaxis for the presence of conjunctivitis among newborns not at risk for gonococcal ophthalmitis. *Pediatrics* 1993;92:755–760.

Crede CSF. Reports from the obstetrical clinic in Leipzig: prevention of eye inflammation in the newborn. *Am J Dis Child* 1971;121:3–4.

Darougar S, Monnickendam MA, Woodland RM. Management and prevention of ocular viral and chlamydial infections. *Crit Rev Microbiol* 1989;16:369–418.

Isenberg SJ, Apt L, Yoshimori R, et al. The source of the conjunctival flora at birth and implications for neonatal prophylaxis. *Am J Ophthalmol* 1988;106:458–462.

Lepage P, Bogaerts J, Kestelyn P, et al. Single-dose cefoxamine intramuscularly cures gonococcal ophthalmia neonatorum. *Br J Ophthalmol* 1988;72:518–20.

Author: Brian J. R. Forbes

Constipation

Database

DEFINITION

Constipation is the passage of infrequent bowel movements, which may be hard or painful. It also may refer to a decrease in frequency of bowel movements compared with the patient's usual bowel pattern. Constipation can result in pain, rectal bleeding, and encopresis or soiling.

CAUSES

• Most patients will have idiopathic or functional constipation with no identifiable cause.

—There is usually an acute event followed by chronicity.

• Hard stools cause anal pain or a fissure, leading to intentional or subconscious withholding.

—This results in rectal dilatation, decreased sensation, shortening of the anal canal, decreased tone of the external anal sphincter, and leaking.

• Precipitating events include the following:

—Transition from breast milk to cow's milk in infants
—Power struggle in toddlers
—Refusal to use toilets outside the home
—Streptococcal infection of the anus and perianal area
—Transient viral illness (diarrhea followed by constipation)
—Zealous toilet training

• Constipation also can be caused by anatomic anomalies in the lower gastrointestinal (GI) tract, decreased propulsion, impaired rectal sensation (primary or secondary), or a functional outlet obstruction (muscular spastic levator ani or impaired relaxation of the puborectalis).
• Neurologic causes (abnormalities of the myenteric plexus, intestinal pseudo-obstruction, congenital aganglionosis, intestinal neuronal dysplasia), muscular diseases (familial and nonfamilial visceral myopathies), and lesions of the spinal cord result in loss of rectal tone and sensation and reduced anal closure, affecting the sacral reflex center (e.g., myelomeningocele, spina bifida occulta, tethered cord).
• Anatomic disorders of anus and rectum (stricture, stenosis, mass, ectopic anus, imperforate anus)
• Endocrine abnormalities (hypothyroidism), drugs, electrolyte Abnormalities

PATHOPHYSIOLOGY

• Retention of stool allows water to move out of stool, increasing size and firmness.
• Decreased motility will lead to retention of stool. See Causes.

GENETICS

• Often a family history of motility disturbances or constipation can be found.

COMPLICATIONS

• Anal fissures: Infrequent hard stools can cause a tear of the anal mucosa, causing pain and withholding.
• Encopresis: Chronic constipation leads to progressive rectal dilatation and decreased rectal sensation. Fecal impaction results with secondary soiling or encopresis.
• Intestinal obstruction manifests as vomiting, abdominal pain, and constipation, with abdominal x-ray (AXR) films showing intestinal obstruction and presence of large amounts of stool.
• Sigmoid volvulus: A chronically constipated child may present with symptoms of acute abdomen, fever, tender abdomen, and palpable mass. AXR shows obstruction in the colon. Barium enema may be both diagnostic as well as therapeutic by achieving reduction.

PROGNOSIS

• For functional constipation, the success rate is variable (45–90%), depending on the treatment and follow-up. Presence of abdominal pain at the time of presentation, close follow-up, and use of mineral oil are good prognostic factors. Presence of soiling, use of Senokot, and lack of follow-up were associated with failure and recurrences.

Differential Diagnosis

• Hirschsprung disease: congenital aganglionic megacolon (i.e., the absence of ganglion cells)
• Neuromuscular causes: tethered spinal cord
• Anal abnormalities: anteriorly displaced anus, ectopic anus, imperforate anus
• Endocrine abnormalities: hypothyroidism and hyperparathyroidism
• Electrolyte imbalance: hypokalemia, hyponatremia, hypomagnesemia, hypercalcemia
• Lead ingestion: can present with anemia, constipation, and abdominal pain
• Infant botulism: constipation, aphonia, and weakness in a previously well infant
• Chronic intestinal pseudo-obstruction syndrome: can present with abdominal distention, diarrhea, and constipation; usually a diagnosis of exclusion
• Abdominopelvic mass: can cause constipation by pressure (i.e., distended bladder or pelvic tumor)
• Surgical conditions: Malrotation, congenital intestinal bands, intestinal stenoses, acquired colonic strictures resulting from inflammatory bowel disease (IBD), necrotizing enterocolitis (NEC), pyloric stenosis
• Drugs: calcium supplements, barium, opiates; always get a careful drug history to avoid missing drug-related constipation.

Data Gathering

HISTORY

Question: What is the timing of the passage of meconium?
Significance: If it is delayed for more than 48 hours, consider Hirschsprung disease.

Question: Is the child able to pass a bowel movement unaided by a suppository or enema?
Significance: If rectal stimulation is required for passage of a bowel movement, think of Hirschsprung disease or habituation to rectal stimulation.

Question: What are the size, frequency, and consistency of bowel movements?
Significance: One to three normal (in size and consistency) painless bowel movements may be passed every 1 to 3 days. The size of bowel movements reflects the caliber of the colon.

Question: Does the child experience frequent urination, bed wetting, or urinary tract infections?
Significance: These are seen frequently with chronic constipation.

Question: Is there soiling?
Significance: Soiling occurs if the stool is impacted or with nerve damage involving the anus.

Question: Is there presence of rectal sensation?
Significance: Patients with long-standing constipation or withholding who develop a dilated rectum will often lose the sensation of rectal distention.

Question: Is there a history of painful bowel movements or rectal fissure?
Significance: This could be the cause of withholding secondary to fear of painful bowel movements.
Some children are too busy playing to take the time to have a bowel movement. Some children do not want to use the toilet in school because of hygiene issues.

Question: Is the child experiencing any stressful events (i.e., new sibling, death in family)?
Significance: Stress can precipitate stool withholding, leading to constipation.

Question: Does the child have an unsteady or clumsy gait?
Significance: This may suggest neuromuscular problems.

Question: Did the child experience difficult toilet training?
Significance: Some children with encopresis have a history of difficult toilet training.

Question: What is the diet history for fluid, milk, caffeine, and fiber intake?
Significance: Excessive amounts of milk (calcium) and caffeine may be constipating in some individuals. Diets low in fiber and fluid can cause constipation.

 ## Physical Examination

- General: Look for evidence of systemic illness.
- Abdomen: Abdominal distention (indicative of the presence of stool or gas), presence of stool masses (size, location), distended bladder and bowel sounds (may be decreased in intestinal pseudo-obstruction).
- Rectal examination: Perianal soiling, size and position of anus (may suggest imperforate or ectopic anus), presence of skin tags and fissures and perianal or anal erythema (streptococcal proctitis), or evidence of child abuse. On digital examination, assess anal tone (in functional constipation, anal tone is decreased; Hirschsprung disease may cause the anal canal to appear very long and tight), amount and consistency of stool, size of rectum (dilated rectum suggestive of chronic constipation; tight and empty anus suggestive of Hirschsprung disease), and presence of blood. Absence of anal wink suggests neurologic abnormalities.
- Neurologic examination: Check reflexes in the lower extremities.
- Back: Check for sacral dimple, tuft of hair (suggestive of underlying sacral abnormality), flat buttocks, and patulous anus.

PITFALLS

- "Grunting baby syndrome": Infants with this syndrome cry, scream, and draw up their legs during a bowel movement. They respond to rectal distention by contracting their pelvic floor. This is not constipation.
- Always rule out an organic cause for constipation.
- In patients with chronic medical conditions, look for medications that could cause constipation.

 ## Laboratory Aids

TESTS

- Abdominal x-ray study: Look for presence and location of stool and evidence of bowel obstruction.
- Barium enema: An unprepped study is useful to diagnose Hirschsprung disease. A prepped study is useful to diagnose a stricture. Most patients with constipation will not require this test.

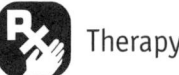 ## Therapy

TREATMENT OF FUNCTIONAL CONSTIPATION

- Clean-out: If patient is impacted, then a series of three to five enemas may be required, depending on the amount of retained stool. In general, children over 2 to 3 years of age require adult-size phosphate enemas. Younger children should get pediatric-size enemas. Oral or nasogastric polyethylene glycol solution (Go-Lytely) given over 6 to 8 hours may be used for clean-out. The solution is given until the effluent is clear. Patients who refuse to drink the above solution because of taste or volume, can be given Miralax (a similar medication) on a daily basis to achieve clean out over 1–2 weeks. Doses are given in 8 ounces of water once or twice a day.
- Stool softeners: Infants up to 1 year of age may be given dark Karo syrup or Maltsupex or barley malt (1 tsp/8 oz of formula) several times a day. Children over 1 year of age may get mineral oil, lactulose, or milk of magnesia several times a day to soften stools and make their passage easier. Patients who refuse to take liquid preparations may be given milk of magnesia (tablets) or lactulose (powder).
- Stimulant laxatives: Senokot may be used as a stimulant for short periods of time. Long-term use has been associated with colonic nerve damage in adults.
- Diet: A high-fiber diet is recommended (toddler: 10–12 g/d; school-aged: 12–16 g/d; adolescent: 16–20 g/d). In some patients, caffeine and excessive milk-product intake may be constipating. Milk intake should be limited to 16 ounces a day.
- Toilet sitting: regular toilet sitting twice a day for 10 minutes, preferably after meals, to help retrain the bowel
- Calendar: It is important to keep a record of stools, accidents, toilet sitting, and medication intake. It is hard for parents to remember details, which may be important in identifying causes of failure.
- Fluid intake: High fluid intake is important.
- Biofeedback is helpful in patients who fail conventional therapy and have the following abnormalities on anorectal manometry: decreased sensory threshold to rectal distention, paradoxical contraction of the external anal sphincter, and puborectalis muscle during simulated defecation.

TREATMENT OF COMPLICATIONS

- Encopresis (soiling or diarrhea): Abdominal tray film shows large amounts of stool in the colon, including a dilated rectum. Disimpaction or clean-out, followed by treatment of constipation, is recommended (see above).

- Intestinal obstruction: vomiting, abdominal pain, and constipation. AXR film shows intestinal obstruction. Make NPO, give IV fluids, and rule out an acute abdomen. Then give enemas and clear out stool from below. Never give oral laxatives or a polyethylene glycol solution in a case of obstruction.
- Sigmoid volvulus: chronically constipated child with symptoms of acute abdomen, fever, tender abdomen, and palpable mass. AXR shows obstruction in the colon. Barium enema may reveal a volvulus and may reduce the volvulus.

 ## Follow-Up

- Schedule regular visits to make sure therapy is maintained.
- Have parents call as soon as problems develop.
- Once patient is doing well, decrease the frequency of visits.
- Compliance and good follow-up are key to successful management of constipation.

PREVENTION

- Dietary measures: high-fiber diet, plenty of fluids, avoidance of excessive caffeine intake, plus regular physical activity.

 ## Common Questions and Answers

Q: When is constipation an emergency?
A: When intestinal obstruction, sigmoid volvulus, or Hirschsprung enterocolitis occur.

ICD-9-CM 564.0

BIBLIOGRAPHY

Abi-Hanna A, Lake AM. Constipation and encopresis in childhood. *Pediatr Rev* 1998;19(1):23–30; quiz 31.

Castoglia PT. Constipation in children. *J Pediatr Health Care* 2001;15(4):200–202.

Loening-Baucke V. Chronic constipation in children. *Gastroenterology* 1993;105:1557–1564.

Seth R, Heyman MB. Management of constipation and encopresis in infants and children. *Gastroenterol Clin North Am* 1994;23(4):621–636.

Staiano GS. The long term follow up of children with chronic idiopathic constipation. *Arch Dis Child* 1992;67:340.

Author: Maria R. Mascarenhas

Contact Dermatitis

 Database

DEFINITION

Contact dermatitis is an eczematous eruption that may result from two different processes: direct irritation to the skin or a delayed hypersensitivity reaction to a contact allergen. Diaper rash is a common form of contact dermatitis (see Diaper Rash).

PATHOPHYSIOLOGY

• Direct irritation to the skin commonly results from harsh soaps, acids, certain foods, saliva, urine, and feces. It does not involve an immunologic response.
• Allergic contact dermatitis first requires exposure and sensitization to an antigen. This sensitization phase lasts at least 5 to 7 days. Repeat exposure to allergens can lead to a dermatitis in 6 to 18 hours. Common allergens resulting in delayed hypersensitivity reactions include:

—Vinyl
—Cosmetics
—Preservatives
—Fragrances
—Dyes
—Metals (particularly nickel)
—Topical medications
—Plasticizers in rubber products
—Poison ivy

• Both processes result in nonspecific findings of intracellular edema and inflammation, indistinguishable from other forms of eczema

GENETICS

Susceptibility to certain contact allergens for delayed hypersensitivity is in part genetically determined. In the past, it was thought that atopic children had a decreased incidence of contact dermatitis; however, recent studies have suggested that it may actually be a predisposing factor.

EPIDEMIOLOGY

Contact dermatitis can occur at any age, although young infant skin is more easily irritated by a primary irritant, but seems to be less likely to develop a delayed hypersensitivity response. It is a very common problem; for example, most children develop diaper dermatitis (a form of contact dermatitis) before 1 year of age.

COMPLICATIONS

Generally, there are no long-term complications, although secondary bacterial infections may occur. Exposure to certain substances, such as latex, can cause reactions ranging from a mild contact dermatitis to life-threatening anaphylaxis.

PROGNOSIS

Complete resolution can be expected after elimination of further exposure to the allergen.

 Differential Diagnosis

• Infection

—Impetigo (bacterial infections of the skin, usually caused by *Staphylococcus* or *Streptococcus*, with characteristic yellow, crusty lesion)
—Scabies: Skin lesions from itching and topical therapies may resemble atopic dermatitis.

• Tumors

—Letterer-Siwe (or Langerhans cell histiocytosis) is an uncommon disease that may present with a rash that begins with a scaly erythematous eruption on the scalp, behind the ears, or in the intertriginous regions, and is differentiated by the presence of small reddish-brown papules or vesicles, purpuric lesions, hepatosplenomegaly, and adenopathy.

• Metabolic

—Acrodermatitis enteropathica (deficiency of zinc, in addition to vesiculobullous lesions of the hands and feet, and surrounding mouth and diaper areas). These patients have failure to thrive, diarrhea, alopecia, and frequent bacterial and candidal infections.

• Immunologic

—Atopic dermatitis usually affects infants at a later onset, is very pruritic, and is often accompanied by a family history of atopy.
—Seborrheic dermatitis: erythematous, scaly, or crusting lesions that are characteristically yellow or salmon-colored and greasy; it tends to involve the scalp, face, and postauricular and intertriginous areas.
—Nummular eczema, named for its characteristic "coin-like" lesions that develop on areas of dry skin, usually begins as tiny papules and vesicles.
—Psoriasis (known for its silvery adherent scale and underlying reddish hue); these lesions have well-delineated margins and usually affect the scalp, extensor surfaces, and genital regions. Guttate (teardrop-shaped) psoriasis is often seen after bacterial and viral infections (especially streptococcal).

 Data Gathering

HISTORY

• The diagnosis is made by determining contact of an offending allergen with the areas of skin involved.
• Obtaining the history of offending allergens is often difficult.
• Depending on the distribution of skin involved, particular allergens may be specifically asked about.
• Having the patient keep a diary may provide clues to other allergens as inciting agents.

 Physical Examination

• Diagnosis is determined by the recognition of the erythematous, edematous, and papular-vesicular eczematous lesions and the distribution of the rash.
• Contact dermatitis commonly shows sharp delimitation or bizarre asymmetric distributions. Rashes localized to one area and those with discrete borders and shapes suggest a contact dermatitis.
• Determining the distribution of the rash may give clues to the etiology. Areas where clothes contact the skin, such as wrist or waist, may suggest detergent or flame-retardant allergies; eruptions on the face and hands suggest a soap dermatitis. Rash on the earlobes or near the umbilicus suggest a nickel allergy. A perioral rash is often from older children repeated licking their lips.
• A perineal rash in an adolescence may be due to the use of perfumed creams or powders, feminine hygiene sprays, or douches. Vulvar skin is irritated more easily than thigh or vaginal skin. Feminine hygiene sprays can lead to either an irritant reaction from the propellant or an allergic contact reaction from perfumes in the spray.
• It is not often possible to differentiate irritant from allergic contact dermatitis by physical examination. Furthermore, pruritus may lead to scratching and secondary infection in both, further confusing the diagnosis. Chronic irritant and allergic dermatitis will result in lichenification (thickening) of the skin.

Laboratory Aids

TESTS

The patch test is the controlled exposure of an antigen to the skin. It should be used only to confirm a suspected allergen. After removal of the patch (generally 48 hours) the skin is examined 20 to 60 minutes later for erythema, papules, vesicles, or bullae.

PITFALLS

- The patch test may be falsely positive if done during times when the skin is acutely inflamed or if it is performed too closely to the previously existing dermatitis.
- The patch test is not well standardized. Most physicians now use adult concentrations of allergens on children.
- The patch test should not be done while the patient is on antihistamines.

 ## Therapy

- Mainstay therapy is eliminating future exposure to the irritant or allergen.
- Application of cool compresses and topical antipruritic lotions such as calamine can be helpful.
- Topical corticosteroids will help with the pruritus but will not accelerate resolution of the rash. For a short period (1–2 weeks), stronger fluorinated topical corticosteroids can be used in areas other than the face, axillae, and groin. The skin of these areas is thinner and more susceptible to side effects from the steroids. A weak steroid cream such as hydrocortisone should be used instead.
- The therapy should be continued for as long as the rash is present. Systemic antihistamines are generally not helpful for treating contact dermatitis.
- In severe cases, systemic corticosteroids may be used for a short course, with a tapering course to avoid a rebound of the dermatitis.
- Use of lotions with potential topical sensitizers, such as benzocaine and antihistamines, should be avoided.

 ## Follow-Up

- Follow-up depends on the severity of the dermatitis and elimination of continued exposure to the allergen.
- Generally, improvement is seen in 5 to 7 days.

PREVENTION

Prevention is the only approach to reduce the incidence of contact dermatitis. Desensitization, using systemic administration of the allergen, is not effective.

 ## Common Questions and Answers

Q: Can the fluid from blisters caused by poison ivy spread the rash to other parts of the body?
A: The contents of the vesicles and bullae from rhus dermatitis are not contagious. After exposure to poison ivy is eliminated, new lesions appear because of the variable sensitivity of various areas of the body to the allergen.

Q: After a picnic at the beach, my child had a red, blistering rash on his face. What was the cause?
A: An interesting contact dermatitis comes from exposure to plant psoralens and ultraviolet light (sunlight). Called phytophotodermatitis, the plants that can cause this include: lime and lemons, celery, dill, parsnip, and carrot juices.

It has been confused with child abuse in the past.

Q: Is it possible to avoid contact dermatitis using protective clothing or skin barrier creams?
A: Proper-fitting protective gloves and clothing are a highly effective means of decreasing irritant exposure. However, gloves permeable to irritants, such as organic solvents, may even increase the exposure to the irritant. Rubber gloves are contra-indicated in individuals with immediate and delayed type allergy to latex and rubber additives. The use of skin protective creams such as skin moisturizers, have not been well studied and have limited usefulness.

ICD-9-CM 692.9

BIBLIOGRAPHY

Beltrani VS, Beltrani VP. Contact dermatitis. *Ann Allergy Asthma Immunol* 1997;78:160–173.

Friedlander SF. Contact dermatitis. *Pediatr Rev* 1998;19:166–171.

Health tips. Allergic contact dermatitis. *Mayo Clin Health Lett* 2001;19(7):3.

Hurwitz S. *Clinical pediatric dermatology*, 2nd ed. Philadelphia: WB Saunders, 1993.

Author: Robert Kamei

Contraception

Database

DEFINITION
Contraception is the prevention of conception or pregnancy. The ideal contraceptive is 100% effective (prevents pregnancy over a 1-year period in all of 100 patients with typical use), has no side effects, can be easily reversed, and can be easily used by adolescents.

CLASSES OF CONTRACEPTIVES AND THEIR HEALTH BENEFITS
• Abstinence
—While many definitions of abstinence are commonly used, most adolescent care providers define it as refraining from vaginal or anal intercourse only.
—Advising teenagers to abstain from all forms of physical intimacy may be counterproductive in the context of the adolescent psychosocial development.
—Refusal, negotiation, and planning skills are necessary for the adolescent to successfully employ this method.
—Primary and secondary abstinence (or celibacy) are the most effective ways to prevent transmission of HIV, viral hepatitis, syphilis, *Neisseria gonorrhea,* and *Chlamydia trachomatis.*
• Barrier methods to sperm entry (male and female condoms, diaphragm)
—Male condoms are 88% effective with typical use. The female condom and diaphragm with spermicide are 75% and 85% effective, respectively.
—Proper use of the male and female condoms can prevent spread of HIV, viral hepatitis, syphilis, *N. gonorrhea,* and *C. trachomatis.* Condoms are not effective in preventing the acquisition of HSV or HPV.
• Spermicidal agents (foam, film, vaginal inserts)
—Nonoxynal-9 is the active agent most widely used.
—Seventy-nine percent effective in preventing pregnancy with typical use.
—Reduced transmission of *C. trachomatis* and *N. gonorrhea.*
—Spermicides used with condoms will increase overall efficacy to 93% with typical use.
• Hormonal agents [oral contraceptives (OCPs), Depo-Provera, and emergency contraception]
—Three categories of OCPs include fixed-dose combination pills, combination phasic preparations, and the progestin-only mini-pill.
—Fixed-dose combination pills and combination phasic preparations contain estrogen *and* a steady or varying dose of progestin, respectively.
—Estrogen/progestin combined OCPs are 94% to 97% effective in preventing pregnancy with typical use (99.9% effective with perfect use).
—Estrogen/progestin combined OCPs have been shown to reduce the incidence of endometrial and ovarian cancers after as little as 3 months of use, protect against salpingitis

(PID) and subsequent ectopic pregnancies, and decrease incidence of benign breast disease and dysmenorrhea, and are effectively used to treat problems such as dysfunctional uterine bleeding and polycystic ovary syndrome.
—The progestin-only mini-pill and Depo-Provera contain progesterone only.
—Progestin-only methods are an option when estrogen-containing preparations are contraindicated (see Complications).
—The mini-pill and Depo-Provera are 99.7% effective in preventing pregnancy.
—An additional benefit of Depo-Provera is that it requires little maintenance on the part of the teenaged girl.
—Emergency contraception, also called postcoital contraception, is a safe method of contraception that employs either combination or progestin-only OCPs.
—Combination pills, containing estrogen and progestin, can reduce the risk of pregnancy by 74% after unprotected intercourse, if taken in correct doses within 72 hours.
—Mechanisms of action include disruption of ovulation, impairment of the endometrium to prevent implantation, and possibly alteration of sperm or ova transport.
• Intrauterine devices, Norplant, tubal ligation, vasectomy, withdrawal, and biofeedback: not currently recommended for the vast majority of teenagers because of increased side effects, irreversibility, high failure rates, or difficulty to maintain.

PATHOPHYSIOLOGY
• The spermicides, nonoxynol-9 and octoxynol-9, act by destroying sperm-cell membranes.
• Most spermicide preparations contain an inert base (foam, cream, or jelly) to support the spermicidal agent and provide a barrier to sperm entry.
• Hormonal therapy suppresses ovulation by directly decreasing release of GnRH from the hypothalamus, and FSH and LH from the pituitary.
• Progesterone causes thickening of the cervical mucus, thinning of the endometrium, and decreased tubal motility.

COMPLICATIONS
Barrier Methods
• Latex allergy: Patients may use polyurethane rather than latex condoms.
• Breakage or permeability: Oil-based lubricants and most intravaginal medications used with latex condoms will increase the risks of these complications. Animal skin condoms are permeable to viral pathogens.
• Irritation, urinary tract infections, and toxic shock syndrome (if left in place longer than 24 hours) may be seen with diaphragm use.

Spermicides
• Local irritation or allergic reaction

Hormonal Contraceptives
• Mortality from gynecologic and related causes of 15- to 19-year-olds was 7.0 (per 100,000 women per year) if no fertility control measures were used, 0.3 in

nonsmoking OCP users, and 2.2 in smoking OCP users.
• Minor side effects of combination OCPs include menstrual spotting, nausea, breast changes, fluid retention, leukorrhea, minor headache, and depression.
• Thromboembolic events and liver disease are extremely rare in nonsmoking adolescents using estrogen-containing OCPs. Patients experiencing severe and sudden head, chest, abdominal, or leg pain, sudden change in vision, severe depression, and jaundice should contact their health provider immediately.
• Contraindications to combination OCPs include history of thromboembolic event, structural heart disease, breast cancer, pregnancy, liver problems, migraine headaches, prolonged immobilization, or severe hypertension. Caution should be taken when prescribing combination OCPs to adolescents with undiagnosed abnormal uterine bleeding, less than 3 weeks postpartum, use of drugs that affect liver enzymes, and gallbladder disease.
• Minor side effects of progestin only methods include weight gain, rapid hair turnover, and menstrual irregularities.
• Nausea and/or vomiting occur in most patients using emergency contraception or "doubling up" on OCPs.
• Prognosis: Poor in teenagers. Within 3 months of OCP use, only 44% to 45% of adolescent patients remain compliant. After 1 year, only 33% are compliant.

Data Gathering

HISTORY
General considerations in method selection include the following:
• What is the teen's sexual history?
• Is sexual activity spontaneous or planned?
• Does the patient feel that she/he can be compliant with a daily pill or barrier methods?
• Does the patient require absolute confidentiality?
• Is the patient comfortable touching genitals?
• Does the patient have open communication with the partner?
• Does the patient desire pregnancy? Does the partner?

Physical Examination

• Obtain baseline weight and blood pressure.
• It is not absolutely necessary to perform a pelvic examination on young women initiating hormonal contraception. Biannual screening for sexually transmitted diseases (STDs) and yearly Papanicolaou smears ideally occur with any sexually active woman.

Laboratory Aids

- Pregnancy test prior to initiating hormonal contraceptives
- Lipid profile if there is a family history of sudden death or cardiovascular disease

Therapy

BARRIER METHODS
Trained personnel can teach the proper technique for application of the diaphragm, and male and female condoms.

SPERMICIDES
- These must be inserted near the time of intercourse; some formulations require 10 to 15 minutes for activation, and most have an unpleasant taste.
- Trained office personnel can teach the proper technique for insertion.

ORAL CONTRACEPTIVES
- OCP monthly packages contain 3 weeks of hormone, followed by 1 week of placebo.
- Menstruation begins after 2 or 3 days of placebo.
- OCPs are taken as a daily pill, preferably at the same time every day (at night with food, to minimize nausea).
- OCPs are usually started on the first Sunday after the menstrual period begins.
- Instructions for missed pills should be explained and given to all adolescents initiating OCPs.
- OCPs may not offer protection during the first cycle; therefore, a backup barrier method should be used.
- Fertility returns, on average, 2 to 3 months after discontinuation. One percent to 2% of patients will experience a delay in fertility for up to 1 year.

OTHER HORMONAL AGENTS
- Depo-Provera is given intramuscularly in the deltoid or gluteus maximus.
—Each shot has a 3-month duration, with subsequent shots occurring every 12 weeks.
—The initial shot should be given within 5 days after the start of the last menstrual period.
—Depo-Provera offers contraceptive protection immediately.
—Fertility (and ovulatory cycles) should return within 6 months of the last injection.
- Since this was revised, two new hormonal formulations are now marketed: 1) injectable estrogen/progesterone, and 2) estrogen/progesterone patch. Their efficacy in adolescents has yet to be determined.

EMERGENCY CONTRACEPTION
- The Yuzpe regimen is safe and well studied. It consists of two fixed-dose combination pills, containing at least 35 μg of estrogen each, taken within 72 hours of unprotected intercourse. This is followed by two additional pills in 12 hours.

- This dose of estrogen will almost always cause nausea and vomiting; therefore, pretreatment with an antiemetic is recommended.
- The FDA has approved two prepackaged preparations: Preven (similar to Yuzpe regimen) and Plan B (progestin only).

DRUG INTERACTIONS
- Drugs that activate the cytochrome P-450 enzyme will diminish the efficacy of hormonal contraceptives. This is of greatest concern with low-dose preparations and can be remedied by using higher doses.
- Drugs that diminish hormonal contraceptive effects include phenobarbital, carbamazepine, primidone, rifampin, griseofulvin, and tetracyclines (including doxycycline). Hormonal contraceptives can increase levels of phenytoins, benzodiazepines, antidepressants, corticosteroids, beta-blockers, theophylline, and alcohol. Hormonal contraceptives can decrease the efficacy of acetaminophen, oral anticoagulants, hypoglycemics, and methyldopa.
- Practitioners should refer to the *Physicians' Desk Reference* for any question about drug interactions.

Follow-Up

- Patients using hormonal contraceptives should be seen within 6 weeks to 3 months of initiation to evaluate compliance and side effects.
- Blood pressure should be monitored at every visit.

PREVENTION
- Inform patients that only male and female condoms offer some protection from HIV, hepatitis B, gonorrheal, chlamydial, or trichomonal infection. They offer only limited protection from HPV or HSV, which are transmitted through skin to skin contact.
- Encourage the consistent use of latex condoms.
- Patients using OCPs must be strongly encouraged to cease tobacco use. Methods of treating nicotine dependence should be employed if indicated.

PITFALLS
- Contraceptive use may lead to patients discontinuing use of condoms. Providers should emphasize at every visit that only condoms protect against *most* STDs.
- Practitioners who are reluctant to use of contraceptives in adolescents should balance the risks of pregnancy with that of the contraceptive method. OCPs are among the most extensively studied and safest medications prescribed for adolescents.

Common Questions and Answers

Q: My patient asks for confidentiality regarding contraception. Should I give it to her?
A: Yes, teenagers have the right to confidentiality regarding contraception and treatment of STDs. It may be in the patient's best interest to have a caring adult involved. Which adult and how he/she is involved should be negotiated with the adolescent.

Q: The FDA recently approved mifepristone (Mifeprex) for use in the United States. Is it safe to use in adolescents?
A: Mifepristone, commonly known as RU486, is used to end an early pregnancy. Therefore, it is not a contraceptive as it does not prevent pregnancy. No age restrictions were described by the FDA; however, as an abortifacient, the use of Mifeprex is subject to state-by-state parental notification or consent statutes.

Q: What should I tell my patient if she misses a dose of her oral contraceptive?
A: If she has missed one pill, she should take it as soon as she remembers; then take the next pill at the regular time. If she has missed two doses, she should take two when she remembers, and then two the next day. She should use a backup method during the cycle in which she had to "double up." If she has missed three or more pills, she will probably menstruate. After discarding the last pack, she should start a new pack on the first Sunday after the start of her next period. She is not protected during the remainder of this cycle.

ICD-9-CM
Family planning advice V025.09
Oral prescription V025.01
Other agents V025.02

BIBLIOGRAPHY
Glasier A. Emergency postcoital contraception. *N Engl J Med* 1997;337(15):1058–1064.

Hatcher RA, Trussell J, Stewart F, et al. *Contraceptive technology*, 17th ed. New York: Ardent Media, 1998.

Nelson A, Neinstein LS. Oral contraceptives. In: Neinstein LS, ed. *Adolescent health care: a practical guide*, 3rd ed. Baltimore: Williams & Wilkins, 1996:695.

Polaneczky M. Adolescent contraception. *Opin Obstet Gynecol* 1998;10(3):213–219.

Trussell J, Rodriguez G, Ellertson C. New estimates of the effectiveness of the Yuzpe regimen of emergency contraception. Contraception 1998;57(6):363–369.

Author: Jonathan R. Pletcher

Cor Pulmonale

 ## Database

DEFINITION

Cor pulmonale is right ventricular (RV) failure secondary to an altered cardiopulmonary process, resulting in excessive pulmonary artery pressure and resistance (PVR). Cor pulmonale is not the result of a primary congenital heart defect.

CAUSES

- Parenchymal lung disease (most common)
- Chronic obstructive pulmonary disease

—Cystic fibrosis
—Asthma

- Restrictive lung disease

—Infectious pulmonary toxins
—Pulmonary fibrosis
—Bronchopulmonary dysplasia (combined)

- Upper airway diseases
- Tonsillar/adenoidal hypertrophy
- Syndromes (Down, Treacher Collins)
- Neuromuscular disorders
- Duchenne muscular dystrophy
- Pulmonary vascular abnormalities
- Collagen vascular diseases
- Pulmonary veno-occlusive diseases
- Pulmonary thromboembolism
- Chest wall deformities
- Primary pulmonary hypertension (PPHN)

PATHOPHYSIOLOGY

Chronic hypoxia is the principal factor, resulting in a cascade of endothelial dysfunction with pulmonary vasoconstriction, followed by the development of pulmonary hypertension. A variety of vasoactive mediators may be responsible for the effect on vasomotor tone. Alveolar hypoventilation, hypoxemia, hypercarbia, and acidemia all result in increased RV afterload and decreased RV systolic function.

EPIDEMIOLOGY

Cor pulmonale may be found at any age, but is typically due to a long-standing pulmonary process. PPHN is most often diagnosed in the second or third decade of life. There is a female predominance, and it is often diagnosed during pregnancy.

COMPLICATIONS

Aside from the underlying lung process, the chronic hypoxia results in anemia, polycythemia-decreased systemic oxygen delivery, and RV failure secondary to the inability of the RV to handle the excessive afterload.

PROGNOSIS

Patients with reversible lung disease usually have a better prognosis. Patients with cor pulmonale are at risk for sudden death because of the inability to augment cardiac output with exercise secondary to a relatively fixed PVR. Numerous medical therapies and lung transplantation may improve long-term survival.

 ## Differential Diagnosis

Congenital heart disease with pulmonary hypertension and right-to-left shunting (Eisenmenger syndrome) should be ruled out.

 ## Data Gathering

HISTORY

- Fatigue
- Dizziness
- Syncope
- Exercise intolerance
- Chest pain (secondary to RV ischemia)
- Palpitations
- Hemoptysis

 ## Physical Examination

- Tachycardia
- Parasternal RV impulse
- Cyanosis may be evident.
- Hepatomegaly, jugular venous distention, peripheral edema
- A loud, narrowly split or single second heart sound (P_2), gallop, holosystolic murmur right of the sternum (tricuspid regurgitation), and diastolic murmur at the left upper sternal border (pulmonary insufficiency)

 ## Laboratory Aids

NONSPECIFIC TESTS

- ECG: may show right atrial enlargement, RV hypertrophy, and T-wave inversion
- Decreased Pao_2, increased $Paco_2$, and a compensatory metabolic alkalosis
- Polycythemia may be consistent with chronic hypoxemia.
- Chest x-ray: cardiomegaly from RV dilation and main pulmonary artery enlargement
- Echocardiography: RV dilation, hypertrophy, pulmonic insufficiency, and if tricuspid regurgitation is present, an RV pressure can be estimated.
- Cardiac catheterization, while invasive, remains the gold standard.

Therapy

- The primary goal is reduction of the abnormally elevated pulmonary artery pressure and the RV workload.
- If at all possible, address the primary etiology (i.e., tonsillectomy/adenoidectomy in a patient with obstructive upper airway disease).
- Oxygen (nocturnal oxygen)
- Diuretics (if pulmonary congestion)
- Bronchodilators (theophylline)
- Digoxin (may improve RV contractility)
- Anticoagulants
- Pulmonary vasodilators

—Nitric oxide
—Prostacyclin
—Calcium channel blockers

- Atrial septostomy (in select cases, may improve cardiac output at the expense of hypoxemia)
- Lung or heart-lung transplantation

 ## Follow-Up

PROGNOSIS

Long-term survival is variable because of the age of onset for pulmonary changes and the underlying conditions (e.g., Down syndrome) that may adversely affect survival. Death often occurs in the second or third decade of life.

PITFALLS

In newborns, the RV muscle mass is comparable to the LV. RV failure from pulmonary hypertension is rare in newborns. RV failure in newborns is usually a consequence of hypoxemia, ischemia, and metabolic acidosis (e.g., persistent fetal circulation).

 ## Common Questions and Answers

Q: Is cardiac catheterization indicated in all patients with cor pulmonale?
A: Yes. While a great deal of information can be learned from echocardiography, direct pulmonary artery pressure/resistance measurements require an invasive procedure. In addition, assessment of the reactivity of the pulmonary vascular bed to various agents (oxygen, prostacyclin, and calcium channel blockers) is best performed in the catheterization laboratory.

Q: Is nocturnal oxygen therapy beneficial?
A: Nocturnal oxygen has been speculated to delay the progression of cor pulmonale in some select patients with obstructive sleep hypoxemia.

ICD-9-CM 416.9

Chronic 415.0

BIBLIOGRAPHY

Bandla HP, Davis SH, Hopkins NE. Lipoid pneumonia: a silent complication of mineral oil aspiration *Pediatrics* 1999;103(2):E19.

Brouillette RT, Fernback SK, Hunt CE. Obstructive sleep apnea in infants and children. *J Pediatr* 1982;100:31.

Perkin RM, Anas NG. Pulmonary hypertension in pediatric patients. *J Pediatr* 1984;105:511.

Wessel DL, Adatia I, Thompson JE, et al. Delivery and monitoring of inhaled nitric oxide in patients with pulmonary hypertension. *Crit Care Med* 1994;22(6): 930–938.

Author: Mitchell I. Cohen

Costochondritis

 Database

DEFINITION

Costochondritis is chest pain that emanates from a costal cartilage and is reproducible on compression of that cartilage.

PATHOPHYSIOLOGY

- Inflammation of unknown etiology (histologic examination is usually normal).
- Infection
  —Complication of median sternotomy
  —Can present months to years after surgery (the costal cartilage is avascular, making it vulnerable to infection if it has been exposed, injured, or denuded of perichondrium)
  —Occurs by spread from adjacent osteomyelitis or may arise de novo during surgery

—Bacterial
  —*Staphylococcus aureus* (especially after thoracic surgery)
  —*Salmonella* (in sickle cell disease)
  —*Escherichia coli*
  —*Pseudomonas* species
  —*Klebsiella* species

—Fungal
  —*Aspergillus flavus*
  —*Candida albicans*

—Posttrauma

EPIDEMIOLOGY

- Costochondritis accounts for 10% to 31% of all pediatric chest pain.
- Peak age for chest pain in children is 12 to 14 years.
- Incidence of sternal wound infections following median sternotomy is 0.1% to 1.6%.

PROGNOSIS

- Inflammatory costochondritis: excellent
- Infectious costochondritis: prognosis relates to:

—Underlying clinical condition of the patient (i.e., immunocompromised, postradiation therapy for cancer, postcardiac surgery)
—Extent of surgery required to reconstruct the area damaged by the infection

 Differential Diagnosis

ETIOLOGIES

- Cardiovascular

—Myocardial infarction
—Pericarditis
—Pericardial effusion
—Myocarditis
—Endocarditis
—Cardiomyopathy
—Premature ventricular contractions
—Supraventricular tachycardia
—Dissecting aneurysm

- Pulmonary

—Asthma
—Exercise-induced bronchospasm
—Pneumonia
—Pleural effusion
—Pneumothorax
—Pulmonary embolism

- Gastrointestinal

—Gastroesophageal reflux
—Esophagitis
—Gastritis
—Achalasia

- Mechanical

—Muscle strain
—Stress fractures
—Precordial catch syndrome
—Trauma

- Rheumatologic

—Rheumatoid arthritis
—Ankylosing spondylitis

- Oncologic

—Rhabdomyosarcoma
—Leukemia
—Ewing sarcoma

- Miscellaneous

—Tietze syndrome
—Psychogenic chest pain
—Breast tissue pain (both sexes)

 Data Gathering

HISTORY

Inflammatory Costochondritis

- Pain usually preceded by exercise or an upper respiratory tract infection
- Description of pain:

—Usually sharp
—Affects the anterior chest wall
—Localized or radiates to the back or abdomen
—Usually unilateral (left side greater than right side)

- The fourth to sixth costochondral junction is the usual site of pain.
- Motion of the arm and shoulder on the affected side elicits the pain.
- Girls are affected more often than are boys.

Tietze Syndrome

- Onset is usually abrupt, but can be gradual.
- Believed to be caused by a minor trauma, though etiology is unknown
- Description of pain:

—Radiates to arms or shoulder
—May last up to several weeks
—Swelling at the sternochondral junction may persist for several months to years.

- Usually affects the second or third costochondral joint
- Pain is aggravated by sneezing, coughing, deep inspiration, or twisting motions of the chest.
- No differences in frequency between sexes

Infectious Costochondritis

- Slow, insidious course
- Usually unimpressive clinical symptomatology

Physical Examination

- Usually normal
- Inspect for evidence of trauma, scars, bruising, and swelling.
- Palpation and percussion of the costochondral and costosternal junctions should reproduce and localize the pain.
- In Tietze syndrome, spindle-shaped swelling is visible at the sternochondral junction.

Laboratory Aids

TESTS

- WBC not helpful (even when infection present)
- ECG (may be helpful if cardiac etiology is being considered)

IMAGING

- Radiologic studies (chest radiography, CT) usually not helpful
- Gallium scan

—May be useful in some cases of infectious origin
—Not highly specific
—May show increased radionuclide uptake
—No evidence of osteomyelitis of the sternum in most cases

- Technetium bone scan

—Not highly specific

Therapy

INFLAMMATORY COSTOCHONDRITIS

- Antiinflammatory and analgesic agents
- Reassurance
- If pain disturbs normal activities and sports, infiltration with local anesthetic may prove useful.

INFECTIOUS COSTOCHONDRITIS

- Prolonged course of IV antibiotics
- Prompt surgical resection of all involved cartilage
- Reconstructive surgery with muscular flaps should be done.

Follow-Up

WHEN TO EXPECT IMPROVEMENT

- Inflammatory costochondritis

—Long-lasting condition
—Follow-up once a year is recommended.

- Infectious costochondritis

—Long-term follow-up after surgery is mandatory.

PITFALLS

- Inflammatory costochondritis

—Important cause of school absence
—Adolescents tend to limit physical activity unnecessarily for long periods.
—Restriction of activities is usually not required.
—Most adolescents still worry about cardiac problems, even after the diagnosis has been made.

- Infectious costochondritis

—Long-term IV antibiotics alone do not resolve the problem; surgical resection and repair also are required.
—There is a tendency for the infection to spread to adjacent costal cartilages and across the sternum to the contralateral chest wall.
—In general, avoid costochondral junctions when performing surgical procedures in the chest (i.e., chest-tube placement).

Common Questions and Answers

Q: Am I having or will I have a heart attack?
A: Chest pain does not imply a heart problem. This pain arises from the chest wall; there is no risk of a myocardial infarction. A cardiac etiology to chest pain in an adolescent is usually uncommon.

Q: Is costochondritis related to arthritis?
A: There is no relation to any form of arthritis.

ICD-9-CM 733.6

BIBLIOGRAPHY

Brown RT. Costochondritis in adolescents. *J Adolesc Health Care* 1981;1:198–201.

Brown RT, Jamil K. Costochondritis in adolescents: a follow-up study. *Clin Pediatr* 1993;32:499–500.

Caruana V, Swayne LC. Gallium detection of salmonella costochondritis. *J Nucl Med* 1988;29:2004–2007.

Chicarilli ZN, Ariyan S, Stahl RS. Costochondritis: pathogenesis, diagnosis and management considerations. *Plast Reconstr Surg* 1986;77:50–59.

Culliford AT, Cunningham JN, Jeff RH. Sternal and costochondral infections following open heart surgery. *J Thorac Cardiovasc Surg* 1976;72:714–726.

Fraz M. *Pediatric respiratory disease: diagnosis and treatment*. Philadelphia: WB Saunders, 1993:162–172.

Kocis KC. Chest pain in pediatrics. *Pediatr Clin North Am* 1999;46:189–203.

Mendelson G, Mendelson H, Horowitz SF, et al. Can ^{99m}technetium methylene diphosphate bone scans objectively document costochondritis? *Chest* 1997;111:1600–1602.

Miller JH. Accumulation of gallium-67 in costochondritis. *Clin Nucl Med* 1980;5:362–363.

Selbst SM, Ruddy RM, Clark BJ, et al. Pediatric chest pain: a prospective study. *Pediatrics* 1988;82:319–323.

Author: Richard M. Kravitz

Crohn Disease

 Database

DEFINITION
Crohn disease is a chronic inflammatory disease that can affect any part of the gastrointestinal tract, but most commonly involves the terminal ileum and proximal colon.

CAUSES
• Multifactorial, please see pathophysiology

PATHOPHYSIOLOGY
• Interaction and combination of environmental factors, genetic susceptibility, host's intestinal flora, and yet unspecified triggering factor may cause a dysregulated immune response, which leads to chronic intestinal inflammation.
• Microscopic inflammation infiltrates all layers of intestine with cryptitis or crypt abscesses, and distortion of crypt architecture, granulomas are found in 20–40% of biopsies and are pathognomonic.
• Normal bowel can exist in continuity with affected bowel (skip areas).
• The intestinal wall is edematous and thickened.
• Mesentery can be thickened, with enlarged lymph nodes, fat extends from the mesentery and "creeps" over the serosal surface of the intestine.
• Matting together of inflamed bowel and organs
• Abscesses/fistulas/strictures

GENETICS
• First-degree relatives have a 5% to 25% higher risk than normal population.
• Family members of patients with Crohn disease have increased risk for both Crohn disease and ulcerative colitis.
• Offspring have an 8.9% and siblings an 8.6% risk of developing inflammatory bowel disease (IBD).
• Concordance in monozygotic twins is 44.4% versus 3.8% in dizygotic twins.
• Susceptibility regions located on different chromosomes (6, 12, 16).

EPIDEMIOLOGY
• The incidence rate in children is 3.5 per 100,000 in North American 10- to 19-year-olds.
• More than a third of patients first present in childhood or adolescence.
• Family history is present in 30% of patients under 30 years old.
• Males and females are equally affected in adulthood, although in childhood it is slightly more predominant in males.
• Highest incidence in the Caucasian population, particularly in Jewish individuals.

COMPLICATIONS
• Obstruction (8–40%) due to strictures, phlegmon, adhesions, giant polyposis, gallstones, lymphoma.
• Abscess due to fistula and perforation.
• Enteroenteric, enterovesical, enterovaginal, and enterocutaneous fistulas
• Perianal disease affects 25% to 50% of patients.
• Malabsorption occurs in small bowel disease. The nutrient affected depends on the site of disease (e.g., vitamin B_{12} deficiency: terminal ileum; iron deficiency: duodenum).
• Incidence of adenocarcinoma is reported to be 4 to 20 times that of the general population.
• Massive hemorrhage is rare (1%). Rectal bleeding is common.
• Growth failure is frequent; final height is reduced and puberty is delayed in Crohn disease affecting prepubertal children.
• Toxic megacolon is a rare but serious complication.

 Differential Diagnosis

• Ulcerative colitis
• Appendicitis
• Infection: *Mycobacteria, Salmonella, Shigella, Campylobacter, Aeromonas, Yersinia, Clostridium difficile, Escherichia coli, Giardia, Cryptosporidium, Strongyloides*
• Hemolytic-uremic syndrome
• Henoch-Schönlein purpura
• Irritable bowel syndrome
• Peptic ulcer disease
• Constipation
• Autoimmune enteropathy, immunodeficiency
• Intestinal tuberculosis
• Lactose intolerance
• Small intestinal lymphoma
• Psychosocial disturbance

 Data Gathering

HISTORY
• Frequency of signs and symptoms
—Weight loss, 85%
—Diarrhea, 80%
—Abdominal pain, 85%
—Rectal bleeding, 50%
—Growth failure, 35%
—Nausea and vomiting, 25%
—Rectal disease, 25%
—Extraintestinal signs, 25%
—Perianal disease, 25%
—Fever, 40%
• Symptoms depend on the site of disease activity.
• The sites most often affected in decreasing frequency are terminal ileum, right colon, isolated colon, proximal small bowel, and upper GI tract (stomach, duodenum, esophagus).

SPECIAL CONCERNS
• Recurrent abdominal pain
• Diarrhea
• Weight loss
• Recent travel (enteric infections)
• Antibiotic use (*C. difficile*)
• Rectal bleeding
• Family history of IBD
• Appendectomy
• Growth failure: Careful charting of recent growth parameters, especially growth velocities from school or medical records, is essential.
—Patients with small bowel disease have emesis, nausea, pain, and diarrhea. Diarrhea is secondary to malabsorption and bacterial overgrowth. Growth retardation is more frequent in these patients.
—Patients with distal disease have symptoms of diarrhea, rectal bleeding, and urgency.
• Extraintestinal disease: arthritis, erythema nodosum, pyoderma gangrenosum, mouth ulcers, episcleritis, uveitis, thromboembolic disease, vasculitis, renal stones, amyloidosis, sclerosing cholangitis, pancreatitis
• Extraintestinal symptoms:
—Aphthous ulcers
—Arthritis
—Erythema nodosum
—Pyoderma gangrenosum

 Physical Examination

• Growth delay and weight loss, delayed puberty
• Abdominal examination: hyperactive bowel sounds, right lower quadrant (RLQ) mass and tenderness, palpable thickened loop of intestine
• Rectal and perianal examination: skin tag, fissure, fistula, hemorrhoids, abscess

 Laboratory Aids

TESTS
Laboratory Tests
• Blood count: microcytosis due to iron-deficiency anemia, normocytic anemia due to anemia of chronic disease, macrocytosis suggesting nutrient deficiency: iron, B_{12}, folate, zinc levels
• ESR (disease activity)
• Electrolytes (hydration, renal function)
• Transaminases, alkaline phosphatase, γ-glutamyl transpeptidase (hepatobiliary disease)
• Perinuclear anti-neutrophil cytoplasmic antibody (pANCA) Crohn disease (19% positive) and ulcerative colitis (UC) (80% positive)
• ASCA (anti–*Saccharomyces cerevisiae* antibody) Crohn disease (60% positive)
• Stool for occult blood and presence of white cells
• Stool cultures, *C. difficile* toxin A and B

Imaging
• Consider plain abdominal radiograph in acute presentation.
• Barium upper GI and small bowel follow-through; this shows extent of disease in small bowel that is not accessible to endoscopy.

- Barium enema has been replaced by colonoscopy in acute colitis; useful in evaluation of complications such as strictures and fistulas.
- CT scan and ultrasound are useful tools for evaluating complications and disease severity.
- Radionuclide tagged white blood cell scan and MRI are increasingly being used.
- Endoscopy with multiple biopsy enables visualization and tissue diagnosis and is the test of choice for initial evaluation of colonic Crohn disease. Upper endoscopy with biopsy is indicated in patients with symptoms of gastroduodenal disease.

 Therapy

DRUGS

- Corticosteroids can control intestinal inflammation. Dosage is 1 to 2 mg/kg/d oral prednisone (maximum, 60 mg). Initially, patient is treated for several weeks and tapered 5 mg weekly to the lowest amount tolerated. Topical hydrocortisone is useful in localized left-sided disease and is available in liquid and foam enemas. Poorly absorbed topical steroids with controlled ileal release, budesonide (9 mg/d) is available in Canada
- Nutritional therapy is frequently used in Europe and Canada as a first-line therapy:
—Elemental and polymeric diet reported to be effective in inducing remission in active disease
—To correct growth failure an increase in caloric intake is recommended and can be given as overnight nasogastric feeding if oral supplements are not tolerated.
- There are many 5-ASA (5-aminosalicylic) preparations used according to their sites of activation to treat diseased bowel:
—Asacol (terminal ileum, colon) 50 to 100 mg/kg/d (maximum 4.8 g/d for active disease and 3.2 g/d to maintain remission)
—Pentasa (duodenum, jejunum, ileum, colon), 50 to 100 mg/kg/d (maximum, 4 g/d for active disease and 3 g/d to maintain remission)
—Dipentum (colon)
—Rowasa, 4-g enemas and 500-mg suppositories qd–b.i.d. PR
- Azathioprine, 2.0 to 3.0 mg/kg/d, and its metabolite 6-mercaptopurine, 1.0 to 1.5 mg/kg/d. Observe for liver toxicity, maintain white cell count greater than 4×10^9/L and platelets greater than 100×10^9/L. Can maintain remission and is steroid-sparing, also used for treatment of fistulas.
- Methotrexate, 25 mg IM q week
- Other immunomodulatory therapy infrequently used: cyclosporine, tacrolimus (FK-506), MMF, thalidomide
- Antibiotics
—Metronidazole (10–20 mg/kg/d)
—Ciprofloxacin (20 mg/kg/d), used for intestinal and perianal disease
- Infliximab, anti–tumor necrosis factor-α antibody (5 mg/kg IV infusion, given

q2–3 months or if medically necessary), approved by FDA in 1998. Recommended for patients unresponsive to the above medical therapies.
- Other therapy currently in clinical trials (IL-10, IL-12, CDP 571, ISIS 2302)

SURGERY
Crohn disease is a chronic recurrent disease with recurrence at sites of anastomosis and ostomies. With obstruction, abscess, fistulas, growth retardation, and bleeding failing to respond to medical therapy, surgery is considered.

 Follow-Up

- The morbidity of this disease is very high. The majority of patients experience recurring disease.
- In adults, 55% of patients will have mild-to-severe disease at any one time, with the remainder in remission.
- Most patients have good general health in between disease and go on to lead productive lives.
- Patients with colonic disease seem to suffer more from extraintestinal disease and are more refractory to treatment.
- Exacerbation of disease in children often follows intercurrent viral illness, such as Epstein-Barr virus (EBV) and adenovirus.
- The cause of poor growth is multifactorial, including anorexia, malabsorption, increased energy expenditure, and prolonged corticosteroid use.
- In terms of risk of neoplasia, incidence of adenocarcinoma of the rectum and colon is reported to be 4 to 20 times that of the general population.
- There are no good population base studies looking at the incidence of lymphoma in IBD. One study of 2,000 patients found that 1 in 300 Crohn disease patients develops lymphoma.
- After 5 and 20 years of disease, the probability of survival was 98% and 89% of expected survival, respectively.
- Death is a rare complication (2.4% in a large series).

 Common Questions and Answers

Q: Should the diet of patients with Crohn disease be restricted?
A: Adequate nutrition is very important, especially in children with Crohn disease. Balanced nutrition is required to assure appropriate growth and development. The only foods not recommended are poorly digestible vegetables (if eaten raw), nuts, and popcorn, which can cause obstruction in the narrowed, inflamed intestine. Patients with secondary lactose intolerance should use lactase supplements, or avoid milk products while ensuring adequate calories and calcium intake.

Q: What is the cause of Crohn disease?
A: Both genetic and environmental factors are important in the development of Crohn disease. Possible environmental factors include aseptic environment in the first few years of life, lack of breast-feeding, frequent use of antibiotics or aspirin, and diet.

Q: Where can I learn more about Crohn disease?
A: The Crohn and Colitis Foundation of America (CCFA at *www.CCFA.org*) is a nonprofit organization dedicated to the care of people with Crohn disease and ulcerative colitis.

Q: What new therapies will be used in the near future?
A: Biologic agents, which use our recently improved knowledge of the immune system, either to downregulate inflammatory mediators or upregulate immunomodulatory mediators. It is hoped that this new class of therapies will greatly improve our care of people with IBD.

ICD-9-CM 558.9

BIBLIOGRAPHY
Chang P, Schwartz RW. Crohn's disease: current concepts in diagnosis and treatment. *Curr Surg* 2001;58(3):288–292.

Greenfield SM, Punchard NA, Teare JP, et al. Review article: the mode of actin of aminosalicylates in inflammatory bowel disease. *Aliment Pharmacol Ther* 1993;7:369–383.

Gryboski JD. Crohn disease in children 10 years old or younger: comparison with ulcerative colitis. *J Pediatr Gastroenterol Nutr* 1994;18(2):174–182.

Hildebrand H, Karlberg J, Kristiansson B. Longitudinal growth in children with IBD. *J Pediatr Gastroenterol Nutr* 1994;18(2): 165–173.

Hofley PM, Piccoli DA. Inflammatory bowel disease in children. *Med Clin North Am* 1994;78(6):1281–1302.

Hyams JS. Extraintestinal manifestations of IBD in childhood (review). *J Pediatr Gastroenterol Nutr* 1994;19(1):7–21.

Pittock S, Drumm B, Fleming P, et al. The oral cavity in Crohn's disease. *J Pediatr* 2001;138(5):767–771.

Seidman E, Leleiko N, Ament M, et al. Nutritional issues in pediatric inflammatory bowel disease. *J Pediatr Gastroenterol Nutr* 1991;12:424.

Spray C, Debelle GD, Murphy MS. Current diagnosis, management and morbidity in paediatric inflammatory bowel disease. *Acta Paediatr* 2001;90(4):400–405.

Walker WA, Durie PR, Hamilton JR, et al. *Pediatric gastrointestinal disease*. Toronto, Canada: BC Decker, 2000.

Author: Petar Mamula and Jonathan Markowitz
Robert Baldassano, 2nd edition

Croup (Laryngotracheobronchitis)

 Database

DEFINITION
- Croup (laryngotracheobronchitis) is an acute viral infection classically characterized by a triad of symptoms: a barking cough, inspiratory stridor, and hoarseness that result from variable degrees of subglottic stenosis.
- *Spasmodic croup* is characterized by the acute onset of inspiratory stridor, usually occurring at night for several hours and recurring over the next several nights. The child is often not ill or has mild upper respiratory symptoms. It may be a variant of viral laryngotracheobronchitis and often recurs.

ETIOLOGY
- Human parainfluenza virus type 1, most commonly identified
- Human parainfluenza virus types 2 and 3
- Respiratory syncytial virus (RSV)
- Adenovirus
- Influenza viruses A and B
- Enteroviruses
- *Mycoplasma pneumoniae* (rare)

PATHOPHYSIOLOGY
- The virus enters the body via respiratory droplets on the epithelium of the nasopharyngeal airway.
- The host defense mechanism is to cause an immune response, resulting in increased mucus production, which leads to airway narrowing.
- Edema and erythema of the mucosa of the subglottic region and vocal cords further narrow the airway.
- Airway narrowing may be severe in the subglottic region because the cricoid cartilage limits the luminal diameter in this area.
- The process of endothelial damage, swelling, and mucus production may extend to the small airways, with resulting atelectasis.

EPIDEMIOLOGY
- Most commonly occurs in the first 3 years of life (6–36 months)
- Peak incidence: second year of life (60 per 1,000)
- The male/female ratio is 3:2.
- Most prevalent in the late fall and winter
- Fewer children are requiring hospitalization.

COMPLICATIONS
- Poor oral intake/dehydration
- Hypoxia
- Upper airway obstruction
- Respiratory failure (rare)

PROGNOSIS
- The vast majority of patients do not require hospitalization.
- Almost all patients go on to complete recovery.

 Differential Diagnosis

- Congenital
—Tracheoesophageal fistula
—Foregut duplication
—Laryngomalacia
—Tracheomalacia
—Vocal cord paralysis
—Arnold-Chiari malformation
—Vascular ring
—Laryngeal web
- Infection
—Epiglottis (although less common since universal HiB vaccine)
—Bacterial tracheitis
—Retropharyngeal abscess
—Adenotonsillitis
—Diphtheria
—Pneumonia
- Toxins
—Foreign-body aspiration
—Caustic material ingestion (very alkaline products)
—Smoke inhalation
- Trauma
—Subglottic edema/stenosis post intubation
—Laryngeal fracture
- Tumor
—Papillomatosis
—Hemangioma
—Cystic hygroma
—Lymphoma
—Rhabdomyosarcoma
—Thymoma
—Teratoma
—Thyroglossal duct cyst
—Branchial cleft cyst
- Genetic/metabolic
—Hypocalcemia
- Allergic/inflammatory
—Asthma
—Angioneurotic edema (anaphylaxis)
—Spasmodic croup
—Microaspiration secondary to gastroesophageal reflux

 Data Gathering

HISTORY

Question: How long have the symptoms been present? Is the process acute or chronic?
Significance: Croup is an acute illness.

Question: Any fever?
Significance: Croup is often associated with fever. If no fever, do not forget foreign-body or caustic ingestions.

Question: When did the stridor begin or occur?
Significance: If the child awakens at night, this supports the diagnosis of croup. If the child is playing at the onset of stridor, consider foreign-body aspiration.

Question: How have the symptoms progressed?
Significance: Ask about URI prodrome, sore throat, change in quality of voice, dysphagia/drooling (consider epiglottitis), dysphonia, particular position of comfort.

Question: Is there a history of previous airway problems or recurrent stridor?
Significance: Recurrence or a prolonged history should lead one to consider subglottic stenosis, gastroesophageal reflux or spasmodic croup.

 Physical Examination

- In general, children with croup are often anxious and ill-appearing. Allow them to sit in a comfortable position and in their caregiver's (parent's) lap, which, it is hoped, will reduce the agitation provoked by examination.
- It is important initially to assess level of consciousness, irritability, color, and respiratory distress.
- Vital signs: Check for pulsus paradoxus (large inspiratory drop in systolic blood pressure because of a fall in pleural pressure secondary to airway obstruction).
- What is the preferred position? Sitting in a tripod position with the neck extended to "sniff" is concerning for epiglottis.
- Assess work of breathing, including respiratory rate, nasal flaring, retractions, abdominal breathing, and head bobbing.
- Assess air entry into the chest.
- Listen for audible stridor at rest.
- Listen for the presence of wheezing.
- Observe for drooling.
- Assess the quality of the voice.
- Neck masses or bruising suggest bacterial infection or trauma.
- The Croup Score (as developed by Westley et al. and modified by Super et al.) is utilized by many clinicians to describe the severity of symptoms (see table Severity Score of Croup Patients).

 Laboratory Aids

TESTS
Laboratory Tests
- In general, laboratory tests are not required to make this diagnosis.
- Blood testing, such as arterial blood gas or complete blood count with differential, is not helpful in diagnosing croup. In fact, the pain and fear of the testing will likely heighten the child's anxiety and worsen respiratory distress.

RADIOGRAPHIC STUDIES
Anteroposterior and lateral view x-rays of the neck: The anteroposterior view classically demonstrates the "steeple" sign in patients with croup. The lateral view is useful in

Severity Score of Croup Patients

INDICATOR OF SEVERITY OF ILLNESS	SCORE
Inspiratory stridor	
None	0
At rest, with stethoscope	1
At rest, without stethoscope	2
Retractions	
None	0
Mild	1
Moderate	2
Severe	3
Air entry	
Normal	0
Decreased	1
Severely decreased	2
Cyanosis	
None	0
With agitation	4
At rest	5
Level of consciousness	
Normal	0
Altered mental status	5
Mild Croup	0–3
Moderate to severe croup	>3

ruling out epiglottis, retropharyngeal cellulitis/abscess (fullness or free air in the retropharyngeal space), and a radiopaque foreign body.

OTHER PROCEDURES
Pulse oximetry: helpful for children in respiratory distress to determine if hypoxia is present.

 ## Emergency Care

- Racemic epinephrine (see below)
- Endotracheal intubation is very rare.

 ## Therapy

- Most do well with conservative management at home or, much less commonly, after a short stay in the emergency department.
- In the child with impending respiratory failure, prompt intubation and direct visualization of the airway *in the operating room* is imperative. Do not wait for x-rays to confirm a diagnosis.
- Humidity: humidified air delivered by tent or face mask in the hospital, or by cool mist vaporizer or a steam-filled bathroom at home. In the cold of winter, walking outside into the crisp, cold air is reported to be very helpful. Most of this evidence is anecdotal and not evidence based.
- Steroids: Utilized in the emergency room and inpatient settings, steroids have resulted in dramatic reduction in the number of admissions and length of hospital stays due to croup.
- Dexamethasone (half-life 36–54 hours) is given intramuscularly (IM) or orally in the setting of moderate-to-severe croup (croup

score ×3). Recent studies have shown that a dose of 0.15 mg/kg is as effective as 0.6 mg/kg as a single-dose treatment. There is no evidence to support additional doses. Oral dexamethasone is the most cost-effective steroid treatment available.
- Budesonide given via nebulizer at a dose of 2 mg given every 12 hours has been shown in recent studies to be as effective as dexamethasone in reducing symptoms. It has a reduced systemic absorption, with maximum deposition of drug in the upper airway.
- Racemic epinephrine: A nebulized racemic epinephrine treatment offers immediate reduction in swelling of the laryngeal airway in children who present in extreme respiratory distress or in whom humidified air does not improve stridor (croup score >3) after 20 to 30 minutes. Dose: 0.5 mL of 2.25% solution (D- and L-isomers) in 2.5 mL normal saline delivered via nebulizer.
- L-epinephrine: If racemic epinephrine is not available, 5 cc of L-epinephrine 1:10,000 delivered via nebulizer is effective.

 ## Follow-Up

- In most cases, the illness is self-limited, lasting 3 to 5 days.
- A "rebound phenomenon" with worsening of stridor and respiratory distress after initial relief with the racemic epinephrine treatment may be seen up to 2 hours posttreatment in some patients. Several studies have shown that children can be safely discharged 3 to 4 hours after racemic epinephrine treatment.

PITFALLS
Recurrent croup may have an underlying anatomic problem associated. In younger children (infants), congenital anomalies and gastroesophageal reflux are more likely contributors.

 ## Common Questions and Answers

Q: Should all children with croup receive steroids in an attempt to prevent hospitalization?
A: The literature certainly is convincing for the use of dexamethasone or budesonide in combination with mist and racemic epinephrine for children with moderate-to-severe croup scores. There is no evidence to date, however, supporting the use of steroids in the mild cases as a preventative measure. Steroids have not been shown to shorten the course of the illness; however, the severity is diminished.

Q: Do children who receive racemic epinephrine for croup require hospitalization?
A: No. Several studies now have shown that after a 3- to 4-hour period of observation and dexamethasone, children can be safely discharged home. Any rebound effects should occur within the first 2 hours.

Q: Do steroids need to be given IM?
A: The bioavailability of steroids is excellent, whether IM or orally administered. The half-life of dexamethasone is much longer (36–54 hours) than that of prednisone (12–36 hours). With croup, many patients have poor oral intake exacerbated by respiratory distress. If oral intake can be assured, dexamethasone at 0.15 mg/kg or 0.6 mg/kg for croup has been proven to be inexpensive and effective. There are no studies evaluating the effectiveness or dosing of prednisolone in croup.

Q: Should we give steroids to any child with a barky cough?
A: In cases where the croup score is less than 3 (i.e., minimal symptoms), there is no evidence to suggest steroids should be used.

Q: Why is budesonide dosed every 12 hours?
A: Like much of our clinical practice, dosing guidelines are based on what the successful studies utilized. Every-12-hour dosing is an interval used in asthma management that was extrapolated to croup.

ICD-9-CM 464.4

BIBLIOGRAPHY
Ausejo M, Saenz A, Pham B, et al. *The Cochrane Library*, Oxford: Update Software, 2001.

Godden CW, Campbell MJ, Hussey M, et al. Double blind placebo controlled trial of nebulised budesonide for croup. *Arch Dis Child* 1997;76:155–158.

Johnson DW, Jacobson S, Edney PC, et al. A comparison of nebulized budesonide, intramuscular dexamethasone, and placebo for moderately severe croup. *N Engl J Med* 1998; 339(8):498–503.

Klassen TP. Croup—a current perspective. *Pediatr Clin North Am* 1999;46(6):1167–1178.

Klassen TP, Craig WR, Moher D, et al. Nebulized budesonide and oral dexamethasone for treatment of croup. *JAMA* 1998;279(20):1629–1632.

Roberts GW, Master VV, Staugas RE, et al. Repeated dose inhaled budesonide versus placebo in the treatment of croup. *Am J Paediatr Child Health* 1999;35:170–174.

Super DM, Cartelli NA, Brooks LJ, et al. A prospective randomized double-blind study to evaluate the effect of dexamethasone in acute laryngotracheitis. *J Pediatr* 1989;115: 323–329.

Westley CR, Cotton EK, Brooks JG. Nebulized racemic epinephrine by IPPB for the treatment of croup. *Am J Dis Child* 1978;132:484–487.

Author: Shannon Connor Phillips

Cryptococcal Infections

Database

DEFINITION
Cryptococcosis is an opportunistic fungal infection caused by *Cryptococcus neoformans*. It can involve several organ systems, including the central nervous system (CNS), lungs, bones, visceral organs, and skin.

PATHOPHYSIOLOGY
- Primary infection occurs through the inhalation of aerosolized soil particles containing the yeast forms. The skin and gastrointestinal tract are also portals of entry.
- Protective immune response requires specific T-cell–mediated immunity.
- CNS involvement with *C. neoformans* results from hematogenous dissemination.

EPIDEMIOLOGY
- Cryptococcal infection is common in patients with impaired cell-mediated immunity and is an occasional pathogen in normal hosts.
- It is a feature of advanced HIV disease; most patients have CD4$^+$ lymphocyte counts <50 cells/mm^3. It occurs in 5% to 15% of HIV-infected adults. It is less common in HIV-infected children, occurring in 0.8% to 2.3% of cases. The infection rate in children reflects their lower exposure to sources of *C. neoformans*. The overall seroprevalence is 0% in neonates and 4.1% in school-age children, compared to 69% in adults.
- There is no person-to-person spread of the infection.

COMPLICATIONS
- CNS involvement occurs in approximately three fourths of patients and is the most serious complication of disseminated cryptococcal infection. There is an increased risk of death when elevated intracranial pressure (ICP) develops. Placement of a ventriculoperitoneal shunt has not been shown to improve the associated mortality. Empiric corticosteroid use is controversial and not generally recommended.
- Pulmonary, cutaneous, and bone involvement may occur (see Associated Diseases).

PROGNOSIS
- In HIV-infected patients untreated cryptococcal infection is usually fatal in 2 to 4 weeks.
- Survival is good with early treatment but, in HIV-infected patients, relapse rates are high (see Prevention).
- Up to 40% of patients with cryptococcal meningitis have residual neurologic deficits.
- In the normal host with cryptococcal meningitis, patients with serum or CSF cryptococcal titers >1:32 or CSF WBCs <20/mm^3 have a worse prognosis. In HIV-infected patients, it is unclear whether the magnitude of titers affects outcome.
- In HIV-infected patients with cryptococcal meningitis, poor prognostic factors include

the presence of hyponatremia, concomitant growth of *C. neoformans* from another site, and any alteration of mental status.
- Patients with isolated pulmonary or cutaneous disease have a favorable prognosis.

ASSOCIATED DISEASES
- Disseminated cryptococcal infection is more common among immunocompromised hosts and children.
- *C. neoformans* is the most common cause of fungal meningitis in the U.S. and is a particular problem in immunocompromised hosts.
- Concurrent *Pneumocystis carinii* pneumonia was detected in 13% of adults with cryptococcal meningitis.
- Pulmonary involvement is asymptomatic in up to 50% of cases and disease may be either focal or widespread.
- Bone involvement occurs in 10% of cases of disseminated cryptococcal infection. Focal pain and swelling are usually present and the diagnosis is made by biopsy.
- Cutaneous involvement mimics acne-type eruptions that ulcerate and results from hematogenous spread of the organism or from direct extension of bone infection.

Differential Diagnosis

- Although cryptococcosis occurs most commonly in HIV-infected patients with low CD4$^+$ lymphocyte counts, the diagnosis warrants consideration in all febrile immunocompromised children.
- Meningitis: Viruses and *Mycobacterium tuberculosis*.
- Pneumonia: Other pulmonary mycoses, including aspergillosis, histoplasmosis, and blastomycosis. Also consider *Mycoplasma pneumoniae* and *M. tuberculosis*.
- Bone: Osteogenic sarcoma.
- Cutaneous: Molluscum contagiosum, HSV infection, pyoderma gangrenosum, and cellulitis.

Data Gathering

HISTORY
- Cryptococcal meningitis may present as either an indolent infection or acute illness.
- Symptoms of cryptococcal meningitis include headache, malaise, and low-grade fever. Nausea, vomiting, altered mentation, and photophobia are less common. Stiff neck, focal neurologic symptoms (i.e., decreased hearing, facial nerve palsy, or diplopia), and seizures are rare.
- Primary pulmonary cryptococcal disease is not well described in children because most cases are disseminated at the time of diagnosis. Fifty percent of adults have cough or chest pain, and fewer have sputum production, weight loss, fever, and hemoptysis.

- In immunocompromised hosts, the onset of infection is more rapid and the course more severe. Pulmonary involvement is minimal when dissemination occurs quickly.

Physical Examination

None of the presenting signs of cryptococcal infection are sufficiently characteristic to distinguish it from other infections, particularly in immunocompromised patients.
- Signs of CNS involvement include nuchal rigidity, photophobia, and focal neurologic deficits.
- Signs of respiratory tract involvement include cough, tachypnea, grunting, and subcostal or intercostal retractions. Decreased breath sounds or dullness to percussion may be present or the lung exam may be normal.
- Cutaneous manifestations are multiple and may include erythematous or verrucous papules, nodules, pustules, acneiform lesions, ulcers, abscesses, or granulomas. Lesions can occur anywhere on the body but are found most often on the face and neck.
- Mucocutaneous findings are present in 10% to 15% of cases of disseminated disease.

Laboratory Aids

TESTS

Test: Lumbar puncture
Significance: Diagnose cryptococcal meningitis.
- CSF should be sent for cell count and differential; protein; glucose; cultures for bacterial, fungal, and viral pathogens; India ink stain; and cryptococcal antigen.
- Examination of the CSF reveals <500 WBCs/mm^3 (usually <100 WBCs/mm^3), mostly mononuclear leukocytes, with minimal changes in protein. CSF glucose is <50 mg/dL in approximately 65% of patients.
- Budding yeast are seen on India ink stain in 50% of cases.
- CSF cultures are positive in approximately 90% of patients.
- The latex agglutination test for cryptococcal polysaccharide antigen is specific, sensitive, and rapid. Titers $\geq$1:4 suggest the diagnosis of cryptococcal infection if appropriate controls (to exclude the presence of rheumatoid factor or other nonspecific agglutinins) are negative.
- HIV-infected patients with pneumonia and CD4$^+$ T-lymphocyte counts <200 cells/mm^3 should be evaluated with sputum fungal culture, blood fungal culture, and a serum cryptococcal antigen test. A lumbar puncture to exclude the possibility of occult meningitis should be considered. If any test is positive for *C. neoformans,* then a lumbar puncture should be performed to exclude cryptococcal meningitis.

Cryptococcal Infections

Test: Blood culture and serum cryptococcal antigen titers
Significance: Diagnose disseminated cryptococcal infection.
Test: Sputum culture
Significance: Diagnose cryptococcal pneumonia.
Test: Skin biopsy
Significance: Diagnose cutaneous cryptococcal infection.
Test: HIV testing
Significance: Evaluation for immunodeficiencies, including HIV, is warranted in any patient with cryptococcosis.
Test: Complete blood count with differential
Significance: May reveal hypereosinophilia (absolute eosinophil count >1,500/mm^3)
Test: Serum electrolytes
Significance: Detect hyponatremia, a complication of cryptococcal meningitis.

RADIOGRAPHIC IMAGING
Test: Chest radiograph (PA and lateral)
Significance: Nodules, diffuse infiltrates, and pleural effusions may be seen in cryptococcal pneumonia.
Test: Head CT
Significance: May demonstrate granulomatous lesions or findings of elevated ICP.

Therapy

Clinical management varies depending on the extent of disease and the immune status of the host.

PULMONARY AND EXTRAPULMONARY DISEASE, HIV-NEGATIVE
• A normal host with isolated pulmonary nodules does not need treatment if the serum cryptococcal antigen is negative and the patient is asymptomatic.
• Patients with extensive pulmonary disease or evidence of extrapulmonary disease require treatment.
• Fluconazole (PO; 6–12 mg/kg/d, max. 400 mg) for 6 to 12 months. Alternate regimen: itraconazole (PO; 4–10 mg/kg/d, max. 400 mg) for 6 to 12 months; or amphotericin B (IV; 0.7–1 mg/kg/d) for 3 to 6 months.
• HIV-negative, immunocompromised hosts with pulmonary or extrapulmonary disease and those with severe symptoms are treated with amphotericin B in the same fashion as patients with CNS disease.
• Due to the high rate of relapse in immunocompromised patients, maintenance therapy with fluconazole should continue as long as the patient is immunocompromised (see Prevention).

CNS DISEASE, HIV-NEGATIVE
• Induction/consolidation: amphotericin B plus flucytosine (PO; 100–150 mg/kg/d divided every 6 hours) for 2 weeks, then fluconazole (PO; see above for dosing) for a minimum of 10 weeks. Alternate regimen: amphotericin B plus flucytosine for 6 to 10 weeks.

PULMONARY AND EXTRAPULMONARY DISEASE, HIV-INFECTED
• Fluconazole (PO) lifelong. Alternate regimen: itraconazole (PO) lifelong.
• Surgery should be considered for patients with persistent or refractory pulmonary or bone lesions.

CNS DISEASE, HIV-INFECTED
• Induction/consolidation: Amphotericin B (IV) plus flucytosine (PO) for at least 2 weeks, followed by fluconazole PO lifelong. Alternate regimen: fluconazole plus flucytosine for 6 weeks followed by fluconazole or itraconazole lifelong (see above for dosing).
• Intrathecal amphotericin B is very toxic but may be used in refractory cases.
• HIV-infected patients require continuation of antifungal drugs indefinitely because of the high recurrence rate of cryptococcosis.
• Lipid formulation of amphotericin B (IV; 3–6 mg/kg/d) may be substituted for amphotericin B.
• Itraconazole for intravenous administration is available but there are insufficient data to guide its current use.
• Flucytosine is used only in combination with amphotericin B and not as a single agent because of the rapid emergence of drug resistance.

Follow-Up

Follow-up is important due to the risk of relapse. Patients should be seen at 3-month intervals for 12 to 18 months following treatment, with cultures obtained for fungal isolation. Immunocompromised patients should be evaluated every 2 to 3 months, even while on suppressive therapy, to monitor clinically for relapse.
• Repeat lumbar punctures documenting a decrease in CSF cryptococcal antigen and sterility of culture are useful in evaluating response to treatment. During therapy for acute meningitis, an unchanged or increased titer of CSF antigen correlates with clinical and microbiologic failure to respond to treatment. Serum antigen titers are not helpful for this purpose.
• Evaluation for neurologic sequelae is essential in patients with cryptococcal meningitis.
• HIV-infected patients require lifelong suppressive antifungal therapy (see Prevention).

PREVENTION
• The dramatic reduction of cryptococcal infections since the introduction of potent antiretroviral therapy suggests that the best prophylaxis for cryptococcosis is effective treatment of HIV.
• In HIV-infected patients with low CD4$^+$ lymphocyte counts, relapse rates are 100% without maintenance antifungal therapy, 18% to 25% with amphotericin B or itraconazole, and 2% to 3% with fluconazole.
• Prophylaxis with fluconazole is also effective in preventing new onset cryptococcal disease. Cryptococcal meningitis occurred once (0.4%)

among 231 HIV-infected children receiving fluconazole 200 mg three times weekly.
• There is no consensus on the duration of fluconazole therapy after acute therapy in HIV-negative immunocompromised patients. Most experts provide suppressive antifungal therapy for at least 1 year after the completion of acute treatment and then reassess its ongoing use based on the level of current immunosuppression.

Common Questions and Answers

Q: What are the sources of *Cryptococcus* in nature?
A: Pigeon droppings and soil. Naturally acquired infections occur in lower mammals, especially cats. However, neither animal-to-human nor human-to-human infections have been reported.
Q: Can "normal" (immunocompetent) children get this infection? How long should it be treated?
A: Yes. Treat for 6 to 10 weeks.
Q: Should all children with *Cryptococcus* be evaluated for immunodeficiency?
A: Yes.

ICD-9-CD 117.5

BIBLIOGRAPHY
Gonzalez CE, Shetty D, Lewis LL, et al. Cryptococcosis in human immunodeficiency virus-infected children. *Pediatr Infect Dis J* 1996;15:796–800.

Harrison TS. *Cryptococcus neoformans* and cryptococcosis. *J Infect* 2000;41:12–17.

Powderly WG. Current approach to the acute management of cryptococcal infections. *J Infect* 2000;41:18–22.

Powderly WG, Cloud GA, Dismukes WE, et al. Measurement of cryptococcal antigen in serum and cerebrospinal fluid: value in the management of AIDS-associated cryptococcal meningitis. *Clin Infect Dis* 1994;18:789–792.

Saag MS, Graybill RJ, Larsen RA, et al. Practice Guidelines for the management of cryptococcal disease. *Clin Infect Dis* 2000;30:710–718.

Singh N, Barnish MJ, Berman S, et al. Low-dose fluconazole as primary prophylaxis for cryptococcal infection in AIDS patients with CD4 cell counts of < or = 100/mm^3: demonstration of efficacy in a positive, multicenter trial. *Clin Infect Dis* 1996;23:1282–1286.

Yogev R. Central nervous system infections in the immunocompromised host. In: Patrick CC, ed. *Clinical management of infections in immunocompromised infants and children*. Philadelphia: Lippincott Williams & Wilkins, 2001:350–370.

Author: Samir S. Shah

Cryptorchidism

Database

DEFINITION

An undescended testis is one that does not remain at the bottom of the scrotum after the cremaster muscle has been fatigued by over-stretching. This is commonly confused with a retractile testis, one that may not always lie in the scrotum, but that will stay in the bottom of the scrotum after overstretching the cremaster.

CAUSES

• A multifactorial mechanism of occurrence involving two types of theories have been postulated:

—Hypogonadotropic hypogonadism
—Abnormal mechanical factors (gubernaculum, epididymis, genitofemoral nerve innervation, intraabdominal pressure)
—While boys with undescended testes do have abnormal attachment of the gubernaculum, the mechanical theories do not consistently explain the testis histology found in cryptorchidism.
—Many boys with cryptorchidism have lower morning urinary LH and a decreased LH/FSH response to GnRH, corresponding to the abnormal germ cell development in both the undescended and contralateral descended testis.
—The normal initial postnatal gonadotropin surge at 60 to 90 days is absent or blunted in some boys with cryptorchidism. Without this surge, Leydig cells do not proliferate, testosterone does not increase, germ cells do not mature, and infertility may result. This suggests that a mild endocrinopathy is responsible and cryptorchidism may be a variant of hypogonadotropic hypogonadism.

• Secondary undescended testes can occur after inguinal surgery, either due to scar tissue or difficulty in diagnosing an undescended testis in a young boy with a hernia.

PATHOLOGY

• The undescended testis fails to show normal maturation at both 3 months and 5 years.

—At 3 months, the fetal gonocytes are transformed into adult dark spermatogonia.
—At 5 years, the adult dark spermatogonia become primary spermatocytes.
—Both of these steps are abnormal in the undescended testis, and to a lesser extent, the contralateral descended testis.
—Previous beliefs that the undescended testis was normal between birth and 1 year are incorrect, since they were derived from counts of all germ cells without taking into account whether maturation was occurring.
—After 2 years of age, thermal effects on the testis being left out of position are seen independent of the endocrinologic effects.

GENETICS

The risk of a male sibling having undescended testis is 1% to 4%; the risk of having a son with undescended testis if the father is affected is 6%.

EPIDEMIOLOGY

• 3% of full-term boys have cryptorchidism.
• This percentage falls to 1% by 3 months.
• Normal descent occurs during the 7th month of gestation.
• The majority of testes that will spontaneously descend do so by 3 months of age, possibly due to the gonadotropin surge that is responsible for maturation of the germ cells.
• Therefore, patients with undescended testes should be referred for surgical evaluation no later than 3 months of age.
• There are two peaks for detection of undescended testes: at birth, and at 5 to 7 years of age. The latter group probably represents those patients with low undescended testes that become apparent with linear growth. Bilateral undescended testes occur in 10% of patients with undescended testicles. Unilateral anorchia is found in 5% of patients. Patients with prune belly, Klinefelter, Noonan, and Prader-Willi syndromes have undescended testes.

Differential Diagnosis

• Retractile testes are commonly confused with undescended testes. The key to distinguishing them from undescended testes is the physical exam. All retractile and many undescended testes can be delivered into the scrotum. The retractile testis will stay in the scrotum after the cremaster muscle has been overstretched. The low undescended testis will immediately pop back to its undescended position after being released.
• Atrophic or "vanishing" testes are found anywhere along the normal path to the scrotum. They are believed to be due to neonatal vascular ischemia. The contralateral testis can be hypertrophied in these boys, but this is not a reliable diagnostic sign.
• Upon evaluation, 80% of nonpalpable testes are present in either the abdomen or in the inguinal canal. A child with bilateral nonpalpable testes should have an endocrine evaluation to rule out anorchia or intersex.
• Cryptorchidism associated with hypospadias should also raise the possibility of intersex states, which occurs in 30% to 40% of patients, mainly consisting of defects in gonadotropin or testosterone synthesis.

Data Gathering

History

• Prematurity
• Exogenous maternal hormones (used in infertility treatments)
• Use of oral contraceptives
• Central nervous system lesions
• Previous inguinal surgery
• Family history for urologic abnormalities
• Neonatal deaths
• Precocious puberty
• Infertility
• Consanguinity

Physical Examination

• The undescended testis may be found at the upper scrotum, in the superficial inguinal pouch, or in the inguinal canal. For treatment purposes, the main distinction that needs to be made is whether or not the testis is palpable.
• The patient should be examined supine in the frogleg position with both legs free.

—With warmed hands, check the size, location, and texture of the contralateral descended testis.
—Begin the examination of the undescended testis at the anterior superior iliac spine.
—Sweep the groin from lateral to medial with the nondominant hand.
—Once the testis is palpated, grasp it with the dominant hand, and continue to sweep the testis toward the scrotum with the other hand.
—With a combination of sweeping and pulling, it is sometimes possible to bring the testis to the scrotum.
—Maintain the position of the testis in the scrotum for a minute, so that the cremaster muscle is fatigued.
—Release the testis, and if it remains in place, it is a retractile testis.
—If it immediately pops back, it is an undescended testis.

• For the difficult-to-examine patient (chubby 6-month-olds or obese youths), the sitting cross-legged position can help relax the cremaster. Wetting the fingers of the nondominant hand with lubricating jelly or soap can increase the sensitivity of the fingers in palpating the small, mobile testis.

Laboratory Aids

TESTS

- For the typical patient with a unilateral palpable or nonpalpable undescended testis, no further laboratory evaluation is necessary.
- For the patient with bilateral undescended testis, with one testis palpable, no further workup is necessary.
- The patient with bilateral nonpalpable testes should have a chromosomal and endocrinologic evaluation, as should the patient with one or two undescended testes and hypospadias.
- If the patient has bilateral nonpalpable testes and is younger than 3 months of age, serum LH, FSH, and testosterone will determine whether testes are present.
- After that age, hCG stimulation will result in a measurable serum testosterone if testes are present. A failure to respond to hCG stimulation in combination with elevated LH/FSH levels is consistent with anorchia.

IMAGING

Ultrasound, CT, and MRI can detect testes in the inguinal region, but this is also the region where they are most easily palpable. They are only 50% accurate in showing intraabdominal testes. Imaging is rarely necessary preoperatively, since for nonpalpable testes, exam under anesthesia, open inguinal exploration, or laparoscopy is necessary to confirm the presence of testes.

 Therapy

HORMONAL THERAPY

- This is widely used in Europe for inducing descent of undescended testes. Both GnRH and hCG are used, with success rates of 30% to 50%. Treatment is most successful for low undescended testes, but there is a 25% relapse rate.
- For these reasons, as well as the fact that GnRH and hCG are not approved for this indication in the United States, most therapy in the U.S. aimed at bringing the testis down to the scrotum is surgical (orchiopexy).
- The use of hormonal therapy after orchiopexy to improve semen analyses in high-risk patients is in its preliminary stages of investigation in Europe and the U.S.

SURGICAL THERAPY

Goals in bringing the testis into the scrotum:

- Prevent ongoing thermal damage to the testis.
- Treat the associated hernia sac.
- Prevent testis torsion/injury against the pubic bone.
- Achieve a good cosmetic result/avoid psychological effects of empty scrotum.
- Show the older child how to perform testicular self-exam for cancer.

PROGNOSIS

- Surgery cannot reverse the maturational failure of the undescended testis, but it can prevent ongoing thermal injury.
- Parents are often concerned about future fertility.

—In patients who have undergone orchiopexy at an early age, it appears that 85% of boys with unilateral cryptorchidism and 50% with bilateral cryptorchidism will achieve paternity.
—Patients who are interested in their risk for infertility may have a semen analysis performed at age 18.

- Surgery also has no effect on the increased risk of testicular cancer (increase from 2–3 to 49/100,000), but it can make the testis easier to examine.

—Approximately 15% of tumors arise in the contralateral descended testis.
—All patients should be taught proper testicular self-exam at the time of puberty. Intraabdominal testes are more at risk than inguinal testes.

 Follow-Up

After successful orchiopexy, patients are examined at 3 months to check on testicular size and position. They are rechecked at puberty to explain the technique and need for testis self-exam. Patients with retractile testes should be examined annually until age 7 because about 5% will be found to have a testis out of the scrotum.

 Common Questions and Answers

Q: If there is only one testicle in scrotum, will fertility be affected?
A: In general, the outlook for paternity is good in a patient with only one testicle.

Q: Are there any herbal treatments that will help bring the testicle into the scrotum?
A: No studies have shown herbal therapy to work in this condition.

ICD-9-CM 752.51

BIBLIOGRAPHY

Berkowitz GS, Lapinski RH, Dolgin SE, et al. Prevalence and natural history of cryptorchidism. *Pediatrics* 1993;92:44–49.

Callaghan P. Undescended testis. *Pediatr Rev* 2000;21(11):395.

Kogan S, Hadziselimovic F, Howards SS, et al. Pediatric andrology. In: Gillenwater JY, Grayhack JT, Howards SS, et al., ed. *Adult and pediatric urology*, 3rd ed. Mosby: St. Louis, 1996.

Lee PA, Coughlin MT. Fertility after bilateral cryptorchidism. Evaluation by paternity, hormone, and semen data *Horm Res* 2001;55(1):28–32.

Pyorala S, Huttunen N-P, Uhari M. A review and meta-analysis of hormonal treatment of cryptorchidism. *J Clin Endocrinol Metab* 1995;80:2795–2799.

Rajfer J. Congenital anomalies of the testes and scrotum. In: Walsh PC, Retik AB, Vaughn ED, et al., ed. *Campbell's urology*, 7th ed. Philadelphia: WB Saunders, 1998.

Authors: Hsi-Yang Wu and Thomas F. Kolon

Cryptosporidiosis

 Database

DEFINITION

In an immunocompetent patient, disease is manifested as a self-limiting gastroenteritis. However, immunocompromised patients can develop protracted severe gastroenteritis, which can lead to severe wasting and ultimately death.

CAUSES

Most commonly, gastrointestinal illness is caused by ingestion of the oocysts of *Cryptosporidium parvum*; a coccidian protozoa that is frequently found in the feces of animals as well as some insects.

PATHOLOGY/PATHOPHYSIOLOGY

- Transmission occurs when oocysts contaminating food or water are ingested or, more commonly, through fecal-oral transmission from person to person.
- The infectious dose for humans is low, estimated at less than 10 oocysts. The incubation period is approximately 5 to 21 days and oocyst shedding may occur for weeks to months.
- Invasion of intestinal epithelial cells of the upper gastrointestinal tract leads to a secretory diarrhea. The exact mechanism by which this occurs is still unclear.

EPIDEMIOLOGY

- Typically children under 5 years of age are most often affected. Severe disease is usually seen in the immunocompromised, such as patients with impaired cell-mediated immunity (in particular those who are HIV positive or taking immunosuppressive medications), those with immunoglobulin deficiencies, as well as interferon-γ deficiencies.
- A significant seasonality has been reported, with peaks occurring in North America during the late summer and early fall.
- Outbreaks have been associated with swimming pools, lakes, water recreation parks, drinking water supplies, day camps, unpasteurized apple cider, exposure to farm animals, and day-care attendance.
- Other risk factors include exposure to dogs, cats, deer, cockroaches, and traveling abroad.

COMPLICATIONS

- In immunocompromised patients, infection can lead to severe protracted diarrhea with malnutrition and wasting. Biliary tract disease and systemic dissemination such as pulmonary disease can also be seen in the immunocompromised.

PROGNOSIS

- For immunocompetent hosts, gastrointestinal disease is self-limited usually lasting 10 to 14 days. Supportive therapy is usually all that is necessary.
- For immunocompromised patients, diarrhea can be severe, debilitating, and often life-threatening. Aggressive supportive therapy is usually required along with a trial of antimicrobial therapy. Unfortunately, there are no agents that are uniformly effective against *Cryptosporidium parvum*.

 Differential Diagnosis

INFECTIOUS

- Viral gastroenteritis including but not limited to:

—Rotavirus
—Adenovirus
—Astrovirus
—Norwalk
—Cytomegalovirus (CMV)

- Bacterial gastroenteritis including but not limited to:

—*Salmonella*
—*Shigella*
—*Yersinia*
—*Campylobacter*
—*Aeromonas*
—*Plesiomonas*
—Enterotoxigenic *Escherichia coli*
—*Vibrio cholerae*

- Parasitic gastroenteritis including but not limited to:

—*Giardia*
—*Entamoeba*
—*Cyclospora*
—*Isospora*
—*Microsporidia*
—*Dientamoeba fragilis*
—*Blastocystis hominis*
—*Clostridium difficile* enterocolitis

NONINFECTIOUS

- Allergic
- Autoimmune
- Anatomic
- Endocrine
- Iatrogenic/medications
- Inflammatory bowel disease
- Malabsorption
- Neoplastic

 Data Gathering

HISTORY

- Onset: Acute onset of watery nonbloody diarrhea, crampy abdominal pain, low-grade fever, and occasionally nausea and vomiting.
- Exposure: Exposure to ill contacts, public swimming pools, lakes or wave parks, animals, day-care attendance, travel history, dietary history such as consumption of unpasteurized beverages and drinking water supply.
- Evidence of immunosuppression: Immunosuppression secondary to disease or medication as well as exposure to immunosuppressed individuals in the household or, if patient is old enough, through occupation.

 Laboratory Aids

Test: Modified acid fast stain
Significance: Diagnosis is made by observing the 4- to 5-μm cysts in preserved stool specimens. Immunofluorescent antibody or rapid (3 minute) direct antigen detection tests are also available. Stool specimens should be performed three times on alternate days to exclude the diagnosis.

Test: Must specifically request that the microbiology lab test for this organism.
Significance: A recent national survey of clinical laboratories revealed only 5% routinely tested for *C. parvum*.

Test: Sputum specimen
Significance: For respiratory infections, diagnosis is made by finding the oocysts in sputum specimens.

Test: H and E staining of small intestinal biopsies
Significance: May show the organism protruding from the microvillus border of enterocytes.

Therapy

• Fluid and electrolyte replacement. For protracted cases, patients will eventually require hyperalimentation.
• The antibiotic paromomycin, an aminoglycoside, can improve symptoms and decrease parasite excretion in the feces of some immunocompromised patients and this has become the treatment of choice for immunosuppressed patients. The dosage is 25 to 30 mg/kg/day three times a day for 7 days. Spiramycin is not effective.
• Some patients have been shown to have improvement in their clinical symptoms with the gastrointestinal hormone octreotide. The dosage is 300 to 500 μg three times a day.
• *Cryptosporidium* is on the CDC recommended reporting list of infectious diseases; however, not all states in the United States mandate reporting *Cryptosporidium*.

Follow-Up

• Since the oocysts can be shed in the stool for a long time after clinical resolution, it is not necessary to check follow-up convalescent stools. However, it is important to realize that asymptomatic patients can still transmit the infection to household and day-care contacts.
• Requiring patients whose diarrhea has resolved to have a negative stool test for *Cryptosporidium* before reentry to day care has not been evaluated as an outbreak control measure. Repeated testing is expensive.

PREVENTION

• Isolation of hospitalized patient

—Contact precautions (i.e., gown and gloves for all patient contact) are recommended for the length of the hospital stay. If possible, a single bedroom would be optimal so that a bathroom does not need to be shared.

• Community prevention

—Public water supplies should be adequately filtered in order to ensure oocyst removal.
—Communities that do not use filtration systems are at increased risk for outbreaks, the most recent of which was the Milwaukee epidemic, where an estimated 400,000 people were affected.
—Homeowners with well water should consider installing drinking water filtration systems.
—Sources of drinking water should be protected from possible fecal contamination.
—Garden hoses should not be used to provide drinking water.
—All juices should be pasteurized. *Cryptosporidium* has been shown to survive in unpasteurized apple cider for up to 4 weeks.

—Symptomatic patients should not be allowed to swim in public pools.
—Good hand washing after contact with animals.

• Control measures

—Hand washing especially after changing diapers.
—Separation of diapering and food handling areas.
—Disinfection of diapering areas after each use, frequent (at least twice daily) disinfection of toys, tabletops, and high chairs during outbreaks is recommended.
—Oocysts can survive for long periods and are resistant to many disinfectants such as pine oil, cresylic acid, ethanol, n-propanol, isopropanol, Lysol, phenol, iodophors, aldehydes, benzalkonium chloride, and quaternary ammonia compounds. Exposure of oocysts to 5.25% sodium hypochloride (full strength bleach) will destroy infectivity after 10 minutes. However, normally used concentrations of bleach have been shown to be poor disinfectants for *Cryptosporidium*. And 3% hydrogen peroxide is felt to be more effective and is recommended for outbreak control; 5% ammonia is also effective; however, it has a strong odor and if mixed accidentally with chlorine containing solutions (such as bleach) can produce hazardous chlorine gas.
—Temporarily excluding or, if possible, cohorting symptomatic children. Since fecal shedding can be quite prolonged, it is generally recommended that once symptoms have resolved children should be allowed to return to their regular settings.

• During an outbreak, screening should be considered for children and caregivers who are in a household or in close contact with immunocompromised persons.
• Swimming pools found to be contaminated with *Cryptosporidium* require closing and hyperchlorination. The level of chlorination required to kill *Cryptosporidium* oocysts is approximately 640 times greater than that required to kill *Giardia* cysts. Maintaining this level of chlorination is not feasible and, therefore, swimming in public pools places an immunocompromised patient at increased risk.

PITFALLS

• Not considering the diagnosis in patients with acute diarrhea.
• Not sending the appropriate number of stool specimens to exclude the diagnosis.
• Assuming the microbiology lab will routinely test for *C. parvum*.
• Forgetting to test for other parasites if *C. parvum* is found in the stool.

Common Questions and Answers

Q: For whom should cryptosporidiosis as a differential diagnosis be considered?
A: For anyone with acute onset of watery diarrhea with any of the mentioned risk factors.

Q: When is it safe for a child with *Cryptosporidium* to return to day care?
A: When the diarrhea has resolved.

ICD-9-CM 559.007.4

BIBLIOGRAPHY

American Academy of Pediatrics. Cryptosporidium. In: *1997 red book: report of the Committee on Infectious Diseases* , 24th ed. Elk Grove Village, IL: American Academy of Pediatrics. 1997:185–186.

Cordel RL, Addiss DG. Cryptosporidiosis in child care settings: a review of the literature and recommendations for prevention and control. *Pediatr Infect Dis* 1994;13:310–317.

LaVia W. Parasitic gastroenteritis. *Pediatr Ann* 1994;(23):556–560.

Outbreak of cryptosporidiosis at a day camp. *MMWR* 1996;45(21):442–444.

Outbreaks of *Escherichia coli* 0157:H7 infection and cryptosporidiosis associated with drinking unpasteurized apple cider. *MMWR* 1997;46(1):4–8.

Author: Jane M. Gould

Cushing Syndrome (Adrenal Excess)

 ## Database

DEFINITION

An excess in the secretion of cortisol by the adrenal cortex. This may be associated with excess production of other adrenal hormones, such as androgens and mineralocorticoids.

PATHOPHYSIOLOGY

- Cushing disease—pituitary ACTH oversecretion, usually due to pituitary adenoma, with resultant bilateral adrenal hyperplasia.

—Adrenal tumors
—Adrenal adenomas—secrete mainly cortisol
—Adrenal cortical carcinomas—usually large, rapidly growing tumors, which produce a variety of hormones including cortisol and androgens.

EPIDEMIOLOGY

- Incidence

—0.1 to 0.5 new pediatric cases per million population/year
—Ten times more common in adults

- Gender

—Cushing disease—female predominance
—Adrenocortical carcinoma—female predominance

- Age

—Cushing disease—accounts for 80% of Cushing syndrome in adults and children greater than 7 years of age.
—Adrenal tumor—adrenocortical carcinomas account for more than 50% of Cushing syndrome in children less than age 7.

- These tumors are less common in adults and children older than 7 years of age.

COMPLICATIONS

- Cushing syndrome

—Growth arrest
—Obesity
—Pubertal arrest
—Glucose intolerance
—Osteoporosis
—Adrenal carcinomas—metastatic spread

PROGNOSIS

- The prognosis for cure is good with Cushing disease and adrenal adenoma.
- The prognosis for adrenal carcinoma is poor because of the frequency of micrometastases and high recurrence rate.

 ## Differential Diagnosis

- Cushing disease
—Pituitary ACTH oversecretion
- Adrenal tumors
—Adrenal adenomas
—Adrenal cortical carcinomas
- Exogenous glucocorticoid treatment

 ## Data Gathering

HISTORY

- Weight gain, gradual onset
- Weakness and fatigue

Question: What emotional/mental changes are seen?
Significance: Cortisol excess can cause emotional changes.

 ## Physical Examination

Finding: Growth arrest
Significance: Most consistent finding

Finding: Obesity
Significance: Cervicodorsal fat (localized: moon facies, truncal obesity)

Finding: Thin skin with striae, facial plethora
Significance: Sign of cortisol excess

Finding: Hirsutism, acne
Significance: Sex hormone effect

Finding: Pubertal arrest/menstrual disorders
Significance: Common finding

Finding: Hypertension
Significance: Mineralocorticoid effect

Finding: Bruising
Significance: Capillary friability

Finding: Hyperpigmentation
Significance: ACTH effect

Finding: Virilization/feminization
Significance: Sex hormone effect

 ## Laboratory Aids

DIAGNOSTIC TESTS

Test: Urinary 24-h free cortisol greater than 90 μg/24 h (preferred test). Correct for creatinine and surface area. Two or three separate collections are preferable.
Significance: Establishes the diagnosis of hypercortisolism

Test: Urinary 24-h 17-hydroxysteroids greater than 6 mg/g creatinine
Significance: Establishes the diagnosis of hypercortisolism

Test: Overnight dexamethasone suppression test (15 μg/kg)
Significance: Screening only; 8:00 A.M. plasma cortisol = 5 μg/L, suspect hypercortisolism

Test: Loss of diurnal variation of plasma cortisol in older children.
Significance: Normally, the 11:00 P.M. cortisol is less than 50% of 8:00 A.M. value. The majority of patients with Cushing syndrome have mean elevated plasma cortisol, without diurnal variation.

DIFFERENTIATE CAUSES

Test: ACTH levels
Significance: Cushing disease: increased ACTH with hypercortisolism. Adrenal tumor: low ACTH and hypercortisolism.

Test: Androgen levels
Significance: Often high in adrenocortical carcinoma. These patients are often virilized. Androgen levels are low in benign cortisol secreting adenomas.

Test: Dexamethasone suppression tests. Low dose (30 μg/kg/day) divided q6h PO × 2 days, followed by high dose (120 μg/kg/day) divided q6h PO × 2 days. A 24-h urine collection for cortisol and 17-hydroxysteroids throughout.
Significance: Non-Cushing states usually suppress urinary-free cortisol and 17 hydroxysteroids to 50% to 90% of baseline values after low dose.

- Majority of pituitary tumors suppressible after high dose.
- Adrenal source: Hypercortisolism will not suppress.

TUMOR LOCATION

Test: Pituitary MRI with gadolinium
Significance: May demonstrate a pituitary adenoma.

Test: Abdominal CT/MRI
Significance: Will demonstrate adrenal carcinoma, adrenal adenomas, or bilateral hyperplasia/nodules resulting from Cushing disease.

Test: Cavernous sinus sampling for ACTH
Significance: Will help to lateralize pituitary microadenomas.

Therapy

CUSHING DISEASE

• Transphenoidal pituitary surgery

—70% to 80% success, may be less in some series
—Perioperative glucocorticoid replacement required

• Pituitary radiation—6 to 18 months for effect

—Remission in 45% to 85% of individuals
—Remission rate improved if combined with o,p'DDD

• Bilateral adrenalectomy

—High rate of surgical complications
—May result in Nelson syndrome—pituitary adenoma growth and hyperpigmentation, long-term glucocorticoid and mineralocorticoid replacement.

• Drug therapy

—Ketoconazole—inhibits multiple adrenal enzymes
—o,p'DDD—adrenolytic agent
—Metyrapone—11-hydroxylase inhibitor
—Aminoglutethimide—20,22-desmolase inhibitor
—Trilostane—3β-hydroxysteroid dehydrogenase inhibitor
—RU-486—Glucocorticoid receptor antagonist
—Drug combinations may lower individual doses and lessen side effects

• Adrenal tumors

—Aggressive surgical resection
—Chemotherapy for carcinoma: Cytoxan, Adriamycin, 5-FU, MTX

• Drug therapy to control hypercortisolism

—o,p'DDD at high doses—may improve recurrence risk in patients with complete tumor resection. In those with residual or recurrent disease, it may improve hypercortisolism, but not survival

• Glucocorticoid and possibly mineralocorticoid replacement.

Follow-Up

• Chronic glucocorticoid replacement 10 to 12 mg/m^{2}day divided as b.i.d. to t.i.d. until recovery of hypothalamic/pituitary function (6–12 months). Triple for stress, fever illness, vomiting. Injectable hydrocortisone for emergency use taper corticosteroid treatment gradually.
• Reassess 24-h urinary cortisol/ketosteroid secretion during the first week after treatment and at 6 weeks.
• In the week after effective pituitary surgery, cortisol should be undetectable and ACTH less than 5 pg/mL, 24 hours after last hydrocortisone dose. Stimulation and suppression tests are performed 6 weeks postsurgery (holding hydrocortisone dose).
• Frequent follow-up to monitor for recurrence. Monitor for cortisol withdrawal symptoms, hypopituitarism. Consider medical treatment for persistent hypercortisolism.

PITFALLS

• False-positive tests for hypercortisolism

—Stress—lack of suppression
—Depression
—Anorexia
—Primary glucocorticoid resistance

• False-negative tests

—Incomplete urine collection
—Periodic hormonogenesis
—Slow metabolism of dexamethasone

• Aberrant renal metabolism
• Repeat if suspicion is strong

Common Questions and Answers

Q: What clinical features help distinguish patients with pituitary Cushing disease from patients with adrenal tumors?
A: Cushing syndrome and hyperpigmentation suggests an ACTH effect. Cushing syndrome and virilization suggests adrenal carcinoma.

Q: What physical characteristics most clearly differentiate children with exogenous obesity from those with Cushing syndrome?
A: Exogenous obesity is associated with robust linear growth while Cushing syndrome is associated with growth failure.

ICD-9-CM 255

BIBLIOGRAPHY

Boscaro M, Barzon L, Fallo F, et al. Cushing's syndrome. *Lancet* 2001;357(9258):783–791.

Cacciari E, Cicognani A, Pirazzoli P, et al. Adrenocortical tumours in children: our experience with nine cases. *Acta Endocrinol Suppl (Copenh)* 1986;279:264–274.

Gomez MT, Malozowski S, Winterer J, et al. Urinary free cortisol values in normal children and adolescents. *J Pediatr* 1991;118(2):256–258.

Leinung MC, Kane LA, Scheithauer BW, et al. Long term-follow-up of transsphenoidal surgery for the treatment of Cushing's disease in childhood. *J Clin Endocrinol Metab* 1995;80(8):2475–2479.

Lindholm J, Juul S, Jorgensen JO, et al. Incidence and late prognosis of cushing's syndrome: a population-based study. *J Clin Endocrinol Metab* 2001;86(1):117–123.

Magiakou MA, Mastorakos G, Oldfield EH, et al. Cushing's syndrome in children and adolescents: presentation, diagnosis, and therapy. *N Engl J Med* 1994;331:629–636.

Papanicolaou DA, Yanovski JA, Cutler GB Jr, et al. A single midnight serum cortisol measurement distinguishes Cushing's syndrome from pseudo-Cushing states. *J Clin Endocrinol Metab* 1998;83(4):1163–1167.

Yanovski JA, Cutler GB Jr, Chrousos GP, et al. The dexamethasone-suppressed corticotropin-releasing hormone stimulation test differentiates mild Cushing's disease from normal physiology. *J Clin Endocrinol Metab* 1998;83(2):348–352.

Yanovski JA, Friedman TC, Nieman LK, et al. Inferior petrosal sinus AVP in patients with Cushing's syndrome. *Clin Endocrinol* 1997;47(2):199–206.

Author: Lorraine Katz

Cutaneous Larva Migrans

 Database

DEFINITION

Infestation of the epidermis by the infectious larvae of certain nematodes. Humans are accidental hosts, with the primary hosts being dogs and cats.

CAUSES

• Most common organism is the dog or cat hookworm, *Ancylostoma braziliense*.
• Other species include *A. canium, Uncinaria stenocephala*, and *Bunostomum phlebotomum*.

PATHOPHYSIOLOGY

• Humans are accidental hosts.
• Filariform larvae penetrate the epidermis either through hair follicles or fissures or through intact skin with the use of proteases.
• Diagnosis is usually clinical. Organisms rarely recovered from biopsy and antibody titers unreliable because symptoms are due to hypersensitivity to the organism or its excreta, and immunity usually does not develop.

ASSOCIATED DISEASES

• Most common manifestation is an intensely pruritic, linear, serpiginous skin lesion known as a "creeping eruption."
• Most common complication is secondary bacterial infection of the involved skin.
• Rare cases of a peripheral eosinophilia with pulmonary infiltrates (Loffler syndrome) occur when dermal penetration by the larvae occurs and the bloodstream is invaded.

EPIDEMIOLOGY

• Contracted from contaminated soil.
• Worldwide distribution, but most frequent in warmer climates, including the Caribbean, Africa, South America, Southeast Asia, and Southeastern United States.
• Occupational exposures occur from crawling under buildings, such as plumbers and pipe-fitters.
• Route of spread

—Primary host (dog or cat) passes eggs to ground through feces.
—Warm, sandy soil acts as an incubator.
—Eggs mature into rhabditiform larvae (noninfectious), which molt in 5 days to filariform larvae (infectious).
—Incubation period from infection to symptoms usually 7 to 10 days, although can range up to several months.

COMPLICATIONS

• Most common complication is secondary bacterial infection of the skin. Self-limited disease—if untreated, larvae die within 2 to 8 weeks but may persist for up to 1 year.
• Rarely, the larvae can invade the dermis and, subsequently, the bloodstream, leading to a peripheral eosinophilia and pulmonary infiltrates (Loffler syndrome).

PROGNOSIS

• This is a self-limited disease and without treatment will resolve when the larvae die.
• There is a 98% response rate to topical thiabendazole and a 99% response rate reported with oral thiabendazole.

 Differential Diagnosis

• Cutaneous larva migrans should be considered in anyone with an intensely pruritic, raised, serpiginous, linear cutaneous eruption.
• Hookworm infections (*Strongyloides stercoralis, Uncinaria stenocephala, Bunostomum phlebotomum, Gnathostoma spinigerum*)
• Free living nematodes (*Pelodera strongyloides*), and insect larvae.
• Other cutaneous eruptions that may mimic cutaneous larva migrans include erythema chronicum migrans of Lyme disease, jelly fish stings, and photosensitivity.

 Data Gathering

HISTORY

Question: What is the incubation period?
Significance: Usual time from infection to symptoms is 7 to 10 days but may last for up to several months.

Question: Is there rash?
Significance: It is intensely pruritic, raised, serpiginous, and linear. Often located on the feet and extremities, buttocks, and genitalia.

Question: Is there pruritus?
Significance: Symptoms typically begin with some tingling in the affected area with the development of the typical rash with intense pruritus.

Question: How fast does rash spread?
Significance: Rash typically lengthens by 2 to 3 cm daily.

Physical Examination

Track under the skin reflects the course of the larvae. The active end is not part of the track.

 ## Laboratory Aids

Test: Biopsy
Significance: Rarely yields organisms

Test: Serologic testing
Significance: Not helpful

Diagnosis based on clinical presentation

 ## Therapy

- First-line treatment is topical thiabendazole, supplied as a 10% suspension of 500 mg/5 mL applied four times per day for 10 days.
- Alternatively, oral thiabendazole in a dose of 25 to 50 mg/kg/day q12h for 2 days
- Albendazole, not approved for use in the United States, is available in other countries and is administered as 400 mg/day for 3 days in adults.

 ## Follow-Up

- Symptoms persist for 8 weeks but up to 1 year in untreated patients.
- Those with extensive involvement should be seen after treatment to be certain of improvement in symptoms.

 ## Common Questions and Answers

Q: Can children spread the infection to each other?
A: The usual spread of infection is from direct contact with the larvae. Spread from one individual to another usually does not occur.

ICD-9-CM 126.9

BIBLIOGRAPHY

Caumes E. Treatment of cutaneous larva migrans. *Clin Infect Dis* 2000;30(5):811–814.

Davies HD, Sakuls P, Keystone JS. Creeping eruption: a review of clinical presentation and management of 60 cases presenting to a tropical disease unit. *Arch Dermatol* 1993; 129(5):588–591.

Jones SK. Cutaneous larva migrans— "recurrens" [letter]. *Br J Dermatol* 1994; 130(4):546.

Jones WB. Cutaneous larva migrans. *South Med J* 1993;86(11):1311–1313.

Uppal A, Liebers D, Tobin EH. Tracking the itch. When to suspect migrating larvae. *Postgrad Med* 1997;101(5):281–282,288.

Van den Enden E, Stevens A, Van Gompel A. Treatment of cutaneous larva migrans. *N Engl J Med* 1998;339(17):1246–1247.

Author: Louis M. Bell
Bret J. Rudy, 2nd edition

Cystic Fibrosis

 Database

DEFINITION
Cystic fibrosis (CF) is an inherited, autosomal-recessive disorder, characterized by chronic obstructive lung disease, pancreatic exocrine insufficiency, and elevated sweat chloride concentration.

PATHOPHYSIOLOGY
• CF transmembrane conductance regulator (CFTR)
—Membrane glycoprotein, which functions as a cyclic AMP-activated chloride channel at the apical surface of epithelial cells.
—An abnormality in CFTR results in defective chloride conductance.
—May have other roles in the regulation of membrane channels and the pH of intracellular organelles.
• In the respiratory system
—Lungs are morphologically normal at birth.
—Increased viscosity of mucus
—Early bacterial colonization despite a robust neutrophilic inflammatory response.
—Mucus plugging and atelectasis
—Bronchiectasis
• In the gastrointestinal tract
—Exocrine pancreatic insufficiency
—Focal biliary cirrhosis of the liver
—Hypoplasia of the gallbladder

GENETICS
• CFTR gene
—Located on the long arm of chromosome 7
—Most common mutation results in deletion of phenylalanine at position 508 in the CFTR glycoprotein. This Δ508 mutation occurs in almost 70% of CF patients.
—Over 1,000 mutations have been reported in the CFTR gene

EPIDEMIOLOGY
• Most common lethal inherited disease in the Caucasian population
• Carrier frequency of mutations in the CFTR gene
—1:29 in Caucasians
—1:49 in Hispanics
—1:53 in Native Americans
—1:62 in African Americans
—1:90 in Asians
• Incidence of CF
—1:3,300 in Caucasians
—1:9,500 in Hispanics
—1:11,200 in Native Americans
—1:15,300 in African Americans
—1:32,100 in Asians

COMPLICATIONS
• Respiratory complications
—Recurrent bronchitis and pneumonia
—Atelectasis
—Bronchiectasis
—Pneumothorax
—Hemoptysis
—Chronic sinusitis and nasal polyps
• Gastrointestinal complications

—Pancreatic insufficiency in 85% to 90% of CF patients
—Patients usually have steatorrhea, poor growth, and nutritional status
—Decreased levels of vitamins A, E, D, and K
—Rectal prolapse
—10% to 15% of patients have meconium ileus
—Distal intestinal obstruction syndrome
—Clinically significant focal biliary cirrhosis hepatobiliary disease in 5% of CF patients
—Esophageal varices
—Splenomegaly
—Hypersplenism
—Cholestasis
• Reproductive complications:
—Sterility in 98% of the males due to absence or atresia of the vas deferens
—Slight decrease in fertility for females secondary to abnormalities of cervical mucus.
• Endocrine complications:
—CF-related diabetes occurs with increasing frequency in CF adolescents and adults.

PROGNOSIS
• Median survival is approximately 30 years of age.
• Variable course of the disease

 Differential Diagnosis

PULMONARY
• Recurrent pneumonia or bronchitis
• Asthma
• Aspiration pneumonia

GASTROINTESTINAL
• Failure to thrive
• Celiac disease
• Protein-losing enteropathy

OTHER
• Metabolic alkalosis
• Immune deficiency

 Data Gathering

HISTORY

Question: Have there been respiratory symptoms?
Significance: The most common presenting respiratory symptoms:
• Chronic cough
• Recurrent pneumonia
• Nasal polyps
• Chronic pansinusitis

Question: Have there been gastrointestinal symptoms?
Significance: Most common presenting gastrointestinal symptoms:
• Meconium ileus (15–20% of patients present with this symptom).
• Pancreatic insufficiency occurs in 85% of patients.
• In infants, fat malabsorption may lead to failure to thrive.
• In older patients, pancreatitis

• Rectal prolapse
—Occurs in 2% of the patients
—Must consider CF until proven otherwise
—Commonly seen between 1 and 5 years
• Meconium ileus equivalent:
—Distal obstruction of the small intestine
—Seen in older children and adults

Question: Evidence of heat intolerance?
Significance: In summer, increased sweating may lead to dehydration with hyponatremia or hypochloremic metabolic alkalosis.

 Physical Examination

Findings: Respiratory findings
Significance:
• Frequent cough, often productive of mucopurulent sputum
• Rhonchi
• Crackles
• Hyperresonance to percussion
• Nasal polyposis

Findings: Other common findings:
• Digital clubbing
• Hepatosplenomegaly in patients with cirrhosis
• Growth retardation
• Hypertrophic osteoarthropathy
• Delayed puberty

 Laboratory Aids

Test: Sweat test
Significance: Keystone for the diagnosis of CF; sweat chloride greater than 60 mEq/L is abnormal.
Other causes of elevated sweat chloride:
• Malnutrition
• Adrenal insufficiency
• Nephrogenic diabetes insipidus
• Ectodermal dysplasia
• Fucosidosis
• Hypogammaglobulinemia
• False-negatives seen in:
—CF Patients with edema

Test: Mutation analysis
Significance: Can detect over 90% of the CF patients. Failure to identify two mutations reduces, but does not eliminate, the possibility of CF.

Collection methods include blood samples or cheek brushings.

Test: Sputum culture
Significance: Frequently recovered organisms include:
• *Haemophilus influenzae*
• *Staphylococcus aureus*
• *Pseudomonas aeruginosa* (nonmucoid and mucoid)
• *Burkholderia cepacia*
• *Stenotrophomonas maltophilia*
• *Aspergillus* species

Test: Pulmonary function tests
Significance: Usually reveals obstructive lung disease, although some patients may have a restrictive pattern.

Test: Analysis of stimulated pancreatic secretions
Significance: Degree of pancreatic exocrine deficiency

Test: 72-hour fecal fat measurement
Significance: Fat malabsorption

Test: Stool trypsin levels
Significance: Correlates with pancreatic insufficiency in infants

IMAGING
- Chest radiology
—Typical features include:
  —Hyperinflation
  —Peribronchial thickening
  —Atelectasis
  —Bronchiectasis
- CT scan
—Early bronchiectasis

Therapy

DRUGS
- Antibiotic therapy (based on sputum culture results)
—Oral antibiotics
—Cephalexin
—Cefaclor
—Trimethoprim-sulfamethoxazole
—Ciprofloxacin
—Inhaled
—Tobramycin or colistin in selected patients
—Intravenous antibiotics
—To treat *S. aureus* consider oxacillin, ticarcillin with clavulanic acid, or vancomycin.
—To treat *P. aeruginosa* and *B. cepacia* consider aminoglycoside plus ticarcillin, ceftazidime, or piperacillin.
—Severe cases with resistant strains may benefit from imipenem or meropenem.
—Synergistic antibiotic studies should be performed in patients with multiresistant organisms.

CLEARANCE OF PULMONARY SECRETIONS
- Chest physiotherapy with postural drainage and vibrations given manually, or with high-frequency oscillatory vest device. Adjunct therapy such as Flutter valve or PEP mask may also be used.
- Bronchodilator: aerosol or MDI
—β_2-agonist
- Mucolytics
—*N*-acetylcysteine
—RhDNase
- Antiinflammatory
—Cromolyn sodium
—Steroid (inhaled or short term oral)

LIVER DISEASE
- Patients with cholestasis may benefit from therapy with ursodeoxycholic acid
- Pancreatic enzyme replacement therapy:
—Used in CF patients who are pancreatic insufficient
—Dosage adjusted for frequency and character of the stools and for growth pattern
—Generic substitutes are not bioequivalent to name brands
—The maximum recommended dose is 2,500 units of lipase/kg/meal
- Vitamin supplements:
—Multivitamin supplement
—Fat-soluble vitamins (usually E and K)

DIET
- High-calorie diet with added salt

DURATION
- Usually lifelong nutritional support required
- Duration of antibiotic therapy is controversial; more frequent use is required as chronic use is required as pulmonary function deteriorates

Follow-Up

CARE PLAN
- Specialized care should be at a CF center
- Frequency of visits depends on severity of illness; usually every 2 to 3 months

PROGNOSIS
- Current median survival is approximately 30 years
- The median survival has been increasing for the past four decades, although the rate of increase in age has slowed in the past decade.

PREVENTION
- Prepregnancy carrier detection

PITFALLS
- Most common pitfall is failure to diagnose.
- Not uncommon to delay making the diagnosis in patients with mild symptoms.

Common Questions and Answers

Q: Should relatives be tested?
A: All siblings should have a sweat test.

Q: How well will a child with CF do?
A: The course of the illness is variable. It is difficult to predict the course of disease in an individual.

Q: How should borderline sweat test be interpreted?
A: Borderline sweat tests should always be correlated with other findings such as physical examination, sputum cultures, pulmonary function, radiographic findings, nutritional evaluation, mutation analysis.

ICD-9-CM 277.0

BIBLIOGRAPHY
Davis PB. *Cystic fibrosis*. New York: Dekker, 1993.

Dezateux C, Walters S, Balfour-Lynn I. Inhaled corticosteroids for cystic fibrosis. Cochrane Database of Systematic Reviews [computer file], issue 2: CD001915, 2000.

Quittner AL. Measurement of quality of life in cystic fibrosis. *Curr Opin Pulmon Med* 1998;4(6):326–331.

Ramsey BW. Management of pulmonary disease in patients with cystic fibrosis. *N Engl J Med* 1996;328:1740–1746.

Robinson CB, Scanlin TF. Cystic fibrosis. In: Fishman EP, ed. *Pulmonary diseases and disorders*. New York: McGraw-Hill, 1997:803–824.

Smyth A, Walters S. Prophylactic antibiotics for cystic fibrosis Cochrane Database of Systematic Reviews [computer file], issue 2: CD001912, 2000.

Welsh MJ, Tsui L-C, Boat TF, et al. Cystic fibrosis, In: Scriber CL, Beaudet AL, Sly WS, et al., eds. *The metabolic and molecular bases of inherited disease*, 7th ed. New York: McGraw-Hill, 1995:3799–3876.

Author: Thomas F. Scanlin

Cytomegalovirus Infection

 Database

DEFINITION

Cytomegalovirus (CMV) is a ubiquitous double-stranded DNA virus that is a member of the herpesvirus family. Establishes latency in peripheral mononuclear cells.

PATHOPHYSIOLOGY

Infection leads to intranuclear inclusions with massive enlargement of cells. Almost any organ may become infected with CMV in severe disseminated infection.

EPIDEMIOLOGY

• Seroprevalence varies with socioeconomic status; 50% of middle and 80% of lower socioeconomic status adults are seropositive.
• Increased rates of primary infection seen in early childhood, adolescence, and childbearing years.
• Transmission may occur via contact with infected respiratory secretions, urine, or breast milk, sexual contact, solid organ transplantation, or infusion of infective blood products.

COMPLICATIONS/PROGNOSIS

Varies with nature of infection (see below).

ASSOCIATED DISEASES

Congenital Infection

• Occurs in 1% of newborns.
• 10% of infected infants are symptomatic at birth, with severe cytomegalic inclusion disease characterized by growth retardation, hepatosplenomegaly, thrombocytopenia, and CNS involvement.
• 10% to 20% of infants who are asymptomatically infected at birth will develop long-term sequelae.
• Most common cause of congenital deafness.

Mononucleosis Syndrome

• CMV can cause a mononucleosis-like syndrome similar to that caused by Epstein-Barr virus (EBV) infection.
• Pharyngitis and splenomegaly may be less severe than that associated with EBV-induced mononucleosis.

Interstitial Pneumonitis

• Primarily seen in immunosuppressed children and adults.
• Usually begins with fever and nonproductive cough, but may progress to dyspnea and severe hypoxia over 1 to 2 weeks.
• Mild, self-limited pneumonitis may occur in immunocompetent patients.

Retinitis

• Seen in approximately 30% of infants with symptomatic congenital infection.
• May complicate CMV disease in patients with severe immunodeficiency.

Hepatitis

• Occurs in healthy individuals with primary infections and immunosuppressed patients with either primary or reactivated disease.
• Characterized by mildly elevated liver function studies, mild hepatomegaly, and fever.
• Jaundice and severe hepatitis uncommon.

Gastrointestinal Disease

• Severely immunosuppressed patients may experience esophagitis, gastritis, colitis, or pancreatitis.

CNS Disease

• Commonly seen in infants with symptomatic congenital infection.
• Characterized by microcephaly, periventricular calcifications, seizures, developmental delay, and sensorineural hearing loss.
• Encephalitis or meningoencephalitis may occur postnatally in either healthy or immunocompromised patients.

 Differential Diagnosis

Congenital Infection

• Congenital rubella syndrome
• Toxoplasmosis
• Syphilis
• Neonatal herpes simplex virus
• HIV
• Enteroviral infection

Mononucleosis Syndrome

• EBV infection
• Toxoplasmosis
• Hepatitis A or B infection

Interstitial Pneumonitis

• Respiratory syncytial virus
• Adenovirus
• Measles
• Varicella
• *Pneumocystis carinii*
• Chlamydia
• Mycoplasma
• Fungal
• Drug/toxin-induced

Retinitis

• Ocular toxoplasmosis
• Candidal retinitis
• Syphilis
• Herpes simplex virus

Hepatitis

• EBV infection
• Hepatitis A, B, or C infection
• Enterovirus
• Adenovirus
• Herpes simplex virus
• Drug/toxin-induced

Gastrointestinal Disease

• Herpes simplex virus
• Adenovirus
• *Salmonella*
• *Shigella*
• *Campylobacter*
• *Yersinia*
• *C. difficile*
• *Giardia*
• *Cryptosporidium*

CNS Disease

• Congenital disease (see Congenital Infection, above)
• Meningoencephalitis in immunocompetent host: herpes simplex virus, EBV, varicella-zoster virus, enterovirus, arbovirus
• Meningoencephalitis in immunocompromised host: in addition to organisms listed previously, differential diagnosis should include HIV encephalitis, fungal meningitis (due to *Cryptococcus, Candida, Aspergillus, Histoplasma*), toxoplasmosis.

 Data Gathering

HISTORY

Question: Day-care attendance?
Significance: Increased risk of infection

Question: Recent blood transfusion?
Significance: Transfusion-associated CMV

Question: Use of immunosuppressive medications?
Significance: Increased use of serious infection

Question: Prolonged fever?
Significance: Mononucleosis-like syndrome

Question: Blurred vision?
Significance: CMV retinitis

Question: Cough, dyspnea, wheezing?
Significance: CMV pneumonitis

Question: Vomiting, abdominal pain, diarrhea (watery or bloody)?
Significance: CMV colitis

Cytomegalovirus Infection

Physical Examination

Finding: Microcephaly
Significance: Congenital infection

Finding: White, perivascular retinal infiltrates and hemorrhage
Significance: Retinitis

Finding: Deafness (may require audiogram, brainstem evoked auditory responses, etc.)
Significance: Congenital infection

Finding: Photophobia, headache, nuchal rigidity
Significance: Meningitis

Finding: Tachypnea, rales
Significance: Pneumonitis

Finding: Hepatomegaly and/or splenomegaly
Significance: Mononucleosis-like syndrome

Finding: Rash
Significance: Petechiae, purpura, "blueberry muffin" lesions, rubelliform rash

Finding: Adenopathy
Significance: Mononucleosis-like syndrome

Laboratory Aids

Test: Viral culture
Significance: Virus may be isolated from nasopharyngeal/oropharyngeal secretions, urine, stool, white blood cells. Isolation of virus may take up to 4 weeks.

Test: Shell-vial assay
Significance: Enhanced viral culture through the use of centrifugation. Allows detection of virus 24 to 72 hours after inoculation.

Test: Direct immunofluorescence
Significance: Detection of CMV-infected cells in specimens from biopsy or bronchoalveolar lavage.

Test: Quantitative antigenemia assay
Significance: Detection of circulating CMV-infected mononuclear cells by indirect immunofluorescence. In an immuno-compromised patient, may monitor response to therapy or identify viral reactivation.

Test: DNA hybridization
Significance: Detection of viral nucleic acid in tissue specimens

Test: Histologic examination
Significance: Presence of typical enlarged cells with intranuclear inclusions ("owl's-eye" nuclear inclusion)

Test: Serology
Significance: ELISA or indirect fluorescent antibody assay to detect the presence of CMV IgM or IgG. CMV IgM usually persists for 6 weeks following primary infection although may persist up to 6 months.

PITFALLS

• Due to frequency of asymptomatic shedding, mere isolation of virus does not necessarily establish an etiologic association.
• Severely immunocompromised patients who are actively infected with CMV may be seronegative.
• Fourfold rise in CMV IgG not diagnostic of primary infection. Increased antibody titers may occur with reactivation.
• False-positive detection of CMV IgM may occur due to production of cross-reactive antibodies.
• Congenital CMV infection should be established by viral isolation from urine or nasopharyngeal secretions within the first 2 weeks of life.

Therapy

DRUGS

• Ganciclovir will suppress replication but not eradicate virus (virostatic agent).

—Indications: CMV chorioretinitis in immunocompromised patients; tissue diagnosis (hepatitis, enteritis, pneumonitis) of CMV infection or isolation of CMV from buffy coat of immunocompromised patient; may consider for neonate with documented CNS disease.
—Side effects: neutropenia (~50%), thrombocytopenia (~5%)

• Foscarnet—virostatic agent

—Indications: CMV chorioretinitis, pneumonitis, hepatitis, enteritis (biopsy-proven) in an immunocompromised patient who has failed to improve on ganciclovir therapy or has experienced significant bone marrow toxicity related to ganciclovir use
—Side effects: renal impairment (25%), headache (25%), seizures (10%)

PREVENTION

• Drainage and secretion, and pregnant women precautions should be instituted for hospitalized patients known to be shedding CMV.
• Seriously ill neonates should receive blood products from CMV-negative donors.
• CMV-seronegative solid organ or bone marrow transplantation recipients should receive organs (and all blood products) from CMV-negative donors whenever possible.
• Controversy exists over role of hyperimmune globulin to prevent disseminated CMV disease in CMV-negative recipient of CMV-positive transplantation.

Common Questions and Answers

Q: Should children with congenital CMV infection be excluded from day-care settings?
A: No. Due to the high frequency of shedding of CMV in the urine and saliva of asymptomatic children, especially under 2 years of age, exclusion from out-of-home care is not justified for any child known to be infected with CMV. Careful attention to hygienic practices, especially hand washing, is important.

ICD-9-CM 078.5

BIBLIOGRAPHY

Boppana SR, Pass RF, Britt WJ, et al. Symptomatic congenital cytomegalovirus infection. *Pediatr Infect Dis J* 1992;11:93–99.

Brown HL, Abernathy MP. Cytomegalovirus infection. *Semin Perinatol* 1998;22(4): 260–266.

Cullen A, Brown S, Cafferkey M, et al. Current use of the TORCH screen in the diagnosis of congenital infection. *J Infect* 1998;36(2): 185–188.

Demmler GJ. Acquired cytomegalovirus infections. In: Feigin RD, Cherry JD, eds. *Textbook of pediatric infectious diseases*, 3rd ed. Philadelphia: WB Saunders, 1992: 1532–1547.

Demmler GJ. Congenital cytomegalovirus infection. *Semin Pediatr Neurol* 1994;1(1): 36–42.

Fowler KB, Stagno S, Pass RF, et al. The outcome of congenital cytomegalovirus infection in relation to maternal antibody status. *N Engl J Med* 1992;326(10):663–667.

Author: Susan E. Coffin

Daytime Incontinence

 Database

DEFINITIONS

- Enuresis—the expulsion of urine beyond the age of anticipated control, generally thought to be 5 years.
- Incontinence—the involuntary leakage of urine in a child older than 5 years.
- Voiding dysfunction—a dysfunction of the lower urinary tract without a recognized organic cause, generally in the form of bladder–sphincter discoordination.

CAUSES

- Neurogenic bladder (e.g., myelomeningocele)
- Anatomic anomalies (e.g., ectopic ureter)
- Obstructive uropathy (e.g., posterior urethral valves)
- Bladder irritability caused by urinary tract infection
- Constipation
- Increased urinary output/polyuria
- Infrequent or deferred voiding
- Low functional bladder capacity, with detrusor instability during filling
- Temperamental factors (short attention span, inattentiveness to body signals) in children who ignore the urge to void
- Developmental differences in age at which toilet training is achieved
- Vaginal reflux with subsequent leakage of urine

EPIDEMIOLOGY

- Of all children who wet, 10% have only daytime wetting, 75% wet only at night, and 15% wet during the day and at night.
- Studies in children 6 to 7 years of age have shown that 3.1% of girls and 2.1% of boys had an episode of wetting at least once per week.
- Spontaneous cure rate of 14% per year without treatment.

GENETICS

- Only anecdotal relationships have been seen in functional daytime incontinence, unlike studies showing genetic tendencies in nocturnal enuresis.
- Increased rates of daytime wetting have been reported in urofacial (Ochoa) syndrome, an autosomal-recessive condition, and Williams syndrome.

COMPLICATIONS

- Local irritation and inflammation of the perineum
- Functional daytime incontinence is primarily a social problem that affects children's self-esteem and interactions with peers.

ASSOCIATED PROBLEMS

- Constipation
- Nocturnal enuresis
- Children with dysfunctional voiding are at greater risk for urinary tract infections due to stasis of urine in the bladder and improper voiding.
- Vesicoureteral reflux is seen frequently in children with voiding dysfunction due to elevated detrusor pressure that overcome a marginal vesicoureteral junction.

 Differential Diagnosis

- Urinary tract infection
- Constipation
- Normal variations in toilet training
- Neurogenic bladder
- Spinal cord abnormality
- Giggle incontinence
- Genitourinary tract abnormality (posterior urethral valve, ectopic ureter)
- Vaginal reflux
- Benign increased urinary frequency (pollakiuria)
- Sexual abuse

 Data Gathering

HISTORY

- Onset (primary vs secondary)
- Frequency of voiding
- Frequency and degree of wetting
- Presence or absence of any dry interval
- Signs of urgency; use of hold maneuvers, waiting until the last minute to void
- Description of stream (strong/weak; continuous/interrupted)
- Straining or pushing during voiding
- Frequency and description of bowel movements/soiling
- History of urinary tract infections, vesicoureteral reflux
- Learning disabilities or developmental delays
- Level of concern on part of child/family
- Medications
- Quality and quantity of fluid intake
- Other medical conditions

 Physical Examination

- Focused PE

—Abdomen—signs of constipation; distended bladder
—Rectal—if constipation is suspected
—Spine—sacral abnormalities
—Genitalia—labial adhesions, erythema, phimosis, stenosis, urethritis
—Neurologic—sensation, reflexes, and gait

 Laboratory Aids

TESTS

- First A.M. urinalysis to check concentrating ability, rule out occult renal disease
- Urine culture to rule out infection

IMAGING

- Renal and bladder ultrasound in children who wet with a history of urinary tract infections and in children with persistent wetting despite regular voiding.
- Kidneys, ureter, and bladder (KUB) x-ray if history/exam suggestive of constipation
- Further imaging generally not indicated if wetting is the only concern.

Therapy

MEDICAL

- Place child on a timed voiding schedule, with voids every 2 to 3 hours.
- Positive reinforcement for regular voiding
- Aggressive management of constipation (see Constipation)
- Avoid consumption of bladder irritants (caffeine, carbonation, chocolate, citrus)
- Hydration
- Local management of perineal irritation/vulvovaginitis to ensure comfort during voiding
- Girls with postvoid dribbling due to vaginal reflux should void with their legs wide apart, sitting backward on the toilet when possible, to minimize backflow of urine into the vagina. Wipe after standing up.

PHARMACOLOGIC

If child continues to wet in spite of medical management, a trial on an anticholinergic medication may be indicated. Extended-release formulations may be tolerated better than short-acting preparations. Common side effects include dry mouth and decreased diaphoresis with flushing. Some patients note blurred vision, dizziness and constipation.

- Oxybutynin (Ditropan/Ditropan XL); 5 to 15 mg/day
- Tolterodine (Detrol/Detrol LA); 2 to 4 mg/day
- Hyoscyamine (Levbid); 0.75 to 1.5 mg/day

REFERRAL TO PEDIATRIC UROLOGIST

When wetting is refractory to behavioral and pharmacologic treatment, child may benefit from:

- Urodynamic study to assess for detrusor instability
- Biofeedback training to learn appropriate relaxation during voiding

 Follow-Up

- Spontaneous cure rate of 14% per year without treatment

PITFALLS

- Failure to recognize and manage constipation, before attempting to manage wetting
- Failure of anticholinergic medication in children with significant postvoid residuals
- Use of anticholinergic medications in children with benign frequency of childhood is generally ineffective.
- Increased risk of urinary tract infections when child is placed on anticholinergic, due to infrequent voiding/incomplete emptying

 Common Questions and Answers

Q: What data can distinguish functional incontinence from an ectopic ureter?
A: An ectopic ureter usually empties below the sphincter or elsewhere such as in the vagina. Therefore, these girls wet all the time with no dry period. They do not have symptoms such as urgency. Since, in most cases, the ureter draining the kidney is duplicated, an ultrasound or intravenous pyelogram (IVP) may provide more information.

Q: What is benign urinary frequency?
A: This condition, commonly seen in both genders around 4 to 5 years of age, is thought to be secondary to stress. It is episodic and may develop temporally after a stressful event such as the beginning of school or an illness in the family. These children may urinate frequently but they do not wet. At night the problem usually disappears. A urinalysis and urine culture are recommended to exclude organic pathology.

ICD-9-CM 788.30

BIBLIOGRAPHY

Bloom DA, Faerber G, Bomalaski MD. Urinary incontinence in girls. *Urol Clin North Am* 1995;22(3):521–537.

Bogaert G, Kogan B. Voiding dysfunction/functional incontinence (daytime wetting) in childhood. In: Baskin LS, Kogan BA, Duckett JW, eds. *Handbook of pediatric urology*. Philadelphia: Lippincott-Raven. 1997

Loening-Baucke V. Urinary incontinence and urinary tract infection and their resolution with treatment of chronic constipation of childhood. *Pediatrics* 1997;100:,228–231.

Rushton H. Wetting and functional voiding disorders. *Urol Clin North Am* 1995;22:75–93.

Schulman SL, Quinn CK, Platcher N, et al. Comprehensive management of dysfunctional voiding. *Pediatrics* 1999;103(3).

Authors: Amanda K. Berry and Seth Schulman

Dehydration

 Database

DEFINITION

- Dehydration is a negative balance of body fluid, usually expressed as a percentage of body weight. Mild, moderate, and severe dehydration correspond to deficits of <5%, 5% to 10%, and >10%, respectively.
- Dehydration is classified into three types based on the serum sodium concentration: isotonic (Na 130–150 mmol/L), hypotonic (Na <130 mmol/L), and hypertonic (Na >150 mmol/L).

PATHOPHYSIOLOGY

Dehydration is caused by either excessive fluid losses or inadequate intake. Some conditions leading to dehydration include:

- Gastrointestinal losses—vomiting, diarrhea (most common cause of dehydration in pediatric patients)
- Renal losses—diabetes mellitus, diabetes insipidus, diuretic agents
- Insensible losses—sweating, fever, tachypnea, increased ambient temperature, large burns
- Poor oral intake—stomatitis, pharyngitis, anorexia, oral trauma, altered mental status

Note that infants and debilitated patients are at particular risk due to lack of ability to satisfy their thirst freely.

EPIDEMIOLOGY

Approximately 10% of children in the United States with acute gastroenteritis develop at least mild dehydration. Although it accounts for 10% of all nonsurgical hospital admissions for children under 5 years of age, up to 90% of cases can be managed on an outpatient basis.

COMPLICATIONS

- Severe dehydration may lead to hypovolemic shock and acute renal failure.
- Hyponatremia is associated with hypotonia, hypothermia, and seizures.
- Overly rapid correction of hypernatremia can produce cerebral edema.

PROGNOSIS

Excellent with appropriate rehydration therapy.

 Data Gathering

HISTORY

Question: Frequency and duration of emesis and/or diarrhea?
Significance: This will give a rough estimate of risk of dehydration.

Question: Amount and type of liquids taken?
Significance: If there were large quantities of water, be alert for hypotonic dehydration. If excessive electrolyte solution used for hydration, may have hypertonic dehydration.

Question: Frequency and quantity of urination (may be difficult to estimate in infants with diarrhea)?
Significance: Decreased urination indicates possibility of dehydration.

Question: Fever?
Significance: Fever increases insensible water loss.

Question: Exertion or heat exposure?
Significance: Increases insensible water loss.

 Physical Examination

Acute change in weight is the best indicator of the fluid deficit. If the child's recent pre-illness weight is not available for comparison, a reasonable estimate of the degree of dehydration may be made from physical findings.

Finding: General appearance
Significance: Lethargy, irritability, thirst

Finding: Vital signs
Significance: Tachycardia; orthostatic increase in heart rate or hypotension; hyperpnea

Finding: Skin
Significance: Prolonged capillary refill at fingertip (<2 seconds is normal in warm environment); mottling; poor turgor

Finding: Eyes
Significance: Decreased or absent tears; sunken eyes

Finding: Mucous membranes
Significance: Dry or parched

Finding: Anterior fontanelle
Significance: Sunken

DIAGNOSTIC PITFALLS

- Physical signs generally appear when the deficit is at least 2% to 3%.
- No single finding is pathognomonic of dehydration. A reasonable guideline is that the presence of three or more findings indicates at least mild dehydration. The number and severity of physical signs increase with the degree of dehydration.
- Urine output decreases early in the course of dehydration, and a history of decreased urination is a nonspecific finding.
- Capillary refill time is a specific indicator, but may be falsely prolonged by cool ambient temperature [<20°C (<68°F)]. It is not affected by fever.
- Children with a deficit greater than 15% will show signs of cardiovascular instability such as severe tachycardia and hypotension.
- Physical findings are more significant for a given degree of dehydration in children with hyponatremia, leading to overestimation of the deficit. Conversely, the clinical picture is somewhat moderated in hypernatremia.

 Laboratory Aids

Diagnosis of dehydration is best made on clinical grounds. The following laboratory tests are sometimes helpful adjuncts.

Test: Serum sodium
Significance: Classifies type of dehydration. Hyponatremia and hypernatremia are uncommon (<5% of cases). Measure sodium levels in cases of clinically severe disease, or if risk factors are present (e.g., young infant, history of excessive free water intake).

Test: Rapid glucose test or serum glucose
Significance: To detect hypoglycemia due to prolonged fasting

Test: Urine specific gravity
Significance: This is elevated early in dehydration, but may not become elevated at all in young infants or children with sickle cell disease.

Test: Serum bicarbonate
Significance: This is frequently low with diarrheal illness, even in the absence of dehydration. Useful to detect significant acidosis when dehydration is clinically severe.

Test: Blood urea nitrogen (BUN)
Significance: Rises only late in dehydration in children.

Dehydration

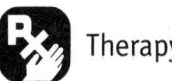

Therapy

ORAL REHYDRATION THERAPY (ORT)

Most children can be successfully managed with ORT.

- Use rehydration solution containing 2% to 2.5% glucose and 75 to 90 mmol/L Na (e.g., WHO solution), or 45 to 50 mmol/L Na [e.g., Pedialyte (Ross Laboratories, Columbus, OH), Infalyte, (Mead Johnson, Evansville, IN)].
- Replace entire deficit in 4 to 6 hours—for mild dehydration, 50 mL/kg; for moderate to severe dehydration, 80 to 100 mL/kg. Include ongoing losses, approximately 5 mL/kg for each diarrheal stool.
- Begin with slow administration, with strict limits when vomiting is present—5 mL every 1 to 2 minutes. For infants, use a syringe or spoon rather than a bottle. After 1 hour, if the oral liquids have been tolerated, increase the volume and rate.
- Have the child's caregiver participate in giving the fluids, and provide education regarding fluid replacement and signs of dehydration.
- Monitor weight, intake and output, and clinical signs. Failure of ORT includes intractable vomiting, clinical deterioration, or lack of improvement after 4 hours.

INTRAVENOUS FLUID THERAPY

Intravenous fluids are required when ORT fails or is contraindicated, such as in severe dehydration or shock, poor gag or suck, depressed mental status, preterm infant, severe hypernatremia (Na >160 mmol/L), suspected surgical abdomen.

- Administer intravenous bolus of normal saline or Ringer lactate, 20 mL/kg, over 10 to 30 minutes. Repeat as needed to restore cardiovascular stability. Avoid dextrose-containing solutions for boluses except to correct documented hypoglycemia.
- Calculate maintenance fluid requirements: 100 mL/kg for the first 10 kg, plus 50 mL/kg for the next 10 kg, plus 20 mL/kg over 20 kg.
- Calculate fluid deficit based on clinical estimate or known weight loss. For isotonic or hypotonic dehydration, give one-third to one-half normal saline with 5% dextrose, at a rate to provide maintenance and replace deficit over 24 hours. For hypertonic dehydration, replace deficit over 48 hours, using one-fifth to one-fourth normal saline with 5% dextrose.
- Monitor weight, intake and output, and clinical signs. With hypernatremia, measure serum sodium every 4 to 6 hours; do not exceed rate of fall of 1 mmol/L/h.

Follow-Up

After rehydration, children with ongoing losses, as in gastroenteritis, should receive a maintenance solution in addition to regular feedings to maintain a positive fluid balance. Recommend 5 to 10 mL/kg for each diarrheal stool. Avoid clear liquids with excessive glucose, such as fruit juices, punches, and soft drinks, as these can promote osmotic fluid losses in the stool. In infants less than 6 months old, do not give large amounts of plain water, which can lead to hyponatremia.

PREVENTION

Many cases of frank dehydration may be prevented by early institution of adequate oral maintenance fluid therapy in children with gastroenteritis, with particular attention to replacement of ongoing stool losses and slow administration of fluids to children with vomiting. Use of appropriate solutions is essential to prevent electrolyte disturbance and worsening of diarrhea.

Common Questions and Answers

Q: How can an oral rehydration solution be prepared at home?
A: An acceptable rehydration solution (2.2% glucose, 70 mmol Na/L) can be prepared with the following: half teaspoon of table salt, half teaspoon of baking soda, and 1 cup of orange juice, added to 3 cups of water. For maintenance solution, decrease the table salt to a quarter teaspoon.

Q: Can commercially available maintenance solutions be used for rehydration as well as maintenance?
A: Data suggest that reduced-osmolarity maintenance solutions, with a sodium concentration of 45 to 50 mmol/L, are equally effective for rehydration as solutions with a higher sodium content.

Q: How can oral rehydration solution be made more palatable?
A: Rehydration solutions may be more palatable if iced, or flavored with apple or orange juice (1 part juice to 4 parts rehydration solution) or unsweetened Kool-Aid powder (2.5 mL powder per 240 mL of solution).

ICD-9-CM 276.5

BIBLIOGRAPHY

American Academy of Pediatrics Provisional Committee on Quality Improvement, Subcommittee on Acute Gastroenteritis. Practice parameter: the management of acute gastroenteritis in young children. *Pediatrics* 1996;97:424–436.

Armon K, Stephenson T, MacFaul R, et al. An evidence and consensus based guideline for acute diarrhea management. *Arch Dis Child* 2001;85(2):132–142.

CHOICE Study Group. Multicenter, randomized, double-blind clinical trial to evaluate the efficacy and safety of a reduced osmolarity oral rehydration salts solution in children with acute watery diarrhea. *Pediatrics* 2001;107(4):613–618.

Gorelick MH, Shaw KN, Murphy KO. Validity and reliability of clinical signs in the diagnosis of dehydration in children. *Pediatrics* 1997;99(5):e6. (*http://www.pediatrics.org/cgi/content/full/99/5/e6*)

Grisanti KA, Jaffe DM. Dehydration syndromes: oral rehydration and fluid replacement. *Emerg Med Clin North Am* 1991;9:565–588.

International Study Group on Reduced Osmolarity ORS Solutions. Multicentre evaluation of reduced-osmolarity oral rehydration salts solution. *Lancet* 1995;345:282–285.

Kallen RJ. The management of diarrheal dehydration in infants using parenteral fluids. *Pediatr Clin North Am* 1990;37:265–286.

Author: Marc H. Gorelick

Dermatomyositis/Polymyositis

 Database

DEFINITION

The dermatomyositis/polymyositis complex includes a number of conditions in which muscle becomes damaged by a nonsuppurative lymphocytic inflammatory process. Juvenile dermatomyositis (JDM) is the most common seen in the pediatric population.

DIAGNOSTIC CRITERIA FOR JDM

Diagnosis requires the presence of the pathognomonic rash plus three additional criteria.

- Progressive symmetric weakness of proximal muscles
- Dermatitis-heliotrope rash over eyelids, Gottron papules over extensor surfaces of joints
- Elevated serum level of muscle enzymes
- Electromyograph (EMG) findings of myopathy and denervation
- Biopsy demonstration of inflammatory myositis
- Although not a criterion, T2-weighted MRI is useful in establishing active myositis.

PATHOPHYSIOLOGY

- Unknown
- Several potential mechanisms include the following:

—Abnormal cell-mediated immunity
—Immune-complex formation
—Immunodeficiency
—Infection
—Toxoplasma gondii
—Coxsackievirus B
—Others

EPIDEMIOLOGY

- Incidence: 1:200,000
- The average age of onset is 7 years
- Overall male/female ratio is 1.0:1.7; however, equal in children under 10 years of age

COMPLICATIONS

- Myositis
- Rash
- Arthritis
- Calcinosis
- Raynaud syndrome
- Dysphagia and dysphonia
- Restrictive lung disease and aspiration pneumonia
- Myocarditis (rare)
- Gastrointestinal tract vasculitis
- Osteoporosis
- Joint contractures
- Skin infections

PROGNOSIS

- Normal to good, 65% to 80%
- Minimal atrophy and joint contractures, 24%
- Calcinosis, 20% to 40%
- Wheelchair dependent, 5%
- Death, 7% to 10%

 Differential Diagnosis

POSTINFECTIOUS

- Influenza A and B, coxsackievirus B, schistosomiasis, trypanosomiasis, toxoplasmosis
- Bacterial/pyomyositis-focal

MYOSITIS WITH OTHER CONNECTIVE TISSUE DISEASES

- Overlap with JRA
- Mixed connective tissue disease
- Systemic lupus erythematosus

CHILDHOOD NEUROMUSCULAR DISEASES

If no rash, consider:

- Muscular dystrophy
- Congenital myopathies
- Metabolic disorders

—Glycogen storage disease
—Carnitine deficiency
—Myoadenylate deaminase

- Neurogenic atrophies

—Spinal muscular atrophy and anterior horn
—Peripheral nerve dysfunction

- Neuromuscular transmission disorders
- Inclusion body myositis

 Data Gathering

HISTORY

Question: Fever?
Significance: Evidence of systemic illness

Question: Anorexia and weight loss?
Significance: Gastrointestinal involvement

Question: Fatigue
Significance: Sign of muscle weakness

Question: Weakness
Significance: Difficulty rising from floor, climbing stairs, swallowing, regurgitation through nose

Question: Dysphonia
Significance: Sign of muscle weakness

Question: Rash
Significance: Clue to diagnosis

 Physical Examination

Finding: Muscle weakness
Significance: Proximal and symmetric tenderness strength

- 0—no contractility
- 1—contracts, no joint movement
- 2—Full range of motion (FROM) without gravity
- 3—FROM against gravity
- 4—complete ROM with some resistance
- 5—normal

Finding: Rash
Significance: 75% have pathognomonic rash, which usually appears several weeks after muscle weakness.

Finding: Facial rash
Significance: Violaceous, heliotropic changes over eyelids

Finding: Extremities
Significance: Gottron papules over extensor surfaces

Finding: Nail-fold telangiectasia
Significance: Simultaneous dilated loops, dropout, and arborized capillary loops

PHYSICAL EXAMINATION TRICKS

- Gower sign: Inability to rise from floor without using hands
- Use ophthalmoscope to examine nail-fold for telangiectasia
- Objective measure of strength: duration of straight leg raise (normal = 20 seconds)

Laboratory Aids

Test: Autoantibodies
Significance:

- Normal RF, complement, and double-stranded DNA (dsDNA)
- ANA: 10% to 50%
- PM-1 60% adult polymyositis; however, rare in children

Test: Muscle enzymes
Significance:

- Elevated in 95% cases
- Creatine kinase
- AST
- Aldolase
- LDH

PATHOLOGY

- Skeletal muscle

—Group atrophy or perifascicular myopathy
—Variation in fiber size due to concomitant degeneration and regeneration
—Inflammatory exudate in perivascular distribution
—Necrotizing vasculitis of arterioles, capillaries, and venules; probably due to immune complex deposition

- Skin

—Epidermal atrophy
—Vascular dilatation
—Lymphocyte infiltration of the dermis

ELECTROMYOGRAPHY

- Myopathic motor units
- Denervation potentials
- High-frequency repetitive discharges
- Do not biopsy same muscle as used for EMG

MRI

- Inflamed muscles are identified by signal enhancement
- Useful to direct biopsy

BARIUM SWALLOW

- To identify palatal or proximal esophageal weakness

PULMONARY FUNCTION TESTS/PEAK FLOW

- To evaluate pulmonary musculature

 ## Therapy

PHYSICAL THERAPY/OCCUPATIONAL THERAPY

- Initially to maintain ROM
- Strengthening only after acute inflammation resolves

DRUGS

- 2 mg/kg of steroids per day for 1 month, taper over 2 years
- Intravenous gamma globulin, controversial, efficacious for rash
- Plaquenil, particularly useful for the rash
- Methotrexate, PO, SC, or IV, avoid IM, which may alter serum levels of muscle enzymes
- Cyclosporine

SUPPORTIVE CARE

- Monitor for swallowing difficulty
- Respiratory compromise/occasionally requires mechanical ventilation
- Treatment of calcinosis may include colchicine, diltiazem, and alendronate

 ## Follow-Up

- Function
- Muscle strength
- Joint ROM
- Development of calcinosis
- Muscle enzyme levels

PITFALLS

- Steroid-induced myopathy
- Insidious onset
- Proximal and distal muscles, often large muscle groups such as hip flexors
- Normal serum muscle enzymes
- Minimal myopathic changes on EMG
- Type II fiber atrophy on muscle biopsy

 ## Common Questions and Answers

Q: Is it mandatory to perform a muscle biopsy to confirm the diagnosis?
A: No.

Q: How long should you treat with prednisone?
A: The usual practice is 2 years minimum.

Q: Is there an associated risk of malignancy as for adults with this disorder?
A: No.

ICD-9-CM 710.3

BIBLIOGRAPHY

Cawkwell GM. Inflammatory myositis in children, including differential diagnosis. *Curr Opin Rheumatol* 2000;12:430–434.

Cron RQ, Sharma S, Sherry DD. Current treatment by United States and Canadian pediatric rheumatologists. *J Rheumatol* 1999;26:2036–2038.

Mukamel M, Horev G, Mimouni M. New insight into calcinosis of juvenile dermatomyositis: a study of composition and treatment. *J Pediatr* 2001;138:763–766.

Pachman LM, Hayford JR, Chung A, et al. Juvenile dermatomyositis at diagnosis: clinical characteristics of 79 children. *J Rheumatol* 1998;25:1198–1204.

Rider LG, Miller FW. Idiopathic inflammatory muscle disease: clinical aspects. *Baillieres Best Pract Res Clin Rheumatol* 2000;14:37–54.

Author: Randy Q. Cron
Emily von Scheven, 2nd edition

Developmental Disabilities

 Database

DEFINITION

Developmental delay is a descriptive term, not a specific diagnosis, comprising many disorders and encompassing a broad category of etiologies. The term describes any situation where a child is not meeting age-appropriate milestones as expected in one or more streams of development. These streams of development include gross motor, fine motor, receptive and expressive language, adaptive, and social. The key feature is that the rate of progress has been slow over time in the area(s) of delay.

PATHOPHYSIOLOGY

This is highly variable depending on etiology, which can include genetic, familial, metabolic, infectious, endocrinologic, traumatic, anatomic brain malformations, environmental toxins, and degenerative disorders as causes. These disorders often result in some neurologic or neuromuscular injury causing the delay. In many cases etiology is never determined.
Prevalence of this group of disorders may vary depending on how inclusive the definition. The milder delays are quite common and can be found in any pediatric practice. Some disorders in this grouping are more prevalent in boys. The long-term outcome depends on the severity and type of delay, with the more involved children usually having lifelong disability.

ASSOCIATED FINDINGS

There are numerous associated findings including, seizures, sensory impairments, feeding disorders, psychiatric disorders (especially depression), and behavioral disorders. Having a child with significant developmental delays also can add stress to the family in terms of time, finances, and emotions.

 Differential Diagnosis

The differential can be extensive and may become more evident with further workup. Broad diagnoses include:

- Mental retardation
- Developmental language disorder
- Autism
- Learning disability
- Cerebral palsy
- Attention-deficit/hyperactivity disorder
- Significant visual or hearing impairment
- Degenerative disorders

Specific etiologies are too numerous to list completely but a partial list of the more common causes would include:

- Genetic/familial—fragile X syndrome

—Trisomy 21 (Down syndrome)
—Other chromosomal abnormalities
—Tuberous sclerosis
—Neurofibromatosis
—PKU
—Muscular dystrophy

- Nervous system anomalies—hydrocephalus

—Lissencephaly
—Spina bifida
—Seizures

- Infections

—Prenatal cytomegalovirus
—Rubella
—Toxoplasmosis
—HIV
—Postnatal bacterial meningitis,
—Neonatal herpes simplex

- Endocrinologic

—Congenital hypothyroidism

- Environmental

—Heavy metal poisoning such as lead

- *In utero* drug or alcohol exposure
- Trauma/injury

—Closed head trauma
—Asphyxia
—Stroke
—Perinatal cerebral hemorrhages

 Data Gathering

HISTORY

A complete and detailed history is needed including:

Question: Pregnancy history?
Significance:

- Maternal age and parity
- Maternal complications (including infections and exposures)
- Medications/drugs used
- Tobacco or alcohol used, along with quantities
- Fetal activity

Question: Birth history?
Significance:

- Gestational age
- Birth weight
- Route of delivery
- Maternal or fetal complications/distress
- Apgar scores

Question: General health?
Significance:

- Significant illnesses, hospitalizations, or surgeries
- Accidents or injuries
- Hearing and vision status
- Medications used
- Known exposures to toxins
- Any new or unusual symptoms

Question: Developmental history?
Significance:

- Current developmental achievement in each stream of development
- Age when developmental milestones were achieved
- Any loss of skills
- Where parents think their child is functioning developmentally

Question: Educational history?
Significance:

- Type of schooling and services received, if any
- Any previous educational/developmental testing

Question: Behavioral history?
Significance:

- Any perseverative or stereotypical behaviors
- Interaction skills
- Attention and activity level

Question: Family history?
Significance: Anyone with developmental delays, neurologic disorders, syndromes, consanguinity

Physical Examination

A complete physical examination including growth perimeters is needed looking for etiology. Key features to include are:

Finding: Observation of interactions and behavior
Significance: Any atypical behaviors and general impression

Finding: Head circumference
Significance: Looking for macro- or microcephaly

Finding: Skin exam
Significance: Looking for neurocutaneous lesions

Finding: Major or minor dysmorphic features
Significance: Any indication of a syndrome or anatomic malformation

Finding: Neurologic examination
Significance: Looking for cranial nerve deficits, neuromuscular status, reflexes, balance and coordination, and any soft signs.

DEVELOPMENTAL TESTING

Although considerable information will already be available on history and observation, a more formal developmental screening or testing should be done. Office tests are the Denver Developmental Screening Test, the CAT/CLAMS, and the ELM. The latter test is basically for language screening. Referral to a specialist or a multidisciplinary team for more detailed testing would be indicated when delay is suspected.

Laboratory Tests

There is no specific laboratory test battery for general developmental delays. The testing needs to be tailored to the individual situation based on the history and physical examination. A high index of suspicion should be maintained for any associated findings and delays in the other streams of development. Listed below are some of the more common studies ordered for developmental delay workup:

Test: Audiologic
Significance: Hearing should be checked in any child with speech and language and/or cognitive delays.

Test: Genetic testing
Significance: Warranted for any dysmorphic features, a family history of delays or genetic disorder. A karyotype and fragile X DNA should be considered particularly for significant cognitive delays.

Test: Metabolic tests
Significance: Tests such as quantitative plasma amino acids, quantitative urine organic acids, lactate, pyruvate, or ammonia should be considered if there is any loss of skills or indication of a metabolic disorder.

Test: Thyroid function tests
Significance: Most infants will have had screening for hypothyroidism shortly after birth. This should be rechecked if symptoms indicate.

Test: Electroencephalogram
Significance: An EEG should be considered if there is any concern about seizures.

Test: Head MRI
Significance: Consider a head MRI for head abnormalities, significant neurologic findings, loss of skills or for workup of a specific disorder such as trauma or leukodystrophy.

Test: Subspecialists
Significance: Referral to other medical specialists may also be indicated. These specialists may include developmental pediatrics, neurology, genetics, orthopedics, or ophthalmology.

 ## Therapy

Therapy should include appropriately treating any medical conditions and associated findings, for example, anticonvulsants for seizures or hearing aids when appropriate for hearing impairment. In addition, traditional therapy has included early intervention or special education services specifically addressing the areas of delay. Therapy could include physical therapists, occupational therapists, speech/language therapists, special educators, psychologists, and audiologists depending on the needs of the child.

 ## Follow-Up

General pediatric care for well-child visits and to monitor any underlying medical conditions is indicated. In addition, these children need ongoing monitoring of their therapy and educational programs to ensure that it is still meeting their individual needs, as these needs change over time. The families will also need ongoing counseling and support in dealing with a child having special needs.

PREVENTION

There is no known prevention of developmental delays, although prevention of some of the underlying etiologies is possible.

PITFALLS

- Children with behavioral problems may also be masking developmental delays.
- Children with delays in one stream of development may also have delays in other areas of development. For example, language delay may be an indication of general cognitive delays.
- Hearing impairment may present as a delay in development

 ## Common Questions and Answers

Q: When do you test a child for delays?
A: A child can have developmental assessments at any age, including infancy. Making a specific diagnosis, for example, level of mental retardation, may need to wait until the child is older.

Q: When can a child start receiving services?
A: Children who qualify can receive therapy services starting at birth and in some cases extending up to age 21 years.

Q: The parents are raising a concern about delays but the general impression in the office is that the child is doing OK. What should be done next?
A: Parents or grandparents may be the first to express concerns, especially in a child with milder delays. A more detailed developmental history and more formal developmental screening or testing would be indicated as an initial step.

ICD-9-CM 315.9

BIBLIOGRAPHY

Gilbride KE. Developmental testing. *Pediatr Rev* 1995;16:338–345.

Johnson CP, Blasco PA. Infant growth and development. *Pediatr Rev* 1997;18:224–242.

Levy SE, Hyman SL. Pediatric Assessment of the child with developmental delay. *Pediatr Clin North Am* 1993;40:465–477.

Liptak GS. The pediatrician's role in caring for the developmentally disabled child. *Pediatr Rev* 1996;17:203–210.

Author: Rita Panoscha

Developmental Dysplasia of the Hip

 ## Database

DEFINITION

A range of congenital hip disorders: from mild acetabular dysplasia to dislocation of the femoral head from the acetabulum.

CAUSES

Mechanical Factors

- Breech position
- Oligohydramnios
- Packing phenomenon (e.g., first born child)
- Postnatal positioning (e.g., swaddling in extension and adduction)

Laxity or Genetic Factors

- Female
- Family history (~20%)
- Certain ethnic groups
- Generalized ligamentous laxity

PATHOLOGY

Due to mechanical forces, abnormal growth, or underlying laxity, the spatial and biomechanical relationship between the femoral head and the acetabulum is altered.

EPIDEMIOLOGY

Incidence of hip dysplasia is 0.5% to 2% of live births; however, true dislocation occurs in 0.1% to 0.2% of live births.

GENETICS

Many patients are first-born females, with familial history of affected first-degree relative.

COMPLICATIONS

- When congenital hip dysplasia results in hip subluxation or dislocation, complaints include limp, pain, and accelerated degenerative disease of the hip.
- Avascular necrosis of the femoral head is a complication of treatment.

 ## Differential Diagnosis

- Infection
- Spastic hip dislocation due to cerebral palsy, closed head injury, or anoxic brain injury.

 ## Data Gathering

HISTORY

Question: Breech delivery?
Significance: Much higher incidence of developmental dysplasia of the hip in breech delivery.

Question: Familial history of hip dysplasia?
Significance: 10–20% of patients have familial history.

 ## Physical Examination

- Infants are tested with the Ortolani and Barlow tests. These maneuvers involve feeling a "clunk" with gentle reduction of the dislocated femoral head with abduction and anterior force (Ortolani) or adduction with posterior force (Barlow).
- Check neck for torticollis, metatarsus adductus, and other "packaging" abnormalities.
- Check for an abnormal sacral dimple.
- Although a baby with a dislocated hip may have asymmetric thigh or gluteal folds, many babies with normal hips have such asymmetry
- Children older than 4 to 6 months may have a negative Ortolani but have limited abduction on the affected hip. Galeazzi sign may be positive (comparing the femoral lengths by flexing the hip and knee in the supine position).
- Walking-age children may have a Trendelenburg gait (lurching to the side) and a leg length inequality.

PHYSICAL EXAMINATION TRICKS

- The infant should be as relaxed as possible—preferably sleeping. Check the hips first—once the baby is active or crying it is difficult to get a good exam.
- The infant should be examined on a firm surface. The pelvis is stabilized with the opposite hand.

Laboratory Aids

IMAGING

Test: X-ray studies
Significance: Generally not very useful prior to 4 to 6 months, and may appear normal because of difficulty determining hip/acetabulum relation in cartilaginous femoral head.

Test: Hip ultrasound
Significance: Can determine hip laxity, subluxation, dislocation, reducibility, presence of interposed tissue, and status of the acetabulum. Can request ultrasound of the lumbosacral spine if there is a deep, abnormal sacral dimple raising concern about tethered cord.

FALSE POSITIVES

Hip "clicks" will be present in 10% of infants; only a small percentage will have hip dysplasia.

PITFALLS

- Examination may be normal initially. Consequently, hip evaluation should be performed as part of infant physical examination through 12 months of age.
- Many babies have "clicks" when their hips or knees are manipulated. These high-pitched snapping sensations should not be mistaken for the instability felt on a properly performed Ortolani or Barlow test.

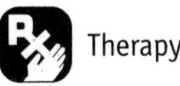 ## Therapy

- Triple diaper: No longer considered to be effective treatment. Expensive for parents.
- Pavlik harness: Up to 95% effective if used prior to 6 months of age. Harness is worn 24 hours per day. Exam or ultrasound should be performed 2 to 3 weeks after initiating the harness for a dislocated hip to prove that the hip is reduced in the harness. Adjust straps every 3 weeks to accommodate growth. After 6 consecutive weeks of treatment, reassess with physical examination and/or ultrasound. Wean if hip is then stable. Complications include avascular necrosis of proximal femur, femoral nerve palsy (resolves spontaneously), skin irritation.
- Closed or open reduction: for patients who present after 6 months of age.

 ## Follow-Up

WHEN TO EXPECT IMPROVEMENT

- Usually after about 6 weeks of treatment in the Pavlik harness.

SIGNS TO WATCH FOR

- A plain radiograph (AP pelvis x-ray) is performed at 6 and 12 months. Measure the acetabular index and check for subluxation or dislocation. Depending on the presence of residual dysplasia, later annual visits may be appropriate.

PROGNOSIS

If diagnosed in infancy, prognosis is generally excellent.

PITFALLS

- Missed early diagnosis can result in more complicated management and less favorable outcome.
- Missing an associated syndrome or condition (e.g., tethered cord, arthrogryposis).
- Mistaking a "click" for instability.

 ## Common Questions and Answers

Q: Why is follow-up needed if the looseness disappears on examination?
A: Follow-up examinations and radiographs periodically detect late instability or acetabular dysplasia.

Q: How effective is the Pavlik harness if used within the first 4 months of life?
A: In patients with reducible hip dysplasia, the current success rate of the Pavlik harness is about 95%.

ICD-9-CM 755.63

BIBLIOGRAPHY

American Academy of Pediatrics. Clinical practice guideline: early detection of developmental dysplasia of the hip (AC0001). *Pediatrics* 2000;105(4):896–905.

Aronsson DD, Goldberg MJ, Kling TF, et al. Developmental dysplasia of the hip. *Pediatrics* 1994;94:201–212.

Bialik V, Bialik GM, Blazer S, et al. Developmental dysplasia of the hip: a new approach to incidence. *Pediatrics* 1999; 103:93–99.

Bond CD, Hennrikus WL, Della Maggiore E. Prospective evaluation of newborn soft tissue hip clicks with ultrasound. *J Pediatr Orthop* 1997;17:199–201.

Clegg J, Bache CE, Raut VV. Financial justification for routine ultrasound screening of the neonatal hip. *J Bone Joint Surg* 1999;81B:852–857.

Hadlow V. Neonatal screening for congenital dislocation of the hip: a prospective 21-year surgery. *J Bone Joint Surg* 1988;70B:740–743.

Tredwell S, Bell H. Efficacy of neonatal hip examination. *J Pediatr Orthop* 1981;1:61–65.

Wynne-Davies R. Acetabular dysplasia and familial joint laxity: two etiological factors in congenital dislocation of the hip: a review of 589 patients and their families. *J Bone Joint Surg* 1970;52:704–716.

Author: John M. Flynn

Diabetes Insipidus

 Database

DEFINITION
Polyuria and polydipsia caused by inability to produce or respond to antidiuretic hormone (ADH) also called arginine vasopressin.

CAUSES

Insufficient ADH Secretion
- Traumatic or postsurgical
- Nonaccidental injury in children
- Related to tumor invasion of posterior pituitary:
- Extension from anterior pituitary/suprasellar: optic glioma, rarely adenomas
- Hypothalamic: germinoma, craniopharyngioma, meningioma
- Lymphoma
- Granulomas: histiocytosis X, sarcoidosis
- Metastatic carcinoma
- Post–severe ischemic or hypoxic injury to the brain
- Familial (autosomal dominant)
- Congenital malformation of central nervous system
- Infection
- Viral encephalitis
- Meningitis
- Tuberculosis
- Increased metabolic clearance of ADH (gestational diabetes insipidus)
- Drug- or toxin-related: snake venom, tetrodotoxin
- Autoimmune disorders; hypophysitis
- Psychogenic: excessive water drinking
- Idiopathic: must observe for many years to exclude slow-growing tumors

Unresponsive to ADH
- Familial or "nephrogenic" (X-linked dominant and autosomal-recessive forms)
- Tumor-related
- Urinary tract obstruction, especially *in utero*
- Renal medullary cystic disease
- Electrolyte disturbances: hypokalemia, hypercalcemia (hypercalciuria)
- Drugs: usually reversible
  - Diuretics
  - Diphenylhydantoin
  - Reserpine
  - Cisplatin
  - Rifampin
  - Lithium: may become permanent
  - Demeclocycline
  - Ethanol
  - Chlorpromazine
  - Volatile anesthetics
  - Foscarnet
  - Amphotericin B
- Loss of the medullary concentrating gradient due to excessive free water intake relative to solute intake

PATHOPHYSIOLOGY
- ADH stimulates the formation of cyclic adenosine monophosphate (cAMP) in the renal collecting ducts, thereby increasing water permeability and increasing reabsorption of free water.
- Lack of ADH effect results in urinary loss of free water.
- Patients with an intact thirst mechanism drink copiously (polydipsia) to compensate for free water loss.
- If the thirst mechanism is not present or if access to free water is limited (e.g., infants or vomiting), severe dehydration can occur.

GENETICS
- Rare cases of autosomal-dominant transmission of ADH deficiency
- Nephrogenic diabetes insipidus (DI) is usually familial (autosomal recessive or dominant and X-linked)

EPIDEMIOLOGY (AGE-RELATED)
Because most cases are secondary to another disease, the incidence depends on the primary causes.

COMPLICATIONS
- Without treatment and without access to water:
- Hypernatremia
- Dehydration
- Coma
- When overdosed with water:
  - Hyponatremia
  - Seizures
  - Cerebral edema

PROGNOSIS
- Generally good, but depends on the primary cause

 Differential Diagnosis

- Psychogenic polydipsia
- Abnormal thirst mechanism (dipsogenic DI)
- Hypernatremic dehydration
- Diabetes mellitus
- Polyuric renal failure (e.g., renal tubulopathy)
- Hypercalcemia
- Adrenal insufficiency
- Cerebral salt wasting

 Data Gathering

HISTORY

Question: Is the child growing normally?
Significance: Abnormal growth can be a sign of DI.

Question: Does the patient wake up during the night to drink or void? If so, what does the patient prefer to drink?
Significance: True DI is associated with polyuria throughout the day and night. Enuresis may be the first sign in a child who previously acquired bladder control. Patients, including infants, prefer water to other liquids such as juice, soda, or milk.

Question: How many hours can the patient go without drinking?
Significance: Patients with complete DI do not voluntarily stop drinking for more than 1 to 2 hours, unless the thirst mechanism is also abnormal.

Question: Does the child drink everything he can including bath and toilet water?
Significance: Patients with DI have such overwhelming thirst, they will drink anything.

Question: Volume of urine output in a day (not just frequency of urination)?
Significance: The daily volume of urine can be as high as 4 to 10 L. Younger or dehydrated children with DI tend to make less urine daily than older or hydrated children with DI.

Question: Familial history of DI?
Significance: Nephrogenic DI will typically affect maternal uncles during infancy and mothers may have a mild form.

Question: Has the child had frequent episodes of dehydration requiring medical attention?
Significance: Families may disregard the polydipsia as normal behavior. Repeated episodes of severe dehydration can damage the brain.

 Physical Examination

Finding: Signs of dehydration
Significance: DI is typically associated with dry, pale skin and mucous membranes. Because this is hyperosmolar dehydration the patient may not look as severely dehydrated as she is.

Finding: Complete neurologic examination
Significance: Check for impaired visual fields that can be the first sign of brain tumor.

Laboratory Aids

SPECIFIC TESTS

Test: Morning urinary osmolality with simultaneous serum sodium and serum osmolality.
Significance: If urine osmolality is at least two times higher than serum osmolality, patient does not have complete DI, but may still have partial DI.

Test: Water-deprivation test
Significance: Though definitive, it requires admission to the hospital for controlled testing under the close supervision of a pediatric endocrinologist. Patient fails test if either:
• Urinary osmolality cannot concentrate more than twice serum osmolality at the same time that serum osmolality exceeds 305 mOsm/kg
• Serum osmolality exceeds 305 mOsm/kg at any time
• Patient loses more than 5% of body weight and becomes symptomatic from hypovolemia

Once patient fails the water deprivation test, a dose of aqueous vasopressin should be given followed by close monitoring of urinary osmolality to document responsiveness to ADH. *Never attempt a water deprivation trial at home.*

NONSPECIFIC TEST

Test: Urinary specific gravity
Significance: Insufficient by itself and nondiagnostic during a water deprivation test.

IMAGING

Test: MRI of the head
Significance: To confirm the "bright spot" normally seen in the posterior pituitary and to search for tumors. Its absence is *not* pathognomonic of DI.

HOME TESTING

Test: 24-hour urine collection
Significance: To obtain accurate urinary volume while patient has free access to water.

Do not restrict water intake unless the patient is in the hospital under close surveillance!

Therapy

DRUGS

• DDAVP: intranasal spray or oral tablets
• Aqueous vasopressin: subcutaneous
• Duration of action of DDAVP is variable from patient to patient. Titration and frequency of dosing should be made by the family under the supervision of an endocrinologist.
• Control of DI in infants is more difficult because these patients may increase fluid intake due to hunger or increase caloric intake due to thirst, thereby causing an imbalance between free water intake and output. Some infants can be treated with diluted formula—the volume and frequency of feedings will be increased, but intake of free water will better match urine output. Strict record keeping of intake/output and accurate daily weighing are usually necessary for infants or patients without an intact thirst mechanism. All infants with DI *must* be treated by people experienced with DI of infancy.
• Nephrogenic DI may be treated with diuretics and solute restriction as these patients are resistant to DDAVP.

SIDE EFFECTS OF DDAVP

• Facial flushing
• Increase in blood pressure
• Headache
• Nasal congestion
• Hyponatremia: caused by water overdose (intoxication), not by overdose of drug. Taking a higher dose of DDAVP will generally extend the period of antidiuresis but will not cause hyponatremia. Drinking too much water in the setting of antidiuresis causes hyponatremia. Water intoxication most often occurs in antidiuresed patients who also are on intravenous fluids, lack an intact thirst mechanism, or have psychogenic polydipsia.

DURATION

Lifelong generally. Some tumors regress with radiation, allowing recovery of ADH secretion.

DIET

• Patients with an intact thirst mechanism should drink only when thirsty.
• Patients without an intact thirst mechanism should drink only a carefully calculated fluid volume.

POSSIBLE CONFLICTS WITH OTHER TREATMENTS

Nasal congestion or gastrointestinal illness can affect the absorption of DDAVP administered.

Follow-Up

Depends on the patient and underlying disease causing DI.

WHEN TO EXPECT IMPROVEMENT

• Effects of DDAVP are immediate.
• Most cases of DI are lifelong. One exception is DI that occurs during the 7 to 10 days immediately after neurosurgery, since this postsurgical DI may resolve spontaneously within 1 to 2 weeks after surgery.

SIGNS TO WATCH FOR

• Lethargy
• Somnolence
• Irritability
• Hyperpyrexia
• Any sign of dehydration
• Seizures

PITFALLS

• Management of patients without an intact thirst mechanism and of newborns is difficult.
• Patients with psychogenic polydipsia may fail a water deprivation test because prolonged excessive water intake can wash out the renal medullary gradient required for concentrating the urine.

• Surreptitious water intake during water deprivation test.
• Idiopathic, acquired DI can be due to slowly growing brain tumors not visible on the initial MRI.

Common Questions and Answers

Q: In a patient with intact thirst mechanism and partial DI is the use of DDAVP necessary?
A: No, as long as the patient has constant access to free water.

Q: How does therapy of DI affect daily life? Is it easily integrated into normal activity and eating patterns?
A: DDAVP is used in a patient with intact thirst mechanism to facilitate the daily routine as well as to allow patients to sleep without the need to void frequently during the night.

Q: Is there a longer acting preparation or an implantable pump for dosing?
A: The longest-acting form of ADH is an injected medication and can have effects for 3 days, increasing the risks of hyponatremia. Home use of the nasal spray or tablets, therefore, is easier and safer than the use of injections.

ICD-9-CM 253.5

BIBLIOGRAPHY

Kirchlechner V, Koller DY, Seidl R, et al. Treatment of nephrogenic diabetes insipidus with hydrochlorothiazide and amiloride. *Arch Dis Child* 1999;80(6):548–552.

Leger J, Velasquez A, Garel C, et al. Thickened pituitary stalk on magnetic resonance imaging in children with central diabetes insipidus. *J Clin Endocrinol Metab* 1999;84(6):1954–1960.

Mootha SL, Barkovich AJ, Grumbach MM, et al. Idiopathic hypothalamic diabetes insipidus, pituitary stalk thickening, and the occult intracranial germinoma in children and adolescents. *J Clin Endocrinol Metab* 1997;82(5):1362–1367.

Robertson GL. Diabetes insipidus. *Endocrinol Metab Clin North Am* 1995;24(3):549–572.

Siegel AJ, Baldessarini RJ, Klepser MB, et al. Primary and drug-induced disorders of water homeostasis in psychiatric patients: principles of diagnosis and management. *Harv Res Psychiatry* 1998;6(4):190–200.

Author: Paul S. Thornton
Robert J. Ferry, Jr., and Paulo F. Collett-Solberg, 2nd edition

Diabetes Mellitus

 ## Database

DEFINITION

Diabetes mellitus (DM) is a disorder of absolute or relative insulin deficiency that results in disruptions in normal energy storage and metabolism. This causes impaired glucose tolerance, hyperglycemia, ketosis, and acidosis, which can ultimately lead to dehydration, shock, and death.

CAUSES

- Type 1 DM: In genetically susceptible individuals, an environmental trigger (believed viral) causes an autoimmune-mediated destruction of pancreatic β cells, leading to absolute insulin deficiency.
- Type 2 DM: Insulin resistance at tissue level in susceptible individuals (impaired β-cell function) leads to relative insulin deficiency.

PATHOLOGY (TYPE 1 DM)

- Induction of expression of DR antigens on β-cell surface following viral infection.
- Recruitment of cytotoxic lymphocytes.
- Production of anti-insulin and anti-islet-cell antibodies.
- Progressive loss of β-cell mass and insulin supply due to inflammatory process, resulting in insulin deficiency.

EPIDEMIOLOGY

- Most common endocrine/metabolic disorder of childhood
- 1 to 2 in 1,000 school-aged children, but increases with age such that:

—1 in 1,500 children by age 5 are affected
—1 in 350 by age 18
—Peak ages of both type 1 and type 2 in early adolescence

- Type 1 DM: More common in Caucasians of Northern European descent
- Type 2 DM: More common in African-Americans, Latino, and Native Americans, usually with strong family history
- Boys and girls equally affected in type 1, female/male ratio 3:2 in type 2
- Incidence: 16 new cases per 100,000 children per year
- Incidence of type 2 DM increasing rapidly, may be as high as 25% to 40% of new cases

GENETICS

- Susceptibility associated with HLA region of chromosome 6 (type 1 DM)
- Fivefold greater risk with MHC antigen types DR3 and DR4 (type 1 DM)
- Genetic defect in type 2 DM unknown
- Maturity-onset diabetes of youth (MODY) is a family of autosomal-dominant syndromes caused by mutations of genes involved in the regulation of pancreatic development or insulin secretion; the syndromes represent a small minority of non–type 1 diabetes in children.

COMPLICATIONS

- Diabetic ketoacidosis (DKA): profound metabolic derangement characterized by hyperglycemia, ketosis, and acidosis, leading to osmotic diuresis, dehydration, shock, and death
- Hypoglycemia: complication of insulin therapy
- Long-term effects:

—Nephropathy—microalbuminuria, proteinuria, chronic renal failure
—Retinopathy—microvascular proliferation, visual loss
—Neuropathy—progressive diminution of nerve conduction velocity
—Vasculopathy—accelerated atherosclerosis, large-vessel disease
—Embryopathy—infants of diabetic mothers at increased risk of birth defects
—Growth failure (Mauriac syndrome) and delayed sexual maturation
—Rate of development of chronic complications related to degree of metabolic control

 ## Differential Diagnosis

- Urinary tract infection (polyuria)
- Renal glycosuria
- Hypercalcemia (polyuria, weight loss)
- Chronic illness (weight loss, malaise)
- Stress-related hyperglycemia
- Drug-induced hyperglycemia (steroids)
- Pneumonia (in DKA)
- Sepsis (in DKA)
- Acute abdominal event (in DKA)

 ## Data Gathering

HISTORY

Question: Polyuria, nocturia, enuresis?
Significance: Related to hyperglycemia.

Question: Polydipsia?
Significance: Increased thirst follows polyuria and dehydration.

Question: Polyphagia?
Significance: Increased appetite related to loss of calories from glucosuria.

Question: Weight loss, poor growth?
Significance: Dehydration, loss of calories

Question: Malaise, weakness?
Significance: Electrolyte disturbance and acidosis.

Question: Changes in behavior, school performance?
Significance: Chronic illness.

 ## Physical Examination

- Usually normal in type 1 DM
- Obesity and acanthosis nigricans (hypertrophic skin pigmentation of the neck and skin folds) in type 2 DM
- In DKA, signs of dehydration and acidosis (Kussmaul respirations)

 ## Laboratory Aids

- Blood glucose more than 200 mg/dL (2-hour postprandial is most sensitive indicator of glucose intolerance)
- Glycosuria, ketonuria (latter is variable in type 2 DM)
- Hemoglobin A_{1c} (gives approximation of average blood glucose level over previous 2–3 months)

Test: Measurement of insulin and C-peptide levels
Significance: Islet cell antibodies may differentiate type 1 from type 2 DM.

Therapy

- Insulin

—Usually given in combination of short-acting and long-acting preparations b.i.d. to t.i.d.
—Total daily dose (TDD) usually about 0.7 to 1.0 U/kg/day, less during "honeymoon period."
—Often given as: two thirds of TDD in morning (one third of that as short-acting and two thirds long-acting), and one third of TDD in evening (with one half of that as short-acting and one half as long-acting, split between dinner and bedtime).
—Oral antidiabetic agents may be effective in type 2 DM
—Sulfonylureas: increase endogenous insulin production and release
—Biguanides: reduce hepatic glucose production
—Thiazolidinediones: improve peripheral insulin sensitivity
—α-Glucosidase inhibitors: competitively inhibit intestinal glucose absorption

DIET

Consistency of amount and timing of meals is important:

- 20% of daily calories from breakfast and lunch
- 30% from dinner
- 10% from snacks evenly spaced between meals and before bedtime
- Balance of source of calories is important:

—55% from carbohydrates (of which 70% complex)
—30% from fats
—15% from protein

- American Diabetes Association system of "exchanges" of different food groups
- Carbohydrate "counting"
- Weight reduction/stabilization critical for most children with type 2 diabetes

EXERCISE

- Regular exercise helps to reduce insulin requirements and reduce blood glucose.
- Regular aerobic activity critical in management of type 2 diabetes

HOME MONITORING

- Checking blood glucose q.i.d. (before meals and bedtime snack), more often if necessary.
- Checking urine for ketones whenever blood glucose more than 240 mg/dL or during intercurrent illnesses.

 ## Follow-Up

- Regular appointments with diabetologist or nurse specialist every 3 months to assess growth and development and trouble-shoot management problems
- Meetings with nutritionist periodically to reassess meal plan
- Meetings with psychologist as needed to address psychosocial and family stressors
- Monitoring of glycosylated hemoglobin every 3 months to assess long-term control and compliance
- Yearly urine collection to evaluate microalbuminuria
- Yearly ophthalmologic examination to evaluate retinopathy
- Yearly cholesterol profile to evaluate hyperlipidemia

 ## Common Questions and Answers

Q: What is the "honeymoon period"?
A: The period of "remission" following initial stabilization of metabolism with exogenous insulin. It is marked by the presence of residual endogenous insulin secretion; insulin doses usually drop to 0.5 U/kg/day or less. The honeymoon phase usually lasts weeks to months, but may persist 1 to 2 years.

Q: What is the risk of diabetes in a sibling or child of a person with type 1 DM?
A: It is 5%–10% in first-degree relatives (siblings, offspring), 40%–50% in identical twins.

Q: What are the goals of glucose control?
A: Preprandial blood glucose 80–120 mg/dL; postprandial blood glucose less than 180 mg/dL; avoidance of episodes of hypoglycemia; maintenance of a reasonably nonrestrictive lifestyle and psychological adjustment.

Q: Does having diabetes necessarily mean that one will develop the long-term complications?
A: The Diabetes Control and Complications Trial showed that intensive management and tight control (average blood sugar <140 mg/dL) reduces the risk of complications (retinopathy, nephropathy, and neuropathy) by 50% to 75%.

ICD-9-CM 250.0

BIBLIOGRAPHY

American Diabetes Association. Standards of medical care for patients with diabetes mellitus. *Diabetes Care* 1994;17:616–623.

Dabelea D, Pettitt DJ, Jones KL, et al. Type 2 diabetes mellitus in children and adolescents: an emerging problem. *Endocrinol Metab Clin North Am* 1999;28:709–730.

Diabetes Control and Complications Trial Research Group. The effect of intensive treatment of diabetes on the development and progression of long-term complications in insulin-dependent diabetes mellitus. *N Engl J Med* 1993;329:977–986.

Kaufman FR. Diabetes in children and adolescents: areas of controversy. *Med Clin North Am* 1998;82:721–738.

Sperling M. Diabetes mellitus. In: Sperling M, ed. *Clinical pediatric endocrinology*. Philadelphia: WB Saunders, 1996:229–263.

Author: Stuart A. Weinzimer

Diabetic Ketoacidosis

 ## Database

DEFINITION

- State of severe metabolic derangement that occurs in patients with insulin-dependent diabetes mellitus secondary to insulin deficiency and stress hormone excess.
- Hyperglycemia (blood glucose >200 mg/dL)
- Ketonemia (>3 mmol in serum) or ketonuria
- Acidosis (pH <7.3 or HCO_3 <15 mEq/L)

CAUSE/PATHOLOGY

- Insulin deficiency and excess of the counterregulatory hormones glucagon, cortisol, and epinephrine lead to unregulated catabolism.
- Glycogenolysis and gluconeogenesis lead to hyperglycemia.
- Lipolysis and ketone production lead to metabolic acidosis.
- Hyperosmolar state leads to osmotic diuresis, dehydration, and electrolyte loss.

EPIDEMIOLOGY

- 30% of new diabetic children present in diabetic ketoacidosis (DKA); higher percentage in children under 5 years.
- Overall mortality ~3% to 5% per episode
- 65% of all hospital admissions in diabetic children under 19 years old
- Most common cause of death (>50%) in diabetic children

COMPLICATIONS

- Cardiovascular collapse

—Caused by osmotic diuresis and dehydration
—Treated with prompt initiation of fluid resuscitation

- Overwhelming acidosis

—From ketoacid accumulation
—Treated with insulin infusion, sodium bicarbonate infusion if necessary

- Hypoglycemia from insufficient dextrose supplementation, treated by increasing dextrose

- Hypokalemia

—Caused by loss of potassium in the urine and correction of acidosis with insulin
—Treated by intravenous potassium supplementation

- Cerebral edema

—Most serious complication of DKA and most frequent cause of death
—Rapid changes in serum osmolarity lead to influx of water into brain tissue
—Occurs 6 to 18 hours after initiation of therapy, often as patient is clinically improving
—Heralded as headache, change in mental status, or abnormal neurologic signs
—May progress rapidly to brain herniation and death
—Treatment is supportive, aimed at reducing intracranial pressure with intravenous mannitol and mechanical hyperventilation

PROGNOSIS

- Overall, 3% to 5% mortality with each episode of DKA

 ## Differential Diagnosis

- Gastroenteritis
- Severe intraabdominal process (e.g., ulcer, pancreatitis, appendicitis)
- Urinary tract infection
- Pneumonia
- Stress hyperglycemia
- Hypercalcemia
- Salicylate ingestion
- Inborn error of metabolism
- Nonketotic hyperosmolar coma

 ## Data Gathering

HISTORY

Question: Polyuria, polydipsia, and polyphagia with weight loss?
Significance: Symptom of hyperosmolar state.

Question: Nausea, vomiting, abdominal pain?
Significance: Related to acidosis and electrolyte disturbance.

Question: Changes in breathing patterns (Kussmaul respirations)?
Significance: Related to acidosis and respiratory correction.

Question: Precipitating event, such as an intercurrent illness or psychosocial stress?
Significance: Increased need for insulin in these states.

 ## Physical Examination

Finding: Vital signs—tachycardia, hypotension
Significance: Seen with dehydration

Finding: Dry mucous membranes, sunken eyes, poor skin turgor, poor distal perfusion, weak pulses
Significance: Dehydration

Finding: Fruity odor to breath
Significance: Ketosis

Finding: Deep, sighing, hyperpneic (Kussmaul) respirations
Significance: Respiratory compensation for primary acid–base disturbance

Finding: Abdominal tenderness
Significance: Related to ketosis, acidosis

Finding: Altered mental status, lethargy, obtundation
Significance: Acidosis, dehydration, and hyperosmolarity

 ## Laboratory Aids

Test: Glucose more than 200 mg/dL
Significance: Indicates insulin deficiency

Test: Urinalysis—glycosuria and ketonuria
Significance: Glucose level exceeds renal threshold

Test: Sodium—serum levels low; from electrolyte losses and artifact of hyperlipidemia; actual Na level = measured Na + 1.6 × [glucose − 200)/100]
Significance: Severity of dehydration

Test: Potassium—serum levels may be elevated, normal, or low; total body is potassium-depleted.
Significance: Potassium depletion from osmotic diuresis. Serum level is dependent on degree of acidosis and dehydration.

Test: Bicarbonate less than 15 mEq/L
Significance: Acidosis

Test: Phosphate—low, secondary to osmotic diuresis
Significance: Acidosis

Test: ABG—low pH (<7.3), low pCO_2, and low HCO_3
Significance: Acidosis

Test: CBC—elevated WBC count even in the absence of infection
Significance: Stress reaction

Therapy

• Resuscitation

—Assess adequacy of airway and breathing.
—Restore circulation if necessary with normal saline bolus of 10 to 20 mL/kg, repeat as needed
—Cannot gauge hydration status initially by urine output because of osmotic diuresis.
—Avoid excessive fluid resuscitation— too-rapid correction of hyperosmolarity increases risk of cerebral edema. However, shock must be treated aggressively.

• Monitoring

—ICU admission for infants, toddlers, initial pH <7.1, hemodynamic or neurologic instability
—ECG monitoring for hypokalemia or hyperkalemia
—Serial neurologic examinations q1h, with special attention to headache, declining mental status, any neurologic symptoms
—Hourly blood sugars
—pH and electrolytes q1–2h until stable

• Fluids

—Assume at least 10% dehydration, 15% in infants.
—Aim to replace losses plus maintenance fluids evenly over 48 hours.
—Replacement fluids should always be normal saline, not $\frac{1}{2}$-normal saline.
—Ongoing renal losses greater than 3 mL/kg/h may be replaced if significant and persistent.

• Electrolytes

—Assume Na and K losses of approximately 5 to 10 mEq/kg.
—Hyponatremia will correct as fluids and insulin are given.
—Continued drop in Na is associated with increased risk of cerebral edema.
—Replace potassium as an equal mixture with chloride and phosphate:
—K+ >5.5, 20 mEq/L in replacement fluids
—K+ = 4.0 to 5.5, 40 mEq/L
—K+ <4.0, 60 mEq/L
—Potassium replacement should never exceed 0.5 mEq/kg/h.

• Acidosis

—Usually corrects once adequate insulin and fluids are given.

—Consider bicarbonate if arterial pH <7.0 or there is inadequate respiratory compensation: rule of thumb, i.e., if $pCO_2 > (1.5 \times [HCO_3])$ + 8). Use of bicarbonate should be judicious, not automatic.

—Give as slow infusion over 1 to 2 hours at dose of 1 to 2 mEq/kg

• Insulin

—Prompt initiation critical in terminating ongoing ketone and acid production.
—Initial dose is 0.1 U/kg/h as continuous intravenous infusion.
—Do not give subcutaneously in DKA, as skin perfusion may be suboptimal.
—Aim to lower serum glucose by 50 to 100 mg/dL/h.

• Glucose

—Add 5% dextrose to intravenous stock when blood glucose <300 mg/dL
—Change to 10% dextrose when blood glucose <200 mg/dL

• Duration

—Stop infusion when pH >7.3, HCO₃ >15, glucose <300, and patient is tolerating oral fluids.

• Convert to subcutaneous therapy by adding up total insulin given over 24 hours and dividing into two to four injections or return to usual home regimen of insulin with frequent monitoring and extra insulin as needed.

Follow-Up

• New diabetic patients should be followed closely after hospital discharge to assess adequacy of insulin regimen.
• Children with recurrent DKA should be evaluated for treatment failure (family dysfunction, knowledge deficits).

PREVENTION

• Timely referral for children with symptoms of polyuria, polydipsia, and weight loss.
• Surveillance with frequent blood sugar and urine ketone monitoring, supplemental insulin dosing; phone contact with pediatrician or endocrinologist should avert almost all episodes of DKA in children known to have diabetes.

Common Questions and Answers

Q: What are the usual triggers for DKA?
A: Intercurrent illnesses, such as gastroenteritis, urinary tract infections, pneumonia; psychosocial stressors; failure to take insulin on schedule.

Q: Does an episode of DKA mean that the insulin regimen is inadequate?
A: DKA always implies insulin deficiency; insulin regimen may be adequate when child is well, but additional stresses of illness or psychosocial factors often require supplemental insulin.

ICD-9-CM 250.1

BIBLIOGRAPHY

Glaser N, Barnett P, McCaslin I, et al. Risk factors for cerebral edema in children with diabetic ketoacidosis. *N Engl J Med* 2001;344:264–269.

Green SM, Rothrock SG, Ho JD, et al. Failure of adjuvant bicarbonate to improve outcome in severe pediatric diabetic ketoacidosis. *Ann Emerg Med* 1998;31:41–48.

Harris G, Fiordalisi I. Physiologic management of diabetic ketoacidemia. *Arch Pediatr Adolesc Med* 1994;148:1046–1052.

Kaufman FR. Diabetes in children and adolescents: areas of controversy. *Med Clin North Am* 1998;82(4):721–738.

Krane E. Diabetic ketoacidosis: biochemistry, physiology, treatment, and prevention. *Pediatr Clin North Am* 1987;34(4):935–960.

Rosenbloom A, Hanas R. Diabetic ketoacidosis (DKA): treatment guidelines. *Clin Pediatr* 1996;35:261–266.

Author: Stuart A. Weinzimer

Diaper Rash

 Database

DEFINITION

Commonly known as diaper or nappy rash, it is a collection of dermatoses defined by its etiology and distribution.

PATHOPHYSIOLOGY

Diaper rashes are the result of several different processes, alone and in combination:

• Friction: Rubbing of wet diapers against exposed skin areas such as the inner surface of the thighs, genitals, buttocks, abdomen; results in an erythematous, shiny rash that spares the intertriginous areas.
• Irritation: Confined to the exposed areas under the diaper, sparing the intertriginous areas, secondary to irritants such as feces/urine, cleaning materials.
• Allergic: Contact allergies may be the result of detergents, topical medicines.
• Atopic: Usually later onset in infants, is pruritic and is often accompanied by a familial history of atopy.
• Seborrhea: Typical yellow-salmon–colored greasy rash especially affecting the intertriginous areas, and may be seen in other areas such as the scalp, face, neck, and flexural areas.
• Candidal: Especially common during or immediately after antibiotic administration, this rash is beefy red, with a raised sharp margin, and characteristic pinpoint erythematous, satellite lesions.

GENETICS

Dependent on the individual causes of diaper dermatitis, such as predisposition for atopy or other allergic-based rashes.

EPIDEMIOLOGY

This dermatitis is by definition exclusive to individuals wearing diapers, and generally resolves when diapers are no longer worn. It is estimated to affect approximately 7% to 35% of the infant population at any given time and is most commonly found in the 9- to 12-month age group.

COMPLICATIONS

Generally none, although secondary bacterial or fungal infections may lead to ulceration. Severe bacterial superinfections in newborns or immune-compromised infants can lead to sepsis.

PROGNOSIS

Diaper rash usually resolves with good skin care. It completely resolves once the child is potty trained and out of diapers.

 Differential Diagnosis

Although any rash under a diaper can be considered a diaper rash, the following are other diseases that may present on the skin of the anogenital region but are not common causes of diaper dermatitis:

• Infection

—Congenital syphilis: Less commonly seen now because of maternal screening, this infection may manifest with a macular, papular, or bullous lesion in the diaper area. The palms and soles may also reveal lesions.
—HIV infection: May first present with erosive and ulcerated lesions, especially in the gluteal cleft. May be associated with other infections such as cytomegalovirus or herpes, may be pruritic. Other findings such as anemia, hepatosplenomegaly are often present.
—Scabies, herpes virus, varicella

• Tumors

—Letterer-Siwe (Langerhans cell histiocytosis) may present as a diaper rash with small reddish-brown papules or vesicles.

• Metabolic

—Acrodermatitis enteropathica: Deficiency of zinc. In addition to vesiculobullous lesions of the hands and feet and surrounding mouth and diaper areas, these patients have failure to thrive, diarrhea, alopecia, and frequent bacterial and candidal infections.
—Biotin deficiency:

• Immunologic

—Psoriasis: Although unusual, may affect the diaper area with dark red, well-marginated plaques with silvery scales. Other areas of the body are usually similarly affected.

• Other

—Granuloma gluteal infantum, the etiology is not well understood, probably an inflammatory response to a variety of irritants. Results in discrete red painless nodules up to 4 cm in size.
—Child abuse, epidermolysis bullosa

 Data Gathering

HISTORY

Question: Any skin disorders at other sites?
Significance: Skin disorders such as atopic dermatitis or seborrhea located elsewhere on the body suggest involvement in the diaper area as well.

Question: Use of medications (especially oral antibiotics, or topical medications)?
Significance: Medications can directly affect the diaper area, or leave it more susceptible to rashes. Oral antibiotics change the normal bowel and skin flora, and may cause diarrhea, which can irritate the skin. Topical medications such as steroid ointments may change the appearance of the rash, or may cause changes in the skin (such as thinning). Some fungal creams contain sensitizers, such as ethylenediamine hydrochloride.

Question: Use of detergents or soaps on skin or clothes?
Significance: These substances are often not recognized by parents as containing irritants (such as perfumes) that can damage the skin, leaving it susceptible to diaper rash.

Question: Any current medical problems (such as diarrhea) that might irritate the skin?
Significance: Many medical problems manifest themselves in the skin, and may affect the diaper rash.

Question: Review skin care techniques: what is put on the skin and how is it used?
Significance: Parents often think a diaper rash represents poor hygiene, and as a result increase the cleaning of the area around the rash. Depending on how it is done and what is used, this cleaning may instead result in further irritation and damage to the skin.

Physical Examination

Finding: Location of the rash should be carefully noted.
Significance: Is it predominately in the exposed surfaces (contact, friction) or in the intertriginous areas (seborrhea, candidal)?

Finding: The margins of the rash should be inspected for satellite lesions.
Significance: Candida classically has satellite lesions.

Finding: Appearance of lesions
Significance: The lesion is dry or moist appearing (candidal); if it has a shiny parchment paper-like appearance (friction or atopic dermatitis).

Finding: A thorough examination of other areas of skin (e.g., looking for atopic or seborrheic dermatitis).
Significance: May give clues to the underlying skin of the diaper area and determine etiologic factors of the rash.

Laboratory Aids

Almost always a clinical diagnosis. Candidal infections may be verified by skin scraping and viewed with potassium hydroxide under a microscope. Other etiologies should be considered with resistant diaper rash and may rarely require skin biopsy.

Therapy

• Proper skin care is the primary treatment modality. When soiled, the skin should be gently washed with a mild soap and patted dry or air-dried.
• The diaper should be kept off and the rash exposed to air as much as possible.
• Any moderate to severe rash will invariably be secondarily infected with *Candida* and should be treated with topical nystatin, miconazole, or clotrimazole.
• If the skin is very inflamed and especially if there is evidence of contact, atopic, or seborrheic dermatitis, a small amount of topical corticosteroid cream (such as 1% hydrocortisone) can be used for a few days.
• Although gentle skin care techniques should be permanently adopted, the use of topical antifungal medication and ointments should be continued until the rash completely resolves.

• Steroid medications should be stopped after a few days, when the intense acute inflammation has improved.
• Sucralfate has been used topically in severe situations, it acts as a physical barrier and may neutralize bile acids and pepsin. It should be considered in children with ostomies who are prone to diaper rashes.

Follow-Up

With proper treatment, the rash should be noticeably better within 4 to 7 days. Failure of resolution of rash indicates that another dermatologic process may be complicating the diaper rash.

PREVENTION

Proper skin care with gentle cleaning and mild soap should be used. Superabsorbent diapers may be suggested, along with frequent diaper changes. Barrier creams such as zinc oxide may help protect the skin from external irritants after resolution of the rash.

PITFALLS

General pitfall to avoid is the use of laboratory aids to help diagnose this disorder, because it is almost always a clinical diagnosis. Topical steroid used alone may worsen a candidal infection.

• Often the caregiver believes the rash is a result of inadequate cleansing of the skin and, subsequently, attempts to wash the skin more. This additionally irritates and exacerbates the rash. Topicals that strongly adhere to the skin do not need to be scrubbed completely clean before putting on another treatment.
• Steroids marketed by drug companies in combination with antifungal creams are often more potent than necessary. In addition, the action of topical steroids is potentiated when used under "occlusion" (the diaper). When topical steroids are used, they are best given as a separate prescription that can be stopped at an earlier time than the antifungal medication.
• Talcum powder can worsen the irritation, and may be aspirated by both baby and caregiver. Its use should be discouraged.
• If a candidal diaper infection is resistant to treatment, and thrush (monilia infection of the mouth) is present, oral nystatin may be added q.i.d. Since an infected mother may reinoculate her infant, an evaluation of the mother for candidal infections of the nipples could be considered.

Common Questions and Answers

Q: Should I switch from cloth to disposable diapers (or vice versa)?
A: This is controversial, although there are some studies that indicate that the superabsorbent disposable diapers may be better for controlling diaper rashes. Cloth diapers used with plastic overpants probably irritate the skin more because they trap moisture against the skin. Frequent changing of diapers is very helpful, along with not wearing diapers at all when practical.

Q: Is the diaper rash due to not keeping the skin clean enough?
A: Although the combination of stool and urine may release enzymes that help break down skin integrity, probably more harmful to skin is vigorous and frequent scrubbing with relatively abrasive materials on the macerated, easily damaged skin typically found in the diaper area. This rough cleaning allows introduction of bacteria and yeast into the skin and results in a diaper rash. Parent should be advised to use soft cleaning materials (such as cotton balls) to gently clean stool from the diaper area. It is not usually necessary to clean the skin of urine every time, rather patting the infant dry with a soft cloth and then replacing the diaper is all that is generally required.

ICD-9-CM 691

BIBLIOGRAPHY

Hurwitz S. *Clinical pediatric dermatology,* 2nd ed. Philadelphia: WB Saunders, 1993.

Kazaks EL, Lane AT. Diaper dermatitis. *Pediatr Clin North Am* 2000;47(4). 909–19.

Singalavanija S, Frieden I. Diaper dermatitis. *Pediatr Rev* 1995;16:142–147.

Wong LD, Brantly D, Clutter LB, et al. Diapering choices: a critical review of the issues. *Pediatr Nurs* 1992;18:41–54.

Author: Robert Kamei

Diaphragmatic Hernia (Congenital)

 Database

DEFINITION

- Herniation of abdominal contents into the thoracic cavity through an opening in the diaphragm causing varying degree of pulmonary hypoplasia
- Two types of congenital diaphragmatic hernia (CDH)
—Bochdalek hernia (posterolateral location)
—Morgagni hernia (retrosternal location)

CAUSES

- True cause: unknown
- Diaphragm forms between 7 and 10 weeks of gestation
- Diaphragm is composed of two parts:
—Pleuroperitoneal folds attach to the chest wall, develop a muscular lining and become the lateral and dorsal portions of the diaphragm.
—Septum transversum, which becomes the central tendon of the diaphragm.
- Anything that interferes with the formation of the diaphragm allows an abdominal hernia to develop.
- Bochdalek hernia develops when:
—Midgut returns to the abdominal cavity prematurely or diaphragmatic development is delayed.
—Bowel is trapped in the thoracic cavity, preventing the pleuroperitoneal folds from connecting with the thoracic wall.
—This allows a communication to exist between the thoracic and abdominal cavities.
- Morgagni hernia develops when:
—A defect develops in the septum transversum.

PATHOPHYSIOLOGY

- Bochdalek hernia
—Usually occurs on the left side (left-sided pleuroperitoneal folds close later than the right)
—Bilateral lung hypoplasia (ipsilateral lung hypoplasia worse than contralateral side)
—Lung abnormal in respect to: morphology, differentiation and maturation
—Abnormal morphology of pulmonary arteries (suggesting primary vascular hypoplasia)
—Possible surfactant deficiency
—Bowel in the thoracic cavity
- Morgagni hernia
—Usually occurs on the right side (left-sided defects are covered by the heart)
—Hernia can contain: liver, bowel, and omentum
—Less lung hypoplasia seen than with Bochdalek hernias

EPIDEMIOLOGY

- Bochdalek hernia
—Accounts for 90% of cases of congenital diaphragmatic hernias
—Incidence: in 1/2000 to 1/5000 live births
—80% to 90% of cases on the left side (2% bilateral)
—More common in males

—40% of cases associated with some type of congenital malformation:
—5% to 16% of cases with chromosomal abnormality (e.g., trisomy 21, 18,13)
—18% associated with a congenital heart disease
—Others: neurologic defects (hydrocephalus, spina bifida, anencephaly)
- Morgagni hernia
—Accounts for 2% of all diaphragmatic hernias; more common in females

GENETICS

- Estimated 2% recurrence rate in first-degree relatives

COMPLICATIONS

- Bochdalek hernia
—Pulmonary hypoplasia
—Persistent fetal circulation
—Pulmonary hypertension
—Right to left shunt
—Pulmonary insufficiency
—Death
- Morgagni hernia
—10% incidence of strangulation of the bowel if not repaired

 Differential Diagnosis

PULMONARY

- Pulmonary cysts
- Cystic adenomatoid malformation
- Pneumatocele
- Congenital lobar emphysema
- Pulmonary sequestration
- Eventration of the diaphragm
- Hiatal hernia
- Laryngotracheal obstruction
- Atelectasis
- Pneumothorax
- Anterior mediastinal mass
- Pneumonia
- Pleural effusion

CARDIAC

- Dextrocardia
- Congenital heart disease

 Data Gathering

HISTORY

Question: Bochdalek hernia?
Significance: Presents at birth; patient frequently presents in severe cardiopulmonary distress.

Question: Morgagni hernia?
Significance: Usually asymptomatic. If symptomatic, usually presents later in life. May have complaints of: vague abdominal discomfort, vomiting, failure to thrive, chest pain, dyspnea, cough, and recurrent respiratory infections.

 Physical Examination

Finding: Bochdalek hernia
Significance: Symptoms are critical in the first 72 hours:
- Severe respiratory distress
- Cyanosis
- Tachypnea
- Decreased breath sounds on the affected side
- Hyperresonance to percussion on the affected side
- Asymmetry of the chest wall (enlarged on the affected side)
- Increased anterior-posterior diameter of the chest
- Occasional bowel sounds heard in the chest
- Tachycardia
- Cardiac point of maximal impulse shifted away from the affected side
- Scaphoid abdomen (abdominal contents in thoracic cavity)

Finding: Morgagni hernia
Significance: Examination may be normal

 Laboratory Aids

TESTS

Test: Arterial blood gas
Significance:
- po_2 shows evidence of severe hypoxia
- pco_2 elevated
- pH, bicarbonate, lactate: reveal significant acidosis (both respiratory and metabolic)

IMAGING

Test: Chest radiograph
Significance:
- Bochdalek hernia
—Mediastinal structures shifted away from the affected side
—Heart shifted away from the affected side
—Decreased lung volumes (ipsilateral lung more than contralateral lung)
—Atelectasis of the contralateral lung
—Unable to visualize the diaphragm on the ipsilateral side
—Loops of bowel in the thoracic cavity
—In left-sided hernias, a nasogastric tube inserted into the stomach will be seen in the thoracic cavity
—Abdominal bowel is usually gasless
- Morgagni hernia
—A mass is seen in the anterior mediastinum: may be solid or gas-filled.

Test: Ventilation/perfusion scan
Significance: Decreased ventilation and perfusion in the hypoplastic lung

Test: Fetal ultrasound
Significance: Abdominal viscera in the thoracic cavity; polyhydramnios

Therapy

- Bochdalek hernia
—Physiologic emergency requiring resuscitation and early stabilization of the patient:
  —Oxygenation
  —Ventilation: permissive hypercapnia has been shown to be the preferred strategy
  —Correction of acidosis
  —Normalization of blood pressure
  —Decompression of the intrathoracic bowel (placement of a nasogastric tube to low suction allows the bowel to decompress, thus letting the ipsilateral hypoplastic lung expand)
—Surgical repair of the defect:
  —Decreased morbidity and mortality if the patient can be stabilized prior to surgical repair
  —ECMO (extracorporeal membrane oxygenation)
  —May prove useful in the perioperative management:
    —Preoperative: for patient stabilization
    —Postoperative: to allow the lungs to fully expand after the compressing intrathoracic bowel has been removed
  —Other: nitric oxide, high-frequency ventilation, liquid ventilation
—Fetal surgical interventions:
  —Fetal tracheal occlusion in some fetuses results in impressive lung growth
  —Consider in severe cases of CDH when diagnosis is made early enough in gestation (i.e., 24–28 weeks' gestation)
- Morgagni hernia
—Surgical repair is indicated, even if the patient is asymptomatic, due to the high rate of strangulation of the intrathoracic bowel (10%).

Follow-Up

WHEN TO EXPECT IMPROVEMENT
Dependent on the extent of pulmonary hypoplasia and pulmonary hypertension.

SIGNS TO WATCH FOR
- The development of pulmonary hypertension in the postoperative period
- Rapid development of hypoxia is associated with the development of a pneumothorax.

PROGNOSIS
- Bochdalek hernias:
—Dependent on the degree of pulmonary hyperplasia and pulmonary hypertension:
—If patient survives the perioperative period: 55% to 65% survival (up to 90% in the most advanced centers)
—Poor prognostic factors:
  —Polyhydramnios *in utero*
  —Liver herniation into the thorax
  —Fetal stomach in the thoracic cavity

—Early presentation (i.e., presenting in the first 6 hours versus after 24 hours)
—Presence of cardiac and chromosomal abnormalities
—Lung-to-head circumference ratio less then 0.6
—Persistent elevated pco_2 and decreased po_2
- Morgagni hernias: excellent

PITFALLS
- Bochdalek hernias
—Not being able to stabilize the patient (suggestive of severe pulmonary hypoplasia and/or pulmonary hypertension)
—Aggressive ventilation causing barotrauma
—Delay in getting the patient to an appropriate medical center
—Not recognizing other congenital malformations or chromosomal abnormalities that may affect the patient's ultimate outcome or which would represent a contraindication for surgical repair (e.g., Trisomy 18)
- Morgagni hernias
—Not considering the diagnosis when abnormalities seen on chest radiograph

LONG-TERM SEQUELAE
- Pulmonary
—Chronic lung disease (60%)
—Diminished perfusion in the hypoplastic lung with progressive improvement in ventilation seen on ventilation/perfusion scan
—Lung function in CDH survivors: spirometry may be normal or indicate mild airway obstruction, slightly reduced lung volumes, normal total lung capacity (TLC) and diffusion capacity
—Recurrent respiratory infections
- Gastrointestinal/nutrition
—Gastroesophageal reflux and delayed gastric emptying (62–81%): may need surgical repair
—Oral aversion (due to prolonged intubation and delay in development of the swallowing reflex)
—Failure to thrive: may need tube feeding
- Neurodevelopmental
—Developmental delays in the first 2 years
—Motor delays tend to improve
—Hearing loss
—Hypotonia
- Chest wall
—Increased incidence of pectus deformity and scoliosis

Common Questions and Answers

Q: What is the long-term pulmonary function in survivors of Bochdalek hernias?
A: Dependent on the degree of pulmonary hypoplasia; pulmonary function testing shows evidence of both obstructive and/or restrictive lung disease. Decreased perfusion on the affected side.

Q: What is the optimal time for surgical repair in neonates with Bochdalek hernias?
A: Delayed surgical repair until the patient is stabilized, avoidance of hyperventilation and alkalization, and pressure-limited ventilation have been shown to significantly decrease mortality in neonates who meet ECMO criteria (up to 90%).

ICD-9-CM 553.3

BIBLIOGRAPHY
Allen JL, Wohl ME. Taussig LM, et al. *Pediatric respiratory medicine.* St. Louis: Mosby, 1999:1154–1178.

Congenital Diaphragmatic Hernia Study Group. Estimating disease severity of congenital diaphragmatic hernia in the first 5 minutes of life. *J Pediatr Surg* 2001;36(1)141–145.

D'Agostino JA, Bernbaum JC, Gerdes J, et al. Outcome for infants with congenital diaphragmatic hernia requiring extracorporeal membrane oxygenation; the first year. *J Pediatr Surg* 1995:30:10–15.

Flake AW, Crobleholme TM, Johnson MP, et al. Treatment of severe congenital diaphragmatic hernia by fetal tracheal occlusion: clinical experience with fifteen cases. *Am J Obstet Gynecol* 2000:183(5):1059–1066.

Ijsselstjin H, Tibboel D. The lungs in congenital diaphragmatic hernia: Do we understand? *Pediatr Pulmonol* 1998;26:204–218.

Katz AL, Wiswell TE, Baumgart S. Contemporary controversies in the management of congenital diaphragmatic hernia. *Clin Perinatol* 1998;25(1):219–248.

Marven SS, Smith CM, Chapman J, et al. Pulmonary function, exercise performance and growth in survivors of congenital diaphragmatic hernia. *Arch Dis Child* 1998;78:137–142.

Muratore CS, Wilson JM. Congenital diaphragmatic hernia: Where we are and where do we go from here? *Semin Perinatol* 2000;24(6):418–428.

Walsh DS, Adzick NS. Fetal surgical intervention. *Am J Perinatol* 2000;17(6):277–283.

Author: Gordana Lovrekovic
Mayra Bustillo and Richard Mark Kravitz, 2nd edition

DiGeorge Syndrome

 Database

DEFINITION

DiGeorge syndrome is characterized by thymic aphasia or hypoplasia resulting in a spectrum of immunodeficiency, absent or hypoplastic parathyroid glands, and cardiac malformations.

- Complete DiGeorge syndrome involves all these abnormalities.
- Partial DiGeorge syndrome occurs when the immune system is intact.

PATHOPHYSIOLOGY

DiGeorge is believed to be a developmental defect of the third and fourth pharyngeal arches.

GENETICS

- Heterogeneous
- Some reported cases of autosomal dominant, autosomal recessive, and X-linked modes of inheritance
- Most common associated chromosomal abnormalities are microdeletions of 22q11.

COMPLICATIONS

In the newborn period, hypocalcemic tetany, manifestation of cardiac abnormality, and recurrent infections. Later on, developmental delay and arthralgias.

PROGNOSIS

Prolonged survival is seen in many patients after the spontaneous improvement of T-cell immunity. These patients are considered to have partial DiGeorge syndrome. However, other patients may have more severe T-cell dysfunction. Complications may include an increase in autoimmune phenomena and neurologic sequelae.

 Data Gathering

HISTORY

- Neonatal hypocalcemia secondary to hypoparathyroidism
- Recurrent infections: diarrhea, candidiasis
- Heart murmurs
- In particular, interrupted aortic arch, septal defects, patent ductus arteriosus, and truncus arteriosus.
- Failure to thrive

 Physical Examination

Finding: Facial dysmorphism
Significance: Small recessed chin; low, rotated ears; "fish-shaped mouth"; micrognathia; short philtrum, anteverted nares, and hypertelorism

- Cleft lip and palate
- Heart murmur
- Hydronephrosis
- Colobomas
- CNS malformations
- Major immunologic features present at birth:

—Lymphopenia
—T-cell dysfunction
—Antibody levels and function are variable

DiGeorge Syndrome

Laboratory Aids

Test: Chest x-ray study
Significance: To evaluate for cardiac malformation and also for the presence of a thymic shadow

Test: CBC
Significance: Immediately after birth, a lymphocyte count of <1,200/mm^3 is suspicious.

Test: Serum levels of calcium and parathormone
Significance: Check for hypocalcemia part of syndrome.

Test: Lymphocyte markers
Significance: To determine absolute numbers of T and B cells and their subsets

Test: Mitogen studies
Significance: To study the functional abilities of T and B cells, often depressed response to phytohemagglutinin, concanavalin A, and pokeweed mitogen

Test: Quantitative immunoglobulins (IgG, IgA, IgM, and IgE)
Significance: Often the humoral system will be abnormal if there is extensive T-cell dysfunction.

Test: FISH (fluorescence *in situ* hybridization) for 22q11 deletion
Significance: Most common chromosomal defect

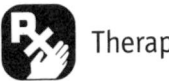

Therapy

Depending on the defects or deficiencies the child manifests, some of the following issues may need to be addressed:

- Cardiology for the cardiac malformations
- Otolaryngology and feeding specialist for cleft palate
- Endocrinology for follow-up of hypoparathyroidism
- Immunology to monitor T-cell disorder and recurrent infections

SPECIAL CONSIDERATION WITH INFECTIONS

Children with the complete DiGeorge syndrome are at increased risk of morbidity and mortality from viral infections either from vaccines such as oral polio or natural infections such as varicella. It is advisable to:

- Avoid live viral vaccines.
- Consider varicella immune globulin in a patient either with unknown humoral immunity status or definitive humoral abnormalities. Intravenous acyclovir may be necessary if varicella develops and patient has a low T-cell count or abnormal mitogens.

SPECIAL CONSIDERATION WITH BLOOD TRANSFUSIONS

Because these patients are at risk for graft-versus-host disease, it is best to use cytomegalovirus-negative, irradiated blood.

Common Questions and Answers

Q: Is there a definitive test to distinguish between partial and complete DiGeorge syndrome?
A: Over time, patients with partial DiGeorge syndrome will reconstitute their T cells and acquire improved function based on mitogen and antigen studies.

ICD-9-CM 279.11

BIBLIOGRAPHY

Amman AJ. T cell immunodeficiency disorders. In: Stites DP, Terr AI, eds. *Basic and clinical immunology.* Norwalk, CT: Appleton & Lange, 1991:335–338.

Conley ME, Beckwith JB, Mancer JF, et al. The spectrum of the DiGeorge syndrome. *J Pediatr* 1979;94:883–890.

Driscoll DA, Budarf ML, Emanuel BS. A genetic etiology for DiGeorge syndrome: consistent deletions and microdeletions of 22q11. *Am J Hum Genet* 1992;50:924–933.

Radford DJ. The DiGeorge syndrome and the heart. *Curr Opin Pediatr* 1991;3:828–831.

Author: Michelle M. Klinek

Diphtheria

 Database

DEFINITION

Diphtheria is an acute infectious disease caused by *Corynebacterium diphtheriae* and affects primarily the membranes of the upper respiratory tract with the formation of a gray-white pseudomembrane.

CAUSES

The causative organism, *C. diphtheriae*, is a gram-positive pleomorphic bacillus.

PATHOPHYSIOLOGY

The initial entry site for *C. diphtheriae* is via airborne respiratory droplets, typically the nose or mouth, but occasionally the ocular surface, genital mucous membranes, or preexisting skin lesions. Following 2 to 4 days of incubation at one of these sites, the bacteria elaborates toxin. Locally, the toxin induces formation of a necrotic coagulation of the mucous membranes (pseudomembrane) with underlying tissue edema. Respiratory compromise may ensue. Elaborated exotoxin may also have profound effects on the heart, nerves, and kidneys in the form of myocarditis, demyelination, and tubular necrosis, respectively.

EPIDEMIOLOGY

- The single known reservoir for *C. diphtheriae* is humans; disease is acquired by contact with either a carrier or a diseased person.
- Though the disease is distributed throughout the world, it is endemic primarily in developing regions of Africa, Asia, and South America. In the Western world, the incidence of diphtheria has changed dramatically in the past 50 to 75 years, as a result of the widespread use of diphtheria toxoid after World War II. The incidence has declined steadily and is now a rare occurrence.
- Recent outbreaks have occurred, most notably in the new independent states of the former Soviet Union, and supply additional evidence that disease occurs among the socioeconomically disadvantaged living in crowded conditions.
- The majority of cases occur during the cooler autumn and winter months in individuals younger than 15 years of age who are unimmunized.

ASSOCIATED ILLNESSES

- Respiratory tract diphtheria:

—Nasal diphtheria starts with mild rhinorrhea that gradually becomes serosanguineous, then mucopurulent, and often malodorous. This form occurs most often in infants.
—Tonsillar and pharyngeal diphtheria begins with anorexia, malaise, low-grade fever, and pharyngitis. A membrane appears within 1 to 2 days. Cervical lymphadenitis and edema of the cervical soft tissues may be severe. Disease course varies with extent of toxin elaboration and membrane production. Respiratory and cardiovascular collapse may occur.
—Laryngeal diphtheria most often represents extension of a pharyngeal infection and clinically presents as typical croup. Acute airway obstruction may occur, and in severe cases the membrane may invade the entire tracheobronchial tree.
—Cutaneous diphtheria occurs in warmer tropical regions. It is characterized by chronic nonhealing ulcers with gray membrane and may serve as a reservoir in endemic and epidemic areas of respiratory diphtheria.

- Other sites: rarely vulvovaginal, conjunctival, or aural forms occur.

COMPLICATIONS

- Cardiac toxicity: myocarditis may develop secondary to elaborated toxin anytime between the first and sixth week of illness. Though cardiac failure can occur, the majority of cases are transient.
- Neurologic toxicity again occurs secondary to toxin elaboration and mainly reflects bilateral motor involvement.
- Paralysis of the soft palate is most common, but ocular paralysis, diaphragm paralysis, peripheral neuropathy of the extremities, and loss of deep tendon reflexes also occur.
- The frequency of all complications, including those listed above, increases with increasing time between symptom onset and antitoxin administration and also with extent of membrane formation.

PROGNOSIS

- Most strongly dependent on the immunization status of the host. Those without prior adequate immunization have significantly higher morbidity and mortality.
- Delay in onset of treatment also increases mortality. When appropriate treatment has been administered on day 1 of illness, mortality may be as low as 1%. When treatment has been delayed until day 4, the mortality rate is up to 20-fold higher.
- Organism virulence: toxigenic strains are associated with more severe disease and a poorer prognosis.
- Location of membrane: laryngeal diphtheria has a higher mortality owing to airway obstruction.

- A megakaryocytic thrombocytopenia and WBC <25,000 are associated with poor outcome.

 Differential Diagnosis

- Nasal diphtheria can present much like the common cold, nasal foreign body, sinusitis, adenoiditis, or snuffles (congenital syphilis).
- Tonsillar or pharyngeal diphtheria may be confused with streptococcal pharyngitis, infectious mononucleosis, primary herpetic tonsillitis, thrush, Vincent angina, posttonsillectomy faucial membranes, or the oropharyngeal involvement caused by toxoplasmosis, cytomegalovirus, tularemia, and salmonellosis.
- Laryngeal diphtheria: differential diagnosis includes croup, acute epiglottitis, aspirated foreign body, peripharyngeal and retropharyngeal abscess, laryngeal papillomas, or other masses.

 Data Gathering

HISTORY

Question: Exposure?
Significance: Exposure to an individual with diphtheria is not necessarily elicited because contact with an asymptomatic carrier may be the only source of infection.

Question: Incubation period?
Significance: The incubation period is 1 to 6 days. Respiratory diphtheria, depending on the site of infection, may begin with nasal discharge alone or with pharyngitis accompanied by mild systemic symptoms. Progression of symptoms thereafter occurs as outlined above (see Associated Illnesses).

 Physical Examination

Finding: Nasal discharge, nasal or pharyngeal membrane, heart rate out of proportion to body temperature, respiratory distress, stridor, cough, hoarseness, palatal paralysis, neck swelling, and cervical lymphadenitis. Attempts to remove any membrane present will result in bleeding.
Significance: Classic findings.

Finding: Conjunctival diphtheria
Significance: Gives palpebral conjunctival involvement with a red, edematous, membranous appearance.

Finding: Aural diphtheria
Significance: Presents as otitis externa with a purulent, malodorous discharge.

Finding: Cutaneous diphtheria
Significance: See Associated Illnesses, above.

SPECIAL QUESTIONS

Previous diphtheria immunization history, diphtheria exposure.

Laboratory Aids

Test: Diagnosis should be on clinical grounds.
Significance: Delay in treatment increases morbidity and mortality.

Test: Culture of material from the membrane or beneath the membrane should be attempted.
Significance: If a strain of *C. diphtheriae* is isolated, additional testing for presence or absence of toxin production should be conducted by a laboratory prepared to conduct an animal neutralization test or, alternatively, neutralization (with antitoxin) in tissue culture.

Test: Examination of a methylene blue-stained lesion
Significance: Metachromatic granules can be helpful, if performed by an experienced technician.

Test: Fluorescent antibody testing and counterimmunoelectrophoresis
Significance: Previously performed in state laboratories; no longer widely available.

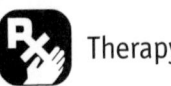

Therapy

DIPHTHERIA ANTITOXIN (DAT)

DAT antiserum, produced in horses, must be administered as soon as possible as follows. (Note: For patients with known horse serum sensitivity, a test dose should be administered first, and if positive, the patient should be desensitized.)

- Pharyngeal or laryngeal disease of <48 hours; duration, 20,000 to 40,000 units IV
- Nasopharyngeal lesions, 40,000 to 60,000 units IV
- Extensive disease of 3 or more days' duration or diffuse neck swelling, 80,000 to 100,000 units IV

ANTIBIOTIC THERAPY

- Antibiotic therapy should be used in addition to DAT, not in place of it, as follows:
- Respiratory diphtheria

—Penicillin G
—Aqueous crystalline, 100,000 to 150,000 U/kg/d in four divided doses × 14 days
—Procaine, 25,000 to 50,000 U/kg/d in two divided doses × 14 days or
—Erythromycin, 40 to 50 mg/kg (maximum 2 g/d) PO or parenterally × 14 days

- Cutaneous diphtheria: requires local care of the lesion with soap and water and administration of antimicrobials for 10 days.

PREVENTION

Active immunization with diphtheria toxoid is the cornerstone of population-based diphtheria prevention. The current recommendations from the Advisory Committee on Immunization Practices (ACIP) of the CDC are:

- Ages 2 months to 7 years: five doses of diphtheria vaccine, the first three given as DTP vaccine 0.5 mL IM at 2-month intervals beginning at 2 months of age. The fourth dose should be either DTaP or DTP at 15 to 18 months of age, and a fifth dose of DTaP or DTP at 4 to 6 years of age.
- Age >7 years: primary immunization of those >7 years should be conducted with adult-type diphtheria and tetanus toxoids, adsorbed (Td) with two doses given IM at least 4 weeks apart and a booster dose 1 year later.
- Booster doses of Td should be given at 10-year intervals to all immunized individuals. Isolation of patients with diphtheria is required until culture from the site of infection is negative on three consecutive specimens.

Follow-Up

- In mild cases of diphtheria, after membrane sloughs off in 7 to 10 days, recovery is usually uneventful.
- In more severe cases, recovery may be slower and serious complications can occur.

Common Questions and Answers

Q: Are there currently places in the world where diphtheria is a problem?
A: Yes. A diphtheria epidemic began in 1990 in Russia, spread in 1991 to Ukraine, and during 1993 and 1994 spread to the remaining new independent states of the former Soviet Union. During 1994, provisional totals of 47,802 cases (39,907 in Russia) and 1,746 deaths due to diphtheria were reported throughout the new independent states.

Q: What is the incidence of diphtheria in the United States?
A: From 1980 to 1993, only 40 cases of diphtheria were reported in the United States, an average of three per year (all respiratory disease).

Q: What precautions should be taken by travelers to areas of the world with diphtheria outbreaks?
A: The ACIP recommends that travelers to such areas should be up-to-date for diphtheria immunization. Infants traveling to areas where diphtheria is endemic or epidemic should receive three doses of DTP or DT before travel.

ICD-9-CD 032.9

BIBLIOGRAPHY

Bisgard KM, Hardy IR, Popovic T, et al. Respiratory diphtheria in the United States, 1980 through 1995. *Am J Public Health* 1998;88(5):787–791.

Enhanced surveillance of non-toxigenic *Corynebacterium diphtheriae* infections. *CDR Weekly* 1996;6(4):29,32.

Feigin RD, Stechenberg BW, Strandgaard BH. Diphtheria. In: Feigin RD, Cherry JD, eds. *Textbook of pediatric infectious diseases*, 3rd ed. Philadelphia: WB Saunders, 1992:1110–1115.

Galazka A. The changing epidemiology of diphtheria in the vaccine era. *J Infect Dis* 2000;181(suppl 1):52–59.

MacGregor RR. Corynebacterium diphtheriae. In: Mandell GL, Douglas RG Jr, Bennett JE, eds. *Principles and practice of infectious diseases*, 3rd ed. New York: Churchill Livingstone, 1990:1574–1581.

Nekrassova LS, Chudnaya LM, Marievskiv F, et al. Epidemic diphtheria in Ukraine, 1991–1997. *J Infect Dis* 2000;181(suppl 1):335–340.

Toxigenic *Corynebacterium diphtheriae*—Northern Plains Indian Community, August—October 1996. *MMWR* 1997;46(22):506–510.

Author: Louis M. Bell
Susan Dibs, 2nd edition

Discoid Meniscus and Sports Injury

 Database

DEFINITION

• A discoid meniscus is a morphologic anomaly of the normal meniscus in which the fibrocartilage is completely or nearly completely disc-shaped, as opposed to the normal shallowed-center, crescent shape.
• A discoid lateral meniscus is more common than a discoid medial meniscus.
• A discoid meniscus can be described as complete, incomplete, or a Wrisberg ligament type. The Wrisberg ligament type lacks a posterior meniscotibial attachment.

CAUSES

• Congenital theories have been postulated with evidence of familial transmission.
• The possibility of a discoid meniscus resulting from an arrest of the normal stages of embryologic development (disc-shaped meniscus fails to resorb *in utero*) has been refuted.
• Clinical manifestations of a discoid meniscus tend to occur when children are old enough to be involved in running, jumping, and pivoting sports.
• Discoid meniscus is not associated with any one particular sport.

PATHOLOGY

• Sports elicit higher repetitive cyclic loading on weight-bearing joints through a greater range of motion. This produces increased shear and compressive forces.
• Shearing forces on the thickened meniscus may cause central delamination with tearing of the central or peripheral portions of the meniscus. These forces may also cause peripheral separation of the capsule from the meniscus.

EPIDEMIOLOGY

• Prevalence of discoid meniscus is 0.4% to 16.6%.
• While some reports have described clinical presentation in infants and toddlers, discoid meniscus is found most frequently in young patients who are old enough to participate in sports.
• A high incidence of discoid menisci has been reported in the Japanese.

COMPLICATIONS

• Although complete and incomplete discoid menisci may be asymptomatic, the Wisberg ligament type often becomes symptomatic.
• Ongoing clicking, pain, swelling, intrameniscal delamination, tearing, and detachment may occur in the persistently symptomatic discoid meniscus.

 Differential Diagnosis

• Torn normal meniscus

—Usually produces more subtle clicking at a discrete location within the meniscus, and can be further distinguished with MRI

• Osteochondral lesion (hinged or displaced)

—More commonly causes tenderness over the femoral condyle

• Patellar subluxation/dislocation

—More commonly associated with anterior knee symptomatology

• Cruciate ligament injury

—Patient complains of the knee's giving way, and examiner will typically find pathologic knee laxity and a more marked effusion.

 Data Gathering

HISTORY

Question: What symptoms do you experience and with what activities?
Significance: The patient may complain of a clunk with knee motion. Discoid meniscus may present during childhood and adolescence as diminished range of motion, locking, swelling, and pain, especially with sports that require twisting and pivoting.

 Physical Examination

Question: Is there any tenderness or effusion?
Significance: Tenderness at the lateral joint line (primarily posteriorly) and mild effusion are indicative of a discoid meniscus. There is usually no pathologic laxity to ligamentous stress testing.

Question: Is there any pain or clunking with special testing?
Significance: While palpating the medial and lateral joint lines, the examiner passively flexes and extends the knee. A palpable and potentially audible "clunk" in the extreme 15 to 20 degrees of flexion and extension is indicative of a discoid meniscus. The clunking sensation is often more pronounced than the subtle click found in a torn meniscus in an adult.

The McMurray test is also useful for identifying a discoid meniscus. With the patient lying supine and the hip and knee flexed, the examiner palpates the associated medial or lateral joint line. Pain or a palpable clunk with valgus/varus stress and circumduction with tibial rotation while extending the knee is suggestive of a discoid meniscus.

 Laboratory Aids

IMAGING

Test: Radiographs (AP and lateral)
Significance: Demonstrate widening of the lateral joint space without evidence of a fracture or osteochondral lesion.

Test: MRI
Significance: Demonstrates a solid rectangular structure traversing the knee joint on three successive sagittal sections, as opposed to the smaller, triangular shapes of a normal meniscus.

Therapy

- Asymptomatic discoid menisci can be managed with observation.
- In general, patients with knee discomfort can benefit from quadriceps strengthening and a stretching program. This includes, for example, 5 minutes of straight leg raise exercises twice daily, beginning with 2 lb of resistance and progressing as symptoms permit up to 10% of the patient's body weight, and hamstrings stretching for 3 minutes, twice a day.
- Surgical arthroscopy is indicated when a symptomatic or torn discoid meniscus is suspected.

SURGERY

- Historically, complete meniscectomies were performed for both complete and incomplete discoid menisci.
- Long-term studies of 20 years' duration have demonstrated a 75% incidence of moderate to severe osteoarthritic changes, despite good subjective results in 90% of patients, following complete meniscectomy.
- Therefore, the authors recommend partial rather than complete meniscectomy and have found more favorable short-term results.

—A partial removal is done to appropriately recontour the shape of the meniscus.
—Care is taken to evaluate the peripheral meniscal capsular attachment, and if there has been any detachment, a portion of the meniscus is repaired to the capsule.
—The knee is flexed and extended to ensure that a portion of the interposed meniscus, which has been clunking and causing mechanical symptoms, is removed and a stable peripheral rim is maintained.

PT/OT

- One day after surgery, the patient is given active range of motion exercises of the hips, including straight leg raises.
- At 2 weeks, a directed knee range of motion and strengthening program is initiated.
- At 9 weeks, walking, submaximal biking, and swimming is allowed.
- At 12 weeks, a progressive return to running, jumping, and pivoting activities is permitted.

 ## Follow-Up

PROGNOSIS

- Without surgical correction, patients with symptomatic discoid menisci with a clunking sensation may develop intrameniscal delamination, horizontal tears, peripheral detachment, and subsequent effusion and pain.
- Patients typically have a good prognosis after partial meniscectomy.
- Asymptomatic patients are encouraged to maintain their strength and flexibility by performing quadriceps strengthening and hamstring stretching.

 ## Common Questions and Answers

Q: Why are discoid menisci problematic in children and adolescents?
A: Discoid menisci do not properly complement the contours of the femoral condyles. This can interfere with normal joint motion and load transmission, and symptoms typically signify a tear of the posterior segment.

Q: Why should total meniscectomy be avoided when possible?
A: Menisci are responsible for absorbing 50% to 70% of the compressive load of the tibiofemoral joint. Therefore, complete removal can lead to osteoarthritic changes. Even a small remnant of meniscus along the tibial condyle has been found to decrease the concentration of compressive forces.

Q: What is the role of the primary care physician?
A: Primary care physicians play an important role in diagnosing discoid menisci, recognizing the need for surgical intervention (effusion, painful clunk, catching, etc.), and in counseling patients to optimize knee strength and flexibility, which can potentially prevent symptoms in patients with partial discoid menisci.

ICD-9 717.5

BIBLIOGRAPHY

Aichroth PM, Patel DV, Marx CL. Congenital discoid lateral meniscus in children. A follow-up study and evolution of management. *J Bone Joint Surg* 1991;73B:932–936.

Dickhaut SC, DeLee JC. The discoid lateral-meniscus syndrome. *J Bone Joint Surg* 1982;64A:1068–1073.

Pellacci F, Montanari G, Prosperi P, et al. Lateral discoid meniscus: treatment and results. *Arthroscopy* 1992;8:526–530.

Washington ER 3rd, Root L, Liener UC. Discoid lateral meniscus in children. Long-term follow-up after excision. *J Bone Joint Surg* 1995;77A:1357–1361.

Woods GW, Whelan JM. Discoid meniscus. *Clin Sports Med* 1990;9:695–706.

Authors: Theodore J. Ganley and Stephan G. Pill

Diskitis

 ## Database

DEFINITION

• Benign, self-limited inflammatory process of an intervertebral disk

CAUSES

• Idiopathic or initiated by low-grade infection

PATHOLOGY

• Probably of infectious etiology by an indolent organism
• Usually none identified; occasionally *Staphylococcus aureus, Moraxella,* or the Enterobacteriaceae are cultured.

EPIDEMIOLOGY

• Over half of cases occur in children younger than 4 years old.
• Peak incidence is between 1 and 3 years of age.

GENETICS

• No specific predispositions identified

COMPLICATIONS

• Occasionally scoliosis or kyphosis
• Rarely, facet joint degenerative disease

 ## Differential Diagnosis

• Infection
—Vertebral osteomyelitis (*Staphylococcus, Salmonella,* etc.)
—Potts disease (tuberculous spondylitis)
• Environmental trauma
—Fracture
—Disk herniation
• Tumors
—Osteoid osteoma
• Vascular
—Avascular necrosis of vertebral body
• Congenital
—Spondylolisthesis
• Immunologic
—Ankylosing spondylitis
• Miscellaneous
—Scheuermann disease (osteochondritis of the vertebral bodies)

 ## Data Gathering

HISTORY

• Uncomfortable child?
• Refuses to walk?
• History of fever?
• Back or abdominal pain?
• Symptoms are of short duration prior to presentation?

 ## Physical Examination

• Usually rigid posture, and pain elicited on movement
• Focal tenderness to palpation
• Most common locations: L4-5 and L3-4

Diskitis

Laboratory Aids

TESTS

- PPD
- WBC
- ESR
- Blood cultures

IMAGING

Test: Plain x-ray studies
Significance: Usually normal, though may demonstrate disk narrowing as illness progresses.

Test: Bone scan
Significance: Demonstrates increased uptake at affected area.

Test: MRI
Significance: Useful in atypical situations to confirm location of pathology (demonstrates disk edema).

Therapy

DRUGS

- Usually quite responsive to NSAIDs
- Rarely, antibiotics are indicated.

DURATION

- Follow CBC and ESR.
- Continue treatment until child is asymptomatic.

PHYSICAL AND OCCUPATIONAL THERAPY

- Patient should be immobilized during acute period.
- Casting may be required.

DIET

- No special changes

Follow-Up

WHEN TO EXPECT IMPROVEMENT

Most patients are asymptomatic in 6 to 8 weeks.

SIGNS TO WATCH FOR

- Recurrence of symptoms due to reactivation of the disease
- Progressive loss of disk height
- Destruction of adjacent vertebral bodies

PROGNOSIS

- Usually excellent
- Scoliosis can occur
- Rarely, facet joint symptoms occur years later.

PITFALLS

- Difficulty separating early vertebral body osteomyelitis from diskitis

Common Questions and Answers

Q: When is a biopsy and tissue culture indicated?
A: If there is bony destruction of adjacent vertebral bodies or if clinical course is prolonged.

Q: When are antibiotics indicated?
A: Obviously in situations with positive cultures, or if course is atypical or prolonged.

ICD-9-CM 722.90

BIBLIOGRAPHY

Brown R, Hussain M, McHugh K, et al. Discitis in young children. *J Bone Joint Surg* 2001;83B:106–111.

Fernandez M, Carrol CL, Baker CJ. Discitis and vertebral osteomyelitis in children: an 18-year review. *Pediatrics* 2000;105:1299–1304.

King HA. Back pain in children. *Orthop Clin North Am* 1999;30:467–474.

Mahboubi S, Morris MC. Imaging of spinal infections in children. *Radiol Clin North Am* 2001;39:215–222.

Ventura N, Gonzalez E, Terricabras L, et al. Intervertebral discitis in children: a review of 12 cases. *Int Orthop* 1996;20(1):32–34.

Authors: Randy Q. Cron
Gregory F. Keenan, 2nd edition

Disseminated Intravascular Coagulation

 ## Database

DEFINITION

Disseminated intravascular coagulation (DIC) is a syndrome characterized by diffuse fibrin deposition in the microvasculature, consumption of coagulation factors, and endogenous generation of thrombin and plasmin in an uncontrolled fashion usually leading to significant bleeding.

PATHOPHYSIOLOGY/PATHOLOGY

- DIC is not a disorder in itself, but occurs as a result of various initiating events.
- DIC is characterized by microvascular hemorrhage and thrombosis.
- DIC may be acute (e.g., meningococcemia) or chronic (e.g., malignancy/leukemia).
- DIC most likely initiated through tissue factor (extrinsic) pathway.
- Most common causes are sepsis (particularly gram-negative sepsis), hypotensive shock, and trauma (particularly head trauma).
- Exact mechanism of DIC is unclear, but in most cases, tissue damage leads to the release of clot-promoting material. Also, all means of anticoagulation are impaired and fibrin is not adequately removed because endogenous fibrinolysis is suppressed by high plasma levels of plasminogen activator inhibitor-1 (PAI-1). The principal cytokine mediator appears to be IL-6.
- Procoagulant factors released in the blood may initiate DIC in acute promyelocytic leukemia.
- Endotoxins released during infections cause activation of coagulation factor XII, endothelial injury, platelet aggregation, and inhibition of fibrinolysis.
- The following disease processes can cause DIC:

- Infections

—Bacterial/septic shock
—Meningococcemia
—Gram-negative and -positive sepsis (e.g., group B streptococcus)
—Parasites—malaria
—Fungal—Aspergillus
—Rickettsial—Rocky Mountain spotted fever
—Viral

- Tissue injury
- Massive head trauma
- Multiple fractures with fat emboli
- Crush injuries
- Profound shock or asphyxia
- Hypothermia or hyperthermia
- Massive burns

- Malignancies

—Acute promyelocytic leukemia
—Acute monoblastic or monocytic leukemia
—Metastatic carcinomas or other widespread malignancies (e.g., neuroblastoma)

- Obstetric causes

—Intrauterine fetal death
—Amniotic fluid embolism
—Abruptio placentae
—Gastrointestinal

- Fulminant hepatitis
- Reye's syndrome
- Severe inflammatory bowel disease
- Neonatal

—Necrotizing enterocolitis
—Congenital viral infections
—Group B streptococcus infection
—Erythroblastosis fetalis
—Small for gestational age newborn

- Miscellaneous

—Acute hemolytic transfusion reaction
—Kasabach-Merritt syndrome
—Snake bite or insect bite
—Severe thrombotic thrombocytopenic purpura
—Hemolytic uremic syndrome
—Homozygous protein C deficiency (purpura fulminans)
—Severe graft rejection
—Severe collagen vascular disease
—Heparin-induced thrombosis
—Infusion of activated prothrombin complex concentrate
—VP shunt
—Kawasaki disease

EPIDEMIOLOGY

- Exact incidence not known.
- Most commonly secondary to infections.
- Snakebite may be most common cause worldwide.

COMPLICATIONS

- Hemorrhage
  —Pulmonary
  —Intracranial

- Renal failure
- Multiorgan system failure

PROGNOSIS

- Poor unless underlying disease is treated.
- The intensity and duration of DIC depend on the degree of activation of the coagulation system, liver function, blood flow, and the ability to reverse underlying etiology that has led to DIC.

 ## Differential Diagnosis

- Prolonged bleeding from venipuncture sites.
- Coagulopathy of liver disease
- Vitamin K deficiency
- Pathologic fibrinolysis
- Microangiopathic disease, e.g., thrombotic thrombocytopenic purpura
- Effects of cardiopulmonary bypass

 ## Data Gathering

HISTORY

- Presence of one of the underlying conditions listed above (see Causes)
- Abrupt onset of bleeding
- Prolonged bleeding from venipuncture sites
- Bleeding from multiple sites, especially venipunctures, cut-down sites, mucous membranes, skin, GI tract, and GU tract
- Pulmonary or intracranial hemorrhage
- Major organ dysfunction—pulmonary, renal, hepatic
- Oliguria

Physical Examination

- Signs of underlying disease.
- Generally a very toxic-appearing patient.
- Ecchymosis and petechiae.
- Bleeding from previously intact venipuncture sites.
- Skin infarctions (purpura fulminans) secondary to thrombosis of dermal vessels.
- Pulmonary hemorrhage, gastrointestinal bleeding, bleeding from surgical wounds, hematuria.
- Intraperitoneal and pleural hemorrhages.

 Laboratory Aids

- There is no single test that can reliably diagnose DIC.
- All these tests should be checked every 4 to 8 hours because they change rapidly.

Test: CBC
Significance: Decreased platelet count, often earliest abnormality.

Test: Peripheral smear
Significance: Schistocytes, microspherocytes (50% of cases).

Test: PT, PTT, and thrombin time
Significance: Prolonged

Test: Fibrinogen
Significance: Decreased

Test: Fibrin degradation products or fibrin split products
Significance: Increased

Test: Soluble fibrin monomer complexes (D-dimers)
Significance: Increased; most sensitive marker for DIC

Test: Antithrombin III or protein C levels
Significance: Decreased

Test: Factor VIII and V
Significance: Decreased; factor VIII is normal in coagulopathy of liver disease.

Therapy

- Treat the underlying disorder.
- Cryoprecipitate, platelets, and fresh frozen plasma to control bleeding.
- Fresh frozen plasma also replaces anticoagulants—protein C and S.
- Heparin used for management of purpura fulminans due to meningococcemia.
- Routine use of heparin for DIC is controversial. It has been used in chronic DIC, arterial thromboses, or large-vessel venous thromboses.
- AT III and protein C concentrates at supraphysiologic dosing have been used rarely but currently are under investigation.

SUPPORTIVE CARE

- Manage other organ system failure.

ICD-9-CM 286.6

BIBLIOGRAPHY

Levi M, ten Cate H. Current concepts: disseminated intravascular coagulopathy. *N Engl J Med* 1999;341(8):586–592.

Levi M, deJonge E, van der Poll T, et al. Novel approaches to the management of disseminated intravascular coagulopathy. *Crit Care Med* 2000;28(9 suppl):S20–S24.

Wintrobe's clinical hematology, 10th ed., vol 2. Baltimore: Lippincott Williams & Wilkins, 1998:1480–1493.

Author: Valerie I. Brown
Sadhna M. Shankar, 2nd edition

Down (Trisomy 21) Syndrome

Database

DEFINITION
- Syndrome consisting of multiple abnormalities, including hypotonia, flat facies, up-slanting palpebral fissures, and small ears
- First described by John Langdon Down in 1866
- Trisomy for chromosome 21

Multiple abnormalities found in Down syndrome:
- Congenital heart disease (40–50%; most not symptomatic as newborn), in decreasing frequency: atrioventricular (AV) canal (60%), ventriculoseptal defect (VSD), patent ductus arteriosus (PDA), atrioseptal defect (ASD), aberrant subclavian artery, tetralogy of Fallot
- Hearing loss (66–75%): sensorineural and conductive.
- Strabismus (33–45%)
- Nystagmus (15–35%)
- Fine lens opacities (by slit-lamp examination 59%), cataracts (1–15%)
- Refractive errors (50%)
- Stenotic nasolacrimal duct
- Delayed tooth eruption
- Tracheoesophageal fistula
- Gastrointestinal atresia (12%)
- Meckel diverticulum
- Hirschsprung disease (less than 1%)
- Imperforate anus
- Renal malformations
- Hypospadias (5%)
- Cryptorchidism (5–50%)
- Thyroid disease (15%): congenital hypothyroidism, hyperthyroidism
- Transient myeloproliferative disorder, neonatal (leukemoid reaction)
- Neonatal polycythemia
- Leukemia (less than 1%; 10 to 30 times greater risk than general population)
- Retinoblastoma and testicular germ-cell tumors (slightly greater risk than general population)
- Infertility, especially in males
- Obesity
- Alopecia areata (10–15%)
- Seizures (5–10%), usually myoclonic
- Alzheimer disease (nearly all over age 40 years)
- Mild to moderate mental retardation (IQ range 25–70)
- Dry hyperkeratotic skin with time (75%)

PATHOPHYSIOLOGY
Specific to the associated findings.

EPIDEMIOLOGY
- Incidence: 1/600 to 1/800 live births
- Male/female ratio is 1.3:1
- For specific maternal ages, incidence is 1 in 1,500 live births for maternal ages 15 to 29 years, 1 in 800 for ages 30 to 34, 1 in 270 for ages 35 to 39, and 1 in 100 for ages 40 to 44
- Best recognized and most frequent chromosomal syndrome of humans
- One of the three most common autosomal trisomies (also trisomy 18 and 13) in humans
- Most common autosomal chromosomal abnormality causing mental retardation
- More than 50% of trisomy 21 fetuses are spontaneously aborted in early pregnancy

GENETICS
- 94% to 97% of cases are due to chromosomal nondisjunction (failure to segregate during meiosis) in the maternal DNA
- Less than 5% of cases are due to paternal nondisjunction
- 2.4% with trisomy 21/normal mosaicism (nondisjunction occurs after conception; two cell lines are present); generally less severely affected
- Remainder due to translocations between chromosome 21 and 14 [t(14q21q)]; rarely between 21 and 13 or 15; 50% of translocations are sporadic *de novo* events; 50% result from balanced translocations in one parent.

COMPLICATIONS
- Serous otitis media (50–70%)
- Conjunctivitis (frequent)
- Sinusitis
- Tonsillar and adenoidal hypertrophy
- Obstructive airway disease with associated sleep apnea (33–75%), cor pulmonale
- Obstructive bowel disease (12%, newborn period)
- Constipation (due to low tone and decreased gross motor mobility)
- Subluxation of the hips (secondary to ligamentous laxity)
- Atlantoaxial instability (10–20%; secondary to ligamentous laxity, which is most severe prior to age 10 years)

PROGNOSIS
- Dependent on the associated findings
- Life expectancy is mildly decreased, with many living into the sixth decade.
- Alzheimer disease affects approximately 15% after the fourth decade.
- Recurrence is approximately 1% if parents are not translocation carriers.
- As adults, the majority of patients with Down syndrome can work in supported positions.

Data Gathering

HISTORY
- Check for previous history of infant with Down syndrome in the family.
- Ask about growth and developmental status.
- Ask about feeding problems.
- Ask about snoring, signs of sleep apnea (e.g., restless sleep).
- Ask about stool habits.
- Ask about hearing concerns.

Physical Examination

The phenotype is variable from person to person.

General: Short stature; hypotonia (80–100%), with an open mouth and a protruding tongue; midface hypoplasia.
Head: Brachycephaly with a flattened occiput, microcephaly, false fontanel (95%).
Eyes: Up-slanting palpebral fissures (98%), inner epicanthal folds, Brushfield spots (speckling of the iris), fine lens opacities on slit-lamp examination, cataracts, refractive error, strabismus, nystagmus.
Ears: Small, prominent; low set; overfolding of upper helix; small canals with difficulty visualizing tympanic membranes.
Nose: Small (85%); flat nasal bridge.
Tongue: Relative but not true macroglossia (tongue mass is normal); fissuring.
Mouth: High-arched or abnormal palate.
Teeth: Missing (50%), small, hypoplastic; irregular placement.
Neck: In infancy, excess skin at the nape; short appearance; occasionally webbed.
Lungs: Check for signs of infection or congestive heart failure.
Heart: Assess for murmur, arrhythmia, cyanosis.
Abdomen: In neonate, distention may be present if obstruction or atresia is present; diastasis recti.
Genital: In adolescents, straight pubic hair; in males, small penis, cryptorchidism.
Extremities: Hands, broad with short metacarpals and phalanges; fifth finger with hypoplasia of the midphalanx (60%) and clinodactyly (50%); simian crease (single transverse palmar crease) in approximately 50%; wide gap between the first and second toes (96%); syndactyly of second and third toes; hyperflexibility of joints. A newborn with a simian crease has a 1 in 60 chance of having Down syndrome.
Skin: Cutis marmorata (43%); in older children, hyperkeratotic dry skin (75%); fine, soft, sparse hair.

Laboratory Aids

Test: Prenatal karyotyping via amniocentesis (16–18 weeks' gestation) or chorionic villus sampling (9–11 weeks' gestation).
Significance: Is typically offered to women >35 years of age given the increased incidence of Down syndrome in the fetus.

Test: Chromosomal karyotype on cultured lymphocytes from peripheral blood
Significance: May be performed postnatally if there is a clinical suspicion of Down syndrome.

Test: Tissue sample other than blood (usually skin)
Significance: To check for mosaicism.

Test: CBC
Significance: In the newborn period to check for polycythemia and transient myeloproliferative disorder; Down syndrome patients may have an increased mean corpuscular volume (MCV) on CBC, making the diagnosis iron-deficiency anemia difficult; repeat in adolescence.

Test: Thyroid-function tests
Significance: To rule out hypo- or hyperthyroidism.

RADIOGRAPHIC STUDIES
Test: Fetal ultrasound
Significance: May show polyhydramnios if bowel obstruction is present. A thickened nuchal fold is associated with an increased risk for Down syndrome.

Test: Echocardiography and chest x-ray study.
Significance: Done in the first month of life to rule out cardiac disease.

Test: Lateral cervical spine x-ray studies in flexion, neutral, and extension
Significance: To rule out atlantoaxial instability, defined as greater than 5-mm space between atlas and odontoid process of the axis. Important measures include (1) the atlantodens interval (ADI; normal <4.5 mm), which is the distance between the posterior surface of the anterior arch of C1 and the anterior surface of the dens; (2) the neural canal width (NCW; normal $\geq$14 mm), which is the distance between the posterior surface of the dens and the anterior surface of the posterior arch of C1; and (3) the distance of subluxation at the occipitoatlantal joint, which is normally $\geq$7 mm.

OTHER STUDIES
Test: Electrocardiogram (ECG)
Significance: Done within the first month of life to rule out cardiac disease.

Test: Auditory brainstem response
Significance: Done within the first 3 months of life to rule out hearing loss.

 ## Therapy

Not applicable except for treatments specific to complications/associated illnesses.

 ## Follow-Up

GROWTH AND DEVELOPMENT
Specific growth charts for Down syndrome are available; average age for acquiring developmental milestones differs from normal population; late closure of fontanelles; consider early intervention program for hypotonia and developmental delay.

GENETICS
Genetic counseling recommended.

CARDIAC
Early evaluation in newborn period, with follow-up until the presence or absence of disease is evident; subacute bacterial endocarditis prophylaxis for patients with certain types of cardiac disease.

OPHTHALMOLOGIC
Early evaluation for cataracts and glaucoma; with visit by 6 months to the ophthalmologist, and then every 2 years.

EAR, NOSE, AND THROAT (ENT)/AUDIOLOGIC
Annual audiologic evaluation in the first 3 years of life, then every other year; ENT referral to visualize tympanic membranes with microscopic otoscope if small narrow external canals.

ORTHOPEDIC
Screen for atlantoaxial instability with x-ray studies in preschool years, then every decade. Prior to participation in contact sports (e.g., Special Olympics), must evaluate for atlantoaxial instability.

ENDOCRINE
Thyroid-function tests in newborn period, age 6 months and 12 months, then yearly.

OTHER
Multiple organizations (e.g., Down Syndrome International) are available to families of children with Down syndrome.

PITFALLS
• Caution with endotracheal intubation if absence or presence of atlantoaxial instability is not known to avoid spinal cord injury, which may be seen in rare cases.
• Hearing loss may be misinterpreted as a behavioral problem.
• Care with atropine and pilocarpine use for ophthalmologic evaluation because of cholinergic hypersensitivity that may be seen.

 ## Common Questions and Answers

Q: Why was Down syndrome referred to as mongolism in the past?
A: There was a mistaken notion about a racial cause for this syndrome due to the facial appearance, which was thought to be similar to that of those from Mongoloid origin.

Q: Do all children with Down syndrome have mental retardation?
A: No. Though all persons with nonmosaic Down syndrome have some degree of cognitive disability, some have IQs greater than 70 and are not considered to have mental retardation.

Q: Do children with this syndrome have an increased susceptibility to infection?
A: The literature on this subject is unclear and has been subject to debate. Midface hypoplasia may contribute to an increased incidence of ear, sinus, and nasolacrimal duct infections. There may be an increased risk of lower respiratory tract infection for children with unrepaired heart disease.

Q: Can a normal cardiac examination rule out the presence of a cardiac anomaly?
A: No, all patients with Down syndrome should have a cardiac evaluation within the first month of life. Timely surgery may be necessary to prevent serious complications.

Q: Are patients with atlantoaxial instability symptomatic?
A: No, most are asymptomatic, but symptoms of cord compression may be seen in 1% to 2% of patients.

Q: I have seen growth charts for Down syndrome patients that allow for plotting of lengths, heights, and weights. Are there special growth charts available for plotting head circumference?
A: Yes. If appropriate growth charts are not used for plotting head circumference, head growth may appear abnormal. Head circumference growth charts are available through the Internet: *http://www.growthcharts.com*.

ICD-9-CM 758.0

BIBLIOGRAPHY
American Academy of Pediatrics. Health supervision for children with Down syndrome. *Pediatrics* 2001;107:442–449.

Brockmeyer D. Down syndrome and craniovertebral instability. Topic review and treatment recommendations. *Pediatr Neurosurg* 1999;31:71–77.

Cooley WC, Graham JM. Down syndrome: an update and review for the primary pediatrician. *Clin Pediatr* 1991;30:233–253.

Cronk C, Crocker AC, Pueschel SM, et al. Growth charts for children with Down syndrome: 1 month to 18 years of age. *Pediatrics* 1988;81:102–110.

Jones KL. Down syndrome. In: Smith DW, ed. *Smith's recognizable patterns of malformation*, 5th ed. Philadelphia: WB Saunders, 1997:8–13.

Saenz RB. Primary care of infants and young children with Down syndrome. *Am Fam Physician* 1999;59:381–390,392,395–396.

Smith-Bindman R, Hosmer W, Feldstein VA, Deeks JJ, Goldberg JD. Second-trimester ultrasound to detect fetuses with Down syndrome: a meta-analysis. *JAMA* 2001;285:1044–1055.

Author: Esther K. Chung

Dysfunctional Uterine Bleeding/Menorrhagia

 Database

DEFINITION
- Endometrial bleeding beyond the range of normal menses: duration of 2 to 8 days, occurring every 21 to 40 days, with blood loss of 20 to 80 mL/cycle.
- Dysfunctional uterine bleeding (DUB) can vary in presentation from heavy, long menses followed by long periods of amenorrhea to short, heavy menses occurring every 1 to 2 weeks.
- Most commonly associated with anovulatory cycles resulting from immature hypothalamic-pituitary-ovarian axis.

PATHOPHYSIOLOGY
- In most cases of DUB presenting within 2 years of menarche, anovulation results in absence of corpus luteum.
- Without the secretory effect of progesterone from the corpus luteum, endometrial proliferation continues due to unopposed estrogen.
- The thickened endometrium eventually outgrows support from basal endometrium, resulting in sloughing of the highest endometrial levels.
- As subsequent levels of endometrium are shed, bleeding increases. Profuse bleeding can result when the basal endometrium is exposed.

GENETICS
- Familial history of anovulatory cycles is common.
- Patients with disorders such as blood dyscrasias and polycystic ovary syndrome (PCOS) usually have familial histories including these disorders.

EPIDEMIOLOGY
- Most commonly occurs within the first 2 years of menarche when more than 50% of cycles are anovulatory.
- Later age at menarche results in greater length of anovulation.
- Most females do not develop DUB during their anovulatory cycles.
- DUB can develop in 20% to 30% of patients with PCOS (Stein-Leventhal syndrome).

COMPLICATIONS
- Mild to severe anemia resulting from blood loss

 Differential Diagnosis

The differential diagnosis can be divided into three categories based on cycle length and timing of bleeding:

CATEGORY I
- Normal cyclic intervals with excess bleeding during each cycle

Infection
- Endometritis due to *Neisseria gonorrhea* or *Chlamydia trachomatis*

- Pelvic inflammatory disease (PID)

Primary Gynecologic
- Intrauterine abnormalities, such as polyps, submucosal myomas, or fibroids
- Endometriosis
- Complication of pregnancy, such as ectopic pregnancy, spontaneous abortion, or placenta previa

Hematologic
- Inborn coagulopathies, such as Von Willebrand disease
- Clotting disorders resulting from systemic disease, such as immune thrombocytopenic purpura, systemic lupus erythematosus, chronic renal failure, hepatic disease, or leukemia
- Medicine or poisons affecting coagulation (e.g., aspirin, Coumadin)

CATEGORY II
- Normal cyclic intervals with bleeding between cycles

Infection
- PID

Primary Gynecologic
- Endometriosis
- Complications of pregnancy

Tumors
- Endometrial adenocarcinoma [exceedingly rare tumor associated with *in utero* exposure to diethylstilbestrol (DES); general usage discontinued in 1974]
- Benign uterine tumors

Trauma
- Vaginal laceration
- Intrauterine device (IUD)
- Foreign body

CATEGORY III
Abnormal cycle intervals or no apparent cycle

Primary Gynecologic
- Premature ovarian failure
- Complications of pregnancy

Tumors
- Craniopharyngioma
- Pituitary adenoma

Endocrine
- Anovulatory cycle
- PCOS (Stein-Leventhal syndrome)
- Thyroid disease
- Pituitary disease, such as prolactinoma
- Adrenal disorders

Psychosocial
- Anorexia nervosa
- Excessive exercise

 Data Gathering

HISTORY
Question: Initial history and evaluation?
Significance: Focus on assessing amount and site of bleeding, and hemodynamic stability.

Question: Complete menstrual history?
Significance: The pattern of DUB in relation to menstrual cycle can help narrow the diagnostic workup (see Differential Diagnosis).

Question: Cramping?
Significance: The presence of cramping suggests ovulation and the presence of progesterone.

Question: Time lapse between menarche and onset of DUB?
Significance: Increased time lapse between menarche and the onset of DUB lessens the likelihood of anovulatory cycles.

Question: Quality of bleeding?
Significance: The presence of clots suggests nonendometrial or basal endometrial bleeding, while brown or prune-colored blood suggests endrometriosis.

Question: Bruising history?
Significance: Easy bruisability, epistaxis, and/or bleeding gums may be suggestive of a clotting disorder.

Question: Should a complete family history be obtained?
Significance: Yes. A family history of thyroid disease, bleeding disorder, PCOS, or DUB can help to guide the laboratory workup.

Question: Should a thorough review of systems be an integral part of the workup?
Significance: Yes. Seemingly unrelated symptoms may reveal cryptic chronic or systemic disease processes.

Question: Should the sexual history also assess the likelihood of sexual abuse?
Significance: Yes. Sexual abuse not only can result in bleeding from trauma, but also can be a source of sexually transmitted diseases and pregnancy.

 Physical Examination

Finding: Vital signs, including orthostatic blood pressures
Significance: Severe blood loss.

Finding: Pelvic examination
Significance: A pelvic examination is essential in determining the source of bleeding. It should include a speculum examination looking for signs of trauma and/or foreign body. The bimanual examination should be performed to assess for ovarian mass, uterine fibroids, signs of PID, or signs of pregnancy.

Finding: Hirsutism and acne
Significance: May indicate a hyperandrogenic state.
- Assessing for signs of thyroid, liver, or hematologic disease.

Laboratory Aids

TESTS

Test: Urine or serum β-HCG should be obtained, regardless of sexual history.
Significance: Urine β-HCG testing can reliably detect pregnancy as early as 2 weeks postconception; however, may be positive for up to 2 weeks following an abortion.

Test: Wet prep and cervical testing for *C. trachomatis* and *N. gonorrhea*
Significance: To test for STDs.

Test: Pap test
Significance: A Papanicolaou smear should be performed to rule out cervical neoplasia as a source of bleeding.

Test: Examination of cervical mucus
Significance: An experienced provider can evaluate cervical mucus in the absence of active bleeding for signs of estrogen or progesterone dominance.

Test: Consider prolactin level and thyroid function tests.
Significance: Hyperprolactinemia can have several causes, including pituitary micro-adenoma, and result in amenorrhea or DUB.

Test: PT, PTT, platelet count, and bleeding time
Significance: To assess for severe bleeding and anemia. Consider in those with a family history of bleeding.

Test: Endometrial biopsy
Significance: Rarely warranted for adolescents.

RADIOGRAPHIC IMAGING

Test: Pelvic ultrasound
Significance: Indicated when ectopic pregnancy is suspected. Should be considered when a pelvic mass is felt, uterine anomaly is being considered, or bimanual examination cannot be completed.

Test: MRI
Significance: Indicated for patients with a suspected pelvic mass when ultrasonography does not clearly define the anatomy.

Therapy

• If attributed to anovulatory cycles, or a complete workup fails to yield a diagnosis, treatment is guided by the severity of DUB and the presence of active bleeding.
• For mild DUB (inconvenient, unpredictable bleeding, and the patient has a normal hemoglobin): Reassurance until ovulatory cycles resume. Encourage maintenance of a menstrual calendar with follow-up in 3 to 6 months.
• Iron supplementation

• If inconvenience and anxiety are unresponsive to reassurance, use of an oral contraceptive should be considered to regulate menstrual cycle. Combination OCPs can be used in sexually active patients, or medroxyprogesterone acetate (Provera), 10 mg daily for 5 to 7 days every 35 to 40 days for patients who are not sexually active.
• For moderate DUB (irregular, prolonged, heavy bleeding with a hemoglobin >10 g/dL); hormonal therapy, as described previously.
• Menstrual calendar with follow-up every 1 to 2 months
• For severe DUB (heavy, prolonged bleeding with a hemoglobin <10 g/dL), treatment depends on the presence of active bleeding.
• If not actively bleeding, hemodynamically stable patients can be started on OCPs, iron supplementation, and have follow-up in 1 to 2 months.
• In the presence of active bleeding:
—Hospitalization of patient to monitor patient during treatment.
—Blood transfusion as necessary.
—Hormonal therapy should be started immediately, and can be either IV or PO. In all but the most severe cases PO therapy is tried first.
—Conjugated estrogen can be given intravenously, 20 to 25 mg every 6 hours for a maximum of 6 doses. Norgestrel/ethinyl estradiol, 1 tablet every 6 hours, should be given concurrently, and then tapered as bleeding resolves. Norgestrel/ethinyl estradiol can be given alone, as described, in the absence of IV estrogen. Tapering can begin when bleeding stops, and can be easily remembered as 150 mg pill q.i.d. for 4 days, 1 pill t.i.d. for 3 days, then 1 pill b.i.d. for 2 weeks.
—After tapering, 30–35 mg OCPs should be continued for 6 to 12 months.
—If hormonal therapy fails, dilation and curettage may be necessary.
—Patients should be monitored monthly after an episode of severe DUB.

POSSIBLE SIDE EFFECTS

• Estrogen, given in high doses, will cause nausea and/or vomiting. An appropriate antiemetic should be used for prophylaxis against these symptoms.
• High-dose estrogen can have vascular side effects and should be used with caution in patients particularly at risk for vascular events (e.g., patients with a history of lupus, strokes, or thrombotic phenomena). In these cases, consult a gynecologist for an alternative progesterone-only therapy.

Follow-Up

WHEN TO EXPECT IMPROVEMENT

• Bleeding usually tapers after the first few doses of hormone therapy.
• After 6 to 12 months have passed, and the patient does not wish to remain on OCPs, a

trial off of medication might reveal normal ovulatory cycles.
• DUB persists for 2 years in 60% of patients, 4 years in 50%, and up to 10 years in 30%.

PITFALLS

• Neglecting to perform testing for pregnancy in an adolescent who denies sexual activity.
• Neglecting to repeat a home pregnancy test.
• If there is a prolonged course of DUB, consider PCOS.

Common Questions and Answers

Q: If most girls have anovulatory cycles, why do only some present with DUB?
A: Most girls do have an irregular menstrual cycle during the first 2 years after menarche. However, in a majority of those girls, the negative-feedback system of estrogen will lead to endometrial shedding and a cyclic pattern.

Q: If DUB from anovulatory cycles is caused by lack of progesterone, why does the initial treatment of severe DUB with active bleeding involve large doses of estrogen?
A: In severe DUB, the exposed endometrial base is bleeding profusely. For progesterone to exhibit its secretory effects, the endometrium in that area must be restored by estrogen.

Q: When hormonal therapy fails, and the basal endometrium continues to bleed, how does a dilation and curettage act as the final treatment?
A: The curettage removes any remaining bleeding vessels and stimulates local prostaglandins to create a uterine contracture that inhibits bleeding.

ICD-9-CM 626.8

BIBLIOGRAPHY

Bayer SR, DeCherney AH. Clinical manifestations and treatment of dysfunctional uterine bleeding. *JAMA* 1993;14:1823–1828.

Bravender T, Emans SJ. Menstrual disorders: dysfunctional uterine bleeding. *Pediatr Clin North Am* 1999;46:545–553.

Edmonds DK. Dysfunctional uterine bleeding in adolescence. *Best Pract Res Clin Obstet Gynecol* 1999;13:239–249.

Neinstein LS. Dysfunctional uterine bleeding. In: *Adolescent health care: a practical guide*, 3rd ed. Baltimore: Williams & Wilkins, 1996.

Wathen PI, Henderson MC, Witz CA. Abnormal uterine bleeding. *Med Clin North Am* 1995;79:329–344.

Authors: Kenneth R. Ginsburg and Jonathan R. Pletcher

Dysmenorrhea

 Database

DEFINITION

• Lower abdominal cramping, spasmodic pain radiating to the lower back and thighs during menstruation
• Primary dysmenorrhea—painful menstruation in the absence of specific pathologic conditions typically presenting within 2 years of menarche. The onset of pain usually occurs within hours of starting menstruation and is most intense during the first 2 days of the cycle.
• Secondary dysmenorrhea—painful menstruation in the presence of pathologic conditions of the pelvic organs, such as endometriosis and salpingitis

CAUSES

• Primary dysmenorrhea is caused by excessive production of prostaglandins that cause uterine contractions and subsequent reduced uterine blood flow.

PATHOPHYSIOLOGY

• Prostaglandin E_2 and $F_{2\alpha}$ are produced in the endometrium from arachidonic acid and are found in higher levels in females with dysmenorrhea.
• Prostaglandin $F_{2\alpha}$ causes myometrial contractions, vasoconstriction, and ischemia, whereas prostaglandin E_2 causes vasodilation and hypersensitivity of the myometrial pain nerve terminals.
• Prostaglandins also mediate associated gastrointestinal symptoms (nausea, vomiting, and diarrhea) via their effect on the intestinal smooth muscle.

EPIDEMIOLOGY

• Most common gynecologic disorder among female adolescents
• Prevalence varies from 43% to 93% among postpubescent females
• Prevalence increases with age and sexual maturity
• Risk factors include:

—Early age of menarche
—Long menstrual periods
—Smoking
—Alcohol intake
—Obesity

• Only 14% to 18% of adolescents seek medical advice and approximately 50% of adolescents take medications for pain relief.

COMPLICATIONS

• School and work absenteeism ranging from 23% to 54%.
• Pain
• Associated systemic symptoms occurring in nearly half of affected females:

—Nausea and vomiting (89%)
—Diarrhea (60%)
—Headaches (45%)
—Dizziness (60%)
—Nervousness (67%)
—Fatigue (85%)

PROGNOSIS

• Dysmenorrhea may decrease with parity though data are limited.

 Differential Diagnosis

INFECTION

• Pelvic inflammatory disease (PID)
• Cervicitis
• Salpingitis

TUMORS

• Uterine fibroids and polyps
• Ovarian neoplasm

TRAUMA

• Intrauterine contraceptive device (IUD)

CONGENITAL

• Congenital obstructive müllerian malformation

PSYCHOSOCIAL

• Functional abdominal pain

MISCELLANEOUS

• Endometriosis
• Cervical stenosis
• Ovarian cysts
• Inflammatory bowel disease

 Data Gathering

HISTORY

• A complete review of systems should elicit any associated systemic symptoms such as nausea, vomiting, or diarrhea.
• Menstrual history should include the severity of pain, the relationship of pain to menstruation, the extent to which the menstrual cramps interfere with daily activities, and the effectiveness of previous therapy.
• Sexual history should include the relationship of pain to sexual activity, the number of sexual partners, and a previous history of sexually transmitted diseases or PID.

 Physical Examination

• No abnormalities are noted on physical exam and on routine pelvic exam for primary dysmenorrhea.
• A pelvic exam is indicated if the adolescent is sexually active, the history is atypical for primary dysmenorrhea, or the symptoms do not respond to standard medical therapy.

 Laboratory Aids

• Not indicated for primary dysmenorrhea
• If PID is suspected:

—CBC
—ESR
—Endocervical cultures

Therapy

• Patient education and reassurance should accompany all therapy.
• Nonsteroidal antiinflammatory drugs (NSAIDs)—first-line therapy; works through inhibition of production and release of prostaglandins; begin 2 to 3 days prior to the onset of menses

—Propionic acids
  —Ibuprofen (Motrin) 400 mg to 600 mg q.i.d.
  —Naproxen sodium (Anaprox) 550 mg once, then 275 mg t.i.d.–q.i.d.
  —Naproxen (Naprosyn) 500 mg once, then 250 mg t.i.d.–q.i.d.

—Fenamates
  —Mefenamic acid (Ponstel) 500 mg once, then 250 mg q.i.d.

—Acetic/salicylic acids
  —Tolmetin (Tolectin) 400 mg t.i.d.
  —Sulindac (Clinoril) 200 mg b.i.d.

• Oral contraceptive pill—second-line therapy unless also needed for birth control; reduces menstrual fluid volume and suppresses ovulation; may take up to three cycles to decrease menstrual pain
• Alternative therapies—increasingly being used and demonstrate some relief of symptoms, though studies are limited in size and length of follow-up.

—Transcutaneous electric nerve stimulation (TENS)
—Laparoscopic presacral neuronectomy
—Acupuncture
—Omega-3 fatty acids
—Transdermal nitroglycerine
—Calcium channel blockers
—Thiamine supplementation
—Magnesium supplements

Follow-Up

• Try one of the NSAIDs for two to three menstrual cycles before changing the class of NSAID.
• When initiating therapy with oral contraceptive pills, consider continuing NSAIDs for breakthrough pain for the next two to three menstrual cycles.

PREVENTION

• Limit caffeine intake and encourage adequate diet.
• Regular exercise can diminish the severity of symptoms.

SIGNS TO WATCH FOR

• Consider a pathologic cause of dysmenorrhea, such as endometriosis, in females who do not respond to appropriate therapy with NSAIDs and/or oral contraceptive pills.
• Many adolescents often do not use the proper doses of medications to relieve severe menstrual pain.

Common Questions and Answers

Q: What circumstances may indicate secondary dysmenorrhea?
A: The diagnosis of secondary dysmenorrhea should be considered in females with the following conditions:

• Late-onset dysmenorrhea (after age 25)
• Progressively worsening dysmenorrhea
• Pelvic abnormality on physical exam
• Heavy menstrual flow or irregular cycles
• Little or no response to therapy with NSAIDs and/or oral contraceptive pills
• Family history of endometriosis
• History of pelvic inflammatory disease
• Dyspareunia and infertility are associated problems

Q: When should I consider referral to a gynecologist for further evaluation?
A: A referral should be initiated if the history and physical are consistent with secondary dysmenorrhea or if the pain remains intractable despite treatment with NSAIDs and/or oral contraceptive pills.

Q: Is acetaminophen an effective adjunct to medical therapy?
A: Acetaminophen is a commonly used over-the-counter medication for adolescent females because of its availability in most households. However, due to its inability to limit prostaglandin synthesis, it cannot effectively relieve the symptoms of dysmenorrhea. Females should be encouraged to use one of the over-the-counter NSAIDs for initial therapy at the maximum daily recommended dose.

Q: How do you approach parents resistant to a trial of OCPs as therapy for their daughter's dysmenorrhea?
A: It is important to explain the noncontraceptive advantages of using hormonal therapy for primary dysmenorrhea, such as decreasing menstrual flow, limiting prostaglandin production, reducing the risk of iron-deficiency anemia, and protecting from endometrial and ovarian cancers. Emphasizing that OCPs are a common, effective medical therapy for dysmenorrhea may relieve the minds of many parents. If the parents or the adolescent patient are uncomfortable with the standard packaging, many pharmacists are willing to repackage the OCPs in a regular medication bottle.

ICD-9-CM 625.3

BIBLIOGRAPHY

Alvin PE, Litt IF. Current status of the etiology and management of dysmenorrhea in adolescence. *Pediatrics* 1982;70(4):516–525.

Banikarim C, Chacko MR, Kelder SH. Prevalence and impact of dysmenorrhea on Hispanic female adolescents. *Arch Pediatr Adolesc Med* 2000;154(12):1226–1229.

Braverman PK, Sondheimer SJ. Menstrual disorders. *Pediatr Rev* 1997;18(1):17–26.

Coco AS. Primary dysmenorrhea. *Am Fam Physician* 1999;60(2):489–496.

Campbell MA, McGrath PJ. Use of medication by adolescents for the management of menstrual discomfort. *Arch Pediatr Adolesc Med* 1997;151(9):905–913.

Kennedy S. Primary dysmenorrhoea. *Lancet* 1997;349(9059):1116.

Neinstein LS. *Adolescent health care: a practical guide*, 3rd ed. Philadelphia: Williams & Wilkins, 1996:766–775.

Schroeder B, Sanfilippo JS. Dysmenorrhea and pelvic pain in adolescents. *Pediatr Clin North Am* 1999:46(3):555–571.

Author: Julieana Nichols

Ehrlichiosis

 Database

DEFINITION

A zoonotic infection caused by four microorganisms of the genus *Ehrlichia*. The two most common clinically described infections are human monocytic ehrlichiosis (HME) caused by *Ehrlichia chaffeensis* and human granulocytic ehrlichiosis (HGE) caused by a species closely related to *E. equi* and *E. phagocytophila*. A new organism, *E. ewingii*, was recently described and clinically indistinguishable from HME. A fourth species, *E. sennetsu*, which causes a mononucleosis-like syndrome, has been described in Japan and Malaysia. The genus *Ehrlichia* is found within the family Rickettsiaceae.

CAUSES

HME and HGE are both carried by tick vectors. HME is thought to be transmitted by *Amblyomma americanum*, the lone star tick. The vector for HGE is believed to be *Ixodes scapularis*, a deer tick, or *Dermacentor variabilis*, a brown dog tick.

PATHOPHYSIOLOGY

- Obligate intracellular, pleomorphic, coccobacilli bacteria
- Transmission to a human by a tick vector
- Incubation period ranges from 1 to 21 days
- HME infects mononuclear phagocytes, while HGE infects granulocytes
- The *Ehrlichia* reside within a leukocyte phagosome (called a morula), where the bacteria divide by binary fission and produce microcolonies.
- The infected cell is destroyed by the morula, thus releasing more organisms into the phagocyte system.

GENERAL EPIDEMIOLOGY OF EHRLICHIOSIS

- Most patients contract illness during April through September, the months of greatest tick and human outdoor activity.
- HME and HGE have been found in Europe.

EPIDEMIOLOGY OF HME

- Males are more often infected (57%).
- Average age is 6.7 (range 7 months to 13.7 years).
- Most children reside in rural areas.
- HME is most commonly found in the southeastern and south central states. Most cases have been reported in Missouri, Tennessee, Oklahoma, Texas, Arkansas, Georgia, and Virginia. Cases have also been found in Maryland.
- HME is found in similar states where Rocky Mountain spotted fever (RMSF) occurs.
- Data from Oklahoma demonstrated that ehrlichiosis was as common as RMSF, with an incidence of 3.3 per 100,000.
- Data from Georgia demonstrated that ehrlichiosis was more common than RMSF, with an incidence of 5.3 per 100,000.
- HME has also been identified in Pennsylvania, Massachusetts, and Washington state.

EPIDEMIOLOGY OF HGE

- Prevalence and incidence are not known.
- HGE is well documented in northeastern and north central states. The states with documented HGE are Minnesota, Wisconsin, New York, Connecticut, New Hampshire, Massachusetts, Pennsylvania, Rhode Island, Delaware, Maryland, Georgia, Florida, Arkansas, and California.
- The majority of HGE infections have occurred in states where Lyme disease is very prevalent: Wisconsin, Minnesota, and Connecticut.
- Congential transmission of HGE has been described.

COMPLICATIONS

Neurologic Sequelae

- Headache, described as severe
- Mental status changes
- Seizures
- Coma
- Focal neurologic findings
- Cognitive learning deficits

Hematologic

- Disseminated intravascular coagulopathy (DIC)
- Thrombocytopenia
- Leukopenia
- Lymphopenia
- Anemia

Gastrointestinal

- Gastrointestinal hemorrhage
- Elevated liver enzymes
- Hepatosplenomegaly

Respiratory

- Pulmonary hemorrhage
- Interstitial pneumonia
- Pleural effusions
- Noncardiogenic pulmonary edema

Infectious

- Fungal superinfection
- Nosocomial infections
- Opportunistic infections

Renal

- Renal failure
- Proteinuria
- Hematuria

Cardiac

- Cardiomegaly
- Cardiac murmurs

Metabolic

- Hyponatremia

PROGNOSIS

- The majority of patients are hospitalized (>60%).
- Case fatality for HME is 2% to 5%, HGE is 7% to 10%.
- Elevated BUN and creatinine have been associated with a more severe course.

- Children appear to have an excellent outcome.
—Blood, renal, and liver abnormalities resolve in 1 to 2 weeks after initiating antibiotics.
- Cognitive and behavioral problems have been reported.
- Neuropathy has also been described.

 Differential Diagnosis

TICK-BORNE INFECTION

- RMSF, tularemia, relapsing fever, Lyme disease, Colorado tick fever, and babesiosis

INFECTION

- Toxic shock syndrome, Kawasaki disease, meningococcemia, pyelonephritis, gastroenteritis, hepatitis, leptospirosis, EBV, influenza, CMV, enterovirus, streptococcus throat

MISCELLANEOUS

- Leukemia, idiopathic thrombocytopenia purpura (ITP), hemolytic uremic syndrome (HUS)

 Data Gathering

HISTORY AND PRESENTING SYMPTOMS

- Tick-bite history or exposure to wooded areas with ticks is very helpful.
- Classic presentation is described as fevers, headache, myalgias, followed by the development of a progressive leukopenia, thrombocytopenia, and anemia.
- Fevers are found in all children.
- Rash occurs in about 66% of patients and is pleomorphic. It has been described as macular, maculopapular, petechial, erythematous, vesicular, scarlet form or in a combination. The distribution is usually located on the trunk and on the extremities.
- Myalgia is found in the majority of children.
- Severe headache is often described.
- Abdominal pain, vomiting, anorexia, and diarrhea are often elicited.
- Arthralgia
- Cough and sore throat is often described.

 Physical Examination

- Mental status changes/irritability
- Nuchal rigidity
- Cardiac murmur (II/VI systolic ejection murmur at the LLSB)
- Hepatosplenomegaly
- Poor perfusion with hypotension (shock) has been described in a few children as a presenting symptom.
- Conjunctival or throat injection
- Rash as described

Laboratory Aids

- CBC with differential (with smear)
—Thrombocytopenia, $<150,000/mm^3$ (77–92% incidence)
—Lymphopenia, $<1,500/mm^3$ (75%)
—Leukopenia, $<4,000/mm^3$ (58–68%)
—Anemia, Hct $<30\%$ (38–42%)
- Electrolytes with BUN and creatinine
—Hyponatremia (33–65%)
- Liver function tests
—Elevated ALT, >55 U/L (90%)
- Coagulation labs, type, and cross as indicated
- Cerebrospinal fluid (CSF)
—Leukocytosis, with an average cell count of $100/mm^3$
—Lymphocytic predominance
—Elevated protein and borderline low glucose
—Microbiology cultures are negative.
—*Ehrlichia* morulae (intraleukocytoplasmic *Ehrlichia* microorganisms) have been described on Gram- and Giemsa-stained CSF smears.
- Bone marrows are usually hypercellular, but normocellularity and hypocellularity have also been found.

SERUM STUDIES
- Titers for *E. chaffeensis* have been developed to diagnose HME, while titers for *E. equi* are being used to diagnose HGE.
- Titers are available through state health departments at the CDC or a reference laboratory.
- Acute and convalescent titers of *Ehrlichia* (a fourfold rise or fall is considered positive), obtained 2 to 4 weeks apart.
- An acute titer of $\geq1:64$ is considered diagnostic.
- Polymerase chain reaction (PCR) has been developed in research laboratories.
- The detection of intraleukocytoplasmic *Ehrlichia* microcolonies (morulae) on peripheral blood monocytes or granulocytes is diagnostic.

Therapy

- Supportive care and medical management
- Volume and blood pressure medications as needed
- Intubation for respiratory failure
- Dialysis for renal failure
- Platelets for thrombocytopenia
- Packed red blood cells for anemia
- Fresh frozen plasma, cryoprecipitate, and vitamin K for DIC
- Antifungal or antibiotics for secondary infections

DRUGS
- Doxycycline is the drug of choice: 3 mg/kg per day in two divided doses (oral or intravenous) regardless of the age of the child.
- Chloramphenicol is effective for HME, but there is little data on the effectiveness with HGE.

- Treatment for a minimum of 5 to 7 days and should continue for 3 days after defervescence.
- Doxycycline is a tetracycline and is associated with permanent dental staining and enamel hypoplasia, although with the short courses of treatment dental staining is unlikely. Other side effects of doxycycline are photosensitivity, hepatotoxicity, nausea, and pseudotumor cerebri.
- Unlike Lyme disease, amoxicillin or ceftriaxone have not been shown to be effective for the treatment of ehrlichiosis.

PREVENTION
- Avoid tick-infested areas.
- Clothes should cover arms and legs.
- Tick repellents, but use with caution in young children.
- A thorough body search should always be done after returning from a tick-infested area. If a tick is found, the area should be cleaned with a disinfectant. To remove the tick, grasp the tick at the point of origin with forceps, staying as close to the skin as possible. Applying steady, even pressure, the tick is slowly pulled off the skin. Once the tick is removed, the skin should be cleaned with a disinfectant.
- Instruct parents to seek medical attention if symptoms develop.
- No vaccine is available.

PITFALLS
- Simultaneous infections have been documented with ehrlichiosis and Lyme disease; therefore, in patients diagnosed with ehrlichiosis, Lyme titers should also be measured to determine if there is a dual infection.
- Failing to consider the diagnosis of ehrlichiosis or a delay in treatment pending confirmatory serum titers

Common Questions and Answers

Q: If a tick is removed from my child, should antibiotics be started?
A: Unlike Lyme disease, there are no data to demonstrate that presumptive treatment with doxycycline will decrease ehrlichiosis sequelae.

Q: What is the most common chief complaint in children with ehrlichiosis?
A: Intense unremitting headache. In patients with headache and flu-like illness in the spring to early fall, consider the diagnosis. Laboratory abnormalities of leukopenia, thrombocytopenia and hepatitis should lead to presumptive therapy until the diagnosis is clear.

ICD-9-CM 066.8

BIBLIOGRAPHY
American Academy of Pediatrics. Ehrlichiosis (human). In: Pickering LK, ed. *2000 red book: report of the Committee on Infectious Disease*, 25th ed. Elk Grove Village, IL: American Academy of Pediatrics, 2000:234–236.

Barton LB, Rathore MH, Dawson JE. Infection with *Ehrlichia* in childhood. *J Pediatr* 1992;120:998–1001.

Berry DS, Miller S, Hooke JA, et al. Ehrlichial meningitis with cerebrospinal fluid morulae. *Pediatr Infect Dis J* 1999;18:552–555.

Buller RS, Arens M, Hmiel P, et al. *Ehrlichia ewingii*, a newly recognized agent of human ehrlichiosis. *N Engl J Med* 1999;341:148–155.

Dumler JS, Bakken JS. Ehrlichial diseases of humans: emerging tick-borne infections. *Clin Infect Dis* 1995;20:1102–1110.

Fichtenbaum CJ, Peterson LR, Weil GJ. Ehrlichiosis presenting as a life-threatening illness with features of the toxic shock syndrome. *Am J Med* 1993;95:351–357.

Harkess JR, Ewing SA, Brumit T, et al. Ehrlichiosis in children. *Pediatrics* 1991;87:199–203.

Horowitz HW, Kilchevsky E, Haber S, et al. Perinatal transmission of the agent of human granulocytic ehrlichiosis. *N Engl J Med* 1999;339:375–378.

Jacobs RF, Schultze GE. Ehrlichiosis in children. *J Pediatr* 1997;131:184–192.

Nadelman RB, Horowitz HW, Heish T, et al. Simultaneous human granulocytic ehrlichiosis and Lyme borreliosis. *N Engl J Med* 1997;337:27–30.

Nadelman RB, Nowakoski J, Fish D, et al. Prophylaxis with single dose doxycycline for the prevention of Lyme disease after an *Ixodes scapularis* tick bite. *N Engl J Med* 2001;345:79–84.

Olson JC, Dalton MJ. Ehrlichia species (ehrlichiosis). In: Long SS, Pickering LK, Prober CG, eds. *Principles and practice of pediatric infectious diseases*, 1st ed. New York: Churchill Livingstone, 1997:1014–1016.

Schutze GE, Jacobs RF. Human monocytic ehrlichiosis in children. *Pediatrics* 1997;100:e10.

Author: Jeffrey P. Louie

Encephalitis

Database

DEFINITION
Encephalitis is an inflammation of the brain parenchyma due to infection. Meningoencephalitis is an inflammation of the brain and the meninges.

PATHOPHYSIOLOGY
• Direct or delayed (postinfectious) reaction by the immune system to a virus, bacteria, fungus, or parasite
• Organisms enter the CNS via the systemic circulation, direct inoculation (trauma), or neural pathways [rabies, herpes simplex virus (HSV)].
• Infiltration of inflammatory cells into the CNS with release of cytokines
• Inclusion bodies [intranuclear; HSV, subacute sclerosing panencephalitis (SSPE), viral, intracytoplasmic; rabies], CSF, and serology changes

EPIDEMIOLOGY
• Depends on age, geographic location, and season
• The most common causes of encephalitis are viruses:
—Summer (enteroviruses)
—Summer and fall (western and eastern equine encephalitis, St. Louis encephalitis, La Crosse encephalitis)
—Winter (varicella)
• Nonviral causes (tuberculosis, Lyme disease, toxoplasmosis, cat-scratch disease, rickettsial disease, tick-borne infections) are sometimes associated with specific environmental or geographic exposure.
• The most common cause of sporadic encephalitis is HSV (rabies and HIV also occur in all seasons).

COMPLICATIONS
Seizure disorders, focal or generalized, quadriparesis/hemiparesis, ataxia, learning disabilities, and aphasias can result from encephalitis.

PROGNOSIS
Outcome can range from complete recovery to coma, persistent vegetative state, and death.

Differential Diagnosis

Several toxic, metabolic, vascular, or epileptic syndromes may resemble encephalitis:
• Ingestions
• Hypothyroid crisis
• Acute electrolyte disturbance, especially hyponatremia
• Reye syndrome
• Noninfectious encephalitides, triggered by immunization or infection include acute hemorrhagic leukoencephalitis and acute disseminated encephalomyelitis (ADEM) (associated *Mycoplasma* or other infection)

• Intracranial hemorrhage
• Pituitary infarction
• Acute obstructive hydrocephalus or ventriculoperitoneal shunt obstruction
• Sinus thrombosis
• Subdural empyema
• Stroke or septic embolization (endocarditis)
• Brain abscess or subdural empyema
• Malignant hyperthermia
• Status epilepticus
• Other considerations include bacterial meningitis (*Neisseria meningitidis, Haemophilus influenzae* type b, group B streptococcus in the neonate, *Escherichia coli* in the neonate) parasites, and vasculitis.
• Diagnosis of specific causes of true encephalitis depends on geographic location, age, and clinical and associated laboratory findings.
• Microbes to consider:
—Herpes viruses (in the child and adult, herpes has preference for the medial temporal lobe)
—Lyme disease; possible coinfection with ehrlichiosis, babesiosis
—Varicella (postinfectious encephalitis)
—Cat-scratch and rickettsial diseases
—Tuberculosis
—Fungal (cryptosporidiosis)
—Parasitic (amoebae, *Toxoplasma,* cysticercosis)
—Toxoplasma
• Meningitis:
—May cause secondary parenchymal inflammation of the brain.
—Mental status changes are more prominent in primary encephalitis compared with meningitis.

Data Gathering

HISTORY
• Ask about a viral prodrome with symptoms such as upper respiratory infection, cough, coryza, malaise, anorexia, decreased enteral intake, diarrhea, nausea, and vomiting.
• Encephalitis is often heralded by headaches, photophobia, a stiff neck, increased sleeping, a change in mental status, irritability, confusion, hallucinations, and seizures.
• Prodromal symptoms can range from hours to weeks; seizures or lapse of consciousness are uncommon as *initial* symptoms of encephalitis
• Inquire about recent travel history, pets, and tick bites.

Physical Examination

• Changing vital signs may suggest impending herniation due to brain swelling (hypertension, bradycardia, apnea).
• Neck: The patient may have meningismus and positive Kernig and Brudzinski signs.
• Adenopathy (especially mycobacterium, cat-scratch encephalitis)
• Chest: signs of pneumonia, rales, rhonchi (especially mycobacteria, *Mycoplasma,* influenza)
• Abdomen: hepatosplenomegaly
• Skin: may show various types of rashes, from petechial (especially rickettsial infection, meningococcemia) to an erythematous or papular rashes (especially Lyme, enteroviridae)
• Neurologic examination: rapid or slow changes in mental status ranging from mild confusion to delirium with hallucinations to stupor and coma
• Aphasia (suggestive of herpes) is distinguished from psychomotor slowing by prominence of grammatic errors and dysarthria and normal alertness.
• There may be pupillary abnormalities with nystagmus: Funduscopic examination may reveal papilledema, a sign of increased intracranial pressure (ICP). Cranial neuropathies, increased muscle tone, pathologic deep tendon reflexes, Babinski sign, clonus, or ataxia (especially varicella) may be encountered.

PITFALLS
A CSF sample without any RBCs does not rule out herpes simplex.
• Never assume that a CSF pleocytosis is secondary to seizures. Institute antiviral and/or antibacterial therapy promptly; it can always be discontinued once an organism is identified or cultures are negative.
• Children with immunodeficiency are at higher risk for fungal meningoencephalitis, which may be missed unless appropriate studies are sent.
• Amebic infection of the brain should be considered in children with exposure to fresh water sources.
• Cysticercosis is common in tropical and underdeveloped areas. Ring-enhancing lesions may point to this diagnosis or to toxoplasmosis.

Laboratory Aids

TESTS

A decision about laboratory testing depends partly on the severity of symptoms.

Radiologic

- CT or MRI of the brain with and without contrast medium should be performed urgently to rule out surgically remediable conditions (empyema, abscess).
- Typical changes in encephalitis include parenchymal, meningeal, and focal or diffuse enhancement of the brain. (HSV has a preference for the medial temporal lobe, with hemorrhagic and cystic changes.)
- Hydrocephalus, obstructive or communicating, may occur as a result of the encephalitis.

Spinal Tap

A CSF spinal tap should be deferred until airway, gas exchange, and circulation has been stabilized. Thereafter, lumbar puncture should be deferred if (a) there is papilledema, or (b) if imaging shows subfalcine herniation (left-to-right shift of lateral ventricles), cerebral edema, obstructive hydrocephalus (lateral ventricles large, fourth ventricle relatively small), or central herniation (asymmetry or effacement of fourth ventricle/basilar cistern).

Lumbar Puncture

If radiologic evidence for increased intracranial pressure has been ruled out, a lumbar puncture should be performed.
- Opening pressure is frequently elevated.
- Pleocytosis is lymphocytic if viral, and usually neutrophilic if bacterial.
- Protein will be increased, glucose will be decreased, and RBCs may be present (particularly in HSV).
- CSF should be sent for bacterial and viral culture. Order a fungal culture if suspected.
- If HSV is suspected, PCR should be obtained, as the virus is difficult to grow *in vitro*. Other PCR-based tests on CSF, including assays for the Lyme spirochete and for enteroviruses, may be considered.
- Gram stain and acid-fast bacillus, cryptococcal antigen, and yeast tests also should be ordered.

Other Routine Tests

- Blood electrolytes, BUN, glucose, calcium, magnesium, phosphorus, blood count with differential, blood and urine culture, and toxicology screen
- An EEG may be helpful, particularly if HSV is suspected; it may show periodic lateralizing epileptiform discharges (PLEDs), which are suggestive, but not diagnostic, of herpes.
- PPD if CSF or other signs suggest the possibility of *Mycobacterium*

 ## Therapy

- General: Patients with encephalitis frequently require ICU care with cardiorespiratory support. Mini-dose subcutaneous heparin is standard for prophylaxis of intravascular thrombosis in acutely ill adults, but is untested in the pediatric age group. Early involvement of physical and occupational therapy is important.
- Treatment of intracranial hypertension includes mannitol and hyperventilation, usually with assistance from intensivists or neurology/neurosurgery consultants; these measures should be reserved for situations in which vital or neurologic signs indicate impending herniation.
- Antiinfective agents: Depending on severity of the illness and clinicians' level of suspicion, initial treatment could include antibacterial and antiviral agents (acyclovir: monitor renal function) until the cause becomes clear or cultures are negative.
- Fluids: Avoidance of fluid overload, which may exacerbate cerebral edema, requires strict attention to fluid/osmotic balance. Normal saline is preferred; electrolytes are closely monitored, anticipating possible SIADH or diabetes insipidus.
- Anticonvulsants are reserved for clinical or electrographic evidence of seizure/epileptic activity; usual choices include phenytoin, phenobarbital, and carbamazepine. Treatment of PLEDs without associated convulsions is controversial. Potential side effects and sedation from anticonvulsants should be considered in this decision.
- A noninfectious encephalitis—ADEM (see above)—may respond to steroids, intravenous immunoglobulins, or both.
- Consultation with an infectious disease specialist, neurologist, or neurosurgeon may be helpful.

 ## Follow-Up

The outcome from encephalitis varies greatly and depends on age and degree of CNS involvement/destruction. Physical and occupational therapy should be consulted early in the course of the hospitalization. Patients who appear to have recovered completely physically may still have cognitive deficits. Neuropsychologic testing is helpful to identify the deficits and to create long-term treatment plans, which will maximize the patient's recovery.

PREVENTION

- Completion of routine immunizations (varicella, H-flu type b, etc.) and routine hygiene (hand washing) are the best preventive measures.
- Other measures should be taken according to the infection (e.g., skin testing contacts in cases of tuberculosis).
- Isolation of hospitalized patient: depends on organism suspected. Airborne, droplet, and contact precautions are frequently used together during the first 24 hours, pending a more specific diagnosis from cultures. The infectious disease department will determine type and duration of isolation and whether family members need to be treated.

 ## Common Questions and Answers

Q: My child has been diagnosed with encephalitis; will he be mentally retarded?
A: The complications following encephalitis vary greatly, from severe mental retardation and cerebral palsy to full recovery. There is a correlation between degree of brain destruction and outcome. However, children frequently recover better than adults with a similar degree of illness.

Q: Do seizures from encephalitis cause permanent damage?
A: Seizures are a symptom of brain inflammation; as long as there are no respiratory complications, there is no reason to anticipate aggravation of the encephalitis from the seizure itself. Once seizures abate, seizure medications can often be withdrawn in the months after recovery from encephalitis.

ICD-9-CM 323.9

BIBLIOGRAPHY

Assa A, Watemberg N, Bujanover Y, et al. Demyelinative brainstem encephalitis responsive to intravenous immunoglobulin therapy. *Pediatrics* 1999;104:301–303.

Balkhy HH, Schreiber JR. Severe La Crosse encephalitis with significant neurologic sequelae. *Pediatr Infect Dis J* 2000;19(1):77–80.

Lovett GD, Tsai T, Thompson A. La Crosse encephalitis in children. *N Engl J Med* 2001;344(11):801–807.

McJunkin JE, de los Reyes EC, Irazuzta JE, et al. Significant neurologic sequelae. *Pediatr Infect Dis J* 2000;19(1):77–80.

Whitley RJ, Kimberlin DW. Viral encephalitis. *Pediatr Rev* 1999;20:192–198.

Author: A. G. Christina Bergqvist

Encopresis

 ## Database

DEFINITION

Encopresis is overflow incontinence resulting from chronic constipation.

PATHOPHYSIOLOGY

Chronic constipation with fecal impaction results in overflow incontinence and reduced sensation secondary to rectal distention. The pattern of holding fecal matter, leading to chronic constipation and overflow incontinence, may result from a variety of etiologies, such as a painful experience from a fissure or refusal to use school bathrooms. However, the history often does not reveal a triggering event.

GENETICS

Monozygotic twins have a fourfold higher incidence than do dizygotic twins.

EPIDEMIOLOGY

The ratio of boys to girls is approximately 6:1. There is no association with family size, ordinal position in the family, age of parents, or socioeconomic status.

COMPLICATIONS

- Social problems
- Urinary tract infections, especially in girls
- Abdominal discomfort
- Decreased appetite

 ## Differential Diagnosis

The physician must determine if stool leakage is due to functional constipation or an underlying anatomic, metabolic, or endocrinologic abnormality.

- Anatomic

—Anterior displaced anus
—Fistula secondary to inflammatory bowel disease
—Stricture (after necrotizing enterocolitis or inflammatory bowel disease)
—Abdominal pelvic mass (sacral teratoma, meningomyelocele)

- Neurologic

—Hirschsprung disease
—Meningomyelocele
—Spinal cord tumor
—Hypotonia (cerebral palsy, amyotonia congenita, familial visceral myopathy)
—Amyloidosis

- Metabolic

—Hypothyroidism
—Panhypopituitarism
—Diabetes mellitus
—Constipating drugs

 ## Data Gathering

HISTORY

- Timing in the neonatal period of meconium passage, as well as past surgeries, medical history, and medications, are relevant.
- The review of systems should be unremarkable, except for possible mild abdominal discomfort and a small amount of blood on the outside of the stool or separate from the bowel movement if a fissure has developed.

 ## Physical Examination

- Demonstrates a dilated rectum but a normally positioned anus
- Should include deep tendon reflexes, anal wink, rectal examination, and documentation of normal growth

Laboratory Aids

No laboratory tests are needed if both the history and physical examination are consistent with functional constipation and associated encopresis. If the patient's history or physical is atypical and Hirschsprung disease is suspected, an unprepped barium enema and rectal suction biopsy may be warranted.

Therapy

Management combines pharmacology, behavioral modification, and dietary alterations.

• Pharmacology

—Remove fecal impaction via enemas, cathartic regimens, including laxatives.
—Stool softener

• Behavior modification

—Decrease family stress.
—Have the child sit on toilet for 5 to 10 minutes one to two times per day (tailored to the age of the child).
—Delay toilet training if the child is in diapers (to reduce stress).
—Motivate
—Biofeedback (reserved for very difficult cases)

• Diet

—High-fiber diet
—Adequate fluid

Follow-Up

The first follow-up is at 2 weeks to ensure compliance and success with the initial management. If the fecal impaction has been successfully removed, a reward system is started. The patient is followed at monthly intervals to ensure motivation and to be supportive. Treatment with stool softeners is needed until behavior and diet have improved and until rectal dilatation has resolved. Medication is often needed for 6 months or longer.

PITFALLS

• Parents may misconstrue stool-withholding behavior as an attempt to defecate.
• Parents think that their child's soiling is deliberate. They do not understand that the child can neither feel the passage of stool nor prevent it. The usual urge to defecate, which comes from stretching of the ampulla and internal anal sphincter, is not felt because the rectal ampulla is massively distended.
• Patients or their parents often stop stool softeners as soon as a normal stool pattern starts. If therapy has been ended prematurely, the patient's constipation and encopresis returns immediately, because rectal tone is still poor and no other behavior or dietary modifications have been made.

Common Questions and Answers

Q: Is the medicine addictive?
A: Stool softeners rather than cathartics are chosen for long-term therapy because the colon does not become dependent.

Q: Will my child become sick if this problem is not resolved?
A: Most children with chronic constipation and encopresis grow well and do not develop other health problems. The major problems are social and should be taken seriously. Social development is crucial for the school-aged child.

ICD-9-CM 787.6

BIBLIOGRAPHY

Wyllie R, Hyams JS. *Pediatric gastrointestinal disease*. Philadelphia: WB Saunders, 1993.

Author: Barbara Haber

Endocarditis

Database

DEFINITION

Infective endocarditis is microbial infection of the endocardium of the heart.

PATHOGENESIS

- Infective endocarditis is primarily seen in patients with preexisting heart disease (congenital or acquired) who develop bacteremia with organisms that are likely to cause infection.
- Intravenous drug abusers and patients with indwelling intravenous catheters may develop endocarditis even in the absence of prior heart disease.
- Local turbulence secondary to the cardiovascular abnormality is thought to result in damage of the endocardial surface.

—The development of a fibrin and platelet network occurs in which bacteria can then become entrapped, causing infection.

- Bacteremia can be a complication of focal infection (e.g., pneumonia, cellulitis, or urinary tract infection) or can be associated with various dental and surgical procedures. Bacteremia, however, can occur spontaneously and has been documented with usual activities such as chewing hard candy and brushing teeth.

MICROORGANISMS

- Gram-positive cocci account for 90% of culture-positive endocarditis.

—α-Hemolytic streptococci (*Streptococcus viridans*) are responsible for most cases of endocarditis in all age groups.
—Staphylococci (*S. aureus* and coagulase-negative staphylococci) are the second largest group.
—Other organisms that can cause endocarditis are β-hemolytic streptococci, pneumococci, enterococci, *Pseudomonas* species, the HACEK bacteria, *Neisseria* species, and *Candida* species.

- Approximately 5% of endocarditis cases are reported as culture-negative.

EPIDEMIOLOGY

- Infective endocarditis is relatively uncommon. Studies have reported incidences between 1 in 1,280 and 1 in 4,500 of all pediatric hospital admissions.
- The overall incidence of endocarditis appears to have decreased with the advent of antibiotics. One might expect, however, an increase in incidence with better survival of patients with congenital heart disease and the wide and often prolonged use of central vascular catheters.

COMPLICATIONS

Despite improvements in diagnosis and treatment of endocarditis, it continues to be a disease with significant morbidity and mortality (approximately 10%).

- Cardiac

—Damage to the valve leaflets may result in valvar regurgitation, heart failure, or conduction abnormalities.

- Embolic

—Embolic events can occur to multiple organ systems (central nervous system, kidneys, spleen, skin, lungs).

PROGNOSIS

If diagnosed in timely fashion and appropriate therapy is instituted, prognosis is relatively good for bacterial endocarditis. Fungal endocarditis, however, is associated with a higher morbidity and mortality.

Differential Diagnosis

- Other infections (e.g., acute rheumatic fever)
- Malignancy
- Connective tissue disorders

Data Gathering

HISTORY

Fever, malaise, anorexia, weight loss, heart failure symptoms, arthralgia, neurologic symptoms, gastrointestinal symptoms, chest pain. Occasionally, a recent infection, dental visit or surgical procedure can be identified.

Physical Examination

- General

—Fever (usually low grade with α-hemolytic streptococci and high grade with *S. aureus*), petechiae (occurring in one third of cases)

- Embolic or immunologic phenomena

—Splinter hemorrhages, retinal hemorrhages, Osler nodes (painful), Janeway lesions (painless), splenomegaly (occurring in about half of cases), clubbing, arthralgia, and arthritis

- Cardiac

—New or change in heart murmur, signs of congestive heart failure

- Neurologic

—Neurologic symptoms can be seen on the basis of central nervous system emboli and hemorrhage, and can sometimes mimic the picture of an abscess, aseptic meningitis, or cerebral infarct.

Laboratory Aids

TESTS

Blood Cultures

- Blood culture is the most important diagnostic test for endocarditis.
- Blood cultures are positive in 85% to 90% of the reported cases of endocarditis
- Three to five sets of blood cultures should be obtained from different sites during the first 24 hours of suspected endocarditis.
- As large a volume as clinically reasonable should be collected.
- The bacteremia of endocarditis is continuous; therefore, it is not necessary to wait to obtain the blood cultures during a fever spike.

Nonspecific Laboratory Data

Elevated ESR (80%), anemia (44%), positive rheumatoid factor (38%), hematuria (35%), leukocytosis, and decreased complement.

Electrocardiogram

- New-onset ECG abnormalities such as AV block (even first degree) may represent conduction system and myocardial involvement from invasive disease.

Echocardiography

- Transthoracic echocardiography is a valuable noninvasive technique in the identification of vegetations.
- The sensitivity and specificity of transthoracic echocardiography, however, is not 100%; therefore, a negative echocardiogram does not rule out endocarditis.
- Transesophageal echocardiography, especially in older or obese patients, provides better visualization of smaller vegetations that may not be readily seen using transthoracic imaging.
- In patients with an inconclusive transthoracic study but a high index of suspicion for endocarditis, transesophageal echocardiography is recommended.

PITFALLS

- The absence of vegetation(s) by echocardiography does not rule out endocarditis.
- In patients with a prosthetic valve, echocardiography is not always helpful, as there is frequently artifact from the prosthetic valve. Abnormal movements of the valve leaflets may suggest a vegetation.
- The ESR may remain elevated for some time, even after cessation of bacteremia.

 ## Therapy

- General

—Rest; antipyretics; optimal nutrition and hydration; careful dental hygiene

- Antibiotics

—Prolonged therapy (at least 4 weeks) with intravenous antibiotics is needed. The choice of antibiotic(s) and the duration of antibiotic treatment depend on the infecting organism and its sensitivity pattern. For fungal SBE, intravenous therapy is given for a minimum of 6 to 8 weeks.

- Surgery: potential indications for surgical therapy (mostly adult data)

—Severe/worsening congestive heart failure with/without embolization or persistent infection
—Aortic valve disease with unstable hemodynamics
—Failing medical therapy
—Large, mobile vegetations
—Fungal endocarditis

 ## Follow-Up

Repeat blood cultures should be obtained after a few days of antibiotic or antifungal therapy to ensure the eradication of bacteria. After completion of a full course of antibiotics, blood cultures should be again obtained in the first 2 months after discontinuation of therapy.

PREVENTION

- Dental hygiene
- Minimal use of central lines
- Correction of the cardiovascular anomaly by surgery or interventional catheterization techniques
- SBE Prophylaxis

SBE PROPHYLAXIS (AHA RECOMMENDATIONS, 1997)

For Dental, Oral, Respiratory Tract, or Esophageal Procedures

- Amoxicillin (50 mg/kg orally 1 hour before procedure; maximum, 2.0 g). If unable to take oral medications, ampicillin (same dose) may be given 30 minutes before the procedure.
- Clindamycin (20 mg/kg orally 1 hour before procedure or same dose IV within 30 minutes of the procedure; maximum, 600 mg) may be used if the patient is allergic to penicillin.

For Genitourinary/Gastrointestinal (Excluding Esophageal) Procedures

- High-risk patients: ampicillin (50 mg/kg; maximum, 2.0 g IM/IV) plus gentamicin 1.5 mg/kg (maximum, 120 mg) within 30 minutes of starting procedure; 6 hours later, 25 mg/kg/IV ampicillin (maximum, 1 g) or amoxicillin 25 mg/kg/PO (maximum, 1 g). Vancomycin plus gentamicin may be used for patients allergic to amoxicillin/ampicillin.
- Moderate-risk patients: amoxicillin (50 mg/kg/PO; maximum, 2.0 g) 1 hour prior to the procedure, or ampicillin 50 mg/kg IM/IV (maximum, 2.0 g) within 30 minutes of starting the procedure. Vancomycin may be used for patients allergic to amoxicillin/ampicillin.

Cardiac Conditions that Require SBE Prophylaxis

- High-risk group: prosthetic valves, previous SBE, cyanotic heart disease, surgically constructed shunts or conduits
- Moderate-risk group: most other congenital heart disease, acquired valvar disease (e.g., rheumatic valvar disease), hypertrophic cardiomyopathy, mitral valve prolapse with regurgitation or thickened leaflets

Cardiac Lesions that Do Not Require SBE Prophylaxis

- Isolated secundum atrial septal defect
- Surgically repaired patent ductus arteriosus
- Ventricular septal defect and atrial septal defect beyond 6 months (without residual)
- Previous coronary artery bypass surgery
- Mitral valve prolapse without regurgitation
- Previous Kawasaki syndrome without valvar dysfunction
- Rheumatic fever without valvar dysfunction
- Pacemakers and defibrillators

Procedures that Require SBE Prophylaxis

- Tonsillectomy, adenoidectomy, surgery of respiratory mucosa, rigid bronchoscopy
- Sclerotherapy for esophageal varices, esophageal dilation, biliary tract and intestinal surgery, endoscopic retrograde cholangiography
- Prostatic surgery, cytoscopy, urethral dilation

- Dental extractions, periodontal procedures, dental implant, endodontic procedures, dental cleaning, intraligamentary injections, initial placements of orthodontic bands, subgingival placement of antibiotic fibers/strips

Procedures that Do Not Require SBE Prophylaxis

These may be recommended in high-risk patients.

- Endotracheal intubation, flexible bronchoscopy, ear tubes, transesophageal echocardiography, GI endoscopy
- Vaginal hysterectomy, vaginal delivery, cesarean section, urethral catheterization, uterine dilation and curettage, abortion, sterilization, intrauterine devices
- Cardiac catheterization
- Circumcision
- Shedding of primary teeth

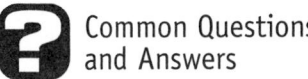 ## Common Questions and Answers

Q: I forgot to give my child antibiotics prior to the procedure. Should I give him a dose afterward?
A: In regard to preventing endocarditis, no data exist on the benefit of administering antibiotics after a procedure.

Q: My child has an innocent heart murmur. Does he need SBE prophylaxis?
A: SBE prophylaxis is not indicated.

Q: My child needs SBE prophylaxis in the appropriate setting and she just fell and scraped her knee. Does she need antibiotics to prevent a heart infection?
A: SBE prophylaxis is not indicated.

ICD-9-CM

421.9–Active or subacute
421.0–Bacterial

BIBLIOGRAPHY

Dajani AS, Taubert KA, Wilson W, et al. Prevention of bacterial endocarditis: recommendations by the American Heart Association. *JAMA* 1997;277:1794–1801.

Feigin RD, Cherry JD, eds. *Textbook of pediatric infectious diseases*, 4th ed. Philadelphia: WB Saunders Company, 1998.

Garson A Jr, Bricker JT, Fisher DJ, et al., eds. *The science and practice of pediatric cardiology*, 2nd ed. Baltimore: Williams & Wilkins, 1998.

Steinberger J, Moller JH, Berry JM, et al. Echocardiographic diagnosis of heart disease in apparently healthy adolescents. Pediatrics 2000;105(4pt1):815–8.

Author: Zev Jacobson
Hae-Rhi Lee, 2nd edition

Enuresis

 Database

DEFINITION

Enuresis is involuntary urination after the age of expected bladder control, and is generally reserved for children 5 to 6 years of age or older.

- In the majority, incontinence occurs only at night (nocturnal enuresis or bed-wetting); a smaller group also is incontinent during the day (diurnal enuresis).
- *Primary enuresis:* Continence is never achieved.
- *Secondary enuresis:* Incontinence recurs after a dry period of at least 6 months.

PATHOPHYSIOLOGY

- For primary nocturnal enuresis (PNE), several theories, with different mechanisms, probably playing greater or lesser roles in specific individuals.

—A maturational delay of neurodevelopmental processes, with bladder emptying at lower volume secondary to smaller functional bladder capacity.
—Other studies suggest that decreased secretion of ADH at night causes some patients to produce urine at the same rate night and day, compared with dry peers, who have decreased rates of urine production at night, due to an increase in ADH secretion.
—Abnormalities of sleep have not been proven to play a role.

- Daytime wetting may be related to detrusor muscle instability, reflux of urine into the vagina with back-seepage after voiding, giggle incontinence, and poor toileting habits.
- Underlying medical or surgical causes are much less common in primary than secondary enuresis.

GENETICS

- Seventy percent of children with enuresis have a parent who was enuretic.
- If both parents were enuretic, 77% of children are enuretic.
- If one parent was enuretic, 43% to 47% of children are enuretic.
- If neither parent was enuretic, only 15% of children are enuretic.
- Incidence in monozygotic twins is twice the incidence in dizygotes.

EPIDEMIOLOGY

- Twenty percent of children have primary nocturnal enuresis at age 5 years, 10% at age 7 years, and 5% at age 10 years; primary nocturnal enuresis persists in approximately 1% of adults.
- Daytime wetting occurs in only 1% of 7- to 12-year-olds.

- Nocturnal enuresis is two to three times more common in males; daytime wetting is more common in females.

COMPLICATIONS

Embarrassment, poor self-esteem, and reluctance to participate in overnight activities with peers

PROGNOSIS

- Prognosis is very good, even without treatment.
- The spontaneous cure rate is 15% per year.

 Differential Diagnosis

Several underlying diseases or conditions can present with enuresis:

- Urinary tract infection
- Diabetes mellitus
- Diabetes insipidus
- Sickle cell disease
- Structural genitourinary tract defects, including ectopic ureter, ureteral duplication, neurogenic bladder
- Spinal cord pathology
- Constipation
- Excessive caffeine, methylxanthines, or other medications
- Any condition causing polyuria can present as enuresis.

 Data Gathering

HISTORY

- Onset (primary versus secondary)
- When it occurs—nighttime, daytime, or both—and how often
- Toileting habits, frequency of voiding and stooling
- Pattern of urination: dribbling, dysuria, hesitancy, urgency (suggest structural defects, dysfunctional voiding, UTI)
- Associated signs and symptoms: stool incontinence, polydipsia, polyuria
- History of other medical problems, including UTIs
- Behavioral/developmental history: age milestones obtained, toilet training methods, behavioral problems
- Medications (especially caffeine or medications with diuretic effects)
- Typical fluid intake (looking for excessive intake in evening)
- Recent environmental stressors (if secondary enuresis)
- Effect of enuresis on child: Does child sleep over with friends or at camp? Is child teased at school?
- Parents' attitude toward the problem

- Family history of enuresis? If positive, is the child aware of it?
- Family history of other diagnoses in differential
- Treatments (or punishments) attempted

 Physical Examination

- Vital signs and growth parameters
- Abdominal examination to rule out masses, renal enlargement, palpable bladder, constipation
- Genitalia: irritation, adhesions, rash, or other signs of constant dampness; balanitis; stenosis; foreign bodies; trauma
- Observe voiding for character of stream, dribbling
- Rectal: perianal sensation, anal sphincter tone, impaction
- Palpate spine for bony defects and cutaneous signs of underlying spinal defects.
- Neurologic: deep tendon reflexes, gait, strength and tone of lower extremities

 Laboratory Aids

TESTS

- Urine for specific gravity, urinalysis (especially glucose), microscopic examination and culture to exclude UTI, diabetes mellitus, and diabetes insipidus. In the majority of cases, this is the only investigation needed.
- If there is a history of UTIs, voiding abnormalities, or voiding symptoms, a voiding cystourethrogram and renal ultrasound should be performed to rule out anatomic defects. The plain scout film can also show constipation or vertebral bony anomalies.
- If findings are suggestive of neurologic dysfunction, urodynamic studies should be performed.

Therapy

- Treat any underlying condition.
- Education, reassurance, and support
- Avoid punishment.
- Encourage positive reinforcement: praise, star charts, and so on.
- Avoid aggressive therapy in those less than 7 years old.
- Fluid restriction in the evenings is unproven but logically appealing.
- Retention training/bladder stretching exercises are controversial.
- Alarm systems: most effective and most cost-effective of all interventions; require several weeks to months to achieve complete dryness
- Desmopressin (DDAVP): remains controversial but is used in PNE when other therapies fail, if use can be monitored appropriately

—Response is generally quick, but enuresis recurs in most subjects after the medication is stopped.
—Concerns remain regarding potential for hyponatremia and volume overload.
—Not recommended in children younger than 9 years of age
—Expensive

- Imipramine: useful but potentially lethal if used inappropriately

—Prescribe only nonlethal quantities to prevent accidental ingestions.

- Oxybutynin: may be useful in the small population of patients with documented detrusor instability
- Night waking exercises and other behavior modification techniques may also be useful in some patients.

Follow-Up

- Timely and regular phone follow-up to answer questions, assess progress, and offer encouragement
- See the patient in the office in 1 month if medications are begun.

PITFALLS

- Remember the natural course of the symptoms, and balance the use of potentially dangerous medications (if used inappropriately) against the social/emotional impact on the individual.
- Do not overdo laboratory studies: Balance risks and costs with the likelihood of yield. Extensive workup of isolated PNE seldom yields an organic etiology; work up should generally be limited to examination of the urine.

Common Questions and Answers

Q: Isn't DDAVP dangerous? What about hyponatremia and volume overload?
A: While the most common side effects noted with DDAVP have been headaches, abdominal pain, and nasal stuffiness, concern remains regarding the potential for hyponatremia and water intoxication. While studies show a safe side-effect profile, there have been scattered reports of serious side effects. Use of DDAVP needs to be monitored carefully, especially since the significance of variations in ADH levels is unclear in the pathophysiology of PNE.

Q: Won't enuresis recur when DDAVP is stopped?
A: While a significant number of children respond to some degree at the initiation of treatment, results of long-term response to prolonged medication use have varied from study to study. In most instances, long-term cure rates have been only slightly better than spontaneous cure rates.

ICD-9-CM 788.30

BIBLIOGRAPHY

Friman PC. A preventive context for enuresis. *Pediatr Clin North Am* 1986;33:871–886.

Ilyas M, Jerkins GR. Management of nocturnal childhood enuresis in managed care: a new challenge. *Pediatr Ann* 1996;25:258–264.

Moffatt ME, Harlos S, Kirshen AJ, et al. Desmopressin acetate and nocturnal enuresis: how much do we know? *Pediatrics* 1993;92:420–425.

Novello AC, Novello JR. Enuresis. *Pediatr Clin North Am* 1987;34:719–731.

Rappaport L. The treatment of nocturnal enuresis-where are we now? *Pediatrics* 1993;92:465–466.

Redsell SA, Collier J. Bedwetting, behaviour and self-esteem: a review of the literature. *Child Care Health Dev* 2001;27(2):149–162.

Robson WLM. Diurnal enuresis. *Pediatr Rev* 1997;18:407–412.

Rushton HG. Evaluation of the enuretic child. *Clin Pediatr* 1993;Special Issue:14–18.

Schmitt BD. Nocturnal enuresis. *Pediatr Rev* 1997;18:183–190.

Schulman SL, Quinn CK, Plachter N, et al. Comprehensive management of dysfunctional voiding. *Pediatrics* 1999;103(3):E31.

Wan J, Greenfield S. Enuresis and common voiding abnormalities. *Pediatr Clin North Am* 1997;44:1117–1131.

Author: Suzette Surratt Caudle

Epiglottitis

 Database

DEFINITION

Epiglottitis is an acute, life-threatening bacterial infection consisting of cellulitis and edema of the epiglottis, aryepiglottic folds, arytenoids and hypopharynx, resulting in narrowing of the glottic opening.

PATHOPHYSIOLOGY

• Etiologic agents include: *Haemophilus influenzae* type B (accounted for >90% of cases prior to the introduction of HiB vaccine), *Staphylococcus aureus, Streptococcus pneumoniae, Streptococcus pyogenes* (group A β-hemolytic streptococcus), and group C β-hemolytic streptococcus (rare). *Candida albicans* may be an etiologic agent in immunocompromised patients. *Pasteurella multocida* has been implicated in a few cases after exposure to nasopharyngeal secretions from a cat. There have been recent reports of epiglottitis due to *Neisseria meningitidis*.
• The inhaled anesthetic, sevoflurane, has been implicated in a few cases of epiglottitis.
• Erythema and edema of the uvula, aryepiglottic folds, arytenoids, epiglottis, and vocal cords include an exudate rich in neutrophils and fibrin, which usually proceed to organization and fibrous scarring.

EPIDEMIOLOGY

• Disease due to *H. influenzae* type B occurs most often between the ages of 2 and 7 years (overall range: infancy to adulthood).
• Epiglottis and other invasive disease (including epiglottitis) secondary to *H. influenzae* have been reduced by 98% since the introduction of the conjugate vaccines in 1989 (approved at 15 months) and 1990 (approved at 2, 4, and 6 months).
• Incidence of epiglottitis due to any organism reduced substantially (e.g., 20.9/100,000/year to 0.9/100,000/year from 1987 to 1996 in Sweden)
• Year-round occurrence
• Affects boys and girls equally
• All geographic areas
• Rare in populations in which the peak incidence of meningitis is shifted toward infancy (e.g., Alaskan Eskimos, Native Americans)
• Occasional secondary cases in households or day-care centers
• May be more frequent in children with sickle cell anemia, asplenia, immunoglobulin defects, or leukemia
• Disease due to *S. pyogenes* occurs most often in early school-age children during the winter and early spring, and has now been seen as a complication of varicella infection.

COMPLICATIONS

• Without prompt medical intervention, complete airway obstruction leading to respiratory arrest, hypoxia, and death
• Necrotizing cervical fasciitis (rarely)
• Therapeutic complications include: aspiration, endotracheal tube dislodgment and extubation, tracheal erosion or irritation, pneumomediastinum, pneumothorax, and pulmonary edema.
• Complications of *H. influenzae* type B bacteremia include: septic shock, pneumonia, cervical lymphadenopathy, and, rarely, arthritis and pericarditis.

PROGNOSIS

• Mortality is estimated at 8% in hospital series.
• Virtually all cases in which arrest occurred prior to transfer to tertiary center resulted in fatality.
• Mortality should approach zero with appropriate airway management.

 Differential Diagnosis

• Viral laryngotracheobronchitis (croup) with or without secondary bacterial tracheitis
• Severe parainfluenza or influenza infection
• Uvulitis
• Peritonsillar, retropharyngeal, or lingual abscess
• Foreign-body aspiration in a child with an upper respiratory infection
• Upper respiratory infection, including croup, in a child with a congenital or acquired airway problem (e.g., premature infant with subglottic stenosis, laryngeal web, vascular ring, tracheal stenosis)
• Diphtheria: rare in United States
• Laryngeal infections, including laryngeal tuberculosis

 Data Gathering

HISTORY

• Abrupt onset of high fever (39°C–40°C), sore throat, and dysphagia
• Very limited or no prodrome of mild upper respiratory illness
• Rapid onset of toxicity and respiratory distress
• Cough and hoarseness are late symptoms, if they occur at all.
• Time from onset of symptoms to presentation with progressive respiratory distress is generally less than 12 hours.
• Has the child been immunized against *H. influenzae* type B?
• How does the child prefer to hold him- or herself (e.g., sitting upright, leaning forward with chin hyperextended)?
• Exposure to cats

 Physical Examination

• Extremely anxious appearance
• Child prefers to remain sitting up.
• Child often leaning forward with chin hyperextended to maintain airway
• Slow and labored respiratory effort
• Drooling is seen as a manifestation of dysphagia.
• Inspiratory stridor, retractions, and late cyanosis
• Diagnosis can be suspected on history and observation of child's appearance alone.
• Do *not* attempt to examine the throat if epiglottitis is a serious consideration.

 Laboratory Aids

TESTS

• CBC: increased white blood cell count with left shift
• Cultures of blood (positive in up to 90%) and epiglottis (only performed in the operating room): may be positive for the causative organism.

IMAGING

• Lateral neck radiograph: showing characteristic "thumb sign" of edematous epiglottis, with narrowing of the posterior airway and ballooning of the hypopharynx (should not be performed until "airway team" is in place)

Therapy

- Airway management: maintain child upright, *never supine*. Personnel experienced in airway management should accompany the child at all times, including during transport and in radiology.
- Rapid assembly of a team, which should include an anesthesiologist, an otolaryngologist, and a pediatrician, if possible.
- Allow the child to assume his or her most comfortable position (usually in the mother's arms).
- Oxygen by mask or blown by face
- Transport to operating room as soon as possible for anesthesia and intubation, followed by positive pressure ventilation as necessary.
- Institute intravenous catheterization and blood collection and culturing of epiglottis only after the airway is secured.
- Perform emergent cricothyrotomy if obstruction occurs prior to controlled airway management.
- Use fluid resuscitation in cases of septic shock.

DRUGS

- Empiric antibiotic coverage to include gram-positive cocci and β-lactamase-producing *H. influenzae* type B. Duration of therapy: 7 to 10 days for all but staphylococcal disease (14–21 days). Switch may be made to oral medication after extubation and resumption of feeding.
- Cefuroxime: 150 mg/kg/d divided every 8 hours
- Ampicillin/sulbactam: 200 mg/kg/d divided every 6 hours
- Chloramphenicol: 75 to 100 mg/kg/d divided every 6 hours
- Ampicillin: 100 to 200 mg/kg/d divided every 6 hours for non-β-lactamase-producing *H. influenzae* type B (approximately 80% of isolates)
- Penicillin: 100,000 to 200,000 U/kg/d divided every 4 to 6 hours for streptococcal disease
- Oxacillin: 100 to 200 mg/kg/d for staphylococcal disease

Follow-Up

- Extubation is usually possible within 24 to 48 hours. Criteria include: decreased epiglottis erythema and edema upon direct inspection, and development of an air leak around the endotracheal tube.
- Defervescence is usually prompt after initiation of appropriate antimicrobial therapy.

PREVENTION

- Rifampin: 20 mg/kg/d in single dose for 4 days to eradicate colonization
- Universal immunization with *H. influenzae* type B capsular polysaccharide conjugate vaccines at 2, 4, and 6 months, with booster at 12 to 18 months

ISOLATION OF HOSPITALIZED PATIENT

Droplet precautions should be continued for at least 24 hours from the initiation of effective therapy.

CONTROL MEASURES

- Prophylaxis for index case and susceptible children in household, child care setting, and intimate contacts

PITFALLS

- A radiograph is indicated only when the diagnosis is in doubt, and should not delay airway management.
- Blood collection should be avoided until the airway has been secured, so as not to upset the child unnecessarily.
- Failure to ensure appropriate airway management prior to any other interventions, including laryngeal examination, radiographs, and laboratory studies

Common Questions and Answers

Q: What is the incidence of epiglottitis since the introduction of conjugate vaccines against *H. influenzae* type B?
A: Because *H. influenzae* type B caused 90% of epiglottitis, and the incidence of all invasive disease due to *H. influenzae* type B has decreased by 98% in children under 5 years of age, one can estimate that the incidence of epiglottitis has been reduced by almost 90%.

Q: Have there been reports of epiglottitis caused by *H. influenzae* type B after complete vaccination?
A: Yes, several cases due to *H. influenzae* type B have been reported both here in the United States and abroad after partial and complete vaccination. Therefore, even a history of having received a full vaccination series does not eliminate the possibility of HiB causing epiglottitis.

Q: How many of the cases of invasive disease due to *H. influenzae* type B occur in children with inadequate vaccination?
A: During 1994 and 1995, 47% of children under 4 years of age were too young (aged 5 months or younger) to have completed a primary series with an HiB-containing vaccine. Among children old enough to be fully vaccinated, 63% of those developing disease were undervaccinated, and the

remainder (37%) had completed a primary series in which vaccine failed. In two more recent reports none of the cases reported in undervaccinated children were due to HiB. In a recent report from Australia 34/412 (8%) cases of invasive HiB disease (including epiglottitis) were reported as vaccine failures. Therefore, HiB cannot be ruled out as a cause of epiglottitis in a fully vaccinated child although the overwhelming majority of cases occur in unvaccinated children.

Q: Should a fully vaccinated child who develops invasive disease due to *H. influenzae* type B be tested for an underlying immunodeficiency?
A: Probably. In one study, about one third of children diagnosed with invasive disease due to *H. influenzae* type B were found to have a previously undiagnosed immunoglobulin deficiency.

Q: Can epiglottitis recur?
A: Yes, but rarely.

Q: Are corticosteroids of any value in the management of epiglottitis?
A: There appears to be no benefit.

ICD-9-CM 464.30

BIBLIOGRAPHY

American Academy of Pediatrics. *Haemophilus influenzae* infections. In: Pickering LK, ed. *Red book 2000: report of the Committee on Infectious Diseases*, 25th ed. Elk Grove, IL: American Academy of Pediatrics, 2000:220–230.

Garpenholt O, Hugosson S, Fredlund H, et al. Epiglottitis in Sweden before and after introduction of vaccination against *Haemophilus influenzae* type B. *Pediatr Infect Dis J* 1999;18:490–493.

Gonzalez-Valdepena H, Wald ER, Rose E, et al. Epiglottitis and *Haemophilus influenzae* immunization : the Pittsburgh experience—a 5-year review. *Pediatrics* 1995;96:424–427.

Herceg A. The decline of *Haemophilus influenzae* type b disease in Australia. *Communicable Dis Intell* 1997;21:173–6.

Hickerson SL, Kirby RS, Wheeler JG, et al. Epiglotittis: a 9-year case review. *South Med J* 1996;89:487–490.

Liptak GS, McConnochie KM, Roghmann KJ, et al. Decline of pediatric admissions with *Haemophilus influenzae* type b in New York State, 1982 through 1993: relation to immunizations. *J Pediatr* 1997;130:923–930.

Midwinter KI, Hodgson D, Yardley M. Paediatric epiglottitis: the influence of the *Haemophilus influenzae* B vaccine, a ten-year review in the Sheffield region. *Clin Otolaryngol Allied Sci* 1999;24:447–448.

Author: Mark L. Bagarazzi

Epstein-Barr Virus (Infectious Mononucleosis)

 Database

DEFINITION

Epstein-Barr virus (EBV) is a double-stranded DNA virus, and was implicated as the causative agent for infectious mononucleosis by 1968.

PATHOPHYSIOLOGY

- EBV replicates initially in the oropharyngeal epithelium.
- Selective infection of B lymphocytes occurs.
- The clinical syndrome of infectious mononucleosis results from proliferation of cells in the tonsils, lymph nodes, and spleen.
- Nonspecific humoral immune responses include the formation of heterophil antibodies and autoantibodies.
- Specific antibodies to EBV antigens are produced.
- Despite humoral responses, cellular immunity is responsible for controlling EBV infection.
- Latent, lifelong infection of B lymphocytes occurs.
- Latent virus can be reactivated during periods of immunosuppression.

EPIDEMIOLOGY

- Worldwide distribution
- Humans are the only known reservoir.
- EBV spreads between individuals in saliva, and occasionally via blood transfusions.
- The incubation period is 30 to 50 days.
- Antibodies to EBV are almost universally present in adult populations.
- Populations with a high population density or low socioeconomic status usually become primarily affected within the first 3 years of life.
- In developed countries, acquisition of EBV is biphasic:

—The initial peak in incidence occurs before the age of 5 years.
—The second peak occurs during adolescence, coinciding with an increased frequency of intimate oral contacts.

COMPLICATIONS

- Dehydration

—Severe pharyngitis often limits fluid intake.
—Is the most common problem requiring hospitalization

- Streptococcal pharyngitis

—Between 5% and 25% of patients with acute EBV infection may have concomitant group A streptococcal pharyngitis.

- Antibiotic-induced rash

—Morbilliform in appearance
—Most common after administration of ampicillin or amoxicillin

—Rare association with penicillin
—Usually benign, resolves with discontinuation of the aminopenicillin

- Splenic rupture

—Incidence of approximately 1 in 1,000 patients
—More common in males
—Half of the cases of splenic rupture are spontaneous; half follow blunt trauma.

- Airway obstruction

—May result from massive lymphoid hyperplasia and mucosal edema

PROGNOSIS

- Most patients with primary EBV infection will recover uneventfully in 1 to 4 weeks.
- Long-lasting immunity generally ensues.
- Prognosis of patients with unusual manifestations of EBV infection depends on the severity of the illness and the organ system involved.
- Patients with inherited or acquired immunodeficiency are at higher risk of complications and neoplasms.

ASSOCIATED ILLNESSES

- Subclinical infection

—The majority of EBV infections in children, and even in adolescents, are clinically inapparent.
—Mild, nonspecific symptoms may include coryza, diarrhea, and/or fever.
—Immunologic seroconversion does occur.

- Infectious mononucleosis ("glandular fever")

—Most commonly observed with late primary acquisition of EBV
—The classically defined illness is characterized by:
    —Fatigue
    —Malaise
    —Fever
    —Tonsillopharyngitis (often exudative)
    —Lymphadenopathy
    —Splenomegaly

—Usually associated with increased numbers of atypical lymphocytes in the peripheral blood

- Rare illnesses of the nervous system have been reported:

—Guillain-Barré syndrome
—Bell palsy
—Aseptic meningitis
—Meningoencephalitis
—Peripheral and/or optic neuritis

- Hematologic disorders have been reported in rare association with EBV:

—Aplastic anemia
—Hemolytic anemia
—Hemolytic-uremic syndrome

- Other illnesses associated with EBV in case reports:

—Hepatitis
—Pancreatitis
—Myocarditis
—Mesenteric adenitis
—Orchitis
—Genital ulcerative disease

- Congenital infection

—Primary EBV infection during pregnancy is uncommon.
—Although rare, TORCH-like congenital defects may conceivably be linked to EBV.

- Lymphoproliferative disorders

—EBV is suspected of occasionally playing a role in the etiology of the lymphoproliferative disorders:
—Burkitt lymphoma
—Nasopharyngeal carcinoma
—Lymphoma and non-Hodgkin lymphoma (in immunocompromised children)
—Virus-associated hemophagocytic syndrome
—Lymphomatoid granulomatosis

- Chronic fatigue syndrome

—EBV, as well as many other infectious and environmental agents, have been proposed to contribute to this vague clinical syndrome.

 Differential Diagnosis

- Infectious mononucleosis is an illness with characteristic clinical features caused by EBV. Other causes of the infectious mononucleosis syndrome include:

—Adenovirus
—Cytomegalovirus
—*Toxoplasma gondii*
—Human herpes virus-6
—Human immunodeficiency virus
—Rubella

 Data Gathering

HISTORY

- A prodrome may occur:

—Commonly lasts 2 to 5 days
—Malaise, fatigue, ± fever

- The following features are common:

—Fatigue
—Malaise
—Anorexia
—Fever
—Sore throat
—"Swollen glands"

- Young children are more likely to have a rash or abdominal pain.

Epstein-Barr Virus (Infectious Mononucleosis)

 Physical Examination

- Tonsillopharyngitis

—May be exudative and mimic streptococcal pharyngitis
—Often accompanied by palatal petechiae

- Lymphadenopathy

—Most prominent in cervical chains
—May be diffuse
—Usually nontender

- Hepatosplenomegaly

—Splenomegaly occurs in over half of cases.
—Even if not palpable, splenomegaly may be demonstrated on ultrasound.
—Most prominent in second to fourth week of illness
—Hepatomegaly is less common

 Laboratory Aids

TESTS

- CBC with differential

—Leukocyte count up to 20,000/mm^3
—Lymphocytosis
—Atypical lymphocytes often comprise more than 10% of total leukocyte count.
—Thrombocytopenia may occur.

- Liver enzymes

—Mild hepatitis often is found.
—Jaundice is rare.

- "Monospot" (mononucleosis rapid slide agglutination test for heterophil antibodies)

—Detects heterophil antibodies (nonspecific IgM antibodies to unrelated antigens)
—Often negative in children under 6 years of age
—Detects 90% of cases in adolescents and adults

- EBV serology

—Usually reserved for heterophil-negative patients where strong clinical suspicion persists
—Antibodies detected by indirect immunofluorescence or ELISA techniques
—Acute or past infection can usually be detected and differentiated.

- Other technology

—Tissue culture of EBV is difficult and therefore not clinically useful.
—Polymerase chain reaction may detect EBV genetic material.

False Positives

- CBC

—Atypical lymphocyte counts greater than 10% of the total leukocyte count also occur with cytomegalovirus and toxoplasmosis infections.

- Monospot

—False-positive tests are infrequent.
—Heterophil antibodies are also produced in serum sickness and neoplastic processes.
—Heterophil antibodies may persist for months after acute infection and be indicative of past illness.

PITFALLS

- Heterophil antibodies may not appear early in the illness.
- Up to 10% of patients with acute EBV infection may have no heterophil response 3 weeks into the illness.
- The heterophil response is less common in infants and children.

 Therapy

- Supportive care and symptomatic treatment will be sufficient for most cases of primary EBV infection.
- Acetaminophen or ibuprofen will reduce fever and provide analgesia.
- Oral, and sometimes IV, rehydration is often indicated.
- Corticosteroids (prednisone, 1 mg/kg/d divided into two doses) may reduce swelling of lymphoid tissues (see Common Questions and Answers, below)

—Indicated for patients with impending airway obstruction
—May be considered for patients with severe tonsillopharyngitis requiring IV hydration
—May be considered for patients with rare, life-threatening manifestations of EBV infection, such as hepatitis, aplastic anemia, and CNS dysfunction

- Acyclovir has not been shown to provide clinical benefit.

PREVENTION

- No vaccine is clinically available.
- Hospitalized patients need not be isolated when rigorous hand washing is employed.
- Restriction of intimate contact with immunosuppressed individuals may be advisable.
- Patients with recent EBV infection, either proven or suspected, should not donate blood.

 Follow-Up

- Immunocompetent individuals usually recover uneventfully in 1 to 4 weeks.
- Recovery is often biphasic, with a worsening of symptoms after a period of improvement.
- Splenomegaly may persist for weeks after primary infection (see Common Questions and Answers, below).
- Fatigue may persist months after recovery.

 Common Questions and Answers

Q: Should all patients with infectious mononucleosis be given corticosteroids?
A: Even though children may feel tired, weak, and ill, symptomatic EBV infection is most often self-limited with only symptomatic care. Long-term effects from the use of steroids to treat EBV are not known. EBV has been linked to certain lymphoproliferative disorders, and theoretical risks to modulating the host immune response with corticosteroids have been proposed.

Q: How long after infectious mononucleosis may a patient return to athletic activity?
A: Over half of patients with "mono" will have a boggy, enlarged spleen. This enlarged spleen is prone to rupture even if it is not palpable. All athletic activity should be restricted until no evidence exists for a clinically enlarged or tender spleen. If this criterion is met, and the patient feels subjectively better, light (noncontact) activities may be resumed. Return to contact sports is not advised until at least 4 to 6 weeks after resolution of all signs and symptoms of illness. Some experts recommend ultrasound study of the spleen before a return to heavy contact sports such as rugby, football, lacrosse, and hockey.

ICD-9-CM 075

BIBLIOGRAPHY

Durbin WA, Sullivan JL. Epstein-Barr virus infection. *Pediatr Rev* 1994;15:63–68.

Hickey SM, Strasburger VC. What every pediatrician should know about infectious mononucleosis and adolescents. *Pediatr Clin North Am* 1997;44:1541–1556.

Jenson HB. Acute complications of Epstein-Barr virus infectious mononucleosis. *Curr Opin Pediatr* 2000;12:263–268.

Peter J, Ray CG. Infectious mononucleosis. *Pediatr Rev* 1998;19:276–279.

Author: Kevin C. Osterhoudt

Erythema Multiforme

 Database

DEFINITION

Erythema multiforme (EM) is an acute self-limited cutaneous eruption with many different or multiform lesions. It is characterized classically as a target or iris lesion, but can appear as erythematous macules, papules, vesicles, and bullae with mucosal involvement. There are many triggers of EM, which is thought to encompass a spectrum of disease from relatively mild disease (EM minor) to severe forms with more than one mucosal surface involved (EM major or Stevens-Johnson syndrome). Some authors include toxic epidermal necrolysis (TEN) as the most severe form of EM, characterized by widespread erythema, bullae, and sloughing of large sheets of skin, with significant morbidity and mortality. However, some debate exists as to whether classical EM minor may represent an entity altogether separate from Stevens-Johnson and toxic epidermal necrolysis.

CAUSES

- The major causes of EM, which is thought to be an immune-mediated reaction, include drugs such as sulfa, penicillin, and phenytoin, and infections such as herpes simplex virus and *Mycoplasma*.
- There are a host of other etiologic factors, including exposure to various chemicals and tumors. The eruption usually occurs 1 to 2 weeks after the initial exposure.
- Often the causative factor is not identified.
- Recurrent EM is generally secondary to herpes simplex virus.

GENETICS

Although simultaneous cases in family members have been reported, the disease is not genetic.

PATHOLOGY

The pathologic findings vary according to the lesion examined. Biopsy reveals necrosis of keratinocytes to varying degrees, depending on the clinical lesion biopsied. There is moderate-to-severe papillary dermal edema with mild-to-moderate perivascular dermal infiltrate composed predominantly of mononuclear cells and also some eosinophils (particularly if drug-related). Subepidermal blistering may be seen. Extravasated blood cells are found, but there is no evidence of vasculitis. Hydropic degeneration of the basement membrane also can be seen, as can epidermal spongiosis.

EPIDEMIOLOGY

- Erythema multiforme is seen in approximately 1% of all dermatology patients and has an equal incidence in men and women. (Some studies suggest a slightly higher incidence of EM minor in women.)
- The disease occurs predominantly in young adults and is believed by some to occur more frequently in spring and summer, with the more severe form of EM major occurring in the winter.

COMPLICATIONS

- Erythema multiforme minor is generally self-limited, with rare complications.
- In EM major, mucosal involvement can lead to stricture formation of the urethra, trachea, and esophagus, as well as conjunctivitis, corneal erosions, and, rarely, blindness.
- Pneumonitis, nephritis, hepatitis, and infection are other reported complications.
- In TEN, mortality and morbidity are high, with death occurring from sepsis.

 Differential Diagnosis

Classic presentation with targetoid lesions and mucosal involvement is generally not a diagnostic challenge; however, given the many forms of presentation, the diagnosis of EM can be difficult. The differential diagnosis can be extensive, depending on the presentation, and includes:

- Viral exanthem
- Bullous impetigo
- Staphylococcal scalded-skin syndrome
- Bullous pemphigoid
- Urticaria
- Urticarial vasculitis
- Systemic lupus erythematosus
- Serum sickness
- Pemphigus vulgaris
- Secondary syphilis
- Chickenpox
- Rocky mountain spotted fever
- Acute neutrophilic dermatosis
- Lyme disease
- Fixed drug eruption

 Data Gathering

HISTORY

The cutaneous findings are sometimes preceded by a prodrome with fever and malaise. A careful drug and exposure history, as well as any signs or symptoms of infection or herpetic lesions, may reveal the etiologic cause. Inquire in detail about the patient's drug history, over-the-counter preparations, and signs or symptoms of infection or herpetic lesions.

Physical Examination

- Erythema multiforme classically appears as target lesions characterized by a dark, dusky center surrounded by a pale zone and then a zone of erythema. The lesions are typically acrally distributed.
- The lesions occur in many forms and can appear as red macules, papules, urticarial lesions, or vesicles and bullae.
- Oral involvement is typically seen. Mucosal involvement with superficial denudation can also occur in the eyes, nasopharyngeal mucosal, or anogenital region.

 ## Laboratory Aids

TESTS

- There are no diagnostic laboratory tests; however, biopsy is often helpful, and other tests may help identify a cause.
- A WBC count with differential, looking for eosinophilia, may help identify a drug as causative.
- Cultures to evaluate for herpes or chest x-ray studies to evaluate for pneumonia or infectious cause of EM
- Cold agglutinins associated with *Mycoplasma*
- Antistreptolysin-O titers and leukocytosis may identify a particular infectious cause.
- ESR may be elevated, but is nonspecific.

 ## Therapy

MILD FORMS

- Mild forms of EM resolve spontaneously without scarring and require only supportive therapy, including antihistamine or topical steroid for pruritus associated with the lesions.
- Oral lesions are often painful, and oral preparations to swish and spit, made of diphenhydramine or viscous lidocaine, may provide relief.
- Treatment of the underlying process is helpful (e.g., acyclovir for herpes simplex virus–associated cases).

ERYTHEMA MULTIFORME MAJOR

- May be life threatening and can require hospitalization
- Supportive care, ophthalmology consultation, monitoring of fluid and electrolyte balance, and vigilant observation for infection are necessary.
- Antibiotics, analgesics, and local care including compresses with acetic acid soaks or saline will help decrease the incidence of infection.
- The use of systemic steroids is controversial, but when helpful, they are given early in the course of disease for approximately 2 weeks when there is no contraindication, such as infection.

TOXIC EPIDERMAL NECROLYSIS

- High associated mortality is often secondary to infection.
- Care is ideally at a burn center, with careful attention to infection and to fluids and electrolytes.
- Antibiotics, local compresses with acetic acid, or saline can help prevent superinfection.
- The use of systemic steroids is controversial, and is most effective when started early. The benefits and risks, including infection, must be weighed.
- Some recent reports demonstrated that IVIG given over 3 to 5 days provided rapid improvement with little to no adverse effects in adult patients with toxic epidermal necrolysis.

 ## Follow-Up

- Mild forms of EM are acute and self-limited, with lesions resolving in 2 to 4 weeks, with postinflammatory hyperpigmentation or hypopigmentation.
- Sequelae due to mucosal scarring can occur.
- Severe forms of EM major or TEN have associated morbidity and mortality.
- When recurrent, EM is often associated with herpes simplex virus.

ICD-9-CM 695.1

BIBLIOGRAPHY

Bondi EE, Jegasothy BV, Lazarus GS. *Dermatology diagnosis and therapy*. Norwalk, CT: Appleton & Lange, 1991.

Duvic M. Erythema multiforme. *Dermatol Clin* 1983;1(2):493–496.

Huff JC, Weston WL, Tonnessen MG. Erythema multiforme: a critical review of characteristics, diagnostic criteria and causes. *J Am Acad Dermatol* 1983;8(6):763–775.

Lever WF, Schaumberg-Lever G. *Histopathology of the skin*, 7th ed. Philadelphia: Lippincott, 1990.

Weston WL, Badgett JT. Urticaria. *Pediatr Rev* 1998;19(7):240–244.

Author: Albert C. Yan
Christen Mowad, 2nd edition

Erythema Nodosum

 Database

DEFINITION

Erythema nodosum is a delayed, cell-mediated hypersensitivity syndrome characterized by red, tender, nodular lesions that are usually on the pretibial surface of the legs and occasionally on other areas of the skin where subcutaneous fat is present.

CAUSES

- Thought to be a result of a host hypersensitivity immune response to circulating immune complexes secondary to infectious and/or inflammatory stimuli, which then results in chronic injury to the blood vessels of the reticular dermis and subcutaneous fat.
- There are many associated triggering/under lying diseases:

—In children
 —Streptococcal infection and tubercular infection are the most common causes.

—In older patients
 —Streptococcus and sarcoidosis are most common.

—Drugs (oral contraceptives, sulfonamides, iodides/bromides, phenytoin)
—Infection (streptococcal infection, tuberculosis, psittacosis, histoplasmosis, yersiniosis, lymphogranuloma venereum, cat-scratch disease, coccidioidomycosis, upper respiratory infection)

- Systemic (sarcoidosis, inflammatory bowel disease, Hodgkin disease, Behçet disease)
- Pregnancy

PATHOLOGY

- Septal panniculitis: lymphocytic perivascular infiltrate in the dermis; lymphocytes and neutrophils in the fibrous septa in the subcutaneous fat
- In older lesions, histiocytes, giant cells, and occasionally plasma cells are seen.
- No fat-cell destruction or vasculitis is present.

EPIDEMIOLOGY

- Girls are affected more often than boys.
- Most cases seen in the third decade, but not uncommon after age 10
- Greatest seasonal incidence in spring and fall

 Differential Diagnosis

- Infection

—Erysipelas/cellulitis
—Superficial or deep thrombophlebitis
—Erythema induratum (nodular vasculitis)
—Deep fungal infection
—Angiitis

- Environmental (poisons)
- Tumors
- Trauma: accidental trauma or child abuse
- Bruise
- Palmoplantar hidradenitis
- Metabolic

—Panniculitis secondary to pancreatic disease
—Congenital

- Immunologic

—Major insect bite reaction
—Psychosocial

- Sarcoidosis
- Polyarteritis nodosa
- Granuloma annulare
- Miscellaneous
- Weber-Christian (thighs and trunk) lesions may suppurate and heal with atrophy/localized depression.

PROGNOSIS

- Most individual lesions will completely resolve in 10 to 14 days.
- In general, erythema nodosum resolves in 3 to 6 weeks with or without treatment, unless the underlying cause is a chronic infection or systemic disorder.
- Aching of legs and swelling of ankles may persist for weeks; rarely, symptoms may persist for up to 2 years.
- In children, the recurrence rate is 4% to 10% and is often associated with repeated streptococcal infection.

 Data Gathering

HISTORY

- In over 50% of patients, a history of arthralgia is noted 2 to 8 weeks prior.
- Prodromal symptoms of fatigue/malaise or upper respiratory infection precedes by 1 to 3 weeks.
- Patients often present with pain and tenderness of extremities, sometimes to the point of difficulty in ambulation.

 Physical Examination

- Red, often tender, nodules on anterior lower legs, 2 to 6 cm in diameter
- Overlying skin is normal except for erythema.
- Initially, lesions are bright to deep red with palpable warmth.
- Later, lesions develop a brownish red or violaceous, bruise-like appearance.
- Smaller lesions are slope-shouldered nodules.
- Larger lesions are flat-topped plaques.

SPECIAL QUESTIONS

- Medication history (oral contraceptives, sulfonamides, iodides/bromides)?
- Last menses (erythema nodosum is seen in pregnancy)?
- History of diarrhea (inflammatory bowel disease or infectious diarrhea)?
- TB exposure?

PHYSICAL EXAMINATION TRICKS

- Erythema nodosum never ulcerates or suppurates.
- Usually, there are no more than six lesions at a time.
- As a rule, both legs are affected.

Laboratory Aids

TESTS

- Throat culture
- Antistreptolysin-O titer
- PPD
- CBC
- ESR
- Stool culture, if history of diarrhea
- Serologic testing, if yersiniosis, histoplasmosis, or coccidioidomycosis suspected
- Chest x-ray study, if diagnosis is in doubt
- Excisional biopsy specimen for histopathology and bacterial and fungal cultures is helpful.

False Positives

Bilateral hilar adenopathy may also be seen with sarcoidosis, coccidioidomycosis, histoplasmosis, TB, streptococcal infection, or lymphomatosis.

 ## Therapy

- Identification and treatment of underlying cause
- Bed rest and leg elevation

DRUGS

- Salicylates or other NSAIDs, such as ibuprofen, naproxen, or indomethacin
- Potassium iodide, 300 mg PO t.i.d. for 3 to 4 weeks, especially for cases diagnosed early in course
- Corticosteroids are effective, but rarely necessary.
- Duration: 2 to 4 weeks

 ## Follow-Up

WHEN TO EXPECT IMPROVEMENT

- Within 2 to 3 days
- Return visit in 1 week

SIGNS TO WATCH FOR

If lesions recur after cessation of treatment, underlying infection may worsen as well.

 ## Common Questions and Answers

Q: Will the lesions leave a scar?
A: Erythema nodosum virtually always heals without scarring.

ICD-9-CM 695.2

BIBLIOGRAPHY

Hurwitz S. *Clinical pediatric dermatology: a textbook of skin disorders of childhood and adolescence*, 2nd ed. Philadelphia: WB Saunders, 1993.

Author: Albert C. Yan
Carmen M. Parrott, 2nd edition

Ewing Sarcoma

 Database

DEFINITION

Ewing sarcoma is the second most common malignant bone tumor in children and adolescents. It represents a family of tumors, including Ewing sarcoma of bone, extraosseus Ewing sarcoma (arises in soft tissue adjacent to bone), and peripheral neuroectodermal tumor (PNET) of bone or soft tissue. The cause of Ewing sarcoma is unknown.

PATHOLOGY

- One of the "small round blue" cell tumors of childhood
- In approximately 90% of cases, the characteristic translocations t(11;22) and the minority t(21;22) can be detected.
- Often a large soft tissue component is present.
- Necrosis and hemorrhage are common.
- The PNET variant has more neural differentiation.

GENETICS

- Majority of cases occur sporadically
- Not associated with familial cancer syndromes

EPIDEMIOLOGY

- Second most common malignant bone tumor of children and young adults
- Approximately 110 new cases are diagnosed in the United States each year.
- Sixty-four percent occur in the second decade of life.
- More common in males than in females
- Ninety-six percent of cases in Caucasian population; extremely rare in Asians and blacks
- Associations (rare): skeletal anomalies (endochondroma, aneurysmal bone cyst), genitourinary anomalies (hypospadias, duplicated renal collecting system), Down syndrome, hereditary retinoblastoma

COMPLICATIONS

- Pathologic fracture
- Cord compression secondary to vertebral involvement
- Metastatic spread is seen in 20% at diagnosis. Sites include lung, bone, and bone marrow; liver and lymph nodes are less often involved.

PROGNOSIS

- Overall, 50% to 70% of patients will be disease free at 5 years from diagnosis.
- Late metastases may occur so that survival rates decrease to 50% 10 years from diagnosis.
- Favorable prognostic features
  —Localized disease
  —Primary site: distal bone, rib
  —Tumor size less than 100 mL or 8 to 10 cm
  —Age less than 10 years
  —Histologic response to chemotherapy: no viable tumor at time of surgical resection

- Unfavorable prognostic features
  —Metastatic disease at diagnosis, especially involving bone or bone marrow (<30% disease-free survival)
  —Primary site: pelvis
  —Elevated LDH
  —Presence of neural differentiation

 Differential Diagnosis

- Malignant
  —Osteosarcoma
  —Neuroblastoma
  —Non-Hodgkin lymphoma
  —Rhabdomyosarcoma

- Nonmalignant
  —Osteomyelitis
  —Trauma/fracture
  —Langerhans cell histiocytosis (eosinophilic granuloma)
  —Benign bone tumor (giant-cell tumor) or cyst

 Data Gathering

HISTORY

- Presenting symptoms and their frequency of occurrence:
- Local pain (85%)
- Local swelling (60%)
- Fever (30%)
- Paraplegia, back pain (2%)
- Systemic symptoms (fever, weight loss) are more common among patients with metastatic disease
- Delay between first symptom and diagnosis is quite common; the duration of symptoms ranges from 4 weeks to 4 years, with an average of 9 months

 Physical Examination

- Can develop in any bone of the body, with equal involvement of flat and long bones (unlike osteosarcoma, which arises more commonly in long bones)
- Distribution of primary sites include the following:

—Extremities (53%): usually begins in the midshaft; lower extremities affected more than upper extremities
—Central axis (47%): pelvis (45%), chest wall (34%), spine or paravertebral (12%), head or neck (9%)

 Laboratory Aids

TESTS

Laboratory Tests

- CBC
- Electrolytes, liver and renal function tests, serum calcium, phosphorus in anticipation of starting chemotherapy

Imaging and Other Tests

To evaluate primary site and confirm diagnosis:

- X-ray (bony destruction with "onion skinning" appearance most often seen)
- CT scan or, preferably, MRI scan
- 99m-Tc-diphosphonate bone scan
- Serum LDH
- Biopsy: In addition to routine morphologic and immunohistochemical stain assessments, analysis of tumor chromosomes by traditional cytogenetics, fluorescent *in situ* hybridization, or reverse transcriptase PCR is helpful in making the diagnosis and may provide information regarding prognosis. Because of the importance of these studies, consultation with a pediatric oncologist before the biopsy is strongly encouraged.

To evaluate for evidence of distant metastases (present in 20% of patients at diagnosis):

- Chest radiograph and CT scan
- 99m-Tc-diphosphonate bone scan
- Bilateral aspiration and biopsy of iliac bone marrow

Ewing Sarcoma

Therapy

- Therapy is a multimodal approach based on location and extent of disease: surgery; chemotherapy (common agents used include vincristine, doxorubicin, cyclophosphamide, etoposide, and ifosfamide); and radiation therapy.
- All patients with localized disease at diagnosis also have tumor cells outside the primary site that cannot be detected by standard measures; chemotherapy is therefore essential for cure.
- Duration of therapy depends on location and extent of disease.
- The surgical trend is toward less radical surgery, with limb preservation.
- Most children are treated according to large cooperative group protocols at pediatric oncology centers.
- Treatment is characterized by significant side effects, including increased susceptibility to infection, severe mucositis, and poor nutritional status.
- Most patients require placement of an indwelling central venous catheter for the duration of their therapy.

Follow-Up

WHEN TO EXPECT IMPROVEMENT

All patients with Ewing sarcoma require approximately 30 to 48 weeks of chemotherapy to prevent recurrence in the original site of tumor or distant spread. However, some improvement in signs and symptoms is usually seen within the first several weeks of therapy.

ACUTE EFFECTS OF THERAPY

Therapy for Ewing sarcoma is intensive. Patients can expect many of the following side effects:

- Frequent admissions to the hospital for chemotherapy or complications of the therapy
- Complications from bone marrow suppressive effects of chemotherapy or radiotherapy:

—Anemia: Blood transfusions are usually necessary; erythropoietin (a stimulator of erythropoiesis) is given to many patients to reduce the number of transfusions required.
—Thrombocytopenia: Platelet transfusions are often necessary to reduce the risk of serious bleeding.
—Neutropenia: Increased risk of bacterial and fungal infections; G-CSF (granulocyte colony-stimulating factor) is usually administered daily following chemotherapy to shorten the duration of neutropenia.

- Complications from the gastrointestinal side effects of chemotherapy or radiotherapy:

—Nausea and vomiting; relieved with ondansetron and other antiemetic agents
—Malnutrition secondary to reduced appetite and mucosal ulcerations; nutritional supplements (oral, nasogastric, gastrostomy tube or parenteral) may be necessary.
—Complications from radiotherapy
  —Skin erythema or breakdown
  —Pathologic fracture or poor function

LATE EFFECTS OF THERAPY

Therapy for Ewing sarcoma is intensive, and is associated with significant long-term adverse effects. Regular follow-up with a pediatric oncologist is strongly recommended. These late effects of therapy include the following:

- Cardiomyopathy
- Anthracyclines (doxorubicin) weaken cardiac muscle, leading to reduced left ventricular function many years after therapy.
- Approximately 5% of patients receiving cumulative doses of doxorubicin greater than 500 mg/m^2 will develop congestive heart failure.
- Radiation to the heart can lower the cumulative dose threshold to 300 mg/m^2.
- Any patient who has received an anthracycline should be cautioned against initiating strenuous physical activity without adequate preparation.
- Pregnant women who have received anthra-cyclines in the past should inform their obstetrician so that appropriate cardiac assessment can be completed prior to vaginal delivery.
- Kidney and bladder damage
- Urinalysis should be performed to detect hemorrhagic cystitis or tubular damage with spilling of sugar, protein, and phosphate into the urine.
- Blood pressure should be monitored in patients who received irradiation to the kidneys; vascular damage and hypertension may develop many years after therapy.
- Infertility and delayed puberty
- Reduced or absent gonadal function is related to high doses of alkylating agents (cy-clophosphamide, ifosfamide): males are at high risk of azoospermia; females may be fertile, but are at risk for premature menopause.
- Low-dose estrogen therapy with oral contraceptive medications may be necessary for amenorrheic women.
- Second malignant neoplasms
- Sarcomas may occur within the radiation field.
- Myelodysplastic syndromes and acute myeloid leukemia may occur secondary to radiation or chemotherapy (cyclophosphamide, ifosfamide, etoposide).
- Growth abnormalities/functional defects at the primary site
- Radiation doses greater than 20 Gy will cause growth retardation in prepubertal children.
- Scoliosis can occur if the vertebrae are involved in the radiation field.

Common Questions and Answers

Q: At what time point is a child with Ewing sarcoma considered cured?
A: Typically, cure is measured as 5-year survival without evidence of disease. However, late relapses or second tumors do occur in children with Ewing sarcoma.

Q: Should a Ewing sarcoma be completely resected at the time of diagnosis?
A: Most times, this is not recommended, as Ewing sarcoma is very sensitive to chemotherapy, facilitating an improved delayed surgical resection.

Q: Should children with Ewing sarcoma take vitamins?
A: There is little information on the necessity and safety of vitamin supplementation during chemotherapy for Ewing sarcoma and other childhood malignancies. In general, supplementation at standard RDA dosing is safe, but high doses are not recommended.

ICD-9-CM 170.4

BIBLIOGRAPHY

Grier HE. The Ewing family of tumors: Ewing sarcoma and primitive neuroectodermal tumors. *Pediatr Clin North Am* 1997;44(4):991–1004.

Womer RB. Problems and controversies in the management of childhood sarcomas. *Br Med Bull* 1996;52(4):826–843.

Author: Kara M. Kelly

Exstrophy of the Bladder

 Database

DEFINITION

Exstrophy of the bladder is an anomaly in which the open bladder is part of the anterior abdominal wall. Bladder exstrophy presents as part of a complex of anomalies consisting of cryptorchidism in males, male and female epispadias, and wide separation of the pubis symphysis. The most severe variant of this complex is cloacal exstrophy where there is a large omphalocele, split bladder, imperforate anus, shortened colon, and multiple upper urinary tract and limb anomalies.

EMBRYOLOGY

- Normal development: The cloacal membrane is located at the caudal end of the infraumbilical abdominal wall by 2 weeks' gestation. Mesenchyme from the primitive streak migrates between the layers of the cloacal membrane to reinforce the abdominal wall as the cloacal membrane regresses.
- Bladder exstrophy: Abnormal thickening of the cloacal membrane prevents medial migration of the mesenchymal tissue and normal lower abdominal wall development. The membrane ruptures as it lacks reinforcement and the timing of this rupture determines the variant of the exstrophy-epispadias complex.
- Cloacal exstrophy: Abnormally large cloacal membrane perforates even prior to division of the cloaca by the urorectal septum.

EPIDEMIOLOGY

- Incidence estimated between 1 in 20,000 to 1 in 40,000 live births.
- Male/female ratio for classic bladder exstrophy is between 1.5 and 2:1.
- Risk of second affected family member is 3.6%.
- Risk of bladder exstrophy in offspring of individuals with bladder exstrophy and epispadias is 1 in 70 births (500-fold greater than the general population).
- Cloacal exstrophy is exceedingly rare with an incidence of 1 in 200,000 births (incidence continues to decrease due to prenatal diagnosis and termination).

 Physical Examination

BLADDER EXSTROPHY

- All cases of exstrophy have widening of the symphysis pubis caused by outward rotation of the innominate bones.
- Triangular defect caused by premature rupture of the abnormal cloacal membrane is occupied by the exstrophied bladder and posterior urethra.

—Located at the upper end of the triangular defect, the distance between the umbilicus and anus is shortened in exstrophy.

- Indirect inguinal hernia and incarceration are common in boys.

—Perineum is short and broad with the anus displaced anteriorly.

- Male genital anomalies

—Penis in boys with exstrophy is short and wide
—Corpora cavernosa are short and widely separated.
—Marked dorsal chordee causes congenital curvature of the penis with a short urethral plate.
—Epispadias is present with the urethral meatus on the dorsum at the penopubic junction.

- Female genital anomalies

—Overall less complex anomalies
—Vaginal orifice is narrowed and displaced anteriorly.
—Uterus may be duplicated; bifid clitoris; divergent labia and mons pubis.
—Epispadias may be less pronounced.

- Urinary defects

—Bladder mucosa at birth usually appears normal. Ectopic bowel mucosa or polyp may be present.
—Exstrophic bladder may exhibit maturational delay that resumes normal development following closure.
—Upper urinary tract usually normal.
—Horseshoe, pelvic, hypoplastic, solitary, or dysplastic kidney occasionally occurs.
—100% of children with exstrophy have vesicoureteral reflux requiring correction.

CLOACAL EXSTROPHY

- Two halves of the exstrophied bladder separated by an exstrophied ileocecal bowel.
- Prolapsed ileum superiorly, and blind-ending colon stump inferiorly.
- Imperforate anus
- Bifid vagina and uterine abnormalities likely.
- Large omphalocele usually present.
- Upper urinary tract anomalies seen in up to 70% of children.
- Vertebral and neurologic abnormalities present in over 50% of children.

 Laboratory Aids

IMAGING

- Prenatal sonographic findings by 20 weeks consistent with absence of a normal fluid-filled bladder, an anterior abdominal mass increasing in size, low-set umbilicus and wide pubic ramus are suggestive of bladder exstrophy.
- Radionuclide scans and ultrasound are required to confirm prenatal findings and diagnose associated anomalies in the neonatal period.

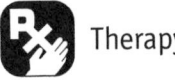 Therapy

POSTNATAL AND NURSERY CARE

- Umbilical cord tied with 2-0 silk to avoid traumatizing the bladder mucosa with an umbilical clamp.
- Bladder covered with plastic wrap to prevent mucosa from sticking to clothing or diapers.
- Occasional warm saline irrigations.
- Immediate transfer to an appropriate center for surgical correction and consultation to a pediatric urologist.
- Broad-spectrum intravenous antibiotics should be started on arrival to a pediatric referral center to sterilize the bladder for surgical manipulation.

SURGICAL TREATMENT

- Goals:

—Provide urinary continence and preserve renal function.
—Surgically reconstruct the male penis to provide an erection straight enough for vaginal penetration and upright voiding.

- Staged repair:

—In the early neonatal period, bladder, posterior urethra, and abdominal wall closure is performed with or without bilateral posterior iliac and anterior innominate osteotomy.
—Epispadias repair at 6 months to 1 year of age.
—Bladder neck reconstruction with an antireflux procedure delayed until 3.5 to 4 years to facilitate adequate bladder growth and development.
—Prophylactic antibiotic therapy should be continued in all children until antireflux procedure completed.

- Combined bladder closure and epispadias repair:

—Only reserved for carefully selected patients. Currently not recommended for children younger than 6 months of age.
—Suitable for children presenting after failed initial closure.

- Results and complications:

—Primary bladder closure followed by bladder neck reconstruction
—Urinary continence following functional bladder closure ranges from 60% to 87%.
—Dehiscence, stone formation, and hydronephrosis requiring urethral dilation or vesicostomy may occur.
—Second attempt at closure delayed 6 months.
—Failed bladder neck repair in 20% to 50% may require further reconstruction including artificial sphincter, augmentation cystoplasty or, rarely, ureterosigmoidostomy.
—Epispadias repair
—Cosmetic and functional success with a straight penis with erections ranges from 60% to 95%
—Urethral strictures and urethrocutaneous fistulas are the most common complications of epispadias repair seen in up to 25% of patients.
—Adenocarcinoma of the bladder occurs in patients with exstrophy 400 times more commonly than in the normal population. This disease is not reported in adults who have had bladder closure after infancy.

- Fertility and pregnancy:

—Sexual function and libido in exstrophy patients is normal.
—Up to 87% of boys have erections following epispadias repair.
—Slow and small volume ejaculation should be expected.
—Successful impregnation achieved with assisted reproductive techniques.
—Pregnancy is commonly achieved in women with bladder exstrophy but uterine and cervical prolapse are common complications.

ICD-9-CM 753.5

BIBLIOGRAPHY

Gearhart JP. The bladder exstrophy-epispadias-cloacal exstrophy complex. In: Gearhart JP, Rink, Mouriquand, eds. *Pediatric urology*. Philadelphia, WB Saunders, 2001:511.

Gearhart JP, Mathew RI, Taylor S, et al. Combined bladder closure and epispadias repair in the reconstruction of bladder exstrophy. *J Urol* 1988;160:1182.

Authors: Aseem Shukla and Douglas Canning

Fetal Alcohol Syndrome

 Database

DEFINITION

Pattern of physical, behavioral, and cognitive abnormalities in individuals exposed to alcohol *in utero*.

DIAGNOSTIC CATEGORIES (INSTITUTE OF MEDICINE)

FAS with Confirmed Maternal Exposure to Alcohol (See below)*

- Characteristic facial anomalies
- Growth retardation
- CNS neurodevelopmental abnormalities

FAS without Confirmed Maternal Exposure

- As above

Partial FAS with Confirmed Exposure

- Confirmed maternal alcohol exposure
- Characteristic facial anomalies
- Either growth retardation, CNS abnormalities, or unexplained behavior/cognitive abnormalities

Alcohol-Related Birth Defects (ARBD)

- Confirmed maternal alcohol exposure
- Birth defects

Alcohol-Related Neurodevelopmental Disorder (ARND)

- Confirmed maternal alcohol exposure
- Either CNS abnormalities or unexplained behavior/cognitive abnormalities
- *Confirmed maternal exposure to alcohol as evidenced by: Substantial regular intake or heavy episodic drinking as evidenced by frequent episodes of intoxication, development of tolerance or withdrawal, social or legal problems related to drinking, engaging in physically hazardous behavior while drinking, or alcohol-related medical problems, e.g., hepatic disease

Note: Some leading dysmorphologists prefer not to use the terms ARBD and ARND. See discussion below (Common Questions and Answers).

DIAGNOSTIC FINDINGS

Facial Anomalies

- Short palpebral fissures
- Premaxillary features (thin upper lip, flat/smooth philtrum, flat midface)
- Ptosis
- Short, upturned nose
- Ptosis and short, upturned nose are not mentioned in IOM criteria, but are commonly seen in children with FAS.

Growth Retardation (At Least One for Diagnosis)

- Low birth weight for gestation
- Growth retardation despite adequate nutrition
- Low weight relative to height

CNS Neurodevelopmental Abnormalities (At Least One for Diagnosis)

- Microcephaly at birth
- Structural brain abnormalities (e.g., agenesis of corpus callosum, cerebellar hypoplasia)
- Neurologic hard or soft signs (e.g., impaired fine motor skills, neurosensory hearing loss, poor tandem gait, poor eye-hand coordination)

Unexplained Behavior or Cognitive Abnormalities

- Learning difficulties
- Poor school performance
- Poor impulse control
- Problems in social perception
- Deficits in higher level receptive and expressive language
- Poor abstract reasoning
- Poor math skills
- Impaired memory, attention, or judgment

Birth Defects

- Cardiac (30%): ASD, VSD(most common), aberrant great vessels, TOF
- Skeletal (18%): clinodactyly, camptodactyly, nail dysplasia, radioulnar synostosis
- Renal: hydronephrosis, renal agenesis, hypoplastic kidney
- Ocular: strabismus, retinal vascular tortuosity, abnormal corneal curvature
- Auditory: hearing loss (conductive—75% of children with FAS; neurosensory—less common)
- Others

PATHOPHYSIOLOGY

Alcohol and its metabolite, acetaldehyde, are embryotoxic and teratogenic, capable of reducing fetal growth and inducing malformations during critical periods in the development of the fetus. Pathophysiology may involve increased susceptibility to cell damage by free radicals in the developing tissues, leading to cell death or decreased cellular proliferation. Exposure in the first trimester affects organogenesis and craniofacial development, resulting in characteristic facial features and birth defects. Exposure at varying times can cause CNS neurodevelopmental effects, since brain formation and neuronal maturation occur throughout pregnancy. Exposure also causes pre- and postnatal growth retardation, probably by inhibiting protein and DNA synthesis.

EPIDEMIOLOGY

Incidence of FAS, ARBD, and ARND range widely from 0.3 to 5 per 1,000 live births. Higher rates reported among selected subgroups, e.g., African Americans and Native Americans, probably relate to lower socioeconomic status rather than race.

GENETICS

Genetic factors contribute to variable susceptibility of individuals to FAS. Evidence: concordance of FAS is higher in monozygotic than dizygotic twins; differential sensitivities to *in utero* alcohol exposure in different strains of mice.

(Other factors that contribute to variable susceptibility include: maternal age/parity, nutritional status, use of other drugs.)

PROGNOSIS

- Fifty percent are mentally retarded (IQ <70). Average IQ in individuals with FAS is in the 60s (mild MR); however, a wide range of IQ exists, from 16 to 115.
- Sixty-two percent have severe behavioral problems, even if a normal IQ exists.
- The major disabilities of FAS caused by the neurocognitive/neurobehavioral effects lead to poor academic performance, legal problems, employment difficulties, and secondary mental health problems.

 Differential Diagnosis

BY PHYSICAL FEATURES

- Aarskog syndrome
- Williams syndrome
- Noonan syndrome
- Dubowitz syndrome
- Bloom syndrome
- Fetal hydantoin syndrome
- Maternal phenylketonuria fetal effects

BY NEUROBEHAVIORAL FEATURES

- Fragile X syndrome
- 22q11 deletion syndromes
- Turner syndrome
- Opitz syndrome

Data Gathering

HISTORY

- Birth history, birth and subsequent growth parameters (weight, height, head circumference)
- Medical history
- Maternal history for alcohol use (binge drinking, average number of drinks per day, timing in pregnancy) and other drug use
- Learning/behavior problems

—Infancy
  —May or may not have EtOH withdrawal as newborn
  —Irritable, irregular sleep, poor feeding, hypotonia, delayed motor function

—Preschool and school age
  —Hyperactive?
  —Slow verbal learning?
  —Slow visual-spatial learning?
  —Poor abstract thinking(planning and organizing)?
  —Perseverates (can't abandon ineffective strategies)?
  —Attention problems?
  —Difficulty with peer interactions?

—Adolescence and adulthood:
  —Substance abuse?
  —Criminal behavior?
  —Unable to work?
  —Unable to live independently?
  —Difficulty managing time and money?

Q: Are siblings affected?
A: Usually younger siblings are affected more severely; if older sibling wasn't previously diagnosed, and shows signs of alcohol-related effects, he/she will also need evaluation and services.

Q: Is child in a high-risk living situation? Who is the caregiver?
A: Keep in mind that external influences such as poverty, unstable home environment, poor emotional support, or educational resources contribute to behavioral problems.

Physical Examination

- Weight, height, head circumference

—Microcephaly persists throughout life
—Some catch-up growth occurs in adolescence, esp. in girls, but adult height attained remains lower than expected for parental height.

- Facial exam (short palpebral fissures, ptosis, flat midface, upturned nose, smooth philtrum, thin upper lip)

—Facial features become less prominent in adolescence and adulthood

- Complete PE, including neurologic exam

—Look for associated defects of the heart, skeletal system

Laboratory Aids

- No laboratory marker exists for FAS.
- Consider chromosome studies if diagnosis is unclear.
- Other laboratory tests as indicated by the child's specific medical problems.

Therapy

The role of the pediatrician is early identification (with help from specialists) resulting in early intervention and appropriate referrals:

- To social and educational resources in the community to support family and child
- For comprehensive neuropsychological evaluation (IQ, achievement, executive function, memory, adaptive function, language, reasoning and judgment, behavior)
- For ophthalmologic exam (consider routine screening prior to school, then every two years)
- For hearing test [consider brainstem auditory evoked response (BAER) at 6–12 months]

Follow-Up

- Growth and nutrition in infancy since failure to thrive is a common problem.
- Regular evaluations of vision and hearing, since these problems occur at a high rate.
- As indicated by other medical/psychological problems.

PREVENTION

FAS is preventable if women of child-bearing age abstain from alcohol prior to conception and throughout pregnancy. Recent FAS prevention research has focused on finding and treating women who drink during pregnancy, e.g., using a screening questionnaire to assess problem drinking in women, and then intervening at a level determined by the level of drinking.

Common Questions and Answers

Q: What is FAE (fetal alcohol effect)?
A: FAE originally described abnormalities seen in animal studies, then was adopted by clinicians, being widely used to refer to behavioral and cognitive problems in children exposed to alcohol *in utero* without the typical diagnostic features. Because of lack of diagnostic criteria for FAE, and the imprecise use of this term, IOM replaced FAE with the terms ARND and ARBD.
Use of these terms (ARND and ARBD) is also controversial in that they imply that confirmed maternal alcohol exposure is causative of the associated abnormalities, which at present is not proven. In summarizing the problem list for an individual who may not meet the criteria for FAS or partial FAS, some leading dysmorphologists recommend listing the elements separately without attribution, rather than using the confusing terms FAE or ARND/ARBD. [Example: Impression: 1. Prenatal alcohol exposure, (mild, moderate, or severe). 2. Cleft lip and palate, complete bilateral. 3. Cognitive deficit, (mild, moderate, or severe).]

Q: How much alcohol does it take to produce damage?
A: Clinically significant effects are more common in children whose mothers consume five or more drinks per occasion per week. (Peak blood alcohol level is more important than a lower sustained blood alcohol level.) However, no minimum safe level of alcohol consumption has been determined.

Q: Do most children with FAS have ADHD?
A: Although hyperactivity appears to be common in FAS, many of these children are misdiagnosed as having ADHD. Instead of difficulty focusing and sustaining attention, children with FAS often have difficulty shifting attention from one task to another. Use of stimulant medication is not routinely supported, although a small proportion may respond to stimulant medication in educational settings.

ICD-9-CM 760.71

BIBLIOGRAPHY

Aase JM, Jones KL, Clarren SK. Do we need the term "FAE"? *Pediatrics* 1995;95:428–430.

Abel EL. *Fetal alcohol abuse syndrome.* New York: Plenum Press, 1998.

American Academy of Pediatrics. Fetal alcohol syndrome and alcohol-related neurodevelopmental disorders. *Pediatrics* 2000;106:358–361.

Dorris M. *The broken cord.* New York: HarperCollins, 1990.

Institute of Medicine. *Fetal alcohol syndrome: diagnosis, epidemiology, prevention, and treatment.* Washington DC: National Academy of Sciences, 1996.

National Institute on Alcohol Abuse and Alcoholism. Fetal alcohol exposure and the brain. *Alcohol Alert* December 2000, no. 50.

Thackray HM, Tifft C. Fetal alcohol syndrome. *Pediatr Rev* 2001;22:47–55.

Author: Janet M. Li-Tempest

Floppy Infant Syndrome

 ## Database

DEFINITION
"Floppy infant" connotes neuromuscular weakness, though central nervous system or nonneurologic problems must also be considered. This syndrome typically presents with decreased movement, abnormal posture due to weakness, or CNS dysfunction.

PATHOPHYSIOLOGY
Two major categories of hypotonia are:
- Hypotonia without significant weakness (nonparalytic)
- Hypotonia with significant weakness (paralytic)

GENETICS
- Numerous genetic, metabolic, and dysmorphic syndromes with varying patterns of inheritance may underlie hypotonia in infancy.
- The most common causes include the "central" causes, involving the cerebellum, brainstem, basal ganglia, and hemispheres.
- Less common are neuromuscular diseases affecting anterior horn cells, peripheral nerves, neuromuscular junction, or muscle.
- Often, central hypotonia that is not due to CNS injury is benign in nature.

COMPLICATIONS
- Respiratory difficulties
- Recurrent pneumonia
- Poor nutritional status resulting from sucking and swallowing difficulties

ASSOCIATED ILLNESSES
- Metabolic disorders
- Hip dislocation
- Gastroesophageal reflux
- Motor delay

 ## Differential Diagnosis

COLLAGEN DISEASES AND SYSTEMIC ILLNESSES
- Ehlers-Danlos syndrome
- Marfan syndrome
- Osteogenesis imperfecta
- Congenital laxity of ligaments

SYSTEMIC DISORDERS
- Sepsis
- Malnutrition
- Cyanotic heart disease
- Renal acidosis
- Hypercalcemia
- Rickets
- Hypothyroidism
- Cystic fibrosis
- Malnutrition
- Sepsis
- Intestinal obstruction (volvulus, intussusception)
- Disorders of connective tissue and other systemic illnesses may produce hypotonia without weakness.

- Hypotonia may be the primary presenting sign in acute infectious or gastrointestinal illness, including GI bleed.
- "Benign congenital hypotonia" denotes a common clinical picture of nonparalytic hypotonia in older infants whose physical examination reveals only hypotonia. These infants have, at most, only mild motor delay and no other neurologic or pertinent physical abnormalities. By definition, the creatine kinase level and other laboratory studies are normal, and prognosis is good.

Disorders Involving Cerebral Cortex, Cerebellum, Brainstem
- Nonspecific mental retardation
- Hypotonic cerebral palsy
- Intracranial hemorrhage
- Malformations
- Infections
- Toxic
- Metabolic encephalopathies
- Hypoxic-ischemic encephalopathies
- Genetic/chromosomal anomalies such as Down and Prader-Willi syndromes
- Aminoacidurias
- Mucopolysaccharidoses
- Organic acidurias
- Sphingolipidoses

Disorders Involving Spinal Cord
- Myelodysplasias (meningomyeloceles, diplomyelia, diastematomyelia)
- Traumatic transection (often seen with breech deliveries)

Paralytic Hypotonia
- Floppy infants whose physical examination reveals significant motor weakness and decreased or absent deep tendon reflexes
- Differential diagnosis in this category involves mainly disorders of anterior horn cell [Hereditary spinal muscular atrophy (Werdnig-Hoffman), Poliomyelitis (polio or other enteroviridae)], peripheral nerve, neuromuscular junction, and muscle

Disorders of Peripheral Nerve
- Dejerine-Sottas disease
- Guillain-Barré syndrome
- Rare causes include giant neuroaxonal dystrophy, congenital hypomyelinating neuropathy, familial dysautonomia (Riley-Day syndrome), metachromatic and Krabbe leukodystrophy, and neonatal Guillain-Barré syndrome.

Disorders of Neuromuscular Junction
- Transient and congenital myasthenia gravis
- Botulism
- Toxic blockade secondary to aminoglycoside antibiotics (especially in infants with renal failure), nondepolarizing neuromuscular blockers (prolonged postoperative hypotonia)
- Hypermagnesemia secondary to treatment of pre-eclampsia in the mother

Disorders of Muscle
- Congenital structural myopathies such as:
—Central core
—Nemaline rod
—Myotubular

—Mitochondrial
—Glycogenosis
—Lipid storage disease
—Congenital myotonic dystrophy
—Congenital muscular dystrophy
—Metabolic myopathies

PITFALLS
- Hypermagnesemia is a common cause of apnea in the intensive care nursery.
- Fasciculations are overdiagnosed and should be included in the clinical picture only when they are noticed at rest.
- Airway protection is of primary concern in hypotonic infants.

 ## Data Gathering

HISTORY
Important factors to obtain in the history include:
- Fetal movements
- Delivery
- Gestational maturity
- Apgar scores
- History of the perinatal period
- Infections, recent illnesses, and medications
- Family history
- Motor milestone achievement

 ## Physical Examination

The physical examination usually indicates whether floppy infant syndrome is due to a neurologic dysfunction, and, if so, whether it is centrally or peripherally based. It should include the following:
- Evaluation of mental status
- Infants with hypotonia secondary to a neuromuscular process often appear very bright and alert despite their weakness.
- Those with CNS dysfunction will likely have cognitive involvement.
- In nonparalytic hypotonia, the infant may initially appear weak and floppy, but spontaneous movements of the limbs occur readily against gravity. Posture and tone should be noted in the supine position, in ventral suspension, and with traction. Look for the presence of a "scarf" sign.
- The presence of brisk tendon reflexes in a hypotonic child almost always signifies that hypotonia is due to cerebral dysfunction. Further development may reveal spastic cerebral palsy.
- Tongue fasciculations are best seen at the lateral margins of the tongue as spontaneous rippling movements with the infant still (not crying). They are most commonly associated with denervation as seen in spinal muscular atrophy.
- Facial weakness (decreased expression) is often seen with congenital myotonic dystrophy, myotubular myopathy, congenital muscular dystrophy, congenital facial diplegia, trauma, or Moebius syndrome.

- Ptosis/ophthalmoplegia suggests myotubular myopathy, mitochondrial myopathy, congenital muscular dystrophy, myasthenia gravis, or congenital fibrosis syndrome.
- Arthrogryposis and contractures are seen in congenital muscular dystrophy, myotonic dystrophy, and neuropathies.
- Hip dislocation should be considered in any hypotonic child. To screen for this, Ortolani maneuver and hip x-ray studies should be done.
- Weakness and respiratory problems are seen in many conditions, such as spinal muscular atrophy, myotonic dystrophy, myotubular myopathy, nemaline myopathy, and congenital muscular dystrophy.
- Swallowing/sucking difficulties can be seen in myotubular myopathy, myotonic dystrophy, nemaline myopathy, and neonatal myasthenia.
- Weakness and loss of tone in the lower extremities with active use of the upper extremities suggests spinal cord injury.

 ## Laboratory Aids

TESTS

- Specifics of the presentation will guide laboratory studies. Initial work-up may include a urinalysis, electrolytes, creatine kinase (CK), thyroid studies, and amino and organic acid screen. Tongue fasciculations and generalized weakness may indicate a DNA test for spinal muscular atrophy. Family history may indicate DNA test for myotonic dystrophy.
- EMG/nerve conduction velocity (NCV) is very useful to localize neuromuscular involvement. If both the CK and EMG/NCV are abnormal, a muscle biopsy should be done to better define the underlying pathology. If the CK and EMG/NCV are normal and the clinical examination points toward CNS involvement, an MRI should be considered.
- A tensilon test may be done if repetitive stimulation on the EMG suggests myasthenia. Acetylcholine receptor antibodies may also be obtained in the work-up of myasthenia.
- Stool samples should be evaluated for *Clostridium* when botulism is suspected.
- A lumbar puncture may be carried out to rule out systemic illnesses, as well as look for increased protein, which may be seen in peripheral nerve disease.
- An MRI or CT with contrast of the spine should be done in a child with a suspected spinal cord injury.
- Elevated lactate and pyruvate levels may be helpful in looking for mitochondrial disease.

 ## Therapy

- Acute respiratory distress or hypoventilation in a weak, hypotonic infant must be anticipated and may require oxygen support as well as aggressive pulmonary toilet, antibiotic therapy, or ventilator assistance.
- Sucking and swallowing difficulties may necessitate nutritional support via NG tube feedings and supplementation.
- Underlying toxic or metabolic causes should be addressed and treated appropriately.
- Spinal cord injury may also cause respiratory embarrassment. Steroid therapy should be considered within the first 8 hours of the injury.
- For transient myasthenia gravis, medical therapy is often not needed. However, anti-cholinesterase medications (pyridostigmine) may be necessary for infants with significant respiratory or feeding difficulties.
- Immunotherapy may also be appropriate for infants with Guillain-Barré syndrome or polymyositis. Immunosuppressive agents used in the acute phase include IV immunoglobulin and plasmapheresis.
- Botulism antitoxin trivalent is used in some centers to treat infantile botulism.
- For many of the congenital myopathies and other neuromuscular disorders, treatment is primarily supportive, and active physical therapy is needed to minimize contractures and maximize strength and mobility. Spinal deformities such as scoliosis should be evaluated on a regular basis, as surgical intervention may be necessary.
- Orthopedic consultation to evaluate hips, and contractures may be helpful.

 ## Follow-Up

- In infants whose hypotonia is secondary to CNS involvement, developmental milestones and early intervention will need to be closely monitored in order to evaluate the degree of motor and cognitive impairment.
- Generally, in infants with spinal muscular atrophy Type I (Werdnig-Hoffman), the earlier the onset, the poorer the prognosis. Approximately 60% die by the age of 2 years, and 80% by the age of 4. Outcome for many of the congenital myopathies and dystrophies depends not only on the specific disease, but also on the age of onset and associated respiratory and feeding difficulties.
- Transient neonatal myasthenia with any of the symptoms listed earlier usually resolves by 8 weeks of age. However, infants with congenital myasthenia gravis usually require long-term therapy, depending on the underlying pathology. Symptoms may persist into childhood and adulthood.

- Infants with botulism may recover completely in weeks to months if adequate medical and supportive therapy is administered.

PITFALLS

- Hypermagnesemia is a common cause of hypotonia in neonates whose mothers were treated for eclampsia. Intensive care monitoring is required because of the risk of apnea.
- Infants with acute/subacute onset of paralytic hypotonia (e.g., botulism, Guillain-Barré syndrome) may lose airway protective reflexes before neurogenic hypoventilation. Pooling of secretions/decreased gag may prompt intubation.
- Intussusception may present with hypotonia. Rectal examination may reveal the diagnosis.

 ## Common Questions and Answers

Q: By what age should one expect resolution of benign congenital hypotonia?
A: Hypotonia should not be evident by the time the infant is walking; a delay in walking beyond 15 months casts doubt on the diagnosis.

Q: When and how should spinal muscular atrophy (SMA) be ruled out?
A: SMA is a consideration in any infant with insidious onset of significant weakness with arreflexia. DNA testing for "SMN deletion" is definitive and may preclude electrophysiologic testing or muscle biopsy.

ICD-9-CM 781.9

BIBLIOGRAPHY

Brooke M. *A clinician's view of neuromuscular diseases*, 2nd ed.Baltimore: Williams & Wilkins, 1986.

Dubowitz V. *Muscle disorders in childhood*. Chicago: Year Book, 1989.

Parush S, Yehezkehel I, Tenenbaum A, Tekuzener E, Bar-Efrat-Hirsch I, Jessel A, Ornoy A. *Dev Med Child Neurol* 1998;40(7):448–452.

Stiefel L. Pediatr Rev 1996;17(3):104–105.

Weiner H, Bresnan M, Levitt L. *Pediatric neurology for the house officer*, 2nd ed. Baltimore: Williams & Wilkins, 1982.

Verrijn Stuart AA, Huisman M, van Straaten HL, Bakker JC, Arabin B. "Shake hands"; diagnosing a floppy infant—myotonic dystrophy and the congenital subtype: a difficult perinatal diagnosis. *J Perinat Med.* 2000;28(6):497-501.

Author: Meena Scavena Baldi

Food Allergy

 Database

DEFINITION

• Food allergy has many manifestations and is estimated to affect 7.5% of the population. Food allergy is overdiagnosed and carries the risk of patients using elimination diets that are nutritionally inappropriate. Food allergies may have systemic, cutaneus, pulmonary, nasal, or GI manifestations. This discussion concentrates on GI manifestations of food allergy and the risk of overdiagnosing, which may lead to extreme elimination diets, placing children at significant nutritional risk.
• Food hypersensitivity is defined as a reproducible response to food in which an immunologic mechanism is incriminated.
• Food intolerance is defined as symptoms that are modulated by nonimmunologic mechanisms (i.e., lactose intolerance).

PATHOPHYSIOLOGY

• The pathophysiology of food allergy is poorly understood and may involve both the classic type I immediate hypersensitivity reaction (linked to IgE) or type IV delayed-type hypersensitivity reaction (non–IgE-mediated). Most of the GI manifestations is non–IgE-mediated.
• The GI mucosal immune system is complex, involving antigen presentation via M cells, macrophages, and dendritic cells to lymphocytes in Peyer's patches, which further subspecialize into B cells, which secrete IgA and IgM, and T cells, which secrete cytokines such as IL-5, which act as eosinophil chemoattractants. Both eosinophils and mucosal mast cells also may play roles in allergic responses to food.

EPIDEMIOLOGY

• The prevalence of *true* food hypersensitivity has been estimated at between 1% and 3%.
• Approximately half of patients with atopic dermatitis had at least one food allergen exacerbating their disease.

 Differential Diagnosis

Rectal bleeding due to cow's milk allergy Any pathologic process leading to colitis in infancy should be considered in the differential diagnosis of allergic colitis, including:

• Infectious colitis
• Hirschsprung enterocolitis
• Inflammatory bowel disease

Systemic or local eosinophilic infiltration, as in patients with eosinophilic gastroenteropathy; the differential includes:

• Inflammatory bowel disease
• Drug allergy
• Hypereosinophilic syndrome
• Celiac disease
• Autoimmune enteropathy
• Parasitic infection

 Data Gathering

• A careful history is important for identifying suspected food allergens; however, it is important to remember that less than half of the reported food reactions will be confirmed on double-blinded placebo-controlled challenges.
• Key pieces of information include type of symptoms, frequency of symptoms, timing of symptoms from ingestion, and quantity of food leading to response.
• In the acute reaction, urticaria, angioedema, exacerbation of atopic dermatitis, and certainly hypotension will lead to supportive evidence for true food allergic response.
• Anaphylaxis is one of the more dramatic presentations of food allergy. It may be systemic or limited to the oropharynx. Systemic anaphylaxis presents with vomiting, pallor, urticaria, listlessness, and respiratory and cardiovascular compromise. Oral allergy syndrome is localized to the oropharynx and consists of urticaria and angioedema. The symptoms of oral anaphylaxis tend to resolve rapidly.

• IgE-mediated reactions:

—Type I reactions are more common in infants, with 50% of these reactions occurring in the first year, 20% in the second, and 10% after 2 years.
—Egg, milk, peanuts, soy, nuts, wheat, and fish account for 90% of food reactions in children.
—Forty percent of these patients developed tolerance to the offending food within 1 to 2 years.

• Non–IgE-mediated reactions:

—Eosinophilic colitis most commonly secondary to cow's milk/soy protein allergy. Infants present with diarrhea associated with blood and mucus in the stool in an otherwise healthy patient. The syndrome has been described in exclusively breast-fed infants who are exposed to antigens transmitted through the breast milk.
—Eosinophilic gastroenteropathy may also occur in patients with cow's milk/soy allergy. These infants often present with protracted vomiting, diarrhea, failure to thrive, iron-deficiency anemia, and hypoalbuminemia. The disease process may involve the mucosa, muscularis, or serosa of the bowel.
—Isolated eosinophilic esophagitis (IEE) presents with gastroesophageal reflux, dysphagia, and poor growth. Intense eosinophilic infiltration of the mucosa is seen on biopsy. Often, pH probe studies are negative or equivocal. The family history may be remarkable for atopy. Both IgE- and non–IgE-related mechanisms for the development of this entity are under investigation.
—Respiratory symptoms as the only manifestation of food allergy are rare. Often, respiratory symptoms accompany other systemic or GI symptoms. No studies at this time have proven a link between food allergy and chronic cough or wheezing.

Laboratory Aids

- In patients with suspected IgE-mediated food hypersensitivity, skin-prick testing may be helpful in defining the offending allergen. A panel of common allergens is often used, including milk, soy, egg, peanuts, fish, and wheat.
- Testing with natural foods may be necessary if there is a high index of suspicion and the commercially prepared extracts do not elicit a response.
- Age is an important factor in interpreting skin-prick tests:

—For patients younger than 1 year of age, a response is highly significant because the presence of IgE in this age group is unusual; a negative skin test will not rule out allergy in this group.

—For patients ≥1 year, skin testing is 90% to 100% sensitive; therefore, a negative test makes IgE-mediated reactions highly unlikely. In non–IgE-mediated food hypersensitivity, skin-prick tests will be negative. The radioallergosorbent test (RAST) does not appear to add to the diagnostic yield when performed with skin testing.

—Open, single-, or double-blinded food challenges are helpful if there is no improvement on elimination of the suspected food allergen from the diet.

—Double-blinded food challenges may be the best way to define a reproducible reaction.

—Further laboratory aids under investigation include lymphocyte proliferation assays and patch skin testing.

 ## Therapy

- For anaphylaxis:

—Full monitoring of vital signs
—Diphenhydramine for milder symptoms
—Epinephrine, if significant respiratory or cardiovascular symptoms persist. All patients at risk for anaphylaxis to foods should have epinephrine for home use and a Medi-Alert bracelet.

- For nonanaphylactic reactions:

—Elimination of the suspected food allergen from the diet. This must be done carefully to maintain adequate nutrition for the child. If the symptoms resolve with elimination, the next step is to reintroduce the allergen to determine if the symptoms are reproducible. If the patient responds to dietary restriction, the elimination diet may be continued for 1 to 3 months. The patient may then be challenged again to determine if tolerance to the offending agent has been established. If the symptoms persist, the pediatrician should consider referral to a specialist for further evaluation and management. Education of the family and caregivers is vital to this therapy. It may be very difficult to identify those foods that may contain the offending allergen. Referral to a dietitian or nutritionist may aid in this education.

- For overdiagnosing and its dietary consequences:

—It is essential for the physician to be aware of the more recent published data regarding nutritional deficiencies even in affluent societies secondary to overdiagnosis of milk protein allergy. There is an increased number of cases of Kwashiorkor even in the U.S. secondary to consumption of rice milk with severe protein depletion (0.3 g/kg/day) and even cases of rickets due to soy milk consumption not enriched with vitamin D in cases with suspected food allergy.

 ## Follow-Up

A prolonged elimination diet is usually not necessary. Tolerance to allergens usually develops over time. In one study, 28% were tolerant at 2 years, 56% by 4 years, and 78% by 6 years. IgE-mediated disease tends to persist longer. Even children with a history of severe allergic reactions will most likely eventually outgrow them.

 ## Common Questions and Answers

Q: Do you recommend elimination diets?
A: No, because doing so often can result in malnutrition without identifying the exact allergen in any specific circumstance. Double-blinded food challenges are the best way to identify the offending agent.

Q: What are the common allergens?
A: Most initial blood tests will screen for allergy to milk, egg, soy, chocolate, fish, nuts, and egg white.

ICD-9-CM 693.1

BIBLIOGRAPHY

Bischoff SC. Mucosal allergy: role of mast cells and eosinophil granulocytes in the gut. *Baillieres Clin Gastroenterol* 1996;10(3):443–459.

Bischoff SC, Herrmann A, Manns MP. Prevalence of adverse reactions to food in patients with gastrointestinal disease. *Allergy* 1996;51:811–818.

Bishop JM, Hill DJ, Hosking CS. Natural history of cow's milk allergy: clinical outcome. *J Pediatr* 1990;116:862–867.

Bock A, Sampson H. Food allergy in infancy. *Pediatr Clin North Am* 1994;41(5):1047–1067.

Burks AW, Sampson HA. Diagnostic approaches to the patient with suspected food allergies. *J Pediatr* 1992;121:S64–S71.

Odze RD, Wershil BK, Leichter AM, et al. Allergic colitis in infants. *J Pediatr* 1995;126(2):163–170.

Sampson HA, McCaskill CC. Food hypersensitivity and atopic dermatitis: evaluation of 113 patients. *J Pediatr* 1985;107:669–675.

Young E, Stoneham MD, Petruchevitch A, et al. A population study of food intolerance. *Lancet* 1994;343:1127–1130.

Author: Dror Wasserman
Donna Zeiter, 2nd edition

Food Poisoning

 Database

DEFINITION

Rapid onset of diarrhea, vomiting, and fever 12 to 72 hours after the ingestion of contaminated food

CAUSES

- See the table Epidemiologic Aspects of Food Poisoning in Section VIII.
- Variety of bacteria: most common are *Campylobacter, Salmonella* (nontyphoid), and *Shigella.*

PATHOLOGY

- Ingestion of preformed toxin
- Elaboration of toxin from bacteria into the gastrointestinal tract
- Direct invasion of mucosa by bacteria

EPIDEMIOLOGY

At least 300 outbreaks of food-borne disease are reported each year.

 Differential Diagnosis

INFECTION

- Parental infections

—Upper respiratory tract
—Urinary tract infections
—Otitis media

- *Escherichia coli*
- *Vibrio*
- *Clostridium difficile*
- *Yersinia enterocolitica*
- *Aeromonas hydrophilia*
- *Giardia lamblia*
- *Entamoeba histolytica*
- Rotavirus
- *Campylobacter jejuni*, most common
- Listerosis
- Vibriosis
- Yersinia

FOOD INTOLERANCE/FOOD ALLERGIES

- Cow's milk protein allergy
- Carbohydrate intolerance (most common is lactose)

MISCELLANEOUS

- Use of antibiotics
- Malnutrition

—Altered mucosal structure
—Defective disaccharidase activity
—Abnormal motility
—Changed intestinal bacterial flora

DIETARY MANIPULATIONS

- Hyperosmolar formulas
- Food additives (dyes, processing materials, coloring)
- Caffeine
- Overfeeding
- Low fat intakes (especially during recovery phase)
- Excessive fluids

 Data Gathering

HISTORY

- Outbreak of illness following ingestion of a meal
- Others in family with similar symptoms
- Time of onset of vomiting after ingestion—relates to type of bacterial toxins (see the table Clinical Aspects of Food Poisoning in Section VIII)
- *E. coli, Campylobacter,* and *Salmonella* are more frequent in summer months

 Physical Examination

- See the table Clinical Aspects of Food Poisoning in Section VIII
- Botulism

—Severity related to host susceptibility and to amount of toxin ingested
—Disease may be so mild that consultation is not obtained; in other cases, it is fatal within a few hours.
—Generalized hypotonia
—Absent deep tendon reflexes
—Dilated, reactive pupils
—Poor suck
—Decreased to absent gag reflex
—Ptosis

 Laboratory Aids

TESTS

- Isolation of the organism from stools and the suspected food
- Demonstrating the toxin in the suspected food
- Identifying 10^5 organisms per gram of suspected food
- Finding 10^6 organisms or spores per gram of patient's stool or vomitus
- Lesions on the hands of food handlers may be the source of contamination and should be cultured.

Botulism

- Toxin in stools is diagnostic.
- Stool culture for *Clostridium botulinum*
- Electromyography with repetitive stimulation
- Lumbar puncture to exclude other diagnoses

Enterohemorrhagic E. coli 0157:H7

- Latex agglutination test

 Therapy

- No specific treatment
- Intramuscular antiemetics
- If clinically dehydrated, rehydration can be accomplished in 4 to 6 hours, using an oral solution containing 75 to 90 mEq Na/L.
- IV fluids for patients unable to be rehydrated via the oral route (because of ileus, circulatory failure, CNS complications), or with stool losses greater than 10 mL/kg/hr
- Most foods (except for lactose) should be tolerated in the pediatric patient recovering from food poisoning.
- The BRATT diet (bananas, rice, applesauce, toast, tea) is inappropriate for the management of acute diarrheal episodes, due to low calorie, protein, and fat contents.
- A balanced, varied diet, providing easily digestible, complex carbohydrates, will promote increased stool consistency.

DRUGS

Antibiotics

Salmonella

- Not used in patients with uncomplicated gastroenteritis
- Does not shorten the duration of the disease
- Can prolong the duration of excretion of *Salmonella* organisms
- Antimicrobial therapy is warranted for *Salmonella* gastroenteritis occurring in patients with an increased risk of invasive disease and other complications:

—Infants under 3 months of age
—Patients with malignancies
—Hemoglobinopathies
—AIDS
—Recipients of immunosuppressive therapy
—Persons with chronic gastrointestinal tract disease
—Patients with severe colitis

- Ampicillin, amoxicillin, trimethoprim-sulfamethoxazole, cefotaxime, or ceftriaxone is recommended for susceptible strains in patients for whom therapy is recommended.

Botulism

- Supportive care
- Monitor cardiac and respiratory function.
- Endotracheal intubation and assisted ventilation
- Avoid aminoglycosides.

 Follow-Up

PROGNOSIS

- Most gastroenteritis secondary to food poisoning is mild and self-limited.
- Recovery is complete in 2 to 5 days in most individuals.
- In the very young, the prognosis is more guarded, because these patients can become dehydrated quickly.
- Once the patient has survived the paralytic phase of botulism, the outlook for complete recovery is excellent.

PREVENTION

- Parenteral vaccines are not recommended for use in children.
- Botulism in infants, 1 year:

—Wash objects placed in infants' mouths (pacifiers, toys, etc.).
—Wash or peel skin of fruits and vegetables.
—Avoid honey.

 Common Questions and Answers

Q: What are the most common causes of food poisoning?
A: Bacteria (*Salmonella, Staphylococcus*).

Q: How are the signs and symptoms of food poisoning different from a viral gastroenteritis?
A: The signs and symptoms of food poisoning and gastroenteritis are similar in that the patient displays diarrhea, vomiting, and fever. Usually, food poisoning occurs after ingestion of a meal, at which time several people can be affected.

Q: Which foods are most likely to be contaminated?
A: Dairy products that are not refrigerated properly and meat that is not cooked at high enough temperatures.

ICD-9-CM 005.9

BIBLIOGRAPHY

Salmonella infections, staphylococcal infections. *2000 red book: report of the Committee on Infectious Diseases* , 25th ed. Elk Grove Village, IL: American Academy of Pediatrics, 2000.

Todd EC. Epidemiology of food-borne diseases: a worldwide review. *World Health Stat Q* 50(1–2):30–50.

Wolfle J, Kowalewski S. Epidemiology of ingestions in a regional poison control center over twenty years. *Vet Hum Toxicol* 1995;37(4):367–368.

Authors: Timothy A. S. Sentongo and Andrew E. Mulberg

Frostbite

 ## Database

DEFINITION
Frostbite is localized injury of the epidermis and underlying tissue resulting from exposure to extreme cold or contact with extremely cold objects. Distal extremities and unprotected areas (fingers, toes, ears, nose, and chin) are most commonly affected. Frostbite is classified according to severity:
- Superficial, first degree: partial skin freezing
- Superficial, second degree: full-thickness skin freezing
- Deep, third degree: full-thickness skin and subcutaneous tissue freezing
- Deep, fourth degree: full-thickness skin, subcutaneous tissue, muscle, tendon and bone freezing

PATHOPHYSIOLOGY
- Tissue damage and cell death result from the initial freeze injury and the inflammatory response that occurs with rewarming.
- Direct cellular damage can occur from frostbite. As the temperature of freezing tissue approaches $-2°C$, extracellular ice crystals form and cause increased osmotic pressure in the interstitium. This leads to cellular dehydration. As freezing continues, these shrinking, hyperosmolar cells die due to abnormal intracellular electrolyte concentrations. With rapid freezing, intracellular ice crystal formation occurs, resulting in immediate cell death.
- Indirect cellular damage results from progressive microvascular insult. Initial tissue response to extreme cold exposure is vasoconstriction. Blood flow to the extremities is reduced as freezing continues. Ice crystals form in the plasma, blood viscosity increases, and cessation of circulation occurs in the distal extremities, resulting in hypoxia and tissue damage.
- Oxygen free radicals and inflammatory mediators, especially prostaglandin F_2 and thromboxane A_2, contribute to tissue injury following rewarming and reperfusion of the damaged tissue.

EPIDEMIOLOGY
- Frostbite is most common in adults aged 30 to 49 years.
- More common in men than women by ratio of 10:1
- The feet and hands account for 90% of frostbite injuries.
- The following groups are at risk:
—Mentally ill patients
—Patients with impaired circulation
—Winter sports enthusiasts and fans
—Homeless persons
—Malnourished people
—Outdoor laborers
—Military personnel exposed to cold, wet climates
—The elderly
—Very young patients

- Risk factors include:
—Alcohol
—Arthritis
—Atherosclerosis
—Constricting clothing
—Diabetes
—Hypothermia
—Immobilization
—Improper use of aerosol sprays
—Previous cold injury
—Smoking
—Vasoconstrictive drugs

COMPLICATIONS
- Amputations
- Arthritis
- Changes in skin color
- Chronic pain
- Digital deformities
- Gangrene
- Growth plate abnormalities (only in children)
- Hyperesthesias
- Squamous cell carcinoma (rare)
- Tetanus
- Tissue loss
- Wound infection

PROGNOSIS
- Dependent on degree of cold injury
- Favorable indicators: sensation in affected area, healthy-appearing skin color, blisters filled with clear fluid
- Unfavorable indicators: cyanosis, blood-filled blisters, unhealthy-appearing skin

 ## Differential Diagnosis

- Frostnip: mild form of cold injury with pallor and painful, tingling sensation. Warming of the cold tissue results in no tissue damage.
- Hypothermia
- Thermal injury: easily excluded based on history, but can result from warming techniques.

 ## Data Gathering

HISTORY
Special Questions
- Was there prolonged exposure to cold environment? In frostbite, there is typically a history of prolonged cold exposure.
- Was there contact with a cold object, especially metal? Metal will drain heat from skin through conduction and increase the risk of frostbite.
- What was the timing and duration of exposure?
- Was there any treatment prior to presentation?
Symptoms depend on severity:
- Superficial, first degree: transient tingling, stinging, and burning followed by throbbing and aching with possible hyperhidrosis
- Superficial, second degree: numbness with vasomotor disturbances in more severe cases

- Deep, third degree: no sensation initially, followed by shooting pains, burning, throbbing, and aching
- Deep, fourth degree: absent sensation and muscle function, pain, and joint discomfort

 ## Physical Examination

- Superficial, first degree: waxy appearance, erythema, and edema of involved area without blister formation.
- Superficial, second degree: erythema, significant edema, blisters with clear fluid within 6 to 24 hours. Desquamation may occur with eschar formation 7 to 14 days after initial injury.
- Deep, third degree: hemorrhagic blisters, necrosis of the skin and subcutaneous tissues, skin discoloration in 5 to 10 days.
- Deep, fourth degree: initially, little edema with cyanosis or mottling; eventually, complete necrosis, then becomes black, dry, and mummifies; occasionally results in self-amputation.

 ## Laboratory Aids

TESTS
Laboratory tests usually are not necessary but may be indicated when infection is suspected.

Radiographic Studies
- No diagnostic studies done immediately after rewarming can accurately predict the amount of nonviable tissue.
- Radionucleotide angiography with 99m-Tc-pertechnetate or bone scanning with 99m-Tc-methylene diphosphonate 1 to 2 weeks after initial injury is advocated by some to assess tissue viability in cases of third- and fourth-degree frostbite.
- MRI and magnetic resonance angiography are being advocated by some as superior techniques. These techniques allow direct visualization of occluded vessels and tissue giving a more clear-cut demarcation of ischemic tissue injury. This may allow for earlier surgical intervention.

 ## Therapy

IMMEDIATE
- Do not rub the area; this may cause mechanical injury.
- Do not expose the area to direct heat; this may cause burn injury.
- Remove wet clothing and constricting jewelry.

MEDICAL CARE
- Check core temperature to rule out hypothermia, which would need to be addressed first.

- Rapid rewarming in warm water (40°–42°C) for 15 to 45 minutes. *Do not* rewarm slowly. Rewarming is complete when skin is soft and sensation returns. Usually this is all that is needed for superficial, first-degree frostbite.
- Apply dry, sterile dressings to affected areas and between frostbitten toes and fingers.
- Drain clear-fluid blisters (thromboxane-containing) to avoid ongoing tissue injury.
- Leave hemorrhagic blisters intact to avoid infection.
- Elevate affected parts to minimize edema.
- Daily hydrotherapy with hexachlorophene or povidone-iodine added to the water.
- Topical application of aloe vera to débrided blisters and intact hemorrhagic blisters to minimize further thromboxane synthesis.
- Tetanus prophylaxis: dT or DT, depending on age, and tetanus immunoglobulin if patient never fully immunized.
- NSAIDs are recommended by some to prevent prostaglandin-induced platelet aggregation and vasoconstriction.
- Analgesics, as indicated.
- Antibiotics: given prophylactically by some, while others recommend waiting for signs of infection.
- High-protein, high-calorie diet to promote healing.
- Prohibit nicotine because of vasoconstrictive properties.
- Physical therapy after edema resolves.

SURGICAL CARE
- Conservative surgical intervention is recommended because it usually takes 6 to 8 weeks for injured tissue to declare viability.
- Escharotomy is performed on digits with impaired circulation or movement.
- Fasciotomy is performed if significant edema causes a compartment syndrome.
- Early amputation and débridement with closure of the wound site are necessary for uncontrolled infection.
- Débridement of mummified tissue is performed after 1 to 3 months.

FUTURE TREATMENT
Experimental work is being done to identify agents that interrupt vasoconstriction, cell injury, and vascular stasis and those that inhibit prostaglandins and free radicals.

 Follow-Up

WHEN TO EXPECT IMPROVEMENT
- Superficial, first-degree frostbite heals in a few weeks.
- More severe frostbite needs to be followed closely for signs of infection.
- Physical therapy and rehabilitation are needed with severe frostbite.

PREVENTION
- Avoid prolonged cold exposure whenever possible.
- Dress appropriately for cold weather. Dress in layers: Undergarments should be made of material that absorbs perspiration and prevents heat loss, and outer garments should be windproof and water repellent/proof. Cover head, ears, and neck. Mittens help conserve heat better than gloves. Footwear should be water repellent and insulated.

PITFALLS
- Refreezing after thawing leads to increased injury.
- Rubbing tissue that is frostbitten increases injury through mechanical injury.

 Common Questions and Answers

Q: How can I protect my child from getting frostbite?
A: Limit the amount of time the child spends outdoors during extremely cold days–especially wet, cold, and windy days. Dress your child appropriately with layers of clothing. Outer garments should be waterproof. Make sure he or she is wearing a hat, scarf, and mittens. Have the child come inside frequently to warm up and for you to check for signs of cold injury.

Q: Can the protective emollients that are sold in Europe prevent frostbite if used on the face and exposed areas?
A: No, research has shown that the use of "protective" emollients and creams leads to a false sense of safety and leads to an increased risk of frostbite. This is thought to be mostly due to the lack of using more efficient protective measures when the emollients and creams are used.

Q: If my child has had frostbite in the past, can she get it again?
A: Yes, children who have had a previous frostbite injury are at increased risk for repeat injury, especially in the location of previous damage. Appropriate clothing and limitation of cold exposure should be strictly enforced.

Q: To prevent frostbite, is there any temperature below which I should not let my child go out to play?
A: Though body tissue freezes more quickly at lower temperatures, the degree of damage from frostbite is related to the length of time tissue remains frozen. Therefore, the amount of time spent outside during cold weather should never be prolonged.

Q: How can I tell if my child has frostbite or just cold fingers?
A: Cold fingers are red and may be painful but do not become numb or white. Frostbitten fingers are painful, white, and waxy prior to rewarming and turn red with rewarming. The sequential development of digital blanching, occasional cyanosis, and erythema of the fingers or toes following cold exposure and subsequent rewarming is known as Raynaud's phenomenon. All types of cold injury should be treated by immersing the fingers in warm water for 15 to 45 minutes. If blisters form or there is no sensation in the fingers, medical care is needed.

Q: If I suspect frostbite in my child and we are stuck outdoors without access to warm water, are there any options for treatment?
A: Of course you would want to get indoors as soon as possible. If that is not possible, you can start to thaw your child's body part by using your body as a warmer, by placing the exposed body part under your armpit and keeping it there until further care can be initiated.

Q: When should I call the doctor?
A: The doctor should be called if, after rewarming, the skin is not soft and/or sensation does not return to normal. Call the doctor immediately if the skin is discolored and cold, blisters develop during rewarming, or there are signs of infection, such as the appearance of red streaks leading from the affected area, pus accumulation, or fever.

Q: What is chilblain?
A: Chilblain is a severe form of cold injury that commonly occurs on the face, anterior tibial surfaces, and dorsum of hands. It is a form of chronic vasculitis of the dermis that is provoked by repeated exposure to cold temperatures above freezing.

Q: Is frostnip the same thing as frostbite?
A: No, frostnip is the mildest form of cold injury that commonly occurs on exposed parts of the body, such as the fingers, nose, and ears. The symptoms of frostnip are numbness and pallor of the involved body parts. Warming of these areas is the only treatment that is needed, and there is no associated tissue damage.

ICD-9-CM 991.3

BIBLIOGRAPHY
Bracker MD. Environmental and thermal injury. *Clin Sports Med* 1992;2:419–436.

Britt LD, Dascombe WH, Rodriguez A. New horizons in management of hypothermia and frostbite injury. *Surg Clin North Am* 1991;71:345–370.

Holmer I. Work in the cold: review of methods for assessment of cold exposure. *Int Arch Occup Environ Health* 1993;65:147–155.

Lehmuskallio E. Emollients in the prevention of frostbite. *Int J Circumpolar Health* 2000;59(2):122–130.

Murphy J, Banwell PE, Roberts AH, et al. Frostbite: pathogenesis and treatment. *J Trauma* 2000;48:171–185.

Reamy BV. Frostbite: review and current concepts. *J Am Board Fam Pract* 1998;11: 34–40.

Author: Denise A. Salerno

Fungal Skin Infections
(Dermatophyte Infections, Candidiasis, and Tinea Versicolor)

 Database

DEFINITION
• Superficial mycoses (fungal infection) involving the skin, hair, or nails

ETIOLOGY
• Dermatophyte infections
—Tinea capitis: >90% *Trichophyton tonsurans* in North America; *Microsporum canis* is a predominant organism in other geographic regions.
—Nonhairy sites: *M. canis, T. tonsurans, T. rubrum, M. audouinii*
• Candidiasis: usually *Candida albicans*
• Tinea versicolor: *Malassezia furfur* (also called *Pityrosporum ovale*)

PATHOPHYSIOLOGY
• Fungal elements penetrate skin, hair shaft, or nail.
• Predisposing factors may include moisture, macerated skin, and immune compromise.
• Fungistatic fatty acids in sebum after puberty may offer protection against tinea capitis.
• Host immune response is usually able to contain infection.
• Inflammatory response is variable; highly inflammatory forms may lead to pustular lesions and kerion (a large inflammatory mass) formation.

GENETICS
• Frequency and severity of infection are possibly determined by unclear genetic factors.
• Increased glycogen granules in the normal skin of patients with tinea versicolor suggest an underlying disorder or genetic predisposition.

EPIDEMIOLOGY
• Dermatophyte infections
—Etiology varies by geographic region.
—Tinea capitis is most common in prepubertal children, peak age about 4 years. More common in African-American children. Incidence has increased over the past decade.
—Tinea corporis is usually seen in younger children; tinea cruris, tinea pedis, and onychomycosis are uncommon in preadolescent children.
—Fomites and pets may be a source of infection. Cats and dogs are a major source of *M. canis*.
• Candidiasis: vast majority of infants colonized with *C. albicans*.
• Tinea versicolor: usually seen in adolescents and young adults

COMPLICATIONS
• Dermatophyte infections
—Secondary bacterial infection (which may obscure the diagnosis of dermatophyte infection)
—Kerion may lead to scarring alopecia.
• Candidiasis
—Scarring in severe disease
—Fungemia in immunocompromised host

 Differential Diagnosis

• Dermatophyte infections
—Dermatologic conditions
—Tinea capitis: seborrheic dermatitis, psoriasis, alopecia areata, trichotillomania, folliculitis, impetigo, atopic dermatitis
—Tinea corporis: herald patch of pityriasis rosea, nummular eczema, psoriasis, contact dermatitis, tinea versicolor, granuloma annulare
—Systemic diseases: cutaneous T-cell lymphoma, histiocytosis, primary skin cancer, sarcoid
• Candidiasis
—Dermatologic conditions: contact dermatitis, seborrheic dermatitis, atopic dermatitis, bacterial infection
—Systemic diseases: acrodermatitis enteropathica, histiocytosis
• Tinea versicolor
—Dermatologic conditions: pityriasis alba, postinflammatory hypopigmentation, vitiligo, seborrheic dermatitis, pityriasis rosea

PROGNOSIS
• Relapses and recurrences are not uncommon.
• Areas with a significant inflammatory component may lead to scarring and permanent alopecia.

 Data Gathering

HISTORY
• Onset is usually gradual, except for candidal diaper rash, which is often abrupt
• Usually pruritic
• Contacts including exposure to pets
• Immunocompromised state
• Medications

Physical Examination

• Dermatophyte infections
—Tinea corporis
—Skin lesions usually annular, hence the term *ringworm*
—May be flesh-colored, erythematous, or violet to brown
—Highly inflammatory forms may be frankly pustular.
—Tinea capitis may have various presentations:
—Round to oval patches of alopecia with erythema
—Seborrheic dermatitis-like pattern with minimal or no alopecia
—Follicular pustules with crusting, resembling bacterial folliculitis
—Boggy, tender plaque with follicular pustules (kerion)
—Diffusely, dry scalp
—Presence of occipital lymphadenopathy may be more likely in tinea capitis.

—Onychomycosis
—White, yellow, or silvery discoloration of lateral border or distal portion of nail
—Nail eventually becomes discolored, thickened, and deformed.
—Affects toes more often than fingers
• Candidiasis
—Diffuse erythema (often "beefy" red)
—Raised edge with a sharp margin
—Pustulovesicular, satellite lesions
—Prefers dark, warm, moist environments; favors skin folds/creases (axillae, groin, below the breasts, and in infants, the diaper area)
• Tinea versicolor
—Scaling, oval macular patches
—Hypopigmented or hyperpigmented, depending on sunlight exposure and complexion
—Distributed on upper trunk, neck, and proximal arms (high amount of sebum and free fatty acids which the organism requires); occasionally occurs on the face

 Laboratory Aids

TESTS
Diagnosis is usually made by characteristic lesions; if in doubt, may do Wood's lamp examination, potassium hydroxide (KOH) preparation, or fungal culture.

Wood's Lamp Examination (Short-Wave Ultraviolet Light)
• Examine in a completely darkened room.
• Dermatophytes: Hair infections caused by *Microsporum* species will give a green fluorescence but *Trichophyton* does not fluoresce; not helpful for skin or nail infections.
• Tinea versicolor: yellow, coppery-orange, or bronze fluorescence.

KOH Preparation
• Clean the site with alcohol.
• Scrape the lesion along the scaling edge with a blade; obtain material from hair follicles and crusts.
• Place material on glass slide with one drop of 10% KOH.
• Warm the slide gently or let it sit for 30 minutes.
• Place a cover slip on the slide.
• Examine the slide under the microscope at low power under low light.

Results
• Dermatophytes: arthrospores around or within hair shaft; long branching hyphae for skin infections
• Candidiasis: budding yeast, pseudohyphae
• Tinea versicolor: hyphae and spores ("spaghetti and meatballs")

Fungal Culture
- Obtain a specimen with scalpel blade as described above.
- For the scalp, a sample obtained by scrubbing a toothbrush over the dry scalp or area of concern can be plated on the appropriate media.
- Results are available in several weeks.
- Some laboratories offer susceptibilities in addition to identification of fungus.
- It may be difficult to distinguish normal skin colonization from infection.

Therapy

DRUGS
Dermatophyte Infections
- Tinea capitis
—First line: griseofulvin 15 to 25 mg/kg once daily, taken with high-fat food (e.g., milk or ice cream) for 6 to 12 weeks; concomitant therapy of 2.5% selenium sulfide shampoo twice weekly will suppress viable spores and decrease spread.
—Second line: itraconazole 3 to 5 mg/kg once daily for 4 to 6 weeks.
—Kerion: treat as tinea capitis; may require oral steroids if significant inflammation present.
- Tinea corporis
—Drug of choice: topical imidazole applied twice daily for 2 to 4 weeks.
—Oral therapy may be used for persistent or extensive involvement.
- Onychomycosis
—Griseofulvin orally for 6 to 18 months (6 months for fingernails and 12–18 months for toenails)
—Itraconazole in weekly pulses for 3 to 4 months is effective; 200 mg twice daily for 7 days, then off for 3 weeks.
—Terbinafine 3 to 6 mg/kg/day for 6 to 12 weeks. May be associated with hepatic failure; should not be used in patients with underlying liver disease. Strongly consider liver enzymes before and after treatment.

Candidiasis
- Topical nystatin three to four times daily for 7 to 10 days

Tinea Versicolor
- Selenium sulfide 2.5% applied to the affected skin for 10 minutes. Wash off thoroughly. Monthly applications may help prevent recurrences.
- Topical imidazoles are effective but more expensive.
- Oral ketoconazole 200 to 400 mg/d for 5 to 10 days, or itraconazole 200 mg/d for 5 to 7 days may be used if extensive, recurrent, or persistent.

POSSIBLE CONFLICTS WITH OTHER TREATMENTS
Many antifungals have drug interactions. Consult a reference (e.g., *Physician's Desk Reference*) when prescribing them to a patient already on medication.

Follow-Up

WHEN TO EXPECT IMPROVEMENT
- Dermatophyte: Inflammation should improve within several days, but may take several weeks to completely resolve; nail infections may take 6 to 12 months to show improvement.
- Candidal skin lesions improve within 24 to 48 hours and resolve by 1 week.
- Tinea versicolor may take weeks to improve; repigmentation may take months and requires exposure to sunlight.

SIGNS TO WATCH FOR
- Watch for signs of secondary bacterial infection.
- Highly inflammatory lesions may require systemic steroids.

PREVENTION
- Children should be discouraged from sharing clothing (especially hats).
- Hair utensils and hats should be washed in hot, soapy water at the onset of therapy.
- Pets should be watched and treated early for any suspicious lesions.
- Isolation of the hospitalized patient is not necessary.

PITFALLS
- Tinea capitis requires systemic therapy.
- Application of topical steroids will decrease inflammation and may mask infection ("tinea incognito"). Use only mild steroids, if necessary.
- Repeated infection may indicate a source that needs to be diagnosed and treated (e.g., family member or pet).
- Systemic therapies associated with elevated hepatic enzymes and hepatic failure. Terbinafine should not be used in patients with underlying liver disease.

Common Questions and Answers

Q: What is the role of topical and systemic steroids in the treatment of dermatophyte infections?
A: Topical corticosteroids may be helpful with antifungal therapy to reduce inflammation for skin infections. Only mildly potent steroids should be used. Combination products containing a potent corticosteroid and an antifungal should be avoided, especially in the diaper area, where absorption may be increased. For tinea capitis, significant inflammation and kerion formation may benefit from a short course of systemic steroids. Reducing the inflammation with steroids may help prevent scarring alopecia.

Q: What can be done to prevent recurrent tinea versicolor in an adolescent?
A: *M. furfur* is a ubiquitous organism and is present on the skin of postpubertal individuals. Humid environments, excessive sweating, and unclear genetic factors result in infection. Recurrences are common and can be prevented by monthly application of selenium sulfide 2.5%.

Q: What is the role of the newer antifungal agents in the treatment of tinea capitis?
A: Griseofulvin has long been considered the gold standard for the treatment of tinea capitis due to its efficacy and safety profile. Development of resistance to griseofulvin has required the use of larger doses and longer courses. This increases the likelihood of noncompliance and treatment failures. In addition, longer courses increase the cost of griseofulvin therapy. The newer antifungals, terbinafine and itraconazole, offer some advantages over griseofulvin. Concentration of these drugs in nails and hair may allow for shorter courses of therapy, with improved compliance and lower cost than griseofulvin. Although still considered by many to be the preferred drug for tinea capitis, griseofulvin is likely to be replaced by these newer antifungals as experience with their uses increases.

ICD-9-CM
Dermatophyte 110.9
Candidiasis 112.9
Tinea Versicolor 111.0

BIBLIOGRAPHY
Elewski BE. Tinea capitis: a current perspective. *J Am Acad Dermatol* 2000;42:1–20.

Friedlander SF. The evolving role of itraconazole, fluconazole and terbinafine in the treatment of tinea capitis. *Pediatr Infect Dis J* 1999;18:205–210.

Goldgeier M. Fungal infections of the skin, hair and nails. *Pediatr Ann* 1993;22:253–259.

Hurwitz S. *Clinical pediatric dermatology*. Philadelphia: WB Saunders, 1993:372–90.

Smith M. Tinea capitis. *Pediatr Ann* 1996;25:101–105.

Suarez S. New antifungal therapy for children. *Adv Dermatol* 1997;12:195–209.

Authors: William R. Graessle and Jill A. Foster

Gastritis

 Database

DEFINITION

Gastritis is inflammation of the mucosa of the stomach. It is the most common cause of upper gastrointestinal tract hemorrhage in older children.

CAUSES

- *Helicobacter pylori* (children more likely to have more severe gastritis, specifically located in antrum of stomach)
- Physiologic stress (e.g., in CNS disease, ICU patients)
- Major surgery, severe burns, renal, liver, respiratory failure
- Idiopathic
- Caustic ingestions (e.g., lye, strong acids, pine oil)
- Drug-induced [e.g., nonsteroidal antiinflammatory drugs (NSAIDs), steroids, valproate]
- Ethanol
- Protein sensitivity (e.g., cow's-milk protein allergy)
- Eosinophilic gastroenteritis
- Crohn disease
- Infection (e.g., tuberculosis, *H. pylori*, cytomegalovirus, parasites)

Less Common Causes

- Radiation
- Vascular injury
- Direct trauma (nasogastric tubes)

EPIDEMIOLOGY

- One of the most frequent GI diagnoses
- 8 out of every 1,000 people
- >2% ICU patients have heavy bleeding secondary to gastritis.

COMPLICATIONS

- Bleeding (from mild to hemorrhagic)
- When gastritis caused by acid/alkali ingestions, outlet obstruction may result from prepyloric strictures.

 Differential Diagnosis

- Peptic ulcer disease
- Gastroesophageal reflux with esophagitis
- Pancreatitis
- Inflammatory bowel disease
- Lactose intolerance

 Data Gathering

HISTORY

- Epigastric pain
- Abdominal indigestion
- Nausea
- Vomiting postprandially
- Vomiting blood, coffee-ground like material
- Diarrhea
- Dark or black stools
- Irritability
- Poor feeding and weight loss
- Less often: chest pain, hematemesis, or melena

 Physical Examination

- Epigastric tenderness upper left quadrant
- Normal bowel sounds

 Laboratory Aids

TESTS

- Heme-test all stools.
- Anemia with other signs of chronic blood loss on CBC (e.g., microcytosis, low reticulocyte count)
- *H. pylori* antibody
- Culture of homogenized gastric biopsy for *H. pylori*
- Silver or hematoxylin and eosin stain of gastric biopsy for *H. pylori*

PROCEDURES

- Upper endoscopy with biopsies: sensitivity greatest
- Edema around small ulcers
- Thickened hyperemic mucosa
- Atrophic mucosa
- When endoscopy not available, upper GI radiography
- Chest x-ray may detect free abdominal air secondary to perforations

Gastritis

 Therapy

DRUGS

• Antacids or H$_2$ blockers to maintain gastric pH greater than 4

—Ranitidine, 2 to 3 mg/kg t.i.d. in children
—Cimetidine, 10 mg/kg q.i.d. (can be used prophylactically for hospitalized patients at risk for physiologic stress)
—Famotidine, 0.5 to 2.0 mg/kg/d divided twice
—Omeprazole, lansoprazole, esomeprazole (Nexium) for resistant cases

• Misoprostol may reduce risk of the progression of gastritis to ulcers in NSAID patients.
• Discontinue NSAIDs.

DIET

• Benefit of changes in diet is inconclusive.
• Eliminate alcohol, tobacco, and caffeine.
• Stress gastritis with hemorrhage
• Vigilant supportive care with close monitoring of hemodynamics, fluids, and electrolytes
• H. pylori

—Triple therapy with proton pump inhibitor, i.e., omeprazole, amoxicillin, and clarithromycin
—If symptoms persist, amoxicillin, bismuth, and metronidazole for 10 days
—Drug regimens change frequently.

 Follow-Up

• Monitor for Hemoccult-positive stools.
• Follow complete blood counts.
• May elect to repeat endoscopy in severe cases.

PITFALLS

• Antacids are not palatable to children and can lead to diarrhea or constipation.
• Ranitidine is less effective and can increase toxicity when given to patients receiving other medicines metabolized by the cytochrome P-450 system (e.g., theophylline).
• Significant relapse rates for H. pylori

 Common Questions and Answers

Q: Will a bland diet help to resolve gastritis?
A: Dietary changes have not been shown to affect the natural course of gastritis.

Q: What is Helicobacter pylori?
A: H. pylori is a bacterium frequently found in the gastric mucosa of patients with gastritis and peptic ulcer disease. Relapse rates for gastritis secondary to this cause are high and can be diagnosed by a combination of upper endoscopy and urea breath tests.

ICD-9-CM 558.9

BIBLIOGRAPHY

Berquist WE. New, improved Helicobacter pylori eradication therapy in children. J Pediatr Gastroenterol Nutr 1998;26(3):360–361.

Cox K, Ament ME. Upper gastrointestinal bleeding in children and adolescents. Pediatrics 1979;63:408–413.

Czinn SJ. Helicobacter pylori gastroduodenal disease in infants and children. In: Wyllie R, Hyams JS, eds. Pediatric gastrointestinal disease. Philadelphia: WB Saunders, 1993:429, 434.

Eule AR. Gastritis. In: Wyllie R, Hyams JS, eds. Pediatric gastrointestinal disease. Philadelphia: WB Saunders, 1993:435–446.

Hassall E, Dimmidk JE. Unique features of Helicobacter pylori disease in children. Dig Dis Sci 1991;36:417–423.

The Merck manual of diagnosis and therapy. Section 3. Gastrointestinal disorders. Chapter 23. Gastritis and peptic ulcer disease. http://www.merck.com/pubs/mmanual/section3/chapter 23/23b.htm.

The Merck manual of medical information, home edition. Whitehouse Station, NJ: Merck Research Labs; 1997:102.

Radiology Museum. Gastritis 72-291. Available at http://www.sbu.ac.uk/~dirt/museum/p72-291.html.

Shayne P. Gastritis and peptic ulcer disease from emergency medicine. February 25, 2001. http://www.emedicine.com/emerg/topic 820.htm.

Authors: Rebecca Kraynak and Andrew E. Mulberg

Gastroesophageal Reflux

 Database

DEFINITION

Gastroesophageal reflux (GER) is defined as effortless regurgitation of gastric contents; it is extremely common in infants. GER occurs physiologically at all ages, and most episodes are brief and asymptomatic. It is important to identify the rare child with pathologic reflux, to perform the appropriate diagnostic studies, and to start effective therapy.

• GER is divided into a pathologic and a physiologic processes. Physiologic reflux (the normal GER of infancy) is the more common form. Most infants eventually outgrow the symptoms by the end of the first year of life. Pathologic reflux is defined by increased number of episodes according to age-accepted norms. Complicated GER is pathologic reflux associated with complications such as irritability, pain, esophagitis, blood loss, esophageal stricture, failure to thrive, reactive airway disease, near-miss SIDS, or aspiration pneumonia.
• GER may be asymptomatic and still carry the risk of complications. GER is the most common cause of vomiting in infancy but many etiologies of vomiting are associated with other conditions and may be associated with medically significant diseases.

 Differential Diagnosis

Not all pediatric vomiting is reflux. Other causes of vomiting in infancy include:

• Infection

—Gastroenteritis
—Urinary tract infection
—Sepsis

• Neurologic

—Meningitis/encephalitis
—Intracranial injury
—Brain tumor
—Hydrocephalus
—Subdural hematoma

• Metabolic

—Uremia
—Aminoacidopathies
—Adrenal hyperplasia
—Phenylketonuria
—Galactosemia

• Food intolerance

—Milk/soy protein allergy
—Celiac disease

• Anatomic malformation

—Gastric-outlet obstruction
—Pyloric stenosis
—Volvulus/malrotation
—Esophageal atresia
—Meconium ileus
—Enteral duplications
—Intussusception
—Trichobezoar

DRUGS THAT AFFECT LOWER ESOPHAGEAL SPHINCTER PRESSURE

• Nitrates
• Nicotine
• Narcotics
• Theophylline
• Anticholinergic
• Estrogen
• Somatostatin
• Prostaglandins

 Data Gathering

HISTORY

• Should identify episodes of near-miss SIDS, aspiration pneumonia, chronic cough, laryngitis, stridor, and reactive airways disease.
• Should exclude bowel obstruction (bile in the emesis, polyhydramnios during pregnancy).
• If the vomiting begins after the first few weeks of life, it is important to rule out infection, metabolic diseases, allergy, and neurologic diseases.
• Pay attention to feeding volume and frequency in addition to weight gain and FTT and irritability.

Special Questions

• Presence of polyhydramnios?
• Bile in emesis?
• Family history of metabolic disease?
• Family history of allergies?
• Perinatal asphyxia (and other neurologic disorders)?
• History of prematurity, skin rash (atopic dermatitis), and reactive airways disease?
• Evidence of overfeeding?

 Physical Examination

• May be normal
• Growth failure
• Blood in the stool
• Reactive airways disease and other manifestations of pulmonary complications
• Anemia

Laboratory Aids

TESTS

Diagnosis of GER is made clinically. Testing is needed to identify potential causes or complications. Evaluation should include:

- Stool Hemoccult
- Growth parameters

Radiographic Studies

- Barium swallow, tracheoesophageal fistulogram
- Chest radiography
- Nuclear medicine studies
- Milk scan
- Gastric emptying study
- Salivagram

pH Probe

The gold standard for the evaluation of reflux; represents 24 hours of patient's life and correlates with symptoms

- Simple (single-channel)
- Double-channel
- pH/Thermistor (apnea) study

Endoscopy

- Esophagogastroduodenoscopy (EGD)
- Laryngoscopy
- Bronchoscopy

Manometric Studies

- Esophageal manometry
- Antroduodenal manometry

 Therapy

Several modes of therapy are available, depending on the severity, duration of reflux, and complications. The treatment should be individualized and should consider cost efficacy.
Most cases will respond to traditional treatment, reduction of overfeeding, positioning, thickening of meals:

- Small frequent feeds
- Thickening of the feeds (approximately 1 tablespoon cereal/ounce of formula)
- Positioning: head elevation
- Consider use of a hypoallergenic formula for patients with associated food allergy.

PROKINETIC THERAPY

- There is no single drug that has great prokinetic effect and minimal side effects:
- Cisapride use has been aborted in the U.S. but some recommendation for its use exist under special circumstances.
- Metoclopramide (Reglan), 0.1 mg/kg/dose q.i.d.
- Antacids

—Require multiple dosing, carry risk of diarrhea, and may also lead to malabsorption of other medications

- H_2 blockers

—Cimetidine (Tagamet), 10 to 12.5 mg/kg/dose q.i.d.
—Ranitidine (Zantac), 2 to 3 mg/kg/dose bid to t.i.d.
—Famotidine (Pepcid), 0.3 to 0.5 mg/kg/dose b.i.d.

- Proton pump inhibitors

—Omeprazole (Prilosec): 1.5 to 2 mg/kg/day divided b.i.d. in children younger than 2 years; ≥2 years: 10 mg starting dose
—Lansoprazole (Prevacid)

- Binding agents

—Sucralfate (Carafate): maximally effective at pH 4 and on mucosal lesions

- Medication interactions

—Reglan may cause oculogyric crisis.
—Antacids may lead to diarrhea and constipation.
—H_2 blockers may cause headache, rash, and diarrhea.

SURGERY AND REFLUX

- The goal of surgery is to increase lower esophageal sphincter tone by wrapping a portion of the cardia around the lower esophagus. This is done to prevent reflux mechanically. Usually, this is associated with a gastric-emptying procedure (i.e., pyloroplasty) and may include placement of a gastric tube.
- The indications for surgery include poor response to medications or in patients with complications (i.e., esophageal stricture, large and symptomatic diaphragmatic hernia, high-grade intestinal metaplastic changes, as in Barrett esophagus).
- Complications of fundoplication include retching, bowel obstruction, dumping syndrome, difficulty in feeding, paraesophageal hernia, sliding of the wrap, and recurrent GER. The surgery has greater morbidity associated with it in the cohort of children with severe physical and mental disabilities.

 Common Questions and Answers

Q: How long will my baby suffer with GER?
A: Most reflux resolve by 9 to 12 months of age. If GER persists after 1 year, it is highly likely that it is associated with an underlying pathology.

Q: Should all babies with reflux be treated with medication?
A: First try basic treatments of thickened feedings, frequent small feeds, and upright head position.

ICD-9-CM 530.81

BIBLIOGRAPHY

Israel DM, Hassall E. Omeprazole and other proton pump inhibitors: pharmacology, efficacy and safety, with special reference to use in children. *J Pediatr Gastroenterol Nutr* 1998;27:568–579.

Jolley S, Halpem L, Tunnell W, et al. The risk of sudden infant death from gastroesophageal reflux. *J Pediatr Surg* 1991;26:691–696.

Orenstein SR. Gastroesophageal reflux. *Curr Probl Pediatr* 1991;May/June:193–241.

Orenstein SR. Gastroesophageal reflux. In: Wyllie R, Hyams J, eds. *Pediatric gastrointestinal diseases*. Philadelphia: WB Saunders, 1993:337–369.

Pashankar D, Blair GK, Israel DM. Omeprazole maintenance therapy for gastroesophageal reflux disease after failure of fundoplication. *J Pediatr Gastroenterol Nutr* 2000;32:145–149.

Vandenplas Y, and the ESPGHAN cisapride panel. Current pediatric indications for cisapride. *J Pediatr Gastroenterol Nutr* 2000;31:480–489.

Author: Dror Wasserman

German Measles (Third Disease Rubella)

 Database

DEFINITION

Rubella is derived from Latin, meaning "little red," and was initially considered a variant of measles. Infection is characterized by mild symptoms (often subclinical), with an erythematous rash progressing from head to toes. Prevention of congenital rubella syndrome (see below) is the main objective of vaccination programs.

CAUSE

Rubella virus is classified in the togavirus family as from the genus *Rubivirus*.

- It is an RNA virus with a single antigenic type.
- It was first isolated in 1962 by Parkman and Weller.

PATHOPHYSIOLOGY

- Respiratory transmission
- Replication in the nasopharynx and regional lymph nodes
- Viremia 5 to 7 days after exposure with spread of the virus throughout the body
- In congenital rubella syndrome (CRS), transplanted infection of the fetus occurs during viremia.

EPIDEMIOLOGY

- Spread person to person via airborne transmission; a worldwide infection
- In temperate regions, incidence peaks in the late winter and early spring.
- Infection is most contagious when rash is erupting. However, the virus may be shed, beginning 7 days before the rash to 14 days after.
- Infants with CRS may shed virus for up to 1 year.
- In the prevaccine era, the incidence of infection in the United States was approximately 58 per 100,000 population.
- Currently, fewer than 1,000 cases per year are reported. In 1993, 192 cases were reported.
- Infection occurs equally in the following age groups: under 5 years, 5 to 19 years, and 20 to 39 years.
- CRS was reported rarely during the 1980s, with fewer than five cases annually. From 1990 to 1991, approximately 30 cases were reported annually.
- The rubella vaccine was licensed in 1969.

COMPLICATIONS

Complications tend to occur in adults, and most are uncommon. They include:

- Arthritis or arthralgia

—Occurs in 70% of adult women, lasting up to 1 month
—Usually affects small joints

- Encephalitis

—1 in 5,000 cases
—May be associated with mortality

- Bleeding

—1 in 3,000 cases
—Occurs in children more than in adults

- Thrombocytopenia is commonly noted.

—Rarely see orchitis and neuritis

- CRS

—In 1964, there were 20,000 newborns with CRS.
—Rubella infection in early gestation can lead to fetal death, premature delivery, and congenital defects.
—The severity of defects is worse the earlier in gestation the infection occurs.
—Eighty-five percent of infants are affected if infection occurs in the first trimester.
—Defects are rare if infection occurs after the 20th week.
—Common defects of CRS include:
   —Deafness: the most common defect
   —Ophthalmologic defects: cataracts, glaucoma, microphthalmia
   —Cardiac defects: patent ductus, arteriosus, ventricular septal defect, pulmonic stenosis, coarctation of the aorta
   —Neurologic defects: mental retardation, microcephalism

—Some manifestations of CRS (diabetes mellitus, progressive encephalopathy) may be delayed for years.

PROGNOSIS

- Quite good. As many as 50% of infections are asymptomatic.
- Rubella infection in a pregnant woman can be devastating for the infant (see above).

ASSOCIATED DISEASES

- Congenital rubella syndrome (see Complications, above)

 Differential Diagnosis

Infections that are sometimes confused with rubella include:

- Modified measles
- Scarlet fever
- Roseola
- Erythema infectiosum (fifth disease, parvovirus B19 infection)
- Enteroviral infections
- Infectious mononucleosis
- Drug eruptions

 Data Gathering

HISTORY

- In children, the prodrome is not often recognized.
- In adults, a 1- to 5-day prodrome of low-grade fever, malaise, and cervical adenopathy may precede the rash.
- Inquire about immunizations and exposures.

German Measles (Third Disease Rubella)

 Physical Examination

- The rash begins on the face, then progresses to the trunk and extremities. The rash does not usually coalesce, and lasts for 3 days.
- Adenopathies, especially postauricular, posterior cervical, and suboccipital, are commonly noted, along with conjunctivitis.
- Arthralgia/arthritis may be seen in adolescents and adults.

 Laboratory Aids

- Viral isolation from throat or urine
- A fourfold or greater rise in specific rubella antibodies, IgG, or a single IgM antibody is diagnostic.

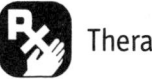 Therapy

- Supportive care

PREVENTION

- The rubella vaccine was licensed in 1969. The current strain of the vaccine (RA 27/3, developed at the Wistar Institute in Philadelphia) was licensed in 1979 and has replaced all other strains.
- Immunity occurs in 95% of vaccines and is thought to be lifelong.
- The vaccine virus is not communicable, except in breast-feedings. Persons who are immunodeficient (except HIV infection) should not receive the vaccine.

PITFALLS

- Not ensuring full vaccination for preschool-aged children
- If suspicious of rubella, it should be reported to the local public health authorities.

 Common Questions and Answers

Q: While pregnancy is a contraindication to rubella vaccination, if a pregnant woman is inadvertently vaccinated, will there be harm to the fetus?
A: Data collected since 1979 by the CDC show no evidence of CRS in 321 susceptible women who were vaccinated while pregnant.

ICD-CM 056.9

BIBLIOGRAPHY

American Academy of Pediatrics. Rubella. In: Peter G, ed. *2000 red book: report of the Committee on Infectious Diseases*, 25th ed. Elk Grove Village, IL: American Academy of Pediatrics, 1994:406–412.

Atkinson W, Furphy L, et al., eds. *Epidemiology and prevention of vaccine-preventable diseases*, 2nd ed. Bethesda, MD: Centers for Disease Control and Prevention, 1995.

Plotkin SA. Rubella vaccine. In: Plotkin SA, Mortimer EA, eds. *Vaccines*. Philadelphia: WB Saunders, 1988:235–262.

Zimmerman L, Reef SE. Incidence of congenital rubella syndrome at a hospital serving a predominantly Hispanic population, El Paso, Texas. *Pediatrics* 2001;107(3):E40.

Author: Louis M. Bell

Giardiasis

 Database

DEFINITION

Giardiasis is the symptomatic infection of the duodenum and jejunum with the flagellated protozoon *Giardia lamblia*.

PATHOPHYSIOLOGY

• *Giardia lamblia* is not a normal inhabitant of the upper small intestine and a frequent cause of diarrhea throughout the world. The life cycle has a multiplying intraduodenal trophozoite and an excreted cyst stage.
• Infection occurs after cyst ingestion from fecally contaminated water or by direct fecal-oral transmission in poor sanitary conditions.

GENETICS

• No confirmed predisposition
• Blood group A, certain human leukocyte antigen alleles are risk factors.

EPIDEMIOLOGY

Direct person-to-person transmission accounts for the very high prevalence rates over the past decade. High prevalence rates have recently been reported in patients with cystic fibrosis as well as Crohn disease. It is the most common nonopportunistic protozoan in AIDS patients.

COMPLICATIONS

• Malabsorption syndrome
• Steatorrhea
• Lactose deficiency
• Deficiencies of iron, folic acid, and vitamins A, B_{12}, and E
• Protein-losing enteropathy
• Urticaria
• Arthralgia

PATHOLOGY AND PATHOGENESIS

• Mucosal lesions vary from normal to subtotal villus atrophy with crypt hyperplasia and proliferation of intraepithelial and lamina propria lymphocytes. Trophozoite may be seen on biopsies as an S-like curled shape on longitudinal sections. Certain factors that could possibly be related to pathogenesis are:

—Small bowel bacterial overgrowth
—Deconjugation of intraluminal bile salts
—Breast milk that has anti-*Giardia* properties related to free fatty acids cleaved from milk triglyceride by a bile salt-stimulated lipase present in human milk

PROGNOSIS

• Remains good for symptomatic patients
• Combination therapy with two medications has been successful when repeated courses of a single drug have failed.

 Differential Diagnosis

• Celiac disease
• Cystic fibrosis
• Lactose intolerance

 Data Gathering

HISTORY

• Exposure to well water
• Living in endemic area
• Asymptomatic infection can occur.
• Common manifestations are watery, foul-smelling diarrhea without blood, abdominal cramps, and bloating.
• A chronic course is associated with weight loss, abdominal distention, anorexia, and flatulence.
• Malabsorption syndrome may include steatorrhea; secondary lactase deficiency; deficiencies of iron, folic acid, vitamins A, B_{12}, and E; and protein-losing enteropathy.

 Physical Examination

• Abdominal distention
• Urticaria
• Arthralgia

 Laboratory Aids

• Stool microscopy for detection of cysts and/or trophozoite
• A commercial ELISA test for detection of *Giardia lamblia* antigen in stools is available.
• In the case of strong suspicion of giardiasis, but in which there are three negative stool samples, a small intestinal sample may be obtained from the duodenum. The string test is the most useful. Consideration of empiric antiparasitic therapy may be recommended in endemic areas.
• If immunodeficiency is suspected, check immune function, especially IgA.

Therapy

DRUGS

• Metronidazole is the most effective and best tolerated. Dose: 15 mg/kg/d divided t.i.d. for 7 days
• Furazolidone has lower efficacy but is better tolerated and is available in liquid suspension.
• For recurrent infection, combination therapy of metronidazole and quinacrine is used.
• Asymptomatic giardiasis, in the absence of risk factors, should not be treated.

INFECTION CONTROL

• Maintenance of good sanitary conditions
• Family members and close contacts should be examined and treated if necessary.
• Examine the water source in endemic areas.

 Follow-Up

• The incubation period is usually 1 to 2 weeks.
• Reinfection is common if the source is not eradicated.
• If symptoms persist, with negative diagnostic studies, consider an alternative etiology or another enteropathogen.

 Common Questions and Answers

Q: Where is a likely place that the infection occurs?
A: Well water is a common place.

Q: What do I do if I suspect *Giardia*, but the stool sample is negative?
A: Three samples are needed. If you are in an endemic area, you may choose to treat empirically.

ICD-9-CM 007.1

BIBLIOGRAPHY

Fraser D. Epidemiology of *Giardia Lamblia* and *Cryptosporidium* infections in childhood. *Isr J Med Sci* 1994;30(5–6):356–361.

Nash TE, Ohl CA, Thomas E, et al. Treatment of patients with refractory giardiasis. *Clin Infect Dis* 2001;33(1):22–28.

Okhuysen PC. Traveler's diarrhea due to intestinal protozoa. *Clin Infect Dis* 2001;33(1):110–114.

Thielman NM, Guerrant RL. Persistent diarrhea in the returned traveler. *Infect Dis Clin North Am* 1998;12(2):489–501.

Author: Helen Anita John-Kelly

Gingivitis

 Database

DEFINITION

Gingivitis is a reversible or chronic inflammation of the gum tissue margin surrounding the teeth. Symptoms may include bleeding, swelling, ulceration, and pain. Gingivitis is usually mild and asymptomatic.

ETIOLOGY

- Poor dental hygiene
- Caries
- Bacterial plaque, calcified and uncalcified
- Mouth breathing
- Orthodontic appliances
- Malocclusion
- Crowded teeth
- Poor nutrition: vitamin deficiencies (e.g., vitamin C deficiency), diet low in coarse detergent-like foods (e.g., raw carrots, celery, apples), high prevalence of anaerobic microflora
- Infections: herpes simplex virus (HSV) type I, *Candida albicans,* HIV, bacterial pathogens
- Drugs: phenytoin, cyclosporine, nifedipine
- Trauma

PREDISPOSING CONDITIONS

- Diabetes mellitus
- Chronic renal failure
- Immunologic deficiency (HIV, Chediak-Higashi, cyclic neutropenia)
- Histiocytosis X
- Scleroderma
- Secondary hyperparathyroidism
- Neurologic problems: cerebral palsy, mental retardation, seizures. Routine dental care is often difficult due to poor cooperation and is often complicated by gingival hyperplasia caused by phenytoin.

PATHOPHYSIOLOGY

- Bacteria and food deposits adherent to the teeth (plaque) may accumulate, eroding the area where the gum and teeth meet.
- Incomplete dental care over time may result in this margin becoming inflamed.
- Inflammation may be more severe in children with altered immune function.
- If allowed to progress, the connective tissue attachment of the teeth and the root surface may become involved, resulting in irreversible periodontal disease.
- Microscopic changes include edema, exudate, ulceration, and proliferation of the epithelium surrounding the tooth.

EPIDEMIOLOGY

- Affects more than 90% of children between the ages of 4 and 13 years, although it is generally low grade.
- Thirteen percent to 40% of children 6 to 36 months of age have eruption gingivitis, which commonly resolves after teeth erupt.
- Boys have more severe and prevalent gingivitis until the early teens.
- Peak incidence is in adolescence, possibly due to hormonal influences and inconsistent dental hygiene.

COMPLICATIONS

- Periodontal disease
- Osteomyelitis
- Tooth decay
- Sepsis, particularly in patients who are immunocompromised

PROGNOSIS

- Good oral hygiene may reverse mild-to-moderate gingivitis within several months.
- Periodontal disease is not reversible; therefore, prevention is essential.

 Differential Diagnosis

- Infection
—Abscess

- Trauma
—Food impaction
—Orthodontic appliances
—Self-inflicted minor injury

- Hematologic
—Gingival bleeding due to hemophilia (factor VIII or IX deficiency)
—Thrombocytopenia

- Immunologic
—Neutrophil disorders
—Leukemia
—HIV
—Graft versus host (infiltrative gingivitis)

- Miscellaneous
—Gingival hyperplasia due to medications, including phenytoin and nifedipine

 Data Gathering

HISTORY

Question: Is there any bleeding along the gum line with routine brushing and flossing?
Significance: This is very common with gingivitis.

Question: Is there any gingival pain, spontaneous bleeding, or loose teeth?
Significance: This may be seen with gingival disease, but one must consider other diagnoses.

Question: Are any dental appliances worn by the patient?
Significance: Orthodontic equipment makes gingiva more difficult to clean, and reactive tissue growth is more common.

Question: Are any regular medications taken?
Significance: As mentioned, phenytoin may result in gingival hyperplasia, and chemotherapeutic agents may result in gingivitis.

Question: Has the patient undergone pubertal changes?
Significance: This seems to worsen gingival inflammation.

- Review significant medical history, asking about bleeding disorders and immunodeficiency.
- Assess the diet of the child to determine if there might be nutritional deficiencies.
- Review the frequency of dental care visits and home dental hygiene regimen.

 Physical Examination

- Examine the face and neck for signs of swelling, erythema, and warmth, which may be signs of more extensive bacterial infection.
- Evaluate the gingival tissue for erythema, swelling, ulceration, fluctuance, or drainage.
- Evaluate the teeth for caries, fractures, looseness, malocclusion, pain, and plaque.
- Assess the patient's oral hygiene technique in the office. This is the single largest contributor to gingivitis.

Gingivitis

Laboratory Aids

TESTS

- Complete blood count with differential: if there is a concern of excess bleeding, which may be due to thrombocytopenia or pancytopenia
- Blood culture: if there is a concern of sepsis complicating the picture
- Direct fluorescent antibody testing for HSV-1: if herpes is suspected (stomatitis is usually present); swab the base of a stoma/vesicle and smear on a slide.
- Biopsy is rarely necessary.

Radiographic Studies

Panoramic or individual tooth radiographic imaging is important to assess the bones for evidence of periodontal extension of the gingivitis.

Therapy

MILD GINGIVITIS

- Mechanical plaque removal
- Careful daily dental hygiene, including meticulous brushing and flossing

MODERATE-TO-SEVERE GINGIVITIS

- Care as outlined for mild gingivitis
- Should be evaluated by a pedodontist (if available) or by a general dentist
- Mouth rinses for plaque inhibition (e.g., chlorhexidine 0.12%)
- Irrigation devices
- Sonic toothbrushes
- Gingivectomies in cases of overgrowth to permit better cleaning
- Antibiotics to cover mouth flora organisms in the more severe cases when bacterial superinfection is suspected

Follow-Up

- Routine dental care with professional cleaning and plaque removal is recommended for all children and adults.
- Appliances to keep gingival growth contained may be used in certain cases.

PREVENTION

- Consistent daily oral hygiene. For infants: gum massage, washcloth to remove plaque; in young children: assistance with brushing with a small amount of fluoridated toothpaste; in school-aged children: supervise brushing and assist if necessary.
- Fluorides: Supplements are appropriate if the water supply is not fluoridated.
- Sealants: adherent plastic coating applied to the pits and fissures of the permanent teeth to provide a mechanical barrier
- Begin regular dental checkups every 6 months at 3 years of age. Children with gingival overgrowth, HIV, or ongoing chemotherapy need visits to the dentist every 3 months to ensure good hygiene. Routine daily care may be inconsistent and often impossible in children with motor and cognitive limitations; these children also need more frequent visits to the dentist.
- Mouth guards for competitive sports
- Counseling about dangers of smoking

PITFALLS

Success in preventing and treating gingivitis requires consistent daily care, which may be very difficult in children and adolescents.

Common Questions and Answers

Q: Are there differences among toothpastes and prevention of gingivitis?
A: Yes. A study demonstrated that stabilized stannous fluoride toothpaste is effective in preventing gingivitis. When essential oil mouthwashes (e.g., Listerine) are added, there is additional reduction in the amount of gingivitis noted.

Q: What dietary changes may improve gingival health?
A: Avoiding frequent carbohydrate intake may reduce gingivitis. Carbonated beverages, sugared chewing gum, and candy often adhere to teeth. When daily dental care is inconsistent, plaque formation is increased and gingivitis is much more likely.

Q: Why do children generally not have the significant periodontal disease that adults get?
A: No one knows for sure; however, it is known that the gingiva of the primary dentition are more rounded and thicker and contain more blood vessels and less connective tissue. Whether these differences mask disease or are helpful is unclear.

ICD-9-CM 523.1

BIBLIOGRAPHY

Abrams, RG, Romberg, E. Gingivitis in children with malnutrition. *J Clin Pediatric Dentistry* 1999;23(3):189–194.

Beiswanger BB, McClanahan SF, Bartizek RD, et al. The comparative efficacy of stabilized stannous fluoride dentifrice, peroxide/baking soda dentifrice and essential oil mouthrinse for the prevention of gingivitis. *J Clin Dentistry* 1997;8(2 spec no):46–53.

Bimstein E. Periodontal health and disease in children and adolescents. *Pediatr Clin North Am* 1991;38(5):1183–1207.

Eaton KA, Rimini FM, Zak E, et al. The effects of a 0.12% chlorhexidine-digluconate-containing mouthrinse versus a placebo on plaque and gingival inflammation over a 3-month period. A multicentre study carried out in general dental practices. *J Clin Periodontal* 1997;24(3):189–197.

Griffen AL, Goepferd SJ. Preventive oral health care for the infant, child, and adolescent. *Pediatr Clin North Am* 1991;38(5):1209–1226.

Ivanovic M, Lekic P. Transient effect of a short-term educational programme without prophylaxis on control of plaque and gingival inflammation in school children. *J Clin Periodontol* 1996;23(8):750–757.

McDonald RE, Avery DR, Weddell JA. Gingivitis and periodontal disease. In: *Dentistry for the child and adolescent*, 6th ed. St. Louis: Mosby-Year Book, 1994:455–502.

Ramberg P, Axelsson P, Lindhe J. Plaque formation at healthy and inflamed gingival sites in young individuals. *J Clin Periodontol* 1995;22(1):85–88.

Author: Shannon Connor Phillips

Glaucoma—Congenital

 Database

DEFINITION

Congenital glaucoma is the improper development of the drainage system for aqueous humor, leading to elevated intraocular pressure with enlargement of the eye and damage to the optic nerve.

CAUSES

• Aqueous humor, a clear fluid produced by the ciliary body at the posterior base of the iris, passes through the pupil and exits through the trabecular meshwork and Schlemm's canal, which are located at the junction of the cornea and the anterior iris.
• Outflow blockage of the aqueous may causes the pressure to build in the eye, resulting in enlargement of the eye in younger children and destruction of fibers of the optic nerve in children with abnormally high intraocular pressures.

PATHOPHYSIOLOGY

• Primary congenital glaucoma caused by structural abnormalities of the aqueous outflow mechanism, which includes the trabecular meshwork, iris, and cornea
• Secondary glaucoma may be associated with systemic abnormalities such as Lowe syndrome, aniridia, rubella, Sturge-Weber
• Glaucoma may also be acquired secondary to an ocular abnormality such as cataract

EPIDEMIOLOGY/GENETICS

• 1:10,000 births
• 2:5 female/male ratio
• Seventy percent bilaterally affected
• Primary congenital glaucoma accounts for approximately one half of all cases of glaucoma in children.

COMPLICATIONS

If glaucoma is undetected or uncontrollable, then severe visual impairment or blindness is the likely result.
If glaucoma is controlled, the following are relatively common:

• Unrecognized and untreated amblyopia (the most serious threat to child's vision)
• High degrees of myopia
• Anisometropia (difference in refractive error between fellow eyes)
• Buphthalmos and corneal scarring

PROGNOSIS

Guarded; even if pressure is well controlled, the child must be carefully followed for amblyopia, abnormal refractive errors, and recurrence of glaucoma.

ASSOCIATED DISEASES

Aniridia, Sturge-Weber, neurofibromatosis, Marfan syndrome, Pierre Robin syndrome, homocystinuria, Lowe syndrome, rubella, chromosomal abnormalities, persistent hyperplastic primary vitreous

 Differential Diagnosis

• Excessive tearing, most commonly due to nasolacrimal duct obstruction
• Megalocornea

—May be associated with high myopia
—Often familial

• Corneal haze
• Birth trauma, forceps
• Congenital corneal dystrophies, developmental anomalies, intrauterine inflammation (rubella, syphilis), mucopolysaccharidoses, cystinosis

 Data Gathering

HISTORY

Question: Is there tearing, light sensitivity, or lid squeezing?
Significance: Epiphora (tearing), photophobia (light sensitivity), and blepharospasm (lid squeezing) may be present due to corneal edema from increased intraocular pressure.

 Physical Examination

• General signs of many systemic syndromes associated with glaucoma (neurofibromatosis, Sturge-Weber)
• Corneal enlargement (11 mm suspicious in patients younger than 1 year)
• Corneal haze from edema and/or scarring, often seen with acute ruptures in Descemet's membrane
• Myopia, often extreme degrees
• Optic nerve cupping develops rapidly in infants but may be reversible with control of glaucoma in very young children.

INTRAOCULAR PRESSURE MEASUREMENT

• An awake child is ideal; use bottle or breast to quiet along with low lighting.
• If examination under anesthesia is needed, check intraocular pressure as soon as possible after induction, as intraocular pressure drops with anesthetic agents.

CORNEAL INSPECTION

• Diameter measure with calipers

—Normal newborn, 10.0 to 10.5 mm
—Over 11.5 mm suspicious
—Watch for asymmetry.

• Clarity

—Haze may be due to edema or breaks in Descemet's membrane (called Haab's striae).

• Refractive error

—High myopia common
—Useful as an office measure of change over time

• Optic disc assessment

—Cupping of nerve head is an early sign.
—May reverse with good intraocular pressure control

 Laboratory Aids

TESTS

• Gonioscopy: evaluation of anterior chamber angle (between iris and cornea)

—In trabeculodysgenesis, the insertion of the iris into the corneoscleral angle is often flat or concave.
—Iris defects may suggest the type of abnormality causing glaucoma.
—Abnormal iris vessels may influence the surgical plan.

• Ultrasound: axial length using A-scan

—Eye usually abnormally long for age
—Longitudinal data very useful in determining continued presence of glaucoma

Therapy

IMMEDIATE

- Medical treatment for glaucoma in children is usually a temporizing measure prior to surgical intervention.
- In other types of glaucoma, medical treatment involves the use of the same medications as those used in adults, such as beta-blockers, adrenergic agents, and carbonic anhydrase inhibitors. In general, miotics are not used because they may cause a paradoxical rise in intraocular pressure.

SURGICAL PROCEDURES

- Goniotomy/trabeculotomy: Both of these procedures open portions of Schlemm's canal (goniotomy approaches Schlemm's canal from inside the eye and trabeculotomy from the outside) into the anterior chamber, allowing easier outflow of aqueous humor to the subconjunctival space.
- Trabeculectomy: This is similar to trabeculotomy but includes excision of a small portion of Schlemm's canal and the trabecular meshwork.
- Seton procedures: Various devices are inserted from the subconjunctival space into the anterior chamber, allowing free flow of aqueous humor from the eye.
- Cyclodestructive procedures: Procedures involving destruction of the ciliary body (which produces aqueous humor) decrease aqueous production.
- Iridectomy: If the mechanism of glaucoma is limited outflow of aqueous humor from posterior to iris through the pupil, then removal of a portion of the iris may eliminate obstruction.

 Follow-Up

EARLY POSTOPERATIVE

- Postoperative steroids and cycloplegic drops are essential to prevent adhesions due to inflammation and to decrease pain.
- Corneal edema clears slowly, but intraocular pressure quickly falls if surgery is successful.
- For young infants, examination under anesthesia may be required frequently in the first 3 to 4 years of life to ensure adequate control of intraocular pressure.
- Contact with social services for blind and visually handicapped individuals must be made for children even if they are only suspected of being visually impaired. Encourage families to make the contact even when the child may be too young to provide objective data on the extent of visual handicap.

PITFALLS

- Even when pressure is well controlled and amblyopia treatment is undertaken vigorously, the child is still at high risk for visual impairment.
- The child and parents must understand that glaucoma may recur at any point and that continued, long-term surveillance is essential.
- Ensure that potential systemic medicines do not raise intraocular pressure.

 Common Questions and Answers

Q: Can glaucoma be painful?
A: If the ocular pressure rises quickly (hours), pain occurs frequently. Very high intraocular pressures may be present without pain if they occur slowly (months to years).

Q: Can glaucoma occur after eye trauma?
A: Yes. This is a very common cause of glaucoma and may be asymptomatic, thus requiring periodic follow-up ophthalmic examinations for early detection and treatment.

ICD-9-CM 743.20

BIBLIOGRAPHY

Dickens CJ, Hoskins HD. Developmental glaucoma. In: Isenberg SJ, ed. *The eye in infancy*, 2nd ed. Chicago: Yearbook Medical, 1994:318–335.

Russell-Eggitt I. Childhood glaucoma. In: Taylor D, ed. *Paediatric ophthalmology*, 2nd ed. Oxford: Blackwell Science, 1997:477–497.

Shields MB. Primary congenital glaucoma. In: Shields MB, ed. *Textbook of glaucoma*. Baltimore: Williams & Wilkins, 1992:220–234.

Author: Graham E. Quinn

Glomerulonephritis

 Database

DEFINITION

- Glomerulonephritis (GN) presents with hematuria, oliguria, hypertension, and volume overload.
- Acute GN (AGN) is associated with inflammation and proliferation of the glomerular tuft. AGN may be rapidly progressive (RPGN).
- Chronic GN (CGN) implies that permanent damage has occurred.

PATHOPHYSIOLOGY

Causes

- Low serum complement level: systemic diseases

—Vasculitis and autoimmune disease, e.g., systemic lupus erythematosus (SLE)
—Subacute bacterial endocarditis (SBE)
—Shunt nephritis
—Cryoglobulinemia

- Low serum complement level: renal diseases

—Acute poststreptococcal GN (APSGN)
—Membranoproliferative glomerulonephritis (types 1, 2, and 3)

- Normal serum complement level: systemic diseases

—Polyarteritis nodose group
—Wegener vasculitis
—Henoch-Schönlein purpura
—Hypersensitivity vasculitis
—Visceral abscess

- Normal serum complement level: renal diseases

—IgA nephropathy
—Idiopathic rapidly progressive glomerulonephritis
—Immune-complex disease
—Pauci-immune glomerulonephritis

PATHOLOGY

In APSGN light microscopy reveals enlarged swollen glomerular tufts, mesangial and epithelial cell proliferation, with polymorphonuclear cell infiltration. There is granular deposition of C3 and IgG on immunofluorescence, and electron-dense subepithelial deposits or humps on electron microscopy. The histology varies in CGN and depends on the cause. RPGN is associated with crescent formation.

EPIDEMIOLOGY

- APSGN can occur in all ages but is most frequent in boys between 5 and 15 years.
- Incidence of APSGN in the United States has declined in the last two decades.
- CGN occurs more often at the end of the first decade of life and in adults.
- Genetic predisposition

—Familial GN (e.g., Alport syndrome, X-linked)
—Autoimmune diseases (e.g., SLE, familial)

COMPLICATIONS

- Acute renal failure
- Hyperkalemia
- Hypertension
- Volume overload (congestive cardiac failure, pulmonary edema, hypertension)
- Chronic renal failure

PROGNOSIS

- Prognosis is excellent in APSGN and variable for other causes of GN in childhood.

 Differential Diagnosis

- Acute postinfectious GN (Lancefield group A β-hemolytic streptococci, pneumococcus, *Mycoplasma*, mumps, Epstein-Barr virus)
- Infection related (hepatitis B and C, syphilis)
- IgA nephropathy
- Membranoproliferative GN
- Autoimmune GN (e.g., SLE)
- Familial GN
- Acute interstitial nephritis
- Hemolytic uremic syndrome
- Pyelonephritis

 Data Gathering

HISTORY

- Macroscopic hematuria (coke-colored urine)
- Sore throat
- Impetigo
- A prior URI of at least 1 week or skin lesions in the proceeding 3 to 4 weeks suggests APSGN.
- An upper respiratory infection URI in the proceeding few days suggests IgA nephropathy.
- Reduced urine output
- Dyspnea, fatigue, lethargy
- Headache
- Seizures (hypertensive encephalopathy)
- Symptoms of a systemic disease such as fever, rash (especially on the buttocks and legs posteriorly), arthralgia, and weight loss

Special Questions

Establish the time relationship between a sore throat and the AGN. The onset of APSGN is usually associated with a time delay of more than 1 week.

 Physical Examination

Look for:

- Hypertension
- Pallor
- Signs of volume overload (edema, jugular venous distention, hepatomegaly, basal pulmonary crepitation, and a triple cardiac rhythm)
- Impetigo or ecthyma (pyoderma)
- Signs of vasculitis such as rash, loss of fingertip pulp space tissue, Raynaud, and vascular thrombosis
- Signs of a systemic disorder (see vasculitis above)
- Signs of chronic renal insufficiency such as short stature, pallor, sallowness, edema, excoriations, pericardial friction rub, pulmonary rales and effusion, uriniferous breath, asterixis, myoclonus, and neuropathy

Laboratory Aids

TESTS

- Throat culture for β-hemolytic streptococcus (positive in 15% to 20% with APSGN)
- Microscopy of the urine for crenated RBCs and RBC casts; CBC is normal in AGN; with chronic renal insufficiency a normocytic normochromic or hypochromic microcytic anemia is found.
- Serum chemistries will reflect the degree of renal failure (raised serum urea and creatinine). The serum potassium and phosphate will be elevated and the calcium decreased.
- ASOT (antistreptolysin O) titer. Positive in 60% of patients with APSGN.
- Streptozyme test. A mixed antigen test for β-hemolytic streptococcus. Together, the ASOT plus streptozyme tests have a greater than 85% sensitivity.
- Complement C3 serum level will be low in APSGN and in other causes of GN as detailed above.
- ECG to assess ventricular size and for hyperkalemia.

Imaging

- CXR to look for pulmonary edema and cardiac size.
- Renal ultrasound if presentation or course not typical of APSGN. The ultrasound is to assess the size and parenchymal texture.

PITFALLS

- Look for and treat hyperkalemia.
- To control seizures treat the hypertension; anticonvulsants have a secondary role.
- Monitor the degree of renal failure.
- Home testing: blood pressure monitoring may be required.

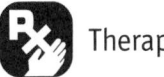 ## Therapy

DIET

Restricted fluid, sodium, potassium, and phosphate are initially required.

DRUGS

The following may be required:

- Loop diuretics (furosemide) for volume, blood pressure, and potassium control
- Antihypertensive agents; vasodilators such as calcium channel blockers (nifedipine, isradipine, amlodipine) and loop diuretics are useful as first-line agents; intravenous hydralazine, labetalol, nicardipine, or nitroprusside may be required to treat severe refractory hypertension.
- Serum potassium-lowering agents (Kayexalate, furosemide, bicarbonate, insulin/glucose, salbutamol). Intravenous calcium is used to stabilize the myocardium in severe hyperkalemia.
- Phosphate binders
- Immunosuppressive agents such as prednisone, cyclophosphamide, and sometimes azathioprine are used in the treatment of vasculitis-associated GN, membranoproliferative GN, and RPGN. Plasmapheresis may be used to treat RPGN. Penicillin is used in APSGN but does not affect the course of the disease.

DURATION

APSGN is a self-limiting disease. Acute therapy is usually sufficient. The therapy of CGN depends on the underlying disease process, may include immunosuppressives and, ultimately, the management of CRF.

 ## Follow-Up

Drug doses may need modification if conflicts with other treatments arise. In APSGN improvement usually occurs within 3 to 7 days, hypertension is not sustained and macroscopic hematuria is transient. Watch for ongoing oliguria, unresolved hypertension, increasing proteinuria, or progressive azotemia.

PITFALLS

- Not checking a serum potassium level stat.
- Not recognizing fluid overload.
- Not recognizing the severity and type of renal failure.

 ## Common Questions and Answers

Q: When does the complement return to normal?
A: Hemolytic complement levels (C3) return to normal within a 6- to 8-week period in APSGN. Persistently low C3 levels suggest a cause other than APSGN.

Q: What are the indications for renal biopsy in AGN?
A: Patients in whom there is sustained hypertension, ongoing or progressive azotemia, or persistent proteinuria of more than 1.5 g/d should be biopsied.

ICD-9-CM 580.9

BIBLIOGRAPHY

Clark G, White RH, Glasgow EF, et al. Post-streptococcal glomerulonephritis in children: clinicopathological correlations and long-term prognosis. *Pediatr Nephrol* 1988;2:381–388.

Cole B, Salinas-Madrigal L. Acute proliferative glomerulonephritis and crescentic glomerulonephritis. In: Barratt TM, Avner ED, Harmon WE, eds. *Pediatric nephrology*, 4th ed. Baltimore: Williams & Wilkins, 1999:669–689.

Jordan S, Lemire JM. Acute glomerulonephritis. Diagnosis and treatment. *Pediatr Clin North Am* 1982;29:857–873.

Madaio MP, Harrington JT. The diagnosis of acute glomerulonephritis. *N Engl J Med* 1984;309:1299–1302.

Author: Kevin E.C. Meyers

Glucose-6-Phosphate Dehydrogenase Deficiency

 Database

DEFINITION

Deficiency of the enzyme glucose-6-phosphate dehydrogenase (G6PD) in the red blood cell, which may result in a hemolytic anemia. Children inherit abnormal G6PD genes that result either in deficient enzyme production or in production of an enzyme with diminished activity.

• Although the majority of patients with G6PD deficiency are never anemic and have mild to no hemolysis, the classic manifestation is acute hemolytic anemia.
• (AHA) World Health Organization (WHO) classification

—*Class 1: Congenital nonspherocytic hemolytic anemia*: a rare form manifesting itself with chronic hemolysis without exposure to oxidative stressors. Most patients have a mild-to-moderate anemia, although some patients are transfusion dependent. Can present as neonatal jaundice, hemolytic anemia, or a secondary manifestation of the chronic hemolysis (e.g., gallstones). Splenomegaly is present in 40% of patients. Affected individuals tend to be white males of Northern European background.
—*Class 2: Severe deficiency* (<5% detectable enzyme activity): oxidative stress-induced hemolysis only. The prototype is G6PD-Mediterranean. Because of severe deficiency, all RBCs are sensitive to stressors, and hemolysis may be severe and persistent.
—*Class 3: Mild deficiency* (approximately 10% enzyme activity): the most common type of G6PD deficiency. Acute hemolytic anemia is uncommon and occurs only with stressors. The prototype is G6PD A—(African or of African descent). Because the enzyme is present and active in young RBCs, the hemolysis preferentially affects older cells and is milder and self-limited (i.e., all cells produced in response to the anemia have adequate G6PD levels).
—*Class 4: Nondeficient variant*: no symptoms, even during oxidant stressors, e.g., G6PD A (variant with normal activity); 20% to 40% allelic frequency in Africans.

• Deficient neonates may have hyperbilirubinemia out of proportion to their anemia. In severe subtypes, this may lead to kernicterus. Elevated bilirubin is only partially due to the hemolysis; the liver plays a role as well.

PATHOPHYSIOLOGY

• G6PD is necessary for the prevention of cell damage during oxidative stress and is critically important in red blood cells because of continuous oxidant stress (from O_2 metabolism) and because anuclear RBCs cannot synthesize more enzyme, unlike cells in other tissues.
• Red blood cells lose G6PD activity throughout their life span, so older cells are more prone to oxidative hemolysis.

• The normal RBC life span of approximately 120 days is unaffected in *unstressed* states, even with severe enzyme deficiency, but may be shortened during oxidant stress.
• G6PD-deficient RBCs are destroyed via *intravascular* hemolysis upon exposure to the oxidative stressor, and acute hemolytic anemia results.
• Oxidant stressors include infections (bacterial, viral, hepatitis) and drugs (mothballs, antimalarials, some sulfonamides, methylene blue, and others).
• Hemolysis usually follows stressor by 1 to 3 days and the nadir occurs 8 to 10 days postexposure. It is therefore necessary to obtain hemoglobins for over a week after the initial exposure.
• Favism, a severe hemolytic anemia in patients with G6PD deficiency related to fava bean ingestion.
• Normal G6PD activity is 7 to 10 IU/g hemoglobin.

GENETICS

• G6PD gene is on the X chromosome (Xq28).
• Males express the enzyme (mutant or normal) from their single X chromosome (hemizygotes). Females inheriting two deficient X chromosomes are considered homozygotes (rare) and are more severely affected than are female heterozygotes. Heterozygote females show variable intermediate expression because of random X inactivation (the Lyon hypothesis).

EPIDEMIOLOGY

• G6PD is the most common of all clinically significant enzyme defects.
• Because it is X-linked it primarily affects males.
• Discovered in 1958 while studying individuals who developed hemolytic anemia when exposed to primaquine, an antimalarial drug
• Over 300 *biochemical* variants of G6PD have been identified, affecting almost 400 million people worldwide.
• The frequency of different G6PD mutations varies from population to population:

—Africans: 20% to 40% of African X-chromosomes are G6PD A (a mutant enzyme with normal activity).
—Sardinians (some regions): 30% have G6PD-Mediterranean.
—Saudi Arabians: 13% have G6PD deficiency.
—African-Americans: 10% to 15% have G6PD A— (a mutant enzyme with decreased activity; see below).
—The high incidence of mutant genes in some regions may relate to a survival advantage conferred against malarial infection (*Plasmodium falciparum*).

COMPLICATIONS

Neonates can be at risk for hyperbilirubinemia requiring treatment.
Severe life-threatening anemia may result after exposure to an oxidant stressor.

• For those with the milder forms, the prognosis is excellent.
• Can cause significant morbidity, but rarely mortality, in those with the more severe forms.

 Differential Diagnosis

Intravascular hemolysis is very rare in children, but other causes include:

• Acute hemolytic transfusion reactions (Coombs test is positive)
• Microangiopathic hemolytic disease, such as hemolytic uremic syndrome, thrombotic thrombocytopenic purpura, and prosthetic cardiac valves
• Physical trauma (e.g., March hemoglobinuria); severe burns (uncommon)
• Other inherited RBC enzyme deficiencies
• Paroxysmal nocturnal hemoglobinuria

Extravascular hemolysis can also be confused with G6PD deficiency and includes:

• Hereditary spherocytosis (spherocytes) seen on smear or detected by osmotic fragility testing
• Autoimmune hemolysis and delayed hemolytic transfusion reactions (both Coombs-positive)
• Hemoglobinopathies (e.g., sickle cell anemia; often apparent from peripheral smear). Having G6PD deficiency and a hemoglobinopathy does not worsen either disease.
• Hypersplenism or severe liver disease
• Gilbert disease may present with intermittent jaundice and indirect hyperbilirubinemia after infections.

 Data Gathering

HISTORY

• Symptoms are generally those of anemia, such as pallor, fatigue, or malaise.
• Children undergoing active hemolysis are often irritable, with nausea, diarrhea, and abdominal or back pain, and they often have low-grade fevers.
• Dark urine ("coca-cola," or tea-colored) may follow moderate-to-severe hemolysis.
• Seek information on recent drug, chemical, or food (fava bean) exposures, as well as recent or current illnesses.
• A detailed family history may reveal chronic anemia or intermittent jaundice or a known G6PD deficiency. Ask about a family history of splenectomy, cholecystectomy, or blood transfusion. Family ethnicity is also very important.

Physical Examination

- Signs include those of anemia, such as tachycardia, a flow murmur, or pallor.
- Significant hemolysis may cause jaundice or scleral icterus.
- Hepatosplenomegaly may occur but is unusual.

Laboratory Aids

TESTS

- CBC usually reveals a normochromic normocytic anemia with an appropriate reticulocytosis. Hemoglobin can drop precipitously and should be monitored closely until stable or a trend upward is seen. Checking a single hemoglobin the day of exposure to the stressor is not sufficient.
- Peripheral blood smear often shows bizarre RBC morphology with marked anisocytosis and poikilocytosis. Can see schistocytes, hemi-ghost cells (uneven distribution of hemoglobin), bite cells, blister cells, and occasional Heinz bodies (on supravital staining).
- Hemoglobinemia can be seen in the plasma (pink-red supernatant) or may be measured as free serum hemoglobin.
- Hemoglobinuria occurs once hemoglobin-binding sites in the plasma (haptoglobin and hemopexin) are saturated and may be visible as hematuria or detected on routine urinalysis.
- Free serum haptoglobin levels decrease.
- Direct and indirect Coombs tests should be done to exclude autoimmune hemolytic anemia. They should be negative in G6PD deficiency.
- Plasma indirect bilirubin, LDH, and AST may be elevated, and hemosiderin may be found in the urine several days after hemolysis. LFTs should be normal.
- Renal functions should be obtained to rule out TTP and HUS.

Diagnostic Tests

- Rapid and relatively simple screening tests for G6PD activity in RBCs are available but are qualitative and will therefore not pick up all female heterozygotes who have a measurable but low enzyme level.
- It is necessary to confirm a deficiency or diagnose a suspected heterozygote with a test to *quantify* G6PD activity. Normal G6PD activity is 7 to 10 IU/g hemoglobin. This will accurately detect deficiency in males and homozygous females with no recent hemolysis and will be helpful with heterozygous women.

PITFALLS

- Measured enzyme levels will be higher immediately after an acute hemolytic event because younger RBCs (reticulocytes) with normal levels of G6PD will have replaced the older, more deficient population. Screening tests may be falsely negative during this time. The most cost-effective approach is to defer screening until 1 to 2 weeks after the resolution of hemolysis.
- Heterozygote female detection: Two RBC populations exist because of mosaicism from random X-inactivation. On average, one half are normal and one half are deficient, but there may be variability. Therefore, quantitative results could be unreliable in extreme cases, which makes family counseling difficult.

Therapy

- Removal of the oxidant stressor is of primary importance. Discontinue the suspected drug and/or treat the infection. In class 3 and 4 patients, essential drug therapy may be continued while monitoring for signs of severe hemolysis.
- Transfusion is rarely necessary (except in some type 1 and 2 deficiencies), but any patient who is symptomatic with anemia or has a low hemoglobin and signs of ongoing brisk hemolysis should be transfused immediately with packed RBCs. Transfused cells should not be G6PD deficient and will not undergo hemolysis.
- Supportive care, evaluation of renal function (risk of atubular necrosis with brisk hemolysis), and monitoring degree of anemia and ongoing hemolysis are important.
- For the affected neonate, one should monitor the bilirubin closely and start bilirubin lights early. Three fourths of affected infants will have clinically apparent jaundice within 24 hours. If necessary, an exchange transfusion should be performed. Phenobarbital has shown some success in decreasing the bilirubin level. Early discharge is not recommended in infants with jaundice and known risk for having G6PD deficiency.

Follow-Up

The majority of G6PD-deficient individuals remain asymptomatic. When hemolysis does occur, it tends to be self-limited and resolves spontaneously, with a return to normal hemoglobin levels in 2 to 6 weeks. The development of renal failure is extremely rare in children, even with massive hemolysis and hemoglobinuria.

PREVENTION

- Avoidance of drugs and toxins known to cause hemolysis is the best prevention.
- Education regarding drug avoidance, signs and symptoms of hemolysis, and family and genetic counseling should be provided.

Common Questions and Answers

Q: Do I need to follow a special diet or avoid medications if I have G6PD deficiency?
A: Though most patients will have no symptoms of their disease, certain medications may cause transient hemolytic anemia, and these should be avoided. When prescribing medications, your physician and pharmacist should know about your G6PD deficiency, but most necessary medications are safe and well tolerated. People with severe variants of the deficiency should also avoid fava beans, but otherwise no dietary restrictions are necessary.

Q: Do I need to know which variant of G6PD deficiency I have?
A: It may be clear which variant you are likely to have based on your clinical symptoms and ethnic background.

Q: Should my family be screened if someone has G6PD deficiency?
A: In families of patients with G6PD deficiency, screening members may help provide meaningful genetic counseling to female carriers and affected but asymptomatic males.

Q: How does G6PD affect sickle cell anemia and vice versa?
A: Having sickle cell disease is somewhat protective in patients with G6PD A— deficiency, because their RBC population is young and therefore higher in enzyme activity. On the other hand, G6PD has no affect on the clinical characteristics of sickle cell disease.

ICD-9-CM 282.2

BIBLIOGRAPHY

Beutler E. G6PD deficiency. *Blood* 1994;84:3613–3636.

Beutler E. Study of glucose-6-phosphate dehydrogenase: history and molecular biology. *Am J Hematol* 1993;42:53–58.

Mason PJ. New insights into G6PDF deficiency. *Br J Haematol* 1996;94(suppl 4):585–591.

Author: Leslie Raffini
Susan Rheingold, 2nd edition

Goiter

Database

DEFINITION

Goiter is enlargement of the thyroid gland.

GENETICS

• The multinodular goiter 1 (MNG1) locus was identified on chromosome 14q by linkage analysis in one large Canadian family and on chromosome Xp22 in an Italian family. Other genes implicated in simple goiter formation include thyroglobulin, TSH-receptor, and Na^+/I^- symporter. Apart from genetic factors, twin and family studies show a modest to major contribution of environmental factors, especially iodine deficiency and cigarette smoking.
• Autoimmune goiters, such as chronic lymphocytic thyroiditis (CLT), occur in children with a genetic predisposition.
• Thyroid cancers are usually sporadic. Medullary carcinoma can be familial (autosomal dominant) as part of multiple endocrine neoplasia (MEN)-2A and -2B, or as isolated malignancy.

EPIDEMIOLOGY

• The most common cause of pediatric goiter in the United States is CLT.
• Prevalence of goiter in the United States is 3% to 7%, though the incidence is much higher in regions of iodine deficiency.
• Thyroid cancers comprise 0.5% to 1.5% of all malignancies in children and adolescents.

COMPLICATIONS

• Depending on gland size, goiters can produce a mass effect on midline neck structures.
• Typically, the child is euthyroid, but clinical hypothyroidism or hyperthyroidism may result from certain types of goiters.
• Therapy for thyroid cancer may induce permanent hypothyroidism.

PROGNOSIS

• Depends on the cause of the goiter.
• Thyroid cancers usually follow an indolent course with excellent prognosis, especially the well-differentiated follicular cell carcinoma. Mortality is most common in medullary and undifferentiated carcinomas, which are relatively rare in children.

Differential Diagnosis

• Immunologic

—Chronic lymphocytic thyroiditis (often referred to as Hashimoto thyroiditis)
—Graves disease

• Infectious

—Acute suppurative thyroiditis (most often *Streptococcus pyogenes, Staphylococcus aureus,* and *Streptococcus pneumoniae*)
—Subacute thyroiditis (often viral)

• Environmental

—Goitrogens: iodide, lithium, amiodarone, oral contraceptives, perchlorate, cabbage, soybeans, cassava
—Iodine deficiency

• Neoplastic

—Thyroid adenoma/carcinoma
—Follicular adenoma: benign
—Follicular, papillary, or mixed carcinoma: well differentiated; follicular 90%
—Medullary carcinoma: 4% to 10% as part of the MEN-2 syndrome
—TSH-secreting adenoma
—Lymphoma

• Congenital

—Ectopic gland
—Unilateral agenesis of gland
—Dyshormonogenesis
—Thyroxine resistance

• Miscellaneous

—Simple colloid goiter
—Multinodular goiter

Data Gathering

HISTORY

• Symptoms of hypothyroidism or hyperthyroidism

—Hypothyroidism: increase in sedentary behavior, lethargy, weight gain, constipation, cold intolerance, dry skin and/or hair, hair loss
—Hyperthyroidism: hyperactivity, irritability, difficulty concentrating or focusing in school, hyperphagia, weight loss, diarrhea, heat intolerance

• Careful dietary and medication history
• History of head, neck, or chest irradiation is associated with increased risk of carcinoma.
• Family history of thyroid carcinoma or MEN syndrome

Physical Examination

• Inspect, palpate, and auscultate the neck.

—Neck extension aids inspection.
—Palpation is best performed standing behind the child. Determine if the thyroid is diffusely enlarged or asymmetric, evaluate gland firmness, and assess for any nodularity. Check for cervical lymphadenopathy.
—Auscultate with the stethoscope diaphragm (while patient holds his/her breath) for a bruit, which is indicative of the hyperthyroidism-associated hypervascularity.

• Pain on palpation suggests acute inflammation.
• Careful examination for signs of hypothyroidism or hyperthyroidism: pulse, linear growth and weight pattern, sexual development, deep tendon reflexes, skin

Procedure

Have patient drink water during inspection of gland. Isthmus of thyroid is just below the cricoid cartilage.

Laboratory Aids

TESTS

• Thyroid function tests: total T_4 and TSH comprise the best screen for hypo- or hyperthyroidism.
• T_3-RIA in cases of suspected hyperthyroidism (note: RIA, which measures total T_3, and *not* resin uptake, which indirectly assesses thyroid hormone binding capacity!)
• In cases of suspected CLT: antithyroglobulin and antimicrosomal (antiperoxidase) antibodies
• In cases of suspected Graves disease: thyroid-stimulating immunoglobulins (or TSH-receptor antibodies)
• Fine-needle aspiration biopsy is not a commonly used procedure in children and should be considered only in the evaluation of low-risk or purely cystic thyroid nodules. (Of all solitary thyroid nodules, the percent that is malignant is much higher in the pediatric age group than in adults).
• Calcitonin levels: elevated in 75% of patients with medullary carcinoma

Imaging

• Ultrasound is useful in determining the number, size, and nature (cystic, solid, or mixed) of nodules.
• ^{123}I thyroid scans should be done in cases of solitary nodules to establish whether or not the nodule concentrates iodide. "Cold" nodules (no I uptake) are suggestive of neoplasia and require immediate evaluation by a pediatric endocrinologist and surgeon.

- Barium swallow studies can reveal a fistulous tract between the left piriform sinus and the left thyroid lobe in children with recurrent acute suppurative thyroiditis. Such fistulas are amenable to surgical resection.

False Positives

- Fat neck: adipose tissue, large sternocleidomastoid muscles
- Thyroglossal duct cysts
- Nonthyroidal neoplasms: lymphoma, teratoma, hygroma

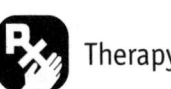 Therapy

Therapy is dictated by the cause of the goiter. Surgery solely to decrease the size of a goiter is indicated only if adjacent structures are compressed.

CANCER

- Surgery is recommended for a non-functioning nodule if there is a history of radiation, rapid growth of a firm nodule, satellite lymph nodes, evidence of impingement on other neck structures, or evidence of distant metastases.
- The affected lobe is removed and sent for frozen section; if this is suspicious, a total thyroidectomy should be performed.
- Following surgery, ^{131}I therapy is administered if a follow-up iodine scan reveals any residual tissue or metastases.
- Suppressive doses of exogenous thyroid hormone are then given to maintain TSH levels below 0.2 μIU/mL.
- Thyroglobulin levels are useful as markers of thyroid tissue; calcitonin level serves as tumor marker for medullary carcinoma.
- Some advocate subtotal thyroidectomy, no irradiation, and suppressive T_4 treatment.

DRUGS

L-thyroxine is indicated for the treatment of goiters with hypothyroidism. In cases of goiter with hyperthyroidism, initial treatment consists of antithyroid drugs (propylthiouracil or methimazole). Please see sections on hypothyroidism and Graves disease for further details.

DURATION

Depends on the cause of the goiter

DIET

Depends on the cause of the goiter. The incidence of iodine deficiency (endemic) goiter has greatly declined since the addition of potassium iodide to table salt. Iodide can also be added to communal drinking water or administered as an iodized oil in isolated rural areas.

POSSIBLE CONFLICTS

In the case of manic-depressive patients on lithium and cardiac patients on amiodarone, medication-induced thyroid abnormalities can be a significant problem that should be addressed by the endocrinologist and appropriate subspecialist.

 Follow-Up

- The potential for goiter regression depends on its cause. Goiters associated with CLT and Graves disease may or may not decrease in size with treatment.
- A goiter patient who is clinically and biochemically euthyroid still requires careful follow-up for the detection of the early signs of developing thyroid dysfunction.
- Potential complications of thyroid surgery include laryngeal nerve damage and hypoparathyroidism.

PITFALLS

Failure to work up solitary thyroid nodules aggressively; remember, incidence of malignancy in these nodules in children is 15% to 40% (less in adults).

 Common Questions and Answers

Q: Does a bigger thyroid gland mean increased thyroid functioning?
A: Goiters can be euthyroid, hypothyroid, or hyperthyroid, depending on cause.

Q: Will the goiter decrease in size with treatment?
A: This again depends on the cause of the goiter. For example, correction of an elevated TSH in CLT with treatment can result in goiter shrinkage. In iodine-deficient states, treatment will cause the *early* hyperplastic goiter to regress.

Q: Does a bigger thyroid gland mean cancer?
A: Most pediatric goiters are benign, and thyroid cancers often are detected as solitary nodules within an otherwise normal gland (in children with solitary nodules, up to 40% are carcinomas). Patients with a history of goiter or benign nodules/adenomas have an increased risk of developing thyroid cancer.

Q: Does thyroid cancer usually present with hyperthyroidism?
A: No. The usual chief complaint is a solitary, hard, painless nodule in a euthyroid patient.

Q: Is there an increased risk of thyroid cancer from diagnostic x-rays (chest x-rays, lateral neck films)?
A: Routine diagnostic x-rays should fall well below the levels of radiation thought to increase risk of thyroid neoplasia. During more prolonged radiologic procedures that might expose the thyroid to higher doses of radiation, a lead neck shield is used.

Q: Should prophylactic thyroidectomy be performed in children identified genetically as having familial medullary carcinoma?
A: Yes, due to the poorer prognosis associated with development of this cancer.

ICD-9-CM 240.9

BIBLIOGRAPHY

Aghini-Lombardi F, Antonangeli Z, Martino E, et al. The spectrum of thyroid disorders in an iodine-deficient community: the Pescopagano survey. *J Clin Endocrinol Metab* 1999;84:561–566.

Alsanea O, Clark OH. Familial thyroid cancer. *Curr Opin Oncol* 2001;13:44–51.

American Academy of Pediatrics Committee on Environmental Health. Risk of ionizing radiation exposure to children: a subject review. *Pediatrics* 1998;101:717–719.

Brix TH, Hegedus L. Genetic and environmental factors in the aetiology of simple goiter. *Ann Med* 2000;32:153–156.

Capon F, Tacconelli A, Giardina E, et al. Mapping of a dominant form of multinodular goiter to chromosome Xp22. *Am J Hum Genet* 2000;67:1004–1007.

Feinmesser R, Lubin E, Segal K, et al. Carcinoma of the thyroid in children—a review. *J Pediatr Endocrinol Metab* 1997;10:561–568.

Franceschi S, Preston-Martin S, Dal Maso L, et al. A pooled analysis of case-control studies of thyroid cancer. IV. Benign thyroid diseases. *Cancer Causes Control* 1999;10:583–595.

From G, Mellemgaard A, Knudson N, et al. Review of thyroid cancer cases among patients with previous benign thyroid disorders. *Thyroid* 2000;10:697–700.

Ladenson PW. Optimal laboratory testing for diagnosis and monitoring of thyroid nodules, goiter and thyroid cancer. *Clin Chem* 1996;42:183–187.

Wang C, Crapo LM. The epidemiology of thyroid disease and the implications for screening. *Endocrinol Metab Clin North Am* 1997;26:189–218.

Yeh SD, La Quaglia MP. 131I therapy for pediatric thyroid cancer. *Semin Pediatr Surg* 1997;6:128–133.

Zimmerman D. Thyroid neoplasia in children. *Curr Opin Pediatr* 1997;9:413–418.

Author: Adda Grimberg
Marta Satin-Smith, 2nd edition

Gonococcal Infections

Database

DEFINITION

Neisseria gonorrhoeae, an aerobic gram-negative diplococcus, is the etiologic agent of gonorrhea. In the U.S., over 1 million new infections are diagnosed each year, usually in sexually active adolescents or adults.

PATHOPHYSIOLOGY

• Transmission results from contact with infected mucous membranes and secretions, usually through sexual activity, parturition, and (very rarely) household contact in prepubertal children.
• The risk of male-to-female transmission is 50% per episode of vaginal intercourse; the risk of female-to-male transmission is approximately 20% per episode. Rectal intercourse is also an effective mode of transmission, but orogenital contact is not.
• Incubation period is 2 to 5 days.
• Immunity is not induced by infection.

ASSOCIATED DISEASES

Pediatric gonococcal infections can be categorized by age group: neonates, prepubertal children, and sexually active adolescents.
• Neonatal gonococcal diseases include ophthalmia neonatorum, scalp abscess (complication of fetal scalp monitoring), and, rarely, vaginitis or systemic disease with arthritis, bacteremia, funisitis, or meningitis.
• Prepubertal gonococcal disease usually occurs in the genital tract. Vaginitis is the most common manifestation. Pelvic inflammatory disease (PID), perihepatitis, urethritis, proctitis, and pharyngitis rarely occur. Sexual abuse must be considered when genital, rectal, or pharyngeal gonococcal infections occur in prepubertal children (see Pitfalls, below).
• Sexually active adolescents have a spectrum of gonococcal disease similar to adults. Orogenital contact may lead to pharyngitis. Asymptomatic or symptomatic anorectal infection occurs in both sexes. In females, genital tract infection may be asymptomatic or cause urethritis, vaginitis, and endocervicitis. Ascending genital tract infection may lead to PID and perihepatitis. In males, acute urethritis is the predominant manifestation. Epididymitis occurs infrequently.

EPIDEMIOLOGY

• In the U.S., the highest attack rates occur in 15- to 24-year-old women and men.
• The black/white incidence ratio of urogenital gonococcal infection is 40:1.
• Gonorrhea is the most common STD found in sexually abused children.
• Gonococcal conjunctivitis is rare in adults, but occurs most often in patients who have anogenital infection; autoinoculation of infected secretions is the most likely mode of transmission.
• PID occurs in 10% to 20% of women with gonorrhea.

COMPLICATIONS

• Gonococcal infection during pregnancy
—Gonococcal PID is associated with spontaneous abortion, preterm labor, and perinatal infant mortality.
• Ophthalmia neonatorum
—Gonococcal ophthalmia neonatorum can have a rapidly destructive course with corneal ulceration or perforation, with subsequent scarring and blindness if not treated early.
• Pelvic inflammatory disease
—Endometritis, salpingitis, tubo-ovarian abscess, and pelvic peritonitis occur as a consequence of untreated vaginal disease.
—Scarring secondary to salpingitis causes sterility in up to 20% of women with a single infection and up to 50% of women after three episodes of infection.
—A woman's risk of ectopic pregnancy increases sevenfold after one episode of PID.
• In males, rare complications include periurethral abscess, acute prostatitis, seminal vesiculitis, and urethral strictures.
• Disseminated disease
—Occurs via hematogenous dissemination of infection.
—Patients with multiple episodes of disseminated gonococcal infection should be tested for complement deficiency.
—In neonates, arthritis is the most frequent systemic manifestation of gonococcal disease. Symptoms develop 1 to 4 weeks after delivery. Involvement of multiple joints is typical, and most of these infants have no evidence of ophthalmia neonatorum.
—In older children and adolescents, septic arthritis (one joint) and a characteristic syndrome of polyarthritis (multiple joints)-dermatitis are predominant manifestations.
—Gonococcal meningitis, endocarditis, and osteomyelitis are very rare in children.

PROGNOSIS

• Good prognosis depends on early diagnosis and effective treatment of infection prior to progression.
• Prognosis has also been improved by treating all forms of infection with a third-generation cephalosporin due to the increased prevalence of penicillin-resistant *N. gonorrhoeae.*

Differential Diagnosis

• Ophthalmia neonatorum: Other causes of neonatal conjunctivitis include *C. trachomatis, S. aureus, S. pneumoniae, Haemophilus* species, and HSV.
• Scalp infection: Gonococcal scalp abscesses may be difficult to distinguish from abscesses caused by staphylococcal species, group B *Streptococcus, H. influenzae,* Enterobacteri-aceae, and HSV.
• Vaginitis: In the prepubertal child, other causes include chemical or environmental irritants, pinworms, foreign body, and infections (i.e., streptococci, other bacteria, *Trichomonas vaginalis*). In cases of sexual abuse, *C. trachomatis* and syphilis may occur.
• Genitourinary tract infection: In adolescents, other causes include *C. trachomatis,* syphilis, and *T. vaginalis.*
• Arthritis: Other bacterial causes of septic arthritis, Reiter's syndrome, and reactive arthritis.
• Abdominal pain: Ectopic pregnancy, appendicitis, cholecystitis, and urinary tract infection.

Data Gathering

HISTORY

Question: Premature or prolonged rupture of membranes (or fetal scalp monitoring)?
Significance: These are risk factors for conjunctival infection caused by *N. gonorrhoeae.* Fetal scalp monitoring places the infant at risk for gonococcal scalp abscess.

Question: Vaginal itching and discharge?
Significance: Signs and symptoms of vaginitis. Prepubertal gonorrheal vaginitis is typically a mild disease that rarely causes ascending or disseminated infection. In adolescents, estrogenization protects the vagina from infection. Instead, the vagina serves as a conduit for cervical exudate.

Question: Purulent urethral discharge and dysuria without urgency or frequency?
Significance: Urethritis.

Question: Abdominal pain?
Significance: Ascending infection is characterized by diffuse lower quadrant abdominal pain, which may cause significant discomfort with ambulation. Low back pain, dyspareunia, and abnormal vaginal bleeding occasionally occur. Fever, chills, nausea, and vomiting may be present. Acute perihepatitis (Fitz-Hugh-Curtis syndrome) causes right upper quadrant pain and results from direct extension of infection from the fallopian tube to the liver capsule.

Question: Symptoms of pharyngitis, arthritis, dermatitis, meningitis, or endocarditis?
Significance: Gonococcal infections may occur outside the genitourinary tract.

Gonococcal Infections

Physical Examination

Finding: Neonatal ophthalmia
Significance: Typical findings include bilateral eyelid edema, chemosis, and copious purulent discharge. Onset may be on the first day of life, if prolonged rupture of membranes has occurred, or as late as several weeks of age.

Finding: Neonatal scalp abscess
Significance: Complication of fetal scalp monitoring.

Finding: Cervical motion tenderness
Significance: Signs of PID include cervical motion tenderness, pelvic adnexal tenderness (usually bilateral), and lower or right upper quadrant abdominal pain (with perihepatitis).

Finding: Purulent vaginal discharge
Significance: Common in both cervicitis and urethritis. Associated bacterial vaginosis may be noted.

Laboratory Aids

Test: Gram stain and culture of infected exudate or body fluid.
Significance: Intracellular gram-negative diplococci on Gram stain. Confirmation is dependent on isolation of *N. gonorrhoeae* from culture. The specimens are inoculated onto Thayer-Martin or chocolate blood agar-based media at room temperature, and placed promptly in an enriched CO_2 environment for incubation. In suspected sexual abuse, genital, rectal, and pharyngeal cultures should be collected

Test: STD panel
Significance: Test for other sexually transmitted diseases in the child in whom sexual abuse is suspected or when evaluating the sexually active adolescent. This includes testing for *C. trachomatis*, syphilis, *T. vaginalis,* and HIV.

Test: Nonculture gonococcal tests
Significance: DNA amplification by polymerase chain reaction or ligase chain reaction (LCR) are comparable to culture in sensitivity and specificity but should NOT be used in investigations of possible sexual abuse (due to the possibility of false-positive results). In nonabuse cases, LCR may be performed on freshly voided urine (95% sensitivity; 100% specificity) and self-administered introital swabs.

Test: CBC, ESR, and C-reactive protein
Significance: Leukocytosis and elevated ESR and C-reactive protein occur in two thirds of patients with PID.

Test: Pelvic ultrasound
Significance: May detect ectopic pregnancy and in PID reveals thick, dilated fallopian tubes or tubo-ovarian abscess.

Test: Synovial fluid cell count and culture
Significance: In septic gonococcal arthritis, synovial fluid has >50,000 WBC/mm^3 and the synovial fluid culture is positive, while the blood culture is usually negative. In arthritis-dermatitis syndrome, the synovial fluid contains <20,000 WBC/mm^3, and the synovial fluid culture is sterile, while the blood culture is positive.

Therapy

• Neonate: Hospitalize and obtain appropriate cultures (blood, CSF, conjunctival, or other site of infection).
—Ophthalmia neonatorum: Ceftriaxone, 25 to 50 mg/kg IV or IM (single dose; up to maximum dose of 125 mg); alternate for infant with hyperbilirubinemia is cefotaxime 100 mg/kg (single dose).
—Disseminated infection: Ceftriaxone daily or cefotaxime b.i.d. for 7 days; continue treatment for 10 to 14 days for meningitis.
• Neonates with gonococcal ophthalmia should have their eyes irrigated with sterile saline at presentation and at frequent intervals until the mucopurulent drainage has ceased.
• Older children and adolescents:
—Uncomplicated gonococcal infection: A single IM dose of ceftriaxone, or an oral dose of cefixime, ciprofloxacin, or ofloxacin. Follow with a treatment regimen for *C. trachomatis*.
—PID: See *Pediatric Red Book 2000* for treatment regimens.
—Disseminated gonococcal infection: Ceftriaxone for 7 days (arthritis), 14 days (meningitis), or 28 days (endocarditis). For arthritis add erythromycin, azithromycin, or doxycycline for 7 days. For meningitis or endocarditis add erythromycin for 7 days.

Follow-Up

INFECTION CONTROL

• Neonatal ophthalmia: Routine use of prophylactic ophthalmic ointment is mandatory in the U.S. Instillation of ointment in both eyes occurs immediately after birth; choice of drugs includes 1% silver nitrate, 1% tetracycline, and 0.5% erythromycin ophthalmic ointments.
• Sexual contacts of persons with gonorrhea should be treated and counseled.
• Evaluate for concurrent infection with other STDs, including syphilis, *C. trachomatis*, *T. vaginalis,* and HIV. Patients beyond the neonatal period should be treated presumptively for *C. trachomatis* infection.
• Routine screening cervical cultures should be performed at the first prenatal visit; repeat at term if high risk.
• All cases of gonorrhea must be reported to public health officials.

ISOLATION OF HOSPITALIZED PATIENT

• Contact isolation precautions for all patients with gonococcal disease in the neonatal and prepubescent age groups are recommended; no special policies are recommended for other patients.

PITFALLS

• Failure to consider the diagnosis of sexual abuse in a child with a gonococcal infection beyond the neonatal period. Cases of transmission via nonsexual contact have been reported (i.e., from freshly infected towels, or other fomites, or by digital transmission from an infected caregiver) but cannot be assumed without first excluding sexual abuse.
• Using DNA amplification methods instead of culture to diagnose infection in cases of suspected abuse.
• Failure to differentiate *N. gonorrhoeae* by culture from other *Neisseria* species, especially in prepubertal children, due to the underlying question of child sexual abuse.
• Failure to consider the diagnosis of acute gonococcal perihepatitis in females with right upper quadrant pain.
• Classic findings of fever, leukocytosis, and elevated ESR or C-reactive protein are absent in one third of patients with laparoscopically documented PID.

ICD-9-CM 098.0

BIBLIOGRAPHY

American Academy of Pediatrics. Pelvic inflammatory disease. In: Pickering LK, ed. *2000 red book: report of the Committee on Infectious Diseases,* 25th ed. Elk Grove Village, IL: American Academy of Pediatrics, 2000:431–435.

Darville T. Gonorrhea. *Pediatr Rev* 1999;20:125–128.

Ingram DM, Miller WC, Schoenbach VJ, et al. Risk assessment for gonococcal and chlamydial infections in young children undergoing evaluation for sexual abuse. *Pediatrics* 2001;107(5):e73.

Koumans EH, Johnson RE, Knapp JS, et al. Laboratory testing for *Neisseria gonorrhoeae* by recently introduced nonculture tests: a performance review with clinical and public health considerations. *Clin Infect Dis* 1998;27:1171–1180.

Sparling PF, Handsfield HH. *Neisseria gonorrhoeae.* In: Mandell GL, Bennett JE, Dolin R, eds. *Principles and practice of infectious diseases.* Philadelphia: Churchill Livingstone, 2000:2242–2258.

Woodin KA. *Neisseria gonorrhoeae.* In: Long SS, Pickering LK, Prober CG, eds. *Principles and practice of pediatric infectious diseases.* New York: Churchill Livingstone, 1997:845–853.

Authors: Samir S. Shah
Molly (Martha) W. Stevens, 2nd edition

Graft Versus Host Disease

 Database

DEFINITION

Graft versus host disease (GVHD) is a multiorgan inflammatory process that develops when immunologically competent T lymphocytes from a histoincompatible donor are infused into an immunocompromised host who is unable to reject the donor T cells. It is divided into acute and chronic forms and is caused by:
- Bone marrow transplantation (BMT)
- Transfusion of nonirradiated blood products (e.g., products containing viable T lymphocytes) to congenitally immunodeficient hosts or to hosts that have received highly immunosuppressive treatment.
- Transfusion of nonirradiated blood products from a donor who is homozygous for one of the recipient's human leukocyte antigen (HLA) haplotypes (usually first- or second-degree relative).
- Intrauterine maternal-fetal transfusions and exchange transfusions in neonates
- Solid organ grafts that contain viable T cells (e.g., small bowel transplants)

PATHOPHYSIOLOGY

- Need three conditions to be met before GVHD can develop:
—The graft must contain immunocompetent cells.
—The host must possess important transplantation alloantigens that are lacking in the donor graft, so the host appears antigenically foreign to the graft-derived T cells.
—The host must be incapable of mounting an effective immune reaction against the graft.
- Acute GVHD: lymphocytic infiltration and epithelial cell necrosis involving the regenerative compartment of the three affected organ systems (e.g., the basal layer of the skin, the crypts of the large and small bowel, and the biliary epithelium of the portal triad).
- Transfusion-associated GVHD also affects the bone marrow.
- Acute GVHD develops within 100 days following allogeneic stem cell transplant.
- Chronic GVHD develops 100 to 500 days following allogeneic stem cell transplant.
- Chronic GVHD is divided into three subsets based on onset:
—Progressive onset—extension of acute GVHD
—Quiescent onset—occurs after resolution of acute GVHD
—De novo onset—no prior acute GVHD

GENETICS

- The major HLA gene complex is found on chromosome 6 and is inherited as a group or haplotype.
- Two full siblings have a 25% chance of being HLA identical.
- Minor histocompatibility antigen differences likely account for GVHD in the HLA identical sibling bone marrow transplant setting.

EPIDEMIOLOGY

- Acute GVHD occurs in 30% to 60% of matched related donor transplants.
- Chronic GVHD occurs 27% to 50% of sibling matched related donor transplants, 42% to 72% of matched related donor transplants, 42% to 72% matched unrelated donor transplants, and 54% to 70% of allogeneic peripheral blood stem cell transplants.
—Chronic GVHD is most common late complication of allogeneic stem cell transplantation.
- Other risk factors include:
—Type of GVHD prophylaxis and history of herpes virus infection in the donor or the recipient
—Prior pregnancies in the marrow donor (which give rise to allosensitization)
—Older donor or recipient age
—Gender mismatch
—Vigorous T-cell depletion decreases the incidence of both acute and chronic GVHD
—Prior acute GVHD increases the risk of developing chronic GVHD

COMPLICATIONS

- Mortality from GVHD after BMT is usually related to infection.
- Rarely, patients die of hepatic failure or abdominal catastrophe.
- In transfusion-associated GVHD, the major cause of death is bone marrow aplasia (usually does not respond to immunotherapy) because of destruction of the host's marrow by donor lymphocytes.

PROGNOSIS

Acute GVHD is graded on a scale from I to IV with percent of total body surface involved (skin), volume of diarrhea (gut), and/or elevation of serum bilirubin (liver).
- Grade I GVHD involves only one organ, usually the skin.
—Patients with grade I GVHD do not have a survival different from those without GVHD.
- Grade II GVHD involves more than one organ; patient can have nausea/vomiting, anorexia, and food intolerance; confirmed by EGD biopsy.
- Grade III GVHD is severe and has multiorgan involvement.
- Patients with grade IV GVHD have a survival of only 10% to 15% as do patients with progressive chronic GVHD (defined as acute GVHD, which does not resolve followed by chronic GVHD).

 Differential Diagnosis

ACUTE GVHD

- Skin: dermal changes from chemoradiotherapy, drug reaction, viral exanthem
- Liver: hepatic veno-occlusive disease (VOD), elevations of liver function tests due to total parenteral nutrition, drug toxicity or infection, especially bacterial sepsis and cytomegalovirus
- Gastrointestinal: diarrhea secondary to the BMT preparative regimen and infectious causes, especially *Clostridium difficile* and cytomegalovirus

 Data Gathering

HISTORY

Acute GVHD

Question: Rash? Itching?
Significance: Pruritus can precede the rash, which in BMT appears as the patient's blood counts are beginning to rise (median time of onset is 19 days posttransplant), and it is usually the first manifestation of acute GVHD. In transfusion-induced GVHD, symptoms usually start 1 week after the transfusion.
Question: Jaundice? Diarrhea? Abdominal pain? Intestinal bleeding?
Significance: GVHD in distal small bowel/colon. Unusual for involvement to precede skin disease.
Question: Anorexia? Nausea? Vomiting? Dyspepsia?
Significance: GVHD proximal to distal small bowel.

Chronic GVHD

Question: Dry eyes? Dry mouth?
Significance: Be sure to ask if the patient forms saliva or tears because sicca syndrome can develop.
Question: Dysphagia?
Significance: Complaints of difficulty swallowing or retrosternal pain may be due to esophageal strictures.
Question: Blurry vision? Eye irritation? Photophobia? Eye pain?
Significance: Keratoconjunctivitis.
Question: Sensitive to mint, spicy foods or tomatoes?
Significance: Mucosal involvement of GVHD
Question: Weight loss?
Significance: GI tract involvement of GVHD
Question: Dyspnea? Wheezing? Cough?
Significance: Bronchiolitis obliterans
Question: Frequent infections?
Significance: GVHD leads to profound immunodeficiency, functional asplenia, and can have variable IgG levels. Patients with chronic GVHD are at high-risk for pneumococcal sepsis, PCP, invasive fungal infections.

Physical Examination

Acute GVHD/Transfusion-Associated GVHD
Finding: Skin
Significance: Often begins as erythema of the palms, soles, and ears. The rash can become confluent erythroderma, and in the most severe cases can lead to bullae formation and even denudation reminiscent of burn injuries.
Finding: Liver
Significance: Jaundice can be seen but painful hepatomegaly, ascites, and rapid weight gain are atypical and are more often seen in VOD.
Finding: Gastrointestinal
Significance: Stool is often watery, green, and bloody (although it may only be guaiac positive).

Chronic GVHD
Characterized as limited (localized skin involvement or hepatic dysfunction) or extensive (diffuse skin and/or multiorgan involvement with a much worse prognosis).

Finding: Skin
Significance: Hyper- or hypopigmentation, patchy erythema, scaling, lichenoid and sclerodermatous changes can be seen. The skin is involved in almost every patient.
Finding: Alopecia
Significance: Scalp and body hair can be thin and fragile.
Finding: Nails
Significance: Vertical ridging and fragile
Finding: Whitish lace-like plaques on cheeks or tongue (resembles lichen planus) or ulcerations that are painful
Significance: Mucosal involvement of GVHD or thrush so should do biopsy for viral and fungal cultures.
Finding: Joints
Significance: Swelling can be seen: a detailed range of motion examination is crucial because contractures can be found in the absence of joint swelling.

Laboratory Aids

The diagnosis of GVHD is often made on clinical grounds.

Test: Laboratory
Significance: In hepatic GVHD isolated elevations of transaminases can be seen without hyperbilirubinemia. In more severe cases, a cholestatic picture is seen. Howell-Jolly bodies can be seen on peripheral blood smear in the functional asplenia of chronic GVHD. Occasionally, patients will have cytopenias, or eosinophilia.
Test: Radiologic
Significance: Although total body irradiation and busulfan used in BMT can lead to pulmonary fibrosis, the picture of bronchiolitis obliterans on CT scan is considered a manifestation of chronic GVHD.
Test: Biopsy
Significance: Skin—localized epidermal

atrophy; liver—bile duct damage reminiscent to primary biliary cirrhosis. Of note, during the first 3 weeks post-BMT, skin and gastrointestinal histologic changes from chemoradiotherapy are indistinguishable from GVHD.
Test: Pulmonary function tests
Significance: Evidence of bronchiolitis obliterans or pulmonary fibrosis
Test: Schirmer's test
Significance: Shows decrease tear production
Test: Fluorescein biomicroscopy
Significance: Punctate keratopathy

Therapy

The best therapy is prevention and includes γ-irradiation of all cellular blood products for patients at risk.
• Treatment of established acute GVHD includes:
—Steroids at a dose of 2 mg/kg/d for 2 weeks followed by a taper over several months
—Cyclosporine or FK506 in those patients who did not receive it as prophylaxis
—Antithymocyte globulin (ATG) for steroid-resistant patients
—Mycophenolate mofetil (MMF), daclizumab (Zenapax) are used as second- line drugs.
• Options in treatment of chronic GVHD include:
—Steroids either alone or in combination with cyclosporine, MMF, daclizumab, or FK506. Because many patients require treatment for months, the goal is alternate-day therapy (e.g., steroids alternating with cyclosporine).
—Psoralen plus ultraviolet A (PUVA) is of some benefit in skin GVHD.
—Oral beclomethasone has been used for treatment of gastrointestinal GVHD.
—Ursodeoxycholic acid may be of benefit for hepatic GVHD.
—Other options include thalidomide and azathioprine. Studies of azathioprine suggested a high infection rate when it was given with steroids.
—Infection is the primary cause of death in patients with chronic GVHD; so all patients should receive PCP and pneumococcal infection prophylaxis.
—IVIG for patients with low serum IgG levels.
• Manage patient's symptoms, e.g., lubricate dry skin with petroleum jelly, protect skin from injury, avoid sunburn, use artificial tears for sicca syndrome, and treat electrolyte imbalances for muscular aches and cramps.
• PT/ROM exercises to help prevent contractures.
• Nutrition consults for malnutrition and wasting

Follow-Up

• Acute GVHD: The institution of steroid therapy should lead to improvement within days in those patients who are destined to respond. However, gastrointestinal symptoms are notoriously slow to respond.

• Chronic GVHD: Acute GVHD, which merges directly into chronic GVHD, is termed progressive and has an extremely poor prognosis (approximately 10% survival at 5 years post-BMT). Thrombocytopenia is another poor prognostic factor. Such patients usually die of infection.
• Of note, patients with limited chronic GVHD have a decreased rate of relapse of leukemia and an increased survival rate.

PITFALLS
• Do not immunize patients with a live vaccine if they have chronic GVHD. This may result in symptomatic infection.
• Take sudden high fevers seriously in a patient with GVHD. Overwhelming bacterial sepsis is not infrequent. Patients with chronic GVHD are often functionally asplenic (even if Howell-Jolly bodies are not seen on peripheral blood smear) and have profound immune function impairment.

Common Questions and Answers

Q: If children get acute GVHD, does that mean they will get chronic GVHD?
A: No. Approximately 30% of patients younger than 10 years of age who receive an HLA identical sibling BMT will get acute GVHD, whereas only 13% will develop chronic GVHD. Of note, chronic GVHD can develop in a patient who did not have acute GVHD. This is termed de novo and is much more favorable than progressive chronic GVHD.
Q: Do patients with severe chronic GVHD all die?
A: No. Occasionally the GVHD will "burn out." This is rare, and the process by which it happens is not understood.

ICD-9-CM 996.85

BIBLIOGRAPHY
Ferrara JLM, Levy R, Chao NJ. Pathophysiologic mechanism of acute GVHD. *Biol Blood Marrow Transplant* 1999;5:347–356.

Gaziev D, Galimberti M, Lucarelli G, et al. Chronic G-V-H disease: is there an alternative to the conventional treatment? *Bone Marrow Transplant* 2000;25:689–696.

Lazarus HM, Vogelsang GB, Rowe JM. Prevention and treatment of acute GVH disease: the old and the new. A report from the Eastern Cooperative Oncology Group (ECOG). *Bone Marrow Transplant* 1997;19: 577–600.

Shivadansani RA, Haluska FG, Dock NL, et al. Brief report: Graft-versus-host disease associated with transfusion of blood from unrelated HLA-homozygous donors. *N Engl J Med* 1993;328:766–770.

Vogelsang GB. How I treat chronic graft versus host disease. *Blood* 2001;27(5):1196–1201.

Author: Valerie I. Brown
Ann Marie Leahey, 2nd edition

Graves Disease

Database

DEFINITION

Multisystem autoimmune disorder that presents with the classic triad of hyperthyroidism (goiter), exophthalmos, dermopathy (rare in children)

PATHOPHYSIOLOGY

- Autoimmune process that includes production of immunoglobulins against antigens in the thyroid, orbital tissue, and dermis.
- IgG_1 anti-TSH receptor-autoantibody (thyroid-stimulating immunoglobulin; TSI) activates the receptor, resulting in constitutive stimulation; thyroid follicular cells hyperfunction, leading to increased production and release of thyroid hormone.
- Fetal and neonatal hyperthyroidism can be caused by transplacental passage of maternal thyroid-stimulating immunoglobulins, activating G_s protein mutations (McCune-Albright syndrome) and activating TSH-receptor mutations.

GENETICS

- No simple hereditary pattern (genetic susceptibility plus environmental factors).
  —Up to 60% of patients have a familial history of autoimmune thyroid disease (hyper- or hypothyroidism).
  —Concordance rates of Graves disease: 30% to 60% in monozygotic twins; 3% to 9% in dizygotic twins.
- Associated with increased frequency of haplotype HLA-DR3.
- Linkage studies identified CTLA-4 (chromosome 2q), TSHR (chromosome 14q), and HLA (chromosome 6p) as susceptibility genes; additional loci have also been reported.

EPIDEMIOLOGY

- 10% to 15% of all childhood thyroid disorders.
- Incidence increases with age, peaking in adolescence and the third to fourth decade.
- Male/female ratio 1:4–5

COMPLICATIONS

- Endocrine disturbances: delayed/early puberty, menstrual irregularity, hypercalcemia
- Ophthalmologic: 3% to 5% of patients develop severe ophthalmopathy, including eye muscle dysfunction and optic neuropathy, requiring specific treatment by an ophthalmologist. Pediatric ophthalmologic findings are more common but usually less severe than in adults.
- Bone: Hyperthyroidism leads to high bone turnover, with osteopenia common at the time of diagnosis. Bone mass corrects with treatment of the Graves disease and return to euthyroid status.
- Fetal/neonatal: IUGR, nonimmune hydrops fetalis, craniosynostosis, intrauterine death, goiter that complicates labor and possibly precipitates life-threatening airway obstruction at delivery, hyperkinesis, FTT, diarrhea, vomiting, cardiac failure and arrhythmias, systemic and pulmonary

hypertension, hepatosplenomegaly, jaundice, hyperviscosity syndrome, thrombocytopenia

PROGNOSIS

- Good, if compliant with treatment.
- Mortality in severe thyrotoxicosis is possible from cardiac arrhythmias or cardiac failure.
- Spontaneous remission occurs in up to 25% of children after 2 years and 50% by 4.5 years. Relapse is not uncommon (3–40%).
- Neonatal hyperthyroidism remits by 48 weeks, and commonly by 20 weeks.

Differential Diagnosis

For other causes of hyperthyroidism, see Goiter

INFECTIOUS

- Acute suppurative thyroiditis (transient thyroxine elevations).
- Subacute thyroiditis after viral illness (also transient hyperthyroidism).

ENVIRONMENTAL

- Thyroid hormone ingestion
- Ingestion of excess iodine (escape from Wolff-Chaikoff effect due to impaired autoregulation)

TUMORS (ALL RARE IN CHILDHOOD)

- TSH-producing pituitary adenoma
- Thyroid adenoma/hyperfunctioning autonomous thyroid nodule (most pediatric cases are euthyroid; incidence of nodule hyperfunctioning rises with increasing patient age).
- Thyroid carcinoma (rarely presents with hyperthyroidism)

CONGENITAL

- Neonatal Graves disease (transplacental antibody transfer from mothers with Graves disease or chronic thyroiditis)

GENETIC AND DEVELOPMENTAL

- Pituitary resistance to thyroid hormones (dominant negative thyroid-receptor gene mutations causing loss of the usual pituitary negative feedback loop and, hence, inappropriately elevated TSH; pituitary resistance can be isolated, with clinical hyperthyroidism, or associated with peripheral thyroid resistance as well, leading to clinical euthyroidism or hypothyroidism).
- TSH-receptor gene mutations (rare; germline activating TSH-receptor mutations cause autosomal-dominant nonautoimmune hereditary hyperthyroidism).
- McCune-Albright syndrome (activating G-protein mutation can lead to indolent hyperthyroidism in addition to the classic features of this syndrome).
- Ectopic thyroid tissue

Data Gathering

HISTORY

Question: Growth acceleration? May also be associated with precocious puberty

Significance: Hyperthyroidism can accelerate the bone age (developmental tempo).
Question: Declining school performance?
Significance: Mind racing, difficulty concentrating; may be mistaken for attention deficit/hyperactivity disorder.
Question: Any symptoms of hyperthyroidism and their duration?

- Restlessness, emotional lability, and nervousness
- Fine tremor
- Insomnia and disturbed sleep pattern; may result in daytime fatigue
- Weight loss, despite increased appetite
- Palpitations and even chest pain with minimal exertion or at rest; diminished exercise tolerance
- Heat intolerance
- Diarrhea
- Muscle weakness (proximal)
- Plummer nails (separation of nail from nail bed)
- Menstrual irregularities
- Increased urination

Significance: If child complains of these symptoms, evaluate for possible hyperthyroidism.
Question: Notice any thyroid gland enlargement? Its duration? Tenderness?
Significance: Goiter can be a presenting sign of Graves. Tenderness suggests an infectious etiology.
Question: Bulging of the eyes or change in facial appearance? Increased staring? Change in vision?
Significance: Exophthalmos due to retro-orbital immune depositions are a hallmark of Graves disease.
Question: Familial history of thyroid disease?
Significance: Increased incidence of Graves disease in families with positive history.

Physical Examination

Finding: Accelerated growth, or height above that expected by genetic potential
Significance: Due to bone age advancement.
Finding: Symmetrically enlarged, smooth, nontender goiter
Significance: More than 95% of cases
Finding: Auscultate the thyroid gland for bruit while patient holds his/her breath
Significance: Due to glandular hyperperfusion associated with hyperthyroidism.
Finding: Resting tachycardia with widened pulse pressure; hyperdynamic precordium
Significance: Cardiac effects of excessive thyroid hormone.
Finding: Slightly elevated temperature
Significance: Thyroid hormone is the main controller of basal metabolic rate and a positive modulator for catecholamine-induced thermogenesis.
Finding: Lid lag/stare; exophthalmos and proptosis
Significance: Severe ophthalmopathy is rare.
Finding: Fine tremor especially visible in hands and tongue

significance: Occurs in about 60% of children with Graves disease

Finding: Proximal muscle weakness
significance: Common but seldom severe
Finding: Exaggerated deep tendon reflexes
significance: Variable
Finding: Skin warmth and moisture
significance: Heat intolerance and excessive sweating occur in more than 30% of children.

Laboratory Aids

TESTS

Test: Total or free T_4
significance: Elevated
Test: T_3 RIA
significance: Elevated (T_3 RIA, as direct measurement of T_3, and not T_3 RU, which indirectly evaluates thyroid hormone binding capacity).
Test: TSH
significance: Significantly suppressed or undetectable
Test: TSI titer
significance: Positive in 90% of children

IMAGING

Test: I-123 scan
significance: Usually not necessary to diagnose Graves disease, show diffuse increased uptake at 6 and 24 hours. If palpation suggests a nodule, however, a scan may be useful to reveal a "hot" nodule within a suppressed gland.

FALSE POSITIVES

• Elevated total T_4 can also be due to conditions of increased protein binding, but does not signify hyperthyroidism.
—Increased estrogen states (e.g., pregnancy and oral contraceptive use) lead to augmented hepatic thyroid binding globulin (TBG) production
—Familial dysalbuminemic hyperthyroxinemia: mutation affecting the binding affinity leads to increased protein-bound pool

Therapy

DRUGS

• First line of therapy in children
• Medications block thyroid hormone synthesis but not the release of already existing hormone.
• Antithyroid medications (thiourea derivatives): 65% to 95% effective
—Methimazole
—Propylthiouracil (PTU)
• Propranolol or atenolol: block β-adrenergic related symptoms; should be used in conjunction with antithyroid medications at the initiation of treatment and whenever cardiac symptoms are prominent.
• Duration of treatment
—Antithyroid medications can be weaned and potentially discontinued after 2 to 3 years of therapy, depending on the patient's course.
—Beta-blockers: used until T_4/T_3 levels are under control (approximately 6 weeks).

• Other therapies should be considered in patients who are unresponsive to drug therapy, who have significant side effects from drug therapy, or who are chronically noncompliant.

I-131 ABLATION THERAPY

• 90% to 100% effective; safe and definitive, with predictable outcome
• Results in permanent hypothyroidism requiring lifelong thyroxine replacement

SUBTOTAL THYROIDECTOMY

• 80% to 100% effective; rapid and definitive
• Expensive and invasive, with risk of significant complications
• Lifelong thyroxine replacement needed

POSSIBLE CONFLICTS

• Antihistamines and cold medications may exacerbate sympathetic nervous system symptoms.
• Treatment for severe ophthalmopathy: must refer to an ophthalmologist
—Three options: high-dose glucocorticoids, orbital radiotherapy, surgical orbital decompression
—Rehabilitative surgery involving the eye muscles or eyelids is commonly needed following ophthalmopathy treatment.
• Radioiodine ablation may exacerbate the ophthalmopathy, but this effect can be prevented with concomitant glucocorticoid administration.

Follow-Up

WHEN TO EXPECT IMPROVEMENT

• Propranolol or atenolol should result in rapid relief of symptoms of sympathetic hyperactivity.
• 4 to 6 weeks of medical treatment should result in normalization of T_4/T_3 levels, though TSH may remain suppressed due to persistent underlying TSI activity.
• Duration and type of treatment depends on remission and relapse pattern.

SIGNS TO WATCH FOR

• Side effects of medications: agranulocytosis (in 0.2—0.5%), rash (the most common side effect), gastrointestinal upset, headache, transient transaminitis/hepatitis with PTU

PITFALLS

• Discontinuation of antithyroid drugs because of low T_4 values while TSH is still suppressed, reflecting continued TSI activity, will likely result in relapse. Antithyroid medication dose should be decreased or L-thyroxine should be added.
• Failure to recognize thyroid storm—an endocrinologic medical emergency.

Common Questions and Answers

Q: Does hyperthyroidism mean my child has thyroid cancer?
A: No. The vast majority of pediatric thyroid cancers are euthyroid because even well-differentiated carcinomas synthesize thyroid hormone much less efficiently than does normal tissue.
Q: Does Graves disease lead to thyroid cancer?
A: No. However, there is an increased incidence of benign thyroid adenoma from 0.6% to 1.9% after use of I-131 ablation.
Q: Does hyperthyroidism affect long-term growth or final adult height?
A: No. Hyperthyroidism can cause tall stature and acceleration of skeletal maturity but does not typically affect final adult height.
Q: Should routine white blood cell counts be monitored while on antithyroid medications due to the risk of agranulocytosis?
A: No. Routine monitoring is not cost-effective due to the acuity and rarity of agranulocytosis. However, white blood cell counts should be checked whenever a patient on antithyroid medication develops a fever.
Q: Will the ophthalmopathy correct with antithyroid treatment?
A: Not necessarily. It may require specific intervention by an ophthalmologist.
Q: Can mothers breast-feed while treated for Graves disease?
A: Yes. PTU has a lower milk/serum concentration ratio than methimazole (0.1 and 1.0, respectively). 3 of 11 infants exclusively breast-fed by women on 300 to 750 mg daily PTU had high TSHs; of these three, one was just above the normal range and the other two completely corrected while the mother was still being medicated.

ICD-9-CM 242.0

BIBLIOGRAPHY

Bartalena L, Pinchera A, Marcocci C. Management of Graves' ophthalmopathy: reality and perspectives. *Endocr Rev* 2000;21:168–199.

Cooper DS. Antithyroid drugs for the treatment of hyperthyroidism caused by Graves' disease. *Endocrinol Metab Clin North Am* 1998;27:225–247.

Kaplan MK, Meier DA, Dworkin HJ. Treatment of hyperthyroidism with radioactive iodine. *Endocrinol Metab Clin North Am* 1998;27:205–223.

Lippe BM, Landau EM, Kaplan SA. Hyperthyroidism in children treated with long term medical therapy: twenty-five percent remission every two years. *J Clin Endocrinol Metab* 1987;64:1241.

Momotani N, Yamashita R, Makino F, et al. Thyroid function in wholly breast-feeding infants whose mothers take high doses of propylthiouracil. *Clin Endocrinol* 2000;53: 177–181.

Raza J, Hindmarsh PC, Brook CG. Thyrotoxicosis in children: thirty years' experience. *Acta Paediatr* 1999;88:937–941.

Zimmerman D. Fetal and neonatal hyperthyroidism. *Thyroid* 1999;9:727–733.

Author: Adda Grimberg
Marta Satin-Smith, 2nd edition

Growth Hormone Deficiency

 Database

DEFINITION

Growth hormone (GH) deficiency is a lack of growth hormone synthesis, release, or effect.

CAUSES

- Idiopathic (the most common form)
- Congenital

—Congenital absence of the pituitary (empty sella syndrome)
—Deletion of the GH gene in familial isolated GH deficiency
—Familial panhypopituitarism
—Growth hormone receptor defect (Laron syndrome)
—Post-growth hormone receptor defect
—Often associated with other midline defects: cleft lip, cleft palate, septo-optic dysplasia, holoprosencephaly

- Acquired

—Trauma: perinatal insult, birth trauma, surgical resection of pituitary gland, surgical damage to pituitary stalk, child abuse
—Infection: viral encephalitis, bacterial or fungal infection, tuberculosis
—Vascular: pituitary infarction, pituitary aneurysm
—Pituitary or hypothalamic irradiation
—Chemotherapy
—Tumors: craniopharyngioma, glioma, pinealoma, primitive neuroectodermal tumor (PNET; medulloblastoma)
—Histiocytosis involving the pituitary gland or sella turcica
—Sarcoidosis
—Psychosocial dwarfism

PATHOPHYSIOLOGY

Lacking GH decreases levels of insulin-like growth factor I (IGF-I) which acts on cartilage to stimulate linear growth.

GENETICS

- Spontaneous
- Autosomal recessive
- Autosomal dominant
- X-linked forms

EPIDEMIOLOGY (AGE RELATED)

- Incidence in the United States is 1 per 4,000
- Males are more commonly diagnosed than females.
- Two peak ages of diagnosis:

—Less than 1 year of age, usually because of associated hypoglycemia
—After 4 years of age, usually because of poor linear growth

COMPLICATIONS

- Short stature
- Lack of self-esteem due to the short stature
- Delay in pubertal changes (sexual characteristics and growth spurt) due to delayed bone age
- Hypoglycemia (in the newborn period)
- Osteopenia

PROGNOSIS

Excellent

 Differential Diagnosis

- Constitutional delay of growth and adolescence
- Familial short stature
- Malnutrition
- Intrauterine growth retardation
- Renal failure
- Inflammatory bowel disease
- Celiac sprue
- Hypo- or achondroplasia
- Turner syndrome
- Russell-Silver syndrome
- Prader-Willi syndrome
- Cystic fibrosis
- Congenital heart disease
- Hypothyroidism
- Hypercortisolism

 Data Gathering

HISTORY

Question: Complications during pregnancy or delivery?
Significance: Growth failure associated with congenital GH deficiency manifests by third trimester; however, you must exclude material factors causing late intrauterine growth retardation such as oligohydramnios.

Question: Birth weight?
Significance: Birth weight is usually normal but birth length below the fifth percentile; length-for-weight at birth will be low.

Question: Hypoglycemia during infancy (the first months of life)?
Significance: GH is important to maintain euglycemia in the first months of life.

Question: Plot previous lengths/heights and characterize growth pattern (velocity)?
Significance: Growth velocity will be low, but the GH-deficient infant may not drop below the third percentile for length until the end of the first year of life.

Question: Signs/symptoms of systemic illness or chronic disease?
Significance: Vomiting, polyuria, loose stools, food-provoked gastrointestinal distress, etc., may suggest a cause other than GH deficiency.

Question: Heights of family members?
Significance: Measure both parents' heights whenever the family history reveals a man below 5'4" or a woman below 4'11" tall.

Question: Family timing of pubertal development: age at menarche or pubertal growth spurt?
Significance: Constitutional delay of growth and development tends to occur in multiple close family members.

Question: Document patient's growth pattern and heights of family members
Significance: Measure height and weight of siblings whenever practical; always review prior growth records for the patient and siblings.

SPECIAL QUESTIONS

Question: Do girls with short stature who are discovered to have a form of Turner syndrome show classic features of Turner syndrome?
Significance: These girls show more subtle features of Turner syndrome such as wide-spaced breasts, scoliosis, marked short stature and commonly delayed puberty. Rarely do such girls show a webbed neck, or lymph edema.

 Physical Examination

- Measure accurate weight and height with wall stadiometer
- Look for signs of syndromes, chronic disease, or malnutrition
- Evaluate Tanner stages of pubertal development
- Check males for micropenis (especially newborns)

Finding: Observe body habitus
Significance: Classic GH-deficient patient has:

- Protrusion of the frontal bones (frontal bossing)
- Midline facial defects such as poor development of nasal bridge and single central maxillary incisor
- Thin hair
- Poor nail growth
- High-pitched voice
- Truncal obesity and relative adiposity
- Cherubic facies

Finding: Observe dental development
Significance: Typically delayed

PROCEDURE

- Calculate dental age based on tooth eruption
- Quantify penile and testicular sizes:

—Small penis in GH deficiency
—Testicular size (volume using Prader beads)

- Palpate for submucosal cleft palate
- Test visual fields

- Calculate growth velocity between growth measurements

Laboratory Aids

SPECIFIC TESTS

Test: Growth factors
Significance: IGF-I and IGFBP-3 (insulin-like growth factor binding protein-3) production is regulated directly by GH

Test: GH provocative testing.
Significance: A random GH level is generally of minimal value to diagnose GH deficiency because beyond the neonatal period, GH is only secreted in brief pulses during deep sleep (at night).

NONSPECIFIC TESTS

Growth factors and the following general tests should be used to screen for common causes of poor growth before embarking on GH provocative testing.

- CBC with differential
- Sedimentation rate: looking for inflammatory processes
- Hepatic and renal function tests
- Chromosomes in females (to exclude Turner syndrome)
- Thyroid function tests

IMAGING

- Bone age: radiography of left hand and wrist
- If proven GH deficient, head MRI to look for central nervous system tumor

REQUIREMENTS FOR TESTING

All blood tests, except GH provocative testing, do not require any form of preparation.

Therapy

DRUGS

- Recombinant human growth hormone (rhGH) by subcutaneous injection daily
- Nutropin depot (long-acting rhGH preparation) by subcutaneous injection every 2 to 4 weeks
- Recombinant human GH-releasing hormone (rhGHRH) by subcutaneous injection

DURATION OF THERAPY

- In children and adolescents:

—Until growth velocity drops to 0.5 cm/year
—Once puberty is complete

- In adulthood:

—GH-deficient adults may benefit from lifelong rhGH therapy due to its effects on body composition, lipids, bone density, and general sense of well-being
—Patient should again undergo GH provocative testing (off rhGH therapy)

DIET

Unrestricted

POSSIBLE CONFLICTS

Usually not given in cancer patients until 1 year has elapsed without recurrence

Follow-Up

Every 3 months by an endocrinologist

WHEN TO EXPECT IMPROVEMENT

- Immediate effect on hypoglycemia
- Growth velocity improves within 3 to 6 months

SIGNS TO WATCH FOR

- Pseudotumor cerebri (headache, vision problems)
- Slipped capital femoral epiphysis (SCFE)
- Theoretically, increased risk of leukemia (though most studies suggest no significant increased risk)

PITFALLS

- Children with constitutional or pubertal delay show poor growth prior to starting puberty mimicking GH deficiency
- GH provocative testing may yield false-positive or false-negative results. 20% of normal children will fail at least one GH provocative test; obese but otherwise normal children are more likely to fail provocative GH testing.
- Malnutrition can cause low IGF-I.
- Psychosocial deprivation mimics GH deficiency. Such deprived patients may have low growth factors and respond poorly to GH provocative testing.
- rhGH therapy is associated with idiopathic intracranial hypertension (pseudotumor cerebri). This side effect is often transient, is usually reversible when the rhGH dose is decreased, and does not require cessation of therapy in all cases.
- Carefully evaluate any limp and knee or hip pain in patients on rhGH therapy because these symptoms may hail the onset of SCFE. SCFE mandates orthopedic consultation.
- There has been a slightly increased incidence of leukemia in rhGH-treated children. It is controversial whether this is due to rhGH or predisposing factors in these children (e.g., selection bias when studying children with growth failure).

Common Questions and Answers

Q: Does growth hormone increase adult height in patients with familial short stature or constitutional delay of growth and adolescence?
A: Clinical studies have not shown that rhGH consistently improves final adult height for these patients.

Q: Does growth hormone cause tumors?
A: Clinical studies have not confirmed an association.

ICD-9-CM 253.3

BIBLIOGRAPHY

Botero D, Lifshitz F. Intrauterine growth retardation and long-term effects on growth. *Curr Opin Pediatr* 1999;11(4):340–347.

Clayton PE, Cohen P, Tanaka T, et al. Diagnosis of growth hormone deficiency in childhood. On behalf of the Growth Hormone Research Society. *Horm Res* 2000;53(suppl 3):30.

Clayton PE, Cowell CT. Safety issues in children and adolescents during growth hormone therapy—a review. *Growth Hormone IGF Res* 2000;10(6):306–317.

Hintz RL. Approaches to the diagnosis and management of growth failure. *Pediatr Ann* 2000;29(9):537–538.

Hintz RL, Attie KM, Baptista J, et al. Effect of growth hormone treatment on adult height of children with idiopathic short stature. Genentech Collaborative Group. Multicenter study. Randomized controlled trial. *N Engl J Med* 1999;340(7):502–507.

Author: Craig A. Alter
Robert J. Ferry, Jr., 2nd edition

Guillain-Barré Syndrome

 ## Database

DEFINITION

Guillain-Barré syndrome (GBS) is an acquired inflammatory demyelinating polyradiculoneuropathy. It affects peripheral nerves, causing progressive weakness in the limbs, face, and respiratory muscles. Paresthesias or loss of sensation in the extremities in a classic stocking-glove distribution may extend proximally.

CAUSES

GBS follows viral infection in over 50% of cases. It has also been associated with bacterial infection (especially *Campylobacter jejuni*), surgery, and vaccination. Often, no precipitating event can be identified.

PATHOPHYSIOLOGY

Inflammatory infiltrate can be seen in areas of demyelination on nerve biopsy; lymphocytes and macrophages likely participate in myelin destruction. Both cell-mediated and humoral immune mechanisms play a role in pathogenesis.

ASSOCIATED DISEASES

- GBS is seen in a higher-than-expected rate in patients with sarcoidosis, systemic lupus erythematosus, lymphoma, HIV infection, Lyme disease, and solid tumors.
- Complications include respiratory failure, autonomic disturbances, aspiration, fluid balance and nutritional deficiencies, deep venous thrombosis, infection susceptibility, muscle atrophy, and joint contractures.

EPIDEMIOLOGY

Overall yearly incidence rate of 0.6 to 1.9 cases per 100,000. Of 95 recently reported pediatric GBS patients, 45 were age 1 to 5, 36 were age 6 to 10, and 14 were age 11 to 15.

GENETICS

Sporadic genetic factors may influence susceptibility to GBS, but there is no clear relationship between GBS and HLA type; few cases of GBS are reported among first-order relatives.

PROGNOSIS

85% have a good recovery; ultimate functional recovery depends on the degree of axonal injury, which can be predicted from electrodiagnostic studies. Death from early respiratory failure, autonomic instability, or other complications occurs in 3% to 6% in modern series.

 ## Differential Diagnosis

- Myasthenia gravis
- Botulism
- Intoxication (heavy metals, organophosphates, etc.)
- Myopathy
- Poliomyelitis and other acute (viral) motor neuron diseases
- Acute cerebellar ataxia
- Transverse myelitis
- Chronic inflammatory demyelinating polyneuropathy (CIDP)
- Vasculitic neuropathy
- Diphtheric neuropathy (rare)
- Porphyric neuropathy
- Locked-in state
- Psychogenic

Approach to the Patient

GBS has a variety of clinical presentations—index of suspicion is critical. Typical features are progressive motor weakness and areflexia, often following distal sensory changes. Common presentations include decreased ambulation (or crawling in toddlers), facial weakness, back pain, or sensory changes in the extremities. Acuity depends on the degree of respiratory involvement. Once respiratory status has been established and stabilized, attention should be directed to managing autonomic dysfunction (including bowel regimen), weakness, and pain.

 ## Data Gathering

HISTORY

Question: Problems walking?
Significance: Most patients first note leg weakness or gait instability that progresses over days to weeks.

Question: Diminished finger and toe sensation?
Significance: Paresthesias and pain frequently appear early in the course. The sensory changes classically occur in a stocking-glove distribution and progress proximally.

Question: Respiratory problems?
Significance: Weakness may lead to respiratory paralysis in 20% to 30% of children with GBS.

Question: Difficulty voiding?
Significance: Urinary retention may complicate course; requires early intervention.

 ## Physical Examination

Finding: Weakness and sensory changes
Significance: Typical signs of GBS, classically with distal greater than proximal involvement. A proximal predominance of symptoms does not preclude the diagnosis.

Finding: Deep tendon reflexes are lost.
Significance: Typical sign of GBS, though it may not occur until several days into the presentation.

Finding: Respiratory difficulty, measured as decreased vital capacity
Significance: Respiratory failure dictates intubation in up to 10% of patients.

Finding: Bilateral facial weakness
Significance: Occurs in up to 50% of cases.

Finding: "Floppy infant"
Significance: Neonates and infants may present as floppy infants.

 ## Laboratory Aids

Test: Lumbar puncture
Significance: Nearly all patients, particularly children, have elevated cerebrospinal fluid protein after the first week of symptoms. Minimal pleocytosis ($\leq$10 WBC/mm^3), comprised largely of mononuclear leukocytes, may occur but disappears in subsequent weeks.

Test: Electrodiagnosis
Significance: EMG findings can support the diagnosis of GBS and are often helpful when clinical or cerebrospinal fluid findings are ambiguous. EMG is abnormal in 50% of patients in the first 2 weeks and in 85% of patients afterward. Features of demyelinating neuropathy in clinically affected areas include slowing of motor conduction, motor conduction block, prolonged distal motor latencies, temporal dispersion of motor responses, and abnormalities of F waves.

Test: MRI of the spine (with gadolinium)
Significance: MRI should be performed if the clinical presentation is suspicious for spinal cord compression syndrome, for example in a child presenting with paraparesis. In patients with GBS, MRI can support the diagnosis if spinal nerve root enhancement is observed.

Test: In atypical cases, consider heavy metal screen, HIV titer, Lyme titer, porphyria screen, acetylcholine receptor antibodies.
Significance: See Differential Diagnosis, above.

Guillain-Barré Syndrome

 ## Emergency Care

The key elements of the emergency care of patients with GBS center around respiratory management, and deciding on the need for hospitalization to monitor and treat possible progressive symptoms.

 ## Therapy

Supportive therapy is the mainstay of treatment, and immunomodulatory therapy may benefit the patient with GBS.

- Regular monitoring of vital capacity is recommended, and patients should be intubated if vital capacity reaches less than 50% of normal.
- Intravenous immunoglobulin (IVIG) has been tried with success in adults and children. One large study showed it to be of equivalent efficacy to plasma exchange in adults. Many investigators have reported an increased rate of relapse in patients treated with IVIG.
- Plasmapheresis has been used successfully in GBS. Total plasma exchange volume of 200 to 250 mL/kg divided in three to five treatments over 7 to 14 days, beginning within 30 days of the onset of weakness significantly hastens recovery in GBS. Plasma exchange has not been studied in large trials in children, but its use in adults is widespread and well tolerated. Comparisons of IVIG with plasma exchange in adults suggest similar efficacy between the two modalities.
- Corticosteroids have not been shown to be helpful and are not used.
- Management in an intensive care unit is usually required. Respiratory vital capacity should be frequently monitored and elective intubation performed when the vital capacity falls below 10 mL/kg or less than 50% of normal for the patient. Particular attention should be given to preventing secondary pressure neuropathies.
- Pain from nerve root inflammation is common in GBS and should be treated aggressively.
- Prevention measures are not known.

 ## Follow-Up

- First improvement typically begins 2 to 3 weeks after onset of symptoms but may not occur for 1 to 2 months in some patients.
- Improvement continues for 1 to 2 years.

PITFALLS

- Respiratory failure may occur quickly.
- Approximately 10% of patients present with a variant syndrome—pure motor GBS, pharyngeal-cervical-brachial weakness, paraparetic form, ataxic form or Miller-Fisher syndrome (ophthalmoplegia, ataxia, and areflexia, associated with anti-GQ1B antibodies in the CSF). An acute syndrome of autonomic dysfunction without motor symptoms is thought to be a variant as well.
- Many patients appear to have psychogenic instability early in the course of GBS.
- Although the loss of deep tendon reflexes is considered a hallmark of the disease, reflexes may be preserved in early stages of illness.
- Though distal onset of symptoms (motor and sensory) is the classic presentation, proximal symptoms may predominate early in the course of illness.
- If a patient first presents with facial weakness, bilateral Bell palsy may be diagnosed if there are no other features of GBS present. Close observation for further development of symptoms or signs of GBS is warranted in these cases.

 ## Common Questions and Answers

Q: Is GBS contagious?
A: No.

Q: Will I get GBS again?
A: Acute relapses occur in 1% to 5% of patients in large series. Chronic inflammatory demyelinating polyradiculoneuropathy (CIDP) can rarely begin with a rapid onset of weakness indistinguishable from GBS.

Q: Do all cases require hospitalization and immunomodulatory treatment?
A: It is reasonable to observe some youngsters who have mild, nondisabling sensory symptoms on an outpatient basis, though hospitalization and pharmacologic intervention is the usual "default" strategy.

ICD-9-CM 357.0

BIBLIOGRAPHY

Abd-Allah SA, Jansen PW, Ashwal S, et al. Intravenous immunoglobulin as therapy for pediatric Guillain-Barre syndrome J Child Neurol 1997;12(6):376–380.

Evans OB, Vedanarayanan V. Guillain-Barre syndrome. Pediatr Rev 1997;18(1):10–16.

Fenichel GM. Clinical pediatric neurology. Philadelphia: WB Saunders, 1997.

Gordon PH, Wilbourn AJ. Early electrodiagnostic findings in Guillain-Barre syndrome. Arch Neurol 2001;58(6):913–917.

Jones HR Jr. Guillain Barre syndrome in children. Curr Opin Pediatr 1995;7(6):663–668.

Kuwabara S, Mori M, Ogawara K, et al. Indicators of rapid clinical recovery in Guillain-Barre syndrome. J Neurol Neurosurg Psychiatry 2001;70(4):560–562.

Author: Ann Poduri
James W. Teener, 2nd edition

Gynecomastia

Database

DEFINITION
Any visible or palpable proliferation of breast glandular tissue, unilateral or bilateral, due to an increase in estrogen action relative to androgen action at the level of the breast.

ETIOLOGY
Physiologic
• Neonatal: transient palpable breast tissue developing in newborns due to the high estrogen levels in the fetoplacental unit. This condition resolves as estrogen levels decline.
• Pubertal: benign transient gynecomastia occurring in otherwise healthy adolescent males. Breast tissue in pubertal gynecomastia measuring less than 4 cm in diameter has a high likelihood of spontaneous regression.
• Involutional: breast enlargement occurring in elderly men.

Pathologic
• Drug-induced
—Hormones: estrogen, androgens, gonadotropins, anabolic steroids, growth hormone, antiandrogens
—Antiinfective agents: ethionamide, isoniazid, ketoconazole, metronidazole
—Antiulcer drugs: cimetidine, ranitidine, omeprazole
—Chemotherapeutic agents: alkylating agents, methotrexate, vinca alkaloids
—Cardiovascular agents: amiodarone, captopril, digitoxin, diltiazem, enalapril, methyldopa, nifedipine, reserpine, spironolactone, verapamil
—Psychotropic agents: diazepam, haloperidol, phenothiazines, tricyclic antidepressants
—Drugs of abuse: alcohol, amphetamines, heroin, marijuana, methadone
—Miscellaneous: metoclopramide, phenytoin, penicillamine, theophylline
• Hypogonadism: primary or secondary
• Tumors: testicular, adrenal, ectopic hCG-producing tumors
• Chronic disease: hyperthyroidism, renal failure, liver disease, malnutrition with refeeding, HIV infection
• Congenital disorders: Klinefelter syndrome, vanishing testes syndrome (also known as anorchia, gonadal agenesis, or testicular regression), androgen resistance syndromes, true hermaphroditism, excessive peripheral tissue aromatase
• Chest wall trauma
• Intercostal nerve damage following surgery or herpes zoster
• Psychological stress
• Spinal cord injury

PATHOPHYSIOLOGY
Any situation that leads to an increase in the net effect of estrogen action relative to androgen action at the level of the breast may lead to gynecomastia. These situations could include:
• Increased estrogen concentration (endogenous or exogenous)

• Normal estrogen levels with decreased androgen concentrations
• Congenital reduction in estrogen receptors
• Pharmacologic blockade of androgen receptors
• Increased breast or peripheral tissue aromatase (aromatase converts androgens to estrogens)
• Testicular dysfunction
• High serum gonadotropins or increased sex hormone binding globulin
• Elevated estrogen levels lead to proliferation of the ducts and surrounding mesenchymal tissue resulting in breast enlargement.
• Mechanism of drug-induced gynecomastia depends on drug type. Reversibility with drug withdrawal is the rule.
If gynecomastia is present for less than 1 year, tissue samples reveal prominent ductules with epithelial hyperplasia embedded in stromal connective tissue, which may spontaneously regress. If present for more than 1 year, tissue samples reveal dense collagen fibers, dilatation of the ducts with significant reduction in epithelial proliferation, which will persist despite hormonal imbalance correction.

GENETICS
Gynecomastia is occasionally familial, following X-linked or sex-limited autosomal-dominant patterns.

EPIDEMIOLOGY
• Two peaks in age distribution occur in the pediatric population: in the neonatal period and in puberty.
• Neonatal gynecomastia occurs in 60% to 90% of all newborns.
• 40% of boys develop transient gynecomastia (measuring ≥0.5 cm) during puberty.
• Peak incidence at 14 years (range 10–16 years)

COMPLICATIONS
• Physical pain, which may interfere with sports
• Psychological pain
• Embarrassment
• Skin erosion of the nipple due to rubbing against clothing
• Breast cancer: patients with Klinefelter syndrome have a 16-fold increased risk of breast cancer; other causes of gynecomastia are not associated with an increased risk of breast cancer

PROGNOSIS
• Overall, good
• Pubertal gynecomastia: 75% disappears spontaneously within 2 years, and 90% within 3 years
• Neonatal gynecomastia usually resolves within the first year of life

Differential Diagnosis

INFECTIOUS
• Breast abscess

NEOPLASTIC
• Breast neoplasm
• Neurofibroma
• Lymphangioma
• Lipoma
• Neuroblastoma metastasis

TRAUMA
• Hematoma

MISCELLANEOUS
• Pseudogynecomastia: excessive adipose tissue only; no discrete subareolar tissue
• Dermoid cyst

Data Gathering

HISTORY
Question: Time of onset relative to puberty?
Significance: Genitalia development will be present for at least 6 months before onset of breast development.
Question: Rate of progression?
Significance: Rapidly enlarging, painful gynecomastia with acute onset is more concerning than long-standing enlargement.
Question: Drug exposures, including alcohol and substance abuse?
Significance: Marijuana and heroin addiction may cause gynecomastia.
Question: Exposure to exogenous estrogen creams?
Significance: Gynecomastia in a prepubertal boy could suggest direct exposure to exogenous estrogens or indirect exposure from an adult.
• Symptoms suggestive of hyperthyroidism? 30% of young men with hyperthyroidism develop gynecomastia.
• Symptoms suggestive of liver disease?
• Symptoms suggestive of renal failure?
• Symptoms suggestive of neoplastic disease? In patients <10 years of age, consider pituitary adrenal or testicular tumor.
• Symptoms suggestive of hypogonadism, such as decreased libido, decreased erectile function, and infertility suggest abnormal estrogen to androgen ratio.

Physical Examination

• Assess height, weight, growth velocity, and blood pressure.
• Assess for malnourishment. Malnourishment may result in hepatic dysfunction causing higher estrogen to androgen ratio.
Finding: Perform a complete breast examination
Significance: With patient in the supine position, grasp the breast between the thumb and forefinger and move digits toward

the nipple: look for a firm, rubbery, mobile, disk-like mound of tissue arising concentrically below the nipple and areola. Measure the diameter of the disk of glandular tissue. Asymmetry and tenderness are common.

Finding: Pseudogynecomastia
Significance: If pseudogynecomastia (fatty enlargement of breasts) is present, no glandular disk will be palpable.

Finding: Check for galactorrhea
Significance: Seen with drug ingestion and pituitary tumor.

Finding: Determine if macrogynecomastia (disk diameter >5 cm with a secondary mound above the level of the breast) is present.
Significance: Macrogynecomastia may be physiologic or pathologic, and is unlikely to regress.

Finding: Examine the thyroid gland for the presence of a goiter
Significance: Gynecomastia seen in puberty and hyperthyroidism.

Finding: Determine the Tanner staging
Significance: Perform a careful testicular examination with measurement of size. Consider Klinefelter's syndrome if testes less than 3 cm in length or 8 mL in volume.

Laboratory Aids

• None indicated for pubertal and neonatal gynecomastia.
• Renal, hepatic, and/or thyroid function tests if indicated.

Test: Karyotype
Significance: Klinefelter syndrome suspected.

Test: Luteinizing hormone (LH), follicle-stimulating hormone (FSH), estradiol, testosterone, dehydroepiandrosterone (DHEA), and human chorionic gonadotropin (hCG).
Significance: To determine if hypogonadism, precocious puberty, testicular tumor or adrenal tumor could be present. An isolated elevated estradiol level in an otherwise normal prepubertal boy may suggest direct or indirect exogenous estrogen exposure.

Test: Prolactin level
Significance: To rule out a prolactin-secreting pituitary tumor: if galactorrhea present or if decreased testosterone with decreased or normal LH.

RADIOGRAPHIC STUDIES

Test: Bone age (radiograph of the left hand and wrist)
Significance: Elevated estrogens may accelerate skeletal maturation.

Test: Testicular ultrasound
Significance: If elevated hCG, elevated estradiol or asymmetric testes on physical examination to rule out testicular tumor.

Test: Chest x-ray with abdominal CT
Significance: If hCG elevated and testicular ultrasound is normal to rule out extragonadal germ cell tumor or hCG-secreting nontrophoblastic neoplasm.

Test: Adrenal CT or MRI

Significance: To rule out adrenal neoplasm, if estradiol elevated, DHEA elevated, LH decreased or normal, and testicular ultrasound normal

Test: Skull x-ray, brain MRI or CT
Significance: If pituitary tumor is suspected.

Therapy

• Reassurance for patients with pubertal gynecomastia measuring less than 4 cm. Treatment guidelines are variable for gynecomastia measuring 4 to 5 cm. Consultation in these patients should be considered.
• Reexamine at 3-month intervals
• Discontinue any drugs known to induce gynecomastia and follow-up in 1 month.
• Correct any underlying disorders (hyperthyroidism, malnutrition, etc.).

DRUGS

• The effectiveness of drugs in the treatment of gynecomastia has been difficult to evaluate due to the high prevalence of spontaneous regression.
• Generally, drug therapy should proceed under the guidance of an endocrinologist.
• Tamoxifen and testolactone (an aromatase inhibitor) have shown some benefit in adolescents with benign pubertal gynecomastia.
• If gynecomastia has been present for more than 1 year, pharmacologic therapy is of little benefit. After 1 year, regardless of the etiology of gynecomastia, epithelial growth becomes less prominent while periductal fibrosis and hyalinization are more evident. Because of the increase in fibrosis, gynecomastia of longer duration is less amenable to medical treatment.
• Surgery is the therapy of choice for macrogynecomastia, or persistent gynecomastia resistant to medical therapy.
• Surgical options include periareolar incision with adjunctive liposuction or glandular tissue removal through two incisions in the anterior axillary regions.

Follow-Up

• Watch for signs of psychological stress.
• Watch for symptoms of chronic disease, abnormal physical changes.

PITFALLS

• Mistaking pseudogynecomastia (i.e., fatty enlargement of the breasts) from true gynecomastia
• Overlooking a potentially drug-related etiology. Drug-related gynecomastia is usually reversible if diagnosed within 1 year of onset.

Common Questions and Answers

Q: When should a patient with gynecomastia be referred to a specialist?

A: If macrogynecomastia is present, if there is an abnormal hormonal workup or an abnormal imaging study, or if there is an abnormal rate of progression.

Q: For how long does neonatal gynecomastia persist?

A: Studies of healthy term infants have shown that the diameter of the breast tissue may actually increase during the first 2 weeks of life. The breast tissue then decreases to an average diameter of 10 mm until about 4 to 6 months of age. The breast tissue of female infants is generally larger and may persist longer than in males. Occasionally, the breast tissue will fail to regress and remain after the first year of life.

Q: Is it normal for a newborn baby's breasts to secrete milk?

A: In the later stages of gestation, the developing breast undergoes a small amount of secretory activity. This produces the so-called witch's milk that is expressed from the breasts of many full-term infants from the fifth to seventh day of life. Witch's milk may persist for 1 to 7 weeks after birth. As fetal prolactin, placental estrogen, and progesterone decline, the breast tissue regresses.

Q: How is gynecomastia distinguished from breast cancer?

A: Breast cancer usually presents as a unilateral, eccentric hard or firm mass that is fixed to underlying tissues. Associated findings can include dimpling of the skin, retraction of the nipple, nipple discharge, or axillary lymphadenopathy. The incidence of breast cancer in the pediatric population is extremely low. Less than 0.1% of all breast cancers occur in patients less than 20 years of age. Benign tumors, such as fibroadenomas, are much more common than malignant breast tumors.

ICD-9-CM 611.1

BIBLIOGRAPHY

Braunstein GD. Gynecomastia. *N Engl J Med* 1993;328(7):490–495.

Felner EI, White PC. Prepubertal gynecomastia: indirect exposure to estrogen cream. *Pediatrics* 2000;105:e55.

Frantz AG, Wilson JD. Endocrine disorders of the breast. In: Wilson JD, Foster DW, eds. *Williams' textbook of endocrinology*, 8th ed. Philadelphia: WB Saunders, 1992:953–975.

Glass AR. Gynecomastia. *Endocrinol Metab Clin North Am* 1994;23(4):825–837.

Mahoney CP. Adolescent gynecomastia: differential diagnosis and management. *Pediatr Clin North Am* 1990;37:1389–1404.

Mathur R, Braunstein GD. Gynecomastia: pathomechanisms and treatment strategies. *Horm Res* 1997;48:95–102.

McKiernan JF, Hull D. Breast development in the newborn. *Arch Dis Child* 1981;56:525–529.

Author: Julie A. Boom

Hand-Foot-and-Mouth Disease

 Database

DEFINITION

Hand-foot-and-mouth disease is a viral illness with the characteristic clinical features of:

- Vesiculoulcerative stomatitis
- Papular or vesicular exanthem on the hands and/or the feet
- Mild constitutional symptoms such as fever and malaise

CAUSES

Coxsackie A16 virus is the most common causative agent. Occasionally, hand-foot-and-mouth disease results from infection with:

- Coxsackie viruses A5, A7, A9, A10, A16, B1, and B3
- Enterovirus 71
- Other enteroviruses
- Herpesviruses

PATHOPHYSIOLOGY

- Enteroviruses are acquired by the oral or respiratory route.
- Lymphatic invasion leads to viremia and spread to secondary sites.
- Viremia ceases with antibody production.
- Direct inoculation of the extremities from oral lesions has been suggested in regard to hand-foot-and-mouth disease.

EPIDEMIOLOGY

- In temperate climates hand-foot-and-mouth disease is most common in the late summer and fall (a pattern common to many of the enterovirus infections).
- Spread primarily by fecal contamination and contact. Oral and respiratory secretions may also transmit the virus.
- Incubation period is 3 to 7 days.
- Highly contagious, afflicting up to one half of those exposed.
- Close household contacts are particularly susceptible.
- May occur as an isolated case or in an epidemic distribution
- Most common in children under 5 years, but may affect adults.

COMPLICATIONS

- Hand-foot-and-mouth disease is usually self-limited and uncomplicated, resolving within 10 days.
- Dehydration is the most frequent morbid complication:

—Oral ulcerations are painful and interfere with feeding.
—Infants and children are at highest risk.

- Rare reports of other complications include:

—Neurologic complications such as aseptic meningitis, encephalitis, and a polio-like paralytic disorder
—Pneumonia
—Myocarditis
—A possible association with first trimester spontaneous abortions in previously infected women

PROGNOSIS

- In the vast majority of instances hand-foot-and-mouth disease will resolve quickly requiring only supportive care.
- Young children bear the closest scrutiny because they suffer the greatest morbidity.
- Careful history and examination should distinguish those individuals with the rare aforementioned complications.
- Rare cases may recur at intervals for up to 1 year.

 Differential Diagnosis

Few infectious diseases have such characteristic clinical findings. Oral ulcerations followed by lesions on the distal extremities are virtually pathognomonic. The most difficult diagnostic dilemmas may be early in the disease course when isolated oral lesions predominate.

- Herpangina

—Also caused by Coxsackie A viruses
—Associated with higher fever
—Usually limited to the posterior oropharynx

- Herpetic gingivostomatitis

—Most common cause of stomatitis in children
—Associated with higher fever
—More frequently associated with lymphadenopathy
—Gingival involvement severe
—Aphthous ulcers
—Generally occurs without fever or upper respiratory symptoms
—Does not occur in "outbreaks"

- Stevens-Johnson syndrome

—Ulcerations frequently coalesce
—Usually affects other mucous membranes
—Often appears with separate cutaneous manifestations

- The "Boston exanthem"

—Caused by echovirus 16
—Mild febrile illness with a macular rash on the palms and soles
—Oral lesions absent

 Data Gathering

HISTORY

Question: History of ill contacts?
Significance: Incubation period may be up to 1 week.

Question: Any fever, pain, or other symptoms?
Significance: A mild prodrome occasionally precedes the characteristic enanthem and exanthem by 1 or 2 days: low-grade fever (usually near 38.3°C), malaise, sore mouth, anorexia, coryza, diarrhea, abdominal pain.

Question: Bone pain?
Significance: Bone and joint aches infrequently accompany this illness.

Question: Lesions in mouth?
Significance: Oral lesions typically occur shortly before the hand and foot manifestations.

Question: Anyone in family sick?
Significance: Family members or close contacts are often similarly affected.

Question: Hydration status?
Significance: Determine quality and amount of oral intake, quality and amount of urine output, recent weight loss, duration of symptoms.

 Physical Examination

Finding: Enanthem
Significance:

- Oral lesions begin as small, red papules.
- Papules quickly evolve to small vesicles on an erythematous base.
- Lesions progress to ulcerations.
- Tongue, buccal mucosa, palate, gingiva, uvula, and/or tonsillar pillars may be involved.
- Usually 2 to 10 lesions.
- Oral lesions may persist up to 1 week.

Finding: Exanthem
Significance:

- Less consistently present than oral lesions (occur in one fourth to two thirds of patients)
- Maculopapular eruptions progress to vesicles.
- Rarely tender or pruritic
- Most frequent on the dorsal aspects of fingers and toes
- May also occur on the palms, soles, arms, legs, buttocks, and face

Finding: Adenopathy
Significance: Enlarged anterior cervical, or submandibular nodes are present in one-fourth of cases.

Hand-Foot-and-Mouth Disease

Finding: Other
Significance: Attention should be given to the patient's vital signs, general appearance, and respiratory, cardiac, and neurologic functioning to help identify the rare patient with a threatening complication of hand-foot-and-mouth disease.

Laboratory Aids

Test: Physical Exam
Significance: Hand-foot-and-mouth disease has rather unique clinical features and a relatively benign course. Laboratory confirmation of the diagnosis is seldom needed or indicated.

Test: Culture
Significance: Causative viruses may be cultured from many sites:

- Oral ulcers
- Cutaneous vesicles
- Nasopharyngeal swabs
- Stool (isolation of an enterovirus from the stool does not confirm it to be the cause of disease; such a result must be paired with clinical suspicion or serologic findings)
- Cerebrospinal fluid (in cases where meningoencephalitis is suspected)

Test: Electron microscopy
Significance: Can identify virus particles from similar sources.

Test: Neutralization technique
Significance: Acute and convalescent specific antibody titers may provide indirect confirmation.

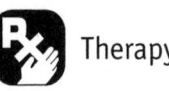

Therapy

- Most cases will spontaneously resolve and require no therapy other than parental reassurance.
- Acetaminophen may relieve malaise and minor discomfort associated with the oral ulcers. It also may be used as an antipyretic in those children with fever.
- Dietary adjustments often improve oral intake and prevent or relieve dehydration:

—Avoid spicy or acidic foods.
—Provide cool or iced liquids in small quantities frequently.

- Symptomatic relief from particularly painful oral ulcers may be accomplished by application of a topical antihistamine or anesthetic directly to the sores (see Common Questions and Answers, below).
- Dehydration should be treated when present. Intravenous fluids may be required in the more severe cases, especially in infants and young children.
- Good supportive care is generally sufficient to treat most complications.

PREVENTION

- Frequent hand washing, especially after changing diapers, and good personal hygiene are the most useful means to prevent spread of enteroviral illnesses.
- Enteric precautions should be maintained with all hospitalized patients.
- The prodromal and enanthem periods appear to be the most contagious; however, some carriers of Coxsackie A16 may shed virus in the stool 3 months after infection (see Common Questions and Answers, below).

Follow-Up

- Hand-foot-and-mouth disease generally resolves spontaneously within 1 week after diagnosis.
- Small children must be followed closely for signs of dehydration.
- The extremely rare complication of myocarditis has been reported to result in at least two fatalities.
- Some patients may become asymptomatic carriers.

Common Questions and Answers

Q: What is in the "magic mouthwash" often used to relieve the pain of stomatitis?
A: Many health care providers will prescribe a "magic mouthwash" for symptomatic relief of oral ulcers, pharyngitis, and teething pain. The most common such treatment consists of an aluminum hydroxide/magnesium hydroxide gel suspension and diphenhydramine elixir (12.5 mg/5 mL) in a 1:1 formulation. It can be applied directly to the sores with a cotton swab or a small syringe before meals. Note: some people will have a reaction to topical diphenhydramine.

Q: Should lidocaine be used topically for symptomatic relief of oral ulcers?
A: The routine use of lidocaine in this situation is not recommended. Lidocaine is an effective topical anesthetic and comes in a 2% viscous suspension. In practice, the pain relief is short-lived, which encourages frequent administration. Lidocaine is absorbed from the mucous membranes (bypassing first-pass liver metabolism) and has been frequently reported to cause poisoning of the cardiovascular and central nervous system. Both pediatric and adult fatalities have occurred. The use of topical viscous lidocaine should be reserved for use by physicians knowledgeable regarding its proper dosage and potential side effects, and by educated, compliant parents or caregivers.

Q: When may children with hand-foot-and-mouth disease return to school?
A: This is a matter of some controversy for this highly contagious, but relatively benign, condition. However, good hygiene will greatly reduce viral transmission. And affected patients are contagious often before the diagnosis is made. Most now suggest isolation from school or day-care contacts while febrile and/or while the enanthem persists. As mentioned, some may shed the virus in their stool for months after symptoms have resolved (again stressing the need for good personal hygiene).

ICD-9-CM 074.3

BIBLIOGRAPHY

Cherry JD. Enteroviruses: polioviruses, coxsackieviruses, echoviruses, and enteroviruses. In: Feigin RD, Cherry JD, eds. *Textbook of pediatric infectious diseases*, 4th ed. Philadelphia: WB Saunders, 1998: 1787–1839.

Enterovirus surveillance—United States, 1997-1999. *MMWR* 2000;49(40):913–916.

Robinson CR, Doane FW, Rhoades AJ. Report of an outbreak of febrile illness with pharyngeal lesions and exanthem: Toronto, 1957-isolation of coxsackie virus. *Can Med Assoc J* 1958;79:615–621.

Slavin KA, Frieden IJ. Picture of the month: hand-foot-and-mouth disease. *Arch Pediatr Adolesc Med* 1998;152:505–506.

Author: Kevin C. Osterhoudt

Hantavirus/Hantapulmonary Syndrome

 Database

DEFINITION

Hantapulmonary syndrome (HPS) is a disease in humans due to a Hantavirus and acquired from certain chronically infected rodent species. When acquired by humans, it results in a syndrome characterized by a flu-like illness followed by rapidly progressive cardiac and respiratory failure with a high mortality.

CAUSE

Original human outbreak recognized in Southwest United States was caused by the *Sin nombre* strain of Hantavirus transmitted from chronically infected deer mice (*Peromyscus maniculatus*). Subsequent cases were recognized throughout the ubiquitous distribution of the deer mouse. Since then, additional strains of Hantavirus have been recognized each with a unique rodent host. The resulting human cases of HPS have now been identified from Canada to Argentina.

EPIDEMIOLOGY

- The host rodent develops a chronic nonfatal infection and excretes virus in urine, feces, and saliva.
- Humans acquire the infection by inhaling virus contaminated airborne particles from the dried rodent excreta. Typically, this occurs when sweeping or otherwise disturbing a rodent-infested building.
- Human cases are more common in the spring and summer and also in years when the population of the rodent host has increased.
- Nosocomial transmission has been observed only with the *Andes* strain in Argentina, never in the U.S.
- In the U.S., HPS has occurred primarily in young healthy adults, although in South America a larger proportion of cases are in children.

PATHOLOGY/PATHOPHYSIOLOGY

- Pathophysiologic changes of most importance are myocardial depression resulting in shock and alveolar capillary leak pulmonary edema resulting in hypoxia.
- The cardiac dysfunction is characterized by a falling cardiac output, increased systemic vascular resistance and normal or low pulmonary artery wedge pressure.
- The pulmonary alveoli are flooded with fluid devoid of red cells but with a protein content similar to serum.

 Differential Diagnosis

- Pneumonic plague
- Influenza
- Bacterial sepsis, especially that caused by pneumococcus and other streptococci
- Other causes of shock and pneumonia or shock and pulmonary edema

 Data Gathering

The clinical symptoms, physical findings and laboratory findings progress in sequence. Early suspicion of the syndrome allows the clinician to prepare for that phase of the illness characterized by the rapid onset of respiratory failure and shock.

HISTORY

Question: Fever and myalgia?
Significance: Usually severe, characterize the prodromal phase lasting 3 to 6 days.

Question: Gastrointestinal complaints?
Significance: Frequently prominent including combinations of nausea, vomiting, diarrhea, or abdominal pain.

Question: Headache?
Significance: Is present in over one half of patients.

Question: Cough?
Significance: Uncommon at the onset of the prodrome but heralds the onset of dyspnea and tachypnea, which is then followed by the rapid progression of cardiorespiratory failure.

Question: Coryza and sore throat?
Significance: Rarely part of the prodrome.

Question: A history of activities that might expose the patient to airborne virus contaminated particles should be sought.
Significance: HPS acquired by inhalation on airborne particles.

 Physical Examination

Tachycardia and hypotension as late findings.

Finding: Fever
Significance: During the prodromal phase, fever is the only finding.

Finding: Cough
Significance: With the onset of the cardiopulmonary phase, there is cough and dyspnea associated with the production of frequently copious amounts of nonpurulent material.

 Laboratory Aids

TESTS

Test: Platelet count
Significance: The platelet count falls on serial testing during the prodromal phase and may be the only laboratory abnormality.

- In addition to leukocytosis, myelocytes and immunoblasts appear in the peripheral blood.
- Liver function tests are mildly abnormal.
- Hypoxemia accompanies the onset of the cardiopulmonary phase.
- Diagnostic serology demonstrates IgM antibody present at the time of clinical presentation.

IMAGING

Test: Chest radiograph
Significance: During the prodrome, chest radiography is normal. With the onset of cardiopulmonary symptoms, chest radiography will show evidence of interstitial fluid manifested by Kerley B lines, hilar indistinctness, and peribronchial cuffing. Alveolar flooding and pleural effusions develop in severe cases. Heart size remains normal.

PITFALLS

- The diagnosis depends on serologic testing, which can take some time.
- Lacking serologic confirmation, one mostly depends on clinical history and serial hematologic tests.
- In anticipation of the rapid progression of the cardiopulmonary phase, it is preferable to have the patient closely observed in the hospital.

Therapy

Because of the rapid progression of the cardiorespiratory failure, all patients with HPS should be managed in an intensive care setting with a pulmonary artery catheter to guide therapy.

- Oxygen, intubation, and mechanical ventilation are frequently needed.
- Use fluids cautiously in view of the capillary leak.
- If the patient develops hypotension, an inotropic agent such as dobutamine should be added; if the patient continues to be hypotensive on maximal doses of dobutamine, vasopressors can be added to maintain blood pressure.
- Use empiric antibiotics because serologic tests confirming HPS are usually delayed and the differential diagnosis includes sepsis from a variety of antibiotic responsive organisms.
- Extracorporeal membrane oxygenation has been used for patients who fail to respond to maximal inotropic and ventilatory support.
- To date, antiviral agents have not been shown to be beneficial.

PREVENTION

- Universal precautions are appropriate in caring for persons with HPS; person-to-person transmission has been demonstrated only with the *Andes* strain in the Southern Hemisphere, not in the United States.
- Preventing infection depends on avoiding contact with airborne particles contaminated by rodent excreta.
- Eliminate rodents and seal off rodent access into the house.
- Reduce rodent shelter and food sources in the immediate vicinity of the home by cutting brush, removing trash, and storing grain and animal feed in rodent-proof containers.
- Wearing gloves, clean up rodent-contaminated areas by spraying nests and droppings with household disinfectants or dilute bleach, and sealing material in bags for burning or burial.
- Ventilate closed areas before initiating cleanup.

 Follow-Up

WHEN TO EXPECT IMPROVEMENT

- Patients who survive the shock phase typically then diurese fluid, which has been third spaced. Recovery is then generally rapid.
- Easy fatigability and mild pulmonary function abnormalities may persist.

PITFALLS

Recognizing the prodrome of HPS is difficult and requires a careful history, evaluation of the risk of exposure, and rapid access to testing.

 Common Questions and Answers

Q: What should I do if I find a dead mouse indoors?
A: Identify if it is a house mouse or a species that could be infected with Hantavirus. If the latter, assume that it is infected and dispose of as described previously and then seal off rodent access to the home and eliminate any still left inside.

Q: What should I do if I find what look like rodent droppings?
A: Clean up with gloves and disinfectant as noted here. Then use traps to catch and identify the rodents involved and proceed as in the answer to the previous question.

Q: Could a patient have HPS without knowing it?
A: In the U.S., asymptotic HPS infections would appear to be uncommon based on serum screening of household contacts of cases and other populations at high risk, which show only infrequent evidence of prior infection.

ICD-9-CM 518.89;09.81

BIBLIOGRAPHY

All About Hantavirus Web page: *http//www.cdc.gov/ncidod/diseases/hanta/hps/index.htm*.

Butler JC, Peters CJ. Hantaviruses and hantavirus pulmonary syndrome. *Clin Infect Dis* 1994;19:387–395.

Duchin JS, et al. Hantavirus pulmonary syndrome: a clinical description of 17 patients with a newly recognized disease. *N Engl J Med* 1994;330:949–955.

Hallin GW, et al. Cardiopulmonary manifestations of hantavirus pulmonary syndrome. *Crit Care Med* 1996;24:252–258.

Author: Bruce Tempest

Headache and Migraine

 Database

DEFINITIONS

Headache may be primary or secondary, symptomatic of a specific oral, dental, cranial, or cervical pathologic process (e.g., trauma or tumor).

- Acute: rapid onset or progression
- Chronic or recurrent: recurring repeatedly over years or persisting relentlessly over days
- Tension headaches, also known as muscle contraction headaches, are thought to be due to simple traction on pain sensors during prolonged contraction of the scalp and neck.
- Migraine is a recurrent, usually throbbing headache with associated gastrointestinal symptoms, photo- or phonophobia. It is usually bilateral in children, unilateral in 75% of adults.

CAUSES OF HEADACHE

- Acute diffuse: trauma, infection (systemic), stress, meningitis, encephalitis, stroke (thrombotic, embolic, hemorrhagic), subarachnoid hemorrhage, toxins (e.g., lead), hypertension, hypoglycemia, postlumbar puncture, collagen vascular disease (arteritis), drug abuse
- Acute focal: trauma, infection (otitis, sinusitis, brain abscess, encephalitis, meningitis), dental process, orbital disease, cranial neuralgias
- Subacute recurrent/progressive: migraine (common and classic), complicated migraine, migraine variants
- Chronic progressive: pseudotumor cerebri, abscess, chronic meningitis, sinus thrombosis, tumor, AVM, hydrocephalus, subdural hematoma, depression, anxiety, drug abuse
- Chronic, nonprogressive: chronic myositis, psychogenic or tension headache, postconcussive syndrome, depression, conversion disorder, cervical osteoarthritis, temporomandibular joint syndrome, atypical facial pain

MIGRAINE TYPES

- Classic migraine

—A visual aura consisting of scintillations, scotomata, or blurred vision precedes the headache followed by a unilateral or bilateral throbbing headache that intensifies over a few hours, can last several hours to days, and often relieved with rest or sleep.
—Nausea, vomiting, nasal congestion, anorexia, abdominal pain, irritability, malaise, fatigue, photophobia, and phonophobia are all common associated symptoms.

- Common migraine

—Most common form of headache in children and adolescents
—Characteristic throbbing headache but without the visual prodrome of classic migraine. Other systemic symptoms, including nasal congestion, gastrointestinal upset, are frequently seen.

- Complicated migraine

—Migraine with transient neurologic deficits such as ophthalmoplegic migraine, hemiplegic migraine, and migraine with aphasia in a patient with known migraine, a patient who develops migraine later, or in a patient who has a family predisposition to migraine.
—Basilar artery migraine is the combination of headache with neurologic dysfunction referable to the posterior circulation: hemianopia, ataxia, dysarthria, stupor.
—Symptoms may include blurred vision, dizziness, vertigo, ataxia, sensory and motor abnormalities, obtundation, and loss of consciousness.
—Acute confusional migraine begins with headache and is followed by confusion, agitation, and altered sensorium and is confused with the confusional state of illicit drug use in adolescents.
—Migraine variants: include paroxysmal vertigo, cyclic vomiting or periodic syndrome, and acephalgic migraine.

EPIDEMIOLOGY OF MIGRAINE

- Migraine occurs in 3% to 5% of children before puberty and increases to 10% to 20% during the second decade.
- Female/male ratio is approximately equal before puberty and increases to 2:1 after puberty.
- Migraine has a strong genetic component; may be autosomal dominant.

PATHOPHYSIOLOGY OF MIGRAINE

The pathogenesis of migraine is believed to involve perivascular inflammatory changes mediated by cytokines. Theories invoke cerebral vasospasm and involvement of bioactive amines such as serotonin and substance P.

 Differential Diagnosis

- Sinusitis
- Trigeminal neuralgia
- Atypical facial pain and factitious pain disorders
- Systemic features of migraine may lead to evaluation for metabolic or cerebrovascular disorders: episodic vomiting (may suggest hyperammonemia), transient ischemic attack, acute/recurrent ataxia-amino acidopathy, channelopathy, mitochondrial disorders, epilepsy.

Other diagnostic considerations are dictated by the temporal characteristics of headache and the presence of focal signs:

- Acute: meningitis, encephalitis, intracranial hemorrhage, sinus thrombosis, dental infection, hydrocephalus
- Chronic: a minority of children with chronic headache have structural brain lesions: brain tumors, hydrocephalus, abscess.
- Pseudotumor cerebri, which is accompanied by papilledema, normal imaging, increased cerebrospinal fluid pressure.
- Postconcussive syndrome should be considered when suggested by the appropriate history.
- Children with psychogenic or tension headaches often lack associated history of social or emotional stress.
- Occipital neuralgia from trauma, shingles, or Lyme disease
- CADASIL: genetic disorder with family history of migraine, early dementia, white matter changes on MRI.

 Data Gathering

HISTORY

Question: Background?
Significance: Important features include duration of the problem, precipitants (menses?), location of the headache, time of onset, mode of onset, precipitating factors, response to medicines, associated symptoms, response to therapy, and family history. Questions regarding sleep, dietary precipitants, and prolonged exposure to TV or video games may be helpful.

Question: Migraine?
Significance: The mode of onset is usually gradual, rarely paroxysmal. The location of the headache is typically bilateral either bifrontal, bitemporal, or bioccipital or diffuse and ill-defined. The quality of the pain may be aching and steady or throbbing.

Question: Stress?
Significance: May exacerbate either migraine or tension headache. Although many adults with migraine are depressed, the prevalence of depression in children with chronic headaches is not known.

Question: Family history?
Significance: Positive family history of migraine is common (60%) and supports the diagnosis of migraine.

Physical Examination

Finding: Blood pressure measurement
Significance: Hypertension alone and in the context of cerebral vasospasm can be associated with headache.

Finding: Auscultation for bruits
Significance: A-V malformations

Finding: Signs of meningeal inflammation
Significance: Meningitis can present with headache meningeal signs, though most commonly with fever.

Finding: Funduscopic examination for papilledema
Significance: Elevated intracranial pressure may be transmitted to the optic disc and suggests the presence of a mass lesion or pseudotumor cerebri.

Finding: Neurologic examination
Significance: Should be normal in primary headache syndromes (migraine, tension), except perhaps during a complicated migraine; focal neurologic deficits suggest a structural basis of headache.

Finding: Examination of jaw (range of motion), teeth, oral cavity, otoscopy, and palpation of maxillary, frontal, and mastoid sinuses.
Significance: TMJ syndrome, dental infection, and sinusitis.

Finding: Trigger points over the trapezius or tender muscles may point to fibromyalgia (generally adolescent or older).

Laboratory Aids

Test: Sinus films or CT
Significance: Indicated if symptoms point to sinusitis. These may not be obvious in sphenoid sinusitis, which may produce unremitting, chronic frontal headache. Migraine may mimic sinusitis and vice versa.

Test: Chronic anemia
Significance: May be associated with headache, although it rarely presents in children as headache.

Test: Neuroimaging studies (CT or MRI)
Significance: Indicated when neurologic examination indicates a focal abnormality; or if the history suggests a specific diagnosis such as a brain tumor, such as association with persistent vomiting. CT should be used in the emergent setting if there is any suspicion for subarachnoid hemorrhage, but otherwise MRI is generally preferable to address possible sinus thrombosis. Neuroimaging may also be indicated for atypical headaches, persistently unilateral headaches, and headaches that are increasing in frequency and severity, or that are refractory to treatment.

Test: EEG
Significance: Should be obtained when headache is associated with focal somatic sensory or motor symptoms; focal slowing may also suggest structural abnormality and the finding necessitates imaging.

Test: Lumbar puncture
Significance: Examination of cerebrospinal fluid to detect infection or elevated pressure may be indicated for evaluation of headache with papilledema (after neuroimaging), or when subarachnoid hemorrhage is suspected (after CT). Opening pressure with patient recumbent should be measured in order to make the diagnosis of pseudotumor cerebri (CSF formula must be normal), and it may be elevated in other conditions such as meningitis as well.

Emergency Care

Emergency evaluation should concentrate on identifying acute processes that require emergent intervention. These include subarachnoid hemorrhage, meningitis, and mass lesions causing elevated intracranial pressure that may lead to herniation. Emergent neuroimaging should be performed if the headache is severe (especially if it is a first or worst headache, that is, the patient's first severe headache or the "worst headache of my life") or if papilledema or focal neurologic are present.

Therapy

- Treatment is similar to that of adult migraine, though on an "off-label" basis. Treatment may be categorized as symptomatic, abortive, or preventive. Rare to occasional migraines may be treated symptomatically with aspirin, NSAIDs, or acetaminophen.
- Abortive therapy: dihydroergotamine (IV), sumatriptan (nasal, oral), zolmitriptan (oral), Maxalt (wafer). Because these medications cause cerebral vasospasm, they should not be used in patients who have a history of complicated migraine (migraine with neurologic deficits) or other risk factors for ischemic stroke. Contraindicated in basilar migraine.
- Antiemetics, including metoclopramide, may help for both migraine pain and GI symptoms.
- Prophylactic therapy includes beta-blockers, cyproheptadine, tricyclic antidepressants, calcium channel blockers, antiinflammatory drugs, and some anticonvulsants (e.g., valproic acid).
- Other treatment modalities may include behavior therapy, relaxation training including biofeedback, avoidance of specific foods or substances that may be migraine triggers. Treatment may also include appropriate psychological counseling.

- Headaches with vomiting may suggest elevated intracranial pressure, not just migraine—look for papilledema.
- Depression and migraine frequently occur together—therapy for depression may help headache.
- Arteriovenous malformation may mimic migraine and should be considered if headache is persistently on the same side of the head or if response to therapy is poor.

Common Questions and Answers

Q: When should migraine be treated?
A: Many children with migraine headaches have attacks so infrequently that daily prophylactic medical therapy is not warranted. Treatment should be considered when attacks occur at least once a month.

Q: What about allergy and headache?
A: Many believe that headache may represent a symptom of hypersensitivity. Headache in the setting of allergic rhinitis/asthma may be due to associated sinusitis/sinus congestion, side effect of treatment (especially theophylline), or muscle tension.

Q: At what age can migraine begin?
A: Even 2- to 3-year-olds may present with headache or migraine equivalent symptoms: episodic vomiting, episodic ataxia that improves after sleep.

ICD-9-CM 346.9

BIBLIOGRAPHY

Annequin D, Tourniaire B, Massiou H. Migraine and headache in childhood and adolescence. *Pediatr Clin North Am* 2000;47(3):617–631.

Forsyth R, Farrell K. Headache in childhood. *Pediatr Rev* 1999;20:39–45.

Hamalainen ML, Hoppu Kalle, Santavuori P. Sumatriptan for migraine attacks in children: a randomized placebo-controlled study. *Neurology* 1997;48:1100.

Holden EW, Levy JD, Deichmann MM, et al. Recurrent pediatric headaches: assessment and intervention. *J Dev Behav Pediatr* 1998;19(2): 109–116.

Lipton RB. Diagnosis and epidemiology of pediatric migraine. *Curr Opin Neurol* 1997;10:231.

Singh BV, Roach ES. Diagnosis and management of headaches in children. *Pediatr Rev* 1998;19:132–135.

Author: Ann Poduri
2nd edition: Patricia Malloy

Heat Stroke and Related Illness

 Database

DEFINITION

Heat stroke results from an imbalance between heat production, absorption, and dissipation. This can result from excessive body heat generation and storage without appropriate dissipation, high ambient temperature, low radiation or convective heat loss, decreased evaporation, medical predisposition, behavioral abnormality, inability to respond to need for environmental change or intervention, or inadequate fluid (sweat or other loss) (water and/or salt) replacement. Heat illness encompasses a spectrum of heat-related disease processes.

PREDISPOSING CONDITIONS

• Environmental predisposition:
Hot and humid without wind, heat wave, hot indoor environment, lack of air conditioning. Social isolation, inability to care for self
• Medical: Cardiac disease, diabetes mellitus, hyperthyroid, parkinsonism, dehydration (gastroenteritis, diuretics, poor fluid intake), vascular disease, skin and sweat gland abnormalities (scleredema, burn scarring), malignancy, concurrent febrile illness, obesity, fatigue, previous occurrence of heat illness.
• Drugs/medications
—Anticholinergics (inhibit perspiration)
—Beta-blockers (unable to increase cardiac output)
—Diuretics
—Phenothiazines
—Psychiatric medications
—Drugs of abuse; hallucinogens, cocaine
—Salicylates
—Sympathomimetics
—MAO inhibitors
—Lithium
—Antihistamines
—Ethanol
• Behaviors
—Lack of recognition of risk factors or warning signs
—Overexertion
—Athletics
—Inappropriate clothing; heavy, dark, tight-fitting, overbundling
—Lack of acclimatization and conditioning
—Inadequate fluid intake
—Children in enclosed space within motor vehicle

PATHOPHYSIOLOGY

• When environmental temperature is greater than body temperature, body gains heat by conduction and radiation and can lose heat by evaporation.
• Heat production increased 10 to 20 times by strenuous exercise
• Heat dissipation (conduction to objects and air, convection, radiation, evaporation)
—If high humidity or little air movement, effectiveness of evaporative heat loss is lessened.

• Heat syncope: venous pooling (redistribution of blood volume) during strenuous or upright event, decreased central venous return, cardiac output, and cerebral perfusion pressure
• Heat exhaustion (prostration): Water depletion: inadequate water replacement in hot environment. Salt depletion: salt (sweat) loss; water, but not salt replacement. Can progress to heat stroke
• Heat stroke: Impaired heat dissipation with extreme elevations of body temperature. Temperature more than 42°C can uncouple oxidative phosphorylation and allow enzyme systems to cease functioning. Cell membrane integrity is lost, proteins denature, and necrosis occurs; leads to dysfunction and organ failure.

ASSOCIATED DISEASES

• Heat cramps/spasms: Related to physical exercise, fluid (sweat) loss, poor sodium repletion (normal body temperature). Usually brief and intermittent in fatigued (used) muscles.
• Heat tetany: Paresthesias and carpopedal spasm help distinguish tetany from heat cramps
• Heat syncope: Alteration of consciousness (dizziness, syncope) at end of strenuous or upright event. Vasodilation, increased dependent, peripheral (decreased thoracic) blood volume. May have prodrome (aura, visual changes, vertigo, nausea, diaphoresis, weakness)
• Heat edema: Swollen feet and ankles (vascular leak, orthostatic pooling). More common in women and nonacclimatized people with prolonged standing or sitting. Self-resolves without complication.
• Heat exhaustion (prostration). Relatively slow onset. Water and/or salt depletion. Headache, nausea, vomiting, malaise, myalgias, pale skin, dizziness, visual disturbances, syncope, temperature 38° to 40°C, dehydration, electrolyte imbalance, hemoconcentration. Can progress to heat stroke
• Heat stroke: Central nervous system (CNS) symptoms (delirium, convulsion, coma), acute, sudden onset (80%), slower onset (minutes to hours in 20%), high fever (>40°–41°C), hypotension, tachycardia, hyperventilation

COMPLICATIONS

• Heat exhaustion: Hypovolemia, hyponatremia, hypernatremia, hypochloremia. Progression to heat stroke.
• Heat stroke: Electrolyte imbalance, seizures, adult respiratory distress syndrome (ARDS), acute renal, liver, cardiac failure, pulmonary edema, rhabdomyolysis (may be delayed 2–3 days), disseminated intravascular coagulation (DIC), coma, death. Severe dehydration if sweating occurred. May have persistent neurologic dysfunction (cerebellar, hemiparesis, dementia)

PROGNOSIS

• Heat illness (heat rash, edema, cramps, tetany, syncope, exhaustion): rapid recovery with supportive care
• Heat stroke: poor prognosis if not recognized and aggressively managed

 Differential Diagnosis

• Heat cramps: rhabdomyolysis, tetany
• Heat edema: thrombophlebitis, lymphedema, congestive heart failure
• Heat stroke: CNS process with fever (CVA, meningitis, encephalitis), other infections, anticholinergic poisoning (dilated pupils), drug induced (medication, recreational), temperature rise, severe dehydration. Chills suggest febrile illness, not heat stroke

 Data Gathering

HISTORY

Question: Initial temperature, if taken at scene?
Significance: The initial temperature can alert one to the potential for and extent of heat-related illness. If the first temperature is not obtained until after cooling interventions, extent of illness may not be fully appreciated, and appropriate therapy may be delayed.
Question: Cooling maneuvers en route to hospital?
Significance: A lower temperature may falsely reassure or mislead caregivers.
Question: History of CNS dysfunction?
Significance: A history of CNS dysfunction in conjunction with an environment consistent with or predisposing conditions conducive to development of heat-related illness should lead one to a presumptive diagnosis of heat stroke.

 Physical Examination

Finding: Heat exhaustion
Significance: Weakness, lethargy, thirst, malaise, diminished ability to work or play, headache, nausea, vomiting, myalgias, pale skin, dizziness, visual disturbances, syncope, mild CNS dysfunction, impaired judgment, cramps, vertigo, hypotension, tachycardia, hyperventilation, paresthesias, agitation, incoordination, psychosis, temperature less than 40°C, sweating, environmental exposure and activity. No coma or seizures.
Finding: Heat stroke
Significance: Temperature more than 40.5°C (may be cooler due to prehospital maneuvers), with or without hot, dry (classic), or clammy (exercise induced) skin, pink or ashen color, weakness, nausea, vomiting, anorexia, headache, dizziness, confusion, drowsiness, irritability, CNS dysfunction, euphoria, combativeness, abrupt or impending alteration of consciousness, obtundation, tachycardia, hypotension or normotension with wide pulse pressure, tachypnea, ataxia, posturing, incontinence, seizures, coma, purpura, or petechia. Two thirds with constricted pupils. May have muscle rigidity with tonic contractions and dystonia that mimic seizures.

Finding: Temperature measurement (continuous is best)
Significance:
- Esophageal thermometry probably the best
- Deep rectal thermometry a good approximation of core temperature
- Tympanic temperature reasonable estimation of CNS temperature
- Oral temperature not as useful due to mouth breathing
- Axillary temperature unreliable, especially with cooling maneuvers

 ## Laboratory Aids

Tests only to confirm diagnosis, evaluate extent of injury, or rule out other processes as treatment should be empiric.

- Heat cramps. Decreased serum and urine sodium and chloride; BUN normal or slightly increased
- Heat exhaustion: May see hyponatremia (salt loss) or hypernatremia (water loss), hypochloremia, low urine sodium and chloride, hemoconcentration. Differentiated from heat stroke by lack of significant liver function test abnormalities
- Heat stroke: Blood chemistries: NaCl normal or high, hypokalemia, increased BUN/CR; hypophosphatemia, hypomagnesemia, hypocalcemia; lactate high; hypoglycemia. Hematologic: CBC (hemoconcentration, leukocytosis, thrombocytosis), coagulation profile for DIC (more likely in exertional than classic heat stroke): PT/PTT, fibrin split products, fibrinogen, malaria evaluation (thick smear), hematuria. Others: LFTs (AST and ALT markedly abnormal and useful to distinguish heat stroke from heat exhaustion), CPK (rhabdomyolysis), ABG (classic heat stroke: respiratory alkalosis and hypokalemia early; lactic acidosis later; exertional heat stroke: lactic acidosis), U/A (casts, brownish color proteinuria, microscopic hematuria, myoglobinuria), CSF, ECG, CXR.

 ## Therapy

- Rapid recognition and cooling imperative
- Specific therapy:
—Heat cramps: Rest, salt and water replacement
—Heat syncope: Self-limited as return to horizontal position is treatment; rest and fluids, salted liquids
—Heat exhaustion: Clinical findings (HR, BP, orthostatic changes, urine output) should direct therapy. Most treated as outpatient with rapid recovery (older patients or those with preexisting illnesses may require hospitalization); rest, rehydration, cooling; mild case: oral electrolyte solution (0.1–0.2% saline = approximately 1/4 to 1/2 teaspoon table salt in 1 quart of water); if CNS/GI dysfunction (nausea, vomiting, inability to drink); IV [0.5% (similar to sweat losses) to

0.9% normal saline solution (NSS)]; avoid rapid overcorrection of hypernatremia (treat as with hypernatremic dehydration); if hyponatremic seizures, treat with 3% saline at approximately 5 mL/kg
—Heat stroke: Immediate cooling. Remove clothing from patient and patient from hot environment; use air conditioning, open vehicle for transport if possible; esophageal or rectal temperature probe (continuous temperature measurements); cooling should exceed 0.1° to 0.2°C/min; slow cooling down at 38.5° to 39°C to avoid overshoot; cooling options (ice bath, cold water bath (15°–16°C) as effective as ice bath without discomfort, shivering or vasoconstriction), massage with ice, ice packs to neck, groin, axilla, wet sheet over patient, moisten skin with water spray, convection increase (fan) to increase evaporative cooling, cooling blankets, cool water lavage (peritoneum, rectum, gastric), cold to room temperature IV fluids, alcohol sponge baths (use with caution due to potential absorption), cardiopulmonary bypass.

NONSPECIFIC
- Heat stroke: Treat empirically, then rule out other causes of presentation. ABCs including securing airway as indicated, supplemental oxygen delivery.
—Fluid replacement: Usually only modest fluid requirements (patients often normovolemic with a distributive shock presentation due to vasodilatation; cooling redistributes volume from periphery to core; aggressive fluid resuscitation can lead to fluid overload and pulmonary edema). IV 0.9% NSS or Ringer's lactate solution. Ensure patient not hypoglycemic.
—Miscellaneous therapies:
  —Foley catheter to monitor urine output
  —Nasogastric tube
  —Chlorpromazine may help with peripheral vasodilatation and prevent shivering [dose: 0.5–1.0 mg/kg (25–50 mg for adult) IV/IM; may cause hypotension];
  —Benzodiazepine for sedation and/or seizures
  —Myoglobinuria therapy (mannitol, bicarbonate, dialysis)
  —Electrolyte replacement if symptomatic from hypokalemia or hypocalcemia
  —Fresh frozen plasma for DIC

MEDICATIONS
Antipyretics not useful because intact hypothalamus required for action. Avoid anticholinergic drugs (atropine), which can inhibit sweating.

PREVENTION
- Recognize and intervene for those at risk in conditions that predispose to heat illness
- Recognize changes (medical or physical conditions, medications) that increase risk of heat illness
- Avoid enclosed spaces (children in closed cars)

- Limit physical activity, keep cool, use shaded areas
- Air conditioning or fans all or part of hot days
- Cool or tepid baths
- Increase fluid intake prior to exercise (400–600 mL in hour prior to exercise in adults), scheduled (not solely based on thirst) fluid replacement during strenuous activity (100–200 mL every 10–15 minutes); cool water and large volumes increase gastric emptying (high osmolality and carbohydrate content decreases gastric emptying), do not usually need glucose
- Fluid replacement during exercise that mimics losses. Carbohydrate concentration of 6% to 8% maximum to avoid delayed gastric emptying
- Loose (avoid occlusive), light-colored clothing, protective hat
- Acclimatization, gradual conditioning to hotter environment (7–14 days)
- Liberal dietary sodium: Avoid sodium chloride tablets: hypernatremia and potassium depletion, gastric irritant, delayed gastric emptying
- Frequently flex leg muscles when standing and avoid prolonged standing in hot environments
- Avoid caffeine and alcohol

 ## Common Questions and Answers

Q: How can one distinguish between heat exhaustion and heat stroke?
A: If CNS abnormalities are present, temperature is greater than 40.6°C and liver function tests (ALT, AST) are markedly elevated, the patient is likely to have heat stroke.
Q: When should heat stroke be suspected?
A: Suspect heat stroke in a patient with or without sweating who demonstrates alterations of CNS function in environment that would be conducive to heat illness.
Q: Does the presence or absence of sweating help with the diagnosis of heat exhaustion versus heat stroke?
A: No. Sweating will be present with heat exhaustion and may or may not be present with heat stroke.

ICD-9-CM 992.0

BIBLIOGRAPHY
Kellermann AL, Todd KH. Killing heat. *N Engl J Med* 1996;335:126–127.

Tek D, Olshaker JS. Heat illness. *Emerg Med Clin North Am* 1992;10:299–310.

Tobin JR, Jason DR, Challa VR, et al. Malignant hyperthermia and apparent heat stroke. *JAMA* 2001;286(2):168–169.

Author: George Anthony Woodward

Hemangioma (Vascular Nevi)

 Database

DEFINITION
- Hemangiomas: nonmalignant neoplasms consisting of vascular endothelial cells
- Vascular malformations: capillaries, veins, lymphatics, or arteries that underwent errors of morphogenesis (i.e., hamartomas); includes port-wine stains (nevus flammeus) and arteriovenous malformations.
- Salmon patches (nevus simplex): distended dermal capillaries (nevus simplex, telangiectatic nevus).

PATHOPHYSIOLOGY
- Hemangiomas: appear in first few weeks of life, grow rapidly in first 6 to 12 months of life, followed by a static period, and then involution. Lesions are made up of proliferating endothelial cells. Markers for angiogenesis are found in lesions.
- Vascular malformations: grow proportionally with the affected individual. Congenital by definition, may not become apparent until adolescence or adulthood. Port-wine stains are apparent at birth. Lesions are dysplastic vessels without endothelial proliferation.
- Salmon patches: Grow proportionally with affected individual. Lesion consists of distended dermal vessels

GENETICS
- Hemangiomas
—Usually no genetic association when isolated finding
—Seen with Klippel-Trénaunay syndrome, Parkes Weber syndrome, Maffucci syndrome, blue rubber bleb nevus syndrome (dominant inheritance), diffuse neonatal hemangiomatosis, Cobb syndrome and PHACES syndrome (posterior fossa malformations, hemangiomas, arterial anomalies, cardiac anomalies, eye anomalies, sternal or abdominal cleft)
—Rarely seen in kindreds with autosomal-dominant inheritance
- Vascular malformations
—Seen with Sturge-Weber syndrome, Cobb syndrome, Wyburn-Mason (or Bonnet-Dechaume-Blanc) syndrome, Klippel-Trénaunay syndrome, Parkes Weber syndrome, Osler-Weber-Rendu syndrome (or hereditary hemorrhagic telangiectasia)
—Most often a sporadic finding
- Salmon patches
—No genetic association

EPIDEMIOLOGY
- Hemangiomas
—Female/male ratio 3:1
—Increased incidence with prematurity
—Ten times increased incidence if chorionic villus sampling was performed during pregnancy
—Present in up to 12% of infants
—80% are single lesions
—60% are found on head and neck
—25% are found on trunk
- Vascular malformations

—Port-wine stains female/male ratio 1:1
- Salmon patches
—Found in 30% to 40% of all newborns

COMPLICATIONS
- Hemangiomas
—Local ulceration, bleeding, superinfection—most common
—Obstruction of important structures including airway, GI tract, eye (even small periorbital lesions have been associated with astigmatism secondary to pressure on the globe).
—Multiple cutaneous hemangiomas may be associated with visceral hemangiomas, including liver, lung, and GI tract. Rarely, the meninges, brain, spinal cord, pancreas, spleen, or adrenals may be involved. Hemangiomas in these organs can result in significant functional impairment.
—Disseminated neonatal hemangiomatosis may have high morbidity and mortality.
—High output cardiac failure in presence of large number of lesions
—Iron-deficiency anemia secondary to hemorrhage from GI lesions
—Liver lesions particularly associated with high mortality
—Kasabach-Merritt syndrome: platelet trapping, coagulopathy, thrombocytopenia; now generally felt only to occur with kaposiform hemangioendothelioma or tufted angiomas (clinically similar to hemangioma but histologically distinct) 20% to 30% mortality
—Rarely cause skeletal overgrowth secondary to increased blood flow
- Vascular malformations
—Port-wine stains can signal underlying developmental defects especially of central nervous system and spine.
—A-V malformations can lead to "steal" causing ischemic necrosis, pain, and increased cardiac output.
—Frequently associated with skeletal abnormalities including hypertrophy (low flow) or destruction (high flow)
—Localized or disseminated intravascular coagulopathy possible, but uncommon
- Salmon patch: none

PROGNOSIS
- Hemangiomas: excellent if cutaneous alone. Association with other syndromes, or visceral involvement worsens prognosis significantly. Superficial scarring varies but can be significant especially with large lesions of the face
- Vascular malformations: varied depending on type of malformation, location, and associated syndromes.
- Salmon patches: excellent.

 Differential Diagnosis

INFECTION
- Bacillary angiomatosis

TUMORS
- Glomus tumor
- Tufted angioma
- Kaposiform hemangioendothelioma

- Angioendothelioma
- Sarcoma

CONGENITAL
- Verrucous hemangioma

MISCELLANEOUS
- Pyogenic granuloma
- Angiokeratomas

Approach to the Patient
The single determination that the primary care provider must make is whether or not specialist referral is necessary. In the great majority of cases, the answer is no. Below lists the situations where specialist consultation is critical:
- Multiple hemangiomas in "beard distribution" frequently associated with airway hemangiomas, these patients require direct visualization of the airway
- Patients with noisy breathing and multiple cutaneous hemangiomas in any distribution should be evaluated for airway involvement, especially when respiratory symptoms appear in the first weeks to months of life, a period of rapid hemangioma growth
- Patients with multiple cutaneous lesions are at risk for visceral involvement. Patient should be referred for imaging studies to assess concealed involvement. Those with hepatic hemangiomas must be monitored very closely as they carry a high mortality rate.
- Those with disfiguring lesions (usually facial) or periorbital lesions should be referred to dermatology and ophthalmology for treatment
- Hemangiomas over the spine, especially in lumbosacral region, require further investigation for spinal dysraphism, tethered cord, and other anomalies.
- Lesions that interfere with function (e.g., periorbital, obstructing ear canal, anogenital region) must be treated aggressively.

 Data Gathering

HISTORY
Question: When did the skin finding appear?
Significance: Diagnosis is generally made by exam rather than history
Question: Hemangioma?
Significance: Present in first few weeks of life, but minimally at birth, rapid growth noted in first year of life.
Question: Vascular malformations?
Significance: Most present at birth, sometimes not noted until adolescence or adulthood.
Question: Salmon patches?
Significance: Noted at birth.

Physical Examination

HEMANGIOMAS
Finding: Lesion with raised, bright red-pink color, sharply demarcated border, stippled surface—hence the term *strawberry hemangioma*
Significance: Young lesion in superficial dermis
Finding: Lesion is bluish in color, raised with smooth overlying skin
Significance: Young lesion in lower dermis or subcutaneous tissue
Finding: Combination of above findings
Significance: Superficial and deep components can be combined in a single lesion
Finding: Lesion develops gray or white areas, usually centrally located, which spread toward periphery
Significance: Involuting hemangioma

VASCULAR MALFORMATIONS
Finding: Apparent at birth, pink-to-red sharply demarcated macule, possibly slightly raised, darkens with age, may develop papules over time
Significance: Port-wine stains
Finding: New lesion in adolescence or adulthood usually soft, easily compressed, and emptied of blood
Significance: Although congenital, vascular malformation other than port-wine stains may appear later in life.
Finding: Port-wine stains including first distribution of the trigeminal nerve
Significance: May reflect presence of anomalies of the choroid plexus and leptomeninges; Sturge-Weber. Specialist referral is often very helpful to determine the need for a brain imaging study.

SALMON PATCHES
Finding: Salmon patches
Significance: Often have more than one lesion; 80% on nape of neck, 45% on eyelids, 33% on glabella.

Laboratory Aids

RADIOGRAPHIC STUDIES
• Occasionally necessary to differentiate hemangiomas from vascular malformations
• Ultrasound is useful to delineate visceral involvement with hemangioma
• Head MRI: performed to rule out anomalies of the choroid plexus and leptomeninges (Sturge-Weber); serious consideration when port-wine stains include first distribution of the trigeminal nerve. Lesions in second and third distribution of trigeminal nerve do not have this risk.
• MRI of spine: performed for hemangiomas overlying spine, especially when lumbosacral, to rule out spinal dysraphism.

Emergency Care

Respiratory compromise can occur with rapidly growing airway hemangioma. Immediate ENT involvement is a must.

Therapy

• Hemangiomas
—For bleeding: direct pressure
—For ulceration: observation or wet compresses and topical antibacterials
—For ulceration that is difficult to manage: pulse dye laser, corticosteroids
—For infection: intravenous antibiotics for cellulitis, topical antibiotics with dressing changes for mild involvement
—Treatment is necessary for lesions that interfere with critical structures (e.g., eye, airway, GI tract) or for serious symptoms, such as consumptive coagulopathy. No therapy indicated in 95%.
—Intralesional or systemic steroids
—Interferon-α-2a or 2b for critically ill steroid nonresponders
—Liquid nitrogen occasionally beneficial, some authors are revisiting sclerotherapy
—Laser therapy beneficial for superficial lesions only
—Surgical resection utilized infrequently
• Vascular malformations
—Port-wine stain: cosmetic camouflage or laser therapy. Flashlamp pulsed dye laser therapy is being continuously improved in terms of quality of outcome and decreased complications as different types of lasers are developed and tested. Multiple laser treatment sessions at 2- to 3-month intervals are usually necessary. Early treatment is advocated because of better outcome, especially children under 1 year of age.

Follow-Up

• Hemangiomas
—50% will spontaneously resolve by 5 years.
—70% will spontaneously resolve by 7 years.
—90% will spontaneously resolve by 9 to 12 years.
—Up to 40% of children are left with residual skin changes including atrophy, redundant skin, discoloration, telangiectasias, and scarring.
• Vascular malformations
—No spontaneous resolution of lesions.
• Salmon patches
—50% on nape of neck spontaneously resolve.
—95% of others spontaneously resolve.
—Tendency toward erythema in affected area may persist after lesions resolve.

PITFALLS
• For hemangiomas, treatment can significantly increase the risk of poor cosmetic outcome.

• α Interferon is associated with spastic diplegia in up to 20%; this does not resolve when interferon therapy is stopped.
• Hemangioma ulceration can result in severe pain.
• For vascular malformations, treatment of port-wine stains may achieve color lightening rather than complete resolution of the lesion.

Common Questions and Answers

Q: What will happen to my child's hemangioma?
A: Expect it to enlarge, get a bluish or gray-ish hue, and then get smaller. In the first year of life, it may enlarge at a rate more rapid than the rest of the child's growth. After that time it will involute, and should resolve by 9 to 12 years of age; most resolve much earlier.
Q: What are the problems of the involuting hemangioma?
A: Infection and ulceration.
Q: What happens to the "stork bite" on the back of the neck?
A: It fades but still may be seen when vessels dilate such as with crying or fever.

ICD-9-CM
Port wine stain 757.32
Hemangioma 228.0

BIBLIOGRAPHY
Brown RL, Azizkhan RG. Pediatric head and neck lesions [tutorial]. *Pediatr Clin North Am* 1998;45(4):889–905.

Burrows PE, Laor T, Paltiel H, et al. Diagnostic imaging in the evaluation of vascular birthmarks. *Dermatol Clin* 1998;16(3): 455–488.

Drolet BA, Esterly NB, Frieden IJ. Hemangiomas in children. *N Engl J Med* 1999;341(3):173–181.

Hurwitz S. Vascular disorders of infancy and childhood. In: *Clinical pediatric dermatology.* Philadelphia: WB Saunders, 1993:242–272.

Metry D, Hebert A. Benign cutaneous vascular tumors of infancy: when to worry, what to do. *Arch Dermatol* 2000;136(7):905–914.

Poetke M, Philipp C, Berlien HP. Flashlamp-pumped pulsed dye laser for hemangiomas in infancy: treatment of superficial vs mixed hemangiomas. *Arch Dermatol* 2000;136(5):628–632.

Powell J. Update on hemangiomas and vascular malformations. *Curr Opin Pediatr* 1999;11(5):457–463.

Winter H, Drager E, Sterry W. Sclerotherapy for treatment of hemangiomas. *Dermatol Surg* 2000;26(2):105–108.

Author: Laura N. Sinai

Hemolytic Disease of the Newborn

Database

DEFINITION

Hemolytic anemia occurring in the newborn due to passive transfer of maternal antibodies (IgG) against fetal red cells.

CAUSES

- Most severe disease due to Rh (D) antigen sensitization
- A and B antigens may also be responsible.
- 1% of cases due to other antigens.
- Other antigens: Kell, Duffy, C, E, and c

PATHOPHYSIOLOGY

- Rh alloimmunization results from passage of fetal red blood cells that express surface Rh (D) antigen across the placenta into the circulation of an Rh-negative mother.
- The passage of fetal Rh positive cells occurs as a result of transplacental hemorrhage
- Initial exposure results in production of maternal IgM antibodies, which do not cross the placenta. This is followed by production of IgG antibodies, which can cross the placenta. On subsequent exposures there is a rapid production of anti-D antibodies
- Rh-negative mothers may have initial sensitization due to transfusion or previous pregnancy.
- Anti-D IgG produced in the maternal circulation crosses the placenta and coats fetal red blood cells (RBC). These cells are then destroyed in reticuloendothelial system, primarily the fetal spleen
- Alloimmunization may lead to severe anemia, hydrops, and hyperbilirubinemia.
- Extramedullary hematopoiesis in the fetal liver and spleen occurs as a response to fetal anemia leading to severe hepatosplenomegaly.
- ABO isoimmunization, usually in case of type O mothers with type A or B fetus, results in a clinically milder hemolysis.

EPIDEMIOLOGY

- 15% of Caucasians are Rh-negative (dd)
- 48% are heterozygous (Dd)
- 35% are homozygous (DD)
- Prevalence of Rh-positive fetus in Rh-negative mother: 15%
- Incidence of Rh hemolytic disease: 6–7/1000 live births
- Of all Rh-sensitized pregnancies:

—50% require no treatment
—31% require treatment after a full-term delivery
—10% delivered early and require exchange transfusion
—9% require intrauterine transfusion

- Reasons for spectrum of clinical severity:

—Rh immunization rarely occurs in first pregnancy
—Many subsequent infants may be Rh-negative
—Only a fraction of women at risk develop antibodies

- 50% of cases of ABO disease occur in first pregnancy

GENETICS

See Epidemiology, above.

COMPLICATIONS

- Hydrops fetalis
- Still births
- Neonatal hyperbilirubinemia and kernicterus
- Fetal anemia

PROGNOSIS

Approximately half the infants have minimal anemia and hyperbilirubinemia and require either no treatment or only phototherapy.

- One fourth will require exchange transfusions.
- Hydropic infants have high mortality.

Differential Diagnosis

- Neonatal hyperbilirubinemia

—ABO incompatibility
—Galactosemia
—G6PD deficiency
—Hypothyroidism
—Pyruvate kinase deficiency
—Crigler-Najjar syndrome
—α-Thalassemia
—Gilbert syndrome
—Spherocytosis
—Breast-milk jaundice

- Hydrops fetalis

—Hematologic: α-thalassemia, severe G6PD deficiency, twin-to-twin transfusion
—Cardiac: hypoplastic left heart syndrome, myocarditis, endocardial fibroelastosis, heart block
—Congenital infections: parvovirus, syphilis, cytomegalovirus (CMV), rubella
—Renal: renal vein thrombosis, urinary tract obstruction, nephrosis
—Placental: umbilical vein thrombosis, true knot of umbilical cord
—Miscellaneous: trisomy 13, 18, 21, triploidy, aneuploidy, diaphragmatic hernia

Data Gathering

HISTORY

- Previous stillbirths, abortions?
- Neonatal hyperbilirubinemia requiring therapy in previous pregnancy?
- Exposure of mother to blood products?
- Father's ABO and Rh type?
- Rh immune globulin given after previous pregnancy or abortion?

Physical Examination

- Pallor, tachycardia, tachypnea due to congestive heart failure (CHF) secondary to severe anemia

—Jaundice developing within 24 hours of birth

- Usually no jaundice at birth
- Generalized edema in cases with severe anemia and hydrops
- Massive hepatosplenomegaly in severe cases
- Milder cases manifest with neonatal hyperbilirubinemia only.
- ABO incompatibility usually manifests jaundice at 24 hours.

Laboratory Aids

ANTENATAL

- ABO and Rh type of all mothers at first prenatal visit
- Zygosity of the father—if the father is Rh+ homozygous, then all children will be Rh positive; if the father is heterozygous, then only 50% of children will be Rh+.
- Fetal Rh D genotyping can be performed on maternal plasma during second trimester.
- Monitor antibody titer by indirect Coombs test in Rh-negative mothers starting at 20 weeks.
- Amniocentesis if maternal antibody titer more than 1:8 at any time
- Spectrophotometric assessment of bilirubin concentration in amniotic fluid
- Amniotic fluid values in Liley's zone 3 and high zone 2 indicative of severe fetal disease (Liley's test measures optical density in amniotic fluid as an indicator for bilirubin levels; do not use for Kell sensitization as it is not a reliable indicator of severity of disease in these patients).
- Fetal blood sampling in severe cases to assess degree of anemia

Hemolytic Disease of the Newborn

NEONATAL

- Cord blood ABO and Rh types
- Cord blood hemoglobin (Hb), hematocrit (Hct), bilirubin (direct and indirect), reticulocyte count
- Direct Coombs test on cord blood—will be positive in immune hemolytic disease
- Indirect Coombs test on cord blood for passively transferred antibody
- Identification of antibody after elution from RBC
- Peripheral smear: nucleated RBC (spherocytes in ABO disease)

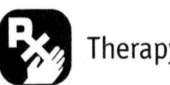 Therapy

- In severely affected fetuses where early delivery is not possible due to lung immaturity, intrauterine intravascular transfusion (IUIVT) is the therapy of choice. Risks if IUIVT include fetal loss (2%), premature labor and rupture of membranes, chorioamnionitis, fetal bradycardia, cord laceration, fetomaternal hemorrhage.
- Early delivery and subsequent resuscitation may be required in severe Rh isoimmunization.
- Phototherapy to start as soon as possible
- Exchange transfusion removes sensitized fetal RBC and circulating bilirubin and is indicated:

—To correct anemia in severely anemic infants
—To prevent or correct hyperbilirubinemia
—To remove circulating antibodies

- Indications for early exchange transfusion:

—Cord blood bilirubin more than 4.5 mg/dL and cord blood Hb less than 10 g/dL
—Bilirubin rising at rate more than 1 mg/dL/h despite optimal phototherapy
—Indirect bilirubin greater than or equal to 20 mg/dL or rising to reach that level
—Lower indirect bilirubin levels are used in preterm or high-risk Infants
—Hb between 11 and 13 g/dL and bilirubin rising at rate more than 0.5 mg/dL/h despite optimal phototherapy

- In hydropic infants, immediate partial exchange may be needed to correct anemia and CHF.
- Double-volume exchanges may be needed for hyperbilirubinemia.
- Type of blood for exchange transfusion:

—As fresh as possible (>72 hours old), CMV negative, and irradiated
—For Rh disease (if prepared before delivery): type O Rh-negative crossmatched against mother's blood; after delivery then O negative crossmatched against infant also
—For ABO disease: type O Rh-negative or Rh-compatible crossmatched against mother and infant

- Risks of exchange transfusion include prolonged neutropenia, thrombocytopenia, late anemia, metabolic abnormalities, arrhythmias, thrombosis, death
- Some studies indicate that administration of IVIG to the neonate diminishes hemolysis and may prevent the need for exchange transfusion
- Most infants with ABO incompatibility require no treatment or phototherapy only.
- Some infants with milder Rh isoimmunization may only have exaggerated physiologic anemia at 12 weeks.
- Avoid drugs that interfere with bilirubin metabolism or its binding to albumin (sulfonamides, caffeine, sodium benzoate).
- Infants who had hemolytic disease of the newborn are at risk for late anemia due to reticulocytopenia from hyporegeneration of persistent high titers of circulating maternal antibody. They should have weekly Hct measured during the first few months of life.

ANTENATAL MANAGEMENT

- Rh immunoglobulin at a dose of 300 μg for the following:

—Unsensitized Rh-negative mother at 28 weeks' gestation and within 72 hours of delivery
—Unimmunized Rh-negative mothers who have undergone spontaneous or therapeutic abortions
—After ruptured tubal pregnancies in Rh-negative mothers

- If previous stillbirth or hydrops and fetus high risk after amniocentesis plan early delivery
- Careful fetal monitoring and induction of pulmonary maturation
- If fetus too immature for delivery, then intrauterine transfusions every 10 to 14 days.

 Follow-Up

- Weekly Hct especially for patients who had exchange transfusion
- Watch for exaggerated physiologic anemia at 12 weeks.
- Assess for neurologic damage.

PREVENTION

Rh hemolytic disease can be prevented by administration of RhoGAM to the Rh-negative women after any exposure to Rh positive blood and prophylactically during pregnancy.

 Common Questions and Answers

Q: Does the condition become worse with each pregnancy?
A: Yes, if the mother is not treated with Rh immunoglobulin after each Rh-positive pregnancy or abortion.

Q: Can maternal blood be used to transfuse the affected baby?
A: It can be used as a lifesaving measure in a situation when there is no other suitable blood available for the baby.

ICD-9-CM 774.6

BIBLIOGRAPHY

Bennebroek J. Diagnosis and treatment of severe alloimmunization. *Vox Sang* 1994;67(suppl 3):235–238.

Bowman JM. Antenatal suppression of Rh alloimmunization. *Clin Obstet Gynecol* 1991;34(2):296–303.

Koenig, Joyce M. Evaluation and treatment of erythroblastosis fetalis in the neonate. In: Christensen RD, ed. *Hematologic problems of the neonate*. Philadelphia: WB Saunders, 2000:185–207.

Nathan DG, Oski FA, eds. *Hematology of infancy and childhood*, 5th ed, vol 1. Philadelphia: WB Saunders, 1998:53–78.

Whittle MJ. Rhesus hemolytic disease. *Arch Dis Child* 1992;67(1 spec no):65–68.

Author: Tammy I. Kang
Sadhna M. Shankar, 2nd edition

Hemolytic Uremic Syndrome

 Database

DEFINITION

The hemolytic uremic syndrome (HUS) is a heterogeneous group of similar entities defined by microangiopathic hemolytic anemia, thrombocytopenia, and acute renal failure. HUS is the most common cause of acute renal failure in childhood.
- Typical (Shiga-toxin, diarrhea-associated) form accounts for greater than 90% of pediatric cases and is characterized by the sudden onset of hemolytic anemia, thrombocytopenia, and acute renal failure after a prodromal illness of acute gastroenteritis, usually with bloody diarrhea.
- Atypical HUS (idiopathic) is a catch-all category for several variants of HUS, including recurrent HUS, inherited HUS, and HUS associated with pregnancy, oral contraceptives, cyclosporine, antitumor drugs, malignancy, and *Streptococcus pneumoniae* infection.

PATHOPHYSIOLOGY

- Common denominator in all forms of HUS is thought to be microvascular endothelial cell injury and dysfunction.
- Typical form usually starts with an infection with a Shiga toxin producing *Escherichia coli*, most commonly *E. coli* 0157:H7.
- Endothelial cell injury ultimately results in local intravascular coagulation and microthrombi formation with microangiopathic hemolytic anemia and thrombocytopenia.
- Pathogenesis of atypical, nonepidemic HUS is not understood.

GENETICS

Atypical HUS has been reported with both autosomal-dominant and autosomal-recessive patterns of inheritance. The pathogenesis and genetics of inherited HUS is unknown.

EPIDEMIOLOGY

HUS has been reported throughout the world.

Typical

- Typical HUS tends to occur in the summer months, and epidemics have been reported in day-care centers and nursing homes.
- Typical HUS occurs mainly in older infants and young children, usually between 6 months and 4 years of age.
- The Shiga toxin producing *E. coli* is found in the intestine of beef cattle. Ground beef may be contaminated throughout with Shiga toxin. If a hamburger is inadequately cooked, infection may ensue.
- In reported outbreaks, the frequency of bloody diarrhea has ranged from 35% to 90%.

Atypical

Atypical HUS has no seasonal variation and may occur at any age.

COMPLICATIONS

GI

- Acute colitis is usually transient.
- Complications include rectal prolapse, toxic megacolon, bowel wall necrosis, intussusception, perforation, and stricture.
- Pancreatic involvement may result in pancreatitis or insulin-dependent diabetes mellitus.

CNS

- Most patients have mild CNS symptoms that include irritability, lethargy, and behavioral changes.
- Major symptoms such as stupor, coma, seizures, cortical blindness, posturing, and hallucinations occur in 20% to 40% of patients.
- Thrombotic or hemorrhagic stroke may occur.
- The risk of seizures is associated with hyponatremia.

PROGNOSIS

Typical HUS

- Improved supportive care and a better understanding of the complications of typical HUS have resulted in a decrease in mortality to an acute fatality rate of 4% to 12%.
- A substantial number of patients develop renal sequelae after typical HUS, and they should be evaluated regularly for many years.
- Persistence of proteinuria after 1 year is a poor prognostic sign and warrants additional evaluation.
- Recurrences of HUS are exceedingly uncommon.
- Chronic renal insufficiency occurs in 4% to 9%. Children who do develop end stage renal disease are good candidates for kidney transplantation.

Atypical HUS

- In general, patients with atypical HUS have a substantially worse prognosis.
- Neurologic symptoms are seen more commonly.
- Hypertension is common during the initial illness and prolonged antihypertensive treatment is required.
- Recurrences have been reported both before and after renal transplantation.
- In familial HUS, relapse, end-stage renal disease, and death are common.

 Differential Diagnosis

- Infectious causes such as *Shigella, Salmonella, Campylobacter, Yersinia enterocolitica, C. difficile,* and *Entamoeba histolytica*
- During the gastrointestinal prodrome, it may be difficult to distinguish HUS from appendicitis, inflammatory bowel disease, diverticulosis, or intussusception.
- Thrombotic thrombocytopenic purpura (TTP) shares many features with HUS.

- Sepsis with disseminated intravascular coagulation may present with acute renal failure and a microangiopathic process.

 Data Gathering

HISTORY

Question: Gastrointestinal prodrome?
Significance: Affected children with typical HUS are usually healthy before the initiation of the gastrointestinal prodrome. The diarrhea is usually watery or bloody and is associated with abdominal discomfort.
Question: Duration?
Significance: The prodrome lasts from 1 to 15 days and often improves before onset of the triad of features inherent to HUS.

 Physical Examination

- Pallor and petechiae
- Dehydration secondary to the gastroenteritis
- May have volume overload secondary to oligoanuric renal failure
- Peripheral edema, congestive heart failure, and hypertension may be present.
- Mild neurologic changes of irritability or behavioral changes

SPECIAL QUESTIONS

Finding: Recent hamburger ingestion.
Significance: Many cases of typical HUS have been associated with inadequately cooked hamburger meat. Epidemics have been reported in fast-food restaurant customers.
Finding: Consumption of unpasteurized milk, cheese, or cider.
Significance: May contain Shiga toxins.

 Laboratory Aids

HEMATOLOGIC

Test: CBC
Significance: The microangiopathic hemolytic anemia may be mild or severe. Leukocytosis is often seen in typical HUS.
Test: Reticulocytes
Significance: Repeated exacerbations of the hemolysis may occur for days or weeks.
Test: Blood smear
Significance: Fragmented red blood cells or schistocytes
Test: Markers of hemolysis
Significance: Elevated lactic dehydrogenase, unconjugated bilirubin, and reticulocyte count are additional evidence of ongoing hemolysis.
Test: Platelets
Significance: The thrombocytopenia may also last for days or weeks.

Test: PT-PTT
Significance: Coagulation studies usually show increased fibrin degradation products with normal prothrombin and partial thromboplastin times.

RENAL
Test: Renal function
Significance: Elevated creatinine and BUN
Test: Electrolytes
Significance: Elevated levels of potassium, phosphorus, hydrogen ion, and uric acid; decreased concentrations of sodium, calcium, and bicarbonate
Test: Urinalysis
Significance: Microscopic hematuria; varying degrees of proteinuria; macroscopic hematuria and RBC casts may be present.

GASTROINTESTINAL
Test: Electrolytes
Significance: Decreased serum potassium
Test: Liver function tests
Significance: Albumen decreased; liver function tests are usually normal.
Test: Amylase, lipase
Significance: Pancreatic involvement may result in hyperglycemia and elevated concentrations of serum amylase and lipase. Exocrine pancreatitis is difficult to evaluate since amylase and lipase are normally cleared by the kidneys.

MICROBIOLOGY
Test: Stool
Significance: All bloody stool samples should be screened for *E. coli* O157:H7. Since the rate of recovery of the organism may decline rapidly after the first 6 days of illness, stool cultures should be obtained as early in the course of illness as possible. The local health department should be notified of any isolates.
Test: Verotoxins
Significance: Serologic evidence of verotoxin may be diagnostic.

IMAGING
Test: Plain film of the abdomen
Significance: Often demonstrates colonic distention. Look for free air as evidence of bowel perforation.

 ## Therapy

• Supportive therapy
—Fluid and electrolyte
—Volume resuscitation initially
—In a euvolemic patient, fluids should provide replacement of ongoing losses with meticulous attention to urine output.
—Hyponatremia is common.
—If the patient is fluid overloaded, fluid intake should be restricted accordingly.

• Dialysis
—If medical management fails to correct hypertension hyperkalemia, hyperphosphatemia, and severe metabolic acidosis, dialysis or hemofiltration may be indicated. Dialysis is required in one half to one third of patients.
• Anemia
—Transfusion of packed red blood cells if the hemoglobin concentration falls below 6.0 to 7.0 g/dL or if there is evidence of cardiac dysfunction. The transfusions should be given slowly since blood pressure occasionally increases during transfusions.
—Platelet transfusions should be reserved for patients with active bleeding or in preparation for an invasive procedure.
—Antibiotics are not prescribed routinely because there is evidence the antimicrobials may increase verotoxin release. Antimotility agents have also been associated with more severe disease and should be avoided.
—Nutrition must be maintained and may require total parenteral nutrition if the intestine is nonfunctional. The degree of renal insufficiency will dictate the need for potassium and phosphorus restriction.
• Specific therapy
—Therapies have not proven to be helpful: plasmapheresis, fresh frozen plasma, intravenous immunoglobulin, heparin, antibiotics, aspirin, vitamin E for typical HUS.
—Plasmapheresis has been advocated for atypical, or idiopathic HUS.

 ## Follow-Up

WHEN TO EXPECT IMPROVEMENT
• Resolution is usually heralded by a rise in platelet count and a gradual decrease in the frequency of blood transfusions.
• During the recovery phase patients may require folic acid and iron supplementation.
• Anuria rarely lasts more than 2 weeks. In general, a longer duration of anuria is a poor prognostic feature.
• Children who sustain structural neurologic damage during the acute phase of HUS may have residual impairment, but there is tremendous potential for improvement and recovery.
• Pancreatic insufficiency may persist requiring long-term insulin therapy beyond resolution of the acute illness.

PREVENTION
Most cases of typical HUS can be avoided by thoroughly cooking all hamburger-containing foods. Other sources of contaminated foods include unpasteurized apple cider or milk.

 ## Common Questions and Answers

Q: What are some predictors of the severity of typical HUS?
A: Predictors include an elevated white cell count, a severe gastrointestinal prodrome, anuria early in the course of illness, and age under 2 years.
Q: In a patient with atypical HUS, what is the chance other siblings will be affected?
A: If there are no other affected family members, it is not possible to determine if the patient has the familial (i.e., autosomal-recessive) form of HUS. Therefore, other siblings may be at no additional risk or may have up to 25% chance of developing HUS.
Q: How many patients with gastroenteritis from *E. coli* O157:H7 will develop HUS?
A: 10% to 20%
Q: What should the family tell the day-care staff and neighbors?
A: If the patient has typical HUS, contacts should be informed that any episodes of gastroenteritis merit close follow-up for evidence of anemia, thrombocytopenia, and renal insufficiency. No prophylaxis is indicated. Exclusion of infected children from day-care centers until two consecutive stool cultures are negative for *E. coli* O157:H7 has been shown to prevent additional transmission.

ICD-9-CM 283.11

BIBLIOGRAPHY
Boyce TG, Swerdlow DL, Griffin PM. Current concepts: *Escherichia coli* O157:H7 and the hemolytic-uremic syndrome. *N Engl J Med* 1995;333:364–368.

Eriksson KJ, Boyd SG, Tasker RC. Acute neurology and neurophysiology of haemolytic-uraemic syndrome. *Arch Dis Child* 2001;84(5):434–435.

Kaplan BS, Meyers KE, Schulman SL. The pathogenesis and treatment of hemolytic uremic syndrome. *J Am Soc Nephrol* 1998;9:1126–1133.

Neuhaus TJ, Calonder S, Leumann EP. Heterogeneity of atypical haemolytic uraemic syndromes. *Arch Dis Child* 1997;518–521.

Romney M. *Escherichia coli* infections and hemolytic-uremic syndrome. *Can Med Assoc J* 2001;164(10):1406.

Siegler RL. The hemolytic uremic syndrome. *Pediatr Clin North Am* 1995;42:1505–1529.

Taylor CM, Monnens LA. Advances in haemolytic uraemic syndrome. *Arch Dis Child* 1998;78(2):190–193.

Author: Mary B. Leonard

Hemophilia

 Database

DEFINITION

Hereditary bleeding disorder caused by the absence, severe deficiency, or defective functioning of plasma coagulation factors VIII (hemophilia A) or IX (hemophilia B) inherited in an X-linked manner.

PATHOPHYSIOLOGY

• Both factors VIII and IX are crucial for normal thrombin generation via the intrinsic pathway. The absence of either protein (or level <25%) severely impairs the ability to generate thrombin and fibrin.
• Hemophilia patients do not bleed more rapidly; rather there is delayed formation of an abnormal clot.
• The friable clot formed has a tendency to ooze and rebleed.
• In closed spaces (e.g., joint), bleeding stops by tamponade; in open spaces (e.g., iliopsoas muscle, open wounds), significant amounts of blood may be lost.
• Repeated joint hemorrhages lead to synovial thickening and joint cartilage erosion. Joint space becomes narrowed and eventually fuses.

GENETICS

• X-linked recessive disorder
• Carrier status and prenatal testing available:
• Hemophilia A:
—Inversion in the factor VIII gene resulting from an intrachromosomal recombination accounts for 40% to 50% of all severe hemophilia A gene abnormalities; detectable by direct gene mutation analysis.
—In families with an unknown mutation, a coagulation-based assay comparing the level of factor VIII with von Willebrand factor can be used to identify carriers.
—Accuracy of screening: 90%
• Hemophilia B (Christmas disease):
—Factor IX genetic mutations are easily identified due to the small size of the factor IX gene.
—Majority of factor IX gene defects are due to single-base pair substitutions, which can be identified in nearly all affected individuals and carriers

EPIDEMIOLOGY

• Most common severe inherited bleeding disorder.
• Distribution
—Hemophilia A: 80% to 85%
—Hemophilia B: 10% to 15%
• Incidence:
—Hemophilia A: 1 per 5,000 male births
—Hemophilia B: 1 per 30,000 male births
• No geographic or ethnic associations

COMPLICATIONS

• Complications of disease
—Hemophilic arthropathy: joint contractures, limited range of motion, and chronic pain
—Intracranial bleeding (can occur without known trauma in severe hemophilia)
—Compartment syndrome

—Airway compromise due to bleeds in the pharynx, tongue, or neck
—Life-threatening hemorrhage due to gastrointestinal, posttraumatic or perioperative bleeds
• Complications of therapy
—Viral transmission (HIV, hepatitis B and C) through clotting factor concentrates derived from pooled plasma preparations (>22000 donors per lot)
—Inhibitors: Antibodies against factor VIII or IX, which can inactivate infused factor
—Anaphylaxis: Continued factor IX replacement in severe factor IX deficient patients with inhibitors may lead to anaphylaxis
—Thromboembolic disease: Use of prothrombin complex concentrates has been associated with thrombus formation, thromboembolic events, and myocardial infarctions in children

 Differential Diagnosis

• Prolonged PTT associated with increased bleeding tendency
—von Willebrand disease
—"Acquired hemophilia" due to development of an inhibitory antibody to factor VIII or IX
—Hereditary factor XI deficiency
—Afibrinogenemia
• Prolonged PTT without increased bleeding tendency
—Factor XII deficiency
—High molecular weight kininogen deficiency
—Prekallikrein deficiency
—Antiphospholipid antibody (lupus anticoagulant)
—Heparin artifact

 Data Gathering

HISTORY

Question: Family history?
Significance: Familial history of hemophilia in male offspring of female blood relatives is present in 30% to 40% of cases.
Question: Excessive bleeding in male neonate?
Significance: Excessive bleeding with circumcision or of the umbilical cord may be an initial presentation of hemophilia; oral bleeding from torn frenulum is also common. 1% to 2% of neonates with hemophilia may present with an intracranial hemorrhage.
Question: Pattern of bleeding?
Significance: Characterized by easy, excessive, and palpable bruising with normal activity, spontaneous joint and muscle hemorrhages, and prolonged and potentially fatal hemorrhage after trauma or surgery.
Question: Age of onset of bleeding?
Significance: Bleeding events occur frequently when the child begins to crawl and walk or with the eruption of teeth.

Question: Location of hemarthroses?
Significance: Large weight bearing joints are most often involved: knees, elbows, ankles, shoulders, and hips.
Question: Early symptoms of a hemarthroses?
Significance: Aura of tingling or warmth, visible swelling, followed by increasing pain and decreasing range of motion.

 Physical Examination

Finding: Joint examination
Significance:
• Acute hemarthrosis: limitation of range of motion of the joint, warmth, swelling, tenderness
• Chronic joint: crepitus, decreased range of motion, proximal muscle weakness; typically occurs in knees, ankles, elbows
Finding: Musculoskeletal examination
Significance:
• Intramuscular hematomas: often little seen on exam; vague feeling of pain with motion
• Discrepancy in limb circumference often earliest sign of intramuscular hematoma
• Distal extremity neurovascular compromise can be a sign of compartment syndrome from bleeding into forearm or calf muscles.

 Laboratory Aids

TESTS

Test: Prothrombin time (PT), activated partial thromboplastin time (PTT), fibrinogen or thrombin time, platelet count, and von Willebrand studies
Significance: Initial screening studies if bleeding disorder suspected.
Test: Assay for factor VIII and factor IX levels
Significance:
• Less than 1%: severe hemophilia. Most common, characterized by spontaneous bleeding; hemarthroses and deep-tissue hemorrhages; will need frequent factor replacement therapy.
• 1% to 5%: moderate hemophilia. Gross bleeding following mild to moderate trauma; some hemarthrosis; seldom-spontaneous hemorrhage.
• 5% to 25%: mild hemophilia. Rare bleeding; requires factor replacement therapy only with significant trauma or surgery.

PITFALLS

• Neonates have a physiologic reduction in the vitamin K–dependent factors, including factor IX, making a determination of the degree of factor IX deficiency difficult in the neonatal period
• Delivery-related stress and other neonatal problems may cause a transient elevation of factor VIII levels.
• Poor venipuncture technique can artifactually shorten or normalize the PTT.

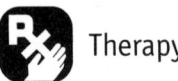 ## Emergency Care

LIFE-THREATENING HEMORRHAGES
- Central nervous system bleeding
- Bleeding into and around the airway
- Exsanguinating hemorrhage
- Prompt therapy with clotting factor concentrate should occur immediately and prior to any diagnostic procedures.

Therapy

ACUTE BLEEDING EPISODES
Factor Replacement
- Factor VIII replacement products
—Recombinant, non–plasma-derived factor VIII
—Plasma-derived, monoclonal antibody-purified factor VIII concentrate; heat or solvent detergent treated for viral inactivation
—Cryoprecipitate (rarely used today)
- Factor IX replacement products
—Recombinant, non–plasma-derived factor IX
—Plasma-derived, immunoaffinity-purified factor IX concentrate; heat or solvent detergent treated for viral inactivation
- Prothrombin complex concentrate (PCC): crude plasma fraction, which contains variable amounts of activated factors II, VII, IX, and X; heat treated for viral inactivation.
- Rarely used: fresh frozen plasma

Calculation of Dose
- Factor VIII dose (units) = % desired rise in plasma factor VIII × body weight (kg) × 0.5
- Factor IX dose = % desired rise in factor IX level × body weight (kg)

Target Factor Levels
- 30% to 40% for 24 to 48 hours for most joint bleeds
- 70% to 100% repeated over 12 to 48 hours for large muscle bleeds
- 100% maintained over 10 to 14 days for life-threatening bleeds or major surgery

DDAVP
- Synthetic vasopressin analog that stimulates release of endogenous factor VIII and von Willebrand factor
- Only suitable for patients with mild or moderate factor VIII deficiency who have shown a response to DDAVP in a trial
- Tachyphylaxis may occur with repeated dosing.
- Hyponatremia may occur in patients receiving repeated doses. Fluid restriction and close monitoring of urine output and serum electrolytes minimize risk of hyponatremic seizure.

Antifibrinolytic Therapy
- Antifibrinolytic therapy is used to stabilize a clot by inhibiting the normal process of clot lysis by the fibrinolytic system.
- Agents used for the treatment of oral hemorrhages and to minimize bleeding from dental procedures
- Epsilon aminocaproic acid (Amicar)—50 to 100 mg/kg/dose PO every 6 hours (max.

5 g/dose), or tranexamic acid (Cyklokarpron)—25 mg/kg/dose PO every 6 to 8 hours (max. 1.5 g/dose)

Immobilization
- Splints, casts, crutches, and/or bed rest
- Prolonged immobilization may reduce recovery of joint range of motion; initiation of physical therapy with factor coverage is recommended, particularly after joint surgery

SPECIAL BLEEDING SITUATIONS
Intracranial Hemorrhage
- Significant bleeding can occur despite the absence of external bruising
- Factor replacement to 100% should be administered immediately
- CT scan of the head is useful but may be negative early in a bleed

Major Surgery
- Factor replacement to 100% pre- and postoperatively
- Regular dosing of factor for a minimum of 1 week postoperatively, even in mild hemophilia

Compartment Syndrome
- Bleeding within the fascial compartments of muscles
- Most often occurs in the forearm and calf
- Neurovascular compromise can lead to Volkmann contracture

Iliopsoas Bleed
- Lower abdominal or upper thigh pain may be first symptom
- Examination is notable for inability to extend hip with preservation of internal and external rotation (allows distinction from hemarthrosis of hip joint)
- Diagnosis confirmed by ultrasound or CT scan
- Large volume of blood can be lost into the retroperitoneal space. Hemoglobin should be monitored.

Oral Bleeding/Epistaxis
- Constant pressure for 15 to 20 minutes
- ϵ-Aminocaproic acid or tranexamic acid
- Topical thrombin directly to the site of bleeding

Dental Care
- Significant dental procedures (e.g., tooth extraction) should be performed by a dentist with experience in treating hemophiliac patients and preferably in a hospital setting where hematology consultation is available.
- Factor replacement is required pre- and postprocedure.

Lacerations
- Sutures should be avoided when possible.
- If sutures are required, factor replacement is necessary at time of placement and removal.

Hematuria
- Increased fluid intake and bed rest as initial treatment
- If hematuria persists 24 to 48 hours, 30% to 40% factor replacement
- Prednisone in HIV-negative patients

 ## Follow-Up

Patients should be followed regularly at a comprehensive hemophilia treatment center, in which care is coordinated by a team including the pediatric hematologist, nurse coordinator, social worker, psychologist, physical therapist, dentist, orthopedic surgeon, and financial counselor.

PREVENTION
Prophylaxis
- Primary prophylaxis: regular dosing in patients with no complications to prevent chronic joint damage. Typically initiated prior to 1 year of age.
- Secondary prophylaxis: regular dosing in patients with target joints to prevent additional damage and facilitate healing and rehabilitation

Anticipatory Guidance and Prevention
- Good dental hygiene
- Immunizations: no intramuscular injections; give subcutaneously with a small-gauge needle and apply direct pressure for several minutes.
- Rapid treatment of hemarthrosis to avoid chronic joint damage
- Avoidance of aggressive contact sports, e.g., football, competitive basketball, lacrosse, hockey, rugby; avoid rollerblading, which puts excessive stress on ankle joints; tennis and baseball are okay, but patients may be prone to small joint bleeds.
- Home infusion therapy as appropriate
- Self-infusion training: usually starts at age 11 years

Common Questions and Answers

Q: Are there any medications contraindicated in a child with hemophilia?
A: Aspirin should not be given, as it interferes with platelet function. Nonsteroidal antiinflammatory agents cause a milder effect on platelets, and should also be avoided when possible.
Q: Can immunizations be given to a child with hemophilia?
A: Immunizations should be given SC (instead of IM) with the smallest-gauge needle; ice or cold packs should be applied to the area to minimize hematoma formation; if excessive bleeding occurs, the child should receive factor replacement.

ICD-9-CM 286.0

BIBLIOGRAPHY
DiMichele D, Neufeld EJ. Hemophilia: a new approach to an old disease. *Heme/Oncol Clin North Am* 1998;12:1315–1341.

Mannucci PM, Tuddenham EGD. The hemophilias: progress and problems. *Semin Hematol* 1999;36:104–117.

Author: Jane E. Minturn
Kara M. Kelly, 2nd edition

Hemoptysis

 ## Database

DEFINITION

Blood loss into the respiratory tract with amounts ranging from mild to massive, which can cause hypoxia or exsanguination

CAUSES

- Cavitary infections (e.g., tuberculosis, abscess, histoplasmosis)
- Tumors (lymphomas)
- Trauma (pulmonary contusion, bronchoscopy, airway manipulation)
- Congenital heart disease with large collateral vessels
- Foreign body aspiration
- Pneumonia
- Hemorrhagic diathesis including anticoagulant therapy
- H-type tracheoesophageal fistula
- Cystic fibrosis
- Tracheostomy-related complications
- Bronchiectasis
- Factitious hemoptysis

PATHOPHYSIOLOGY

- Related to the underlying pulmonary disease
- The vascular origin of hemoptysis is from two sites—pulmonary arteries or bronchial arteries.

EPIDEMIOLOGY

- Large series of pediatric patients with massive hemoptysis have not been described.
- Most instances of massive hemoptysis take place in older children.

COMPLICATIONS

- Respiratory insufficiency
- Hypovolemic shock

 ## Differential Diagnosis

- Infections: pneumonia, pulmonary abscess, tuberculosis
- Pulmonary disease: cystic fibrosis, bronchiectasis, foreign body, arteriovenous malformation, congenital lung malformation, pulmonary emboli, pulmonary hemosiderosis
- Cardiovascular disease
- Collagen vascular disease: lupus, vasculitis, Goodpasture disease
- Trauma
- Coagulation disorder
- Munchausen syndrome
- Complications: anemia, pneumonia

 ## Data Gathering

HISTORY

- Familial history of pulmonary disease or bleeding disorder?
- Exposure to environmental toxins?
- Exposure to tuberculosis?
- Drug use: cocaine, marijuana?

Question: Recurrent episodes of hemoptysis with significant spectrum production and cyst formation on chest x-ray?
Significance: Suggests a diagnosis of bronchiectasis

Question: Acute pleuritic chest pain?
Significance: Raises the possibility of pulmonary embolism with infarction or some other pleurally based lesion. A pleural friction rub may be present.

Physical Examination

Finding: Pleural friction rub
Significance: May be associated with pulmonary embolism

Finding: Pulmonary hypertension
Significance: Raises the diagnostic possibilities of primary pulmonary hypertension, mitral stenosis, and Eisenmenger syndrome

Finding: Localized wheeze over a major lobar airway
Significance: Suggests an intramural lesion such as a foreign body or carcinoma

Finding: Presence of a murmur over the lung fields
Significance: May suggest pulmonary arteriovenous malformation

 Laboratory Aids

Test: Complete blood count, reticulocyte count, and coagulation profile
Significance: May reveal the volume of blood loss, chronicity, and evidence of bleeding diathesis

Test: Sputum and PPD
Significance: Tuberculosis is suspected.

Test: Drug screen
Significance: If appropriate

Test: Chest x-ray both AP and lateral
Significance: May reveal pleural effusion, bronchiectasis, foreign bodies, or consolidation

Test: Bronchoscopy
Significance: Usually performed to localize the site of bleeding and at times may be therapeutic (e.g., in foreign body removal). Fiberoptic bronchoscopy performed acutely (during hemoptysis or within 48 hours after) is more likely to visualize active bleeding or its site than delayed bronchoscopy.

Test: CT
Significance: High-resolution CT may identify source of bleeding especially if bronchiectasis and arteriovenous malformation are suspected.

Test: Angiogram
Significance: Used to detect bleeding from arteriovascular malformation.

 Therapy

• Initial management should follow the lines of basic life support.
• Support intravascular volume by packed red blood cells or fresh frozen plasma.
• Methods used to stop localized bleeding include tamponade with balloon-tipped catheters, ice water lavage, catheter-directed umbilication, intravenous pitressin, and surgical resection. The last option is usually reserved for most difficult cases such as extensive collateralization of bronchial arteries or arteriovenous malformations not responsive to embolization.

PROGNOSIS

It depends on the etiology and the nature of hemoptysis. Immediate management of airway central decreases the morbidity and mortality.

ICD-9-CM 786.3

BIBLIOGRAPHY

Blumer JL. Pulmonary hemorrhage. *Practical guide to pediatric intensive care*, 3rd ed. 1991:359–361.

Gong H Jr, Salvatierra C. Clinical efficacy of early and delayed fiberoptic bronchoscopy in patients with hemoptysis. *Am Rev Respir Dis* 1981;124:221.

Thompson AB, Teschler H, Rennard SI. Pathogenesis, evaluation and therapy for massive hemoptysis. *Clin Chest Med* 1992;13(1):69–82.

Author: Helen Anita John-Kelly

Henoch-Schönlein Purpura

 Database

DEFINITION
• Henoch-Schönlein purpura (HSP) is an immunologically mediated, nonthrombocytopenic, purpuric, and systemic vasculitis involving the small blood vessels of the skin, gastrointestinal (GI) tract, joints, and kidneys.
• Defined by the presence of two of the following:
—Palpable purpura
—Age of onset less than 20
—Abdominal pain
—Granulocytic infiltration of vessel walls
• In children, only palpable purpura with normal platelet count need be documented. While most children do have purpura, colicky abdominal pain and arthritis, up to one half may present with symptoms other than purpura.

PATHOPHYSIOLOGY
• No single etiologic agent has been identified.
• Most cases associated with preceding upper respiratory infections, usually group A β-hemolytic streptococci, but also reported following infections with parvovirus, adenovirus, *Helicobacter pylori*, and *Mycoplasma pneumoniae*. Also reported after drug ingestion (e.g., thiazides) and insect bites.
• Capillaries, arterioles, and venules are affected in HSP as opposed to polyarteritis nodosa, Wegener and systemic lupus erythematosus (SLE), where small arteries are affected.
• Biopsy of skin lesions show leukocytoclastic vasculitis with perivascular infiltration of small vessels with polymorphonuclear and mononuclear cells. Eosinophils, granular deposits of IgA1, C3, and fibrin may also be present.
• Biopsy of the involved kidneys show endocapillary proliferative glomerulonephritis involving endothelial and mesangial cells. Crescent formation may also be present. IgA, IgG, C3, and fibrin are commonly found in the mesangial regions.
• Considered to be an immune-mediated vasculitis disorder involving primarily IgA, specifically subclass IgA1. This is indirectly suggested by the elevation of serum IgA levels, circulating IgA immune complexes, IgA rheumatoid factor, IgA-fibronectin complexes, and immunoregulatory abnormalities involving IgA production.
• IgA from mucosal B cells interacts with IgG to form immune complexes that activate the alternate pathway of the complement system. Circulating IgA is deposited in the affected organs causing the inflammatory process.
• Investigation is continuing in the study of O-glycosylation abnormalities of IgA1 and the IgA receptor interactions that may be responsible for the findings in HSP.

GENETICS
• There is only anecdotal evidence of genetic predisposition.
• Familial history of IgA-related disorders or inherited defects in complement (C2, C4 deficiency) may predispose to HSP.

EPIDEMIOLOGY
• Incidence of 13.5 cases per 100,000 school-aged children per year (90% of patients are younger than 10 years old)
• Slightly more common in males (e.g., male/female ratio of 58:42 in one study).
• Year round occurrence, but more common in spring, winter, and fall.
• Most common in Caucasians, Japanese, and Native Americans. Low incidence in blacks, both in Africa and North America.

COMPLICATIONS
• Persistent hypertension
• End-stage kidney disease (acute or as a late sequela)
• Intussusception (most common GI complication; affecting 1% to 5% of patients)
• Protein-losing enteropathy
• Pancreatitis
• Hydrops of the gallbladder
• Strictures of the esophagus and ileus
• Bowel perforations and infarctions
• Pseudomembranous colitis
• Appendicitis
• Skin necrosis
• Subarachnoid, subdural, and cortical hemorrhage and infarction
• Peripheral mono- and polyneuropathies (Guillain-Barré)
• Pulmonary hemorrhage (uncommon, but may result in death)
• Torsion of the testis and appendix epididymis

PROGNOSIS
• Generally excellent
• Better prognosis associated with younger age
• Recurrence within the first 6 weeks in up to 33%
• Most have only one to three episodes of purpura; however, a few will continue to experience symptoms for months or years. These patients have a poor prognosis and are more likely to develop severe nephritis.
• Renal involvement is the cause of the most serious long-term morbidity. Microscopic hematuria alone or with mild proteinuria generally has a good outcome. A nephritic and nephrotic combination is more guarded, and those patients with a high percentage of crescent formation do less well.

 Differential Diagnosis

• Petechial and purpuric rashes seen in thrombocytopenia from:
—Idiopathic thrombocytopenic purpura (ITP)
—Sepsis/infection: meningococcemia, Rocky Mountain spotted fever
—Leukemia
—Hemolytic uremic syndrome (HUS)
—Coagulopathies
• Vasculitic rashes may result from primary and secondary vasculitides:
—Polyarteritis nodosa
—Wegener granulomatosis
—Infection-related
—Connective tissue diseases (e.g., SLE), Berger disease (IgA nephropathy): glomerulonephritis similar to HSP both clinically and immunologically, but not associated with the skin, GI, or joint manifestations of HSP streptococcal glomerulonephritis
—Infantile acute hemorrhagic edema: vasculitis that presents with urticarial or maculopapular rash that then becomes purpuric. It is differentiated from HSP in that it usually affects children from 4 months to 2 years of age, is more common in the winter, and is not associated with systemic symptoms. On biopsy, IgA deposits are not a consistent finding as they are with HSP.
—Rheumatoid arthritis
—Rheumatic fever

 Data Gathering

HISTORY
Question: Previous disease?
Significance: Especially infections such as hepatitis, URI, and streptococcal infections
Question: Abdominal pain?
Significance: This is the most common GI symptom. Emesis and melena are also reported.
Question: Transient, nondeforming, nonmigratory arthritis of knees, ankles, wrists, elbows, and digits?
Significance: Frequent problem
Question: Presence of testicular pain or scrotal swelling, headache, cough, edema of the ankles or periorbital region, and hematuria?
Significance: Vasculitic lesion in the associated system

Physical Examination

Finding: Particular attention to blood pressure.
Significance: Hypertension is common.
Finding: Low-grade fever is present in 50% of the cases.
Finding: Rash that is petechial or purpuric in a pressure-dependent, symmetric distribution, usually around the lateral malleoli of the ankles, on the ventral surfaces of the feet and on the buttocks.
Significance: Purpura may be briefly preceded by maculopapular or urticarial lesions.
Finding: Joints should be examined for swelling and limitation of motion.
Significance: Redness and warmth are not common. Symptoms precede the rash by up to 2 weeks in 25% of patients.

Finding: Nonpitting subcutaneous edema of the scalp, periorbital region, hands, and feet is often noted.
Significance: Generalized edema is more common in children under 2 years of age.
Finding: Abdomen is often tender to palpation, but without rebound tenderness. Hepatosplenomegaly may be found.
Significance: Abdominal symptoms may precede the rash by up to 2 weeks.
Finding: Orchitis, where affected testicle may be tender and swollen. Swelling and bruising may be noted on the scrotum.
Significance: Testicular torsion has also been reported in HSP and may mimic orchitis.
Finding: Neurologic changes
Significance: CNS involvement may present with headaches, seizures, or behavioral changes.

 ## Laboratory Aids

There are no definitive tests to confirm the diagnosis of HSP.

Test: CBC: Hemoglobin is usually normal; leukocytosis; eosinophilia especially may be present; platelet count is normal or elevated.
Significance: Normal platelet count differentiates from thrombocytopenic purpura
Test: ESR
Significance: Normal or elevated
Test: PT and PTT
Significance: Normal
Test: IgA
Significance: Often elevated in the acute phase of illness, with normal or increased IgG and IgM
Test: C3
Significance: Normal (decreased in poststreptococcal glomerulonephritis and SLE)
Test: Antinuclear antibody
Significance: Negative (elevated in SLE)
Test: Throat swab for group A β-hemolytic streptococci
Significance: Positive in up to 75% of cases
Test: Elevated BUN and creatinine, decreased protein and albumin, and urinalysis with RBC, WBC, casts, or protein are seen with renal involvement
Test: Urinalysis
Significance: Microscopic hematuria is consistent with nephritis. Gross hematuria and proteinuria are present in many patients. Proteinuria alone is rare.
Test: Urinalysis
Significance: It is uncommon for nephritis (as opposed to GI and joint findings) to precede the rash.
Test: Stool guaiac
Significance: GI involvement may present as guaiac positive stools, bloody stools or melena.
Test: Renal biopsy
Significance: With severe renal failure, a biopsy should be performed to determine the extent of disease

RADIOGRAPHIC STUDIES
Test: Chest radiograph
Significance: May show interstitial lung disease
Test: Abdominal ultrasound
Significance: Barium enemas are NOT indicated for suspected intussusception. They will not reduce the ilio-ileal intussusception common to HSP (idiopathic intussusception is usually iliocolic in location) and may damage or perforate the inflamed bowel.

 ## Therapy

HSP usually resolve spontaneously without specific therapy.

- Analgesics and NSAIDs may be used for control of joint pain and inflammation, but salicylates and other agents that affect platelet function should be avoided if GI bleeding is present.
- Steroids are used for painful cutaneous edema, arthritis, and abdominal pain (2 mg/kg/d of prednisone until clinical resolution); however, steroids have not been shown to affect purpura or to decrease duration of disease or frequency of recurrences.
- No consensus on management of GI and renal involvement. Oral prednisone at 2 mg/kg/d has shown faster resolution of abdominal pain, while other studies indicate the symptoms will resolve similarly without intervention.
- In nephritis, immediate treatment with steroids may prevent more serious renal disease; however, the majority will improve spontaneously. Treatment should be considered for children at high risk for chronic renal insufficiency or failure (those presenting with nephrotic syndrome or renal insufficiency).
- More than 50% crescentic glomerulonephritis on renal biopsy has a greater risk of future renal failure and should be considered for aggressive therapy with pulse or oral steroids and/or immunosuppressants (azathioprine, cyclophosphamide, cyclosporine) or plasmapheresis, IVIG, danazol, or fish oil.
- Treatment of hypertension may delay or prevent progression of renal disease in patients with glomerulonephritis.

 ## Follow-Up

- Patients should be seen weekly during the acute illness. Visits should include history and physical exam, along with blood pressure measurement and urinalysis.
- All patients, even those who did not present with renal involvement, should have urine checked for blood weekly for 6 months, and then monthly for 3 years as deterioration or renal function has been observed years after presentation in some patients.
- Women with a history of HSP should be monitored for proteinuria and hypertension during pregnancy

 ## Common Questions and Answers

Q: When should I consider hospitalization?
A: Often it is not necessary. Severe complications may require admission. These include GI hemorrhage, protein-losing enteropathy requiring TPN, decreased GFR or hypertension, and pulmonary hemorrhage.
Q: Is there a use for prophylactic penicillin?
A: In patients with frequent relapses, where group A β-hemolytic streptococci is often the inciting agent, administration of penicillin may be helpful.
Q: Who are Henoch and Schönlein?
A: The clinical finding of joint pain associated with purpura was named "purpura rheumatica" in 1837 by Schönlein. Henoch, a student of Schönlein's, later described the association of GI and renal involvement. However, the first report was by Heberden in 1801. Of note, it has been speculated that Mozart—whose symptoms included fever, vomiting, exanthem, arthritis, anasarca, and coma—died of HSP.

ICD-9-CM 287.0

BIBLIOGRAPHY
Cuttica RJ. Vasculitis in children: a diagnostic challenge. *Curr Probl Pediatr* 1997;27: 309–318.

Egan CA, Taylor TB, Meyer LJ, et al. IgA1 is the major IgA subclass in cutaneous blood vessels in Henoch-Schonlein purpura. *Br J Dermatol* 1999;141:859–862.

Kraft DM, McKee M, Scott C. Henoch-Schonlein purpura: a review. *Am Fam Physician* 1999;58(2):405–408.

Piette WW. What is Schönlein-Henoch Purpura, and why should we care? *Arch Dermatol* 1997;133:515–518.

Saulsbury FT. Henoch-Schönlein purpura. *Curr Opin Rheumatol* 2001;13:35–40.

Saulsbury FT. Henoch-Schönlein purpura in children: report of 100 patients and review of the literature. *Medicine* 1999;78(6):395–409.

Szer IS. Henoch-Schönlein purpura: when and how to treat. *J Rheumatol* 1996;23: 1661–1665.

Author: Blaze Robert Gusic

Hepatic Encephalopathy

 Database

DEFINITION

Hepatic encephalopathy (HE) is any brain dysfunction that occurs as a result of acute hepatocyte failure.

CAUSES

Acute changes in mental status in a patient with chronic liver disease should prompt investigation for a precipitating factor.

- Gastrointestinal hemorrhage (secondary to varices, ulcers, gastritis)
- Intracranial hemorrhage (secondary to coagulopathy)
- Infections, including spontaneous bacterial peritonitis
- Dehydration (often secondary to aggressive diuresis)
- Administration of sedatives (benzodiazepines and barbiturates)
- Placement of a porta-systemic shunt—surgical or transjugular intrahepatic portosystemic shunt (TIPS) procedure

PATHOPHYSIOLOGY

The appearance of HE depends on the interactions of three factors:

- Porta-systemic shunting—shunting can occur around the liver through collateral vessels or through the liver as the blood passes by damaged or necrotic hepatocytes.
- Changes in the blood–brain barrier—Increased permeability of blood–brain barrier has been demonstrated with increased uptake of markers (e.g., horseradish peroxidase) during acute liver failure. Toxic metabolites of liver failure (ammonia and mercaptans) have been shown to increase blood–brain barrier permeability.
- Interactions of toxic metabolites with the CNS

—Ammonia hypothesis—ammonia, produced by the bacterial metabolism of amino acids, is usually detoxified in the liver by the urea cycle. Measures to decrease dietary protein and decrease serum ammonia (e.g., lactulose and neomycin) can improve the clinical status in HE. Ammonia does not correlate with the stage of HE, and is not the sole mediator of HE.
—False neurotransmitter hypothesis—excessive production of brain "false" inhibitory neurotransmitters (serotonin and octopamine) that are usually not found in the brain or systemic circulation, and a deficiency of excitatory neurotransmitters (dopamine and norepinephrine).

—γ-Aminobutyric acid (GABA) inhibitory neurotransmitter hypothesis—GABA is an inhibitory neurotransmitter produced in the brain by decarboxylation of glutamic acid. GABA, benzodiazepines, and barbiturates activate the GABA receptor in the brain. Increased GABA-like agents and endogenous benzodiazepines are produced from intestinal bacterial metabolism, reaching the brain and promoting inhibitory neurotransmission.
—Synergistic neurotoxin hypothesis—HE may result from the combined accumulation of several neurotoxins, each of which alone would be insufficient to cause HE. These would include substances such as ammonia, mercaptans, short- and medium chain fatty acids. This occurs in the setting of incomplete detoxification of potentially neurotoxic intestinal metabolites (secondary to impaired hepatocyte function and porta-systemic shunting) and increased permeability of the blood–brain barrier.

 Differential Diagnosis

- Infection: meningitis, encephalitis
- Tumors: intracranial lesions
- Trauma: cerebral hemorrhage, cerebral hematoma
- Metabolic: inborn errors of metabolism, lactic acidemias, urea cycle deficiencies
- Immunologic: AIDS dementia

 Data Gathering

HISTORY

Question: Alteration in mental status and personality?
Significance: Classic feature. Often first noted by family members or a child's teacher.

 Physical Examination

Central nervous system manifestations—the initial manifestations can be very subtle, especially in children.
Four clinical stages of hepatic coma are described, based on changes in conscious intellectual functioning and behavior. Any neurologic function can be impaired in HE.

- Changes in consciousness—hypersomnia, reversal of sleep patterns, slowing of speech, and eventually coma.
- Personality changes—irritability, inattentiveness, apathy, childishness, regressive behaviors, emotional outbursts. Any child with acute onset of combative or irrational behavior in the classroom should be evaluated for HE.

- Intellectual deterioration—worsening of school performance secondary to inattentiveness and confusion.
- Constructional apraxia—a defect in visual spatial skills, demonstrated with age-appropriate tasks, such as writing, drawing, and coloring.
- Neuromuscular dysfunction—muscle tone and deep-tendon reflexes may be exaggerated in early HE, but in later stages the muscles become flaccid and reflexes disappear.
- Signs of end-stage liver failure—varices, ascites, spider angiomata, palmar erythema, caput medusa.
- Asterixis—ask the patient to stand with both arms raised horizontally in front of him, wrists dorsiflexed, and fingers held apart for at least 15 seconds. A flapping tremor of the fingers and wrists will be present with voluntary movement, but absent at rest. This is characteristic of hepatic encephalopathy, although it may also be seen with uremia, respiratory failure, and congestive heart failure.

STAGES

Four clinical stages of HE are described. These are useful for assessing HE in older patients, but have less value in assessing neonates and younger children, especially in the early stages of HE.
Stage I—alert, irritable, sleep rhythm reversal, poor handwriting, inattentive to tasks, slowness of mentation.
Stage II—lethargic, confused, combative, inappropriate behavior, disorientation, mood swings, tremor, asterixis.
Stage III—stuporous but arousable, marked confusion, delirious, hyperreflexia, positive Babinski sign.
Stage IV—comatose, no motor activity, decerebrate or decorticate, may respond to painful stimuli.

 Laboratory Aids

TESTS

- No specific lab test, including serum ammonia, correlates well with the stage of HE.
- EEG—may show a slowing from the normal alpha frequency to the delta range. Nonspecific and may be seen in other disease processes.
- Visual evoked potentials—may become more useful than EEGs.
- Neuropsychiatric testing—must be age-appropriate testing. In older children, can use subtraction of serial sevens, number connection test, handwriting, and event recall. In younger children, can use task of coloring within the lines, if this is a skill that the child had previously developed.

IMAGING

- Head CT scan—assess for signs of increased intracranial pressure or cerebral edema. These do not help with diagnosis but may indicate severity of encephalopathy and suggest prognosis.
- Proton magnetic resonance spectroscopy—characteristic changes have been identified in HE. Has not yet proven helpful in diagnosing subclinical HE.

Emergency Care

HE necessitates immediate hospital admission, usually to an intensive care unit, for close observation. It is imperative to promptly identify and treat any precipitating factor of HE.

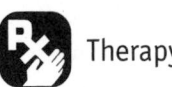

Therapy

SUPPORTIVE CARE

- Fluids and electrolyte monitoring, vital signs, paying close attention to development of infection (respiratory, urinary).
- Avoid administration of sedatives, which can worsen or confound the clinical neurologic status in HE.
- Frequent, repeated neurologic examinations. The clinical course typically fluctuates in HE, and patients can deteriorate within hours or days.

DRUGS

- Lactulose, a nonabsorbable disaccharide that is metabolized by colonic bacteria, which results in acidified fecal contents (pH <6.0) that trap ammonia. Lactulose has also been shown to change colonic flora, increasing *Lactobacillus* species. Complications include diarrhea and dehydration.
- Neomycin reduces the amount of bacterial urease available by directly suppressing ammonia-forming bacteria. Systemically absorbed, and long-term use has been associated with ototoxicity.
- Acidifying enemas (lactulose or lactitol) can help lower serum ammonia, and are helpful after a GI bleed.
- Flumazenil, a benzodiazepine receptor antagonist, can block the GABA receptor in the brain, and temporary reversal of the electrophysiologic and clinical abnormalities in HE. Results are conflicting, and require randomized controlled trials.
- Branched-chain amino acids (BCAAs) may reverse the altered ratio of branched-chain to aromatic amino acids, and decrease muscle protein breakdown. Conflicting results in adults with chronic encephalopathy.
- Levodopa and bromocriptine, a dopamine agonist, have resulted in temporary reversal of HE in a few patients.

DIET

- Avoid hypoglycemia, which can further aggravate HE.
- Protein restriction is recommended during acute HE to avoid further increases in ammonia levels.
- In children, need to balance that protein restriction that can result in growth failure.

SURGERY

- Placement of a porto-systemic shunt before the onset of the acute development of neurologic deterioration may suggest that the shunt is not allowing enough circulation through the liver. Reversal of the shunt, by either surgical or balloon occlusion, may improve the clinical picture.
- Liver transplantation

Follow-Up

WHEN TO EXPECT IMPROVEMENT

Often, improvement (a change in the level of HE by 1 or 2 stages) is seen 2 to 3 days after initiation of therapy.

SIGNS TO WATCH FOR

- Progression of neurologic status through the stages of HE. Passage through the stages of HE can be very rapid (e.g., in fulminant hepatic failure) or more gradual in the setting of chronic liver disease.

PROGNOSIS

Depends to some degree on stage of encephalopathy. Prognosis is better if a precipitating factor can be promptly identified and treated effectively. Orthotopic liver transplantation should be performed in children with severe and worsening encephalopathy before the development of radiographically apparent cerebral edema. Cerebral edema with brainstem herniation is the major cause of mortality (frequency between 25% and 81% in various studies) in patients with fulminant hepatic failure in stage III or IV. Patients with HE and underlying chronic liver disease have a much lower incidence of cerebral edema. In one study, on multiple logistic regression analysis, presence of GI hemorrhage ($p = .005$), degree of coma ($p = .02$), and serum bilirubin level (p = 0.025) were identified as independent predictors of mortality.

Common Questions and Answers

Q: My child has chronic liver failure and has experienced two episodes of hepatic encephalopathy managed in the ICU. Is there any special diet I should be providing him?
A: Because dietary intake of protein can lead to accumulation of nitrogenous waste that can accumulate into ammonia, it is best to keep your child on a low-protein diet.

ICD-9-CM 572.2

BIBLIOGRAPHY

Butterworth RF. Complications of cirrhosis III: hepatic encephalopathy. *J Hepatol* 2000; 32(1 suppl):171.

Hawkins RA, Mans AM. Brain metabolism in hepatic encephalopathy and hyperammonemia. In: Felipo V, Grisola S, eds. *Cirrhosis, hyperammonemia, and hepatic encephalopathy*. New York: Plenum, 1994: 13–19.

Jones EA. Pathogenesis of hepatic encephalopathy. *Clin Liver Dis* 2000;4(2):467.

Riordan SM, Williams R. Treatment of hepatic encephalopathy. *N Engl J Med* 1997;337(26): 1921.

Rodes J. Clinical manifestations and therapy of hepatic encephalopathy. In: Felipo V, Grisola S, eds. *Cirrhosis, hyperammonemia, and hepatic encephalopathy*. New York: Plenum, 1994:39–44.

Suchy FJ, Sokol RJ, Balistreri WF. *Liver disease in children*. Philadelphia: Lippincott, Williams & Wilkins, 2001.

Author: Lynette A. Gillis

Hereditary Spherocytosis

 Database

DEFINITION

Hemolytic anemia with shortened red cell survival due to selective trapping of osmotically fragile spherocytic red blood cells in the spleen secondary to an inherent defect of the red cell membrane

PATHOPHYSIOLOGY

The most common biochemical abnormality is a combined deficiency of ankyrin and spectrin, two major proteins of the erythrocyte membrane skeleton. The membrane skeletal defect results in red cell membrane instability and loss of membrane surface. The sequelae are as follows:

- Loss of cell surface area relative to volume (spherocytosis) causing a decrease in cellular deformability.
- The spleen detains and "conditions" the nondeformable spherocytic red cells.
- Conditioning of cells involves depletion of ATP, increased glycolysis, increased influx and efflux of sodium, and loss of membrane lipid.
- Ultimately, the events lead to premature red cell destruction.

GENETICS

- Approximately 75% of cases are inherited in an autosomal-dominant pattern.
- The other 25% are autosomal-recessive forms, dominant disease with reduced penetrance, or new mutations.

EPIDEMIOLOGY

- Most common in people of Northern European extraction (about 1:2000)

COMPLICATIONS

- Gallstones: most common complication of hereditary spherocytosis (HS), pigment stones can lead to cholecystitis and/or biliary obstruction.
- Cholelithiasis in HS manifests in second and third decades of life.
- Aplastic crises: can result in severe life-threatening anemia. Often caused by parvovirus B19 infection.
- Hyperhemolysis: increased red cell destruction, often precipitated by infection.
- Postsplenectomy sepsis: lower risk of infection if postponed until 4 to 5 years of age, and immunized with pneumococcal vaccine (50–70% sepsis due to *Streptococcus pneumoniae*)
- Folate deficiency: caused by insufficient dietary intake of folic acid for increased bone marrow requirement.
- Other rare complications: gout, indolent leg ulcers, or chronic erythematous dermatitis on legs.

PROGNOSIS

Severity of disease is extremely variable ranging from extremely mild to severe anemia.

 Differential Diagnosis

- Hemolysis secondary to intrinsic RBC defects

—Membrane defects secondary to inherited disorders of membrane skeleton (hereditary spherocytosis and elliptocytosis) and red cell cation permeability and volume (stomatocytosis and xerocytosis)
—Enzyme defects: Embden-Meyerhof pathway (i.e., pyruvate kinase deficiency) and hexose monophosphate pathway (i.e., G6PD deficiency)
—Hemoglobin defects: heme, congenital erythropoietic porphyria; globin, qualitative (e.g., HbS, C, H, M); quantitative (e.g., thalassemias)
—Congenital dyserythropoietic anemias

- Hemolysis secondary to extracorpuscular RBC defects

—Immune-mediated (important in differential because spherocytes are present on smear): isoimmune (e.g., hemolytic disease of the newborn, blood group incompatibility) and autoimmune (e.g., cold agglutinin disease, warm auto immune hemolytic anemia)
—Non–immune-mediated: idiopathic and secondary to underlying disorder (e.g., HUS, TTP)

 Data Gathering

HISTORY

Question: Anemia, jaundice, dark urine, fatigue?
Significance: Signs of hemolysis

Question: Requiring phototherapy in newborn period (50% of cases)?
Significance: Hyperbilirubinemia due to hemolysis

Question: Positive familial history (for disease, gallstones, or splenectomy)?
Significance: Autosomal-dominant inheritance

Physical Examination

Finding: Splenomegaly, icterus/jaundice, pallor
Significance: All increased with hemolysis

Finding: Linear growth, weight gain, and sexual development may be delayed
Significance: Delayed growth is indication for splenectomy.

 ## Laboratory Aids

Test: CBC
Significance: Mild to moderate anemia; MCV usually normal; MCHC elevated (useful screening test with high specificity)

Test: Reticulocyte count
Significance: Level usually >6%; often accompanied with an elevated red blood cell distribution width (RDW).

Test: Indirect hyperbilirubinemia
Significance: Present in 50% to 60% of cases

Test: Peripheral smear
Significance: Microspherocytes, polychromasia

Test: Coombs test
Significance: Negative. Important differential test in a patient with hemolytic anemia

Test: Urinalysis
Significance: Hemoglobinuria, increased urobilinogen.

SPECIAL TESTS

Test: Osmotic fragility (most useful test in diagnosis)
Significance: Spherocytes are more fragile; therefore, less resistant to osmotic stress and lyse in higher concentration of saline than normal red cells. This test can result in a false negative, especially in newborns whose red blood cells may be more dehydrated. It is important to use an age-matched control if possible.

 ## Emergency Care

A patient with hereditary spherocytosis may become extremely anemic during an aplastic crisis, hyperhemolysis or folic acid deficiency requiring transfusion.

 ## Therapy

- Folic acid supplement
- Penicillin prophylaxis (if splenectomized)
- Pneumococcal and *H. influenza* B vaccines (if splenectomized)

SPLENECTOMY

- High response rate (most patients normalize their blood counts)
- Indications: moderate-to-severe anemia with significant hemolysis (reticulocyte count repeatedly >5%) resulting in transfusion dependence, decreased exercise tolerance, skeletal deformities, or delayed growth.
- Complications: risk of postsplenectomy sepsis

CHOLECYSTECTOMY

- Indications: symptomatic gallbladder disease. Sometimes done concomitantly with splenectomy if gallstones evident by ultrasound.
- Complications: morbidity of surgical procedure and postoperative period.

 ## Follow-Up

- Physical examination: splenomegaly, follow growth curves for FTT
- CBC with reticulocyte count as needed—if patient develops fatigue, pallor, increased jaundice
- Penicillin prophylaxis if splenectomy

PITFALLS

- False-negative osmotic fragility tests can occur in several situations; therefore, index of suspicion must be high to follow the clinical course and repeat test (e.g., in neonatal period, during megaloblastic crisis, and recovery from aplastic crisis after transfusion).
- 20% to 25% of HS patients have normal unincubated osmotic fragility (incubated test almost always positive; therefore, may need both).
- Spherocytes are often present in immune-mediated hemolysis.

 ## Common Questions and Answers

Q: Will my child require blood transfusions?
A: It depends on the clinical severity of his/her disease.

Q: If a parent has HS, how should the newborn be followed?
A: The infant has a 50% chance of having HS. In infants with HS the CBC is usually normal in the first 72 hours of life but then drops because of an inability to mount an appropriate erythropoietic response to increased destruction. Therefore, infants at risk should have a CBC with reticulocyte count after 72 hours. These infants also need to be monitored more closely for hyperbilirubinemia.

Q: What are the risks and benefits of splenectomy:
A: Splenectomy is almost always successful in ameliorating anemia, but adds the risk of postsplenectomy infections.

ICD-9-CM 282.0

BIBLIOGRAPHY

Becker PS, Lux SE. Disorders of the red cell membrane. In: Nathan DG, Oski FA, eds. *Hematology of infancy and childhood*, 5th ed. Philadelphia: WB Saunders, 1998:578–601.

Delhommeau F, Cynober T, Schischmanoff P, et al. Natural history of hereditary spherocytosis during the first year of life. *Blood* 2000;95(2):393–397.

Hassoun H, Palek J. Hereditary spherocytosis: a review of the clinical and molecular aspects of the disease. *Blood Rev* 1996;10:129–147.

Michaels LA, Cohen AR, Huaqing Z, et al. Screening for hereditary spherocytosis by use of automated erythrocyte indexes. *J Pediatr* 1997;130(6):957–960.

Miraglia del Giudice E, et al. High frequency of de novo mutations in ankyrin gene (ANK1) in children with hereditary spherocytosis. *J Pediatr* 1998;132(1):117–120.

Schroter W, Kahsnitz E. Diagnosis of hereditary spherocytosis in newborn infants. *J Pediatr* 1983;103:460–463.

Author: Leslie Raffini

Heroin Intoxication

 Database

DEFINITION
- Heroin is a semisynthetic derivative of opium.
- The opioid family includes:
—Drugs that occur naturally in opium (from the poppy plant)
  —Codeine
  —Morphine
—Semisynthetic derivatives (e.g., hydromorphone, oxycodone)
—Synthetic compounds (e.g., meperidine, methadone)

PHARMACOLOGY/PATHOPHYSIOLOGY
- Well-absorbed from GI tract, nasal mucosa, pulmonary capillaries, and subcutaneous and intramuscular injection sites
- Oral dose less potent than parenteral because of first-pass hepatic metabolism
- IV heroin peaks in less than 1 minute; intranasal and IM heroin peak in 3 to 5 minutes
- Very lipid soluble; crosses blood–brain barrier within 15 to 20 seconds
- Extensive distribution into skeletal muscle, kidneys, liver, intestine, lungs, spleen, brain, and placenta
- Rapidly crosses the placenta, entering fetal tissues within 1 hour
- Crosses into breast milk in quantities sufficient to cause addiction
- Excreted in urine as morphine
- Receptor types
—Mu (or OP_3)
  —Located in CNS, GI tract, sensory nerve endings
  —Effect: analgesia, euphoria, respiratory depression, physical dependence, gastrointestinal dysmotility, miosis, pruritus, bradycardia
—Kappa (or OP_2)
  —Located in CNS
  —Effect: analgesia, miosis, diuresis, dysphoria
—Delta (or OP_1)
  —Located in CNS
  —Effect: spinal analgesia, modulation of mu receptors/dopaminergic neurons

EPIDEMIOLOGY
Neonatal
- Prevalence of fetal exposure <1% to 3.7%
- Fetal exposure commonly involves polysubstance abuse
- 60% to 80% of heroin exposed infants develop withdrawal—dependent on maternal dosing and length of use

Adolescents
- Use peaked among U.S. adolescents in the 1970s and then declined.
- Use is increasing again because a more pure product allows for smoking or snorting as well as injecting.
- Most use experimentally or intermittently; few become addicted and use daily.

Overdose
- Up to one third of heroin users experience nonfatal overdose.
- The majority occur in the home and with other people present.

Deaths
- Most heroin deaths occur when drug administered IV.
- Most deaths in patients in their late 20s or 30s, with significant drug dependence.
- Multiple drug use common in heroin-related deaths.

COMPLICATIONS
Intoxication/Overdose
- Respiratory arrest
- Noncardiogenic pulmonary edema
- CNS depression/coma
- Hypotension
- Aspiration pneumonia

Pregnancy
- No known teratogenic effects
- Poor prenatal care
- Preterm labor
- Premature rupture of membranes
- Breech presentation
- Antepartum hemorrhage
- Toxemia
- Anemia
- Uterine irritability
- Infection (e.g., HIV, Hep B)
- Infantile dependence

Naloxone Use
- May precipitate withdrawal syndrome in opioid dependent patients
- Symptoms: agitation, hypertension, tachycardia, emesis
- See below for dosing recommendations
- May cause acute severe withdrawal in infants born to addicted mothers

PROGNOSIS
Neonatal
- Long-term morbidity from neonatal heroin dependence unclear due to confounding variables (e.g., developmental environment)

Intoxication/Overdose
- With adequate early treatment, patients with uncomplicated overdoses do well—key is to prevent respiratory arrest

Addiction
- Dependent on involvement in other risky behaviors (polydrug use, high-risk sexual practices, school failure, delinquency, etc.)
- Longer treatment likely produces a better outcome
- Majority relapse; require lifetime of therapy

 Differential Diagnosis

NEONATAL EXPOSURE
- Sepsis
- Hypoglycemia
- Central nervous system abnormality
- Metabolic disorder
- Withdrawal from other maternal drug use

INTOXICATION/OVERDOSE
- Other pharmacologic agents:
—Clonidine
—Sedative-hypnotics
—Barbiturates
—Antipsychotics
—GHB
- Hypoglycemia
- Hypothermia
- Hypoxia
- Heatstroke
- Pontine or subarachnoid hemorrhage

 Data Gathering

HISTORY
Neonate
- Maternal history of heroin or other drug use
- Extent of prenatal care
- Time from most recent use to delivery
- Breast-feeding

Older Child/Adolescent
- History of heroin use
- Observed overdose
- Found in setting consistent with possible drug use

 Physical Examination

NEONATE WITH IN UTERO EXPOSURE
- Prematurity
- Low birth weight
- Perinatal depression with 5-minute Apgar <5
- Hypotonia

INTOXICATION/OVERDOSE
- Classic toxidrome
—Depressed level of consciousness
—Very decreased respiratory effort
—Miotic pupils
—±Diminished bowel sounds
- More severe overdose
—Bradycardia
—Hypotension

WITHDRAWAL
Early Signs (8–24 Hours)
- Anxiety
- Restlessness
- Insomnia
- Yawning
- Rhinorrhea
- Lacrimation
- Diaphoresis
- Stomach cramps
- Mydriasis

Late Signs (Up to 3 Days)
- Tremor
- Muscle spasms
- Vomiting
- Diarrhea
- Hypertension
- Tachycardia
- Fever
- Chills
- Piloerection
- Seizures

Additional Neonatal Withdrawal Signs and Symptoms
- Hyperirritability
- Hypertonicity
- Posturing
- Exaggerated startle
- Tachypnea
- Hyperpyrexia
- Poor suck/swallow coordination
- High-pitched cry
- Poor weight gain

 Laboratory Aids

- Therapy should not be withheld pending laboratory results
- Urine toxicology screen (heroin easily detected)
- Serum toxicology screen for acetaminophen level, etc., if suspect polydrug use
- Serum tests to rule out other etiologies, if needed (e.g., glucose)
- Meconium testing in neonates

 Therapy

INTOXICATION/OVERDOSE
- Start with the ABCs (airway, breathing, circulation)
- Antidote is naloxone (Narcan)
- Assessment of respiratory status/adequacy of ventilation
- If adequate respiratory effort, observe until normal level of consciousness
—Consider naloxone as diagnostic challenge
- If inadequate respiratory effort:
—Bag-valve-mask ventilation
—Intravenous naloxone (or subcutaneous, intramuscular, endotracheal)
—0.1 mg/kg if <20 kg; 2 mg if >20 kg. Can repeat to 10 mg total dose
—If suspect dependence, start with lower dose (0.4 mg amp)

—If no response to large dose, question diagnosis of heroin toxicity—heroin exquisitely sensitive to naloxone
—Naloxone loses efficacy in 20 to 40 minutes; may need repeat dosing
—Can give as continuous infusion if necessary; dosing recommendations vary
  —One method: two thirds of effective dose given over 1 hour with gradual wean
—Endotracheal intubation if no response to naloxone in 5 to 10 minutes, or other reason for invasive airway management
- Observe in ED for minimum 2 to 3 hours for respiratory status stabilization
- Consider chest x-ray

WITHDRAWAL
- Standard treatment methadone maintenance (adolescents/adults)
—Blocks euphoria and prevents withdrawal symptoms
—Patients generally treated in established methadone maintenance programs
—Stabilize with 20 to 40 mg/day ; wean by 2 to 5 mg/week over several months
—Adjust wean if signs of withdrawal appear
- Clonidine (0.2 mg q4–6h for 7–10 days) can control acute withdrawal symptoms
- Diazepam (10–15 mg q4–6h for 3–4 days), an alternative to clonidine
- Rapid and ultrarapid detoxification (using opioid antagonist with or without general anesthesia) a possibility in selected patients; research ongoing
—Should be used only by experienced team with appropriate resources
- In neonates:
—Paregoric (0.4 mg/mL) not recommended due to high alcohol content (45%) and toxic compounds such as camphor, anise oil, benzoic acid, and glycerin
—Tincture of opium (10 mg/mL) best diluted 25-fold to a concentration equal to paregoric (0.4 mg/mL)
—0.1 mL/kg (2 drops/kg) q4h; increase 0.1 mL/kg q4h as needed to control symptoms. After 3 to 5 days wean dose by 0.1 ml/kg/day. Observe infant for 3 to 5 days after stopping therapy.
—May need IV morphine in severe cases
—Methadone has been used occasionally.
—Clonidine gaining favor for use in infants; pharmacokinetic data not available.
—Phenobarbital not a first-choice agent due to long half-life, CNS depression, induction of drug metabolism, and rapid tolerance to sedative effect.

 Follow-Up

- Developmental follow-up for exposed neonates
- Most patients with overdose warrant hospitalization
- Social services and referral to substance abuse program
- Consider referral for testing for HIV, hepatitis B and C

 Common Questions and Answers

Q: Is nalmefene an appropriate substitute for naloxone in a heroin overdose?
A: Nalmefene, a long-acting specific narcotic antagonist, has not proved to be as effective as naloxone in a randomized, double-blind trial. It also may result in prolonged, dangerous withdrawal. It therefore has limited usefulness in this setting.

BIBLIOGRAPHY

AAP Policy Statement. Neonatal drug withdrawal. *Pediatrics* 1998;101(6): 1079–1088

Alderman EM. Opiates. *Pediatr Rev* 1997;18(4):122–126.

Bauer CR. Perinatal effects of prenatal drug exposure. *Clin Perinatol* 1999;26(1):87–106.

Bishai R, Koren G. Maternal and obstetric effects of prenatal drug exposure. *Clin Perinatol* 1999;26(1):75–86.

Chamberlain JM, Klein BL. A comprehensive review of naloxone for the emergency physician. *Am J Emerg Med* 1994;12(6): 650–660.

Hans SL. Demographic and psychosocial characteristics of substance-abusing pregnant women. *Clin Perinatol* 1999;26(1):55–74.

Kandall SR. Treatment strategies for drug-exposed neonates. *Clin Perinatol* 1999;26(1): 231–244.

Nelson LS. Opioids. In: Goldfrank LR, ed. *Goldfrank's toxicologic emergencies*, 6th ed. Stamford: Appleton & Lange, 1998:975–995.

O'Connor PG, Kosten TR. Rapid and ultrarapid opioid detoxification techniques. *JAMA* 1998;279(3):229–234.

Sporer KA. Acute heroin overdose. *Ann Intern Med* 1999;130(7):584–590.

Authors: Cynthia J. Mollen and Thomas J. Mollen

Herpes Simplex Virus (HSV)

 Database

DEFINITION

Herpes simplex virus (HSV) is a moderately large double-stranded DNA virus. There are two serologically distinguishable subtypes: HSV-1 and HSV-2. HSV produces a wide spectrum of illness ranging from fever blisters to fatal viral encephalitis.

PATHOPHYSIOLOGY

- Initial viral replication occurs at the portal.
- Vesicular fluid contains infected epithelial cells.
- After primary HSV infection, the virus remains latent in sensory neural ganglia innervating portions of the skin or mucous membranes originally involved. The virus can be reactivated by an appropriate stimulus such as sunlight or immune suppression.
- HSV can be replicated easily in the laboratory in tissue cultures.

EPIDEMIOLOGY

- HSV-1 usually causes infections of the upper torso, head, and neck.
- HSV-2 usually causes genital infection. However, both forms can infect either oral or genital cells and thus the virus type is not a reliable indicator of the anatomic site of infection.
- Neonatal HSV infections are acquired from maternal strains and 75% to 85% are caused by HSV-2.
- After the neonatal period, HSV-1 infections predominate and 40% to 60% of children are seropositive for HSV-1 by age 5 years.
- During puberty and early adolescence, the prevalence of HSV-2 increases and 20% to 35% of adults are seropositive for HSV-2.
- Route of spread is usually by close bodily contact or trauma such as teething or a break in the skin.
- Incubation period is 2 to 12 days (average, 6 days).

ASSOCIATED DISEASES

- Neonatal infection is usually acquired from the maternal genitourinary tract and causes serious disease with high mortality and morbidity.
- Gingivostomatitis is the most common form of HSV primary infection in children.
- Encephalitis due to HSV accounts for 2% to 5% of all encephalitis in the United States.
- Vulvovaginitis due to primary infection with HSV-2 and sometimes HSV-1 has increased markedly in the past 2 years.

 Differential Diagnosis

- Neonatal HSV infection must be distinguished from viral or bacterial sepsis especially in the first 4 weeks of life.
- HSV infection should be considered in all neonates with vesicular rash, chorioretinitis, microcephaly, or hepatosplenomegaly. It must be distinguished from other congenital viral infections such as rubella or CMV.
- Herpes gingivostomatitis must be distinguished from herpangina, an enteroviral infection usually presenting as posterior pharyngeal ulcers, and sometimes as hand-foot-and-mouth disease.
- HSV encephalitis must be distinguished from other viral encephalitis and from the HSV-induced aseptic meningitis syndrome, which is a complication of primary genital infection.
- HSV vulvovaginitis must be distinguished from chancroid and syphilis. Syphilis lesions are usually nonpainful hard ulcers. Chancroid lesions are multiple purulent ulcers from which *Haemophilus ducreyi* can be cultured.

 Data Gathering

HISTORY
Neonatal Infection

- HSV-2, the most common cause of neonatal infection, is usually acquired from maternal labial lesions, but a history of previous or current genital HSV infection is only present in 20% to 30% of mothers who deliver infected infants. HSV-2 can be transmitted to the infant without rupture of the amniotic membranes or after delivery by cesarean section.
- HSV-1 can be transmitted to a neonate by any adult with active herpes labialis.
- A vesicular rash or bullae are present at birth or within a few days in almost all infants.
- Disseminated infection (32% of cases) involves the liver, lungs, adrenals, and sometimes the central nervous system (CNS).
- Localized CNS infection (33% of cases) presents with irritability, bulging fontanelle, or seizures.
- Localized skin, eye, or mouth infection (35% of cases) present with rash alone, or keratitis or chorioretinitis.

Gingivostomatitis

- Fever and irritability precede the development of vesicular lesions on the lips, gingiva, and tongue. The vesicles then break down and become gray ulcers that are friable and bleed easily.
- Children refuse to drink because of the mouth pain and are at risk of dehydration.
- The child usually starts to improve in 3 to 5 days and recovers in 14 days.
- Latent virus causes recurrent stomatitis or labiitis.

Encephalitis

- The illness begins with fever malaise and irritability that last 1 to 7 days and progress to mental status changes, seizures, and coma. Meningeal signs are not common.
- Patients can develop hemiparesis, cranial nerve palsy, and visual field defects.
- No presence of oral or genital lesions

Vulvovaginitis

- 35% to 50% of patients with the first episode of genital herpes will be able to give a history of genital HSV infection in their contact.
- The primary illness is characterized by fever, headache, malaise, and myalgias. Local genital symptoms include severe pain, itching, dysuria, vaginal or urethral discharge, and tender inguinal adenopathy. The genital lesions begin as vesicles and progress to ulcers before they crust over. Lesions last for 2 to 3 weeks.
- An aseptic meningitis syndrome occurs in 1% to 35% of cases. Patients will have fever, headache, meningismus, and photophobia.
- Latent virus causes recurrent episodes, which are painful but less severe than in primary infections.

 Laboratory Aids

Neonatal Infection

- Samples for viral isolation can be obtained from viral transport media.
- Serologic tests are not useful for diagnosis of maternal or neonatal herpes during the acute phase of the disease.
- PCR testing of the CSF is now recommended, and in some studies is proving to be quite useful in making the diagnosis.
- Cells from the base of freshly unroofed vesicles can be smeared on a slide for monoclonal antibody immunofluorescence.

Encephalitis

- Cerebrospinal fluid (CSF) reveals a pleocytosis with up to 2000 WBC/mm^3 and usually over 60% of the cells are lymphocytes.
- In an atraumatic lumbar puncture red blood cells, indicating hemorrhagic necrosis occur in 75% to 85% of cases.
- CSF protein is elevated (median, 80 mg/dL).
- HSV almost never grows from CSF.
- Electroencephalogram (EEG) can reveal a "typical pattern" of unilateral or bilateral focal spikes.
- A focal abnormality on EEG, CT, or MRI is highly suggestive of HSV encephalitis.
- The only definitive way to make the diagnosis is to perform a brain biopsy, which is essential to provide appropriate therapy.

Gingivostomatitis
Physicians usually make this diagnosis clinically since it is so common in young children.

Vulvovaginitis
• A Tzanck preparation from the base of a lesion will show multinucleate giant cells in 60% of cases.
• Viral culture obtained by unroofing a vesicle and rubbing a sterile swab over the base of the vesicle to have a sensitivity of 94% for early lesions. Sensitivity decreases to 27% for crusted lesions.
• Immunofluorescence has a sensitivity of 90%.

 ## Therapy

Neonatal Infection
Intravenous acyclovir (60 mg/kg/d in 3 divided doses) is the drug of choice. The recommended minimal duration of therapy is 14 days (if the disease is limited to the skin, eye, and mouth), and 21 days if disease is disseminated or involves the CNS. Infants with ocular involvement due to HSV infection should receive a topical ophthalmic drug (1–2% trifluridine, 1% iododeoxyuridine, or 3% vidarabine) in addition to parenteral antiviral therapy.

Encephalitis
Intravenous acyclovir (30 mg/kg/d) three times a day for 21 days is appropriate therapy for HSV encephalitis after the neonatal period. In addition to parenteral antiviral therapy, appropriate management of fluids, intracranial pressure, and seizures is essential.

Gingivostomatitis
Most patients are managed with symptomatic therapy including antipyretics and oral fluids like popsicles. Oral anesthetics can be harmful and result in self-injury when children chew on anesthetized lips. Topical acyclovir is often used in the treatment of recurrent HSV oral herpes. It decreases the duration of HSV shedding but has minimal effect on the symptoms.

Vulvovaginitis
Acyclovir (Zovirax) is the appropriate therapy for genital herpes infection. Oral acyclovir is used for patients with primary genital HSV infection. Intravenous acyclovir is used for patients with severe local or systemic or complications like aseptic meningitis syndrome.

 ## Follow-Up

PREVENTION
• Neonatal infection
• Cesarean section in a mother with active genital herpes at the time of delivery is the main way to prevent neonatal infection. The risk of HSV infection in an infant born vaginally to a mother with a first-episode primary genital infection is high (33–50%). The risk to an infant born to a mother with recurrent HSV infection at delivery is much lower (3–5%). However, this does not prevent all cases since 60% to 80% of mothers of infected infants are asymptomatic or have unrecognized infection.
• Postnatal infection
—Universal body substance precaution policies
—Adults with oral herpes must be particularly careful to use appropriate hygiene.
—Wrestlers with skin lesions suggestive of herpes
—Patients with genital lesions from HSV should not have intercourse until the lesions heal.
—Condoms can prevent the spread of virus.

PROGNOSIS
• Neonatal infection
—Overall mortality from untreated neonatal HSV infection is 50% and only 26% of survivors are normal.
—Combined treatment with vidarabine and acyclovir lowers mortality to 17% and increases survival.
—Infants with disseminated disease or localized CNS disease have the worst prognosis to 67%.
—The major sequelae in survivors are brain damage, seizures, and blindness.

 ## Common Questions and Answers

Q: What about recurrent cutaneous eruptions in a neonate? Should they be treated?
A: The need for re-treatment of infants with recurrent skin lesions is undetermined and under study. Because of concerns about silent CNS recurrent infection, some experts are recommending acyclovir, 300 mg/m^2 in three doses for 6 to 12 months. One needs to look for neutropenia, which will occur in 25% of patients.

Q: Is prophylactic therapy for recurrent herpes genitalia helpful? When is it indicated?
A: Antiviral therapy has minimal effect on recurrent genital herpes. Oral acyclovir initiated within 2 days of onset of symptoms shortens the course. Topical acyclovir is not helpful.

Q: What steps should be taken in the nursery for an infant born to an HSV-positive mother?
A: Neonates with documented perinatal exposure to HSV may be in the incubation phase of infection and should be observed carefully. Infants of mothers with active HSV

should be isolated if they have been delivered vaginally or by cesarean section after membranes were ruptured for more than 4 to 6 hours. The risk of HSV infection in possibly exposed infants (e.g., those born to a mother with a history of recurrent genital herpes) is low, and isolation is not necessary.

Q: Is a repeat lumbar puncture necessary at the end of therapy for neonates or for children with HSV encephalitis?
A: Some experts recommended repeating the lumbar puncture at the end of the planned course of therapy to determine whether the virus is still present by PCR assay. If there is a positive test, prolonging therapy may be considered.

ICD-9-CM 054.9

BIBLIOGRAPHY
American Academy of Pediatrics. Herpes Simplex. In: Pickering LK, ed. *2000 red book: report of the Committee on Infectious Diseases*, 25th ed. Elk Grove Village, IL: American Academy of Pediatrics, 2000:309–318.

Corey L, Adams HG, Brown ZA, et al. Genital herpes simplex virus infections, clinical manifestations, course, and complications. *Ann Intern Med* 1983;98:958–972.

Corey L, Spear PG. Infections with herpes simplex virus. *N Engl J Med* 1986;314: 686–691,749–757.

Emans SJ, Goldstein DP. *Vulvovaginal complaints in the adolescent in pediatric and adolescent gynecology*, 3rd ed. Boston: Little, Brown, 1990:307–343.

Kohl S. Postnatal herpes simplex virus infection. In: Feigin RD, Cherry JD, eds. *Pediatric infectious diseases*, 3rd ed. Philadelphia: WB Saunders, 1992:1558–1583.

Marshall GS. Epidemiology and clinical manifestations of herpes infections in infants and children. *Semin Pediatr Infect Dis* 1997;8:151–168.

Nahmias AJ, Keyserling HL, Kevich GM. Herpes simplex. In: Remington JS, Klein JU, eds. *Infectious diseases of the fetus and newborn infant*, 2nd ed. Philadelphia: WB Saunders, 1983:636–678.

Nahmias AJ, Whitley RJ, Herpes simplex virus encephalitis in pediatrics. *Pediatr Rev* 1981;2:259–266.

Toltzis P. Infectious encephalitis. In: Jenson HB, Baltimore RS, eds. *Pediatric infectious diseases, principles and practice*, 2nd ed. Philadelphia: WB Saunders, 2002:669–673.

Whitley RJ, Kimberlin DW. Treatment of viral infections during pregnancy and the neonatal period. *Clin Perinatol* 1997;24(1):267–283.

Author: Louis M. Bell
Jane M. Gould, 2nd edition

Hiccups

Database

DEFINITION

• Known medically as singultus, from the Latin "singult" (a sob or speech punctuated by sobs), hiccups are a result of involuntary spasm of the diaphragm and intercostal muscles, leading to inspiration and abrupt closure of the glottis. Hiccups affect nearly everyone at one time or another.
• Hiccup bouts may last up to 48 hours. Persistent hiccups last from 48 hours up to 1 month, and intractable hiccups last for longer than 1 month.

PATHOPHYSIOLOGY

• Hiccups serve no physiologic function and are often simply a benign affliction.
• A hiccup reflex arc has been postulated, although the exact anatomic mechanism remains unknown. The arc consists of:

—The afferent limb: phrenic and vagus nerves, the pharyngeal plexus from C2 to C4 and the thoracic sympathetic chain from T6 to T12
—The efferent limb: phrenic nerve to the diaphragm and the external intercostal nerves to the intercostal muscles
—A central connection: a nonspecific location incorporating the medulla but independent of the respiratory center, the hypothalamus, and the phrenic nerve nuclei

• Hiccups have negligible effect on ventilation and usually involve only unilateral diaphragmatic contraction, most frequently on the left.
• Hiccups serve no respiratory function, despite activation of inspiratory musculature far more than during normal respiration.

CAUSES

• Hiccup bouts may be precipitated by a number of benign causes including:

—Gastric distention: aerophagia, ingestion of excessive food, carbonated beverages or alcohol, and gastric insufflation during endoscopy
—Changes in the ambient or gastrointestinal temperature: cold showers, ingestion of hot or cold beverages
—Sudden excitement or stress
—Tobacco use

• Persistent and intractable hiccups have many causes, which can be characterized as psychogenic, organic, or idiopathic:
• Psychogenic

—Stress
—Conversion reactions
—Anorexia nervosa
—Malingering
—Personality disorders

• Organic

—Central nervous system disorders: V-P shunts, hydrocephalus, A-V malformations, stroke, temporal arteritis, CNS trauma, encephalitis, meningitis, brain abscess
—Peripheral nervous system disturbances: irritation of the phrenic or vagus nerve, from a variety of causes, including:
  —Goiter, tumors or cysts of the neck, hiatal hernia, esophagitis, pneumonia, bronchitis, asthma, mediastinal lymphadenopathy, pericarditis, peptic ulcer disease, pancreatitis, inflammatory bowel disease, appendicitis, cholecystitis, and renal and hepatic disorders (stones or infections)
  —Infectious etiologies: sepsis, influenza, herpes zoster, malaria and tuberculosis
  —Metabolic or pharmacologic causes: anesthesia, IV methylprednisolone, barbiturates, diazepam, methyldopa, uremia, hypocalcemia, and hyponatremia

EPIDEMIOLOGY

• There is no male or female predominance for hiccup bouts; however, persistent and intractable hiccups have been shown to have a greater frequency in males, and are seen predominantly in adults.
• There is no racial, geographic, seasonal, or socioeconomic variability.
• Fetal hiccups are common in the third trimester of pregnancy.

COMPLICATIONS

Adverse effects that have been associated with intractable hiccups include malnutrition and dehydration, weight loss, insomnia, and fatigue. Rarely, cardiac dysrhythmia, reflux esophagitis, and even death may occur.

PROGNOSIS

• Self-limited and resolves without complications

Differential Diagnosis

• Hiccups are not often mistaken for any other entity
• The differential diagnosis for persistent and intractable hiccups is outlined above (see Definition)

Data Gathering

HISTORY

• Severity, duration, and characteristics of hiccups?
• Medication and alcohol use?
• Hiccups persisting during sleep suggests an organic etiology.

Physical Examination

Finding: Head and neck examination
Significance: May reveal evidence of trauma, foreign body in the ear, nuchal rigidity, masses, cervical lymphadenopathy, or an enlarged thyroid.

Finding: Assess the chest.
Significance: Evidence of pneumonia, bronchitis, or pericarditis

Finding: Assess the abdomen.
Significance: Evidence of appendicitis, intestinal obstruction, ruptured viscus, pancreatitis, or hepatobiliary disease

Finding: Neurological examination
Significance: Evidence of trauma, meningitis, encephalitis, V-P shunt malfunction, or neoplasm

Laboratory Aids

Tests should be chosen based on historical and physical findings.

- CBC
- Renal function and electrolytes
- LFTs and calcium
- Toxicology screen and blood gas

RADIOGRAPHIC STUDIES

Test: Chest x-ray
Significance: May rule out phrenic, vagal, and diaphragmatic irritation by pulmonary, cardiac, and mediastinal abnormalities.

 ## Therapy

- Directed at the underlying disease.
- If etiology is unknown, empiric therapy may be necessary.

DRUGS

- Studies confined to adult populations. Pharmaceuticals rarely recommended for children.
- Chlorpromazine widely used in adults in IV preparations. Intramuscular haloperidol has also been effective in adults.
- Anticonvulsants, including diphenylhydantoin, valproic acid, and carbamazepine reported effective.
- Combination of cisapride, omeprazole, and baclofen has been reported to be effective and is considered the mainstay for idiopathic chronic hiccups.
- Gabapentin has been shown to be effective as a substitute for baclofen or as an additional agent in the above regimen.

NONPHARMACOLOGIC MODALITIES

- Interruption of respiratory function: sneezing, coughing, breath holding, hyperventilation, sudden pain or fright.
- Disruption of phrenic nerve transmission: tapping over the fifth cervical vertebra, ice applied to the skin over the area of the phrenic nerve, and even transecting the phrenic nerve.
- Behavioral modification, hypnosis, and acupuncture.
- Nasopharyngeal stimulation: traction of the tongue, stimulation of the pharynx with a cotton swab, lifting the uvula with a spoon.
- Old-fashioned home remedies such as sipping ice water, swallowing granulated sugar, drinking water from the far side of a glass, and biting on a lemon.

 ## Follow-Up

No specific follow-up is indicated unless a specific organic cause has been identified.

PREVENTION

Avoid precipitating factors.

PITFALLS

Failure to recognize a serious underlying condition and assigning the label of idiopathic or psychogenic hiccups to an otherwise serious illness

 ## Common Questions and Answers

Q: Does breathing into a paper bag really work?
A: As a fall in pco$_2$ can increase frequency of hiccups, rebreathing air will increase pco$_2$ and thus terminate hiccups.

Q: Will hiccups harm my baby?
A: Hiccups alone are harmless. If they are truly persistent, intractable, or disrupt sleep, they may have the side effects as mentioned. Premature babies have been observed to spend 2.5% of their time having hiccups.

ICD-9-CM 786.8

BIBLIOGRAPHY

Kahrilas PJ, Shi G. Why do we hiccup? *Gut* 1997;41(5):712–713.

Pelig R, Shvartzman P. Hiccup. *J Fam Pract* 1996;42(4):424.

Petroiano G, Hein G, Petroiano A, et al. Idiopathic chronic hiccup: combination therapy with cisapride, omeprazole and baclofen. *Clin Ther* 1997;19:1031–1038.

Petroianu G, Hein G, Stegmeier-Petroianu, et al. Gabapentin "add-on therapy" for idiopathic chronic hiccup. *J Clin Gastroenterol* 2000;30(3):321–324.

Rousseau P. Hiccups. *South Med J* 1995;88(2): 175–181.

Author: Blaze Robert Gusic

Hirschsprung Disease

 Database

DEFINITION

• Intestinal abnormality of abnormal innervation of the distal bowel beginning at the anus and extending proximately for a variable distance, causing partial or complete intestinal obstruction, difficulty in passing stools, and in some cases enterocolitis.
• Also known as congenital megacolon and was first reported by Harold Hirschsprung in 1886.
• Present as complete obstruction, delayed passage of meconium, "chronic constipation," or enterocolitis.

PATHOPHYSIOLOGY

• Basic histologic finding is the absence of Meissner and Auerbach plexuses, hypertrophied nerve bundles between the circular and the longitudinal muscles and in the submucosa.
• Defect considered as a failure of caudal migration of the neural crest cells.

GENETICS

• Possible gene locus on the long arm of chromosome 10. Recent mouse models suggest a defect in the endothelin receptor.

EPIDEMIOLOGY

• Most common cause of lower intestinal obstruction in neonates: 1 in 5,000 births
• Overall rate of male/female patients is 2.8:1; in long-segment disease, it is 2.8:1, and in total colonic aganglionosis, it is 2.2:1.
• No racial predilection
• Familial incidence in total colonic aganglionosis: 75% of cases, rectosigmoid involved; 14%, descending colon involved; 8%, colon involved; 3%, small bowel affected.

ASSOCIATED DISEASES

In 3% of the patients, there has been an association with Down syndrome, cardiac anomalies, and coexistent multiple neuroblastomas.

 Differential Diagnosis

Chronic constipation

 Data Gathering

HISTORY

Question: Age of presentation
Significance: 80% of the time patients present in the neonatal period.

Question: Typical symptoms
Significance: Failure to pass meconium by 48 hours of life; delayed passage of meconium after 24 hours of life; history of constipation; history of chronic laxative use, abdominal distention, bilious vomiting, diarrhea in 22% of patients.

Question: Growth pattern
Significance: Neonates usually have normal weight, but growth retardation may occur when the disease is severe.

Question: Type of stools
Significance: Children with Hirschsprung disease usually have small volume and small diameter stools. Some may have overflow diarrhea as well.

 Physical Examination

Finding: On rectal examination, the sphincter tone is usually normal or increased.
Significance: Removal of the finger may be followed by explosive diarrhea; transition zone is usually not felt in infants under 2 months of age.

Finding: Stool in rectum.
Significance: In most instances, especially in older children, the rectum is empty.

Finding: Anemia?
Significance: Patients are usually anemic due to chronic blood loss from the large bowel secondary to infection.

 Laboratory Aids

TESTS

Test: Complete blood count
Significance: Anemia, leukocytosis in the presence of enterocolitis.

Test: Plain film of abdomen
Significance: May show distended loops of colon. Small bowel air is usually present in the bowel proximal to the obstruction. Diffuse intestinal pneumatosis has been reported as a rare presentation.

Test: Barium enema
Significance: Useful but not diagnostic; transition zone is a funnel-shaped area of intestine with normal distal area and dilated proximal area. Barium enema reveals large mucosal pattern, prominently thickened folds, and irregular margins secondary to ulceration.

Test: Anorectal manometry
Significance: Diagnostic but usually reserved for those cases causing diagnostic difficulties, as in the ultrashort segment disease.

Test: Biopsy
Significance: Suction biopsy should be done approximately 2 to 4 cm from the anal verge depending on the age of the patient. The biopsies must have adequate submucosa to demonstrate neurofibrils detected using acetylcholinesterase as a stain. With the absence of ganglion cells, biopsy is diagnostic. If the suction biopsies are not conclusive, a full-thickness biopsy is mandatory.

COMPLICATIONS

Enterocolitis is the most important complication:

• Secondary to obstruction causing an increase in intraluminal pressure and decreased intramural capillary blood flow.
• Affects the protective mucosal barrier enabling fecal breakdown products, bacteria, and toxins, to enter into the bloodstream.
• Usually present with fever, diarrhea, and frequent, bloody, bilious vomiting.

Therapy

- Stabilizing treatment is fluid resuscitation, nasogastric decompression, broad-spectrum antibiotics, and saline enemas.
- The initial operation is a defunctionalizing colostomy or an ileostomy for total colonic aganglionosis. This is performed to avoid the hazards of enterocolitis. If the child has already developed enterocolitis, colostomy is deferred until the general condition improves.
- Definitive surgery is performed 6 months to a year after the initial colostomy. The various surgical procedures performed are:

—Endorectal pull-through: widely used. Basic principle is to strip the aganglionic rectum of its mucosa and then to bring normally innervated colon through the residual rectal muscular cuff, thereby bypassing the abnormal bowel from within. Advantages: sphincter function is preserved and minimal danger of injury to pelvis.

—Retrorectal transanal pull-through (Duhamel procedure): The normally innervated bowel is brought behind the abnormally innervated rectum approximately 1 to 2 cm above the pectinate line and an end-to-side anastomosis is performed. This procedure creates a neorectum with the anterior one-half having normal sensory receptors and a posterior one-half with normal propulsion. Advantages: reduces pelvic dissection to a minimum and retains the sensory pathway of rectal reflexes. Disadvantages: incontinence if anastomosis is too low and obstructive symptoms if anastomosis is too high or if the aganglionic segment is too long.

- Other procedures include the Soave (endorectal pull through).
- In total colonic aganglionosis, the modified Lester Martin technique is performed. It involves the anastomosis of the cecum and ascending colon as an onlay patch graft in the more distal normal small bowel, which is then pulled through the amputated rectum that has been stripped of its mucosa and a primary anastomosis is performed.
- These procedures can now be performed laparoscopically.

PITFALLS

Early recognition is of utmost importance in reducing the morbidity and mortality of Hirschsprung disease.
Fecal incontinence could occur after surgery.

Follow-Up

Most children are followed on a regular basis for the first decade after surgery.

Common Questions and Answers

Q: Will the bowel movements be normal after surgery?
A: Studies have shown that 83% of children have three or fewer stools per day at a mean follow-up of 4.1 ± 2.5 years.

Q: Are laxatives required after surgery?
A: In about 20% of children some sort of laxative therapy or rectal irrigation may be required.

ICD-9-CM 751.3

BIBLIOGRAPHY

Abi-Hanna A, Lake AM. Constipation and encopresis in childhood. *Pediatr Rev* 1998;19(1):23–30.

Athow AL, Filipe MI, Drake DP. Problems and advantages of acetyl cholinesterase histochemistry of rectal suction biopsies in Hirschsprung's disease. *J Pediatr Surg* 1990;25(5):520–526.

Diseth TH, Egeland T, Emblem R. Effects of anal invasive treatment and incontinence on mental health and psychosocial functioning of adolescents with Hirschsprung's disease and low anorectal anomalies. *J Pediatr Surg* 1998;33(3):468–475.

Fitzgerald CJ. New concepts of the etiology, diagnosis, and treatment of congenital megacolon (Hirschsprung's disease), by Orvar Swenson, MD, et al., *Pediatrics* 1949;4: 201–209. *Pediatrics* 1998; 102(1 Pt 2): 205–207.

Hsieh WS, Yang PH, Huang CS, Wang CR. Hirschsprung's disease presenting with diffuse intestinal pneumatosis in a neonate. *Acta Paediatr Taiwan* 2000;41(6):336–338.

Lyonnet S, Bolino A, Pelet A, et al. A gene for Hirschsprung's disease maps to the proximal long arm of chromosome 10. *Nature Genet* 1993;4(4):346–501.

Mahboubi S, Schnaufer L. The barium enema and rectal manometry in Hirschsprung's disease. *Radiology* 1979;130:643–647.

So HB, Becker JM, Schwartz DL, et al. Eighteen years' experience with neonatal Hirschsprung's disease treated by endorectal pull-through without colostomy. *J Pediatr Surg* 1998;33(5):673–675.

Teitelbaum DH, Cilley RE, Sherman NJ, et al. A decade of experience with the primary pull-through for Hirschsprung disease in the newborn period: a multicenter analysis of outcomes. *Ann Surg* 2000;232(3):372–380.

Van der Zee DC, Bax KN. One-stage Duhamel-Martin procedure for Hirschsprung's disease: a 5-year follow-up study. *J Pediatr Surg* 2000;35(10):1434–1436.

Authors: Helen Anita John-Kelly and Andrew E. Mulberg

Histiocytosis

 ## Database

DEFINITION
Clinical conditions resulting from or associated with proliferation of the mononuclear phagocytic system.

CLASSIFICATION
• Dendritic cell-related disorders (e.g., Langerhans cell histiocytosis)
• Macrophage-related disorders (e.g., hemophagocytic lymphohistiocytosis)
• Malignant histiocytic disorders

LANGERHANS CELL HISTIOCYTOSIS

 ## Database

DEFINITION
• Reactive disorder of unknown etiology in which cells similar to Langerhans cells of the skin cause damage to organs by excessive production of cytokines and prostaglandins
• Previously known as histiocytosis X, eosinophilic granuloma, Hand-Schüller-Christian syndrome, Letterer-Siwe disease, and Hashimoto Pritzker syndrome

PATHOPHYSIOLOGY
• Lesions have proliferation of abnormal Langerhans cells in locations where they are not typically found; electron microscopy reveals tennis racquet-shaped inclusions (Birbeck granules).
• May arise as a result of an underlying immunodeficiency or as an abnormal response to a viral infection
• Monoclonal histiocytes have been detected in all forms of disease.

GENETICS
Generally not an inherited disease. There are rare reports of recurrence within families.

COMPLICATIONS
• Single-system disease
—Some patients with bone involvement will have a chronic remitting and relapsing course.
• Multisystem disease
—Approximately 20% risk of fatal progression, especially in patients with liver, bone marrow or lung involvement and a slow response to initial therapy.
—Risk of diabetes insipidus, especially in patients with orbital, facial bone or sinus based lesions
—Chronic disabilities including pulmonary fibrosis, hepatic fibrosis, deafness, orthopedic problems, short stature, permanent ataxia or poor dentition.

PROGNOSIS
• Majority of patients have no recurrence.
• Approximately 20% to 35% of patients with single system disease will have a remitting and relapsing course.

• Tendency for the disease to "burn out" by the end of childhood. Approximately 5% will continue to have exacerbations as adults.
• 30% to 50% of patients with multisystem disease will not respond to initial therapy and are at higher risk for death.
• For patients with liver, bone marrow, or lung involvement who have not responded to initial therapy, the risk for fatal outcome is approximately 75%.

 ## Differential Diagnosis

• Other histiocytic disorders:
—Hemophagocytic lymphohistiocytosis
—Sinus histiocytosis with massive lymphadenopathy (cervical nodes grossly enlarged)
—Malignant histiocytosis
—Bone/soft tissue lesions
—Metastatic neuroblastoma
—Osteosarcoma
—Ewing sarcoma
—Rhabdomyosarcoma
—Craniopharyngioma
—Organomegaly/pancytopenia
—Acute leukemias
—Metastatic neuroblastoma

 ## Data Gathering

HISTORY
• Swelling or pain, from soft tissue or bone lesion
• Persistent otitis.
• Early loss of teeth.
• Failure to thrive. Bloody diarrhea.
• Fever of unknown origin. Anorexia.
• Polydipsia or polyuria. (Diabetes insipidus from posterior pituitary gland involvement).
• Dyspnea. Persistent cough. History of spontaneous pneumothorax.

 ## Physical Examination

Growth: Height, weight, and head circumference, <5%.
Skin: Brownish red papules often involving creases, seborrheic dermatitis of the scalp ("cradle cap"), purpura, petechial rash especially at areas of skin contact (e.g., top of diaper)
Ears: Otorrhea, deafness
Head: Skull swelling or mass, often very tender to palpation
Teeth: Gingivitis, "floating teeth"
Eyes: Orbital swelling, cranial nerve palsies
Lungs: Tachypnea, intercostal retractions
GI: Hepatosplenomegaly, ascites, edema, jaundice. Stool with blood or mucus
Neuro: Ataxia

 ## Laboratory Aids

MANDATORY INITIAL INVESTIGATIONS
• CBC with differential
• PT, PTT, fibrinogen
• Electrolytes, liver function tests
• Chest x-ray
• Skeletal survey (radionuclide bone scan is not as sensitive as the skeletal radiograph survey in most patients)
• Urine osmolarity in early AM as a screen for diabetes insipidus

OTHER INVESTIGATIONS
• Pulmonary involvement: High-resolution chest CT scan, pulmonary function tests, bronchoalveolar lavage to exclude infection
• Colon involvement: endoscopic biopsy of small and large colon
• Liver dysfunction: hepatic ultrasound, liver biopsy (to exclude sclerosing cholangitis)
• Neurologic involvement: MRI brain with gadolinium
• Diabetes insipidus: endocrine evaluation including water deprivation test, evaluation of anterior pituitary hormone production, MRI brain with gadolinium
• Gingival involvement, loose teeth: panoramic dental radiography, CT scan of mandible and maxilla
• Aural involvement, deafness: audiogram, ENT evaluation, MRI brain with gadolinium

 ## Therapy

SINGLE SYSTEM
• Observation
• Local therapy
—Surgery
—Intralesional steroids (bone lesions)
—Radiotherapy is not recommended unless there is compromise to vital structures (optic nerve, spinal cord)
—Topical nitrogen mustard for refractory skin lesions
• Systemic therapy
—Low-dose chemotherapy is used for some patients with multifocal bone disease or multiply recurrent single bone lesions.
—Indomethacin may be effective for refractory bone lesions for both its analgesic and antiprostaglandin effects.
—The biphosphonate pamidronate has been used in a few patients with refractory bone lesions.

MULTISYSTEM
• Chemotherapy: often a 6 to 12 month course; most commonly used agents: prednisone, vinblastine, etoposide, methotrexate, 6-mercaptopurine, 2-chlorodeoxyadenosine
• Immunotherapy: cyclosporin A, antithymocyte globulin
• Radiation therapy

- Stem cell transplantation for high-risk patients with organ dysfunction
- Most patients are treated at pediatric oncology centers. There is an international clinical trial in progress to identify the most effective treatment strategies.

 ## Follow-Up

As the course is quite variable, patients need to be followed closely at a center experienced in the management of histiocytosis. Multidisciplinary care with expertise in pediatric oncology and stem cell transplantation, orthopedics, dermatology, otolaryngology, dentistry, neurology, ophthalmology, hepatology, gastroenterology, pulmonary, and endocrinology may be required.

 ## Common Questions and Answers

Q: Is Langerhans cell histiocytosis a form of cancer?

A: Although the abnormal Langerhans cells have been found to be derived from a single cell (i.e., monoclonal), the natural history of the disease is not typical of a malignant disorder, and therefore it is not classified as a type of cancer.

HEMOPHAGOCYTIC LYMPHOHISTIOCYTOSIS

 ## Database

DEFINITION
Reactive disorder characterized by an accumulation of erythrophagocytic histiocytes:
- Primary (also known as familial erythrophagocytic lymphohistiocytosis)
—Immunodysregulatory disorder
—Classically an inherited disease
- Infection associated:
—Microorganisms implicated include: cytomegalovirus, Epstein-Barr virus (EBV), herpes simplex virus, HIV, adenovirus, tuberculosis, brucellosis, typhoid fever, leishmaniasis

PATHOPHYSIOLOGY
- Characterized by an accumulation of phagocytic histiocytes and lymphocytes in the reticuloendothelial system, skin, and central nervous system (CNS)
- Immune system dysregulation with defective T-cell function, low or absent natural killer cell activity, and elaboration of large amounts of inflammatory cytokines

GENETICS
- Primary:
—Autosomal recessive
—History of consanguinity may exist
—Familial history frequently negative
- Infection associated:
—Sporadic

EPIDEMIOLOGY
- Primary:
—Incidence is 0.12 per 100,000 children
—Males and females equally affected
—70% present in the first year of life
—Occurs in all races
- Infection associated:
—Incidence variable
—Patients often have an underlying immunodeficiency disorder or are medically immunosuppressed (e.g., cancer chemotherapy

PROGNOSIS
- Primary:
—Usually fatal secondary to bleeding, infection (usually gram-negative sepsis) or progressive cerebral damage from CNS involvement
—Untreated the median survival is 2 to 3 months, 12% live more than 6 months
—Allogeneic stem cell transplantation has resulted in some long-term survivors
- Infection associated:
—Mortality rates; immunocompromised 40%, immunocompetent 20%
—Improved recovery in cases associated with bacterial infections; EBV-associated has the worst prognosis

 ## Differential Diagnosis

- Langerhans cell histiocytosis
- Sepsis with disseminated intravascular coagulation
- Syphilis
- Leishmaniasis
- Encephalitis
- Hepatitis
- Acute monoblastic leukemia
- Malignant histiocytosis
- Systemic juvenile rheumatoid arthritis
- Degenerative cerebral disorders
- Severe combined immunodeficiency disorder
- X-linked lymphoproliferative syndrome
- Chediak-Higashi syndrome

 ## Data Gathering

HISTORY
Question: History of a rapid progression of symptoms or a viral prodrome for 2 to 6 weeks followed by constitutional symptoms, especially fever?
Significance: Evidence of systemic involvement
Question: Irritability, seizures, vomiting?
Significance: CNS involvement

 ## Physical Examination

- Fever
- Splenomegaly
- Hepatomegaly
- Lymphadenopathy

- Seizure, irritability, bulging fontanel, neck stiffness, cranial nerve palsy, hypertonia or hypotonia, blindness, hemiplegia, coma and increased intracranial pressure

 ## Laboratory Aids

Test: CBC with differential
Significance: Thrombocytopenia, anemia, and, to a lesser extent, neutropenia, are observed.
Test: Fibrinogen, prothrombin time, activated partial thromboplastin time
Significance: Low fibrinogen, prolonged PT, and aPTT are signs of active disease
Test: Serum triglycerides, bilirubin, AST, ALT
Significance: Triglycerides classically very high; other liver function tests may be elevated
Test: Bone marrow aspirate/biopsy
Significance: Activated histiocytes with hemophagocytosis, particularly of erythrocytes
Test: Liver biopsy
Significance: Prominent histiocytes, many with hemophagocytosis
Test: Cerebrospinal fluid cell count
Significance: Moderate pleocytosis $(5–50 \times 10^6/L)$ with mainly lymphocytes

 ## Therapy

- Primary
—Cytotoxic drugs: etoposide, intrathecal methotrexate, corticosteroids
—Immunosuppressive therapy: cyclosporin A, antithymocyte globulin
—Plasmapheresis or exchange blood transfusions
—Allogeneic stem cell transplantation is necessary for cure
- Infection associated
—Withdrawal of immunosuppression if possible
—Antimicrobial therapy
—Corticosteroids
—Intravenous immunoglobulin
—Plasmapheresis
—For patients with uncontrolled fever, progressive pancytopenia, DIC, or impending organ failure, cytotoxic therapy (as used for primary hemophagocytic lymphohistiocytosis) should be instituted.

ICD-9-CM 277.8

BIBLIOGRAPHY
Arico M, Egeler RM. Clinical aspects of Langerhans cell histiocytosis. *Hematol Oncol Clin North Am* 1998;12:247–258.

Janka G, Imashuku S, Elinder G, et al. Infection- and malignancy-associated hemophagocytic syndromes. *Hematol Oncol Clin North Am* 1998;12:435–443.

Author: Kara M. Kelly

Histoplasmosis

 Database

DEFINITION
A spectrum of illness, ranging from primary pulmonary to disseminated infection, caused by the dimorphic fungus *Histoplasma capsulatum*.

CAUSES
• Inhalation of *H. capsulatum* spores
• The dimorphic fungus exists in mycelial form in the environment at 25°C and in yeast form in tissues at 37°C

PATHOPHYSIOLOGY
• Micronidia or mycelial fragments inhaled into alveoli and transform to yeast phase
• Phagocytosis followed by lymphatic and hematogenous spread
• T-cell response follows in 10 to 21 days after infection; number of T-suppressor cells decreases while number of T-helper cells increases, resulting in delayed-type hypersensitivity.
• Localized mononuclear cell infiltrates may develop into a tuberculoid granuloma with multinucleated giant cells.
• Lesions can undergo caseation necrosis, fibrosis, and, ultimately, calcification.
• Lesions usually localized to the lungs, though dissemination can occur.

EPIDEMIOLOGY
• The most common systemic fungal infection in the United States
• Organism has been found in nitrogen-rich soil contaminated by animal droppings, especially those of bats and birds.
• Outbreaks reported in pigeon breeders or cleaners of chicken coops, explorers of caves with bats, and populations living close to construction.
• Endemic in the eastern and central United States, more specifically in the St. Laurence, Mississippi, and Ohio River valleys, the Rio Grande, Texas, Oklahoma, Kansas, Pennsylvania, Maryland, and Virginia
• 80% to 90% of adults in endemic areas are skin test positive.
• No human-to-human or animal-to-human transmission
• The incubation period is variable, between 1 and 3 weeks.
• Severity of symptoms depends on the immunologic status of the host and the size of the inoculum:
• Asymptomatic in 50% to 95% of cases
• With heavy inoculum, 50% to 100% develop symptoms. Of these, 80% develop flu-like symptoms: fever, chills, headache, myalgia, anorexia, nonproductive cough, pleuritic chest pain, lasting about a week. 10% to 20% develop pericarditis, arthritis, or erythema nodosum, resolving after a few weeks.

• Risk factors for severe disease (progressive disseminated histoplasmosis, PDH) include very old and very young (less than 2 years) age, and cellular immunocompromise, e.g., AIDS

GENETICS
No genetic implications

COMPLICATIONS
In general, complications are rare, and usually indicate disseminated disease.
• Symptoms include:
—Prolonged fever, malaise, cough, weight loss, hepatosplenomegaly, diarrhea
—Patients may also develop DIC, ARDS, renal failure, endocarditis, Addison's disease.
• Disseminated disease can involve:
—Skin
—Eyes (uveitis)
—Liver
—Spleen
—Bone marrow
—Heart
—Central nervous system
• Other complications include:
—Tracheobronchial compression
—Mediastinal granuloma formation or fibrosing mediastinitis
—Fistula formation
—Pericarditis
—Obstruction of the superior vena cava, esophagus, or pulmonary arteries
—Chronic cavitary pulmonary disease very similar to tuberculosis

 Differential Diagnosis

• Infections
—Pneumonia (viral, bacterial)
—Influenza and other viral syndromes
—Tuberculosis
—Other fungal diseases: aspergillosis, blastomycosis, coccidioidomycosis
—Sarcoidosis
• Malignancy

 Data Gathering

HISTORY
Question: Environmental exposures (pigeon breeding, construction, cave exploration, travel in endemic areas)?
Significance: Epidemiologically suggestive of histoplasmosis.

Question: Upper respiratory symptoms, low grade fever, cough, pleuritic chest pain?
Significance: Suggestive of mild disease lasting 1 to 5 days

Question: Arthritis, more severe chest pain, skin lesions?
Significance: Suggestive of pericarditis or pleural effusion, moderate disease lasting approximately 15 days

Question: High fever, night sweats, weight loss, cough, chest pain, shortness of breath, hoarseness lasting more than 2 to 3 weeks?
Significance: Suggestive of disseminated disease and underlying immune suppression

Question: Chronic cough, dyspnea, disabling respiratory dysfunction?
Significance: Suggestive of chronic cavitary pulmonary disease

 Physical Examination

Finding: Flu-like signs and symptoms
Significance: Common presentations, mild disease
• Fever
• Cough
• Physical examination may be normal

Finding: Less usual manifestations
Significance: Suggestive of moderate or disseminated disease
• Hepatosplenomegaly
• Adenopathy
• Pneumonitis
• Skin lesions (erythema nodosum)
• Pericardial friction rub
• Pallor, petechiae
• CNS findings

 Laboratory Aids

Test: Culture of the organism in sputum, tissue specimens, peripheral blood, or bone marrow
Significance: Definitive method of diagnosis, but requires 2 to 6 weeks. Sputum cultures positive in two thirds of patients with cavitary disease and one third of patients with non cavitary disease. In PDH in patients with AIDS, bone marrow and blood cultures positive in 80% to 90% of patients, bronchoscopic cultures positive in 80% to 90% of patients with abnormal chest radiographs.

Test: Identification of organism by microscopy
Significance: Histologic identification from sputum, blood (buffy coat—50% positive in PDH), bone marrow, biopsy specimens, and/or cerebrospinal fluid. Staining methods: hematoxylin and eosin (H&E), Wright, Giemsa, periodic acid-Schiff (PAS). Gomori methenamine silver (GMS) more likely to detect sparse organisms

Test: Skin testing
Significance: A positive delayed hypersensitivity reaction (48 h) to the histoplasmin test may become reactive 2 to 6 weeks after infection. This test is not recommended for diagnostic purposes in adults: it is very often indicative of past infection in endemic areas (see Epidemiology, above). In children younger than 5, only 0.5% from endemic areas are skin test positive, making it more useful. 50% of immunocompromised patients may have false-negative skin tests. False positive in blastomycosis and coccidioidomycosis. Skin testing can falsely elevate antibody levels in 15% to 25% of patients, and therefore should only be done *after* serologic testing if done at all.

Test: Radioimmune and hemagglutinin assays for H capsulatum antigen
Significance: Radioimmunoassay is a specific, sensitive and rapid method for diagnosing PDH. Hemagglutinin found in urine or blood in 50% to 80% of patients with PDH, and in bronchoalveolar lavage fluid in 70% of AIDS patients with pulmonary histoplasmosis. Antigen tests generally useful only in first month of infection, but can persist for much longer in AIDS patients. DNA probes are being increasingly used.

Test: Serologic studies for antibodies
Significance: Titers become positive 4 to 6 weeks after infection, peak at 2 to 3 months and decline over a period of 2 to 5 years. Positive titers in 90% of patients with symptomatic disease. False positives in patients with coccidioidomycosis, blastomycosis, tuberculosis and paracoccidioidomycosis. False negatives in immunocompromised patients with PDH.

Test: Complement fixation
Significance: A single titer 1:32 (1:8 in nonendemic areas) is diagnostic; a fourfold increase in titers is diagnostic. This test is more sensitive than the immunodiffusion test, which is more specific.

Test: Precipitating antibodies by immunodiffusion
Significance: H band suggests active infection, M band less specific, presence of H and M bands highly diagnostic

IMAGING
Test: Chest radiograph
Significance: Normal in 75% of the patients with histoplasmosis, 40% to 50% of immunocompromised patients with disseminated disease
- Most common radiologic changes include:
—Small 2- to 5-mm infiltrates in the lung bases
—Lobar or diffuse infiltrates
—Enlarged or calcified hilar nodes
—Buckshot calcifications seen in patients with large inoculum
—Cavitary lesions
—Pleural effusions in 10% of adult x-rays
—Calcified nodules in the liver and spleen

 ## Therapy

DRUGS
- The uncomplicated cases of primary histoplasmosis of the lungs may not require drug therapy
- Patients with more severe or disseminated disease or the immunocompromised may require treatment with antifungal agents. Treatment regimens can vary.
—Amphotericin B, 0.5 to 1.0 mg/kg/d for 4 to 6 weeks, or 35 mg/kg, total. Recommended for disseminated disease or patients with respiratory compromise and hypoxemia
—Ketoconazole, 3.3 to 6.6 mg/kg/d PO (400 mg/d is maximum dose) for 3 to 6 months. Should be used with caution in patients receiving H2 blockers, because absorption is decreased in achlorhydric state. Levels can also be reduced by rifampin and phenytoin.
—Other effective agents include fluconazole and itraconazole. Although the latter has not been approved for the use in children, it is effective in the treatment of HIV patients with histoplasmosis
—In patients with AIDS, lifelong suppressive therapy is recommended
—Adjunct therapy with corticosteroids may be added in patients with life-threatening airway obstruction secondary to hilar adenopathy

 ## Follow-Up

WHEN TO EXPECT IMPROVEMENT
- In mild-to-moderate cases not requiring drug therapy, usually 1 to 2 weeks
- In cases requiring therapy, improvement is usually noted within 2 weeks.
- Response to therapy is more variable in AIDS patients.

PROGNOSIS
- In most cases, prognosis is excellent.
- 90% mortality within 3 months in patients with acute disseminated histoplasmosis if left untreated.
- High relapse in AIDS patients if not treated with chronic suppressive therapy.

PITFALLS
Can be difficult to distinguish between active disease and previous exposures in patients from endemic regions. Skin testing not recommended for adults in endemic regions, and may cause false-positive serology. May be confused with TB and other fungal diseases. Isolated pulmonary nodule on CXR may be difficult to distinguish from malignancy

PREVENTION AND CONTROL MEASURES
- Investigation for the common source of infection in outbreaks. Limit exposure to soil and dust from areas contaminated with bat and bird droppings.

- For occupational exposure to *H. capsulatum*-contaminated soil
—Use of wetting agents to prevent aerosolization of contaminated dust
—NIOSH approved respirators, gloves and dispensable clothing (see NIOSH Web site in bibliography)
- Isolation of the hospitalized patient
—Standard precautions recommended

 ## Common Questions and Answers

Q: What are the most common clinical presentations of histoplasmosis?
A: Asymptomatic, mild primary pulmonary (1–2 weeks), moderate (2–3 weeks), disseminated, and cavitary

Q: How is histoplasmosis best diagnosed?
A: Skin test generally not useful, culture and serologic testing recommended

Q: Does histoplasmosis need to be treated with antifungal therapy?
A: Primary mild disease—no; more severe or disseminated disease—yes

Q: How can histoplasmosis be prevented?
A: Prevention can only be achieved by controlling the environmental factors in the affected areas; there are no vaccines for the prevention of histoplasmosis.

Q: Do patients with histoplasmosis need to be isolated?
A: No isolation of infected patients is required.

ICD-9-CM 115.90

BIBLIOGRAPHY
Afghani B, Marks MI. Other fungal infections: Histoplasmosis. In: Taussig L, Landau L, eds. *Textbook of pediatric respiratory medicine.* St. Louis: Mosby, 1999:753–755.

American Academy of Pediatrics. Histoplasmosis. In: Pickering LK, ed. *2000 red book: report of the Committee on Infectious Diseases,* 25th ed. Elk Grove Village, IL: Academy of Pediatrics, 2000:319–321.

Bosso JA. Fungal infections in pediatric patients. *Pharmacotherapy* 1990;10:150S–153S.

Maxson S, Jacobs RF. Community acquired fungal pneumonia in children. *Semin Respir Infect* 11:196–203, 1996.

National Institute for Occupational Safety and Health (NIOSH) web site:
http://www.cdc.gov/niosh/97-146.html.

Walsh TJ, Gonzalez C, Lyman CA, et al. Invasive fungal infections in children: recent advances in diagnosis and treatment. *Adv Pediatr Infect Dis* 1996;11:187–290.

Author: Julian L. Allen
Hector L. Flores-Arroyo, 2nd edition

Hodgkin Lymphoma

 Database

DEFINITION

A malignant enlargement of lymph nodes characterized by a pleomorphic cellular infiltrate with multinucleated giant cells (Reed-Sternberg cells)

PATHOPHYSIOLOGY

• Exact cause unknown
• Reed-Sternberg cells are the malignant cells of Hodgkin lymphoma; however, their normal counterparts have not been definitively identified. They may originate from activated B or T lymphocytes or from an antigen-presenting cell. Histologically, Reed-Sternberg cells are dispersed among apparently normal reactive cells including lymphocytes, plasma cells, and eosinophils.
• The Rye classification histologically divides the disease into four categories: lymphocyte predominant, mixed cellularity, lymphocyte depleted, and nodular sclerosis. Most common subtype in children is nodular sclerosis (approximately 50% of cases).
• Unicentric in origin with spread mostly by contiguity from one chain of lymph nodes to another.

GENETICS

• Familial clustering suggests the role of both genetic and environmental factors in pathogenesis:
—Three- to sevenfold increased risk of disease among siblings.
—Affected parent–child pairs have been reported.

EPIDEMIOLOGY

• Incidence shows bimodal age distribution:
—Early peak, before adolescence in developing countries, mid- to late 20s in United States
—Second peak, late adulthood, >50 years of age
—Childhood cases, rare before 5 years of age
—More common in white race in patients >15 years of age
• Infections with Epstein-Barr virus (EBV), cytomegalovirus, and herpesvirus-6 may play role in transmission of disease.
—Patients with history of EBV infection have a threefold increased risk of disease.
• Male predominance

COMPLICATIONS

• Acute toxicity of treatment
—Radiation effects are generally reversible and not serious. Includes erythema with or without hyperpigmentation of involved skin, nausea, fatigue, and possibly myelosuppression. Lhermitte syndrome, a sensation of "electric shock" radiating down the back into the extremities, may occasionally be seen.
—Chemotherapy regimens will cause nausea, vomiting, and reversible alopecia to some degree. Transfusions may be required for anemia and thrombocytopenia. Each individual agent also has a list of toxicities

that must be reviewed before using alone or in combination. Most important of these include cardiac toxicity with Adriamycin, neurotoxicity with vincristine, and pulmonary toxicity with bleomycin.
• Infection
—Most common dose-limiting acute toxicity of chemotherapy is myelosuppression. Patients may have to be admitted for antibiotics if fever develops during neutropenia. Prophylactic antibiotics and vaccines have reduced the incidence of serious bacterial infections in the splenectomized host.

PROGNOSIS

• With current therapy including chemotherapy and/or radiation, 5-year disease-free survival ranges from:
—88% to 100% in low-stage disease
—54% to 94% in advanced-stage disease

 Differential Diagnosis

• Infection is most common cause for acute lymphadenopathy.
—Bacterial (*Staphylococcus aureus*, β-hemolytic streptococcus, TB, atypical mycobacterium)
—Other (EBV, CMV, cat-scratch disease, toxoplasmosis, HIV, histoplasmosis)
• Malignancy is more common with chronic adenopathy.
—Non-Hodgkin lymphoma, neuroblastoma, leukemia, rhabdomyosarcoma
• Mediastinal masses divided anatomically:
—Anterior: lymphoid and thyroid tumors, bronchogenic cysts, aneurysms, lipomas
—Middle: lymphoid tumors, angiomas, pericardial cysts, teratomas, esophageal lesions, hernias
—Posterior: neurogenic tumors, cysts, thoracic meningocele, sarcomas

 Data Gathering

HISTORY
Signs/Symptoms
• Fatigue, anorexia, weight loss in one third of patients
• "B" symptoms (part of staging classification) include one of the following:
—Unexplained fever with temperature >38°C for at least 3 days
—Unexplained weight loss >10% body weight in previous 6 months
—Drenching night sweats
• "A" disease (asymptomatic)
—Pruritus or pain that worsens with ingestion of alcohol seen in some patients
• History relative to possible EBV or HIV infection should be recorded as well as any history suggesting immunodeficiency

 Physical Examination

• Painless lymphadenopathy most common
—Nodes are usually firmer and less mobile than inflammatory nodes; cervical chain is most frequently involved.
—Mediastinal mass in two thirds of patients, may cause nonproductive cough or difficulty breathing.
—Hepatosplenomegaly and bone tenderness in advanced stages
—Unusual signs and symptoms: nephrotic syndrome, dermatomyositis, and acute dysautonomia

 Laboratory Aids

• CBC, ESR
• Liver and renal function studies
• Baseline thyroid functions (preradiotherapy)
• Baseline electrocardiogram, echocardiogram, and pulmonary function tests

PATHOLOGY
• Lymph node biopsy for definitive diagnosis

RADIOLOGIC STUDIES
• Chest x-ray (PA and lateral) to look for mediastinal mass
• CT scan (chest, abdomen, pelvis) to rule out disseminated disease
• CT or MRI of spine (if bony tenderness or symptoms of cord compression suspected)

SPECIAL TESTS
• Bone marrow biopsy
• Gallium scan (detects residual disease in the mediastinum)
• Bone scan (evaluates bone involvement, optional)
• Lymphangiogram (evaluates retroperitoneal adenopathy, optional)
• Cardiac troponin-T levels (elevated after myocardial damage possibly due to therapy, investigational)

STAGING
• Staging laparotomy is indicated in patients with equivocal abdominal findings from clinical staging or in patients with radiotherapy treatment only.
—I: Involvement of a single lymph node region (I) or of a single extralymphatic organ or site (IE) by direct extension
—II: Involvement of two or more lymph node regions on the same side of the diaphragm (II) or localized involvement of an extralymphatic organ or site and one or more lymph node regions on the same side of the diaphragm (IIE)

Hodgkin Lymphoma

—III: Involvement of lymph node regions on both sides of the diaphragm (III), which may be accompanied by involvement of the spleen (IIIS) or by localized involvement of an extralymphatic organ or site (IIIE) or both (IIIES)
—IV: Diffuse or disseminated involvement of one or more extralymphatic organs or tissues with or without associated lymph node involvement
• Staging is further subclassified "A" or "B" according to absence or presence of symptoms (listed above), respectively.

RISK GROUPS
• Low risk
—IA–IIA, no bulk mediastinum
—No extranodal extension or B symptoms
—No more than two involved regions
• Intermediate risk
—IA–IIA with bulk mediastinum or extranodal extension or three or more involved nodal sites
—IB–IIB–IIIA
• High risk
—IIIB, IVA-B

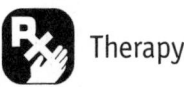 ## Therapy

RADIOTHERAPY (XRT)
• Exquisitely responsive to XRT
• Decisions to use XRT based on patient age, tumor burden, and potential complications
• Standard dose XRT, 3,500 cGy; low dose, 2,500 cGy; total dose given to all involved areas
• Doses administered in fractions, 150–200 cGy per day/five times a week

CHEMOTHERAPY
Multiple agents allow different mechanisms of action (to circumvent resistance) and nonoverlapping toxicities so that full doses can be given.
• MOPP: mechlorethamine + vincristine (Oncovin) + procarbazine + prednisone
• COPP: cyclophosphamide substituted for mechlorethamine in MOPP (favored over MOPP, less AML, less sterility)
• COMP: methotrexate substituted for procarbazine in COPP
• ABVD: doxorubicin (Adriamycin) + bleomycin + vinblastine + dacarbazine
• DBVE: doxorubicin + bleomycin + vincristine + etoposide
• DBVE-PC: DBVE + prednisone + cyclophosphamide
• Each cycle consists of 21 to 28 days, dependent on toxicity. Some regimens alternate therapy (i.e., COPP alternating with ABVD), or use growth factor support to intensify schedule.
• Stages IA, IIA
—Attained full growth; no unfavorable signs: standard-dose XRT alone
—Still growing, bulky disease, or E lesions: (see staging) low dose XRT + two to four courses multiagent chemotherapy
• Stages IB, IIB, IIIA/B, IVA/B

—Attained full growth; no unfavorable signs: combined modality therapy with three to five courses multiagent chemotherapy + low-dose XRT
—Still growing or large mediastinal mass: low-dose XRT + chemotherapy (same as above)

 ## Follow-Up

• Office visits monthly with CBC
• CT scan of involved areas every 3 months for first 2 years, then every 6 months for 3 years
• Relapse of disease usually occurs within first 3 years. Some may relapse as late as 10 years after initial diagnosis.
• Special studies as needed for toxicity-related complications. For example:
—Yearly thyroid function tests if history of irradiation
—Regular self–breast examination for females treated with chest radiation
—Mammograms beginning by the age of 25 or 10 years post–chest radiation (whichever is earlier) in females
—Regular electrocardiograms, echocardiograms, and Holter monitors if treated with radiation or anthracyclines

LATE EFFECTS
• Radiation
—Pulmonary damage (radiation-induced)—pneumonitis, pulmonary fibrosis, decreased pulmonary function, pneumothorax
—Cardiac damage (XRT-induced)—cardiomyopathy resulting in CHF, pericarditis, valvular damage, coronary heart disease, and myocardial infarction
—Radiation nephritis
—Radiation-induced ovarian damage can be avoided by performing oophoropexy during laparotomy.
—Hypothyroidism, thyroid nodules, thyroid cancer
—Growth retardation with high doses of XRT (>3,500 cGy), resulting in a disproportionate alteration in sitting height versus standing height. Risk is highest during active bone growth (under 6 years of age and puberty).
—Secondary malignant neoplasms are a major concern in selecting therapy. One study showed the risk of second neoplasm 15 years after diagnosis was 7%, with breast cancer as the most common solid tumor. Other secondary neoplasms associated with treatment are thyroid and skin carcinomas, brain tumor, and malignant fibrous histiocytoma.
• Chemotherapy
—Pulmonary damage (bleomycin): pulmonary fibrosis, decreased pulmonary function
—Cardiac damage (Adriamycin): cardiomyopathy resulting in CHF, arrhythmias with conduction defects, pericarditis
—Azoospermia induced by alkylating agents is almost always permanent in postpubertal boys.

—Amenorrhea occurs in 20% of patients under 25 years using the MOPP regimen.
—Secondary malignant neoplasms—the risk of developing leukemia (AML) is highest when both radiotherapy and alkylating agents are used.
• Laparotomy, splenectomy
—Obstruction, sepsis

 ## Common Questions and Answers

Q: Is my child at risk for other cancers?
A: Yes. Although the incidence is low, children with Hodgkin disease are primarily at risk for cancers resulting from their treatment. Breast cancer is the most common solid tumor and can occur decades after therapy. Therefore, long-term follow-up is essential.

Q: Will my child be infertile following treatment?
A: It depends on the therapy he/she received. Certain chemotherapy agents are associated with a higher risk of infertility (alkylating agents). Radiation to the gonads is also associated with infertility.

BIBLIOGRAPHY
Aviles A, Soto B, Guzman R, et al. Results of a randomized study of early stage Hodgkin's disease using ABVD, EBVD, or MBVD. *Med Pediatr Oncol* 1995;24:171–175.

Bhatia S, Robinson LL, Oberlin O, et al. Breast cancer and other second neoplasms after childhood Hodgkin's disease. *N Engl J Med* 1996;334:745–751.

Bunin N, Meadows AT. Lymphomas in children. In: Holland JF ed. *Cancer medicine*, 3rd ed. Philadelphia: Lea & Febiger, 1993:2197–2206.

Leventhal BG, Donaldson SS. Hodgkin disease. In: Pizzo PA, Poplack DG, eds. *Principles and practice of pediatric oncology*, 2nd ed. Philadelphia: JB Lippincott, 1993:577–594.

Louw G, Pinkerton CR. Interventions for early stage Hodgkin's disease in children. *Cochrane Database of Systematic Reviews* 2000;2: CD002035.

Mack TM, Cozen W, Shibata DK, et al. Concordance for Hodgkin's disease in identical twins suggesting genetic susceptibility to the young-adult form of the disease. *N Engl J Med* 1995;332:413–418.

Ottlinger ME, Sallan SE, Rifai N, et al. Myocardial damage in doxorubicin-treated children: a study of serum cardiac troponin-T. *Proc Am Soc Clin Oncol* 1995;14:345.

Author: Jill P. Ginsberg
Deborah Kramer, 2nd edition

Human Immunodeficiency Virus Infection

 Database

DEFINITION

- HIV-1 and HIV-2 are the etiologic agents of HIV infection and the acquired immunodeficiency syndrome (AIDS).
- HIV infection is lifelong.
- For most infected individuals, a long clinically asymptomatic period (5–15 years in adults, frequently shorter in children), is followed by the development of generalized nonspecific signs and symptoms (weight loss, adenopathy, hepatosplenomegaly) and mild clinical immunodeficiency.
- Eventually, after progressive immunologic deterioration, patients are susceptible to a wide variety of opportunistic infections and cancers, which represent the clinical syndrome known as AIDS.

PATHOLOGY

- The HIV outer envelope protein has a strong affinity for cells that express the CD4 molecule, a protein that coats the surface of various normal cells, including specific T lymphocytes and macrophages. The virus attaches to the CD4 molecule, as well as a cytokine co-receptor. The virus then penetrates these cells, followed by transcription (using viral reverse transcriptase) of viral RNA into double-stranded DNA. This viral DNA is then integrated into the host cell genome and will remain there for the lifetime of the cell.
- Active viral replication continues after the primary infection. Even during the clinically latent period, more than 10^6 viral particles are produced daily. Over time, the host immune system loses the ability to contain viral replication and replace lost CD4 cells.

EPIDEMIOLOGY

- HIV infection is transmitted via:
—Sexual contact: male to female transmission more efficient than female to male; anal receptive sex more likely to transmit than vaginal sex.
—Exposure to infected blood: almost always involves parenteral exposure to infected blood (via transfusions or sharing needles). In occupational exposure, the risk of transmission from percutaneous exposure to needle contaminated with HIV-infected blood is 1/300.
—Breast milk: the overall risk of breast-feeding is about 15%. In countries where breast-feeding is the norm, up to 40% of perinatally acquired HIV infections occur through breast-feeding.
—Perinatally, either *in utero* or during labor and delivery. Of perinatally infected infants, 5% to 20% are believed infected *in utero*; the rest acquire the infection around the time of birth. The risk of an HIV-infected mother giving birth to an infected infant is approximately 20%, with increased rate of transmission for women with low CD4 counts or higher viral titers, and for those who were previously diagnosed with AIDS. In addition, vaginal delivery, especially with rupture of

membranes longer than 8 hours, appears to increase the risk of infant infection. The presence of untreated STDs, chorioamnionitis, and prematurity also all increase the risk of mother-to-child transmission of HIV.
- HIV is not believed to be transmitted by:
—Bites
—Sharing utensils, bathrooms, bathtubs
—Exposure to urine, feces, vomitus (except where these fluids may be grossly contaminated with blood, and even then transmission is rare, if at all)
—Casual contact in the home, school, or day-care center

COMPLICATIONS

- *Pneumocystis carinii* pneumonia (PCP): With a peak age of 3 to 9 months, PCP is the most common early fatal illness in HIV-infected children. In infancy, the mortality is 30% to 50% for the acute episode, with a median survival after first episode of less than 24 months. A high index of suspicion necessary for prompt diagnosis (by lavage) and initiation of therapy. 40% of new cases of HIV-related pediatric PCP involve infants not previously recognized as HIV-infected.
- Lymphocytic interstitial pneumonitis (LIP): Frequently asymptomatic, LIP can lead to slow onset of chronic respiratory symptoms. LIP causes a distinctive diffuse reticulonodular pattern on chest radiographs. Usually diagnosed between 2 and 4 years of age, LIP is related to dysfunctional immune response to EBV infection. Definitive diagnosis is made by lung biopsy. For symptomatic patients, prednisone is effective.
- Recurrent invasive bacterial infections: The risk of bacteremia is approximately 10%/year in HIV-infected children. Pneumococcal bacteremia is the most common invasive bacterial disease. Bacterial pneumonia, sinusitis, and otitis media are common among infected children.
- Progressive encephalopathy: Generally diagnosed between 9 and 18 months of age, the hallmark is progressive loss of developmental milestones or neurologic dysfunction. Cerebral atrophy is noted on CAT scan.
- Disseminated *Mycobacterium avium-intracellulare* (DMAC): DMAC occurs in older children, usually older than 5 years of age, with severe immunodeficiency (CD4 <100). Symptoms include prolonged fevers, abdominal pain, anorexia, and diarrhea.
- *Candida* esophagitis: As with DMAC, seen in older children with severe immunodeficiency. Patients usually present with dysphagia or chest pain. Oral thrush is noted on examination. Diagnosis suggested by findings on barium swallow. Definitive diagnosis made by biopsy.
- Disseminated CMV disease: Retinitis less common in HIV-infected children than in adults. CMV may also cause pulmonary disease, colitis, and hepatitis.
- HIV-related cancers: Non-Hodgkin lymphoma most common cancer, with primary site usually located in the CNS.

- Other organ dysfunction associated with HIV-infection in children: cardiomyopathy, hepatitis, renal disease, thrombocytopenia/ITP.

PROGNOSIS

Prior to the advent of aggressive combination therapies, data suggested a bimodal survival curve, with 25% of perinatally infected infants developing early symptomatic disease, with an AIDS diagnosis by 1 to 2 years of life and frequently dying by 3 years of age. The remaining 75% have a delayed onset of symptoms, usually after 5 years of age, and the median survival of this group was to 8 to 12 years old. Since the use of combinations of three or more drugs have become standard, morbidity and mortality are both greatly decreased. The median survival is now clearly into adolescence. In addition, the incidence of new opportunistic infections (AIDS signal illnesses) has decreased greatly, as have hospital admissions.

 Differential Diagnosis

- Neoplastic disease: lymphoma, leukemia, histiocytosis X
- Infectious: congenital/perinatal CMV, toxoplasmosis, congenital syphilis, acquired EBV
- Congenital immunodeficiency syndromes: Wiskott-Aldrich syndrome, chronic granulomatous disease

 Data Gathering

HISTORY

- Parental risk factors?
- Intravenous drug use?
- Noninjectable drug use?
- Sexually transmitted diseases, especially syphilis?
- Bisexuality?
- Transfusions before 1986?
- Frequent infections?
- Sinopulmonary infections?
- Recurrent pneumonia/invasive bacterial disease?
- Severe acute pneumonia (PCP)?
- Recurrent or resistant thrush, especially after 12 months of age?
- Congenital syphilis?
- Presence of STDs in an adolescent?
- Acquired microcephaly?
- Progressive encephalopathy, loss of developmental milestones?
- History of ITP/thrombocytopenia?
- Failure to thrive?
- Recurrent/chronic diarrhea?
- Recurrent/chronic enlargement of parotid gland?

Physical Examination

May be entirely normal in the first few months of life; 90% will have some physical findings by age 2. The most common findings are:
- Adenopathy, generalized
- Hepatosplenomegaly
- Failure to thrive
- Recurrent/resistant thrush, especially after 1 year of age
- Recurrent or chronic parotitis

Laboratory Aids

Test: ELISA antibody screen
Significance: For children over 18 months of age, repeatedly reactive ELISA antibody screen, followed by confirmation with Western blot analysis, is diagnostic of HIV infection. Any positive test should always be repeated before a definitive diagnosis is discussed with family. In first year of life, positive HIV ELISA and Western blot antibody tests simply confirm maternal infection, because the antibody test is IgG based, and maternal anti-HIV antibodies readily cross placenta. Maternal antibodies may remain detectable until 15 months of age.
Test: HIV blood culture and/or PCR DNA testing
Significance: Most reliable way of diagnosing HIV infection in infancy. The PCR test has slightly more false positives and false negatives; the blood culture is more expensive, takes longer to run, and is technically more difficult. Both tests have sensitivities and specificities greater than 95% when performed after 4 weeks of age.
Test: Elevated IgG levels
Significance: First observed immune abnormality noted in HIV-infected infants, generally reaching twice the normal values by 9 months of age.
Test: CD4 counts
Significance: Obtained at diagnosis and every 1 to 3 months. Results need to be evaluated on the basis of age-adjusted normal values. Absolute CD4 counts are elevated in childhood, with normal median values greater than 3,000/mm^3 in the first year of life, which then gradually decline with age, reaching values comparable with adult levels (800–1,000/mm^3) by age 7.
Test: Quantitative viral RNA PCR assays
Significance: Termed "viral loads," results are reported in a range from "undetectable," usually less than 40 copies/milliliter, to upper values over 10 million. Long-term prognosis is closely related to viral loads. Viral loads that remain over 100,000 are associated with poor short-term (2–5 year) outcomes. Also used as a marker of drug therapy, the goal is to suppress viral replication to the undetectable range, for as long as possible. About 40% to 50% of pediatric patients presently followed at tertiary sites have an undetectable viral load. Test is done at time of diagnosis, twice,

to establish baseline, and then 1 month after initiating, or changing therapies, and every 1 to 3 months thereafter.
Test: Neurologic evaluation, with psychometric testing, and an initial CAT scan/MRI screening for cerebral atrophy.
Significance: Should be repeated at yearly intervals.
Test: Postimmunization antibody levels
Significance: Assess B cell function.

Other frequent lab abnormalities include thrombocytopenia, anemia, and elevated liver enzymes.

Therapy

- Immunizations: All infected children receive standard childhood immunizations, including the recently approved pneumococcal conjugate vaccine. Infected children should receive yearly influenza A/B immunizations and the pneumococcal vaccine at age 2. Symptomatic children should not receive the varicella vaccine, and those with low CD4 counts should not receive the MMR.
- Antiretroviral therapy: Specific combination antiretroviral therapy delays progression of illness, promotes improved growth, and improves neurologic outcome. The standard of care now involves the administration of combination (usually three or more drugs) therapy. The most potent agents are those that inhibit viral protease (termed protease inhibitors). Drug regimens are complex, with as many as nine doses of medication a day. Adherence to prescribed schedules is critical. When patients miss even 20% to 25% of doses, the durability of response is short.
- Immune enhancement
—Passive: Recent studies suggest that monthly gamma globulin infusions decrease, somewhat, febrile episodes and pneumococcal bacteremia. The children who benefit the most are those with CD4 counts greater than 200/mm^3 and not on antibiotic prophylaxis for PCP or otitis media.
—Active: Studies continue on reconstitution of the immune system. Intravenous interleukin-2, given for 5 days every 8 weeks, has proven efficacy in increasing CD4 counts (above that achieved with antiretroviral therapy alone).
—Prophylaxis: One of the major advances in the care of HIV-infected children and adults has been the ability to offer prophylaxis against the most common opportunistic infections.

PREVENTION
- HIV infection is almost completely preventable. Educational efforts aimed at achieving behavior change is a key component of HIV-directed work.
- It is now possible to significantly decrease the risk to newborns of HIV-infected women. Prenatal ZDV therapy, followed by continuous IV ZDV therapy during labor, and treatment of the infant for the first 6 weeks of life have

been shown to decrease the risk of HIV infection in the infant from 20% to 8%. With the newer combination therapies, and delivery via elective cesarean section for selected cases, perinatal transmissions rates have now fallen below 2% to 3% in HIV-specialty care sites. Partly in response to these results, in 1995 both the CDC and AAP recommended that all pregnant women should receive counseling about the benefits of HIV testing, including the possibility of preventing fetal or infant infection, and should be offered HIV testing at the first prenatal visit.

Follow-Up

Psychosocial support for the family is critical. Because of the complexity of, and the rapidly changing, therapies available to treat pediatric HIV-infection, all infected patients should be co-managed with an HIV specialty care site.

PITFALLS
The result of failing to screen for HIV infection is the inability to offer antiretroviral therapy for pregnant women, therefore possibly preventing infant infection, and also the inability to prescribe PCP prophylaxis to infected newborns.

Common Questions and Answers

Q: Once the HIV-exposed infant has seroreverted to antibody negative status, how sure are we that he/she is uninfected?
A: With today's technology, if the child has also been PCR and/or HIV blood culture negative at least twice, and is clinically well, the chance that the child still harbors HIV is very low and appears to be less than 1/5,000. The child should continue to be followed by a health care provider aware of his/her past HIV antibody status. If clinical conditions warrant, retesting would be an option at a later date.

BIBLIOGRAPHY
Mofenson LM, and the Committee on Pediatric AIDS. Technical report: perinatal human immunodeficiency virus testing and prevention of transmission. *Pediatrics* 2001;106:1–12.

Perinatal HIV Guidelines Working Group. PHS Task Force recommendations for use of antiretroviral drugs in pregnant HIV-1 infected women for maternal health and interventions to reduce perinatal transmission in the United States. Revised May 4, 2001. Available at *http://www.hivatis.org*.

Working Group on Antiretroviral Therapy and Medical Management of HIV-1 infected children. Guidelines for the use of antiretroviral agents in pediatric HIV infection. *HIV Clin Trials* 2000;1:58–99. (Also available, and updated, on line, at *http:www.hivatis.org*.)

Author: Richard M. Rutstein

Hydrocephalus

 Database

DEFINITION

Hydrocephalus is the accumulation of cerebrospinal fluid (CSF) in the ventricles and subarachnoid spaces, leading to their enlargement.

CAUSES

• Developmental

—Chiari malformation, type II (associated with myelomeningocele; small posterior fossa; inferior displacement of medulla and cerebellum)
—Primary aqueductal stenosis
—Dandy-Walker malformation (absence of cerebellar vermis, small cerebellar hemispheres, enlarged posterior fossa, often with cystic fourth ventricle)
—Idiopathic

• Tumors of any histologic type located near the foramina or the aqueduct, or within the ventricular system
• Infection (meningitis) can lead to leptomeningeal adhesions and granulations.
• Intraventricular hemorrhage of prematurity or trauma-related) may result in a blood clot, meningeal adhesions, or granular ependymitis.

PATHOPHYSIOLOGY

• Normal pathway of CSF: choroid plexus, lateral ventricles, foramina of Monro, third ventricle, aqueduct of Sylvius, fourth ventricle, foramina of Luschka and Magendie, subarachnoid space, arachnoid granulations, venous circulation
• Hydrocephalus *often* involves obstruction to CSF flow or inadequate reabsorption, even in the rare case of choroid plexus papilloma (overproduction of CSF).
• Noncommunicating (obstructive) hydrocephalus: the obstruction is in the ventricular system.
• Communicating hydrocephalus: the problem is outside of the ventricular system; generally there is a problem with reabsorption.
• Although the noncommunicating/communicating distinction has traditionally been fundamental in the literature, it has no prognostic significance; the value of the distinction concerns choice of a site for palliative drainage, and etiologic considerations.

COMPLICATIONS

• Acute hydrocephalus

—*Herniation syndromes may be fatal*

• Chronic hydrocephalus

—Macrocephaly
—Spastic paraparesis may lead to gait and motor problems.
—Developmental delay

 Differential Diagnosis

• Other causes of macrocephaly:

—Familial macrocephaly
—Pericerebral effusions
—Congenital anomalies of intra- or extracerebral veins
—Achondroplasia
—Tumors, intracranial cysts
—Neurocutaneous syndromes
—Dysmorphic syndromes
—Primary megalencephaly
—Some leukodystrophies
—GM2 gangliosidosis
—Mucopolysaccharidoses
—Head-sparing intrauterine growth retardation (relative macrocephaly)
—Rapid catch-up growth following prolonged malnutrition

• Other causes of ventriculomegaly include brain atrophy and chronic ethanol or corticosteroid exposure (reversible)
• In "benign external hydrocephalus," both the ventricles and extraaxial CSF spaces are proportionately enlarged, and macrocephaly is common. A better nomenclature for this entity is "benign extraaxial collections of infancy" since they almost always a symptomatic and resolve spontaneously.

 Data Gathering

HISTORY

• Hydrocephalus is more common in preterm neonates in the intensive care nursery.
• Infants and children may also present to the primary pediatrician with new-onset hydrocephalus.
• Concerning complaints, especially in infants, include:

—Behavioral changes (especially decreased feeding and increased somnolence or irritability)
—Enlarging head (most often revealed by serial head circumference measurements)
—Vomiting

 Physical Examination

• Vital signs: The Cushing triad (hypertension, bradycardia, respiratory irregularities), which is characteristic of increased intracranial pressure, may be present in acute hydrocephalus (generally not in infants prior to sutural closure).
• HEENT: Increasing head circumference in infants. Fullness of the anterior fontanelle is neither sensitive nor specific for the diagnosis, but should be noted.
• Mental status: irritability in infants, behavioral changes in children (acute or chronic)
• Cranial nerves: Parinaud syndrome (setting-sun sign, paralysis of upward gaze), papilledema or optic atrophy, visual changes (chronic only)
• Motor: spastic paraparesis in chronic hydrocephalus
• Reflexes: increased in chronic hydrocephalus

 Laboratory Aids

TESTS

Imaging

• Head ultrasound

—Standard screening test for neonates with suspected hydrocephalus or intraventricular hemorrhage
—The anterior fontanelle must be patent for this test.
—Shows size of ventricles and presence or absence of blood; associated structures and anomalies

• Unenhanced CT of the brain

—Mainly used in infants and children whose anterior fontanelles have closed and postshunting
—Advantage compared to ultrasound: better visualization of fourth ventricle/brainstem, calcifications; standardized technique and better availability than ultrasound, especially in the emergency room setting.

• MRI

—Definitive test for analyzing brain anatomy
—Can identify developmental malformations such as Chiari and Dandy-Walker
—Rarely helpful in the early stage of diagnosis and management

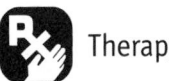 ## Therapy

Neurosurgeons' use of therapeutic lumbar or ventricular puncture has decreased in recent years. These procedures must be weighed against risk of herniation (decreased when sutures are open).

VENTRICULAR SHUNT

- Indication: progressive hydrocephalus
- Contraindications: active central nervous system infection, active intraventricular hemorrhage, and poor overall prognosis
- Components: ventricular catheter, reservoir (target of "shunt taps"), valve, distal catheter
- Distal sites: The peritoneum is the most common choice, pleura, ureter, and right atrium are other choices.
- Siphon effect: drop in ventricular pressure on sitting or standing, alleviated in newer shunt systems, such as the *Delta shunt*, by antisiphon devices that close the valve when there is excessive negative pressure in the distal catheter; rarely a problem in infants and children due to short distance between head and abdomen
- Complications:
- Obstruction is the most common, approximately 60% revision rate in first year; presents with same signs and symptoms as hydrocephalus
- Infections occur at a rate of 5+%/shunt manipulation and rarely present before 2 weeks or after 2 months relative to shunt operation; low-grade persistent fever and signs and symptoms of shunt malfunction predominate; rarely present with wound infections of following sepsis.

THIRD VENTRICLE FENESTRATION (THIRD VENTRICULOSTOMY)

- Background: An old procedure that had fallen out of favor with development of modern shunt systems
- Current status: New endoscopic techniques make this procedure useful in cases of isolated intraventricular obstruction.
- Pitfall: don't assume hydrocephalus is "cured." Although most failures occur shortly after procedure, delayed, unrecognized failures have resulted in death from acute hydrocephalus-related herniation.

 ## Follow-Up

- When the etiology or need for shunt placement may not be clear, it is important to follow clinical status, head circumference, and ventricular size (by head ultrasound or CT).
- Chronic hydrocephalus is often accompanied by spastic paraparesis, visual problems, and developmental delay.
- Most important interventions are supportive, including physical therapy, occupational therapy, and orthopedic therapies for spasticity; interdisciplinary cerebral palsy clinics can be critical in providing easy access to these resources. Special education programs may be appropriate for children with severe developmental delay.

PITFALLS

- It is important for long-term patients in intensive care nurseries to have head circumferences recorded at least twice weekly. Macrocephaly is not always obvious on visual inspection.
- Papilledema is a sign of chronic increased intracranial pressure, but its absence does not rule out this possibility.

—Head CT often will not show developmental malformations that may accompany hydrocephalus. MRI is the imaging procedure of choice.

—Timing of shunt placement is critical. A shunt placed too early may become infected or obstructed, while waiting too long may worsen permanent brain damage.

 ## Common Questions and Answers

Q: When does an infant need a head ultrasound?
A: Preterm infants below a certain gestational age or birth weight (varies from hospital to hospital) should all receive screening head ultrasounds while in the intensive care nursery, as well as any infant (inpatient or outpatient) whose head circumference crosses two percentile lines on the growth chart.

Q: When should an infant or child receive an MRI first rather than an ultrasound or CT?
A: Although MRI may be superior in many cases, the logistics of ordering the proper sequences and the need for sedation or anesthesia for long studies must be strongly considered. Consultation with a neurologist or neurosurgeon is generally advised.

Q: What is the workup for shunt obstruction and shunt infection?
A: Symptoms and signs of increased intracranial pressure should lead to a neurosurgical evaluation; frequently acquired studies include head CT (to assess ventricular size and placement of ventricular catheter), and shunt series (plains films of the entire shunt system to check for disruptions) and a tap of the shunt reservoir to ascertain pressures and patency. Fever is the most important indication for a shunt infection evaluation (shunt tap with CSF cell count, protein, glucose, Gram stain, and culture). Often patients will be evaluated for both complications.

ICD-9-CM 741.0

BIBLIOGRAPHY

Aicardi J. *Diseases of the nervous system in childhood.* Oxford: Blackwell Scientific, 1992.

Boockvar JA, Loudon W, Sutton LN. Development of the Spitz-Holter valve in Philadelphia. *J Neurosurg.* 2001;95(1):145–147.

Drake JM, Kestle J. Determining the best cerebral fluid shunt valve design: the Pediatric valve design trial. *Neurosurgery* 1996;38:604–607.

Guertin SR. Cerebrospinal shunts: evaluation, complications and crisis management. *Pediatr Clin North Am* 1987;34:203–217.

McLone DG, ed. *Pediatric neurosurgery.* Philadelphia: WB Saunders, 2000:455–559.

Veyrac C, Couture A, Saguintaah M, et al. Brain sonography in 2001. Evaluation of macrocrania in the infant. *J Radiol* 2001;82 (6 suppl):717–725.

Author: Peter B. Kang
Peter Bingham, 2nd edition

Hydronephrosis

 Database

DEFINITIONS
- Hydronephrosis—Dilation of the renal pelvis (pelviectasis) and calyces (calyectasis) due to excess urine in the collecting system of the kidney
- Hydroureteronephrosis—Dilation of the renal collecting system and the ureter to the level of the bladder

ETIOLOGIES
- Ureteropelvic junction (UPJ) obstruction: Hydronephrosis caused by either an intrinsic narrowing of the UPJ or external compression of the UPJ from accessory renal vessels. For more information see Ureteropelvic Junction Obstruction.
- Ureterovesical junction (UVJ) obstruction: Hydroureteronephrosis caused by either an intrinsic narrowing or an aperistaltic segment of distal ureter. These are also called megaureters. These ureters enter the bladder in a normal position on the trigone.
- Vesicoureteral reflux (VUR): The reflux of urine from the bladder into the ureter during filling or voiding. In primary reflux (grades I–V depending on the severity) it is due to an insufficient flap valve type mechanism at the ureterovesical junction. Hydroureteronephrosis is usually seen only with higher grades of reflux (grades III–V) or secondary reflux. Secondary reflux is reflux in the presence of an abnormal bladder, in which the reflux is often due to high storage or voiding pressures within the bladder. Secondary reflux is not graded.
- Ureterocele: Hydroureteronephrosis due to obstruction of the ureter from a cystic dilation of the intravesical portion of the distal ureter. These are most often associated with the upper pole ureter in a duplicated collecting system. They are less frequently associated with a single system. The ureterocele is further classified as an intravesical (contained completely within the bladder) or ectopic (extending down the bladder neck and often into the urethra).
- Ectopic ureter: A ureter that drains into an abnormal location away from the trigone. The hydroureteronephrosis can be the upper pole ureter of a duplicated collecting system or a single system. Ectopic ureters can drain at various sites along the lower urinary tract depending on the sex of the child. In boys they can be located in the bladder neck, prostatic urethra, vas deferens, seminal vesicle or epididymis. In girls they can be located in the bladder neck, urethra, introitus, and vagina. The ectopic locations often require passage through the bladder neck or urogenital diaphragm, which produces obstruction of the distal ureter.
- Stone disease: Obstructing calculi often produce dilation of the urinary tract proximal to its location. Stone disease is rare in infancy. The hydronephrosis is nearly always associated with renal colic.
- Posterior urethral valves (PUV): Hydroureteronephrosis, nearly always bilateral, produced by outflow obstruction of the bladder from valve leaflets in the prostatic urethra. Since both kidneys are affected, there is a significant risk of chronic renal insufficiency and development of end-stage renal disease.
- Triad syndrome (TS): Hydroureteronephrosis, often with massively dilated ureters, and a large bladder. The disorder is also known as prune belly syndrome or Eagle-Barrett syndrome. These boys have a triad of hypoplastic abdominal wall musculature (leading to a prune-like appearance), bilateral undescended testes, and a dilated urinary tract. Many have associated urethral atresia, which imparts a worse prognosis for renal function. The exact cause of TS remains elusive. There is a significant risk of renal insufficiency in these patients. A similar syndrome may occur in girls with a prune-like appearance to the abdomen and anomalies of the urogenital tract; however, it is very rare.
- Other rare causes—retrocaval ureter, pelvic tumor, ureteral valves, and cloacal malformation with hydrocolpos.

EPIDEMIOLOGY
- Incidence of genitourinary abnormalities noted on routine prenatal ultrasound is 0.2%.
- 87% of these are antenatally detected hydronephrosis/hydroureteronephrosis.
- 75% of fetuses with hydronephrosis are due to UPJ obstruction.
- Perinatal mortality associated with hydronephrosis has ranged from 13% to 72%, but is most strongly correlated with the presence of chromosomal abnormalities, multiple system abnormalities, detection earlier in gestation, oligohydramnios, and evidence of infravesical obstruction.
- PUV and TS account for 6% of cases.

 Differential Diagnosis

- Cystic renal tumor—most commonly Wilms tumor. These should be distinguished from hydronephrosis by ultrasound or CT scanning.
- Multicystic dysplastic kidney—can be difficult to distinguish from severe hydronephrosis with marked parenchymal thinning. A renal scan will show no function or perfusion with a multicystic dysplastic kidney.

 Data Gathering

HISTORY
Newborns
- Antenatal hydronephrosis: presence of hydronephrosis or hydroureteronephrosis.
- Whether unilateral or bilateral and timing during gestation. If unilateral, timing and severity of hydronephrosis and the status of contralateral kidney.
- Presence of bladder wall thickening, bladder enlargement, bladder emptying, or a

dilated posterior urethra (keyhole sign) may indicate PUV or TS.
- If oligohydramnios is present, pulmonary hypoplasia is a concern. The presence of oligohydramnios, increased renal echogenicity, and cystic changes in the kidneys point toward poor renal function postnatally.

Older Children
- History of urinary tract infections or gross hematuria
- General health and growth (poor growth with chronic renal insufficiency)
- Daytime incontinence, poor urinary stream, or symptoms of voiding dysfunction may be an indicator of bladder dysfunction due to PUV.
- History of episodic abdominal (which may not lateralize well), flank, or back pain in the presence of hydronephrosis is often due to symptomatic UPJ obstruction (see Ureteropelvic Junction Obstruction).

 Physical Examination

- Neonate: Signs of oligohydramnios (Potter facies, lateral patellar dimples, clubfeet, and other limb deformities) and respiratory distress.
- Palpable abdominal mass. Palpable walnut-shaped bladder (PUV). Patent urachus. Development of abdominal wall musculature (wrinkled prune-like appearance in TS).

Older Children
- Presence of abdominal mass. Abdominal or flank tenderness.

 Laboratory Aids

LABORATORY TESTS
Newborn
- Hydronephrosis or hydroureteronephrosis with a normal contralateral kidney does not require any immediate laboratory testing.
- If both kidneys are affected or a solitary kidney is affected, there is a need for serial assessments of renal function (serum electrolytes and creatinine).

Older Children
- Urinalysis to detect hematuria or pyuria.
- Culture if infection suspected. In cases where both kidneys are affected or there is a solitary kidney, renal function should be evaluated.

IMAGING
Antenatally Hydronephrosis
- Infants with antenatally detected hydronephrosis typically are evaluated with three imaging studies:
—Renal/bladder ultrasound
—Voiding cystourethrogram
—Renal scan
- The timing can be elective for a unilateral lesion with a normal contralateral kidney, but if both kidneys are affected or a solitary kidney is involved, then prompt evaluation of the newborn should be undertaken.

- Renal/bladder ultrasound
—Because of a period of relative oliguria of a newborn in the first 24 to 48 hours of life, an ultrasound may underestimate the degree of hydronephrosis during this time and thus should be postponed until the infant is at least 48 hours old. This should not preclude evaluating an infant during this time as long as a normal study is repeated in 4 to 6 weeks.
—In cases where both kidneys were affected or there is a solitary affected kidney, the evaluation should not be delayed. Ultrasound of the kidneys should reveal the severity of dilation of the renal pelvis and calyces, changes in the amount and echogenicity of the parenchyma, and presence of cortical cysts. The evaluation of the full bladder is important as well. It will show dilated distal ureters, which may indicate a UVJ obstruction, VUR, or hydroureteronephrosis from PUV or TS.
- Voiding cystourethrogram (VCUG)
—Evaluates for the presence of VUR
—Allows for the grading of the severity of reflux as well
—The shape of the bladder, presence of diverticulum, and trabeculations may indicate hypertrophy from PUV, neurogenic bladder dysfunction, or voiding dysfunction (in older children).
—Test can be delayed until after discharge from the nursery unless there is concern about posterior urethral valves, in which case it should be performed in the early postnatal period.
- Renal scan: The two most commonly used radionuclides are 3-mercaptoacetyl triglycine (MAG-3) and diethylenetriamine pentaacetic acid (DTPA). MAG-3 (excreted by the tubules) is a better choice for the immature kidneys in infants.
—Very useful in detecting a kidney with significantly reduced function in the presence of a normal contralateral kidney. If both kidneys are affected, this information is less reliable, since both kidneys can have reduced function yet have a differential split of close to 50% each.
—In addition to the ability to detect diminished function, the drainage of the kidney can be quantitatively assessed. If there is poor drainage of the affected kidney, furosemide is given when the radiotracer reaches its maximum level of accumulation in an attempt to wash out the radiotracer. The time for washing out half of the accumulated radiotracer ($T_{1/2}$) is often given in the report. A prompt $T_{1/2}$ (less than 10 minutes) washout time is indicative of a nonobstructed kidney. A slower washout time may be indicative of obstruction when it is greater than 20 minutes. An intermediate time (10–20 minutes) is indeterminate. Many factors affect the reliability of the $T_{1/2}$ for indicating obstruction such as the hydration status, presence of VUR, and the overall function of the kidney (very poorly functioning kidneys have a poor response to diuretics).
- Intravenous pyelogram (IVP)
—This study is most useful for evaluating the anatomy of the kidney and the ureters.

—Also a useful test for evaluating an older child with intermittent symptoms of abdominal or flank pain
—Can be diagnostic of an intermittent UPJ obstruction as the cause of the child's pain
- CT scan: Most commonly done in cases where the hydronephrosis is symptomatic. A noncontrast spiral CT is the most sensitive way to detect stones, as even those radiolucent stones on plain films (uric acid) will be detected.
- MRI: Currently has a limited role in evaluating hydronephrosis, but gadolinium-enhanced MRI has been used with increasing frequency, primarily in pilot studies.

 Therapy

- Neonates with hydronephrosis are started on prophylactic antibiotics (one fourth the therapeutic dose given once a day) of amoxicillin. When the baby is 3 months old the antibiotic can be changed to trimethoprim/sulfamethoxazole or nitrofurantoin.
- UPJ obstruction: After initial evaluation, the infants are usually followed with serial studies, either ultrasound or renal scans, depending on the degree of functional impairment, the severity of the hydronephrosis, and the pattern of drainage on the renal scan. From more information see Ureteropelvic Junction Obstruction.
- UVJ obstruction: After initial evaluation these children are followed with serial studies as with UPJ obstruction. These lesions are much less common than UPJ obstruction and the majority of the time the affected kidneys have normal function and can be followed conservatively. If the function of the kidney is significantly diminished (differential function of 35–40%), surgical relief of the obstruction is indicated. Depending on the age of the child and the size of the distal ureter the child will be treated with a temporary cutaneous ureterostomy followed by reimplantation or a ureteral reimplantation alone.
- Vesicoureteral reflux: Infants with reflux are kept on prophylactic antibiotics. In the absence of breakthrough infections they are reevaluated annually. If persistent high-grade reflux continues or breakthrough infections are a problem, surgical correction is performed. For more information see Vesicoureteral Reflux.
- Ureterocele: Since ureteroceles are obstructive lesions, they are generally treated surgically early in life. Most commonly, the ureterocele is endoscopically punctured for decompression. If there is little to no function of the affected renal unit and there is no reflux, either nephrectomy or heminephrectomy (depending on single vs. duplex collecting system) may be alternatively performed. A subset of patients, especially those with reflux, may need a bladder level procedure at a later date (usually excision of the ureterocele with ureteral reimplantation).

- Ectopic ureter: obstructive lesion is treated surgically. If there is a reasonable amount of function in the affected unit reconstruction can be performed by either a temporary ureterostomy followed by ureteral reimplantation or, if there is a duplicated collecting system, a uretero-ureterostomy (anastomosing the ectopic ureter to the nonectopic one). If there is very poor to no function, then a nephrectomy or heminephrectomy (depending on single vs. duplex collecting system) may be alternatively performed.
- Posterior urethral valves (PUV): Full-term infants undergo valve ablation, whereas preterm infants may require a temporary vesicostomy until endoscopic treatment is feasible. These boys require careful follow-up from a pediatric urologist and nephrologist as they grow up. For more information see Posterior Urethral Valves.
- Triad syndrome (TS): Typically these boys will undergo bilateral orchiopexy with or without an abdominoplasty depending on the severity of the hypoplasia of the abdominal wall during the first 6 to 12 months of life.

 Common Questions and Answers

Q: If my baby has hydronephrosis affecting only one kidney, will he need a kidney transplant?
A: In the absence of oligohydramnios and bilateral hydroureteronephrosis, it would be a very rare event that a child would develop renal failure requiring transplantation.
Q: My unborn baby has hydronephrosis in only one kidney, and the other kidney is normal. What are the chances that it is a UPJ obstruction?
A: The chances are about 75% that isolated hydronephrosis will be due to a UPJ obstruction.
Q: My male unborn baby has bilateral hydroureteronephrosis but a "normal" bladder. Is there still a chance that he has PUV?
A: Yes. Although it is less likely to be due to PUV than if a thick-walled, enlarged, poorly emptying bladder were seen, ultrasound could miss dilated ureters and more subtle bladder abnormalities.

BIBLIOGRAPHY
Bauer SB. Anomalies of the kidney and ureteropelvic junction. In: Walsh PC, Retik AB, Vaughan ED, et al., eds. Philadelphia: W.B. Saunders. *Campbell's urology*. 1998: 1708–1755.

Mandell J, Peters CA, Retik AB. Perinatal urology. In: Walsh PC, Retik AB, Vaughan ED, et al., eds. *Campbell's urology*. 1998:1601–1618.

Roth JA, Diamond DA. Prenatal hydronephrosis. *Curr Opin Pediatr* 2001;13(2):138–141.

Authors: J. Christopher Austin and Michael C. Carr

Hyperimmunoglobulinemia E Syndrome

 Database

DEFINITION

Hyperimmunoglobulinemia E syndrome is a rare disorder characterized by markedly elevated serum IgE levels, chronic eczematoid dermatitis, and recurrent infections.

PATHOPHYSIOLOGY

The syndrome is poorly understood; the following abnormalities have been noted in subgroups of patients:

- Phagocytic: impaired chemotaxis
- T cell: impaired proliferative response to antigens
- B cell: variable heterogeneity of ability to form antibodies to antigens

 Differential Diagnosis

- Atopic dermatitis
- Wiskott-Aldrich syndrome
- Chronic granulomatous disease

 Data Gathering

HISTORY

- Recurrent infection: otitis media, pneumonia, sinusitis, subcutaneous abscesses, pneumatoceles
- Organisms that cause infection: *Staphylococcus aureus, Candida, Haemophilus influenzae, Streptococcus pneumoniae,* group A streptococcus
- Severe eczematoid dermatitis as early as 1 week of age

 Physical Examination

- Coarse facial features, broad nasal bridge, prominent nose
- Growth retardation can occur with recurrent illnesses.
- Osteoporosis complicated by recurrent fractures

Laboratory Aids

TEST

- Eosinophilia: peripheral eosinophils, >500 cells/mL
- Quantitative immunoglobulins: IgG, IgA, IgM usually normal, but IgE elevated, usually >5,000 IU/mL
- IgE antibodies against *S. aureus*
- Functional antibodies to diphtheria, tetanus, HIB, and pneumococcus results are variable, but there is a subgroup of patients who are unable to mount an appropriate antibody response to these antigens.
- Pulmonary function tests to evaluate extent of lung disease from infections such as pneumatoceles

 Therapy

- Supportive, based on clinical and laboratory findings
- Lifelong use of antistaphylococcal therapy (i.e., dicloxacillin or Augmentin at therapeutic doses)
- Surgical intervention for management of pneumatoceles for drainage or secondary to compression of nearby parenchyma
- IVIG as replacement therapy for abnormal functional antibodies is usually given at 400 g/kg on a monthly basis.

 Follow-Up

Long-term outcome is unknown; it depends on a timely diagnosis that allows for close monitoring and aggressive treatment of infections. Sequelae from recurrent infections such as pneumonias and pneumatoceles can result in a debilitating course. An increased chance of malignancy has been reported in some cases.

 Common Questions and Answers

Q: Is this disease also referred to as Job syndrome?
A: Yes, because Job suffered from difficulties with boils and other skin manifestations.

ICD-9-CM 279.3 (UNSPECIFIED)

BIBLIOGRAPHY

Amman AJ. Phagocytic dysfunction diseases. In: Stites DP, Terr AI, eds. *Basic and clinical immunology*. Norwalk, CT: Appleton & Lange, 1991:356–360.

Douglas SD, Campbell DE. The hyperimmunoglobulinemia E-recurrent infection syndrome. *Clin Immunol Newsletter* 1984;5:86–87.

Lavoie A, Rottem M, Grodofsky MD, et al. Anti-staphylococcus aureus IgE antibodies for diagnosis of hyperimmunoglobulinemia E-recurrent infection syndrome in infancy. *Am J Dis Child* 1989;143:38–104.

Leung DYM, Geha RS. Clinical and immunologic aspects of the hyperimmunoglobulin E syndrome. *Hematol Oncol Clin North Am* 1988;2(1):81–97.

Marone G, Florio G, Triggiani M, et al. Mechanisms of IgE elevation in HIV-1 infection. *Crit Rev Immunol* 2000;20(6):477–496.

Sheerin KA, Buckley RH. Antibody response to protein, polysaccharide, and Ox174 antigens of the hyperimmunoglobulinemia E syndrome. *J Allergy Clin Immunol* 1991;87(4):803–811.

Author: Michelle M. Klinek

Hyperinsulinism/Hypoglycemia

 Database

DEFINITION

Hyperinsulinism (HI) is a disorder of dysregulated insulin secretion characterized by excessive and/or inappropriate insulin secretion resulting in hypoglycemia.

CAUSES

Mutations in four genes that lead to defects in early signaling events in beta cells have now been identified as being associated with HI: the sulfonylurea receptor (*SUR1*) or its associated inwardly rectifying potassium channel (*Kir6.2*), glucokinase, and glutamate dehydrogenase. These mutations result in uncoupling of insulin secretion from the glucose-sensing machinery of the pancreatic beta cell, and inappropriate insulin secretion even in the face of low blood glucose. The most common and severe forms of HI arise from *SUR1* and/or *Kir6.2* mutations, which can manifest in focal or diffuse disease. Transient HI may be caused by perinatal stress (maternal hypertension, precipitous delivery, or hypoxia).

PATHOLOGY

The histologic appearance of the pancreata from affected children can be subdivided into two major forms:

• Diffuse HI, which bears some characteristics of nesidioblastosis (increased number of beta cells arising from ductular epithelium), and also demonstrates nuclear enlargement.
• Focal HI, generally easily recognized as a discrete region of adenomatous hyperplasia, with a surrounding normal-appearing pancreas.

Normal histology can also be found in cases of HI.

GENETICS

• Autosomal recessive form: defect of sulfonylurea receptor (SUR) or KATP channel (*Kir6.2*) at chromosomal locus 11p14-15.1 resulting in diffuse involvement throughout the pancreas (diffuse disease).
• A nonmendelian mode of inheritance through loss of short arm of maternal chromosome 11 in a patient carrying a mutant *SUR1* on the paternal allele. The loss of maternally expressed tumor suppressor genes creates the first "hit," and expression of a mutant paternal allele creates the second "hit," resulting in clonal expansion of abnormally regulated beta cells, focal areas of adenomatosis (focal disease).
• Autosomal-dominant variant: some may have an activating mutation in the glucokinase gene
• Hyperinsulinism with hyperammonemia variant: autosomal-dominant and sporadic forms, due to activating mutations of glutamate dehydrogenase (GDH) enzyme at regulatory guanosine triphosphate (GTP)-binding site

EPIDEMIOLOGY

• Most common cause of persistent or recurrent hypoglycemia in children beyond the immediate neonatal period
• Annual incidence estimated at about 1:40,000–50,000 live births
• May be as high as 1:2,500 in select populations (Saudi Arabians, Ashkenazi Jews)

COMPLICATIONS

• Severe refractory hypoglycemia
• Cognitive deficits, especially short-term memory, visual-motor integration, and arithmetic skills
• Seizures
• Coma
• Permanent brain damage
• Glucose intolerance or frank diabetes mellitus after treatment

PROGNOSIS

• Historically, over 50% patients sustained severe brain damage from hypoglycemia.
• Today the prognosis is somewhat more favorable, provided hypoglycemia is avoided.
• Glucose intolerance: diabetes may develop later in life, especially postpancreatectomy.

 Differential Diagnosis

• Sepsis
• Congenital heart disease
• Infant of diabetic mother (IDM)
• Beckwith-Wiedemann syndrome (BWS)
• Panhypopituitarism
• Respiratory distress syndrome
• Erythroblastosis fetalis
• Other inborn errors of metabolism

 Data Gathering

HISTORY

Symptoms of hypoglycemia in the infant:

• Poor feeding
• Hypotonia
• Lethargy
• Cyanosis
• Tachypnea
• Tremors
• Seizures
• Early-morning irritability that responds to feeding

 Physical Examination

Finding: Macrosomia
Significance: Suggests autosomal-recessive SUR defect variant

Finding: Absence of macroglossia, umbilical hernia, visceromegaly
Significance: Suggest BWS

Finding: Normal palate and genitalia
Significance: Cleft palate or micropenis suggests hypopituitarism.

Laboratory Aids

Finding: Inappropriately elevated insulin level (>2 μU/mL on newer assays) at time of hypoglycemia
Significance: Indicates uncoupling of insulin secretion from ambient glucose concentration

Finding: Suppressed levels of free fatty acids and ketones at time of hypoglycemia:

- Free fatty acid level <0.5 mM
- β-Hydroxybutyrate level <1.1 mM

Significance: Indirect signs of excessive insulin action

Finding: Glycemic response to glucagon (blood sugar rise >30 mg/dL) at time of hypoglycemia
Significance: Sign of inappropriately stored glycogen at time of hypoglycemia (sign of excessive insulin action)

Finding: Suppressed insulin-like growth factor binding protein-1 (IGFBP-1) level
Significance: IGFBP-1 production is inhibited by insulin (sign of excessive insulin action)

Finding: Abnormal response to insulin secretagogues calcium, leucine, and tolbutamide during acute insulin responses.
Significance: Patients with mutations in the *SUR1/Kir6.2* genes respond to calcium; diffuse form does not respond to tolbutamide, whereas focal disease typically does. Patients with hyperinsulinism/hyperammonemia syndrome demonstrate abnormal response to leucine.

Finding: Elevated ammonia levels
Significance: Suggests hyperinsulinism/hyperammonemia syndrome

Finding: Normal growth hormone, cortisol, and thyroxine levels
Significance: Excludes hypopituitarism

 ## Therapy

- The major goal is prevention of brain damage by controlling blood glucose.

—Parenteral dextrose infusions to stabilize blood sugar acutely
—Supplemental oral or nasogastric feeds
—Diazoxide, a suppressant of insulin secretion, at 10 to 15 mg/kg/d divided q12h
—Octreotide, a long-acting somatostatin analog, at 5 to 20 μg/kg/d divided q6h or given by continuous subcutaneous infusion
—Glucagon, at 0.5–1.0 mg/day by continuous intravenous infusion, may stabilize blood glucose levels in preparation for surgery.
—Subtotal pancreatectomy in those children refractory to medical therapy or in those with focal lesions

- Diet

—Frequent feedings and avoidance of long fasts
—Avoidance of protein loads in those with hyperinsulinism/hyperammonemia, as high-protein diets may stimulate insulin secretion.

 ## Follow-Up

- Home blood glucose monitoring, especially with longer fasts or intercurrent illnesses
- Hospitalizations for intravenous glucose infusions may be necessary during intercurrent illnesses with vomiting.
- Follow-up fasting studies may be needed to evaluate safety and/or disease regression.
- Close observation of linear growth is necessary, because octreotide can suppress GH secretion

 ## Common Questions and Answers

Q: What is the chance of hyperinsulinism in the sibling of an affected child?
A: Twenty-five percent in the autosomal-recessive type; as high as 50% in the autosomal-dominant type.

Q: How low and for how long can glucose go before brain damage occurs?
A: Hypoglycemia is traditionally defined as glucose less than 40 mg/dL, but glucose concentrations should be maintained greater than 55 to 60 mg/dL, the level at which symptoms of hypoglycemia typically occur. The duration of hypoglycemia necessary for brain damage to occur is unknown.

Q: What is the chance that it will eventually resolve without surgery?
A: Only approximately 40% to 50% of cases are controlled with medication alone. Patients with mutations in *SUR1* and/or *Kir6.2* genes may be more likely to require surgery, and in those patients with focal disease, surgery may be curative.

ICD-9-CM 251.1

BIBLIOGRAPHY

De Lonlay P, Fournet J-C, Rahier J, et al. Somatic deletion of the imprinted 11p15 region in sporadic persistent hyperinsulinemic hypoglycemia of infancy is specific of focal adenomatous hyperplasia and endorses partial pancreatectomy. *J Clin Invest* 1997;100: 802–807.

Ferry RJ, Kelly A, Grimberg A, et al. Insulin responses to peripheral intravenous and intrahepatic arterial calcium stimulation in diffuse vs. focal forms of congenital hyperinsulinism due to mutations of the SUR1 sulfonylurea receptor. *J Pediatr* 2000;137: 239–246.

Glaser B, Kesavan P, Heyman M, et al. Familial hyperinsulinism caused by an activating glucokinase mutation. *N Engl J Med* 1998;338(4):226–230.

Grimberg A, Ferry RJ, Kelly A, et al. Dysregulation of insulin secretion in children with congenital hyperinsulinism due to sulfonylurea receptor mutations. *Diabetes* 2001;50:322–328.

Nestorowicz A, Inagaki N, Gonoi T, et al. A nonsense mutation in the inward rectifier potassium channel gene, Kir6.2, is associated with familial hyperinsulinism. *Diabetes* 1997;46:1743–1748.

Stanley CA. Hyperinsulinism in infants and children. *Pediatr Clin North Am* 1997;44: 363–374.

Stanley CA, Baker L. Hyperinsulinism in infants and children: Diagnosis and therapy. *Adv Pediatr* 1976;23:315–355.

Stanley CA, Lieu YK, Hsu BY, et al. Hyperinsulinism and hyperammonemia in infants with regulatory mutations of the glutamate dehydrogenase gene. *N Engl J Med* 1998;338:1352–1357.

Thomas PM, Cote GJ, Wohlik N, et al. Mutations in sulfonylurea receptor gene in familial persistent hyperinsulinemic hypoglycemia of infancy. *Science* 1995;268: 426–429.

Thornton PS, Satin-Smith MS, Herold K, et al. Familial hyperinsulinism with apparent autosomal dominant inheritance: clinical and genetic differences from the autosomal recessive variant. *J Pediatr* 1998;132:9–14.

Verkarre V, Fournet JC, de Lonlay-Debeney P, et al. Paternal mutation of the sulfonylurea receptor (SUR1) gene and maternal loss of 11p15 imprinted genes lead to persistent hyperinsulinism in focal adenomatous hyperplasia. *J Clin Invest* 1998;102: 1286–1291.

Weinzimer SA, Stanley CA, Berry GT, et al. A syndrome of congenital hyperinsulinism and hyperammonemia. *J Pediatr* 1997;130: 661–664.

Authors: Stuart A. Weinzimer and Diva D. Ng

Hyperlipidemia

 Database

DEFINITION

Hyperlipidemia refers to serum elevations of cholesterol, triglycerides, and lipoprotein. Total cholesterol consists of very low density lipoprotein (VLDL), low-density lipoprotein (LDL), and high-density lipoprotein (HDL).

• Normal serum concentrations:

—Total cholesterol: 170 mg/dL (borderline, 170–199 mg/dL)
—LDL cholesterol: 110 mg/dL (borderline, 110–129 mg/dL)
—Total triglycerides: 100 mg/dL (borderline, 100–140 mg/dL)

• Primary hypercholesterolemia or hypertriglyceridemia (hyperlipidemia): elevation in serum cholesterol as a result of an inherited disorder of lipid metabolism (i.e., familial hypercholesterolemia)
• Secondary hypercholesterolemia or hypertriglyceridemia: elevation in serum cholesterol as a result of another disease process (i.e., nephrotic syndrome)

PATHOPHYSIOLOGY

Primary hypercholesterolemia:

• Familial hypercholesterolemia (FH): defect of LDL receptor, resulting in the body's inability to properly utilize circulating LDL cholesterol
• Familial hypertriglyceridemia (FHTG): a severe elevation in serum triglycerides; can be associated with lipoprotein lipase deficiency or apolipoprotein C-II deficiency

GENETICS

• Familial hypertriglyceridemia (FHTG): dominantly inherited disorder
• Familial hypercholesterolemia (FH): dominantly inherited defect of LDL receptor
• Familial combined hyperlipidemia (FCHL): dominantly inherited lipid disorder

EPIDEMIOLOGY

The incidence of familial hypercholesterolemia homozygotes is 1 in 1,000,000; heterozygotes, 1 in 500, with unknown cause resulting in hypercholesterolemia and/or hypertriglyceridemia occurring in 2% of the population

COMPLICATIONS

Hypercholesterolemia has been linked to premature coronary artery disease and vascular disease. Severe hypertriglyceridemia can cause pancreatitis. The presence of significant atherosclerotic vessel disease is unusual in most children; however, it can occur in the first decade of life in children with homozygous familial hypercholesterolemia.

PROGNOSIS

• Familial hypercholesterolemia:

—Homozygotes: coronary artery disease in first or second decade of life
—Heterozygotes: 50% of males develop premature heart disease by age 50 (females, age 60)

• Familial combined hyperlipidemia: occurs in 1% to 2% of the population and accounts for 10% of all premature heart disease. A reduction of LDL cholesterol by 1% reduces risk by 2%.

 Differential Diagnosis

• Hypercholesterolemia

—Primary hypercholesterolemia (see above)
—Hypothyroidism
—Nephrotic syndrome
—Liver disease (cholestatic)
—Renal failure
—Anorexia nervosa
—Acute porphyria
—Myelomatosis
—Medications (antihypertensives, estrogens, steroids, microsomal enzyme inducers, cyclosporine, diuretics)
—Pregnancy
—Dietary: excessive dietary intake of fat, cholesterol and/or calories

• Hypertriglyceridemia

—Primary hypertriglyceridemia (see above)
—Acute hepatitis
—Nephrotic syndrome
—Chronic renal failure
—Medications (diuretics, retinoids, oral contraceptives)
—Diabetes mellitus
—Alcohol abuse
—Lipodystrophy
—Myelomatosis
—Glycogen storage disease
—Dietary: excessive dietary intake of fat and/or calories

 Data Gathering

HISTORY

Question: Is there a family history of premature heart disease?
Significance: Almost all cases of primary hyperlipidemia are of dominant inheritance; thus, questions should be asked regarding the occurrence of premature heart disease and hyperlipidemia in parents and grandparents.

Question: Does your child smoke?
Significance: Smoking reduces HDL cholesterol levels and increases the risk of vascular disease.

Question: Does your daughter use oral contraceptives?
Significance: Birth control pills have been shown to cause elevations in lipoprotein levels and, when coupled with already elevated lipid levels, can increase the risk of atherosclerosis.

Question: Does your child exercise regularly?
Significance: Lower levels of cholesterol and triglycerides are generally found in children and adolescents who are physically fit.

 Physical Examination

• Eye examination:

—Arcus corneae: deposits of cholesterol, resulting in a thin, white circular ring located on the outer edge of the iris

• Skin examination:

—Tendon xanthomas: thickened tissue surrounding the Achilles' and extensor tendons
—Xanthelasma: yellowish deposits of cholesterol surrounding the eye
—Palmar xanthomas: pale lines in creases of palms
—Eruptive xanthomas: characteristic of hypertriglyceridemia; papular yellowish lesions with a red base that occur on the buttocks, elbows, and knees.

Laboratory Aids

TESTS

• Fasting serum lipoprotein levels: total cholesterol, HDL cholesterol, and triglycerides

—Determine the type of hyperlipidemia

• Calculated LDL cholesterol: LDL cholesterol = total cholesterol − [HDL cholesterol + triglycerides/5]

—Determines the level of LDL cholesterol chemistry panel (ALT, AST, Bili, BUN, creatinine, urinalysis)
—Screening test for liver and kidney disease

• Thyroid evaluation (T_4, TSH)

—Determines the presence of hypothyroidism
—Three-day diet history
—Evaluates dietary intake of calories and cholesterol with 3-day diet

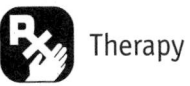

Therapy

GENERAL MEASURES

Outpatient management unless secondary hyperlipidemia caused by liver or renal failure, which would necessitate inpatient management of primary illness
Note: The cause of secondary hyperlipidemia should be treated with disease-specific therapy to affect a reduction in elevated lipid levels.

FOR PRIMARY HYPERLIPIDEMIA

Dietary management (recommended dietary intake):

• Total calories: age-appropriate to promote normal growth (do not limit children <3 years)
• Total fat: <20% total fat <30% of calories
• Saturated fat: 10% of calories
• Cholesterol: up to 100 mg/1,000 calories
• Protein: approximately 15% to 20% of calories
• Carbohydrates: approximately 55% of calories

NOTE: Hypertriglyceridemia almost always responds to strict dietary management (10–15 g/d of fat) and weight loss.

RISK FACTORS

The following are factors that contribute to heart disease:

• Smoking
• Excessive weight gain: <110% ideal body weight
• Hypertension
• Diabetes mellitus
• Low HDL cholesterol (35 mg/dL)
• Physical inactivity (bedridden)
• Family history of premature heart disease (55 years of age)

Patient education: Instruct patients on risk factors of premature heart disease, American Heart Association STEP I diet, and the need for adequate exercise and routine follow-up. *Note:* Therapy is indicated if hyperlipidemia is caused by a dominantly inherited lipid disorder and the child is over 10 years of age and either LDL cholesterol greater than 190 mg/dL after dietary trial (6 months) or LDL cholesterol greater than 160 mg/dL after dietary trial and two or more additional risk factors exist. When drug therapy is considered, a referral to a pediatric lipid specialist is necessary.

DRUG OF CHOICE

Cholestyramine (bile acid resins) is the drug of choice for the initial treatment of primary hypercholesterolemia. It is not indicated for hypertriglyceridemia. It is contraindicated in patients with biliary obstruction or in patients with prior allergic reaction. All causes of secondary hyperlipidemia should be ruled out before starting therapy. Side effects include foul taste, constipation, nausea, and possible vitamin K deficiency. Cholestyramine may reduce or delay the absorption of concomitant oral medications secondary to drug binding.

ALTERNATIVE DRUGS

• Statin group of drugs—Pravachol, lovastatin, Zocor etc. (HMG-CoA reductase inhibitor)—is an effective drug in adults and may prove to be beneficial in children in the future. Side effects include hepatitis and myositis.
• Niacin in megavitamin doses has been effective in the reduction of both serum LDL cholesterol and triglycerides; however, side effects occur in more than 50% of individuals, including flushing, itching, and headache.
• Experimental gene therapy has been shown to be effective in an animal model for familial hypercholesterolemia and may be the treatment of choice in the future for genetic disorders of lipid metabolism; it has been used recently in adult patients.

Follow-Up

For patients with primary hyperlipidemia who are off medication, follow-up should be performed every 1 to 2 years with lipoprotein profile evaluation. For those patients on medication, follow-up should be conducted every 3 months.

PREVENTION

• Avoid other risk factors (see above).
• Limit dietary intake of fat and cholesterol (see above).
• Increase exercise.
• Become educated about heart disease and atherosclerosis.

POSSIBLE COMPLICATIONS

• Hypercholesterolemia

—Premature heart disease
—Stroke
—Carotid artery disease

• Hypertriglyceridemia

—Pancreatitis

CLINICAL PEARLS

Serum total cholesterol is inaccurate when serum triglycerides are greater than 400 mg/dL.

ICD-9-CM 272.4

BIBLIOGRAPHY

Havel RJ. Approach to the patient with hyperlipidemia. *Med Clin North Am* 1982;66:319.

National Cholesterol Education Program. Report of the Expert Panel on Blood Cholesterol Levels in Children and Adolescents. *Pediatrics* 1992;89(suppl): 525–584.

Newman WP, Freedman DS, Voors AW, et al. Relation of serum lipoprotein levels and systolic blood pressure to early atherosclerosis: the Bogalusa Heart Study. *N Engl J Med* 1986;314:138.

Poskitt EME, ed. *Practical paediatric nutrition.* London: Butterworths, 1988.

Shamir R, Lerner A, Fisher EA. Hypercholesterolemia in children. *Isr Med Assoc J* 2000;2(10):767–771.

Author: Chris A. Liacouras

Hypertension

Database

DEFINITION

Hypertension is average systolic and/or diastolic blood pressures above the 95th percentile for age and gender as defined by the Second Task Force on Blood Pressure Control in Children. References now include norms based on the patient's age, gender, and height percentile. The final determination should be based on at least three measurements obtained on separate occasions. The significance of this definition with regard to morbidity and mortality is unclear.

PATHOPHYSIOLOGY

Hypertension is either primary (essential) or secondary. Secondary causes, with examples, include:

- Renal: acute glomerulonephritis, chronic renal failure, polycystic kidney disease, reflux nephropathy
- Renovascular: fibromuscular dysplasia, neurofibromatosis, vasculitis
- Cardiac: coarctation of the aorta
- Endocrine: pheochromocytoma, neuroblastoma, glucocorticoid-remediable aldosteronism
- Neurologic: increased intracranial pressure, Guillain-Barré syndrome
- Drugs: corticosteroids, oral contraceptives, sympathomimetics, illicit drugs (cocaine, phencyclidine)
- Other: obesity, burns, traction

GENETICS

Primary hypertension is more likely to develop in individuals when there is a strong family history. The genetics of secondary causes depend on the condition (e.g., polycystic kidney disease: autosomal dominant, autosomal recessive; neurofibromatosis: autosomal dominant; glucocorticoid-remediable aldosteronism: autosomal dominant).

EPIDEMIOLOGY

Primary hypertension is the most common cause of hypertension in adolescents and adults. Various rates of hypertension in children have been reported, from 1.2% to 13%, but less than 1% appear to require medication. African-American adults have a greater incidence of hypertension. Racial differences in children, however, are not seen until after age 12. Tracking (i.e., determining the risk of adult hypertension based on earlier blood pressure measurements) is not reliable in children.

COMPLICATIONS

- Congestive heart failure
- Renal failure
- Encephalopathy (seizures)
- Retinopathy

PROGNOSIS

The patient's prognosis depends on the underlying cause of the hypertension. It is excellent if the blood pressure is well controlled.

Differential Diagnosis

The initial objective after diagnosing hypertension in children is distinguishing primary from secondary causes. Generally, the younger the child and more elevated the blood pressure measurements, the more likely the cause of hypertension is secondary.

Data Gathering

HISTORY

Question: Is there a family history of hypertension?
Significance: Hypertension may be familial.

Question: Do you have symptoms of headache or blurry vision?
Significance: These are signs of increased intracranial pressure.

Question: Do you have chest pain?
Significance: This may indicate hypertensive heart disease or decreased coronary blood flow.

Question: Do you have epistaxis, weight gain or loss?
Significance: These are other signs of hypertension.

Question: Salt intake?
Significance: Excessive salt in diet may contribute to hypertension.

Question: Do you have flushing?
Significance: Flushing may be a sign of pheochromocytoma.

Question: Do you have a history of urinary tract infections?
Significance: Infections can be associated with reflux nephropathy and hypertension.

SPECIAL QUESTIONS

- Medical history: umbilical artery line, urinary tract infection
- Medications: corticosteroids, cold preparations, oral contraceptives, illicit drugs
- Family history: hypertension, phakomatosis, endocrinologic disorders
- Trauma: AV fistula, traction
- Review of symptoms: other systemic diseases

Physical Examination

- Body habitus: thin, obese, growth failure, virilized, stigmata of Turner or Williams syndrome
- Skin: café-au-lait spots, neurofibromas, rashes
- Head: moon facies, cranial bruits
- Eyes: funduscopic changes, proptosis
- Lungs: rales
- Heart: rub, gallop, murmur
- Abdomen: mass, hepatosplenomegaly, bruit
- Genitalia: ambiguous, virilized
- Neurologic: Bell palsy

Laboratory Aids

TESTS

Ambulatory blood pressure monitoring may be helpful in cases where the diagnosis of hypertension is uncertain (white-coat hypertension, labile hypertension).
The laboratory evaluation to determine the etiology of hypertension should proceed in a stepwise fashion.

- All patients should have:

—Urinalysis, urine culture
—Serum electrolytes, BUN, creatinine, calcium, uric acid, cholesterol
—CBC
—Echocardiogram: the most sensitive study to monitor end-organ changes
—Renal ultrasound

- Further evaluation, based on history, physical examination, and/or to prove secondary causes, includes:

—Voiding cystourethrogram
—DMSA renal scan
—Urine for catecholamines and metanephrines
—Plasma renin activity
—Aldosterone levels

- More invasive studies include:

—Renal angiogram
—Renal vein renin concentrations
—MIBG (metaiodobenzylguanidine) scan
—Renal biopsy

Therapy

- Mild primary hypertension may be managed with nonpharmacologic treatment: weight reduction, exercise, sodium restriction, avoidance of certain medications.
- Pharmacologic therapy should be directed to the cause of secondary hypertension when this is known or for severe, sustained hypertension. Medications may be needed in children with mild-to-moderate hypertension if nonpharmacologic therapy has failed or if end-organ changes are present.
- Classes of antihypertensive agents include alpha- and beta-blockers, diuretics, vasodilators (direct and calcium channel blockers), and angiotensin-converting enzyme (ACE) inhibitors.
- Other *specific therapies* include surgery (renovascular hypertension, coarctation of the aorta), percutaneous transluminal angioplasty (renovascular hypertension), and dialysis (chronic renal failure).

Follow-Up

The reduction of blood pressure with medication should be gradual to avoid side effects. The medications themselves cause adverse effects, such as exercise intolerance (beta-blockers), headaches (vasodilators), cough, angioedema, and renal insufficiency (ACE inhibitors), and hypokalemia (diuretics). Certain classes of medication should be avoided in patients with specific conditions, such as asthma and diabetes (beta-blockers) and bilateral renal artery stenosis (ACE inhibitors).

PITFALLS

- Use the proper cuff size. The inflatable bladder should completely encircle the arm and cover approximately 75% of the upper arm. A cuff that is inappropriately small will artifactually increase the measurement.
- ACE inhibitors and beta-blockers alter plasma renin activity levels.
- Several medications, such as labetalol, can affect an MIBG scan.
- Avoid multiple medications with the same mechanism of action.
- Elicit a history of adverse effects and adjust medications accordingly.
- If patients feel the medication is making them feel ill, they will discontinue it themselves.
- Attempt to wean medication intermittently.

Common Questions and Answers

Q: How does licorice cause hypertension?
A: British licorice contains glycyrrhizinic acid, a mineralocorticoid-like substance that causes sodium retention, potassium wasting, and hypertension. This substance is not found in most commercially available licorice in the United States.

Q: What percentage of children have renovascular causes for their hypertension?
A: Studies looking at the etiology of hypertension indicate that 10% to 24% of children may have a renovascular cause. Children under 5 years of age are four times more likely to have renal artery stenosis than are adolescents.

Q: What are the indications for invasive studies such as angiography?
A: This decision should be individualized and based on the severity of the hypertension, response to medication, the clinical presentation (e.g., neurofibromatosis), and results of other studies. In general, young children and all children with severe, unexplained hypertension should be completely evaluated.

Q: Can adolescents with elevated blood pressure compete in sports?
A: Adolescents with hypertension should be encouraged to participate in athletics if their blood pressures are well controlled. The use of stress testing in this population is controversial.

ICD-9-CM 401.9 (UNSPECIFIED)

BIBLIOGRAPHY

Bartosh SM, Aronson AJ. Childhood hypertension. An update on etiology, diagnosis, and treatment. *Pediatr Clin North Am* 1999;46:235–252.

Daniels SR. Hypertension in childhood. *Pediatr Rev* 1997;18:331.

Fivush B, Neu A, Firth S. Acute hypertensive crises in children. *Curr Opin Pediatr* 1997;9:233–236.

Rosner B, Prineas RJ, Loggie JMH, et al. Blood pressure nomograms for children and adolescents, by height, sex, and age, in the United States. *J Pediatr* 1993;123:871–876.

Sinaiko AR. Hypertension in children. *N Engl J Med* 1996;335:1968–1973.

Sorof JM. Portman RJ. Ambulatory blood pressure monitoring in the pediatric patient. *J Pediatr* 2000;136:578–586.

Author: Seth L. Schulman

Hypoparathyroidism

 Database

DEFINITION

Hypoparathyroidism is decreased parathyroid hormone (PTH) effect.

PATHOPHYSIOLOGY

- Diminished or absent PTH activity results in:

—Hypocalcemia and hyperphosphatemia
—Reduced vitamin D activation to $1,25(OH)_2$-vitamin D
—Hypocalcemia leads to increased neural excitability.

- Hypoparathyroidism

—Transient
  —Fetal parathyroid suppression: maternal hypercalcemia, diabetic mother
  —Hypomagnesemia: direct effects (suppressed PTH secretion, increased PTH resistance)
  —Alcohol intoxication

—Congenital
  —Familial: X-linked recessive, autosomal dominant, autosomal recessive
  —Sporadic and isolated
  —DiGeorge syndrome: parathyroid gland hypoplasia, thymic hypoplasia/aplasia, facial abnormalities, aortic arch and cardiac defects

—Acquired
  —Postsurgical
  —Postirradiation
  —Following severe burns
  —Type 1 polyglandular autoimmune disease (Blizzard syndrome): hypoparathyroidism associated with chronic mucocutaneous candidiasis and autoimmune adrenal insufficiency; can also have diabetes mellitus, lymphocytic thyroiditis, hypogonadism, pernicious anemia, chronic hepatitis
  —Iron deposition: thalassemia, hemochromatosis
  —Copper deposition: Wilson disease
  —Metastatic carcinoma
  —Miliary tuberculosis

- Pseudohypoparathyroidism: resistance to PTH

—Albright hereditary osteodystrophy: G protein mutation

GENETICS

- X-linked recessive: neonatal onset
- Autosomal-dominant and autosomal-recessive forms

—Chromosome 3q13: mutations in the calcium-sensing receptor gene
—Chromosome 11p: mutations in the PTH gene
—Chromosome 22q11: DiGeorge syndrome
—Chromosome 21q22: Type 1 polyglandular autoimmune disease
—Chromosome 20q13: Albright hereditary osteodystrophy

- Mitochondria diseases: Kearns-Sayre syndrome (hypoparathyroidism and deafness)

EPIDEMIOLOGY

Many normal neonates can have hypocalcemia (serum calcium less than 8 mg/dL) during the first 3 weeks of life due to physiologic transient hypoparathyroidism.

- Parathyroid gland immaturity can lead to deficient PTH release and exaggerated normal fall in serum calcium concentration during the first 3 days of life.
- Relative immaturity of renal phosphorus handling and response to PTH can lead to late neonatal hypocalcemia precipitated by a high phosphate diet (cow's milk–based formulas).

COMPLICATIONS

- Hypocalcemia can cause tetany, arrhythmias, seizures, and respiratory arrest.
- Long-standing untreated hypoparathyroidism and pseudohypoparathyroidism can lead to intracranial calcifications, especially in the basal ganglia. These may cause extrapyramidal signs (e.g., chorioathetosis, dystonic spasms, parkinsonism). Cognitive impairment and psychiatric disturbances can also be seen.

PROGNOSIS

Fair; long-term outcome: development of nephrocalcinosis resulting in renal insufficiency

 Differential Diagnosis

HYPOCALCEMIA

- Vitamin D deficiency
- Vitamin D–dependent rickets type I and II
- Hyperphosphatemia
- Prematurity
- Acute pancreatitis
- Malignancy: osteoblastic metastases, tumor lysis syndrome
- Medication: citrated blood products, phenobarbital, Dilantin, phosphate

 Data Gathering

HISTORY

- In neonates: maternal calcium and magnesium abnormalities, maternal diabetes
- Family history of calcium disorders
- Medications
- Recurrent infections
- Recurrent muscle cramps
- Paresthesias

 Physical Examination

- Chvostek sign: Facial nerve stimulation (tapping anterior of external auditory meatus) causes contraction of orbicularis oris, producing upper lip or mouth twitch.
- Trousseau sign: Inflation of blood pressure cuff reduces the blood flow to peripheral motor nerves and thereby can elicit carpopedal spasm in latent tetany.
- Carpopedal spasm
- Laryngeal stridor
- Mental status changes
- Irritability
- Papilledema
- Cataracts
- Bradycardia, hypotension
- Dry skin, coarse hair, brittle nails
- Albright hereditary osteodystrophy (pseudohypoparathyroidism type Ia): short stature, round face, thick neck, barrel chest, obesity, subcutaneous calcifications, brachydactyly (short 4th metacarpal bones)

Laboratory Aids

TESTS

Laboratory Tests

- Total and ionized serum calcium concentrations: low
- Serum phosphorus concentration: elevated in hypoparathyroidism; low in rickets
- Serum magnesium concentration: rule out hypomagnesemia
- Albumin: assess calcium binding (if cannot get ionized calcium)
- Intact PTH levels
- 25-OH- and 1,25(OH)$_2$-vitamin D levels: distinguish hypoparathyroidism from rickets
- Urinary calcium-to-creatinine ratio: low in idiopathic hypoparathyroidism, higher (almost equal to normocalcemic controls) in calcium ion-sensing receptor gain-of-function mutations
- Urinary cyclic AMP response to PTH: diagnostic test if concerned about pseudohypoparathyroidism; otherwise, not routinely done

Imaging

- Chest x-ray: rachitic rosary (rickets), absence of thymus (DiGeorge syndrome)
- Head CT: intracranial calcifications are associated with chronic hypoparathyroidism and pseudohypoparathyroidism

False Positives

- Hypomagnesemia

Therapy

DRUGS

Titrate therapy to maintain serum calcium concentrations greater than 8.0 mg/dL. In cases requiring lifelong therapy, compromise for serum calciums in the 8- to 9-mg/dL range to decrease the long-term risk for developing nephrocalcinosis.

- 1,25(OH)$_2$-vitamin D: less than 1 year: 0.04 to 0.08 μg/kg/d; 1 to 5 years: 0.25 to 0.75 μg/d; greater than 6 years and adults: 0.5 to 2.0 μg/d.
- Calcium: Dose depends on preparation and on patient needs.

DURATION

For life

DIET

Unrestricted

Follow-Up

Regularly with the endocrinologist

WHEN TO EXPECT IMPROVEMENT

Immediately

SIGNS TO WATCH FOR

- Patients with acute, severe hypocalcemia should be placed on telemetry to monitor for cardiac arrhythmias (especially prolonged QTc).
- Muscle cramps
- Carpopedal spasms
- Seizures

Common Questions and Answers

Q: Is the thyroid also involved?
A: No.

Q: Are seizures common?
A: Yes, seizures are a common presentation of hypoparathyroidism in childhood, and physiologic transient hypoparathyroidism is the most common cause of neonatal seizures.

Q: Can hypoparathyroidism be associated with other abnormalities?
A: Yes. Investigate neonates at the time of diagnosis for cardiac defects and thymic aplasia (DiGeorge syndrome), and monitor patients with hypoparathyroidism for development of other autoimmune endocrinopathies and chronic mucocutaneous candidiasis (type 1 polyglandular autoimmune disease).

Q: When should IV versus oral calcium supplementation be used?
A: IV calcium supplementation provides the quickest correction of hypocalcemia and is therefore useful in severe cases (seizures, stridor, tetany, cardiac arrhythmias) or in the initiation of therapy (as you await establishment of adequate vitamin D levels, which are necessary for enteral calcium absorption). Switch to oral calcium supplementation as soon as possible to reduce the risk of potential IV calcium-mediated venous sclerosis and tissue extravasation.

ICD-9-CM 252.1

BIBLIOGRAPHY

Bassett JH, Thakker RV. Molecular genetics of disorders of calcium homeostasis. *Baillieres Clin Endocrinol Metab* 1995;9:581–608.

Betterle C, Greggio NA, Volpato M. Clinical review 93: autoimmune polyglandular syndrome type 1. *J Clin Endocrinol Metab* 1998;83:1049–1055.

Cuneo BF, Driscoll DA, Gidding SS, et al. Evolution of latent hypoparathyroidism in familial 22q11 deletion syndrome. *Am J Med Genet* 1997;69:50–55.

Eronocodelu Y, Bober E, Tunnessen W Jr. Picture of the month. Albright hereditary osteodystrophy. *Arch Pediatr Adolesc Med* 1997;151:1263–1264.

Gertner JM. Disorders of calcium and phosphorus homeostasis. *Pediatr Clin North Am* 1990;6:1441–1465.

Guise TA, Mundy GR. Evaluation of hypocalcemia in children and adults. *J Clin Endocrinol Metab* 1995;5:1473–1478.

Klein GL, Langman CB, Herndon DN. Persistent hypoparathyroidism following magnesium repletion in burn-injured children. *Pediatr Nephrol* 2000;14:301–304.

Kowdley KV, Coull BM, Orwoll ES. Cognitive impairment and intracranial calcification in chronic hypoparathyroidism. *Am J Med Sci* 1999;317:273–277.

Levine MA. Pseudohypoparathyroidism: from bedside to bench and back. *J Bone Miner Res* 1999;14:1255–1260.

Marx SJ. Hyperparathyroid and hypoparathyroid disorders. *N Engl J Med* 2000;343:1863–1875.

Yamamoto M, Akatsu T, Nagase T, et al. Comparison of hypocalcemic hypercalciuria between patients with idiopathic hypoparathyroidism and those with gain-of-function mutations in the calcium-sensing receptor: is it possible to differentiate the two disorders? *J Clin Endocrinol Metab* 2000;85:4583–4591.

Author: Adda Grimberg
Paulo F. Collett-Solberg, 2nd edition

Hypoplastic Left Heart Syndrome

 Database

DEFINITION

Hypoplastic left heart syndrome (HLHS) is a continuum of congenital cardiac defects resulting from severe underdevelopment of the structures of the left side of the heart: left atrium, mitral valve, left ventricle, aortic valve, and ascending aorta.

PATHOPHYSIOLOGY

The etiology of HLHS appears multifactorial, most likely resulting from either an *in utero* reduction of left ventricular inflow or outflow (mechanisms postulated include premature closure of the foramen ovale and fetal cardiomyopathy). As a result, the right ventricle (RV) must supply both the pulmonary and the systemic (via the ductus arteriosus) circulations before and after birth. The reduction in pulmonary vascular resistance that occurs with lung expansion at birth reduces the proportion of RV output to the systemic circulation. If the ductus arteriosus closes, shock may occur.

GENETICS

• Familial inheritance:

—Sibling recurrence risk (0.5%), although some kinships have a frequency approaching autosomal-dominant transmission.
—Other forms of congenital heart disease (CHD) (13.5%)

• Male predominance (67%)
• Definable genetic disorder (10–28%)

—Turner syndrome, Noonan syndrome, Smith-Lemli-Opitz syndrome, Holt-Oram syndrome
—Trisomy 13, 18, 21, or other microdeletion syndromes
—Major extracardiac anomalies (diaphragmatic hernia, omphalocele, and hypospadias)

EPIDEMIOLOGY

• 0.16 to 0.36 per 1,000 live births
• 8% of CHD; third most common cause of critical CHD in the newborn
• 23% of all neonatal mortality from CHD

COMPLICATIONS (NEONATAL PRESENTATION)

• Circulatory collapse with resultant metabolic acidosis
• Multiorgan system failure (i.e., necrotizing enterocolitis, renal failure, liver failure, CNS injury)

PROGNOSIS

• Fatal if untreated (95% within the first month of life)
• 90% early survival after stage I palliation if treated in a timely fashion at experienced institutions
• 5% mortality at hemi-Fontan (bidirectional cavopulmonary) procedure
• Recently, 1% to 3% mortality at Fontan operation (with the addition of a fenestration to allow right-to-left shunting)
• Excluding infants that die waiting for a donor organ, 5-year actuarial survival for either staged palliation (Fontan) or heart transplantation is similar, approximately 70% to 75%.

 Differential Diagnosis

• Cardiac: other causes of circulatory collapse in the neonate include critical aortic stenosis and coarctation of the aorta, cardiomyopathy (infectious, metabolic, or hypoxic), intrauterine supraventricular tachycardia, obstructive cardiac neoplasms, and large arteriovenous fistulae.
• Noncardiac: infant septicemia, respiratory distress syndrome

 Data Gathering

HISTORY

• Respiratory distress (tachypnea, grunting, flaring, retractions)
• Cyanosis
• Cardiovascular collapse and profound metabolic acidosis when the ductus closes

 Physical Examination

• Congestive heart failure (tachycardia, hepatomegaly, gallop)
• Normal S_1 and single S_2 (A_2 absent), a murmur of tricuspid regurgitation may be auscultated
• Varying degree of cyanosis
• Decreased perfusion and weak peripheral pulses

 Laboratory Aids

TESTS

• CXR: varying degree of cardiomegaly with increased pulmonary vascular markings (if atrial septum is intact, lungs will appear hazy with pulmonary venous obstructive pattern)
• ECG: right axis deviation (+90 to +210 degrees), RVH with qR pattern in right precordial leads, paucity of left ventricular forces with rS pattern in left precordial leads
• Echocardiogram: diagnostic procedure, demonstrating varying degrees of hypoplasia or atresia of the mitral valve, left ventricle, aortic valve, ascending aorta, and aortic arch; PDA with right-to-left shunt in systole and diastolic flow reversal; ± ASD with left-to-right flow
• Cardiac catheterization: no longer routinely performed; similar findings as with echocardiography

Hypoplastic Left Heart Syndrome

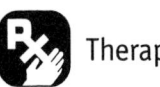 Therapy

MEDICAL

- The preoperative goal is to balance the systemic and pulmonary circulation provided by the right ventricle to a Qp/Qs (ratio of pulmonary to systemic blood flow) of about 1:1, usually achieved with a pulse oximetry measurement of 75%.
- Prostaglandin E_1 infusion: 0.05 to 0.1 $\mu g/kg/min$
- Aggressive treatment of metabolic acidosis with fluid boluses, bicarbonate, and/or THAM
- 21% Fio_2, goal Pao_2 of 35 to 40 mm Hg
- Careful use of small amount of inotropic agents (in cases of sepsis or RV failure). Aggressive use of inotropic agents (alpha effect) may worsen systemic perfusion.

SURGICAL

- Palliative surgery is generally performed in three stages:

—Stage I (Norwood) palliation (performed in first few days of life or soon after presentation): involves transection of main pulmonary artery with anastomosis of the augmented aortic arch to the pulmonary valve stump to form a neo-aortic valve and arch, placement of an aortic-to-pulmonary shunt (modified Blalock-Taussig shunt) and often an atrial septectomy. The RV continues to provide both systemic and pulmonary blood flows.
—Hemi-Fontan procedure: involves anastomosis of the superior vena cava to the pulmonary artery, resulting in volume unloading of the RV. All prior shunts are usually removed.
—Modified-Fontan procedure: baffling the inferior vena cava to the pulmonary artery with placement of a small fenestration in the baffle, permitting a small residual right-to-left shunt. The RV is now supplying only systemic blood flow

- There are many surgical modifications on these three procedures. In addition, these procedures may be performed at different ages based on an institution's experience. Our approach has been to perform the hemi-Fontan operation around 6 months of age and the Fontan operation near the age of 2 years.
- Orthotopic heart transplantation may be performed either as an initial approach or after a stage I palliation.

SUPPORTIVE

While surgical intervention has become the medical standard, supportive measures are sometimes offered especially when multiple noncardiac congenital anomalies exist or when serious multiorgan system damage is present.

 Follow-Up

Interval pediatric evaluations should include careful consideration of growth parameters, cardiovascular symptoms, and developmental milestones. Examinations should focus on the presence or absence of cyanosis, edema, pleural effusions, and arrhythmia.
For Fontan patients, frequent echocardiograms and intermittent cardiac catheterizations may be needed to assess:

- RV dysfunction
- Aortic arch obstruction
- Branch pulmonary artery narrowing
- Collateral formation causing excessive cyanosis
- Protein-losing enteropathy
- Sinus node dysfunction
- Atrial arrhythmias

If the patient instead underwent heart transplantation, other lifelong issues should be addressed:

- Graft rejection and/or coronary vasculopathy
- Infection
- Hypertension
- Lymphoproliferative diseases

PITFALLS

During initial resuscitation and stabilization of a newly diagnosed infant:

- *Avoid using oxygen despite low pulse oximetry saturation.* Increasing Fio_2 will lower pulmonary vascular resistance and increase blood flow to the lungs, which are already "overcirculated," shunting blood away from the systemic circulation and worsening systemic perfusion.
- *Avoid overventilating the infant.* Carbon dioxide is a pulmonary vasoconstrictor and may improve systemic perfusion by decreasing pulmonary perfusion. Maintain mildly elevated $Paco_2$ levels (40–50 mm Hg).

 Common Questions and Answers

Q: What is the usual pulse oximetry reading for a child with HLHS?
A: 75% to 80% after stage 1 palliation, 80% to 85% after a hemi-Fontan, and 92% to 95% after the fenestrated Fontan.

Q: What is the usual medical therapy employed at various stages?
A: Lifelong SBE prophylaxis. Digoxin and furosemide are generally used until the hemi-Fontan. Afterload reduction (i.e., captopril) may be used to reduce the workload on the heart at any stage. Antiplatelet (i.e., aspirin) and anticoagulant (i.e., Coumadin) therapy are used by most physicians after stage 1 and later in light of the low-flow state of the cavopulmonary connections. For transplant patients, immunosuppressive regimens are managed differently according to institution preferences.

ICD-9-CM 746.7

BIBLIOGRAPHY

Barber G. The hypoplastic left heart syndrome. In: Garson A, Bricker TJ, Fisher DJ, et al., eds. *The science and practice of pediatric cardiology*, 2nd ed. Baltimore: Williams & Wilkins, 1998:1625–1645.

Bove EL. Current status of staged reconstruction for hypoplastic left heart syndrome. *Pediatr Cardiol* 1998;19(4):308–315.

Mahle WT, Clancy RR, McGaurn SP, et al. Impact of prenatal diagnosis on survival and early neurologic morbidity in neonates with the hypoplastic left heart syndrome. *Pediatrics* 2001;107(6):1277–1282.

Tworetzky W, McElhinney DB, Reddy VM, et al. Improved surgical outcome after fetal diagnosis of hypoplastic left heart syndrome. *Circulation* 2001;103(9):1269–1273.

Williams DL, et al. Hypoplastic left heart syndrome: Valuing the survival. *J Thorac Cardiovasc Surg* 2000;119:720–731.

Author: Michael P. Mulreany
David Bush, 2nd edition

Hypospadias

 Database

DEFINITION

Hypospadias is the incomplete development of the anterior urethra due to a failure of the urethral folds to unite over and cover the urethral groove.

GENETICS

- Increased incidence in monozygotic twins (8.5-fold that in singletons).

—Reported mutations include defects in the androgen receptor, 5α-reductase II defects, alterations in homeobox genes, although these are found only in a minority of patients.

ETIOLOGY

- Polygenic/multifactorial
- Higher familial incidence
- Proposed theories include:

—Estrogenic environmental contamination
—Pressure of the fetal limbs on developing penis
—Insufficient HCG in placenta
—Abnormality in androgen metabolism as a local manifestation of a systemic endocrinopathy

EPIDEMIOLOGY

- 1/250 to 1/300 live male births

—Incidence
    —With affected father—8%
    —With affected brother—14%
    —With 2 or more affected family
    members—21%

—Unexplained increase in incidence since the 1970s
—Higher prevalence in Italian and Jewish populations

 Differential Diagnosis

- Ambiguous genitalia, namely severely masculinized female pseudohermaphroditism

Approach to the Patient

HISTORY

- Important to inquire about

—Other affected family members
—Other congenital anomalies

- Increased incidence of cryptorchidism, inguinal hernia

—May be associated with an enlarged utricle, complicating urethral catheter placement.

 Physical Examination

- Incomplete foreskin
- Distal urethral pit on glans
- Chordee (ventral curvature of penis)

—Localize meatal position by pulling outward on ventral penile shaft skin. Record position as glanular; coronal; distal, middle, or proximal shaft; penoscrotal; or perineal
—Important to document position of testes

 Laboratory Aids

- Karyotype in patients with bilateral undescended testes and hypospadias, may also be obtained in cases of unilateral undescended testis and hypospadias.

IMAGING

- If there is a question of ambiguous genitalia, pelvic ultrasound or cystography may be indicated.
- There is no need for imaging in cases of routine, isolated hypospadias.

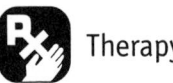 ## Therapy

• If the patient has a very small penis, he may benefit from hormonal stimulation preoperatively.

—Surgical repair is usually performed in the first year of life.
—Mild glandular hypospadias may not need surgery.
—Type of repair depends on position of meatus and degree of chordee.
—Tubularized incised plate
—Meatal advancement
—Onlay island flap
—Tubularized island flap
—90% success rate for all one-stage repairs
—Potential complications include
  —Urethrocutaneous fistula
  —Urethral diverticulum
  —Urethral stricture
  —Unacceptable cosmetic outcome

 ## Follow-Up

• Compressive dressing for 2 days, removed by parents at home
• Indwelling urethral catheter/stent remains for about 2 weeks
• Postoperative visit at 2 weeks to remove catheter

PITFALLS

Newborn circumcision is absolutely contraindicated

 ## Common Questions and Answers

Q: Does the patient with hypospadias routinely have other anatomic problems?
A: No. The majority of patients with hypospadias have no other problems.

Q: Why is there no need for routine imaging?
A: These studies have been done and show that without symptoms or problems, patients with hypospadias have no other congenital problems.

ICD-9-CM 752.61

BIBLIOGRAPHY

Baskin L. Hypospadias and urethra development. *J Urol* 2000;163:951.

Fisch M. Urethral reconstruction in children. *Curr Opin Urol* 2001;11(3):253–255.

Kelalis P, King K, Belman A, eds. *Clinical pediatric urology*. Philadelphia: WB Saunders, 1992:619–652.

Author: Michele Clement and Douglas Canning

Idiopathic Thrombocytopenic Purpura

 ## Database

DEFINITION

Idiopathic thrombocytopenic purpura (ITP) is a syndrome characterized by:
- Isolated thrombocytopenia (platelet count $<100,000/mm^3$)
- Shortened platelet survival
- Presence of circulating platelet autoantibodies.
- Increased number of megakaryocytes in the bone marrow
- Acute ITP resolves (platelet count $>150,000/mm^3$) within 6 months after diagnosis, without relapse
- Chronic ITP is defined by persistent thrombocytopenia ($<150,000/mm^3$) greater than 6 months after initial presentation.
- Recurrent ITP exhibits an intermittent pattern of thrombocytopenia after an initial recovery to normal count.

PATHOLOGY/PATHOPHYSIOLOGY
- Thrombocytopenia results from increased destruction of antibody-coated platelets by phagocytic cells in the reticuloendothelial system, particularly the spleen.
- It is hypothesized that antibodies generated in response to foreign antigen or drug cross-react with platelet membrane glycoproteins (most commonly IIb/IIIa and Ib/IX).
- Compensation for platelet destruction occurs by increased platelet production from megakaryocytes in the bone marrow. Typical bone marrow aspirate shows increased numbers of immature megakaryocytes.

EPIDEMIOLOGY
- ITP is the most common acquired platelet disorder of childhood.
- Incidence is approximately 4 per 100,000 children per year (<15 years of age).
- Greater than 80% of childhood ITP is acute.
- Males and females equally affected in childhood ITP (female/male ratio is 3:1 in adult and chronic ITP).
- Median age at diagnosis is 4 years (range: 2 to 10 years for acute ITP). Children younger than 1 year or older than 10 years are more likely to develop chronic ITP.

COMPLICATIONS
- Intracranial hemorrhage (ICH) is a rare but often fatal event in acute ITP. It occurs in approximately 1 per 1,000 cases.
- Platelet count at time of ICH always below $20,000/mm^3$ in published literature (80% of cases below $10,000/mm^3$); may be spontaneous without antecedent trauma
- Traditionally thought to occur early in disease course, but more recently shown to occur at any time
- Mucosal bleeding from nose, gums, lower gastrointestinal tract, or kidneys is not uncommon. Hematemesis and melena are rare. Menorrhagia may be severe.
- Retinal hemorrhage is rare.

PROGNOSIS
- Acute ITP: 80% of children will have normal platelet count in 2 months, 95% at 1 year from diagnosis.
- Chronic ITP is more difficult/resistant to treat and therefore has an increased risk of bleeding complications. Platelet count tends to be higher at $40,000-80,000/mm^3$. Remissions can continue to occur many years after diagnosis (predicted spontaneous remission rate—61% after 15 years).
- Cannot predict who will resolve acute ITP and who will persist with chronic ITP.
- Patients with chronic ITP must be evaluated for secondary ITP associated with underlying diseases such as systemic lupus erythematosus, HIV infection, or Evans syndrome.

 ## Differential Diagnosis

- Destructive thrombocytopenias (normal or increased megakaryocytes in marrow)
- Immunologic: ITP, infection (HIV, CMV, EBV, VZV, parvovirus B19), drug-induced, post-transfusion purpura, autoimmune hemolytic anemia (Evans syndrome), lymphoproliferative disorders, SLE, hyperthyroidism
- Nonimmunologic: microangiopathic hemolytic anemia, hemolytic-uremic syndrome, DIC, thrombotic thrombocytopenic purpura, Kasabach-Merritt syndrome (giant hemangioma), cardiac defects (left ventricular outflow obstruction, prosthetic heart valves, repaired intracardiac defects), malignant hypertension
- Impaired or ineffective production (decreased or absent megakaryocytes in marrow)
- Marrow infiltrative processes (leukemias, myelofibrosis, lymphomas, neuroblastoma, other solid tumor metastases, osteopetrosis, storage diseases), drug- or radiation-induced, aplastic anemia, nutritional deficiency states (iron, folate, vitamin B_{12}), viral-induced suppression (e.g., hepatitis, EBV, HIV), thrombocytopenia absent radii (TAR) syndrome, Fanconi anemia, trisomy 13 and 18, Bernard-Soulier syndrome, Wiskott-Aldrich syndrome, May-Hegglin anomaly, inherited thrombocytopenias (X-linked or AD), metabolic disorders (e.g., methylmalonic acidemia)
- Clumping of platelets in the laboratory or giant platelets can artificially decrease a machine-generated platelet count. Review the smear to confirm.

 ## Data Gathering

HISTORY
- Onset is acute in an otherwise well child, sometimes with overnight development of bruising, petechiae, and purpura without history of trauma. Not associated with pallor, fatigue, weight loss, or persistent fevers.
- Half of cases are preceded by a viral infection 1 to 3 weeks before onset (particularly varicella; also EBV, CMV)
- Ask about unusual bruising, rashes (petechiae or purpura), blood in urine or stool, epistaxis, gum bleeding with tooth brushing, and any change in neurologic status.
- Recent immunizations, especially MMR vaccine
- Drug history focusing on drugs with antiplatelet effects (e.g., ASA, seizure medications, heparin)
- Evidence of other autoimmune diseases (e.g., rheumatoid or collagen vascular symptoms, thyroid disease, hemolytic anemia)
- Family history is usually negative for bleeding disorders. Inquire about autoimmune disease in the family.

SPECIAL QUESTIONS
Risk factors for HIV should be elicited, because ITP-like thrombocytopenia may be a presentation of HIV in children.

 ## Physical Examination

- Clusters of petechiae or large bruises readily apparent on skin.
- Purpura in the oropharynx and dried blood or clots in the nares.
- The physical examination should otherwise be normal.
- Consider other diagnoses if there is pallor, jaundice, adenopathy, bone pain, arthritis, or organomegaly (mild splenomegaly may occur in 5–10%)
- A funduscopic examination should be performed on all patients (retinal hemorrhage)

 ## Laboratory Aids

TESTS
Diagnosis based on isolated thrombocytopenia with no other abnormal laboratory values or physical signs (other than bleeding).
- CBC shows thrombocytopenia with a normal WBC count and hemoglobin (mild anemia in proportion to amount of blood loss).
- Mean platelet volume (MPV) is typically increased.
- Peripheral blood smear should always be reviewed to differentiate platelet clumps from true thrombocytopenia. The few platelets present on smear are large. Smear otherwise normal, with no red-cell fragmentation, no spherocytes, and no blasts.
- Platelet counts are frequently less than $20,000/mm^3$ (tend to be $>30,000/mm^3$ in chronic ITP).
- PT and PTT are normal. Bleeding time would be prolonged, but testing is unnecessary.
- A direct antiglobulin test (DAT) to exclude coexisting autoimmune RBC hemolysis (Evans syndrome).
- ANA in subset of patients for whom acute childhood ITP is an unusual diagnosis: including older girls, patients with chronic ITP, and with suspicion of autoimmune disease.
- HIV testing if risk factors are identified

- Need for bone marrow aspirate is controversial. It is safe to perform with a low platelet count.
- Bone marrow aspirate is indicated if anemia, abnormal WBC counts, leukemic blasts on peripheral smear, organomegaly, jaundice, or lymphadenopathy is present.
- Most hematologists examine bone marrow before initiating corticosteroids or if child fails to remit within 2 to 3 weeks (with or without treatment).
- Marrow shows normal to increased numbers of megakaryocytes with otherwise normal morphology and cellularity.
- Assays for platelet-associated antibodies (either direct or indirect) are not established as clinically useful.
- Demonstration of platelet-associated IgG may be useful in more complicated patients in whom chronic ITP is a possible diagnosis.

 ## Therapy

Which patients need treatment remains controversial. Though the eventual duration of ITP in children is not affected by therapy, the platelet count can often be increased rapidly to a safer level by treatment. Guidelines put forth by the American Society of Hematology include:
- Any patient with life-threatening bleeding
- Any patient with a platelet count less than 10,000/mm^3 with minor or "wet" purpura should be hospitalized and treated.
- Any patient with a platelet count of 10,000–20,000/mm^3 plus "wet" purpura should be treated.
- Active toddlers or children at risk for trauma are usually treated.
- Medical treatment interferes with the antibody-mediated platelet clearance and raises platelet counts acutely, but does not alter the long-term course.
- Observation alone is acceptable for older children without serious bleeding and in whom adequate supervision and follow-up are assured.
- Avoid medications that affect platelet function, such as aspirin, ibuprofen, and cold medications with antihistamines.
- Precautions to prevent trauma: limited activity, helmet and pads around bed.
- Parental education should be for signs and symptoms of acute ICH and ICP.

CHOICE OF THERAPY FOR ACUTE ITP
- Corticosteroids: 80% respond with platelet counts over 20,000/mm^3 by 72 hours.
—Oral prednisone at 2 mg/kg/d tapered over 2 to 4 weeks is a typical course.
—Advantages: ease of dosing (oral, outpatient) and low cost.
—Side effects: moodiness, increased appetite, weight gain, hypertension.
—Disadvantage: most pediatric hematologists require a bone marrow aspirate before steroid therapy is begun to exclude leukemia.
—Prolonged steroid treatment has serious side effects.

- Intravenous immunoglobulin G (IVIgG): 94% to 97% of children will have a rise in platelet count >20,000/mm^3 by 72 hours with IVIgG.
—The usual dose is 0.8 to 1 g/kg over 6 to 8 hours, and often repeated if slow or no response.
—Advantages: faster time to platelet count over 20,000/mm^3 (24 hours); marrow aspirate may be deferred.
—Disadvantages: high cost, long infusion time, allergic reactions, 10% to 30% have evidence of aseptic meningitis with severe headache and stiff neck, 50% to 75% have headache, nausea, vomiting, or fever.
- Premedicate with acetaminophen and diphenhydramine.
- Anti-Rh D immunoglobulin (Win-Rho): Rh D immunoglobulin coats Rh D-positive erythrocytes and causes an immune clearance of the antibody-coated autologous red blood cells (transient hemolysis); blocking Fc receptors of splenic macrophages prolongs the survival of platelets in ITP.
—Platelet count typically rises after 48 hours.
—Patient must be Rh(+) and nonsplenectomized.
—Dose is 50 to 75 μg/kg IV over 3 to 5 minutes.
—Advantages: Anti-D is less expensive than IVIgG but more costly than steroids.
—Lower rate of allergic side effects (10%) than IVIgG and does not cause aseptic meningitis.
—Disadvantages: mild hemolysis with a transient hemoglobin decrease of 1 to 3 g/dL.

CHOICE OF THERAPY FOR CHRONIC ITP
In general, children with chronic ITP have few bleeding manifestations, and observation alone is often justified.
- Splenectomy: approximately 60% of patients will respond with complete remission. No presurgical predictors of response have been found.
—Disadvantages: surgical morbidity and risk of postsplenectomy sepsis with encapsulated organisms (management should include vaccination against *Haemophilus influenzae*, pneumococcus, and meningococcus, and lifelong prophylactic penicillin).
- Medical therapy: IVIG, corticosteroids, anti-D immunoglobulin, immunosuppressives (azathioprine, cyclophosphamide, cyclosporine), vincristine, danazol, and monoclonal anti-Fc receptor have been used.
—Plasmapheresis and staphylococcal protein A column adsorption for antibody removal have been used with limited success in refractory cases.

LIFE-THREATENING HEMORRHAGE
The goal is to stop bleeding. Transfused platelets are destroyed like native platelets but may help with hemostasis. IVIG may be given concomitantly. Multimodality therapy is frequently necessary during life-threatening hemorrhage. Emergent splenectomy is sometimes necessary. Plasmapheresis may also be beneficial.

 ## Follow-Up

- Spontaneous recovery is the norm (60% by 3 months, 80% by 6 months, and 90% by 1 year). The incidence of significant bleeding-related morbidity and mortality is extremely low (<5%).
- Of patients with chronic ITP, 50% to 60% eventually stabilize without need for ongoing therapy or need for splenectomy. Spontaneous resolution of thrombocytopenia can be as long as 10 to 20 years after diagnosis.

 ## Common Questions and Answers

Q: Why aren't platelet transfusions used to increase the platelet count?
A: Transfused platelets are rapidly consumed and no increase in platelet count is observed.
Q: Will the ITP recur after another viral infection?
A: Only a minority of recovered patients have recurrence in the setting of a viral illness.
Q: How should activities be limited until the platelet count returns to normal?
A: A commonsense approach to activities for children with low platelet counts is to avoid any activity in which one foot is not on the ground at all times (e.g., bicycle riding, swinging, jungle gym). Also, avoid all contact sports.
Q: How often should platelet counts be obtained?
A: Initially, quite frequently to follow the response to therapy and until count is >20,000/mm^3 and stable. Thereafter, get counts during times of high risk of relapse (e.g., after steroid taper) and monthly until a normal platelet count is consistently seen. After resolution, platelet counts only for clinical suspicion of recurrent thrombocytopenia.
Q: Can IVIgG or anti-Rh D immunoglobulin be given repeatedly if the platelet count falls as the treatment wears off (4–5 weeks)?
A: Yes. Some patients with chronic ITP have been on monthly IVIG for years without problems. Steroids also may be resumed if there is a fall in the platelet count.

ICD-9-CM 287.3

BIBLIOGRAPHY
Blanchette V, Carcao M. Approach to the investigation and management of immune thrombocytopenic purpura in children. *Semin Hematol* 2000;37:299–314.

Bolton-Maggs PHB. Idiopathic thrombocytopenic purpura. *Arch Dis Child* 2000;83:220–222.

Chong BH, Keng TB. Advances in the diagnosis of idiopathic thrombocytopenic purpura. *Semin Hematol* 2000;37:249–260.

De Matta D, et al. Acute childhood idiopathic thrombocytopenic purpura: AIEOP consensus guidelines for diagnosis and treatment. *Haematologica* 2000;85:420–424.

Author: Jane E. Minturn
Susan R. Rheingold, 2nd edition

Immunoglobulin A Deficiency

 Database

DEFINITION

Patients are considered IgA deficient if they have a serum IgA less than 5 mg/dL and a normal serum IgG and IgM, and they are older than 1 year.

PATHOPHYSIOLOGY

Increased incidence of the following:

- Atopy
- Sinopulmonary infections
- Gastrointestinal infections (especially *Giardia lamblia*)
- Crohn disease
- Ulcerative colitis
- Sprue
- Autoimmune illnesses

—Arthritis
—Lupus
—Immune endocrinopathies
—Autoimmune hematologic conditions

- Chronic active hepatitis

GENETICS

Most commonly autosomal-dominant mode of inheritance with variable expressivity, but the following rare associations also occur:

- 18q syndrome
- Partial deletions in the long or short arm, and ring forms of chromosome 18
- Also associated with: HLA-A1, HLA-A2, B8, and Dw3.

EPIDEMIOLOGY

The prevalence is between 1 in 600 and 1 in 800 in a normal population.

COMPLICATIONS

Increased incidence of the following:

- Respiratory tract infections
- Gastrointestinal tract infections
- Atopy

PROGNOSIS

Survival into the seventh decade is common.

 Differential Diagnosis

- Toxic, environmental, drugs

—Penicillamine and anticonvulsants can induce IgA deficiency.

- Genetic/metabolic

—X-linked agammaglobulinemia (Bruton)
—Common variable immune deficiency
—Severe combined immune deficiency
—Ataxia telangiectasia
—DiGeorge syndrome
—Chronic mucocutaneous candidiasis
—Nezelof syndrome
—Selective IgG2 deficiency

- Miscellaneous

—Patients may be completely healthy and IgA deficiency may be an incidental finding.

- Common causes: may be the result of decreased synthesis or impaired differentiation of IgA B lymphocytes into IgA plasma cells

 Data Gathering

HISTORY

Question: Does the patient have frequent sinopulmonary infections?
Significance: Patients with IgA deficiency can have frequent sinopulmonary infections.

Question: Does the patient have frequent gastrointestinal infections?
Significance: Patients with IgA deficiency can have frequent gastrointestinal infections.

Question: Does the patient have allergies?
Significance: Patients with IgA deficiency tend to be allergic.

Question: Does the patient have any autoimmune diseases?
Significance: Patients with IgA deficiency have an increased incidence of autoimmune diseases.

Question: Can healthy patients have IgA deficiency?
Significance: Approximately 30% of patients with IgA deficiency are completely healthy.

 Physical Examination

The physical examination should look for signs of recurrent infection and atopy.

Finding: Cobblestoning of the conjunctiva
Significance: Cobblestoning of the conjunctiva is caused by allergic inflammation in the eyes. Allergies are associated with IgA deficiency.

Finding: Allergic shiners
Significance: Allergic shiners are the result of allergies. Allergies are associated with IgA deficiency.

Finding: Serous otitis media
Significance: Serous otitis may be the result of recurrent ear infections. Increased ear infections can be seen in IgA deficiency. Furthermore, serous otitis media can be secondary to allergies, which is also associated with IgA deficiency.

Finding: Pain on palpation of the sinuses
Significance: Recurrent sinus infections are associated with IgA deficiency.

Finding: Pneumonia
Significance: An increased frequency of pneumonia is associated with IgA deficiency.

Finding: Swollen joints
Significance: An increased frequency of autoimmune diseases are associated with IgA deficiency.

Immunoglobulin A Deficiency

 Laboratory Aids

GENERAL GOAL

Decide whether the patient's complaints are consistent with IgA deficiency (frequent upper respiratory and gastrointestinal infections, or allergies).

- Measure serum IgA level.
- If the patient is IgA deficient, exclude other conditions associated with IgA deficiency.

Test: Serum IgA level
Significance: A patient is considered deficient if the serum IgA level is less than 5 mg/dL.

Test: Total immunoglobulins
Significance: If normal, this study would help rule out X-linked agammaglobulinemia (Bruton), common variable immunodeficiency, and severe combined immunodeficiency.

Test: IgG subclasses
Significance: This study would help rule out an associated IgG2 subclass deficiency.

Test: Lymphocyte mitogens
Significance: This is a functional lymphocyte study. If normal, this study would help rule out common variable immunodeficiency, severe combined immunodeficiency, ataxia telangiectasia, DiGeorge syndrome, and Nezelof syndrome.

Test: Lymphocyte *Candida* antigen stimulation
Significance: No response to *Candida in vivo* is consistent with chronic mucocutaneous candidiasis.

ISSUES FOR REFERRAL

Factors that may help alert you to make a referral include:

- Suggestion that IgA deficiency may be part of a more complex immune deficiency. An allergist/immunologist can assist with an appropriate immunologic evaluation.
- IgA deficiency associated with autoimmune disease. Evaluation and treatment by a rheumatologist would be indicated.
- Patient likely to need a blood transfusion. There is an increased incidence of anaphylaxis to IgA-containing blood products when administered to IgA-deficient patients. The allergist can help select appropriate blood products for these patients.

 Therapy

There is no specific drug therapy.

- Recurrent infections should be treated aggressively with broad-spectrum antibiotics.
- Antibiotic prophylaxis to prevent recurrent sinopulmonary infections is often indicated.
- Intravenous gamma globulin is not indicated.

CONFLICTS WITH OTHER TREATMENTS

Patients with IgA deficiency may develop antibodies against IgA in transfused blood products. These patients are at risk for anaphylactic (or anaphylactoid) transfusion reactions. To avoid these reactions, these patients may receive packed red blood cells (only if these cells have been washed three times), or they may receive plasma products from IgA-deficient donors, or they may receive autologous banked blood.

 Follow-Up

Patients should be observed for:

- Sinopulmonary infections
- Gastrointestinal infections
- Autoimmune diseases
- Inflammatory bowel disease

Note: It is important to manage infectious complications aggressively, and to intervene promptly when the associated conditions present.

 Common Questions and Answers

Q: What is the recurrence risk for a couple with an affected child?
A: It depends on the mode of inheritance. Most commonly, the mode of inheritance is autosomal dominant and the risk would be 50%. However, the expressivity is variable and the patient's phenotype may not be that of an IgA-deficient person.

Q: Does the patient take any medications?
A: IgA deficiency can be induced by some anticonvulsants and by penicillamine.

Q: Should IgA patients wear medical alert bracelets?
A: Yes. These patients can have anaphylaxis if administered blood products containing IgA. In an emergency situation, this is important information for the caregivers to know.

BIBLIOGRAPHY

Burrows PD, Cooper MD. IgA deficiency. *Adv Immunol* 1997;65:245–276.

Middleton E, Reed CE, Ellis EF, et al. *Allergy principles and practice*, 4th ed. Philadelphia: Mosby, 1993.

Rankin EC, Isenberg DA. IgA deficiency and SLE: prevalence in a clinic population and a review of the literature. *Lupus* 1997;6(4):390–394.

Sites DP, Terr AI, Parslow TG. *Basic and clinical immunology*, 8th ed. Englewood Cliffs, NJ: Prentice Hall, 1994.

Smith CA, Driscoll DA, Emanuel BS, et al. Increased prevalence of immunoglobulin A deficiency in patients with the chromosome 22q11.2 deletion syndrome (DiGeorge syndrome/velocardiofacial syndrome). *Clin Diagn Lab Immunol* 1998;5:415–417.

Author: Christopher A. Smith

Imperforate Anus

 Database

DEFINITION

Imperforate anus is a congenital abnormality whereby the bowel fails to perforate or only partially perforates the pelvic muscular floor and/or the epidermal covering.

CAUSES

Not determined

PATHOLOGY

• The hindgut comes in contact with the cloacal membrane during the sixth week of fetal development. At this time, the hindgut is divided into a ventral urogenital and dorsal rectal component. By the eighth week, the dorsal half perforates to the exterior. In imperforate anus, the process is arrested during this critical period.
• There are many anatomic variants of imperforate anus. From the prognostic point of view, the most important is classification, distinguishing two main types: supralevator (high) and translevator (low). Separate is a group of cloacal malformations in which the urinary genital and digestive systems drain to a common channel that communicates with the perineum.
• A fistula communicating from the gut to the urogenital system or to the external opening is present in 90% of cases. In females, most commonly the fistula leads to the opening in the posterior fourchette of the vagina (in low lesions) or to the upper vagina (in high lesions). In males, the fistula leads to the raphe of the scrotum (in low lesions) or to the urethra (in high lesions).

GENETICS

• Imperforate anus can be an isolated defect or part of the syndrome or association.
• Syndromic disorders that contain imperforate anus are associated with defects on chromosomes 6, 7, 10, and 16.

EPIDEMIOLOGY

Incidence is estimated between 1 in 3,000 to 1 in 9,000. High lesions are more common in males (2:1). Low lesions occur with equal frequency in both sexes.

COMPLICATIONS

• Other anomalies are present in one third of patients with an imperforated anus.
• Imperforate anus can be associated with vertebral and cardiac anomalies, tracheoesophageal fistula and, renal and limb anomalies (VACTERL).
• Other anomalies associated with imperforate anus include intestinal atresia, malrotation, omphalocele, annular pancreas, urologic anomalies, spinal anomalies, duplicate uterus, septate vagina, vaginal atresia, and absence of rectal muscles.

PROGNOSIS

Continence can be attained in 90% if patients have low lesions. Less than 50% of patients with high lesions are continent before school age, but most of them continue to improve and achieve continence by adolescence.

 Differential Diagnosis

There are no disorders that can mimic imperforate anus. The task is to define the location of the termination of the bowel and the opening of the fistula.

 Data Gathering

HISTORY

• A majority of children are diagnosed in the first days of life by abnormal findings on physical examination.
• Failure to pass meconium, a history of constipation, and signs of low intestinal obstruction (abdominal distention and vomiting) should mandate reexamination of perianal area.

 Physical Examination

• Lesion presents as either no opening, an inadequate caliber of anus, or an anterior malposition of the opening.
• Physician should attempt to localize the opening of the fistula and look for associated anomalies.
• Evaluation for lumbosacral neurologic function should be done. Anal wink can usually be elicited, because a vertiginous external anal sphincter is present in a majority of the cases.

Laboratory Aids

TESTS

• Invertogram: After sufficient time for a transit of gas (>12 hours after birth), the child is placed in an upside-down position for 3 minutes, after which a lateral view of the pelvis is obtained.
• Lumbosacral films to evaluate for vertebral anomalies.
• An MRI of the spine should be considered to look for a tethered cord.
• Renal ultrasound, voiding cystoureterogram, and IVP can be used to evaluate for urinary tract anomalies.

 ## Therapy

• Surgery should be performed by an experienced surgeon.
• High lesions require an emergent diverting colostomy and pull-through procedure with a Pena midsagittal anorectoplasty at 3 to 9 months of age. The colostomy is closed after the anoplasty has healed and any necessary secondary dilations have been completed.
• Complications of surgery include stricture of the anocutaneous anastomosis, rectourinary fistula, mucosal prolapse, constipation, and incontinence.

 ## Common Questions and Answers

Q: Is this an isolated defect in my child?
A: Often, imperforate anus can be associated with multiple other anomalies and not necessarily isolated. Renal and vertebral anomalies must be excluded.

Q: What is the genetic basis for this defect?
A: Imperforate anus can be associated with chromosomal anomalies or can be an isolated problem.

BIBLIOGRAPHY

Bill AH, Hatch EI. Neonatal obstruction of the intestinal tract: patterns and management. In: Kelley VC, ed. *Practice of pediatrics*. Philadelphia: Harper & Row, 1987:27–32.

Chen CJ. The treatment of imperforate anus: experience with 108 patients. *J Pediatr Surg* 1999;34(11):1728–1732.

Javid PJ, Barnhart DC, Hirschl RB, et al. Immediate and long-term results of surgical management of low imperforate anus in girls. *J Pediatr Surg* 1998;33(2):198–203.

Jona JZ. Advances in neonatal surgery. *Pediatr Clin North Am* 1998;45(3):605–617.

Pena A, Hong A. Advances in the management of anorectal malformations. *Am J Surg* 2000; 180(5):370–376.

Raffensperger JG. *Swenson's pediatric surgery*, 4th ed. New York: Appleton-Century-Crofts, 1980:538–578.

Author: Gregorz Telega

Impetigo

 ## Database

DEFINITION

Impetigo is a superficial skin infection involving almost any part of the body. It occurs in two forms: bullous and nonbullous.

CAUSES

• Bullous: always *Staphylococcus aureus*, usually toxin producing, 80% by phage group 2 type strains
• Nonbullous: still predominantly *S. aureus*, but may also be group A β-hemolytic streptococcus, gram-negative bacteria, and miscellaneous anaerobes.
• Associated illnesses: any condition that disrupts the integrity of the skin (varicella, tinea capitis/corporis, scabies, contact dermatitis, eczema, herpes simplex virus) could result in impetigo occurring as a secondary bacterial infection.
• Predisposing conditions: warm temperature, high humidity, prior antibiotic use (altering normal skin flora), and altered host immunity (e.g., IgA deficiency and defect in cellular immune system).
• Factors that expose fibronectin receptors in the skin, enhancing bacterial binding: underlying skin disease (atopic dermatitis, fungal skin infections), minor trauma (scratches, insect bites, burns).

PATHOPHYSIOLOGY

• Organisms colonize the skin surface and then invade superficially in areas of minor trauma (e.g., an insect bite). Bacteria are transferred from a colonized area (e.g., under the fingernails) to another area (e.g., the nares).
• Microscopic findings: vesicle formation in the subcorneal or granular region with acantholytic cells, spongiosis, edema of the papillary dermis, infiltration of lymphocytes and neutrophils around the blood vessels (the nonbullous form will have little or no vesicle formation)

EPIDEMIOLOGY

• Most common in warm, humid areas
• Most common during warm, humid seasons
• Associated with socioeconomic disadvantage, especially crowding
• Most common bacterial skin infection in children; bacterial skin infections account for up to 17% of clinical visits
• Rare under 2 years of age; most common between 2 and 7 years of age; seen in older groups more often as part of an epidemic

COMPLICATIONS

• Suppurative

—Cellulitis
—Lymphadenitis
—Lymphangitis
—Guttate psoriasis
—Osteomyelitis
—Pyogenic arthritis
—Endocarditis
—Pneumonia
—Sepsis

• Nonsuppurative

—Staphylococcal scalded skin syndrome
—Toxic shock syndrome
—Scarlet fever
—Acute poststreptococcal glomerulonephritis

PROGNOSIS

• Lesions left untreated resolve spontaneously in most cases.
• Treatment primarily prevents spread and speeds healing.
• Unless there is extension of infection beyond impetigo to cellulitis or abscess (uncommon), the infection is superficial and there is no scarring.

 ## Differential Diagnosis

• Varicella
• Eczema herpetiformis
• Staph scalded-skin syndrome
• Tinea corporis
• Scabies
• Contact dermatitis
• Nummular eczema
• Linear IgA bullous dermatosis
• Burns (thermal and chemical)

 ## Data Gathering

HISTORY

• Systemic symptoms are rare.
• Bullous impetigo develops in previously untraumatized skin.
• Nonbullous impetigo is frequently associated with predisposing mild trauma.

 ## Physical Examination

• Bullous: transparent bullae that rupture easily, leaving a rim surrounding a shallow ulcer, a "collarette"; normal surrounding skin; regional adenopathy rare
• Nonbullous: papule or vesicle progression to a honey-crusted plaque; erythema of surrounding skin; regional lymphadenopathy common (up to 90%)
• May see fever, lymphadenopathy
• Frequently the face, extremities, and trunk are affected.

 ## Laboratory Aids

TESTS

• None needed in most cases: clinical diagnosis
• Gram stain and culture are indicated for recurrent or systemic illness; obtain needle aspirate from bulla or by "unroofing" crust and obtaining sample of the purulent material beneath. If positive, it may represent colonization rather than infection; it should be used to identify the organism, not to make a diagnosis.
• CBC: in the presence of systemic symptoms, leukocytosis is common in nonbullous form but not necessarily clinically significant
• Blood culture: in the presence of systemic symptoms
• A skin biopsy may be indicated if diagnosis is in question.
• In outbreaks, use of microbial sensitivity patterns, plasmid typing, or pulsed field gel electrophoresis may be helpful for epidemiologic investigation

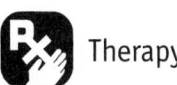
Therapy

SUPPORTIVE

Cleansing and debriding lesions is not necessary.

DRUGS

- Antibiotic resistance patterns in the community will guide choice of antibiotic.
- Most community-acquired cases of *S. aureus* are not methicillin-resistant but may occur in households with IV drug users or in someone who works or lives in a nursing home.
- Many infections, even with organisms resistant *in vitro*, will still have a good clinical response.
- Topical treatment with mupirocin (Bactroban) three times per day for 7 days will not prevent nonsuppurative complications and is not appropriate when lesions are extensive, around the mouth, or there is propylene glycol hypersensitivity. Cream is preferred over the ointment unless there is so much crusting that the cream will not penetrate.
- Other topical antibacterials (bacitracin, polysporin) are *not* effective.
- Oral agents should be used when topical agents are contraindicated, when compliance with a topical agent is doubtful, and/or when lesions are widespread:

—First line: cephalexin 50 mg/kg/d in two divided doses or erythromycin ethylsuccinate 50 mg/kg/d in three to four divided doses for 7 to 10 days (compliance with cephalexin is better because of erythromycin's gastrointestinal side effects)
—Second line: dicloxacillin 50 mg/kg/d (very effective, but unpalatable in liquid form), amoxicillin/clavulanic acid 40 mg/kg/d (very effective, with high cost and higher incidence of gastrointestinal side effects); clindamycin 15 mg/kg/d (very effective, but with greatest alteration of GI flora), azithromycin [very effective and fewer days (only 5 days) of dosing, but with higher cost], extended-spectrum cephalosporins (probably no more effective than first-generation, but at higher cost)

- Failed treatment: Add rifampin 20 mg/kg/d and use mupirocin in nose four times per day to decrease staphylococcal carriage
- Alternative health/complementary medicine remedies: tea ointment (made from a concentrate of brewed tea) has been found effective in a study done in Iraq and is used by some in the U.S.

Follow-Up

- Nonbullous: If untreated, lesions progress slowly over several weeks and then heal spontaneously; occasionally ulcer forms, even when properly treated.
- Bullous: They usually rupture spontaneously (based on size and body location) and then heal over a period of several days to 1 week when properly treated.

SIGNS TO WATCH FOR

- Surrounding skin, for development of deeper infection with abscess or cellulitis
- Fever is unusual and should prompt investigation for deeper infection or another cause.
- Recurrence suggests an *S. aureus* carrier state or inadequate initial therapy.

PREVENTION

- Patient/school education (hand washing of paramount importance): very contagious; spread throughout household not unusual; easily spread via physical contact and fomites, especially on athletic teams
- Trim fingernails to prevent scratching; use gloves at night.
- Separate sleeping quarters and clothing until lesions resolved.
- Treat underlying (predisposing) skin diseases and infestations.

PITFALLS

- Spread throughout a household is not uncommon, with children frequently reinfecting themselves and other family members. Children with underlying skin disease (e.g., eczema) are difficult to treat because of heavy bacterial skin colonization and mechanical trauma to skin associated with itching.
- When cultures reveal both staph and strep, there is no way to determine which is causing the infection; both must be treated empirically.

Common Questions and Answers

Q: How do you decide to treat topically or systemically?
A: Many factors influence this decision. It is impractical to treat a large number of lesions topically, and it is "overkill" to treat a few small lesions with a systemic course of antibiotics. Individual therapy should be tailored to the number and extent of lesions, caregivers' preference for type of therapy, and prior experience with infections in this patient.

Q: What should be done with a patient who continues to have impetigo despite repeated courses of antibiotics?
A: A search for a household source who is reinfecting the patient is probably most important. Culture with sensitivities should be performed to determine if treatment is adequate, but in most cases this is not the problem. Eliminating patient carriage of the organism (with rifampin and mupirocin) should be considered. Underlying skin diseases and irritants should be eliminated if possible. Other diagnoses should be entertained in the truly recalcitrant cases.

Q: Should the child be isolated from other family members and kept home from school?
A: Until the lesions are treated, close contact of the child with other people should be discouraged through both sleeping and play.

Q: What is the difference between mupirocin cream and ointment?
A: The cream with a water base will be absorbed into the skin at a higher concentration in most cases and therefore be more effective. However, if there is significant crusting, the ointment with its oil base may penetrate better.

ICD-9-CM 684

BIBLIOGRAPHY

Bass JW, Chan DS, Creamer KM, et al. Comparison of oral cephalexin, topical mupirocin, and topical bacitracin for treatment of impetigo. *Pediatr Infect Dis J* 1997;16(7):708–710.

Kakar N, Kumar V, Mehta G, et al. Clinico-bacteriological study of pyodermas in children. *J Dermatol* 1999;26(5):288–293.

Mancini AJ. Bacterial skin infections: the common and the not so common. *Pediatr Ann* 2000;29(1):26–35.

Sadick NS. Current aspects of bacterial infections of the skin. *Dermatol Clin* 1997;15(2):341–349.

Scales JW, Fleischer AB, Krowchuk DP. Bullous impetigo. *Arch Pediatr Adolesc Med* 1997;151(11):1168–1169.

Author: Jill A. Foster

Inappropriate Antidiuretic Hormone Secretion

 Database

DEFINITION

Inappropriate antidiuretic hormone (ADH) or ADH-like peptide secretion in the presence of low serum sodium, low serum osmolality, and high urine osmolality, but in the absence of renal or adrenal pathology

CAUSES

- Idiopathic
- CNS pathology, causing increased secretion of ADH or ADH-like peptides: meningitis, head trauma, neurosurgical procedures, encephalitis, Guillain-Barré syndrome, brain tumor, brain abscess, hydrocephalus, hypoxia, subarachnoid hemorrhage, cerebral venous thrombosis
- Non-CNS tumor with independent secretion of ADH or ADH-like peptides: bronchogenic carcinoma, pancreatic carcinoma, Hodgkin disease, prostatic cancer
- Pulmonary disease (leading to secondary elevation in ADH secretion or ADH-like peptides): tuberculosis, pneumonia, asthma, cystic fibrosis, positive-pressure ventilation
- Drugs (which mimic ADH or stimulate its release): vincristine, cyclophosphamide, carbamazepine, chlorpropamide, phenothiazines, clofibrate, nicotine, fluoxetine, sertraline

PATHOPHYSIOLOGY

- ADH is synthesized within neurons of the hypothalamus, transported in conjunction with neurophysin down the supraoptico-hypophyseal tract and stored in the posterior pituitary.
- ADH acts on the renal collecting ducts.
- Interaction of ADH with its receptors forms intracellular cyclic AMP (cAMP).
- cAMP increases water permeability through aquaporins (water channels) of the ducts and consequently reabsorption of free water.

The syndrome of inappropriate ADH (SIADH) results when elevated levels of ADH or ADH-like peptides cause free water retention and hypervolemia leading to hyponatremia. Three possible mechanisms include:

- Direct stimulation of the posterior pituitary (e.g., CNS disorders)
- Independent production of ADH or ADH-like substances from ectopic sources (e.g., oat-cell carcinoma, tuberculosis)
- Decreased venous return that stimulates atrial volume receptors and thereby leads to ADH release (e.g., pulmonary and intrathoracic diseases)

EPIDEMIOLOGY

SIADH can occur at any age. Its incidence depends on the various possible etiologies.

COMPLICATIONS

Severe hyponatremia can cause seizures and, rarely, brain damage. Correcting hyponatremia too quickly can lead to central pontine myelinolysis, which impairs vital functions such as breathing.

PROGNOSIS

Based on the primary cause

 Differential Diagnosis

- Hyponatremic dehydration
- Congestive heart failure
- Adrenal insufficiency
- Cirrhosis
- Nephrotic syndrome
- Renal failure
- Severe potassium depletion
- Water intoxication
- Cerebral salt wasting (CSW): excess production or effects of atrial and/or brain natriuretic peptide hormones
- Hypothyroidism
- Reset hypothalamic osmostat
- Rocky Mountain spotted fever

 Data Gathering

HISTORY

- Unusual water intake (suspicious for psychogenic polydipsia)
- Review of intake and output for inpatients
- Changes in urine output
- Anorexia, lethargy
- Weight gain or weight loss
- Renal disease
- Vomiting
- Diarrhea
- Use of diuretics
- Burns
- Heart disease
- Liver disease
- Brain injury: trauma, surgery, hypoxia, toxin

 Physical Examination

- No signs of dehydration
- Signs of fluid overload
- Lack of edema
- No hyperpigmentation of skin creases/gums
- Due to hyponatremia, the patient may be lethargic or irritable with muscle cramps. In severe cases, patients may lose deep tendon reflexes, seize, or be comatose.

PITFALL

Failure to distinguish SIADH from various forms of salt wasting such as cerebral salt wasting or adrenal insufficiency

PROCEDURE

A complete neurologic and physical examination must be performed. Classically, patients with SIADH manifest signs of hypervolemia but without increased urine output and without edema.

 Laboratory Aids

TESTS

Specific Tests

- Urinary osmolality and sodium with simultaneous serum osmolality, sodium, and uric acid
- Typically, serum sodium is less than 125 mEq/L, serum osmolality is less than 260 mOsm/L, and serum uric acid is less than 2.4 mg/dL, while simultaneous urinary osmolality is greater than 260 mOsm/L and urine sodium >30 mmol/L
- Plasma ADH concentration: diagnostic but not helpful for rapid diagnosis

Nonspecific Tests

- Fractional renal excretion of sodium: Net sodium loss is normal or elevated and is dependent on sodium intake.
- Urinary specific gravity
- Urine output in cc/kg/hr. SIADH usually <1 cc/kg/hr, cerebral salt wasting >2–3 cc/kg/hr)
- Blood glucose
- Triglycerides

Imaging

Head MRI if indicated

Home Testing

Timed urinary volume is helpful.

Therapy

The most important aspects of therapy for SIADH are diagnosis and treatment of the underlying cause.

DIET

- Fluid restriction. Complete until Na >130, insensible losses only until >135 mEq/dL

DRUGS

- For emergency use only: hypertonic saline (1.5–3% NaCl).
- Diuretics should be avoided because they worsen hyponatremia.
- ADH antagonists: Available only through research trials now but expected to soon become standard of care
- Demeclocycline (for chronic SIADH)

DURATION

- Varies with different etiologies and between patients

POSSIBLE CONFLICTS

- Use of other medications that require a large volume for administration

 Follow-Up

WHEN TO EXPECT IMPROVEMENT

Slowly, but usually during the first 48 to 72 hours

SIGNS TO WATCH FOR

Changes in neurologic status

PREVENTION

Clinicians should have a high index of suspicion when administering certain medications, in order to serially monitor serum sodium and fluid status carefully.

 Common Questions and Answers

Q: Is the use of diuretics beneficial?
A: No. Although diuretics may relieve the effects of volume overloading, they also worsen hyponatremia. Overall, diuretics usually cause more detriment than benefit.

Q: What distinguishes SIADH from hyponatremic dehydration?
A: The history of dehydrated patients reveals excessive water loss (e.g., vomiting and diarrhea). Dehydrated patients are thirsty and have lost weight. Patients with SIADH have a history of underlying disease and weight gain. On physical examination, patients with dehydration have signs of hypovolemia in contrast to patients with SIADH who do not. Dehydrated patients have elevated blood urea nitrogen (BUN) and serum creatinine, whereas patients with SIADH have low BUN, creatinine, and albumin.

Q: What distinguishes SIADH from cerebral salt wasting (CSW)?
A: Salt wasters appear dehydrated due to decreased plasma volume, but SIADH patients do not. CSW is associated with very high urine output in contrast to SIADH, which has low urine output. Net sodium loss is very high in CSW, but SIADH has normal to slightly elevated net sodium loss. Distinguishing laboratory features of CSW include suppressed plasma aldosterone concentration and normal serum uric acid concentration. Note that plasma ADH concentration is high in both SIADH and CSW.

Q: Why is it important to distinguish SIADH from CSW (and other causes of hyponatremic dehydration)?
A: Therapies differ dramatically for these conditions. Unlike the water restriction used to treat SIADH, treatment of dehydration, such as that seen in CSW, requires replacement of ongoing salt and water losses.

ICD-9-CM 253.6

BIBLIOGRAPHY

Deen PM, Knoers NV. Physiology and pathophysiology of the aquaphorin-2 water channel. *Curr Opin Nephrol Hypertens* 1998;7(1):37–42.

Gross P, Wehrle R, Bussemaker E. Hyponatremia: pathophysiology, differential diagnosis and new aspects of treatment. *Clin Nephrol* 1996;46(4):273–276.

Kappy MS, Ganong CA. Cerebral salt wasting in children: the role of atrial natriuretic hormone. *Adv Pediatr* 1996;43:271–308.

Olson BR, Gumowski J, Rubino D, et al. Pathophysiology of hyponatremia after transphenoidal pituitary surgery. *J Neurosurg* 1997;87(4):499–507.

Soupart A, Decaux G. Therapeutic recommendations for management of severe hyponatremia: current concepts on pathogenesis and prevention of neurologic complications. *Clin Nephrol* 1996;46(3): 149–169.

Author: Paul S Thornton
Robert J. Ferry, Jr. and Paulo F. Collett-Solberg 2nd edition

Infantile Spasms

 Database

DEFINITION

Infantile spasms are myoclonic seizures, usually occurring in clusters, associated with a typical EEG pattern: high voltage, chaotic slowing, multifocal spikes, and marked asynchrony (known as hypsarrhythmia). Flexor, extensor, mixed flexor/extensor, and arrest/akinetic fits occur. The combination of infantile spasms, hypsarrhythmia, and mental retardation is known as West syndrome. Infantile spasms are classified as *symptomatic* if a specific etiology can be identified and *cryptogenic* if no underlying cause is found.

CAUSES

- Tuberous sclerosis (TS)
- Down syndrome
- Aicardi syndrome
- Metabolic disorders (congenital lactic acidoses, PKU)

Almost any cause of pre- or perinatal brain injury may lead to infantile spasms, including meningitis, hypoxic-ischemic injury, uremia, and congenital infection.

GENETICS

Families of probands have a higher incidence of epilepsy, suggesting multifactorial inheritance. Tuberous sclerosis may be sporadic or autosomal dominant.

EPIDEMIOLOGY

Incidence is 0.25 to 0.42 per 1,000 live births. Peak age of onset is 4 to 9 months; onset usually occurs before 1 year of age. Boys are more often affected than girls.

ASSOCIATED CONDITIONS

- Intrauterine infection
- Cerebral malformations
- Perinatal asphyxia
- Prenatal/perinatal stroke
- Lennox-Gastaut syndrome
- Traumatic brain injury
- CNS infections
- Intraventricular hemorrhage
- Kernicterus
- Genetic conditions noted above
- 40% of infantile spasms are idiopathic

PROGNOSIS

Infantile spasms carry a poor developmental prognosis. Approximately 65% to 90% of patients are developmentally delayed at the time of initial diagnosis, and perhaps 10% of these children will achieve normal cognitive, physical, and educational development. Approximately 55% to 65% of children with infantile spasms go on to develop other seizure types, and 23% to 50% develop Lennox-Gastaut syndrome. Prognosis is better in the cryptogenic group, with up to 40% having normal cognitive development and freedom from seizures on long-term follow-up.

 Differential Diagnosis

- Nonepileptic disorders: benign myoclonus, posturing related to gastroesophageal reflux, shuddering spells
- Myoclonic epilepsy of infancy

—Benign
—Severe myoclonic epilepsy (early infantile epileptic encephalopathy, EIEE)

 Data Gathering

HISTORY

- Prenatal and perinatal history, including:

—Maternal age
—Pregnancy complications
—Perinatal difficulties

- Family history of TS or previous children with infantile spasms should be elicited.
- A detailed developmental history is needed to establish any preexisting developmental delay.
- A detailed description of spells may be useful in differentiating spasms from nonepileptic seizures, though these may be visually indistinguishable from infantile spasms.

 Physical Examination

- Check general growth parameters, specifically head circumference, because microcephaly suggests preexisting brain abnormality and a poorer prognosis.
- On general physical examination, look for dysmorphisms (Down stigmata, retinal defects as in Aicardi syndrome), suggesting genetic abnormalities, and hepatomegaly, suggesting inborn errors of metabolism or congenital infection.
- Careful skin examination, including a Wood's lamp examination, should be performed for evidence of neurocutaneous disorders, specifically the hypopigmented macules associated with TS.
- On neurologic examination, particular attention should be given to level of alertness, attainment of age-appropriate developmental milestones, and motor tone.

 Laboratory Aids

TESTS

- Diagnosis depends on EEG: high voltage, chaotic slowing, multifocal spikes, marked asynchrony known as hypsarrhythmia.
- Routine blood studies should include electrolytes, calcium, and glucose (though generally unrevealing). Chromosomal analysis; metabolic screening, including blood lactate and pyruvate, serum amino acids, and urine organic acids; and TORCH titers may be helpful in identifying underlying etiology.
- If no cause is found, lumbar puncture to look for evidence of CNS infection or lactic acidosis
- Neuroimaging studies are most helpful test to determine etiology. MRI is preferred because of higher resolution for heterotopias and focal anatomic abnormalities; however, the intracranial calcifications associated with intrauterine infections and TS may be more apparent on CT.
- Infants with cutaneous signs of TS should undergo cardiologic evaluation, renal ultrasound, genetic consultation for genetic counseling, and evaluation of other family members.
- Infantile spasms can be an atypical presentation of pyridoxine-dependent seizures (see Therapy).

Therapy

DRUGS

• Adrenocorticotropic hormone (ACTH) is generally considered the most effective therapy for infantile spasms. Treatment is generally initiated at 150 units/m^2/d IM for 1 to 2 weeks, and then gradually tapered over a period of 1 to 6 months.

—Side effects of ACTH therapy include cushingoid appearance, irritability, sleep disturbance, hyperglycemia, hypertension, electrolyte abnormalities, hypertrophic cardiomyopathy, immunosuppression, gastritis/GI bleeding, osteoporosis, and growth failure.
—ACTH therapy has not been proved to affect outcome in infants whose spasms are due to prenatal or perinatal brain abnormalities (symptomatic infantile spasms).
—Alternative therapies include:
—Topiramate (at dosages up to 20–60 mg/kg/d),
—Zonisamide (5–15 mg/kg/d)
—Clonazepam (0.1–0.15 mg/kg/d)
—Nitrazepam (0.5–3.5 mg/kg/d)
—Tiagabine (0.3–1.3 mg/kg/d)
—Valproate (at dosages up to 100 mg/kg/d)
—Phenobarbital (3–6 mg/kg/d)
—Prednisone (2 mg/kg/d).

—Valproate should be used with caution because of the increased rate of fatal hepatotoxicity in this age group.
—A trial of pyridoxine (100 mg IV) should be given to all to rule out pyridoxine-deficiency or dependency. There are also reports (primarily from Japan) of successful treatment of infantile spasms with daily high-dose pyridoxine (200–300 mg/d).
—Vigabatrin (100–150 mg/kg/d) is considered the initial treatment of choice in Europe, but is not currently available in the U.S., and may not become available due to concerns regarding visual-field constriction associated with its use.

 ## Follow-Up

Institution of ACTH therapy necessitates weekly follow-up to monitor blood pressure, glucose, electrolytes, BUN/creatinine, stool guaiac and signs of infection. Weight gain, cushingoid appearance, and irritability/insomnia associated with ACTH resolve as the medicine is tapered.

PITFALLS

• *Hypertension and hemorrhagic gastritis* may occur in infants on ACTH therapy and must be anticipated by weekly follow-up visits.
• *Other seizure disorders* may supervene after infantile spasms have remitted and may require alternate anticonvulsant therapy.

 ## Common Questions and Answers

Q: Do infantile spasms ever remit spontaneously?
A: Spontaneous remission of infantile spasms has been reported but appears to be rare.

Q: What predictions can be made about prognosis of the child with idiopathic infantile spasms?
A: Periodic evaluation by a child neurologist or child developmentalist helps to detect delays in motor or cognitive development; neither the EEG nor any other laboratory test contributes prognostic information in cryptogenic infantile spasms.

ICD-9-CM 345.6

BIBLIOGRAPHY

Baram TZ, Mitchell WG, Tournay A, et al. High-dose corticotrophin (ACTH) versus prednisone or infantile spasms: a prospective, randomized, blinded study. *Pediatrics* 1996;97(3):375–379.

Chugani HT. Infantile spasms. *Curr Opin Neurol* 1995;8(2):139–144.

Kramer U. Epilepsy in the first year of life: a review. *J Child Neurol* 1999;14(8):485–489.

Wong M, Tevathan E. Infantile spasms. *Pediatr Neurol* 2001;24(2):89–98.

Author: Amy R. Brooks-Kayal

Influenza

Database

DEFINITION
Influenza is an acute febrile illness characterized by respiratory, gastrointestinal, and systemic symptoms.

CAUSES
Influenza is caused by the orthomyxoviruses influenza types A, B, and C. Influenza C virus has not been reported as a cause of influenza epidemics.

PATHOLOGY/PATHOPHYSIOLOGY
- The incubation period of influenza virus is approximately 2 to 3 days.
- Pneumonia is a result of direct invasion of the organism as well as secondary bacterial infection.
- Persons are considered contagious on the day before symptoms, and remain so until 5 days after illness onset. This period can be longer for children.

EPIDEMIOLOGY
- Although influenza affects persons of all ages, the highest morbidity and mortality occurs in infants and the elderly.
- Epidemics of influenza occur almost exclusively during winter months, peak approximately 2 weeks after the index case, and last 4 to 8 weeks. Up to 75% of schoolchildren in the epidemic region may be affected.
- Transmission of influenza virus occurs by aerosol droplets as well as by direct or indirect contact.
- Infants <6 months old with influenza are hospitalized at a rate of 1,040 per 100,000 population. These rates are much lower for children ages 5 to 14 years (20–40 per 100,000); however, they can increase more than tenfold for children with high-risk conditions (see Special Questions, below).

COMPLICATIONS
- Secondary bacterial infections (10% of children): bacterial pneumonia (pneumococcal or staphylococcal), otitis media, sinusitis
- *Primary progressive viral pneumonia*: pulmonary hemorrhage, high morbidity and mortality rates
- *Acute myositis* during convalescent period is most commonly associated with influenza B infection: rhabdomyolysis, myoglobinuria, elevated transaminase levels
- *Reye syndrome*: fatty degeneration of the liver and diffuse encephalopathy; more commonly associated with influenza B infection, although can occur after influenza A infection as well; association between aspirin use during acute illness
- *Febrile convulsions*
- *Drug toxicity*: Influenza infection may result in increased serum levels of certain medications that are metabolized by the liver (i.e., theophylline).
- Rare sequelae in severe cases of influenza infection include focal and diffuse myocarditis, diffuse cerebral edema, mediastinal lymph node necrosis, sudden death, and encephalitis.

ASSOCIATED ILLNESSES
- Pharyngitis
- Laryngotracheitis (croup)
- Bronchitis
- Bronchiolitis
- Pneumonia
- Gastroenteritis
- Conjunctivitis

Differential Diagnosis

INFECTION
- Viral infections, including but not limited to respiratory syncytial virus (RSV), parainfluenza, adenovirus
- *Streptococcus pyogenes* infection
- Bacterial sepsis in young infants

Data Gathering

- Infection with the influenza virus causes distinct clinical pictures based on the age of the affected individual.
—Infants and young children may suffer higher fevers and more severe respiratory symptoms.
—Many older children and adults infected with influenza are diagnosed with a "viral respiratory infection," without specific reference to the viral etiologic agent.
—The diagnosis of influenza infection is more commonly made in light of previously identified index cases or specific findings such as myositis.

HISTORY
- Abrupt onset of illness, beginning with dry cough, coryza
- Fever, headache, anorexia, malaise, myalgias, sore throat, irritability
- Respiratory complaints range from mild cough to severe respiratory distress (infants).
- Gastrointestinal complaints in younger children may include vomiting, diarrhea, and severe abdominal pain.

Physical Examination

- Cough is the predominant respiratory sign. Infants and small children may exhibit a "barky" cough (croup).
- Nasal congestion and conjunctival and pharyngeal infections are common.
- Cervical adenopathy is more common in children than in adults.
- Neonates may appear septic: apnea, circulatory collapse, petechiae.
- A generalized macular or maculopapular rash is sometimes observed.
- The myositis that accompanies the convalescent phase of influenza infection is commonly limited to or most severe in the gastrocnemius and soleus muscles. These patients may present with inability to walk or toe-walking.

SPECIAL QUESTIONS
- Patients considered to be at high risk for severe disease include those with asthma or other chronic pulmonary disease, hemodynamically significant cardiac disease, immunosuppressed children including those with HIV infection, sickle cell anemia, chronic renal disease, and diabetes mellitus or other chronic metabolic disease.
- Persons ≥50 years (formerly 65 years) are recommended for annual vaccination.
- Infection with the influenza virus may trigger exacerbations of asthma.

Laboratory Aids

TESTS
All specimens should include a throat swab and nasopharyngeal washing.

- Viral culture from nasopharyngeal secretions will be positive within 2 to 6 days.
- Rapid immunofluorescent tests utilizing monoclonal antibodies have variable sensitivity (70–100%), but high specificity (100%). These are more reliable for influenza A. Polymerase chain reaction (PCR) assays are also available.
- Serologic evidence of infection involves comparison of acute and convalescent serum antibody titers (6 months). ELISA testing is now available for influenza.

IMAGING
- The chest radiographs in patients with lower airway involvement are indistinguishable from other viral lower respiratory infections.
- Chest radiographs may be normal despite significant respiratory involvement.

FALSE POSITIVES
The specificity of 100% for both the fluorescent antibody tests and culture ("gold standard") for influenza virus renders false-positive tests almost nonexistent.

PITFALLS
- The leukocyte count in patients with influenza may be high, low, or normal.
- The differential count is too variable to be of help in diagnosis.
- Evaluation of arterial oxygenation by arterial blood gas analysis or, preferably, pulse oximetry may be required in severe cases of influenza infection. Occasional infants without roentgenographic evidence of lower respiratory tract infection have experienced apnea or rapid decrements in pulmonary function.

HOME TESTING
An ELISA kit is available for diagnosing influenza A in the office setting; however, sufficient data are not available at this time to comment on the efficacy of this test.

Therapy

- Most patients with influenza infection require supportive oral hydration, antipyresis, and routine decongestant therapy.
- Antitussive medications should be used cautiously, and should be appropriate to the age of the child.
- Neuraminidase inhibitors, are not approved for use in children under age 12 years

IMMEDIATE

With the exception of the young infant, previously healthy children with influenza infection rarely require emergency treatment.
- Humidified air, with oxygen as needed, will be helpful to most patients with respiratory symptoms of influenza.
- Supplementary airway maneuvers, including endotracheal intubation, may be required for severe laryngotracheitis or patients with hypoxia that is unresponsive to high-flow oxygen administration.
- Hypovolemic and distributive causes of poor peripheral circulation respond well to intravascular volume repletion.

DRUGS

- Symptom severity and duration may be reduced if antiviral medications are administered within 2 days of symptom onset.
- No antiviral medications have been proven to reduce serious complications of influenza infection.
- Amantadine hydrochloride (<9 years of age or <40 kg: 5 mg/kg/day in 1–2 divided doses; $\geq$40 kg: 200 mg/day in 1–2 divided doses) has *in vitro* activity against influenza A. Rimantadine (5 mg/kg/day in 2 divided doses, maximum 150 mg/day), a synthetic analog of amantadine, can be used as well. Neither medication is approved for use in infants younger than 1 year of age or for influenza B infection.
- Zanamivir (two 5-mg inhalations twice daily for 5 days), is approved for use in children $\geq$12 years old.
- Ribavirin has been used successfully as an aerosol medication in the treatment of both influenza A and influenza B; however, it is not currently approved for treatment of influenza in children.

DURATION

Therapy should be given until 1 to 2 days after the disappearance of signs and symptoms. Zanamivir should be used for 5 days.

POSSIBLE CONFLICTS

- Amantadine dose should be reduced in patients with renal insufficiency, similarly for rimantadine and severe hepatic insufficiency. The side effects of these drugs include insomnia, lightheadedness, and difficulty concentrating.
- Patients with epilepsy have a higher risk of seizure activity when receiving amantadine.

- Inhalation of zanamivir can cause bronchospasm in those patients prone to this symptom.

PREVENTION
Vaccination

- It is necessary to provide annual vaccination to high-risk individuals and persons likely to transmit influenza infection to high-risk individuals. These groups are delineated in the types of patients listed above (see Special Questions).
- Children who are receiving chronic aspirin therapy should be considered for vaccination because of the associations between aspirin use, influenza infection, and Reye syndrome.
- Children <10 years old receiving influenza vaccination for the first time should receive two doses of vaccine administered at least 1 month apart.
- Influenza vaccine is recommended for women who will be in the first trimester of pregnancy during the influenza season. Vaccination is safe during any stage of pregnancy and during breast-feeding.
- Persons with a known anaphylactic hypersensitivity to eggs should consult a physician before receiving influenza vaccination.
- Young children are particularly at risk for attenuated flu-like symptoms beginning 6 to 12 hours after vaccination and lasting up to 2 days.

Chemoprophylaxis

- Prophylactic administration of amantadine or rimantadine is recommended for certain subgroups of patients:
—High-risk children who are exposed to influenza A infection less than 2 weeks after the final dose influenza vaccination was given (see Special Questions, above)
—Immunocompromised patients (poor response to vaccine)
—High-risk patients who cannot receive the vaccine (anaphylactic reaction to chicken or eggs)
—Control of outbreaks in institutions housing high-risk persons
- The dosages for prophylaxis are the same as those used for treatment.
- Daily therapy should be given during periods of peak influenza activity in a community.
- The neuraminidase inhibitors, zanamivir and oseltamivir, are not yet approved for prophylaxis

Follow-Up

WHEN TO EXPECT IMPROVEMENT

- Fever associated with influenza infection usually lasts up to 5 days. Recrudescence of fever does not necessarily signify the onset of a secondary bacterial infection.
- Cough may last up to 2 weeks.
- Lethargy or malaise may persist for up to 2 weeks.

- Influenza A infection usually lasts longer than influenza B or influenza C infections.

SIGNS TO WATCH FOR

- Clinical signs of secondary bacterial infection (see Complications, above)
- Deteriorating mental status or respiratory status after initial improvement
- Myoglobinuria in the face of muscle pain

PITFALLS

The patient presenting with benign acute viral myositis might have an elevated creatinine phosphokinase (CPK). However, the presence of myoglobinuria might suggest acute viral rhabdomyolysis, which can be more damaging to the kidney. These patients should be hospitalized and monitored for adequate hydration.

Common Questions and Answers

Q: When is it safe for a child with influenza to return to daycare or school?
A: Older children with influenza may shed the virus in nasal secretions for up to 7 days from onset of symptoms, and younger children even longer. Therefore, older children with influenza may return to school 1 week after the onset of symptoms, and infants and toddlers should remain home for 10 to 14 days.
Q: Can a child on chronic steroid therapy be immunized against influenza?
A: In general, children who require maintenance steroid therapy for their underlying illness should still receive influenza immunization. If possible, immunize while the child is on the lowest possible dose of steroids and not during a period of high-dose therapy.
Q: What are the chances of acquiring influenza despite annual vaccination?
A: Vaccination against influenza is greater than 70% to 90% effective in preventing disease and greater than 90% effective in preventing death from the infection.

ICD-9-CM 487.1

BIBLIOGRAPHY

American Academy of Pediatrics. Influenza. In: *Red book: report of the Committee on Infectious Diseases*. Washington, DC: American Academy of Pediatrics, 2000:351–359.

Cifu A, Levinson W. Influenza. *JAMA* 2000;284:2847–2849.

Prevention and control of influenza: recommendations of the Advisory Committee on Immunization Practices (ACIP). *MMWR* 2000;49(RR-03):1–38.

Author: Joel A. Fein

Inguinal Hernia

 Database

DEFINITION

Hernia is a protrusion of an organ outside the compartment of the anatomic location. *Inguinal hernia* is a protrusion of a portion of the abdominal content in the area on the inguinal canal.

CAUSES

The processus vaginalis is the outpouching of the peritoneum entering the inguinal canal during testicular migration into the scrotum. The processus vaginalis is normally obliterated after the birth but in some people remains a potential space for herniation. Local weakness of muscles and ligaments in the inguinal area and increased intraabdominal pressure predispose to this hernia.

PATHOLOGY

- The herniated contents are lined by a pouch of peritoneum and accompany the spermatic cord blood vessels and nerves in the canal.
- In girls, there may be an ovary in the hernia sac.

EPIDEMIOLOGY

Inguinal hernias are present in 1% to 3% of children; 90% of inguinal hernias are present in males. Predisposing factors:

- Prematurity
- Ascites
- Chronic lung disease
- Congenital anomalies of the pelvis and perineum
- Ehlers-Danlos syndrome

COMPLICATIONS

- Intestinal obstruction
- Incarceration
- Testicular infarction
- Bowel ischemia
- Skin ulceration
- Cryptorchidism (association)

 Differential Diagnosis

- Seminoma, teratoma, and other testicular tumors
- Scrotal trauma
- Hydrocele
- Undescended testis
- Lymphadenopathy

 Data Gathering

HISTORY

Question: Where is the location of the bulge?
Significance: Hernia presents as a swelling in the inguinal region. Hernia descending to the scrotum or labial area is known as *complete*. Hernia not entering the scrotum (labia) is known as *incomplete*.

Question: What makes the bulge larger?
Significance: The hernia can increase in size with maneuvers increasing intraabdominal pressure (coughing, crying, voiding, defecation).

Question: Is there any pain?
Significance: Uncomplicated hernias usually do not cause pain. Presence of inguinal pain in the absence of incarcerated hernia should raise the suspicion of hip disease.

Question: Are there signs of obstruction?
Significance: Question symptoms of obstruction (emesis, abdominal distention), bowel ischemia (pain, emesis, abdominal distention, fever, irritability, lethargy), reducibility, and traumatic attempts to reduce.

Physical Examination

- Ensure an empty bladder.
- Older children should be in a standing position for the examination. Ensure that your hands are warm.
- If the hernia is not present at the time of examination, maneuvers increasing intraabdominal pressure can reveal suspected hernia (Valsalva maneuver, coughing, crying, voiding, defecation).
- Transillumination is achieved by shining light behind the scrotum anteriorly. Hernias as opposed to hydrocele generally do not transluminate.
- Always consider testicular torsion, epididymitis, orchitis, and trauma when examinations reveal a tender mass in the scrotum.
- Try to reduce the hernia with the child in the supine or head-down position so that gravity assists the maneuver. Use a pacifier to calm the infant. Do not force a difficult incarcerated hernia.

Therapy

- Herniorrhaphy is the definitive treatment. Ten percent of patients will return with contralateral hernia after a unilateral repair. Surgical exploration of the contralateral inguinal canal in patients with unilateral hernia is controversial.
- The underlying cause should be addressed when present (ascites, Ehlers-Danlos syndrome).

PITFALLS

- *Richter hernia:* herniation of only part of the bowel wall, resulting in bowel ischemia without bowel obstruction; rare occurrence
- Failure to consider possibility of ovary in inguinal hernia in girls

Common Questions and Answers

Q: Is surgery of great urgency in childhood?
A: Irreducible incarceration is common in infants less than 1 year of age, and surgery is recommended early. Surgery for uncompli-cated hernia can be postponed in the premature infant or when other medical conditions need to be treated prior to surgery. An irreducible hernia requires urgent surgery.

Q: What are concerns regarding inguinal hernias in girls?
A: Of all inguinal hernias, only 10% are present in girls. The ovary is the most common organ to herniate. Detection is more difficult than in boys and is commonly mistaken for lymphadenopathy. One percent of phenotypic females with inguinal hernia have testicular feminization syndrome with a testicle present in the inguinal canal.

BIBLIOGRAPHY

Kelly RE Jr, Wenger A, Horton C Jr, et al. The effects of a pediatric unilateral inguinal hernia clinical pathway on quality and cost. *J Pediatr Surg* 2000;35(7):1045–1048.

Ozbey H, Ratschek M, Schimpl G, et al. Ovary in hernia sac: prolapsed or a descended gonad? *J Pediatr Surg* 1999;34(6):977–980.

Tackett LD, Breuer CK, Luks FI, et al. Incidence of contralateral inguinal hernia: a prospective analysis. *J Pediatr Surg* 1999;34(5):684–687; discussion 687–688.

Author: Gregorz Telega

Intersex

 Database

DEFINITION

Chromosomal sex is established at fertilization, which then directs the undifferentiated gonads to develop into testes or ovaries. Phenotypic sex results from the differentiation of internal ducts and external genitalia under the influence of hormones and transcription factors. If there is any discordance among these three processes (i.e., chromosomal, gonadal, or phenotypic sex determination), then ambiguous genitalia (intersex) develop.

CAUSES

Currently, four main categories of intersex are described:
- Female pseudohermaphroditism (FPH)
- Male pseudohermaphroditism (MPH)
- Gonadal dysgenesis [pure (PGD) or mixed (MGD)]
- True hermaphroditism (TH)

FPH is the most common intersex disorder. The ovaries and müllerian derivatives are normal and the sexual ambiguity is limited to virilization of the external genitalia. A female fetus is masculinized only if exposed to androgens and the degree of masculinization is determined by the stage of differentiation at the time of exposure. Virilization may also be secondary to exogenous maternal steroids. Congenital adrenal hyperplasia (CAH) accounts for the majority of FPH patients (most commonly 21α-hydroxylase or 11β-hydroxylase deficiencies).

MPH is a heterogeneous disorder in which testes are present but the internal ducts and/or the external genitalia are incompletely virilized. The phenotype ranges from completely female external genitalia to mild male ambiguity (such as hypospadias or cryptorchidism). MPH can result from eight basic etiologic categories:
- Testicular unresponsiveness to hCG and LH (Leydig cell agenesis/hypoplasia due to hCG/LH receptor defect)
- Enzyme defects in testosterone biosynthesis, some of which are common to CAH (StAR, HSD3B2, CYP17, 17βHSD3)
- Defects in androgen-dependent target tissues (androgen insensitivity syndrome, AIS)
- A defect in the enzymatic conversion of testosterone (T) to DHT (5α-reductase deficiency)
- Defects in the synthesis, secretion, or response to antimüllerian hormone (AMH) or müllerian inhibiting substance (MIS) resulting in persistent müllerian duct syndrome
- Aberrations in testicular gonadogenesis (testicular dysgenesis)
- Primary testicular failure (vanishing testes)
- Exogenous insults (maternal ingestion of progesterone/estrogen or environmental hazards).

Gonadal dysgenesis disorders comprise a spectrum of anomalies ranging from complete absence of gonadal development to delayed gonadal failure. Complete GD or PGD includes failed gonadal development in genetic males and females due to abnormalities of sex or autosomal chromosomes. Partial gonadal dysgenesis refers to disorders with partial testicular formation at some point in development including MGD, dysgenetic MPH, and some forms of testicular or ovarian regression.

TH requires the presence of both ovarian and testicular tissue in the individual. TH can result from sex chromosome mosaicism, chimerism, or Y chromosomal translocation. This uncommon condition may be classified into three groups: lateral—testis and ovary (usually left); bilateral—ovotestis and ovotestis; and unilateral (most common)—ovotestis and testis or ovary. The genital development is ambiguous with hypospadias, cryptorchidism, and incomplete fusion of labioscrotal folds. Genital duct differentiation generally follows that of the ipsilateral gonad.

PATHOLOGY

- A testis that is poorly formed is called a dysgenetic testis
—A dysgenetic testis usually has discontinuity of the tunica albuginea with hilar disorganization, hypoplastic or disordered tubules, and fibrotic stroma.
- An ovary that is poorly formed is called a streak gonad.
—Streak gonads contain ovarian-like stroma with occasional primordial follicles.
—A patient with a Y chromosome is at high risk to develop a tumor in a streak or dysgenetic gonad. Gonadoblastoma is the most common tumor. Although it is a benign growth, it can give rise to a malignant tumor called a dysgerminoma. The risk of tumor formation is about 20% and is age-related (older more at risk).
- An ovotestis has evidence of both seminiferous tubules and ovarian stroma and follicles.

EPIDEMIOLOGY

Low birth weight is a well-established risk factor for cryptorchidism and hypospadias but associations with low maternal parity and low socioeconomic status are still uncertain. Ambiguous genitalia are also part of the Denys-Drash syndrome (Wilms tumor, hypertension, nephropathy).

GENETICS

- Inactivating or loss of function mutations in five genes involved in steroid biosynthesis can cause CAH: CYP21, CYP11B1, CYP 17, HSD3B2, and StAR. Each of these genetic defects is inherited in an autosomal-recessive pattern.

- MPH can result from Leydig cell unresponsiveness to hCG-LH since the production of testosterone by the Leydig cells is critical to male differentiation of the wolffian ducts and the external genitalia. Familial studies are consistent with autosomal-recessive transmission. Multiple cases have been described and conversion and nonsense mutations have been identified in homozygous and compound heterozygous individuals.
- 47XXY males may develop through nondisjunction of the sex chromosomes during the first or second meiotic divisions in either parent or, less commonly, through mitotic nondisjunction in the zygote at or after fertilization. These abnormalities almost always occur in parents with normal sex chromosomes
- Categories of 46XX sex reversal include classic XX male individuals with apparently normal phenotypes, nonclassic XX males with some degree of sexual ambiguity, and XX true hermaphrodites; 80% to 90% of 46XX males result from an anomalous Y to X translocation involving the SRY gene during meiosis. However, 8% to 20% of XX males have no detectable Y sequences, including SRY.
- XY gonadal dysgenesis (XY sex reversal or Swyer syndrome) is a heterogeneous condition that can result from deletions of the short arm of the Y chromosome, SRY gene mutations, alterations in autosomal genes, or duplications of the DSS locus on the X chromosome.
- A 45X karyotype may be due to nondisjunction or chromosome loss during gametogenesis in either parent resulting in a sperm or ovum without a sex chromosome. 45X/46XX mosaicism may be present in up to 75% of Turner syndrome patients.
- In TH, the most common karyotype is 46XX followed by 46XX/46XY chimerism, mosaicism, and 46XY. Most 46XX TH are SRY-negative and the genes responsible have not yet been identified. A mutated downstream gene in the sex determination cascade likely allows for testicular determination.

 Differential Diagnosis

The differential diagnosis initially depends on the palpability of gonads on presentation.
- If no gonads are palpable, all four categories are possible (FPH, MPH, GD, TH). Of these, FPH is most commonly seen followed by MGD.
- If one gonad is palpable, FPH and PGD are ruled out because ovaries and streak gonads do not descend. MGD, TH, and MPH remain possibilities.
- If two gonads are palpable, MPH and rarely TH are the most likely diagnoses.
- In 46XY boys, hypospadias and cryptorchidism without an underlying intersex etiology would be a diagnosis of exclusion after a full evaluation.

HISTORY

- Prematurity
- Exogenous maternal hormones (used in infertility treatments)
- Use of oral contraceptives
- Central nervous system lesions
- Family history for urologic abnormalities
- Neonatal deaths
- Precocious puberty
- Infertility
- Consanguinity

 Physical Examination

- Any abnormal virilization or cushingoid appearance of the child's mother should be noted.
- Note any dysmorphic features including a short, broad neck or widely spaced nipples.
- The patient should be examined supine in the frogleg position with both legs free.
—Abnormal phallic size should be documented by width and stretched length measurements.
—Describe the position of the urethral meatus and amount of chordee (ventral curvature).
—Note the number of orifices: three in normal girls (urethra, vagina, and anus) or two in boys (urethra, anus).
- A rectal exam should always be performed for palpation of a uterus.
- With warmed hands, begin the inguinal examination at the anterior superior iliac spine. Sweep the groin from lateral to medial with the nondominant hand. Once a gonad is palpated, grasp it with the dominant hand, and continue to sweep toward the scrotum with the other hand to attempt to bring the gonad to the scrotum.
—Check the size, location, and texture of both gonads if palpable. Wetting the fingers of the nondominant hand with lubricating jelly or soap can increase the sensitivity of the fingers.
—The undescended testis may be found in the inguinal canal, the superficial inguinal pouch, at the upper scrotum, or, rarely, in the femoral, perineal, or contralateral scrotal regions.
—For differential diagnosis and treatment purposes, the distinction needs to be made whether or not the testis is palpable. Unless associated with a patent processus vaginalis, ovaries and streak gonads do not descend, while testes, and rarely ovotestes, may be palpable.
- Document development and pigmentation of the labioscrotal folds.

 Laboratory Aids

TESTS

All patients require:
- Serum electrolytes
- 17-OH progesterone
- T
- LH
- FSH
- Karyotype
- If 17-OHP is elevated, 11-deoxycortisol and DOC will help differentiate 21α- from 11β-hydroxylase deficiency.
- If 17-OHP is normal, T/DHT ratio along with androgen precursors pre/post-hCG stimulation (if older than 3 months) will help elucidate the MPH etiology.
- A failure to respond to hCG in combination with elevated LH/FSH levels is consistent with anorchia.

IMAGING

- Ultrasound can detect gonads in the inguinal region, (where they are also most easily palpable) but are only 50% accurate in showing intraabdominal testes. These tests are also helpful in identifying a uterus.
- A genitogram should be performed to evaluate a urogenital sinus including the entry of the urethra and vagina.
- A cervical impression can be identified on the vaginogram.
- CT and MRI may also help to delineate the anatomy, although they are more expensive.

SURGERY

Infants in whom TH, MGD, or MPH is considered will require an open or laparoscopic exploration with bilateral deep longitudinal gonadal biopsies for histologic evaluation.

 Therapy

Much current research is aimed at understanding the influence of androgens on the fetal/newborn brain and its relationship to gender identity. Diagnosis and management of these children is very individualized and should always involve a "team effort" including the pediatric urologist, endocrinologist, geneticist, and the child's parents immediately after birth.

MEDICAL THERAPY

- Treatment on the newborn with CAH involves correction of dehydration and salt loss by electrolyte and fluid therapy with mineralocorticoid replacement. Glucocorticoid replacement is generally added on confirmation of the diagnosis.
- Estrogen replacement is begun after puberty in girls with complete AIS.
- Testosterone replacement may be needed in some cases of MPH (partial AIS, testicular dysgenesis, primary testicular or Leydig cell failure) to aid in pubertal changes and for maintenance through adulthood.

SURGICAL THERAPY

- Until further data are available, the current recommendation for a girl with CAH is to continue a female sex of rearing and perform a feminizing genitoplasty. This surgery has three main aims: reducing the size of the enlarged, masculinized clitoris; reconstructing the female labia; and increasing the opening and possibly length of the vagina. Many surgeons advocate early surgery for technical and psychological reasons, realizing that vaginal revision may be needed after puberty.
- Some gonads need to be removed due to the risk of tumor formation. Controversy exists concerning the best time to perform orchiectomies in a child with complete AIS reared female (at diagnosis vs. after puberty). Streak gonads in the presence of a Y chromosome and dysgenetic abdominal testes should be removed. All other undescended testes need to be anchored in the scrotum by abdominal or inguinal orchidopexy. Dysgenetic testes in the scrotum need to be followed closely.
- Urethral reconstruction of hypospadias is performed in all children raised as boys at about 6 months of age.

PROGNOSIS

- The overall prognosis for somatic, sexual, and psychosocial growth and development is good with careful management of most of these children. Any thoughts of gender reassignment should only be entertained after thoughtful discussion with the child's parents and all medical staff involved.
- Except for girls with CAH, most of these patients are infertile.

 Follow-Up

- Long-term management of mineral and glucocorticoids is managed by the pediatric endocrinologist. The vaginal introitus in CAH is reexamined after puberty to assess adequacy of width and depth.
- Undescended testes, especially dysgenetic testes, have an increased risk of tumor formation even after orchidopexy. These boys need to learn testis self-exam after puberty.
- Hypospadias repairs are followed at least through potty-training to ensure good voiding habits and absence of meatal stenosis or urethrocutaneous fistulae.

ICD-9-CM 752.7

BIBLIOGRAPHY

Aaronson I. Sexual differentiation and intersexuality. In: Gillenwater JY, Grayhack JT, Howards SS, et al., ed. *Adult and pediatric urology*, 3rd ed. St. Louis: Mosby, 1996.

Kolon T, Lamb D. The molecular basis of intersex conditions. *AUA Updates* 2001;20: lesson 14.

Mandell J. Sexual differentiation: normal and abnormal. In: Walsh PC, Retik AB, Vaughn ED, et al., ed. *Campbell's urology*, 7th ed. Philadelphia: WB Saunders, 1998.

Author: Thomas F. Kolon

Intestinal Obstruction

 Database

DEFINITION

Intestinal obstruction is pathologic blockage of aboral progression of intestinal contents, which can be secondary to mechanical or paralytic etiologies.

CAUSES

Of the various etiologies that have been cited as acquired causes of intestinal obstruction, authors cite the following in decreasing order of prevalence:

- Pyloric stenosis, 25%
- Intussusception, 18%
- Atresia of the intestine, 15%
- Imperforate anus, 11%
- Hirschsprung disease, 6%
- Postoperative adhesions, 5%
- Meconium ileus, plug, 5%
- Malrotation, 5%
- Annular pancreas, 3%
- Meckel diverticulum, 3%

Generally, etiologies can be classified as:

- Intraluminal: polyp, mass, bezoar, foreign body, parasites, and tumor
- Intramural: stricture, tumor, hematoma
- Extrinsic: postoperative adhesions, adhesions from peritonitis, hernia, volvulus, and tumor

Paralytic Ileus

- Caused by a failure of intestinal motor function resulting from drugs, i.e., vincristine, hypokalemia, systemic sepsis, uremia, myxedema, and diabetic ketoacidosis. Usually this is self-limiting and acute, characterized by an absence of bowel sounds and air throughout the intestine. Conservative therapy usually resolves the latter.
- Differential diagnosis must include *chronic intestinal pseudo-obstruction,* a syndrome of altered intestinal and colonic motility of undefined etiology.

Mechanical

Mechanical obstructions can be either simple or strangulating and may be caused by congenital or acquired diseases. The latter impair intestinal blood flow and may cause intestinal necrosis, resulting in higher morbidity and mortality than caused by simple obstructions.

GENETICS

No genetic predisposition to intestinal obstruction in general cases

EPIDEMIOLOGY

- The different causes of intestinal obstruction have their own identified epidemiologic patterns: small bowel obstruction secondary to *Ascaris lumbricoides* in Calcutta, India; colonic volvulus secondary to aerophagia and constipation in mentally retarded children; or meconium ileus equivalent in children with cystic fibrosis.
- Down syndrome with a higher prevalence of duodenal atresia

COMPLICATIONS

Perforation and peritonitis as secondary phenomena are classically the most common complications of intestinal obstruction if not corrected in the initial stages.

PROGNOSIS

Excellent in cases of simple intestinal obstruction without strangulation

 Differential Diagnosis

Intestinal obstruction is a final common pathway for multiple etiologies, including those that lead to simple or strangulated obstruction.

- Metabolic: meconium ileus, electrolyte disturbance
- Congenital: esophageal atresia, intestinal atresia, duplication of bowel, malrotation, diaphragmatic hernia, Hirschsprung disease, imperforate anus, annular pancreas, pyloric stenosis
- Miscellaneous: adhesive bands, intussusception, meconium plug, volvulus, postoperative adhesions

 Data Gathering

HISTORY

- Pain is one of the cardinal manifestations of intestinal obstruction, resulting from distention of the intestine, producing visceral pain that is poorly localized, with nausea and vomiting.
- Pain that is well localized and associated with tenderness and rigidity results from peritonitis.
- A history of bilious emesis and feculent characteristics confirm obstruction.
- Passage of bloody stool and mucus may suggest strangulation.
- Elicit any family history of cystic fibrosis, polyps, and previous abdominal surgery, as well as recent weight loss or spinal surgery.

 Physical Examination

- Palpation may reveal the presence of a hernia, a mass suggestive of feces or intussusception, and tenderness or rigidity.
- Presence of scoliosis or kyphosis should be recognized.
- Rectal examination will reveal, at times, a palpable polyp or intussusceptum. The latter have been unusual presentations of Peutz-Jeghers syndrome, a classic polyposis syndrome in children, characterized by features including pigmentation of the lips and buccal mucosa.

Laboratory Aids

TESTS

• Electrolyte abnormalities, including sodium, chloride, bicarbonate, and potassium, are necessary to identify for the proper assessment of hydration and third-spacing of fluids.
• No particular laboratory test will confirm the diagnosis, other than imaging techniques, as described below.

IMAGING

• Plain abdominal radiographs in the supine and erect views will identify the classic features of a gasless abdomen, with air-fluid levels and distended loops of intestine.
• Paralytic ileus may present with dilation of the small and large intestines.
• Ultrasonography has been used to identify a mass (i.e., perforated appendix) as the cause of the obstruction.
• In isolated cases, contrast examinations may be helpful in making a diagnosis (e.g., barium enema to confirm intussusception or Hirschsprung disease, and upper GI series to exclude malrotation or volvulus).

 ## Therapy

MANAGEMENT

• Initial stages:

—Hold oral intake.
—Decompress the stomach with a nasogastric tube.
—Hydration IV and correct electrolyte imbalance.
—Identify etiology of obstruction and establish definitive repair.

• Surgical:

—In cases of strangulation, immediate surgical options may be needed in cases of perforation and peritonitis. In isolated cases of distal obstruction secondary to intussusception, surgery is avoided with the institution of hydrostatic or air reduction of the mass effect.

 ## Common Questions and Answers

Q: Will my child need surgery for this problem?
A: Most likely; surgical treatment is necessary to correct the cause of intestinal obstruction except in a few cases, such as intussusception, pseudo-obstruction, and paralytic ileus.

Q: What is the most common cause of this problem in my 3-day-old son?
A: In an infant, the most common causes are atresias of the intestine, which are absences of the normal amount of large or small intestine in the abdomen. Other causes are defects in the large intestine, such as Hirschsprung disease. Other notable risk factors include cystic fibrosis and diabetes in the mother.

ICD-9-CM 560.9

BIBLIOGRAPHY

Madonna MB, Boswell WC, Arensman RM. Acute abdomen. *Semin Pediatr Surg* 1997;6(2):105–111.

Villamizar E, Mendez M, Bonilla E, et al. *Ascaris lumbricoides* infestation as a cause of intestinal obstruction in children: experience with 87 cases. *J Pediatr Surg* 1996;31(1): 201–206.

Wesson D. Acute intestinal obstruction. In: Walker W, Durie P, Hamilton JR, et al., eds. *Pediatric gastrointestinal disease*. Philadelphia: BC Decker, 1994:486–494.

Author: Andrew E. Mulberg

Intoeing—Tibial Torsion

 Database

DEFINITION

- Tibial torsion—twisting the tibia (can be associated with femoral torsion)
- Medial or internal tibial torsion (MTT) associated with intoeing (most common).
- Lateral or external tibial torsion associated with out-toeing.
- Normal defined as within 2 standard deviations of mean.

CAUSES

- Normal fetal development
- Intrauterine position
- Heredity-familial tendency
- Posturing (sitting position)—cause or effect?
- Associated pathology (e.g., spasticity, fracture malunion, or DDH)

PATHOLOGY

- Tibial torsion—twisting the tibia; usually medial or internal; associated with intoeing.
- If associated with increased femoral anteversion, may be associated with patellofemoral malalignment (knee cap subluxation)

EPIDEMIOLOGY

Common and usually normal (i.e., within 2 standard deviations of the mean)

GENETICS

No strong evidence to suggest that this is an inherited condition (heredity-familial tendency)

COMPLICATIONS

None proven

PROGNOSIS

Good; usually not painful, cosmetically unattractive, or dysfunctional

 Differential Diagnosis

Look for DDH, spasticity (e.g., mild cerebral palsy)

 Data Gathering

HISTORY

Question: Birth history?
Significance: Firstborn common

Question: Pain, limping?
Significance: May indicate other diagnosis

Question: Other "packaging" conditions?
Significance: Metatarsus adductus, torticollis, DDH

Question: When first noticed? Getting better or worse? Functional limitations (i.e., trips and falls frequently)?
Significance: Functional limitations may suggest other diagnosis such as mild cerebral palsy, especially if abnormal birth history or developmental milestones.

 Physical Examination

Finding: If ambulatory, watch gait and assess for foot progression angle
Significance: The angle formed between the axis of the foot and the axis of forward progression of gait.

Finding: Also assess other aspects of gait.
Significance: Stride, heel-toe gait, cadence, limping, other abnormalities. Unilateral or bilateral torsion.

Finding: Leg length discrepancy, hip abnormalities, contractures, spasticity, thigh foot axis (TFA).
Significance: With the child prone, the knee flexed to 90 degrees, and the ankle at neutral, measure the difference between the axis of the foot and the axis of the femur. If the thigh-foot axis is internal, this suggests internal tibial torsion; if external, external tibial torsion.

Finding: Transmalleolar axis
Significance: With the child seated and the knee flexed to 90 degrees, assess the malleolar axis in reference to the coronal plane (less reliable than TFA).

Finding: Look for abnormalities of the feet.
Significance: Metatarsus adductus or clubfoot may be a primary cause of intoeing. Significant calcaneovalgus may be a component of out-toeing.

Finding: Careful neurologic examination
Significance: To see if intoeing is related to a mild neurologic abnormality, such as mild spastic diplegic cerebral palsy.

SPECIAL QUESTIONS

Physical Examination Tricks

- Normal torsional alignment
- "Torsional profile"

—Foot-progression angle
—Medial hip rotation in extension
—Lateral hip rotation in extension
—Thigh-foot angle
—Transmalleolar axis
—Configuration of the foot

- "Kissing patellae"

—Occurs when bilateral increased femoral anteversion causes the patellae to face one another, giving the appearance of kissing patellae.

Laboratory Aids

Usually not helpful.

IMAGING STAGES

Usually not needed. Physical examination gives information needed.

Test: Hip x-ray
Significance: If hip pathology (i.e., DDH) is suspected, then may be indicated.

Test: CT
Significance: CT is an accurate way of measuring tibial and femoral torsion but there is radiation exposure. An occasional indication may be a patient who is being evaluated for surgery.

Test: MRI
Significance: Techniques for using MRI and ultrasound have also been described, but in general are less accurate than CT.

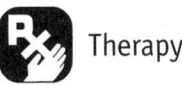 ## Therapy

- Observation and familial and patient reassurance (almost always the treatment of choice).
- Devices such as casts, shoe wedges, twister cables, splints, Denis Brown bars have no proven benefit (i.e., they will not change the natural history). They may in fact cause problems such as ligamentous damage to hip, knee, ankle, and foot.
- Reassurance is usually enough. The condition improves spontaneously. Usually corrects enough by 8 years of age.
- Surgery seldom needed.
- Tibial osteotomy: when done is usually a distal supramaleolar osteotomy.

GENERAL TREATMENT MODALITIES

- Observation
- Physical therapy: will not change natural history (it may help with associated patellofemoral malalignment pain)
- Devices (casts, shoe wedges, twister cables, splints, Denis Brown bars): no proven benefit
- Tibial osteotomy is seldom, if ever, needed.

 ## Follow-Up

WHEN TO EXPECT IMPROVEMENT

Usually corrects enough by 8 years of age

SIGNS TO WATCH FOR

Should improve with growth and development. There is no substantial evidence that increased femoral anteversion will cause arthritis of the hip or knee (chondromalacia patella).

PROGNOSIS

Overall, good prognosis for the majority of patients

 ## Common Questions and Answers

Q: When are special shoes or braces indicated for tibial torsion?
A: Almost never. The situation will improve without treatment in most. There is no strong evidence that any of these treatments truly alter the natural history of the condition.

Q: Why do patients with torsional pathology occasionally have knee pain?
A: Children can have increased femoral anteversion with associated external tibial torsion (i.e., an external rotation of the tibia that matches and, in effect, balances the internal rotation of the femur). This can be diagnosed by observing the above rotational profile and by noting increased Q-angle. This situation is sometimes a "setup" for patellofemoral pain.

ICD-9-CM 736.89

BIBLIOGRAPHY

Schoenecker PL, Rich MM. The lower extremity. In Morrissy RT, Weinstein SL, eds. Lovell and Winter's pediatric orthopaedics, 5th ed. Philadelphia: Lippincott Williams & Wilkins. 2001:1059–1104.

Staheli LT. Lower positional deformity in infants and children: a review. *J Pediatr Orthop* 1990;10:559.

Staheli LT. Torsional deformities. *Pediatr Clin North Am* 1977;24:799.

Author: John P. Dormans

Intracranial Hemorrhage

 Database

DEFINITION

Intracranial hemorrhage is extravasation of blood from intracranial vessels to the epidural, subdural, intraparenchymal, or intraventricular space within the cranial vault.

CAUSES

- Trauma
- Prematurity
- Birth trauma
- Coagulopathies related to vitamin K deficiency, hemophilia, idiopathic thrombocytopenic purpura, protein C or S deficiency, hemolytic-uremic syndrome, disseminated intravascular coagulation, leukemia
- Brain tumors
- Encephalitis, especially herpes simplex infection
- Intracranial aneurysms
- Arteriovenous malformations
- Hypertension
- Cocaine use
- Cerebral infarction

PATHOPHYSIOLOGY

- Epidural hematoma (blood between the dura mater and the skull) is frequently from arterial bleeding related to skull fracture, typically middle meningeal artery bleeding following temporal bone fracture. However, approximately one fourth of epidural hematomas in children are from venous bleeding.
- Subdural hematoma (blood between the dura mater and the arachnoid membrane) is frequently from venous bleeding resulting from trauma or coagulopathy.
- Subarachnoid hemorrhage (blood between the arachnoid membrane and brain) is frequently from a ruptured intracranial aneurysm or trauma.
- Blood within the brain parenchyma can be the result of trauma, infections such as herpes simplex encephalitis, brain tumors, venous sinus thrombosis, or cerebral infarction.
- Subependymal germinal matrix hemorrhage occurs in newborns, more commonly in premature infants who are born at less than 34 weeks gestational age.
- Intraventricular hemorrhage most commonly occurs when either an intraparenchymal or subependymal germinal matrix hemorrhage extends into the ventricular system. The grading system is as follow:
- grade I—isolated germinal matrix hemorrhage;
- grade II—intraventricular hemorrhage without ventricular dilatation;
- grade III—intraventricular hemorrhage with ventricular dilatation; and
- grade IV—intraventricular hemorrhage with ventricular dilatation and hemorrhage into parenchymal tissue.

GENETICS

Increased frequency with hereditary disorders of coagulation, congenital heart disease, and polycystic kidney disease associated with intracranial aneurysms.

COMPLICATIONS

- Increased intracranial pressure
- Hydrocephalus
- Vasospasm
- Seizures
- Motor, visual, and cognitive deficits
- Death

 Differential Diagnosis

- Stroke
- Brain tumor
- Migraine headache

APPROACH TO THE PATIENT

Intracranial hemorrhage should be suspected in any patient presenting with a history of head injury. Other presentations include change or loss of consciousness, seizure, headache, meningismus (since blood is an irritant), or sudden focal neurologic deficit. Expeditious history, examination, and emergent CT should occur whenever intracranial hemorrhage is suspected. While the bleeding itself may not cause permanent damage to the brain, rapidly increasing intracranial pressure is a life-threatening situation that may arise from intracranial hemorrhage.

 Data Gathering

HISTORY

- Head trauma
- Head trauma during delivery, especially with prolonged labor and a large infant
- Headache, with attention to severity, quality (worrisome if different from prior headaches)
- History of a "warning leak" from a ruptured arterial aneurysm (headache, stiff neck, low-grade fever)
- Change in level of consciousness
- Seizures, especially new-onset
- Visual problems
- Focal neurologic deficits
- Epistaxis (may occur with leakage of CSF if skull fracture is present)
- Meningeal symptoms
- History in patient or family of coagulopathy
- Risk factors for cerebral venous sinus thrombosis: dehydration, coagulopathy, polycythemia, sepsis, and asphyxia (especially in newborns)
- Risk factors for arterial aneurysms: polycystic kidney disease, coarctation of the aorta

 Physical Examination

- Signs of increased intracranial pressure or herniation, such as Cushing triad (hypertension, bradycardia, abnormal respiratory pattern), papilledema, pupils that do not constrict to light, ophthalmoparesis, decorticate or decerebrate posturing. Intraventricular blood may present with signs of increased intracranial pressure caused by communicating hydrocephalus.
- Meningeal signs
- If associated with trauma, intraventricular hemorrhage may be:

—Leakage of cerebrospinal fluid from the ear or nose
—Battle sign: bruising over the mastoid process suggestive of basilar skull fracture
—Macewen sign: percussion of the skull gives a cracked pot sound suggestive of skull fracture
—Raccoon eyes: periorbital ecchymosis suggestive of recent head trauma
—Retinal hemorrhages

- Herpes simplex type 1 encephalitis: frequently presents with fever, cognitive impairment, seizures
- Germinal matrix hemorrhages are frequently clinically silent but may present with apnea in the newborn.
- Intracranial hemorrhage should be suspected in the septic-appearing neonate, especially if there are no obvious risk factors for sepsis.
- Subarachnoid hemorrhage frequently presents as the worst headache ever experienced, subhyaloid hemorrhages, and signs of meningeal irritation.

Laboratory Aids

TESTS

Imaging

• CT of the head is the most important study to obtain when considering intracranial hemorrhage in the differential diagnosis because of its relative convenience, speed, and low false-negative rate. Acute blood appears as areas of increased density on head CT; however, after approximately 3 days, the blood will appear progressively less dense.
• MRI is frequently less useful for diagnosing acute hemorrhage unless signal sequences are specifically adjusted to look for blood.
• MRI is the diagnostic study of choice for venous sinus thrombosis.
• Lumbar puncture, if not contraindicated because of increased intracranial pressure, thrombocytopenia, or skin infection, will show RBCs and xanthochromia if the blood is contiguous with the ventricular system. If there is a high suspicion for subarachnoid hemorrhage and CT does not show evidence of hemorrhage, it is important to continue to try to rule out the condition by spinal fluid evaluation. The presence of several hundred RBCs or xanthochromia (best observed in natural light by the clinician taking the CSF sample) raises the likelihood that a small subarachnoid hemorrhage is present.
• Angiography, either with conventional dye or using magnetic resonance angiography, is helpful when looking for vasospasm and arterial venous malformations. It also helps to identify aneurysms that may have ruptured and may require neurosurgical intervention (e.g., insertion of clips or thromboembolic coils).
• Head ultrasound is the most convenient method for diagnosing germinal matrix and intraventricular hemorrhages in infants. Infants born at gestational age of <32 weeks, with birth weight <1,800 g, or infants at high risk due to low Hct, low platelets, unstable BP, cardiopulmonary arrest, or pneumothorax. If hemorrhage is identified or until approximately 32 weeks gestational age, serial ultrasound examinations are warranted.

 Therapy

• Acyclovir therapy should be instituted if herpes simplex type 1 encephalitis is considered, because, if untreated, there is a high rate of mortality.
• Intracranial aneurysms are frequently amenable to neurosurgical intervention to decrease the likelihood of rebleeding; in addition, careful control of increased intracranial pressure, decreasing vasospasm with nimodipine, and prompt attention to hydrocephalus may be necessary.
• Neurosurgical intervention is frequently necessary for subdural and epidural hematomas. Frequent serial neurologic examinations and CT scans should be performed on all patients undergoing treatment for intracranial hemorrhage.

 Follow-Up

• Patients should be observed long-term for evidence of hypoxic-ischemic injury including cognitive deficits, focal motor weakness, and seizures. Since in some cases of intracranial hemorrhage there is no damage to the underlying brain parenchyma, good neurologic recovery is possible.

PREVENTION

• Automobile seat belts; bicycle, skating, and skateboarding helmets; child abuse prevention; diving safety practices; preventing falls; maintaining safe driving speeds; keeping children away from firearms.

PITFALLS

• Epidural hematoma may present in a delayed fashion after head trauma. A typical scenario would consist of head trauma with or without brief loss of consciousness followed by complete resolution to normal neurologic baseline, a "lucid interval" of approximately 24 hours, and then the sudden hemorrhage accompanied by change in consciousness, headache, and other neurologic symptoms and signs.
• Early subarachnoid hemorrhage may not be apparent on CT and may require LP (if safe to perform) or serial CT evaluation while a patient is under clinical observation.
• Intracranial hemorrhage, especially in young infants and children without an obvious etiology, should raise the suspicion of nonaccidental trauma.
• Patients with concussion without intracranial hemorrhage may still develop cerebral edema, and these patients should be observed closely for signs of increasing intracranial pressure.

ICD-9-CD 432.9

BIBLIOGRAPHY

Adams RJ. Stroke prevention and treatment in sickle cell disease. *Arch Neurol* 2001;58(4): 565–568.

deVeber G. Cerebrovascular disease in children. In Swaima KF and Aswall S, eds. *Pediatric Neurology*, 3rd ed. St. Louis: Mosby, 1999.

Fenichel GM. *Clinical pediatric neurology.* Philadelphia: WB Saunders, 1997.

Medeiros D, Buchanan GR. Major hemorrhage in children with idiopathic thrombocytopenia purpura: immediate response to therapy and long term outcome. *J Pediatr* 1998;133(3): 334–339.

Proust F, Toussaint P, Garnieri J, et al. Pediatric cerebral aneurysms. *J Neurosurg* 2001;94(5):733–739.

Tabori U, Kornecki A, Sofer S, et al. Repeat computed tomographic scan within 24–48 hours of admission in children with moderate and severe head trauma. *Crit Care Med* 2000;28(3):840–844.

Wear WE. Index of suspicion. Case presentation. *Pediatr Rev* 1997;18(7): 248,250–251.

Author: Ann Poduri
Douglas Hyder, 2nd edition

Intussusception

 Database

DEFINITION

• Intussusception is the telescoping of one part of the bowel into itself and leads to significant morbidity if diagnosed late. It is the most common abdominal emergency of early childhood. Telescoping of the bowel causes diminished venous blood flow due to venous ischemia. This results in edema and hemorrhage, leading to decreased arterial flow and ischemia and infarction. Male/female ratio is 3:2. Peak age of presentation is the first year of life.
• Ileocolic accounts for 90% of intussusceptions.
• Ileoileal and colocolic types do occur.
• Ischemia of the bowel occurs later in the course of disease and rarely in the first 24 hours of intussusception.

There are two subtypes of the disease associated with age at diagnosis and underlying lead point; in younger patients it is idiopathic and in older patients (after 3rd year of life) an underlying lead point should be looked for (Meckel's diverticulum; lymphoma).

EPIDEMIOLOGY

• Male/female ratio 3:2
• Most common from 6 to 12 months

COMPLICATIONS

• Bowel necrosis secondary to local ischemia
• Gastrointestinal bleeding
• Bowel perforation
• Sepsis, shock

PROGNOSIS

• Timely diagnosis results in a highly favorable prognosis.
• Hydrostatic reduction by air or barium enema is therapeutic in 50% to 90%.
• Risk of recurrence is approximately 10% after reduction, 1% after manual reduction, and not reported after intestinal resection.

 Differential Diagnosis

• Infection: parasites (*Enterobius*)
• Tumors: The association of lymphoma and intussusception is known.
• A series of 1,200 intussusceptions reported 11 lymphomas; all patients were over 3 years of age. Only one lymphoma was reduced, and a filling defect was noted in the cecum.
• Congenital: Hirschsprung disease
• Immunologic: Henoch-Schönlein purpura: often found at the same time
• Miscellaneous:

—Meckel diverticulum: usually painless rectal bleeding
—Incarcerated hernia
—Incarcerated malrotation (midgut volvulus)
—Obstruction: adhesions, hernia, volvulus, stricture, bezoar, foreign body, fecal impaction, polyp

 Data Gathering

HISTORY

• Intermittent abdominal pain with emesis and blood and mucous stools is considered the classic presentation.
• A complete classic presentation is only found in 20% of cases.
• Colicky pain is the major symptom.
• "Currant-jelly" stools appear in about 50% of cases.

 Physical Examination

• A mass effect in the right upper quadrant may be noted.
• Absence of bowel contents in right lower quadrant (Dance sign)
• Occasionally, the intussusception can be felt on rectal examination.
• A bowel sound may be absent.

Laboratory Aids

TESTS

- CBC, electrolytes
- Plain abdominal films: obstruction, air-fluid levels, paucity of distal gas, soft tissue mass; may result in false-negative reading
- Barium enema: "cervix-like mass" or "coiled spring" on evacuation film

PITFALLS

- Some of the classic symptoms may be absent on presentation, and suspicion must be sufficient to act upon.
- Hypovolemic patients will be worsened with high osmotic contrast agents.

 ## Therapy

- The bowel should be decompressed by use of NG tube.
- An intravenous line should be placed, and fluid and electrolyte losses should be corrected.
- Contraindications to reduction by BE include peritonitis, shock, and perforation.
- Caution should be used when symptoms have been present more than 5 days and when radiologic evidence of obstruction, fever, or leukocytosis are present.
- A barium enema may miss a lead point.
- A surgical consultation should be obtained before the reduction attempt; because reduction may cause perforation, and failed reduction requires surgical correction.
- Perforation during reduction occurs in 1% of cases, mostly in the transverse colon.

 ## Follow-Up

Recurrence after nonoperative reduction has been reported in up to 10% and usually is seen within 24 hours of the reduction, so hospitalization and observation are appropriate.

 ## Common Questions and Answers

Q: Can my child have a recurrent intussusception?
A: Yes, the risk, though, is very low, probably below 10% if the child has had a nonsurgical reduction or removal of the lead point.

Q: Can my child with constipation get this problem?
A: This is doubtful, although in severe cases it might be possible.

Q: What are the common ages for presentation?
A: Six months to 3 years is the age range associated with the greatest risk of intussusception, but it can occur at any age. The prevalence of pathologic conditions rises with the age of a child diagnosed with intussusception.

ICD-9-CM 560.0

BIBLIOGRAPHY

Chang HG, Smith PF, Ackelsberg J, et al. Intussusception, rotavirus diarrhea, and rotavirus vaccine use among children in New York State. *Pediatrics* 2001;108(1):54–60.

Ein SH, Stephens CA, Shandling B, et al. Intussusception due to lymphoma. *J Pediatr Surg* 1986;21:786–788.

Fujimoto T, Fukuda T, Uetani M, et al. Unenhanced CT findings of vascular compromise in association with intussusceptions in adults. *AJR* 2001;176(5):1167–1171.

Petit P, Pracros J. Role of ultrasound in children with acute abdominal pain. *J Radiol* 2001;82(6 suppl):764–778.

Stringer DA, Ein SH. Pneumatic reduction: advantages, risks and indications. *Pediatr Radiol* 1990;20:475–477.

Tamanaha K. Air reduction of intussusception in infants and children. *J Pediatr* 1987;3:733–736

Author: Dror Wasserman

Iron Deficiency Anemia

 Database

DEFINITION

A decrease in hemoglobin production due to an insufficient supply of iron that results in a microcytic, hypochromic anemia.

PATHOPHYSIOLOGY

• Iron is required for oxygen transport by hemoglobin.
• Iron homeostasis is regulated by gastrointestinal absorption (duodenum and upper jejunum).
• Causes of iron depletion include:

—Dietary deficiency
—Malabsorption
—Blood loss. Most commonly secondary to cow's milk enteropathy (seen in infants).

• Other etiologies include perinatal loss, inflammatory bowel disease, pulmonary hemosiderosis, hematuria, and menorrhagia.
• Increased requirements. Seen with rapid growth. Low birth weight infants and adolescents are particularly susceptible.
• Sequential stages of iron deficiency:

—Depletion of iron stores. Reflected by low serum ferritin. Increase iron absorption when possible.
—Iron deficient erythropoiesis. Near-normal number of red blood cells produced, but have abnormal hemoglobin synthesis with wide distribution in red blood cell size.
—Iron deficiency anemia. Microcytosis evident. May lead to impaired tissue oxygenation.

EPIDEMIOLOGY

• Leading cause of anemia among infants and children in the United States. Most commonly seen in children ages 9 months to 3 years and in teenage girls. Prevalence is variable depending on socioeconomic status, availability of iron-fortified formulas, prevalence and duration of breast-feeding, and the way that iron deficiency is defined. Prevalence is generally between 1% and 8% of children in the United States.

COMPLICATIONS

• Impaired cognitive and motor development in infants and toddlers.
• Positive correlation between cognitive and motor deficits and severity and duration of anemia.
• Impaired lymphocyte and neutrophil function leading to an increased risk of infection.
• Short-term memory impairment and poor exercise performance in adolescents

PROGNOSIS

• Anemia readily corrected with iron replacement.
• Developmental delay may be long lasting or irreversible.

 Differential Diagnosis

• Recent infection
• Lead poisoning
• Thalassemia trait
• Anemia of chronic disease (JRA, IBD, renal failure)

 Data Gathering

HISTORY

• Evaluate dietary intake of iron, including breast- or formula feeding and type of formula
• Age of introduction of cow's milk
• Daily intake of cow's milk
• Birth history for prematurity or blood loss
• Pica
• Lead exposure
• Blood loss from urine, stool, menorrhagia
• Decreased exercise tolerance in adolescents

 Physical Examination

• Usually normal exam
• Pallor, irritability
• Tachycardia, flow murmur
• Koilonychia
• Glossitis or stomatitis
• Test for occult blood in stool and urine.

 Laboratory Aids

• Low hemoglobin. Hemoglobin less than 2 standard deviations below the age specific mean.
• Low MCV (red cell volume) and MCH (hemoglobin concentration) for age.
• High red cell distribution width (RDW) >14.5%. Measures the variation in red cell size. Often increased before anemia present.
• Low serum ferritin reflects tissue iron stores. Earliest laboratory abnormality. May be normal or increased with concurrent infection.
• Low serum iron
• Increased transferrin (total iron binding capacity)
• Low transferrin saturation; measures the iron available for hemoglobin synthesis
• Increased soluble transferrin receptor. Indicator of increased tissue iron demand. Also increased in thalassemia syndromes.
• Increased free erythrocyte protoporphyrin (FEP), a precursor molecule to hemoglobin synthesis. Also increased in lead poisoning and chronic inflammation.
• Thrombocytosis (500,000–700,000 cells/fL)
• Peripheral blood smear with microcytosis, hypochromia, poikilocytosis, and anisocytosis
• Hypercellular bone marrow with erythroid hyperplasia and poor hemoglobinization. Decreased iron stores by hemosiderin staining. Bone marrow rarely needed to establish diagnosis.

Therapy

• Oral replacement with ferrous iron, 4 to 6 mg/kg/day of elemental iron divided into two or three doses. Iron should be given on an empty stomach or with a vitamin C–containing juice to increase absorption.
• Family education regarding age-appropriate diet and iron-containing foods
• May require initial inpatient observation in cases of severe anemia
• Red cell transfusion only if evidence of cardiovascular compromise (rarely indicated)
• Parenteral (IM or IV) iron dextran indicated only for severe noncompliance, malabsorption, or if ongoing loss exceeds absorption capacity. Administration may be associated with pain at injection site or anaphylaxis.

Follow-Up

• Reticulocyte count should double in 1 to 2 weeks.
• Hemoglobin concentration should be increased at least 1.0 g/dL in 2 to 4 weeks.
• Check CBC and reticulocyte count at 2 weeks to assess response.
• Continue iron for 3 months to replete body stores.

PREVENTION

• Maintain breast-feeding for the first 5 to 6 months of life when possible. Although the concentration of iron is lower in breast milk than in formula, iron in breast milk is more bioavailable (50% vs. 10%).
• Iron supplementation (1 mg/kg/day) for infants who are exclusively breast-fed beyond 6 months.
• Iron-fortified formula for the first 12 months of life for infants who are not breast-fed.
• Iron supplementation after 2 months of life for low birth weight and premature infants because of decreased iron stores and increased growth rate.
• Encourage iron-enriched cereal when infants are started on solid food.
• Avoid whole cow's milk during the first year of life to prevent occult GI bleeding.
• Screen hemoglobin level at periodic intervals. (AAP recommends 9 months, 5 years, and 14 years.)

PITFALLS

• Causes of poor response to oral iron supplementation include:

—Noncompliance (most common)
—Ongoing blood loss
—Insufficient duration of therapy
—High gastric pH
—Concurrent lead intoxication
—Incorrect diagnosis (thalassemia trait and anemia of chronic disease are not iron responsive.)

Common Questions and Answers

Q: What dietary changes can help prevent the reoccurrence of iron deficiency?
A: Limit milk to not more than 24 ounces a day so that your child has a better appetite for iron-containing foods. Foods rich in iron include meats, fish, and poultry. Other foods that contain iron are raisins, dried fruit, sweet potatoes, lima beans, chili beans, green peas, peanut butter, and enriched foods. Give iron on an empty stomach along with an ascorbic acid-containing juice to increase absorption of iron. Foods that decrease iron absorption include bran, vegetable fiber, tannins found in tea, and phosphates. Antacids may also decrease iron absorption.

Q: What are the side effects of iron therapy?
A: Iron can cause temporary staining of the teeth, which can be decreased by diluting the iron with a small amount of juice. Iron will also change the color of bowel movements to greenish black and may be associated with constipation.

Q: What are the most important tests to do to establish the diagnosis of iron deficiency?
A: For patients with a history of dietary deficiency or known blood loss, a complete blood count that shows a low Hgb and MCV and an elevated RDW is very suggestive of iron deficiency. A therapeutic trial of iron without further laboratory testing is an appropriate next diagnostic step. An increase in the hemoglobin concentration of 1 g/dL or greater after 1 month of therapy confirms the diagnosis. If this does not occur, further laboratory testing is necessary and other diagnoses should be considered.

Q: How does a concurrent infection affect the diagnosis of iron deficiency?
A: Common childhood infections can be associated with a mild microcytic anemia that resembles iron deficiency. Laboratory tests to diagnose iron deficiency can be misleading while a child is acutely ill. Acute infection is associated with a shift of iron from serum to storage sites causing a decrease in serum iron and an increase in ferritin. It is therefore more helpful to screen a child for iron deficiency 3 to 4 weeks after an acute infection.

ICD-9-CM 280

BIBLIOGRAPHY

Booth I, Aukett MA. Iron deficiency anaemia in infancy and early childhood. *Arch Dis Child* 1997;76:549–554.

Graham EA. The changing face of anemia in infancy. *Pediatr Rev* 1994;15:175–183.

Griffin IJ, Abrams SA. Iron and breastfeeding. *Pediatr Clin North Am* 1001;48:401–413.

Lozoff B, Jimenez E, Wolf AW. Iron deficiency anemia and infant development: effects of extended oral iron therapy. *J Pediatr* 1996;129:382–389.

Lozoff B, Jimenez E, Wolf AW. Long-term developmental outcome of infants with iron deficiency anemia. *N Engl J Med* 1991;325:687–694.

Nathan DG, Orkin SH, eds. *Nathan and Oski's hematology of infancy and childhood*, 5th ed. Philadelphia: WB Saunders, 1998.

Oski FA. Iron deficiency anemia in infancy and childhood. *N Engl J Med* 1993;129:190–193.

Pappas DE. Iron deficiency anemia. *Pediatr Rev* 1998;19:321–322.

Wharton BA. Iron deficiency in children: detection and prevention. *Br J Hematol* 1999;106:270–280.

Author: Suzanne Shusterman

Iron Poisoning

 Database

DEFINITION

Iron poisoning is the result of the ingestion of >20 mg/kg of elemental iron.
Toxic doses of elemental iron and usual effects:

- <20 mg/kg—usually nontoxic
- 20 to 30 mg/kg—self-limited abdominal pain, vomiting, diarrhea
- 40 to 60 mg/kg—shock, coma
- >60 mg/kg—potentially lethal

PATHOPHYSIOLOGY

- Direct corrosive effect on gastric mucosa causes hemorrhagic necrosis and perforation.
- Absorbed iron causes multisystem cellular dysfunction by two postulated mechanisms:

—Uncoupling mitochondrial oxidative phosphorylation
—Disruption of the lipid peroxidase system through the generation of ferrous ions, which are free radicals

EPIDEMIOLOGY

- Most common cause of fatal poisonings in children.
- Most cases in children 4 years old and younger.
- The victim of an accidental ingestion has a 25% chance of sustaining another within 1 year.

COMPLICATIONS

- Hemorrhagic shock
- Hypovolemic shock
- Coagulopathy
- Hepatic failure
- Renal failure
- Myocardial dysfunction
- Yersinia sepsis
- Acute respiratory distress syndrome (ARDS)
- Seizures
- Gastric outlet obstruction
- Small bowel obstruction
- Coma
- Death

PROGNOSIS

- If asymptomatic for 6 hours postingestion and WBC, glucose, and abdominal x-ray normal, then prognosis is excellent.
- Serum iron >500 μg/dL is a poor prognostic sign.

 Differential Diagnosis

INGESTIONS

- Drain cleaners (sulfuric acid)
- Oven cleaners (sodium hydroxide)
- Dishwasher detergents (tripolyphosphates)

GASTROINTESTINAL

- Gastroenteritis
- Hemolytic uremic syndrome
- Esophagitis
- Gastritis
- Mallory-Weiss tear
- Vascular malformation

 Data Gathering

HISTORY

- Ask about form of iron ingested
- Approximate number of cc's or pills
- Determine amount (in mg) of elemental iron ingested
- Also inquire about other medicines (including OTC medications and herbals) in home

 Physical Examination

- Assess mental status (parents often very helpful here)
- Assess for cardiovascular stability (tachycardia suggests early shock, hypotension suggests severe shock)
- Test stool and emesis for occult blood

Phases of Acute Iron Poisoning

PHASE	TIME RANGE	DESCRIPTION
Phase I	0–6 hours	Nausea, vomiting, diarrhea, GI hemorrhage, metabolic acidosis, leukocytosis, hyperglycemia, seizures, lethargy, shock, coma
Phase II	2–6 hours	Apparent recovery
Phase III	6–48 hours	Recurrence of GI bleeding, anion gap metabolic acidosis, coagulopathy, renal failure, myocardial depression, shock, coma
Phase IV	2–5 days	Hepatic failure with jaundice, hypoglycemia
Phase V	2–6 weeks	Pyloric scarring, small bowel obstruction

Laboratory Aids

TESTS

- Serum iron at 4 hours after ingestion
- CBC to help quantify and follow blood loss
- PT, PTT at presentation and to follow for evolving coagulopathy
- Electrolytes, glucose, BUN, Cr, transaminases at presentation and to follow for renal/liver damage
- Consider ABG to assess severity of metabolic acidosis when present.
- Consider type and cross if significant GI bleeding or any cardiovascular instability.
- TIBC generally felt to be unreliable

RADIOGRAPHIC STUDIES

- Always obtain abdominal x-ray—useful to visualize pill fragments before and after lavage

 Therapy

- If asymptomatic, check 4-hour iron level, electrolytes, and abdominal x-ray. Observe for 6 hours. If still no symptoms, then discharge patient.
- Supportive care (airway, fluid, etc.)
- Syrup of ipecac if not already vomiting
- Consider gastric lavage with normal saline if ingestion known to be >60 mg/kg and/or pill fragments seen on abdominal x-ray.
- Whole bowel irrigation with polyethylene glycol electrolyte lavage solution if pill fragments visible on abdominal x-ray after initial emesis or lavage, or if severe symptoms present.
- Hemodialysis/hemoperfusion only for renal failure for removing deferoxamine-iron complex
- Activated charcoal is ineffective.
- Cathartics are not recommended.
- Deferoxamine IV if more than transient, minor symptoms or serum iron >500 μg/dL. Monitor urine for orange color of chelated complex. When urine returns to normal or when serum iron normalizes, treatment may be stopped.

 Follow-Up

Repeat serum iron level and abdominal x-ray until normal.

PREVENTION

- Encourage safe storage of all iron containing medicines (especially prenatal vitamins).
- Counsel family about preventing future ingestion and other home safety issues.

PITFALLS

- Iron is rapidly cleared from the serum and deposited in the liver, so the peak level may be missed and iron levels may be deceptively low within a few hours of a substantial ingestion.
- An iron bezoar of partially digested pill fragments may need to be removed from the stomach by endoscopy or gastrostomy.
- Missing the diagnosis in a patient in phase 2 of iron ingestion.
- Rapid infusion of deferoxamine IV can cause hypotension.
- Compazine and deferoxamine given simultaneously can cause coma.

 Common Questions and Answers

Q: Above what serum iron level is systemic toxicity generally seen?
A: 350 μg/dL

Q: For how long should a patient with iron ingestion of unknown quantity be observed for symptoms?
A: Six hours.

ICD-9-CM 964.0

BIBLIOGRAPHY

Fine JS. Iron poisoning. *Curr Probl Pediatr* 2000;30(3):71–90.

Litovitz T, Manoguerra A. Comparison of pediatric poisoning hazards: an analysis of 3.8 million exposure incidents. *Pediatrics* 1992;89(6):999–1006.

Morris CC. Pediatric iron poisonings in the United States. *South Med J* 2000;93(4):352–358.

Osterhoudt KC, Shannon M, Henretig FM. Toxicologic emergencies. In: Fleisher GR, Ludwig S, eds. *Textbook of pediatric emergency medicine,* 4th ed. Philadelphia: Lippincott Williams & Wilkins, 1999:914–917.

San Francisco Bay Area Regional Poison Control Center. *Poisoning and drug overdose.* Norwalk: Appleton & Lange, 1994:189–191.

Author: Deirdre Bernard-Pearl

Irritable Bowel Syndrome

 Database

DEFINITION

• Irritable bowel syndrome (IBS) describes a cluster of symptoms that include abdominal distention and pain, improvement in the abdominal pain after a bowel movement, an increasing number of stools with the start of the pain, and looser stools with mucus associated with the onset of pain. These symptoms need to occur on a recurrent basis in order for IBS to be considered.
• Terms such as *spastic colon, nervous colon*, or *spastic colitis* have also been used to describe IBS. Spastic colitis, however, is inaccurate because these patients do not have evidence of inflammation of their colon (colitis) at colonoscopy.

PATHOPHYSIOLOGY

• Most commonly, IBS is thought to be a problem with the motility of the gastrointestinal tract.
• There are no actual histologic, microbiologic, or biochemical abnormalities noted in patients with IBS.
• A variety of investigators have hypothesized that IBS may represent an altered perception of normal gastrointestinal motility.
• A variety of other mechanisms for IBS have been proposed and include:

—Altered electric response in the colon to food
—Motility studies that in some cases demonstrated certain differences (attributed to abnormal smooth muscle function) between patients with IBS and normal controls, including poor antral contractility, high pressure/poorer contracting duodenal contractions, disrupted migrating motor complexes, and prominent duodenal contractions at inappropriate times.

EPIDEMIOLOGY

• IBS is thought to occur in 15% to 30% of the general population.
• In adults, IBS is the seventh most common cause of visits to primary care physicians and the most common cause of referral to a gastroenterologist.
• 50% of patients present with symptoms before age 35, and 33% can trace their symptoms back into childhood.
• Female/male ratio ranges from 1.5 to 2.0:1.
• There is no known genetic predisposition for developing IBS.

COMPLICATIONS

• A large number of the complications that arise from IBS are psychologically based. A large number of these patients may show evidence of depression and have increased anxiety.
• Patients with IBS show a significant amount of absenteeism from both school and work.

 Differential Diagnosis

• The diagnosis of IBS is based on a clinical spectrum of symptoms and, as a result, remains a diagnosis of exclusion.
• Common disorders that need to be considered include lactose intolerance, inflammatory bowel disease, constipation, urinary tract infection, esophagitis, gastritis, duodenitis, antibiotic usage (Augmentin, erythromycin), chronic pancreatitis, chronic aspirin use, and nonsteroidal antiinflammatory drug use.
• Less common disorders that need to be considered include giardiasis, celiac disease, ureteropelvic junction obstruction, kidney stones, gallstones, cystic fibrosis, endometriosis, porphyria, duplication/mesenteric cysts, and abdominal migraines.

 Data Gathering

HISTORY

• The initial evaluation of these patients needs to include a careful and detailed history, including a description of the symptoms, with assessment if they recur on a regular basis.
• A detailed diet and travel history can be important to focus the differential.
• Careful questioning about inciting and exacerbating factors
• Clinically, patients with IBS have abdominal pain as their most common presenting complaint. This pain can be sharp, dull, crampy, or burning. It is usually periumbilical or lower abdominal in nature, but not necessarily. The pain starts after a meal and rarely awakens a patient from sleep. Patients, especially children, describe associated symptoms, such as nausea, anorexia, and fatigue with the abdominal pain.
• Another very common complaint at presentation in patients with IBS is abdominal distention and increased belching and/or flatulence.
• Patients with IBS frequently present with a change in their bowel habits. These changes appear to be progressive and at times can lead to bouts of alternating diarrhea and constipation. Patients appear to have one predominant form consistently. Most patients experience relief of pain after a bowel movement. In patients with constipation, they may go several days to a week without any stool passage.
• In some instances, mucus can be described in this group of patients. However, blood is a rare finding and is usually associated with local/anal irritation or fissure secondary to diarrhea or constipation.
• Patients with IBS rarely have other systemic complaints, such as pallor, fever, anorexia, and weight loss.
• Commonly, patients with IBS report that they can identify certain events that exacerbate or trigger an episode. These triggers may include stress, anxiety, certain foods (wheats, milk, alcohol, caffeine), and cigarette smoking.

 Physical Examination

• Findings are usually completely normal, including the abdominal and rectal examinations.
• There is usually no evidence of weight loss or growth failure.
• May have large air pockets

Laboratory Aids

TESTS

- There are no laboratory tests that are diagnostic for IBS. There are some routine laboratory tests that may be helpful in the initial evaluation. These include a CBC, ESR, urinalysis, electrolytes, and albumin. An abdominal x-ray may help to rule out an intraabdominal process, and a lactose breath test will assess lactose intolerance. Stool cultures for routine specimen, *Clostridium difficile* and ova and parasites may also be obtained.
- In certain instances, further testing may include both an upper endoscopy and a colonoscopy.

 ## Therapy

- The best, but at times the most difficult, treatment for IBS is reassurance of both the parents and the child.
- The symptoms should be addressed, but the patient and/or parents should be made aware that the symptoms are not dangerous to the child.
- A variety of interventions have been attempted to decrease the severity of the symptoms.

—Fiber supplementation in the diet is a usual first step in therapy. This is an attempt to prolong stool transit time and then allow for more water absorption. Some also feel that this decreases the high pressure seen in the rectosigmoid region.
—There are a large number of medications that have been used in patients with IBS. Some that may be helpful include the anticholinergics and/or antispasmodics, such as dicyclomine (Bentyl), hyoscyamine (Levsin), Donatal, and mebeverine. Other agents, such as amitriptyline and lorazepam, have been tried in rarer cases.

- Psychotherapy may be tried. Patients are taught a variety of techniques and exercises to use during the episodes of pain that allow them to focus on other subjects, not on the pain.

 ## Follow-Up

There is no standard or specific follow-up needed for patients with IBS. They should continue with routine care, and one should review the clinical symptoms on a regular basis to avoid the misdiagnosis of an underlying problem.

PITFALLS

- Avoid downplaying the clinical symptoms of patients because it will make their acceptance of the treatment plan more difficult.
- Confine testing to basic screening tests so that patients are not left with the impression that there is a significant organic disease present.

 ## Common Questions and Answers

Q: Is there a genetic inheritance with IBS?
A: Although family inheritance patterns exist, no specific data are available.

Q: Are there any personality traits identified that cause certain people to be more likely to develop IBS?
A: Adult studies suggest a predilection for certain types, but no studies have been done on children.

ICD-9-CM 564.1

BIBLIOGRAPHY

Campo JV, Di Lorenzo C, Chiappetta L, et al. Adult outcomes of pediatric recurrent abdominal pain: do they just grow out of it? *Pediatrics* 2001;108(1).

Friedman G. Irritable bowel syndrome I. A practical approach. *Am J Gastroenterol* 1989;84:863–867.

Hyams JS. Recurrent abdominal pain in children. *Curr Opin Pediatr* 1995;7(5): 529–532.

Mezoff AG. Irritable bowel syndrome. In: Wyllie R, Hyams JS, eds. *Pediatric gastrointestinal disease*. Philadelphia: WB Saunders, 1993:724–731.

Milla PJ. Irritable bowel syndrome in childhood. *Gastroenterology* 2001;120(1): 287–290.

Staiano A, Corazziari E. Irritable bowel syndrome: contrasts and comparisons between children and adults. *J Pediatr Gastroenterol Nutr* 2001;32(suppl 1):S32–4.

Talley NJ. Irritable bowel syndrome and health care seeking: do we pass our bad habits onto our children? *Am J Gastroenterol* 2000;95(2):340–341.

Thompson WG. A strategy for management of the irritable bowel. *Am J Gastroenterol* 1986;81:95–100.

Authors: Edisio Semeao and Andrew E. Mulberg

Kawasaki Disease (Mucocutaneous Lymph Node Syndrome)

 Database

DEFINITION

• An idiopathic, multisystem disease of young children characterized by vasculitis of the small- and medium-sized blood vessels.
• Diagnosis of Kawasaki disease (KD) requires a fever for greater than 5 days and four of the following criteria:
—Nonexudative conjunctival injection
—Polymorphous, nonvesicular rash
—Mucosal involvement of the upper respiratory tract that may include erythema, fissures of the lips, crusting of the lips and mouth, or a strawberry tongue. Exudative pharyngitis and discrete oral lesions (e.g., vesicles, etc.) are rare.
—Edema or erythema of the hands and feet
—Cervical adenopathy of at least 1.5 cm in diameter, which is often unilateral
• Atypical KD
—Patients may present with less than four of the five diagnostic criteria and still develop aneurysms.
—Atypical disease is more common in children younger than 1 year of age.

CAUSES

• Etiology is uncertain. Epidemiologic and clinical features suggest an infectious cause.
• Association with recent use of rug cleaners or having had rugs shampooed has not been substantiated.

EPIDEMIOLOGY

• Median age of cases is 2.3 years with 80% of cases in children younger than 4 years of age, 5% of cases in children older than 10 years of age, and almost unheard of in children over age 15. Recurrence is low, approximately 0.8%.
• In the United States, incidence seems to be increasing, approximately 11% in incidence per year in the period 1984–1990.

GENETICS

There is no clear genetic pattern to this disease.

COMPLICATIONS

• Aneurysms usually first noted 12 to 28 days after onset of the disease. Rarely appear more than 28 days after onset.
• Aneurysms may thrombose leading to myocardial infarction and death.
• Rarely, aneurysms may rupture acutely.
• A pancarditis is often present in the first 10 days of the illness. Pericardial effusions may accompany this.

PROGNOSIS

• Without treatment with intravenous immunoglobulin (IVIG) 15% to 25% of patients develop coronary aneurysms.
• Use of IVIG decreased the incidence of coronary artery aneurysms to 4% to 8%.
• Death occurs secondary to cardiac disease in 0.3% to 2% of cases; approximately 10% is related to early myocarditis, and the remainder due to myocardial infarctions.

• Myocardial infarction can occur several years after the initial illness.
• Patients who are younger than 1 year, older than 8 years, male, and whose fevers persist for greater than 14 days are more likely to develop aneurysms.
• Mortality rates are much higher in males and patients who develop giant coronary artery aneurysms (diameter of greater than 8 mm).
• Patients with a history of KD may have a worse cardiovascular risk profile in later life, indicative of an increased risk of atherosclerotic heart disease compared to the general population.

ASSOCIATED ILLNESSES

• Diarrhea and abdominal pain may be seen.
• Patients may develop arthralgias or even frank arthritis.
• Pancarditis may present as myocardial dysfunction early in the course of disease with signs of congestive heart failure.
• Infantile periarteritis nodosa (PAN) is a previously described entity in which the pathologic findings of coronary artery aneurysms are indistinguishable from those seen in KD. Most patients with PAN do not have the other findings of KD.

 Differential Diagnosis

• Infections
—In one series, measles and group A β-hemolytic streptococcal infections most closely resembled KD and accounted for 83% of patients referred who did not have KD.
—Severe staphylococcal infections with toxin release (e.g., toxic shock syndrome) may also resemble KD, although there is usually renal involvement (extremely rare in KD) and low platelets.
—Other infections that must be considered include adenovirus, Epstein-Barr virus, roseola, enterovirus, Rocky Mountain spotted fever, and leptospirosis.
• Immunologic
—Juvenile rheumatoid arthritis and unusual variants of acute rheumatic fever
—Hypersensitivity reactions and Stevens-Johnson syndrome
—In Stevens-Johnson syndrome the conjunctivitis is more likely to be exudative, the rash is more likely to be vesicular with crusting, and there is often a history of drug ingestion.

 Data Gathering

HISTORY

Typical presentation proceeds through three recognizable phases:
• Acute phase (1–2 weeks from onset):
—Highly febrile, irritable, toxic appearing
—Fever usually greater than 40°C and may be as high as 41.6°C
—Oral changes usually quickly follow and also may last 1 to 2 weeks.

—Rash prone to occur in perineal area
—Edema and erythema of the feet are usually painful and limit ambulation.
• Subacute phase (from 2 to 8 weeks after onset)
—Without treatment gradual improvement occurs; fever decreases and there is desquamation of the perineal area, palms, soles, and/or periungual areas.
—Coronary artery aneurysms often appear during the early portion of this phase and acute myocardial infarction may be seen.
—May have persistent arthritis or arthralgias
• Convalescent phase (from months to years after)
—Resolution of remaining symptoms
—Laboratory values return to normal (see subsequent text).
—Aneurysms may resolve or patients may have persistent aneurysms, persistent cardiac dysfunction, or even myocardial infarction.

 Physical Examination

Finding: High, unremitting fevers that last 1 to 2 weeks
Significance: Fever
Finding: Rash is polymorphous and not vesicular.
Significance: Seen in 99% of cases; predilection for perineum. Often prominent on trunk, usually maculopapular, may coalesce and may be petechial.
Finding: Conjunctivitis
Significance: Bilateral and nonexudative (96% of cases)
Finding: Oral changes may be erythema, fissures, and crusting of lips, diffuse oropharyngeal erythema, or the presence of a strawberry tongue or any combination of these findings.
Significance: Usually not exudative
Finding: Extremity changes may include erythema of the palms and soles and/or induration of the hands and feet (99% of cases).
Significance: Desquamation, especially periungual, usually occurs in subacute phase. Transverse grooves across the fingernails (Beau lines) may be seen 2 to 3 months after onset.
Finding: Adenopathy is usually cervical and often unilateral.
Significance: Least often seen of the major criteria (75–82% of cases). May be fleeting and easily missed.
Finding: Aseptic meningitis
Significance: Is common and patients are extremely irritable and may show signs of encephalopathy or ataxia.
Finding: Pancarditis during the acute phase
Significance: May present with tachycardia, gallop rhythms, muffled heart sounds, signs of congestive heart failure, and murmurs consistent with aortic and mitral insufficiency.
Finding: Abdominal exam
Significance: Patients may have a right upper quadrant mass (hydrops of gallbladder), diarrhea, hepatosplenomegaly, or jaundice.

Kawasaki Disease (Mucocutaneous Lymph Node Syndrome)

Finding: Meatitis and vulvitis
Significance: May be seen in association with urethritis and sterile pyuria.
Finding: Arthralgias are common; frank arthritis is seen in approximately one third of patients.
Significance: May involve large and small joints; is nondeforming. Onset may be as late as second or third week. Usually resolves in approximately 1 month.
Finding: Uveitis
Significance: During acute phase, slit lamp examination may reveal anterior uveitis in approximately 80% of KD cases.

 ## Laboratory Aids

Test: Complete blood cell
Significance: WBC usually increased with a left shift; greater than 20,000 in 50% of cases and greater than 30,000 in 15%. Hemoglobin less than 10 mg/dL is an independent predictor of poor response to IVIG.
Test: Increased erythrocyte sedimentation rate; increased CRP
Significance: ESR often greater than 100 mm; CRP greater than 10 predicts a poor response to IVIG.
Test: Platelet count
Significance: Platelets may be low, normal, or high at presentation but increase rapidly after the second week of illness; during subacute phase platelet counts may increase to 1 to 2×10^6.
Test: Lactate dehydrogenase level (LDH)
Significance: LDH greater than 590 IU/L predicts poor response to IVIG.
Test: Other laboratory abnormalities include:
• Sterile pyuria and mild proteinuria on urinalysis
• Mild increases in hepatic transaminases
• A cerebrospinal fluid pleocytosis with a normal protein and glucose
• Mild anemia
• Mild hypoalbuminemia
• Hyponatremia
• Hypophosphatemia
• Severe hemolytic anemias

Test: ECG
Significance: During acute phase may show prolonged PR interval, decreased QRS voltage, flat T waves, and ST changes.
Test: Chest x-ray
Significance: May show dilated heart during acute phase.
Test: Echocardiogram
Significance: During acute phase can show a decreased shortening fraction and effusion. Aneurysms may be detected as early as 6 days into the illness, and peak onset is between 3 to 4 weeks.
Test: Increased BUN or creatinine
Significance: If laboratory indicators of renal involvement are present, then illnesses other than KD should be considered (e.g., toxic shock syndrome).

 ## Emergency Care

• Maintain high suspicion so that cases of KD are not missed in the emergency department.
• If KD is suspected, assess for cardiac dysfunction with an ECG and obtain a cardiology consult.
• Good supportive care should be provided including fluid therapy and possibly inotropes to treat shock when present (rare presentation).
• Admission for definitive treatment and monitoring is imperative.

 ## Therapy

DRUGS
• Intravenous immunoglobulin (IVIG)
—Usual dose is 2 g/kg as a one-time dose over 10 hours.
—Efficacy of IVIG after the 10th day of illness is unclear.
—Patients who fail to respond to an initial dose of IVIG or who have a recrudescence of their symptoms should be retreated (up to two thirds may have a good response to repeat doses).
—Side effects: Patients may develop signs of fluid overload and congestive heart failure.
• Aspirin
—High-dose aspirin was the mainstay of therapy; still used in conjunction with IVIG, although no data look at IVIG with aspirin versus IVIG alone.
—Usual initial dose is 80 to 100 mg/kg/d in divided doses. High dose required to overcome malabsorption of aspirin seen during acute phase of KD.
• Corticosteroids
—New data suggest IV pulse methylprednisolone may be useful.
—Methylprednisolone has been given in conjunction with early doses of IVIG or as rescue therapy in patients who don't respond to two or three doses of IVIG. It may need to be tapered to prevent recrudescence of symptoms.
• Cyclophosphamide has also been reported to be useful in some patients who do not respond to repeated doses of IVIG.

DURATION
• Aspirin is continued at high dose until day 14 of the illness or when the child has been afebrile for 48 hours.
• Aspirin dose is then decreased to 30 mg/kg/d until 4 weeks after onset and additionally decreased to 3 to 10 mg/kg/d for 6 to 8 weeks or until the platelet count returns to normal.
• If there are coronary artery abnormalities dipyridamole at 3 to 5 mg/kg/d should be added to the aspirin for its vasodilatory effect. Aspirin and dipyridamole should be continued for 1 year or until coronary artery aneurysms resolve.

ACTIVITY
• Children with KD should be kept at bed rest until the second or third week of illness or when they have been afebrile for over 72 hours due to the possibility of myocardial involvement during the acute phase.
• Isolation of patients is not indicated.
• Even asymptomatic patients should be restricted from strenuous activities.

 ## Follow-Up

WHEN TO EXPECT IMPROVEMENT
• The natural course is a gradual improvement during the subacute phase.
• With IVIG children usually defervesce and show significant resolution of clinical symptoms within 2 to 3 days of treatment (70–80%).
• Two thirds of patients who receive a repeat dose of IVIG will respond to this dose.

SIGNS TO WATCH FOR
• White blood cell count, platelet count, and ESR should be followed weekly to biweekly until they return to normal.
• Weekly echocardiograms should be done to rule out the development of coronary artery aneurysms from weeks 2 to 6 of the illness.
• If aneurysms are present, cardiology follow-up should include coronary artery catheterization and imaging at some time (usually 8–12 weeks after onset of illness).
• Symptoms of cardiac insufficiency (fatigue, chest pain, dyspnea on exertion, etc.) should be respected and an evaluation for myocardial dysfunction undertaken when these are present.
• In patients with aneurysms, ECG, CXR, echocardiogram, and exercise myocardial perfusion studies should be done at regular intervals.

Common Questions and Answers

Q: Do coronary artery aneurysms associated with KD ever resolve?
A: Most coronary artery aneurysms do resolve. Even some giant aneurysms (those greater than 8 mm in diameter) will resolve; there is concern, however, that even if aneurysms resolve, these patients may be at risk for the early development of atherosclerosis.

ICD-9-CD 446.1

BIBLIOGRAPHY
Momenah T, Sanatini S, Potts J, et al. Kawasaki disease in the older child. *Pediatrics* 1998;102(1):e7.

Rowley AH, Shulman ST. Kawasaki syndrome. *Pediatr Clin North Am* 1999;46(2): 313–329.

Silva AA, Maeno Y, Hashmi A, et al. Cardiovascular risk factors after Kawasaki disease: a case-control study. *J Pediatr* 2001;138(3):400–405.

Author: James M. Callahan

Kwashiorkor

 Database

DEFINITION

• Extreme expression of protein-energy malnutrition
• Characterized by edema, growth failure, hypoalbuminemia, fatty infiltration of the liver, and specific dermatosis
• First described in West Africa by Cecily Williams. The word *kwashiorkor* in Ghanian means "red or yellow boy."

CAUSES

Diet deficient in protein and a low protein-to-energy ratio are important factors in the development of kwashiorkor. Other factors postulated include:

• Carbohydrate overloading of a severely malnourished child
• Aflatoxin poisoning
• Imbalance between the production of toxic free radical and its disposal
• Essential fatty acid deficiency
• Deficiency of trace minerals (e.g., zinc, copper, manganese, and selenium)
• Oxidative and nitrosative stress

PATHOPHYSIOLOGY

• Hypoalbuminemia reduces colloid osmotic pressure, leading to edema.
• Reduction in renal blood flow and glomerular filtration rate due to decreased plasma volume and decreased cardiac output as a consequence of hypoalbuminemia.
• Increase in ferritin stimulates release of antidiuretic hormone and subsequent fluid retention.

EPIDEMIOLOGY

• Most common age group are children younger than 2 years of age.
• Prevalent in Third World countries; occurs in developed countries secondary to nutritional ignorance rather than food deprivation
• Other contributory factors include misconception concerning the use of foods, unstable home environment, high prevalence of alcoholism, poor sanitary conditions, and societal beliefs that prohibit the use of many nutritious foods.

COMPLICATIONS

• Fluid and electrolyte disturbances

—Hypoosmolality with moderate hyponatremia
—Mild-to-moderate metabolic acidosis
—Hypocalcemia
—Decreased body potassium without hypokalemia
—Decreased body magnesium with or without hypomagnesemia

• Infections

—Gram-positive and gram-negative organisms; the latter is more common in severe protein-energy malnutrition

• Cardiac failure

—May occur in the midst of severe anemia, during rehydration, and shortly after the introduction of high-protein and high-energy feedings

• Severe anemia

—Hemoglobin levels usually improve with proper dietary management.
—Blood transfusion should be reserved for patients with hemoglobin less than 4 g/100 mL, hypoxia, or impending cardiac failure.

• Hypothermia and hypoglycemia

—Secondary to either impaired nonregulatory mechanisms, reduced fuel substrate, or severe infection

• Severe vitamin deficiency

—Vitamin A deficiency is common

 Differential Diagnosis

Protein energy malnutrition due to the impairment in protein absorption or metabolism

 Data Gathering

HISTORY

Question: Dietary history?
Significance: Assess for adequacy of protein and total calories.

Question: Cultural beliefs about feeding?
Significance: May contribute to low protein intake.

Question: Breast-feeding?
Significance: May protect infant but expose older sibling to protein deficiency.

Question: Possible protein loss, diarrhea, renal disease?
Significance: Nondietary cause of decreased serum protein.

Question: Skin rash?
Significance: See Physical Examination, below.

Question: Growth records?
Significance: Decreased growth velocity commensurate with poor protein intake.

Physical Examination

- Children appear apathetic, irritable, and sad.
- Predominant soft, pitting, painless edema of the soft tissues usually in the feet and legs, perineum, upper extremities, and face.

Finding: Dyspigmentation of the skin
Significance: Hair develops a red-brown color, loses its luster, becomes fragile and easily pluckable. Alternating bands of depigmentation and normal hair known as the "flag sign."

Finding: Characteristic dermatosis of kwashiorkor
Significance: Also known as "flaky" dermatosis. Appears in areas of the body subject to friction or pressure, notably the flexures, groin, buttocks, behind the knees, or at the elbows. It is described as patchy areas of darkly pigmented skin with a clear margin and a slightly raised edge. As the lesions progress, these lesions peel or desquamate. In severe cases, the skin peels away in patches leaving pale, ulcerated lesions lacking pigmentation. The borders of these lesions may have new highly pigmented dark plaques. These severe peeling lesions may resemble second-degree burns, but unlike burns, the dermatosis of kwashiorkor lacks a surrounding of erythema and is accompanied by edema.

Finding: Vesiculations of skin
Significance: Resulting in weeping lesions

Finding: Height
Significance: May be normal or retarded, depending on the chronicity of the illness.

Finding: Pale, cold, and cyanotic extremities
Significance: Decreased vascular volume secondary to decreased protein concentration.

Finding: Abdomen is frequently protuberant secondary to poor peristalsis.
Significance: Leading to distended stomach and intestinal loops.

 Laboratory Aids

Test: Common biochemical findings
Significance:

- Significant reduction in serum concentration of total protein and albumin.
- Hemoglobin and hematocrit are usually low.
- Ratio of nonessential to essential amino acids in plasma is elevated in kwashiorkor and usually normal in marasmus.
- Increased serum elevation of free fatty acids
- Low serum and urine carnitine levels

 Therapy

Treatment protocol is usually divided into three stages:

- Resolving life-threatening conditions

—Restoration can be achieved by oral rehydration solution. As soon as the patient improves, liquid elemental feeds can be initiated. Intravenous fluids must be used when there is persistent vomiting or abdominal distention. Electrolyte imbalances should be treated.

- Restoring nutritional status

—Nutritional status can be improved by nasogastric feeds with 6 to 12 feedings per day. High-protein, high-energy formulas are used. Initial treatment should provide average energy and protein requirements, followed by a gradual increase to 1.5 times the energy and 3 to 4 times the protein requirements by the seventh day. No change in weight or a decrease caused by loss of edema, accompanied by large diuresis, can occur.

- Ensuring nutritional rehabilitation

—Intravenous alimentation is rarely justified in primary protein-energy malnutrition and can increase mortality rates.
—Introduction of traditional home food and therapy can continue on an outpatient basis. Emotional and physical stimulation must be provided. Emphasizing nutritious use of household foods, personal and environmental hygiene, and dietary management of diarrhea and other diseases is also an aspect of management.

PROGNOSIS

Early recognition is important in treating kwashiorkor. Treatment corrects the acute signs of the disease, but catch-up growth in height may never be achieved. A higher mortality rate is associated with severe anthropometric deficits. Mortality rate in kwashiorkor can be as high as 40%, but adequate treatment can reduce it to less than 10%. Some of the factors that indicate poor prognosis are:

- Age of less than 6 months
- Infections
- Dehydration and electrolyte abnormalities
- Persistent tachycardia, signs of heart failure
- Total serum protein less than 3 g/100 mL
- Elevated serum bilirubin
- Severe anemia with hypoxia
- Hypoglycemia and/or hypothermia

ICD-9-CM 260

BIBLIOGRAPHY

Carvalho NF, Kenney RD, Carrington PH, et al. Severe nutritional deficiencies in toddlers resulting from health food milk alternatives. *Pediatrics* 2001;107(4):E46.

Latham MC. The dermatosis of kwashiorkor in young children. Ithaca, NY: Cornell University, 1991.

Liu T, Howard RM, Mancini AJ, et al. Kwashiorkor in the United States: fad diets, perceived and true milk allergy, and nutritional ignorance. *Arch Dermatol* 2001;137(5):630–636.

Ocal B, Unal S, Zorlu P, et al. Echocardiographic evaluation of cardiac functions and left ventricular mass in children with malnutrition. *J Paediatr Child Health* 2001;37(1):14–17.

Rossouw JE. Kwashiorkor is North America. *Am J Clin Nutr* 1989;49:588–592.

Author: Helen Anita John-Kelly

Lacrimal Duct Obstruction

 Database

DEFINITION

Congenital or acquired blockage of the distal portion of the tear drainage system extending from the lacrimal sac to opening of the nasolacrimal duct in the inferior meatus in the nose. This results in chronic tearing.

PATHOPHYSIOLOGY

- Congenital obstruction occurs from incomplete canalization of the nasolacrimal duct
- Acquired obstructions result from scar tissue occluding the duct. This usually results from chronic inflammation or trauma.

EPIDEMIOLOGY

Approximately 5% of newborns, most of which resolve spontaneously.

COMPLICATIONS

- Acute dacryocystitis (acute infection of the lacrimal sac), which rapidly appears as red subcutaneous nodule and surrounding cellulitis in the inferior medial canthal area and medial lower eyelid
- Chronic low-grade dacryocystitis manifested by subtle mucopurulent discharge from the eye

PROGNOSIS

- Spontaneous resolution in approximately 95% of patients by 12 months of age in children with congenital obstruction
- Acquired obstruction requires surgical intervention

 Differential Diagnosis

- Causes of increased tear production: congenital glaucoma, reflex tearing secondary to dry eye, seventh nerve palsies, trichiasis, entropion.
- Causes of decreased drainage: imperforate puncta or canaliculi, ectropion, lateral canthus dystopia, traumatic injury to the nasolacrimal drainage system

 Data Gathering

HISTORY

Determine when the onset of symptoms occurred. Congenital obstruction usually manifests itself within the first few months of life. Patients with acquired obstruction usually have a history of chronic or acute dacryocystitis or trauma to the drain system. Both present with symptoms including tearing, crusting of eyelashes particularly upon awaking, and discharge from eye. Finally clarify which eye is involved and how often the tearing is present.

 Physical Examination

Finding: Increased tear meniscus, maceration of eyelid skin, mucopurulent discharge, crusted debris on the eyelashes, and occasionally conjunctival hyperemia
Significance: Common symptoms

Finding: Palpation of lacrimal sac
Significance: Expression of mucopurulent material from the puncta with pressure on the lacrimal sac

 Laboratory Aids

Test: Dye disappearance test (DDT)
Significance: Fluorescein is applied to the conjunctival cul de sac and the patient is observed for 5 minutes. In a negative test (normal) the tear meniscus will become relatively unstained as the tears flow through the drainage system. In a positive test the height of the stained tear meniscus will either increase or fail to decrease due to the obstruction.

Therapy

- Initially, in congenital obstruction lacrimal sac massage and either ophthalmic antibiotic drops or ointment are applied when ocular discharge increases. This conservative approach is applied for the first year of life.
- If symptomatic at 12 months of age, probing and irrigation of the nasolacrimal system are performed. Occasionally inferior turbinate infracture is performed to increase the space in the inferior meatus.
- If probing and irrigation fail, then the procedure is repeated with Silastic tube intubation or stretching of the lacrimal duct with balloon dacryoplasty.
- If all else fails, a dacryocystorhinostomy (permanent surgical connection between the lacrimal sac and the nose) is performed to prevent recurrent infections (dacryocystitis) and maceration of the eyelids from tearing.
- Patients with acquired obstructions require surgery. Probing and irrigation are performed to determine where the obstruction is located. These patients require Silastic tube intubation if possible or dacryocystorhinostomy surgery if the obstruction is complete and cannot be relieved.

 Follow-Up

Children with congenital obstruction should be reevaluated at 12 months of age and referred for probing and irrigation if still symptomatic. Children with acquired obstruction should be referred to an ophthalmologist for surgical treatment.

PITFALLS

Referral for probing and irrigation is delayed until patient is about 12 months of age; the probing and irrigation should be performed in a timely fashion to ensure a good outcome.

 Common Questions and Answers

Q: Is my child in any danger while the nasolacrimal duct remains obstructed?
A: Not usually. The obstruction presents more of a nuisance. However, occasionally the contents of the sac can become infected and will require oral or parenteral antibiotics.

Q: Why not wait longer to do the probing and irrigation in congenital nasolacrimal duct obstruction?
A: The failure rate of the initial procedure increases with age: if performed before 13 months of age, 96% success rate; between 13 and 18 months of age, 77% success rate; and between 18 and 24 months, 54% success rate.

ICD-9-CM 375.56

BIBLIOGRAPHY

Granet DB, Olitsky S, Burke MJ. Nasolacrimal duct obstruction. *J Pediatr Ophthalmol Strabismus* 2000;37(2):103–106.

Katowitz JA, Welsh MG. Timing of initial probing and irrigation in congenital nasolacrimal duct obstruction. *Ophthalmology* 1987;94:698–705.

Kushner BJ. The management of nasolacrimal duct obstruction in children between 18 months and 4 years old. *J AAPOS* 1998; 2:57–60.

Author: Scott M. Goldstein
Katrinka L. Heher, 2nd edition

Lactose Intolerance

 Database

DEFINITION

Lactose is a disaccharide built from glucose and galactose. It is the major carbohydrate in infant's food (breast milk or milk-based formula). Lactose is important as a source of energy and it promotes the absorption of calcium, phosphorus, and iron. It has a prebiotic effect on the gut flora.

Inability to digest the disaccharide lactose secondary to deficiency of the enzyme lactase, resulting in clinical symptoms and possible subsequent malabsorption. Three types of deficiency have been noted:

1) • Congenital lactase deficiency is extremely rare. It presents during the newborn period, often with the first feeding of lactose-containing formula. Will cause severe diarrhea, failure to thrive and risk the newborns' life.
• Acquired lactase deficiency can be divided to two subtypes:
2) • Secondary to an insult/damage to the small bowel mucosa.
3) • Secondary to developmental loss of enzyme activity due to genetic predisposition and aging.

PATHOLOGY

• Disaccharide activity can be measured in biopsy specimens of the small bowel and compared to normal values.
• Small bowel biopsy will often be normal (unless the reason is insult/damage to the small bowel mucosa).

EPIDEMIOLOGY

• After the lactation period there is gradual reduction of the enzyme activity—with genetic predisposition.
• Deficiency is found in up to 80% of native Australians, Americans, tropical Africans, and East and Southeastern Asians. It is also highly prevalent in African Americans.
• It can be clinically evident in many African Americans by 3 years of age.
• In Caucasians the clinical pictures starts in the second decade of life

GENETICS

• Adult lactase production is a dominant trait; lactase deficiency is a recessive trait with single mendelian locus.
• The gene for lactase-phlorizin-hydrolase has been localized on chromosome 2.

PROGNOSIS

Prognosis is excellent as elimination and enzyme replacement are possible; with lactose avoidance or with enzyme supplementation, the child can control and eliminate symptoms.

 Differential Diagnosis

Lactose intolerance may be secondary to a generalized small bowel mucosal dysfunction; the presence of other symptoms should prompt an evaluation. The differential diagnosis includes:

• Infection

—Viral and bacterial infections can cause secondary lactose intolerance. Most common pathogen is rotavirus.
—Parasitic infections can mimic lactose intolerance (giardiasis).

• Inflammatory

—Small intestine Crohn disease can have associated lactose intolerance.

• Congenital

—Other carbohydrate enzyme deficiencies can mimic lactose intolerance. This includes sucrase-isomaltase or glucose-galactose malabsorption.
—Cystic fibrosis, Shwachman syndrome can mimic lactose intolerance.

• Allergic/immune

—Celiac disease often is associated with lactose intolerance due to small intestinal damage.
—Protein intolerance can cause secondary lactose intolerance.

 Data Gathering

HISTORY

Question: Symptoms?
Significance: Classic symptoms include bloating, gaseousness, colicky abdominal pain, and diarrhea after digestion of lactose-containing meal.

Question: Diet history?
Significance: Provides important information.

Question: A detailed history of symptoms.
Significance: Blood or mucus in the stools, failure to thrive, fat malabsorption, or any extraintestinal symptoms strongly suggest different etiologies.

Question: Lactose ingestion.
Significance: Symptoms vary in severity and with dose of lactose.

Question: Milk ingestion?
Significance: Association with milk ingestion may not be evident.

 Physical Examination

Finding: Height and weight
Significance: Should be measured and plotted against age-appropriate norms; any deviation should not be evaluated as lactose intolerance alone.

Finding: Abdomen percussion
Significance: Abdomen may be distended.

Finding: Blood in the stool
Significance: Must be evaluated, because lactose intolerance does not cause bleeding.

Lactose Intolerance

 Laboratory Aids

Test: Stool-reducing substances and fecal acidity
Significance: A positive result indicates malabsorption of carbohydrates. A pH less than 6.0 or reducing substances greater than 0.5% are interpreted as a positive result. This is a very reliable test in the presence of diarrhea; however, it is not specific for lactose intolerance alone.

Test: Lactose hydrogen breath test
Significance: Is used for lactose intolerance. It is noninvasive and highly sensitive. It is based on the fact that in the human, the only source of hydrogen is fermented unabsorbed carbohydrates. A rise of breath H_2 concentration of greater than or equal to 20 ppm over baseline appears to correlate better with subsequent symptom development than does a concentration of greater than or equal to 10 ppm. However, the frequently poor association between symptoms of lactose intolerance and breath H_2 excretion suggests caution in the interpretation of the clinical significance of the breath hydrogen test.

False-positive test results occur due to inadequate fasting before the test, rapid intestinal transit, toothpaste, smoking, and bacterial overgrowth.
False-negative results occur due to diarrhea, hyperventilation, recent antibiotics exposure, and delayed gastric emptying. Up to 10% of the population are colonized with bacteria unable to produce hydrogen and will give a negative result.

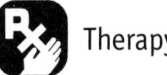 Therapy

- Removal of lactose from the diet is effective in eliminating symptoms. However, a milk-free diet may result in calcium deficiency and other nutritional issues.
- Predigestion of lactose can be done by the addition of commercially available enzyme supplementation. Multiple products are available over the counter. Liquid preparations, capsules, and chewable tablets can be obtained.
- Some acquired deficiencies, particularly those associated with infection, may resolve over time. The majority of patients with lactose intolerance will not recover the ability to digest lactose.

PITFALLS

Care must be taken to determine if the lactose intolerance is secondary to a primary pathologic process (i.e., Celiac disease, Crohn disease, or giardiasis).

 Common Questions and Answers

Q: When is the usual time for presentation of lactose intolerance?
A: In whites, the age of presentation is after 5 years of age. In blacks, 2- to 3-year-old children may present. The differential diagnosis must distinguish primary from secondary causes.

Q: Does lactose intolerance prevent the child from ever eating lactose?
A: No, the patient can take smaller amounts of lactose in the diet, or have the enzyme supplemented.

Q: Does this problem ever get better?
A: No, it is a lifelong problem, but seems to become less symptomatic for adults, in light of their individual desire to tolerate symptoms.

ICD-9-CM 271.3

BIBLIOGRAPHY

Auricchio S. Genetically determined disaccharidase deficiencies. In: Walker WA, Durie PR, Hamilton JR, et al., eds. *Pediatric gastrointestinal disease*. Philadelphia: BC Decker, 1991:657–660.

de Vrese M, Stegelmann A, Richter B, et al. Probiotics—compensation for lactase insufficiency. *Am J Clin Nutr* 2001;73 (2 suppl):421S–429S.

Kokkonen J, Tikkanen S, Savilahti E. Residual intestinal disease after milk allergy in infancy. *J Pediatr Gastroenterol Nutr* 2001;32(2):156–161.

Rose S. Milk consumption for the lactose intolerant: a clarification. *J Am Diet Assoc* 2000;100(9):1007; discussion 1007–1008.

Shulman RJ. Enzyme and transport defects. In: Oski FA, DeAngelis CD, Feigin RD, et al., eds. *Principles and practice of pediatrics*, 2nd ed. Philadelphia: JB Lippincott, 1994:1895–1899.

Suarez FL, Saviano DA, Levitt MD. A comparison of milk or lactose hydrolyzed milk by people with self-reported severe lactose intolerance. *N Engl J Med* 1995;333:1–5.

Veligati LN, Treem WR, Sullivan B, et al. Delta 10 ppm versus delta 20 ppm: a reappraisal of diagnostic criteria for breath hydrogen testing in children. *Am J Gastroenterol* 1994;89(5):758–761.

Vesa TH, Marteau P, Korpela R. Lactose intolerance. *J Am Coll Nutr* 2000;19 (2 suppl):165S–175S.

Author: Dror Wasserman

Lead Poisoning

 Database

DEFINITION

- The most common pediatric environmental health problem involves a systemic intoxication by the heavy metal lead; most commonly this is with inorganic lead.
- Children in the U.S. are predominantly exposed to lead through ingestion of contaminated house dust, and soil and paint chips from deterioration of pre-1980 housing and buildings.
- The CDC considers a blood lead level of 10 μg/dL or higher to represent undue lead exposure and absorption; a level of 20 μg/dL or higher is generally considered to constitute lead poisoning.

PATHOPHYSIOLOGY

- Lead adversely affects many organ systems including the neurologic (e.g., encephalopathy, peripheral neuropathy in adults, subtle neuropsychological effects), hematologic (e.g., anemia due to several mechanisms), gastrointestinal (e.g., abdominal colic), renal (e.g., proximal renal tubular injury leading to Fanconi syndrome), and reproductive systems.
- Many of the toxic effects result from inhibition of enzymes involved in heme biosynthesis, as the electropositive metal binds to the negatively charged sulfhydryl groups on the active sites of δ-aminolevulinic acid dehydratase (ALA-D), ferrochelatase, porphobilinogen synthase, coproporphyrinogen oxidase, and other enzymes. Divalent lead also acts competitively with calcium in various biologic systems and lead affects nucleic acids.
- Children absorb lead more efficiently from the gastrointestinal tract and are more likely to ingest lead through hand-to-mouth activity as compared to adults.
- As the developing, immature central nervous system is susceptible to the toxic effects of lead, the neuropsychological effects of lead poisoning on young children have been of particular concern.

EPIDEMIOLOGY

- Prevalence of elevated lead levels and geometric mean blood lead level (BLL) have decreased significantly in the last 20 years.
- Almost 1 million American children aged 1 to 5 years (4.4% of a representative national sample) are estimated to have BLL of 10 μg/dL or higher.
- Higher prevalence occurs among children aged 1 to 3 years, those living in older housing, those from lower income families, and those living in metropolitan areas with populations of 1 million or greater.
- Approximately 86% of American pre-1980 publicly owned housing units and 83% of privately owned units contain some lead-based paint.

COMPLICATIONS

- Acute encephalopathy
- Seizures
- Coma
- Death (predominantly due to cerebral edema)
- Mental retardation
- Cognitive, behavioral, attentional, and neurodevelopmental impairment
- Anemia
- Fanconi syndrome

PROGNOSIS

- In general, there is an increased risk for long-term neuropsychological sequelae, which increases with lead exposure and absorption that is more intense, of longer duration, and begins at an early age when the central nervous system is still maturing.
- Recurrent episodes of symptomatic lead poisoning increase the risk for permanent sequelae.
- More subtle effects may not be detected until school entry.

 Differential Diagnosis

- Most lead poisoning in children is asymptomatic.
- Lead encephalopathy should be considered in the differential diagnosis of a child presenting with seizures, altered mental status, and/or coma.
- Lead poisoning should also be considered in the differential diagnosis of mental retardation, behavioral disorders, and anemia.

 Data Gathering

HISTORY

Question: Exposure to a source of lead?
Significance: The most common sources of lead include residence in or visitation of older, deteriorated housing, a parental occupation or hobby involving lead exposure, use of remedies or cosmetics containing lead, and ingestion of contaminated water, food, or beverages.
Question: Typical symptoms?
Significance: Although many of the clinical manifestations of symptomatic lead poisoning are nonspecific, a cluster of complaints including anorexia, intermittent abdominal pain, constipation, sporadic vomiting, change in mental status (such as irritability or lethargy), decreased play activity, and change in developmental status (particularly with regression of developmental milestones) may herald this condition.
Question: Lead encephalopathy?
Significance: Can present with change in consciousness, ataxia, persistent vomiting, seizures, and coma; often this presents after a prodrome of the previous symptoms.
Question: Anemia or developmental delay?
Significance: Result of lead poisoning.

 Physical Examination

- Not generally helpful at lower lead levels. Symptomatic and/or encephalopathic patients may have acute gastrointestinal, neurologic, hematologic, and systemic manifestations.
- Assess for clinical evidence of developmental delay.
- Burton gum lead line: a blue-gray discoloration at the gum–tooth interface typically along the lower incisors rarely can be seen in the setting of chronic, fairly high lead exposure and poor dental hygiene.

 Laboratory Aids

SPECIFIC TESTS

Test: Blood lead test, either venous or capillary.
Significance: Compare result with CDC classification system. Results may be reportable to local health authorities. Is a measure only of recent lead exposure; does not indicate total body burden of lead.

NONSPECIFIC TESTS

Test: Complete blood count
Significance: To assess for anemia. Anemia is seen in lead poisoning starting at about 60 μg/dL from globin and heme synthesis inhibition and hemolysis. Iron deficiency anemia is often seen concomitantly. Anemia related to lead toxicity is typically normocytic and normochromic; a microcytic, hypochromic anemia may be seen with a mixed etiology. Basophilic stippling is sometimes seen on peripheral blood smear.
Test: Free erythrocyte protoporphyrin (FEP) and other blood and urine markers
Significance: Markers of lead-induced inhibition of heme synthesis. FEP can be useful clinically to follow the recovery from heme synthesis inhibition during management.

RADIOGRAPHIC STUDIES

Test: Abdominal radiograph
Significance: Look for radiopaque foreign material suggestive of ingestion of lead paint chips or other lead-containing foreign body.
Test: Long bone x-rays
Significance: Look for "lead lines" or metaphyseal sclerosis, characterized by increased density along transverse lines in the metaphyses of growing long bones representing increased mineralization due to interference with the metabolism of bone matrix. If present, this implies a more chronic lead exposure.
Test: X-ray fluorescence for estimation of body lead burden
Significance: Used mainly in experimental settings

Therapy

- Environmental management, which includes removing children from the lead source(s), should occur when venous lead levels are recurrently 15 to 19 $\mu g/dL$ (CDC class IIB) and when levels are greater than or equal to 20 $\mu g/dL$ (CDC class III).
- Chelation therapy should complement environmental management in all children with venous levels of 45 $\mu g/dL$ (CDC class IV) or higher, using parenteral calcium disodium ethylenediamine tetraacetate (EDTA; also calcium disodium versenate) or oral agents such as meso 2,3-dimercaptosuccinic acid (DMSA, succimer, Chemet). Chelation of children with levels in the 25- to 45-$\mu g/dL$ range may be considered in certain cases, although it is not routinely recommended and evidence suggests it may not be beneficial. Outpatient therapy can take place if a lead-safe environment has been identified and compliance is expected. Succimer is given at 10 mg/kg/dose (or 350 mg/m^2/dose) every 8 hours for 5 days, then every 12 hours for 14 more days. Weekly monitoring for neutropenia, platelet abnormality, and increased liver enzymes is recommended. Succimer is more lead-specific than other chelators and causes less mineral depletion.
- Children with symptomatic lead poisoning or with levels of 70 $\mu g/dL$ (CDC class V) or higher should be admitted immediately to a hospital for parenteral chelation with both intramuscular dimercaprol (British anti-lewisite, BAL) and intravenous or intramuscular calcium disodium EDTA. As there are many issues involved with administration of both chelating agents, consultation of appropriate guidelines and pharmacologic information is recommended. Children with encephalopathy constitute a medical emergency and should receive the preceding treatment in an intensive care setting with attentive neurosurgical support. Consultation with a clinician experienced in lead toxicity treatment is advised for these patients.
- Ingested lead-containing foreign bodies should be evacuated with whole bowel irrigation using a high molecular weight glycol solution.
- Nutritional support with calcium and iron supplementation should be given if intake is inadequate; deficiencies of these increase lead absorption from the gastrointestinal tract. Iron supplementation should be withheld during chelation therapy.

Follow-Up

- Prompt environmental follow-up of current lead exposure situations and vigilance for additional exposure (with family moves, visitation of new residences, etc.) should occur.

- Follow-up of elevated venous levels from 10 to 19 $\mu g/dL$ (CDC class IIA, IIB) approximately every 3 to 4 months.
- Follow-up of venous levels of 20 $\mu g/dL$ or higher at 1 to 2 month intervals until no additional lead exposure is present and levels have decreased.

PREVENTION

- Primary prevention: removal of potential environmental lead hazards.
- Secondary prevention: screening for elevated lead levels. Since 1997, the CDC has recommended that state and local health departments make the determination for a universal versus targeted screening approach. Screening is recommended by use of a blood lead test for children at ages 1 and 2 and for those of 36 to 72 months of age without previous screening.
  —Universal screening for communities where the risk for lead exposure is widespread and where 12% or more of children aged 12 to 36 months have lead levels of 10 $\mu g/dL$ or higher and/or 27% or greater of the housing stock was built prior to 1950.
  —Targeted screening for communities not meeting above criteria. Screening would be indicated for children meeting local criteria for screening such as residence in a specified geographic area, membership in a high-risk group, or a high-risk status as determined by the use of a personal-risk questionnaire.
- Tertiary prevention: case management and environmental remediation for children with lead poisoning. Closer attention to the first two modes of prevention should obviate the need for this.

CONTROL MEASURES

- Abatement of building-based (residential) lead hazards by removal or enclosure of lead-containing structures.
- Control of environmental lead dust exposure and ingestion by good housekeeping (wet dusting and mopping of household dust) and personal hygiene (cleaning of child's hands, toys, personal items, etc.).
- Removal of any other known lead source from the child's environment.

PITFALLS

- Delay in checking a blood lead test in the presence of clinical signs or symptoms of lead poisoning or neuropsychological disorders.
- Failure to inquire about lead exposure possibilities, especially of non-urban children.

Common Questions and Answers

Q: What is lead abatement?
A: Lead abatement is removal of a lead hazard from the environment either by replacing it (e.g., installing a new window), enclosing the area with the lead source (e.g., installing paneling), removing the lead-based paint from a surface (burning or dry sanding methods should never be used), or encapsulating the area (placement of a

specific coating over the lead-containing surface, which prevents access to the lead hazard).
Q: Is lead abatement permanent?
A: Often the lead paint that is chipping or peeling is removed from a home. Any areas with intact lead-based paint may become deteriorated with aging, leading to new lead hazards, although ongoing maintenance and repair may prevent this.
Q: Why didn't my child's brother or sister get lead poisoned at the same age, as he/she lived in the same house?
A: Children are different; some do much more hand-to-mouth activity than others, which is the main way that children get lead into their bodies. Also, your home may not have had the same lead dangers (hazards) when the sibling was younger.

ICD-9-CM 984.9

BIBLIOGRAPHY

American Academy of Pediatrics Committee on Drugs. Treatment guidelines for lead exposure in children. *Pediatrics* 1995;96:155–160.

American Academy of Pediatrics Committee on Environmental Health. Screening for elevated blood lead levels. *Pediatrics* 1998;101:1072–1077.

Centers for Disease Control and Prevention. *Screening young children for lead poisoning: guidance for state and local public health officials.* U.S. Dept. of HHS, 1997.

Centers for Disease Control and Prevention. Update: blood lead levels—United States, 1991–94. *MMWR* 1997;46:141–146.

Chisolm JJ, O'Hara DM, eds. *Lead absorption in children: management, clinical, and environmental aspects*, 1st ed. Baltimore: Urban & Schwarzenberg, 1982.

Lanphear BP, Matte TD, Rogers J, et al. The contribution of lead-contaminated house dust and residential soil to children's blood lead levels. *Environ Res* 1998;79(section A):51–68.

Pueschel SM, Linakis JG, Anderson AC, eds. *Lead poisoning in childhood*. Baltimore: Paul H. Brookes, 1996.

Rogan WJ, Dietrich KN, Ware JH, et al. The effect of chelation therapy with succimer on neuropsychological development in children exposed to lead. *N Engl J Med* 2001;344(19):1421–1426.

Rosen JF, Mushak P. Primary prevention of childhood lead poisoning—the only solution. *N Engl J Med* 2001;344(19):1470–1471.

Author: Carla Campbell

Lice (Pediculosis)

 Database

DEFINITION

Infestation of the head, body, or anogenital region with one of three species of lice

CAUSES

Three species of ectoparasites (6-legged, wingless, 1- to 4-mm insects that live on humans, feeding on human blood):
- *Pediculus humanus capitis:* head louse
- *Pediculus humanus corporis:* body louse
- *Phthirus pubis:* pubic or crab louse

PATHOPHYSIOLOGY

- Head lice
—Survives for several weeks on scalp
—Typical infestation, 12 to 24 live insects per patient
—Single louse produces up to 120 eggs
—Ova (nits) laid close to the scalp; firmly attached to hair shaft by chitinous ring (usually clustered in the parietal and occipital areas)
—Ova hatch after 8 days, leaving shell of nit on hair (readily visible to examiner).
—Transmitted by personal contact, or fomites (e.g., combs, hats, upholstery, clothing, headsets)
—Prefer to feed on scalp skin; hook onto scalp, pierce skin to feed
—Release poisonous saliva that causes pruritus, dermatitis
—Survive 1 to 2 days off human host
- Body lice
—10% to 20% larger than head lice
—Prefer to live on clothing, visiting human only to feed
—Lay eggs along seams of clothing, which hatch when warmed by wear
—Transmitted through contact with infested clothing or bedding
—Viable off of human for 10 to 21 days
- Pubic lice
—Crab-like appearance with predilection for pubic hair
—Transmitted almost exclusively by sexual contact
—Uncommonly spread by fomites (e.g., toilet seats, bedding)
—Occasionally will infest axillary hair, beard, or eyelashes
—May infest eyebrows/lashes (pediculosis palpebrarum) in young children (associated with maternal infestation; but one must consider possible sexual abuse)

EPIDEMIOLOGY

- Head lice
—Common in day-care setting and elementary school children
—Affects all socioeconomic groups
—Not indicative of poor hygiene
—Slightly higher incidence in girls
- Body lice
—Found on persons with poor hygiene
—More common in extreme conditions such as crowding, homelessness, wars, famine, flood, and earthquakes
—Highest incidence in the Sudan and Ethiopia
- Pubic lice
—Most common in adolescents and young adults

COMPLICATIONS

- Head lice
—Secondary dermatitis, impetigo, or furunculosis
- Body lice
—Secondary eczema, impetigo (from scratching)
—Postinflammatory hyperpigmentation
—Known vector for disease; *Rickettsia prowazekii* (epidemic typhus), *Rickettsia quintana* (trench fever), *Borrelia recurrentis* (relapsing fever).

ASSOCIATED ILLNESSES

- These lice are not responsible for the spread of any disease.
- Pubic lice: up to 50% of patients have another sexually transmitted disease, particularly gonorrhea, or syphilis.

 Differential Diagnosis

- Seborrheic dermatitis
- Contact dermatitis
- Eczema
- Impetigo

 Data Gathering

HISTORY

Question: Pruritus?
Significance: Itching is the most common symptom, however some patients are asymptomatic.
Question: Secondary skin lesion (from scratching)?
Significance: May be chief complaint
Question: Symptoms?
Significance: Review of symptoms (if body lice) to detect symptoms of rickettsial or spirochetal illness.

SPECIAL QUESTIONS

Question: Contacts?
Significance: Possible infested contacts (home, school, or sexual).
Question: Special living circumstances?
Significance: Crowding or institutionalization.

 Physical Examination

Finding: Lice (difficult to find) on the scalp, in the pubic hair or in the seams of clothing.
Significance: Diagnostic.
Finding: Nits clustered in parietal and occipital regions, in the perianal region or in the seams of clothing.
Significance: Diagnostic.
Finding: Use of Wood's light.
Significance: Live nits fluoresce under Wood's light.
Finding: Primary skin lesion
Significance: Pinpoint, erythematous macule, papule, or urticarial wheel. These can be obliterated by scratching.

OTHER FINDINGS

- Secondary skin lesions; dermatitis of the neck, shoulder area.
- Examine eyelashes, eyebrows for secondary infestation.
- Posterior occipital lymphadenopathy
- Body lice
- Postinflammatory hyperpigmentation
- Maculae cerulae (bluish/slate macules, 0.5- to 1-mm diameter), from heavy infestation in pubic, trunk, and thigh areas.

PROCEDURES

- Nits only behind patient's ears in early infestation
- Nits difficult to flick away (unlike dandruff); need to be pulled along entire length of hair shaft to remove.

 Laboratory Aids

Test: Rarely necessary
Significance: Can examine louse or nit under microscope to confirm characteristic appearance. Dandruff is a false-positive finding.
Test: Home testing
Significance: Parents can be instructed how to examine all family members for infestation.
Test: School testing
Significance: Schools should perform examinations during epidemics.

Lice (Pediculosis)

 Therapy

DRUGS
Head and Pubic Lice
• Permethrin (Nix) 1% creme rinse; drug of choice
—Acts on nerve cell membranes causing paralysis/death of insect
—10-minute application, followed by second application 7 to 10 days later.
—High ovicidal activity; continued activity up to 12 days after application
—High cure rate, prevalence to resistance in the U.S. is unknown.
—Over-the-counter preparation, low toxicity
• Pyrethrins (Rid, A-200)
—Neurotoxin also, low ovicidal activity
—No resistance documented in the U.S.
—10-minute shampoo application, second application in 1 week
—Over-the-counter preparation
—Some develop contact dermatitis to natural chrysanthemum base.
• Lindane (Kwell) 1% lotion
—4-minute shampoo application, second application 7 to 10 days
—Low ovicidal activity, neurotoxic if not used correctly
—Contraindicated in premature infants, persons with known seizure disorders and known hypersensitivity
—Use with caution in children <2 years of age, and in pregnant or nursing women
—Used primarily for persons who have not responded to other therapies.
—Lindane-resistant strains of pediculosis have been reported in some countries.
• Malathion (Ovide) 0.5%
—Better ovicidal activity, highly effective
—Requires 8- to 12-hour application, repeat at 7 to 9 days
—Less toxicity than lindane and pyrethrins
—Alcohol base of product causes patient to be flammable while product is on.
• Other considerations:
—Cortisone creams for secondary dermatitis; decreases pruritus
—Antibiotics for impetiginized lesions

GENERAL
Head Lice
• Examine household members and treat those who are infested.
• Prophylactically treat bed mates.
• Wash bedding, clothes, and cloth toys in hot water (>128°F).
• Treat combs by washing in hot water, and soaking in pediculicide.
• Seal anything not washable in plastic bags for 10 to 14 days.
• Nit removal not necessary, especially if pediculicide reapplied 1 week later
• If nit removal desired, soak hair with white vinegar for 30 to 60 minutes, followed by combing with a fine-toothed nit comb.
• Environmental insecticide is not helpful in the control of head lice.

Body Lice
• Pediculicide not necessary (insects live in clothing)
• Improve hygiene.
• Wash clothing and bedding in hot water.
• Dry cleaning is effective, as is hot ironing (particularly along seams of clothing).

Pubic Lice
• Treat sexual contact to prevent reinfestation: pediculosis palpebrarum
• Petrolatum ointment applied to lashes three to four times per day for 8 to 10 days
• Removal of nits with fine-toothed comb helpful from pubic hair or by hand from the eyelashes.

DURATION
• The pediculicide kills the lice shortly after application; therefore, living lice after treatment is indicative of incorrect use of the pediculicide, very heavy infestation, reinfestation or resistance to therapy. Re-treatment with a second pediculicide with reapplication 7 to 10 days later is recommended.

PREVENTION
Head lice is not preventable.

 Follow-Up

WHEN TO EXPECT IMPROVEMENT
Risk of transmission promptly reduced after single application, so child should be allowed to return to school or day care. Removal of nits is not necessary to reduce spread. Pruritus may persist for 2 weeks after therapy.

SIGNS TO WATCH FOR
Recurrence of symptoms represents improper use of the treating agent, reinfestation, failure to recognize and treat other sites of infestation, such as perianal hair, axillary hair, or sexual contacts: pediculosis pubis.

PROGNOSIS
Excellent

PITFALLS
Pediculosis palpebrarum: pediculicides are oculotoxic and must be avoided. Use lindane cautiously in patients with seizure disorder.

 Common Questions and Answers

Q: Did my child get head lice because my house or my child is not clean enough?
A: No, head lice is unrelated to personal hygiene. Some experts even believe lice prefer a clean scalp.
Q: Should I cut my child's long hair to get the lice out?
A: No, meticulous application of the pediculicides to the entire scalp and pulled through all hair shafts is adequate treatment. Urgently cutting a child's hair to alleviate parental anxiety can be traumatizing to the child.
Q: Can infants become infested with pubic lice (*Phthirus pubis*)?
A: Yes. Although the primary mode of transmission of the crab louse is via sexual contact, it can be transmitted through close personal contact with an infested individual. Small children become infested on the eyebrows or lashes with crab lice.
Q: If children are infested with the head louse, how can items such as stuffed animals or other cloth toys be decontaminated?
A: Machine washable items can be washed in hot water at temperatures >128°F. An alternative method of decontamination is sealing the items in a plastic bag for 10 to 14 days.
Q: Is removal of nits necessary to prevent spread?
A: No. They can be removed from a cosmetic standpoint by using a fine-toothed comb or by soaking the hair in a solution of white vinegar followed by wrapping the head with a towel soaked in the same solution for 30 to 60 minutes.
Q: What is appropriate treatment of infestation of the eyelashes?
A: A petroleum-based ocular ointment should be applied three to four times daily for a period of 10 days. Nits should be removed mechanically from the lashes.

ICD-9-CM 132.9

BIBLIOGRAPHY
Harwitz S, ed. *Clinical pediatric dermatology*, 2nd ed. Philadelphia: WB Saunders, 1993.

Hogan D, Schachner L, Tanglertsaman C. Pediatric dermatology. *Pediatr Clin North Am* 1991;38(4):953–957.

Meinking TL, Taplin D. Infestations: pediculosis. *Curr Probl Dermatol* 1996;24: 157–163.

Red Book 2000: Report of the Committee on Infectious Diseases, 25th ed. Elk Grove Village, IL: American Academy Of Pediatrics, 2000.

Authors: Jane Lavelle and Catherine B. Sullivan

Lupus Erythematosus

 Database

DEFINITION

Multisystem, autoimmune disease characterized by the production of antibodies to various components of the cell nucleus, in conjunction with a variety of clinical manifestations. Four of the following 11 criteria, developed by the American College of Rheumatology, must be met to classify a patient with systemic lupus erythematosus (SLE):

- Malar (butterfly) rash
- Discoid rash
- Photosensitivity
- Oral or nasal ulcers
- Arthritis
- Cytopenia: anemia, leukopenia, lymphopenia, or thrombocytopenia
- Neurologic disease: seizures or psychosis
- Nephritis: >0.5 g/d proteinuria or cellular casts
- Serositis: pleuritis or pericarditis
- Immunologic disorder: antibodies to double-stranded DNA (dsDNA) or Sm nuclear antigen, LE cell prep, or false-positive serologic test for syphilis
- Positive ANA

CAUSE

Although the exact etiology is unknown, lupus is an autoimmune disease, with genetic, environmental, and hormonal factors playing a role.

PATHOLOGY

- Immune complex-mediated vasculitis, which can occur in almost any organ system.
- Cutaneous lesions in SLE are very variable. They include the erythematous malar or "butterfly" rash, maculopapular rashes (which can occur anywhere on the body), periungual erythema, and mucosal membrane vasculitis.
- Arthritis in SLE can affect large and small joints and is usually symmetric and nonerosive.

- Hematologic pathology in lupus includes a hemolytic anemia, anemia of chronic disease, leukopenia, lymphopenia, and thrombocytopenia.
- Neurologic impairments in SLE include psychosis, depression, seizures, organic brain syndromes, and peripheral neuropathies.
- Renal pathology includes mesangial changes and glomerulonephritis (focal, diffuse, proliferative, or membranous). The first signs of renal disease in a lupus patient are often proteinuria and an active urinary sediment. Hypertension, nephrotic syndrome, and renal failure can also occur.
- Serositis is usually seen as pericarditis or pleuritis, but peritonitis can also occur.

EPIDEMIOLOGY

- Approximately 15% of lupus patients have their onset of symptoms in childhood.
- Peak incidence of SLE is between the ages of 15 and 40.
- It has been estimated that 5,000 to 10,000 children in the United States have SLE.
- Female/male ratio is between 5:1 and 10:1.

GENETICS

- Increased frequency of lupus in first-degree family members of patients with SLE
- Approximately 10% of patients have at least one affected relative.
- Concordance rate of 25% to 50% in monozygotic and 5% in dizygotic twins

COMPLICATIONS

- Renal disease
- Central nervous system (CNS) involvement
- Infections secondary to the treatments used to control the disease
- Myocardial infarctions at a young age

 Differential Diagnosis

- Systemic juvenile rheumatoid arthritis
- Oncologic disease (leukemia, lymphoma)
- Other vasculitic disorders
- Dermatomyositis
- Fibromyalgia
- Drug-induced lupus

 Data Gathering

HISTORY

Question: Photosensitive?
Significance: A history of photosensitivity or a malar rash is common but not necessary in SLE.

Question: Systemic complaints?
Significance: Many patients have systemic complaints, such as fevers, fatigue, and malaise.

Question: Other complaints?
Significance: Some patients complain of joint pains, Raynaud phenomenon, or alopecia.

 Physical Examination

- Rash: may be malar, discoid or vasculitic. Periungual erythema may also be seen.
- Oral or nasal ulcers (usually on the hard or soft palate) that are painless and often go unnoticed by the patients.
- Arthritis of the large and small joints
- Pericardial friction rub if the patient has pericarditis
- Edema may be present secondary to renal disease.
- CNS changes, such as personality changes, psychosis, seizures

Laboratory Aids

Test: Antinuclear antibodies (ANA)
Significance: Found in over 95% patients with SLE, but a positive ANA can occur in many diseases (and in 10–15% of the normal population).

Test: Anti-dsDNA and anti-Sm.
Significance: Very specific to lupus. In many patients, the anti-DNA levels vary with the activity of disease, so it can be used as a sign for flares.

Test: CBC
Significance: Anemia, leukopenia, lymphopenia, and/or thrombocytopenia may be seen.

Test: Urinalysis
Significance: May show proteinuria or an active urinary sediment if there is renal dysfunction.

Test: Complement levels
Significance: Can fall very low during a lupus flare (C3 and C4).

Test: PTT
Significance: Patients may also have a prolonged PTT, as the result of antiphospholipid (APL) antibodies, which are often seen in SLE. Patients with APL antibodies are at an increased risk for thrombotic events, such as deep venous thromboses, strokes, and fetal losses during pregnancies.

 Therapy

• Avoid excessive sun exposure and use sunscreen liberally.
• Nonsteroidal antiinflammatory drugs may be used for the musculoskeletal and mild systemic complaints, although ibuprofen has been noted to cause an aseptic meningitis in a small number of patients with SLE.
• Hydroxychloroquine is often used to help control the cutaneous manifestations of lupus, and steroids are often necessary to control the systemic and renal problems.
• Patients with renal disease often need immunosuppressive agents, such as cyclophosphamide (usually given as monthly intravenous boluses). Mycophenolate mofetil or azathioprine may also be used.

PITFALLS

Overdiagnosis; a positive ANA in the absence of clinical signs or symptoms of SLE is not lupus.

PROGNOSIS

• Extremely variable. Renal disease and CNS involvement are poor prognostic signs, whereas systemic complaints and joint findings are not.
• The 10-year survival in a child presenting with SLE is over 80%.

 Common Questions and Answers

Q: If a patient has a positive ANA but no clinical signs of SLE, how often should the ANA be followed?
A: A positive ANA will usually remain positive indefinitely, but it has no real significance in the absence of clinical or other laboratory disturbances. Up to 15% of the normal population may have a positive ANA, so there is no need to repeat the test frequently.

Q: Can SLE patients with end-stage renal disease obtain renal transplants?
A: Yes, and SLE usually does not recur in the new kidney.

Q: What is neonatal lupus (NLE)?
A: Neonatal lupus is due to maternal autoantibodies (usually SS-A or SS-B antibodies), that cross the placenta and can cause rashes, congenital heart block, cytopenias, and/or hepatitis in the newborn baby. Many mothers of babies with NLE are asymptomatic and unaware that they have these autoantibodies. The rash, erythema annulare, can begin a few days after delivery and usually resolves within 6 to 9 months. Topical steroids can minimize the lesions. Congenital heart block is due to damage of the conducting system of the developing fetal heart. Bradycardia may be noted by 22 weeks' gestation and congestive heart failure with nonimmune hydrops fetalis may ensue.

ICD-9-CM 710.0

BIBLIOGRAPHY

Lehman TJA, McCurdy DK, Bernstein BH, et al. Systemic lupus erythematosus in the first decade of life. *Pediatrics* 1989;26:235.

Schumacher HR, ed. *Primer on the rheumatic diseases*, 10th ed. Atlanta: Arthritis Foundation, 1993.

Author: Elizabeth Candell Chalom

Lyme Disease

 ## Database

DEFINITION

Multisystemic illness caused by the spirochete *Borrelia burgdorferi*

CAUSE

The tick-borne spirochete *B. burgdorferi*

PATHOLOGY

- *B. burgdorferi* is injected into the skin with the saliva of the deer tick. The spirochetes first migrate within the skin, forming the typical rash, erythema migrans. The rash starts as a red macule or papule and then expands to an annular lesion up to 30 cm in diameter with partial central clearing. The spirochetes then spread hematogenously to other organs, including the heart, joints, and nervous system.
- Joints: Early on, the patient may experience migratory joint pain (often without frank arthritis), myalgias, and painful tendons and bursae. Months later, 60% of untreated patients will develop mono- or pauciarticular arthritis of the large joints, especially the knees. Joint fluid can have a white blood count anywhere from 500 to 110,000 cells/mm^3, and the cells are mostly neutrophils.
- Neurologic: 14% of untreated patients will develop neurologic symptoms of Lyme disease several weeks after the initial rash. These symptoms include aseptic meningitis, cranial nerve palsies (especially facial nerve palsies), mononeuritis, plexitis, and myelitis. Months to years later, chronic neurologic symptoms may occur, including a subtle encephalopathy, memory, mood, and sleep disturbances.
- Cardiac: Approximately 8% of untreated patients develop cardiac disease several weeks after the initial Lyme rash. The most common cardiac lesion is atrioventricular block (primary, secondary, or complete). Pericarditis, myocarditis, or pancarditis can also develop. Most of the cardiac manifestations will disappear with or without treatment in a short time (3–4 weeks), but they may later recur. Severe cardiac involvement rarely may be fatal.

EPIDEMIOLOGY

- Lyme disease can affect people of all ages, but one third to one half of all cases occur in children and adolescents.
- Male/female ratio is 1:1 to 2:1.
- Lyme disease has now become the most common tick-borne disease in the United States with over 16,000 cases reported each year.
- Onset is most often in the summer months, and the endemic areas are in the northeast, north central, and Pacific Coast states.

GENETICS

Chronic Lyme arthritis seems to be associated with an increased incidence of HLA-DR4 and less so with HLA-DR2.

COMPLICATIONS

- Chronic arthritis occurs in approximately 2% of children with the disease.
- Other complications arise from the treatment of Lyme disease, such as cholecystitis secondary to treatment with ceftriaxone, and infections from indwelling catheters used for intravenous antibiotics.

 ## Differential Diagnosis

- Viral arthritis/arthralgias
- Septic arthritis
- Juvenile rheumatoid arthritis
- Postinfectious arthritis
- Primary fibromyalgia
- Systemic lupus erythematosus

 ## Data Gathering

HISTORY

Question: Tick bite?
Significance: A history of a tick bite can only be elicited in one third of patients with Lyme disease, and most people with tick bites do not develop Lyme disease. Even in endemic areas, the risk of developing Lyme disease after a tick bite is less than 5%.

Question: Rash?
Significance: 50% to 80% will have or will recall the typical rash, which is not painful or pruritic, but does feel warm.

Question: Other Symptoms
Significance: Many patients will complain of fatigue, headaches, fevers, chills, myalgias, and arthralgias early on in the disease.

Question: Joint pain?
Significance: Many patients will complain of painful joints early on, and later will develop joint swelling.

 ## Physical Examination

- The rash of erythema migrans, if seen, is virtually pathognomonic for Lyme disease. If the patient does not have the rash, there is no physical finding that gives a definitive diagnosis of Lyme.
- The physical examination may be completely normal early in the course of the disease.
- The patient may have arthritis, a cranial nerve palsy, or an irregular heart beat.

 ## Laboratory Aids

Test: ELISA
Significance: Several weeks after the tick bite, antibodies to *B. burgdorferi* can be detected by ELISA. This test, however, has a relatively high false-positive rate and occasionally false-negative results.

Test: Western blot analysis
Significance: A much more specific test. After 4 to 8 weeks of the infection, at least five of the following IgG bands must be present for the test to be positive: 18, 21, 28, 30, 34, 39, 41, 45, 58, 66, and 93 kd. During the first 2 to 4 weeks of the infection, 2 IgM bands may establish the diagnosis.

Test: A positive ELISA with a negative Western blot
Significance: Usually means the patient does not have Lyme disease and the ELISA was a false positive.

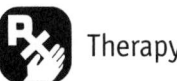 Therapy

- Initial therapy for early Lyme disease consists of oral antibiotics. For patients over 8 years old, doxycycline is the drug of choice. For younger children or for people who do not tolerate tetracyclines, amoxicillin is preferred, but penicillin (PCN) V is also acceptable. For PCN-allergic patients, erythromycin may be used, but it is less effective.
- For patients with only the skin rash, 14 days of oral antibiotics is usually sufficient. If other symptoms are present, 30 days are recommended.
- For persistent arthritis unresponsive to oral medications, severe carditis, or neurologic disease (other than an isolated seventh nerve palsy), intravenous antibiotics become necessary. Ceftriaxone is the drug of choice, but intravenous PCN V may also be used. Treatment should be given for 14 to 21 days.
- Recent studies suggest that a single dose of doxycycline after a tick bite will prevent Lyme Disease.

PROGNOSIS

In general, the prognosis for children with Lyme disease is much better than that for adults. Only 2% of children have chronic arthritis at 6 months.

PITFALLS

Incorrect diagnosis: Many patients with vague systemic complaints (fatigue, headaches, arthralgias) are incorrectly diagnosed with Lyme disease, even though their Lyme tests are negative (or the ELISA is mildly positive and the Western blot is negative). These patients are then treated with multiple courses of oral antibiotics; if they do not respond, they are often treated with intravenous antibiotics, sometimes for prolonged periods of time. This delays diagnosing the true problem and subjects the patient to the unnecessary risks of long-term antibiotic use and occasionally of central venous lines.

 Common Questions and Answers

Q: What does the deer tick look like?
A: The deer tick is flat, very small (about the size of a pin head), and has eight legs. The adult male is black and the female is red and black. They can grow to three times their normal size when they are engorged with blood.

Q: Do all bites from infected deer ticks cause Lyme disease?
A: No. Even infected ticks will not cause Lyme disease if they are attached to the skin for a short period of time. If the tick is attached for less than 24 hours, the chances of transmitting the disease are very low. The longer the tick is attached, the higher the probability of disease transmission.

Q: Should all patients be retested for Lyme disease after a full course of treatment?
A: No. Lyme titers will remain elevated for months to years after adequate treatment for Lyme disease. If the patient's symptoms have resolved, there is no point in rechecking the titer. If the patient is still symptomatic, titers and a Western blot may be checked before starting intravenous antibiotic therapy, to look for a rising titer and to be sure the patient truly has Lyme disease. If symptoms remain after intravenous therapy, other diagnoses should be considered.

ICD-9-CM 088.81

BIBLIOGRAPHY

Culp RW, Eichenfield AH, Davidson RS, et al. Lyme arthritis in children. *J Bone Joint Surg* 1987;69B:96.

Dressler F, Whalen JA, Reinhardt BN, et al. Western blotting in the serodiagnosis of Lyme disease. *J Infect Dis* 1993;167:392–400.

Lyme disease surveillance. *MMWR* 1991;40:417.

Pachner AR, Steere AC. The triad of neurologic manifestations of Lyme disease: meningitis, cranial neuritis, and radiculoneuritis. *Neurology* 1985;35(1):47–53.

Shapiro ED. Lyme disease. *Pediatr Rev* 1998;19(5):147–154.

Steere AC, Bartenhagen NH, Craft JE, et al. The early clinical manifestations of Lyme disease. *Ann Intern Med* 1983;99:76.

Steere AC, Bratsford WP, Weinberg M, et al. Lyme carditis: cardiac abnormalities of Lyme disease. *Ann Intern Med* 1980;93:8–16.

Steere AC, Schoen RT, Taylor E. The clinical evolution of lyme arthritis. *Ann Intern Med* 1987;107:725–731.

Williams CL, Strobino B, Lee A, et al. Lyme disease in childhood: clinical and epidemiologic features of ninety cases. *Pediatr Infect Dis J* 1990;9:10–14.

Author: Elizabeth Candell Chalom

Lymphadenopathy

 Database

DEFINITION
- Enlargement of a lymph node larger than 10 mm.
- Additional differentiation should be made between lymphadenopathy, which is enlargement alone, and lymphadenitis, which is enlargement plus signs of inflammation such as erythema and tenderness.

PATHOPHYSIOLOGY
- Lymphadenitis
—Organisms enter the lymph node (either through hematogenous spread of a systemic infection or through the lymphatic drainage of an infected area) and establish a local infection with microabscess formation and suppuration.
- Etiology
—Direct invasion of node with regional bacterial organism (*Streptococcus* species, *Staphylococcus aureus, Haemophilus influenzae,* anaerobes).
—Systemic or locally draining pathogens
—Mycobacterium (tuberculous and nontuberculous)
—Cat-scratch disease (*Bartonella henselae*)
- Lymphadenopathy, enlargement may occur by:
—Follicular proliferation as a response to an infectious trigger or as a malignant process.
—Infiltration by metastatic tumor cells or metabolic products
—Reactive lymphadenopathy: proliferation of node in response to infectious trigger in adjacent site or systemically

INFECTIOUS
- Systemic viral
—Epstein-Barr virus (EBV)
—Cytomegalovirus
—Herpes simplex virus
—Varicella zoster virus
—Adenovirus
—Human immunodeficiency virus
- Fungal
—Histoplasmosis
—Coccidioidomycosis
—Blastomycosis
- Bacterial
—Syphilis
—Brucellosis
—Tularemia
—Yersiniosis
- Parasitic
—Toxoplasmosis
—Leishmaniasis
—Malaria

NEOPLASTIC
- Primary lymphoid
—Hodgkin disease
—Non-Hodgkin lymphoma
- Metastatic
—Leukemia
—Neuroblastoma
—Rhabdomyosarcoma
- Immunologic
—Vasculitis syndromes (systemic lupus erythematosus, rheumatoid arthritis, miscellaneous vasculitides)
—Systemic immune responses (serum sickness, autoimmune hemolytic anemias)
—Chronic granulomatous disease

METABOLIC
- Infiltrative
- Gaucher disease
- Niemann-Pick disease

DRUGS
- Phenytoin
- Isoniazid

MISCELLANEOUS
- Kawasaki syndrome
- Sarcoidosis
- Histiocytosis
- Dermatopathic lymphadenitis
- Kikuchi histiocytic necrotizing lymphadenitis

EPIDEMIOLOGY
- Adenitis is most common in children younger than 5 years old.
- Age distribution for reactive adenopathy follows the pattern for each etiology.
- Hodgkin disease is rare younger than 7 years old with incidence increasing until early adulthood, more frequent in whites.

COMPLICATIONS
- Lymphadenitis
—Suppuration may progress to abscess formation and rupture through skin.
—Bacteremia, especially in immunocompromised host.
- Lymphadenopathy
—Compression of adjacent structures, including vascular structures and airways.

PROGNOSIS
- Related to the prognosis of the underlying illness.
- In simple bacterial adenitis, most recover completely with no sequelae.
- May have scarring if drains.

 Differential Diagnosis

Consider the anatomy at each site and whatever variants may occur that would mimic an enlarged node (e.g., a femoral hernia may look like an enlarged inguinal node).

INFECTIOUS
- Abscess in soft tissue site near a node group
- Parotitis

ENVIRONMENTAL
- Insect bite/sting

TRAUMA
- Soft tissue swelling from blunt trauma
- Hematoma

METABOLIC
- Thyroid nodule

CONGENITAL
- Branchial cleft cyst
- Cystic hygroma
- Thyroglossal duct cyst
- Inguinal hernia

 Data Gathering

HISTORY
An appropriate history includes a general screening history, as well as anything that would be pertinent for diseases common to the age group (e.g., mononucleosis in an adolescent), body site (e.g., sexual history in inguinal adenopathy), or geography.

DIRECTED REVIEW OF SYSTEMS
Question: Systemic complaints?
Significance: Fever, chills, sweats, weight loss, myalgias, arthralgias, rash

Question: Dental problems?
Significance: Tooth pain, foul taste, hot/cold sensitivity

Question: Respiratory problems?
Significance: Upper respiratory infection symptoms, cough, dyspnea, hoarseness

Question: Gastrointestinal problems?
Significance: Vomiting, diarrhea, dysphagia

Question: Endocrine?
Significance: Heat/cold intolerance

Question: Musculoskeletal?
Significance: Joint stiffness, pain, swelling

Question: Social?
Significance: Pets (especially kittens for cat-scratch disease); travel (especially foreign, but domestic travel for certain diseases is important, e.g., Southern California for coccidioidomycosis); hobbies (hunting and skinning wild animals); ill contacts; sexual history (unprotected intercourse, prior sexually transmitted diseases).

Physical Examination

Finding: Vital signs, including temperature, heart rate, respirations, blood pressure
Significance: May help determine if process is localized or systemic

Finding: Enlarged lymph nodes
Significance:
• Examine not just the most noticeably enlarged node, but all other regions as well to determine if this is a localized or systemic process; measure the size of each enlarged node(s) and characterize as hard or soft, fixed or mobile, and tender or nontender. Serial measurements of nodes that are not of an obvious infectious etiology should be made weekly.
• When palpating for lymphadenopathy, gently roll the node under your fingertips to best appreciate texture and mobility.
• Have the patient in as relaxed a position as possible to appreciate nodes that are associated with large muscle groups (e.g., the neck).

Finding: Pharyngitis
Significance: Pharyngitis commonly gives lymphadenopathy.

Finding: Swellings in the neck.
Significance: Careful exam is necessary for congenital anomalies, such as associated skin dimples that may be suspicious for branchial cleft cysts.

Finding: Adventitious sounds in the chest.
Significance: May indicate a systemic process such as histoplasmosis.

Finding: Hepatosplenomegaly
Significance: The liver and spleen, as part of the reticuloendothelial system, are usually enlarged when there is a systemic process leading to lymphadenopathy

Finding: Abdominal masses
Significance: May be a clue that the enlarged nodes contain metastatic disease.

 ## Laboratory Aids

None needed in most cases initially. In cases where the lymphadenopathy does not resolve or improve within a week, more specific testing should be guided by risk factors as assessed by the history and physical.

Test: Complete blood count and blood culture
Significance: In cases where the patient appears systemically ill and a bacterial infection is suspected.

Test: EBV serology (preferred over the heterophile antibody test)
Significance: In a patient with fever, pharyngitis, and splenomegaly.

Test: Toxoplasmosis serology
Significance: In a patient with a cat and the appropriate clinical presentation.

Test : Bartonella serology
Significance : In a patient with a cat and the appropriate clinical presentation.

Test: Lymph node biopsy
Significance: To rule out malignancy, indicated when:
• No obvious infectious etiology (e.g., lymphadenitis present or EBV serologies not suggestive of acute infection), especially if rapidly enlarging.
• Persistent supraclavicular adenopathy
• Adenopathy associated with weight loss or persistent fever and sweats
• Fixation of the lymph node to the overlying skin
• Presence of other symptoms suggesting malignancy (e.g., Horner syndrome suggestive of neuroblastoma)

RADIOGRAPHIC STUDIES
In general, imaging techniques are not helpful in defining lymphadenopathy.
• CXR is helpful to look for hilar nodes in association with regional adenopathy.
• CT is helpful to look for hilar, other thoracic, abdominal, and pelvic adenopathy. These are indicated only if the etiology is not able to be determined through history, physical, and laboratory workup or if malignancy is suspected.

 ## Therapy

• Incision and drainage: may be required if nodes with suppuration, especially if the patient is toxic appearing, there has been no response to antibiotics, or lymph node abscess is suspected.
• Simple aspiration: may lead to formation of fistulous tracts if there is a strong suspicion for a mycobacterial etiology, either tubercular or nontubercular; therefore, the patient should be referred to a surgeon for complete excision.

DRUGS
• Lymphadenitis
—If underlying disorder is present, guide your antibiotic choice accordingly (i.e., documented staphylococcal infection distal to node group should be treated with an antistaphylococcal agent)
—Empiric therapy: cephalexin 50 mg/kg/d in 4 divided doses or cefadroxil 30 mg/kg/d in 2 divided doses
—Penicillin-allergic patients: erythromycin 50 mg/kg/d in 4 divided doses
• Lymphadenopathy
—Treat underlying disease if treatable (e.g., penicillin for syphilis)

 ## Follow-Up

Patients without persistent adenopathy should be followed monthly for examination (and measurement) of lymph node size, change in character of node, presence of other nodes, and hepatosplenomegaly.

 ## Common Questions and Answers

Q: In an otherwise well child, who presents with isolated cervical adenopathy, how extensive an initial workup should be done?
A: Assuming that the node is soft, small, mobile, and without inflammation, the initial evaluation would be a baseline measurement and a thorough history and physical exam to uncover underlying causes. If this is unrewarding, a plan should be made for follow-up in several weeks. Acceptable alternatives other than waiting are a trial of empiric antibiotics and a complete blood count. The parent should be reassured that this may be normal and advised to return sooner if there is any worsening.

Q: How soon should I see a child with adenitis for follow-up?
A: In a child who is non–toxic appearing, but has significant inflammation, since the physical examination findings may worsen within the first 24 hours, it is best to see the child in 48 to 72 hours if the node is not improving. Parents should be instructed to return sooner if the child develops worsening systemic symptoms or appears toxic.

ICD-9-CM 785.6

BIBLIOGRAPHY
Marcy S. Infections of the lymph nodes of the head and neck. *Pediatr Infect Dis J* 1983; 2:397–405.

Margileth A. Sorting out the causes of lymphadenopathy. *Contemp Pediatr* 1995; 12:23–40.

Suskind DL, Handler SD, Tom LH, et al. Nontubercular mycobacterial cervical adenitis. *Clin Pediatr* 1997;36(7)403–409.

Author: Jill A. Foster

Lymphedema

 Database

DEFINITION

• Accumulation of interstitial fluid in part of the body (usually an extremity) secondary to malformation or malfunction of the lymphatic system.
• Divided into primary and secondary forms (although other classification tools exist):

—Primary: usually an isolated finding, thought to result from abnormal development of the lymphatics. Deep tissues and muscles not affected. Primary lymphedema often divided into:
  —Congenital lymphedema: presenting in the first few months of life
  —Lymphedema praecox: presenting from late in first year of life to early adulthood (20–35 years of age)
  —Lymphedema tarda: presenting in adulthood (after 20–35 years of life)

• Secondary: the etiology of lymphatic damage has been identified, causes include surgery, neoplasm (primary or metastatic), parasitic infestation, infection, irradiation, and trauma.

PATHOPHYSIOLOGY

• Represents state of overproduction or decreased removal of lymph.
• Initially edema is pitting. Chronic edema may result in fibrosis.

GENETICS

• In 1998 a defect in the long arm of chromosome 5 (5q35) was identified to cause dominantly inherited congenital lymphedema
• Many genetic disorders are associated with lymphedema: Fabry disease, Milroy (congenital familial lymphedema with ocular findings), Meige disease (familial lymphedema praecox), and Down, Turner, Noonan, yellow nail, Klippel-Trenaunay-Weber, pes cavus, and other syndromes.
• Inheritance can be autosomal dominant, recessive, or sex-linked.
• No increased rate of congenital anomalies of other organ systems, but may be associated with other vascular malformations.

EPIDEMIOLOGY

• Most lymphedema in childhood is primary lymphedema.
• Congenital lymphedema comprises 10% of primary lymphedema cases; lymphedema praecox, 71%; and lymphedema tarda, 19%.
• Incidence of 1.5 per 100,000 in children less than 20 years.
• Female/male ratio in congenital lymphedema close to 1:1; in praecox and tarda, 2:1 to 9:1 (64–90% female).
• Case reports of recurrent lymphedema secondary to herpes virus 2 exist

COMPLICATIONS

• Cellulitis and lymphangitis occur in one fourth to one half of patients over long-term follow-up
• Lymphangiosarcoma extremely rare
• Enormous psychological burden; nearly universal
• Limitations in job-related and leisure activities
• Fibrosis

PROGNOSIS

• Edema persists throughout life.
• Natural history: plateau in severity of edema after an initial few years of progression in 50%, slow constant progression in 50%.
• Edema of contralateral extremity (usually leg) develops in up to 10% over prolonged follow-up.
• Chronic inflammation and edema ultimately lead to fibrosis and induration of the involved area.

 Differential Diagnosis

INFECTION

• Cellulitis
• Lymphangitis
• Herpes virus 2

TUMORS

• Pelvic mass

METABOLIC

• Cushing disease

ANATOMIC

• Venous stasis
• Deep venous thrombosis
• Hemihypertrophy
• Atrioventricular fistula

MISCELLANEOUS

• Heart failure
• Nephrosis
• Cirrhosis
• Hypoproteinemia
• Reflex sympathetic dystrophy
• Multiple enchondromatosis

 Data Gathering

HISTORY

Question: Is there a history of cellulitis or trauma?
Significance: Many report prior history of cellulitis or trauma of the limb later affected with lymphedema.

Question: Unilateral edema often of long-standing history?
Significance: Subacute or chronic painless swelling of one leg in an otherwise healthy pubertal female is classic for lymphedema praecox.

Question: History of surgery?
Significance: Painless swelling in an extremity distal to surgical or trauma site is common for secondary lymphedema.

 Physical Examination

• Subcutaneous tissue filled with fluid resulting in pitting edema
• Chronic inflammation leads to fibrosis, which corresponds to a change from pitting to nonpitting edema and induration.
• Hair loss and hyperkeratosis of the affected limb develop over time.
• Pain in affected limb uncommon

 Laboratory Aids

Test: Urine protein
Significance: Rule out nephrosis

Test: Serum total protein and albumin
Significance: Rule out hypoproteinemia

RADIOGRAPHIC STUDIES

Test: Ultrasound, CT, or MRI of pelvis
Significance: Useful when evaluating lower extremity edema as obstructive pelvic lesions may be otherwise inapparent.

Test: Doppler ultrasound
Significance: Helpful when deep venous thrombosis is diagnostic possibility

Test: Lymphangiography or radionuclide lymphangiography
Significance: When history and physical examination yield a diagnosis of uncomplicated primary lymphedema in childhood, it is controversial as to whether or not these tests are necessary. Most feel it adds little to diagnosis and treatment.

Test: Venography and biopsy
Significance: Considered unnecessary for diagnosis.

Lymphedema

 Therapy

- Therapy should be instituted as soon as possible and before fibrosis develops.
- Goals: maintain or possibly decrease status of swelling, decrease risk of infections, minimize skin changes
- Extremity elevation and compression (e.g., Jobst stocking, Ace wrap) recommended long-term for all patients.
- Meticulous skin care
- Pneumatic machines or manual massage: short-term recommendation to achieve greatest reduction of edema
- Exercise (walking and swimming) thought to enhance lymphatic return
- Cellulitis and lymphangitis treated with hospitalization and intravenous antibiotics
- Complete decongestive physiotherapy is a comprehensive treatment program offered at few selected centers, but seems to be effective in reducing swelling and maintaining the reduction.
- Diuretics: not used in children and adolescents; efficacy debated
- Surgery has one of two goals: removal of excess edematous tissue or attempts to restore lymph drainage; both may decrease the rate of infections but have poor cosmetic results and are recommended only for those with uncontrolled swelling with significant disability.
- Prophylactic antibiotic use is indicated for patients with recurrent cellulitis or lymphangitis.
- Compression and elevation are lifelong measures.

 Follow-Up

Some edema reduction achieved with pneumatic compression or massage over short term, but persistent use of elevation and compression stockings necessary to maintain benefit.

SIGNS TO WATCH FOR

Fever, chills, red streaks on the extremity, inflamed lymph nodes all point to cellulitis or lymphangitis.

PREVENTION

- Primary disease cannot be prevented, but progression should be minimized with therapies listed here.
- Secondary disease can be prevented by altering surgical approaches to diseases that emphasize sparing of lymphatics and nodes.
- Skin care and properly fitting shoes must be emphasized to avoid skin breakdown, which can lead to cellulitis and/or lymphangitis.

PITFALLS

- Systemic reactions to lymphangiography are not uncommon.
- Compliance with compression stockings is poor because they are often hot and uncomfortable.

 Common Questions and Answers

Q: Is the swelling going to go away?
A: No, this is a lifelong disorder in most cases.

Q: Could this have been prevented?
A: No, primary lymphedema is most likely due to abnormal embryologic development.

Q: If the lymph channels have been abnormal since birth, why does the swelling present during adolescence?
A: No one really knows; hormones may affect lymphedema.

ICD-9-CM 457.1

BIBLIOGRAPHY

Butler DF, Malouf PJ, Batz RC, et al. Acquired lymphedema of the hand due to herpes simplex virus type 2 [letter]. *Arch Dermatol* 1999;135(9):1125–1126.

Child AH, Beninson J, Sarfarazi M. Cause of primary congenital lymphedema. *Angiology* 1999;50(4):325–326.

Greenlee R, Hoyme H, Witte M, et al. Developmental disorders of the lymphatic system. *Lymphology* 1993;26:156–168.

Johansson K, Albertsson M, Ingvar C, et al. Effects of compression bandaging with or without manual lymph drainage treatment in patients with postoperative arm lymphedema. *Lymphology* 1999;32(3):103–110.

Ko DSC, Lerner R, Klose G, et al. Effective treatment of lymphedema of the extremities. *Arch Surg* 1998;133:452–458.

Miller AJ, Bruna J, Beninson J. A universally applicable clinical classification of lymphedema. *Angiology* 1999;50(3):189–192.

Smeltzer DM, Stickler GB, Schirger A. Primary lymphedema in children and adolescents: a follow-up study and review. *Pediatrics* 1985;76:206–218.

Wright NB, Carty HML. The swollen leg and primary lymphedema. *Arch Dis Child* 1994;71:44–49.

Author: Laura N. Sinai

Malaria

Database

DEFINITION

- Malaria was described by the earliest medical writers in China, Assyria, and India, and by the fifth century B.C., Hippocrates was able to describe the characteristic fever patterns and clinical manifestations of the disease.
- Malaria is a febrile illness due to the *Plasmodium* species of protozoan parasites. *P. vivax, P. malariae, P. falciparum,* and *P. ovale* are the species that infect humans.
- Severe malaria is defined as parasitemia >5% with CNS and other end-organ dysfunction (shock, acidosis, renal failure, and/or hypoglycemia).

PATHOPHYSIOLOGY

- Two discrete stages of the *Plasmodium* life cycle: sexual stage, which develops in the female *Anopheles* mosquito providing the sporozoites to the host; and asexual stage, which occurs in the human, first in the liver producing merozoites and then in the erythrocytes as trophozoites. Trophozoites cause red cell hemolysis, therefore, releasing more merozoites to infect other erythrocytes.
- With the exception of infants with the disease, the cycle is characteristically synchronous and periodic, giving the typical tertian periodicity seen in *P. falciparum, vivax,* and *ovale* and the quartan periodicity seen in *P. malariae.*
- Infection from a contaminated blood transfusion or needle can occur; congenital malaria has also been reported.
- Hemolytic anemia, the most common disease finding, can be severe, especially in *P. falciparum;* the predominant mechanism is due to intravascular hemolysis from fragile erythrocytes rather than solely rupture from infected cells.
- Cerebral malaria, the most serious consequence of malaria noted in *P. falciparum* infection, is caused by occlusion of the cerebral microvasculature from infected red cells. Prognosis often depends on the management of other complications, e.g., acidosis, renal failure.
- Tropical splenomegaly syndrome seen in chronic infections caused by *P. malariae* produces splenomegaly, hepatomegaly, portal hypertension, and pancytopenia. In *P. vivax* malaria, acute splenomegaly can induce rupture.
- Blackwater fever is due to acute renal failure caused by accumulation of hemoglobin in the renal tubules resulting in hemoglobinuria with dark urine. This often occurs after repeated attacks of *P. falciparum.*
- Other diseases such as pulmonary edema, distributive shock, dysentery, and nephrotic syndrome have been described.

GENETICS

- Sickle cell disease and trait confers protection against malaria by two postulated mechanisms: release of a toxic form of heme from these erythrocytes that possess antimalarial properties; the hemoglobin S erythrocyte tends to lose potassium required for adenosine triphosphatase (ATPase) activation, thereby depriving the parasites of nutrients.
- Thalassemia and G6PD deficiency may also provide innate resistance to malaria.

EPIDEMIOLOGY

- High-risk areas of the world for malaria include parts of Central and South America, Africa, and Asia under tropical climates.
- Malaria is a major cause of infant death in the tropical regions of the world.
- Infection transmission is acquired through the life of the female *Anopheles* mosquito but can also occur through contaminated blood transfusions or needles as well as be acquired congenitally.
- The most common infecting species are *P. falciparum* and *P. vivax.*
- *P. vivax* and *P. ovale* are associated with relapsing disease because of the persistent hepatic stage of the infection.

COMPLICATIONS

- *P. falciparum* tends to cause more severe disease, and morbidity is significantly increased due to the multiorgan system involvement.
- Chronic relapses occur from *P. vivax* and *P. ovale* infections and can occur during periods ranging from every few weeks to a few months.
- In the pregnant patient, increased perinatal mortality has not been reported with malaria in stable, endemic regions. However, for semi-immune or nonimmune mothers, transplacental antibodies may be lacking, and the risk of congenital infection may be higher in this subgroup.

PROGNOSIS

- The prognosis is dependent on the *Plasmodium* species, relapsing nature of the disease, chloroquine resistance, and age of the patient. The infant with *P. falciparum* infection accounts for most of the mortality due to malaria.

Differential Diagnosis

Because there are few clearly distinctive clinical features of malaria, it can be easily overlooked if a good travel history is not obtained in any child with prolonged fever.

Data Gathering

HISTORY

- Travel
- Dark urine
- Fevers
- Pattern of fevers
- Headaches
- Malaria prophylaxis

Physical Examination

- High fevers, headache, chills, sweating, and rigors are common presenting findings.
- Other features such as cough, irritability, anorexia, vomiting, abdominal pain, back pain, and arthralgias may also be present.
- Periodicity of fever is less commonly seen in young children and is dependent on the *Plasmodium* species.
- Hepatosplenomegaly may be present and is more likely observed in chronic infections due to *P. falciparum.*
- Cerebral malaria will manifest with signs of increased intracranial pressure with encephalopathy and seizures.

Laboratory Aids

Test: Hemoglobin
Significance: Hemolytic anemia due to intravascular hemolysis as well as direct red cell infection is present initially as mild then more severe, depending on the *Plasmodium* species.

Test: WBC
Significance: Leukocyte counts are usually normal or low; there is no eosinophilia. Thrombocytopenia due to liver and splenic sequestration occurs in the more severe cases.

Test: Peripheral smear
Significance: Thick and thin peripheral blood smears are required for definitive diagnosis (thick smears enable better sensitivity if the parasitemia is low; thin smears provide for species identification). If initial smears are negative, repeat specimens should be obtained every 8 to 12 hours during a 72-hour period to confirm a truly negative result.

Test: Quantitative buffy coat (QBC) analysis
Significance: Available as a rapid screening test, but confirmation by blood smears is still necessary.

Test: Serologic tests
Significance: Using indirect immunofluorescent assays may be helpful but have a low sensitivity in the early phases of acute infections.

Test: Polymerase chain reaction (PCR)
Significance: Other tests using PCR techniques are being studied and may be useful in the near future.

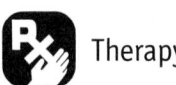

Therapy

• For all *Plasmodium* species except chloroquine-resistant *P. falciparum,* chloroquine phosphate is recommended at a dose of 10 mg/kg PO (maximum 600 mg), then 5 mg/kg PO in 6 hours (maximum 300 mg), then 5 mg/kg PO in 24 and 48 hours (maximum 300 mg).
• If parenteral therapy is necessary, treatment with quinidine gluconate, 10 mg/kg IV initial dose (maximum 600 mg) over 2 hours followed by 0.02 mg/kg/min infusion until oral therapy can be started.
• For chloroquine-resistant *P. falciparum,* quinine sulfate, 8 mg/kg/d PO three times a day for 3 days plus tetracycline, 5 mg/kg PO four times a day for 7 days (maximum 1 g/d) is recommended.
• A safe alternative for children is mefloquine, 15 mg/kg PO followed by 10 mg/kg PO 8 to 12 hours later.
• Other alternatives include pyrimethamine-sulfadoxine (Fansidar), quinine sulfate plus doxycycline, or atovaquone plus proguanil.
• Primaquine phosphate is used for the prevention of *P. vivax* and *P. ovale* relapses but should not be used in patients with G6PD deficiency or in pregnancy.
• Consultation with a pharmacist is recommended to identify other possible contraindications and warnings associated with these medications.

Follow-Up

• Delay in the diagnosis of malaria has been shown to increase the morbidity and mortality up to 20-fold compared with diagnosis and treatment within 24 hours of presentation.
• If treated promptly, even *P. falciparum* malaria will respond well to current treatment options.

PREVENTION

• In the hospital setting, universal precautions should be followed.
• Control measures are targeted toward control of the *Anopheles* mosquito population, and protective measures such as remaining in well-screened areas, and wearing protective clothing should be advised. Use of insect repellents such as DEET is recommended. However, in children younger than 2 years, concentration of less than 10%, and concentrations less than 35% for the older child is recommended.
• Chemoprophylaxis for travelers in endemic areas should begin 1 week before arrival, once weekly during the period of exposure, and then 4 weeks after leaving the endemic region.
• Chloroquine is the drug of choice except in resistant areas (500 mg once a week or 5 mg/kg once a week); in chloroquine-resistant areas, mefloquine is recommended (250 mg once a week; if <15 kg, 5 mg/kg; if 15–19 kg, 1/4 tablet; if 20–30 kg, 1/2 tablet; if 31–45 kg, 3/4 tablet). Contraindications to mefloquine use include patients taking beta-blockers or other drugs altering cardiac conduction, patients with seizures or psychosis, and patients requiring fine motor skill performance. Doxycycline or chloroquine plus proguanil are alternatives to mefloquine.
• Travelers should use pyrimethamine-sulfadoxine (Fansidar) if a febrile illness occurs while on chloroquine and access to medical care is not readily available.

PITFALLS

Failure to obtain a thorough travel history to determine exposure risk to developing malaria can delay the diagnosis and appropriate therapy.

Common Questions and Answers

Q: What is the optimal drug regimen for the young infant or child or the lactating or pregnant female?
A: The only drug not contraindicated in any of these patients is chloroquine. In chloroquine-resistant areas, mefloquine has been shown to be safe in the second and third trimesters. Limited data suggest safety in the first trimester also. Mefloquine is excreted in breast milk; however, limited data suggest safety young infants.

Q: Is there a vaccine available to prevent malaria?
A: Although the possibility of vaccination against malaria continues to attract interest, no adequate vaccination is available. Recent advances in the technology for introducing malarial DNA coding into bacteria may lead to an effective vaccine in the future.

Q: How can I determine if the area my patient is traveling to has chloroquine-resistant malaria?
A: The CDC has an automated traveler's hotline accessible from a touch-tone phone 24 hours a day, 7 days a week: (404) 332-4559. Questions can also be faxed to (404) 332-4565. The Internet address for information is *www.cdc.gov*.

ICD-9-CM 084.6

BIBLIOGRAPHY

Emanuel B, Aronson N, Shulman S. Malaria in children in Chicago. *Pediatrics* 1993;92:83–85.

Fitch CD. Malaria. In: Feigin RD, Cherry JD, eds. *Pediatric infectious diseases*, 3rd ed. Philadelphia: WB Saunders, 1992:2042–2057.

Katz M. Treatment of protozoan infections: malaria. *Pediatr Infect Dis J* 1983;2:475–480.

Kramer MH, Lobel HO. Antimalarial chemoprophylaxis in infants and children. *Paediatr Drugs* 2001;3:113–121.

Newton CR, Hien TT, White N. Cerebral malaria. *J Neurol Neurosurg Psychiatry* 2000;69:433–441.

Peter G, Halsey NA, Marcuse EK, et al. Malaria. In: *2000 red book: report of the Committee on Infectious Diseases* , 25th ed. Elk Grove Village, IL: American Academy of Pediatrics, 2000:381–385.

Silver HM. Malarial infection during pregnancy. *Infect Dis Clin North Am* 1997;11:99–107.

Steele RW. Malaria in children. *Adv Pediatr Infect Dis* 1997;12:325–349.

White NJ, Miller KD, Churchill FC, et al. Chloroquine treatment of severe malaria in children. *N Engl J Med* 1988;319:1493–1500.

Author: Philip V. Scribano

Mammalian Bites

 Database

DEFINITION

Injury to the human skin and/or subcutaneous tissues caused by bite, causing usually local, and in some cases systemic, effects.

CAUSES

- Animal bites

—Dogs
—Cats
—Rodents
—Wild animals

- Human bites

PATHOPHYSIOLOGY

- Animal bites

—Crush and tear injuries can result from dog maulings, sometimes even involving bone.
—Cat bites are generally puncture-type wounds, penetrating deeper and carrying a higher risk of infection.

- Human bites generally only violate skin, although penetration into joint and tendon sheath spaces can occur (especially bites overlying the metacarpal-phalangeal areas).

EPIDEMIOLOGY

- Animal bites

—Dogs are responsible for 90% to 95% of cases, while the remainder of cases are divided as follows: cats, 3% to 8%; rodents or rabbits, 1%; and raccoons and other animals, 1%.
—Ninety percent of the offending animals are well known to the victim.
—Children are the most common victims. Boys are twice as likely as girls to be bitten by dogs; girls are more likely to be bitten by cats.

- Human bites

—Incidence is unknown due to lack of reporting.
—Most common in children of ages 2 to 5 years.
—In older children may occur accidentally during sports activities or intentionally during altercations or abusive situations.

PROGNOSIS

- Animal bites

—Most injury from animal bites is trivial, but infections, and rarely deaths, do occur.

- Human bites over metacarpals (clenched fist) can penetrate tendon sheaths, become infected, and result in a tenosynovitis.

HISTORY

- Animal bites

—Type of animal?
—Apparent health of the animal?
—Any provocation for the attack?
—Location of the bite or bites?
—Is animal available to undergo observation (i.e., it is a known animal as opposed to a stray or wild animal)?
—Rabies immunization status of the animal?
—Tetanus immunization status of the child?

Physical Examination

- Carefully assess neurovascular integrity.
- Location of bite: If bite is located over a joint, assess for violation of joint capsule.
- Examine entire patient to ensure that all wounds are identified and treated.
- Older wounds: assess for signs of infection such as erythema, induration, purulence, regional adenopathy, and elevated temperature.

DIAGNOSTIC AIDS

- No tests routinely done.
- In significant dog bites, consider radiography to evaluate for presence of fracture, foreign body (e.g., tooth), air within joint.
- Blood culture if fever, systemic toxicity

 ## Therapy

- Wound care: copious irrigation to remove visible debris; cleanse but do not irrigate puncture wounds.
- Human bites over metacarpals (clenched-fist injuries) require orthopedic evaluation for possible surgical exploration and irrigation.
- Debride devitalized tissue.
- Primary closure of larger wounds by suturing unless wound is old or has evidence of infection. Hand wounds may be an exception due to high propensity for infection.
- Antibiotics: Data are often contradictory. In general:

—All cat bites should be treated with prophylactic antibiotics due to high risk of infection with *Pasteurella multocida*. Amoxicillin-clavulanic acid is drug of choice (50 mg/kg/day divided b.i.d. or t.i.d. for 5 days).
—All human bites should be treated with antibiotic prophylaxis. Infections are often polymicrobial including *Streptococcus viridans*, *Staphylococcus aureus*, *Eikenella corrodens*, and *Bacteroides* species. Amoxicillin-clavulanic acid is drug of choice (50 mg/kg/day divided b.i.d. or t.i.d. for 5 days).
—Bites to the hand, deep puncture wounds, and wounds in immunocompromised hosts may be treated empirically.
—Skin and soft tissue infections requiring hospitalization: ampicillin/sulbactam 150 mg/kg/day in 4 divided doses. For penicillin allergic patients, third-generation cephalosporin. Antibiotics with poor activity against *Pasteurella* include penicillinase-resistant penicillins, clindamycin, and aminoglycosides.

- Tetanus prophylaxis if indicated
- Rabies prophylaxis if indicated (unknown dog or cat); dogs or cats with unknown immunization status that cannot be observed for 10 days; bites from wild animals including raccoons, bats, skunks, foxes, coyotes. Rabies is unlikely if the child was bitten by an immunized dog or cat, other pet (e.g., hamsters, guinea pigs, gerbils, rabbits), squirrels, mice, or rats.

PREVENTION

- Educate children about the safe handling of animals.
- Ensure children and family pets are routinely immunized against tetanus and rabies, respectively.
- Local regulations dictate the reporting of animal bites to health departments.

BIBLIOGRAPHY

Goldstein EJC. Current concepts on animal bites: bacteriology and therapy. *Curr Clin Top Infect Dis* 1999;19:99–111.

Griego RD, Rosen T, Orengo IF, et al. Dog, cat, and human bites: a review. *J Am Acad Dermatol* 1995;33:1019–1029.

Author: Jill C. Posner

Mastoiditis

 Database

DEFINITION

Mastoiditis is an infection of the mastoid air cells that can range from an asymptomatic illness to a severe life-threatening disease.

CAUSES

- Acute mastoiditis is caused by an extension of the inflammation of acute otitis media into the mastoid air cells.
- The bacteria causing acute mastoiditis are usually *Streptococcus pneumoniae*, group A β-hemolytic streptococci, and *Staphylococcus aureus*.
- Chronic mastoiditis is usually caused by *S. aureus*, anaerobic bacteria, enteric bacteria, and *Pseudomonas aeruginosa*. Chronic mastoiditis is often a multiple organism infection.
- Unusual agents of chronic mastoiditis include *Mycobacterium tuberculosis*, atypical mycobacterium, *Nocardia asteroides*, and *Histoplasma capsulatum*.
- Cholesteatomas may contribute to the development of mastoiditis by impeding mastoid drainage or erosion of underlying bone.

PATHOLOGY

- The mastoid process is the posterior portion of the temporal bone and consists of interconnecting air cells that drain superiorly into the middle ear. Because these mastoid air cells connect with the middle ear, all cases of acute otitis media are associated with some mastoid inflammation.
- Acute mastoiditis develops when the accumulation of purulent exudate in the middle ear does not drain through the eustachian tube or through a perforated tympanic membrane but spreads to the mastoid.
- Acute mastoiditis can progress to a coalescent phase when the air cells are destroyed and may then progress to subperiosteal abscess or to chronic mastoiditis.

EPIDEMIOLOGY

- At the start of the 20th century, about half the cases of otitis media developed into a coalescent mastoiditis. The routine use of antibiotics for otitis media and aggressive management of treatment failures has decreased this incidence to 0.2% to 0.4%.
- Some recent studies have documented increasing incidence of mastoiditis at their centers.
- Most patients are between 6 and 24 months old.
- It is unusual to see mastoiditis in the very young because of incomplete pneumatization of the mastoid air cells.

COMPLICATIONS

- The mastoid's proximity to many important structures can result in serious complications from extension of infection or as a response to the inflammatory process.
- Intracranial complications include meningitis and extradural, subdural, or brain parenchymal abscesses.
- Venous sinus thrombophlebitis results from extension of disease to the sigmoid or lateral sinus. Sepsis, increased intracranial pressure, or septic emboli may result.
- Facial nerve palsy is usually unilateral and can be permanent.
- Labyrinthitis or osteomyelitis may result from extension of the infection into adjacent bones.
- Subperiosteal abscess
- Hearing loss can occur from destruction of the ossicles or from labyrinthine damage.
- Bezold abscess is a deep neck abscess along the medial sternocleidomastoid muscle that develops when the infection erodes through the tip of the mastoid bone and dissects down tissue planes.

PROGNOSIS

- Mastoiditis has a good prognosis if it is treated early. However, intracranial extension of mastoiditis can lead to permanent neurologic deficits and death.
- Chronic mastoiditis can lead to irreversible hearing loss.

 Differential Diagnosis

- Parotitis
- Postauricular lymphadenopathy or cellulitis
- Otitis externa or an ear canal furuncle
- Neoplastic disease: leukemia, lymphoma, rhabdomyosarcoma, histiocytosis X
- Branchial cleft anomaly

 Data Gathering

HISTORY

- Symptoms include fever, ear pain, and postauricular swelling.
- Past medical history usually may include a recent or a chronic history of treatment for otitis media.
- Intracranial extension should be suspected if there is lethargy, a stiff neck, headache, focal neurologic symptoms, seizures, visual changes, or persistent fevers despite appropriate antibiotic treatment.
- Labyrinthitis initially presents with tinnitus and nausea, which can progress to vomiting, vertigo, nystagmus, and loss of balance.

 Physical Examination

- The ear may protrude away from the scalp. In infants, the ear protrudes out and is displaced down.
- The tympanic membrane is hyperemic with decreased mobility.
- The mastoid process is tender with soft tissue swelling and erythema and sometimes postauricular fluctuance.
- In chronic mastoiditis, the fever and postauricular swelling are often not present and the patient presents with ear pain, persistent drainage, or hearing loss.

Laboratory Aids

Test: Middle ear aspirate obtained by myringotomy
Significance: Gram stain and cultures for aerobic and anaerobic bacteria should be done. There is some correlation between middle ear bacterial cultures and mastoid cultures.

Test: Radiographs
Significance: Reveal haziness of the mastoid air cells and can show bony destruction in more advanced disease. However, radiographs are unreliable and can be falsely normal as well as falsely abnormal.

Test: CT
Significance: Helpful in the confirmation of the diagnosis, identification of coalescence or a subperiosteal abscess, and evaluation for concomitant intracranial complications. However, intracranial complications are best seen with MRI.

Test: Lumbar puncture
Significance: Must be performed in any child with symptoms of meningitis.

Test: Complete blood count with differential
Significance: May show a leukocytosis with a neutrophil predominance.

Test: Erythrocyte sedimentation rate
Significance: May be elevated in acute mastoiditis but is usually normal in the chronic stage.

Test: Purified protein derivative (PPD)
Significance: Should be done if tuberculosis is suspected.

 ## Therapy

- Middle ear drainage is essential, and therefore a myringotomy with or without tube placement should be performed early.
- Parenteral antibiotics are chosen on the basis of the most likely organisms. In acute mastoiditis, oxacillin (150 mg/kg/d in 4 doses) or cefotaxime (150–200 mg/kg/d in 4 doses) can be used. Broad-spectrum coverage such as oxacillin and gentamicin is recommended for chronic mastoiditis. If *M. tuberculosis* is suspected, then antituberculosis therapy should be started.
- Indications for surgical intervention include subperiosteal abscess, coalescence, facial nerve palsy, meningitis, intracranial abscess, venous thrombosis, or persistent symptoms despite adequate antibiotic treatment.

PREVENTION

- Appropriate early treatment of otitis media as well as timely follow-up to identify treatment failures.
- Avoid factors that predispose to otitis media, including smoking and bottle feeding.
- Early recognition of mastoiditis decreases the risk of intracranial complications.
- Streptococcal vaccination may help decrease the occurrence of otitis media.

 ## Follow-Up

- If patients respond quickly to parenteral therapy, they can complete a 3-week course with oral antibiotics and weekly follow-up visits.
- Audiograms should be performed later to screen for hearing loss.

 ## Common Questions and Answers

Q: Do all children with mastoiditis need a CT scan of the head if mastoiditis is suspected?
A: No, in general if the child with mastoiditis has mild swelling, no fluctuance of the mastoid, and responds to therapy, no CT scan is needed. A patient who appears toxic, is not responding to appropriate antibiotic therapy, or one suspects is a surgical candidate should undergo additional imaging studies.

Q: Should all children with mastoiditis be admitted to the hospital?
A: Yes, in general, admission with intravenous antibiotics and ENT evaluation is warranted to rule out complications.

ICD-9-CM

383.00 (acute)
383.1 (chronic)

BIBLIOGRAPHY

Alford BR, Cohn AM. Complications of suppurative otitis media and mastoiditis. In: Paparella MM, Shumrick DA, eds. *Otolaryngology*, 2nd ed. Philadelphia: WB Saunders, 1980:1490–1509.

Antonelle PJ, Dhanani CM, et al. Impact of resistant pneumococcus on rates of acute mastoiditis. *Otolaryngol Head Neck Surg* 1999;121:190–194.

Bitar CN, Kluka EA, Steele RW. Mastoiditis in children. *Clin Pediatr* 1996; 35:391–395.

Lewis K, Cherry JD. Mastoiditis. In: Feigin RD, Cherry JD, eds. *Textbook of pediatric infectious diseases*. Philadelphia: WB Saunders, 1992: 189–195.

Spiegel JH, Lustig LR, Lee KC, et al. Contemporary presentation and management of a spectrum of mastoid abscesses. *Laryngoscope* 1998;108:882–888.

Author: Frances M. Nadel

Measles (Rubeola-First Disease)

Database

DEFINITION

Measles is an exanthematous disease that has a relatively predictable course, making diagnosis clinically possible. The disease involves fever, cough, conjunctivitis, or coryza with an erythematous rash, which has a characteristic progression.

CAUSES

Measles is a paramyxovirus, genus *Morbillivirus*. It was first isolated in 1954 in human and monkey kidney tissue cultures.

PATHOPHYSIOLOGY

The infection is probably acquired by inoculation of the nose or conjunctivae.

EPIDEMIOLOGY

- Measles is a highly contagious disease in nonimmune persons.
- Transmission of measles is thought to occur mainly by microaerosolized droplets of respiratory secretions.
- Hospital or clinic waiting rooms (especially pediatric emergency department waiting rooms) have been identified as a major risk accounting for up to 45% of the known exposures in this setting.
- Prior to the 1963 licensure of vaccine, approximately 500,000 cases of measles (330 cases per 100,000) population were reported annually.
- In 1983, there were only 0.7 cases per 100,000 population. However, in 1990, 27,672 cases were reported with 89 deaths.
- The reason for the 1989–1991 outbreak was failure to adequately vaccinate preschool-aged children.
- Patients are contagious from 1 to 2 days before onset of symptoms until 5 days after the appearance of the rash.
- The incubation period is generally 8 to 12 days from exposure to onset of symptoms and about 14 days until the appearance of rash.
- With adequate vaccinations, measles could be eliminated as a disease.
- In 1999 only 86 cases of measles were reported to the CDC.

COMPLICATIONS

- Complication rates in 1989–1990 outbreaks that occurred throughout the country was 23% and included diarrhea (9%), otitis media (7%), pneumonia (6%), and encephalitis (0.1%). Encephalitis, which can lead to permanent neurologic sequelae, occurs in 1 of every 1,000 cases reported in the United States.
- In 1990, approximately 18% to 20% of patients required hospitalization, many for either dehydration or pneumonia.
- In patients with poor nutrition, such as found in developing countries, mortality is higher.
- Croup, pneumonia, myocarditis, pericarditis, encephalitis, and disseminated intravascular coagulation (black measles)
- Subacute sclerosis panencephalitis (SSPE) occurs in 1 per 100,000 children with naturally occurring measles. After an incubation period of several years (mean 10.8), a progressive encephalopathy develop among unvaccinated children. Patients with SSPE are not infectious.

PROGNOSIS

- Mortality in the modern outbreak of 1989–1990 occurred in 3 of every 1,000 cases in the United States.
- Case-fatality rates are increased in immunocompromised children.

ASSOCIATED DISEASES

- Typical measles
- Modified measles

—Occurs naturally in infants younger than 9 months of age because of the presence of transplacental antibody or as a result of administration of immunoglobulin to an exposed susceptible child.
—The illness is similar to typical measles but is generally mild. The patient may be afebrile and the rash may last only 1 to 2 days.

- Atypical measles

—Occurs as a result of a hypersensitivity reaction to measles infection in those who received killed virus vaccine between 1963 and 1967 and are subsequently exposed to wild virus.
—This group of young adults (second and third decade of life) become quite ill, with sudden onset of fever from 103° to 105°F associated with headache. The rash, unlike typical measles, appears first on the distal extremities and progresses in a cephalad direction.
—Virtually all patients with atypical measles have respiratory distress with clinical and radiographic signs of pneumonia often with pleural effusions.
—Diagnosis depends on recognition and on acute and convalescent measles antibody titers.
—The differential diagnoses included meningococcemia, Rocky Mountain spotted fever (RMSF), and toxic shock syndrome.

Differential Diagnosis

- Steven-Johnson syndrome
- Kawasaki disease
- Viral exanthem
- With a careful history and physical examination it is almost always possible to rule in measles and rule out other possibilities.

Data Gathering

HISTORY

- Case definition from the CDC includes:

—Generalized rash lasting 3 days or longer
—A temperature of 101°F or higher and cough, coryza, or conjunctivitis

- The mean incubation period is 10 days (range: 8–21 days)
- The prodrome of measles lasts 2 to 4 days and begins with symptoms of upper respiratory infection and fever up to 104°F. General malaise, conjunctivitis with photophobia, and cough increasing in severity over this period.
- During the prodrome, Koplik spots (white spots on the buccal mucosa) appear.
- The rash appears on the face (often the nape of the neck, initially) and abdomen 14 days after exposure. The rash is erythematous and maculopapular and spreads from the head to the feet.
- After 3 to 4 days, the rash begins to clear, leaving a brownish discoloration and fine scaling.
- Fever usually resolves by the fourth day of rash.

Physical Examination

- The rash appears on the face (often the nape of the neck, initially) and abdomen 14 days after exposure. The rash is erythematous and maculopapular and spreads from the head to the feet.
- Pharyngitis, cervical lymphadenopathy, and splenomegaly may accompany the rash.

Laboratory Aids

- The course of typical measles follows a predictable pattern and, therefore, laboratory studies to confirm infection are rarely indicated.
- At the beginning of a suspected case, confirmation of the index cases is important.
- Nasopharynx culture: Virus may be cultured from the nasopharynx if inoculated into tissue culture within 24 hours of the onset of rash.
- Monoclonal antibody immunofluorescence cells test: Rapid detection of measles virus from nasal secretions is also possible. Measles infected with epithelial cells will demonstrate fluorescence. However, after the third day of rash, detection of virus by the method becomes increasingly difficult.
- Blood sample: Measles-specific IgM titers will confirm infection but blood samples should be drawn no sooner than 5 days after the rash first appears. Prior to this IgM titers will be negative.
- Blood sample: A comparison of IgG titers obtained during the acute and convalescent stages can be done. Blood samples must be taken at least 7 to 10 days apart.

Therapy

SPECIFIC

- There is no specific therapy for this infection other than supportive care. Antipyretics, plenty of oral fluids, and room humidification to help reduce cough are usually all that is needed.
- In April 1993, the American Academy of Pediatrics issued a policy statement concerning vitamin A treatment of measles.

—The use of vitamin A should be considered for children 6 months to 2 years of age who are hospitalized with measles or its complications; and
—Children over 6 months of age who have an immunodeficiency, ophthalmologic evidence of vitamin A deficiency, impaired intestinal absorption, or moderate to severe malnutrition, or who are recent immigrants from areas of high mortality from measles.
—Children 6 months to 1 year should receive 100,000 IU of water-miscible vitamin A.
—The recommended dosage for children over 1 year of age is a single dose of 200,000 IU of water-miscible vitamin A on admission, a second dose the following day.
—The higher dose may be associated with vomiting and headache for a few hours.
—For children with ophthalmologic evidence of vitamin A deficiency, a third dose at 4 weeks is indicated.
—Vitamin A is available in 50,000 IU/mL solution and may be given orally.

PREVENTION

- Vaccine recommendations

—Routine vaccination against measles, mumps, rubella (MMR) for children begins at 12 to 15 months with a second MMR vaccination at entrance to elementary school, age 4 to 6 years or middle school, age 11 to 12 years.
—With the recent resurgence of measles, aggressive employee immunization programs should be pursued for all health care workers.
—Health care workers born in 1957 or after who have no documentation of vaccination or other evidence of measles immunity should be vaccinated at the time of employment and revaccinated no sooner than 1 month later.

- Infection control measures

—Any patient suspected of having measles should be in a negative-pressure isolation room, in respiratory isolation.
—All health care workers involved with the patient must wear masks, gloves, and gowns.
—Isolation is required until 5 days after the first appearance of the rash, except for immunocompromised patients, who require isolation for the course of the illness.
—All suspected cases of measles should be reported immediately to the local health department.

Follow-Up

In uncomplicated measles infection the patient begins feeling better with a fading of rash on the third and fourth day.

PITFALL

Misdiagnosis is the biggest problem with measles infection. Because it is rare and may occur in outbreaks, initially cases are often misdiagnosed as Kawasaki disease or Stevens-Johnson syndrome.

Common Questions and Answers

Q: If a health care worker has had a natural measles infection or measles immunization, should one be concerned about infection following exposure?
A: Those persons born prior to 1957 who had a "wild measles virus" infection are usually immune from reinfection. However, in a report in 1993, four health care workers who were previously vaccinated with positive preillness measles antibody levels developed modified measles following exposure to infected patients. Therefore, all health care workers should observe respiratory precautions in caring for patients with measles.

Q: During an outbreak of measles, should children younger than 12 months be vaccinated?
A: In an outbreak of measles, public health officials may recommend vaccination of infants 6 months to 11 months with a single antigen measles vaccine; children initially vaccinated before their first birthday should be revaccinated at 12 to 15 months of age. A second dose should be administered during the early school years.

ICD-9-CM 056.9

BIBLIOGRAPHY

American Academy of Pediatric Measles. In: Peter G, ed. *1994 red book: report on the Committee on Infectious Diseases* , 23rd ed. Elk Grove Village, IL: American Academy of Pediatrics, 1994:308–323.

Arrieta AC, Zaleska M, Stutman HR, et al. Vitamin A levels in children with measles in Long Beach, California. *J Pediatr* 1992;121:75.

Atkinson W, Wolfe C, Humiston S, Nelson, R (eds). Epidemiology and prevention of vaccine preventable diseases, 6th edition, January 2000. Department of Health & Human Services, Public Health Foundation.

Bell LM. Update on measles. *Cortlandt Forum* 1993;6:131–134.

Farizo KM, Stehr-Green PA, Simpsons DM, et al. Pediatric emergency room visits: a risk factor for acquiring measles. *Pediatrics* 1991;98:74.

Hussey GD, Klein M. A randomized controlled trial of vitamin A in children with measles. *N Engl J Med* 1990;323:169.

Author: Louis M. Bell

Meckel Diverticulum

Database

DEFINITION

• Meckel diverticulum is a congenital anomaly that is part of the group known as the omphalomesenteric duct remnants.
• A remnant of the embryonic yolk sac found in 1% to 3% of all infants; the most common congenital gastrointestinal anomaly.
• This diverticulum originates from the antimesenteric border of the bowel approximately 40 to 50 cm from the ileocecal valve and is between 3 and 6 cm in length.

CAUSES

• Meckel diverticulum results from a partial or complete failure or involution of the omphalomesenteric duct.
• The omphalomesenteric duct is the portion of the yolk sac that becomes incorporated into the ventral wall of the primitive gut.

PATHOLOGY

• Meckel diverticulum contains all three layers of the intestinal wall.
• The majority of these diverticuli are lined with ileal mucosa, but ectopic tissue is often present. The variety of ectopic tissue that may be present includes gastric (which is the most common), duodenal, colonic, and pancreatic.
• Of the symptomatic cases of Meckel diverticulum, 40% to 80% have some type of ectopic tissue, including gastric or pancreatic type.

EPIDEMIOLOGY

• In asymptomatic and incidentally discovered cases of Meckel diverticuli, there is no sex ratio difference. In cases in which the diverticulum is symptomatic there is a 3:1 male predominance.
• The risk of developing complications from Meckel diverticulum is approximately 4%.
• The development of symptoms seems to be age related, with the peak incidence being 2 years of age.
• 80% of all patients requiring surgery were less than 10 years of age and nearly 50% were under 2 years of age.
• There have been reports of a higher incidence of Meckel diverticulum in patients with esophageal atresia (12%), imperforate anus (11%), and minor omphalocele (25%).

Differential Diagnosis

• The differential diagnosis for Meckel diverticulum is based on its two main clinical symptoms: bleeding and obstruction.
• The causes of a lower gastrointestinal hemorrhage include milk protein colitis, gastroenteritis, intussusception, Henoch-Schönlein purpura, polyps, inflammatory bowel disease (IBD), volvulus, lymphonodular hyperplasia, hemolytic uremic syndrome, pseudomembranous colitis, and arteriovenous malformation.
• The differential for obstruction includes malrotation, volvulus, intussusception, atresias, adhesions, and strictures.

Data Gathering

HISTORY

Question: Bleeding?
Significance: The most common presentation for a Meckel diverticulum is intermittent, painless rectal bleeding secondary to peptic ulceration that arises at the junction of the ectopic gastric mucosa and the normal ileal mucosa. The bleeding can be excessive if the erosion is at the site of the remnant vitelline artery. The bleeding, even in the most severe cases, tends to be self-limiting, because of constriction of the splanchnic vessels secondary to hypovolemia. Bleeding is most commonly seen in children younger than 5 years of age.

Question: Small bowel obstruction?
Significance: A second common clinical presentation is partial or complete small bowel obstruction. The mechanism of the obstruction can be secondary to intraperitoneal bands, volvulus, intussusception (which is the most common), or an internal herniation.

Question: Similarity to appendicitis?
Significance: Meckel diverticulum may present with signs and symptoms of appendicitis (inflammatory) with right lower quadrant pain, vomiting, and low-grade fever. This occurs when the diverticulum becomes acutely inflamed secondary to an obstruction or peptic ulceration. Approximately one third of Meckel diverticulum may progress to perforation before exploration.

Physical Examination

Finding: None
Significance: Usually normal; may be anemic from blood loss.

 Laboratory Aids

Diagnosis of Meckel diverticulum depends on clinical presentation and suspicion. There are no specific laboratory evaluations that aid in the diagnosis of a Meckel diverticulum.

Test: Standard abdominal x-rays
Significance: No value in diagnosing a Meckel diverticulum.

Test: Meckel scans
Significance: An important advance in making the diagnosis, but they are only 85% sensitive and 95% specific. During the scan, the technetium-99m pertechnetate is taken up by the ectopic gastric tissue (mucous neck secreting cells). Certain substances enhance the detection of the ectopic gastric tissue including pentagastrin, glucagon, and cimetidine.

Test: Red cell tagged scans
Significance: Not specific for a Meckel diverticulum, but may be useful in localizing the site of bleeding.

Test: Superior mesenteric angiography
Significance: Have been used in making the diagnosis but are rarely indicated.

 Therapy

• The therapy for a Meckel diverticulum is removal, in cases in which the patient is symptomatic. The important factors in the removal are to remove all ectopic tissue during the surgery and to ensure that the closure of the bowel wall does not cause a narrowing of the lumen.
• In some cases a Meckel diverticulum is found incidentally. Some believe that if found, it should be removed secondary to the potential complications of hemorrhage, perforation, and obstruction. Others feel that the lifetime risk for developing these complications is low, and therefore they would not remove the diverticulum.
• The current favored practice is to examine the diverticulum for evidence of ectopic tissue, which includes either a thickening or a mass within the wall of the diverticulum. If present, then removal is indicated. A second feature that may lead to removal is a narrowing at the base of the diverticulum, therefore increasing the risk for obstruction and perforation.

 Follow-Up

• Once the Meckel diverticulum is removed, standard postoperative care is undertaken. No specific follow-up is indicated.
• In cases in which the diverticulum is found incidentally but not removed, one should be aware of its existence. No other specific follow-up or surveillance is needed.

 Common Questions and Answers

Q: What are the reasons for resection of a Meckel diverticulum?
A: Narrowing at base of diverticulum or presence of ectopic tissue

Q: What is the most common ectopic tissue present in Meckel diverticulum?
A: Gastric

Q: What is the most common presentation of a Meckel diverticulum?
A: Intermittent, painless rectal bleeding

ICD-9-CD 751.0

BIBLIOGRAPHY

Anderson GF, Sfakianakis G, King DR, et al. Hormonal enhancement of technetium-99m pertechnetate uptake in experimental Meckel's diverticulum. *J Pediatr Surg* 1980;15:900–905.

Cullen JJ, Kelly KA. Current management of Meckel's diverticulum. *Adv Surg* 1996;29: 207–214.

Emamian SA, Shalaby-Rana E, Majd M. The spectrum of heterotopic gastric mucosa in children detected by Tc-99m pertechnetate scintigraphy. *Clin Nucl Med* 2001;26(6): 529–535.

Lobe TE. The role of laparoscopy. *Semin Pediatr Surg* 1997;6(2):81–87.

Soltero MJ, Bill AJ. The natural history of Meckel's diverticulum and its relation to incidental removal. *Am J Surg* 1976;132: 168–173.

Stuvil O, Brandt ML, Panic S, et al. Meckel's diverticulum in children: a 20 year review. *J Pediatr Surg* 1991;26:1289–1292.

Yahchouchy EK, Marano AF, Etienne JC, et al. Meckel's diverticulum. *J Am Coll Surg* 2001;192(5):658–662.

Author: Edisio Semeao

Megaloblastic Anemia

 Database

DEFINITION

Anemia characterized by megaloblastic red blood cells (RBC; large cells with abundant cytoplasm) in the bone marrow and hypersegmented neutrophils on peripheral blood smears.

PATHOPHYSIOLOGY

• Abnormal DNA synthesis in hematopoietic precursors
• Anemia is due to ineffective hematopoiesis and hemolysis
• Overall causes are numerous, but the following are the most common general etiologic categories:

—Vitamin B_{12} (cobalamin) deficiency
—Folate (folic acid) deficiency
—Refractory dyserythropoietic anemias—rare in children

• Other disorders may be associated with an increased mean corpuscular volume (MCV) other than megaloblastic anemias, e.g., reticulocytes (young red blood cells), which are increased in hemolytic anemias; liver disease; pregnancy; aplastic anemia; hypothyroidism.

EPIDEMIOLOGY

• Exact incidence and prevalence figures in American children are unknown, but overall the disease is rare.
• In adults, pernicious anemia is a common cause.

COMPLICATIONS

• Mild congestive heart failure may develop due to anemia but this is uncommon due to the insidious onset of megaloblastic anemia in general.
• Neurologic complications from vitamin B_{12} deficiency.
• Folate deficiency may complicate vitamin B_{12} deficiency.

PROGNOSIS

Prognosis depends on etiology of megaloblastic anemia; usually good if dietary deficiency. Poor prognoses may be associated with inborn errors of metabolism that sometimes present with megaloblastic anemia.

 Differential Diagnosis

Macrocytic anemias must be differentiated from megaloblastic anemias. In macrocytic anemias, the MCV is increased but without megaloblastic bone marrow changes.

 Data Gathering

HISTORY

• Insidious onset of anemia and associated symptoms such as increased pallor, increased fatigue, poor appetite, irritability, etc.
• Gastrointestinal history may include:

—Malabsorption/diarrhea
—Special diets: particularly strict vegan diets
—Prior gastrointestinal surgery

• Medications such as anticonvulsants and chemotherapeutic agents that interfere with folate metabolism.
• Neurologic symptoms most commonly associated with vitamin B_{12} deficiency; symptoms may include:

—Difficulty walking
—Numbness/tingling in hands and/or feet

 Physical Examination

• Pallor and other associated signs of anemia
• Smooth and sometimes tender tongue
• Neurologic findings: abnormal position and vibratory sensation, ataxia, muscular weakness, peripheral neuropathy, positive Babinski sign

 Laboratory Aids

Test: Complete blood count (CBC)
Significance:

• Decreased hemoglobin
• Increased MCV
• Increased red cell distribution width (RDW)
• Normal to decreased white blood count (WBC) and platelets

Test: Peripheral blood smear
Significance:

• Macro-ovalocytes
• Hypersegmented neutrophils
• Increased anisocytosis (variation in RBC size)
• Increased poikilocytosis (variation in RBC shape)

Test: Reticulocyte count
Significance: Low reticulocyte count

Test: B_{12}
Significance: Low serum vitamin B_{12}

Test: Folate
Significance: Low serum and RBC folate

Test: Bone marrow and biopsy examination
Significance:

• Large RBC, WBC, and platelet precursors with nuclear-to-cytoplasmic dissociation prominent in red cell line.
• Increased iron stores
• Multiple bi- and trinucleate RBC precursors and multiple mitotic Figures

Test: Schilling test
Significance: Assesses B_{12} absorption

• Part 1 evaluates vitamin B_{12} absorption by measuring urine radioactivity after oral radioactive vitamin B_{12}. (Note: This test may be performed after the patient has been treated, but the test involves administration of vitamin B_{12} so that all other tests, particularly bone marrow examination, should be performed beforehand or shortly thereafter.)
• If the urinary excretion is lower than expected, then abnormal absorption is present; this may be due to malabsorption or intrinsic factor disorders.
• Part 2 should be performed if part 1 is abnormal; this involves oral intrinsic factor. If part 2 is normal and part 1 is abnormal, then pernicious anemia is highly suspected. If part 2 remains abnormal, then a malabsorption syndrome is the most likely diagnosis.

Test: Barium studies
Significance: May be needed to evaluate gastric, small bowel, and large bowel anomalies.

Therapy

- General considerations: the following three categories should be addressed for all patients:

—Adequate replacement of deficient substance, vitamin B_{12}, or folate at adequate doses for an adequate duration
—Treatment/management of underlying disorder, such as malabsorption syndromes, chronic hemolytic anemias
—Monitoring response to therapy

- Treating undiagnosed vitamin B_{12} deficiency with high doses of folate may worsen neurologic complications, although a hematologic response may occur.
- Folic acid deficiency: folic acid at 1 to 5 mg oral daily dose for at least 2 to 3 months; parenteral preparation also available if needed.
- Vitamin B_{12} deficiency: acutely, daily doses of 25 to 100 mg IM; long-term, 200 to 1,000 mg monthly IM. Most patients with vitamin B_{12} deficiency require lifelong treatment because most cases are due to abnormal absorption.

 ## Follow-Up

- The reticulocyte count should increase within the first 2 weeks of therapy, whereas the hemoglobin will take longer, in some cases months, to increase.
- If the hemoglobin fails to rise in 2 months, then other causes of anemia including iron deficiency and anemia of chronic disease should be considered.

PITFALLS

- Microcytic anemias such as iron deficiency, thalassemia, and anemia of chronic disease may obscure the diagnosis of megaloblastic anemias by falsely lowering the MCV; however, hypersegmented neutrophils should be present to aid in the correct diagnoses.
- Serum B_{12} and folate rise rapidly after beginning supplements; therefore, diagnostic levels should be drawn prior to administration of supplements or normal diets.

 ## Common Questions and Answers

Q: What are common dietary sources of vitamin B_{12}?
A: Meat, eggs, and milk; liver contains the greatest amount of vitamin B_{12}.

Q: What are common dietary sources of folate?
A: Vegetables (primarily green, leafy vegetables), citrus fruits and berries, liver.

Q: Can food preparation destroy vitamin B_{12} and folate?
A: Food preparation cannot destroy vitamin B_{12}, but excessive heating can destroy folate.

ICD-9-CM 281.9

BIBLIOGRAPHY

Rosenblatt DS, Whitehead VM. Cobalamin and folate deficiency: acquired and hereditary disorders in children. *Semin Hematol* 1999;36:19–34.

Snow C. Laboratory diagnosis of vitamin B12 and folate deficiency: a guide for the primary care physician. *Arch Intern Med* 1999;159:1289–1298.

Author: Kim Smith-Whitley

Meningitis

 Database

DEFINITION
Meningitis is inflammation of the membranes of the brain or spinal cord usually caused by bacteria, viruses, fungi, and rarely parasites. It is almost always a result of hematogenous spread.

CAUSES
- Bacterial
—Bacteria causing meningitis differ depending on age:
    —Less than 1 month: Group B streptococcus, *Escherichia coli,* other enteric, *Listeria monocytogenes, Streptococcus pneumoniae*
    —4 to 6 weeks: *Haemophilus influenzae* type b, *E. coli, S. pneumoniae,* group B streptococcus
    —6 weeks to 6 years: *S. pneumoniae, Neisseria meningitides, H. influenzae* type b
    —Older than 6 years: *S. pneumoniae, N. meningitis*
- Viral
—Approximately 70 different strains of enteroviruses, which include polioviruses, Coxsackie A, Coxsackie B, and echoviruses. Enteroviruses discovered recently are not placed in the above four groups but simply numbered (e.g., enterovirus 68), arboviruses (e.g., eastern equine encephalitis), mumps, herpes simplex virus
- Fungal
—Fungi most commonly isolated include *Candida* spp., *Aspergillus, Cryptococcus neoformans*
- Aseptic meningitis
—Agents not easily cultured in the viral or microbiology laboratory can cause meningitis and include *Borrelia burgdorferi* (Lyme disease), *Treponema pallidum* (syphilis)
—Tuberculous meningitis

EPIDEMIOLOGY
- Bacterial meningitis
—Most bacterial meningitis (80%) occurs in patients younger than 24 months of age.
—*S. pneumoniae* isolates are becoming more resistant to penicillin. Currently, approximately 20% of isolates causing invasive disease are at least relatively resistant to penicillin.
- Viral meningitis
—85% are due to enteroviruses that tend to occur in outbreaks in summer and early fall.
- Fungal meningitis
—Cryptococcus neoformans is a budding encapsulated yeast-like organism found in soil and avian excreta.
—Although associated with meningitis in immunocompromised adults (especially those with AIDS), this is rare in children with AIDS. Thirty percent of patients with cryptococcal meningitis have no underlying immunodeficiency.

—Meningitis caused by *Candida* spp. occurs in ill premature infants and other immunocompromised individuals.
- Tuberculous meningitis
—The incidence of disease due to *Mycobacteria tuberculosis* (TB) is on the rise throughout the world.
—TB meningitis occurs in 1 of every 300 primary TB infections.
—This is most commonly seen in children ages 6 months to 6 years.
—Meningitis will accompany miliary TB in approximately 50% of cases.
—There are increasing concerns about antimycobacterial resistant strains of TB requiring four to five antimycobacterial drugs and close follow-up for patient compliance (see Treatment, below).

COMPLICATIONS
- Bacterial meningitis
—Acute complications
—Syndrome of inappropriate ADH secretion (SIADH)
—Seizures: focal neurologic signs occur in 15% to 20%.
- Long-term complications
—Neurologic sequelae: mental retardation
—Hearing defects
- Viral meningitis
—SIADH in 10%
—Long-term sequelae
—It is unusual to have any complication from viral meningitis. The exception to this occur in neonates (<1 month of age) or older agammaglobulinemic children with sepsis/meningitis from enterovirus infections.
- Tuberculous meningitis
—Acute complications
—The most common early on are cranial nerve findings, especially 6th cranial nerve palsy affecting the eyes.

PROGNOSIS
- Bacterial meningitis
—Approximately 500 to 1,000 deaths each year
—Sequelae from the infection including hearing deficits and neurologic damage may occur in up to 25% of children.
- Viral meningitis
—Prognosis for enteroviral meningitis is quite good.
- Aseptic meningitis
—Lyme disease: prognosis with diagnosis and treatment is quite good (see Lyme Disease).
- Tuberculous meningitis
—The long-term prognosis in children with tuberculous meningitis depends on the stage of disease in which treatment is begun (for staging, see Data Gathering, History, and Physical Examination, below).
—Complete recovery occurs in 94% of those whose treatment was started in stage 1, but only 51% and 18% for those whose treatment began in stage II or stage III, respectively.

 Data Gathering

HISTORY
Bacterial Meningitis
- Children older than 12 months of age will often complain of neck pain, headache, or back pain.
- Nausea and vomiting are commonly associated.
- Nuchal rigidity in children over 12 months. Common chief complaints by the infants' caregivers include:
—Irritable or "sleeping all the time"
—"Won't take to bottle"
—"Not acting right"
—"Cries when moved or picked up"
—"Won't stop crying"
—"Soft spot bulging out"
- Kernig and Brudzinski signs may be present. Brudzinski sign is positive: if the neck is passively flexed, flexion of legs occur. Kernig sign is positive: complete extension of the leg causes neck pain and flexion.
- In children younger than 12 months symptoms are often nonspecific. They may not have nuchal rigidity. Kernig and Brudzinski signs may not be present.

Other historical information that may affect management:

Question: Is the patient immunocompromised?
Significance: This makes unusual pathogen more likely.
Question: Recurrent meningitis
Significance: Recurrent meningitis with *S. pneumoniae* or *Enterococcus* may indicate a skull fracture or cribiform plate fracture with contamination of the cerebral spinal fluid (CSF) by nasopharyngeal secretions.

Viral Meningitis
Question: Early symptoms
Significance: Headache and fever may precede signs of meningitis such as stiff neck, vomiting, photophobia.
Question: Duration
Significance: The illness lasts 2 to 6 days.

Fungal Meningitis
Question: Symptoms
Significance: Cryptococcal meningitis is often indolent with complaints of worsening headaches and vomiting for days to weeks.
Question: Exposure
Significance: Exposure to pigeon droppings or other bird droppings can be a valuable clue to etiology if present.

Tuberculous Meningitis
- Symptoms often are nonspecific initially with fever, nausea, and vomiting progressing to anorexia, irritability, and lethargy (stage I disease).
- Stage II disease is characterized by focal neurologic signs (most often involving the cranial nerves, III, VI, VII).
- Stage III disease is characterized by coma and papilledema.

Physical Examination

- Stiff neck in older children but not infants with poor neck muscle tone
- Classically, there may be "paradoxical" crying, crying increases when child is picked up.
- Tache cerebri—flaring of skin when stroked.

Laboratory Aids

Test: Lumbar puncture with analysis of the CSF
Significance: Depending on the presentation, age, history, and physical examination, some or all of the following tests should be requested for CSF analysis.
- Opening pressure: normal is less than 200 mm H_2O in lateral recumbent position.
- Cell count and differential
- Glucose: To be compared with the serum glucose; normal is more than 40 mg/dL or one half to two thirds of the serum glucose.
- Protein: Normal 5 to 40 mg/dL except in newborns who may have protein levels of 150 to 200 mg/dL.
- Cultures: For bacteria, fungi, viruses, and mycobacteria. Approximately 80% of blood cultures are positive in children with bacterial meningitis.

Test: PCR
Significance: TB, HSV
Test: Antibody studies
Significance: Lyme disease, HSV
Test: Other laboratory studies
- CBC: platelet count, PT/PTT, electrolytes, BUN, creatinine, glucose, arterial blood gas
- Blood culture

Therapy

- Assure adequate ventilation and cardiac function (the ABCs).
- Initiate hemodynamic monitoring and support by achieving venous access and treat shock syndrome, if present.
- Monitor serum sodium concentrations because inappropriate ADH secretion is a frequent complication during the first 3 days of treatment.
- Glucose should be given intravenously if <50 mg/dL at a dose of 0.25 to 1 g/kg.
- Acidosis should be corrected if pH is less than 7.2 with 1 to 2 mEq/kg of sodium bicarbonate.
- Coagulopathy should be treated with platelet concentrates (0.2 units per kg) if platelets are less than 50,000/mm³ and fresh frozen plasma (10 mL/kg) if PT/PTT is prolonged.
- Steroids are used commonly in the initial therapy of TB meningitis along with antibiotic drugs. Use in child with bacterial meningitis is controversial.

Bacterial Meningitis
- Antimicrobial agents: <6 weeks: ampicillin IV (200 mg/kg/d); cefotaxime IV (100–200 mg/kg/d); ≥6 weeks: vancomycin IV (60 mg/kg/d) in four divided doses; cefotaxime IV (180 mg/kg/d) in four divided doses.
- Note: Vancomycin and cefotaxime should be considered for presumptive therapy for bacterial meningitis until a resistant *S. pneumoniae* meningitis is ruled out including infants (0 to 2 months of age); also, vancomycin and rifampin PO or IV 10 to 20 mg/kg/d in one dose is an alternative.

Fungal Meningitis
- Amphotericin B ± 5-flucytosine depending on the type of fungi isolated.

Tuberculous Meningitis
- Treatment is generally with four drugs for 2 months followed by two drugs for 10 months.
- Initially, treatment can start with isoniazid, rifampin, parazinamide, and streptomycin.

Viral Meningitis
- Enterovirus: no specific therapy other than supportive
- HSV: acyclovir for neonate and older child

PREVENTION
H. *influenzae* type b (HIB) vaccine has significantly reduced the incidence of meningitis and other invasive HIB infections. A seven-valent streptococcus pneumoniae protein conjugate vaccine (PCV 7) has shown greater than 90% efficacy in preventing invasive diagnosis and is recommended for use in all infants given at 2, 4, 6, and 12 to 15 months of age.

Follow-Up

- Most children with bacterial meningitis become afebrile by 7 to 10 days after starting therapy with gradual improvement in activity with less irritability.
- Evaluation for neurologic sequelae, such as hearing and vision testing, is essential.
- Prophylaxis (for family and for patient before discharge): rifampin should be given if the child had *H. influenzae* meningitis (20 mg/kg/dose, maximum 600 mg) once daily for 4 days or *N. meningitidis* (10 mg/kg/dose, maximum 600 mg) twice daily for 2 days.

PITFALLS
- If no etiology is discovered after the first lumbar puncture and the child is not responding to therapy, then a repeat lumbar puncturing should be performed at 36 to 48 hours.
- Remember that in tuberculous meningitis, up to 10% of children will not react to the five tuberculin unit Mantoux tests. Therapy should be started if suspicious; do not rely on the skin testing.
- Be aware that the isolation of resistant strains of *S. pneumoniae* is increasing (currently it is approximately 5%); therefore, antibiotics such as vancomycin and cefotaxime should be used until antibiotic sensitivity data are available.

Common Questions and Answers

Q: Is lumbar puncture required before starting antibiotics in the patient with suspected meningitis with unstable vital signs requiring resuscitation?
A: No. In the unstable patient it is contraindicated to perform a lumbar puncture. Appropriate intravenous antibiotic should be started. When resuscitated, a lumbar puncture should be performed. A latex agglutination along with routine analysis is then performed.

ICD-9-CM 322.9

BIBLIOGRAPHY
Agarwal R, Emmerson AJ. Should repeat lumbar punctures be routinely done in neonates with bacterial meningitis? Results of a survey into clinical practice. *Arch Dis Child* 2001;84(5):451–452.

Feign RD, McGracken GH, Klein JO. Diagnosis and management of meningitis. *Pediatr Infect Dis J* 1992;11:785–814.

Lebel MH, Freij BJ, Syrogiannopoulos GA, et al. Dexamethasone therapy for bacterial meningitis: results of two double-blind, placebo-controlled trials. *N Engl J Med* 1988;319(15):964–971.

Saez-Llorens X, Ramilo O, Mustafa MM, et al. Molecular pathophysiology of bacterial meningitis: current concepts and therapeutic implications. *J Pediatr* 1990;116(5):671–684.

Wald ER, Kaplan SL, Mason EO Jr, et al. Dexamethasone therapy for children with bacterial meningitis. Meningitis Study Group. *Pediatrics* 1995;95:21–28.

Author: Louis M. Bell

Meningococcemia

 Database

DEFINITION

• Meningococcemia is a systemic infection with the bacterium *Neisseria meningitidis,* a gram-negative diplococcus that is relatively fastidious. Despite treatment with appropriate antibiotics, this disease may have a fulminant course with a high likelihood of mortality.
• Thirteen serogroups have been described on the basis of capsular polysaccharide antigens; A, B, and C produce 90% of disease.
• Fifteen serotypes have been described on the basis of outer membrane proteins; type 2 is found in 50% of cases in United States and Canada.

PATHOPHYSIOLOGY

• Colonization and infection of the upper respiratory tract occurs after inhalation of, or direct contact with, the organism, usually in oral secretions.
• Disseminated disease occurs when the organism penetrates the nasal mucosa and enters the bloodstream, where it replicates.
• Fulminant disease is signified by diffuse microvascular damage and disseminated intravascular coagulation (see Septic Shock).
• Death results from effects of endotoxic shock including circulatory collapse and myocardial dysfunction.
• Bacteremia without sepsis presents with fever, malaise, myalgias, and headache. Patients may clear the infection spontaneously, or it may invade meninges, joints, lungs, etc.
• Meningococcemia without meningitis occurs after initial bacteremia with systemic sepsis. A rash erupts, which may be nonspecific maculopapular, morbilliform, or urticarial. Progression to petechiae or purpura signifies evolution of disease.
• Fulminant disease is signified by hypotension, oliguria, disseminated intravascular coagulation (DIC), myocardial dysfunction, and vascular collapse. Death occurs in approximately 20% of these patients.

GENETICS

Inherited deficiency of terminal complement may be found in 5% to 10% of patients during epidemics. The frequency increases to 30% in patients with recurrent disease.

EPIDEMIOLOGY

• Patients with deficiency of a terminal complement component (C5–9), asplenia, or properdin deficiency are at increased risk for invasive and recurrent disease.
• Children younger than age 5 years are most often affected, with peak incidence between 3 and 5 months.
• During epidemics, more school-aged children may be affected.
• The disease occurs most commonly in winter and spring months.
• Increased disease activity may follow an influenza A outbreak.

COMPLICATIONS

• Complications may result directly from the infection or be classified as allergic immune complex mediated.
• Meningococcemia may be complicated by myocarditis, arthritis, hemorrhage, and pneumonia.
• Meningococcal meningitis is most commonly complicated by deafness in 5% to 10% of survivors.
• Other complications of meningitis include seizures, subdural effusions, and cranial nerve palsies.
• Allergic complications include arthritis, vasculitis, pericarditis, and episcleritis.

PROGNOSIS

• Fatality rate of meningococcemia is 20%, even when recognized and treated.
• Fatality rate of meningococcal meningitis is 5%. The most severe cases often have a rapid progression from onset of symptoms to death over a matter of hours. At the time of hospital admission, the following signs predict poor survival:

—Lack of meningitis
—Shock
—Coma
—Purpura
—Neutropenia
—Thrombocytopenia
—DIC
—Myocarditis

 Differential Diagnosis

• Meningitis due to *N. meningitidis* is indistinguishable from that of other causes, except for one third of children who have a petechial rash.
• Sepsis from other microbial causes may appear identically, including the petechiae or purpuric rash.

 Data Gathering

HISTORY

Time of onset of fever, malaise, and rash?

Physical Examination

- Recognition of abnormal vital signs and lethargy is necessary.
- Careful examination of the skin for petechiae is important.
- Nuchal rigidity, lethargy, and irritability should be carefully evaluated.

Laboratory Aids

The organism can be cultured from blood, cerebral spinal fluid (CSF), and skin lesions.

Test: Gram stain of CSF or scraped petechia (pressed against a glass slide)
Significance: Revealing gram-negative diplococci will give a presumptive diagnosis.

Test: Rapid test for antigen detection
Significance: Best found in CSF but not sensitive for serogroup B.

Therapy

- Patients with acute onset of petechial rash and fever should receive a prompt initial dose of antibiotics (preferably after blood culture)
- Close monitoring of vital signs and clinical status should follow, preferably in an ICU setting.
- Cefotaxime or ceftriaxone can be initiated as presumptive therapy. Once sensitivity is confirmed, penicillin is preferred.
- After isolate is proven to be sensitive to penicillin, treatment of choice is aqueous penicillin G IV at a dose of 300,000 IU/kg/d every 4 to 6 hours for 5 to 7 days.
- In penicillin-allergic patients, third-generation cephalosporins or chloramphenicol are acceptable alternatives.

Follow-Up

Patients with bacterial meningitis should have hearing test as a follow-up.

PREVENTION

- Isolation of the hospitalized patient.
- Hospitalized patients require respiratory isolation until 24 hours after appropriate antibiotic therapy.

CONTROL MEASURES

- Exposed contacts, including household, day care, and nursery school, should receive rifampin, 10 mg/kg (maximum 600 mg) every 12 hours for four doses.
- Ceftriaxone administered intramuscularly is effective prophylaxis. Its safety profile is preferred for pregnant women.
- Medical personnel should receive prophylaxis only if they had close contact with respiratory secretions.
- Vaccines for types A, C, 4, WBS are available and produce an immune response in 10 to 14 days.

PITFALLS

- Public health officials should be notified of *N. meningitidis* cases.
- Physical examination of a child with fever should include careful evaluation of the skin for petechiae and signs of early shock (tachycardia, delayed capillary refill, abnormal mental status, etc.).

Common Questions and Answers

Q: How long should antibiotic therapy be given in a patient with septic shock?
A: 7 days.

Q: When is meningococcal vaccine indicated?
A: In asplenic, or functionally asplenic patients, in patients with terminal complement deficiency, and in epidemics in conjunction with chemoprophylaxis.

Q: When should one test for complement deficiency?
A: In patients with recurrent disease.

Q: Which hospital personnel should receive prophylaxis?
A: Only those with close contact with secretions.

ICD-9-CM 036.2

BIBLIOGRAPHY

American Academy of Pediatrics. Meningococcal infections. In: Pickering LK, ed. *2000 red book: report of the Committee on Infectious Diseases*, 25th ed. Elk Grove Village, IL: American Academy of Pediatrics, 2000:396–401.

Apicella MA. Neisseria meningitidis. In: Mandell GL, Douglas GR, Bennet JE, eds. *Principles and practice of infectious diseases*, 3rd ed. New York: Churchill Livingstone, 1990:1600–1613.

Baker CJ, Edwards MS. Meningococcemia. In: Oski FA, ed. *Principles and practice of pediatrics*. Philadelphia: JB Lippincott, 1990:1097–1101.

Beaty HN. Meningococcemia. In: Fauci A, Braunwald E, Isselbacher KJ, eds. *Harrison's principles of internal medicine*. New York: McGraw-Hill, 1998:574–576.

Glode MP, Smith AL. Meningococcemia. In: Feigin RD, Cherry JD, eds. *Textbook of pediatric infectious diseases*. Philadelphia: WB Saunders, 1997:1211–1224.

Author: Louis M. Bell
Janet H. Friday, 2nd edition

Mental Retardation

Database

DEFINITION
• Mental retardation essentially means slow rate of learning or slow cognitive processing abilities. By definition there are significant cognitive and adaptive delays first evident in childhood. Significant cognitive delays are defined as two standard deviations below the population mean on a standard cognitive or IQ test. This usually indicates an IQ score of less than 70 to 75. Adaptive skills are the functional skills of everyday life, including communication, social skills, daily living/self-care skills, and the ability to safely move about the home and community.
• Mental retardation is typically subdivided into mild, moderate, severe, and profound categories depending on the severity of the delays. A more recent definition by the American Association on Mental Retardation (AAMR) puts more emphasis on the level of functioning and amount of supports required of an individual.

CAUSES
• The cause of mental retardation is usually an insult to the brain or abnormal development of the central nervous system. The exact pathophysiology may differ depending on the etiology, which can include:
—Genetic
—Familial
—Metabolic
—Endocrinological
—Infectious
—Environmental toxins
—Traumatic
—Anatomic brain malformation
• The etiology is not evident in many cases of mental retardation.

EPIDEMIOLOGY
• Prevalence of mental retardation is generally listed as 2% to 3% of the population.
• It is found in both sexes and all racial and socioeconomic groups.
• Of the different subcategories of mental retardation, the mild form is the most prevalent at 85% of the mental retardation population.
• Profound mental retardation is least prevalent at about 1% of this group.
• Associated findings are more common in the more severe forms of mental retardation. The prognosis for longevity varies with the associated findings and overall health, but individuals with mental retardation can live to adulthood and old age. An individual's level of functioning is variable depending on the level of retardation, special individual skills, and family or community supports. In general the following applies:
• Mild mental retardation (IQ 55–70): Formerly called educable. May be in school with extra help and may achieve roughly a fourth grade level in reading and math. May

be employed in an unskilled to semiskilled job. May live in a group home or independently. Some marry.
• Moderate mental retardation (IQ 40–54): May learn to recognize basic words and learn basic skills. May work in a sheltered workshop or with supported employment in an unskilled job. May live with family or in a group home doing much of their own care.
• Severe mental retardation (IQ 25–39): May live with family, or in a group home or institution. Some may be in a sheltered workshop. May be able to do some daily self-care or chores with supervision.
• Profound mental retardation (IQ <25): Live with family, or in a group home or institution. Usually require full care.
Mental retardation has many associated findings including seizures, autism, cerebral palsy, communication disorders, failure to thrive, sensory impairments, and psychiatric disorders. Behavioral disorders also can be seen including attention deficit hyperactivity disorder, self-injurious and self-stimulating behaviors. Families often face additional stressors when caring for a child with mental retardation.

Differential Diagnosis

The differential can include several other developmental diagnoses, including:
• Borderline cognitive abilities
• Developmental language disorder
• Autism
• Learning disability
• Cerebral palsy
• Significant visual or hearing impairment
• Degenerative disorders
Specific etiologies are too numerous to list completely but a partial list of the more common causes would include:
• Genetic/familial
—Fragile X syndrome
—Trisomy 21 (Down syndrome)
—Other chromosomal abnormalities
—Tuberous sclerosis
—Neurofibromatosis
—Phenylketonuria (PKU)
—Other inborn errors of metabolism
• Nervous system anomalies
—Hydrocephalus
—Lissencephaly
—Seizures
• Infections
—Prenatal cytomegalovirus, rubella, toxoplasmosis, HIV
—Postnatal bacterial meningitis, neonatal herpes simplex
• Endocrinologic—congenital hypothyroidism
• Environmental
—Heavy metal poisoning such as lead
—In utero drug or alcohol exposure, including fetal alcohol syndrome
• Trauma/injury
—Closed head trauma
—Asphyxia

Data Gathering

HISTORY
A complete and detailed history is needed including:

Question: Pregnancy history?
Significance:
• Maternal age and parity
• Maternal complications (including infections and exposures)
• Medications/drugs used
• Tobacco or alcohol used, along with quantities
• Fetal activity

Question: Birth history?
Significance:
• Gestational age
• Birth weight
• Route of delivery
• Maternal or fetal complications/distress
• Apgar scores

Question: General health?
Significance:
• Significant illnesses, hospitalizations, or surgeries
• Accidents or injuries
• Hearing and vision status
• Medications used
• Known exposures to toxins
• Any new or unusual symptoms

Question: Developmental history?
Significance:
• Current developmental achievement in each stream of development
• Age when developmental milestones were achieved
• Any loss of skills
• Where parents think their child is functioning developmentally

Question: Educational history?
Significance:
• Type of schooling and services received, if any
• Any previous educational/developmental testing

Question: Behavioral history?
Significance:
• Any perseverative or stereotypical behaviors
• Interaction skills
• Attention and activity level

Question: Family history?
Significance: Anyone with developmental delays, neurologic disorders, syndromes, inherited disorders or consanguinity

Physical Examination

A complete physical examination including growth perimeters is needed looking for etiology. Key features to include are:

Finding: Observation of interactions and behavior
Significance: Any atypical behaviors and general impressions
Finding: Head circumference
Significance: looking for macro- or microcephaly
Finding: Skin examination
Significance: Looking for neurocutaneous lesions
Finding: Major or minor dysmorphic features
Significance: Any indication of a syndrome or anatomic malformation
Finding: Neurologic examination
Significance: Looking for cranial nerve deficits, neuromuscular status, reflexes, balance and coordination, and any soft signs.

DEVELOPMENTAL TESTING
When developmental delays are present and mental retardation is suspected, more formal developmental screening or testing should be done. Possible testing for the pediatrician would be the Denver Developmental Screening Test or the CAT/CLAMS. The diagnoses need to be made on standardized tests, usually done by a clinical psychologist. Such standardized testing might include the Stanford Binet Intelligence Scale, the Wechsler scales, or the Vineland Adaptive Behavior Scales. A referral to a clinical psychologist for the formal diagnosis is indicated.

LABORATORY TESTS
There is no specific laboratory test battery for mental retardation. The testing needs to be tailored to the individual situation based on the history and physical examination. A high index of suspicion should be maintained for any associated findings and delays in the other streams of development. Listed below are some of the more common tests ordered for mental retardation workup.

Test: Audiologic testing
Significance: Hearing should be checked in any child with speech and language and/or cognitive delays.
Test: Genetic testing
Significance: Warranted for any dysmorphic features, a family history of delays or genetic disorder. A karyotype and fragile X DNA should be considered particularly for significant cognitive delays.
Test: Metabolic tests
Significance: Tests such as quantitative plasma amino acids, quantitative urine organic acids, lactate, pyruvate, or ammonia should be considered if there is any loss of skills or indication of a metabolic disorder. More specific metabolic tests may be indicated depending on symptoms.

Test: Thyroid function tests
Significance: Most infants will have had screening for hypothyroidism shortly after birth. This should be rechecked if symptoms indicate.
Test: Electroencephalogram
Significance: An EEG should be considered if there is any concern about seizures.
Test: Head MRI
Significance: Consider a head MRI for head abnormalities, significant neurologic findings, loss of skills or for workup of a specific disorder such as trauma or leukodystrophy.
Test: Subspecialists
Significance: Referral to other medical specialists may also be indicated. These specialists may include developmental pediatricians, neurologists, geneticists, or ophthalmologists.

Therapy

There is no specific cure for mental retardation. Therapy should consist of appropriate treatment for any underlying or associated medical condition. Early intervention and special education programs are available for an individualized education program based on the child's needs and abilities. Behavior management programs or selected use of medications is available for patients with severe behavioral problems. The ultimate goal of all therapies is to help the child reach his/her full potential.

Follow-Up

Children with mental retardation will need regular pediatric preventative care in addition to management of any underlying medical conditions. Ongoing monitoring of the educational programs, to ensure that they are still meeting the child's needs, is important. The family will also need ongoing counseling and support in dealing with a child having special needs.

PREVENTION
There is no specific prevention for mental retardation, but prevention of some underlying causes may be possible. Immunization programs and early detection of metabolic disorders as well as education programs for head injury/asphyxia prevention may be useful in some of cases. Avoidance of alcohol and some drugs during pregnancy may also decrease some brain insults.

PITFALLS
- Children with behavioral problems may also be masking cognitive delays.
- Hearing impairment may present as a delay in development.
- Children with mild mental retardation may not be picked up until they are having difficulties keeping up in elementary school.

Common Questions and Answers

Q: Will my child be "normal" by adulthood?
A: Generally, mental retardation is considered a lifelong condition. Some individuals, usually with the milder form of mental retardation, can function well in the community, especially when given added supports.
Q: Can my child learn?
A: Except for the severest forms of mental retardation, children do learn. This learning may not be as rapid or as extensive as that of a typically developing child.
Q: But my child looks fine and has had appropriate motor development. How can he/she be mentally retarded?
A: Mental retardation is a slowed rate of cognitive development. Many children with mental retardation do not have obvious dysmorphic features. Other streams of development, such as gross motor skills, may be reached on time or nearly so, yet the cognitive developmental streams can be significantly delayed.

ICD-9-CM

Mild mental retardation 317
Moderate mental retardation 318.0
Severe mental retardation 318.1
Profound mental retardation 318.2
Unspecified mental retardation 319

BIBLIOGRAPHY
American Psychiatric Association. *Diagnostic and statistical manual of mental disorders*, 4th ed. Washington, DC: American Psychiatric Association, 1994.

Batshaw ML. Mental retardation. *Pediatr Clin North Am* 1993;40:507–521.

Gilbride KE. Developmental testing. *Pediatr Rev* 1995;16:338–345.

Palmer FB, Capute AJ. Mental retardation. *Pediatr Rev* 1994;15:473–479.

Author: Rita Panoscha

Mesenteric Adenitis

 Database

DEFINITION

Inflammation of the mesenteric lymph nodes

CAUSES

- Infection

—Viral: echovirus 1 and 14, Coxsackie B1 and B5
—Bacterial: tuberculosis, streptococcus
—Inflammation or hypersensitivity reaction to a foreign protein

PATHOPHYSIOLOGY

- Lymph nodes involved are those draining the ileocecal area.
- Absorption of toxic products or bacterial products secondary to stasis of the intestinal contents
- Nodes are enlarged, discrete, soft, and pink, and with time become firm. Calcification and suppuration are rare.
- Cultures of the nodes are negative.
- Reactive hyperplasia: the adenitis results from a reaction to some material absorbed from the small intestine, reaching the intestine from the blood or lymphatic system.
- Hypersensitivity reaction to a foreign protein

EPIDEMIOLOGY

- Age related, most common in patients under 18 years of age
- Previous history of recent sore throat or upper respiratory tract infection
- Most common cause of acute abdominal pain in young adults and children
- Self-limiting condition
- Can be diagnosed accurately at laparotomy
- True incidence is not known
- Probably most common cause of inflammatory adenopathy; even more common than tuberculosis.
- Can mimic acute appendicitis.

COMPLICATIONS

- Suppuration
- Rupture of lymph nodes
- Peritonitis
- Abscess formation

 Differential Diagnosis

- Infection:

—Acute appendicitis: 20% of patients treated for possible acute appendicitis had mesenteric adenitis.
—Infectious mononucleosis: associated lymphadenopathy more generalized than in mesenteric adenitis. Look for associated splenomegaly; can check for cold agglutinins and screen for positive mono or EBV titers.
—Tuberculosis: Look for associated intestinal involvement, positive PPD.
—Pelvic inflammatory disease: a consideration in sexually active adolescents; vaginal examination useful
—Urinary tract infections: urinalysis is helpful.
—Abscess: related to missed acute appendicitis, IBD
—Yersinia enterocolitica infection: bloody diarrhea, arthropathy present; stool culture is diagnostic
—Typhlitis: transmural inflammation of the cecum seen in patients with neutropenia and chemotherapy.

- Tumors: lymphoma; can get more generalized adenopathy; may need to get CT scan of the abdomen and even laparotomy to make or confirm the diagnosis
- Trauma: hematomas of the abdominal wall and intestines; history of trauma will be present.
- Metabolic: acute intermittent porphyria; cyclical episodes of acute abdominal pain and vomiting; appropriate metabolic workup diagnostic
- Congenital: duplication cysts; may present with abdominal pain due to rupture, bleeding, intussusception, or volvulus
- Psychosocial: irritable bowel syndrome; alternating diarrhea and constipation with crampy abdominal pain
- Miscellaneous:

—Crohn disease: associated mesenteric adenitis but also intestinal involvement
—Intussusception: acute abdominal pain with currant jelly stools; barium/air enema is diagnostic and therapeutic
—Ovarian cysts: may need abdominal/pelvic ultrasound to differentiate between the two
—Volvulus: acute, severe abdominal with vomiting. No fever or prodrome. Acute surgical abdomen on physical examination.

 Data Gathering

HISTORY

Question: Abdominal pain?
Significance: Ache to severe colic; is the first symptom, due to stretch on the mesentery.

Question: Location of pain?
Significance: May initially be in the upper abdomen/right lower quadrant (RLQ) or generalized. If generalized, eventually becomes localized to RLQ. An important point is that the patient cannot localize the exact point of the most intense pain, unlike appendicitis.

Question: Spasms?
Significance: Between spasms the patient feels well and can walk without any difficulty. One third of patients have nausea and vomiting.

- Anorexia and fatigue are uncommon.

 Physical Examination

- Patient flushed: Early in the attack fever may be 38° to 38.5°C.
- May have an associated rhinorrhea or acute pharyngitis.
- Approximately 20% of patients will have cervical adenopathy.
- Abdominal examination shows tenderness of the RLQ: It may be a little higher, more medial, and less severe than acute appendicitis.
- Point of maximal tenderness may vary from one examination to the next.
- Some patients may have diffuse or periumbilical tenderness as well. There is no rigidity.
- Voluntary guarding and rebound tenderness may be seen.

Laboratory Aids

Test: CBC
Significance: One half of the patients may have WBC counts over 10,000.

IMAGING

Test: Abdominal ultrasound
Significance: Will differentiate between acute appendicitis, pelvic inflammatory disease, ovarian pathology, and mesenteric adenitis.

Test: An upper GI with small bowel follow-through series
Significance: May be diagnostic for inflammatory bowel disease.

 ## Therapy

Mainly supportive

 ## Follow-Up

WHEN TO EXPECT IMPROVEMENT

Acute symptoms may take days to resolve and generally last a few days after the associated viral symptoms have resolved.

SIGNS TO WATCH FOR

- Increasing abdominal pain
- Vomiting
- Fevers
- Toxic appearance
- Severe tenderness that is persistent
- Guarding
- Rigidity
- Decreasing bowel sounds

PROGNOSIS

- Very good. Most patients recover completely without any specific treatment.
- Death is very unusual and may occur only when secondary specific infection occurs with bacteria (e.g., hemolytic strep leading to suppuration, rupture of the nodes with resulting abscess and peritonitis).

PITFALLS

Can be difficult to differentiate from acute appendicitis clinically, and many patients may have a laparotomy before the right diagnosis is made.

 ## Common Questions and Answers

Q: Can one clinically differentiate between acute appendicitis and nonspecific mesenteric adenitis?
A: Patients with nonspecific mesenteric adenitis cannot localize the exact point of the most intense pain, unlike appendicitis. Between spasms patients with nonspecific mesenteric adenitis feel well and can walk without any difficulty. Abdominal examination shows tenderness of the RLQ that is a little higher, more medial, and less severe than in acute appendicitis. Point of maximal tenderness may vary between examinations in patients with nonspecific mesenteric adenitis. There is no rigidity on abdominal examination in patients with nonspecific mesenteric adenitis. However, it is clinically difficult to differentiate the two.

Q: What are the two investigations that can be diagnostic for RLQ pain?
A: An ultrasound of the RLQ can differentiate between acute appendicitis, ovarian pathology, and lymphadenopathy. An upper GI with small bowel follow-through series can be diagnostic for inflammatory bowel disease.

ICD-9-CM 089.2

BIBLIOGRAPHY

Adams JT. Abdominal wall, omentum, mesentery and retroperitoneum. In: Schwartz SI, Shires GT, Spencer FC, eds. *Principles of surgery*. New York: McGraw-Hill, 1989:1491–1524.

Bell TM, Steyn JH. Viruses in lymph nodes of children with mesenteric adenitis and intussusception. *Br Med J* 1962;2:700–702.

Cherry JD. Enteroviruses: poliovirus, Coxsackie virus, echovirus and enterovirus. In: Feigin RD, Cherry JD, eds. *Textbook of pediatric infectious diseases*, 3rd ed, vol 2. Philadelphia: WB Saunders 1997;157:1705–1752.

Swischuk LE. Periumbilical pain and fever. *Pediatr Emerg Care* 1998;14(2):159–160.

Author: Dror Wasserman

Metabolic Disease in Newborns

 Database

DEFINITION

Inborn errors of metabolism of amino acids, carbohydrates, fats, or of energy harvesting processes within the mitochondria can present in the neonatal period. Milder forms present later with less severe manifestations. Symptoms may be incorrectly attributed to perinatal insults. Signs and symptoms suggest neonatal sepsis and may include vomiting, poor feeding, lethargy or depressed consciousness, hypo- or hypertonia, hyperreflexia, hypothermia, and the presence of odors in urine or body secretions.

PATHOPHYSIOLOGY

- Central nervous system (CNS) accumulation of lipid soluble neurotoxic metabolites
- Failure of neuronal energy production
- Severe metabolic acidosis
- Hepatic dysfunction

GENETICS

Majority are autosomal recessive; mitochondrial disease may have a maternal inheritance pattern.

COMPLICATIONS

- Developmental delay and neurologic dysfunction
- Recurrent acidosis or hyperammonemia, especially with fasting or infection
- Death
- Pancreatitis can occur in association with metabolic decompensation

 Differential Diagnosis

Metabolic disorders can mimic almost any acute disease of the neonate. Any full-term infant sick enough to warrant a blood culture, because of possible neonatal sepsis, should also have several chemical studies performed (see Laboratory Aids, below).

- Sepsis (bone marrow suppression by toxins)
- Hyperammonemia (with respiratory alkalosis)
- Encephalopathy with metabolic acidosis
- Encephalopathy without metabolic acidosis

 Data Gathering

HISTORY

Question: Have any members of your family died early in life? What was the diagnosis?
Significance: Because these disorders are genetic, a sibling or relative who died in infancy may have been an undiagnosed case. Quite often, the stated diagnosis is sepsis or meningitis.

Question: What is the dietary intake?
Significance: Feeding history (breast-feeding with lower protein content may delay presentation); lactose-containing formula will increase symptoms of galactosemia. Most present in the first 2 weeks of life. Protein feeding may hasten clinical presentation but normal turnover of proteins will cause symptoms in a neonate with an inborn error of amino acid catabolism.

Question: Are there any signs of sepsis?
Significance: Septic-appearing neonate with associated hepatic, renal, hematologic, or gastroenterologic abnormalities should prompt search for metabolic disorder.

SPECIAL QUESTIONS

Question: Gestational age?
Significance: Most patients are full-term.

Question: Did any sibling die in the neonatal or early infancy period?
Significance: Positive family history of previous sibling deaths, without a clear diagnosis, is an important clue.

 Physical Examination

GENERAL

Finding: Odors in urine (warm tube in hand to volatilize organic acids), cerumen, saliva
Significance: Organic acidurias

Finding: Hepatomegaly without splenomegaly
Significance: Urea cycle defects

Finding: Facial dysmorphic features
Significance: Various storage and peroxisomal diseases

Finding: Very large fontanelle
Significance: Peroxisomal diseases

NEUROLOGIC

Finding: Level of consciousness and effect of feeding
Significance: Possible intoxication because of blocked metabolism

Finding: Seizures
Significance: CNS toxicity

Finding: Hypotonia and hypertonia
Significance: CNS toxicity

Finding: Abnormal reflexes
Significance: CNS toxicity

Laboratory Aids

Test: ABG
Significance: Acidosis

Test: Blood glucose
Significance: Hypoglycemia

Test: Blood ammonia
Significance: 1° or 2° hyperammonemia

Test: Electrolytes
Significance: Determine anion gap

Test: Urine or serum ketones
Significance: Specialized laboratory testing will probably be required and includes plasma amino acid quantitation, urinary organic acid quantitation, analysis for sulfites, very long chain fatty acids, cerebrospinal fluid examination for lactate/amino acids.

Test: Hyperammonemia without metabolic acidosis
Significance: Urea cycle defects

Test: Acidosis with ketosis
Significance: With or without secondary hyperammonemia suggests organic acidurias

Test: Ketosis with minimal acidosis
Significance: Consider maple syrup urine disease (MSUD)

Test: Ketosis with lactic acidemia
Significance: Mitochondrial defects

Test: Hepatic dysfunction
Significance: Galactosemia, tyrosinemia, gluconeogenic defects, α_1-antitrypsin deficiency

Test: Disorders with normal routine blood chemistry
Significance: Nonketotic hyperglycinemia, peroxisomal diseases

 Therapy

GENERAL

Temporizing measures while arranging transfer to a center equipped to care for a neonate with an inborn error of metabolism include:

- Caloric support: glucose 10% to 12.5% to blunt catabolism
- Restore normal acid-base balance
- Remove CNS toxins with hemofiltration or hemodialysis
- If pyruvate dehydrogenase defects suspected, ketogenic diet is preferable to high glucose.

SPECIFIC THERAPEUTIC MEASURES

- Consult a specialist in inherited metabolic disease.
- Admit to intensive care unit pending transfer to a center expert in the care of such patients.
- Pyridoxine responsive seizures respond to 100 to 300 mg IV pyridoxine.
- For hyperammonemia drugs to increase waste nitrogen excretion such as Na benzoate and Na phenylbutyrate (these agents are not innocuous and should be administered by someone experienced in their use).

 Follow-Up

- Prognosis depends on early diagnosis and treatment.
- Recurrent episodes of metabolic decompensation occur with intercurrent illness and fasting.
- Follow-up for their metabolic disorder should be at a center familiar with all aspects of these diseases.

PRENATAL DIAGNOSIS

When possible it may permit therapy at or before birth (requires close association with metabolic experts who will take care of the newborn).

PITFALLS

- Failure to consider the diagnosis of one of these rare disorders may delay appropriate therapy.
- Do not delay therapy until a definitive diagnosis is made—it may be too late.
- Failure to consult with expert in inborn errors once such a diagnosis is suspected.

 Common Questions and Answers

Q: If an infant dies before a diagnosis is established, what can be done to provide information for genetic counseling?
A: Explain to the family why a postmortem examination would be helpful for additional counseling. Notify the pathologist immediately that a possible inborn error was the cause of the infant's demise. Collect body fluids, skin for fibroblast culture, and tissue (to be frozen) for enzymatic assays.

Q: Does the degree of developmental disability depend on the severity of the neonatal presentation?
A: Not entirely, as the number and severity of subsequent episodes of metabolic decompensation influence the developmental outcome.

ICD-9-CM

Hyperaminoaciduria 270.9
Hyperammonemia 270.6

BIBLIOGRAPHY

Brusilow SW, Maestri NE. Urea cycle disorders: diagnosis, pathophysiology, and therapy. *Adv Pediatr* 1996;43:127–170.

Greene C, Goodman. Catastrophic metabolic encephalopathies in the newborn period. *Clin Perinatol* 1997;24:773–786.

Leonard JV, Morris AA. Inborn errors of metabolism around time of birth. *Lancet* 2000;356:583–587.

Stone DL, Disransky E. Hydrops fetalis: lysosomal storage disorders in extremis. *Adv Pediatr* 1999;46:409–440.

Author: Robert M. Cohn

Metabolic Disorders with Hepatic Dysfunction

 Database

DEFINITION

Some metabolic diseases present throughout the life span from infancy to adulthood with signs/symptoms of hepatic dysfunction including:

- Hepatomegaly
- Jaundice
- Hypoglycemia
- Elevations of hepatic enzymes
- Hyperammonemia
- Failure to thrive
- Protein/food intolerances
- Anorexia, vomiting, diarrhea

Adverse effects of hepatic dysfunction on the central nervous system (CNS) include ataxia, stupor, coma, and hypoglycemic seizures. Examples of inborn errors with hepatic dysfunction:

- Urea cycle enzyme defects (failure to remove ammonia, a potent neurotoxin)
- Organic acidurias
- Fatty acid oxidation disorders
- Tyrosinemia type I
- Hepatic glycogen storage diseases (GSD I, III)
- Transferase deficient galactosemia
- Hereditary fructose intolerance
- Wilson disease
- Various storage diseases (see Metabolic Disorders with Neurologic Dysfunction)

PATHOPHYSIOLOGY

- The liver is the major organ for removal of ammonia and other toxins and carries out glucose production, glycogen storage, fat metabolism, and the synthesis of plasma proteins.
- Liver failure hampers detoxification and energy balance, adversely affecting the function of other organs.

GENETICS

Almost all of the disorders are autosomal recessive with incidences of 1:10,000 to 1:500,000.

EPIDEMIOLOGY

- Some diseases are detected by screening before any signs or symptoms are present.
- Hyperammonemic states and organic acidurias can occasionally present with hepatic more than CNS findings.

COMPLICATIONS

- Neurotoxins can cause seizures, motor and developmental delay
- Hypoglycemia
- Hepatic disease: fibrosis, cirrhosis; transplantation may have to be considered
- Pancreatitis

 Differential Diagnosis

Precious time can be lost if the diagnosis of an inborn error is not considered, and hepatopathy and CNS symptoms are attributed to perinatal insults:

- Infections: TORCH
- Toxins (history is key): heavy metals, acetaminophen, heterocyclic compounds, alcohol and substances of abuse
- Pancreatitis
- Congenital hepatic and bile duct malformations
- Malrotation/volvulus
- Ketotic hypoglycemia
- Reye syndrome (associated with salicylates

 Data Gathering

HISTORY

Question: Is there a family history of death in early infancy or undiagnosed severe liver disease?
Significance: Metabolic diseases involving the liver are mainly autosomal recessive.

Question: Is there any pattern to the illness?
Significance: Tip-off may be episodic nature of signs and symptoms.

- Metabolic deterioration to fasting or childhood infection
- Association of symptoms with ingestion of protein, lactose, or sucrose (fruits)
- Avoidance of sweets (hereditary fructose intolerance, protein in urea cycle defects, anorexia)
- Salicylates and viral infection
- Inability of patient to fast for longer than 8 to 12 hours: consider glycogenoses and fatty acid oxidation defects.
- Pancreatitis may be a presenting sign of organic acidurias.

 Physical Examination

Finding: Tachypnea/hyperpnea
Significance: Caused by metabolic acidosis or respiratory alkalosis (hyperammonemia)

Finding: Telltale odors on breath, in urine, saliva, cerumen
Significance: Maple syrup urine disease (MSUD) (syrup odor), isovaleric acidemia and glutaric aciduria type I (sweaty socks odor), tyrosinemia (cabbage odor), ketones (fruity odor)

Finding: Hepatomegaly
Significance: Storage diseases; urea cycle defects

Finding: Jaundice
Significance: Common in galactosemia, also in tyrosinemia and hereditary fructose intolerance

Finding: CNS findings
Significance: Lethargy after feeding, developmental delay, ataxia. In some disorders the findings are episodic.

Finding: Failure to thrive (FTT)
Significance: Most inborn errors cause FTT

Metabolic Disorders with Hepatic Dysfunction

 Laboratory Aids

ROUTINE STUDIES

Test: Blood glucose, ammonia, electrolytes, liver functions
Significance: Look for increased unconjugated bilirubin fraction

Test: Lactate; urine ketones
Significance: Organic acidemias

Test: Increased anion gap in organic acidurias.
Significance: Acid ion accumulation

Test: Reducing substances in urine
Significance: Galactosemia, hereditary fructose intolerance

Test: Amylase, lipase with findings compatible
Significance: Pancreatitis

SPECIAL

In consultation with an expert in inherited metabolic diseases the following should be considered:

Test: Plasma amino acid quantitation, copper, ceruloplasmin, urinary organic acid quantitation, urinary orotate
Significance: Amino acid, organic acid disorders, Wilson disease

Test: Enzyme studies
Significance: When glycogen storage diseases are suspected

Test: Provocative testing
Significance: Should only be performed in hospital under close observation and after consultation with expert in inborn errors. Tests like prolonged fasting and fructose challenges are best done in a center familiar with the vagaries of such protocols.

CONFIRMATION

Test: Cultured skin fibroblasts or liver biopsy
Significance: May require enzyme assays

Test: DNA analysis
Significance: May be diagnostic

SCREENING

Test: Some states screen for galactosemia and tyrosinemia
Significance: Early diagnosis but result may arrive after *Escherichia coli* sepsis occurs

Test: Blood by blood spot card
Significance: Screening possible of acylcarnitines

IMAGING

Test: MRI
Significance: In organic aciduria and other inborn errors which affect the CNS, MRI may shown lesions, especially in the basal ganglia.

 Therapy

- Acute detoxification to protect CNS—may require hemofiltration or hemodialysis
- Restore acid/base balance.
- Administer intravenous glucose at 5 to 9 mg/kg/min to prevent catabolism.
- Removal of ammonia: agents to shunt ammonia into minor metabolic pathways, may require dialysis
- Acute illness may be associated with cerebral edema.
- Long-term therapy requires a diet deficient in the offending dietary component (such a prescription should be developed by an expert in inborn errors). Examples of dietary measures:

—Organic acidurias: protein restriction, high carbohydrate, glycine (in isovaleric acidemia), carnitine
—Urea cycle disorders: protein restriction and agents that foster waste nitrogen removal: Na benzoate and Na phenylbutyrate
—Hypoglycemic disorders: avoidance of fasting, uncooked starch to release carbohydrate over a prolonged period, continuous night feeds by NG tube
—Hereditary fructose intolerance: avoidance of fructose and sucrose in all foods including fruits

 Follow-Up

- Clinical improvement in acute states may take a short time (acidosis) to days (stupor, coma)
- In galactosemia, jaundice may improve in several days
- These disorders are signified by episodic relapses

PITFALLS

Failure to consider these disorders may result in fatal outcome

 Common Questions and Answers

Q: Can episodic vomiting be the only symptom of an inborn error?
A: Yes, vomiting can be the only symptom in organic acid disorders, urea cycle disorders, and fatty acid oxidation disorders.

Q: What are the characteristics of ketotic hypoglycemia?
A: Hypoglycemia in a child 18 to 72 months of age, often symptomatic in the morning after overnight fast; laboratory: absence of abnormal levels of organic acids (including lactate) in urine or plasma; response to glucose alone; exclusion of other causes of hypoglycemia.

ICD-9-CM

Galactosemia 270.1
Tyrosinemia 270.2
Wilson 275.1

BIBLIOGRAPHY

Clarke JTR. *A clinical guide to inherited metabolic diseases.* Cambridge, MA: Cambridge University Press, 1996.

Cohn R, Roth K. *Biochemistry and disease: bridging basic science and clinical practice.* Baltimore: Williams & Wilkins, 1996.

Cuthbert JA. Wilson's disease: update of a systemic disorder with protean manifestations. *Gastroenterol Clin North Am* 1998;27:655–681

Fernandez J, Saudubreay JM, Van den Berghe G, eds. *Inborn metabolic diseases prognosis and treatment,* 3rd ed. New York: Springer-Verlag, 2000.

Sokol RJ, Treem WR. Mitochondria and childhood liver disease. *J Pediatr Gastroenterol Nutr* 1999;28:4–16.

Author: Robert M. Cohn

Metabolic Disorders with Neurologic Dysfunction

 Database

DEFINITION

Neurodegenerative disorders (NDDs) may target gray matter (poliodystrophy), or white matter (leukodystrophy), or both (many inborn errors including mitochondrial encephalomyopathies). Hepatosplenomegaly or cardiomyopathy is also an early finding.

PATHOLOGY

Many of these disorders are lysosomal storage diseases, which cause dysfunction or death of neurons. Some of these disorders have an unrelenting downhill course marked by inanition, respiratory failure, seizures, and worsening central nervous system (CNS) function. Biopsy of tissue outside the CNS may provide a clue to the nature of material stored.

EPIDEMIOLOGY

Different variants of these storage diseases may present at different ages. Often the disorder is not suspected until significant nervous system symptoms and signs are present.

GENETICS

- Autosomal recessive

—PKU
—Many lysosomal storage diseases
—Leukodystrophies
—Organic acidurias
—Aminoacidopathies

- Dominant

—Ataxias
—Huntington disease
—Some of the porphyrias

- X-linked

—Lesch-Nyhan
—X-linked adrenoleukodystrophy
—Ornithine transcarbamylase deficiency

- Maternal

—Several of the mitochondrial encephalomyopathies

COMPLICATIONS

- Neurologic dysfunction can lead to infection
- Respiratory failure
- Decubiti

 Differential Diagnosis

Loss of previously acquired skills or slowdown in cognitive/motor development is the sign of these disorders; this requires a painstaking history and neurologic examination. NDD must be distinguished from:

- Nonneurologic disorders that may retard motor or language development:

—Hypothyroidism
—Deafness
—Osteodystrophies, Ehlers-Danlos, and other connective tissue disorders
—Rheumatoid disorders
—Prematurity or birth trauma
—Psychiatric–depression, schizophrenia, conversion

- Genetic causes of nonprogressive CNS dysfunction

—Down syndrome (premature Alzheimer-type dementia occurs in adults with Down syndrome)
—Fragile X
—Duchenne or myotonic muscular dystrophy
—Tuberous sclerosis, neurofibromatosis

- Multifactorial/acquired neurologic disorder

—Autism and other developmental language disorders
—Attention-deficit hyperactivity disorder
—Congenital infection (TORCH)
—CNS migrational disorders: lissencephaly/pachygyria (chromosome 17)

 Data Gathering

HISTORY

Question: Developmental history?
Significance: Decrease in development may occur rapidly or very slowly. Compounding the difficulty in recognition, many of these disorders progress very slowly until an intercurrent infection causes metabolic decompensation (e.g., organic acidurias, urea cycle defects).

Question: Is there a familial history of any other affected members?
Significance: These disorders are familial (see Genetics, above).

SPECIAL QUESTIONS

Question: Personality changes?
Significance: May be a feature

Question: Ethnic origin?
Significance: May furnish clues

Question: How has individual performed in school?
Significance: Obtain input from teachers, standardized tests to document deterioration.

FINDINGS

Question: Leukodystrophies?
Significance: Associated with dysarthria, ataxia, visual loss, spasticity (X-linked adrenoleukodystrophy, metachromatic leukodystrophy, Krabbe).

Question: Poliodystrophies?
Significance: Associated with seizures, cognitive decline, personality change (Rett syndrome, mitochondrial disease, Wilson disease, Alper disease, Lafora body disease, Huntington disease).

Question: Mitochondrial disorders?
Significance: Associated with sensorineural hearing loss, cardiac and skeletal myopathy, failure to thrive, marrow dysfunction, diabetes mellitus.

Question: Renal stones?
Significance: Lesch-Nyhan may present with renal stones.

Question: Hepatic porphyrias?
Significance: Present with abdominal pain, vomiting, weakness, sensory loss, altered mental state, seizures, liver disease.

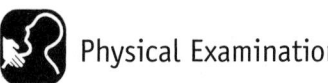 Physical Examination

Finding: Obtain height, head circumference
Significance: Also measure family members for comparison.

Finding: Microcephaly
Significance: Lactic acidoses, ceroid lipofuscinoses, Rett syndrome

Finding: Macrocephaly
Significance: MPS, Canavan, Zellweger, glutaric aciduria type I

Finding: Short stature
Significance: Mitochondrial disorders, storage disorders.

SKIN/HAIR

Finding: Doughy, puffy skin
Significance: Found in many storage disorders.

Finding: Hyperpigmentation
Significance: Adrenoleukodystrophy

Finding: Light complexion
Significance: In comparison to other family members: PKU

Finding: Friable hair
Significance: Menkes disease, argininosuccinic aciduria

Finding: Erythematous rash
Significance: Biotinidase deficiency, Hartnup

EYES

Finding: Retinal pigmentary changes
Significance: Ceroid lipofuscinosis, abetalipoproteinemia, MPS, Kearns-Sayre

Finding: Cherry-red macular spots
Significance: Tay-Sachs, sialidoses, Niemann-Pick, mucolipidosis I.

Finding: Nystagmus
Significance: Pelizaeus-Merzbacher, ataxias, mitochondrial disorders

FACIAL FEATURES

Finding: Coarsening
Significance: Storage diseases, except MPS III (Sanfilippo disease)

THORAX/ABDOMEN

Finding: Visceromegaly
Significance: Storage disorders, Zellweger disease

Finding: Scoliosis
Significance: Homocystinuria

EXTREMITIES

Finding: Arthropathy
Significance: Storage diseases

Finding: Arachnodactyly
Significance: Homocystinuria

NEUROLOGIC

Finding: Peripheral nervous dysfunction
Significance: Some leukodystrophies

Finding: Myopathy
Significance: Mitochondrial diseases

 Laboratory Aids

COMMON ABNORMALITIES

Test: Blood glucose
Significance: Hypoglycemia

Test: Blood ammonia
Significance: Hyperammonemia

Test: Electrolytes
Significance: Persistent anion gap

Test: Hepatic function
Significance: Elevated liver enzymes

SPECIAL TESTS

Test: Amino acid quantitation
Significance: Amino acid disorders

Test: Urine organic acid quantitation
Significance: Organic acidemias

Test: Lysosomal enzyme studies
Significance: Storage diseases

Test: Carnitine levels
Significance: Depleted in organic acidurias, mitochondrial disorders

Test: Cholesterol and 7-deoxycholesterol
Significance: Smith-Lemli-Opitz

Test: Plasma very long chain fatty acids
Significance: Peroxisomal disorders

Test: *N*-acetylaspartate in urine or plasma
Significance: Canavan disease

Test: Urate elevation
Significance: Lesch-Nyhan

Test: Serum transferrin isoelectric focusing
Significance: Carbohydrate-deficient glycoprotein disease

Test: Muscle biopsy
Significance: In suspected mitochondrial disorders

Test: Porphyrins in blood, urine, stool
Significance: Various porphyrias

Test: MRI
Significance: Abnormal white matter signal in leukodystrophies; cortical atrophy in poliodystrophies; caudate atrophy in Huntington disease

Test: Basal ganglia abnormalities
Significance: Wilson, mitochondrial (Leigh's disease), organic acidurias

 Therapy

• Supportive

—Correct acidosis
—Muscle relaxants, chloral hydrate, or benzodiazepines may help relieve hypertonicity and spasticity
—Anticonvulsants for epilepsy
—Gastrostomy feeding may be required to provide adequate calories in the face of anorexia or swallowing dysfunction

• Treatment of underlying disease

—Dietary manipulation and megavitamin supplementation in vitamin dependent disorders
—Na benzoate and Na phenylbutyrate in hyperammonemic disorders
—Erucic acid ("Lorenzo's oil") may delay onset of symptoms in X-linked adrenoleukodystrophy.
—Coenzyme Q, vitamin K, vitamin C, riboflavin, electron acceptors for respiratory chain defects
—Biotin in holocarboxylase deficiency
—Pyridoxine (B6) in some cases of neonatal/infantile epilepsy
—Folate in folate reductase deficiency
—Betaine, pyridoxine, and folate in some cases of homocystinuria
—Vitamin E in abetalipoproteinemia
—Cholesterol supplementation in Smith-Lemli-Opitz
—Allopurinol in Lesch-Nyhan

• Treatment of porphyria

—Avoid stress triggers: certain drugs precipitate attacks
—Increase carbohydrate intake
—Protect skin from exposure to sun, use of powerful sun blocks, oral β-carotene

 Follow-Up

• Arrange for genetic counseling and consultation with metabolic expert.
• Seek out nutritional support group.

PITFALLS

• Risk of recurrence requires making a specific diagnosis.
• Occasionally a static encephalopathy may represent the aftermath of an unrecognized neurodegenerative process.
• Lactate and pyruvate levels can be normal in individuals with lactic acidosis because compensation waxes and wanes.
• Consult an expert before arranging for enzyme assays.

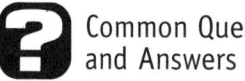 Common Questions and Answers

Q: Why put the patients and families through a costly and long workup when so few of these disorders are treatable?
A: Accurate diagnosis is essential for genetic counseling for the family, will help predict the clinical course, and may identify other affected family members.

Q: Can seizure medications ever be dangerous in children with inborn errors?
A: Yes. Valproate can cause hepatotoxicity in some children with abnormal carbohydrate metabolism. Many anticonvulsants/sedatives can precipitate an acute porphyric attack.

ICD-9-CM

Lesch-Nyhan 277.2
PKU 270.1
Tay-Sachs 330.1

BIBLIOGRAPHY

Berry G, Bennett M. A focused approach to diagnosing inborn errors of metabolism. *Contemp Pediatr* 1998;15(11):79–102

Lyon G, Adams R, Kolodny EH. *Neurology of hereditary metabolic diseases of children*. New York: McGraw-Hill, 1996.

Pourmand R, ed. Metabolic myopathies. *Neurol Clin* 2000;28:1–271.

Swaiman K, Ashwal S. *Pediatric neurology principles and practice*, 3rd ed. St. Louis: Mosby, 1999.

Author: Robert M. Cohn

Milia

 Database

DEFINITION

White papules that occur commonly and spontaneously on the face, and frequently elsewhere; after healing of blisters when present on mucous membranes; referred to as Epstein pearls

PATHOPHYSIOLOGY

• Retention of keratin and sebaceous material within the pilosebaceous duct, eccrine sweat duct, or sebaceous collar surrounding vellus hair.
• Lamellated keratin deposits are found in the superficial papillary dermis.

EPIDEMIOLOGY

• Common in all age groups.
• Up to 40% of newborns have milia on the skin.
• In older patients, most often related to trauma, site of irradiation or reepithelializing blister

COMPLICATIONS

• Primarily of cosmetic concern.
• Rare potential for foreign body reaction to occur.
• If persistent milia in an unusual or widespread distribution when seen with other defects: hereditary trichodysplasia (Marie-Unna hypotrichosis) or oral-facial-digital syndrome type I. Often seen in healed areas of dystrophic forms of epidermolysis bullosa.

PROGNOSIS

• Spontaneous regression of milia occurs in infants.
• In older individuals the lesions are usually chronic unless treated.
• Lesions uncommonly recur.

 Differential Diagnosis

• Infection

—Flat warts
—Molluscum contagiosum
—Impetigo (pustules)
—Herpes simplex (clouded vesicles)
—Environmental (poisons)

• Tumors

—Sebaceous gland hyperplasia

• Miscellaneous

—Neonatal acne
—Keratosis pilaris

Data Gathering

HISTORY

- Asymptomatic
- Recent trauma?
- History of blistering diseases?

 ## Physical Examination

- 1- to 2-mm bright white papules with smooth surface: Most often found on cheeks, nose, chin, forehead, but occasionally on dorsal surface of hands and over knees, especially if related to trauma.
- Occasionally, lesions may be seen on upper trunk, extremities, penis, or mucous membranes.
- Distinguish from pustules by palpation

 ## Laboratory Aids

Milia are firm and, when incised, reveal solid keratin rather than liquid contents.

 ## Therapy

- No need for treatment in infants because they are benign, asymptomatic, and often resolve on their own.
- Alternatively, cyst contents may be expressed by squeezing or with a comedone extractor after incision of the overlying epidermis with a needle or no. 11 scalpel blade.

SPECIAL QUESTIONS

If present periocularly, ask about history of atopy/allergic conjunctivitis.

 ## Follow-Up

Without treatment, most lesions resolve in 1 to 2 weeks in infants.

 ## Common Questions and Answers

Q: Will the lesions get bigger before they go away?
A: No, there is no tendency to enlarge with time.

ICD-9-CM 706.2

BIBLIOGRAPHY

Hurwitz S. *Clinical pediatric dermatology: a textbook of skin disorders of childhood and adolescence*, 2nd ed. Philadelphia: WB Saunders, 1993.

Author: Albert C. Yan
William J. Alms and Carmen M. Parrott, 2nd edition

Milk Protein Allergy

 Database

DEFINITION

Milk protein allergy describes an entity in which symptoms affecting the gastrointestinal tract, skin, and respiratory tract result from ingestion cow's milk protein. This condition is usually a temporary disorder of infancy, leading to abnormalities of the intestinal mucosa in the presence of ingested cow's milk.

• Predisposing factors include:

—Age (diagnosis usually before 2 years)
—Immune deficiency (immaturity of the mucosal immune system, immaturity or damage of mucosal barrier function, low IgA)
—History or presence of atopy
—Early milk protein–based formula feeding
—Allergenicity of formula supplied
—Gastrointestinal infection

PATHOPHYSIOLOGY

• Unprocessed cow's milk protein is 80% casein and 19% whey. The whey fraction contains over 20 types of antigenic proteins, including:

—β-lactoglobulin
—α-lactalbumin
—Bovine serum albumin
—Orosomucoid
—Folate-binding protein
—β_2-microglobulin
—Transferrin
—Lactoferrin

• Infants ingesting cow's milk appear to always develop an immune response to the proteins with the formation of circulating IgG antibodies and mucosal IgA antibodies, which is thought to be protective.
• If children are allergic to cow's milk, they develop clinical symptoms associated with an abnormal immune response.
• Exclusively breast-fed infants may also develop milk protein allergy through exposure to allergen that has been transported from the maternal diet into the breast milk.
• Most children appear to be allergic to multiple cow's milk protein fractions; rarely are patients allergic to only one fraction. Although β-lactoglobulin is suspected to be a major antigenic stimulus, no single protein fraction has been proven to be the major allergen.
• There is 30% cross-reactivity between milk proteins and soy proteins.

EPIDEMIOLOGY

The prevalence of this entity has been estimated at between 2.0% and 7.5% of otherwise normal infants.

 Differential Diagnosis

Any disease process that presents with diarrhea, abdominal pain, and blood in the stool should be considered. One should always exclude infections (dysentery, *Clostridium*) and celiac disease in the differential diagnosis.

 Data Gathering

History and physical examination are important in raising the suspicion of cow's milk protein allergy; however, these tools have not been proven to have a positive predictive value. Additionally, no single laboratory test appears to have significant sensitivity for detecting this syndrome. RAST testing and skin testing may be used with limited value, with positive predictive value of 50%.

HISTORY

• The diagnosis is implied if clinical symptoms resolve upon removal of cow's milk protein–containing food products.
• Most patients will present in the first few months of life. Symptoms include:

—Failure to thrive
—Chronic diarrhea
—Vomiting
—Abdominal distention
—Occult blood loss with anemia
—Hypoproteinemia

• Infants with allergic colitis present with diarrhea associated with red blood and mucus.
• Often, the infants otherwise appear to be well.
• Rarely, infants may present with hemorrhage and shock.

 Laboratory Aids

• Occasionally, peripheral blood and stool eosinophilia may be documented.
• Certain infectious etiologies of enteropathy may mimic these histologic findings; therefore, infection should be ruled out with stool cultures and duodenal fluid cultures, if available.
• Biopsy is not routinely performed.
• Histologic changes in bowel mucosa tend to be nonspecific.
• Grossly, the mucosa appears friable and inflamed, rarely with erosions or gross ulcerations.
• Pathologic findings may include:

—Partial villous atrophy with reduction in villous height
—Moderate increase in intraepithelial lymphocytes
—Prominent eosinophilic infiltrate

 Emergency Care

In the rare situation of severe food allergy with shock-like picture and acidosis fluids and elimination of food should be given in the hospital.

Milk Protein Allergy

Therapy

- Removal of cow's milk protein–containing products from the diet is the cornerstone of treatment.
- Because approximately 10% to 30% of children allergic to cow's milk will also be allergic to soy, hydrolyzed formulas (Pregestimil, Nutramigen, Alimentum) are the formulas of choice for infants with cow's milk protein intolerance.
- Resolution of bloody stools usually occurs within 24 to 72 hours, but guaiac-positive stools may continue for 2 to 6 weeks.
- Newer therapies have included the Neocate and Elecare formulas, which are amino acid, simple carbohydrate, and fat-based formulas that have been more effective in recalcitrant cases of allergy.

Follow-Up

- Tolerance to cow's milk protein usually develops between the ages of 1 and 2 years, and reintroduction of a normal diet can be safely done at that time.
- Occasionally, symptoms of intolerance may persist past the third year of life, and approximately 20% will have symptoms that persist at 6 years of age.
- Cow's milk protein challenge with RAST testing, skin testing and possible gastrointestinal biopsies can help to monitor the degree of allergic response in these older children.
- If there is a history of severe anaphylactic reactions or acute urticaria, the cow's milk challenge should be performed in a hospital under medical supervision.
- Gastrointestinal intolerance seems to persist in a certain proportion of subjects, with intestinal symptoms and increased prevalence of lactose intolerance.

Common Questions and Answers

Q: What are the newer formulas for treating milk protein allergy?
A: The newest formulas are Neocate and Elecare. These are amino acid–based formulas that are made with single amino acids and have the least allergic potential.

Q: When does this problem usually resolve?
A: In most infants who develop minimal symptoms the problem will resolve by the first year of life, but the range can be several years. Some reports of residual gastrointestinal disease exist.

ICD-9-CM 995.67

BIBLIOGRAPHY

Justinich C. Food allergy and allergic enteropathy. In: Hyams JS, Wyllie R, eds. *Pediatric gastrointestinal disease: pathophysiology, diagnosis, and management.* Philadelphia: WB Saunders, 1998.

Kokkonen J, Tikkanen S, Savilahti E. Residual intestinal disease after milk allergy in infancy. *J Pediatr Gastroenterol Nutr* 2001;32:156–161.

Sampson HA, Anderson JA. Summary and recommendation: classification of gastrointestinal manifestations due to immunologic reactions to foods in infants and young children. *J Pediatr Gastroenterol Nutr* 2000;30:S87–S94.

Savilahti E, Kuitunen M. Allergenicity of cow milk proteins. *J Pediatr* 1992;121:S12–S20.

Vinton N. Gastrointestinal bleeding in infancy and childhood. *Gastroenterol Clin North Am* 1994;23(1):93–122.

Walker-Smith JA. Cow milk-sensitive enteropathy: predisposing factors and treatment. *J Pediatr* 1992;121:S111–S1115.

Author: Dror Wasserman
Donna Zeiter, 2nd edition

Mumps/Parotitis

 Database

DEFINITION

Mumps is an acute viral disease characterized by painful enlargement of the parotids and other salivary glands.

CAUSES

- Parotitis is usually caused by mumps, a paramyxovirus.
- Other viral causes of parotitis include influenza, parainfluenza, and enteroviruses.
- Bacterial cases are usually secondary to *Staphylococcus* (suppurative parotitis).
- Recurrent parotitis is an idiopathic, rare, recurrent swelling of the parotids, without suppuration or external inflammatory changes.
- Rare childhood cases may be secondary to an obstructing calculus, foreign body (sesame seed), or various drugs (antihistamines, phenothiazines, iodine-containing drugs/contrast media).

PATHOPHYSIOLOGY

- The mumps virus enters via the respiratory tract, and a viremia ultimately ensues.
- The viremia spreads to many organs, including the salivary glands, gonads, pancreas, and meninges.

EPIDEMIOLOGY

- Humans are the only known host for mumps.
- Spread is via the respiratory route.
- Incidence of this once very common disease has declined dramatically since the advent of universal childhood immunization. Outbreaks, however, continue to occur.
- Period of communicability: 7 days before to 5 days after onset of parotid swelling
- Most communicable period: 1 to 2 days before the parotid swelling
- Incubation period: 12 to 25 days after exposure
- Mumps is most common in the late winter and spring.
- One attack of mumps (clinical or subclinical) confers lifelong immunity.

COMPLICATIONS

- Meningitis: most frequent childhood complication; this "aseptic meningitis" is usually benign.
- Encephalitis: rarely causes permanent sequelae
- Oophoritis, nephritis, thyroiditis, myocarditis, mastitis, arthritis, transient ocular involvement, deafness, and sterility (all rare)

PROGNOSIS

Complete recovery in 1 to 2 weeks is the rule.

ASSOCIATED ILLNESSES

- Salivary adenitis: This is the most common manifestation of mumps, but one third occur subclinically.
- Epididymo-orchitis: Up to 35% of adolescent and adult mumps is complicated by orchitis. It most commonly occurs in adolescents. Orchitis develops within 4 to 10 days of the onset of the parotid swelling.
- Pancreatitis: Mild inflammation is common; serious involvement is rare.

 Differential Diagnosis

- Mumps parotitis can be distinguished from the other viral causes by clinical presentation along with specialized laboratory studies (see below).
- Bacterial parotitis is usually caused by *Staphylococcus aureus,* but streptococci, gram-negative bacilli, and anaerobes are also possible.
- Cases of tuberculous and nontuberculous (atypical) mycobacterial parotitis are rare, but have been reported.
- Parotid enlargement can be an initial sign in HIV-infected children.
- A salivary calculus can be diagnosed by sialogram.
- Recurrent childhood parotitis is a rare disorder in which symptoms initially manifest in children 3 to 6 years of age; it is largely a diagnosis of exclusion.
- Cervical or preauricular adenitis may simulate parotitis; close anatomic localization should be diagnostic.
- Infectious mononucleosis and cat-scratch disease are other considerations.
- Drug-induced parotid enlargement occasionally occurs.
- Malignancies of the parotid are extremely rare.
- Pneumoparotitis is seen in those with a history of playing a wind instrument, glass blowing, scuba diving, and even general anesthesia.

 Data Gathering

HISTORY

- Prodromal symptoms are uncommon in children with mumps but may include fever, anorexia, myalgia, headache, and malaise.
- Onset of mumps is usually pain and swelling in front of and below the ear.
- Swelling usually starts with one ear and then rapidly progresses to the other ear.
- Mild fever usually accompanies parotid swelling.
- Dysphagia and dysphonia are common.
- Testicular pain and swelling, along with constitutional symptoms, usually begin approximately 1 week after the parotid swelling of mumps.
- Epigastric pain and constitutional symptoms with pancreatic involvement
- Fever, headache, and stiff neck with meningitis
- Behavioral changes, seizures, and other neurologic abnormalities are rare.
- Other symptoms are analogous to the particular organ involved.

 Physical Examination

- Nonerythematous, tender parotid swelling (erythema seen with suppurative parotitis)
- Swelling ultimately obscures the mandibular ramus.
- The ear is often displaced upward and outward.
- Submaxillary and sublingual glands also may be swollen.
- Inflammation may be noted intraorally at the orifice of Stensen duct.
- Presternal edema is occasionally noted.
- Mumps are infrequently associated with truncal rash.
- Tender, edematous testicle in mumps orchitis (usually unilateral)

SPECIAL QUESTIONS

Ask the patient if the pain (at the parotid) intensifies with the tasting of sour liquids.

PROCEDURE

Have the patient suck on a lemon drop or lemon juice, and note any discharge from Stensen duct.

Laboratory Aids

- Uncomplicated parotitis: mild leukopenia with lymphocytosis
- Suppurative parotitis and mumps orchitis: leukocytosis
- Pancreatic involvement: hyperamylasemia and elevated serum lipose.
- Salivary adenitis without pancreatic involvement: isolated hyperamylasemia
- Meningitis: CSF pleocytosis (predominately mononuclear)
- Gram stain and culture of pus expressed from Stensen's duct is diagnostic in suppurative parotitis.
- Sialography is useful to evaluate for stones or strictures, but is contraindicated in acute infection.
- Serologic confirmation of mumps parotitis: complement fixation, neutralization, hemagglutination inhibition, or enzyme immunoassays
- Definitive laboratory diagnosis of mumps parotitis: body fluid isolation of mumps virus in tissue culture

PITFALLS

Skin tests should not be used for test of immunity; serologic studies are more reliable.

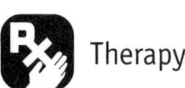 ## Therapy

- Supportive therapy is all that is required in mumps parotitis.
- Antibiotics directed against *S. aureus* should be used in cases of suppurative parotitis.

 ## Follow-Up

- Most children have resolution of glandular swelling by about 1 week.
- Disappearance of testicular pain and swelling can be expected 4 to 6 days after onset.
- Testicular atrophy is common, though infertility is rare.
- Markedly elevated pancreatic enzymes should be monitored until they improve.
- Children should not return to school until at least 9 days after the onset of parotid swelling.

PREVENTION

- A single 0.5-mL subcutaneous injection of live mumps vaccine (usually given together with measles and rubella, the "MMR") at 12 to 15 months usually confers long-lasting immunity.
- Primary vaccine failure and waning vaccine-induced immunity have been reported.
- A second vaccination is recommended between 4 and 6 years of age.
- The first dose of MMR vaccine sometimes causes fever and rash, usually 7 to 10 days after immunization. The measles component is usually the culprit.
- Links of the MMR vaccine to autism have not been substantiated.
- Vaccine should not be administered to children who are immunocompromised by disease or pharmacotherapy, or to pregnant women.
- Children with symptomatic AIDS who are to be vaccinated against measles through the MMR, however, may (and should) receive the live virus vaccine.

 ## Common Questions and Answers

Q: Should immunization be deferred in children with intercurrent illness?
A: No, children with minor illnesses, even with fever, should be vaccinated.

Q: Should vaccination be withheld in children living with immunocompromised hosts?
A: No, vaccinated children do not transmit mumps vaccine virus.

BIBLIOGRAPHY

American Academy of Pediatrics. Mumps. In: Pickering LK, ed. *2000 red book: report of the Committee on Infectious Diseases*, 25th ed. Elk Grove Village, IL: American Academy of Pediatrics, 2000:405–408.

Casella R, Leibundgut B, Lehman K, et al. Mumps orchitis: report of a mini-epidemic. *J Urol* 1997;158(6):2158–2161.

Chitre VV, Premchandra DJ. Recurrent parotitis. *Arch Dis Child* 1997;77(4):359–363.

Elliman D, Bedford H. MMR vaccine: the continuing saga. *BMJ* 2001;332:183–184.

Galazka AM, Robertson SE, Kraigher A. Mumps and mumps vaccine: a global review. *Bull WHO* 1999;77(1):3–14.

Gold E. Almost extinct diseases: measles, mumps, rubella, and pertussis. *Pediatr Rev* 1996;17(4):120–127.

Taylor B, Miller E, Farrington CP, et al. Autism and measles, mumps, and rubella vaccine: no epidemiologic evidence for a causal association. *Lancet* 1999;353:2026–2029.

Virtanen M, Peltola H, Paunio M, et al. Day to day reactogenicity and the healthy vaccinee effect of measles-mumps-rubella vaccination. *Pediatrics* 2000;106(5). URL: *http://www.pediatrics.org/cgi/content/full/106/5/e62*.

Watson JC, Hadler SC, Dykewicz CA, et al. Measles, mumps, and rubella—vaccine use and strategies for elimination of measles, mumps, rubella, and congenital rubella syndrome and control of mumps. *MMWR* 1998;47(RR-8):1–57.

Whitelaw CC, Kallis JM. Pediatric facial swelling. *Acad Emerg Med* 1998;5(2):146,198–202.

Author: Nicholas Tsarouhas

Munchausen Syndrome by Proxy

 Database

DEFINITION

Munchausen syndrome by proxy (MSBP) describes an illness in a child that is fabricated by someone else (usually the parent). This results in repeated interactions with the medical care system, often leading to multiple medical procedures. The perpetrator denies the cause of the child's illnesses. Symptoms decrease when the child is separated from the perpetrator.

CAUSES

It is the parent, commonly the mother, who fabricates the illnesses.
Little is known. The parent may have Munchausen syndrome. They may be seeking secondary gain from the attention of medical staff or financial gain by having the child be disabled.

EPIDEMIOLOGY

- Varies with presentation
- Of infants monitored in apnea programs, 0.27% are believed to be secondary to MSBP.
- 5% of allergy patients in some clinic settings are estimated to be MSBP.
- Mortality is approximately 9%.

PROGNOSIS

If undiagnosed, mortality has been estimated at 9%. Some children go on to develop Munchausen syndrome themselves. The long-term consequences to the child are unknown.

 Differential Diagnosis

Diagnosis depends on presentation. MSBP should be considered in unusual presentations of:

- GI bleeding
- Apnea/apparent life-threatening event
- Asthma
- Seizures
- GU bleeding
- Unexplained abnormalities in electrolytes
- Chronic diarrhea or vomiting
- Infections with multiple organisms found in blood or urine culture.

PITFALLS

- Delay in making the diagnosis: The average length of time to diagnosis is 14 months.
- Physicians and nursing personnel may be reluctant to suspect the parent because of their own involvement with the family.

 Data Gathering

HISTORY

- Unexplained or unusual illness, symptoms, and signs that are incongruous or present only when the perpetrator is present
- Usual medical treatment is ineffective in treating the presenting symptom.
- The perpetrator may not be concerned about the patient, may be constantly present while the patient is in the hospital, or may form unusually close relationships with the hospital staff.

SPECIAL QUESTIONS

- A history of frequent moves, other siblings who have either died or had unusual medical illnesses may suggest MSBP.
- In the context of divorce, repeated allegations of sexual abuse may represent MSBP.

 Physical Examination

- Examination of the patient with apnea presentation may indicate evidence of intentional suffocation.
- Patients who present with unusual bleeding may have lacerations on other parts of the body.
- The perpetrator also may have lacerations.
- Note the presence of indwelling intravenous, CSF, or bladder catheters.
- The patient may have evidence of old fractures.

 Laboratory Aids

TESTS

Workup is dictated by presentation:

- Pneumogram to rule out apnea
- If bleeding is the major presentation, identify the blood as the patient's (as opposed to that of the perpetrator or an animal).
- A toxicology screen may be helpful for unusual presentations of poisoning.
- Separating the perpetrator from the patient, with resultant decrease in symptoms, may suggest the diagnosis.
- Suspect MSBP when there is blood or urine culture with many organisms.
- If GI bleeding is the presenting symptom, use endoscopy or a Meckel scan to rule out anatomic causes of bleeding.
- Video monitoring of a patient's room may demonstrate the perpetrator harming the child.
- Ensure that the perpetrator cannot tamper with testing.

Munchausen Syndrome by Proxy

 Therapy

- If MSBP is documented, the patient must be separated from the perpetrator. Psychotherapy for the perpetrator is warranted.
- As long as the perpetrator is in need of intensive psychotherapy, the patient should be protected.

 Follow-Up

If the perpetrator agrees to seek help, improvement usually occurs, but long-term follow-up is necessary.

SIGNS TO WATCH FOR

- Recurrence of original presentation, unusual new symptoms

 Common Questions and Answers

Q: Is it legal to use video surveillance or to separate the parent from the patient?
A: If suspicions of MSBP are high and other laboratory tests are negative, it is important to make the diagnosis. Hospital administration and/or risk management should be consulted on how to proceed.

Q: Should this be reported to child abuse authorities?
A: If documented, this should be reported to protect the child.

ICD-9-CM 301.51

BIBLIOGRAPHY

Anderson J, McKane JB. Munchausen syndrome by proxy and apnea. *Br J Hosp Med* 1996;56(1):43–45.

Babcock J, et al. Rodenticide-induced coagulopathy in a young child. A case of Munchausen syndrome by proxy. *Am J Pediatr Hematol Oncol* 1993;15(1):126–130.

Berg B, Jones DP. Outcome of psychiatric intervention in factitious illness by proxy. *Arch Dis Child* 1999;81(6):465–472.

Bools CN, Schreirer HA, Libow JA, et al. Co-morbidity associated with fabricated illness (Munchausen syndrome by proxy). *Arch Dis Child* 1992;67:77–79.

Bryk M. Siegel PT. "My mother caused my illness": The story of a survivor of Munchausen by proxy syndrome. *Pediatrics* 1997;100(1):1–7.

D'Avanzo M, et al. Concealed administration of furosemide simulating Bartter syndrome in a 4.5 year old boy. *Pediatr Nephrol* 1995;9(6):749–750.

Hall DE, et al. Evaluation of covert video surveillance in the diagnosis of Munchausen syndrome by proxy: lessons from 41 cases. *Pediatrics* 2000;105(6):1305–1312.

Light MJ, Sheridan MS. Munchausen syndrome by proxy and apnea. *Clin Pediatr* 1990;29:162–168.

Magen D, Skorecki K. Extreme hyperkalemia in Munchausen-by-proxy syndrome. *N Engl J Med* 1999;340:1293–1294.

Meadow R. Munchausen syndrome by proxy: the hinterland of child abuse. *Lancet* 1977;2:343–345.

Meadow R. Management of Munchausen syndrome by proxy. *Arch Dis Child* 1985;60:385–393.

Meadow R. Non-accidental salt poisoning. *Arch Dis Child* 1993;68(4):448–452.

Meadow R. False allegations of abuse and Munchausen syndrome by proxy. *Arch Dis Child* 1993;68(4):444–447.

Schreir HA, Libow JA. Munchausen syndrome by proxy: diagnosis and prevalence. *Am J Orthopsychiatry* 1993;63:318–321.

Author: Cheryl L. Hausman

Muscular Dystrophies

 Database

DEFINITION

Muscular dystrophies (MDs) are hereditary diseases that cause progressive weakness and degeneration of muscle. MDs frequently involve proximal muscles and may also involve cardiac and smooth muscle. These diseases share similar electromyographic (EMG) and muscle pathologic findings and usually show an elevated creatine kinase (CK). The availability of genetic tests for most forms of MDs has changed the diagnostic approach for these disorders.
Forms of MDs include:
- Duchenne muscular dystrophy (DMD)
- Becker muscular dystrophy (BMD)
- Myotonic dystrophy (MyD)
- Congenital myotonic dystrophy (CMyD)
- Emery-Dreifuss muscular dystrophy (EDMD)
- Facioscapulohumeral muscular dystrophy (FMD)
- Limb-girdle muscular dystrophy (LGMD)
- Congenital muscular dystrophies (CMDs): Fukuyama-type, merosin-deficient type, others

CLASSIFICATION

MDs have been classified by clinical criteria such as inheritance pattern, age of onset, pattern of muscle involvement, severity of the disease, and associated conditions. Revised classifications based on mutation analysis are evolving.

PATHOPHYSIOLOGY

Slowly, progressive weakness involves all muscle groups—some worse than others—in a symmetric fashion.
Common pathologic findings:
- Loss of muscle cells and residual muscle fibers have variability in size.
- Segmental necrosis of the muscle fiber and some regenerative activity
- Accumulation of lipocytes and collagen between muscle fibers
- Smooth muscle and heart are also affected.
- In some types (MyD, EDMD, DMD, BMD, FMD), innervation of the muscle is also affected.
- Brain pathology:
—For an unknown reason, deficiency of membrane-associated cytoskeletal proteins (e.g., in DMD) interferes with brain development.
—The milder clinical course in BMD corresponds to a milder degree of dystrophin deficiency that can be measured in muscle.

GENETICS

- DMD and BMD are X-linked recessive. One third of cases are sporadic and are due to new mutations in the dystrophin gene.
- MyD is autosomal dominant.
- EDMD is X-linked recessive (chromosome Xq28), autosomal dominant or autosomal recessive (chromosome 1q21).
- FMD is autosomal dominant, due to deletions on chromosome 4q35.

- LGMD: Autosomal-recessive types: mutations in α-sarcoglycan gene (17q); β-sarcoglycan gene (4q); γ-sarcoglycan gene (13q); δ-sarcoglycan gene (5q); calpain-3 gene (15q); dysferlin gene (2q); telethonin gene (17q).
- Autosomal-dominant type: mutation in caveolin-3 gene (3q)
- CMDs are autosomal recessive. To date these mutations have been identified:
—Laminin-α-2 gene (6q22): primary merosin deficiency CMD type
—Fukutin gene (9q): Fukuyama CMD type (mostly in Japan)

EPIDEMIOLOGY

- The incidence of DMD is 1 in 3,500 live male births.
- The estimated minimum incidence of MyD is 1 in 8,000, and BMD is 3 to 6 per 100,000 male births.
- Other forms of MD are less common.

COMPLICATIONS

- Patients with DMD usually die in their 20s of heart failure or pneumonia.
- MyD patients frequently die of cardiomyopathy and respiratory failure.
—Posterior capsular cataracts, ptosis, and ophthalmoplegia are common in adults.
—Gastrointestinal dysmotility is common in all age groups.
—Hyperinsulinemia with peripheral resistance to insulin, testicular and ovarian atrophy, and hypersomnolence also occur.
- Severe and potentially fatal cardiac arrhythmias are common in EDMD.
- CMDs are often fatal by the end of the first decade because of respiratory failure.
—Cerebro-ocular muscular dystrophy (muscle-eye-brain disease) has ocular anomalies and cerebral malformations (also known as Walker-Warburg syndrome).
- Orthopedic complications, such as arthrogryposis, contractures, kyphoscoliosis, and lumbar lordosis, frequently occur in CMDs, CMyD, EDMD, DMD, and BMD.
- Retinal telangiectasias are common in FMD.

ASSOCIATED CONDITIONS

- MR or learning difficulty, except in Becker dystrophy, LGMD, FMD, some cases of CMD.
- Seizures: occasional in DMD and CMD
- Sensorineural deafness: some cases of FMD
- A variant of malignant hyperthermia with general anesthesia may occur in MDs.

 Differential Diagnosis

- Nonneurologic disorders that may superficially appear to cause muscle weakness include factitious weakness and any disorder causing pain with movement.
- Electrolyte disturbance may acutely produce muscle weakness (hypercalcemia, hypokalemia).
- Weakness due to other neurologic disorders that may mimic muscular dystrophy:

—Polyneuropathy: hereditary neuropathy, such as Charcot-Marie-Tooth disease or acquired neuropathy (chronic inflammatory demyelinating polyneuropathy)
—Spinal dysraphism
—Motor neuron disease
—Myasthenia gravis
—Motor degenerative disorders or acquired structural CNS lesions (neoplastic, vascular, or demyelinating)
—Muscle diseases (electromyography usually abnormal) such as inflammatory myopathies, periodic paralyses, and congenital myopathies
—Metabolic myopathies
- Disorders causing creatine kinase isoenzyme elevation: infectious, inflammatory, and metabolic myopathies, hypothyroid myopathy, muscular trauma, and malignant hyperthermia
- Myopathy and medication: steroids, Mevacor (lovastatin), alcohol, penicillamine, antimalarials, and antiparasitic medication

 Data Gathering

HISTORY

- Age and rapidity of symptom onset
- Symptoms progressive or static
- Disability indicates symmetric, usually proximal, pattern of involvement.
- Pre- and perinatal history is important: paucity of fetal movements, polyhydramnios, neonatal hypotonia, or respiratory failure could be the first sign of MD.
- Pain, fasciculations, rash, or marked fluctuation in weakness are not features of MD.
- Exposure to certain medications (diuretics, steroids, Mevacor) or toxins may suggest alternative causes of muscle weakness (see Differential Diagnosis, above).
- Detailed developmental and family histories are essential.
- DMD is usually apparent by the third year of life, with frequent falls, waddling gait, lumbar lordosis, difficulty climbing stairs, and difficulty arising from the floor. Most boys are wheelchair-bound by 13 years of age and die of cardiac or respiratory failure in their 20s.
- BMD appears usually beyond age 6 years. Progression is slower, and death usually occurs beyond the third decade. Sometimes presents with discolored urine (myoglobinuria).
- CMyD presents with generalized hypotonia, respiratory distress, facial diplegia, distal limb weakness, and skeletal deformities at birth. The long-term prognosis poor: 50% survive into their 30s. Requirement of mechanical ventilation beyond 1 month of age is a poor indicator. Adults with MyD may be diagnosed when CMyD appears in the family, because of weakness during immobilization or during workup for arrhythmias.
- EDMD presents between ages 5 and 15 years with weakness of upper arms and peroneal muscles. Flexion contractures are common in the elbows, neck, and calf muscles. Progression is slow, but some patients have fatal cardiac arrhythmias.

- FMD has onset between ages 5 and 25 years, with weakness of facial, shoulder, and upper arm musculature. There is an inability to close the eyes, whistle, drink through a straw, and raise the arms above the head. Progression is slow, often with periods of nearly complete arrest.
- Autosomal-recessive LGMD has a DMD phenotype in girls and boys and begins between ages 5 and 10 years. In contrast to DMD, the cognitive function is normal.
- Autosomal-dominant LGMD begins in the second or third decade with complaints similar to those of DMD.
- CMDs have neuromuscular symptoms similar to those of CMyD, but may also have brain or ophthalmologic disease as well. Progression is variable, but most die in the first decade.

Physical Examination

- Resting tachycardia may be an early sign of cardiomyopathy in DMD and CMyD.
- The respiratory pattern may reflect hypoventilation from weakness of respiratory muscles.
- Children with decreased vital capacity may have a rapid, shallow breathing pattern.
- Check for contractures, scoliosis/lordosis, and pseudohypertrophy.
- There is frontal balding and testicular atrophy in MyD.
- Neurologic
—Cognitive developmental milestones, weakness of facial and shoulder girdle muscles. Functional testing may be most helpful in documenting extremity weakness: The ability of the child to raise the arms over the head, write, stand from a seated position, run, squat, and so on, may be more reproducible, especially when different examiners are involved in follow-up. Myotonia, seen in CMyD and MyD, is a sustained contraction of skeletal muscle in response to voluntary contraction or percussion. It is clinically apparent as an inability to release a hand grip or jaw clench. Deep tendon reflexes are diminished.
—Muscle enlargement also may be seen in motor neuron disease, glycogen storage diseases, hypothyroidism, and amyloidosis. The calf muscles in DMD feel rubbery (pseudohypertrophy).
—Toe walking is also seen in spastic diplegia, spinal tumors, spinal dysraphism, hereditary neuropathies, benign/developmental.
—The Gower sign (propping hands on thighs upon rising) and a waddling gait suggest pelvic weakness. The patient stands and walks on a wide base.
—Infants with CMDs and CMyD are hypotonic, with frog-leg posture and head lag: They may be indistinguishable on examination from spinal muscular atrophy, except that MD does not cause tongue fasciculations.

Laboratory Aids

TESTS
- Chemistry: creatine kinase (CK), aspartate aminotransferase (SGOT), alanine aminotransferase (SGOT), lactate dehydrogenase (LDK), and aldolase. Of these, the CK MM isoenzyme is the most sensitive and specific for primary muscle disease.
—CK measurement should be done before EMG, which might raise the level.
—DMD and the Fukuyama-type CMD have the highest CK level. CK level falls with progression of disease as muscle mass decreases. CK level is usually elevated in female carriers of DMD and BMD.
- Molecular genetics: DNA-based mutation studies using polymerase chain reaction (PCR) and Southern blot assay are available for DMD, BMD, EDMD, FMD, LGMD, primary merosin- and Fukuyama-type CMDs.
- The role of traditional diagnostic tests such as electromyography (EMG), nerve conduction studies (NCS), and muscle biopsy has diminished in the era of molecular DNA testing. These tests are now performed in patients with negative genetic analysis, atypical presentation, or when immunohistochemistry is necessary to make the diagnosis.
- Immunologic: Muscle biopsy tissue can be immunostained specifically for the presence of dystrophin, emerin, sarcoglycans, dysferlin, calpain-3, telethonin, merosin, and fukutin. These proteins can be quantified by Western blot analysis. Dystrophin is measured in fetal muscle biopsies in difficult cases.
- Electrophysiologic: EMG/NCS helps to differentiate anterior horn cell disease, peripheral neuropathy, and neuromuscular junction disorder from myopathy. In myopathic conditions, nerve conduction velocity is normal, but motor unit action potentials have shortened duration and lower amplitude.
—Spontaneous trains of discharges by inserting the EMG needle are characteristic for myotonia.
- Electrocardiography (ECG) may reveal tall R waves and a deep Q wave in DMD and A-V block in EDMD.
- Prenatal diagnosis possible

Emergency Care

- Respiratory failure: DMD, MyD, CMyD, and CMDs.
- Cardiac or arrhythmias in DMD, MyD, and EDMD.

Therapy

- Mainly supportive. Passive muscle stretching and night splinting delay contractures. Maintenance of upright posture delays scoliosis. Major surgery or long bed rest should be avoided while the patient is still walking. Cataract surgery is recommended in MyD. Attention to healthy diet to avoid obesity; exercise as tolerated; swimming is useful; intubation and mechanical ventilation in infantile forms; pacemakers for arrhythmias.
- Vitamin therapies or specific diets have not proved beneficial.
- Dilantin (phenytoin) and Tegretol (carbamazepine) may be helpful for myotonia, but the myotonia of MyD is usually not troublesome. Metoclopramide is useful in gastroparesis.
- Gene therapy is not currently available for any of these disorders.

PITFALLS
- Pain is usually not present in MDs, but polymyositis, dermatomyositis, and infectious myositis may be painful.
- Dermatomyositis has a typical rash not seen in MD.

Follow-Up

- Best done in multidisciplinary neuromuscular clinics.

Common Questions and Answers

Q: What is the recurrence risk in DMD?
A: Because of new mutations, the mothers of probands may not be carriers. Each time a carrier (heterozygous woman) has a child, there is a 25% chance it will be an affected male. Each time a heterozygous mother has a son, the chance that she will transmit the abnormal gene is 50%. Each time a daughter is born, she will have a 50% chance of being a carrier. Affected males transmit the gene to all of their daughters.

ICD-9-CM 359.1

BIBLIOGRAPHY
Basil BT, Jones HR Jr. Diagnosis of pediatric neuromuscular disorders in the era of DNA analysis. *Pediatr Neurol* 2000;23:289–300.

Birch JG. Orthopedic management of neuromuscular disorders in children. *Semin Pediatr Neurol* 1998;5(2):78–91.

Bushby K. Genetics and the muscular dystrophies. *Dev Med Child Neurol* 2000;42:780–784.

Author: Olafur Thorarensen

Myasthenia Gravis

 Database

DEFINITION

Myasthenia is a disorder caused by a disruption in signal transmission from the motor neuron to the muscle. It presents as intermittent weakness that worsens with exercise and improves with rest. The majority of patients present with ptosis and diplopia alone or in combination with swallowing difficulties and generalized weakness. There are no sensory or cognitive symptoms.

PATHOPHYSIOLOGY

In a healthy person, the motor nerve terminal lies in close proximity to the end plate, a region of the muscle cell membrane with a high concentration of acetylcholine receptors. When stimulated, the motor nerve terminal releases vesicles of acetylcholine that traverse the synaptic cleft and bind to the receptors, causing contraction of the muscle. The cleft contains acetylcholinesterase, an enzyme that breaks down acetylcholine and helps terminate the muscle contractions. In the common autoimmune form of myasthenia, an autoantibody binds to the acetylcholine receptor, and blocks its activity. The rate of receptor breakdown also increases and fewer receptors are present, resulting in decreased muscle contraction.

EPIDEMIOLOGY

There are three types of myasthenia gravis seen in childhood: neonatal transient, congenital myasthenia, and juvenile myasthenia.

• Neonatal transient: 10% to 20% of infants born to mothers with autoimmune myasthenia have maternal-fetal transmission of antibodies against the acetylcholine receptor and are born with weakness and hypotonia. The severity of maternal symptoms does not predict the likelihood of an affected infant. Occasional arthrogryposis (joint contractures) reflects *in utero* paralysis from transplacental transmission of the antibody. High levels of maternal antibodies against the fetal form of the acetylcholine receptor correspond to an increased risk of disease. A previous pregnancy with an affected infant places future pregnancies at much higher risk. In rare cases, the mother is asymptomatic, despite placental transmission of maternal antibody.
• Congenital myasthenia: rare; less than 10% of all childhood myasthenia. Weakness usually starts in the first year of life and is caused by an inherited disorder in neuromuscular transmission. Mutations have been described in the presynaptic nerve terminal, acetylcholinesterase, acetylcholine receptors, and postsynaptic proteins.

• Juvenile myasthenia: an autoimmune disorder caused by aberrant production of antibodies against the acetylcholine receptor. It is relatively rare, with one new diagnosis per million patients per year. The average age of onset is 10 to 13 years, with a female predominance of 2:1 or 4:1, depending on the study. Thymic pathology is believed central to the pathogenesis of autoimmune myasthenia; hyperplasia is present in most children who undergo thymectomy.

PROGNOSIS

• Neonatal transient: a self-limited disorder that resolves spontaneously over the first few months of life as maternal antibodies disappear. The infant may require ventilatory and nutritional support during the first few months of life. Infants with arthrogryposis multiplex congenita (born to mothers with antibodies against the fetal form of acetylcholine receptors) may gain mobility with time.
• Congenital myasthenia: Prognosis varies, depending on the specific defect. Autosomal-recessive disorders tend to be more severe than the dominant disorders. Weakness shows variable response to cholinesterase inhibitors. Immunosuppressants are not helpful. In general, these are indolent disorders. Ptosis and fatigability resemble the juvenile type, but are more stable over time.
• Juvenile myasthenia: Most patients do extremely well with treatment. Longitudinal studies suggest that the rate of spontaneous remission is approximately 2% per year and can occur throughout the lifetime of the patient. Patients with generalized weakness are slightly less likely to experience remission. The mortality rate from myasthenia is near that of the general population in patients under 50 years of age.

ASSOCIATED ILLNESSES

In juvenile myasthenia, other autoimmune disorders may occur: Hyperthyroidism is present in 3% to 9% of patients, and there is a small increase in the incidence of rheumatoid arthritis and diabetes. Some reports suggest an increased incidence of seizures in autoimmune myasthenia. Screening for thymoma at initial diagnosis is appropriate (by chest CT scan)—children appear to have a lower incidence of this tumor than adults in the setting of autoimmune myasthenia.

 Differential Diagnosis

• In specific endemic areas, generalized botulism may cause generalized weakness in infants. It is caused by a *Clostridium* toxin that blocks the release of acetylcholine from the nerve terminal. The infant usually presents with generalized hypotonia and a

poor suck for days (or weeks). Prominent symptoms unique to botulism are constipation and pupillary dilation. Nerve conduction studies and stool tests for the botulism toxin confirm the diagnosis.
• Guillain-Barré syndrome, or acute inflammatory demyelinating polyneuropathy, is a frequent cause of rapidly progressive generalized weakness. Unlike myasthenia, there are often sensory symptoms, and areflexia occurs even with minimal weakness.
• Acute spinal cord compression can present as generalized weakness of the extremities. If facial and extraocular muscles are not weak, then it is important to look for a sensory level, bowel or bladder dysfunction, and hyperactive reflexes.
• Organophosphate ingestion or an overdose of Mestinon (pyridostigmine bromide) can cause profound weakness. Symptoms of parasympathetic hyperactivity, such as hypersalivation, miosis, diarrhea, and bradycardia, will usually be present.
• Penicillamine is used for the treatment of autoimmune disorders and can induce autoantibodies that bind the acetylcholine receptor, causing myasthenia gravis. The weakness usually resolves when the drug is stopped.

 Data Gathering

HISTORY

• Transient neonatal: The infant is usually born to a mother with known autoimmune myasthenia or a history of weakness, ptosis, or dysphagia.
• Congenital myasthenia: The patient usually presents in the first year of life (though a later age of presentation can occur) with hypotonia and delayed motor milestones. Poor feeding and ptosis are common. There may be a family history of similar weakness. There is no response to thymectomy or immunosuppressant medications.
• Juvenile myasthenia: There is usually a gradual onset of weakness over weeks, months, or even years. The symptoms are worse after prolonged activity or late in the day. Intermittent ptosis, diplopia, dysphagia, and dysphonia are common.

 Physical Examination

• Neonatal: From birth, the infant is hypotonic, with a weak suck, a weak cry, and ptosis.

- Congenital and juvenile myasthenia:

—Weakness of neck flexion
—Ptosis and ophthalmoplegia are often the earliest findings of myasthenia.
—Generalized weakness may be asymmetric in the limbs. The weakness is more pronounced with endurance tasks.
—Shallow, rapid respirations suggest impending ventilatory failure. Vital capacity of less than 50% of predicted (in older children) indicates a danger of respiratory failure.

Laboratory Aids

JUVENILE MYASTHENIA

- Nerve conduction and electromyography studies: Repetitive stimulation of a nerve will demonstrate a rapid decremental response. The decreased number of acetylcholine receptors limits the response to a nerve impulse. Single-fiber electromyography measures the variability in firing rates of two muscle fibers innervated by different branches of the same motor neuron. A large variability, "jitter," suggests a higher threshold for activation because of a limited number of acetylcholine receptors.
- Acetylcholine receptor antibody levels (most specific): Acetylcholine receptor antibody levels are elevated in approximately 80% of patients with generalized myasthenia. Only 50% of patients with isolated ocular myasthenia have an elevated level.
- Tensilon (edrophonium chloride) is a fast-acting acetylcholinesterase-blocking agent. A patient with myasthenia often has an immediate transient improvement in muscle strength after the IV infusion of Tensilon. A measurable weakness should be present prior to testing, and a placebo dose of saline should be given initially. Though the risk of a hyperreactive cholinergic response with muscle weakness and bradycardia is low, atropine should always be available, and the patient's vital signs should be closely monitored during a Tensilon test. A Tensilon test should not be performed if the patient has a known history of heart disease. Cranial nerve findings, such as ptosis, are often responsive to Tensilon and are easily measured.
- Children receive 20% of a 0.2-mg/kg dose of Tensilon over 1 minute; if there is no response after 45 seconds, the rest of the dose is then given, up to a maximum of 10 mg. Have atropine and epinephrine readily available.

 Emergency Care

Respiratory failure is a rare but serious complication of juvenile myasthenia gravis. Shallow breathing, a vital capacity of less than 50% predicted, or a rapidly worsening vital capacity suggests impending respiratory failure.

Therapy

- Neonatal myasthenia: severity of disability should be used to guide the aggressiveness of therapy. Respiratory or swallowing impairment: pyridostigmine syrup, 60 mg/5 mL, 7 mg/kg, 30 minutes before feeds. 1 mg intramuscular = 30 mg oral dose.
- **Juvenile myasthenia:** Most patients benefit from pyridostigmine bromide given three to four times per day. A long-acting component prior to bedtime may alleviate obstructive hypoventilation during sleep. Mestinon improves strength by blocking acetylcholinesterase activity. A normal starting dosage is approximately 7 mg/kg/d. The dosage is slowly titrated upward by following symptoms at several-day intervals. Common side effects are hypersalivation, blurry vision, and diarrhea. Most patients can take Robinul (glycopyrrolate) 1 mg by mouth to decrease diarrhea.
- Prednisone considered in patients with disabling symptoms and inadequate response to pyridostigmine. Watch for transient worsening in up to 50% of patients. Start daily dose at 2 mg/kg, watch for improvement in 3 to 6 weeks, taper toward 1.5 mg/kg/day on alternate-day schedule for 4 months. Taper slowly thereafter by 5 mg/week. Monitor for side effects, including growth stunting—critical in children. Calcium and every-other-day dosing limit the bone deterioration from chronic steroids.
- Azathioprine induces remission in 30% of patients and results in significant improvement in another 25% to 60%. Azathioprine is a useful adjunctive to steroids and thymectomy; however, it takes 3 to 12 months for its suppressant effects to occur. In one long-term study of juvenile myasthenia, there was no increased risk of cancer or infection with the use of azathioprine.
- Thymectomy generally results in a 20% to 60% remission, and another 15% to 30% of patients show a marked improvement after surgery. As surgical techniques for thymectomy have improved, the complications and recovery times have decreased. Thymectomy earlier in the course of illness appears to produce a higher rate of remission. There are no studies in children, looking at CT or MRI studies of the thymus, that can predict which patients will benefit from thymectomy. On pathology, 80% to 90% of patients undergoing thymectomy have thymic hyperplasia. There are scant data about thymectomy and the risk of infection and other autoimmune disorders during childhood.
- Juvenile myasthenics with profound weakness and respiratory failure should undergo immediate therapy to decrease the number of circulating receptor antibodies. Plasmapheresis or intravenous immunoglobulin can be effective within a few days by decreasing or diluting, respectively, the acetylcholine receptor antibodies. Steroids will diminish antibody production within weeks to months. There may be a paradoxical worsening of symptoms in some patients in the weeks following an increase in steroid dosage.

 Follow-Up

- Penicillamine is the only drug that has been shown to induce production of antiacetylcholine receptor antibodies.
- The following medications can exacerbate myasthenia gravis and should be avoided:

—Corticosteroids may worsen symptoms, but usually only briefly, after increasing the dose.
—Aminoglycosides
—Ciprofloxacin
—β-adrenergic blocking agents, including eyedrops
—Lithium
—Procainamide
—Quinidine
—Phenytoin

- Nondepolarizing neuromuscular blocking agents may cause lasting (eventually reversible) weakness.
- Always start new medications cautiously.

ICD-9-CM 358.0

Neonatal 775.2

BIBLIOGRAPHY

Abul Matin M, Alam K, O'Driscoll K, et al. Acute inspiratory stridor: a presentation of myasthenia gravis. *J Laryngol Otol* 1999;13:1114–1115.

Gardnerova M, Eymard B, Morel E, et al. The fetal/adult acetylcholine receptor antibody ration in mothers with myasthenia gravis as a marker for transfer of the disease to the newborn. *Neurology* 1997;48:50–54.

Lindner A, Schalke B, Toyka VK. Outcome in juvenile-onset myasthenia gravis: a retrospective study with long-term follow up. *J Neurol* 1997;244:515–520.

Rodriguez M, Gomez MR, Howard F, et al. Myasthenia gravis in children: long term follow-up. *Ann Neurol* 1983;13:504–510.

Selcen D, Dabrowski ER, Michon AM, et al. High-dose intravenous immunoglobulin therapy in juvenile myasthenia gravis. *Pediatr Neurol* 2000;22:40–43.

Wittbrodt ET. Drugs and myasthenia gravis: an update. *Arch Intern Med* 1997;157(4): 399–408.

Authors: Brenda E. Porter and Grant T. Liu

Myocarditis

Database

DEFINITION

Myocarditis is defined as inflammation of the myocardium in association with myocellular necrosis.

PATHOLOGY

- Infective myocarditis may be caused by viral, bacterial, rickettsial, fungal, or parasitic organisms. Viruses, particularly the enteroviruses (coxsackievirus, echovirus), are the predominant causative agents. Group B coxsackieviruses are the most frequent viral agents associated with myocarditis.
- Other etiologic categories include hypersensitivity drug reactions (rare), toxic myocarditis (drug ingestion), and autoimmune or collagen vascular diseases (systemic lupus erythematosus, rheumatic fever, rheumatoid arthritis, sarcoidosis, peripartum myocarditis, and Kawasaki disease).
- "Idiopathic" myocarditis (unknown etiology) is the most common form encountered in North America.
- While some cases of myocarditis, particularly fulminant ones involving infants and children, may be the result of direct viral cytopathic effect, there is increasing evidence that most cases of myocarditis reflect immunologically mediated cellular injury in response to prior cardiotropic virus infection in genetically predisposed individuals.
- Pathologic specimens reveal lymphocytic infiltration and focal myocardial necrosis during the acute phase of myocardial inflammation. A minority of patients will have persistent lymphocytic infiltrate and ongoing focal necrosis. Rare patients will have diffuse pleomorphic infiltration and necrosis.

PATHOPHYSIOLOGY

- Seventy percent to 80% present with mild-to-moderate congestive heart failure. The vast majority of these children will fully recover in a rapid fashion. A small minority of these patients will have chronic lymphocytic infiltration and focal myocardial necrosis and progress to a dilated cardiomyopathy.
- Twenty percent to 30% present with acute left ventricular failure and shock. One third of these patients make a full recovery, one third develop dilated cardiomyopathy, and one third die at presentation or require cardiac transplantation.
- Left ventricular dysfunction results in pulmonary venous hypertension and pulmonary edema.

EPIDEMIOLOGY

- Enteroviruses such as coxsackievirus and echovirus are ubiquitous and very common in children.
- Enteroviral infection is most common in the summer months.
- Cardiovascular sequelae occur in less than 1% of reported enteroviral infections.
- The incidence increases to approximately 4% when coxsackievirus (group B) is considered.

PROGNOSIS

- Seventy percent of patients with acute myocarditis recover completely.
- Twenty percent of patients develop dilated cardiomyopathy.
- Ten percent of patients die during the acute phase or have cardiac transplantation.

Differential Diagnosis

- Anomalous origin of the left coronary artery from the pulmonary artery
- Critical aortic stenosis
- Critical coarctation of the aorta
- Interrupted aortic arch
- Dilated cardiomyopathy 2% to non-myocarditis cause

Data Gathering

HISTORY

- Tachypnea
- Dyspnea
- Fatigability
- Malaise
- Anorexia and/or emesis (especially in children)

Note: Antecedent, nonspecific "flu-like" illness or an episode of gastroenteritis?

Physical Examination

- Pulmonary

—Rales
—Tachypnea

- Cardiovascular

—Sinus tachycardia (at rest)
—Arrhythmias (atrial fibrillation, supraventricular or ventricular ectopy)
—Gallop
—Murmur (mitral and/or tricuspid insufficiency)
—Jugular venous distention (difficult to detect in infants)

- Abdomen

—Hepatomegaly

- Extremities

—Weak pulses
—Poor capillary refill
—Cool extremities

Note: Not all findings are present.

Laboratory Aids

TESTS

- Chest radiograph: cardiomegaly and varying amounts of pulmonary edema
- Electrocardiogram: Findings are highly variable and may include low QRS voltages, ST changes, T-wave flattening or inversion, prolongation of the QT interval, and arrhythmias, especially premature atrial or ventricular contractions.
- Echocardiogram

—Cardiac chamber enlargement
—Impaired left ventricular function
—Segmental wall abnormalities
—Global hypokinesis
—Valvar insufficiency (particularly mitral regurgitation)
—Pericardial effusion
—Left ventricular thrombi (occasionally found)

- Endomyocardial biopsy: gold standard for the diagnosis of myocarditis in both adults and children. However, the incidence of "biopsy proven" myocarditis in patients presenting with acute-onset congestive heart failure and dilated cardiomyopathy is approximately 10%. In most cases, virus is not recovered from myocardial biopsy specimens.
- Radionuclide imaging: Gallium-67 scintigraphy is a screening technique that is used routinely to detect chronic inflammatory processes. It has been shown to be sensitive, but it is limited by its low specificity and predictive accuracy in myocarditis. Similarly, indium-111 antimyosin antibody cardiac imaging has been shown to have high sensitivity for myocardial necrosis, but low specificity.
- Viral identification: Viral cultures of the blood, stool, and nasopharynx should be done. Acute and convalescent serum should be sent to the lab for serologic titer rise.
- Laboratory tests: The erythrocyte sedimentation rates (ESR), and creatinine kinase–MB fraction (CK-MB), and troponin I level are variably elevated. The degree of elevation depends on the stage of disease, degree of cardiac failure, and extent of myocardial necrosis.

Note: One must rule out structural causes of severe left ventricular dysfunction (see Differential Diagnosis, above).

Therapy

- Bed rest and limited activity (during acute phase)
- Anticongestive therapy

—Diuretics
—Inotropic agents (e.g., dobutamine, dopamine, or digoxin)
—Afterload reduction (e.g., milrinone or captopril)

- High-dose gamma globulin (2 g/kg over 24 hours) therapy during the acute phase has been associated with improved recovery of left ventricular function and with a tendency to better survival during the first year after presentation.
- The role of immunosuppression is unclear.
- Corticosteroids are effective in rheumatic carditis.

 Follow-Up

- The patient who presents with mild-to-moderate congestive heart failure should be followed every 3 to 6 months, until full myocardial recovery is noted.
- The patient who progresses to dilated cardiomyopathy should have interval follow-up every 3 months. If myocardial function is depressed but stable, the patient may be followed expectantly. If myocardial function progressively deteriorates, cardiac transplantation may be needed.

 Common Questions and Answers

Q: What can parents expect of children who have had myocarditis?
A: Most children present with only minimal signs of heart failure and recover completely (two thirds). Of the remaining one third who present in shock and LV failure, one third recover, one third develop a cardiomyopathy, and one third go on to transplantation.

Q: Is there a role for steroids?
A: In addition to bed rest, inotropic support, diuretics, and gamma globulin, the use of steroids is controversial and has not been prospectively studied in a large pediatric population.

ICD-9-CM

Secondary to rheumatic fever 398.0
Acute myocarditis 422.90

BIBLIOGRAPHY

Drucker NA, Colan SD, Lewis AB, et al. Gammaglobulin treatment of acute myocarditis in the pediatric population. *Circulation* 1994;89:252–257.

Drucker NA, Newburger JW. Viral myocarditis: diagnosis and management. *Adv Pediatr* 1997;44:141–171.

Feldman AM, McNamara D. Myocarditis [see comments]. *N Engl J Med* 2000;343(19): 1388–1398.

Gajarski RJ, Towbin JA. Recent advances in the etiology, diagnosis, and treatment of myocarditis and cardiomyopathies in children. *Curr Opin Pediatr* 1995;7:587–594.

Levi D, Alejos J. Diagnosis and treatment of pediatric viral myocarditis. *Curr Opin Cardiol* 2001;16(2):77–83.

Modlin JF. Update on enterovirus infections in infants and children. *Adv Pediatr Infect Dis* 1996;12:155–180.

Author: Bradley S. Marino

Near Drowning

 Database

DEFINITION

Near drowning, or submersion injury, is survival, at least temporarily, after suffocation by submersion in water. Near drowning may be described by the water temperature and tonicity—warm water ($\geq 20°C$), cold water ($<20°C$), or very cold water ($<5°C$)—and as "freshwater" versus "saltwater" near drowning.

CAUSES

- "Wet drowning": aspiration of fluid into the trachea and lungs with either denaturation of surfactant by freshwater or washout of surfactant due to saltwater, which results in intrapulmonary shunting and hypoxemia.
- "Dry drowning": hypoxemia from prolonged severe laryngospasm as water enters the larynx when the near-drowning victim becomes hypercapnic and takes an involuntary gasp of air. No fluid is aspirated into the lung.

PATHOPHYSIOLOGY

- Grossly, the lungs are edematous, but not filled with aspirated fluid, with focal hemorrhages.
- Microscopically, there is thinning of the alveolar septum with emphysematous changes and frothy fluid in the airways.

EPIDEMIOLOGY

- Second only to motor vehicle accidents as the most common cause of death due to injury in childhood
- Children younger than 5 years of age, especially toddlers and boys, who cannot swim and have direct access to swimming pools are at highest risk.
- Bathtub drowning and near drowning are common in babies, and child neglect or abuse should be considered.
- Adolescent near drowning usually involves substance abuse or risk-taking behavior.
- Children with seizure disorders are at higher risk of near drowning.

COMPLICATIONS

- Brain injury secondary to hypoxia
- Pulmonary injury with intrapulmonary shunting secondary to damage of the alveoli
- ARDS
- Metabolic acidosis secondary to hypoxemia
- Ischemic injury to organs such as liver, kidneys, and intestines
- Disseminated intravascular coagulation (DIC) secondary to ischemia
- Electrolyte abnormalities uncommon; may occur if a large volume of freshwater is in the stomach and not removed
- Hypothermia in cold water near drowning

PROGNOSIS

- Most children (60%–95%) recover with intact neurologic survival.
- Brain injury and death correlate with degree of hypoxia/anoxia.
- Children with warm water submersion time longer than 4 minutes, who do not receive CPR at the scene and who have absent vital signs or a Glasgow Coma Scale (GCS) score less than 5 in the emergency department, usually have a poor prognosis.
- Victims who have prolonged submersions in very cold water may have good prognosis because of "core" cooling with a concomitant decrease in metabolic rate while the brain is still being perfused.
- A good prognostic indicator is continuing improvement in the neurologic examination over the first several hours.

ASSOCIATED CONDITIONS

- C-spine injuries should be considered in older children with diving accidents.
- Signs of child abuse or neglect (burns, whip marks, bruises) should be sought in young children.
- Toxicology screens should be done for adolescents.

 Differential Diagnosis

Children with smoke inhalation or hydrocarbon ingestion may have similar presentations. However, the history and physical examination should easily determine the diagnosis.

 Data Gathering

HISTORY

- Mechanism: history of diving injury, intoxication, seizure disorder, child abuse
- Prognostic indicators: length of submersion, vital signs and examination at scene, CPR done at scene, temperature of water

 Physical Examination

- Vital signs with temperature
- Neurologic: pupillary response, cranial nerve findings, GCS score
- Respiratory: lower airway findings (rales, tachypnea, wheezing, retractions)
- Circulation: perfusion, strength of distal pulses, capillary refill, urine output
- GI: abdominal distention from swallowed water or ventilation

Glasgow Coma Scale

RESPONSE	POINTS
1. Eye Opening	
Spontaneous	___ 4
To voice	___ 3
To pain	___ 2
None	___ 1
2. Verbal Response	
Oriented	___ 5
Confused	___ 4
Inappropriate words	___ 3
Incomprehensible words	___ 2
None	___ 1
3. Motor Response	
Obeys commands	___ 6
Purposeful movement (pain)	___ 5
Withdraw (pain)	___ 4
Flexion (pain)	___ 3
Extension (pain)	___ 2
None	___ 1
Total GCS points	___ (1 + 2 + 3)

Question: Was the child apneic, cyanotic, or pulseless at the scene?
Significance: If so, the child requires admission and close observation even if he or she appears well at presentation to the hospital.

Question: Did the child fall through ice?
Significance: Very cold water near drowning may have a good prognosis despite submersion time longer than 5 minutes.

Question: What was the estimated time of submersion, and when was CPR begun?
Significance: Shorter time periods (<2–5 minutes) for each answer correlate with better prognosis.

- Near-drowning victims may have deteriorating pulmonary involvement, despite an initially normal examination. Watch closely for signs of lower airway involvement, such as tachypnea, retractions, or rales.
- Serial neurologic examinations with pupillary response should be performed to access neurologic outcome. Children with a GCS score less than 5 after resuscitation usually have a poor neurologic outcome.

Near Drowning

Laboratory Aids

TESTS

• Pulse oximetry is a critical aid in assessment of pulmonary involvement in the near-drowning victim. An oxygen saturation less than 97% within 4 hours after the near drowning indicates pulmonary involvement and need for admission.
• Arterial blood gases to detect and treat metabolic acidosis and hyperpnea should be done in the child with respiratory distress or apnea.
• An initial chest x-ray is indicated for endotracheal tube placement in the intubated child and as a baseline film for those with pulmonary involvement.
• Cervical spine films are indicated in the diving accident victim.
• Renal electrolytes are not indicated unless a large volume of water has been swallowed and not evacuated from the stomach.
• Anticonvulsant levels for victims with seizure disorders
• Toxicology screening when suspected
• ECG to document normal function and evaluate for prolonged QTC if indicated by history

False Positives

Initial pulse oximetry and chest x-rays may be normal in the near-drowning victim. Victims should be monitored with pulse oximetry for 4 to 6 hours for progressive respiratory distress.

Therapy

• Airway: Protect the C-spine if indicated by history. Ensure a patent airway in the arrested or comatose victim.
• Breathing: supplemental oxygen for oxygen saturations by pulse oximetry less than 95%. The near-drowning victim should be intubated and positive end-expiratory pressure (PEEP) and ventilation given if apneic or unable to maintain a Pao2 greater than 60 or a pco2 less than 50 in 50% supplemental oxygen. Prophylactic antibiotics or steroids are not indicated.
• Circulation:

—For the victim with cardiopulmonary arrest, asystole protocol should be followed, using epinephrine via the ET tube or intravenously and chest compressions done.
—Since capillary leak may occur after an ischemic/anoxic episode, isotonic fluids (e.g., normal saline solution or Ringer's lactate) (10-mL/kg aliquots) should be given for signs of intravascular volume depletion (tachycardia, poor perfusion) until normalized.

—ECG monitoring should be provided with appropriate response to dysrhythmias, especially for the hypothermic, cold water near-drowning victim. For core temperature less than 29.5°C, attempts at electrical defibrillation are not likely to be successful, and "chemical defibrillation" with amiodarone or lidocaine and aggressive rewarming are tried.

• Disability: maintenance of eucapnia and adequate oxygenation to prevent further hypoxemia. There is no indication for measures to reduce ICP (hyperventilation, barbiturates, mannitol, fluid restoration, ICP monitoring, or steroids) because the brain injury and swelling is secondary to hypoxic cell injury as opposed to a traumatic lesion.
• Exposure: The near-drowning victim should be dried and warmed: for core temperatures 32°C to 35°C, active rewarming with heating blankets or radiant warmers; for less than 32°C, active internal rewarming added (heated aerosolized oxygen and intravenous fluids, gastric lavage with warm saline); for severe very cold water drowning cases and where available, peritoneal or hemodialysis, mediastinal irrigation, and cardiac bypass

DURATION

• The cold water near-drowning victim with hypothermia must be rewarmed to greater than 32°C before CPR is terminated. Remember: "The patient is not dead until he is warm and dead."
• Pulmonary treatment is provided as needed (see Breathing, above). Complications may include pneumonia; pneumothorax or pneumomediation in the ventilated patient; and ARDS.

Follow-Up

• Long-term follow-up of apparently neurologically intact survivors has shown mild coordination or gross motor deficiencies.
• The victim may be at increased risk for chronic lung disease, depending on the degree of pulmonary involvement.

PITFALLS

• Failure to observe near-drowning victim for signs of pulmonary involvement, since late deterioration can occur 24 to 48 hours postincident.
• The hypothermic patient who is a warm water near-drowning victim does not have a good prognosis or need vigorous rewarming.

PREVENTION

• Most drownings are preventable.
• Legislation to require adequate fencing and rescue equipment for public and residential pools

• Restriction of sale and consumption of alcohol in boating areas, pools, and beaches
• Parental education regarding adequate supervision during bathing and around swimming pools

Common Questions and Answers

Q: Should the near-drowning victim who arrives at the hospital with cardiopulmonary arrest be resuscitated?
A: Yes, a brief (10–15 minutes) attempt at resuscitation is indicated until circumstances of the near drowning and core temperature are known. Warm water near-drowning victims who require CPR in the emergency department may rarely (0%–25%) have good neurologic recovery but usually respond quickly (<15 minutes) to therapy.

Q: Is artificial surfactant useful in near-drowning victims?
A: Although useful in neonates, surfactant has not been well studied in near-drowning victims. In a dog model and in addicts with ARDS, it has not been beneficial. Further investigation is needed before it can be recommended for clinical use.

ICD-9-CM 994.1

BIBLIOGRAPHY

Barkin S, Gelberg L. Sink or swim—clinicians don't often counsel on drowning prevention. *Pediatrics* 1999;104:1217–19.

Biggarat MJ, Bohn D. Effect of hypothermia and cardiac arrest on outcome of near-drowning accidents in children. *J Pediatr* 1990;117:179–183.

Bratton SL, Jardine DS, Morra JF. Serial neurologic examination after near drowning and outcome. *Arch Pediatr Adolesc Med* 1994;148:167–170.

Diekma DS, Quan L, Holt VL. Epilepsy as a risk factor for submersion injury in children. *Pediatrics* 1993;91(3):512–616.

Lavelle JM, Shaw KN. Near drowning: is emergency department cardiopulmonary resuscitation or intensive care unit cerebral resuscitation indicated? *Crit Care Med* 1993;21(3):368–373.

Lavelle JM, Shaw KN. Ten year review of pediatric bathtub near-drownings: evaluation for child abuse and neglect. *Ann Emerg Med* 1995;25:344–348.

Modell JH. Drowning: current concepts. *N Engl J Med* 1993;328(4):253–256.

Spack L, Rainer G, Gedeit R, et al. Failure of aggressive therapy to alter outcome in pediatric near-drowning. *Pediatr Emerg Care* 1997;13(2):98–102.

Author: Kathy N. Shaw

Neck Masses

Database

To diagnose and appropriately manage the wide range of problems associated with neck masses, one must consider the history and combine it with a careful examination of the mass. The major task of the differential diagnosis is to distinguish infections from congenital and malignant causes.

Differential Diagnosis

- Infectious

—Reactive hyperplasia: self-limited, usually viral enlargement of bilateral minimally tender nodes
—Bacterial lymphadenitis: usually staphylococcal or streptococcal infection of unilateral, tender, swollen, warm, erythematous node. In neonates, a cellulitis-adenitis syndrome is usually caused by group B streptococcus.
—Cat-scratch disease: sometimes protracted illness caused by the gram-negative bacillus *Bartonella henselae,* which starts as a papule at a cat-scratch site and then progresses to tender, regional adenopathy
—Tuberculosis (TB): acute or insidious onset of fever and firm, nontender adenopathy in children exposed to adult infected with the acid-fast bacillus *Mycobacterium tuberculosis*
—Atypical mycobacterial disease: infection usually caused by *Mycobacterium avium* complex or *M. scrofulaceum* (ubiquitous agents found in the soil). Rapidly enlarging mass of firm, nontender nodes in 1- to 4-year-olds with no known exposure to TB. Nodes often occur with overlying skin discoloration and thinning; some spontaneously drain
—Infectious mononucleosis: Epstein-Barr viral infection most commonly seen in older children who present with fever, exudative pharyngitis, adenopathy, and hepatosplenomegaly
—Retropharyngeal abscess: suppurative adenitis of the retropharyngeal nodes that presents in children under 5 years of age with fever, toxicity, dysphagia, respiratory distress, drooling, and stridor
—Peritonsillar abscess: suppurative sequelae of a severe tonsillopharyngitis, usually caused by group A β-hemolytic *Streptococcus,* which commonly presents in older children and adolescents with trismus, "hot potato" voice, and uvular deviation from a bulging palatal abscess

- Congenital

—Thyroglossal duct cyst: remnant of the embryonic thyroglossal sinus, which presents as a nontender (unless infected) mobile, anterior midline mass near the hyoid bone
—Branchial cleft cyst: remnant of the second branchial cleft, which presents as a nontender (unless infected) cyst at the anterior border of the sternocleidomastoid
—Cystic hygroma (lymphangioma): complex, multiloculated mass of lymphatic tissue, which presents in the first year of life as a large, soft, compressible neck structure
—Dermoid cyst: small, firm, nontender mass, usually high in the midline
—Hemangioma: bluish purple, blanching mass appearing in first year of life

- Malignant

—Hodgkin lymphoma: slowly enlarging, unilateral, firm, nontender neck malignancy, which usually presents in previously well adolescents
—Non-Hodgkin lymphoma: presents in young adolescents as a painless, rapidly growing, firm collection of lymph nodes
—Neuroblastoma: most commonly presents in toddlers as a large, nontender, abdominal mass, often associated with a myriad of signs and symptoms as a result of its propensity for metastasis
—Rhabdomyosarcoma: head and neck malignancy that usually presents as a rapidly enlarging mass

- Thyroid

—Chronic lymphocytic thyroiditis (Hashimoto thyroiditis): autoimmune childhood goiter that may be euthyroid, hypothyroid, or hyperthyroid
—Thyrotoxicosis (Graves disease): clinically hyperfunctioning thyroid caused by circulating thyroid cell-stimulating antibodies
—Thyroiditis: painful bacterial infection of the thyroid caused by *Staphylococcus* or *Streptococcus*

- Miscellaneous

—Kawasaki disease: idiopathic vasculitis distinguished by fever, conjunctivitis, oral involvement, extremity changes, rash, and adenopathy
—Sinus histiocytosis with massive lymphadenopathy (Rosai-Dorfman disease): benign form of histiocytosis that presents as massive, painless enlargement of cervical nodes
—Sternocleidomastoid tumor of infancy (congenital muscular torticollis): benign perinatal fibromatosis, often associated with difficult deliveries or abnormal uterine positioning, that results in a hard, immobile, fusiform mass in the sternocleidomastoid
—Hematoma: secondary to trauma
—Hypersensitivity reaction: secondary to bites, stings, or other allergens

Data Gathering

HISTORY

Question: Fever?
Significance: Infection, Kawasaki disease, malignancy

Question: Noticed with intercurrent infection?
Significance: Reactive hyperplasia, mononucleosis, adenitis, abscess, congenital cyst

Question: Increasing size?
Significance: Infection, malignancy

Question: Sore throat?
Significance: Mononucleosis, peritonsillar abscess

Question: Swallowing problems?
Significance: Retropharyngeal or peritonsillar abscess, thyroglossal duct cyst

Question: Cats?
Significance: Cat-scratch disease

Question: History of scratch or papule on face?
Significance: Cat-scratch disease

Question: Recurrently infected same neck mass?
Significance: Thyroglossal duct cyst, branchial cleft cyst

Question: Recurrently infected different neck mass?
Significance: Immunodeficiency

Question: Noticed at or shortly after birth?
Significance: Cystic hygroma, hemangioma, sternocleidomastoid tumor of infancy

Question: Weight loss, cough, or other chronic constitutional symptoms?
Significance: Malignancy, tuberculosis

Question: Hypo- or hyperthyroid symptoms?
Significance: Thyroglossal duct cyst, thyroidal diseases

Physical Examination

Finding: Tender, erythematous, indurated mass
Significance: Cervical adenitis, infected congenital lesion

Finding: Nontender, enlarged lymph nodes(s)
Significance: Reactive hyperplasia, malignancy

Finding: Fluctuant
Significance: Adenitis with abscess, cystic hygroma

Finding: Drainage
Significance: Adenitis with abscess, atypical mycobacterial disease, infected thyroglossal duct or branchial cleft cyst

Finding: Regional adenopathy
Significance: Reactive hyperplasia, cat-scratch disease

Finding: Exudative pharyngitis
Significance: Mononucleosis

Finding: Asymmetric soft palate with uvular deviation
Significance: Peritonsillar abscess

Finding: Pulmonary findings
Significance: Tuberculosis, malignancy

Finding: Midline
Significance: Thyroglossal duct cyst, dermoid cyst, thyroidal disease

Finding: Moves with tongue protrusion
Significance: Thyroglossal duct cyst

Finding: Sinus opening
Significance: Thyroglossal duct, branchial cleft, or dermoid cyst

Finding: Multiloculated
Significance: Cystic hygroma

Finding: Matted down
Significance: Malignancy

Finding: Posterior to sternocleidomastoid muscle
Significance: Malignancy, infectious

Finding: Inferior deep cervical nodes (scalene and supraclavicular)
Significance: Malignancy

Finding: Generalized adenopathy
Significance: Malignancy

Finding: Hepatosplenomegaly
Significance: Malignancy, infectious mononucleosis

Finding: Skin discoloration
Significance: Trauma, abscess, atypical mycobacterial disease

Finding: Conjunctivitis, oral involvement, extremity changes, rash
Significance: Kawasaki disease

Laboratory Aids

Test: CBC
Significance: Leukocytosis in infections; atypical lymphocytosis in mononucleosis; thrombocytosis after 1st week in Kawasaki disease; usually normal CBC in most patients with neck malignancies

Test: Epstein-Barr virus titers, mononucleosis spot test
Significance: "Monospot" test less reliable in children younger than 4 years old; therefore, titers more useful

Test: Indirect fluorescent antibody titers for *Bartonella*
Significance: Reliable test to confirm clinical suspicion of cat-scratch disease

Test: PPD
Significance: Negative or only weakly positive in atypical mycobacterial infections

Test: Chest x-ray
Significance: Cavitary lesions and infiltrates in TB; adenopathy in malignancies and TB

Test: Lateral neck x-ray
Significance: Prevertebral soft tissue space at C2-C3 should be $\frac{1}{2}$ adjacent vertebral body diameter, otherwise, suspect retropharyngeal abscess

Test: Ultrasound
Significance: Often the first imaging modality for neck masses; provides immediate, noninvasive information on location, size, and composition of mass (cystic versus solid)

Test: CT or MRI scan
Significance: Useful in evaluating deep neck infections and complex or extensive neck masses

Test: Thyroid scintigraphy
Significance: Useful in evaluating thyroid lesions, especially when malignancy is a concern

Test: Gram stain and culture of specimen after needle aspiration or incision and drainage
Significance: Diagnostic as well as therapeutic procedure when infection suspected

Test: Histologic evaluation of specimen after fine-needle aspiration or biopsy
Significance: Diagnostic to distinguish malignant causes from congenital and infectious ones

Therapy

- Infectious—antibiotics; drainage for abscesses.
- Congenital—antibiotics if infected; ENT referral for surgical excision
- Malignancy—oncology referral for chemotherapy/radiation
- Thyroidal—endocrine referral for pharmacotherapy
- Miscellaneous

—Kawasaki disease—IVIG, aspirin; cardiology referral for echocardiography
—Sternocleidomastoid tumor of infancy—massage, range of motion, and stretching exercises

Follow-Up

Close follow-up is essential for all neck masses; consider referral for biopsy in the following cases:

- Failure of antibiotics
- Toxic illness/systemic symptoms
- Clinical signs of malignancy
- Nodes that are firm, nontender, and fixed to skin/deep tissues; nodes located posterior to the sternocleidomastoid or in the lower cervical/supraclavicular regions
- Increasing size after 2 weeks without diagnosis
- No decrease in size after 4 to 6 weeks without diagnosis
- Not back to normal size after 8 to 12 weeks

ICD-9-CM 784.2

BIBLIOGRAPHY

Armstrong WB, Giglio MF. Is this lump in the neck anything to worry about? *Postgrad Med* 1998;104(3):63–78.

Brown RL, Azizkhan RG. Pediatric head and neck lesions. *Pediatr Clin North Am* 1998;45(4):889–905.

Chesney PJ. Cervical adenopathy. *Pediatr Rev* 1994;15:276–285.

Connolly AAP, MacKenzie K. Paediatric neck masses—a diagnostic dilemma. *J Laryngol Otol* 1997;111(6):541–545.

Kelly CS, Kelly RE. Lymphadenopathy in children. *Pediatr Clin North Am* 1998;45(4):875–888.

McGuirt WF. The neck mass. *Med Clin North Am* 1999;83(1):219–234.

Park YW. Evaluation of neck masses in children. *Am Fam Physician* 1995;51(8): 1904–1912.

Ponder TB, Smith D, Ibrahim R. Lymphadeno-pathy in children and adolescents: role of fine-needle aspiration in management. *Cancer Detect Prevent* 2000;24(3):228–233.

Swischuk LE, John SD. Neck masses in infants and children. *Radiol Clin North Am* 1997;35(6): 1329–1340.

Torsiglieri AJ, Tom LW, Russ AJ, et al. Pediatric neck masses: guidelines for evaluation. *Int J Pediatr Otorhinolaryngol* 1988;16:199–210.

Weber AL, Siciliano A. CT and MR imaging evaluation of neck infections with clinical correlations. *Radiol Clin North Am* 2000;38(5):941–968.

Wetmore RF, Mahboubi S, Soyupak SK. Computed tomography in the evaluation of pediatric neck infections. *Otolaryngol Head Neck Surg* 1998;119(6):624–627.

Author: Nicholas Tsarouhas

Necrotizing Enterocolitis

 Database

DEFINITION

Necrotizing enterocolitis (NEC) is a necrotizing inflammatory bowel disorder affecting the premature infant; only 10% of cases occur in term infants. NEC, the most common and most serious acquired gastrointestinal disorder among hospitalized preterm infants, is associated with significant acute and chronic morbidity and mortality.

CAUSES

NEC is a disease of unknown etiology. There are, however, several hypotheses that are believed to act in a multifactorial way to initiate the disease process.

- Hypoxia/ischemia: alterations in blood flow to mucosal surfaces secondary to hypoxic injury and other systemic factors, such as polycythemia, drug exposure, cardiac defects, and exchange transfusions
- Enteral alimentation: Since 95% of infants who develop NEC have been enterally fed, the act of initiation of feeds has been implicated as a possible cause of NEC. The composition of the formula, the rate of volume increase, and the immaturity of the mucosa have all been implicated as factors that may increase the risk of NEC.
- Because of the frequent report of epidemic, cluster-type episodes, a variety of microorganisms have been implicated in the development of NEC. In the majority of cases no identifiable organism is recovered, but at times certain microbes, such as *Escherichia coli, Klebsiella, Salmonella,* and *Staphylococcus epidermidis,* have been recovered. Blood cultures may be positive in 20% to 30% of cases.
- As a result of the type of injury that is seen, a cytokine-mediated cascade has also been proposed to play a role in the disease process. In some patients, there have been elevations in serum tumor necrosis factor-α and platelet-activating factor.

PATHOLOGY

- The traditional pathologic features of NEC that are most commonly seen include varying degrees of inflammation and coagulation necrosis of the colonic and intestinal mucosa.
- NEC can be transmural in nature in the most severe cases.
- The most common sites for NEC include the terminal ileum, ileocecal region, and ascending colon.
- Fifty percent of infants have both colonic and small intestine disease, while the other 50% is divided fairly equally between isolated ileal or colonic involvement.

GENETICS

There is no known genetic predisposition or component in the development of NEC.

EPIDEMIOLOGY

- The prevalence for NEC is approximately 4%, and the incidence ranges from 1 in 2,000 to 4,000 live births.
- The incidence is highest in infants with birth weights between 500 and 750 g (13–20%) and decreases to approximately 2% in infants greater than 750 g.
- NEC usually has an onset within the first 2 weeks of life (3–12 days) and after enteral feeds have been initiated. The more premature the infant, the longer the child is at risk for developing NEC, and cases have been reported 3 months after birth.
- There is no association between NEC and sex or race.
- The overall mortality for infants with NEC is between 20% and 40%.
- Mean gestational age is 31 weeks.

COMPLICATIONS

- NEC is associated with significant morbidity and mortality.
- A variety of complications may occur in infants with this disease process, including gastrointestinal perforation, acquired short bowel syndrome, DIC, sepsis and shock, intestinal strictures, enterocolic fistulae, and abscess formation.

 Differential Diagnosis

The clinical spectrum of signs and symptoms that can be seen in a patient with NEC leads to a variety of other disease processes that must be considered. Some processes can be related to the gastrointestinal tract, while others may be systemic in nature:

- Systemic

—Sepsis with ileus
—Pneumothorax causing a pneumoperitoneum
—Hemorrhagic disease of the newborn
—Swallowed maternal blood
—Postasphyxia bowel necrosis

- Gastrointestinal

—Volvulus
—Malrotation
—Pseudomembranous colitis
—Hirschsprung colitis
—Intussusception
—Spontaneous bowel perforation
—Stress ulcer
—Meconium ileus
—Milk protein allergy
—Umbilical arterial thromboembolism

 Data Gathering

HISTORY

- The clinical presentation is variable in this group of patients, but the triad of abdominal distention, bloody stools, and bilious emesis is frequently seen shortly after initiating enteral feeds.
- A number of more subtle, nonspecific findings may be the initial sign of NEC and include apnea and/or bradycardia, lethargy, diarrhea, acidosis, and temperature instability.
- Patients who have more advanced disease may present with more serious problems: coagulopathy, increased fluid requirements and shock.

 Physical Examination

- Clinical symptoms that are helpful in raising suspicion include abdominal distention, increased stool output, heme positive stools, emesis, increased gastric residuals, decreased bowel sounds, and mottling of the extremities.
- Patients who have more advanced disease may present with more serious problems: vital sign instability (shock), ascites, and peritonitis.

PITFALLS

The major pitfall occurs when there is a delay in making the correct diagnosis and in the institution of appropriate therapy. This leads to a rapid progression of symptoms and usually a worse outcome.

 Laboratory Aids

TESTS

- The diagnosis of NEC is confirmed by the presence of pneumatosis intestinalis or hepatic venous gas on x-ray. Perforation in the setting of other clinical symptoms is also indicative of NEC.
- Laboratory evaluation may be helpful in assessing the severity of the episode but is not enough to make the diagnosis.
- Laboratory abnormalities may include thrombocytopenia, disseminated intravascular coagulopathy, metabolic acidosis, anemia, neutropenia, and peripheral eosinophilia.
- Other radiologic findings may include ileus, isolated dilated intestinal loop, ascites, and free air.

Therapy

- For patients who develop NEC, therapy is based on the severity and progression of the symptoms.
- Initial management of all patients with suspected or proven NEC needs to include NPO status, intravenous fluids, NG tube placement for decompression, and intravenous antibiotics.
- Patients need to have blood and stool cultures sent and need to have frequent evaluation of CBC, fluid status, and abdominal x-ray. These should be evaluated every 6 hours to once a day, depending on the severity of the episode.
- Length of therapy and reinstitution of feeds tend to be based on the severity of the episode and on clinical, laboratory, and radiologic abnormalities.
- If the infant responds immediately to therapy and there are no laboratory or radiographic abnormalities, feeds may be started as early as 72 hours after the episode.
- If mild abnormalities arise and the patient remains only mildly ill, a 10-day course of therapy is considered.
- In cases in which laboratory and radiologic abnormalities include pneumatosis intestinalis, acidosis, and/or thrombocytopenia, a 14-day course is indicated.
- Overall, the best therapy for NEC is prevention. Although several small studies have attempted to use immunoglobulin therapy and steroid therapy as a way to decrease the incidence of NEC in premature infants, no significant change in prevalence has been reported. The best way to decrease the possibility of NEC in the premature infant is the use of slow enteral feeding protocols.
- Surgical intervention is required in 25% to 50% of all cases.

 Follow-Up

- Despite early recognition and intervention, NEC is associated with a significantly high morbidity and mortality.
- Mortality results from perforation, sepsis, shock, and DIC.
- Morbidity may be related to anemia, intravenous access difficulties, and the risk for infection. The other most common, long-term sequelae seen in 25% to 30% of infants with NEC are intestinal strictures and short gut syndrome if the patient undergoes surgical resection of bowel.

 Common Questions and Answers

Q: What is the most common complication of NEC?
A: Not recognizing the problem and the development of a short gut syndrome.

Q: Is this preventable?
A: The development of NEC is not clearly preventable, but clinicians are careful to start feeding extremely premature infants slowly with elemental diets.

ICD-9-CM 557.0

BIBLIOGRAPHY

Bell MJ, Ternberg JL, Feigin RD. Neonatal necrotizing enterocolitis: therapeutic decisions based upon clinical staging. *Ann Surg* 1978;187:1B7.

Engum SA, Grosfeld JL. Necrotizing enterocolitis. *Curr Opin Pediatr* 1998;10(2):123–130.

Kleigman RM. Neonatal necrotizing enterocolitis. In: Wyllie R, Hyams JS, eds. *Pediatric gastrointestinal disease.* Philadelphia: WB Saunders, 1993:788–798.

Kliegman RM. Neonatal necrotizing enterocolitis: bridging the basic science with clinical disease. *J Pediatr* 1990;117:833–853.

Ladd AP, Rescorla FJ, West KW, et al. Long-term follow-up after bowel resection for necrotizing enterocolitis: factors affecting outcome. *J Pediatr Surg* 1998;33(7):967–972.

Udall JN. Gastrointestinal host defense and necrotizing enterocolitis. *J Pediatr* 1990;117:533–543.

Author: Edisio Semeao

Neonatal Alloimmune Thrombocytopenia

Database

DEFINITION

Neonatal alloimmune thrombocytopenia (NAIT) is analogous to hemolytic disease of the newborn.

PATHOPHYSIOLOGY

• Caused by maternal antibodies directed against fetal platelet antigens, inherited from the father, which cross the placenta and enter the fetal circulation
• Antibody-coated platelets in the fetus or newborn are destroyed at an increased rate.

EPIDEMIOLOGY

• Occurs in 1 in every 1,000 to 5,000 live births, including first-born offspring
• The most common antigens responsible are human platelet antigen-1a (HPA-1a, formerly PL^{A1}), responsible antigen in over 75% of cases, HPA-5b (formerly Br^a), and HPA-3 (formerly Bak); however, many other antigens can be responsible and vary in frequency according to ethnic group.
• Severe thrombocytopenia (platelet counts <50,000/μL) due to HPA-1a antibodies occurs in 1 in 1,100 births
• Mothers who are HPA-1a negative and HLA-DR3, -B8, or -DR52a positive form platelet antibodies at increased rates and are more likely to have severely affected neonates
• Less commonly, maternal antibodies directed against fetal histocompatibility antigens may cause thrombocytopenia or neutropenia.

COMPLICATIONS

• Abnormal bleeding: primarily skin and mucous membrane bleeding, including but not limited to:

—Petechiae and ecchymoses: These lesions are progressive and not confined to areas of birth trauma, such as the head and shoulders.
—Prolonged bleeding from the umbilical stump, phlebotomy sites, and/or at circumcision sites
—Cephalohematomas
—Hematuria
—Gastrointestinal bleeding
—Intracranial hemorrhages: reported in 2% to 20% of cases; 50% of these occur *in utero*.

PROGNOSIS

• The overall prognosis is fair, as the majority of patients will experience little morbidity or mortality associated with bleeding; however, the risk of bleeding is higher than in infants of mothers with ITP, and reported mortality is 10% in some series.
• The majority of future pregnancies are equally or more severely affected, but this is controversial.

Differential Diagnosis

• Infection: primarily related to disseminated intravascular coagulation (DIC)

—Bacterial: sepsis
—Viral: congenital rubella or cytomegalovirus
—Spirochetal: syphilis
—Protozoal: toxoplasmosis

• Tumor/malignancy

—Bone marrow disease: congenital leukemia, neuroblastoma

• Metabolic

—Methylmalonic or isovaleric acidemia

• Congenital

—Thrombocytopenia with absent radii (TAR) syndrome
—Wiskott-Aldrich syndrome
—May-Hegglin anomaly
—Hemangiomata with Kasabach-Merritt syndrome

• Immunologic

—Autoimmune neonatal thrombocytopenia: primarily seen in infants of mothers with a history of idiopathic thrombocytopenia purpura (ITP)
—Infants of mothers with systemic lupus erythematosus

• Miscellaneous

—Catheter-associated thrombosis with increased platelet consumption
—Renal vein and other large-vessel thromboses
—DIC
—Necrotizing enterocolitis

Data Gathering

HISTORY

• Family history of bleeding disorders, particularly a history of thrombocytopenia or ITP in the mother
• Medications used during pregnancy or in the newborn
• Infectious diseases in mother and/or newborn

Special Questions

Affirmative answers to the following questions increase the likelihood of NAIT in the thrombocytopenic newborn:

• Is there no history of maternal ITP or SLE?
• Is the mother's platelet count presently normal?
• Has the mother had prior newborns with thrombocytopenia, NAIT, or *in utero* intracranial hemorrhage?
• Has the mother ever been told that she was HPA-1a- or PL^{A1}-negative?

Physical Examination

• Most neonates with NAIT are well appearing unless they have already experienced an intracranial hemorrhage.
• Skin and mucous membrane bleeding, petechiae, and ecchymoses are common findings.
• Less commonly, if significant hemorrhaging occurs, the following signs may be noted: irritability, pallor, and signs of intracranial hemorrhage, including those related to increased intracranial pressure.
• If congenital anomalies, hepatosplenomegaly, or masses are present, causes of thrombocytopenia, other than immune-mediated, should be investigated.

PITFALLS

NAIT is a difficult diagnosis to confirm and often requires expensive tests, the results of which are often not available to guide the acute management of the newborn; however, a complete workup is necessary for management of future pregnancies in the affected neonate's mother.

Laboratory Aids

TESTS

• Complete blood count (CBC) in newborn

—Low platelet count: less than 150,000 often below 50,000
—Hemoglobin and hematocrit should be normal: Infants with low values may have experienced perinatal blood loss or could have active bleeding.
—White blood cell (WBC) should be normal in uncomplicated NAIT.

• Consider a PT/PTT to evaluate for DIC, particularly if the infant is ill-appearing or has a complicated pre- and/or perinatal history.
• Maternal platelet count: This is usually normal in NAIT, but a normal maternal platelet count does not rule out autoimmune thrombocytopenia.
• Maternal serum for antiplatelet antibody analysis: To confirm the diagnosis of NAIT, the antibody detected should be specific for a known platelet antigen.
• Maternal and paternal platelet antigen typing: This is crucial for counseling regarding future pregnancies.
• Newborn platelet antigen typing: Use only when absolutely necessary to make the diagnosis, as large amounts of blood are required for this test.

• Consider urine and stool for detection of occult blood.
• Head ultrasound to rule out intracranial hemorrhages

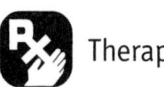

Therapy

• Therapy primarily involves close monitoring for severe bleeding, including intracranial hemorrhage
• Daily platelet counts at minimum during the first several days of life
• If significant bleeding occurs, the neonate should receive a platelet transfusion with the first available product, in order of preference:

—Washed, irradiated maternal platelets
—Platelets cross-matched with maternal serum
—Irradiated PL^{A1}-negative platelets
—Irradiated random donor platelets: often very limited success in increasing platelet count, as 98% of the U.S. population is PL^{A1}-positive

• Platelet transfusions, when needed, are usually required only once.
• The treatment of severely thrombocytopenic neonates without evidence of significant bleeding is controversial, because of the small but real risk of intracranial hemorrhages.
• Often transfusions are performed at platelet counts of 20,000 to 30,000.
• Other therapies have been reported with limited success, such as steroids, intravenous gamma globulin, and exchange transfusions.

Follow-Up

• The thrombocytopenia of NAIT usually resolves within 3 to 4 weeks but can be present for up to 12 weeks.
• Family counseling regarding management of future pregnancies after a thorough diagnostic evaluation is strongly recommended.

SIGNS TO WATCH FOR

If the thrombocytopenia persists after 3 months, other etiologies of thrombocytopenia should be investigated.

PREVENTION

Although the disease cannot be prevented, mothers of infants with NAIT can be monitored and possibly treated during subsequent pregnancies.

ISOLATION OF HOSPITALIZED PATIENTS

Isolation of hospitalized patients is not required.

Common Questions and Answers

Q: What is the HPA-1a- or PL^{A1}-negative mother's risk of having other affected newborns?
A: This depends on the genotype of the father:

• If the father is homozygous for HPA-1a or PL^{A1}, all offspring will be heterozygous PL^{A1}-positive and at great risk for developing NAIT.
• If the father is heterozygous for HPA-1a or PL^{A1}, 50% of offspring will be at risk for developing NAIT.

Q: What is the management of future pregnancies in mothers known to be HPA-1a- or PL^{A1}-negative?
A: This depends on the risk of having an affected child and the clinical course of past affected children. Some perinatal monitoring and therapeutic techniques have shown limited success but not without risks. However, if the risk of having an affected child is 100% and the clinical course of prior affected newborns was associated with significant morbidity and/or mortality, consider the following perinatal management:

• Percutaneous umbilical blood sampling for a platelet count
• Maternal intravenous gamma globulin therapy
• Maternal low-dose prednisone
• Weekly intrauterine platelet transfusions
• Early elective cesarean section to avoid birth trauma

Q: Will the affected neonate be at increased risk for other bleeding problems later in life?
A: If the neonate has confirmed NAIT, there is no increased risk for bleeding problems later in life relative to the general population.

BIBLIOGRAPHY

Bussel J, Kaplan C, MacFarland J, et al. Recommendations for the evaluation and treatment of neonatal autoimmune and alloimmune thrombocytopenia. *Thromb Haemost* 1991;65:631–634.

Bussel JB, Zabusky MR, Berkowitz RL, et al. Fetal alloimmune thrombocytopenia. *N Engl J Med* 1997;337:22–26.

Glader BE, Buchanan GR. The bleeding neonate. *Pediatrics* 1976;58:548–555.

Lanzkowsky P. *Manual of pediatric hematology and oncology*. New York: Churchill Livingstone, 1995.

Ouwehand WH, Smith G, Ranasinghe E. Management of severe alloimmune thrombocytopenia in the newborn. *Arch Dis Child Fetal Neonatal Edition* 2000;82:F173–175.

Pramanik AK. Bleeding disorders in neonates. *Pediatr Rev* 1992;13:163–173.

Author: Kim Smith-Whitley

Neonatal Apnea

 Database

DEFINITION

• Apnea is the cessation of breathing for 15 seconds or longer. It may be associated with cyanosis, pallor, hypotonia, or bradycardia.
• Apnea of prematurity is a specific diagnosis that occurs in premature infants without other identifiable causes of apnea. It usually develops after the first 24 hours of life and persists throughout the first postnatal month of life. Some infants continue to have apnea until >42 weeks postconceptional age.
• Periodic breathing is a breathing pattern that demonstrates inspiratory and expiratory cycles for 10–20 seconds followed by respiratory pauses of 3 or more seconds in length. The breathing pattern may indicate hyperventilation followed by breathing pauses. It is a normal phenomenon.
• Apnea of infancy occurs in term infants with respiratory cycle pauses of 15 seconds or more that may become clinically apparent when pallor, choking, or cyanosis is evident.

CAUSES

Apnea itself may be idiopathic, as in premature infants, or it may be a sign of other medical problems that include:
• Infection: bacteremia, fungemia, viremia, meningitis, NEC
• Pulmonary/cardiopulmonary disease: RDS, PDS, increased pulmonary blood flow due to other left-to-right shunts
• Birth trauma: spinal cord injury, intracranial hemorrhage, asphyxia
• Maternal medications: maternal opiate addiction, hypermagnesemia, narcotic use/anesthesia during labor
• Neuromuscular disease: congenital myasthenic syndromes, infantile form of spinal muscular atrophy, myotonic dystrophy, central hypoventilation syndrome
• Metabolic disease: electrolyte disturbances, hypoglycemia, hyperammonemia, inborn errors of metabolism
• Anemia been thought to cause apnea of prematurity, although there continues to be debate on this subject.
• Congenital anomalies: tracheoesophageal fistula, Pierre Robin sequence, velopalatal insufficiency, choanal atresia, airway obstruction

PATHOPHYSIOLOGY

• Neonatal apnea has three patterns.
—Central apnea has no chest wall movement or air flow movement and results from blunted responses from chemoreceptors and decreased activity of respiratory centers of the brain.
—Obstructive apnea has chest wall movement, but no air flow movement.
—Mixed episodes demonstrate both obstructive and central apnea, and usually involve obstructive episodes progressing toward central apnea.

• Hypoxemia in premature infants may cause apnea by blunting the response of chemoreceptors to changes in carbon dioxide levels.
• Apnea may occur through abnormal reflexes triggered by suctioning, feeding, and lung hyperinflation.

GENETICS

• Apnea itself has no genetic component, although some of the causes of apnea, such as neuromuscular disease, may have genetic correlates.
• Siblings of infants who were victims of SIDS often receive home apnea monitors. This is based on several cases of recurrent SIDS in families that have seemed to demonstrate a familial element to this entity, although recent investigations have reclassified these cases as homicides.

EPIDEMIOLOGY

• Apnea of prematurity occurs in 25% of infants less than 1,800 g at birth and 85% of infants less than 1,000 g at birth.
• Typically presents after first 24 hours of life, but can occur in first 24 hours of life if other causes of apnea are excluded.
• Apneic events decrease in frequency in most infants in first month of postnatal life to 37 weeks postconceptional age, although some infants demonstrate obstructive events during feeds until 42 to 44 weeks postconceptional age or longer.

COMPLICATIONS

• Persistent, severe apnea and bradycardia that is unremitting may have neurologic consequences.
• Recent trends in neonatal care, however, permit many apneic events before resorting to invasive ventilatory techniques, in attempts to avoid ventilator associated lung injury. No neurologic sequelae are specifically reported from this practice.
• SIDS may not be a complication related to apnea.

PROGNOSIS

• Apnea of prematurity has no long-term morbidity associated with it.
• Apnea of term infants may demonstrate morbidity or mortality that is associated with the underlying etiology of the apnea.

 Differential Diagnosis

INFECTION
• Pneumonia
• NEC
• Systemic infection—bacteria or fungal
• Meningitis

CONGENITAL
• Tracheoesophageal fistula
• Pierre Robin sequence
• Velopalatal insufficiency
• Choanal atresia

RESPIRATORY
• Respiratory distress syndrome
• BPD exacerbation
• Airway obstruction

CARDIAC
• PDA/left to right shunts

TRAUMA
• Intracranial hemorrhage
• Spinal cord injury
• Asphyxia

NEUROMUSCULAR
• Congenital myasthenic syndromes
• Infantile form of spinal muscular atrophy
• Myotonic dystrophy
• Central hypoventilation syndrome

METABOLIC
• Electrolyte disturbances
• Hypoglycemia
• Hyperammonemia
• Inborn errors of metabolism
• Hypermagnesemia

TOXINS
• Maternal opiate addiction
• Narcotic use/anesthesia during labor

 Data Gathering

HISTORY
• Is the mother colonized with group B streptococcus?
• How long were the membranes ruptured?
• Were there any maternal illnesses during pregnancy, such as hypertension or preeclampsia?
• Were any instruments used to deliver the infant?
• Is there maternal chorioamnionitis? Maternal fever?
• What medications has the mother received?
• When did the infant last feed?
• How did the infant appear during the apneic event?
• Was there any evidence of rhythmic muscle activity, color changes, back-arching?
• Any evidence of spitting-up formula or emesis after feeds?
• What is the amount and frequency of feeds?
• Have any siblings died during infancy?

Physical Examination

• General appearance of the infant may suggest signs of infection, such as respiratory distress, pallor, lethargy.
• Vital signs may indicate hyperthermia or hypothermia, both of which increase the likelihood of apnea.
• Abnormal growth parameters suggest genetic syndromes.
• Ascertain patency of the nares.
• Identify palatal sufficiency or macroglossia and obstruction (such as with the Pierre Robin sequence).

- Identify murmurs, a hyperdynamic precordium, or increased peripheral pulses to evaluate for the presence of a PDA or other left-to-right shunt.
- Identify the presence or absence of reflexes throughout the infant's neurologic exam to evaluate for the presence of neuromuscular disease and trauma.
- Abdominal distention may indicate the presence of NEC.
- Observe the infant's tone and identify hypotonia, lethargy, and weakness.
- If apnea occurs with feeds, feed the infant or observe the infant feeding to evaluate whether the infant has difficulty with oral motor control.

 Laboratory Aids

TESTS
- Complete blood count, blood culture to evaluate for infection
- Serum electrolytes, serum calcium, serum glucose
- Arterial blood gas
- A polysomnogram may help elucidate the etiology of the apnea, such as obstructive apnea vs. central apnea

RADIOGRAPHIC STUDIES
- Chest x-ray
- Head ultrasound for premature infants
- CT or MRI of head for term infants
- Barium swallow
- Echocardiogram
- Video swallowing study, if history and evaluation of infant indicate this (assists in the assessment of oral motor coordination)

 Therapy

Therapeutic interventions depend on the etiology of the apnea.

Apnea of Prematurity
- Infant positioning may help maximize mechanical actions of respiratory muscles.
- Pharmacologic intervention is typical. Methylxanthines can be used to stimulate respiratory centers in the brainstem. Caffeine, theophylline, and aminophylline are examples of this class of drug. Caffeine is the most popular since it has a very wide therapeutic index and side effects are rare. Caffeine also has a long half-life in premature infants, allowing once daily dosing.
- Side effects of methylxanthines are tachycardia, emesis, dysrhythmias, seizures, and agitation.
- Serum levels of these drugs need to be monitored for therapeutic efficacy and toxicity.

Obstructive Apnea Secondary to Reflux
- Prone positioning may be valuable in reflux-associated apnea. The infant typically has his head of bed elevated 45 degrees.
- Feeds are typically thickened with rice cereal. Some infant formulas are now available that thicken when the formula reaches gastric acid, such as Enfamil AR. Feeds may be decreased in volume and increased in frequency.
- Pharmacologic intervention may be of assistance. H2-receptor antagonists decrease acidity of gastric contents and decrease reflux-associated pain and abnormal vagal responses to esophageal burning. Side effects include renal toxicity, elevated transaminases, and CNS depression. Metoclopramide and bethanecol promote gastric emptying. Metoclopramide is known to cause dystonic reactions, although this is extremely rare in infants.

 Follow-Up

- Home monitors: infants with apnea often receive home monitors. Most home monitors today have a memory that records events when the infant is being monitored. Infants who are discharged from the nursery have home monitor downloads that are evaluated by a pediatrician, who may decide to end home monitoring 1 to 2 months after no events have been recorded. CPR training for the infant's caregivers is required before the infant can be discharged from the hospital.
- Few infants are discharged home on caffeine, but this is usually discontinued gradually as the infant gains weight and the dose of the caffeine remains the same. Some pediatricians will discontinue the caffeine after 1 to 2 weeks of no apneic events.
- All infants who are discharged on caffeine must have home monitors.
- All infants should be placed to sleep in the supine position.

PITFALLS
- Epidemiologic studies do not demonstrate that home apnea monitoring has any impact on the incidence of SIDS.
- Failure to identify an infant's airway obstruction, such as nasal secretions and swollen nasal turbinates, often leads to unnecessary investigations and interventions.
- Some infants with severe apnea during feedings have poor oral motor control and this may persist despite advanced postconceptional age. These infants should also be evaluated by a video swallowing study to determine whether formula aspiration is a concurrent phenomenon, warranting enteral feeds through a nasogastric tube.

 Common Questions and Answers

Q: What is the role of the polysomnogram in evaluating apnea?
A: The polysomnogram can assist in the identification of the type of apnea (central, obstructive, or mixed), and with a pH probe can diagnose reflux-associated apnea. The follow-up polysomnogram can assist in the evaluation of a particular intervention's efficacy. A polysomnogram cannot predict the infant at risk for SIDS and should not be used in the evaluation of the infant for home monitoring.
Q: What caffeine levels are efficacious in preventing apnea in the premature infant?
A: Frequently, caffeine levels needs to be as high as 20 to 25 mg/dL for an infant to respond to this drug.
Q: Can premature infants less than 24 hours old develop apnea of prematurity?
A: Premature infants less than 24 hours old typically are influenced enough by the neurochemical/adrenocortical changes of birth and are less likely candidates to have apnea of prematurity. However, as neonatal practice has embraced early extubation and noninvasive respiratory support for the extremely low birth weight infant, this entity is more common in the first 24 hours after birth, particularly in the most premature of infants.

ICD-9-CM 770.8
BIBLIOGRAPHY
Bhatia J. Current opinions in the management of apnea of prematurity. *Clin Pediatr* 2000;39:327–336.

Comer AM. Caffeine citrate: a review of its use in apnea of prematurity. *Paediatr Drugs* 2001;3:61–79.

Morris P. Pharmacology of respiratory control in neonates and children. *Paediatr Pulmonol Suppl* 1997;16:222–224.

Praud JP. Larynx and neonatal apnea. *Paediatr Pulmonol Suppl* 1999;18:190–193.

Thach BF. Reflux-associated apnea in infants: evidence for a laryngeal chemoreflex. *Am J Med* 1997;103:1205–1245.

Author: Daniel H. Conway

Nephrotic Syndrome

 Database

DEFINITION

Nephrotic syndrome (NS) applies to any glomerular disorder associated with heavy proteinuria, hypoproteinemia, edema, and hypercholesterolemia. Nephrotic-range proteinuria is found when there is 4+ protein on the urine dipstick, which correlates with proteinuria of more than 40 mg/kg/d.

PATHOPHYSIOLOGY

Causes

• Most pediatric cases are primary; 10% are secondary to other diseases.
• The most common primary cause of NS in childhood is minimal change nephrotic syndrome (MCNS). It is characterized by minimal histologic changes on light microscopy, usually responds to steroid therapy, and follows a relapsing course.
• Other causes of primary nephrotic syndrome include focal segmental glomerulosclerosis and membranous and membranoproliferative glomerulonephritis (GN).
• Secondary causes of NS include infections, vasculitis, diabetes, drugs, and hereditary disorders.

Immunologic Abnormalities

A number of immunologic abnormalities are seen with NS that predispose to infection. These include defective opsonization, decreased serum levels of complement factors D and B, abnormal humoral immunity, decreased delayed hypersensitivity and proliferative responses, and increased suppressor-cell activity and suppressor lymphokine levels.

Pathology (in MCNS)

• The glomerular tuft and size are normal. Mesangial expansion is absent or minimal.
• Immunofluorescence is usually negative, although scanty staining for C3, IgM, and IgA may occasionally be found; these patients are usually steroid dependent.
• Electron microscopy reveals widening and effacement of the visceral epithelial foot processes, which are reversible, occur in association with proteinuria, and are not specific for MCNS.

EPIDEMIOLOGY

• The peak age of onset is 3 years.
• The incidence of new cases is 2 to 7 per 100,000 in children less than 16 years of age.
• The prevalence is 16 per 100,000 in children less than 16 years of age.
• Boys are more commonly affected than girls (3:2).
• A positive family history is present in 3.5% of patients.
• Atopy and MCNS have an association.
• The most common MHC haplotype associated with MCNS is HLA-DR7.
• African-American children have a higher incidence of focal glomerulosclerosis (FSGS) than do Caucasian and Asian children.
• Examples of congenital NS are Finnish, mesangiosclerotic, and syphilitic nephrosis.

COMPLICATIONS

• Most complications are secondary to steroid therapy and include growth retardation, glaucoma, posterior lens cataracts, obesity, mood changes, hirsutism, osteoporosis, and infection.
• Primary peritonitis and cellulitis may occur de novo or with steroid therapy.
• Diarrhea and vomiting may result in rapid severe hypovolemia.
• Vascular thromboses are found with NS in relapse, especially if hypovolemia is present.
• Acute reversible renal failure is an uncommon complication of NS of childhood.
• MCNS does not result in chronic renal failure.

PROGNOSIS

The prognosis for MCNS is excellent, with a mortality rate of less than 1%.

 Differential Diagnosis

• Edema

—Congestive cardiac failure
—Liver failure
—Protein-losing enteropathy
—Protein energy malnutrition (Kwashiorkor)

• Nephrotic syndrome

—Focal glomerulosclerosis (FSGS)
—Membranous GN
—Membranoproliferative GN
—Diffuse mesangial proliferation

 Data Gathering

HISTORY

• Fatigue and general malaise
• Reduced appetite
• Weight gain and facial swelling
• Abdominal swelling or pain
• Urine that is foamy
• Atopy

 Physical Examination

• Pitting-dependent edema
• Fluid accumulation in body spaces (ascites, pleural effusions, scrotal swelling)
• White nails, lusterless hair, soft ear cartilage
• Hepatomegaly
• Mild hypertension

SPECIAL QUESTIONS

• Inquire about known atopy or food intolerance.
• Inquire about drug exposure (especially nonsteroidal antiinflammatory agents).
• Inquire about any infections or hernias.

PROCEDURE

Look for edema in the most dependent area of the child.

Laboratory Aids

TESTS

- The urine dipstick usually shows 2,000 mg/dL (4+) of protein.
- Timed or spot urine protein collection: The 24-hour urine shows more than 40 mg/kg/d, and the spot urine protein/creatinine ratio is above 1.

IMAGING

In complicated cases, renal ultrasound to look at the kidney size and parenchymal architecture

PITFALLS

- In small children with NS, the urine dipstick may be less than 4+.
- Failure to monitor complications of glucocorticoid therapy. Growth failure, especially, must be monitored for.

HOME TESTING

The first morning urine is tested for protein.

REQUIREMENTS

Educate the family about urine testing, complications, diet, and therapy.

 ## Therapy

DRUGS

- Corticosteroids used as first-line agents
- Alkylating agents (cyclophosphamide, chlorambucil)
- Cyclosporine
- Diuretics
- Albumin

DURATION

There are a number of similar regimens.

- On presentation: daily corticosteroids for 4 weeks, followed by alternate-day therapy for 4 weeks
- On relapse: daily corticosteroids until in remission, followed by alternate-day therapy for 8 to 12 weeks

DIET

Restrict salt intake while in relapse or on daily corticosteroids.

POSSIBLE CONFLICTS

- Live vaccines are contraindicated while daily corticosteroids or alkylating agents are being given.
- Children in relapse, on corticosteroids, or on alkylating agents and who are nonimmune and exposed to varicella should receive VZIG.
- Albumin and/or Lasix must be used cautiously to prevent fluid overload or intravascular dehydration.

 ## Follow-Up

WHEN TO EXPECT IMPROVEMENT

Remission occurs 2 to 4 weeks after starting corticosteroids in MCNS.

SIGNS TO WATCH FOR

Fever, abdominal pain, oliguria

PITFALLS

Recognize situations in which hypovolemia may occur.

 ## Common Questions and Answers

Q: Will the MCNS recur?
A: The clinical course tends to be one of multiple remissions and relapses. Relapses usually stop about the time of puberty.

Q: Can the NS return in adult life?
A: Although uncommon, this does occur.

Q: Is macroscopic hematuria ever found with MCNS?
A: Gross hematuria suggests a renovascular event or a diagnosis other than MCNS. Microscopic hematuria occurs in approximately 25% of cases.

Q: What other agents are used to treat NS?
A: Cyclosporin A is used in children with steroid-dependent or -resistant NS.

ICD-9-CM 581.9

BIBLIOGRAPHY

Barratt TM, Clark G. Minimal change nephrotic syndrome and focal segmental glomerulosclerosis. In: Holliday M, Barratt TM, Avner ED, eds. *Pediatric nephrology*, 3rd ed. Baltimore: Williams & Wilkins, 1994:767–787.

Chesney RW. The idiopathic nephrotic syndrome. *Curr Opin Pediatr* 1999;11(2):158–161.

Hodson EM, Knight JF, Willis NS, et al. Corticosteroid therapy for nephrotic syndrome in children. *Cochrane Database of Systematic Reviews* 2000;4:CD001533.

McEnery PT, Strife CF. Nephrotic syndrome in childhood. *Pediatr Clin North Am* 1982;89(4):875–885.

Meyers KEC, Kujubu DA, Kaplan BS. Minimal-change nephrotic syndrome. In: Neilson EG, Couser WG, eds. *Immunologic renal diseases*. Philadelphia: Lippincott-Raven, 1997:975–992.

Robson WLM, Leung AKC. Nephrotic syndrome in childhood. *Adv Pediatr* 1993;40:287–323.

Vande Walle JG, Donckerwolcke RA. Pathogenesis of edema formation in the nephrotic syndrome. *Pediatr Nephrol* 2001;16(3):283–293.

Author: Kevin E. C. Meyers

Neural Tube Defects

 Database

DEFINITION

Neural tube defects (NTDs) include a range of defects, including some subclinical defects, resulting from failure of neural tube closure between the third and fourth week of gestation. NTDs include anencephaly, encephalocele, myelomeningocele, and occult spinal dysraphism.

PATHOPHYSIOLOGY

- Neural tube closure begins midway along the neural axis, continues like a zipper in both rostral and caudal directions, and is completed in a few days. Failure of neural tube closure most often occurs in the lumbosacral region.
- The defect itself may be only the "tip of the iceberg," since the total extent of the malformation may involve the entire central nervous system. This includes disorganized brainstem nuclei or brainstem herniation (Chiari II malformation).

GENETICS

Most cases are due to a combination of genetic, environmental, and dietary factors. Five percent of patients are born to a couple with a family history of NTD. After one NTD, the recurrence rate is 2% to 4% for subsequent pregnancies. Some cases are due to a specific genetic syndrome that may be sporadic, recessive, or dominant.

EPIDEMIOLOGY

- One per 1,000 live births in the United States (not including occult defects, for which no accurate epidemiologic data are available)
- Anencephaly: 0.2 per 1,000
- Myelomeningocele: 0.2 to 0.4 per 1,000

COMPLICATIONS

- Encephalocele: hydrocephalus (50%), intellectual deficits (40%), motor and cognitive deficits, seizures likely due to dysplastic cortex surrounding the encephalocele
- Myelomeningocele: hydrocephalus (80%); Chiari II malformation (80%), with some exhibiting feeding difficulties, stridor, and apnea due to lower cranial nerve dysfunction; neurogenic bladder (80%) with risk of renal damage; orthopedic deformities; seizures (25%); below average intelligence (15–20%); and tethered spinal cord later in childhood
- Occult dysraphism: progressive lower extremity motor or sensory deficit, gait dysfunction, sphincter dysfunction, foot deformities, scoliosis

PROGNOSIS

- Anencephaly is uniformly fatal
- Encephalocele: Prognosis is largely dependent on the size of the defect, the amount of brain tissue contained within the sac, and any associated brain malformations.
- Myelomeningocele: prognosis for ambulation depends on the location of the lesion. The lower the lesion, the more likely the patient will walk. Cognitive outcome depends in part on associated brain malformations and treatment of hydrocephalus.

 Differential Diagnosis

Diagnosis reflects the embryogenesis and anatomy of each defect.

- *Encephalocele* is a more limited failure of anterior neural tube closure. Abnormal brain tissue protrudes through a skull defect usually covered by skin. Seventy percent to 80% are occipital, 20% are frontal. Ten percent to 20% of occipital defects are meningoceles and contain no brain tissue. Frontal encephaloceles, unless accompanied by craniofacial abnormalities, may not be identified unless a neuroimaging study is performed for an associated symptom (such as developmental delay or seizures).
- *Myelomeningocele* is a failure of posterior neural tube closure. Abnormal neural tissue protrudes through a vertebral column defect. Eighty percent are thoracolumbar, lumbar, or lumbosacral. By definition, this is an open defect, and the diagnosis is obvious at birth.
- *Occult spinal dysraphism* includes a variety of lesions, all with intact skin over the defect. The wide spectrum of defects includes dermal sinus tracts, cysts, lipomas, other tumors, diastematomyelia (bifid spinal cord), tethered spinal cord, and sacral agenesis (caudal regression syndrome).
- A *syndromic basis* for dysraphism should be considered when nonneural congenital defects are present (e.g., telecanthus-Waardenburg syndrome; conotruncal defect-chromosome 22q11 deletion).

 Data Gathering

HISTORY

- Family history of NTD
- NTDs are also associated with maternal folic acid deficiency, gestational diabetes, maternal hyperthermia during days 20 to 28 of gestation, and use of valproic acid, carbamazepine, or alcohol during pregnancy.
- Polyhydramnios may signal swallowing difficulty due to neurologic dysfunction

- Occult frontal encephaloceles may come to attention because of a history of developmental delay, seizures, or focal neurologic signs.
- Occult spinal dysraphism presents with lower extremity weakness or sensory loss, gait abnormalities, bowel and bladder dysfunction, foot deformities, and, rarely, recurrent meningitis.

 Physical Examination

- Plot head circumference as a marker of developing hydrocephalus.
- Note other dysmorphic features because NTDs are found in various syndromes and chromosomal abnormalities.
- Neurologic exam of the lower extremities in a myelomeningocele outlines the functional level of the lesion and provides an estimate of future ambulatory potential. Intact hip flexion (L1-L2) and knee extension (L3-L4) are favorable signs for future ambulation.
- Flaccid paralysis is present below the level of the lesion, and ultimate limb growth may be asymmetric. Sensory level may not correspond to motor level. Cranial neuropathies, such as strabismus, laryngeal paresis, and stridor, may be present at birth or may develop in the first months of life.
- Local signs of occult spinal dysraphism include a dimple, sinus, lipoma, skin pigment change, or tuft of hair in the lumbosacral area. Examination may show arthrogryptic foot deformities, tight heel cords, unequal leg or foot length, decreased sphincter tone, lower extremity weakness, or sensory changes.

 Laboratory Aids

TESTS

- Maternal serum α-fetoprotein (MSAFP) testing, done at 16 to 18 weeks' gestation, can identify 88% of cases of anencephaly and 79% of cases of myelomeningocele.
- Ultrasonography can diagnose more than 99% of cases of anencephaly and 90% of cases of myelomeningocele. Since most encephaloceles are skin covered, they are more likely to be diagnosed by ultrasound than by MSAFP testing.
- After delivery, serial cranial ultrasounds or CT scans can evaluate hydrocephalus, which can occur without rapid head growth in patients with NTDs.
- MRI can outline other brain anomalies, including areas of cortical dysplasia, found in 92% of patients in one neuropathologic study.
- EEG is useful in apparent or suspected seizures.
- Urodynamic evaluation can identify infants with high-pressure bladders and sphincter dyssynergia, who are at risk for renal damage.

• Suspected occult spinal dysraphism can be initially evaluated with spine x-rays and ultrasound (in the newborn period). CT scan provides more detail of bony anatomy, and MRI more detail of spinal cord anatomy.

Therapy

• Route of delivery: One study concluded that women with known NTD pregnancies should have a scheduled cesarean section before the onset of labor, since infants delivered in this fashion may have improved neurologic outcome compared with infants delivered vaginally or by cesarean section after onset of labor. Other studies have not confirmed this finding.
• Neurosurgical closure of a myelomeningocele is done within the first few days of life to prevent infection and for cosmetic reasons. Prophylactic antibiotics given to patients awaiting surgery decrease the incidence of meningitis and ventriculitis. Closure of the defect in the first hours of life is no longer felt to be necessary, as long as the defect can be kept clean and moist.
• Fetal surgery is being explored as a new option for the repair of myelomeningoceles.
• An encephalocele with adequate skin covering can be repaired less urgently.
• V-P shunts should probably be placed in infants with NTDs with any degree of hydrocephalus, because early treatment of hydrocephalus may improve cognitive outcome.
• Infants with high bladder pressure typically are treated initially with anticholinergics and clean intermittent catheterization.
• Occult spinal dysraphism should be referred to neurosurgery for evaluation.

Follow-Up

• Children with NTDs benefit from a multidisciplinary approach, involving a primary pediatrician, neurosurgeon, urologist, orthopedist, neurologist, physiatrist, and others.
• Prognosis for ambulation is dependent on the location of the myelomeningocele. Virtually all children with sacral lesions are able to ambulate; 95% of adolescents and 40% of younger children with low lumbar lesions will ambulate; 30% of adolescents with high lumbar or thoracic lesions will ambulate.
• Approximately 80% of children with myelomeningocele will have a neurogenic bladder, which can be characterized by urodynamic testing. The goal of therapy is urinary continence and control of high bladder pressure.

• Many children can ultimately achieve bowel control with bowel programs involving high-fiber, low-fat foods; enemas; stool softeners; and biofeedback.
• Approximately 60% of children with encephalocele and 80% to 85% with myelomeningocele are of normal intelligence.
• Risk of epilepsy generally corresponds to the degree of mental retardation and is particularly high with frontal encephaloceles. Routine EEG cannot substitute for directed history to identify possible seizure activity.
• Anticipation of skin breakdown, decubitus ulcers, and leg injuries are important, since sensory deficits impair protective reflexes.
• In an older child with a myelomeningocele, loss of motor function in the legs, increased spasticity, gait difficulties, pain, bladder dysfunction, and scoliosis may be signs of a tethered cord.

PREVENTION

• Folic acid supplementation in early pregnancy can reduce the incidence of NTDs by 50% in the general population, and by 70% in women with a history of NTD in a previous pregnancy.
• Since many pregnancies are not discovered until after the fourth week of gestation, when neural tube closure occurs, the CDC recommends that all women of childbearing age receive a minimum of 0.4 mg of folic acid daily.
• The American Academy of Pediatrics recommends women with a history of NTD in a previous pregnancy receive 4 mg of folic acid daily, starting 1 month before and through the first 3 months of pregnancy.
• Women who are taking anticonvulsants and other medications linked to NTDs may also benefit from receiving 4 mg of folic acid daily.
• Some authors recommend spine imaging when there are midline lesions of the spine such as tufts of hair, masses, or sinus tracts that may signal underlying dysraphism, since tethered cord could be identified presymptomatically.

PITFALLS

• The neurologic status of a patient with a repaired neural tube defect should not deteriorate with time, unless something else is wrong. Have a high index of suspicion for worsening hydrocephalus, syringomyelia, and tethered spinal cord—all treatable conditions that may develop over time.
• *Tethered cord* may accompany occult dysraphism and is a surgically treatable cause of acquired neurogenic bladder/cauda equina syndrome in young children.
• *Vocal cord paralysis* may appear episodically, resembling croup, in children with myelomeningocele.
• *Shunt blockage or infection* must be diagnosed early and may be heralded by subtle symptoms of irritability, increased sleep, or low-grade fever.

Common Questions and Answers

Q: Will my child have learning problems?
A: At least 50% of those with myelomeningocele have normal intelligence. Cognitive outcome appears improved with the advent of early shunting of hydrocephalus.

Q: Could my baby have other problems besides neurologic problems?
A: Infants with NTDs need to be checked periodically for signs of bladder problems. Some develop problems with control of eye movements (strabismus), but this is often correctable.

Q: Do the child's uncles or aunts have an increased risk of having a child with a birth defect?
A: Though some families do seem to carry an increased risk for NTDs, the increase is small and seems to affect the immediate, not the extended, family.

Q: Should I stop taking anticonvulsants during pregnancy to reduce my risk of NTDs?
A: Not unless your doctor recommends doing so. In general, continuing the lowest dose of the medication that best controls your seizures is recommended during pregnancy. There are risks to the fetus from poorly controlled seizures during pregnancy. The overall risks and benefits of medications must be weighed. Any woman of childbearing age who is taking anticonvulsants should receive at least 0.4 mg of folic acid daily (and taking 4 mg daily is often recommended).

ICD-9-CM

Myelomeningocele 741.9
Anencephaly 740.0

BIBLIOGRAPHY

American Academy of Pediatrics, Committee on Genetics. Folic acid for the prevention of neural tube defects. *Pediatrics* 1993;92:493–494.

Blum RW, Pfaffinger K. Myelodysplasia in childhood and adolescence. *Pediatr Rev* 1994;15:480–484.

Drolet B. Birthmarks to worry about. Cutaneous markers of dysraphism. *Dermatol Clin* 1998;16:447–453.

McComb JG. Spinal and cranial neural tube defects. *Semin Pediatr Neurol* 1997;4:156–166.

Olutoye OO, Adzick NS. Fetal surgery for myelomeningocele. *Semin Perinatol* 1999;23:462–473.

Volpe JJ. *Neurology of the newborn*, 4th ed. Philadelphia: WB Saunders, 2001:3–21.

Author: Dennis J. Dlugos

Neuroblastoma

Database

DEFINITION
Neuroblastoma is tumor derived from neural crest cells that form the sympathetic ganglia and adrenal medulla.

PATHOPHYSIOLOGY
- Etiology unknown
- Neuroblastoma should be distinguished from ganglioneuroma and ganglioneuroblastoma, which, in general, show features of differentiation or maturation.
- Included in the category of small, round blue-cell tumors of childhood
- Metastatic spread by lymphatic and hematogenous routes

GENETICS
- Familial neuroblastoma has been reported but is rare (autosomal dominant with variable penetrance, 1% of patients)
- Neuroblastoma cells may acquire specific genetic alterations, which are of prognostic importance (i.e., amplification of the N-*myc* gene).

EPIDEMIOLOGY
- Most common extracranial solid tumor of children; 7% to 10% of all childhood cancers
- Prevalence: 1 in 7,000 live births in the United States; 600 new cases a year
- Majority of children are younger than 4 years of age and have disseminated disease at diagnosis
- Fifty percent of tumors arise from the adrenal gland.
- Eighty percent of tumors occur below the diaphragm; 20% occur in cervical and thoracic sites.

COMPLICATIONS
Common sites of metastases include:
- Liver
- Bone marrow
- Skin: nontender subcutaneous nodules with a bluish hue
- Lymph nodes
- Bone, particularly the skull and facial bones as well as long bones
- Mass effect at the site of the primary lesion (i.e., spinal cord compression, Horner syndrome)

Paraneoplastic syndromes
- VIP syndrome: due to VIP (vasoactive intestinal peptide) production by tumor; watery diarrhea, abdominal distention, and electrolyte imbalances usually resolve with treatment.
- Opsoclonus-myoclonus: etiology unknown but thought to be due to an autoimmune process; associated with chaotic eye movements ("dancing eyes") and myoclonic jerks ("dancing feet") with or without cerebellar ataxia; may not resolve with treatment of tumor. Specific therapy includes high-dose steroids and IVIG.

- Catecholamine excess: flushing, sweating, tachycardia, headache, hypertension (hypertension more commonly of renal origin than catecholamine excess)

PROGNOSIS
- Most important adverse prognostic factors are N-*myc* amplification, metastatic disease, and age over 1 year
- The following biologic properties have prognostic significance:
  —Histology: "favorable" versus "unfavorable"
  —N-*myc* amplification: Amplification is associated with more aggressive, higher stage tumors (22% of patients).
  —Serum ferritin: High levels are associated with more aggressive tumor.
  —DNA index (ploidy): Hyperdiploid tumors are associated with less aggressive tumors than diploid tumors (in infants).
  —Chromosome analysis: chromosome 1 deletions associated with more advanced stage tumors.
  —Lactate dehydrogenase (LDH): High levels associated with more aggressive tumors.
  —Neuron-specific enolase (NSE): may be elevated in pediatric tumors other than neuroblastoma.
  —Children with low-risk disease, such as those younger than 1 year with low-stage tumors, have an overall cure rate of greater than 90%.
  —Older children with advanced-stage tumors have historically significantly lower cure rates of 15% to 30%. With intensive multimodal therapies, including high-dose therapy with stem cell rescue and *cis*-retinoic acid, long-term survival may approach 50% to 60%.

Differential Diagnosis

- Depends on the presentation of the patient and the site of the primary tumor
- Included in the differential diagnosis of abdominal or thoracic mass:
  —Abdominal primaries include Wilms tumor, Burkitt lymphoma, and germ-cell tumor.
  —Thoracic primaries include lymphoma (usually non-Hodgkin), leukemia with bulky disease, and germ-cell tumors.
- The differential diagnosis of a "small, round, blue-cell tumor" should include neuroblastoma, lymphoma, Ewing sarcoma, and rhabdomyosarcoma.

Data Gathering

HISTORY
- Presenting signs and symptoms of neuroblastoma depend on the primary site of the tumor and the degree of dissemination.
- General well-being: Ask about activity level, change in appetite, irritability, specific areas of discomfort, and so forth. This may give some indication of the extent of disease. Patients with neuroblastoma may present appearing either well or sick, though those

with disseminated disease generally appear both chronically and acutely ill.

Physical Examination

ABDOMINAL MASS
- Abdominal mass is usually firm, fixed, irregular, and frequently crosses the midline.
- Abdominal distention with or without tenderness
- Mass effect
- Signs of bowel obstruction: anorexia, vomiting, low stool output
- Hypertension
- Genital and lower extremity edema from obstruction of venous and lymphatic drainage

CERVICAL/THORACIC MASS (POSTERIOR MEDIASTINAL)
- Respiratory distress or stridor with thoracic masses
- Horner syndrome with cervical or high thoracic masses: ptosis, myosis, and anhydrosis
- Anisocoria
- Superior vena cava syndrome with large mediastinal tumors

PARASPINAL MASS
- Vertebral body involvement and nerve root compression
- Bladder and bowel dysfunction, paraplegia, and back pain due to spinal cord compression

METASTATIC DISEASE
- Liver: hepatomegaly
- Bone: with or without bony pain, periorbital ecchymoses and/or proptosis
- Bone marrow: cytopenias, pain from marrow expansion
- Lymph nodes: adenopathy
- General: fever, irritability, failure to thrive
- Periocular ecchymosis

Laboratory Aids

TESTS
- Office evaluation should include CBC, a basic chemistry panel to assess electrolyte imbalance, and a radiographic study of the suspected primary tumor site (generally an ultrasound or CT scan; MRI may be necessary for paraspinal tumors).
- Further studies should be obtained at the referral center where the patient will receive treatment; this will avoid repeating expensive tests.

Laboratory Tests
- CBC: decreased hemoglobin, platelets, and/or white blood cell counts may indicate bone marrow involvement.
- Urine catecholamines: homovanillic acid (HVA); vanillylmandelic acid (VMA); secreted by some neuroblastomas
- Liver function tests: may indicate liver involvement when elevated

- Lactate dehydrogenase (LDH): may have prognostic value
- Serum ferritin: may have prognostic value
- Bone marrow aspirate and biopsy: to evaluate bone marrow involvement

IMAGING
- Plain films of the primary site (calcification suggests neuroblastoma)
- US, CT, and/or MRI of the primary site and possible metastatic sites
- Skeletal survey or bone scan to rule out bone lesions
- MIBG scan: can detect both bone and soft tissues that are involved

STAGING
- The International Neuroblastoma Staging System (INSS) is the commonly used, current staging system.
- Low-risk groups usually have localized disease.
- High-risk groups have disseminated disease often involving the bones, bone marrow, liver, and/or skin. Biologic characteristics of the tumor can also help stratify risk (i.e., N-*myc* amplification).
- Stage 4S (IVS or D) are patients younger than 12 months of age who have a localized primary mass (stage 1 or 2) with disseminated disease involving the liver, skin, or (minimal) bone marrow but sparing the bones.

PITFALLS
Do not use the spot VMA or HVA to screen for neuroblastoma. False positives (excretion due to other sources) and false negatives (nonsecreting tumors) are both possible.

Therapy

Treatment protocols are based on prognostic categories:
- Patients with low-risk disease, such as stage 4S or stage 1, may only require surgery alone, particularly if surgical resection is complete and the biologic characteristics of the tumor are favorable.
- Patients with advanced-stage disease, such as stage 4 (extensive metastases), usually require a combination of surgery, chemotherapy, and radiation therapy with or without high-dose therapy and stem-cell rescue (HDT/SCR).

SURGERY
- Total surgical resection is attempted but not aggressively; if gross total resection is risky, partial resection or biopsy alone is indicated.
- After a histologic diagnosis has been established, chemotherapy and radiation therapy can be instituted to obtain tumor shrinkage for a later attempt at total gross resection.

CHEMOTHERAPY
- Multiagent chemotherapy is often used in patients who are not low risk.
- Common chemotherapeutic agents for neuroblastoma include cyclophosphamide (Cytoxan), doxorubicin (Adriamycin), etoposide (VP-16), vincristine, ifosfamide, cisplatin, and carboplatin.

RADIATION
- Radiation therapy is used for control of local disease and/or for palliation.
- Total body radiation may be a component of preparative regimens for bone marrow transplantation (BMT).

BIOLOGIC THERAPY
- 13-*Cis*-retinoic acid: cellular differentiating agent that has shown improved survival when used posttransplant

BONE MARROW TRANSPLANTATION
- Autologous bone marrow transplantation (ABMT) or peripheral SCR after intensive chemotherapy is used in high-risk protocols. Tandem transplants, using high-dose chemotherapy with or without total body irradiation, are currently being explored.

DURATION
- Depends on stage of disease, response, and complications: generally under 12 months. Prolonged maintenance chemotherapy does not play a role in therapy, although biologic response modification therapy may be given in the second year after diagnosis.

SIGNS TO WATCH FOR
- Patients are often followed by radiographic studies of the primary site and sites of metastases as well as laboratory tests and bone marrow studies, depending on the presentation and staging of the patient—for example, urine catecholamines, serum ferritin, and abdominal CT for a patient with an adrenal primary without metastases.
- Complications depend on the primary site of the tumor and the therapy received; acute and late effects of chemotherapy and radiation therapy require close monitoring.

ISOLATION OF HOSPITALIZED PATIENTS
- Patients with neuroblastoma should take measures to avoid contact with persons known to have active varicella.
- Neutropenic patients do not require special isolation precautions except in the transplant setting.

Common Questions and Answers

Q: Are siblings of children with neuroblastoma at increased risk for neuroblastoma compared with the general population?
A: No, except in rare families with a known history of neuroblastoma (<1%).
Q: Can neuroblastoma spontaneously regress?
A: Yes; however, this is usually seen only in children under 1 year of age with lower stage disease.
Q: What are the biggest risks during therapy?
A: The risk of infection is quite high due to the presence of an indwelling catheter and severe neutropenia secondary to aggressive chemotherapy. Platinum-containing regimens can cause significant hearing loss that may worsen the higher the cumulative dose.
Q: What therapy is available to patients who either fail to go into remission or relapse following aggressive therapy?
A: There is no standard approach to a refractory or relapsed patient with neuroblastoma. Generally, phase I or II therapies may be offered, although the outcome for these patients is generally very poor.

ICD-9-CM 194.0

BIBLIOGRAPHY
Brodeur AE, Brodeur GM. Abdominal masses in children: neuroblastoma, Wilms tumor, and other considerations. *Pediatr Rev* 1991;12(7):196–206.

Castleberry RP. Biology and treatment of neuroblastoma. *Pediatr Clin North Am* 1997;44:919–937.

Caty MG, Shamberger RC. Abdominal tumors in infancy and childhood. *Pediatr Surg* 1993;40(6):1253–1271.

Finklestein JZ. Neuroblastoma: the challenge and the frustration. *Hematol Oncol Clin North Am* 1987;1(4):675–694.

Grupp SA, Stern JW, Ross AA, et al. Tandem high dose therapy in rapid sequence for children with high-risk neuroblastoma. *J Clin Oncol* 2000;18(13):2567–2575.

Reynolds CP, Villablanca JG, Stram DO, et al. 13-cis-retinoic acid after intensive consolidation therapy for neuroblastoma improves event-free survival: a randomized Children's Cancer Group (CCG) study. *Proc Am Soc Clin Oncol* 1998.

Author: Julie W. Stern
Kim Smith-Whitley, 1st edition

Neurofibromatosis

Database

DEFINITION

Neurofibromatosis type 1 (NF1) is a neurocutaneous syndrome in which tumors grow along various types of nerves, both internal and external. Neurologic features include cognitive disability, intra- and extracranial tumors of the nervous system, and stroke (rare). The diagnosis is based on the presence of any two of the following physical/familial criteria:

- Two or more cutaneous neurofibroma(ta) or one plexiform neurofibroma
- Two or more Lisch nodules (see Physical Examination)
- Inguinal or axillary freckling
- Six or more (smooth-edged) café-au-lait spots, at least 1.5 cm in diameter in postpubertal individuals or 0.5 cm in diameter in prepubertal individuals
- Optic nerve glioma
- Osseous lesions, including sphenoid wing dysplasia, pseudarthrosis
- A first-degree relative (parent, sibling, or offspring) with NF

Tumors may be cosmetically disfiguring and physically limiting; they rarely undergo sarcomatous transformation.

GENETICS

- NF1 is an autosomal-dominant disorder; half of the cases are inherited, and half occur as a sporadic mutation.
- NF1 is one of the most commonly inherited autosomal- dominant disorder (approximately 1 in 4,000), with no known gender or ethnic predisposition.
- The NF1 gene is located on chromosome 17.
- Expression of NF1 varies widely within and among families, from mildly affected to severely impaired.
- The course of NF1 is impossible to predict; even a relative's disease will not be an indication of progression.

EPIDEMIOLOGY

- The frequency is 1 in every 3,000 to 4,000 live births.
- NF1 affects 100,000 Americans.
- Occurrence appears to be independent of sex, race, or environmental factors.

COMPLICATIONS

- Oncologic

—Neurofibromas are benign tumors of Schwann cells, nerve fibers, and fibroblasts that arise along the nerves.
—Plexiform neurofibromas occur in approximately 15% of patients with NF1; these are extensive tumors that grow along the nerve root and may invade adjacent structures, threatening vital structures (especially in the neck and throat) or cause gross disfigurement. Approximately 10% of these tumors undergo sarcomatous degeneration.
—CNS tumors include optic nerve/pathway gliomas or gliomas elsewhere in the brain.

- Neurologic: learning disability, language disorders, autism, seizures, retardation, and attention deficit occur with higher than background frequency in NF.
- Renal: hypertension
- Circulatory: moyamoya, stroke
- Endocrine: pheochromocytoma
- Hematologic: leukemia

ASSOCIATED CONDITIONS

- Head circumference greater than the 98th percentile
- Developmental speech delay, motor incoordination, learning disorders, attention-deficit disorder
- Hypertension
- Brain tumor, moyamoya disease
- Sarcoma, leukemia, Wilms tumor, pheochromocytoma
- Headaches, scoliosis
- Abnormalities in growth, hemihypertrophy

Differential Diagnosis

- Café-au-lait spots are most often benign findings unrelated to NF.
- NF2 may resemble NF1.
- NF1 versus NF2: NF2 is also known as central bilateral acoustic NF, a rare disorder characterized by multiple tumors on the cranial and spinal nerves, and by other lesions of the brain and spinal cord.
- NF2 is genetically and clinically distinct from NF1. The NF2 gene is located on chromosome 22.
- The diagnosis of NF2 is made if the individual has the following:

—Bilateral acoustic neuromas OR
—A first-degree relative with NF2 and either
  —A unilateral acoustic neuroma OR
  —Two of the following:
  —Meningioma
  —Glioma
  —Schwannoma
  —Juvenile posterior subcapsular lenticular opacity

- Sotos syndrome features macrosomia, hypertelorism, ventriculomegaly, and cognitive difficulties.
- McCune-Albright syndrome has large café-au-lait spots with irregular margins and polyostotic fibrous dysplasia
- Tuberous sclerosis (TS) may share autosomal-dominant transmission, Café-au-lait spots (CAL), and hypopigmented lesions in common with NF; features distinctive for TS include adenomal sebaceum, cardiac and renal tumors, and prominent epilepsy. Genetic testing for TS may soon be available.

Data Gathering

HISTORY

- A family history is from a first-degree relative, mother, or father of the proband. The disorder shows 100% penetrance.
- Vision: optic path tumors generally occur between the ages of 2 and 6 years.
- Development: learning problems and ADHD are common.
- Seizures: also more common in NF
- Joint/extremity pain: neuropathic pain or abrasion due to neurofibroma
- Back pain: could signal potentially serious cord or root compression
- Headache: hydrocephalus; migraine also common in NF
- Respiratory problems: neurofibromas may encroach upon the airway; sexual development, abnormalities due to hypothalamic disease, psychiatric concerns, and depression are common.

Physical Examination

- Café-au-lait spots are noted at birth or within the first year of life; the macules are generally flush and circular, although they may have jagged edges or areas of hypertrichosis. Café-au-lait spots result from collection of heavily pigmented melanocytes of neural crest origin in the epidermis. The macules will appear for the first 5 years of life and then slow or stop, although they will grow with the child.
- Axillary and inguinal freckling are generally seen by puberty. The freckling is a cluster often seen in the skin folds.
- Lisch nodules are best assessed by slit-lamp examination. The Lisch nodules are small bumps on the iris that do not interfere with vision. They are uncommon during infancy, but by age 20, 99% of NF1 patients will have Lisch nodules.

Neurofibromatosis

- Optic pathway tumors (OPTs) are present in 20% of patients with NF1, although only approximately 20% of those will require intervention. Treatment should be limited to those patients who have uncorrectable visual acuity, a change in visual fields, and/or endocrine abnormalities, or to those patients with lesions that extend to the hypothalamus.
- Bony dysplasias occur in approximately 3% of patients with NF1. Dysplasias frequently occur in the tibia or the sphenoid wing. A pseudarthrosis will occur due to thinning of the long bone and its inability to heal after it breaks.

GENERAL

- Blood pressure
- Review of palpable tumors for extension or "stoney" feel that could signal cancerous change
- Abdominal examination for masses
- Funduscopy and acuity check for evidence of optic pathway tumor
- Neck and spine palpation/mobility
- Reflexes for evidence of nerve root tumor
- Growth parameters (including head circumference) for evidence of hydrocephalus, hypothalamic disturbance
- Scoliosis screen

Laboratory Aids

TESTS

- In some families, the mutation causing NF1 can be detected by DNA testing. DNA-based testing of the NF1 gene is rarely utilized for diagnosis or prenatal diagnosis, because of the difficulty in identifying the individual mutations.
- Renal studies may be indicated for persistent hypertension or difficulty with urine flow.

IMAGING

- Bright areas in cerebral white matter on T2-weighted MRI are common in NF1, and their clinical significance is uncertain. Indications for neuroimaging depend on findings that may warrant it, such as progressive macrocrania, sensory deficits (especially visual), new-onset seizure, and chronic headaches. Some clinicians obtain a scan as a baseline on all new cases, but this is controversial.

Therapy

- Presently, there is no treatment for tumor growth, except surgical interventions; tumors cannot be predicted based on their occurrence in another member of the family with NF. Interventions are palliative and supportive.
- Surgical intervention is performed on those tumors that are medically compromising, painful, or cosmetically disfiguring. Subcutaneous nodules are flesh-colored, raised, pea-like nodules that may be present during childhood; these commonly appear and grow during puberty or pregnancy and do not grow into plexiform tumors.
- Family counseling regarding genetic implications, possible genetic testing using linkage, or, in some cases, mutation testing of the gene neurofibromin.
- Vigilance/anticipatory care regarding common psychological and developmental issues, such as speech delay, incoordination, hyperactivity/attention deficit, and learning disabilities. Early educational assessment and interventions may improve developmental outcome.

Follow-Up

- Anticipatory care issues (see Data Gathering, above) are all pertinent to follow-up: monitoring for the development of tumors, hypertension, and psychological and developmental disabilities.
- Continuous yearly ophthalmologic examinations: Goldman visual field perimetry is suggested in those with any question of an optic nerve tumor. Some practitioners use yearly visual field testing (by an ophthalmologist) in lieu of MRI scanning.
- Orthopedic, oncologic, endocrine, surgery, and plastic surgery consultants may be helpful, depending on individual issues.
- Blood pressure checks are increasingly important in adolescents and adults with NF.
- Deaths have been associated with cancer, heart disease, and strokes, similar to the general population.
- Optimism: natural history studies indicate that people with NF1 can live long, full lives.

PITFALLS

- Macrocrania is a common feature of NF, but growth curve for the head is necessary to determine whether it signifies a concern.
- Regrowth of plexiform neurofibromas: even after apparent total resection, regrowth is common, and should be discussed before surgery.
- The possibility of nerve injury after surgery on plexiform neurofibromas should also be considered with the family/individual before surgery.

Common Questions and Answers

Q: Can neurofibromatosis develop into cancer?
A: Most tumors caused by NF are benign and remain benign (even large tumors). In rare cases, they may become malignant.

Q: My child has NF1. What specialists must he see?
A: Your child should have yearly checkups with a physician familiar with the issues of NF (could be a family physician, pediatrician, child neurologist, or geneticist) who will know when to refer to other specialists. Otherwise, periodic visits to an ophthalmologist with experience in NF is the only routine recommendation.

ICD-9-CM 237.70

BIBLIOGRAPHY

American Academy of Pediatrics Committee on Genetics. Health supervision for children with neurofibromatosis. *Pediatrics* 1995;96:368–372.

Gabriel KR. Neurofibromatosis. *Curr Opin Pediatr* 1997;9(1):89–93.

Gutman DH, Aylsworth A, Carey JC, et al. The diagnostic evaluation and multidisciplinary management of neurofibromatosis 1 and neurofibromatosis 2. *JAMA* 1997;278:51–57.

North KN, Riccardi V, Samango-Sprouse C, et al. Cognitive function and academic performance in neurofibromatosis 1: consensus statement from the NF1 Cognitive Disorders Task Force. *Neurology* 1997;48:1121–1127.

Author: Leah Burke
Sheila Vaughn, 2nd edition

Neutropenia

Database

DEFINITION

A decrease in the number of circulating neutrophils (both segmented and band forms), strictly defined as an absolute total neutrophil count (ANC) of less than 1,500/mm^3. To calculate ANC, multiply the total WBC count by the percentage of segmented neutrophils and band forms. For example: WBC count 5,200 with 15% segs/polys, 4% bands, 76% lymphocytes, 5% monocytes: ANC = 5,200 × [0.15 + 0.04] = 988).

PATHOPHYSIOLOGY

Causes include:

- Decreased production in the bone marrow (congenital and acquired)
- Immune-mediated destruction
- Increased utilization (usually with overwhelming infection)
- Sequestration in the spleen

GENETICS

Some neutropenia syndromes can be inherited (i.e., Kostmann syndrome: autosomal recessive).

EPIDEMIOLOGY

- Normal values for total WBC counts and ANCs vary with age and race.
- African-American children have lower total WBC counts and lower ANCs than do Caucasian children.
- Infants have a higher total WBC count and a higher percentage of lymphocytes in their differential counts.

COMPLICATIONS

- Systemic bacterial infection or localized infections such as cellulitis, labial abscesses, perirectal abscesses, oral mucosal ulceration, thrush

PROGNOSIS

- Varies
- Death from overwhelming infection does occur.
- Neutropenia resulting from infection or drug use is usually short-lived, but the congenital neutropenia syndromes may result in chronic lifelong neutropenia.
- Immune-mediated neutropenia frequently improves with age.

Differential Diagnosis

- Neutropenia associated with infection

—Bacterial: Group B streptococcal disease, tuberculosis, brucellosis, tularemia, typhoid, paratyphoid
—Viral: hepatitis A and B, parvovirus, respiratory syncytial virus (RSV), influenza A and B, rubeola, rubella, varicella, cytomegalovirus (CMV), Epstein-Barr virus (EBV), human immunodeficiency virus (HIV)
—Other: malaria, visceral leishmaniasis, scrub typhus, sandfly fever

- Drug-induced

—Antibiotics: sulfonamides (trimethoprim-sulfamethoxazole is a common offender), penicillin, chloramphenicol (may be irreversible)
—Chemotherapy agents: alkylating agents, antimetabolites, anthracyclines
—Antipyretics: aspirin, acetaminophen (uncommon)
—Sedatives: barbiturates, benzodiazepines
—Phenothiazines: chlorpromazine, promethazine
—Antirheumatic agents: gold, penicillamine, phenylbutazone

- Tumors

—Leukemia
—Solid tumors that invade bone marrow

- Metabolic

—Nutritional: malnutrition, copper deficiency, megaloblastic anemia secondary to folate or vitamin B$_{12}$ deficiency
—Inborn errors of metabolism: hyperglycinemia, isovaleric acidemia, propionic acidemia, methylmalonic acidemia

- Congenital

—Kostmann syndrome (severe congenital neutropenia)
—Cyclic neutropenia (regular oscillations in the number of circulating neutrophils: periodicity every 7–36 days; duration of neutropenia, 3–10 days)
—Chronic benign neutropenia of childhood (diagnosis of exclusion)
—Schwachman-Diamond syndrome (neutropenia and exocrine pancreatic insufficiency)
—Cartilage—hair hypoplasia (neutropenia, dwarfism, abnormal cellular immunity)
—Reticular dysgenesis

- Immunologic

—Neutropenia associated with primary immunodeficiencies (abnormalities in T and B lymphocytes)
—Autoimmune neutropenia: idiopathic (common in childhood; onset usually before age 2 years; diagnosis established by demonstrating antineutrophil antibodies; typically a benign course with resolution within several years; steroids may help in severe cases); Felty syndrome (neutropenia, splenomegaly, and rheumatoid arthritis); secondary to drugs, infection, or rheumatologic process
—Isoimmune neonatal neutropenia

- Miscellaneous

—Hypersplenism
—As part of evolving aplastic anemia (idiopathic, Fanconi anemia, familial aplastic anemia, dyskeratosis congenita)
—Bone marrow infiltration (tumor, osteopetrosis, Gaucher disease)
—Radiation injury

Data Gathering

HISTORY

- Current or recurrent history of fever, skin abscesses, infection, or oral ulceration (helps establish duration of neutropenia)
- Medication use (many medications can cause neutropenia)
- Results of prior CBC with differential (a prior normal WBC count and ANC essentially rule out Kostmann syndrome)
- Symptoms of systemic infection: fever, rash, upper respiratory symptoms, jaundice
- Diet (looking for evidence of nutritional deficiency)
- Family history of neutropenia, recurrent infection, or early death (points to an inherited condition)

Physical Examination

- Fever (temperature should not be taken rectally), tachycardia, and hypotension may indicate systemic infection.
- Oral ulceration, gingival irritation, pharyngitis, thrush
- Cellulitis, perirectal, or labial abscesses
- Hepatomegaly or splenomegaly
- Bruises, petechiae, pallor (other cell lines may be involved)
- Phenotypic abnormalities (thumb anomalies, dwarfism, joint findings)

Laboratory Aids

TESTS

- CBC with differential count (serial testing two to three times a week for 3 to 4 weeks may be necessary to evaluate for cyclic neutropenia)
- Bone marrow aspirate and biopsy [may be normal or may reveal a decrease in the number of myeloid precursors or a maturational arrest of the myeloid line (usually in the later stages), depending on the cause of neutropenia]
- Antineutrophil antibodies (present in autoimmune and isoimmune neutropenia) both on the neutrophils (direct) and in the serum (indirect)
- Cultures

Therapy

GENERAL

- Correction of underlying cause of neutropenia (discontinue drug, treat infection, correct nutritional deficiency)
- Treatment of fever and suspected infection when neutropenic. Initially, broad-spectrum antibiotics are indicated; once the diagnosis has been established, this may not be necessary (i.e., individuals with chronic benign neutropenia).
- Prophylactic antibiotics are not usually beneficial and may predispose to systemic fungal infection.
- Stool softeners may be helpful in the profoundly neutropenic patient at risk for constipation to prevent development of a perirectal abscess.

SPECIFIC

- Hematopoietic growth factors

—Granulocyte colony-stimulating factor (G-CSF): drug of choice for Kostmann syndrome
—Granulocyte-macrophage colony-stimulating factor (GM-CSF)

- Granulocyte transfusions (rarely indicated)
- Corticosteroids and/or plasmapheresis (most helpful in immune-mediated neutropenia)
- No therapy may be required if neutropenia is not severe and there are no serious or recurrent infections (often the case in autoimmune neutropenia and chronic benign neutropenia).

Follow-Up

- CBCs and physical examinations at regular intervals while the patient is neutropenic
- Management of febrile episodes: prompt evaluation by a physician, obtain blood culture, hospitalize, and treat with intravenous antibiotics

PREVENTION

Neutropenia syndromes are not predictable and thus are not preventable.

ISOLATION OF HOSPITALIZED PATIENT

Isolation would be prudent until the etiology of the neutropenia is identified.

PITFALLS

Factitious causes of a low WBC count:

- Long time period between when blood sample is drawn and when it is tested
- Excessive leukocyte clumping (in presence of certain paraproteins)
- Leukocyte fragility secondary to leukemia or medication use

Common Questions and Answers

Q: Do all episodes of fever and neutropenia require antibiotics?
A: In severe neutropenia syndromes (i.e., Kostmann syndrome) or when the etiology of the neutropenia is unclear, it is prudent to promptly evaluate the child, draw a blood culture, and administer intravenous broad-spectrum antibiotics. Certain neutropenia syndromes are not associated with an increased risk of infection (i.e., chronic benign neutropenia of childhood); children with these syndromes should be evaluated when they have fever but probably do not require intravenous antibiotics if they look well.

Q: Should a child with neutropenia be allowed to go to school?
A: Yes.

Q: Do they need to wear a mask?
A: No.

Q: When should a hematologist be consulted?
A: With any of the following:

- Chronic or profound neutropenia
- History of recurrent skin infections
- When bone marrow examination is indicated
- When hematopoietic growth factors, plasmapheresis, or granulocyte transfusion are being considered

ICD-9-CM 288.0

BIBLIOGRAPHY

Alexander SW, Pizzo PA. Current considerations in the management of fever and neutropenia. *Curr Clin Topics Infect Dis* 1999;19:160–180.

Bernini JC. Diagnosis and management of chronic neutropenia during childhood. *Pediatr Clin North Am* 1996;43:773–792.

Calhoun DA, Christensen RD. Recent advances in the pathogenesis and treatment of nonimmune neutropenia in the neonate. *Curr Opin Hematol* 1998;5(1):37–41.

Christensen RD, Calhoun DA, Rimsza LM. A practical approach to evaluating and treating neutropenia in the neonatal intensive care unit. *Clin Perinatol* 2000;27(3):577–601.

Dale DC. Immune and idiopathic neutropenia. *Curr Opin Hematol* 1998;5(1):33–36.

Dinauer MC. The phagocyte system and disorders of granulopoiesis and granulocyte function. In: Nathan DG, Orkin SH, eds. *Hematology of infancy and childhood*. Philadelphia: WB Saunders, 1998.

Hughes WT, Armstrong D, Bodey GP, et al. 1997 guidelines for the use of antimicrobial agents in neutropenic patients with unexplained fever. *Clin Infect Dis* 1997;25(3):551–573.

Rolston KV. New trends in patient management: risk-based therapy for febrile patients with neutropenia. *Clin Infect Dis* 1999;29(3):515–521.

Welte K, Gabrilove J, Bronchud MH, et al. Filgrastim (r-metHuG-CSF): the first 10 years. *Blood* 1996;88:1907–1929.

Author: Cynthia F. Norris

Non-Hodgkin Lymphoma

 Database

DEFINITION

Non-Hodgkin lymphoma (NHL) is a malignant proliferation of cells of lymphocytic or histiocytic lineage that spread in a pattern similar to the migration of normal lymphoid cells.

PATHOPHYSIOLOGY

The exact cause is unknown. In contrast to adult lymphomas, childhood NHL is almost never nodular alone and rarely occurs in peripheral nodal areas.

Pediatric NHL can be divided into three major categories according to the NCI Formulation:

- Small noncleaved-cell lymphomas
—40% to 50% of childhood NHL
—Subdivided into Burkitt and Burkitt-like based on the degree of pleomorphism
—A variety of B-cell markers are usually present (e.g., CALLA, CD20).
—Express surface immunoglobulins, majority bearing IgM of either kappa or lambda light-chain subtype
—Terminal deoxyribonucleotidyl transferase (TdT) is negative.
—Characteristic chromosomal translocation, usually t(8;14), rarely t(8;22) or t(2;8); all translocations involve the c-*myc* proto-oncogene.
- Lymphoblastic lymphomas
—Comprise 30% of childhood NHL
—Predominantly of thymocyte (T-cell) origin: Morphologically identical to acute leukemia T lymphoblasts. Bone marrow involvement of >25% blasts is considered leukemia.
—T-cell lymphomas are positive for TdT and have a T-cell immunophenotype (e.g., CD7).
—Majority lack chromosomal translocations; seldom involve T-cell receptor genes on chromosomes 7 and 14q.
- Large-cell lymphomas
—20% of childhood NHL
—The large noncleaved or cleaved type is of B-cell origin.
—Immunoblastic types are primarily of B-cell origin except for the Ki-1 antigen-positive type (anaplastic), which is of T-cell origin.

EPIDEMIOLOGY

- Third most common childhood malignancy (approximately 12% cancers in children <20 years of age in developed countries)
- Incidence is approximately 1.0 to 1.5 per 100,000 children.
—Higher frequency of endemic Burkitt type in equatorial African countries (10–15 per 100,000 children under 5–10 years of age)
—Incidence increases steadily with age; in children, usually occurs in first two decades of life (unusual <3 years of age)
- Sex: male to female ratio is 3:1

- Genetic predisposition: increased risk in patients with immunologic defects (e.g., Bruton agammaglobulinemia, ataxia-telangiectasia, Wiskott-Aldrich, severe combined immunodeficiency)
- Environmental factors
—Drugs: immunosuppressive therapy and diphenylhydantoin
—Radiation: atomic-bomb survivors and ionizing radiation
—Viruses: Epstein-Barr virus (EBV), human immunodeficiency virus (HIV); EBV present in greater than 95% of cases of endemic Burkitt's versus fewer than 20% cases of sporadic

COMPLICATIONS

- Tumor lysis syndrome
—Combination of hyperuricemia, hyperkalemia, and hyperphosphatemia with hypocalcemia, resulting in uric acid nephropathy that leads to renal failure
—Correct before starting chemotherapy.
- Gastrointestinal obstruction, perforation, bleeding, intussusception
- Inferior vena cava obstruction and venous thromboembolism
- Neurologic (e.g., paraplegia, increased intracranial pressure)
- Superior vena cava (SVC) and superior mediastinum syndrome (SMS)
—Associated with lymphoblastic lymphomas that invade the thymus and nodes surrounding the vena cava and airways
- Massive pleural effusion
- Cardiac tamponade or arrhythmia

PROGNOSIS

Important prognostic factors for outcome include tumor burden at presentation.
- Favorable: stages I and II with primary site being head and neck (nonparameningeal), peripheral nodes, or abdominal site (80% or greater 2-year survival).
- Unfavorable: stage III or IV, parameningeal stage II, stage IV with CNS involvement (worst); incomplete initial remission within 2 months (60%–80% 2-year survival)

 Differential Diagnosis

- Abdominal masses
—Newborns: hydronephrosis, renal cysts, Wilms' tumor, or neuroblastoma.
—Older children: constipation, full bladder, hamartoma, hemangioma, cysts, leukemic or lymphomatous involvement of the liver and/or spleen, Wilms tumor, or neuroblastoma
- Mediastinal masses
—Anterior: masses of thymic origin, teratomas, angiomas, lipomas, or thyroid tumors
—Middle: metastatic or infection-related lesions involving the lymph nodes, pericardial or bronchogenic cysts, esophageal lesions, or hernias
—Posterior: neurogenic tumors (e.g., neuroblastoma, ganglioneuroma, neurofibroma), enterogenous cysts, thoracic meningocele, or hernias

 Data Gathering

A diagnosis needs to be made expeditiously, as pediatric lymphomas generally have a rapid growth rate.

HISTORY

- B-cell lymphomas
—Systemic manifestation (e.g., fever, weight loss, anorexia, fatigue) if disseminated; less likely if tumor localized
—Lump in neck that does not respond to antibiotics
—Abdominal mass with pain, swelling, change in bowel habits, nausea, or vomiting
- T-cell lymphomas
—Mediastinal tumor symptoms include cough, hoarseness, dyspnea, orthopnea and chest pain, anxiety, confusion, lethargy, headache, distorted vision, syncope, and a sense of fullness in the ears.
—Marrow involvement
—Bleeding and/or bruising, bone pain, pallor, fatigue

 Physical Examination

- Small non–cleaved-cell lymphomas
—Intraabdominal mass (up to 90%): involving ileocecal region, appendix, ascending colon, or some combination of these sites. Lymphadenopathy may be present in inguinal or iliac region; hepatosplenomegaly. Acute abdomen with intussusception, peritonitis, ascites, and acute GI bleeding. Lymphoma is the most frequent cause of intussusception in children over age 6 years.
—In endemic Burkitt lymphoma, jaw tumors are the most frequent; orbital involvement in infants; abdominal masses in 50%.
—Other sites: testis, unilateral tonsil hypertrophy, peripheral lymph nodes, parotid gland, skin, bone, CNS, and marrow
- Lymphoblastic lymphoma
—Mediastinal mass (50–70%) with pleural effusion present with decreased breath sounds, rales, and cough with or without SVC or SMS syndrome. Signs include swelling, plethora, and cyanosis of the face, neck, and upper extremities; diaphoresis; and stridor and wheezing.
—Lymphadenopathy (50–80%) is primarily above the diaphragm.
—Abdominal involvement is uncommon, likely to involve only liver and spleen.
—Cranial nerve involvement is rarely seen.
- Large cell lymphomas
—Sites involved include mediastinum, bone, inguinal nodes, and skin.
—Bone marrow and CNS involvement are rarely found at diagnosis.

Laboratory Aids

TESTS
The diagnosis should be established with the least invasive method possible. A bone marrow aspirate and biopsy may establish the diagnosis without further testing. Fluid from ascites in patients with abdominal disease, or pleural fluid should be obtained for cytology, immunophenotyping and cytogenetics. Biopsy of an enlarged lymph node may be performed.

Laboratory Tests
- CBC
- Liver and renal function studies
- Serum LDH and uric acid
- Adequate surgical biopsy

Imaging
- Abdominal ultrasound
- Chest PA and lateral
- CT scan of chest, abdomen, and pelvis
- Gallium scan
- Bone scan (optional or if gallium scan suggests bone involvement)
- MRI (especially for bone involvement)

Special Tests
- CSF examination
- Peritoneal or pleural fluid examination
- Bone marrow aspiration and biopsy
- Cytogenetics and immunophenotyping of tumor

STAGING
No uniform staging system exists for childhood NHL. The St. Jude Children's Research Hospital staging system is as follows:
Stage I: single-tumor (extranodal) or single-nodal area, excluding mediastinum or abdomen
Stage II: single tumor with regional nodal involvement, two or more tumors or nodal areas on one side of the diaphragm, or a primary GI tract tumor (resected) with or without regional node involvement
Stage III: tumors or lymph node areas on both sides of the diaphragm, any primary intrathoracic or extensive intraabdominal disease (unresectable), or any primary paraspinal or epidural tumors
Stage IV: bone marrow or CNS disease regardless of other sites; marrow involvement defined as 0.5% to 25% of malignant cells.

 Therapy

A multidisciplinary approach is imperative to ensure the best therapy.

RADIOTHERAPY (XRT)
- Radiation adds no therapeutic benefit in children with limited disease.
- Increases both short- and long-term toxicity
- XRT used as emergent treatment for SVC obstruction, CNS, or testicular involvement.

SURGERY
- Performed if total resection can be achieved
- Additional indications: intussusception, intestinal perforation, suspected appendicitis, or serious GI bleeding
- It is important to avoid extensive surgery in patients with NHL.

PRECHEMOTHERAPY MANAGEMENT
Allopurinol, hydration, and urinary alkalinization to prevent tumor lysis syndrome. Monitor uric acid, BUN, creatinine, K^+, Ca^{2+}, and PO_4^-.

CHEMOTHERAPY
- Histology and stage determine choice of a particular protocol.
- Because of a high-conversion rate of lymphomas to leukemias, prophylactic CNS treatment is given (except in patients with totally excised intraabdominal tumor).
- Duration: 6 to 18 months
- Drugs: cyclophosphamide, vincristine, methotrexate (IV + IT), prednisone, daunorubicin, asparaginase, cytarabine, thioguanine, carmustine, hydroxyurea, hydrocortisone, doxorubicin, mercaptopurine, etoposide
- Common side effects: hair loss, myelosuppression with transfusions required, nausea/vomiting

IMMUNOTHERAPY
- Rituximab is a chimeric monoclonal antibody directed against the CD20 antigen, which is almost universally expressed on tumor cells in pediatric B-cell NHL.
- This is a new active agent for patients with lymphoma. It has been used successfully in patients with relapsed/refractory B-cell NHL.
- There is a lack of significant overlapping side effects with the combination of rituximab and conventional chemotherapeutic agents.

MANAGEMENT OF RELAPSE
- Relapse indicates extremely poor prognosis.
- No uniform approach to rescue therapy
- In patients refractory to or relapsing after initial therapy, different chemotherapy combinations may induce a new response, but long-term survival is rarely seen.
- Allogeneic or autologous bone marrow transplant should be considered.
- For patients with chemosensitive relapse, salvage therapy followed by high-dose therapy with stem cell support is recommended, since this may result in prolonged survival.

 Follow-Up

- Patient monitoring weekly to monthly with CBC and examination.
- Radiologic imaging at intervals during and off therapy.
- Monitor for toxicity-related complications

PITFALLS
Late effects from therapy:
- Cardiomyopathy from anthracyclines
- Impaired reproductive function or infertility from alkylating agents
- Second malignant neoplasms from etoposide and alkylators
- Psychological consequences of life-threatening illness

 Common Questions and Answers

Q: Did I do something to cause this?
A: No. The majority of cases are sporadic and not associated with diet, underlying immune dysfunction, or viral illness.
Q: When will my child be "cured"?
A: For patients with small- or large-cell lymphomas, relapse most commonly occurs in the first 10 months. Therefore, a child may be considered cured if he or she remains in remission after the first year off therapy. A patient with lymphoblastic lymphoma is considered cured if he or she remains in remission after about 3 years from onset of therapy.
Q: Is this contagious?
A: No. Siblings may have slightly higher inherent risk than the general population, but they are not at risk from the affected child.

ICD-9-CM 200

BIBLIOGRAPHY
Coiffier B, Haioun C, Ketterer N, et al. Rituximab (anti-CD20 monoclonal antibody) for the treatment of patients with relapsing or refractory aggressive lymphoma: a multicenter Phase II study. *Blood* 1998;92:1927–1932.

Kelly K, Lange B. Oncologic emergencies. *Pediatr Clin North Am* 1997;44(4):809.

Magrath I. Lymphocyte differentiation pathways—an essential basis for the comprehension of lymphoid neoplasia. *J Natl Cancer Inst* 1981;67:501.

Murphy SB, Fairclough DL, Hutchison RE, et al. Non-Hodgkin's lymphomas of childhood: an analysis of the histology, staging and response to treatment of 338 cases at a single institution. *J Clin Oncol* 1989;7(2):186–193.

Pinkerton CR. The continuing challenge of treatment for non-Hodgkin's lymphoma in children. *Br J Haematol* 1999;107(2):220–234.

Shad A, Magrath I. Diagnosis and treatment of non-Hodgkin's lymphoma in childhood. In: Wernik P, Canellos G, Putcher J, eds. *Neoplastic diseases of the blood*, 3rd ed. New York: Churchill Livingstone, 1996:925.

Author: Jill P. Ginsberg
Deborah Kramer, 2nd edition

Nosebleeds (Epistaxis)

 Database

DEFINITION

Epistaxis is bleeding from the nose. Bleeding may be evident anteriorly through the nares or posteriorly through the nasopharynx.

CAUSES

• Inflammation of, or trauma to, the nasal passages account for most nosebleeds:

—Viral upper respiratory infections, allergic rhinitis, bacterial rhinitis
—Nose picking, external trauma, foreign bodies, postsurgical bleeding, chemical or caustic agents/inhalants

• Local structural abnormalities may predispose to epistaxis:

—Rhinitis sicca, or environmental drying of the nasal mucosa, commonly promotes epistaxis (see Common Questions and Answers, below).
—Nasal polyps, telangiectasias, meningoceles, angiofibromas, vascular malformations

• Less commonly, nosebleeds may herald, or accompany, systemic illnesses:

—Hematologic diseases such as leukemias, thrombocytopenias, hemophilias (and von Willebrand disease), and hemoglobinopathies
—Clotting disorders due to infection, hepatic failure, or poisoning/envenomation
—Hypertension

PATHOPHYSIOLOGY

• The nasal mucosa has a rich blood supply originating from both the internal and external carotid arteries.
• Blood vessels of the nasal septum and lateral nasal walls have little anatomic support or protection. The thin mucosal surface is prone to drying.
• Blood vessels of the nose form many plexiform networks. Especially important is Kiesselbach plexus in the anterior nasal septum, the most common site of nosebleeds in children.
• The nose is subject, by position, to traumatic injury.

EPIDEMIOLOGY

• Nosebleeds occur in all ages throughout the year.
• Children aged 2 to 10 years are most commonly affected.
• Nosebleeds are more common in the winter.

COMPLICATIONS

• Nosebleeds are most commonly uncomplicated.
• Rare complications include significant blood loss, airway obstruction, aspiration, and vomiting.

PROGNOSIS

• Uncomplicated epistaxis is most often self-limited or resolves with simple first-aid techniques.
• Refractory or recurrent epistaxis may require more specialized techniques, surgical intervention, and/or otorhinolaryngologic intervention.

ASSOCIATED ILLNESSES

Hemoptysis, hematemesis, or melena may be the presenting concerns in individuals with bleeding from the nasopharynx.

 Differential Diagnosis

Epistaxis is a common event in normal children. A careful history and physical examination should identify those children with unusual predisposing causes for nosebleeds.

 Data Gathering

HISTORY

• Frequency of occurrence
• Persistence of bleeding
• Nose-picking behavior/traumatic injury
• Nasal congestion, discharge, obstruction
• Allergies
• Medications or drugs of abuse (especially cocaine)
• Previous or concurrent bruising or bleeding
• Menstrual history
• Family history of systemic disease or hemorrhagic disorder

 Physical Examination

• Vital signs with blood pressure determination
• Inspection of nose, nasopharynx, and oropharynx
• General examination with attention to lymph nodes, liver and spleen size, rashes, icterus, pallor

PROCEDURE

• Examination of the nose may be facilitated by application of a topical vasoconstricting agent and/or anesthetic agent.
• Anxiety may interfere with examination and treatment of children. Sedation and analgesia may be beneficial in some circumstances.

 Laboratory Aids

TESTS

• Laboratory evaluation is not indicated in healthy children with readily controlled epistaxis from an anterior site.
• Recurrent or refractory nosebleeds, or suspicious findings from the history and physical examination, may warrant a directed laboratory evaluation (such as platelet count, prothrombin and partial thromboplastin times, complete blood count, and/or bleeding time) and/or consultation.

Nosebleeds (Epistaxis)

 Therapy

- Elevate the head of the bed.
- Direct pressure, applied by gently squeezing the nostrils, is usually sufficient to stop most nosebleeds.
- Ice to the nasal dorsum may be combined with application of direct pressure.
- A cotton pledget beneath the upper lip may aid hemostasis by compressing the labial artery.
- Vasoconstricting agents (0.25% phenylephrine, 0.05% oxymetazoline, 1:1,000 epinephrine, or 1–5% cocaine) will help reduce bleeding as well as improve visualization.
- Application of topical thrombin with a cotton swab may be used when direct visualization of the bleeding site is achieved.
- Once identified, an offending vessel may be cauterized with a silver nitrate stick or a swab dipped in trichloroacetic acid.
- An anterior nasal packing with oxycellulose or petroleum jelly gauze may be required to control refractory epistaxis when the site of bleeding cannot be precisely identified.
- Otorhinolaryngologic consultation may be needed for severe nosebleeds or when posterior nasal packing, fracture reduction, and/or surgery are required.
- Parental reassurance is an important, but often neglected, aspect of therapy.

PREVENTION

- Vaporizers, humidifiers, or saline sprays prevent desiccation of the nasal mucosa.
- Petroleum jelly applied to the anterior nasal septum aids healing of inflamed nasal mucosa.
- Antigen avoidance and medical therapy should be used to reduce allergic symptoms.
- Fingernails should be cut short, and nose-picking behavior should be discouraged.
- Protective athletic equipment should be worn.

 Follow-Up

- Nosebleeds are easily controlled and self-limited in most instances.
- Families should be given instructions in basic first aid for nosebleeds, because minor insults, such as sneezing or excessive manipulation, may cause nosebleeds to recur.
- Referral to an otorhinolaryngologist is indicated for patients with specific local abnormalities, such as polyps, tumors, or vascular malformations.
- Severe nosebleeds, recurrent nosebleeds, and/or posteriorly located nosebleeds may warrant evaluation by an otorhinolaryngologist.
- Identification of systemic illness may require referral to the appropriate specialist.
- Postsurgical nosebleeds can be particularly problematic.

PITFALLS

- Blood clots in the nasopharynx should be removed because they may obscure engorged, bleeding vessels.
- Failure to detect a posterior location within the nasal cavity as the source of bleeding may interfere with measures to control bleeding.
- After nasal packing, it is essential to examine the oropharynx to confirm adequate hemostasis.
- Absorbable-type packings should be used, if required, in patients with bleeding disorders. Standard packings are prone to rebleeding upon removal.
- Impregnation of nasal packings with antibiotic ointment reduces the risk of toxic shock syndrome.

 Common Questions and Answers

Q: How should the patient with nosebleeds be positioned?
A: When possible, patients with nosebleeds should be kept erect. The upright position decreases vascular congestion. Recumbent patients may appear to have less bleeding, but this is due to redirection of blood flow through the posterior pharynx.
Q: How does rhinitis sicca contribute to epistaxis, and why does it occur?
A: The nose warms, humidifies, and filters inspired air. Many modern heating systems and air-conditioning units reduce household humidity to unnaturally low levels. Rhinitis sicca is the direct result of inhaling dry air and results in friable nasal mucosa. Turbulent airflow from a septal deformity also promotes drying.

ICD-9-CM 784.7

BIBLIOGRAPHY

Alvi A, Joyner-Triplett N. Acute epistaxis: How to spot the source and stop the flow. *Postgrad Med* 1996;99:83–96.

Guarisco JL, Graham HD III. Epistaxis in children: causes, diagnosis, and treatment. *Ear Nose Throat J* 1989;68:522–538.

Tan LS, Calhoun KH. Epistaxis. *Med Clin North Am* 1999;83:43–56.

Author: Kevin C. Osterhoudt

Obesity

 Database

DEFINITION

Obesity is defined as excess body fat. However, body fat assessment is not easily available and there are no widely recognized age-specific cutoff points for obesity based on body fat. Therefore, body mass index (BMI) is considered an appropriate alternative.

• Children with a BMI above the 95th percentile are considered overweight.
• Children with a BMI between the 85th and the 95th percentile are considered at risk for overweight.
• For international comparisons, the BMI cutoff points of the International Obesity Task Force are recommended.

CAUSES

• Positive energy balance:

—Excessive energy intake: sugar-containing drinks, high-fat food, large portion size
—Excessive inactivity: television, video, and computer games
—Low level of physical activity
—Low resting energy expenditure (controversial)

EPIDEMIOLOGY AND RISK FACTORS

• In the U.S. in 1999, 13% of children ages 6 to 11 years, and 14% of children aged 12 to 19 years were overweight (BMI >95th percentile), which makes overweight status the most frequent pediatric chronic condition.
• Dramatic increase compared to 1971–74, when 4% of children aged 6 to 11 years, and 6% of children aged 12 to 19 years were overweight.
• Risk factors:

—Family history of obesity: shared genetic factors, shared environment
—Female sex
—Low income for European Americans

COMPLICATIONS

Immediate:

• Pulmonary: asthma, sleep apnea, sudden death
• Endocrine: insulin resistance and type 2 diabetes, hypercholesterolemia, early menarche, polycystic ovarian syndrome
• Hypertension
• Gastroenterologic: gallstones, liver steatosis, liver fibrosis, and cirrhosis
• Orthopedic: femoral head damage
• Neurologic: pseudotumor cerebri
• Psychosocial: decreased self-esteem, discrimination, depression

Long-term, all of the above as well as:

• Persistence of obesity
• Ischemic heart disease
• Cerebrovascular disease
• Osteoarthritis, gout
• Some cancers
• Increased mortality from all causes in adulthood

PROGNOSIS

• Poor for long-term maintenance of weight loss, but usually better for children than for adults
• Better prognosis for children with good adherence to self-monitoring (see Behavior Modification, below)
• Significant health benefits from modest decrease in BMI, which can be achieved by weight maintenance with normal growth in height
• Importance of realistic expectation in treatment to avoid disappointment, decrease in self-esteem, and weight cycling

 Differential Diagnosis

• The overwhelming majority of obesity cases are exogenous. If the child has a height appropriate for his age and parental height, a normal neurologic development and physical examination, with no dysmorphic signs, then an underlying medical disorder is very unlikely.
• The medical conditions that unusually underlie obesity include:

—Down Syndrome
—Prader-Willi syndrome
—Hypothalamic dysfunction
—Brain tumor
—Excessive tube feeding in mental retardation and cerebral palsy
—Cushing syndrome: iatrogenic and spontaneous
—Hypothyroidism
—Hyperinsulinism
—Growth hormone deficiency

HISTORY

• Level of concern, readiness to change, weight loss expectation
• General medical history
• Review of systems, including potential complications (see Complications, Immediate, above)
• Psychosocial history: school, family support, counseling, depression, eating disorders
• Dietary history: 3-day diet record, portion size
• Dietary pattern: number of meals and snacks, eating in front of the television, family meals
• Physical activity: type and duration of physical activity
• Duration of inactivity: television, computer and video games, Internet, telephone

Physical Examination

- Anthropometric measurements: height, weight, BMI, possibly waist circumference, skinfold thickness
- Blood pressure
- General physical examination
- Dysmorphic signs, xanthoma, acanthosis nigricans
- Funduscopic examination

LABORATORY TESTS

- Total cholesterol or lipid profile if family history of hypercholesterolemia or early heart disease (less than 55 years)
- Fasting glucose if risk factors (family history, African American) or acanthosis nigricans
- Thyroid status: TSH, T_4 if short stature
- Genetic studies if clinical signs compatible with an underlying genetic cause

Therapy

- As in other chronic conditions, the objective of the treatment should be to control obesity, and to prevent complications, rather than to eliminate obesity.
- When possible, a multidisciplinary team approach is recommended, including a pediatrician, a nutritionist, a psychologist, and a social worker.
- Family involvement, as well as recognition of the difficulty of weight management, is critical for success.

DRUGS

None presently approved for children. Clinical trials underway.

BEHAVIOR MODIFICATION

- Goal-setting, contracting, reward system
- Self-monitoring of time of inactivity, time of physical activity, sometimes food intake and body weight
- Environmental control to reduce cues and opportunities for energy intake and inactivity and to increase cues and opportunities for physical activity
- Management of high-risk situations, such as parties or vacations
- Improvement of parenting skills

DIETARY CHANGES

- Encourage structured family meal
- Encourage eating slowly
- Eliminate eating or snacking in front of the television
- Eliminate sugar-containing drinks
- Decrease portion size
- Replace high-energy density foods with an increased variety of fruits and vegetables
- Consider the use of the "stoplight diet," where foods are categorized as red (stop), yellow (caution), or green (go), based on their nutrient content (Epstein et al., 1998)
- In cases where a rapid weight loss is necessary, consider the use of a protein-sparing modified fast under medical supervision

PHYSICAL ACTIVITY AND INACTIVITY

- Monitor and limit time of physical inactivity: television, computer and video games, Internet, telephone
- Establish and monitor regular physical activities that the child feels comfortable with and enjoys: family walks, biking, skating, dancing, home exercise, stair climbing, rope skipping, rowing machine, hiking, jogging, snowshoeing, soccer (not goalie), squash, swimming, tennis.
- Establish healthy lifestyles: using stairs, walking to the store, visiting friends rather than talking on the phone

Follow-Up

- Initially frequent, every 4 to 6 weeks
- After healthy habits have been established, less frequent follow-up

Common Questions and Answers

Q: Is childhood obesity due to a slow metabolism or hormonal problems?
A: Hormonal and metabolic causes of obesity are unusual. Most often, obesity is due to exogenous causes, such as physical inactivity and excessive food intake.

Q: Can childhood obesity be treated despite parental obesity?
A: Familial obesity results from a genetic predisposition, but also from a shared environment that can be modified.

Q: How can obesity be prevented in high-risk children?
A: By limiting television watching, establishing healthy lifestyles, regular physical activities, and a healthy balanced diet.

ICD-9-CM

Obesity 278.0
Morbid obesity 278.01

BIBLIOGRAPHY

BMI growth charts: http://www.cdc.gov/nchs/about/major/nhanes/growthcharts/clinical_charts.htm

Cole TJ, Bellizzi MC, Flegal KM, et al. Establishing a standard definition for child overweight and obesity worldwide: international survey. *BMJ* 2000;320: 1240–1243.

Epstein LH, Myers MD, Raynor HA, et al. Treatment of pediatric obesity. *Pediatrics* 1998;101:554–570.

Epstein LH, Paluch RA, Gordy CC, et al. Decreasing sedentary behaviors in treating pediatric obesity. *Arch Pediatr Adolesc Med* 2000;154:220–226.

Epstein LH, Valoski A, Wing RR, et al. Ten-year outcomes of behavioral family-based treatment for childhood obesity. *Health Psychol* 1994;13:373–383.

Kuczmarski RJ, Flegal KM. Criteria for definition of overweight in transition: background and recommendations for the United States. *Am J Clin Nutr* 2000;72: 1074–1081.

Must A, Strauss RS. Risks and consequences of childhood and adolescent obesity. *Int J Obes* 1999;23(suppl 2):s2–11.

Robinson TN. Behavioural treatment of childhood and adolescent obesity. *Int J Obes* 1999;23(suppl 2):s52–57.

Robinson TN. Reducing children's television viewing to prevent obesity: a randomized controlled trial. *JAMA* 1999;282:1561–1567.

Author: Nicolas Stettler

Omphalitis

 Database

DEFINITION

Omphalitis is an infection of the umbilical stump. It begins in the neonatal period as a superficial cellulitis but may progress to necrotizing fasciitis, myonecrosis, or systemic disease.

CAUSES

- Most (85%) cases of omphalitis are polymicrobial.
- Aerobic bacteria are involved in 85% of infections. The most common aerobic organisms include Gram-positive cocci (*Staphylococcus aureus,* group A *Streptococcus*) and Gram-negative enteric bacilli (*Escherichia coli, Klebsiella pneumoniae,* and *Proteus mirabilis*).
- Gram-positive organisms predominated in the past; however, the introduction of antistaphylococcal cord care (triple dye) has led to an increase in colonization and infection with Gram-negative organisms.
- Anaerobic bacteria are isolated in 30% to 39% of infections. The most common anaerobic organisms are *Bacteroides fragilis* and *Clostridium perfringens*.
- *Clostridium tetani* and *Clostridium sordellii* have been reported when deliveries have occurred outside a medical facility and when the cultural practice of placing cow dung on the umbilical stump after delivery was observed.
- Gram-negative organisms are more likely in hospitalized preterm infants compared to term infants (69% vs. 52%).
- Anaerobic organisms are more likely to be isolated from infants with necrotizing fasciitis or myonecrosis than from infants with superficial abdominal wall cellulitis.

PATHOPHYSIOLOGY

- The umbilical stump is normally colonized with potential bacterial pathogens during or soon after birth.
- These bacteria invade the umbilical stump, leading to omphalitis.
- The presence of established aerobic bacterial infection, necrotic tissue, and poor blood supply facilitate the growth of anaerobic organisms.
- Infection may also extend beyond the subcutaneous tissues to involve fascial planes (fasciitis), abdominal wall musculature (myonecrosis), and the umbilical and portal veins (phlebitis).

EPIDEMIOLOGY

- The incidence varies from 0.2% to 0.7% in industrialized countries.
- The incidence is higher in hospitalized preterm infants compared to term infants.
- Episodes of omphalitis are usually sporadic, but rare epidemics have been reported.
- The mean age of onset is day of life 5 to 9 in term infants and day of life 3 to 5 in preterm infants.
- There is no gender difference in the incidence of omphalitis, although males may have a worse prognosis.
- Risk factors for the development of omphalitis include low birth weight, prior umbilical catheterization, septic delivery, and prolonged rupture of membranes.

COMPLICATIONS

- Necrotizing fasciitis, a bacterial infection of the subcutaneous fat, and superficial and deep fascia, complicates 8% to 16% of cases of omphalitis. It is characterized by rapidly spreading infection, often with systemic toxicity.
- Myonecrosis refers to infectious involvement of the muscle. The rapid development of edema may constrict the muscle within its fascia and cause a superimposed ischemic myonecrosis. Extensive areas of necrotic tissue facilitate the growth of anaerobic organisms.
- Portal vein thrombosis or septic embolization may arise from infected umbilical vessels.
- Sepsis complicates omphalitis in 13% of cases.

PROGNOSIS

- The outcome of infants with uncomplicated omphalitis is generally good. The mortality rate among all infants with omphalitis, including those who develop complications, is 7% to 15%. The mortality rate is significantly higher (38–87%) with necrotizing fasciitis or myonecrosis.
- Risk factors for poor prognosis include male gender, prematurity, low birth weight, and septic delivery, including delivery outside a medical facility.

ASSOCIATED DISEASES

- Omphalitis may be the initial manifestation of an underlying disorder of neutrophil migration such as leukocyte adhesion deficiency, a rare immunologic disorder with an autosomal-recessive pattern of inheritance. These infants present with leukocytosis, delayed separation of the umbilical cord, and recurrent infections.
- Omphalitis may also be a manifestation of neutropenia in the neonate.

—In neonatal alloimmune neutropenia, maternal IgG antibodies cross the placenta and result in an immune-mediated destruction of fetal neutrophils bearing antigens that differ from the mother's. The resultant neutropenia can last for several weeks to as long as 6 months. Antineutrophil antibodies are found in the serum of the mother and the infant. Affected infants may also present with other cutaneous bacterial infections, pneumonia, sepsis, and meningitis.

—Causes of neutropenia associated with immune dysfunction include autoimmune neutropenias, X-linked agammaglobulinemia, hyper-IgM immunodeficiency syndromes, and HIV.

—Other causes of neutropenia include metabolic disorders such as hyperglycinemia, isovaleric acidemia, propionic acidemia, methylmalonic acidemia, tyrosinemia, and glycogen storage disease type IB.

- Omphalitis complicated by sepsis can also be associated with neutropenia. Therefore, the underlying disease process producing neutropenia may not be immediately appreciated in affected newborns.
- Rarely, an anatomic abnormality such as a patent urachus or patent omphalomesenteric duct may be present.

 Differential Diagnosis

- The clinical picture of omphalitis is characteristic and the diagnosis is made on clinical grounds. It is important to determine whether associated complications, such as necrotizing fasciitis, myonecrosis, or systemic infection, are present. It is also important to consider an underlying immunologic or metabolic disorder.

 Data Gathering

HISTORY

- A detailed review of pregnancy, labor, delivery, and neonatal course is important.
- Poor feeding or feeding intolerance may be an early indication of infection.
- A history of change in mental status such as irritability, lethargy, somnolence, or decreased level of activity may indicate systemic dissemination of the infection.
- A history of urine or stool discharge from the umbilicus suggests an underlying anatomic abnormality.
- Family history may reveal individuals with metabolic disorders or recurrent infections.

Physical Examination

Physical signs vary with the extent of disease. Signs of localized infection include the following:

- Abdominal tenderness
- Periumbilical edema and erythema
- Purulent or malodorous discharge from the umbilical stump

The following indicate more extensive local disease such as necrotizing fasciitis or myonecrosis:

- Periumbilical ecchymoses or gangrene
- Abdominal wall crepitus
- Progression of cellulitis despite antimicrobial therapy

Signs of systemic disease are nonspecific and include thermodysregulation and evidence of multiorgan dysfunction:

- Fever or temperature instability
- Tachycardia, hypotension, delayed capillary refill
- Apnea, tachypnea, flaring of the alae nasi, grunting, intercostal/subcostal retractions, hypoxemia
- Abdominal distention, diminished bowel sounds
- Cyanosis, petechiae, jaundice
- Lethargy, hypotonia

Laboratory Aids

LABORATORY STUDIES

Test: Umbilical stump Gram stain and culture for aerobic and anaerobic organisms
Significance: Identify potential organisms and antimicrobial susceptibility patterns. While suggestive, cultures of umbilical discharge may reflect only colonization of the stump and are not proof of an etiologic role in the underlying process. Therefore, if myonecrosis is suspected, specimens of muscle should be sent for culture.

Test: Blood culture
Significance: There is a risk of systemic dissemination of infection in the neonate.

Test: Complete blood count
Significance: Neutropenia or neutrophilia may be present. An immature-to-total neutrophils ratio >0.2 is suggestive of systemic infection. Thrombocytopenia may be present.

Test: Prothrombin time, partial thromboplastin time, fibrinogen, fibrinogen split products
Significance: Indicated if sepsis or disseminated intravascular coagulation is suspected.

Test: Lumbar puncture
Significance: Indicated if sepsis is suspected.

RADIOLOGIC IMAGING (CASE DEPENDENT)

Test: Abdominal radiographs
Significance: Portal venous or intramural air require immediate surgical consultation.

Test: Abdominal CT
Significance: Confirms involvement of fascia and muscle and delineates the extent of infection.

Emergency Care

Immediate evaluation, antimicrobial therapy, and supportive care is essential to survival.

Therapy

- A combination of an antistaphylococcal penicillin and an aminoglycoside is recommended due to concern for both Gram-positive and Gram-negative organisms.
- Anaerobic coverage is indicated for complicated infections, including the presence of necrotizing fasciitis or myonecrosis. The addition of metronidazole provides anaerobic coverage. Clindamycin also provides anaerobic coverage and may be substituted for the antistaphylococcal penicillin.
- As with antimicrobial therapy for other infections, consider local antibiotic susceptibility patterns.
- Early and complete surgical debridement of affected tissue and muscle is important. Delay in diagnosis or surgical intervention allows local progression of infection and worsening systemic toxicity.
- The role of hyperbaric oxygen in the treatment of anaerobic necrotizing fasciitis and myonecrosis is controversial. No prospective data are available. The delivery of high concentrations of oxygen to marginally perfused tissues may have a detrimental effect on the growth of anaerobic organisms and improve phagocytic function. However, surgical therapy remains the highest priority.

PREVENTION

- Antimicrobial agents applied to the umbilicus decrease bacterial colonization and prevent omphalitis.
- Effective methods of umbilical cord care include:

—Triple dye daily until cord separation
—Triple dye once and then alcohol daily until cord separation
—Triple dye once and no further treatment
—Povidone-iodine daily until cord separation
—Silver sulfadiazine daily until cord separation
—Bacitracin daily until cord separation
—There are no significant differences in the incidence of omphalitis with these regimens. However, the duration of umbilical cord attachment is significantly longer with triple dye daily compared to the other regimens (17 days vs. 10–13 days).

Follow-Up

- Infants developing associated portal vein thrombosis require follow-up for complications due to portal hypertension.

Common Questions and Answers

Q: Do all infants with omphalitis require IV antibiotic therapy?
A: Yes, the relative immune-compromised status of the newborn infant, the high risk of systemic dissemination of focal bacterial infections, and the morbidity and mortality associated with complicated omphalitis necessitate parenteral antimicrobial therapy, close monitoring of cardiovascular and respiratory stability, and early surgical intervention.

Q: Do all infants who develop omphalitis require evaluation for immunologic disorders?
A: No, particularly if predisposing factors such as an umbilical catheter are present. Infants requiring further evaluation include those with persistent neutropenia, recurrent infections, delayed separation of the umbilical cord, or a family history of immunologic disorders.

Q: Is surgical consultation required for all infants with omphalitis?
A: No, surgical consultation is not required for uncomplicated omphalitis. However, a high degree of suspicion should exist for associated complications. The presence of necrotizing fasciitis or myonecrosis requires immediate surgical consultation.

ICD-9-CM 771.4

BIBLIOGRAPHY

Bradley JS. Wound and deep-tissue infections. In: Jenson HB, Baltimore RS, eds. *Pediatric infectious diseases: principles and practice.* Norwalk: Appleton and Lange, 1995:723–732.

Cushing AH. Omphalitis: a review. *Pediatr Infect Dis J* 1985;4:282–285.

Gladstone IM, Clapper L, Thorpe JW. Randomized study of six umbilical cord regimens. *Clin Pediatr* 1988;27:127–129.

Mason WH, Andrews R, Ross LA. Omphalitis in the newborn infant. *Pediatr Infect Dis J* 1989;8:521–525.

Author: Samir S. Shah

Osteogenesis Imperfecta

 Database

DEFINITION

Osteogenesis imperfecta (OI) is a group of genetically heterogeneous connective tissue disorders affecting bone and soft tissue, causing abnormal fragility of bone, resulting in recurring fractures and deformity.

CAUSES

Abnormality of collagen production and organization; failure of maturation of procollagen to type 1 collagen and failure of normal collagen cross-linking

PATHOLOGY

- In general, both enchondral and intramembranous bone formation are disturbed.

—Osteoid seams are wide and crowded by osteoblasts (woven bone).
—Osteoclasts are normal. Collagen fibrils are disorganized (by EM).

- Physis broad and irregular

—Osteopenia
—Long bones are slender and smaller.
—Fractures (recent or healed)
—Deformities
—Spine: scoliosis, compression fractures, kyphosis
—Skull: multiple centers of ossification, wormian bones

GENETICS

- Sillence classification:

—Type 1: autosomal dominant, blue sclera, onset preschool
   —A: teeth involved
   —B: teeth not involved
—Type II: autosomal recessive, lethal, blue sclera
—Type III: autosomal recessive, severe, normal sclera
—Type IV: autosomal dominant, normal sclera, mild form
   —A: teeth involved
   —B: teeth not involved

- Some cases of OI occur as spontaneous mutations.

EPIDEMIOLOGY

Approximately 1 in 20,000

PROGNOSIS

- In general, the earlier the fractures occur, the more severe the disease.
- For moderate and mild types, there is a gradual tendency to improvement, with the incidence of fractures decreasing after puberty.

 Differential Diagnosis

- Severe: congenital hypophosphatasia, achondroplasia, camptomelic dwarfism
- Mild: cystinosis, pyknodysostosis, child abuse, leukemia, idiopathic juvenile osteoporosis, steroid treatment, rickets in very-low-weight infants, Menkes' kinky-hair syndrome [newborn male (X-linked recessive) with failure to thrive, metaphyseal corner fractures, and abnormal hair]

 Data Gathering

HISTORY

Variable; family history

 Physical Examination

- Severe congenital forms: multiple fractures, limbs deformed and short, skull soft
- Mild and moderate forms

—General: short stature, hernias
—Extremities: bowing, coxa vara deformity, cubitus varus, hypermobility of joints: subluxations and dislocations
—Pelvis: trefoil pelvis, protrusio acetabuli
—Spine (cause: osteoporosis, compression fractures, and ligamentous laxity): kyphoscoliosis (30–40%), platybasia
—Skin: thin skin, subcutaneous hemorrhages, wide surgical scars
—Eyes: blue sclera caused by thin collagen layer, Saturn's ring (white sclera immediately) hyperopia, embryotoxon or arcus juvenilis occasionally, retinal detachment occasionally
—Teeth: dentinogenesis imperfecta, enamel normal, both deciduous and permanent teeth affected, teeth easily broken, discoloration
—Deafness: either conduction or nerve type

Laboratory Aids

TESTS

Blood Tests

- Serum calcium and phosphorus is normal.
- Alkaline phosphatase may be elevated.
- There is no widely available specific laboratory test that is diagnostic of this abnormality.
- Collagen testing is becoming more available.

Radiographs

- Osteopenia
- Fractures: new, healing, or healed; malunions
- Deformity
- Metaphyseal ends of long bones: honeycomb appearance of ends of long bones, popcorn calcifications, Erlenmeyer flask appearance, acetabular protrusio
- Spine: atlantoaxial subluxation, spondylolisthesis, scoliosis, compression fractures

Emergency Care

- For unstable fractures, such as femur fractures
- Depends on location of fracture and details of individual situation

 ## Therapy

DRUGS

None (gene therapy possibly in future). Sex hormones, fluoride, magnesium oxide, calcitonin, and special diets have all been tried; bisphosphonates are being used currently in clinical trials for children with severe involvement.

ORTHOPEDIC

- Fracture treatment: Fractures heal at a normal rate; splinting, orthoses, casting, operations (intramedullary rod)
- Education: fracture prevention is key
- Scoliosis: seen in approximately 50%; orthoses usually ineffective; spinal fusion for curves greater than 50 degrees
- Correction of deformities (e.g., realignment osteotomies with intramedullary fixation most common for long bone deformity)

 ## Follow-Up

PROGNOSIS

- Depends on severity of OI
- Spranger scoring system
- Moderate and mild types: gradual tendency to improvement, with incidence of fractures decreasing after puberty

PITFALLS

- Hyperplastic callus formation may be confused with osteogenic sarcoma.
- Education and injury prevention are key.

ICD-9-CM 756.51

BIBLIOGRAPHY

Minch CM, Kruse RW. Osteogenesis imperfecta: a review of basic science and diagnosis. *Orthopedics* 1998;21(5):558–567, 568–569 (quiz).

Sillence DO. Osteogenesis imperfecta: an expanded panorama of variants. *Clin Orthop* 1981;159:11.

Spanger JW, Cremin B, Beighton P. Osteogenesis imperfecta congenita. *Pediatr Radiol* 1982;12:21.

Tosi LL. Osteogenesis imperfecta. *Curr Opin Pediatr* 1997;9(1):94–99.

Zaleske DJ. Metabolic and endocrine abnormalities. In: Morrissy RT, Weinstein SL, eds. *Lovell and Winter's paediatric orthopaedics*, 4th ed. Philadelphia: Lippincott–Raven, 1996:164–170.

Author: John P. Dormans

Osteomyelitis

 Database

DEFINITION

Osteomyelitis is infection of the bone.

CAUSE

- *Staphylococcus aureus:* causes 90% of osteomyelitis in otherwise healthy children of all ages
- *Streptococcus pyogenes* or *Haemophilus influenzae* can also be the etiologic agent.
- Group B streptococci and *Escherichia coli* are often isolated in children under 1 month of age.
- *Salmonella* can be the cause in children with sickle cell anemia.
- *Pseudomonas aeruginosa* can be found in puncture wounds to the foot.

PATHOLOGY

- Usually, osteomyelitis begins as bacteremia with hematogenous spread to the bone, but direct inoculation of bacteria into the bone by trauma is also possible.
- Most bacteria that enter the bone are phagocytosed, so that no infection develops. When bacteria enter areas of the bone with low blood flow, however, such as the metaphysis directly beneath the physeal plate, they may not be phagocytosed, and an infection may develop.
- The first changes noted in osteomyelitis are the death of the osteoblasts in the infected area and resorption of trabeculae. Inflammation develops, which further compromises blood flow, and microabscesses are formed within the bone. Pus can spread through the bone and between the bone and the periosteum. This pus can lift the periosteum, causing point tenderness.

GENETICS

Increased incidence in patients with sickle cell disease and other immunodeficiencies

EPIDEMIOLOGY

Incidence of 0.016% per year. The femur and tibia are most often affected.

COMPLICATIONS

Permanent damage to the growth plate, septic arthritis, fracture in a weakened bone

 Differential Diagnosis

- Cellulitis
- Septic arthritis
- Inflammatory arthritis or JRA
- Malignancy
- Trauma
- Sickle cell crisis
- Toxic synovitis

 Data Gathering

HISTORY

A child with osteomyelitis usually complains of sudden onset of bone or joint pain and fever. A younger child may refuse to bear weight on or move the extremity that is involved.

 Physical Examination

- Physical examination usually reveals a febrile child with point tenderness over the area of infected bone. The child is often unwilling to move the involved extremity.
- As the infection progresses, swelling, warmth, and erythema of the skin overlying the infection may be noted.
- An infant with osteomyelitis may appear septic.

Laboratory Aids

TESTS

- Patients usually have an elevated white blood cell count and a high sedimentation rate.
- C-reactive protein levels are usually elevated and are useful for monitoring response to therapy.
- Blood cultures are positive in over 50% of patients.
- Aspiration of the infected bone, even in the absence of débridement, is useful to determine the etiologic organism.

IMAGING

- Plain films begin to show the changes of osteomyelitis 10 to 14 days into the infection, with periosteal elevation and bone destruction.
- ^{99}Tc bone scans are 80% accurate, and gallium scans are thought to be 91% accurate in diagnosing osteomyelitis.
- MRI can be useful in defining abscesses and extent and anatomy of bone sequestra; it is also the most useful imaging study to delineate chronic osteomyelitis.

 ## Therapy

- Antibiotic therapy for 4 to 6 weeks is usually required for osteomyelitis. Intravenous oxacillin is usually the empiric drug of choice until an organism can be isolated. Gram-negative coverage should be added for neonates, and *Salmonella* coverage is needed in sickle cell patients. If a recent foot puncture wound was experienced, coverage for *Pseudomonas* is recommended.
- Once the organism is known and sensitivities are established, the patient may be switched to oral antibiotics, as long as the serum bactericidal titer can be maintained.
- If an abscess is present in the bone, surgical débridement may also be necessary.

 ## Follow-Up

Patients should be followed to ensure adequate treatment of infection and continued growth of the extremity involved.

PITFALLS

Delayed diagnosis, difficulty distinguishing osteomyelitis from a sickle cell crisis

 ## Common Questions and Answers

Q: Do you need to surgically débride osteomyelitis?
A: This is a very controversial topic. Many physicians feel that all osteomyelitis should be surgically débrided, while others believe that in the absence of an abscess, antibiotic therapy alone is adequate. Most agree, however, that if an abscess is present, it should be drained.

Q: Will osteomyelitis cause permanent damage in the bone?
A: If the growth plate is not damaged and the infection is adequately treated, there should be no permanent sequelae of osteomyelitis. If the growth plate is damaged, however, the affected limb may not grow evenly, or at all, even after the infection is treated.

Q: Is CRP a more useful laboratory study than ESR for osteomyelitis?
A: The CRP level is known to respond more quickly to changes in the inflammatory state than the ESR, reflecting changes in as short a period as 6 to 8 hours. Studies have shown that the CRP normalizes sooner in osteomyelitis than does the ESR, and studies have also shown that a persistently high CRP is a better indicator than ESR of inadequate therapy, the need for repeated drainage procedures, worsened radiographic appearance, and symptoms of greater duration.

ICD-9-CM 730.2

BIBLIOGRAPHY

Barron SA. Index of suspicion. Case 1. Diagnosis: osteomyelitis. *Pediatr Rev* 1998;19(2):51,52.

Dirschl DR. Acute pyogenic osteomyelitis in children. *Orthop Rev* 1994;May:305–312.

Fink CW, Nelson JD. Septic arthritis and osteomyelitis in children. *Clin Rheum Dis* 1986;12:423.

Roine IR, et al. Serial serum C-reactive protein to monitor recovery from acute hematogenous osteomyelitis in children. *Pediatr Infect Dis J* 1995;14:40–44.

Roy DR. Osteomyelitis. *Pediatr Rev* 1995;16(10):380–384, 385 (quiz).

Wall EJ. Childhood osteomyelitis and septic arthritis. *Curr Opin Pediatr* 1998;10(1):73–76.

Author: Elizabeth Candell Chalom

Osteosarcoma

 Database

DEFINITION

Osteosarcoma is a tumor of the bone composed of spindle cells that produce malignant osteoid.

CAUSES

- The etiology of most cases is unknown.
- There is an association of osteosarcoma with exposure to ionizing radiation.
- Secondary osteosarcoma is seen in up to 5% of patients who received radiation therapy for an initial malignancy.
- Children with hereditary retinoblastoma are at increased risk of developing osteosarcoma with and without prior exposure to radiation.
- Osteosarcoma can arise in patients with Paget disease of the bone, Rothman-Thompson syndrome, enchondromatosis, hereditary multiple exostoses, and fibrous dysplasia.

PATHOLOGY/PATHOPHYSIOLOGY

- Osteosarcoma most often involves the medullary region of bone.
- Two rare clinical subtypes, periosteal and parosteal osteosarcoma, rarely metastasize and carry a better prognosis.
- Rarely, osteosarcoma occurs in soft tissue separate from underlying bone.
- Classic or conventional osteosarcoma, the largest group of osteosarcomas, is composed of connective tissue stroma containing highly malignant spindle-shaped cells as well as areas of osteoid production and calcification.
- Four microscopic subtypes are osteoblastic, chondroblastic, fibroblastic, and telangiectatic. These variants are rare in the pediatric population, and lack prognostic significance at present.

EPIDEMIOLOGY

- Osteosarcoma is the most common malignant bone tumor of childhood, representing 60% of all bone tumors in the pediatric age group.
- Overall, it accounts for less than 1% of all malignant neoplasms.
- Peak incidence is in adolescence and early adulthood, with a median age of 18 at diagnosis. Osteosarcoma is thought to begin during the adolescent growth spurt.
- Approximately 90% of tumors occur at the metaphyseal ends of long tubular bones, but any portion of the skeleton may be involved.
- The most frequent site is the distal femur, followed by the proximal tibia and the proximal humerus.

COMPLICATIONS

Ten percent to 20% of patients have pulmonary metastases at the time of diagnosis; a smaller proportion have metastases to other bones.

PROGNOSIS

The majority of patients with osteosarcoma involving an extremity without pulmonary metastases can be cured. Five-year survival for nonmetastatic disease ranges from 60% to 70%. The following have been associated with a poorer prognosis:

- Pulmonary metastases
- Disseminated bone metastases
- Poor response of the tumor to preoperative chemotherapy
- Inability to achieve a total surgical excision of the tumor

 Differential Diagnosis

- Infection: osteomyelitis, septic arthritis
- Trauma: stress fracture
- Tumors

—Benign: unicameral bone cyst, osteoblastoma, eosinophilic granuloma, giant-cell tumor, aneurysmal bone cyst, osteochondroma
—Malignant: Ewing sarcoma, chondrosarcoma, fibrosarcoma
—Metastatic lesions of other primary tumors

 Data Gathering

HISTORY

- Pain at the site of the tumor is the most common presentation.
- Swelling over the involved area is also reported.
- The duration of symptoms varies.
- A history of recent trauma is common, but unrelated. Trauma often brings the affected area to the patient's or parents' attention, but does not actually cause osteosarcoma.
- Weight loss is rare but may occur in advanced disease.
- If fever is present, it may indicate osteomyelitis rather than osteosarcoma.

 Physical Examination

- A tender, soft tissue mass and increased warmth may be present in the involved area.
- Localized erythema is uncommon.
- Unless there exists an underlying fracture range of motion of the limb is normal and there is no difficulty weight bearing.
- Regional lymphadenopathy is rare.

 Laboratory Aids

TESTS

- Laboratory tests are not generally helpful in osteosarcoma. Serum lactate dehydrogenase (LDH) and alkaline phosphatase may be elevated.
- The prognostic significance of alkaline phosphatase is controversial.
- An elevated WBC or sedimentation rate may suggest osteomyelitis.

IMAGING

- Radiographic examination should include the primary tumor site as well as areas of potential metastases. A chest CT and bone scan should be done to assess for pulmonary and bone metastases.
- A plain radiograph of the involved area always reveals some abnormality. Most commonly, one sees a lytic or blastic region of the bone with ill-defined borders. Other findings may include periosteal elevation adjacent to the primary lesion, a sunburst appearance of the primary lesion caused by neoplastic spicules adjacent to the bony cortex, or a pathologic fracture.
- An MRI should be done to better evaluate the extent of the tumor. It should include the joint above and below the involved bony area. MRI can delineate the intra- and extraosseus extent of the tumor as well as evaluate the neurovascular structures involved.

REFERRAL AND STAGING

- When a malignant bone tumor is suspected, the patient should be referred immediately to a pediatric cancer center. Children's cancer centers can provide the multidisciplinary team needed to diagnose, biopsy, treat and rehabilitate children with bone tumors.
- A staging workup should include a bone scan to look for bone metastases and local skip lesions, as well as a chest x-ray and CT to detect macroscopic pulmonary metastases.
- The diagnosis of osteosarcoma can be confirmed only by a biopsy, which should be done by an experienced pediatric orthopedic surgeon in conjunction with a pediatric oncologist and pediatric pathologist.
- Certain surgical incisions at the time of biopsy may make patients ineligible for limb-sparing procedures.

Osteosarcoma

 Therapy

DRUGS

- At present, therapy incorporates preoperative chemotherapy followed by surgical resection.
- The goals of adjuvant chemotherapy are treatment of pulmonary micrometastases and shrinkage of the primary tumor mass, particularly when limb-salvage procedures are surgical options.
- Groups such as the Children's Oncology Group (COG) have developed chemotherapy protocols for osteosarcoma. The majority of children with osteosarcoma are treated on these chemotherapy protocols.
- The mainstays of treatment are cisplatin and doxorubicin, with many protocols also using high-dose methotrexate and ifosfamide.

—The duration of chemotherapy varies from 8 to 12 months according to the extent of the tumor at diagnosis, tumor response to therapy, and the individual protocol.

SURGERY

In the past, when osteosarcoma was managed by surgery alone, the majority of patients subsequently developed pulmonary metastases and died of progressive disease. Surgical options depend on the primary site of the tumor and the extent of tumor involvement. Complete surgical resection with wide margins is necessary for cure. Surgical options for osteosarcomas of the extremities include:

- Amputation
- Limb salvage with allograft or prosthetic reconstruction
- Rotationplasty

Macroscopic pulmonary metastases should be resected at the time of initial surgery if still visible by radiographic examination. Localized pulmonary recurrences that develop after treatment also should be resected, as this can result in long-term cure or a prolonged symptom-free period.

RADIATION

Osteosarcoma is a radiation-insensitive tumor, but radiation has been used in individual cases.

PHYSICAL THERAPY/REHABILITATION

All patients need to work with specialists to learn how to adapt to their surgically induced disability. The duration of physical therapy and rehabilitation is dependent on the disability and the individual patient's needs.

 Follow-Up

SIGNS TO WATCH FOR

- Wound infections may develop in surgical sites in the initial postoperative period. Significant pain, fever, swelling, discharge, and foul odor from the surgical site should be evaluated, preferably by the surgeon. Poor healing of the surgical site may be a problem, particularly in patients receiving chemotherapy or in those with poor nutrition. May require intravenous antibiotics, supplemental feeding or surgical revision of the wound.
- If prostheses are required, skin breakdown and fitting difficulties with prosthetic devices, such as adjustments for changes in height and weight, should be diagnosed and corrected. Scoliosis and back pain may develop in patients using improperly adjusted crutches and/or prosthetic devices after lower extremity or pelvic procedures. This requires expertise in prosthetic devices for children.
- "Phantom" pain is a normal phenomenon after amputation. Patients and their families should be reassured if this occurs. Sometimes medication can reduce the pain.

All children need to be followed by an oncologist regularly after treatment is completed to monitor for recurrence as well as long-term side effects of the chemotherapy, such as cardiac toxicity, infertility, or secondary malignancy.

 Common Questions and Answers

Q: How does one differentiate osteosarcoma from Ewing sarcoma, the second most common bone tumor of childhood?
A: Ultimately, only a biopsy can differentiate the two. In general, Ewing sarcoma is seen in younger children and tends to affect the axial bones, such as the pelvis. When found in the long bones, it is usually in the diaphyseal regions. Symptomatology does not differ, but Ewing sarcoma is metastatic to the bone marrow, as well as the bones and lungs.

Q: Is there an increased risk of osteosarcoma in the contralateral limb?
A: No.

Q: Does limb salvage incur a greater risk of recurrence than does amputation?
A: Recent studies have shown that there is no increase in recurrence if wide margins are achieved at the time of surgery.

ICD-9-CM 170.9

BIBLIOGRAPHY

Arndt CAS, Crist WM. Medical progress: common musculoskeletal tumors of childhood and adolescence. *N Engl J Med* 1999;341(5): 342–352.

Himelstein BP, Dormans JP. Malignant bone tumors of childhood. *Pediatr Clin North Am* 1996;43(4):967–984.

Rougraff BT, Simon MA, Kneisl JS, et al. Limb salvage compared with amputation for osteosarcoma of the distal end of the femur. A long-term oncologic, functional, and quality-of-life study. *J Bone Joint Surg* 1994;76(5):649–656.

Author: Susan R. Rheingold

Otitis Externa

 Database

DEFINITION

Otitis externa is inflammation or infection of the external auditory canal and/or the auricle. May be categorized as follows:

- **Acute diffuse:** also known as swimmer's ear; usually an acute bacterial infection of the external auditory canal.
- **Acute localized:** also known as furunculosis; usually a local infection of the lateral third of the posterosuperior aspect of the external auditory canal; due to blocked apopilosebaceous units.
- **Chronic:** persistent, low-grade infection and inflammation of the external ear.
- **Eczematous:** encompasses otitis externa due to atopic dermatitis, seborrheic dermatitis, psoriasis, and other inflammatory conditions.
- **Fungal:** occurs more commonly in patients with diabetes mellitus or an immunodeficiency.
- **Malignant:** severe otitis externa; seen more commonly in patients with diabetes mellitus or immunodeficiency; may progress to invasive disease of the surrounding structures.

Infectious agents that cause otitis externa include:

- **Bacteria:** *Pseudomonas aeruginosa, Staphylococcus aureus,* other staphylococcal species, *Streptococcus pyogenes, Streptococcus pneumoniae, Escherichia coli, Haemophilus influenzae, Klebsiella,* and other gram-negative species
- **Fungal:** *Candida albicans, Aspergillus niger, Aspergillus versicolor*
- **Viral:** herpes simplex virus (acute infection and herpes zoster) and varicella

PATHOPHYSIOLOGY

- Cerumen provides an acidic layer, which prevents infection of the external auditory canal. Warm, humid air (i.e., in the summer time) can disrupt the integrity of cerumen.
- Trauma to the squamous epithelium of the external auditory canal or an increase in the pH of the external auditory canal increases the risk of inflammation and infection.
- Cleaning or removal of cerumen, or introduction of water into the canal (i.e., from swimming, playing water sports) can lead to maceration of the canal and the onset of infection.

EPIDEMIOLOGY

- Occurs more commonly in summer months
- 10% of the population has acute otitis externa
- 90% of cases are unilateral
- Risk factors include increased environmental temperature, high humidity, local trauma, and exposure to water with high bacterial counts.

COMPLICATIONS

- Cellulitis of adjacent tissues (facial or auricular)
- Lymphadenitis of upper neck or parotid lymph nodes
- Otitis media and rarely mastoiditis
- Facial nerve neuritis
- Canal stenosis (usually in chronic otitis externa that results in hypertrophy of the canal walls)
- Hearing loss, if there is significant edema of the canal walls

PROGNOSIS

Very good, with rapid response to treatment

 Differential Diagnosis

INFECTIOUS

- Otitis media
- Mastoiditis

TUMORS

- Squamous cell carcinoma
- Basal cell carcinoma
- Acoustic neuroma
- Other metastatic tumors

MISCELLANEOUS

- Foreign body
- Cerumen impaction

 Data Gathering

HISTORY

- Ask about known risk factors, including swimming, ear cleaning, history of atopic or seborrheic dermatitis.
- Has there been any hearing loss, pain that is worse with chewing or activities that result in motion of the ear, pruritus, and/or ear discharge?
- The presence of fever may suggest a more severe infection.

 Physical Examination

- Pain with traction of pinna or with applied pressure to the tragus
- Canal appears macerated with erythema, purulent discharge, and/or edema
- Look for the presence of foreign bodies, including pieces of cotton from cleaning with cotton swabs
- Tympanic membrane should appear intact with normal landmarks. If not, there may be a simultaneous otitis media.
- In cases of fungal infection, "mold" or black or white fungal hyphae with spores may be seen.
- In viral infections, vesicles may be present.
- In eczematous otitis externa, the skin is dry and flaky with crust. Excoriation may be visible as well.
- A somewhat fruity smell can be associated with infections due to *Pseudomonas*.

 Laboratory Aids

- In simple, uncomplicated otitis externa, testing is generally not indicated.
- In more severe infections, recalcitrant infections or immunocompromised patients, bacterial culture with Gram stain and fungal cultures should be obtained. Viral cultures should be considered if there is a vesicular component.
- Herpes has been described as an etiologic agent; therefore, direct fluorescence antibody (DFA) testing for herpes may be helpful.

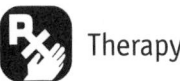 Therapy

GENERAL MANAGEMENT

• Hydrogen peroxide or 3% hypertonic saline may be used to clean the ear. Be sure to use a cotton swab to dry the canal after cleansing.
• Pain can usually be managed with mild analgesics, such as acetaminophen or ibuprofen.
• If there is significant edema of the canal, using ophthalmic drops (which tend to be less viscous than otic drops) in combination with a wick to facilitate introduction of medication into the ear canal may be useful.

SPECIFIC THERAPIES, DEPENDING ON THE PRESENTATION

• Remove foreign body if present
• For acute localized otitis externa (furunculosis), incision and drainage of the abscess in combination with antistaphylococcal penicillins or first-generation cephalosporins.
• For fungal otitis externa, antifungal drops such as clotrimazole 1% solution are used.
• For eczematous otitis externa, appropriate management of the underlying dermatologic condition is appropriate along with the topical application of corticosteroid to the affected parts of the ear.
• For cellulitis, lymphadenitis, or otitis media, oral antimicrobials are used.
• For malignant otitis media or mastoiditis, intravenous antimicrobials and consultation with an otolaryngologist are indicated.
• In the case of chronic otitis externa, surgical intervention is rare, and occurs only when there is failure of long-term medical therapy.
• In the case of malignant otitis externa, or when pseudomonal infection is suspected, an antipseudomonal agent, such as a third-generation cephalosporin should be used.

TOPICAL ANTIBIOTICS/ ANTIINFLAMMATORY AGENTS

• Cortisporin (polymyxin B, neomycin, and hydrocortisone in an acidic medium) otic solution or suspension can be used to treat a simple infection. It is used three to four times a day for 7 to 10 days.
• Other topical agents include gentamicin sulfate drops.

Topical ophthalmic antimicrobial/steroid drops may be tolerated better if there is severe maceration of the canal since they are less acidic.

 Follow-Up

• Reevaluation if there is no symptomatic improvement 24 to 48 hours after starting treatment.
• Fever or progression of symptoms in spite of treatment warrants more aggressive therapy.
• Immunocompromised or relatively immunocompromised patients (i.e., those with diabetes mellitus) should be followed closely—daily or every other day—depending on severity, to ensure improvement.

PREVENTION

• Earplugs that prevent water from entering the ear canal should be used prior to swimming or participation in other water sports.
• Acetic acid drops (which can be made at home with one part vinegar to two parts rubbing alcohol) followed by wicking away moisture with cotton can be used to restore the acidic pH of the ear canal and decrease moisture to prevent otitis externa after swimming.
• Discourage removal of cerumen with vigorous ear cleaning.

 Common Questions and Answers

Q: How should I clean my child's ear?
A: Only the external tragus, pinna, and visible parts of the ear should be cleaned with a cotton ball or washcloth. No foreign object should be placed in the canal.

Q: When can my child swim again?
A: After completion of the prescribed therapy, your child may resume water sports. He/she should use waterproof earplugs and acetic acid drops to prevent another infection.

Q: When should otitis externa be referred to an otolaryngologist?
A: In refractory cases, chronic otitis externa, or persistent hearing loss after treatment, and when there are severe complications (e.g., malignant otitis externa, mastoiditis).

ICD-9-CM 380.10

BIBLIOGRAPHY

Bojrab DI, Bruderly T, Abdulrazzak Y. Diseases of the external auditory canal: otitis externa. *Otolaryngol Clin North Am* 1996;29(5): 761–782.

Cantor RM. Pediatric emergencies: otitis externa and otitis media. A new look at old problems. *Emerg Med Clin North Am* 1995;13(2):445–455.

Hughes E, Lee JH. Otitis externa. *Pediatr Rev* 2001;22(6):191–197.

Mirza N. Otitis externa: management in the primary care office. *Postgrad Med* 1996;99(5):153–158.

Author: Lee R. Atkinson

Otitis Media

Database

DEFINITION
Otitis media refers to inflammation of the middle ear. A distinction is usually made between otitis media with effusion and acute otitis media. Acute otitis media implies that infection is present.

ETIOLOGY
- *Streptococcus pneumoniae:* up to 40%
- Nontypeable *Haemophilus influenza:* 25% to 30%
- *Moraxella catarrhalis:* 10% to 20%
- Other organisms include group A streptococci, *Staphylococcus aureus* and gram-negative organisms, such as *Pseudomonas*. Respiratory viruses are often noted as part of acute otitis media.

PATHOPHYSIOLOGY
- Dysfunction of the eustachian tube is the most important factor.
—The eustachian tube in younger children is shorter, more compliant, and more horizontal than in older children and adults.
—Children with craniofacial anomalies have an increased risk of eustachian tube dysfunction and subsequent otitis media.
- Viral upper respiratory infection often precedes or coincides with acute otitis media. Viral infections may lead to development of otitis by several mechanisms:
—Inducing inflammation in the nasopharynx and eustachian tube
—Enhancing nasopharyngeal bacterial colonization
—Impairing host immune system and increasing susceptibility to secondary bacterial infection
- Interaction of viruses and bacteria may lead to increased inflammation and delay in clearance of bacteria from the middle ear fluid.

GENETICS
- Otitis media is more common in Native-American and Native-Eskimo children.
- Genetic predisposition appears to play a role.

EPIDEMIOLOGY
- Reported frequency of otitis media has increased over the past two decades.
- Increased incidence in those younger than 2 years of age, with the peak at age 6 to 12 months
- More common in fall and winter, and less common in spring and summer
- Risk increased with exposure to large numbers of children (day care). Additive factors include hours spent in child care, number of children, younger age at entry, and center vs. home child care.
- Inverse relationship with breast-feeding duration
- More common in males
- Exposure to environmental tobacco smoke is an independent risk factor.

COMPLICATIONS
Suppurative complications of otitis media much less common with current antibiotic therapy. The recent increase in resistant organisms could lead to a resurgence of suppurative complications.
- Hearing loss—acute conductive hearing loss is common and usually resolves with the effusion. Fluid of long-standing duration may lead to permanent conductive hearing loss. Sensorineural hearing loss may result from spread of infection into labyrinth.
- Tympanic membrane perforation
- Chronic suppurative otitis media
- Tympanosclerosis
- Cholesteatoma
- Acute mastoiditis
- Petrositis
- Labyrinthitis
- Facial nerve paralysis
- Bacterial meningitis
- Epidural abscess
- Subdural empyema
- Brain abscess
- Lateral sinus thrombosis

PROGNOSIS
- Symptoms of acute infection (fever and otalgia) relieved within 24 hours in most patients. Treatment failures more likely with increased severity of disease and younger age.
- Development of another infection within 30 days usually represents a recurrence caused by a different organism rather than a relapse.
- Recurrences are frequent and are more common in younger children and if initial episode is more severe.
- 30% to 70% of treated children will have an effusion at 2 weeks. Middle ear effusion may persist for weeks to months.

Differential Diagnosis

- Other causes of fever including pharyngitis, pneumonia, meningitis, urinary tract infections, and bone and joint infections.
- Pharyngitis and dental pain may be mistaken for otalgia.

Data Gathering

HISTORY
- History of current episode with presence of ear pain, fever, and associated symptoms
- Past medical history, including underlying disorders (e.g., cleft palate, Down syndrome), immune deficiency, and previous history of otitis media
- Recent treatment with antibiotics
- Exposure to large numbers of children (school, day care, large family)

Physical Examination

- Physical exam of the patient should look for other causes of fever and irritability in children: upper respiratory infections, pharyngitis, lymphadenitis, meningitis, urinary tract infection, and bone and joint infections.
- Physical examination of the ear is best done with pneumatic otoscopy.
—The patient should be adequately restrained if uncooperative.
—Cerumen in the canal should be removed if view of tympanic membrane is inadequate.
—The tympanic membrane is visualized still and with gentle positive and negative pressure.
- The presence of a middle ear effusion is determined by the characteristics of the tympanic membrane:
—Contour: normal, retracted, full, or bulging
—Color: gray, pink, yellow, white, or red
—Translucency: translucent or opaque
—Mobility: normal, decreased, or absent
- The presence of a middle ear effusion is suggested by abnormal color, opacification, decreased mobility or visible fluid bubbles. A diagnosis of acute otitis media is suggested if a middle ear effusion is present along with ear pain, erythema, fullness, or bulging.

Laboratory Aids

TESTS
Tympanometry
- A tympanogram is easily performed by office personnel.
- Provides information on middle ear pressure and tympanic membrane compliance
- Sensitive in detecting middle ear effusion, but poor positive predictive value
- May help make follow-up of middle ear effusions more objective

Tympanocentesis
- For episodes of acute otitis media that are resistant to antibiotic therapy, tympanocentesis and culture and sensitivity of the middle ear fluid may help guide antibiotic therapy.
- Tympanocentesis or myringotomy may also be required as part of the treatment of suppurative complications.

Therapy

DRUGS
Note: Since many patients who have physical findings consistent with diagnosis of otitis media may recover without treatment, some experts recommend withholding treatment for 48 to 72 hours before starting antibiotics.

First-Line Therapy

• Amoxicillin (45 mg/kg/d divided t.i.d.) is still the drug of choice for most episodes of acute otitis media. Reasons for this include cost, safety profile, and its activity against the common organisms causing otitis media. Recent FDA approval allows for b.i.d. dosing, which should improve adherence.

• Using higher doses of amoxicillin (80–90 mg/kg/d) will cover many of the moderately resistant strains of *S. pneumoniae*. Increasing the dose of amoxicillin should be considered when the risk of resistant *S. pneumoniae* is increased:
—Children less than 2 years of age
—Recent β-lactam use
—Exposure to day care
—Communities with a high incidence of resistant organisms

• Azithromycin may be used in patients who are allergic to penicillin.

Second-Line Therapy

• Failure of antibiotic therapy may be related to bacterial resistance or a viral etiology. The choice of a second-line antibiotic depends on suspected mechanism of resistance. *H. influenzae* and *M. catarrhalis* produce β-lactamase. *S. pneumoniae* alters penicillin binding proteins.

• In cases where resistant *S. pneumoniae* is likely, treatment with higher doses of amoxicillin (80–90 mg/kg/d) is recommended if not done initially.
—Amoxicillin-clavulanate, cefuroxime axetil, and intramuscular ceftriaxone are also effective against resistant strains.
—The macrolides, cephalosporins, and trimethoprim-sulfa do not provide reliable coverage for resistant *S. pneumoniae*.

• Amoxicillin-clavulanate or a second-generation cephalosporin may be used if *H. influenzae* or *M. catarrhalis* is suspected.

• Intramuscular ceftriaxone is not recommended for routine treatment of otitis media. It may be considered when oral therapy is impossible or when appropriate first- and second-line therapy for *S. pneumoniae* has already failed. When used for treatment of resistant organisms, ceftriaxone 50 mg/kg should be given every 1 to 3 days for three doses.

Duration of Therapy

• Usual duration of therapy is 10 days, but may be shortened to 5 to 7 days in children over 2 years of age who are not otitis-prone.

Adjunctive Therapy

• Fever relief may be provided with acetaminophen.

• Pain may be treated with acetaminophen, ibuprofen, or topical anesthetic drops.

 Follow-Up

• Expect symptomatic improvement within 48 to 72 hours of treatment. May need to switch antibiotic therapy and/or reevaluate for complications.

• Tympanic membrane may appear abnormal for some time after treatment. Initial follow-up exam should be scheduled 3 to 4 weeks after completion of antibiotic therapy. If effusion present, follow monthly. For persistent effusions of more than 3 months duration, a hearing evaluation is recommended.

• Consider ENT referral:
—Persistent otitis media not responding to antibiotic therapy. Tympanocentesis may be helpful.
—Recurrent otitis media with more than four episodes during a respiratory season, especially if earlier in the season. Prior to ENT referral some clinicians recommend prophylactic antibiotic therapy with once-daily amoxicillin.
—Persistent and/or recurrent otitis with abnormal hearing

SIGNS TO WATCH FOR

• Watch for signs of persistent infection including persistent fever, persistent or severe otalgia, or ear discharge.

• Signs of complications include posterior auricular swelling or erythema, headache, and meningismus

PREVENTION

• Breast-feeding protects against otitis media in the first year of life.

• Preventing exposure to environmental tobacco smoke can decrease the risk of otitis media.

• Decreasing exposure to multiple respiratory pathogens by delaying entrance to group child care or choosing settings with fewer numbers of children.

• Vaccines
—Influenza vaccine can decrease incidence of otitis media by preventing the preceding viral illness.
—In addition to preventing invasive disease, conjugated pneumococcal vaccine significantly reduces the risk of otitis media.
—Other vaccines being developed against both viruses and bacteria [*Moraxella*, nontypeable *H. influenzae,* respiratory syncytial virus (RSV)] may help to prevent episodes of otitis media.

 Common Questions and Answers

Q: When should children with otitis media be treated?
A: The presence of a middle ear effusion may occur commonly with an upper respiratory infection. The presence of an effusion is suggested by fluid bubbles or a dull tympanic membrane with decreased mobility. An effusion that is likely to be complicated by infection, and therefore represents acute otitis media, shows significant pressure with a bulging and immobile tympanic membrane. This may be accompanied by fever and ear pain. The presence of infection usually warrants treatment with antibiotics, especially in children less than 2 years of age,

those who are prone to infection, and during the winter season.
Q: What is the current strategy for dealing with resistant *S. pneumoniae*?
A: *S. pneumoniae* develops resistance by alteration of penicillin binding proteins. *H. influenza* and *M. catarrhalis* produce β-lactamase. A previous strategy to deal with these resistant organisms was to use antibiotics resistant to β-lactamase, such as second-generation cephalosporins. This strategy is not effective for resistant strains of pneumococcus. The most effective strategy is to increase the dose of amoxicillin, bringing the concentration of antibiotic in the middle ear fluid above the MIC. These higher doses of amoxicillin, 80 to 90 mg/kg/d, are recommended when initial treatment has failed and resistant organisms are suspected. It is also recommended as initial therapy if resistant strains are likely in the community or in younger children, those in day care, and those treated with β-lactam antibiotics recently.
Q: What can be done to prevent the development of otitis media in an individual child?
A: A number of factors appear to put children at risk for otitis media, including genetic, immune, environmental, and exposure to viral upper respiratory infections. Breast-feeding during the first year of life decreases the risk of otitis media and is recommended. Eliminating exposure to environmental tobacco smoke may also be helpful. Development of upper respiratory infections at an early age is probably the most important factor in the development of otitis media. Limiting the exposure to large numbers of children by delayed entry to child care or by choosing a setting with smaller numbers of children should decrease a child's risk of otitis media.

ICD-9-CM 382.9

BIBLIOGRAPHY

Bluestone CD. Clinical course, complications and sequelae of acute otitis media. *Pediatr Infect Dis J* 2000;19:S37–46.

Butler CC, MacMillan H. Does early detection of otitis media with effusion prevent delayed language development? *Arch Dis Child* 2001;85(2):96–103.

Daly KA, Giebink GS. Clinical epidemiology of otitis media. *Pediatr Infect Dis J* 2000;19:S31–35.

Hoberman A, Paradise JL. Acute otitis media: diagnosis and management in the year 2000. *Pediatr Ann* 2000;10:609–620.

Wetmore RF. Complications of otitis media. *Pediatr Ann* 2000;10:637–646.

Author: William R. Graessle

Pancreatic Pseudocyst

 Database

DEFINITION

Pancreatic pseudocysts, are part of a larger group of pancreatic cysts. These are fluid-containing structures, which result as an exudative reaction to inflammation and do not communicate with the pancreatic ductular system. Pancreatic cysts come in many forms, which include:

- True cysts
- Pancreatic pseudocysts
- Pseudo-pseudocysts
- Pancreatic sequestra
- Primary cystic neoplasms
- Parasitic cysts

Among them, pancreatic pseudocysts are most common and do not have epithelial lined capsule. This discussion addresses only pseudocysts.

PATHOPHYSIOLOGY

- Pancreatic pseudocysts develop when the pancreatic ductular system has been disrupted, resulting in the extravasation of pancreatic exocrine secretions including proenzymes and active enzymes such as amylase, lipase, and ribonucleases.
- These enzymes stimulate an inflammatory reaction, which ultimately leads to the formation of a fibrous capsule, which does not have a true epithelial lining.
- If these cysts remain in communication with the pancreatic ductular system, enzyme and proenzyme levels remain elevated and the cyst will persist.
- A capsule, if present, is not lined by epithelium.
- These cysts usually develop earlier in the course of acute pancreatitis and lack a fully formed fibrous capsule.
- Because there is no ductular communication, the cysts do not have persistently elevated enzyme and proenzyme concentrations.

EPIDEMIOLOGY

- Approximately 30% to 50% of patients with severe pancreatitis develop pseudocysts.
- Pseudocysts are the most common form of pancreatic cyst, accounting for 75% of the pancreatic cystic lesions.
- In children, 60% of pseudocysts form as a result of blunt abdominal trauma (bicycles).
- The second most common etiology is acute pancreatitis. The cyst fluid contains plasma concentration of electrolytes and high concentration of pancreatic enzymes. The cyst forms over a period of several weeks after ductal disruption.
- Approximately 5% to 15% of patients with acute pancreatitis progress to developing a pseudocyst.

PROGNOSIS

The natural history of these cysts is to ultimately resolve over time.

DIFFERENTIAL DIAGNOSIS OF PANCREATIC CYSTS

- Congenital

—Congenital cysts
—Simple cysts
—Polycystic kidney disease
—von Hippel–Lindau

- Infections

—Parasitic
—Echinococcal (hydatid) cyst
—Taenia solium cyst

- Toxic
- Trauma
- Tumor

—Serous cystadenoma
—Cystadenocarcinoma
—Mucinous cystadenoma
—Cystic islet cell tumors
—Cystic teratoma
—Angiomatous cystic neoplasms

- Angiomas

—Lymphangiomas
—Hemangioendotheliomas

- Genetic/metabolic

—Cystic fibrosis

- Inflammatory

—Postinflammatory cystic fluid collections
—Pancreatic sequestrum

- Miscellaneous

—Pancreatic polycystic disease
—Enterogenous cyst
—Endometriosis
—Extrapancreatic cysts
—Paraduodenal duplication cysts
—Splenic cyst
—Adrenal cyst

 Data Gathering

HISTORY

Question: When does one suspect pancreatic pseudocyst?
Significance: Pancreatic pseudocyst formation should be suspected in patients recovering from acute pancreatitis who develop recurrence or persistence of abdominal pain (a presenting symptom in 90% of pseudocyst cases), abdominal mass or elevated pancreatic enzymes.

Question: What is the patient presenting with?
Significance:

- Nausea and vomiting (70%)
- Weight loss (35%)
- Jaundice (10–15%)
- Palpable abdominal mass
- Persistently elevated amylase

Question: Other presenting complaints?
Significance:

- Sepsis from cyst infection
- Splenic or portal vein obstruction leading to portal hypertension.
- Intraabdominal hemorrhage from pseudoaneurysms in adjacent vessels.

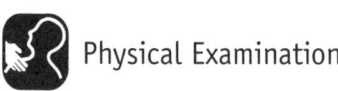 Physical Examination

- Abdominal mass
- Abdominal tenderness
- Lower extremity edema from compression of the inferior vena cava.

Laboratory Aids

- Laboratory evaluations are nonspecific in defining the presence of a pancreatic pseudocyst.
- Many patients will have an elevated serum amylase.
- Radiographic studies
- CT is considered to be the best means of visualizing pseudocysts because it permits a more accurate visualization of the entire pancreas in addition to providing vital information on other intraabdominal structures and a more sensitive means of following the natural history of the pseudocyst.
- Ultrasonography will visualize pancreatic pseudocysts; however, this test is more useful in following patients for changes in cyst size.
- Endoscopic retrograde cholangiopancreatography (ERCP): Though controversial, may be important in decision making concerning additional intervention. ERCP may define whether the pseudocyst is in communication with the pancreatic ductular system, which, if present, many consider to be an indication for an internal drainage procedure. ERCP may also detect other abnormalities of the pancreatic duct or intrapancreatic common bile duct, which will affect the type or extent of procedure performed. ERCP may be performed safely if done within 24 hours of the definitive procedure and with broad-spectrum antibiotic coverage.

Therapy

- Prior to the development of current radiologic procedures, surgical treatment was recommended for clinically detected pseudocysts, and a high rate of serious complications was reported. Currently, approximately half of patients with asymptomatic pseudocysts can be managed safely without any intervention (approximately 60% having complete resolution by 1 year). Factors that must be taken into account when managing patients with pseudocysts include the presence of symptoms, age and size of the pseudocyst, and presence of complications.
- In patients with acute asymptomatic pseudocysts, most surgeons recommend a 4- to 6-week period of observation to permit maturation of the pseudocyst.
- If the pseudocyst remains less than approximately 6 cm, continued period of observation, imaging, and anticipation for complications is justified.

- If the pseudocyst is greater than 6 cm in size and increasing, an internal drainage procedure is indicated. For those patients who develop complications while being observed, an external drainage procedure should be considered. In patients with chronic pseudocysts greater than 6 cm, internal drainage or excision should be considered.
- Nonoperative treatment options include:

—Percutaneous cyst aspiration (which has an overall success rate of approximately 44%)
—Percutaneous catheter drainage (which has an overall success rate of approximately 81%).

- Endoscopic treatment options include endoscopic transmural cystenterostomy and, in those patients where the pseudocyst communicates with the pancreatic duct, transpapillary stent placement. These endoscopic procedures carry the risk of bleeding (especially in patients with pseudoaneurysm formation), retroperitoneal perforation, and infection. To date, there is minimal experience with these techniques in children.

Surgical options include:

- Internal drainage to adjacent organs

—Recurrence rate of 5%
—Mortality of less than 5%
—Cystojejunostomy
—Cystogastrostomy
—Cystoduodenostomy (usually small cysts in the head of the pancreas)

- External drainage

—Recurrence rate of 22%
—Mortality rate of 6%
—Preferred when the cyst is infected or has an immature fibrous capsule
—Development of a persistent pancreatic fistula may occur in approximately 10%

- Excision

COMPLICATIONS

- Infection (incidence reported between 1% and 20% in the literature)

—Infected pseudocysts require immediate, surgical external drainage
—Incidence of approximately 1% to 10% in acute pancreatitis
—Mortality of 80%

- Arterial hemorrhage (incidence of approximately 7%)
- Obstruction (esophagus, stomach, duodenum, jejunum, colon, portal venous system, inferior vena cava, urinary system, biliary tree)
- Rupture (least common, <3%)

Common Questions and Answers

Q: What is the most common cause of pancreatic pseudocyst?
A: Trauma leading to pancreatitis and the subsequent development is the most common.

Q: Which therapy has the lowest incidence of recurrence?
A: Surgical drainage and excision.

ICD-9-CM 577.2

BIBLIOGRAPHY

Canty TG Sr, Weinman D. Management of major pancreatic duct injuries in children. *J Trauma* 2001;50(6):1001–1007.

Gilchrist JA, Broadley PS, Shawis RN. Pancreatic trauma in a child. *Emerg Med J* 2001;18(2):146.

Grace PA, Williamson RC. Modern management of pancreatic pseudocysts. *Br J Surg* 1993;80(5):573–581.

Guelrud M. Endoscopic therapy of pancreatic disease in children. *Gastrointest Endosc Clin North Am* 1998;8(1):195–219.

Howell DA, Elton E, Parsons WG. Endoscopic management of pseudocysts of the pancreas. *Gastrointest Endosc Clin North Am* 1998;8(1): 143–162.

Wyllie R, Hyams J. *Pediatric gastrointestinal disease: pathophysiology, diagnosis, management.* Philadelphia: WB Saunders, 1993.

Yeo CJ, Sarr MG. Cystic and pseudocystic diseases of the pancreas. *Curr Probl Surg* 1994;31(3):165–243.

Author: Dror Wasserman

Pancreatitis

Database

DEFINITION
Pancreatitis, an inflammation of the pancreas, represents a wide spectrum of inflammatory conditions of the pancreas, ranging from severe to mild and even subclinical forms. In addition, pancreatitis may be acute (where pancreatic function and morphology are restored) or chronic (where there is irreversible pancreatic insufficiency). The clinical spectrum includes abdominal pain that is aggravated by eating, nausea, and vomiting.

CAUSES
• In children the most common etiologic factors are trauma, multisystem disease and viral infection, and drugs.
• In 25% of cases of acute pancreatitis, no cause is identified.

PATHOPHYSIOLOGY
Chronic pancreatitis is characterized by progressive and irreversible destruction of the pancreas and leads to exocrine and endocrine pancreatic insufficiency. Chronic pancreatitis leading to strictures, dilatations of the ducts, sclerosis, and destruction of pancreatic acini.

COMPLICATIONS
• The complications of pancreatitis may be divided into local and systemic complications.
• They are associated with significant risk for morbidity and mortality.

LOCAL COMPLICATIONS
• Pancreatic phlegmon/abscess/pseudocyst/hemorrhagic pancreatitis
• Pancreatic ascites

SYSTEMIC COMPLICATIONS
• Pulmonary
—Atelectasis
—Pleural effusion
—Pneumonitis
—ARDS
• Cardiovascular
—Hypotension
—Pericardial effusion
—Myocardial infarction
—Sudden death
—Circulatory collapse
• Hematologic
—Hemoconcentration
—Disseminated intravascular coagulation
• Gastrointestinal
—Paralytic ileus
—Gastritis
—Ulcer
—Upper gastrointestinal bleeding
—Portal vein thrombosis/splenic vein thrombosis/obstruction
• Renal
—Oliguria
—Azotemia
• Neurologic
—Psychosis
—Stupor
—Coma
• Metabolic
—Hyperglycemia
—Hypertriglyceridemia
—Hypocalcemia

Differential Diagnosis

CAUSES
Mechanical/Structural
• Bile reflux
• Outflow obstruction (congenital or acquired, commonly gallstones)
• Trauma (abdominal/child abuse)

Multisystem Disease
• Infection/sepsis
—Bacterial/mycoplasma
—Viral (measles, mumps, Epstein-Barr virus, Coxsackie B, rubella, influenza, echovirus, hepatitis A and B)
—Parasites (*Ascaris lumbricoides, Echinococcus granulosus, Cryptosporidium parvum, Plasmodium falciparum*)
• Shock/hypoxemia
• Hemolytic uremic syndrome
• Crohn disease
• Celiac disease
• Kawasaki disease
• Metabolic
—Hyperlipidemia
—Hypercalcemia
—Uremia
—α_1-Antitrypsin deficiency
—Organic acidemias
• Cystic fibrosis
• Malnutrition/refeeding/bulimia
• Diabetes mellitus
• Mitochondropathy
• Hemochromatosis
• Vasculitis
—Systemic lupus erythematosus
—Henoch-Schönlein purpura
—Kawasaki disease
• Drug
—L-asparaginase, azathioprine, sulfonamides, thiazides, furosemide, tetracyclines, valproic acids, estrogens, procainamide, ethacrynic acid
• Pancreatic and biliary disorders
—Cystic fibrosis
—Pancreatic divisum
—Anomalies of the pancreatic duct
—Cholelithiasis
—Choledochal cyst
—Postendoscopic retrograde cholangiopancreatography (ERCP)
• Toxins
—Alcohol
—Organophosphates
—Yellow scorpion sting
• Unknown
—Hereditary: Recently described genetic mutation on chromosome 7, leading to recurrent acute pancreatitis and cell death. Described in family cohorts and associated with increased risk of development of insulin-dependent diabetes mellitus and pancreatic cancer.
—Idiopathic

PROGNOSIS
• Ranson's criteria can help to assess the severity of the disease. The prognosis in the pediatric age group is good with a low mortality rate even in severe cases.
• Acute pancreatitis rarely progresses to chronic pancreatitis.
• In pediatric populations, the most common etiologies of chronic pancreatitis are hereditary pancreatitis and obstructive pancreatitis secondary to structural anomalies.
• History reveals that repeat episodes of acute pancreatitis, which may also be asymptomatic, may lead to destruction of the pancreas and diminished pancreatic function.
• Pain may exist but is not essential for diagnosis; however, most patients with chronic pancreatitis complain of chronic severe abdominal pain.
• Physical examination is remarkable for weight loss and wasting.
• Laboratory tests may indicate fat and protein malabsorption when the exocrine pancreatic capacity has decreased to approximately 10%.
• Insulin-dependent diabetes mellitus may accompany the diseases, in some cases.

Data Gathering

HISTORY
Question: Abdominal pain?
Significance: In the acute presentation, patients may present with abdominal pain radiating to the back and associated with nausea and vomiting.
Question: Febrile?
Significance: If the patient is febrile, the temperature is usually below 38.5°C. Higher temperatures are suggestive of infection. Special attention should be made to a previous history of episodes of abdominal pain.
Question: History of abdominal trauma?
Significance: Evaluate for history of abdominal trauma and consider the possibility of child abuse.

Physical Examination

Finding: Evaluate for epigastric tenderness, decreased bowel sounds, abdominal distention, tachycardia, hypotension, hypoxemia, and shock in severe cases.
Significance: Complications of pancreatitis.
Finding: Abdominal tenderness, paralytic ileus, ascites, blueish discoloration of the flanks (Grey-Turner sign) or around the umbilicus (Cullen sign).
Significance: Indicate severe necrotizing pancreatitis.
Finding: Auscultation of lungs.
Significance: Other signs include pleural effusion and adult respiratory distress syndrome (ARDS).
Finding: Palpable pancreatic mass
Significance: Suggestive of a pancreatic pseudocyst.

 Laboratory Aids

PROGNOSTIC FACTORS
Test: CBC
Significance: Hemoconcentration or decreased hemoglobin in hemorrhagic pancreatitis. Evaluate for elevated white blood cell count (with left shift).
Test: Glucose
Significance: Transient hyperglycemia
Test: Calcium
Significance: Hypocalcemia (in 15% of patients)
Test: Liver function tests
Significance: Increased liver enzymes and bilirubin
Test: Amylase level
Significance: An elevated serum amylase is most commonly suggestive of pancreatitis; however, increased serum amylase may be associated with other etiologies. The amylase level has low sensitivity and specificity. Measuring the fractionated pancreatic amylase may help to differentiate the etiology of the elevated amylase.

CAUSES OF ELEVATED SERUM AMYLASE
- Pancreatic origin
—Pancreatitis
—Pancreatic tumors
—Pancreatic duct obstruction
—Pseudocyst
—Perforated ulcer
—Bowel obstruction/infarction
—ERCP–postprocedure
- Salivary/others
—Infection (mumps)
—Trauma
—Salivary duct obstruction
—Lung carcinoma
—Ovarian tumor/cysts
—Prostate tumors
- Diabetic ketoacidosis
- Mixed (unknown)
- Cystic fibrosis

- Renal insufficiency
- Pregnancy
- Cerebral trauma
- Burns
- Macroamylasemia

IMAGING
Test: Abdominal radiographs
Significance: May identify ileus, sentinel loop, and colonic dilatation.
Test: Abdominal ultrasound
Significance: Most commonly used and can measure pancreatic size, contour, and echo texture of stones. The measures of these parameters are not accurate and overlap with normal.
Test: CT
Significance: Procedure of choice for evaluating complications of pancreatitis such as pseudocyst and hemorrhagic pancreatitis. CT can also be helpful in providing anatomic information prior to surgery.
- Ranson's criteria are used to define the severity of pancreatitis, risk of systemic complication, and prediction of mortality. These criteria include:
—Age
—White blood cell count on presentation
—Elevated blood glucose
—Elevation of lactate dehydrogenase
—Elevated AST
—Decreased hemoglobin (hemorrhagic pancreatitis)
—Increased BUN
—Hypocalcemia
—Hypoglycemia
—Acidosis
—Hydration status

 Therapy

Supportive care in an intensive care unit and anticipating complications before they occur are the major cornerstones of treatment. Management includes:
- NPO
- Placement of nasogastric tube
- Hyperalimentation (use intralipids only if triglycerides are normal)
- Antibiotic if infection suspected
- Oxygen as needed
- Pain control
- Measurement of vital signs
- Urine output and specific gravity
- Frequent labs
- Intravenous fluids (consider third spacing of intravascular fluids)
- Intravenous colloid and blood products as needed
- Treatment of disseminated intravascular coagulation
- Intravenous H_2 blockade to prevent additional gastrointestinal complications

DURATION
Dictated by the severity of the pancreatitis and clinical improvement of the patient

 Common Questions and Answers

Q: What tests are available for detecting genetic causes of pancreatitis?
A: Cystic fibrosis gene testing and hereditary pancreatitis testing are available on special request or directly through the genetics department at the University of Pittsburgh in Pennsylvania.
Q: What is hereditary pancreatitis?
A: This has been described specifically in families with a strong history of pancreatic cancer, diabetes mellitus, and recurrent pancreatitis. It is a rare diagnosis but must be considered in the right circumstances.
Q: My child has asthma, recurrent sinusitis, and has chronic abdominal pain. Can she have cystic fibrosis?
A: Yes, these is definitely a concern of cystic fibrosis that should be excluded by appropriate genetic and sweat testing.

ICD-9-CM 577.0

BIBLIOGRAPHY
Greenfeld JI, Harmon CM. Acute pancreatitis. *Curr Opin Pediatr* 1997;9(3):260–264.

Hirohashi S, Hirohashi R, Uchida H, et al. Pancreatitis: evaluation with MR cholangiopancreatography in children. *Radiology* 1997;203(2):411–415.

Mader T, McHugh T. Acute pancreatitis in children. *Pediatr Emerg Care* 1992;8(3):157.

Somogyi L, Martin SP, Venkatesan T, et al. Recurrent acute pancreatitis: an algorithmic approach to identification and elimination of inciting factors. *Gastroenterology* 2001;120: 708–717.

Tagge EP, Tarnasky PR, Chandler J, et al. Multidisciplinary approach to the treatment of pediatric pancreaticobiliary disorders. *Surgery* 1997;32(2):158–165.

Weitzman Z. Acute pancreatitis. In: Wyllie R, Hyams JS, eds. *Pediatric gastrointestinal diseases*. Philadelphia: WB Saunders, 1993:873.

Author: Dror Wasserman

Panhypopituitarism

 Database

DEFINITION
Deficiency of multiple pituitary hormones

CAUSES
- Idiopathic
- Congenital
—Absence of the pituitary (empty sella syndrome)
—Pituitary malformations (ectopic posterior pituitary, hypoplastic infundibular stalk)
—Familial panhypopituitarism
- Acquired
—Birth trauma or perinatal insult
—Surgical resection of the gland or damage to the stalk
—Child abuse
- Infection
—Viral encephalitis
—Bacterial or fungal infection
—Tuberculosis
- Vascular
—Pituitary infarction
—Pituitary aneurysm
- Cranial irradiation
- Chemotherapy
- Tumors
—Craniopharyngioma
—Germinoma
—Glioma
—Pinealoma
—Primitive neuroectodermal tumor (medulloblastoma)
—Histiocytosis
—Sarcoidosis

PATHOPHYSIOLOGY
Pathology is based on specific deficiency:
- Growth hormone: hypoglycemia in newborns and poor growth in other patients
- ACTH: hypocortisolism
- TSH: hypothyroidism
- LH/FSH: hypogonadism
- ADH: diabetes insipidus
- Prolactin: hyperprolactinemia

GENETICS
There are rare cases of autosomal-recessive, autosomal-dominant, and X-linked forms.

EPIDEMIOLOGY
Congenital forms affect both sexes equally and are diagnosed at a young age.
The incidence of secondary forms depends on the underlying cause.

COMPLICATIONS
- Hypoglycemia in the newborn period
- Short stature
- Adrenal crisis
- Dehydration

PROGNOSIS
- Prognosis for congenital forms is excellent.
- Prognosis for secondary forms depends on the primary disease.

 Differential Diagnosis

- Hyperinsulinism in newborns
- Isolated growth hormone deficiency in newborns

 Data Gathering

HISTORY
Question: Birth history?
Significance: Hyperinsulinemic infants are typically large for gestational age, which can be associated with shoulder dystocia; hypopituitary babies are not large.

Question: Complications during pregnancy or delivery?
Significance: Birth trauma may be associated with pituitary injury. Breech delivery or vacuum extraction has been associated.

Question: Birth weight?
Significance: Hypopituitary infants are usually normal or small for gestational age in contrast to hyperinsulinemic infants who are typically large.

Question: History of hypoglycemia during the neonatal period?
Significance: Ask about symptoms of lethargy, poor feeding, irritability, or seizures, which could suggest hypoglycemia.

Question: History of surgeries and previous diseases?
Significance: Congenital hypopituitarism is often associated with midline facial defects (such as bifid uvula or cleft palate), which require repair.

Question: Growth pattern?
Significance: Plot previous heights and look for growth pattern. GH deficiency usually manifests as poor linear growth by the end of the first year of life.

Question: Delayed puberty?
Significance: Children with delayed puberty show further growth failure in adolescence. Sense of smell should be assessed to rule out Kallmann syndrome (isolated central hypogonadism and anosmia).

Question: Increased thirst and urination?
Significance: Children with hypothalamic disorders may present with symptoms of diabetes insipidus.

Special Questions

Question: Any complaints of headache?
Significance: Headache can be a symptom of a brain tumor.

Question: Any neurologic signs or symptoms?
Significance: Focal neurologic symptoms are highly suggestive of CNS pathology.

 Physical Examination

Finding: Actual height and weight
Significance: Patients with panhypopituitarism have normal size in the newborn period. Patients with hyperinsulinism are typically large for gestational age.

Finding: Prolonged indirect hyperbilirubinemia
Significance: May be first sign of hypothyroidism. Some state newborn screens will not detect central hypothyroidism.

Finding: Micropenis in males
Significance: Neonatal penis should be at least 2.5 cm in length; micropenis suggests gonadotropic deficiency.

PHYSICAL EXAMINATION TRICKS
Finding: Penile and testicular size
Significance: Measure stretched phallic length (from pubic ramus to glans) with patient lying supine and phallus at 90° to the body; use Prader beads to assess testicular volume.

Finding: Midline defects
Significance: Palpate for submucosal cleft palate.

Finding: Visual field testing
Significance: Visual field defects suggest a brain tumor.

ASSOCIATIONS
- Midline defects (e.g., cleft lip/palate, hypotelorism, single central maxillary incisor)
- Septo-optic dysplasia (de Morsier syndrome)
- Holoprosencephaly

 Laboratory Aids

SPECIFIC TESTS
Test: Liver function tests
Significance: Typically elevated liver enzymes in the newborn period.

Test: Thyroid function tests including free thyroxine (T_4)
Significance: Total T_4 and TSH may be normal, but free T_4 will be low.

Test: TRH stimulation test
Significance: Delayed, normal, or exaggerated TSH response is consistent with a hypothalamic lesion.

Test: Serum IGF-I and IGFBP-3
Significance: May be low but normal growth factors do not exclude GH deficiency in children with brain tumors.

Test: Free thyroxine by equilibrium dialysis
Significance: Must measure, not calculate, the free T_4 concentration in serum.

Test: Growth hormone stimulation tests
Significance: Should be performed by a pediatric endocrinologist, but such testing is seldom indicated clinically.

Test: Cortrosyn stimulation test
Significance: More helpful in the diagnosis of primary adrenal insufficiency than secondary (ACTH) or tertiary (CRH) deficiency.

Test: Metyrapone or CRH stimulation test
Significance: The definitive tests for ACTH or CRH deficiency but must be performed by a pediatric endocrinologist.

Test: Water deprivation test
Significance: The definitive test for ADH deficiency but must be performed by a pediatric endocrinologist.

IMAGING
Test: Bone age
Significance: Typically delayed in GH deficiency or hypothyroidism.

Test: MRI with contrast of brain with fine cuts through the pituitary hypothalamus
Significance: Look for tumors and presence of normal "bright spot" in posterior pituitary.

COMMENTS ON TESTING
Test: Measurement of water intake and urine output over 24 hours at home.
Significance: Can help diagnosis diabetes insipidus.

Baseline serum tests
Can all be done in a nonfasting state.

Stimulation tests
Need to be performed by a pediatric endocrinologist.

 ## Emergency Care

If ACTH deficient, stress dosing of glucocorticoids is necessary

 ## Therapy

DRUGS
• Recombinant human growth hormone (rhGH) by subcutaneous injection daily: 0.3 mg/kg/wk
• Levo-thyroxine orally: 25 to 150 μg daily, based on weight, age, and free thyroxine levels
• Hydrocortisone
—At replacement doses if needed: 8 to 15 mg/m^2/d orally, divided q8h (or three times daily)
—At stress doses for surgery, major illness, vomiting, etc.: 50 to 100 mg/m^2/d IV or PO
—Intravenous doses should be divided q4h; oral stress doses should be divided q8h
—To calculate hydrocortisone dose, estimate body surface area (BSA) using a nomogram or the following formula: BSA (m^2) = ((height (cm) × weight (kg))/3600)
—DDAVP: available in oral and intranasal formulations

DURATION
• Long-term therapy: monitored by a pediatric endocrinologist
• Recombinant human growth hormone (rhGH)
—In children and adolescents:
  —Until growth velocity drops to 0.5 cm/year
  —Once puberty is complete
—In adulthood:
  —GH-deficient adults may benefit from lifelong rhGH therapy due to the impact of GH on body composition, lipid profile, and cardiac function
  —Patient should again undergo GH provocative testing (off rhGH therapy, of course)
• Levo-thyroxine: for life
• Hydrocortisone
—Replacement dose based on individual's need
—Stress dose coverage for life
• DDAVP: for life as needed to control symptoms of polyuria/polydipsia

DIET
There are no restrictions; it is important to know if patient has intact thirst mechanism.

POSSIBLE CONFLICTS WITH OTHER TREATMENTS
There is a theoretical risk that growth hormone might stimulate tumor growth due to its mitogenic effect. Current data generally argue against growth hormone as a tumor stimulant.

 ## Follow-Up

Initially, every 3 months by a pediatric endocrinologist

WHEN TO EXPECT IMPROVEMENT
• Immediately, if hypoglycemic
• Growth velocity should increase within 3 to 6 months
• The growth response to thyroid hormone replacement is slow, but free T$_4$ levels should normalize within 4 to 6 weeks.

SIGNS TO WATCH FOR
• Headache
• Vision problems
• Seizures
• Changes in activity level
• Limp, knee, or hip pain

PITFALLS
• rhGH therapy is associated with idiopathic intracranial hypertension (pseudotumor cerebri), which typically improves whether or not medication is stopped.
• rhGH deficiency/therapy is associated with slipped capital femoral epiphysis (SCFE). Carefully evaluate any limp or knee or hip pain in patients on rhGH therapy. SCFE mandates orthopedic consultation.
• Growth hormone is a mitogenic factor so there has been a theoretical potential for increasing the incidence of leukemia. Clinical studies have not confirmed this hypothesis.

• The family and the patient must understand the importance of taking stress doses of steroid appropriately (e.g., with surgery, vomiting, or febrile illnesses).
• You must consider the diagnosis of panhypopituitarism in patients with hypoglycemic seizures.
• Normal children can fail to respond to growth hormone provocative testing.
• Ordering a TSH level is generally not helpful when evaluating pituitary/hypothalamic causes of hypothyroidism. The unbound thyroxine level (free T$_4$ by equilibrium dialysis) is the most useful test in these cases both to establish the diagnosis and to monitor L-thyroxine replacement therapy.

 ## Common Questions and Answers

Q: When do I give the stress dose of steroid and for how long?
A: Whenever the patient has fever, vomiting, serious illness, or surgery. Continue until 24 hours after stress resolves (e.g., the day after fever breaks or vomiting stops).

Q: What are the chances of cretinism if hypopituitarism is congenital?
A: Minimal, if medication is taken properly.

ICD-9-CD 253.2

BIBLIOGRAPHY
Maghnie M, Cosi G, Genovese E, et al. Central diabetes insipidus in children and young adults. *N Engl J Med* 2000;343(14):998–1007.

McGauley G, Cuneo R, Salomon F, et al. Growth hormone deficiency and quality of life. *Horm Res* 1996;45(1–2):34–37.

Radovick S, Cohen LE, Wondisford FE. The molecular basis of hypopituitarism. *Horm Res* 1998;49(suppl 1):30–36.

Romeo JH. Hyperfunction and hypofunction in the anterior pituitary. *Nurs Clin North Am* 1996;31(4):769–778.

Sklar CA, Constine LS. Chronic neuroendocrinological sequelae of radiation therapy. *Int J Radiat Oncol Biol Phys* 1995;31(5):1113–1121.

Soule SG, Jacobs HS. The evaluation and management of subclinical pituitary disease. *Postgrad Med J* 1996;72(847):258–262.

Weinzimer SA, Homan SA, Ferry RJ Jr, et al. Serum ICF-1 and IGFBP-3 concentrations do not accurately predict growth hormone deficiency in children with brain tumors. *Clin Endocrinol* 1999;51:339–345.

Authors: Robert J. Ferry, Jr. and Paulo F. Collett-Solberg

Parvovirus B19 (Erythema Infectiosum, Fifth Disease)

 Database

DEFINITION

Parvovirus B19 (B19) is a common viral infection of school-aged children that is most commonly associated with an erythematous macular rash in a patient whose appearance remains well.

CAUSES

- B19 is a single-stranded DNA virus, one of the smallest of the human viruses.
- It was first isolated from asymptomatic blood donors in 1975.

PATHOPHYSIOLOGY

- Parvovirus B19 replicates in the red blood cell precursors in the bone marrow and is associated with a number of different diseases ranging from benign to severe.
- There is no practical *in vitro* system for isolation or culture of the virus.

ASSOCIATED DISEASES

- Aplastic crisis secondary to B19 in patients with hereditary hemolytic anemias or any condition that shortens the red blood cell life span, such as sickle cell disease or spherocytosis, may cause severe anemia.
- Fifth disease or erythema infectiosum caused by B19 occurs in up to 35% of school-aged children.
- Human parvovirus arthropathy, symmetrical joint pain, and swelling especially of the hands, knees, and feet, is seen in adults much more frequently than children; among women with B19 infection, 80% to 100% develop polyarthritis.
- Hydrops fetalis may develop following maternal B19 infection and intrauterine involvement.
- Chronic bone marrow failure due to persistent B19 infection in immunocompromised patients has been reported.
- Extremity numbness and tingling, hemophagocytic syndrome, and Henoch-Schönlein purpura has recently been sporadically reported as being associated with B19 infection.

EPIDEMIOLOGY

- Most B19 infections occur in school-aged children.
- Seroprevalence of B19 IgG antibodies:

—<5 years, 2% to 9%
—5 to 18 years, 15% to 35%
—Adults, 30% to 60%

- Route of spread includes exposure to:

—Nasal secretions
—Aerosolized large-droplet respiratory secretions
—Blood (10^{11} virions per mL or serum in patients with hereditary hemolytic anemias)

- Attack rates range from 15% to 60% of susceptibles (i.e., seronegative) will become infected on exposure.
- 40% of susceptible health care workers were infected in a Philadelphia outbreak in 1989.

COMPLICATIONS

- Parvovirus B19 during pregnancy

—Fetal loss or hydrops fetalis may occur if infected with B19 during pregnancy.
—50% of women are susceptible to B19 infection.
—The infection is not a teratogen to the fetus.
—Fetal death occurs in 3% to 9%.
—The greatest risk for B19 infection to affect the fetus exists in the first 20 weeks of gestation.
—There is no indication for elective abortion in cases of maternal infection.
—The risk of fetal death after exposure, if antibody status is unknown, is from 0.05% to 1%.

- Aplastic crisis

—Transfusions may be necessary to treat symptoms of severe anemia.

- Arthritis/arthropathy

—Although most cases of polyarthritis resolve within 2 weeks, persistent symptoms for months to even years (rarely) have been reported.

PROGNOSIS

The prognosis is quite good for all manifestations of B19 infections; in general, they require supportive care only until spontaneous recovery.

 Differential Diagnosis

B19 infection should be considered in all patients with arthritis or viral exanthems with a history and examination that is consistent.

 Data Gathering

HISTORY

Question: Asymptomatic infection?
Significance: May occur in approximately 20% of children and adults.

Question: Erythema infectiosum?
Significance: The most common form of parvovirus infection recognized. The incubation period is 4 to 14 days; prodromal symptoms are mild and include headache, sore throat, lethargy, and low-grade fevers lasting 1 to 4 days. A facial rash that is erythematous (slapped cheeks) is noticed next, which spreads to the body and extremities. The body rash is macular erythematous and lacy appearing. It may become more intense with exercise and may be pruritic. Occasionally, it involves the palms and soles and rarely can be papular, vesicular, or purpuric. It may last for approximately 7 days but can persist more than 20 days. The child is usually unaffected and remains active and playful. Symptoms in adults are similar although often more severe. During the illness, 80% of adults have arthralgias or arthritis.

Question: Aplastic crisis
Significance: Prodromal symptoms in B19-infected children with sickle cell disease or other hereditary hemolytic anemias are nonspecific and consist of fever, malaise, and headache. Laboratory testing confirms the diagnosis.

Question: Chronic marrow suppression
Significance: In immunocompromised patients, B19 infection may persist for months, leading to chronic anemia with B19 viremia. Low-grade fever and neutropenia may accompany anemia.

Parvovirus B19 (Erythema Infectiosum, Fifth Disease)

 Physical Examination

- Fifth disease

—A facial rash that is erythematous (slapped cheeks) is noticed next, which spreads to the body and extremities.
—The body rash is macular erythematous and lacy appearing. It may become more intense with exercise and may be pruritic.
—Occasionally, it involves the palms and soles and rarely can be papular, vesicular, or purpuric.

 Laboratory Aids

The diagnosis of B19 infection depends on recognition of typical symptoms and the following tests:

Test: Specific antibodies
Significance: Presence of specific IgM or IgG antibodies as determined by EIA and/or detection of virus. In patients with symptoms of erythema infectiosum or aplastic crisis, the presence of B19-specific IgM antibodies is diagnostic. IgM- and IgG-specific antibodies are detected in 90% of such patients by 3 to 7 days of illness. B19-specific IgG antibodies persists for years, while specific IgM antibodies begin to fall 30 to 60 days after onset of illness.

Test: Polymerase chain reaction (PCR) techniques
Significance: Immunocompromised patients with chronic marrow may be unable to produce B19-specific IgG or IgM antibodies. In such cases, B19 viral DNA can be detected using nuclear and hybridization or PCR techniques. Such techniques are also useful for detecting infection in fetuses.

Test: Hematocrit and reticulocyte count in patients with aplastic crisis
Significance: Laboratory studies reveal reticulocytopenia, usually with counts of <1%. During the illness, the patient's hematocrit may fall as low as 15%.

 Therapy

- There is no specific therapy for this infection other than supportive care.
- Intravenous immunoglobulin therapy has been given with some success to a few patients with chronic marrow suppression secondary to B19 infection.

PREVENTION INFECTION CONTROL

In the hospital environment, secondary attack rates approaching 40% were reported in susceptive health care workers exposed to two children with sickle cell disease and unsuspected B19 infections. In response, all patients with suspected aplastic crisis secondary to B19 should be placed in contact isolation. No measures are needed for normal hosts with rash. In addition, pregnant teachers who are at risk for infections should consider a leave of absence during community outbreaks of B19.

 Follow-Up

EXPECTED COURSE OF ILLNESS

- During aplastic crisis secondary to B19 the reticulocytopenia usually remains low (often <1%) for approximately 8 days before spontaneous recovery.
- The rash of erythema infectiosum in the child or adult may last up to 20 days. It may, at times, fade and/or intensify depending on sunlight exposure, exercise, or body surface temperature changes (bathing).

 Common Questions and Answers

Q: When may children with B19 infection return to school?
A: Children are not infectious when the rash appears. Therefore, they may return to school or day care. The infectious period is only during the prodromal phase of illness, which is often unrecognized.

Q: What can be done to reduce risk of fetal infection?
A: Because B19 infections during pregnancy may result in fetal death, and B19 infections often occur in community outbreaks, fetal risks following maternal exposure to persons with recognized B19 infection are a frequent concern. Among pregnant women of unknown antibody status, the risk of fetal death after exposure to B19 is estimated to be <1.5%. Risk to the fetus appears to be greatest if the infection occurs prior to the 20th week of gestation. Pregnant teachers who are at risk for infection should consider a leave of absence during community outbreaks of B19.

ICD-9-CM 057.0

BIBLIOGRAPHY

Anderson LJ, Tsou C, Parker RA, et al. Detection of antibodies and antigens of human parvovirus B19 by ELISA. *J Clin Microbiol* 1986;24:522–526.

Bell LM. Parvovirus B19 infection: a decade of discovery. In: Long SS, Starr SE, eds. *The report on pediatric infectious diseases.* 1992;2:6.

Bell LM, Naides SJ, Stoffman P, et al. Human parvovirus B19 infection among hospital staff members after contact with infected patients. *N Engl J Med* 1989;321:485–491.

Cherry JD. Parvovirus infections in children and adults. *Adv Pediatr* 1999;46:245–269.

Kerr JR. Pathogenesis of human parvovirus B19 in rheumatic disease. *Ann Rheum Dis* 2000;59(9):672–83.

Török TJ. Parvovirus B19 and human disease. *Adv Intern Med* 1992;37:431–455.

Ware R. Human parvovirus infection. *J Pediatr* 1989;114:343–348.

Author: Louis M. Bell

Patent Ductus Arteriosus

 Database

DEFINITION

• Patent ductus arteriosus (PDA) is the persistence in postnatal life of the normal fetal vascular conduit between the central pulmonary and systemic arterial systems. Normally, the ductus arteriosus (DA) functionally closes by 18 hours of life. Structural closure is usually completed by the third week of life. If the DA remains patent beyond 3 months of life, it is considered abnormal and is unlikely to close spontaneously (spontaneous closure rate 0.6% per year).

• In the infant with a normal left aortic arch, the DA connects the main pulmonary artery at the origin of the left pulmonary artery to the descending aorta, distal of the origin of the left subclavian artery.

• Many variations can occur although they are less common. The main, proximal right or left pulmonary artery may be connected to virtually any location on the aortic arch or proximal portions of the brachiocephalic vessels.

• There are five distinct clinical conditions associated with PDA:

—Isolated cardiovascular lesion in premature infants.

—Isolated cardiovascular lesion in otherwise healthy term infants and children.

—Incidental finding associated with more significant structural cardiovascular defects.

—Compensatory structure in cases of neonatal persistent pulmonary hypertension (PPHN) without congenital heart disease.

—Critical compensatory structure in some cyanotic or left-sided obstructed lesions.

In this chapter only the issue of PDA as an isolated cardiovascular lesion is discussed.

CAUSES

• Prematurity
• Rubella infection in the first trimester
• Genetic or familial factors
• High altitude
• Idiopathic

EPIDEMIOLOGY

• As an isolated defect, PDA is the sixth most common congenital cardiovascular lesion.
• Incidence 1:2,000 (5% of all types of CHD).
• Female/male ratio 2:1
• The incidence increases with the degree of prematurity (15–80% in preterm infants <26 weeks' gestation). The incidence varies significantly depending on management style (e.g., amount of maintenance fluids prescribed, surfactant administration, use of phototherapy), coexisting diseases (e.g., RDS, hypoxemia, fluid overload, NEC, sepsis, hypocalcemia), and environmental factors (altitude).

PATHOLOGY

In premature infants and term infants with PPHN, delayed closure represents an impaired developmental process while in the full-term infant a PDA probably reflects a structural abnormality of the ductal tissue.

PHYSIOLOGY

Fetal blood flows from the MPA to the DA to the aorta, thus bypassing the pulmonary vascular bed and supplying systemic blood flow. With the first postnatal breaths, the pulmonary arteriolar resistance falls abruptly, the DA constricts, and pulmonary blood flow is directed into the lungs. With a PDA, excessive blood flow will continue from the aorta into the pulmonary artery causing pulmonary vascular flooding and volume load on the left side of the heart.

COMPLICATIONS

• Pulmonary edema and congestive heart failure
• Pulmonary hemorrhage
• Pulmonary vascular obstructive disease
• Increased chronic lung disease
• Failure to thrive
• Recurrent respiratory infections
• Lobar emphysema or collapse
• Infective endarteritis
• Thromboembolism of cerebral arteries
• Aneurysm of the ductus
• Intracranial hemorrhage
• Necrotizing enterocolitis
• Renal dysfunction

 Differential Diagnosis

• Aortopulmonary window
• Systemic or pulmonary arteriovenous communications
• Ruptured sinus of Valsalva
• Coronary artery fistula
• Truncus arteriosus
• Venous hum in older children
• Pulmonary atresia with collaterals
• Ventricular septal defect with aortic regurgitation
• Ventricular septal defect in infancy

 Data Gathering

Clinical features depend on:

• The clinical condition associated with the PDA
• The magnitude of the left-to-right shunt
• Anatomic and physiologic features of the PDA in each individual
• Reaction to the increased pulmonary blood flow

HISTORY

Premature Infants

• Variable, ranging from asymptomatic to complete cardiovascular collapse.
• Increased ventilatory support, pulmonary hemorrhage, respiratory or metabolic acidosis from low cardiac output and excessive pulmonary blood flow.
• Tachypnea, feeding intolerance, apnea, bradycardia, necrotizing enterocolitis, and decreased urine output.

Infants and Older Children

• Small PDA: usually asymptomatic with incidental heart murmur found on routine exam.
• Moderate PDA: Possible congestive heart failure, poor feeding, and poor weight gain.
• Large PDA: Symptoms as above and also recurrent respiratory infections.

Patent Ductus Arteriosus

 ## Physical Examination

PREMATURE INFANTS

Findings:

- Tachypnea, rales, tachycardia (±S3 gallop)
- Hyperdynamic precordium and bounding pulses with wide pulse pressure (due to "run off" of the aorta).
- The typical PDA murmur in a premature infant is a pansystolic murmur audible at the left upper or midsternal border.
- With a large PDA and equalization of pressure between the MPA and the aorta, no murmur may be heard.
- Hepatomegaly may exist with heart failure (late sign).

INFANTS AND OLDER CHILDREN

Findings: Varies with size of shunt.

- Small PDA

—A pansystolic murmur may be heard at second left intercostal space. Murmur becomes continuous (i.e., extends into diastole) as the pulmonary vascular resistance decreases over the first months of life.

- Moderate or large PDA

—The murmur is louder, has a harsh quality, and acquires a machinery quality often being heard posteriorly. In that case, a systolic thrill may be felt at the left upper sternal border.
—Tachycardia, bounding pulses with a wide pulse pressure and a mid-diastolic low-frequency rumbling murmur may be audible at the apex in a large PDA.
—With severe left ventricular failure the classic PDA signs may disappear, but there will be findings consistent with CHF (tachycardia, third sound at the apex, hepatomegaly, tachypnea, rales), although this is a very late finding.
—In extreme cases, pulmonary hypertension may occur with the murmur shortening, the diastolic component disappearing, and S2 becoming accentuated. At advanced stages of irreversible pulmonary vascular disease cyanosis begins to appear with reversal of shunting, often more pronounced in the lower limbs.

 ## Laboratory Aids

Test: ECG—usually normal in small PDA; LAE and LVH with moderate and large PDA; biventricular hypertrophy in later stages

Test: Chest x-ray—usually normal with small PDA, although occasionally prominence of main and peripheral pulmonary arteries may be seen. In moderate and large PDA these findings become more pronounced along with an enlarged heart and prominence of the ascending aorta. Increased pulmonary vascular markings are proportionate to the left-to-right shunt. Pulmonary edema can be seen if CHF develops. In premature infants with respiratory distress syndrome there is evidence of deteriorating lung disease with unclear cardiac borders.

Test: ECHO—diagnostic procedure. Delineates the PDA and assesses the size of dilated LA and LV. Doppler techniques assess the ductal flow pattern and may be useful for estimating the pulmonary artery pressure.

Test: Cardiac catheterization—most often not essential for diagnosis; indicated for suspected pulmonary hypertension; also can be performed for treatment via transcatheter closure techniques

 ## Therapy

PREMATURE INFANT

- Supportive treatment (careful use of O_2, respiratory assistance, correction of metabolic acidosis)
- Management of CHF with fluid restriction and diuretics
- If PDA persists despite above management or patient is symptomatic, closure of PDA is indicated.
- Medical closure: indomethacin (or ibuprofen) dosing schedules
- Contraindications to medical management include: renal failure (creatinine >1.8 mg/dL), thrombocytopenia (platelets <100,000), associated conditions (NEC, IVH grade IV)
- Surgical closure indicated if medical treatment fails or use of indomethacin is contraindicated

INFANTS AND OLDER CHILDREN

- Medical management of CHF with digoxin and diuretics.
- Endocarditis prophylaxis for any at-risk procedures.
- Spontaneous closure rate low and response to indomethacin not effective in this group of patients.
- Closure is indicated whenever a symptomatic PDA exists.
- For asymptomatic PDA, the closure can be performed electively after the first year of age and is mainly performed to reduce the risk of endocarditis. Recommendations for closure of an asymptomatic, incidentally found ("silent" ductus) vary by cardiologist.
- Closure of ductus can be achieved by one of three means:

—Open surgical ligation or division
—Videoscopically assisted ligation
—Transcatheter coil occlusion

 ## Follow-Up

PROGNOSIS

- Outcome in treated premature infants is generally good but mostly depends on the degree of prematurity and the presence of associated conditions.
- Outcome in term infants and older children is excellent if no complications have previously occurred or occurred at the time of treatment.
- PDA among adults may be associated with significant mortality with or without surgery.
- Postclosure of PDA no endocarditis prophylaxis is needed if complete obliteration of flow is achieved.

ICD-9-CM 747.0

BIBLIOGRAPHY

Cowley CG, Lloyd TR. Interventional cardiac catheterization advances in nonsurgical approaches to congenital heart disease *Curr Opin Pediatr* 1999;11(5):425–432.

Emmanouilides GC, Riemenschneider TA, Allen HD, et al., eds. *Moss and Adams' heart disease in infants, children and adolescents including the fetus and the young adult.* Baltimore: Williams & Wilkins, 1998:746–765.

Knight DB. The treatment of patent ductus arteriosus in preterm infants. A review and overview of randomized trials. *Semin Neonatol* 2001;6(1):63–73.

Mullins CE. Patent ductus arteriosus. In: Garson A, Bricker TJ, Fisher DJ, et al., eds. *The science and practice of pediatric cardiology*, 2nd ed. Baltimore: Williams & Wilkins, 1998:1181–1197.

Author: Michael P. Mulreany
Lazaros Kochilas, 2nd edition

Pelvic Inflammatory Disease (PID)

 Database

DEFINITION

An ascending, polymicrobial, genital tract infection of sexually active females. It includes an array of inflammatory disorders, including endometritis, parametritis, salpingitis, oophoritis, tubo-ovarian abscess (TOA), peritonitis, and perihepatitis.

PID is a clinical diagnosis. The CDC has established the following clinical criteria. If the following minimum criteria are present and no other cause can be identified, empiric therapy for PID should be initiated in sexually active young women:

- Uterine adnexal tenderness or
- Cervical motion tenderness.

The additional criteria can be used to enhance the specificity of the diagnosis of PID in women with more severe clinical signs:

—Oral temperature higher than $101°F$ ($38.3°C$)
—Abnormal cervical or vaginal mucopurulent discharge
—Presence of white blood cells (WBCs) on saline microscopy of vaginal secretions
—Elevated erythrocyte sedimentation rate (ESR)
—Elevated C-reactive protein (CRP)
—Laboratory documented evidence of infection with *Neisseria gonorrhoeae* or *Chlamydia trachomatis*

- Definitive criteria

—Histopathologic evidence of endometritis on endometrial biopsy
—Transvaginal sonography or other imaging techniques showing thickened fluid-filled tubes with or without free pelvic fluid or TOA
—Laparoscopic abnormalities consistent with PID

ETIOLOGY

Although a polymicrobial infection, cervical infection or vaginal bacterial overgrowth with the following organisms can lead to acute PID:

- *N. gonorrhea* cervicitis
- *C. trachomatis* cervicitis: tends to be associated with less fever, pain, and systemic symptoms than PID due to gonococcus
- Bacterial vaginosis: *Bacteroides, Mobiluncus,* and *Peptostreptococcus* species

PATHOPHYSIOLOGY

- Direct spread of bacteria to ascending structures, via migration, sperm transport, refluxed menstrual blood, or intrauterine device (IUD) string
- Direct migration may be facilitated by menstrual flow, as there is loss of protective cervical mucus
- Microbes invade epithelial cells, mucosa, and serosa, causing inflammation with subsequent scarring
- Adolescents exhibit increased susceptibility due to increased cervical ectopy (more exposed columnar epithelium), relative lack of local immunity, increased high-risk sexual behaviors, and lower compliance with barrier contraceptives.

EPIDEMIOLOGY

- Affects more than 1 million American women per year
- Estimated cost over $4.2 billion per year
- Adolescent cases account for 20% to 30%, and have a 10-fold risk when compared to adults.
- Risk increases with failure to use condoms, the number of lifetime partners, new partners within 3 months, past history of STDs, and the presence of IUD.
- Oral contraceptive (OCP) use decreases the risk of PID, but does not reduce the risks of vaginal or cervical infections.

COMPLICATIONS

- Chronic pelvic pain or dyspareunia
- Ectopic pregnancy: suspicion should be high in any adolescent early in pregnancy with a history of PID
- Infertility: risk increases with number of episodes of PID
- Tubo-ovarian abscess (TOA): occurs in up to one-third of all patients with PID; risk increases with time between infection and treatment; associated with higher mortality and increased rates of infertility and other sequelae
- Fitz-Hugh-Curtis syndrome (perihepatitis) results from tracking of pus along the paracolic gutters yielding inflammation of the hepatic capsule and diaphragm
- Other STDs may occur concomitantly, including HIV, syphilis, trichomoniasis, HSV, or vaginal warts

PROGNOSIS

- Excellent if adequate treatment obtained early and acute complications absent
- One episode is associated with a 13% to 21% risk of infertility, two episodes with a 35% risk, and three or more episodes with a 55% to 75% risk.
- Dyspareunia or chronic pelvic pain has been reported by up to 18% of women treated for PID.
- Long-term sequelae are present in 25% of affected women, with a higher likelihood in adolescents due to later presentation, delay in diagnosis, and inadequate treatment.

 Differential Diagnosis

INFECTION

- Cervicitis
- Vulvovaginal candidiasis, trichomoniasis, or bacterial vaginosis: commonly associated with malodorous discharge originating from vaginal walls
- Tubal ovarian abscess
- Pyelonephritis or cystitis
- Appendicitis, appendiceal abscess
- Tuberculosis
- Viral or bacterial enteritis
- Acute cholecystitis
- Mesenteric lymphadenitis
- Pelvic thrombophlebitis

GYNECOLOGIC

- Dysmenorrhea

- Pregnancy, intrauterine or ectopic
- Ovarian cyst or torsion
- Chronic pelvic pain
- Endometriosis
- Teratoma or other mass

MISCELLANEOUS

- Foreign body or pelvic trauma
- Functional pain

 Data Gathering

HISTORY

Assessment begins with sensitive, private interview with a practitioner who can assure confidentiality.

Question: Review of systems.
Significance: Presentation may be "silent," with relatively few or mild symptoms.
Question: Ask about pain, fever, and gynecologic symptoms.
Significance: Classic presentation of PID includes:

- Lower abdominal pain
- Abnormal vaginal discharge or bleeding
- Fever

Question: Take complete menstrual, sexual, gastrointestinal, and urinary histories.
Significance: Associated symptoms may include:

- Dysmenorrhea
- Dyspareunia
- Vomiting, diarrhea, or constipation

Question: Past medical history, including gynecologic, should be obtained.
Significance: Supportive historical data include:

- Recent menstruation
- Use of IUD or douche
- Inconsistent condom use
- Multiple or new sexual partners
- Prior history of PID

 Physical Examination

- Perform a thorough abdominal exam, noting tenderness, rebound or guarding, and signs of perihepatic involvement

Finding: Pelvic examination
Significance: Document the following:

- Presence of external or vaginal lesions
- Origin, quality, and quantity of discharge (e.g., "copious, mucopurulent cervical discharge," or "scant, thin vaginal discharge")
- Signs of cervical inflammation (e.g., erythema, friability)
- Cervical motion tenderness
- Adnexal tenderness and/or fullness
- Blot away discharge to better assess the source of new fluid accumulation

 Laboratory Aids

SPECIFIC TESTS

- Urine β-HCG, regardless of sexual history

- Complete blood count with differential
- ESR or CRP
- Wet prep of discharge for trichomonads, hyphae, or clue cells
- Gram stain of cervical discharge
- Testing for *N. gonorrhea* and *C. trachomatis*
- Culture is technique dependent, yielding an 80% sensitivity.
- Antigen detection tests (e.g., DFA, ELISA) have lower sensitivities.
- Genetic amplification (LCR) requires a single specimen for both organisms, has a 24-hour turnaround time, and has 90% to 95% sensitivity.
- Syphilis serology (RPR) and HIV testing with appropriate counseling and follow-up
- Test of cure examination and laboratory testing should be done for all patients 6 to 8 weeks after diagnosis.

RADIOGRAPHIC STUDIES
Test: Pelvic ultrasound
Significance: To rule out TOA or other pelvic pathology
Test: Laparoscopy
Significance: Not routinely used, but considered the "gold standard" for diagnosis.

 ## Emergency Care

- TOA rupture, which requires immediate surgical or gynecologic consultation, can present as acute peritonitis.
- If an IUD is in place, it must be removed immediately.

 ## Therapy

Inpatient treatment has been the standard of care, and should be done if:
- Suspected TOA
- Patient has failed outpatient treatment
- Patient is clinically ill or is at high-risk for sequelae
- Patient is immunocompromised or suppressed

When choosing outpatient treatment:
- Repeat bimanual exam must be done within 72 hours of initiating therapy.
- Patient must be compliant with medications and follow-up.
- The patient should be given a full course of doxycycline (or other oral medications) and tolerate the first dose under supervision.
- All patients with PID should receive intensive education about STD prevention.

DRUGS
Inpatient Management
- CDC regimen A:
—Cefotetan (2 g IV every 12 hours) or cefoxitin (2 g IV every 6 hours)
—Plus, doxycycline (100 mg PO twice a day for 14 days)
- Regimen B:
—Clindamycin (900 mg IV every 8 hours)
—Plus, gentamicin (loading dose 2 mg/kg IV or IM, followed by maintenance dose 1.5 mg/kg every 8 hours)

- Alternative parenteral regimens include:
—Ofloxacin (400 mg IV every 12 hours) plus metronidazole (500 mg IV every 8 hours), or
—Ampicillin/sulbactam (3 g IV every 6 hours) plus doxycycline (100 mg IV or PO every 12 hours), or
—Ciprofloxacin (200 mg IV every 12 hours) plus doxycycline (100 mg IV or PO every 12 hours)
—Plus metronidazole (500 mg IV every 8 hours)

The choice between parenteral regimens A or B is based on availability and the drug allergy history of the patient. Data to support the use of alternative regimens are limited.
- Regimen A should be continued for at least 48 hours after clinical improvement, and is followed by the completion of a 14-day course of doxycycline (100 mg PO twice a day).
- Regimen B should be continued for at least 24 hours after clinical improvement, and is followed by completion of a 14-day course of either doxycycline or clindamycin (450 mg PO twice a day).

Outpatient Management
- Regimen A
—Ofloxacin (400 mg PO twice a day for 14 days) (approved for ages >16 years)
—Plus, metronidazole (500 mg PO twice a day for 14 days)
- Regimen B
—Ceftriaxone (250 mg IM once) or cefoxitin (2 g IM with probenecid 1 g PO once) or other parenteral third-generation cephalosporin
—Plus doxycycline (100 mg PO twice a day for 14 days)
- The choice between oral regimens is based on availability, cost, and patient history of drug allergy.

 ## Follow-Up

- For inpatients, substantial clinical improvement should occur within 3 to 5 days if the patient has been properly diagnosed and treated.
- Outpatients should have significant improvement after 48 to 72 hours of treatment.

PREVENTION
- Primary prevention involves early education and aggressive screening for STDs.
- Abstinence and barrier contraceptive use should be advocated and facilitated.
- Screening and treatment of sexual partners should be encouraged and facilitated.

PITFALLS
- Doxycycline lowers the efficacy of oral contraceptives.
- Most bacteriologic studies are technique-dependent. Therefore, the clinician should be trained in the technique for the specific method being used.
- All home pregnancy tests should be repeated.
- Pelvic ultrasound requires a full urinary bladder, unlike transvaginal ultrasound.

- Overzealous education concerning possible sequelae or future infertility may lead to the patient "testing" fertility in the future.

 ## Common Questions and Answers

Q: A patient states she is not sexually active. Should I continue to consider PID?
A: Yes. Because of the risk and severity of sequelae, PID should always be considered. Continue considering alternative diagnoses.
Q: A patient does not meet the criteria for PID; however, it is still the most likely diagnosis. Should I start therapy while other studies are pending?
A: Yes, appropriate therapy for PID may be initiated while other workups are in progress. Delay in therapy results in increased risk of sequelae from PID. When considering other diagnoses, the most life-threatening processes, including ectopic pregnancy, septic abortion, and appendicitis, should be considered first. Always consider ovarian torsion high among the differential diagnoses because it must be corrected in a timely fashion to maintain ovarian function.
Q: An adolescent patient with PID has inquired about fertility. What should I tell her?
A: Many clinicians would argue that an episode of PID could serve as a "wake-up" call to teenagers, inspiring them to abstain or comply with barrier contraception. However, a young woman who is told that she may have impaired fertility might try testing it through unprotected sex. Regardless, information about future sequelae must be given in a sensitive manner, taking into account the young woman's developmental status and her support network.
Q: Does the absence of cervical motion tenderness exclude the diagnosis of PID?
A: No, cervical motion tenderness is one of three major diagnostic criteria that are recommended by the CDC. The presence of all three major, or two major and two minor, criteria is needed to make the clinical diagnosis of PID. If adnexal and abdominal tenderness are present along with two of the minor criteria described above, then the absence of cervical motion tenderness does not exclude the diagnosis of PID.

ICD-9-CM 614.9

BIBLIOGRAPHY
Centers for Disease Control and Prevention. 1998 sexually transmitted disease guidelines. *MMWR* 1998;47(RR-1):79–86.

Pletcher JR, Slap GB. Pelvic inflammatory disease. In: Neinstein LS ed. *Adolescent health care: a practical guide,* 4th ed. Baltimore: Lippincott Williams & Wilkins, in press.

Rome ES. Pelvic inflammatory disease: the importance of aggressive treatment in adolescents. *Cleve Clin J Med* 1998;65:369–376.

Authors: Jonathan R. Pletcher and Kenneth R. Ginsburg

Penile and Foreskin Problems

 Database

DEFINITION

Complaints relating to problems with retracting the foreskin, discharge from the foreskin, and problems relating to circumcision. These are common causes for concern in male infants. The most common diagnoses are listed below.

• Phimosis—two types:

—Physiologic attachment of the prepuce to the glans, which it protects and gradually separates from as desquamated cells (smegma) accumulate and separate the two layers
—Ring of fibrotic scar tissue that which prevents the foreskin, which has already separated from the glans, from being retracted.

• This probably results from recurrent bouts of irritation of the foreskin from improper hygiene habits such as voiding through the foreskin.
• It is important that all parents of uncircumcised boys teach them proper hygiene habits during potty training.
• Penile adhesions—Attachments of the foreskin back to the glans after circumcision.

—Physiologic adhesions, where the prepuce has stuck back down onto the glans after it was separated during the circumcision
—Surgical adhesions, between the raw surface where the foreskin was removed (the junction between the inner preputial skin and the skin of the penis) and the glans.

• Sometimes referred to as skin bridges
• Meatal stenosis—narrowing of the urethral meatus due to recurrent irritation of the meatus, likely from rubbing against moist diapers. Occurs almost exclusively in circumcised boys. Significant narrowing will produce an upwardly deflected stream, which is tiny and strong. In severe cases straining and prolonged voiding.
• Epidermal inclusion cysts—small, enlarging white bumps occurring at the scar from circumcision. These are caused by small islands of epithelium buried beneath the skin surface that progressively accumulate desquamated skin cells. These may also occur from congenital rests of skin cells buried during development but these are rare and occur along the median raphae of the penis.
• Balanitis—infection of the glans. May also involve the prepuce (balanoposthitis).

—Probably overdiagnosed due to physiologic drainage of smegma or urea dermatitis from failure to retract foreskin during voiding in potty trained boys.
—When infections do present, there can be significant cellulitis of the penis and fever.
—Most common causative organisms are gram positive. Yeast is another causative organism.

 Data Gathering

HISTORY

• Problems associated with newborn circumcision, when the changes occurred, character of urinary stream, presence of fever, or discharge in cases of balanitis. Retraction of foreskin in uncircumcised males during voiding. Ballooning of the foreskin with voiding.
• In older boys inquire about sexual activity or masturbation.

 Physical Examination

• Circumcised males—size and position of meatus, redundancy of inner preputial skin, presence of adhesions to the glans, and whether or not they involve the scar line between the shaft skin and the inner preputial skin. Lesions or erythema of glans or shaft. Watch patient void if meatal stenosis is suspected.
• Uncircumcised males—ability to retract foreskin with gentle retraction, presence of phimotic ring. Lesions or erythema of prepuce. Do not try to forcefully retract the foreskin. It can take 8 to 10 years before the foreskin is able to be retracted.

Laboratory Aids

In cases of balanitis with drainage, cultures may be taken. If urethral discharge is present, culture for gonorrhea and chlamydia.

Therapy

• Phimosis

—Physiologic—no need for intervention. Good hygiene practices should be encouraged such as pulling the foreskin back to expose the meatus when voiding and not voiding through the foreskin. Pamphlets that explain the care of the penis for uncircumcised males are helpful to give to the parents.
—Fibrotic ring—If there is a fibrotic ring of scar tissue preventing the retraction of the foreskin, a trial of betamethasone cream 0.05% applied to the foreskin b.i.d. for 4 weeks with daily gentle retraction may soften the scar tissue enough to resolve the phimosis. In cases where conservative measures fail, a circumcision is indicated.

• Penile adhesions:

—Physiologic—Practices in the past have included separation using eutectic mixture of local anesthetics (EMLA) cream. If there is redundancy of the foreskin or a prominent suprapubic fat pad that can tend to hide the penis in infants, adhesions often recur or require constant application of barrier creams or ointments to the penis and manual retraction of the redundant foreskin by the parents to prevent recurrence. In many cases no treatment is necessary, as the adhesions will break down with time over a period of years. If there are extensive adhesions with significant redundancy of foreskin, then consideration should be given to revision of the circumcision if the adhesions are to be treated.

—Surgical—These adhesions or skin bridges are due to scar tissue formation between the raw cut edge where the foreskin was removed to the raw surface of the glans. As this represents true scarring and not two epithelial surfaces stuck together, the surfaces cannot be simply pulled apart like physiologic adhesions. They will not resolve with time, and if left in place, with growth, penile skin will be transferred to the glans, resulting in discoloration, especially in patients with darker skin tones. These adhesions need sharp division either in the office with EMLA cream anesthesia or under general anesthesia if they are extensive.

• Meatal stenosis—When the narrowing at the meatus is producing an upwardly deflected, narrow stream (which can make aiming into the toilet tricky) or is causing straining and prolonged voiding, treatment is indicated. A meatotomy can be done in the office using EMLA anesthesia or as an outpatient surgical procedure.
• Epidermal inclusion cysts—These subcutaneous islands of skin cells will progressively enlarge over time. Complete excision under general anesthesia is nearly always curative.
• Balanitis—When the inflammation and irritation seem to be from chronic dampness and exposure to urine, treat with barrier creams or ointments. Keeping the area clean and dry will help prevent future episodes. If there are small whitish plaques (not smegma), associate with redness, yeast may be present and an antifungal cream such a 1% clotrimazole can be used to help speed the healing. In cases where there is purulent drainage and cellulitis of the penis, which can often be rapidly spreading over 24 hours, treatment with antibiotics is recommended. If the child is afebrile, oral antibiotics such as a first-generation cephalosporin would be the first line of treatment. If the child develops fever or there is progression of cellulitis despite 24 to 48 hours of antibiotics, then admission and treatment with intravenous antibiotics (ampicillin/sulbactam is a good choice) should be considered. Genital infections of this nature should be taken quite seriously, and if treatment as an outpatient is attempted, close follow-up (return visit in 24 to 48 hours) is prudent.

Common Questions and Answers

Q: The foreskin stuck back down to my son's penis. Does that mean he needs another circumcision?
A: Not necessarily. If there is minor redundancy and a small physiologic adhesion, then no treatment at all may be needed.

Q: My uncircumcised son had some thick white drainage from his foreskin. Is that from an infection?
A: Probably not. The thick white material is probably shed skin cells, which have been slowly separating the foreskin from the glans.

BIBLIOGRAPHY

Bartholomew TH, McIver B. Other disorders of the penis and scrotum. In: Gonzales ET, Bauer SB, eds. *Pediatric urology practice.* Baltimore: Lippincott Williams & Wilkins. 1999:533–546.

Elder JS. Congenital anomalies of the genitalia. In: Walsh PC, Retik AB, Vaughan ED, et al., eds. *Campbell's urology.* Philadelphia: W.B. Saunders. 1998:2120–2143.

Orsola A, Caffaratti J, Garat JM. Conservative treatment of phimosis in children using a topical steroid. *Urology* 2000;56:307–310.

Authors: J. Christopher Austin and Stephen A. Zderic

Pericarditis

 Database

DEFINITION

Inflammation of the pericardium, usually resulting in the accumulation of fluid in the pericardial space between the visceral (intimately related to the myocardium) and parietal (several layers of elastic fibers and collagen) pericardium; may be serous, fibrinous, purulent, hemorrhagic, or chylous.

CAUSES

- Infectious: viral (coxsackie B, Epstein-Barr, adenovirus, influenza, HIV), bacterial (streptococcus, pneumococcus, staphylococcus, meningococcus, mycoplasma, tularemia, *Haemophilus influenzae* type B), tuberculosis, fungal (histoplasmosis, actinomycosis), parasitic (toxoplasmosis, echinococcus)
- Rheumatologic: acute rheumatic fever, rheumatoid arthritis, systemic lupus erythematosus, systemic sclerosis, sarcoidosis, and familial Mediterranean fever
- Metabolic/endocrine: hypothyroidism, uremia (chemical irritation)
- Neoplastic disease: lymphoma, lymphosarcoma, leukemia, metastatic disease to the pericardium, radiotherapy induced
- Postoperative: postpericardiotomy syndrome (after cardiac surgery), chylopericardium
- Other: trauma, drug-induced (hydralazine, isoniazid, procainamide), aortic dissection, idiopathic

PATHOPHYSIOLOGY

Fine deposits of fibrin develop next to the great vessels and this leads to altered function of the membranes of the pericardium, including changes in oncotic and hydrostatic pressure with subsequent accumulation of fluid in the pericardial space. In postpericardiotomy syndrome, there appears to be a nonspecific hypersensitivity reaction to the direct entrance into the pericardial space.

EPIDEMIOLOGY

- Infectious pericarditis is more frequently seen in children younger than 13 years, with predominance in children younger than 2 years.
- Can occur in any age group.
- Overall incidence is slightly higher in males.
- Postpericardiotomy syndrome occurs in approximately 5% to 10% of children after uncomplicated cardiac surgery, particularly when the atrium has been entered.

COMPLICATIONS

- Cardiac tamponade: Intrapericardial pressure rises at a rapid rate secondary to decreased compliance of the pericardial membranes, resulting in restriction of ventricular filling and eventual decrease in stroke volume and cardiac output. The compliance of the pericardium is influenced by the disease process itself (i.e., the pericardium is thickened and stiff in bacterial and tuberculin pericarditis). During cardiac tamponade, ventricular end-diastolic, atrial, and venous pressures are all equal. In acute pericarditis, tamponade may occur with small amounts of fluid because of rapid increase in the intrapericardial pressure. In contrast, large amounts of fluid may be tolerated if the accumulation is a chronic, slow process.
- Constrictive pericarditis: Thick, fibrotic and often calcified pericardium is seen, usually a late result of purulent or tuberculous pericarditis; it can occur months to years after the initial infection. It can also be seen in oncology patients with direct invasion of tumor into the pericardium or with significant radiation to the chest. Poor compliance of the pericardium leads to diminished diastolic filling of the ventricle. Patients may complain of exercise intolerance and fatigue. Additionally they may have signs of right heart failure. This entity may be difficult to distinguish from restrictive cardiomyopathy.

PROGNOSIS

Most children recover fully from pericarditis, even if it is bacterial in etiology. However, there is a small but significant morbidity and mortality associated, especially in young infants when the diagnosis is delayed and/or when *Staphylococcus aureus* is the etiologic agent. Pericarditis can also recur in as many as 15% of patients. The prognosis varies with the other causes of pericarditis, but generally is directly related to the primary disease.

 Differential Diagnosis

- Acute myocarditis
- Restrictive cardiomyopathy
- Other nonspecific causes of chest pain

 Data Gathering

HISTORY

Question: Fever, cough, precordial chest pain, and shoulder pain (which is aggravated by changes in position)?
Significance: Most common symptoms.

Question: Respiratory distress?
Significance: Seen if there is rapid accumulation of fluid.

Question: Pain?
Significance: Often relieved if the child sits leaning forward.

Question: No symptoms?
Significance: Slow, chronic accumulation may be associated with no symptoms at all. Other symptoms are dependent on the etiology of the pericarditis.

Question: Recent upper respiratory infection or gastroenteritis?
Significance: With viral pericarditis, there may be a preceding history of a recent upper respiratory infection or gastroenteritis.

 Physical Examination

Finding: Pericardial friction rub is the pathognomonic finding
Significance: It may be heard if only a small amount of fluid is in the pericardial space.

Finding: Quiet precordium, tachycardia, and muffled heart sounds
Significance: May be heard when there is a large amount of fluid and/or tamponade

Finding: Right-sided heart failure
Significance: Tamponade, including peripheral edema, jugular venous distention, and hepatomegaly

Finding: Pulmonary edema
Significance: Rare because the heart is underfilled, and left atrial pressure, though elevated, does not exceed right atrial pressure

Finding: Pulsus paradoxus
Significance: An exaggerated decrease in systolic blood pressure with inspiration

Finding: Kussmaul sign
Significance: Paradoxical rise in jugular venous pressure during inspiration, often considered diagnostic of tamponade

Laboratory Aids

Test: Chest roentgenogram
Significance: Often shows enlargement of the cardiac silhouette ("water bottle") usually in association with normal pulmonary vascular markings. However, heart size may appear normal in acute pericarditis. Calcification may be seen in constrictive pericarditis.

Test: Echocardiography
Significance: Most sensitive and specific test for pericardial thickening and fluid in the pericardial space. In the presence of a large effusion, the heart may appear to swing within the pericardial cavity. In tamponade, diastolic collapse of the right atrium and ventricle may be seen as well.

Test: Electrocardiogram
Significance: Nonspecific but generally demonstrates low-voltage QRS complexes secondary to dampening of the signal from the pericardial fluid. One can also see ST segment elevation throughout the leads with possible T wave inversion as well, and these findings may be secondary to inflammation of the myocardium. Electrical alternans can be seen with large effusions.

Test: Pericardiocentesis
Significance: Fluid obtained should be sent to the lab for cell count, cytology, and culture (including bacteria, viruses, *Mycobacterium tuberculosis*, and fungi).

Therapy

- Treatment depends on etiology.
- However, no matter the cause, pericardiocentesis is required if there is an effusion that causes hemodynamic compromise and it may be lifesaving in patients with bacterial pericarditis.
- This procedure may also be indicated for diagnostic purposes when etiology of the effusion is in question.
- Complications of pericardiocentesis include myocardial puncture, coronary artery/vein laceration, hemopericardium, and pneumothorax.
- Echocardiographic or fluoroscopic guidance is useful for this procedure but is not required if there is impending cardiovascular collapse.

THERAPY BY DIAGNOSIS

- **Viral pericarditis** usually resolves spontaneously in 3 to 4 weeks with bed rest and analgesics.
- **Bacterial pericarditis** can potentially be life threatening and requires immediate decompression of the pericardial space, most often with open drainage and possible pericardial window, intravenous antibiotic

therapy for at least 4 weeks, and supportive therapy (i.e., volume expansion, inotropes).
- **Rheumatologic** causes of pericardial inflammation usually respond to corticosteroids and/or salicylates and rarely require pericardiocentesis.
- **Uremic pericarditis** usually responds to dialysis but pericardiotomy (surgical removal of the pericardium) may be necessary if it becomes a chronic problem.
- **Neoplastic pericarditis**, the primary disease, is treated and pericardiocentesis is performed if indicated for diagnostic and/or hemodynamic reasons.
- **Hemorrhagic pericarditis** secondary to trauma should be drained because of the risk of developing constrictive pericarditis.
- **Constrictive pericarditis** is treated with complete stripping of the pericardium (pericardiectomy). Often, immediate clinically improvement is not seen because there has been myocardial damage as well, but full recovery is the norm.
- **Postpericardiotomy syndrome** occurs 1 to 4 weeks after cardiac surgery and is usually treated with antiinflammatory drugs, bed rest, and occasionally steroids. Pericardiocentesis is indicated if tamponade develops.

Follow-Up

WHEN TO EXPECT IMPROVEMENT

Most forms of pericarditis resolve on their own or with antiinflammatory medication over the course of several weeks. Follow-up is necessary to be sure that effusions have resolved and to assess for recurrence (up to 15% relapse). Patients with bacterial pericarditis require long-term therapy and close follow-up to assess for the development of constrictive pericarditis.

SIGNS TO WATCH FOR

All cardiac surgical patients need an evaluation 2 to 4 weeks after surgery to assess for postpericardiotomy syndrome, with treatment and follow-up as necessary. Signs of low cardiac output and right heart failure indicate impending cardiac tamponade. Constrictive pericarditis may present with a rapidly decreasing cardiac silhouette and calcifications seen on chest roentgenogram, as well as the onset of signs and symptoms of right heart failure.

PREVENTION

Viral and rheumatologic pericarditis cannot be prevented. The incidence of bacterial pericarditis has decreased with immunization for such bacterial infections as *H. influenza* type B.

PITFALLS

The history, physical examination, and laboratory findings of acute pericarditis can be quite similar to those found in acute myocarditis. In addition, myocarditis can be a

component of pericardial disease and vice versa. Echocardiography is an excellent tool to help differentiate between these two entities.

Common Questions and Answers

Q: How does cardiac tamponade present?
A: Patients with impending tamponade appear quite ill with tachycardia, chest pain, and signs of right heart failure including jugular venous distention, hepatomegaly, and peripheral edema/ascites. They may also have signs of poor systemic perfusion secondary to low cardiac output. The chest x-ray may or may not show evidence of enlarged cardiac silhouette depending on how acutely the process occurs. It takes much less fluid to cause tamponade in an acute process than in a chronic long-standing one. Echocardiography is the standard tool to make the diagnosis and pericardiocentesis is the treatment.

Q: What is pulsus paradoxus and how does one measure it?
A: Pulsus paradoxus is an exaggerated response of the systolic blood pressure to the normal respiratory cycle. Normally with inspiration, the systolic blood pressure drops approximately 5 mm Hg secondary to the increased capacitance of the pulmonary veins from the increased systemic venous return. In tamponade, this response becomes more profound (>10 mm Hg), most likely secondary to diminished filling of the left heart. Pulsus paradoxus can also be seen in patients with severe respiratory distress such as in asthma and emphysema.

To assess for pulsus paradoxus, measure the systolic blood pressure first in expiration; then allow it to fall to the place where it is heard equally well in inspiration and expiration. The difference is the degree and paradox and greater than 10 mm Hg is considered abnormal.

ICD-9-CM 420.91, 420.90, 423.20

BIBLIOGRAPHY

Dupuis C, Gonnier P, Kachaner J, et al. Bacterial pericarditis in infancy and childhood. *Am J Cardiol* 1994;74:807–809.

Fyler DC. Pericardial disease. In: Fyler DC, ed. *Nadas' pediatric cardiology*. Philadelphia: Hanley and Belfus, 1992:1590–1599.

Pinsky WW, Friedman RA. Pericarditis. In: Garson A, Bricker JT, McNamara D, eds. *The science and practice of pediatric cardiology*. Kent, UK: Lea and Febiger, 1990:1531–1540.

Rheuban KS. Disease of the pericardium. In: Emmanoulides GC, Allen HD, Riemenschneider TA, et al., eds. *Heart disease in infants, children, and adolescents: including the fetus and young adult*, 5th ed. Baltimore: Williams & Wilkins, 1995.

Author: Meryl S. Cohen

Periodic Breathing

 Database

DEFINITION

Periodic breathing is a respiratory pattern in which three or more apneas lasting 3 or more seconds in duration occur separated by less than 20 seconds of respiration

CAUSES

• Periodic breathing can be seen in healthy infants, children, and adults.
• Periodic breathing in infants is associated with:

—Apnea of prematurity or infancy
—Familial history of sudden infant death syndrome (SIDS)
—Anemia of prematurity
—Hypoxemia
—Hypochloremic alkalosis

• Periodic breathing with adults is associated with:

—Cardiac abnormalities (congestive heart failure)
—Neurologic dysfunction (meningitis, encephalitis, brainstem dysfunction)
—Also referred to as Cheyne-Stokes respiration

• Abnormalities in any component of the breathing control system may result in an increased amount of periodic breathing
• Possible etiologies for periodic breathing include:

—A delay in detecting changes in blood gas values by the chemoreceptors
—Increased chemoreceptor gain

PATHOLOGY

• There is no common pathologic finding
• Abnormalities, when they exist, are related to the underlying disorder causing the periodic breathing

EPIDEMIOLOGY

• Usually absent in the first 48 hours of life
• More frequent during REM (active) sleep versus non-REM (quiet) sleep
• Less common in prone versus supine position
• In full term infants:

—Amount of periodic breathing usually, <4% of their sleep time
—Amount gradually decreasing through the first year of life
—By 1 year of age, the mean amount of periodic breathing is <1% of total sleep time.

• In premature infants:

—Amount of periodic breathing higher than in full-term infants
—Amount correlates inversely with the gestational age

• Incidence among healthy children and adults is unknown.

COMPLICATIONS

Relationship between periodic breathing and SIDS is controversial.

PROGNOSIS

• In otherwise normal premature or term infants: excellent
• With an underlying cardiac or neurological disorder, the prognosis is governed by this primary process

 Differential Diagnosis

• Other forms of apnea:

—Central apnea
—Obstructive apnea

• Other forms of periodic breathing:

—Cheyne-Stokes respiration
—Biot breathing
—Kussmaul respiration

• Normal irregular respiration seen in infants

 Data Gathering

HISTORY

• In most cases, parents notice periodicity in the respiration of the child.
• An apparent life-threatening episode (ALTE) might precipitate an evaluation on which periodic breathing is thereafter documented.
• In otherwise healthy premature or term infants, there are no other symptoms.

 Physical Examination

In otherwise healthy premature or term infants, the physical examination is normal.

 Laboratory Aids

TESTS

Polysomnography

• Assesses the extent of periodic breathing episodes
• Determines if there is accompanying hypoxemia, hypercarbia, or bradycardia with events
• Distinguishes between periodic breathing and obstructive and/or central apnea
• Useful for following response to treatment (i.e., normalization of polysomnography)
• Variables to be monitored include:

—EEG, EOG, and EMG (for sleep state determination)
—O_2 saturation
—End-tidal CO_2 tension
—Respiratory movements (abdomen, chest)
—Airflow
—pH probe (if gastroesophageal reflux is suspected)

• Record for a minimum of 6 hours

2-Channel Pneumogram

• Gives less information than polysomnography
• Can document periodic breathing, but may miss episodes of obstructive apnea
• Variables to be monitored include:

—Heart rate
—Respiratory effort
—O_2 saturation

IMAGING

• Chest radiograph

—Usually normal

Therapy

- Therapy should be directed to treating any underlying primary disease.
- If periodic breathing is associated with apnea, hypoxemia, and/or other sleep disturbances, appropriate treatment should be instituted.

DRUGS

Stimulants

- Caffeine

—Loading dose: 10 mg/kg
—Maintenance dose: 2.5 mg/kg daily
—Therapeutic level: 5 to 20 mg/L

- Theophylline

—Loading dose: 4 to 5 mg/kg
—Maintenance dose: 3 to 5 mg/kg/day divided t.i.d.
—Therapeutic level: 6 to 10 mg/L

- Supplemental oxygen

—Useful if periodic breathing is secondary to hypoxemia

- Nasal CPAP

—Very effective in eliminating periodic breathing

- Home monitoring

—Indicated when:

 —The amount of periodic breathing is significant.
 —There is accompanying apnea.
 —There is associated hypoxia and/or bradycardia.

Duration

- Dependent on the underlying cause of the periodic breathing
- Treatment does not change the natural course of periodic breathing in otherwise healthy infants.
- Therapy should continue until the periodic breathing resolves or is no longer clinically significant.

 ## Follow-Up

WHEN TO EXPECT IMPROVEMENT

- Dependent on the underlying cause of the periodic breathing
- Improvement is anticipated as the infant ages.
- When treatment is started, a decrease in the amount of periodic breathing should be seen almost immediately.

PITFALLS

Confusing periodic breathing with obstructive or central apnea

 ## Common Questions and Answers

Q: What is the risk of the patient dying of SIDS?
A: The relationship between periodic breathing and SIDS is not clear, although most studies have not found a higher frequency of SIDS among patients with periodic breathing.

ICD-9-CM 786-09

BIBLIOGRAPHY

Glotzbach SF, Ariagno RL. *Respiratory control disorders in infants and children*. Baltimore: Williams & Wilkins, 1992:142–160.

Horemuzova E, Katz-Salamon M, Milerad J. Breathing patterns, oxygen and carbon dioxide levels in sleeping healthy infants during the first nine months after birth. *Acta Paediatr* 2000;89:1284–1289.

Hunt CE, Corwin MJ, Lister G, et al. Longitudinal assessment of hemoglobin oxygen saturation in healthy infants during the first six months of age. *J Pediatr* 1999;134:580–586.

Kelly DH, Stellwagen LM, Katz E, et al. Apnea and periodic breathing in normal full-term infants during the first twelve months. *Pediatr Pulmonol* 1985;1:215–219.

Lieber C, Mohsenin V. Cheyne-Stokes respiration in congestive heart failure. *Yale J Biol Med* 1992;65:39–50.

Shannon DC, Carley DW, Kelly DH. Periodic breathing: quantitative analyses and clinical description. *Pediatr Pulmonol* 1986;4:98–102.

Author: Richard M. Kravitz

Periorbital Cellulitis

 Database

DEFINITION

Periorbital cellulitis is an acute infection of the superficial skin and subcutaneous tissues of the eyelids. It is also known as preseptal cellulitis because the inflammation is localized in the tissues anterior to the orbital septum. Thus the eyeball and orbital tissue are not involved.

PATHOPHYSIOLOGY

• Preseptal cellulitis is an infection caused by a variety of bacteria. The most common pathogens are *Staphylococcus aureus*, *Streptococcus pneumoniae*, *Staphylococcus epidermis*, and *Haemophilus influenzae*.
• Predisposing factors that may lead to infection include skin trauma, insect bites, and upper respiratory infections with paranasal sinusitis.

EPIDEMIOLOGY

This infection usually occurs in young children, commonly under the age of 5.

COMPLICATIONS

Orbital extension (2.5–17%), skin abscess (8%), eyelid necrosis (1–2%), sepsis, intracranial extension (2–3%)

PROGNOSIS

Excellent with minimal incidence of long-term sequelae unless complication encountered

 Differential Diagnosis

• Infectious

—Early orbital cellulitis
—Dacryocystitis
—Stye
—Severe adenoviral conjunctivitis

• Allergic

—Periocular allergic reaction
—Insect bite
—Angioneurotic edema

• Other

—Periocular trauma
—Rhabdomyosarcoma
—Idiopathic orbital inflammation

 Data Gathering

• Clinical examination will provide the necessary information to make the appropriate diagnosis.
• It is important to inquire about the time course of the swelling as the cellulitis occurs acutely over a few days.
• Any history of trauma or underlying respiratory infection may be helpful, although these types of questions have a low yield.
• The presence of pain would support cellulitis while complaints of itching are more suggestive of an allergy.
• Quantify systemic symptoms such as fever and lethargy as these indicate a more severe, disseminated infection.

 Physical Examination

• The lids will be edematous, erythematous, warm to the touch, and usually, but not always, tender. The findings can start in one eyelid but both the upper and lower eyelids are usually swollen.
• The globe should be carefully examined. In preseptal cellulitis, the ocular exam is normal. The eye is almost always white, although patients can have some conjunctival edema. Any change in vision or pupillary function, or limitations in motility suggest orbital involvement.
• Many patients with preseptal cellulitis appear to have proptosis but actually do not. The presence of proptosis suggests deep orbital involvement.
• Finally, signs of fever, respiratory infection, and sepsis should be identified.

PHYSICAL EXAM TRICKS

Occasionally the eyelids are so swollen it is difficult to examine the globe. To do so, place anesthetic eyedrops on the eye and fashion a paperclip into a lid retractor to lift the eyelid.

Laboratory Aids

- Lab tests are usually not helpful or indicated.
- CBC is warranted only if bacteremia is suspected.
- Skin cultures and blood cultures have a low yield. Blood cultures are only obtained when the child is febrile or appears septic.

IMAGING

- CT scanning is a helpful modality to rule out sinus and orbital disease. It is important to obtain imaging studies if orbital cellulitis is suspected and in cases that do not respond to treatment.
- Of note, CT scan findings will lag behind clinical findings by several days. Thus serial CT scanning should only be done if the child is not improving with treatment.

 ## Therapy

GENERAL MANAGEMENT

- New antibiotics are constantly being introduced to replace older medications, so it is hard to give a specific list of drugs. Antibiotics that cover *Staphylococcus*, *Streptococcus*, and *Haemophilus*, such as second-generation cephalosporins or β-lactamase–resistant penicillins, should be started as soon as possible.
- Children under the age of 2 years should be hospitalized for intravenous therapy and very close observation.
- Children between the age of 2 and 5 should be watched closely. Mild cases may be managed on an outpatient visit.
- Children over the age of 5 years can usually be treated with an oral regimen as long as they do not appear toxic.

DRUGS

- In nontoxic children, oral antibiotics (Augmentin, cefaclor, Pediazole, etc.) are started on an outpatient basis and the child should be seen again in within 24 hours.
- Children who do not improve or who worsen, as well as children who present with fever or septic symptoms, should be admitted for intravenous antibiotic (Unasyn, ceftriaxone, etc.) and close observation.

SURGERY

- Surgical intervention is usually required when an abscess or a foreign body is present.

 ## Follow-Up

WHEN TO EXPECT IMPROVEMENT

- Patients usually take 24 to 48 hours to respond to therapy.
- Patients should be seen daily until a definite improvement is noted.

SIGNS TO WATCH FOR

Watch patients closely for signs of orbital extension, bacteremia, or other forms of disseminated infection.

PITFALLS

- Neonates and infants can become septic very quickly, so they need to be closely monitored.
- Periorbital cellulitis may be a secondary extension of another process like sinusitis
- CT scans will lag behind clinical findings once treatment is started. In fact, a repeat scan 24 to 48 hours after starting antibiotics will usually look worse than the pre-antibiotic scan.

ICD-9-CM 376.01

BIBLIOGRAPHY

Donahue SP, Schwartz G. Preseptal and orbital cellulitis in childhood. A changing microbiologic spectrum. *Ophthalmology* 1998;105:1902–1905.

Foster JA, Katowitz JA. Pediatric orbital and periocular infections. In: Katowitz JA, ed. *Pediatric oculoplastic surgery*. Springer-Verlag, 2001.

Lessner A, Stern GA. Preseptal and orbital cellulitis. *Infect Dis Clin North Am* 1992;6:933–952.

Powell KR. Orbital and periorbital cellulitis. *Pediatr Rev* 1995;16:163–167.

Author: Scott M. Goldstein

Perirectal Abscess

 Database

DEFINITION

Abscess in the perirectal area, which may extend into surrounding soft tissues

- Most common cause of anorectal suppuration
- May or may not be associated with a fistula
- Infection usually starts in the intersphincteric space, probably in one of the small anal glands.

CAUSES

- Nonspecific anal gland infection
- Crohn disease
- Perforation by a foreign body
- External trauma
- Tuberculosis
- Carcinoma
- Immune deficiency (e.g., AIDS, neutropenia, diabetes mellitus)

PATHOPHYSIOLOGY

- Majority of anal abscesses and fistulas originate from infected anal glands.
- Infection from the anal glands penetrate through the internal sphincter and end in the intersphincteric space.
- Abscess formation is the acute phase; fistula is the chronic phase.

EPIDEMIOLOGY

- Can occur in any age group
- No racial predilection

COMPLICATIONS

- Fulminant sepsis
- Fistulas can occur if abscesses are not drained as soon as possible.

PROGNOSIS

Prognosis is good if there is early detection and drainage of abscesses.

 Differential Diagnosis

- Pilonidal infection
- Hidradenitis suppurativa
- Crohn disease
- Gangrenous hemorrhoids
- Foreign body
- Tuberculosis

 Data Gathering

HISTORY

- History of constipation?
- Fevers?
- Painful defecation?
- Refusing to walk?
- Rectal pain?
- Weight loss, diarrhea, abdominal pain, and poor growth are symptoms associated with Crohn disease.
- Foreign body?
- Trauma?

 Physical Examination

The various types of anorectal abscesses give rise to the following presentations:

Finding: Intersphincteric abscess
Significance: Is limited to the primary site in the intersphincteric space between the internal and external sphincters associated with throbbing pain on defecation and continues for hours thereafter; severe enough to prevent sleep. It often does not cause perianal skin changes.

Finding: Perianal abscess
Significance: Result of distal vertical spread of the infection to the anal margin. Presents as tender, red swelling; often misdiagnosed as an external anal thrombosis.

Finding: Intermuscular abscess/supralevator abscess
Significance: Results from two different sources. One source is a proximal vertical spread of infection from the gland through the intersphincteric space to the supralevator space. The other source is an abscess resulting from a pelvic pathology such as Crohn's disease. Patients usually complain of vague pelvic discomfort, fever, and sometimes urinary retention; rectal exam usually reveals an indurated swelling above the anorectal ring.

Finding: Ischiorectal abscess
Significance: Due to horizontal spread of infection across the external anal sphincter into the ischiorectal fossa. Sometimes infection may track across the internal anal sphincter into the anal canal. Patients may complain of pain and fever before a swelling is visible. Induration then occurs under the skin over the ischiorectal fossa and eventually a typical red fluctuant abscess is seen.

Finding: Circumferential spread
Significance: May occur from one side to the other in the intersphincteric space and can present with pain

Laboratory Aids

- CBC
- Culture
- CT scan

 Therapy

- Abscesses should all be drained as soon as diagnosed. Lack of fluctuation should not delay treatment.
- Pus should be sent for culture, and use of antibiotics is usually reserved for an infection that does not respond to drainage or if gut organisms are present. The most common organism is *Escherichia coli*.
- At times, a repeat exploration of the abscess/fistula under general anesthesia may be performed to drain residual abscess.
- Sitz baths may be helpful postprocedure.

 Follow-Up

EXPECTED COURSE OF ILLNESS

- Patients usually recover well after surgical drainage of abscess.
- Fistulae may occur after aspiration of abscess.
- Additional follow-up to determine the cause of the abscess formation is crucial in attempting to prevent recurrence.

 Common Questions and Answers

Q: What are complications of this problem?
A: Fistula formation is seen in up to 25% of patients with a predilection for males.

Q: What is the most common organisms of the abscess?
A: *Staphylococcus.*

Q: What other disease may my child have if he has perirectal abscess?
A: Crohn disease must be excluded. If there is exposure to tuberculosis, this also must be excluded.

Q: Will the abscess recur after surgery?
A: Yes, if the disease process is secondary to a chronic disease-like inflammatory bowel disease.

Q: What treatments can be done other than surgery?
A: Antibiotics, sitz baths, and warm compresses can give symptomatic improvement.

ICD-9-CM 566

BIBLIOGRAPHY

al-Salem AH, Qaisaruddin S, Qureshi SS. Perianal abscess and fistula in ano in infancy and childhood: a clinicopathological study. *Pediatr Pathol Lab Med* 1996;16(5):755–764.

Bassford T. Treatment of common anorectal disorders. *Am Fam Physician* 1992;45(4):1787.

Festen C, van Harten H. Perianal abscess and fistula-in-ano in infants. *J Pediatr Surg* 1998;33(5):711–713.

Rosen L. Anorectal abscess-fistulae. *Surg Clin North Am* 1994;74(6):1293.

Seon-Choen F, Nicholls RJ. Anal fistula. *Br J Surg* 1993;80(12):1626.

Authors: Helen Anita John-Kelly and Andrew E. Mulberg

Peritonitis

Database

DEFINITION

Peritonitis is defined as inflammation of the peritoneal cavity. This inflammation may be categorized as spontaneous bacterial peritonitis (no intraabdominal source of infection) or secondary bacterial peritonitis (intraabdominal source of infection present).

PATHOPHYSIOLOGY

Spontaneous bacterial peritonitis (SBP) occurs when pathogenic bacteria are cultured from peritoneal fluid but no intraabdominal surgical treatable source of infection is identified. This disease entity has gained increasing recognition as a complication in patients with ascites as a result of cirrhosis of any etiology. There have also been isolated patients reported with noncirrhotic ascitic diseases:

- Budd-Chiari syndrome
- Congestive heart failure
- Nephrotic syndrome
- Systemic lupus erythematosus
- Rheumatoid arthritis

Secondary bacterial peritonitis results from any process leading to perforation of the gastrointestinal tract including:

- Necrotizing enterocolitis
- Volvulus with ischemia
- Intussusception with ischemia
- Trauma
- Perforation from duodenal/gastric ulcers

Translocation of organisms from the gut into the portal veins or lymphatics or, less likely, directly into the ascites may account for the source of the infection; however, other sites have been found to be infected in patients with SBP.
Therefore, the ascitic infection may be secondary to seeding from generalized bacteremia. Clearance of bacteria from the bloodstream may be impaired in patients with cirrhosis and ascites because of diminished phagocytic activity of the hepatic reticuloendothelial system (RES), which may be linked to either intrinsic cellular functional defects or shunting of blood away from the liver.
Complement, necessary for the opsonization of bacteria and ultimately clearance by phagocytes, is decreased in the ascitic fluid of patients with ascites.

EPIDEMIOLOGY

Infectious organisms include:

- Aerobic-gram negative organisms: *E. coli* (approximately 50%), *Klebsiella* (approximately 13%).
- Aerobic gram-positive organisms: *Streptococcus* (approximately 19%), *Enterococcus* (5%).
- Anaerobes rarely cause SBP and polymicrobial infections occur in relatively few patients (approximately 8%).
- Urine cultures have been found to be positive for the same organism in approximately 44% of patients.
- Pneumonias and soft tissue infections have also been suggested as sources.
- In secondary bacterial peritonitis, the underlying bacterial infection tends to be a complex polymicrobial infection with an average of 2.9 to 3.9 different isolates.
- The most commonly isolated combination of organisms is *E. coli* and *Bacteroides fragilis*.
- The most common gram positive organism is nonenterococcal streptococci and enterococci.

Predisposing Factors to SBP

- Advanced liver disease
- Decreased RES activity
- Decreased serum complement levels
- Decreased ascitic protein and complement levels
- Presence of gastrointestinal hemorrhage

PROGNOSIS

- SBP is associated with a high mortality, with 37% to 77% of patients dying during hospitalization. The combination of underlying disease and the infection causes acute decompensation in a marginally compensated host—hence the high mortality rate.
- Retrospective studies have indicated that SBP appears to be recurrent with 51% of patients who survive the first episode going on to develop one or more recurrences.

Data Gathering

HISTORY

Clinical features depend on the stage at which peritonitis is diagnosed.

- Fever, chills?
- Generalized abdominal pain with rebound tenderness?
- Decreased bowel sounds? In SBP, approximately 10% of cases are entirely asymptomatic.

Other rare findings include:

- Hypothermia?
- Hypotension?
- Diarrhea?
- Increased ascites despite diuretics?
- Encephalopathy?
- Unexplained decrease in renal function?

Physical Examination

- Painful palpation of abdomen
- Decreased bowel sounds
- Evidence of chronic liver disease
- Evidence of ascites

Laboratory Aids

• Diagnosis may be confirmed with paracentesis.

—To improve culture yield, culture bottles should be inoculated immediately at the bedside in large volume blood culture bottles.
—An elevated ascitic PMN count is important in the early diagnosis of SBP and is considered the most important laboratory indicator of SBP.

• Diagnostic criteria for SBP include:

—Polymorphonuclear leukocyte counts of greater than $250/mm^3$
—Ascitic fluid culture usually for a single organism

• Diagnostic criteria for secondary bacterial peritonitis include:

—Ascitic fluid culture positive for polymicrobial infection
—Total protein greater than 1 g/dL
—Glucose less than 50 mg/dL
—LDH greater than 225 mU/mL

 ## Therapy

• Support the patient's cardiovascular and respiratory systems.
• Control the underlying infection with antibiotics or surgery (in secondary bacterial peritonitis). Empirical antibiotic coverage should be directed primarily toward enteric gram-negative aerobes and gram-positive cocci.
• In SBP, cefotaxime, a third-generation cephalosporin, has been shown to have higher resolution of infection and lower hospital mortality than the traditional ampicillin and an aminoglycoside as empiric coverage.
• Once the organism is identified, the antibiotic coverage may be optimized.
• For patients at significant risk for SBP, selective intestinal decontamination is effective in preventing bacterial infections. Antibiotics that have been studied for this use in adults include:

—Norfloxacin
—Ciprofloxacin
—Trimethoprim-sulfamethoxazole

In SBP, surgery is the primary management tool with control of the source of the intraabdominal infection. No particular antibiotic regimen has been shown to be superior in controlled clinical trials. Both single agents and combination regimens have been used. For mild to moderately severe infections, single-drug regimens have included:

• Cefoxitin
• Cefotetan
• Cefmetazole
• Ticarcillin

Combination regimens that have been used include:

• Flagyl or clindamycin plus aminoglycoside
• Flagyl or clindamycin plus a third-generation cephalosporin
• Clindamycin plus aztreonam
• For severe infections, imipenem-cilastin has been used.

COMPLICATIONS

• Hypovolemia results from extravascular extravasation and sequestration from the inflamed peritoneal membrane, and the intravascular volume must be supported with crystalloids and blood products.
• Respiration may be impaired via mechanical mechanisms through diaphragmatic spasm and reflex abdominal rigidity and through increased permeability of the pulmonary vasculature in response to systemic inflammation.
• The role of surgery is to gain control of the underlying source of the abdominal infection by repairing the affected bowel through laparotomy/laparoscopy. The degree of contamination may be decreased through intraoperative peritoneal lavage, and debridement of loculations and abscesses. Adding antibiotics to lavage fluid has lost favor after the discovery that this procedure appears to impair neutrophil chemotaxis, inhibit neutrophil bacteriocidal activity, and increases the formation of adhesions. Catheters may be placed to drain well-defined abscess cavity, form a controlled fistula, or provide access for continuous postoperative peritoneal lavage.

 ## Common Questions and Answers

Q: Is peritonitis common in children with ascites?
A: Despite the frequency of ascites from many different causes, peritonitis occurs rarely. In the setting of children with chronic liver disease and ascites, spontaneous bacterial peritonitis may occur rarely.

Q: What are the most useful laboratory aids for this diagnosis?
A: Analysis of the fluid for pH, glucose content, and amount of inflammatory cells provides the most useful information regarding the diagnosis of peritonitis.

ICD-9-CM 567.9

BIBLIOGRAPHY

Farber MS, Abrams JH. Antibiotics for the acute abdomen. *Surg Clin North Am* 1997;77(6):1395–1417.

Gilbert J, Kamath P. Spontaneous bacterial peritonitis: an update. *Mayo Clin Proc* 1995;70:365–370.

Guarner C, Soriano G. Spontaneous bacterial peritonitis. *Semin Liver Dis* 1997;17(3):203–217.

Nathans AB, Rotstein OD. Therapeutic options in peritonitis. *Surg Clin North Am* 1994;74(3):6577–6592.

Author: Dror Wasserman

Peritonsillar Abscess

 Database

DEFINITION

Infectious complication of tonsillitis or pharyngitis resulting in an accumulation of purulence in the tonsillar fossa. Also referred to as "quinsy."

CAUSE

- Group A β-hemolytic *Streptococcus* (GABHS)
- α-Hemolytic streptococci
- Miscellaneous anaerobic bacteria
- *Staphylococcus aureus*

PATHOPHYSIOLOGY

- Infectious tonsillopharyngitis progresses from cellulitis to abscess.
- Purulence collects within one, and sometimes both, tonsillar fossa.
- Tonsillar and peritonsillar edema may lead to compromise of the upper airway.

EPIDEMIOLOGY

Seen most commonly in adolescents, but occasionally in younger children

ASSOCIATED ILLNESS

- Tonsillitis or pharyngitis usually precedes its development.
- Peritonsillar cellulitis is often associated with infectious mononucleosis.

COMPLICATIONS

- Upper airway obstruction is the most feared complication.
- Dehydration, from decreased oral intake, is the most common complication.

PROGNOSIS

- Complete swift recovery can be expected with appropriate therapy.
- Recurrence of peritonsillar abscesses are not uncommon

 Differential Diagnosis

- Peritonsillar cellulitis: the most common diagnostic consideration; can be distinguished by its lack of peritonsillar space "fullness," uvular deviation, dysphonia, and trismus
- Retropharyngeal abscess: Minimal peritonsillar findings, along with a widened prevertebral space on lateral neck x-ray is diagnostic of this airway-compromising disease, which almost always occurs in preschool children.
- Epiglottitis: This life-threatening airway emergency presents abruptly with fever, stridor, increased work of breathing, and drooling; usually occurs in toxic-appearing children 3 to 7 years of age but becoming a rare entity since the advent of the *Haemophilus influenzae* type B vaccine.
- Other infectious etiologies of severe tonsillopharyngitis: Epstein-Barr virus (infectious mononucleosis), coxsackievirus (herpangina), *Corynebacterium diphtheriae, Neisseria gonorrhoeae*

 Data Gathering

HISTORY

Question: Fever and sore throat?
Significance: Most common initial complaints

Question: Trouble swallowing, pain with opening the mouth (trismus), muffled ("hot-potato") voice?
Significance: Classic presenting symptoms

Question: Unilateral neck or ear pain?
Significance: Other common presenting symptoms

 Physical Examination

Finding: Unilateral peritonsillar fullness, or bulging of the posterior, superior, soft palate
Significance: Diagnostic physical exam finding

Finding: Uvular deviation
Significance: Another classic physical exam finding

Finding: Palpable fluctuance of palatal swelling
Significance: Calls for urgent aspiration

Finding: Erythematous, edematous pharynx, with enlarged and exudative tonsils
Significance: Coexisting tonsillopharyngitis is common.

Finding: Cervical adenopathy
Significance: Common

Finding: Drooling
Significance: Often present

Finding: Torticollis
Significance: Sometimes seen

 Laboratory Aids

Test: White blood cell count
Significance: Usually elevated with prominent "left shift"

Test: Rapid streptococcal throat antigen studies
Significance: Helpful to diagnose GABHS infection

Test: Gram stain and culture of aspirate specimen
Significance: Confirms causative microorganism

Test: CT scan or ultrasound
Significance: Differentiation of peritonsillar cellulitis from peritonsillar abscess (rarely indicated).

Therapy

- True abscesses should be urgently/ emergently drained via either needle aspiration or surgical incision and drainage.
- Antibiotic therapy can be initiated with high-dose intravenous penicillin.
- Clindamycin, nafcillin, oxacillin, cefazolin, and ampicillin/sulbactam (Unasyn), are acceptable, broader-spectrum alternatives.
- Surgical drainage with tonsillectomy should be considered in children not responding to parenteral antibiotics within 24 to 48 hours.
- Appropriate analgesia and adequate hydration should be ensured.

 Follow-Up

- Patients may be discharged on oral antibiotics to complete a 10- to 14-day course when afebrile and peritonsillar swelling has subsided.
- Tonsillectomy should be considered after severe or recurrent peritonsillar abscesses.

PREVENTION

Abscess formation can often be prevented if appropriate antimicrobial therapy is initiated while the infection is still at the cellulitis stage.

PITFALLS

Treating a true abscess without incision and drainage is inadequate and can have airway-threatening implications.

 Common Questions and Answers

Q: Are radiographs necessary to make the diagnosis of peritonsillar abscess?
A: No. The physical examination is diagnostic; a lateral neck radiograph is useful only if retropharyngeal abscess or epiglottitis are diagnostic concerns.

Q: Is surgical consultation necessary in cases of peritonsillar abscess?
A: Yes. Otorhinolaryngology consultation is indicated for both acute as well as chronic management.

ICD-9-CM 475

BIBLIOGRAPHY

Blotter JW, Yin L, Glynn M, et al. Otolaryngology consultation for peritonsillar abscess in the pediatric population. *Laryngoscope* 2000;110:1698–1701.

Friedman NR, Mitchell RB, Pereira KD, et al. Peritonsillar abscess in early childhood. Presentation and management. *Arch Otolaryngol Head Neck Surg* 1997;123(6): 630–632.

Herzon FS. Peritonsillar abscess: incidence, current management practices, and a proposal for treatment guidelines. *Laryngoscope* 1995;105(8 pt 3 suppl 74):1–17.

Herzon FS, Nicklaus P. Pediatric peritonsillar abscess: management guidelines. *Curr Probl Pediatr* 1996;26(8):270–278.

Kieff DA, Bhattacharyya N, Siegel NS, et al. Selection of antibiotics after incision and drainage of peritonsillar abscesses. *Otolaryngol Head Neck Surg* 1999;120:57–61.

Passy V. Pathogenesis of peritonsillar abscess. *Laryngoscope* 1994;104(2):185–190.

Savolainen S, Jousimies-Somer HR, Makitie AA, et al. Peritonsillar abscess. Clinical and microbiologic aspects and treatment regimens. *Arch Otolaryngol Head Neck Surg* 1993;119:521–524.

Scott PMJ, Loftus WK, Kew J, et al. Diagnosis of peritonsillar infections: a prospective study of ultrasound, computerized tomography, and clinical diagnosis. *J Laryngol Otol* 1999;113: 229–232.

Szuhay G, Tewfik. Peritonsillar abscess or cellulitis? A clinical comparative pediatric study. *J Otolaryngol* 1998;27(4):206–212.

Weinberg E, Brodsky L, Stanievich J, et al. Needle aspiration of peritonsillar abscess in children. *Arch Otolaryngol Head Neck Surg* 1993;119:169–172.

Author: Nicholas Tsarouhas

Persistent Pulmonary Hypertension of the Newborn (PPHN)

 Database

DEFINITION
- Persistent pulmonary hypertension of the newborn (PPHN) is a neonatal physiologic entity in which the pulmonary vascular resistance either fails to decline after delivery of the infant or rises several hours after delivery.
- PPHN manifests as severe hypoxemia.
- Severe pulmonary parenchymal disease may or may not be present.
- Patients with PPHN have a structurally normal heart; however, right to left shunting of blood through the ductus arteriosus and the foramen ovale is clearly present on echocardiography.

CAUSES
Asphyxia
Hypoxemia and acidosis, either fetal or neonatal in origin, leads to the processes of PPHN.

Infection
Sepsis, particularly group B streptococcal septicemia, leads to mediators promoting PPHN.

Parenchymal Lung Disease
- RDS and inborn causes of surfactant deficiency, such as surfactant protein B (SP-B) deficiency, lead to PPHN.
- Meconium aspiration pneumonitis leads to PPHN.

Pulmonary Hypoplasia
- Primary pulmonary hypoplasia, or as a result of oligohydramnios, leads to PPHN.
- Bronchopulmonary malformations that cause space-occupying chest lesions, such as congenital cystic adenomatoid malformation (CCAM), can lead to PPHN.
- Congenital diaphragmatic hernias are often associated with elements of PPHN.

Maternal Drug Therapy
Prostaglandin synthesis inhibitors, such as ibuprofen or naproxen, in pregnant women have been implicated in PPHN.

Congenital Heart Disease
- Pulmonary venous flow obstruction, as in myocardial failure or left-sided obstructive lesion, can lead to PPHN.
- Congenital heart disease therapy such as tricuspid atresia or total anomalous pulmonary venous return may result in PPHN.

PATHOPHYSIOLOGY
- The primary pathophysiologic defect in PPHN lies within the pulmonary vascular system. Elevated pulmonary artery and arteriole resistances normally exist in the fetus, allowing only 10% to 20% of the circulating blood to perfuse the pulmonary vessels. Pulmonary artery pressures in the fetus have been measured to be 60 to 70 mm Hg. In normal transition of the fetus to extrauterine life, the pulmonary artery pressures fall to 33 mm Hg within 3 hours of delivery. Normal transition to extrauterine life involves multiple biochemical and cellular processes that remodel the pulmonary vessels and muscular arterioles, and involve the production of local vasodilators, such as bradykinins, prostacyclins, and nitric oxide.
- Infants who develop PPHN and fail this normal transition have abnormally hypertrophied pulmonary arteriole musculature. Abnormal musculature is likely to be a cause of PPHN in patients with primary or secondary causes of pulmonary hypoplasia.
- In some causes of PPHN, particularly infectious causes, vasoconstriction occurs through the action of mediators such as thromboxane.
- Furthermore, pathophysiologic consequences of poor pulmonary perfusion, such as hypoxemia, acidosis, and hypercarbia, contribute to the increased pulmonary vascular resistance.

GENETICS
- PPHN is not typically considered to possess a pattern of inheritance.
- Underlying causes of PPHN may be inherited, as in SP-B deficiency, autosomal-recessive polycystic kidneys (leading to pulmonary hypoplasia and oligohydramnios), and congenital malformations (like CDH).

EPIDEMIOLOGY
- Incidence: 1 to 2 in 1,000 newborns.
- Typically affects term newborns. All newborns with a fetal pattern of acidemia or hypoxia are susceptible, as well as all newborns with severe bacteremia or pulmonary parenchymal disease.
- Infants with meconium aspiration pneumonitis are at particular risk.

COMPLICATIONS
Short Term
- Pneumothorax
- Seizures
- Hypoxic ischemic encephalopathy
- Right-sided heart failure
- Hypotension
- Pulmonary barotrauma
- Feeding intolerance
- Opioid dependence

Long Term
- Feeding difficulties and gastroesophageal reflux
- Cerebral palsy and mental retardation
- Seizure disorder
- Sensorineural deafness
- Asthma
- Chronic pulmonary insufficiency

PROGNOSIS
- Greater than 90% of all infants with this entity survive. Overall extracorporeal membrane oxygenation (ECMO) survival for PPHN is 85%. Underlying disease etiology best predicts outcome.
- As a pathophysiologic process, PPHN usually resolves in 3 to 5 days.
- Patients with pulmonary hypoplasia and PPHN often have longer disease courses.

 Differential Diagnosis

CYANOTIC CONGENITAL HEART DISEASE
- Transposition of the great arteries
- Total anomalous pulmonary venous return
- Tetralogy of Fallot
- Pulmonary stenosis
- Truncus arteriosus
- Tricuspid atresia

PARENCHYMAL LUNG DISEASE
- RDS
- Pneumonia
- Surfactant protein B (SP-B) deficiency
- Meconium aspiration pneumonitis
- Hydrops fetalis

PULMONARY HYPOPLASIA
- Primary pulmonary hypoplasia, or as a result of oligohydramnios
- Bronchopulmonary malformations that cause space-occupying chest lesions, such as congenital cystic adenomatoid malformation
- Congenital diaphragmatic hernias
- Bronchogenic cysts
- Mediastinal masses

 Data Gathering

HISTORY
Question: Were there any difficulties with the pregnancy?
Significance: Data concerning gestational age, congenital malformations, poly- or oligohydramnios, and maternal drug ingestion can help to identify the underlying etiology of PPHN.
Question: Were there any difficulties during labor?
Significance: Signs of fetal distress, meconium-stained amniotic fluid, late decelerations of fetal heart rate, and prolonged active labor are associated with the development of PPHN.
Question: What are the risk factors for sepsis?
Significance: Risk factors for group B streptococcal disease (rupture of membranes greater than 18 hours, maternal chorioamnionitis, maternal fever) are associated with PPHN.

 Physical Examination

GENERAL
- Cyanosis
- Poor perfusion, pallor
- Signs of respiratory distress—grunting, intercostal/subcostal/supraclavicular retractions, nasal flaring

CHEST
- Increased AP diameter
- Breath sounds depend on etiology: may be decreased unilaterally with congenital diaphragmatic hernia, pneumothorax, effusions. May be normal also.

Persistent Pulmonary Hypertension of the Newborn (PPHN)

CARDIAC
Normal or murmur of tricuspid regurgitation.

FACIES
Typical facies of Potter syndrome and fetal compression may be evident.

 Laboratory Aids

TESTS
Test: Arterial blood gas
Significance: Postductal hypoxemia is the hallmark of this process. Increases in blood Pao_2 values greater than 150 mm Hg with 100% inspired oxygen makes the presence of cyanotic heart disease unlikely. Hyperventilation may demonstrate an increase in Pao_2. Frequent monitoring of blood gases is necessary to monitor the neonate's therapy.
Test: Complete blood count
Significance: Anemia and thrombocytopenia need rapid correction. Correction of these abnormalities may improve systemic perfusion. Leukocytosis and leukopenia are present in sepsis.
Test: Blood culture
Significance: Sepsis may be the underlying etiology of the patient's PPHN.
Test: Electrolytes
Significance: Fluid and electrolyte abnormalities, including hypocalcemia, may complicate this disease entity as a result of therapy and require correction.
Test: PT/PTT
Significance: Coagulopathies may result from sepsis or severe acidosis. Administration of these blood products further enhances systemic perfusion.
Test: Blood type and cross-match
Significance: Infants with PPHN usually require blood products to correct pathologic processes.

RADIOGRAPHIC STUDIES
Test: Chest x-ray
Significance: Decreased presence of pulmonary vasculature is hallmark of classic PPHN. Otherwise, a primary pulmonary parenchymal disease pattern is present, such as RDS or meconium aspiration pneumonitis. It is important to identify the presence of air leak syndromes, such as pneumothorax.
Test: Echocardiography
Significance: This is important to evaluate the patient for structural heart disease. In many patients, pulmonary arterial pressures can be estimated from the tricuspid regurgitation jet seen on cardiac echocardiograms. An echocardiogram can evaluate right heart function for presence of failure, and need for further escalation of care.

 Therapy

- Proper airway management and monitoring is critical.
- Central arterial and venous access is imperative.
- The infant should receive 100% inspired oxygen. Arterial Po_2 levels should be maintained at greater than 70 mm Hg. While successful oxygenation of an infant may demonstrate high blood Po_2 levels, only very slow reductions in percentage of inspired oxygen levels (1%/hour) after the establishment of several hours of clinical stability is advisable.
- Infants most severely affected by this process will require mechanical ventilation.
- Correct any acidosis, metabolic or respiratory. Even mild acidosis promotes severe pulmonary hypertension.
- Metabolic alkalosis (pH maintenance greater than 7.5) has been suggested to provide further vasodilation, although use of this technique has been correlated with an increased need for ECMO.
- Underlying etiologies of PPHN should be rapidly treated. Empiric antibiotics are warranted for presumed neonatal septicemia. Surfactant should be used for RDS. Surfactant lavages for meconium aspiration have been suggested, although efficacy is unproven.
- Systemic perfusion must be maintained. Maintenance of systemic perfusion with colloid or crystalloid boluses will raise systemic blood pressures, decreasing right-to-left shunting. Infusions of dopamine and dobutamine are particularly helpful. The goal of this therapy is to treat underlying systemic hypoperfusion and increase the systemic vascular resistance.
- Frequent laboratory monitoring of blood gases, chest radiographs, and hematologic values are imperative for the care of the infant with PPHN.
- Ventilatory support should be weaned only very slowly with the establishment of successful correction of the pathophysiology.
- High frequency oscillatory ventilation (HFOV) has a place in the management of PPHN, particularly in the delivery of nitric oxide. One downside of this therapeutic modality is decreased cardiac output due to reduced end-diastolic filling of the right atrium (decreased preload).
- Nitric oxide (NO) administration has been demonstrated to decrease the need for ECMO in patients with PPHN by one third.
- ECMO is used in severe PPHN for infants with reversible disease processes. This form of long-term cardiopulmonary bypass is used only in those infants with the severest disease and high predicted mortality.

 Follow-Up

Infants with PPHN, particularly those receiving NO or ECMO, require frequent evaluation by a developmental pediatrician every 3 months for the first 2 years of life. Hearing screens should be done prior to discharge of these patients from the nursery.

PITFALLS
- Anomalous pulmonary venous return frequently is mistaken for PPHN and requires careful echocardiographic evaluation to eliminate the possibility of this diagnosis.
- Rapid reductions in inspired oxygen levels frequently result in severe hypoxemia, and a return to severely elevated pulmonary vascular resistance.
- Lower Pco_2 levels are a risk factor for sensorineural hearing loss.

 Common Questions and Answers

Q: What are the long-term complications of PPHN?
A: This depends on the underlying etiology. Patients with congenital diaphragmatic hernia have a 40% to 50% mortality rate, and complications include pulmonary sequelae with chronic respiratory insufficiency, and developmental delay. Meconium aspiration has a survival rate greater than 95%. Of infants who receive ECMO, 80% have a normal developmental outcome.

Q: When should the patient be referred to an ECMO center?
A: Patients who do not achieve adequate oxygenation in the first hours of life should be immediately referred to an ECMO center. Referral to a center that can provide NO therapy, if not ECMO, is advisable early in the infant's course. Declining right heart function is a sign of worsening clinical status as well as refractory hypotension, an increased Aa gradient, and a declining ability to oxygenate. Early referral to an ECMO center is advisable, since it takes time to mobilize transport and to assemble the center's ECMO team, which must be figured into the patient's care.

ICD-9-CM 416

BIBLIOGRAPHY
Finer NN, Barrington KJ. Nitric oxide and respiratory failure in the newborn infant. *Semin Perinatol* 1997;21:426–440.

Kinsella JP, Abman SH. Inhaled nitric oxide: current and future uses in neonates. *Semin Perinatol* 2000;24:387–395.

Montgomery V, Buchino JJ. Clinical pathologic conference: A newborn with pulmonary hypertension. *J Pediatr* 1998;133:157–161.

Author: Daniel H. Conway

Perthes Disease

 Database

DEFINITION

Self-limited osteonecrosis of the proximal femoral epiphysis of unknown etiology.

CAUSES

Unknown; related to a combination of trauma and vascular insult (recent evidence suggests thrombophilia).

PATHOLOGY

- Four stages

—Initial: bone necrosis
—Fragmentation: fragmentation of necrotic bone with early revascularization
—Reossification: revascularization, resorption, and repair via creeping substitution
—Healing: remodeling

EPIDEMIOLOGY

- Seen most commonly between ages 4 to 8 years
- Boys affected more than girls, with ratio of 4.5:1
- 10% bilateral
- Majority have delayed bone age
- More common in lower socioeconomic groups

GENETICS

No strong evidence to suggest that Perthes is an inherited condition.

COMPLICATIONS

- Osteoarthritis
- Mild limb length discrepancy
- Restriction of hip range of motion
- Pain, limping

PROGNOSIS

- Based on the following factors:

—Age of the patient at onset of the disease; if onset older than 8 years of age, poorer prognosis than if onset at younger age
—Extent of femoral head involvement; if more than one half of epiphysis involved, poorer prognosis
—Subluxation of femoral head, poorer prognosis
—Growth disturbance of the physis, poorer prognosis

 Differential Diagnosis

- Toxic synovitis
- Chondrolysis
- Infection
- Juvenile rheumatoid arthritis
- Rheumatic fever
- Tuberculosis of the hip
- Tumors
- Meyer dysplasia
- Bone dysplasias

—Multiple epiphyseal dysplasia
—Trichorhinophalangeal syndrome
—Spondyloepiphyseal dysplasia

- Hypothyroidism, juvenile cretinism
- Sickle cell disease, hemophilia
- Gaucher disease

 Data Gathering

HISTORY

Question: Age at onset of symptoms/signs?
Significance: Older age at onset implies worse prognosis.

Question: Limping?
Significance: Weeks to months duration

Question: Hip, thigh, or knee pain?
Significance: Hip pathology may cause referred pain at thigh or knee.

 Physical Examination

Finding: Limitation of range of motion
Significance: Especially internal rotation and abduction

Finding: Irritability and tenderness of hip joint area
Significance: Usually early—related to synovitis from early repair

Finding: Atrophy of thigh
Significance: Late finding

Finding: Slight shortening of affected limb
Significance: Due to collapse (real) or contracture (apparent)

Finding: True hip joint irritability
Significance: Early finding indicating intraarticular synovitis

Finding: Trendelenburg gait
Significance: Leaning over affected leg during stance, due to mechanical disadvantage from collapse

SPECIAL QUESTIONS

Finding: Distribution of pain may follow the sensory distribution of the obturator nerve.
Significance: Medial thigh and knee (i.e., referred pain).

PHYSICAL EXAMINATION TRICKS

The Trendelenburg test is positive when a patient stands on the affected side and the pelvis drops on the opposite side.

 Laboratory Aids

Test: Laboratory tests
Significance: Generally are not helpful, but may be necessary to rule out other conditions such as infection.

IMAGING STAGES

- Incipient stage (1st)
- Aseptic or avascular stage (2nd)
- Fragmentation stage (3rd)
- Residual or remodeling stage (4th)
- The first radiographic sign of Perthes is smaller size of the femoral head epiphysis and a widened articular cartilage space compared with the other side; the second sign is the subchondral fracture.

Perthes Disease

Therapy

- Most do not need surgery
- Treatment needed generally for those with more severe involvement (one half of head involved or late onset).
- Two basic treatment principles:

—Restoration of range of motion
—Containment of the femoral head epiphysis in the acetabulum

- General treatment modalities

—Weight relief early during collapse
—Bed rest early during collapse
—Physical therapy to maintain range of motion
—Traction—less popular now
—Bracing
—Surgery

DRUGS

NSAIDs for pain and inflammation

DURATION

Generally continues until patient enters the reossification phase

Follow-Up

WHEN TO EXPECT IMPROVEMENT

- The magnitude and duration of symptoms depends on the age of the patient at onset of the disease and the degree of involvement of the disease process. Most patients show improvement in symptoms by 6 months after the onset of disease.
- Patients with Perthes disease should be seen and followed by a pediatric orthopedic surgeon.

SIGNS TO WATCH FOR

- Stiffness—loss of range of motion
- Limping
- Pain
- Subluxation of the hip joint

PROGNOSIS

Overall, good prognosis for the majority of patients

PITFALLS

The majority of patients with Perthes disease do not need surgery. For those who do, early recognition and appropriate early referral are key.

Common Questions and Answers

Q: How long do you observe a patient with hip pain before ordering an x-ray?
A: It depends on the presence or absence of abnormalities on the physical examination. If any of the signs mentioned above are seen in conjunction with significant hip pain, an x-ray is indicated. An x-ray should be done early to establish the diagnosis and rule out other abnormalities.

Q: Why do patients with hip pathology have knee pain?
A: This is because the nerves that innervate the hip joint also have cutaneous sensory distributions. Both the obturator and femoral nerves innervate the hip joint and both also have cutaneous sensory distribution in the region of the thigh and knee joint.

ICD-9-CM 732.1

BIBLIOGRAPHY

Harrison MH. Bassett CA. The results of a double-blind trial of pulsed electromagnetic frequency in the treatment of Perthes' disease. *J Pediatr Orthop* 1997:17(2):264–265.

Kaniklides C, Lonnerholm T, Moberg A, et al. Legg-Calve-Perthes disease. Comparison of conventional radiography, MR imaging, bone scintigraphy and arthrography. *Acta Radiol* 1995;36(4):434–439.

Salter RB. The present status of surgical treatment of Legg-Perthes disease: current concept review. *J Bone Joint Surg* 1984;66A:961.

Weinstein SL. Legg-Calve-Perthes disease. In: Morrissy RT, Weinstein SL, eds. *Lovell and Winter's pediatric orthopaedics*, 4th ed. Philadelphia: Lippincott Raven, 1996:951–992.

Author: John P. Dormans

Pertussis

Database

DEFINITION

- *Bordetella pertussis* is a small, nonmotile, fastidious, gram-negative rod.
- The first description of the disease appeared in 1578 during an epidemic in Paris, France.

PATHOPHYSIOLOGY

- Replicates only in association with ciliated epithelium, causing congestion and inflammation of the bronchi; peribronchial lymphoid hyperplasia followed by a necrotizing process occurs and results in a bronchopneumonia; atelectasis can occur due to bronchiolar obstruction from accumulated secretions.
- Filamentous hemagglutinin (FHA), lymphocytosis promoting factor (LPF), and adenylate cyclase play a role in the organism's attachment and adversely affect immune cell function.
- The long incubation period (7–21 days) reflects the time necessary for *B. pertussis* to increase in numbers needed for progressive spread of infection in the respiratory tract and produce enough toxin for eliciting damage and dysfunction of the respiratory epithelium.
- Respiratory illness characterized as a bronchopneumonia.
- Apnea is a common manifestation in the young infant, <6 months of age. The characteristic "whoop" is typically absent.

EPIDEMIOLOGY

- One of the most highly communicable diseases with attack rates close to 100% in susceptible individuals.
- A disease of young children; the infant either nonimmunized or partially immunized is at greatest risk.
- Approximately one third of cases reported to the CDC are in infants, <6 months of age.
- Disease in adolescents and adults is not usually recognized as pertussis despite a cough that is paroxysmal and may last for weeks. Despite improved vaccination rates in the U.S., pertussis infection rates have steadily risen since the early 1980s. This is thought to be attributed to the growth of a susceptible adult population, and these patients are the major source of pertussis infection in children.
- Route of spread includes aerosolized respiratory droplets, direct contact with nasal secretions, and indirect contact with secretions through hand contact.

COMPLICATIONS

- Pneumonia, the most frequent complication, is responsible for more than 90% of deaths in young children with pertussis, and is usually owing to secondary bacterial disease rather than *B. pertussis* itself.
- Superinfections due to viruses (adenovirus, respiratory syncytial virus, cytomegalovirus) or bacteria (*Streptococcus pneumoniae, Staphylococcus aureus*) and gram-negative iatrogenic infections can complicate pneumonias.
- Other pulmonary complications include atelectasis, pneumothorax, pneumomediastinum, and subcutaneous emphysema.
- Seizures (3%) and encephalopathy (0.9%) have been observed in infants with pertussis, although these findings may be related to fever causing febrile convulsions and cerebral hypoxia due to the pulmonary complications.

PROGNOSIS

The prognosis is directly related to patient age; the highest mortality is observed in infants, <6 months of age. Infants have a 0.5% to 1% risk of death, whereas, in the older child, prognosis is good.

Differential Diagnosis

- *B. parapertussis* and adenoviruses
- *B. pertussis*
- Bronchiolitis
- Bacterial pneumonia
- Cystic fibrosis
- Tuberculosis
- Foreign body aspiration should also be considered.

Data Gathering

HISTORY

Question: What are clinical stages of pertussis infection?
Significance:

- Three stages:

—Catarrhal stage (1–2 weeks) with symptoms of an upper respiratory infection
—Paroxysmal stage (2–4 weeks or longer) characterized by paroxysmal cough with increased severity and frequency producing the characteristic whoop during the sudden forceful inspiratory phase; post-tussive vomiting is also observed during this stage.
—The convalescent stage begins and lasts 1 to 2 weeks but cough can persist for several months. In the adolescent or adult, long-standing cough of 2 to 3 weeks is the hallmark symptom. Most patients report a paroxysmal or staccato quality to the cough.

Physical Examination

- Rhinorrhea, lacrimation, conjunctival hyperemia, and fever seen in the early stage of disease
- Cyanosis observed during the paroxysmal stage

- Lung auscultatory examination is usually normal unless significant atelectasis or pneumonia has occurred.

Laboratory Aids

Test: CBC
Significance: Leukocytosis with predominant lymphocytosis (77%) is commonly observed at the end of the catarrhal stage and throughout the paroxysmal stage of illness, although this phenomenon is not frequently observed in infants.

Test: Chest radiographs
Significance: May reveal perihilar infiltrates or a "shaggy right heart border," although these findings can be seen with other respiratory infections.

Test: Culture of *B. pertussis*
Significance: Achieved using calcium alginate or Dacron swabs of the nasopharynx and plated onto selective media such as Regan-Lowe or Bordet-Gengou and incubated for 7 days.

Test: Culture isolation of *B. pertussis*
Significance: Most frequently successful during the catarrhal or early paroxysmal stages and is rarely found beyond the 4th week of illness. The overall sensitivity is 60% to 70%.

Test: Direct immunofluorescent assays of nasopharyngeal specimens
Significance: Can provide a rapid and specific diagnosis but is limited by the experience of the laboratory personnel for interpretation

Test: Polymerase chain reaction (PCR) techniques
Significance: Available in most centers, and have been shown to have a higher sensitivity than culture in the detection of *B. pertussis* from nasopharyngeal specimens

Test: Recently developed monoclonal immunofluorescent antibody (BL-5)
Significance: Has been shown to be at least as sensitive and specific as culture but needs additional investigation

Test: Serology
Significance: Has excellent sensitivity and specificity when the acute serum is collected early in the course of illness and compared to the convalescent serum specimen

Therapy

- Patients with more severe disease manifestations (apnea, cyanosis, feeding difficulties) or other complications require hospitalization for supportive care.

- If antibiotic treatment is initiated during the catarrhal stage, it can prevent disease from progressing. Antibiotics have not been shown to shorten the course of illness if begun during the paroxysmal stage, although it will eliminate the organism from the nasopharynx within 3 to 4 days, thus shortening the potential for contagion.
- Erythromycin (50 mg/kg/d) in four doses for 14 days is recommended; an alternative dose with 40 mg/kg of erythromycin estolate twice a day for 14 days has shown equal efficacy. Note, an association between oral erythromycin use and hypertrophic pyloric stenosis has been reported in infants younger than 6 weeks of age. Given the limited study of this causal relationship, the American Academy of Pediatrics continues to recommend erythromycin for treatment and prophylaxis against *B. pertussis*.
- Newer macrolides, azithromycin and clarithromycin, may be effective in shorter courses of 5 to 7 days, however, their efficacy has not been fully studied.
- Trimethoprim-sulfamethoxazole is another alternative to erythromycin, although its efficacy is unproved.
- Infants under 6 months may develop apnea from fatigue secondary to excessive coughing. They need close observation, preferably in the hospital.

Follow-Up

- The paroxysmal stage can last up to 4 weeks and the convalescent stage up to several months and can be quite problematic for patient and family.
- The complications of pertussis are more likely to occur in the younger infant and therefore tend to have a more serious, protracted course.

PITFALLS

The most likely source of pertussis in young infants is from the adolescent or adult with mild symptoms of pertussis. Therefore, a high index of suspicion must exist in this population before adequate control of exposure to the partially or unimmunized infant can be successful.

PREVENTION

Infection Control

- Isolation of hospitalized patient: respiratory isolation for 5 days after starting erythromycin therapy or until at least 3 weeks after the onset of the paroxysmal stage, if antibiotics were not given, is recommended.
- Control measures: exposed individuals (all household contacts, other close contacts, other children in child care) should receive erythromycin chemoprophylaxis to limit secondary transmission, regardless of immunization status.

Immunizations

- Vaccinations available in the United States include acellular vaccines in combination with diphtheria and tetanus toxoids as the preferred vaccination product over previous whole cell products. Universal immunization of the preschool child is paramount to control the rate of infection.
- Combination DTaP and HiB vaccine is available with the benefit of fewer injections and immunization visits; however, lower antibody responses have been reported.
- The DTaP licensed vaccines in the U.S. have variable efficacy, and further study of the immunity data is necessary to determine the optimal pertussis vaccine.
- It seems prudent to vaccinate adults with periodic booster vaccinations given the risk they create for young infants.

Common Questions and Answers

Q: Why is the transmission of pertussis difficult to control in the young infant?
A: Unfortunately, many physicians do not consider pertussis in an adolescent or adult because they assume that childhood immunization will protect adults against pertussis. In addition, delays in antimicrobial treatment are common in adults due to the lack of index of suspicion of pertussis by their providers. The immunity protection by pertussis immunization is limited and, due to the poor tolerability of booster immunizations in adults, this has not been a universal recommendation.

Q: Are there any risks associated with the pertussis vaccine?
A: The rates of local reactions, fever, and other common systemic symptoms of somnolence, fussiness, and loss of appetite, are significantly lower with the acellular pertussis vaccine than with whole-cell pertussis vaccine. Moderate to severe systemic reactions, including high temperature, persistent, inconsolable crying for more than 3 hours, seizures, and collapse, have rarely been reported with DTaP, and the frequency is much lower than DTP immunization. Because of the temporal relation between administration of pertussis vaccine and severe adverse events such as death, encephalopathy, developmental delay with learning, and behavioral problems or onset of seizures, much publicity has been given to this vaccine, yet causation has not been established.

Q: What are the contraindications to pertussis vaccination?
A: Contraindications to avoid initial or subsequent doses of pertussis vaccine (DTP and DTaP) include the following: an immediate anaphylactic reaction, encephalopathy within 7 days of a prior injection or a seizure within 3 days or persistent crying, a shock-like state

or fever greater than 104.9°F within 48 hours of a prior injection. A progressive neurologic disorder or history of seizure disorder is a contraindication also.

ICD-9-CM 033.9

BIBLIOGRAPHY

Bass JW, Wittler RR. Return of epidemic pertussis in the United States. *Pediatr Infect Dis J* 1994;13:343.

Black S. Epidemiology of pertussis. *Pediatr Infect Dis J* 1997;16:S85–S89.

Cherry JD, Olin P. The science and fiction of pertussis vaccines. *Pediatrics* 1999;104: 1381–1384.

Cromer BA, Goydos J, Hackell J, et al. Unrecognized pertussis infections in adolescents. *Am J Dis Child* 1993;147: 575–577.

Edwards KM. Pertussis in older children and adolescents. *Adv Pediatr Infect Dis* 1998;13:49–77.

Eskola J, Ward J, Dagan R, et al. Combined vaccination of Haemophilus influenzae type B conjugate and diphtheria-tetanus-pertussis containing acellular pertussis. *Lancet* 1999;354:2063–2068.

Feigin RD. Pertussis. In: Feigin RD, Cherry JD, eds. *Textbook of pediatric infectious diseases*, 3rd ed. Philadelphia: WB Saunders, 1990:1208.

Gordon M, Davies HD, Gold R. Clinical and microbiologic features of children presenting with pertussis to a Canadian pediatric hospital during an eleven year period. *Pediatr Infect Dis J* 1994;13:617–622.

He Q, Mertsola J, Soini H, et al. Sensitive and specific polymerase chain reaction assays for detection of Bordetella pertussis in nasopharyngeal specimens. *J Pediatr* 1994;124:421–426.

Hewlett EL. Pertussis: current concepts of pathogenesis and prevention. *Pediatr Infect Dis* 1997;16:S78–S84.

Hoppe JE. Comparison of erythromycin estolate and erythromycin ethylsuccinate for treatment of pertussis. *Pediatr Infect Dis J* 1992;11:189–193.

Hoppe JE. Neonatal pertussis. *Pediatr Infect Dis J* 2000;19:244–247.

Muller FMC, Hoppe JE, Wirsing Von Konig CH. Laboratory diagnosis of pertussis: state of the art in 1997. *J Clin Microbiol* 1997;35: 2435–2443.

Peter G, Halsey NA, Marcuse EK, et al. Pertussis. In: *2000 red book: report of the Committee on Infectious Diseases*, 25th ed. Elk Grove Village, IL: American Academy of Pediatrics, 2000:435–448.

Author: Philip V. Scribano

Pharyngitis

 Database

DEFINITION

Pharyngitis (i.e., sore throat) is inflammation of the mucous membranes and underlying structures of the pharynx and tonsils, usually secondary to viral or bacterial infection.

EPIDEMIOLOGY

• Streptococcal pharyngitis is most common in children 5 to 15 years of age; peak incidence is in the winter.
• Viral disease is more common in younger children during the winter months.
• Day-care attendance is a risk factor.

COMPLICATIONS

• Streptococcal pharyngitis—suppurative complications include peritonsillar abscess, cervical lymphadenitis, and mastoiditis. The most significant nonsuppurative complication is acute rheumatic fever.
• Infectious mononucleosis (IM) due to Epstein-Barr virus (EBV): complicated by upper airway obstruction due to tonsillar hypertrophy and splenic rupture due to associated splenomegaly. Postanginal sepsis: can also occur in adolescents or young adults following IM.

 Differential Diagnosis (in Approximate Order of Frequency)

VIRAL

• Adenovirus types 1 through 7, 7a, 9, 14, 15, and 16 are the most common causes of nasopharyngitis overall.
—Often a follicular exudative pharyngotonsillitis
—May occur in association with conjunctivitis (pharyngoconjunctival fever)
• Epstein-Barr virus (EBV)
• Influenza A, B: usually associated with more severe systemic complaints
• Parainfluenza 1, 2, and 3
• Enteroviruses
—Often with ulcerative lesions (herpangina or hand-foot-and-mouth disease)
—Characteristic enanthem consists of two to 14 ulcers and vesicles (1 to 2 mm in size) in the posterior pharynx.
—May be caused by Coxsackie A, B, and echoviruses.
• Measles and rubella and coronavirus, cytomegalovirus
• Herpes simplex virus (HSV)
—Usually associated with ulcers on anterior oropharynx (gingivostomatitis) but also causes an exudative pharyngitis in adolescents that may be difficult to differentiate from streptococcal or EBV pharyngitis.
• Rhinovirus and RSV: not usually associated with pharyngeal inflammation.
• Human immunodeficiency virus (HIV): pharyngitis associated with primary HIV infection (acute retroviral syndrome),
accompanied by systemic complaints simulating mononucleosis.

BACTERIAL

• *Streptococcus pyogenes* (group A β-hemolytic *Streptococcus*)
—Most common in children 5 to 15 years old, causing at least 15% to 20% of cases of pharyngitis in this age group.
—Usually exudative with only 10% complaining of cough or rhinorrhea
• Group C or G streptococci
—Less common, but cause outbreaks associated with contaminated foods
• *Arcanobacterium hemolyticum*
—More commonly recognized in United Kingdom and Scandinavia
—Exudative pharyngitis in adolescents, young adults; can give scarlatiniform rash.
• *Corynebacterium diphtheriae* (diphtheria)
—Characterized by membrane formation that may extend from the tonsils, uvula, and pharyngeal walls to the larynx and trachea. Often foul or sweet odor to breath.
—Lymphadenitis may be so severe to create "bull neck" appearance.
• *Corynebacterium hemolyticum*
—More common in adolescents and adults
• *Neisseria gonorrhea* and *N. meningitidis*
• *Mycoplasma pneumoniae, M. hominis, Chlamydia pneumoniae, C. psittaci*
• *Yersinia enterocolitica* may occur with the enterocolitis.
• *Francisella tularensis* (tularemia)
—Associated with undercooked meat, pet rabbits; may have membrane similar to diphtheria
—Cervical nodes may suppurate.
• *Treponema pallidum* (syphilis)
—Usually subacute in secondary syphilis.
• Oral anaerobes (Vincent angina)

FUNGI

• *Candida* species (oral thrush)
—In infants or immunosuppressed individuals

 Data Gathering

HISTORY

Question: Is the pharyngitis associated with the sudden onset of fever with headache, nausea, and vomiting?
Significance: Frequent in streptococcal pharyngitis
Question: Is the pharyngitis associated with rhinorrhea, cough, hoarseness, conjunctivitis, and ulcerative pharyngeal lesions?
Significance: More likely to be a viral etiology
Question: Has the patient been swimming in an inadequately chlorinated pool?
Significance: Consider adenoviral pharyngoconjunctival fever.
Question: Appearance of papular eruption after administration of ampicillin or amoxicillin?
Significance: Consider EBV.
Question: Ingestion of undercooked meat or handling of rabbits?
Significance: Consider tularemia.

 Physical Examination

Finding: Moderate to severe pharyngeal erythema and tonsillar enlargement.
Significance: Erythema may be associated with petechiae, exudate, or ulceration.
Finding: Scarlatiniform rash
Significance: Strongly suggests diagnosis of GAS
Finding: Varying degrees of cervical adenopathy
Significance: Tender anterior lymphadenopathy is more likely associated with streptococcal disease.
Finding: Presence of an adherent membrane in pharynx extending to uvula
Significance: Suggests diphtheria
Finding: Splenomegaly and/or generalized adenopathy
Significance: Suggests EBV
Finding: Presence of more than six palatal petechiae
Significance: Strongly associated with streptococcal pharyngitis

 Laboratory Aids

Because of the importance of its complications, streptococcal disease should be confirmed or excluded by laboratory testing, except in presentations suggestive of viral or other etiology of pharyngitis (e.g., a toddler with conjunctivitis and rhinorrhea, presence of gingivostomatitis, findings consistent with IM, etc.).

SPECIFIC TESTS

Test: Rapid streptococcal antigen detection tests (RADTs)
Significance: Are effective as initial tests with greater than 95% specificity and 50% to 80% sensitivity. Cultures should be performed when rapid test is negative. (Hint: culture throat using two swabs initially, keeping one for culture if the rapid test is negative.) Positive rapid tests do not require culture confirmation.
Test: Throat culture
Significance: The "gold standard" with best sensitivity ($>$90%) for group A β-hemolytic streptococci.
Test: Monospot (heterophile antibody) test or Epstein-Barr virus serology
Significance: For IM

 Therapy

• Usually no therapy indicated, except for streptococcal pharyngitis (and other rare cases of bacterial or fungal pharyngitis)
• May withhold treatment for GAS pharyngitis until throat culture result is available

Pharyngitis

DRUGS

- Oral penicillin V: is the drug of choice for GAS pharyngitis except in penicillin-allergic individuals. Resistant strains have not been documented *in vitro*.
—Children: use 400,000 units (250 mg) b.i.d. or t.i.d. for 10 days.
—Adolescents/adults: use 800,000 units (500 mg) b.i.d. for 10 days or 400,000 units (250 mg) t.i.d. or q.i.d. for 10 days.
- Intramuscular benzathine penicillin G: ensures compliance, useful in outbreaks
—Children (<60 lbs): 600,000 units IM (1 dose)
—Children (≥60 lbs) and adults: 1,200,000 units IM (1 dose); bringing to room temperature reduces discomfort; also procaine penicillin combinations are less painful.
- Oral erythromycin is indicated in penicillin-allergic individuals. Erythromycin ethyl succinate (40 to 50 mg/kg/d in 2–4 divided doses). Resistance is rare in the United States (<5% of isolates).
- Amoxicillin, clindamycin, and first-generation oral cephalosporins (up to 15% of penicillin-allergic persons are also allergic to cephalosporins) are reasonable alternatives to penicillin in GAS pharyngitis.
- Tetracyclines and sulfonamides should *not* be used due to resistance of group A streptococci.
- Newer agents such as azithromycin, and various oral cephalosporins have also been shown to eradicate streptococci; however, because of the broad spectra of these antibiotics and the increasing incidence of antibiotic-resistant bacteria, they are not recommended.

DURATION OF THERAPY

Recent trials comparing 10-day courses of penicillin with newer oral cephalosporins or azithromycin used for 5 days have shown similar bacteriologic and clinical cure rates, but efficacy in prevention of nonsuppurative sequelae is unknown, and these agents have broad spectra and greater expense.

 Follow-Up

PATIENTS WITH STREPTOCOCCAL PHARYNGITIS

- Clinical improvement is usually rapid.
- Cure rate is excellent except in noncompliant patients, *rare* co-infection with pathogens that elaborate β-lactamase (consider therapy with clindamycin), or in cases of a new infection acquired from family or classroom contact (also rare).
- No need to perform posttreatment cultures for GAS in asymptomatic patients in areas where incidence of ARF is low (e.g., United States, Canada, Western Europe).

PREVENTION

- Long-term penicillin prophylaxis for patients with a history of rheumatic fever.
- Immunization with diphtheria toxoid (DPT, DaPT, or dT) has dramatically decreased childhood mortality from diphtheria.

ISOLATION OF HOSPITALIZED PATIENT

- Isolation of hospitalized patients with respiratory viruses and pharyngitis
- Droplet precautions for hospitalized children with streptococcal pharyngitis until 24 hours after initiation of therapy

CONTROL MEASURES

- Children with GAS pharyngitis can return to school or day care 24 hours after starting antimicrobial therapy.
- Cultures of asymptomatic contacts of patients with streptococcal pharyngitis are not indicated except in outbreak situations in school or day care (where treatment of patients with positive RADT or culture is indicated) or in contacts with a history of nonsuppurative complications.

PITFALLS

- Swabbing the throat from anywhere other than the tonsils and posterior pharyngeal wall
- Even experienced clinicians may overestimate the diagnosis of GAS pharyngitis using clinical grounds alone by up to 80%.
- About 20% of children with GAS pharyngitis that have mild symptoms may go unrecognized if cultures are not done.
- Reliance on Monospot test in young children (<5 years) because of a high incidence of false negatives (consider EBV serology instead).
- Positive throat culture or RADT in patients with viral pharyngitis may represent streptococcal carrier state. Diagnostic tests for GAS should be utilized in patients suspected to have streptococcal disease on clinical and epidemiologic grounds, not on all patients who complain of a "sore throat."
- Overtreatment of patients who are streptococcal carriers—asymptomatic patients (or patients with intercurrent viral infections) who have a positive test for GAS are at low or no risk of developing suppurative or nonsuppurative complications and unlikely to spread the organism to close contacts.

Common Questions and Answers

Q: Are rapid antigen detection tests (RADTs) alone adequate for the diagnosis of GAS pharyngitis?
A: No, only if it is positive; a negative RADT result should be confirmed by the more sensitive culture.
Q: How many days after onset of GAS pharyngitis will therapy be effective in preventing ARF?
A: Therapy started as late as 9 days after illness onset has been shown to be effective in preventing ARF.
Q: Is there any benefit to starting therapy while waiting for culture results?
A: Immediate therapy probably shortens the symptomatic period, but waiting for a positive test result avoids overuse of antibiotics.

Q: Does an asymptomatic patient with a positive test for GAS from the pharynx require therapy?
A: Usually not. Between 8% and 20% of children in school or day care will have asymptomatic carriage of GAS and generally do not require therapy. Exceptions are those with a history of ARF, outbreak situations, or to achieve eradication in families with recurrent episodes of GAS pharyngitis.
Q: Is there any evidence of GAS resistance to penicillin and other β-lactam antibiotics?
A: No, GAS has never been found to be resistant to penicillin but some studies suggest tolerance to penicillin where penicillin is bacteriostatic rather than bactericidal. However, 2% to 8% of GAS strains are resistant to macrolides.
Q: Is tonsillectomy indicated for recurrent GAS pharyngitis?
A: Rare patients in whom multiple symptomatic episodes of laboratory-confirmed GAS pharyngitis occur despite appropriate therapy may be considered for tonsillectomy.
Q: Is continuous antimicrobial prophylaxis for recurrent GAS pharyngitis recommended?
A: No, there is insufficient evidence to show that it is effective, except for preventing recurrences of acute rheumatic fever.
Q: What is the association of pharyngitis and recurrent fever?
A: There is an increasingly recognized syndrome of periodic fever, aphthous stomatitis, pharyngitis, and adenitis, dubbed PFAPA by some. The fever is usually high, recurs at fixed intervals of 2 to 8 weeks, and resolves spontaneously within 4 days. It does not appear to be familial, begins before the age of 5 years, the patient is well between episodes, and there are no known sequelae or cause.

ICD-9-CM

Pharyngitis (Streptococcal) 034.0
Pharyngitis (acute, viral, infective) 462.0
Pharyngitis (influenza) 487.1
Pharyngitis (Coxsackie) 074.0, and others

BIBLIOGRAPHY

Bisno AL, Gerber MA, Gwaltney JM, et al. Diagnosis and management of group A streptococcal pharyngitis: a practice guideline. *Clin Infect Dis* 1997;25:574–583.

Bisno AL, Gerber MA, Gwaltney JM, et al. Diagnosis and management of group A streptococcal pharyngitis: a practice guideline. *Clin Infect Dis* 1998;26:1020–1021.

Pichichero ME. Sore throat after sore throat after sore throat—Are you asking the right questions? *Postgrad Med* 1997;101:205–225.

Shulman ST. Evaluation of penicillins, cephalosporins, and macrolides for therapy of streptococcal pharyngitis. *Pediatrics* 1996;97(suppl):955–959.

Author: Mark L. Bagarazzi

Photosensitivity

 Database

DEFINITION

Adverse or abnormal reaction of the skin to sunlight

CAUSES

• Combination of sunlight with some abnormality in the skin such as loss of pigment, a chemical agent, a metabolic product, another skin disorder, a genetic disease, or an unknown factor, produces a cutaneous abnormality.
• Specific wavelengths of the radiant energy emitted by the sun and reaching the earth are usually responsible for each photosensitivity disorder, most commonly ultraviolet B (UVB, 290–320 nm), ultraviolet A (UVA, 320–400 nm), and visible light (400–800 nm).

PATHOLOGY

Findings are diverse for the different disorders and rarely diagnostic.

EPIDEMIOLOGY

• Variable for each disorder
• Photosensitivities with onset in childhood include albinism, hydroa aestivale, hydroa vacciniforme, the porphyrias (e.g., erythropoietic, erythropoietic protoporphyria, hepatoerythropoietic), and genetic disorders (e.g., xeroderma pigmentosa, Hartnup disease, poikiloderma congenitale, Bloom syndrome, and Cockayne syndrome).
• Photosensitivities that occur frequently in adults but can occur in childhood are vitiligo, chemically induced photosensitivities, polymorphous light eruption, and connective tissue disease.

GENETICS

• The genetic disorders include the porphyrias and others as previously listed.
• The various porphyrias have variable inheritance patterns, while most of the other genetic disorders are inherited in an autosomal-recessive pattern.
• There is a positive familial history in many cases of polymorphous light eruption.

 Differential Diagnosis

• Photosensitivity resulting from pigment loss:

—Albinism
—Vitiligo

• Idiopathic photosensitivity:

—Polymorphous light eruption
—Solar urticaria

• Chemically induced reactions

—Topical agents: perfumes, plant-associated phytophotodermatitis (e.g., lemons, limes, celery, parsnips, carrots, dill, parsley, figs, meadow grass, giant hogweed, mangos, wheat, clover, cocklebur, buttercups, Shepherd's purse, and pigweed), blankophores (e.g., optical brighteners in detergents), sunscreens, topical retinoids (e.g., tretinoin, adapalene)
—Systemic agents: tetracyclines, sulfonamides, nalidixic acid, griseofulvin, phenothiazines, oral hypoglycemic agents, amiodarone, quinine, isoniazid, and thiazide diuretics

• Metabolic disorders:

—Porphyrias: disorders of hemoglobin synthesis producing various porphyrins that are photosensitizers

• Genetic disorders:

—(see Epidemiology, above)

• Cutaneous diseases aggravated by sunlight:

—Connective tissue diseases

 Data Gathering

HISTORY

• Age of onset of rash?
• Occurrence in spring and summer?
• Occurrence after sun exposure?
• How long after sun exposure?
• Occurrence after exposure to sun through glass?
• Any oral medications? May be related to oral contraceptives, sulfa drugs, iodines/bromides, or phenytoin.
• Any new topical agents (e.g., perfumes, lemons, limes, sunscreens, etc.)? Photosensitivity may occur on neck or places where agents were placed on skin.

 Physical Examination

Finding: Distributed lesions
Significance: The distribution of lesions is the main sign of photosensitivity reactions. Lesions are prominent on sun-exposed skin such as the face, pinnae of the ears, the V of the neck, the nuchal area, and the dorsa of the hands. Often, sparing of the philtrum, the area below the chin, the eyelids, and other covered areas is seen. In phytophotodermatitis, linear or bizarre shapes can occur, including, as an example, hand prints if a caregiver has been squeezing limes and then picks up a child and the child is then exposed to sunlight.

Finding: Lesion characteristics
Significance: The characteristics of individual lesions vary with the particular disease and can include papules, vesicles, and plaques (polymorphous light eruption), sunburn (chemical reaction to a systemic agent), linear areas of hyperpigmentation (chemical reaction to a topical agent), skin cancers (xeroderma pigmentosum), vesicles (porphyria). In some cases, scarring can also be seen related to severe burns (porphyria).

PHYSICAL EXAMINATION TRICKS

Careful examination reveals accentuation of the rash on the nose, cheeks, and forehead with sparing of the eyelids and the submental portion of the chin. There is often a sharp cutoff in the nuchal area at the collar line.

 Laboratory Aids

Test: Phototesting
Significance: Using an artificial source of light, can confirm the presence of certain photosensitivities. Procedures are of two types. The first is exposure of skin to increasing doses of ultraviolet A and ultraviolet B to determine the erythema response (present at lower exposures than usual) and possibly reproduce lesions in certain diseases.
The second is photopatch testing in which photoallergic chemicals are applied under patches in duplicate, and one set is subsequently exposed to UVA. Patients who have photoallergic contact dermatitis develop a reaction under only the exposed patch of the agent causing the problem.

Test: Biochemical tests
Significance: Helpful for the diagnosis of the porphyrias with elevated levels of various porphyrins specific to each type in the urine, blood, or stool

SPECIALIZED TESTS FOR GENETIC DISEASES

- Cell culture: to evaluate DNA repair for xeroderma pigmentosum, or demonstrate chromosomal breaks in Bloom disease
- Measurement of specific amino acid and indole excretion patterns in Hartnup disease
- Measurement of antinuclear antibodies are helpful in connective tissue diseases.

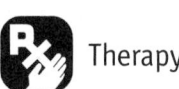 Therapy

- Protection against sun exposure is necessary.

—Avoiding the sun, particularly between 10 A.M. and 3 P.M., and wearing protective clothing is important.
—Sunscreens are helpful for those sensitive to UVB.
—Sunscreens should be waterproof and reapplied every 2 hours.
—The higher the sun protection factor (SPF—ratio of minimal erythema dose of sunscreened skin to minimal erythema dose of unprotected skin), the better.
—Sunscreens are less effective for blocking UVA and therefore less effective in helping patients with sensitivities to longer wavelengths.
—Sunscreens that contain both UVA and UVB blocking capabilities offer better protection than most. These include sunscreens containing avobenzone (Parsol 1789), titanium dioxide, and zinc oxide.
—Opaque formulations such as zinc oxide and titanium dioxide block ultraviolet and visible light but may be less cosmetically appealing.
—Patients with severe photosensitivities may have to avoid any significant light exposure.

- Removal of the offending agent is necessary in chemically induced photosensitivities.

—Any severe and acute eruptions may require a short course of oral prednisone.
—Antimalarial agents have been used for polymorphous light eruption, lupus erythematosus, solar urticaria, and porphyria cutanea tarda and require the experience of a specialist.

DURATION

Most patients require chronic protection against sun exposure. However, the problem is generally more acute in spring and summer months.

 Follow-Up

WHEN TO EXPECT IMPROVEMENT

Variable, depending on the specific condition

PROGNOSIS

With the exception of chemically induced photosensitivities, most of the conditions are chronic.

PITFALLS

If possible, it is important to accurately document the specific wavelength of light and the degree of photosensitivity in order to accurately advise the patient. This requires phototesting by a specialist.

 Common Questions and Answers

Q: What is the best sunscreen to use?
A: It depends on your particular problem. If you are sensitive to UVB, use a sunscreen with the highest SPF. If you are sensitive to UVA, sunscreens containing avobenzone, titanium dioxide, or zinc oxide are best.

Q: I have heard that sunscreens with an SPF above 15 are not necessary?
A: This is definitely not true for patients with photosensitivities, who have abnormal responses to light and require excessive protection. Even for the normal person, it is often not true. An SPF of 15 suggests that someone may receive 15 times more sun exposure with the sunscreen applied than without and not become sunburned. Some physicians have suggested that this is more than anyone should need. However, this number is calculated by testing in a controlled laboratory. Normal outdoor conditions, such as wind, reflection from water and sand, perspiration, and water exposure, can significantly decrease the effectiveness of the sunscreen.

Q: What is "sun allergy"?
A: This is a lay term for polymorphous light eruption, one of the most common photosensitivities presenting with papules, vesicles, and plaques 1 to 2 days after sun exposure. It usually recurs every spring and most patients learn to avoid sun exposure. However, ironically, it can improve with slow gradual sun exposure.

Q: Can I become allergic to sunscreens?
A: Certain active agents in sunscreens can produce an allergic response in rare individuals. If the rash recurs with each use, switch to another sunscreen with different ingredients. If the problem continues, it is necessary to consult a specialist for evaluation.

ICD-9-CM 692.72

BIBLIOGRAPHY

Harber LC, Bickers DR. *Photosensitivity diseases: principles of diagnosis and treatment*, 2nd ed. Toronto: BC Decker, 1989.

Hurwitz S. Photosensitivity and photoreactions. In: *Clinical pediatric dermatology a textbook of skin disorder of childhood and adolescence*, 2nd ed. Philadelphia: WB Saunders, 1993:83.

Author: Albert C. Yan
Cynthia Guzzo, 2nd edition

Pinworms

 Database

DEFINITION

Severe perianal pruritus, usually nocturnal or early morning and associated with difficulty sleeping; caused by deposition of pinworm eggs around the anus.

ETIOLOGY

Infection by *Enterobius vermicularis*

PATHOPHYSIOLOGY

- Adult worms inhabit the cecum, migrate to the anus, and deposit eggs on the perianal skin, which causes pruritus.
- Minimal inflammatory response in lower bowel mucosa correlates with few gastrointestinal symptoms.
- Ectopic locations (e.g., peritoneum, endometrium) are associated with granuloma formation.
- Pruritus in anal region may be associated with mucosal mastocytosis and histamine production.

EPIDEMIOLOGY

- Humans are the only natural host
- Spread by hand-to-mouth transmission
- Unrelated to personal hygiene
- Close contact is required for transmission
- Infection rates in the United States are 10% to 40%
- Late fall and winter infection most common
- Preschool- and school-aged children (5 to 10 years) predominantly

COMPLICATIONS

- Urethritis
- Vaginitis
- Salpingitis
- Pelvic peritonitis

PROGNOSIS

- Recurrence is common.
- Symptoms should resolve within a few days of treatment.

 Differential Diagnosis

INFECTION

- Other parasites
- Bacterial or fungal vulvovaginitis

ENVIRONMENTAL

- Irritative diaper dermatitis
- Chemical dermatitis
- Vulvitis from soaps or lotions

MISCELLANEOUS

- Habit (escalating itch-scratch cycle)
- Anal fissures (pain misinterpreted as pruritus)

 Data Gathering

HISTORY

Question: Is there a familial history of pinworms?
Significance: If yes, there may be spread between family members, so treatment of one patient will not clear the problem.

Question: When is the itching greatest?
Significance: Typically pinworm infections cause perianal itching at night or early morning.

Question: Have you seen any evidence of tiny white worms?
Significance: It may be possible to see small, white worms in the perianal area or stool at nighttime.

Physical Examination

- Few physical findings present
- Excoriation from scratching around anus
- Pinworms may be visible around anus

 ## Laboratory Aids

Test: "Scotch-tape" slide test
Significance: Parents press sticky side of clear tape to the perianal area in the morning before child rises; apply tape to a microscope slide and examine for pinworm ova; may need to be repeated several times.

 ## Therapy

- Mebendazole (Vermox), 100 mg chewable tablet by mouth, once; may repeat in 2 weeks, if necessary.
- Second-line drugs: pyrantel pamoate (11 mg/kg, maximum 1 g) and piperazine citrate (65 mg/kg, maximum 2.5 g for 7 days)

 ## Follow-Up

Generally not necessary

PREVENTION

- Treat all affected family members.
- Decontamination of the environment (wash sheets, towels, clothing; vacuum household)

PITFALLS

Reinfection is common if all close contacts are not treated.

 ## Common Questions and Answers

Q: Is this caused by poor hygiene?
A: No.

Q: Is infection with pinworms usually associated with other parasitic infections?
A: No.

Q: Can they be spread at day care?
A: Yes.

ICD-9-CM 127.4

BIBLIOGRAPHY

American Academy of Pediatrics. Pinworm infestation. In: Peter G, ed. *2000 red book: report of the Committee on Infectious Diseases*, 25th ed. Elk Grove, IL: American Academy of Pediatrics, 2000:448–450.

Cook GC. Enterobius vermicularis infection. *Gut* 1994;35(9):1159–1162.

Grencis RK, Hons BS, Cooper ES. Enterobius trichuris, Capillaria and hookworm including Ancylostoma caninum. In Weinstock JV, ed. Parasitic disease of the liver and intestines. *Gastroenterol Clin North Am* 1996;25(3):579–597.

Katz M, Hotez PJ. Parasitic nematode infections. In: Feigin RD, Cherry JD, eds. *Textbook of pediatric infectious diseases*, 4th ed. Philadelphia: WB Saunders, 1998:2503–2505.

Wu ML, Kuksuk LK, Olinger EJ. Enterobius vermicularis. *Arch Pathol Lab Med* 2000;124(4):647–648.

Author: Deborah L. Silver

Plague

 Database

DEFINITION

The bubonic plague is an enzootic infection that results in lymphadenitis and fever. Severe constitutional, gastrointestinal, neurologic, and respiratory symptoms (pneumonic plague) can also occur. "The black death" has a secure place in history as a devastating epidemic that affected one third of the population of Europe during the 14th century.

CAUSES

The illness commonly known as the plague is caused by *Yersinia pestis*, a gram-negative pleomorphic bacillus that is part of the Enterobacteriaceae family.

PATHOLOGY/PATHOPHYSIOLOGY

Dermatologic Portal of Entry

• *Y. pestis* is most commonly transmitted from fleas to humans via the regurgitation of the organism into the skin tissue during the flea's blood meal. Rodents, as well as dogs, cats, and rabbits, can thereby act as reservoirs of infection.
• Lymphatic spread of infection to the regional lymph nodes creates a localized inflammatory response. If antibody response prevents additional spread, this condition is known as *pestis minor*.
• Subsequent hematogenous spread of the organism to other organs results in the production of greater levels of bacterial endotoxin. This endotoxin is responsible for the systemic manifestations, as well as the high mortality rate, of the untreated illness.

Respiratory Portal of Entry

Pneumonic Plague

• Acquired via contact with the saliva or respiratory droplets
• Replication of the organism within the alveolar spaces results in a fulminant localized infection and endotoxemia.

Other Organ Systems Involved

• Liver
• Spleen
• Kidney
• Meninges

EPIDEMIOLOGY (AGE RELATED)

• More than half of the contemporary cases of plague occur in persons under 20 years of age, possibly because of an increased tendency for children to come into contact with small animals and rodents.

• An outbreak of the pneumonic plague has been reported recently in India; however, the identification of the specific causative organism has been called into question.
• A large proportion of the cases in the United States has occurred in the Southwest.
• No cases of person-to-person transmissions of plague pneumonia have been reported in the United States since 1925.

ASSOCIATED ILLNESSES

• Bubonic plague: lymphadenitis (usually inguinal); systemic manifestations; 75% of plague cases worldwide
• Pneumonic plague: pneumonia; systemic manifestations; rapidly progressive, often fatal
• Septicemic plague: tachycardia, hypotension, other organ involvement; either bubonic or pneumonic plague may progress to this condition.

 Differential Diagnosis

• Diagnosis of plague follows a high index of suspicion and a thorough review of the patient's lifestyle, travel history, and recent activities.
• The appearance of septicemia and endotoxin-mediated shock includes a large differential diagnosis that includes sepsis due to other bacteria or viruses, as well as distributive shock resulting from toxic ingestion or anaphylaxis.

INFECTION

• Recent reports of plague-like illnesses have been associated with infections by other organisms such as *Pseudomonas pseudomallei* (melioidosis) and *Francisella tularensis* (tularemia).
• *Pestis minor*, which involves exquisitely tender lymph nodes, may be confused with bacterial adenitis, tularemia, lymphogranuloma venereum, chancroid, or cat-scratch disease.

 Data Gathering

HISTORY

Question: What is the incubation period for this disease?
Significance: There is usually 2 to 6 days between exposure and first presentation of symptoms, but this period can be shorter for pneumonic plague.

Question: In the context of exposure to *Y. pestis*, what are the initial symptoms of exposure?
Significance: Initial symptoms include abrupt onset of fever, weakness, malaise.

Question: What are the initial symptoms of bubonic plague?
Significance: The patient may complain of pain in the groin or axillae prior to lymph node swelling.

 Physical Examination

• Patients may present initially with suppurative lymphadenitis in the groin, axillae, or neck regions.
• Patients with rapidly progressive illness are tachycardic, hypotensive, and toxic in appearance. Rashes and fever are more likely to be the initial presentation of patients with an initial pneumonic focus of infection.
• Other organ system involvement is common.

—Gastrointestinal: Abdominal pain, nausea, and diarrhea are usually due to the presence of inflammatory mediators. Hepatosplenomegaly is a common finding.

—Neurologic: Weakness, delirium, and coma are due to the effects of the endotoxin of *Y. pestis*.

• Patients with septicemia can experience renal (glomerular and parenchymal damage), hematologic (disseminated intravascular coagulation), and hepatic necrosis.

SPECIAL QUESTIONS

• A thorough travel history is imperative in order to raise the index of suspicion for diagnosing plague.
• Environmental history should include the presence of rats, ground squirrels, or prairie dogs in the patient's locale.

 Laboratory Aids

Test: Total white blood count
Significance: Usually 10,000 to 20,000, but may be as high as 100,000

Test: *Y. pestis* culture
Significance: Can be cultured on blood agar plates from lymph node aspirate, blood, cerebrospinal fluid, or sputum from patients with pneumonic plague.

Test: Gram stain, Wayson stain, Giemsa stain, or fluorescent antibody staining of the specimen.
Significance: May reveal the bipolar organisms.

Test: Comparison of acute and convalescent sera
Significance: Taken 3 to 4 weeks apart, show at least a fourfold increase in antibody titers by passive hemagglutination

Test: ELISA or direct fluorescent antibody (DFA) for *Y. Pestis*
Significance: Detects F1 antigen in blood or bubo during the acute phase of illness

Test: PCR assay for *Y. Pestis* (not available in commercial laboratories)
Significance: Detects, through amplification methods, dead bacteria from bubo aspirate

 Emergency Care

For septicemic patients, initial attention should be given to airway management and fluid resuscitation.

 Therapy

DRUGS

• In the acutely ill patient suspected of *Y. pestis* infection, streptomycin (30 mg/kg/d) can be administered by the intravenous or intramuscular route.
• Tetracycline (20–30 mg/kg IV per day), or chloramphenicol (75–100 mg/kg per day IV), should be added in severe cases or if meningitis is present.
• For the patient who does not require hospitalization, streptomycin (30 mg/kg/d), tetracycline (20–30 mg/kg/d) or chloramphenicol (75–100 mg/kg/d) may be administered enterally after cultures are obtained.
• Drainage of affected lymph nodes or abscesses, if necessary, should wait until at least 24 hours after initiation of therapy to prevent unnecessary spread of infected drainage.

DURATION

Therapy continued for at least 10 days. Severely ill patients may require a substantially longer course of therapy. Patients treated with streptomycin can be switched to other medications a few days after improvement is noted.

POSSIBLE CONFLICTS WITH OTHER TREATMENTS

To avoid permanent dental staining, patients younger than 8 years of age should not receive tetracycline unless absolutely necessary.

PREVENTION

• General prevention: Suppression of the rodent population in endemic areas, as well as de-infestation of cats and dogs, may reduce the prevalence of disease considerably.
• Hospital isolation (negative pressure) should be continued for 3 days after initiation of therapy.

—Pneumonic plague patients require strict respiratory and secretion isolation precautions.
—Bubonic plague patients with no evidence of pneumonia require drainage and secretion precautions.

• Exposed persons: All contacts of patients thought to suffer from plague should undergo:

—De-infestation of all clothing, pets, bedding, and homes
—Observation for fever or symptoms of disease for 7 to 10 days (inpatient or outpatient)

• Persons who have had contact with a patient with pneumonic plague require antimicrobial prophylaxis with tetracycline (15 mg/kg/d). For children under 8 years old, use trimethoprim-sulfamethoxazole (40 mg/kg/d), or IM streptomycin (20 mg/kg/d) for a total of 7 days.
• State public health authorities should be notified in cases of suspected plague.
• Vaccination with a five-vaccine regimen (three primary and two boosters) of inactivated whole-cell product is indicated for:

—Persons who intend to travel to or reside in endemic regions in which the domestic rats are infested.
—Laboratory workers or other professional who will be in contact with potentially infected rodents or their fleas.
—Booster doses should continue every 1 to 2 years as long as the exposure exists.

 Follow-Up

WHEN TO EXPECT IMPROVEMENT

Resolution of symptoms should begin in the first 3 days after initiation of therapy; however, the rate of clinical improvement depends on the initial severity of illness.

SIGNS TO WATCH FOR

Neurologic sequelae of the plague often manifest during the course of treatment for the illness.

PITFALLS

• Certain strains of *Y. pestis* are resistant to streptomycin. In general, these organisms are sensitive to chloramphenicol.

• A high index of suspicion is needed to diagnose plague. Patients who present with fever, tachycardia, or tachypnea, rather than lymphadenitis, are at higher risk for delayed diagnosis and serious sequelae.

 Common Questions and Answers

Q: Can one determine the risks of being exposed to plague during international travel?
A: Yes. The CDC provides a service that contains updated information for international travel. This automated traveler's hotline is accessible from a touch-tone telephone at all hours. The telephone number is (404) 332-4559. Similar information is available by facsimile at (404) 332-4565.

Q: Does persistent fever during treatment for plague warrant altering the antibiotic regimen?
A: No, fever can persist for up to 2 weeks after appropriate antibiotic therapy for plague.

ICD-9-CM 020.9

BIBLIOGRAPHY

American Academy of Pediatrics. Plague. In: *2000 red book: report of the Committee on Infectious Diseases*, 25th ed. Elk Grove IL: American Academy of Pediatrics, 2000.

Centers for Disease Control and Prevention. Fatal human plague—Arizona and Colorado, 1996. *MMWR* 1997;46:617–620.

Centers for Disease Control and Prevention. Human plague—United States, 1993–1994. *MMWR* 1994;43:242–246.

Centers for Disease Control and Prevention. Update: human plague—India, 1994. *MMWR* 1994;43:722–723.

Cleri DJ, Vernaleo JR, Lombardi LJ, et al. Plague pneumonia disease caused by *Yersinia pestis. Semin Respir Infect* 1997;12:12–23.

Crook LD, Tempest B. Plague: a clinical review of 27 cases. *Arch Intern Med* 1992;152:1253.

Gage KL, Dennis DT, Orloski KA, et al. Cases of cat-associated human plague in the western US, 1977–1998. *Clin Infect Dis* 2000;30: 893–900.

Gomez NF, Cleary TG. Yersinia species. In: Long SS, Pickering LK, eds. *Principles and practice of pediatric infectious diseases*. New York: Churchill Livingstone, 1997:935–939.

Perry RD, Featherston JD. Yersinia pestis—etiologic agent of plague. *Clin Microbiol Rev* 1997;10:35–66.

Rahalson L, Vololonirina M, Ratsitornahina M, et al. Diagnosis of bubonic plague by PCR in Madagascar under field conditions. *J Clin Microbiol* 2000;38:260–263.

Author: Joel A. Fein

Pleural Effusion

 Database

DEFINITION
Accumulation of fluid in the pleural cavity

CAUSES
- There is normally 1 to 15 mL of fluid in the pleural space.
- Alterations in the flow and/or absorption of this fluid leads to its accumulation.
- Mechanisms influence this flow of fluid:
—Increased capillary hydrostatic pressure (e.g., congestive heart failure, overhydration)
—Decreased pleural space hydrostatic pressure (e.g., post-thoracentesis, atelectasis)
—Decreased plasma oncotic pressure (e.g., hypoalbuminemia, nephrosis)
—Increased capillary permeability (e.g., infection, toxins, connective tissue diseases, malignancy)
—Impaired lymphatic drainage from the pleural space (e.g., disruption of the thoracic duct)
—Passage of fluid from the peritoneal cavity through the diaphragm to the pleural space (e.g., hepatic cirrhosis with ascites)

PATHOPHYSIOLOGY
- Dependent on the underlying disease
- Two types of pleural effusion:
—Transudate: Mechanical forces of hydrostatic and oncotic pressures are altered, favoring liquid filtration.
—Exudate: Damage to the pleural surface occurs that alters its ability to filter pleural fluid; lymphatic drainage is diminished
- Stages associated with parapneumonic effusions (infectious exudates):
—Exudative stage: free flowing fluid; pleural fluid glucose, protein, LDH, and pH are normal
—Fibrinolytic stage: loculations are forming; increase in fibrin, polymorphonuclear leukocytes, and bacterial invasion of pleural cavity are occurring; pleural fluid glucose and pH falls while protein and LDH increase
—Organizing stage (empyema): fibroblasts grow; pleural peal forms; pleural fluid parameters worsen

EPIDEMIOLOGY
- Dependent on underlying cause
—Pneumonia (most common cause effusion)
—For parapneumonic effusion, the most common organisms include:
  —*Staphylococcus aureus*: 28%
  —*Streptococcus pneumoniae*: 20%
  —*Haemophilus influenzae*: 13%
—Congenital heart disease
—Malignancy

COMPLICATIONS
- Hypoxia
- Respiratory distress
- Persistent fevers
- Decreased cardiac function
- Malnutrition (seen in chylothorax)
- Shock (secondary to blood loss in cases of hemothorax)
- Trapped lung

PROGNOSIS
- Dependent on underlying disease process:
—Properly treated infectious etiology: excellent prognosis
—Malignancy: poor prognosis

 Differential Diagnosis

TRANSUDATE
- Cardiovascular
—Congestive heart failure
—Constrictive pericarditis
- Nephrotic syndrome with hypoalbuminemia
- Cirrhosis
- Atelectasis

EXUDATE
- Infection
—Bacterial effusions (*S. aureus* is most common organism)
—Tuberculous effusion
—Viral effusions: adenovirus; influenza
—Fungal effusions: most not associated with effusions; *Nocardia* and *Actinomyces* are most common
—Parasitic effusions
- Neoplasm
—Seen mostly in leukemia and lymphoma
—Uncommon in children
- Connective tissue disease
—Rheumatoid arthritis
—Systemic lupus erythematosus
—Wegener granulomatosis
- Pulmonary embolus
- Intraabdominal disease
—Subdiaphragmatic abscess
—Pancreatitis
- Others
—Sarcoidosis
—Esophageal rupture
—Hemothorax
—Chylothorax
—Drugs
—Chemical injury
—Postirradiation effusion

 Data Gathering

HISTORY
- Underlying disease determines most of systemic symptoms
- The patient may be asymptomatic until the amount of fluid is large enough to cause cardiorespiratory distress
- Dyspnea and cough are associated with large effusions
- Fever
- Pleuritic pain (pneumonia may cause irritation of the parietal pleura causing pleural pain; as the effusion increases and separates the pleural membrane, the pain may disappear)

 Physical Examination

- Decreased thoracic wall excursion on the ipsilateral side
- Fullness of intercostal spaces on the ipsilateral side
- Trachea and cardiac apex displaced toward the contralateral side (may produce a mediastinal shift that can reduce venous return and compromise the cardiac output)
- Dull or flat percussion on the ipsilateral side (suggesting the presence of consolidation of pleural effusion)
- Decreased tactile and vocal fremitus
- Decreased whispering pectoriloquy
- Pleural rub during early phase (may resolve as fluid accumulates in the pleural space)
- Decreased breath sounds

 Laboratory Aids

- Tests
—Thoracentesis: indicated whenever etiology is unclear or effusion is symptomatic
—Pleural biopsy: if thoracentesis is nondiagnostic; most useful for diseases that cause extensive involvement of the pleura (e.g., tuberculosis, malignancies); confirms neoplastic involvement in 40% to 70% of cases
—Serology values (to follow the degree of inflammation and the response to therapy): Erythrocyte sedimentation rate (ESR); C reactive protein (CRP)
- Imaging
—Chest radiograph (upright film): anteroposterior projection can see pleural fluid when there is >400 mL; lateral projection can see pleural fluid when there is >200 mL
—Chest radiograph (lateral decubitus film): can evaluate for free-flowing pleural fluid; can identify as little as 50 mL of pleural fluid
—Ultrasound: can diagnose small (3–5 mL) loculated collections of pleural fluid; useful as a guide for thoracentesis; can distinguish between pleural thickening and pleural effusion
—CT scan: can clearly identify effusions/ empyemas, abscess, or pulmonary consolidations; useful for defining the extent of loculated effusions

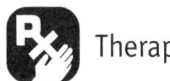 Therapy

OVERVIEW
- Supportive measures
—Maintain adequate oxygenation, fluid status, and nutritional balance
—Antipyretic agents when febrile
—Pain control

Pleural Fluid Analysis

TEST	TRANSUDATE	EXUDATE
pH	7.4	<7.3
Protein (g/100 mL)	<3.0	≥3.0
Pleural/serum protein	<0.5	≥0.5
LDH (IU)	<200	≥200
Pleural/serum LDH	<0.6	≥0.6
Pleural/serum amylase	<1	≥1
Glucose (mg/dL)	>40	≤40
RBC	<5000	≥5000
WBC	<1000 (mostly mononu-clear cells)	≥1000 (mostly PMNs)

—Note: pleural fluid glucose of less than 40 mg/dL suggests a parapneumonic, tuberculosis, malignant, or rheumatic etiology to the effusion.
• Treat the underlying disease
—Antibiotics for infections
—Cardiac medications for congestive heart failure
—Chemotherapeutic agents for malignancies
—Antiinflammatory agents (e.g., steroids) for connective tissue diseases
—Medium-chain triglycerides and low-fat diet for chylothorax
• Effective drainage of pleural fluid
—Thoracentesis
—Chest tube drainage
—Surgical drainage

DRAINAGE METHODS
• Thoracentesis
—For diagnosis (to distinguish between a transudate and an exudate; for culture material if infection is suspected)
—For relief of dyspnea or cardiorespiratory distress
• Chest tube thoracostomy
—Reduce reaccumulation of fluid
—Drain empyema
• Intrapleural fibrinolytics
—Adjunct to complete drainage in complicated (e.g., multiloculated empyema) pleural effusions
—Streptokinase and urokinase are agents of choice

SURGICAL MANAGEMENT
• Video-assisted thoracic surgery (VATS)
—Alternative to more invasive procedures (e.g., open thoracotomy/decortication)
—Débridement through pleural visualization and lysis of adhesions/loculations
—Useful when initial drainage is delayed, when loculations prevent adequate drainage, or patient is failing more conservative therapy
• Open thoracotomy with rib resection
—Encapsulated empyema

• Decortication
—Symptomatic chronic empyema
—Relief of thick fibrous peal
• Pleurectomy
—Chylothorax
—Malignant effusions
• Pleurodesis
—For recurrent effusions
—Chemical agents frequently used: tetracycline, doxycycline, talc, quinacrine
—Surgical methods include mechanical abrasion, pleurectomy via VATS, or open thoracotomy route

ANTIBIOTICS
• Used when effusion is caused by an infection
• Specific antibiotics dictated by organism identified
• If effusion is sterile, broad-spectrum antibiotics are indicated to cover for the usual organisms.

DURATION OF THERAPY
• Drainage
—Stopped when patient is asymptomatic (afebrile, no distress) and drainage <50 mL/h
—Thick, loculated empyema requires prolonged drainage (and possibly a VATS procedure if not improving).
• Antibiotics
—Clinical improvement usually occurs in 48 to 72 hours
—Dependent on organism and degree of illness (total duration is controversial):
 —*Staphylococcus aureus:* 3 to 4 weeks minimum
 —*Streptococcus pneumoniae:* 2 weeks minimum
 —*Haemophilus influenzae:* 2 weeks minimum
—Should remain on IV antibiotics until afebrile
—Complete remainder of therapy on oral antibiotics

DIET
• Chylothorax
—Medium-chain triglycerides
—Nutritional replacement
—(At least) 4 to 5 weeks on this regimen

Follow-Up

WHEN TO EXPECT IMPROVEMENT
• Clinical improvement usually within 1 to 2 weeks
• With empyemas, may have fever spikes for up to 2 to 3 weeks after improvement noted

PITFALLS
• Cytologic examination
—Fresh and heparinized specimen should be refrigerated at 4°C until it can be processed.
—Fixatives should not be added.
• Malignant effusions
—Sclerosing procedures usually ineffective
—Chest tube drainage can create a pneumothorax because the lung is incarcerated by the tumor.

Common Questions and Answers

Q: How long of a treatment course of antibiotics is required for empyemas?
A: Dependent on the underlying organism; usually between 2 to 4 weeks total of IV/PO.
Q: When will the chest x-ray normalize?
A: May take up to 6 months (or longer) to normalize.
Q: When will the pulmonary function tests normalize?
A: Dependent on extent of effusion, it may take up to 6 to 12 months.

ICD-9-CM 511.9

BIBLIOGRAPHY
Alkrinawi S, Chernick V. Pleural infection in children. *Semin Respir Infect* 1996;11:148–154.

Bouros D, Schiza S, Patsourakis G, et al. Intrapleural streptokinase vs. urokinase in the treatment of complicated parapneumonic effusions: a prospective, double blind study. *Am J Respir Crit Care Med* 1997;155:291–295.

de Benedictis FM, De Giorgi G, Niccoli A, et al. Treatment of complicated pleural effusion with intracavitary urokinase in children. *Pediatr Pulmonol* 2000;29(6):438–442.

Doski JJ, Lou D, Hicks BA, et al. Management of parapneumonic collections in infants and children. *J Pediatr Surg* 2000;35:265–268; discussion 269–270.

Givan DC, Eigen H. Common pleural effusions in children. *Clin Chest Med* 1998;19:363–371.

Kern JA, Rodgers BM. Thorascopy in the management of empyema in children. *J Pediatr Surg* 1993;28:1128–1132.

Kogut KA, Lobe TE. Urokinase in the management of complicated parapneumonic effusions in children *Clin Pediatr* 1999;38(6):378–379.

Kornecki A, Sivan Y. Treatment of loculated pleural effusion with intrapleural urokinase in children. *J Pediatr Surg* 1997;32:1473–1475.

Merino JM, Carpintero I, Alvarez T, et al. Tuberculous pleural effusion in children. *Chest* 1999;115(1):26–30.

Montgomery M. Air and liquid in the pleural space. In: Chernick V, ed. *Kendig's disorders of the respiratory tract in children*. Philadelphia: WB Saunders, 1998:389–411.

Ramnath RR, Heller RM, Ben-Ami T, et al. Implications of early sonographic evaluation of parapneumonic effusions in children with pneumonia. *Pediatrics* 1998;101(1 pt 1):68–71.

Sahn SA. The pleura. *Am Rev Respir Dis* 1988;138:184–234.

Author: Richard M. Kravitz

Pneumocystis Carinii Pneumonia

 Database

DEFINITION

Opportunistic lung infection caused by *Pneumocystis carinii* (PC). This organism is currently considered a primitive fungus. It has two developmental forms: a cyst containing sporozoites and an extracystic one named trophozoite.

- *P. carinii* pneumonia (PCP) occurs almost exclusively in the immunocompromised host. Children with congenital or acquired immune deficiency syndrome (AIDS), and recipients of suppressive therapy in the treatment of malignancies or after organ transplantation are at high risk.
- Sporadic cases have been reported in patients with hematologic disorders, rheumatoid arthritis, nephrosis leading to hypoproteinemia, and chronic infectious diseases.
- PCP is an AIDS-defining illness. It is the most common opportunistic life-threatening lung infection in infants with perinatally acquired HIV disease.
- PC causes a diffuse pneumonitis characterized by fever, tachypnea, hypoxemia, and bilateral diffuse infiltrates in the roentgenogram. It is a severe condition frequently leading to respiratory failure necessitating intubation and mechanical ventilation.
- Chemoprophylaxis against this microorganism has proven successful. Therefore, early identification of the HIV-infected mother becomes essential.
- Despite the advances in therapy, its infection continues to carry severe morbidity and mortality.

PATHOPHYSIOLOGY

- In the immunodeficient child the pathologic changes occur predominantly in the alveoli. Cysts and trophozoites are seen adhering to the alveolar lining cells or in the cytoplasm of macrophages.
- As infection progresses, the alveolar spaces are filled with a pink, foamy exudate containing fibrin, abundant desquamative cells, and large number of organisms. Alveolar septal thickening with mononuclear cell infiltration is also seen.

EPIDEMIOLOGY

- Mode of transmission is unknown.

—Airborne person-to-person transmission is possible, but case contacts are rarely identified.
—Environmentally acquired.

- Asymptomatic infection appears early in life, more than 70% of healthy individuals have antibodies by age 4.
- Primary infection is likely to be the prominent mechanism in infants, whereas reactivation of latent disease may play a significant role later in life.

- PCP in the HIV patient can occur at any time, but usually presents during the first year of life. The higher incidence is between 3 and 6 months of age.
- In leukemic patients, the incidence of PCP has been directly related to the degree of immunodeficiency resulting from chemotherapy.
- Epidemics of PCP were reported in premature and malnourished infants during wartime. This type has been termed the infantile form.

COMPLICATIONS

High rate of respiratory failure necessitating intubation and mechanical ventilation (about 60%)

PROGNOSIS

- 10% to 40% mortality in treated patients
- Near 100% mortality if patient is untreated
- About 35% of the patients will have reoccurrence unless lifetime prophylaxis is instituted.

 Differential Diagnosis

VIRAL INFECTIONS

- Common viral respiratory pathogens
- Cytomegalovirus
- Epstein-Barr virus

BACTERIAL INFECTIONS

- *Mycobacterium tuberculosis*
- *Mycobacterium avium-intracellulare*

OTHER

Lymphocytic interstitial pneumonitis

 Data Gathering

HISTORY

Question: Malnourished?
Significance: Infantile form has a subacute onset with nonspecific manifestations:

- Poor feeding, weight loss, and restlessness
- Chronic diarrhea
- Usually without fever
- After 1 to 2 weeks, the patient develops progressive tachypnea, respiratory distress, and cough.

Question: Sporadic or immunocompromised host?
Significance: This form has a more abrupt onset, even a fulminant one:

- Fever (>38.5°C)
- Nonproductive cough
- Dyspnea at rest

These listed forms are general clinical guidelines. Symptoms may be superimposed and can be seen in infants, children, and adolescents.

 Physical Examination

Finding: Fever and significant tachypnea
Significance: Are characteristic

Finding: Hypoxemia
Significance: Early in the course of disease that seems disproportionate with the auscultatory findings

Finding: Rapidly progressive respiratory distress with cyanosis
Significance: Respiratory failure early in course

Finding: Absence of crackles
Significance: A common initial finding

Finding: Chest auscultation
Significance: Can reveal decreased breath sounds, crackles, and rhonchi

Finding: Coryza and wheezing
Significance: Have infrequently been reported

 Laboratory Aids

Test: Arterial blood gas
Significance:

- pH is usually increased
- Reduced Po_2 in room air (<70 mm Hg)
- Alveolar-arterial oxygen gradient (>30 mm Hg)
- Decreased Pco_2

OTHER TESTS

- Chest radiograph

Test: Lactate dehydrogenase (LDH)
Significance: Can be elevated in patients with AIDS and PCP, but this finding is nonspecific.

Test: White blood count
Significance: Is usually normal

PATHOLOGY

- Definitive diagnosis can be obtained by demonstration of PC in pulmonary specimens:

—Induced sputum
—Bronchoalveolar lavage (90% sensitivity), usually through flexible bronchoscopy
—Open lung or transbronchial biopsy

Test: Staining
Significance:

- Cysts stain with Gomori methenamine-silver nitrate or toluidine blue-O stains
- Sporozoite and trophozoites are identified with polychrome stains (Giemsa, Wright, polychrome methylene blue)
- Immunofluorescent monoclonal antibodies (high sensitivity)

- May appear normal (4% of cases)
- Most common radiologic presentation is diffuse bilateral alveolar infiltrates:

—Initially of perihilar distribution, spreads to the periphery
—Apices are the least affected
—Interstitial infiltrates and air bronchograms can be seen
—Rapid progression to whole lung consolidation

- Presence of a hilar or mediastinal adenopathy may indicate other process such as *M. tuberculosis*, *M. avium-intracellulare*, fungal infections, cytomegalovirus, or lymphoma.

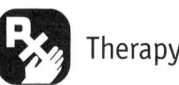 ## Therapy

ANTIBIOTICS

- Trimethoprim-sulfamethoxazole (TMP-SMX) is the drug of choice.

—TMP (15–20 mg/kg/d) and SMX (75–100 mg/kg/d) IV PO divided every 6 hours.
—Follow-up of serum levels may be considered. Target values are 3 to 5 μg/mL TMP and 100 to 150 μg/mL SMX.
—Minimum 2 weeks, sometimes 3 weeks of therapy is required.

ALTERNATIVE THERAPY

- Pentamidine isothionate

—4 mg/kg/d IV (or IM) given in a single daily dose for minimum 2 weeks.
—Total daily dose should not exceed 300 mg.
—Used in patients who cannot tolerate TMP-SMX or unresponsive after 5 to 7 days of therapy.
—Same effectiveness as TMP-SMX, but with higher incidence of side effects. Concomitant use with didanosine increases the risk of pancreatitis.

- Atavaquone is approved for adults who cannot tolerate TMP-SMX.

—Limited pediatric experience. Suggested dose is 40 mg/kg daily divided bid.

SUPPORTIVE THERAPY

- Supply oxygen as necessary to keep Pao_2 above 70 mm Hg
- Mechanical ventilation must be considered if Pao_2 is less than 60 mm Hg on Fio_2 of 0.5
- Corticosteroids

—May be beneficial in HIV patients with moderate to severe PCP
—Not systematically evaluated in children

- Consider when Pao_2 is less than 70 mm Hg or the alveolar-arterial gradient is greater than 35 mm Hg
- In patients over 13 years of age suggested dose: prednisone 40 mg PO b.i.d. for days 1 to 5, 40 mg PO qd for days 6 to 10, 20 mg PO qd for days 11 to 21 with tapering. Younger patients may receive 2 mg/kg/d during days 7 to 10 with weaning over 10 to 14 days.

PROPHYLAXIS

- During specially high-risk periods, PCP can be effectively prevented in the immunodeficient host by chemoprophylaxis in the following groups:

—HIV-exposed: 4 to 6 weeks to 4 months
—HIV-infected or indeterminate: 4 to 12 months
—HIV-infected: 1 to 5 years if $CD4^+$ T-lymphocyte count is less than 500 cells/μL or percentage less than 15%
—HIV-infected: more than or equal to 5 years if $CD4^+$ T-lymphocyte count is less than 200 cells/μL or percentage less than 15%
—Severely symptomatic HIV patient or with rapidly declining CD4 count
—High-risk periods of children with congenital immunodeficiencies, cancer, or organ transplants
—HIV patients who had previous episode of PCP
—HIV-exposed: birth to 4 to 6 weeks require no prophylaxis

RECOMMENDED STRATEGY

- TMP (150 mg/m^2/d) with SMX (750 mg/m^2/d) PO divided b.i.d. daily on 3 consecutive days per week, or
- TMP (5 mg/kg/d) and SMX (25 mg/kg/d) PO divided b.i.d. daily on 3 consecutive days per week.

ALTERNATIVE REGIMEN

- Dapsone 2 mg/kg (100 mg maximum) PO once daily
- Aerosolized pentamidine (>5 years old)

—300 mg via Respigard II inhaler once monthly

- If neither dapsone nor pentamidine is tolerated, IV pentamidine 4 mg/kg administered every 2 or 4 weeks is recommended.

 ## Follow-Up

WHEN TO EXPECT IMPROVEMENT

- After 5 to 7 days of treatment
- If no improvement, TMP-SMX should be replaced with pentamidine.

ISOLATION OF HOSPITALIZED PATIENT

Standard precautions required. Isolation from other immunodeficient patients is recommended.

PITFALLS

- HIV-infected patients have a higher rate of adverse reactions to TMP-SMX than in the general population, approximately in 15% of patients. One half of them will develop rash, fever, or neutropenia.
- Prophylactic medication protects the patient as long as the drug is administered. Does not eradicate PC.
- Aerosolized pentamidine prophylaxis failure usually demonstrates organisms in the upper lobes. BAL of this area becomes the procedure of choice.

 ## Common Questions and Answers

Q: Which are the most common side effects of pentamidine?
A: They include hypoglycemia, impaired renal or liver function, anemia, thrombocytopenia, neutropenia, hypotension, and skin rashes. Can be expected in 50% of the patients.

Q: How frequently is prophylaxis failure seen?
A: Adequate TMP-SMX treatment has only a 3% failure rate.

Q: Adverse reactions to TMP-SMX during PCP therapy?
A: Continuation of treatment, if the reactions are not severe, is recommended.

ICD-9-CM 136.3

BIBLIOGRAPHY

Abrams EJ. Opportunistic infections and other clinical manifestations of HIV disease in children. *Pediatr Clin North Am* 2000;47:79–103.

American Academy of Pediatrics. *2000 red book: report of the Committee on Infectious Diseases*, 25th ed. Elk Grove Village, IL: American Academy of Pediatrics 2000:460–465.

Hughes WT. Pneumocystis carinii pneumonitis. In: Chernick V, ed. *Kendig's disorders of the respiratory tract in children*, 46th edition. Philadelphia: W.B. Saunders. 1998;503–511.

Authors: Danna Tauber
Roberto V. Nachajon, 2nd edition

Pneumonia—Bacterial

 Database

DEFINITION

Inflammation and infection of the lung due to a bacterial pathogen: classified by anatomy such as lobar, interstitial, or broncho-pneumonia, or by microbiologic pathogen

ETIOLOGY

- *Streptococcus pneumoniae*
- *Haemophilus influenzae*
- *Staphylococcus aureus*
- Group B streptococcus (neonates)
- Anaerobic bacteria (aspiration pneumonia)
- *Legionella pneumophila*
- Group A streptococcus
- *Neisseria meningitidis*
- Gram-negative enteric bacilli
- *Mycoplasma pneumoniae*
- *Chlamydia pneumoniae*
- *Pneumocystis carinii*
- Other infections can be source of local infection or result in hematogenous spread to the lungs: sinusitis, otitis media, epiglottitis, meningitis, osteomyelitis
- Predisposing conditions include cerebral palsy, altered mental status, seizure disorder, and congenital disorders.

PATHOPHYSIOLOGY

- Hematogenous spread is rare.
- Acquired immunodeficiency may result in decreased host defense against infectious agents.
- Impairment in any one of these areas may result in infection: epiglottal reflex (prevents aspiration), cough reflex (expulsion of infected secretions), protective epithelial lining with cilia and mucus-producing cells, alveolar macrophages (bacterial killing), immune response (includes antibodies, complement, opsonins), and lymphatic drainage (affects host's susceptibility to infection).
- Nasogastric tube and filtration in nares may also predispose one to infection.

GENETICS

Predisposing genetic conditions:

- Congenital anomalies (cleft palate, tracheoesophageal fistula, pulmonary sequestration, Kartagener syndrome)
- Congenital defects of immune system, sickle cell disease
- Defect in quality of secretions (cystic fibrosis)

EPIDEMIOLOGY

- Children younger than 2 years of age more susceptible than older children
- Male/female ratio is 2:1
- May follow epidemics of viral infections
- Human transmission via droplet spread, more rarely airborne
- All seasons; winter and spring, most common

COMPLICATIONS

- Respiratory failure and cardiorespiratory collapse
- Pleural effusion
- Empyema
- Lung abscess
- Pneumothorax
- Pneumatoceles
- Pericarditis
- Bacteremia
- Sepsis
- Antibiotic resistance

PROGNOSIS

- Excellent: 1% mortality rate in uncomplicated cases of pneumococcal pneumonia
- Longer recovery, but still good outcome with other pathogens
- Uncomplicated pneumonias will recover in 1 to 5 days

 Differential Diagnosis

INFECTION

- Viral pneumonia (adenovirus, influenza, parainfluenza, respiratory syncytial virus, echovirus, and coxsackievirus)
- Fungal infections (histoplasmosis, blastomycosis, *Candida*)
- Rickettsia
- Tuberculosis
- Parasites

ENVIRONMENTAL

- Aspiration of foreign body
- Inhalation of toxin
- Drug reaction

TUMORS

- Metastatic (leukemia, lymphoma, solid tumors)
- Primary lung malignancy (rare in children)

TRAUMA

- Pulmonary contusion
- Traumatic airway obstruction

CONGENITAL

- Cystic fibrosis
- Pulmonary sequestration
- Congenital heart disease

IMMUNOLOGIC

- Collagen vascular disease
- Sarcoidosis

MISCELLANEOUS

- Reactive airways disease
- Pulmonary hemosiderosis
- Intraabdominal pathology causing splinting or reactive effusion
- Atelectasis

 Data Gathering

HISTORY

- Recent upper respiratory tract is often part of the presenting history.
- Fever, headache, malaise, lethargy, chills
- Anorexia with dehydration is common.
- Cough, shortness of breath, trouble breathing
- Chest pain
- Nausea, vomiting, diarrhea, abdominal pain
- Underlying medical conditions
- Duration of symptoms
- Ill contacts
- History of previous pneumonias

 Physical Examination

- Tachypnea, dyspnea, cough, grunting, intercostal retractions, nasal flaring, splinting of affected side, abdominal distention
- Decreased breath sounds, rales, and dullness to percussion
- Lung examination may be normal.
- Friction rub may be heard over an effusion.
- Wheezing is rare in bacterial pneumonia (exception: *Mycoplasma pneumoniae* pneumonia).
- Observe bare-chested child in parent's arms from a distance to determine respiratory rate and work of breathing.

Laboratory Aids

Test: CBC
Significance: White blood cell count of 15,000 frequently found; low white blood cell counts (e.g., <5,000) sometimes associated with severe and overwhelming infection

Test: Blood culture
Significance: Positive in 10% to 15% of cases of *H. influenzae, S. pneumoniae,* and *S. aureus* pneumonias

Test: Pleural fluid studies
Significance: Gram stain, culture, cell count, glucose, protein, LDH, and pH may be helpful if effusion present

Test: Gram stain and culture of sputum
Significance: Almost impossible to acquire in children without bronchoscopy; if obtained, may identify pathogen

Test: Pulse oximetry
Significance: Less than 92% oxygen saturation indicates significant hypoxia.

Test: Arterial blood gas
Significance: Evaluate for hypoxia, hypercarbia, and respiratory acidosis in patient with respiratory distress.

RADIOGRAPHIC IMAGING

Test: Chest radiograph, two views (PA and lateral; AP for children too young to cooperate and sit upright)
Significance: Lobar consolidations are common in *S. pneumoniae* and *H. influenzae;* patchy infiltrates are nonspecific in infancy; hilar adenopathy is a red flag for tuberculosis; pneumatoceles suggest *S. aureus* or gram-negative organisms.

Test: Decubitus chest films
Significance: May be needed to determine the size and nature of effusions

Test: CT scans of the chest
Significance: Allow one to differentiate parenchymal consolidation from pleural fluid when an effusion is suspected

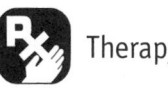

Therapy

- ABCs (airway, breathing, circulation); life support measures including mechanical ventilation may be required
- Supplemental humidified oxygen as needed
- Intravenous fluid rehydration is often necessary
- Bronchodilator inhalation therapy (Albuterol) may be used if wheezing is present
- Drainage of pleural effusions (therapeutic) and chest tube placement may be necessary.
- Bronchoscopy to determine pathogen or rule out foreign body or tumor indicated when

illness is protracted, recurrent, or not responding to therapy.

DRUGS

- Neonates

—Intravenous ampicillin *and*
—Aminoglycoside (gentamicin) *or*
—Third-generation cephalosporin (cefotaxime)

- Older children

—Inpatient—intravenous ampicillin, second- or third-generation cephalosporins. Complicated pneumonias with effusion and/or abscess formation require 14 to 21 days of IV therapy.
—Outpatient—amoxicillin (high dose, 80 mg/kg/d, if resistance suspected), amoxicillin/clavulanate, second- or third-generation cephalosporins, erythromycin, semisynthetic macrolides. Treat for 7 to 10 days if uncomplicated.

- Organism-specific therapy

—*S. aureus:* Use penicillinase-resistant penicillin (nafcillin, oxacillin)
—Resistant *S. pneumoniae* (know prevalence in your area). If infection is life threatening, consider vancomycin until sensitivities are available.
—*H. influenzae* infections should be treated with cephalosporins.
—Anaerobic infections (aspiration pneumonia) should be covered with penicillin or clindamycin.
—Gram-negative pneumonia should be treated with a regimen that includes an aminoglycoside with broad activity such as amikacin or tobramycin.
—*M. pneumoniae* and *C. pneumonia* require therapy with erythromycin, a macrolide, or tetracycline (in children older than 8 years of age).

- Therapeutic procedures

—Thoracentesis (diagnostic or therapeutic) in presence of effusion
—Chest tube placement for empyema
—Surgical drainage of lung abscess may be indicated

Follow-Up

- Radiograph may be abnormal for up to 6 weeks; therefore, serial x-rays are not recommended.
- Complicated pneumonias may be associated with restrictive or obstructive lung disease.
- Pulmonary function tests should be done on a case-by-case basis.

PREVENTION

- Pneumococcal vaccine should be given to immunocompromised patients and those with sickle cell disease.

- Children with sickle cell disease should take prophylactic penicillin for protection against encapsulated organisms, including pneumococcus.
- Pneumococcal 7-valent conjugate vaccine (Prevnar) now recommended at 2, 4, 6, and 12 to 15 months of age and for older, unvaccinated children following a schedule depending on age.

PITFALLS

- Dehydration or very early detection may correspond to x-ray findings lagging behind the clinical course.
- Bacterial resistance and poor response to antimicrobial require attention and reevaluation.
- Hydration and nutritional status are sometimes overlooked.

Common Questions and Answers

Q: When should a child with pneumonia be admitted to the hospital?
A: When any of the following conditions are present: dehydration, hypoxia, significant respiratory distress, failure of outpatient management (worsening or no response in 24–72 hours), very young age (<6 months), concern for compliance with treatment, or secondary complications (e.g., effusions, empyema, pneumothorax, etc.).

Q: Who should get a follow-up chest radiograph?
A: Any child with recurrent pneumonias, persistent symptoms, severe atelectasis, unusually located infiltrates, pneumothorax, or large effusions.

ICD-9-CM 482.9

BIBLIOGRAPHY

Arquedas AG, et al. Bacterial pneumonias. In: Chernick V, Kendig EL, eds. *Disorders of the respiratory tract in children.* Philadelphia: W.B. Saunders. 1990:371–380.

Lerou PH. Lower respiratory tract infections in children. *Curr Opin Pediatr* 2001;13(2): 200–206.

McCracken GH Jr. Diagnosis and management of pneumonia in children. *Pediatr Infect Dis J* 2000;19(9):924–928.

McCracken GH Jr. Etiology and treatment of pneumonia. *Pediatr Infect Dis J* 2000;19(4): 373–377.

Author: Deborah L. Silver

Pneumothorax

 Database

DEFINITION

Air in the pleural space

PATHOPHYSIOLOGY

- Air can enter the pleural space via:

—Chest wall (e.g., penetrating trauma)
—Intrapulmonary (e.g., ruptured alveoli)

- Usually collapse of the lung on the affected side seals the leak.
- If a ball valve mechanism ensues, however, air can accumulate in the thoracic cavity, causing a tension pneumothorax (a medical emergency).

CAUSES

- Spontaneous (secondary to rupture of apical blebs)
- Mechanical trauma

—Penetrating injury (e.g., knife or bullet wound)
—Blunt trauma

- Barotrauma

—Mechanical ventilation
—Cough (if severe enough)

- Iatrogenic

—Central venous catheter placement
—Bronchoscopy (especially with biopsy)

- Infection: most common organisms:

—*Staphylococcus aureus*
—*Streptococcus pneumoniae*
—*Mycobacterium tuberculosis*
—*Bordetella pertussis*
—*Pneumocystis carinii*

- Airway occlusion

—Mucus plugging (asthma)
—Foreign body
—Meconium aspiration

- Bleb formation (e.g., idiopathic, secondary to cystic fibrosis)
- Malignancy

EPIDEMIOLOGY

- Dependent on the underlying lung disease
- Spontaneous pneumothorax:

—Incidence: 7.4 to 18/100,000
—Male/female ratio 6:1
—Peak incidence: 10 to 30 years old

- Cystic fibrosis

—Incidence: 20% of patients more than 18 years old
—Risk increases as pulmonary function deteriorates

COMPLICATIONS

- Pain
- Hypoxia
- Respiratory distress
- Tension pneumothorax

—Hypoxia
—Hypercarbia with acidosis
—Respiratory failure

- Pneumomediastinum with subcutaneous emphysema
- Bronchopulmonary fistula

PROGNOSIS

- Dependent on the underlying etiology of the pneumothorax
- If simple, spontaneous pneumothorax recovery is excellent

 Differential Diagnosis

PULMONARY

- Congenital lung malformations

—Cysts (e.g., bronchogenic cysts)
—Cystic adenomatoid malformation
—Congenital lobar emphysema

- Acquired emphysema
- Hyperinflation of the lung
- Postinfectious pneumatocele
- Bullae formation

MISCELLANEOUS

- Diaphragmatic hernia
- Infections (e.g., pulmonary abscess)
- Muscle strain
- Pleurisy
- Rib fracture

 Data Gathering

HISTORY

- Patient may be asymptomatic (pneumothorax discovered on chest film obtained for other reasons)
- Cough
- Shortness of breath
- Dyspnea
- Pleuritic chest pain that is usually sudden in onset and localized to apices (referred pain to shoulders)
- Respiratory distress

SPECIAL QUESTIONS

Question: Does the patient have any underlying medical problems that are associated with an increased risk for pneumothoraces?
Significance: Patients with asthma, cystic fibrosis, pneumonia, or collagen vascular

diseases have an increased risk for developing a pneumothorax.

Question: Did the patient do anything prior to developing symptoms that might have caused the pneumothorax?
Significance: Heavy lifting or increased coughing

 Physical Examination

- May be normal
- Decreased breath sounds on the affected side
- Decreased vocal fremitus
- Hyperresonance to percussion on the affected side
- Tachypnea
- Tachycardia
- Shortness of breath
- Respiratory distress
- Shifting of the cardiac point of maximal impulse away from the affected side
- Shifting of the trachea away from the affected side
- Subcutaneous emphysema
- Cyanosis
- Scratch sign: listening through the stethoscope, a loud scratching sound is heard when a finger is gently stroked over the area of the pneumothorax

 Laboratory Aids

Tests:

- Arterial blood gas

—Po$_2$ can frequently be decreased
—Pco$_2$: elevated with respiratory compromise; decreased from hyperventilation

- Pulse oximetry

—Useful for assessing oxygenation

- Electrocardiogram (ECG)

—Diminished amplitude of the QRS voltage
—Rightward shift of the QRS axis (if left-sided pneumothorax)

IMAGING

- Chest radiograph

—Radiolucency of the affected lung
—Lack of lung markings in the periphery of the affected lung
—Collapsed lung on the affected side
—Possible pneumomediastinum with subcutaneous emphysema

- Chest CT

—Useful for finding small pneumothoraces
—Can help distinguish a pneumothorax from a bleb or cyst

—Helpful for locating small apical blebs associated with spontaneous pneumothoraces

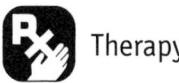

Therapy

OVERVIEW

- Stabilization of the patient
- Evacuation of the pleural air

—Should be done urgently if tension pneumothorax is suspected
—In small asymptomatic pneumothoraces, observation of the patient indicated

- Treat the underlying condition predisposing for the pneumothorax:

—Antibiotics for infection
—Bronchodilators and antiinflammatory agents for asthma attacks

DRUGS

- Oxygen

—Used to keep $Sao_2 \geq 95\%$
—Breathing 100% O_2 can speed the intrapleural air's reabsorption into the bloodstream (useful for treating smaller pneumothoraces, especially in neonates) hastening lung reexpansion

SURGERY

- Needle thoracentesis

—Useful for evacuation of the pleural air in simple, uncomplicated spontaneous pneumothorax

- Chest tube drainage

—Used for evacuation of the pleural air in recurrent pneumothoraces, complicated pneumothoraces, and cases with significant underlying lung disease
—Thoracotomy versus video-assisted thoracoscopic surgery (VATS)

- Surgical removal of pulmonary blebs

—Blebs have a high rate of rupturing with resultant pneumothorax.
—In patients with established pneumothoraces, the blebs should be removed or oversewn to prevent reoccurrence of the pneumothorax (blebs have a high rate of reoccurrence if not repaired).

- Pleurodesis

—Used to attach the lung to the intrathoracic chest wall to prevent reoccurrence of a pneumothorax
—Useful in cases of recurrent pneumothorax or if the pneumothorax is unresponsive to chest tube drainage (e.g., cystic fibrosis, malignancy)
—Mechanism of action: the surface of the lung becomes inflamed and adheres to the chest wall via the formation of scar tissue.

—Two commonly used methods:
1. Surgical pleurodesis
—Mechanical abrasion of part of the lung or pleurectomy
—Advantages: very effective: low reoccurrence rate; site specific (limits affected area)
—Disadvantages: requires surgery and general anesthesia; contraindicated if unstable
2. Chemical pleurodesis
—Chemicals are used to cause inflammation
—Chemicals commonly used: tetracycline, minocycline, doxycycline, quinacrine, talc
—Advantages: requires no surgery or general anesthesia
—Disadvantages: less effective than surgery; generalized inflammation (rather than site-specific; makes future thoracic surgery more difficult; painful)

DURATION

- Chest tube should be left in until:

—Majority of the air is reabsorbed
—No reaccumulation of air is seen on sealing of the chest tube

- Usually 2 to 4 days

Follow-Up

WHEN TO EXPECT IMPROVEMENT

Symptomatic relief within seconds of the air being evacuated

SIGNS TO WATCH FOR

Unable to remove the chest tube without reaccumulation of air (suggestive of a bronchopulmonary fistula; requires surgical exploration if no improvement in 7–10 days)

PITFALLS

- Not considering the diagnosis in otherwise healthy patients
- Confusing the symptoms with those of an underlying lung disease
- Inserting a needle into a cyst or bleb (can cause a tension pneumothorax with rapid respiratory compromise)

Common Questions and Answers

Q: Can a pneumothorax reoccur?
A: Reoccurrence is dependent on the underlying cause of the pneumothorax.

- Spontaneous pneumothorax (reoccurrence rates):

—Observation alone: 20% to 50%
—If thoracentesis performed: 25% to 50%

—If chest tube drainage performed: 32% to 38%
—Overall reoccurrence rate: 16% to 52%

- Chemical pleurodesis:

—25% for tetracycline
—8% to 10% for talc

- Surgical pleurodesis:

—13% for VATS
—3% for thoracotomy
—0% to 4% for thoracotomy with pleurectomy

- Cystic fibrosis (reoccurrence rates):

—If no drainage attempted: 60%
—Thoracentesis alone: 79%
—Chest tube drainage alone: 63%
—Chemical pleurodesis:
  —42% to 86% for tetracycline
  —11% to 12.5% for quinacrine

- Surgical pleurodesis:
  —0–4% for thoracotomy with pleurectomy

ICD-9-CM 512.8

BIBLIOGRAPHY

Baumann MH, Strange C. Treatment of spontaneous pneumothorax: a more aggressive approach? *Chest* 1997;112:789–804.

Boutin C, Astoul P, Rey F, et al. Thoracoscopy in the diagnosis and treatment of spontaneous pneumothorax. *Clin Chest Med* 1995;16:497–503.

Briassoulis GC, Venkataraman ST, Vasilopoulos AG, et al. Air leaks from the respiratory tract in mechanically ventilated children with severe respiratory disease. *Pediatr Pulmonol* 2000;29(2):127–134.

Cook CH, Melvin WS, Groner JI, et al. A cost-effective thoracoscopic treatment strategy for pediatric spontaneous pneumothorax. *Surg endosc* 1999;13(12):1208–1210.

Genc A, Ozcan C, Erdener A, et al. Management of pneumothorax in children. *J Cardiovasc Surg* 1998;39(6):849–851.

Jantz MA, Pierson DJ. Pneumothorax and barotrauma. *Clin Chest Med* 1994;15:75–91.

Montgomery M. Air and liquid in the pleural space. In: *Kendig's disorders of the respiratory tract in children*. Philadelphia: WB Saunders, 1998:389–411.

Sahn SA, Heffner JE. Primary care: spontaneous pneumothorax. *N Engl J Med* 2000;342:868–874.

Schidlow DV, Taussig LM, Knowles MR. Cystic fibrosis foundation consensus conference report on pulmonary complications of cystic fibrosis. *Pediatr Pulmonol* 1993;15:187–198.

Warick WJ. Pneumothorax. In: *Pediatric respiratory disease: diagnosis and treatment*. Philadelphia: WB Saunders, 1993;575–578.

Author: Richard M. Kravitz

Polyarteritis Nodosa

 Database

DEFINITION

An inflammatory process of small and medium-sized muscular arteries resulting in dysfunction of affected organs.

CAUSES

- Idiopathic
- Postinfectious (streptococcal, hepatitis B)

PATHOLOGY

Necrotizing arteritis of small- and medium-sized arteries resulting in segmental fibrinoid necrosis

EPIDEMIOLOGY

- Extremely rare in childhood
- Prevalence equal in boys and girls

GENETICS

No specific HLA types known to be at increased risk

COMPLICATIONS

- Hypertension
- Renal failure
- Digital necrosis
- Intestinal infarction

 Differential Diagnosis

INFECTION

- Bacterial endocarditis
- Brucellosis

TUMORS

- Left atrial myxoma

METABOLIC

- Homocystinuria

CONGENITAL

- Immunologic

—Systemic necrotizing vasculitis
—Systemic lupus erythematosus
—Kawasaki disease
—Systemic juvenile rheumatoid arthritis
—Wegener granulomatosis
—Takayasu arteritis
—Cryoglobulinemia
—Antiphospholipid antibody syndrome

PSYCHOLOGICAL

- Munchausen syndrome

MISCELLANEOUS

- Degos disease (malignant atrophic papulosis)

 Data Gathering

HISTORY

- Moderate constitutional symptoms?
- Abdominal pain?
- Weight loss?
- Unexplained fever?
- Headache?
- Arthralgia/myalgia?
- Rashes?
- Seizures?
- Weakness?

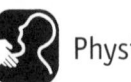 Physical Examination

- Assess BP and pulses
- Check skin for livedo reticularis, splinter hemorrhages, erythema nodosum, and necrotic digits
- Neurologic examination for findings consistent with neuropathy (mononeuritis multiplex)

PHYSICAL EXAMINATION TRICKS

Finding: The lacy network of superficial vessels of livedo reticularis
Significance: Does not blanch and is somewhat tender. Mottling of the skin seen in fair-skinned individuals will blanch and is not tender, and disappears with warming.

Laboratory Aids

Test: ESR
Significance: Usually extremely elevated; leukocytosis and thrombocytosis are seen.

Test: Urine analysis
Significance: Proteinuria and hematuria can be present.

Test: Cr and BUN
Significance: May be elevated

Test: ANA and RF
Significance: Usually negative

Test: Antineutrophil cytoplasmic antibody (ANCA)
Significance: Detectable in some; usually perinuclear (p) type, rarely cytoplasmic (c) type

Test: Hepatitis B serologies
Significance: Hepatitis B has been associated in some series of PAN patients.

Test: Biopsy of affected tissue/organ
Significance: As indicated, usually skin, kidney, nerve, testicle

Test: Streptococcal titers
Significance: Polyarteritis nodosa may develop following streptococcal infections in children.

Test: MRA (magnetic resonance angiography)
Significance: Can demonstrate vessel wall stenoses and aneurysm.

FALSE POSITIVES

Elevated ESR is seldom due to PAN. Consequently, a vigorous search for alternate explanations should be sought prior to making this diagnosis.

PITFALLS

The detection of ANCA, previously thought to be highly specific for vasculitis, now appears to be less so. Hence, it remains important to confirm the diagnosis of PAN with biopsy or angiography.

HOME TESTING

May wish to have patients monitor blood pressure periodically if renal involvement suspected

 Therapy

DRUGS

- Corticosteroids are mainstay; usually start at dose of 1 to 2 mg/kg/d and adjusting based on response.
- Immunosuppressives such as methotrexate, azathioprine, and cyclophosphamide may be necessary.
- Hypertension should be managed aggressively, especially with calcium channel blockers.

DURATION

May require long-term therapy

DIET

- If renal system involved, low in sodium and potassium
- Possible conflicts with medications

 Follow-Up

WHEN TO EXPECT IMPROVEMENT

Initiation of steroid therapy may bring response in 1 to 2 weeks; however, management of specific organs affected during acute stage is essential.

SIGNS TO WATCH FOR

- Rising creatinine and BUN
- Abdominal pain
- Uncontrolled hypertension

PROGNOSIS

- May be extremely poor over the long term
- Risk high for renal failure, hypertension, myocardial infarction, bowel infarction, and death
- Due to low incidence/prevalence, precise data not available

PITFALLS

Initiation of therapy prior to efforts to clinch the diagnosis

 Common Questions and Answers

Q: What is the difference between PAN and systemic necrotizing vasculitis?
A: PAN has a fairly strict definition. There are many children who clearly have vasculitis of the small and medium-sized arteries who do not fit precisely into the description of PAN. In most ways the search for organ involvement and therapy is the same.

Q: Who should manage the patient with PAN?
A: Usually one discipline provides comprehensive management plan (either the pediatrician or rheumatologist). Subspecialist(s) of the affected organ systems provide management guidelines for specific organ issues.

ICD-9-CM 446.0

BIBLIOGRAPHY

Cassidy JT, Petty RE. *Textbook of pediatric rheumatology*, 4th ed. Philadelphia: WB Saunders, 2001.

Cuttica RJ. Vasculitis in children: a diagnostic challenge. *Curr Probl Pediatr* 1997;27(8): 309–318.

Fink CW. The role of the streptococcus in poststreptococcal reactive arthritis and childhood polyarteritis nodosa. *J Rheumatol Suppl* 1991;29:14–20.

Ozen S, Besbas N, Saatci U, et al. Diagnostic criteria for polyarteritis nodosa in childhood. *J Pediatr* 1992;120:206–209.

Author: Randy Q. Cron
Gregory F. Keenan, 2nd edition

Polycystic Kidney Disease

 Database

DEFINITION

Polycystic kidney disease (PKD) is a heritable disorder with diffuse cystic involvement of both kidneys without other dysplastic elements.

There are two forms with considerable overlap in the pediatric population:

• Autosomal-dominant polycystic kidney disease (ADPKD):

—Characterized by the presence of cysts at any point along the nephron or collecting duct
—Occasionally associated with characteristic cardiovascular and gastrointestinal manifestations
—Referred to as adult polycystic kidney disease because it usually presents with clinical symptoms in the third to fifth decade
—May present in early childhood

• Autosomal-recessive polycystic kidney disease (ARPKD):

—Cystic dilation of renal collecting ducts
—All cases accompanied by hepatic abnormalities such as biliary dysgenesis and periportal fibrosis (congenital hepatic fibrosis)
—Was called infantile polycystic kidney disease but can present at any time from the prenatal period through adolescence

• Diffuse cystic disease occurs in several other conditions in children and adults. Examples include tuberous sclerosis, multicystic dysplastic kidney, and a variety of malformation syndromes.

PATHOPHYSIOLOGY

• ARPKD

—In the infant and young child the kidneys are enlarged, spongy, and reniform. The cystic cortical collecting ducts are grossly visible as pinpoint dots on the capsular surface. The dilated ducts are 1 to 2 mm in diameter.
—Microscopic examination reveals medullary ductal ectasia, which is the characteristic feature of ARPKD. The glomeruli and remaining tubular structures are decreased in number.
—In older patients larger renal cysts and fibrosis develop.
—Hepatic involvement is invariably present.

• ADPKD

—Kidneys are enlarged with numerous round protuberances on their surfaces, and cysts are irregularly dispersed through the parenchyma. The cysts may measure from a few millimeters to many centimeters.

GENETICS

• ARPKD

—Sexes involved equally
—Gene recently localized to chromosome 6

• ADPKD

—Each offspring has a 50% chance of inheriting the gene.
—Expression may vary among affected individuals in terms of age of presentation, severity of involvement, and frequency of associated abnormalities.
—Causative gene is on the short arm of chromosome 16 (PKD1) in the majority.
—Second locus on chromosome 4 has been reported, which is responsible for a clinically indistinguishable form of ADPKD (PKD2).

EPIDEMIOLOGY

• Estimated incidence of ARPKD is 1:10,000 to 1:40,000.
• ADPKD is one of the most common hereditary disorders and accounts for 8% to 10% of cases of end-stage renal disease. Prevalence rates range from 1:200 to 1:1,000.

COMPLICATIONS

• ARPKD

—Most patients present in infancy.
—Severely affected infants may have the oligohydramnios sequence at birth, with pulmonary hypoplasia and Potter phenotype.
—As renal function diminishes, the child may develop growth failure, anemia, and renal osteodystrophy.
—In the older child, complications of hepatic fibrosis and portal hypertension predominate. Hepatosplenomegaly, bleeding esophageal varices, and hypersplenism causing thrombocytopenia, anemia, and leukopenia may occur.

• ADPKD

—Patients may present with hypertension, urinary tract infection, abdominal pain, hematuria, or a palpable abdominal mass.
—The extrarenal complications seen in adults with ADPKD such as hepatic cysts, pancreatic cysts, colonic diverticula, cardiac valvular abnormalities, and intracranial aneurysms are very rarely seen in pediatric patients.

PROGNOSIS

• ADPKD

—Patients who are symptomatic at birth may die from pulmonary insufficiency.
—In ARPKD, those who survive to 1 year have a much better prognosis.
—Renal insufficiency begins in early childhood and the progression is extremely variable.
—Causes of death outside of the neonatal period include renal failure, sepsis, hypertension, and complications of bacterial cholangitis and portal hypertension.
—Treatment with renal transplantation and liver transplantation may increase longevity.

• ADPKD

—Patients who present during infancy with symptomatic renal involvement may have an ominous prognosis and up to 50% die in the neonatal period.
—Presentation of ADPKD in the older child has a better prognosis.
—Control of hypertension and urinary tract infection improves the prognosis.

 Differential Diagnosis

• Multicystic dysplastic kidney (MDK)

—Congenital condition with multiple large cysts of various sizes with no overall structural pattern to the kidney and no functional tissue, rarely bilateral renal involvement; often associated with cardiac, gastrointestinal, and CNS abnormalities

• Glomerular cystic kidney disease (GCKD)

—Consists of bilateral cystic dilations of Bowman space with lack of significant tubular involvement and may have clinical and radiologic features consistent with ARPKD or ADPKD.

• Malformation syndromes
• Renal cysts occur in many hereditary syndromes in the form of peripheral cortical microcysts:

—Examples include trisomy 9, trisomy 13, Meckel syndrome, Jeune syndrome, Ivemark syndrome, Zellweger syndrome, and Bardet-Biedl syndrome.
—Acquired cystic disease may occur in patients with end-stage renal disease.

 Data Gathering

HISTORY

ARPKD

• Patients usually present in infancy.
• Prenatal ultrasound may reveal oligohydramnios, large renal masses, or absence of urine in the bladder.
• Patients may present during the neonatal period with flank masses or respiratory distress.
• May present older children with symptoms of enlarged kidneys or hepatosplenomegaly.
• A concentrating defect may result in polydipsia and polyuria.
• Hypertension is common and may result in cardiac hypertrophy and congestive heart failure.

ADPKD

• The most common presenting complaint in adults is pain.
• Older children may present with hypertension, abdominal pain, abdominal mass, hematuria, or urinary tract infection.
• Cerebral vessel aneurysms are rarely detected before age 20.

Physical Examination

ARPKD

- Flank mass most common.
- May also reveal evidence of portal hypertension (hematemesis, hepatosplenomegaly) or hypersplenism (pallor, petechiae).

ADPKD

- The clinical spectrum of disease is highly variable.
- Most common presentation in neonates is flank masses or palpable kidneys
- Older children may present with hypertension, abdominal pain, abdominal mass, hematuria, urinary tract infection, or renal insufficiency.

 ## Laboratory Aids

Patients should undergo evaluation for renal insufficiency including BUN, creatinine, electrolytes, calcium, phosphorus, and CBC.

IMAGING

ARPKD

Test: Ultrasound
Significance:

- Will reveal, in patients with ARPKD, bilateral, enlarged kidneys with increased echogenicity of the parenchyma, and loss of corticomedullary differentiation
- Occasional macrocysts may be present, >2 cm in diameter.
- The liver is enlarged and hyperechoic but usually less echogenic than the kidney. Dilated intrahepatic biliary ducts or decreased visualization of peripheral portal veins due to fibrous tissue may be seen.
- The disease may be diagnosed after 24 to 30 weeks' gestation by ultrasonographic evidence of hyperechogenic enlarged kidneys, oligohydramnios, and no evidence of bladder filling.

Test: Intravenous pyelogram (IVP)
Significance:

- Usually shows the classic finding of medullary streaking (radial striations) corresponding to accumulation of contrast in dilated collecting ducts.
- In older children with ARPKD the kidneys may be less enlarged, with evidence of macrocysts and loss of radial striations.

ADPKD

Test: Ultrasound
Significance:

- The kidneys of ADPKD may be enlarged with macrocysts of varying size. In children, renal involvement is frequently asymmetric and occasionally unilateral. However, the renal enlargement and macrocysts may not develop until adulthood. In children at risk, even single cysts in normal-sized kidneys are highly predictive of future ADPKD.
- Extrarenal cysts may also be seen in the liver, pancreas, ovary, or spleen, although rarely in children.
- May not always distinguish ADPKD and ARPKD

Test: IVP
Significance:

- Will reveal enlarged, lobular kidneys
- The calyces are stretched and distorted.
- Numerous cysts of various sizes are seen in the parenchyma.

False Positives/Negatives

- The sonographic features of ADPKD and ARPKD may be present in the second trimester but usually are not manifested until after 30 weeks. Both false positives and false negatives have been reported.
- Although the combination of renal collecting tubule ectasia and biliary ectasia with periportal fibrosis is unique to ARPKD, portal duct fibrosis and bile duct proliferation may be seen in a variety of renal diseases such as Jeune and Zellweger syndromes and trisomy 9 and 13.

 ## Therapy

- Medical management of PKD is supportive.

—Hypertension is common in ADPKD and ARPKD. Patients may require antihypertensive therapy such as calcium-channel blockers.

- Supplemental bicarbonate may be indicated for metabolic acidosis.

—Urinary tract infections or bacterial cholangitis require aggressive antibiotic therapy.
—Infection of hepatic cysts may require drainage.

- Overall, renal replacement therapy with maintenance dialysis and renal transplantation is at least as successful in PKD as in non-PKD patients.

DIET

The degree of renal insufficiency will dictate the need for a low potassium or low phosphorus diet.

 ## Follow-Up

SIGNS TO WATCH FOR

- Asymptomatic children in families with ADPKD are at risk and should be followed closely for hypertension, hematuria, and the development of an abdominal mass and the extrarenal manifestations.
- Routine screening with cerebral arteriography for evidence of possible intracranial aneurysms in pediatric ADPKD patients is not recommended.

 ## Common Questions and Answers

Q: What can be done to slow the progression of renal insufficiency in ADPKD?
A: Well-controlled blood pressure and rapid treatment of urinary tract infections may decrease the progression of renal failure.

Q: Should asymptomatic, older siblings of an infant with ARPKD be evaluated?
A: Yes. An older child may have congenital hepatic fibrosis with minimal renal involvement.

Q: Should one screen ADPKD-affected family members for the presence of cerebral vessel aneurysms if other family members have berry aneurysms?
A: Although routine screening is not recommended, intrafamilial clustering of aneurysms has been reported and it may be advisable to screen children with MRI or cranial CT in a family with aneurysms.

ICD-9-CM 753.1

BIBLIOGRAPHY

Gabow PA. Medical progress: autosomal dominant polycystic kidney disease. *N Engl J Med* 1993;329(5):332.

Grantham JJ. The etiology, pathogenesis, and treatment of autosomal dominant polycystic kidney disease: recent advances. *Am J Kidney Dis* 1996;28:788–803.

Kaplan BS, Kaplan P, Rosenberg HK, et al. Polycystic kidney disease in childhood. *J Pediatr* 1989;115(6):867.

Author: Mary B. Leonard

Polycystic Ovary Syndrome

 Database

DEFINITION

Polycystic ovary syndrome (PCOS) is an endocrinologic disorder characterized by chronic anovulation, excessive androgen production, and noncyclical gonadotropin secretion. It begins perimenarcheally, and its clinical manifestations include hirsutism, amenorrhea or oligomenorrhea, and obesity.

CAUSES

- The characteristic polycystic ovary emerges when a state of anovulation persists for any length of time.
- Although the ovaries of these women produce excessive amounts of androgens, there is no inherent endocrinologic abnormality in the ovaries.
- The tonically elevated levels of luteinizing hormone (LH) cause the ovarian stromal tissue to produce more androgens, which in turn produce premature follicular atresia.
- Because there are many causes of anovulation, there are many causes of polycystic ovaries.
- It has been suggested that heredity, central catecholamine abnormalities, psychological stress, insulin resistance, and obesity may be involved.
- At least one group of patients with this condition inherits the disorder, possibly by means of an X-linked dominant transmission.

PATHOPHYSIOLOGY

- The ovaries of most women with PCOS are enlarged as much as 5 cm in diameter, and the ovarian capsule is smooth, white, and thickened.
- Beneath the capsule are numerous small follicular cysts.
- For years it was erroneously believed that the thick sclerotic capsule acted as a mechanical barrier to ovulation.
- Instead of the characteristic picture of fluctuating hormone levels in the normal menstrual cycle, a steady state of gonadotropin and sex steroids are produced in association with persistent anovulation.
- There is an increased pulse amplitude of gonadotropin-releasing hormone (GnRH) and tonically elevated levels of LH.
- The polycystic ovary is a sign of these underlying endocrinologic abnormalities, not a disease intrinsic to the ovary.

EPIDEMIOLOGY

PCOS is relatively common and usually begins soon after menarche.

COMPLICATIONS

- The elevated levels of androgens that are produced are associated with hirsutism.
- The lack of a normal menstrual cycle leads to irregular bleeding, amenorrhea, and infertility.
- Because of the increased levels of unopposed estrogens, there is a threefold increased risk of endometrial cancer, and a 34-fold greater risk of breast cancer appearing in the postmenopausal years.

 Differential Diagnosis

- Congenital adrenal hyperplasia
- Cushing syndrome
- Adrenal androgen-producing tumors
- Ovarian androgen-producing tumors
- Extragonadal sources of androgens

 Data Gathering

HISTORY

- Complete menstrual history
- Amenorrhea or irregular vaginal bleeding
- Infertility

 Physical Examination

HIRSUTISM

- Most patients with this syndrome are obese.
- Obesity probably enhances the syndrome because of the decrease in sex hormone—binding globulin, but is probably not important in its pathogenesis, because the syndrome occurs in some thin women and because many obese women do not have PCOS.

Polycystic Ovary Syndrome

Laboratory Aids

- Because FSH levels are normal or low, an LH/FSH ratio greater than 3 (provided the LH level is not lower than 8 mIU/mL) may be used to suggest the diagnosis in women with clinical features of PCOS.
- Androgen levels are elevated. Serum testosterone levels are usually between 70 and 120 ng/dL, and androstenedione levels are usually between 3 and 5 ng/mL.

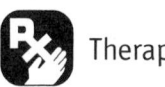

Therapy

- The best treatment for PCOS is oral contraceptives, unless pregnancy is desired, because these agents inhibit LH, decrease circulating testosterone levels, and increase levels of sex hormone–binding globulin, which binds and inactivates more of the testosterone in the circulation.
- Use oral contraceptives that contain less than 50 μg estrogen and a progestin other than norgestrel, which is the most androgenic progestin in current use.
- Patients who desire fertility should be treated with ovulation-inducing agents, starting with clomiphene citrate and proceeding to human menopausal gonadotropin or GnRH agonists if unresponsive.

- If adrenal androgens (DHEAs) are elevated, dexamethasone (0.25–0.5 mg at bedtime) should be given along with the oral contraceptive to reduce adrenal androgens to normal.
- Patients with amenorrhea or irregular bleeding should be treated with monthly progestins, such as oral medroxyprogesterone acetate 10 mg daily for the first 10 days of the month, to prevent the effects of unopposed estrogens.
- Spironolactone 50 to 100 mg twice daily causes regression of the hirsutism in women with PCOS by decreasing androgenic action in the target organs.
- Ovarian wedge resection was advocated in the past for treatment of androgen excess, but the decrease in circulating androgens occurred for only a short time, and this therapy should no longer be used.

Follow-Up

In the patient who has long-standing anovulation, an endometrial biopsy, with extensive sampling, should be done because of the link between unopposed estrogen and endometrial cancer.

Common Questions and Answers

Q: Can I still get pregnant if I have this syndrome?
A: Yes. Although the best treatment for this syndrome is oral contraceptives, those patients who desire to become pregnant can be treated with ovulation-inducing agents.

Q: I've noticed increased facial hair recently. Is there anything I can do about this?
A: Yes. In most cases, the oral contraceptives will decrease circulating androgen levels sufficiently so that this will regress, but if increased body hair (hirsutism) persists, another drug, called spironolactone, that blocks the action of androgens, can be added to more effectively treat this.

ICD-9-CM 256.4

BIBLIOGRAPHY

DeVane GW, Czckala NM, Judd HL, et al. Circulating gonadotrophins, estrogens, and androgens in polycystic ovarian disease. *Am J Obstet Gynecol* 1975;121:496.

Givens JR, Andersen RN, Wiser WI, et al. The effectiveness of two oral contraceptives in suppressing plasma androstanedione, testosterone, LH and FSH and stimulating plasma testosterone binding capacity in hirsute women. *Am J Obstet Gynecol* 1976;124:333.

Goldzieher JW. Polycystic ovarian syndrome. *Fertil Steril* 1981;35:371.

Kazar AR, Kessel B, Yen SSC. Circulating luteinizing hormone pulse frequency in women with polycystic ovary syndrome. *J Clin Endocrinol Metab* 1987;65:233.

Lobo RA, Goebelsmann U. Effect of androgen excess on inappropriate gonadotropin secretion as found in polycystic ovary syndrome. *Am J Obstet Gynecol* 1982;142:394.

Author: Ernest M. Graham

Polycythemia

 Database

DEFINITION

• Polycythemia is elevated hemoglobin and hematocrit owing to an absolute increase in red-cell mass. Polycythemia can be divided into subcategories, as follows:

—Primary polycythemia: primary defect of bone marrow erythropoiesis, resulting in overproduction of red cells
—Secondary polycythemia: stimulation of red-cell production by increased levels of erythropoietin (EPO), which may be appropriately secreted in response to tissue hypoxia, or may be inappropriately secreted because of renal disease or from a tumor
—Relative polycythemia: increased hematocrit without true increase in red-cell mass

PATHOPHYSIOLOGY

Primary Polycythemias

• Polycythemia vera (PCV): myeloproliferative disease with abnormal multipotent progenitor cells with abnormally high sensitivity to EPO; EPO levels are normal.
• Primary familial and congenital polycythemia (PFCP): red-cell precursors highly sensitive to EPO. Usually autosomal dominant; some families have mutations in the EPO receptor (EPOR).

Secondary Polycythemias

Relative tissue hypoxia resulting from deficiency of oxygen delivery, due to:

• Chronic lung disease and inadequate oxygenation due to a defect in gas exchange
• Cyanotic heart disease: desaturation of arterial blood because of admixture of oxygen-poor venous blood due to right-to-left shunt
• Circulatory: right-to-left shunting outside the heart
• Hemoglobinopathy: abnormal oxygen transport to tissues because of a mutant hemoglobin with higher than normal oxygen affinity.
• At the partial pressure of oxygen of the tissues, high oxygen-affinity hemoglobins release less oxygen than normal, resulting in hypoxia.
• Tissue hypoxia leads to supernormal secretion of EPO by the kidney, and increased production of red cells from the marrow.
• 2,3-bisphosphoglycerate (2,3-BPG) deficiency: increased oxygen affinity of hemoglobin because of reduced level of red-cell 2,3-BPG
• Inappropriate EPO secretion associated with kidney disease (not end stage, where EPO is usually deficient)
• Malignant tumor, which secretes EPO

GENETICS

• High oxygen-affinity hemoglobins: autosomal dominant
• Primary familial and congenital polycythemia: usually autosomal dominant; Finnish and Chuvash Republic (former USSR republic) clusters described
• 2,3-BPG mutase deficiency: autosomal recessive

EPIDEMIOLOGY

• Uncorrected cyanotic congenital heart disease: most common cause of polycythemia
• PCV: Fewer than 50 reported childhood cases; 0.1% of cases of PCV are in children.
• High oxygen-affinity hemoglobins; 2,3-BPG dismutase deficiency; EPOR mutations, primary familial and congenital polycythemia: all rare

COMPLICATIONS

• Hyperviscosity: Blood viscosity increases dramatically when hematocrit >65%. Decreased exercise tolerance, dyspnea, and mental status changes are due to slowed microcirculation in the CNS.
• Thrombosis: Budd-Chiari syndrome from hepatic vein thrombosis, deep vein thrombosis, pulmonary embolus; seen especially in PCV
• Stroke: Cerebral thrombosis due to hyperviscosity
• Malignant transformation of PCV; not seen in PFCP

PROGNOSIS

Depends on underlying condition:

• High oxygen-affinity hemoglobinopathies: very good for normal life
• PCV: guarded, as may progress to myelodysplastic syndrome
• Eisenmenger syndrome (see below): poor; progressive pulmonary hypertension and cor pulmonale

 Differential Diagnosis

PRIMARY POLYCYTHEMIA

• PCV
• Myeloproliferative disease
• May have thrombocytosis or leukocytosis
• Primary familial and congenital polycythemia

SECONDARY POLYCYTHEMIA

• Cyanotic congenital heart disease
• Eisenmenger syndrome
• Pulmonary hypertension from long-standing uncorrected congenital heart disease with left-to-right shunting (acyanotic) leads to elevated right-sided pressures and reversal of shunt to flow right to left, leading to cyanosis
• Extreme high altitude

• Compensation for low O_2 pressure includes an increase in red-cell mass.
• Alveolar hypoventilation: neuromuscular
• Muscular dystrophy
• Poliomyelitis
• Pickwickian syndrome
• Central hypoventilation
• End-stage lung disease
• Abnormal hemoglobins with high O_2 affinity
• 2,3-BPG mutase deficiency
• Inappropriate EPO secretion may occur in:

—Renal disease
—Iatrogenic
—Excessive red-cell transfusion, possible in trauma, resuscitations, neonatal blood exchange

• Excessive exogenous dosing of EPO
• Neonatal polycythemia
• Twin-to-twin or placental transfusion
• Cobalt poisoning

RELATIVE POLYCYTHEMIA

• May be seen in smokers
• Dehydration or diuretic use

 Data Gathering

HISTORY

• Diagnosis of congenital heart disease, uncorrected or partially corrected
• History of cyanosis
• Delivery history
• Baby held below placenta
• Delayed clamping of cord
• Twins of disparate size
• Transfusion history
• Headache, paresthesias, dizziness, syncope
• Transient blindness
• Decreased exercise tolerance, respiratory distress, dyspnea on exertion, oxygen requirement
• Pruritus
• Lethargy
• Cigarette smoking
• Prolonged time spent at extremely high altitude
• Family history of cyanosis, high hematocrit, need for phlebotomy
• Cobalt poisoning: Homemade beer and magnets may contain cobalt.

Physical Examination

• Central and acral cyanosis
• Signs of dehydration: dry mucous membranes, no tears, poor skin turgor
• Heart murmur
• Clubbing
• Plethora: conjunctival, mucous membranes, nailbeds
• Splenomegaly: present in 75% of PCV

Polycythemia

 Laboratory Aids

TESTS

Initial

- CBC
- Serum EPO: Distinguish 1° from 2° polycythemia.
- Pulse oximetry: to determine percent saturation of hemoglobin
- Arterial blood gas: Po_2 low in lung disease or right-to-left shunt

To Investigate High Oxygen-Affinity Hemoglobin

- Hemoglobin electrophoresis
- Whole-blood P50 and red-cell 2,3-BPG level
- Met-hemoglobin level: apparent cyanosis

To Investigate PCV

- Total red-cell mass measurement by chromium 51–tagged red cells: top normal range (adults) is less than 36 mL/kg in men, less than 32 mL/kg in women; gold standard test for true polycythemia
- Bone marrow aspirate with chromosomes: morphologic evidence of myelodysplastic syndrome; abnormal clone by karyotype
- Serum B12, unsaturated B12-binding capacity (UB12BC): markedly elevated in PCV

Other Testing

- Total blood viscosity: rarely measured
- Iron studies: serum Fe, TIBC, ferritin
- BUN, creatinine, urinalysis: underlying renal disease

IMAGING

- Echocardiography: to evaluate shunting
- Chest radiograph: to evaluate chronic lung disease, lung malignancies
- Abdominal ultrasound: to evaluate renal disease, spleen size, abdominal tumors
- Sleep study: looking for nighttime airway obstruction and desaturation

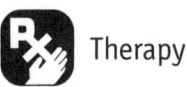 Therapy

OBSERVATION ONLY

Many patients require no therapy.

THERAPEUTIC PHLEBOTOMY

- Removal of red cells every 3 to 4 weeks to maintain hematocrit below threshold for symptoms; usually below 50% to 55%
- Patients with Eisenmenger syndrome and symptoms of hyperviscosity may not tolerate intravascular volume reduction if a large volume of blood is removed at one time.
- Patients on a chronic phlebotomy program may require iron supplementation.

DRUGS

- Hydroxyurea, alkylating agents, ^{32}P (in adults) to suppress red-cell production in PCV
- Interferon-α for PCV

SUPPLEMENTAL OXYGEN

Helpful for secondary polycythemia due to underlying lung disease; may not help in right-to-left shunt

SURGERY

Correction of underlying cardiac disease

DIET

- No specific recommendation
- Dietary restriction of water and salt intake may be required for underlying renal disease.

 Follow-Up

SIGNS TO WATCH FOR

- Insufficient phlebotomy
- Headache
- Dizziness
- Syncope
- Decreased exercise tolerance between phlebotomies
- Progression of myelodysplastic disease
- Thrombocytopenia
- Bleeding
- Thrombosis
- Stroke
- Severe headache
- Jaundice
- Ascites

PREVENTION

- There are no preventive measures for primary conditions such as PCV, hemoglobinopathies, or PFCP
- Treatment of the underlying condition, such as correction of a cyanotic heart lesion, will prevent the development of secondary polycythemia.

PITFALLS

- Fingerstick CBC: Squeezing the finger to collect a specimen may give a falsely elevated hematocrit.
- Arterial blood gas: cannot interpret low Po_2 if specimen is mixture of venous and arterial blood
- Relative polycythemia: red-cell mass normal
- Decreased plasma volume with normal red-cell mass; seen in adult cigarette smokers
- Dehydration; elevated hematocrit due to hemoconcentration
- Hemoglobin electrophoresis does not identify all high-affinity hemoglobins.

—Many co-migrate with normal hemoglobins
—Hemoglobin electrophoresis cannot be interpreted if the patient has been transfused within the past 3 months.

- Whole blood P50

—Fresh specimen required; normals different from red cell lysates, purified hemoglobin

 Common Questions and Answers

Q: Can a child with uncorrected cyanotic congenital heart disease be supported indefinitely with phlebotomy?
A: No. Phlebotomy relieves the symptoms of hyperviscosity, but does not stop the progression of pulmonary hypertension.

Q: When should a child with polycythemia be referred to a pediatric hematologist?
A: If the high hematocrit is persistent and not clearly related to dehydration or neonatal causes (e.g., placental transfusion), then the child should be referred to a pediatric hematologist. Unexplained cyanosis is also a reason for referral. In the case of congenital heart disease, the pediatric cardiologist may be comfortable managing polycythemia without consultation with a hematologist.

ICD-9-CM 238.4

BIBLIOGRAPHY

Danish EH, Rasch CA, Harris JW. Polycythemia vera in childhood: case report and review of the literature. *Am J Hematol* 1980;9:421.

Kralovics R, Prchal JT. Congenital and inherited polycythemia. *Curr Opin Pediatr* 2000;12:29.

Pearson TC, Messinezy M. Investigation of patients with polycythemia. *Postgrad Med J* 1996:519–524.

Prchal JF, Prchal JT. Molecular basis for polycythemia. *Curr Opin Hematol* 1999;6:100.

Prchal JT, Sokol L. "Benign erythrocytosis" and other familial and congenital polycy-themias. *Eur J Haematol* 1996:57:263–268.

Author: David F. Friedman

Porencephaly Cortical Dysplasia/Neuronal Migration Disorders—Malformations of Cortical Development

 Database

DEFINITION

Malformations of cortical development (MCD) are a heterogeneous group of development brain malformations that are highly associated with epilepsy, developmental delay, and mental retardation. Associated features may include autism, learning difficulties, hypotonia, and spasticity. In some cases, there is global neurodevastation and failure to thrive. The key histological feature of MCD is that the structural organization of the cerebral cortex is abnormal. MCD may affect focal regions of the brain as in focal cortical dyslasia, tuberous sclerosis complex, or porencephaly or may affect more widespread regions of the brains such as in lissencephaly or hemimegalencephaly. As a general rule, the more extensive the malformation, the greater the degree of neurological impairment.

MCD Affecting Wide Regions of Cortex

• Etiologic agent likely before 20 weeks' gestation
• *Lissencephaly* (smooth brain): loss of cerebral cortical convolutions (sulci) and cortical laminations; may occur in combination with agyria-pachygyria (see below).
• *Agyria-pachygyria:* a more heterogeneous pathologic classification in which there are broad regions of cortex without gyri (similar to lissencephaly), but, in addition, focal areas of thickened cortical gyri also may be present.
• *Hemimegalencephaly:* a rare condition in which one cerebral hemisphere is enlarged and may exhibit concomitant agyric-pachygyric features. The normal-sized hemisphere may also contain subtle, focal abnormalities.

MCD Affecting Focal Regions of Cortex

• Etiologic agent likely after 20 weeks' gestation
• *Dysplastic cortical architecture:* focal regions of disorganized cortical architecture and abnormally shaped neurons
• *Heterotopia:* clusters of neurons found within the white matter (where neurons are not typically found); may be nodular and confined to small region in cortex or adjacent to the ependyma (nodular forms); may extend across portions of a hemisphere (laminar heterotopia)
• *Schizencephaly:* nonloculated cavities or clefts (uni-or bilateral) in the brain that communicate with the system and/or subarachnoid space

Recent Classification Scheme for MCD (Barkovich et al., 2001)

Disorders of Cell Proliferation
• Tuberous Sclerosis Complex
• Focal Cortical Dysplasia
• Hemimegalencephaly
• Microcephaly syndromes
• DNET (Dysembryoblastic neuroepithelial tumors)

• Ganglioglioma
• Gangliocytoma

Disorders of Neural Migration
• Lissencephaly Type I (Classical)
—Miller-Dieker syndrome
—X-linked lissencephaly (XLIS)
• Lissencephaly Type II (Cobblestone)
—Walker-Warburg syndrome
—Muscle-eye-brain disease
—Fukuyama Congenital Muscular Dystrophy
• Subcortical Band Heteropia ("Double cortex syndrome")
• Periventricular Nodular Heterotopia

Disorders of Brain Organization
• Polymicrogyria
• Schizencephaly
• Taylor Type I dysplasia
—Microdysgenesis

Malformations, not otherwise classified
• Mitochondrial disorders
• Peroxisomal disorders (e.g., Zellweger syndrome)

CAUSES

CD/NMDs result from a variety of in utero causes, including infectious, toxic-metabolic, ischemic insults. Several MCDs result from single gene mutations.
• Genetic
—Lissencephaly may occur as a sporadic syndrome but has been associated with mutations in select genes
—Miller-Dieker lissencephaly syndrome
  —Chromosome 17p13.3
—Lissencephaly with cerebellar hypoplasia
  —Chromosome 7q22
—XLIS
  —Chromosome Xq22
—Periventricular nodular heterotopia
  —Chromosome Xq28
—Subcortical band heterotopia
  —Chromosome Xq22
—Tuberous Sclerosis Complex
  —Chromosome 9q34
  —Chromosome 16p13
—Fukuyama Congenital Muscular Dystrophy
  —Chromosome 9q31
• Other lissencephaly-associated syndromes, including the Norman-Roberts, Neu-Laxova, and Walker-Warburg syndromes, are believed to have an autosomal-recessive pattern of inheritance.
• The HARD syndrome (hydrocephalus, agyria, retinal dysplasia and encephalocele is autosomal recessive.
• Cortical cytoarchitectural abnormalities may also occur in trisomy 13, 18 and 21.
• Infectious
—*Polymicrogyria, pachygyria-agyria,* and *heterotopias* may occur in the setting of toxoplasmosis, other agents, rubella, cytomegalovirus, and herpes virus (TORCH) infections of the central nervous system during early development. They may also occur as a consequence of intrauterine hypoxic-ischemic injury.

• Ischemic
—*Polymicrogyria* and *heterotopia* may occur in the setting of *in utero* hypoxic-ischemic injury.
—*Schizencephaly* may reflect intrauterine infarction and is characterized by a large cleft in one or both hemispheres. Whether schizencephaly is truly an MCD remains to be shown.
—*Porencephaly* (porencephalic cysts) are intraparenchymal cavities that communicate with the ventricular system, which also result from intrauterine hypoxic-ischemic injury.
• Toxins
—Ethanol
—Ionizing radiation
—Carbon monoxide
—Isotretinoin
—Methyl mercury
• Metabolic
—CD/NMDs have been reported in association with Zellweger syndrome, neonatal adrenoleukodystrophy, Menkes disease, and GM_2 gangliosidoses.
• Miscellaneous
—MCDs may occur in syndromes characterized by numerous other congenital anomalies, such as the Smith-Lemli-Opitz, Potter, and Meckel syndromes.

PATHOLOGY

The most characteristic feature is disruption of normal cerebral cortical architecture. In lissencephaly, there are few cerebral convolutions (sulci and gyri) in the entire brain, and the normal layering of cortex is abnormal. Neurons are often abnormally shaped and are oriented incorrectly within the cortex. In heterotopias, clusters of neurons are located inappropriately in the subcortical white matter. A large bilateral subcortical heterotopia is found in patients with "double cortex syndrome" and clusters of heterotopic neurons line the ventricles in periventricular nodular heterotopia. Disruption of the synaptic connections between various brain regions likely accounts for epilepsy and other neurologic problems such as mental retardation or autism associated with MCDs. (See above definitions.)

GENETICS

See Causes, above.

EPIDEMIOLOGY

• Incidence varies according to syndrome.
• Some children die at birth or in early childhood, owing to global devastation.
• Epilepsy may be associated with MCD in as many as 70–90% of cases. MCD are also a common cause of infantile spasms (especially tuberous sclerosis complex and lissencephaly).
• Approximate estimates are that from 20% to 40% of specimens resected during epilepsy surgery contain MCD.

Porencephaly Cortical Dysplasia/Neuronal Migration Disorders—Malformations of Cortical Development

PROGNOSIS
Most patients with CD/NMDs will continue to suffer from seizures and cognitive impairment as well as other neurological and behavioral abnormalities.

 Differential Diagnosis

In patients presenting with either overt or subtle neurologic symptoms or signs, consider a developmental central nervous system abnormality. Seizures and/or developmental delay are especially common manifestations of MCDs. Epilepsy in pediatric patients may be a manifestation of a neurocutaneous disorder such as TSC. Tumors, vascular malformations, and *in utero* ischemic insults also should be considered.

 Data Gathering

HISTORY
- Important questions include family history of genetic or chromosomal syndromes, family members with mental retardation, neurologic dysfunction or seizures, and infant deaths associated with profound neurologic impairment.
- Ask about parental consanguinity.
- Subtle manifestations of neurocutaneous syndromes may be identified in family members with skin lesions or, in more overt cases, as individuals with CNS or other cancers, as in TSC. Inquire about head or truncal flexion movements suggestive of infantile spasms.

 Physical Examination

- Many children with MCDs have no overt signs of dysfunction, while others have global neurologic impairment.
- Developmental delay, seizures (especially infantile spasms), and focal neurologic signs may be observed.
- Microcephaly or macrocephaly also may be identified.
- Some children will have dysmorphic facies characterized by hypotelorism, malformed skull, and midline deformities.
- Characteristic facies of the Miller-Dieker lissencephaly syndrome include a thin upper lip and microcephaly.
- Cutaneous manifestations such as hypomelanotic lesions ("ash leaf spots"), facial angiofibromas, a shagreen patch, or other regions of hyper/hypo pigmentation may identify patient with neurocutaneous disorders such as tuberous sclerosis.
- Funduscopic examination may reveal retinal hamartomas in TSC.
- A linear sebaceous nevus on the forehead is associated with hemimegalencephaly.

- Hypomelanosis of Ito is also associated with MCDs.

PHYSICAL EXAMINATION TRICKS
- Cutaneous examination with a Wood's lamp may be useful in identifying ash leaf or café-au-lait spots.
- Tooth enamel pits may be identified in TSC.

 Laboratory Aids

TESTS
- Most routine blood tests and cerebrospinal fluid will be normal.
- Metabolic derangements characteristic of disorders such as gangliosidoses may be identified with specific blood tests.
- Chromosomal karyotyping analysis (genetic screening) for Miller-Dieker syndrome, and various trisomies can be performed to aid in both diagnosis and further genetic counseling.
- Screening for select gene mutations is available through several research labs and will become commercially available.
- EEG is critical in diagnosing seizures and assessing the degree of underlying brain dysfunction. Characteristic findings may be sharp waves, spikes, hypsarrhythmia (in infantile spasms), and slow spike-wave discharges (Lennox-Gastaut syndrome). In children with developmental delay, formal neuropsychiatric assessment may be useful.

IMAGING
- Brain MRI with and without gadolinium contrast is essential in identifying and classifying MCDs. Brain CT may be useful but has lower resolution that does MRI.
- Functional brain imaging with *single-photon emission computed tomography* (SPECT) and *positron-emission tomography* (PET) is gaining popularity in assessing regional changes in glucose or oxygen metabolisms within regions of dysplasia.

 Therapy

DRUGS
In general, neurological consultation is recommended to help manage children with MCD and epilepsy. Virtually all children with MCD and seizures will require anticonvulsants drugs for adequate seizure control. These regimens must be tailored to account for drug interactions, potential side effects, and long-term efficacy in seizure control. Children with infantile spasms may respond to ACTH or vigabatrin therapy.

Epilepsy Surgery
A significant proportion of children with MCD and seizures will not respond to medications and will require epilepsy surgery to remove the seizure focus within the MCD. In some cases, the surgery is a small focal resection while in others, removal of a brain hemisphere is indicated. Some cases are not amenable to epilepsy surgery and other treatment modalities include the vagal nerve stimulator or the ketogenic diet.

 Follow-Up

WHEN TO EXPECT IMPROVEMENT
Adequate seizure control may be difficult in MCD patients. Cognitive and other neurologic deficits may benefit somewhat from neuropsychological intervention, education, and physical therapy. In children with a documented MCD and refractory seizures, resective epilepsy surgery provides a safe and often successful alternative to conventional anticonvulsant medications.

SIGNS TO WATCH FOR
Most worrisome would be a persistent change in mental status, which could indicate status epilepticus. Other worrisome signs include development of new neurologic symptoms in patients with TSC, suggesting hydrocephalus.

ICD-9-CM LISSENCEPHALY 742.2

BIBLIOGRAPHY
Barkovich AJ, Kuzniecky RI, Jackson GD, Guerrini R, Dobyns WB. Classification system for malformations of cortical development: update 2001. *Neurology* 2001;57:2168–78.

Barkovich AJ, Kuzniecky RI. Gray matter heterotopia. *Neurology* 2000;55:1603–1608.

Crino PB, Chou K. Epilepsy and Cortical Dysplasias. *Curr Treat Options Neurol* 2000;2:543–552.

Crino PB, Henske EP. New developments in the neurobiology of the tuberous sclerosis complex. *Neurology* 1999;53:1384–1390.

Eller KM, Kuller, JA. Fetal porencephaly: a review of etiology, diagnosis and prognosis. *Obstet Gynecol Surv* 1995;50:684–687.

Ho SS, Kuzniecky RI, Gilliam F, et al. Congenital porencephaly: MR features and relationship to hippocampal sclerosis. *AJNR* 1998;19(1):135–141.

Author: Peter B. Crino

Portal Hypertension

 ## Database

DEFINITION

Portal hypertension (HTN) is elevation of portal blood pressure above 10 to 12 mm Hg (normal, approximately 7 mm Hg).

PATHOPHYSIOLOGY

- Portal HTN is the result of a combination of increased portal blood flow and increased portal resistance.
- The portal vein carries blood from the stomach, spleen, pancreas, gallbladder, small intestine, and large intestine.
- Since no valves exist in the portal venous system, direction of flow reflects the pressure gradient and patency.
- All the major sequelae result from decompression of the venous pressure through portosystemic collaterals.
- The collaterals that develop are areas of decreased vascular resistance that become congested and lead to splenomegaly, esophageal varices, rectal varices, and caput medusae (periumbilical varices).

COMPLICATIONS

- The clinical manifestations of engorged collateral vessels include:

—Hemorrhage from esophageal varices
—Malabsorption due to congestion of the intestinal mucosa
—Ascites due to increased venous congestion with weeping of the mesentery
—Hypersplenism from splenic engorgement.

- Hemorrhage from esophageal varices is the most common presenting symptom (70%).

 ## Differential Diagnosis

Portal HTN can be seen in many different diseases. Conceptually, it is easiest to divide the causes of increased portal pressure by location of the underlying lesion.

- Suprahepatic (6% of cases)

—Budd-Chiari (associated with congenital web, tumor, trauma, clotting disorder, contraceptives)
—Congestive heart failure
—Veno-occlusive disease

- Intrahepatic (60% of cases)

—Cirrhosis from any disorder (biliary atresia, cystic fibrosis liver disease, autoimmune hepatitis, chronic hepatitis, tyrosinemia, Wilson disease, α_1-antitrypsin
—Schistosomiasis (parasitic eggs located in the hepatic venule)
—Peliosis hepatitis (associated with androgens)
—Vitamin A toxicity (Ito-cell hyperplasia)
—Congenital hepatic fibrosis

- Subhepatic (34% of cases)

—Splenic vein thrombosis
—Portal vein thrombosis

 ## Data Gathering

HISTORY

- History of umbilical catheterization
- History of hepatitis, abdominal trauma, clotting disorder, contraceptive pills, underlying medical problem such as cystic fibrosis, tyrosinemia, Wilson disease
- Ingestion of vitamin A
- Hematemesis

—Upper GI bleed from varices may be the first sign of long-standing silent liver disease or previously undiagnosed portal vein thrombosis.
—In patients with a stoma and portal HTN, life-threatening stomal variceal bleeds can develop.

 ## Physical Examination

- Splenomegaly (although size of spleen does not correlate with pressure)
- Hemorrhoids
- Prominent vascular pattern on the abdomen
- The direction of flow through these veins can be indicative of the site of obstruction.

—For example, with inferior vena cava obstruction, the blood flow of the abdominal surface vessels is cephalad.
—Another clue may be the lack of a caput medusa. This typically occurs with portal vein obstruction due to obliteration of the umbilical vein. Physical examination of the liver may also provide information about the etiology.

- Hepatomegaly is commonly present with suprahepatic processes and may or may not be present for intrahepatic disease; for example, Budd-Chiari is associated with a large, tender liver; chronic intrahepatic liver disease may have a shrinking liver and an enlarging spleen.
- Prehepatic processes may have either a normal or atrophied liver, depending on the adequacy of blood flow.

 ## Laboratory Aids

TESTS

- CBC and smear (will detect hypersplenism, GI blood loss, and chronic liver disease)
- PT, PTT
- Liver function tests
- Ultrasound with Doppler: used to identify whether the portal HTN results from a prehepatic, intrahepatic, or subhepatic process

—Can investigate liver echogenicity, biliary tree, spleen size, renal abnormalities associated with cystic disease of the liver, vessel diameter, and direction of blood flow
—Hepatofugal flow in the left gastric, paraduodenal, or paraumbilical veins is consistent with portal HTN.
—Sonographically engorged collateral vessels can be identified; can see if there are esophageal varices

- Esophagogastroduodenoscopy (EGD): used for definitive determination of the presence of esophageal varices and identification of bleeding source in the patient who presents with bleeding
- Barium swallow: rarely useful because it is an insensitive measure of varices (only 70% detection in adults)
- Liver biopsy and/or appropriate serologic tests: may be needed to identify the underlying cause of the portal hypertension
- Hepatic venous wedge pressure gradient is used in adults because of the correlation of pressure with bleeding risk. However, it is not used in pediatrics because of a lack of well-documented pediatric measurements.

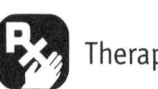

Therapy

ACUTE MANAGEMENT OF VARICEAL BLEED

- Lavage

—Use room temperature saline until clear.

- Blood products

—Replace blood products as needed
—Coagulopathy should be corrected with parenteral vitamin K and FFP.

- Medications

—Vasopressin: increases splanchnic vascular tone
—Somatostatin
—Nitroglycerin

- Endoscopy

—Sclerotherapy
—Ligation

- Direct tamponade

—Sengstaken-Blakemore tube

- Surgical intervention

—Portosystemic shunt
—Esophageal devascularization and/or transection
—Liver transplantation
—TIPS (transjugular intrahepatic portosystemic shunting)

CHRONIC MANAGEMENT

- Beta-blockade: Nonselective blockers lower portal pressure by a combination of two mechanisms. β_2-blockade will increase splanchnic tone and subsequently decrease portal perfusion, and β_1-blockade will lower cardiac output and portal perfusion. Propranolol may have a specific effect in decreasing collateral circulation. Beta-blockade has been shown to be effective in preventing both initial and recurrent bleeds. It is unclear if its administration changes survival. In pediatrics it is rarely used in patients prior to adolescence for fear of lack of adaptive response if the patient should bleed.
- Sclerotherapy: not used prophylactically because of the lack of consistent data demonstrating a benefit. However, it has been successfully used to prevent recurrence of bleeding.
- Shunt: infrequently used in pediatrics. Portosystemic shunting has not been shown to improve long-term survival in patients with intrahepatic disease.
- Liver transplantation: A number of studies have established that long-term survival is better for transplanted patients than for patients treated with any other mode of therapy for bleeding. Therefore, the current approach at most institutions is liver transplantation for those patients with life-threatening bleeds not amenable to beta-blockade or sclerotherapy.

Follow-Up

- Depends on the etiology of the disease
- Most patients are followed closely for hepatic compensation.
- Growth failure, poor quality of life, and life-threatening bleeds not controllable with prophylactic intervention are indications for transplantation.

PITFALLS

- The site of bleeding needs to be identified and managed appropriately.
- Not all GI bleeding in a patient with portal HTN is upper.
- NG tube lavage, as well as being therapeutic, will help determine if the problem is from the upper tract. In some cases, the GI bleeding is from hemorrhoids or another area of the GI tract.
- The second most common pitfall is to overestimate the hemoglobin, because equilibration may not have taken place at the time of presentation with an acute bleed.

Common Questions and Answers

Q: What is my child's long-term prognosis?
A: The prognosis depends on the underlying etiology. Upper GI bleeding associated with portal vein thrombosis typically becomes less problematic as the child ages. Therefore, this group of patients will most likely not require a shunt and may be easily managed with sclerotherapy. Similarly, the group of patients with congenital hepatic fibrosis also does very well, because the underlying disease is nonprogressive and bleeding may be easily managed with sclerotherapy. In contrast, progressive liver disease and uncorrectable suprahepatic problems have a worse prognosis, and discussion needs to be tailored to the underlying pathology.

Q: Should I restrict my child's activities?
A: Limit contact sports if splenomegaly is present or use a spleen guard. Avoid aspirin and NSAID-containing products.

ICD-9-CM 306.2

BIBLIOGRAPHY

Gitnick G, LaBrecque DR, Moody FG. *Diseases of the liver and biliary tract*. St. Louis: Mosby-Year Book, 1992.

Mowat AP. *Liver disorders in childhood*. Boston: Butterworth-Heinemann, 1987.

Suchy F. *Liver disease in children*. St. Louis: Mosby, 1994.

Wyllie R, Hyams JS, eds. *Pediatric gastrointestinal disease*. Philadelphia: WB Saunders, 1993.

Author: Barbara Haber

Posterior Urethral Valves

Database

DEFINITION

Valvular obstruction of the posterior urethra that results in variable dysfunction of all segments of the urinary tract, including the bladder, ureters, and renal parenchyma

PATHOPHYSIOLOGY

• The embryogenesis of posterior urethral valves (PUVs) is unclear.
• PUVs may arise from abnormal insertion and persistence of the distal end of the mesonephric duct.
• The valve is a fold of mucosa and fibrous tissue that usually forms a diaphragm with a slit-like orifice.
• Children with PUVs commonly have renal parenchymal dysplasia.
• With flow of urine from the bladder in patients with PUVs, the valves balloon into the urethra, causing obstruction. As a result of the increased work of voiding, the bladder hypertrophies, with trabeculation and diverticulum formation. The bladder develops poor compliance, decreased capacity, increased pressure, and spastic hyperreflexia.
• The segment of the urethra proximal to the obstruction dilates and elongates.
• Obstructive uropathy produced by PUVs is the result of transmission of high bladder pressures to the ureters and kidneys.
• Hydroureteronephrosis, vesicoureteral reflux, perirenal urinoma, or urinary ascites may occur.
• Renal parenchymal damage may result.

GENETICS

• The genetic basis of PUVs remains unclear.
• The majority of cases are sporadic, although rare cases in siblings have been reported.

EPIDEMIOLOGY

• PUVs is the most common cause of lower urinary tract obstruction in male infants.
• There are rare reports of obstructive valves in the female urethra; however, they differ embryologically from PUVs seen in males.
• The majority of boys with PUVs present in the first year of life.

COMPLICATIONS

• Severe cases may suffer the effects of intrauterine oligohydramnios, including Potter syndrome and pulmonary hypoplasia.
• The renal parenchymal damage results in the sequelae of progressive renal failure, such as anemia, acidosis, fluid and electrolyte abnormalities, and failure to thrive.
• Urinary tract infections and vesicoureteral reflux are common complications.
• Urinary incontinence may result from uninhibited bladder contractions, bladder noncompliance, and polyuria.

PROGNOSIS

• The prognosis for infants with severe PUVs has improved due to earlier recognition and improved management of pulmonary hypoplasia and fluid and metabolic derangements. Pulmonary hypoplasia and renal dysplasia account for most causes of death in infants with PUVs.
• Measures of renal function at the time of presentation may not correlate with ultimate outcome. Rather, the rate of improvement following relief of obstruction is more indicative of prognosis. An early nadir creatinine below 1.0 mg/dL does not preclude renal failure, as the child attains greater body mass.
• During the course of many years, many children who seem to do well initially will suffer progressive renal failure and require renal transplantation.
• Patients with an abnormal serum creatinine at 2 years of age often develop end-stage renal disease by adolescence or young adulthood.
• Children with significant bilateral reflux, renal dysplasia, and/or bladder dysfunction are more likely to eventually develop renal insufficiency and hypertension.

Differential Diagnosis

• Nonobstructive urinary tract dilation may occur secondary to:

—Vesicoureteral reflux
—Prune-belly syndrome
—Detrusor-sphincter dyssynergia
—Polyuria
—Urinary tract infection

• Other entities that may mimic PUVs include:

—Urethral strictures
—Primary vesical neck contractures
—Anterior urethral valves

Data Gathering

HISTORY

• The clinical presentation depends on the age of presentation and the severity of the obstruction.
• Many severe cases are diagnosed postnatally as the result of evaluation of hydronephrosis detected antenatally on maternal ultrasound.
• Severely affected infants may present with respiratory distress and other sequelae of oligohydramnios, azotemia, sepsis, dehydration, acidosis, and electrolyte disorders.
• Patients may present with palpable bladder, urinary tract infection, abnormal urinary stream, or failure to thrive as a result of renal failure.
• Toddlers may present with urinary tract infection or voiding symptoms such as dysuria and a weak urinary stream.
• Older boys may present with daytime incontinence, nocturnal enuresis, or urinary frequency as a result of bladder hypertrophy coupled with polyuria secondary to a renal concentrating defect.
• A strong urinary stream does not exclude the diagnosis of PUVs because an adequate flow may be generated by the hypertrophied bladder.

Physical Examination

Palpably enlarged bladder and kidneys are the most common physical finding.

Laboratory Aids

Infants with severe PUVs may have urinary tract infections and/or azotemia and fluid and electrolyte abnormalities such as dehydration, acidosis, hyperkalemia, and hyponatremia.

IMAGING

- The *voiding cystourethrogram* (VCUG) is the most important study in the diagnosis of PUVs. VCUG will reveal a sharply defined lucency in the posterior urethra and bladder hypertrophy. Bladder trabeculation, diverticuli, and vesicoureteral reflux may also be demonstrated.
- *Abdominal ultrasound* may demonstrate hydroureteronephrosis, evidence of renal dysplasia, dilation of the posterior urethra, a thickened bladder, and urinary ascites.
- Hydronephrosis is present in 90% of infants with PUVs.
- Definitive diagnosis requires *endoscopic examination*.

Therapy

SUPPORTIVE

- Initial management in the neonate consists of inserting a fine urethral catheter into the bladder and treating any fluid and electrolyte disturbances and/or urinary tract infection.
- A large postobstructive diuresis may occur, requiring ongoing management of fluids and electrolytes.

SPECIFIC

- Valve ablation (destruction of the obstructive valve leaflet) is the definitive treatment of the primary lesion. The most common approach is to incise the valves transurethrally through an endoscope.
- *In utero* drainage of the fetal bladder, with unclear benefits, has been attempted at a few medical centers.
- Unless the patient has renal insufficiency that does not improve after fluid resuscitation and catheter drainage, the next step is endoscopic ablation of the valves.
- If the infant's urethra is too small for the endoscope, cutaneous vesicostomy may be necessary.
- If rapid recovery does not occur following placement of the catheter or after valve ablation, vesicostomy or supravesical urinary diversion (such as ureterostomy or nephrostomy) may be required. The optimal anatomic level of urinary diversion remains controversial.
- Following valve ablation, the posterior urethra will appear less dilated on VCUG. However, improvement in hydroureteronephrosis and vesicoureteral reflux occurs more slowly, over years.

Follow-Up

- Growth problems, renal insufficiency, and end-stage renal disease can occur at any time during childhood, puberty, or beyond.
- Patients who require extensive urinary diversion, such as vesicostomy, pyelostomy, or ureterostomy, will require long-term reconstruction, including possible bladder reconstruction.
- Delayed obstruction may occur owing to urethral stricture.
- Patients with persistent incontinence require urodynamic evaluation to determine the case and individualized therapy.
- All children with PUVs should have careful follow-up through childhood and puberty. Each visit should include imaging for renal function and upper tract dilation and drainage, urodynamic studies of bladder function, assessment of growth, blood pressure, urinary protein, and serum creatinine.

PITFALLS

When a catheter is passed into the bladder, the valves flatten and are nonobstructive. This may give the misleading impression that there is no obstruction.

Common Questions and Answers

Q: What can be done for children with long-term bladder dysfunction and incontinence?
A: Voiding dysfunction may occur as the result of myogenic failure, detrusor hyperreflexia, and bladder hypertonia. Patients may require a combination of clean intermittent catheterization (CIC), pharmacologic therapy, and bladder augmentation. Approximately 20% of patients with PUVs have secondary bladder pathology that is not reversible by primary therapy of the valves.

Q: Are patients with PUVs good candidates for renal transplantation?
A: Patients with valves have a 5-year graft survival rate of only 50%, compared with 75% for patients with other diagnoses. The main adverse factor is poor bladder function. Better results may follow more aggressive correction of the bladder anomalies. Transplantation has been successful in patients with bladder augmentation and in patients using clean intermittent catheterization.

Q: Do patients with PUVs have impaired sexual and reproductive function?
A: In a small study, patients had good sexual function and some were fertile. Ninety-five percent had normal erections and were able to achieve penetration. Thirty-four percent and 50% had normal and slow ejaculation, respectively. Approximately one half had normal semen.

ICD-9-CM 753.6

BIBLIOGRAPHY

Churchill BM, McLorie GA, Khoury AE, et al. Pediatric renal transplantation into the abnormal urinary tract. *Urol Clin North Am* 1990;17:343.

Holmes N, Harrison MR, Baskin LS. Fetal surgery for posterior urethral valves: long-term postnatal outcomes. *Pediatrics* 2001;108(1).

Parkhouse HF, Woodhouse CRL. Long-term status of patients with posterior urethral valves. *Urol Clin North Am* 1990;17:373.

Radhakrishnan J. Obstructive uropathy in the newborn. *Clin Perinatol* 1990;17:215–239.

Roth KS, Carter WH Jr, Chan JC. Obstructive nephropathy in children: long-term progression after relief of posterior urethral valve. *Pediatrics* 2001;107(5):1004–1010.

Author: Mary B. Leonard

Premature Adrenarche

 Database

DEFINITION

Premature adrenarche is characterized by the appearance of small amounts of pubic hair before age 8 in girls and age 9 in boys. However, recent data suggest that the onset of normal sexual development in girls is younger than previously recognized. Puberty is starting 2 years earlier in African-American girls and 1 year earlier in white girls. With premature adrenarche, axillary hair, acne, and apocrine sweat gland secretion are not always present. No other signs of sexual development are exhibited.

PATHOPHYSIOLOGY

- Dehydroepiandrosterone (DHEA) and dehydroepiandrosterone sulfate (DHEAS) from the adrenal glands rise earlier than typically seen in normal puberty.
- Zona reticularis of the adrenals normally begins to increase androgen secretion at age 7 to 8 years.

GENETICS

- A familial pattern suggesting either recessive or dominant inheritance has been described.
- Occurs more frequently in African Americans

COMPLICATIONS

Can be the first sign of true precocious puberty (i.e., development of breast tissue and advancement of bone age) and thus warrants careful observation

PROGNOSIS

- Undergo puberty appropriately with normal fertility
- Ovarian hyperandrogenism is more common in some girls with premature adrenarche. Insulin resistance, a common finding in ovarian hyperandrogenism, has been reported in some children and adolescents with a history of premature adrenarche.
- Final adult height is normal.

 Differential Diagnosis

- Tumors

—Androgen-secreting tumors can arise in the gonads or adrenal glands.

- Congenital

—Nonclassic congenital adrenal hyperplasia (CAH)

- Miscellaneous

—Central precocious puberty
—Familial male precocious puberty (testotoxicosis)
—Exogenous male hormone ingestion

 Data Gathering

HISTORY

- Careful attention to presence of any other signs of sexual precocity as well as temporal nature of the adrenarche (i.e., rate of progression)
- Family history of pubertal development, infertility, irregular menses, hirsutism, premature male pattern balding

 Physical Examination

- The presence of pigmented, curly hairs in the pubic area is consistent with the androgen effect.
- In girls, clitoromegaly suggests CAH or androgen-secreting tumors.
- The finding of acanthosis nigricans suggests that insulin resistance and the risk of developing ovarian hyperandrogenism are present.

PITFALLS

Failure to differentiate between true pubic hair (curly and short) and dark lanugo hair (straight and long)

Laboratory Aids

TESTS

• Adrenal steroids: DHEA and DHEAS are often in the early pubertal range, but testosterone and 17α-hydroxyprogesterone (17-OHP) should be in the prepubertal range.
• GnRH stimulation test: not routinely recommended but would have a normal prepubertal response
• Children with systemic signs of virilization (such as a significantly advanced bone age) or elevated adrenal steroids (17-OHP or DHEA) should have ACTH stimulation testing to exclude CAH and other hyperandrogen syndromes.

IMAGING

• Bone age usually is normal (not significantly advanced).
• CT scan or MRI should be considered if there are other signs of significant virilization; look for intracranial or intraabdominal masses, especially if androgens are markedly elevated.

Therapy

• No treatment
• Reassure parents and children that this is a benign process.
• Reassess every 6 months to look for signs of virilization and pubertal progression.

Follow-Up

WHEN TO EXPECT IMPROVEMENT

Regression does not occur.

SIGNS TO WATCH FOR

• Watch for other signs of puberty, such as breast development or testicular enlargement (= 4 mL), that suggest onset of true precocious puberty.
• Increasing virilization suggests nonclassic CAH or early polycystic ovarian syndrome.

Common Questions and Answers

Q: Is there a dietary cause of excess adrenal hormones?
A: No.

Q: Does premature adrenarche mean puberty will be early?
A: The onset of puberty in these children is within the normal range and should follow the familial pattern.

Q: Can anything be done to reverse the changes?
A: This is a benign process that does not have long-term sequelae. Antiandrogen drugs are available but are not recommended.

ICD-9-CM 255.3

BIBLIOGRAPHY

Herman-Giddens ME, Slora EJ, Wasserman RC, et al. Secondary sexual characteristics and menses in young girls seen in office practice: a study from the pediatric research office in settings network. *Pediatrics* 1997;99:505–512.

Ibanez L, Potau N Virdis R, et al. Postpubertal outcome in girls diagnosed of premature pubarche during childhood: increased frequency of functional ovarian hyperandrogenism. *J Clin Endocrinol Metab* 1993;76:1599–1603.

Kaplowitz P, Oberfield SE, and the Drug and Therapeutics and Executive Committees of the Lawson Wilkins Pediatric Endocrine Society. Reexamination of the age limit for defining when puberty is precocious in girls in the United States: Implications for evaluation and treatment. *Pediatrics* 1999;104:936–941.

Karth-Schutz S, Levine LS, New MI. Serum androgens in normal prepubertal and pubertal children and in precocious adrenarche. *J Clin Endocrinol Metab* 1976;42:117.

Kornreich L, Horev G, Blaser S, et al. Central precocious puberty: evaluation by neuroimaging. *Pediatr Radiol* 1995;25(1):7–11.

Morris AH, Reiter EO, Geffner ME, et al. Absence of non-classical congenital adrenal hyperplasia in patients with precocious adrenarche. *J Clin endocrinol Metab* 1989;69:709.

Oppenheimer E, Linder B, DiMartino-Nardi J. Decreased insulin sensitivity in prepubertal girls with premature adrenarche and acanthosis nigricans. *J Clin Endocrinol Metab* 1995;80:614–618.

Pere A, Perheentupa J, Peter M, et al. Follow up of growth and steroids in premature adrenarche. *Eur J Pediatr* 1995;154(5):346–352.

Styne DM. New aspects in diagnosis and treatment of pubertal disorders. *Pediatr Clin North Am* 1997;44(2):505–529.

Authors: Andrea Kelly and Robert J. Ferry, Jr.

Premature Thelarche

 Database

DEFINITION

Premature thelarche is breast development before age 8 years in girls with no other signs of pubertal development.

CAUSE

Intermittent estrogen secretion by ovarian cysts

PATHOPHYSIOLOGY

- Low levels of estrogen secretion by normal follicular cysts
- Increased sensitivity of breast tissue to low levels of estrogen (surmised to be environmental)
- Ovarian response to transient increases in FSH levels and possibly to variations in ovarian sensitivity to FSH

EPIDEMIOLOGY

Sixty percent noted between 6 months to 2 years of age

COMPLICATIONS

May be the first sign of precocious puberty

PROGNOSIS

- No known effects on growth or fertility
- Onset after age 2 years may be associated with increased risk of progression to precocious puberty.

 Differential Diagnosis

- Environmental

—Exposure to exogenous estrogens in form of creams or birth control pills
—Intake of food with high estrogen levels (e.g., chicken liver)

- Tumors

—Benign lipomas

- Congenital

—Neonatal breast hyperplasia (*ICD-9-CM 778.7*) is benign breast enlargement in newborn boys or girls that is apparent shortly after birth and is due to gestational hormones. This form of breast development usually regresses.

- Severe acquired hypothyroidism: High levels of TSH may cross-stimulate gonadal FSH and/or LH receptors.
- McCune-Albright syndrome: triad of precocious puberty, café-au-lait spots, and polyostotic fibrous dysplasia
- True precocious puberty

 Data Gathering

HISTORY

- Careful assessment of onset and progression of breast tissue
- Family history of early puberty
- Exposure to estrogens

Special Questions

Ingestion of foods with high estrogen levels?

 Physical Examination

- Areolar enlargement is usually not present.
- Galactorrhea is not present.
- Look carefully for other signs of puberty:

—Menstrual blood
—Dull, gray-pink, or rugose vaginal mucosa (versus prepubertal appearance: shiny, bright red, and smooth)
—Pubic or axillary hair

- Inspect skin for birthmarks suggestive of McCune-Albright syndrome (café-au-lait spots in a "coast of Maine" pattern)
- Evaluate for signs of hypothyroidism: goiter, short stature.

PROCEDURE

Palpate carefully to distinguish fat from true breast tissue.

 Laboratory Aids

TESTS

No test is specific. Serum FSH and estradiol may be slightly higher than age-matched controls but are not consistently elevated.

IMAGING

- Bone age is not significantly or very mildly advanced (<1 year ahead of chronologic age). Useful in guiding the need for more intensive evaluation of true precocious puberty
- Pelvic sonography: may demonstrate presence and regression of small ovarian cysts (1–15 mm)

Therapy

- Observation
- Reassurance that this is a benign process

 Follow-Up

WHEN TO EXPECT IMPROVEMENT

Regression may occur up to 6 years after onset.

SIGNS TO WATCH FOR

Evidence of pubertal progression should prompt additional evaluation by an endocrinologist:

- Rapid increase in size of breast tissue
- Vaginal bleeding
- Growth spurt
- Development of pubic and axillary hair

PITFALLS

- Must distinguish fat from breast tissue in obese girls
- Removal of a breast bud will result in failure of that breast to develop during adolescence.

 Common Questions and Answers

Q: Does premature thelarche predispose the child to abnormalities in pubertal development?
A: If onset occurs after age 2 years, the girl may be more likely to enter puberty earlier. However, the majority of girls with premature thelarche will have normal pubertal development and fertility.

Q: Is my child susceptible to breast cancer?
A: There are no data to suggest that premature thelarche increases the risk of breast neoplasia.

Q: Can it happen in boys?
A: Many newborn male and female infants have breast buds as a result of exposure to maternal estrogen *in utero*. This neonatal gynecomastia usually resolves quickly.

Q: My daughter has breast development on only one side. Is this a tumor?
A: Asymmetric breast development is quite common in the early stages of normal pubertal development. Malignant tumors of the breast during childhood are extremely rare. As mentioned earlier, any removal of breast tissue prior to or during puberty must be avoided if possible.

ICD-9-CM 259.1

BIBLIOGRAPHY

Haber HP, Wollmann HA, Ranke MB. Pelvic ultrasonography: early differentiation between isolated premature thelarche and central precocious puberty [see comment in *Eur J Pediatr* 1997;156(1):78–79]. *Eur J Pediatr* 1997;154(3):182–186.

Herman-Giddens ME, Slora EJ, Wassermn RC, et al. Secondary sexual characteristics and menses in young girls seen in office practice: a study from the pediatric research office in settings network. *Pediatrics* 1997;99:505–512.

Kaplowitz P, Oberfield SE, and the Drug and Therapeutics and Executive Committees of the Lawson Wilkins Pediatric Endocrine Society. Reexamination of the age limit for defining when puberty is precocious in girls in the United States: implications for evaluation and treatment. *Pediatrics* 1999;104:936–941.

Klein Ko, Mericq V, Brown-Dawson JM, et al. Estrogen levels in girls with premature thelarche compared with normal prepubertal girls as determined by an ultrasensitive recombinant cell bioassay. *J Pediatr* 1999;134(2):190–192.

Mills JL, Stolley PD, Davies J, et al. Premature thelarche. Natural history and etiologic investigation. *J Dis Child* 1981;135(8):743–745.

Pasquino AM, Pucarelli I, Passeri F, et al. Progression of premature thelarche to central precocious puberty [see comment in *J Pediatr* 1995;127(2):336–337]. *J Pediatr* 1995;126(1):11–14.

Salardi S, Cacciari E, Mainetti B, et al. Outcome of premature thelarche: relation to puberty and final height. *Arch Dis Child* 1998;79(2):173–174.

Styne DM. New aspects in the diagnosis and treatment of pubertal disorders. *Pediatr Clin North Am* 1997;44(2):505–529.

Authors: Andrea Kelly and Robert J. Ferry, Jr.

Premenstrual Syndrome (PMS)

 Database

DEFINITION

Premenstrual syndrome (PMS) is a poorly defined constellation of emotional, behavioral, and physical symptoms restricted to the luteal phase of the menstrual cycle. Symptoms may begin around ovulation and continue through the first few days of menses. The symptoms completely resolve after menses. Premenstrual dysphoric disorder (PMDD): PMDD is the most severe form of PMS. The *Diagnostic and Statistical Manual of Mental Disorders* (DSM-IV) defines the diagnostic criteria for PMDD.

PATHOPHYSIOLOGY

- PMS appears to be secondary to abnormal physical responses to normal menstrual cycle hormonal changes.
- The pathogenesis of PMS has not been fully explained. The variable nature of PMS makes it likely that the underlying cause is multifactorial.
- Hypersensitivity to normal ovarian function rather than hormonal imbalance is being investigated as a factor in PMS. It has been postulated that normal biochemical events trigger psychoneuroendocrine events within the central nervous system resulting in the array symptoms found in PMS.
- Serotonin has also been investigated in the pathogenesis of PMS. Reduced platelet serotonin content and reuptake during the luteal phase, and decreased serum serotonin levels have been found in patients suffering from premenstrual dysphoric disorder (PMDD). Additionally, the serotonin 5-HT receptor may be subsensitive in affected patients.

GENETICS

- PMS is cross-cultural and has been documented in all ethnic groups.
- Twin studies have shown greater concordance in monozygotic than in dizygotic twins.
- Women with PMS generally have a greater number of relatives with PMS than controls without PMS.

EPIDEMIOLOGY

- PMS is only seen in menstruating females during ovulatory cycles.
- As many as 80% of adolescent females experience one or more premenstrual symptom(s).
- Forty-four percent of adolescent females experience symptoms severe enough to interfere with school attendance.
- Fifty-nine percent of adolescents self-reported PMS symptoms to be severe and 43% reported their symptoms to be "extreme."
- Studies in adolescents have shown a significant correlation between severe dysmenorrhea and premenstrual symptoms.

COMPLICATIONS

- No physical sequelae.
- Psychologic symptoms, when severe, can affect family, relationships, and school attendance.

PROGNOSIS

Good for overall health; however, symptoms tend to worsen through adolescence.

 Differential Diagnosis

PSYCHIATRIC

- Premenstrual magnification (PMM): An underlying psychiatric disease may be magnified in the luteal phase of the menstrual cycle. This phenomenon is referred to as PMM.
- Major depression
- Psychosis
- Dysthymia
- Anxiety disorder
- Physical, sexual, or emotional abuse
- Substance abuse

ENDOCRINOLOGIC

- Cushing disease
- Diabetes mellitus
- Thyroid disease
- Hyperprolactinemia
- Panhypopituitarism

GYNECOLOGIC

- Dysmenorrhea
- Pregnancy
- Premenopause
- Postpartum
- Oral contraceptive use
- Endometriosis

IMMUNOLOGIC/HEMATOLOGIC

- Fibromyalgia
- Anemia
- Lupus
- Chronic fatigue syndrome

MISCELLANEOUS

- Irritable bowel syndrome
- Migraine headaches
- Cancer

 Data Gathering

HISTORY

Medical and gynecologic history should confirm regular menses, determine if the woman is postpartum or perimenopausal, or has any prior mental health diagnosis. Data gathering in the form of a calendar of daily symptoms can be instrumental in

making the diagnosis. Several calendars have been published and validated including the Calendar of Premenstrual Experiences (COPE) and the Prospective Record of the Impact and Severity of Menstruation (PRISM). Common symptoms can be separated into two categories.

Physical

- Fatigue
- Breast tenderness
- Abdominal bloating
- Decreased energy
- Insomnia
- Hypersomnia
- Headaches
- Muscle pain
- Weight gain

Emotional

- Irritability
- Mood swings
- Depressed mood
- Anxiety
- Feeling out of control
- Feeling overwhelmed
- Increased appetite
- Food cravings
- Avoidance of social activities
- Difficulty concentrating
- Decreased efficiency

 Physical Examination

Physical examination aids in ruling out other diseases in the differential diagnosis. There are no physical findings specific to PMS. There is no minimum number of symptoms that must be present in order to make the diagnosis, nor must there be functional impairment.

SPECIAL QUESTIONS

- Are the symptoms limited to the luteal phase of the menstrual cycle?
- Is there any indication of a preexisting psychiatric illness?
- Are the DSM-IV criteria for PMDD met?

 Laboratory Aids

None

EMERGENCY CARE

Emergency hospitalization may be necessary in the case of severe psychiatric symptoms when the patient is believed to be a danger to herself or the public.

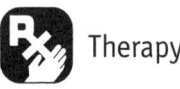 ## Therapy

NONPHARMACOLOGIC

Diet

- Increasing complex carbohydrates and fiber in the diet may lead to increased serotonin availability by helping with L-tryptophan uptake.
- Avoidance of caffeine, nicotine, alcohol, chocolate, salt, and sugar
- Calcium supplements: 1,000 mg per day. Calcium is a cofactor in the conversion of serotonin and may help reduce dysphoric mood, water retention, and food cravings.
- Pyridoxine (vitamin B_6): 50 to 100 mg per day. Studies suggest reduced headaches, water retention, irritability, and depression with up to 100 mg of vitamin B_6 per day. The data, however, are inconclusive. Doses greater than 117 mg daily may cause sensory neuropathy.

Behavioral Therapy

- Anger management
- Stress management
- Relaxation techniques
- Aerobic exercise
- Education about PMS
- Self-help groups
- Light therapy and homeopathic remedies. There are no research data to support any benefit to these options. Their use should be based on the individual patient and the potential for adverse side effects.

Pharmacologic

First Line

- Nonsteroidal antiinflammatory drugs relieve premenstrual cramping, migraine, and body aches. Side effects include gastrointestinal upset and renal problems.
- Ibuprofen: 400 mg every 6 to 8 hours
- Mefenamic acid: 500 mg once, then 250 mg every 4 to 6 hours
- Naproxen: 500 mg twice daily for 10 days prior to menses
- Diuretics aid in reducing bloating, swelling, and weight gain.
- Furosemide: 20 to 40 mg daily
- Spironolactone: 25 mg four times per day
- Oral contraceptives suppress ovulation but may exacerbate depressive symptoms. Some studies have shown improvement in a subset of women. May consider in adolescents at risk for pregnancy.
- Selective serotonin reuptake inhibitors (SSRIs) are the treatment of choice for women with significant premenstrual impairment. Improvement can be seen as early as the first menstrual cycle after the initiation of treatment. Side effects for SSRIs include gastrointestinal upset, sleep disturbances, lethargy, dry mouth, dizziness, and sexual dysfunction.
- Fluoxetine: 10 to 20 mg daily

- Paroxetine: 20 mg daily
- Sertraline: 50 to 100 mg daily

Second Line

- Androgens should be titrated to amenorrhea. May cause acne, renal problems, weight gain, and hirsutism.
- Danazol: 200 mg twice daily. Danazol has been shown to significantly improve cyclic mastalgia.
- Benzodiazepines relieve anxiety associated with PMS and should be used only during the luteal phase of the cycle. Sedation, tiredness, and respiratory depression are common side effects.
- Lorazepam: 0.5 to 1 mg twice daily
- Alprazolam: 0.25 to 0.5 mg three to four times per day. Alprazolam has few side effects. It does, however, have substantial addictive potential and may need to be tapered once menstruation begins.
- Gonadotropin-releasing hormone (GnRH) agonists can be given intranasally, intramuscularly, or subcutaneously. GnRH agonists produce a hypoestrogenic amenorrheic state. Side effects include symptoms similar to menopause such as hot flashes and vaginal dryness. Long-term use may result in accelerated bone loss.
- Leuprolide: 3.75 to 7.5 mg intramuscularly once per month.
- Tricyclic antidepressants tend to have worse headaches, dry mouth, dizziness, and gastrointestinal upset than SSRIs and may trigger mania.
- Clomipramine: 25 to 75 mg daily during the luteal phase only. Clomipramine has some serotonin and noradrenaline reuptake inhibiting properties.
- Buspirone: 25 to 60 mg in the luteal phase.
- Bromocriptine at 1.25 to 7.5 mg per day during the luteal phase can help relieve mastalgia and bloating.

PREVENTION

None

 ## Follow-Up

- Follow for improvement within two menstrual cycles after initiating treatment.
- Follow for significant side effects of treatment especially second-line therapy.

SIGNS TO WATCH FOR

- Worsening psychiatric symptoms.
- Sensory neuropathy in patients treated with pyridoxine.

 ## Common Questions and Answers

Q: Is it necessary to use a calendar to diagnose PMS?

A: It is not necessary to use a calendar to diagnose PMS. However, daily tracking with a symptom rating scale is extremely helpful in making the diagnosis of PMS. The calendar tracks cycle length, qualifies and quantifies symptoms, and determines if symptoms are truly limited to the luteal phase.

Q: Are there any diagnostic clues to help determine if the patient truly has PMS?
A: Yes, patients whose symptoms are not due to PMS may not have a symptom-free period during the follicular phase of the menstrual cycle.

Q: When should I consider moving from nonpharmacologic therapy to pharmacologic therapy?
A: Patients with significant impairment who do not improve with behavioral and dietary intervention should be considered for pharmacologic treatment.

Q: How does exercise help in premenstrual syndrome?
A: Exercise alleviates premenstrual symptoms by increasing endorphin release, which has a positive effect on mood.

ICD-9-CM 625.4

BIBLIOGRAPHY

American Psychiatric Association. *Diagnostic and statistical manual of mental disorders*, 4th ed. (DSM-IV). Washington, DC: American Psychiatric Association, 1994.

Cleckner-Smith CS. Premenstrual symptoms: prevalence and severity in an adolescent sample. *J Adolesc Health* 1998;22(5):403–408.

Kessel B. Premenstrual syndrome advances in diagnosis and treatment. *Obstet Gynecol Clin North Am* 2000;27(3):625–639.

Korzekwa MI, Steiner M. Premenstrual syndromes. *Clin Obstet Gynecol* 1997;40(30): 564–576.

Mortola JF, Girton L, Beck L, et al. Diagnosis of premenstrual syndrome by a simple prospective and reliable instrument: the calendar of premenstrual experiences. Obstet Gynecol 1990;72(2):302–307.

Pearlstein T, Stone AB. Premenstrual syndrome. *Psychiatr Clin North Am* 1998;21(3):577–590.

Thys-Jacobs S, Starkey P, Bernstein D, et al. Calcium carbonate and the premenstrual syndrome: effects on premenstrual and menstrual symptoms. Premenstrual Syndrome Study Group. *Am J Obstet Gynecol* 1998;179(2):444–452.

Wyatt PM, Dimmock PM, Jones PW, et al. Efficacy of vitamin B6 in the treatment of premenstrual syndrome: systematic review. *BMJ* 1999;318(7195):1375–1381.

Author: Krystal Revai

Primary Adrenal Insufficiency

 Database

DEFINITION

Primary adrenal insufficiency is a deficiency in the secretion of cortisol by the adrenal glands, which may also be associated with deficiencies of other hormones, including aldosterone and adrenal androgens.

PATHOPHYSIOLOGY

• Addison disease: primary hypoadrenalism due to bilateral destruction of the adrenal cortices; autoimmune destruction (isolated or part of polyendocrine autoimmune syndromes), tuberculosis, hemorrhage, fungus, neoplastic infiltration, AIDS
• Adrenoleukodystrophy: inherited disorders of impaired peroxisomal degradation of very long chain fatty acids, resulting in adrenal insufficiency and progressive neurologic deterioration
• ACTH unresponsiveness: an inherited defect in the ACTH receptor, resulting in isolated glucocorticoid deficiency with hypoglycemia in infancy and hyperpigmentation
• Congenital adrenal hypoplasia

GENETICS

• Addison disease: autoimmune adrenal insufficiency may be isolated or part of polyendocrine autoimmune syndromes. Familial and sporadic cases have been reported. An association exists between idiopathic Addison disease and HLA-138 and -Dw3.
• Adrenoleukodystrophy: X-linked recessive disorder of very long chain fatty acid metabolism. An autosomal-recessive form of the disease exists, with presentation during infancy.
• ACTH unresponsiveness: autosomal-recessive ACTH receptor defect
• Congenital adrenal hypoplasia—X-linked mutation in DAX-1 gene

EPIDEMIOLOGY

Age

• Addison disease is uncommon in children and usually presents between ages 20 and 50 years. In the pediatric population, it is most often seen in late childhood and adolescence.
• Adrenoleukodystrophy typically presents late in the first decade of life with neurologic symptoms. Signs and symptoms of adrenal insufficiency may present at any age.
• ACTH unresponsiveness presents in late infancy or the toddler period.
• Congenital adrenal hypoplasia presents in infancy or early childhood.

Sex

• Addison disease is more common in females.
• Adrenoleukodystrophy, an X-linked disorder, predominantly affects males.
• ACTH unresponsiveness affects both sexes equally.
• Congenital adrenal hypoplasia, an X-linked disorder, predominantly affects males.

COMPLICATIONS

• If not diagnosed and/or treated properly, a significant physical stress such as surgery or illness may result in a life-threatening adrenal crisis.
• Adrenoleukodystrophy results in severe neurologic impairment and death.
• Unrecognized ACTH unresponsiveness is associated with recurrent hypoglycemia, seizures, mental retardation, and death.
• Pubertal delay or hypogonadotropic hypogonadism is seen with congenital adrenal hypoplasia due to DAX-1 mutations.

PROGNOSIS

• The long-term prognosis of isolated adrenal insufficiency is good, provided adequate hydrocortisone is provided, particularly in times of illness.
• The diagnosis of adrenoleukodystrophy carries a poor prognosis.

 Differential Diagnosis

• Autoimmune adrenal cortical destruction
• Infectious adrenal cortical destruction

—Tuberculous
—Fungal
—AIDS

• Adrenal hemorrhage
• Neoplastic adrenal infiltration
• Adrenoleukodystrophy
• ACTH unresponsiveness
• Congenital adrenal hypoplasia

 Data Gathering

HISTORY

• Weakness and fatigue
• Anorexia, weight loss
• Headache
• Nausea, vomiting, diarrhea, abdominal pain
• Postural dizziness
• Muscle or joint pains
• Emotional lability
• Salt craving
• Hyperpigmentation, especially on lip borders, buccal mucosa, nipples, and over creases
• Decreased axillary or pubic hair in females due to lack of adrenal androgens
• Amenorrhea in females

 Physical Examination

• Hyperpigmentation
• Weight loss
• Hypotension
• Evaluate for other signs of autoimmune disease (e.g., thyromegaly, vitiligo).
• Pubertal staging

Laboratory Aids

TESTS

Specific

- Cortrosyn stimulation test: Administer cosyntropin (synthetic ACTH) 250 μg IV and measure cortisol at 30 and 60 minutes. A normal rise is a final cortisol exceeding 18 μg/dL. An insufficient cortisol response is diagnostic of adrenal insufficiency.
- A baseline ACTH greater than 200 pg/mL with inadequate cortisol is seen in primary adrenal insufficiency
- Serum adrenal antibodies may be positive in autoimmune Addison disease.
- Very long chain fatty acids are elevated in adrenoleukodystrophy.
- Hypogonadotropic hypogonadism may be seen with DAX-1 mutations causing congenital adrenal hypoplasia.

Nonspecific

Electrolytes

- Hyponatremia: result of the mineralo-corticoid defect and glucocorticoid deficiency; combination sodium loss from kidneys and the inability to excrete a water load
- Hyperkalemia and acidosis: chronic mineralocorticoid deficiency with the inability to excrete potassium and acid
- Hypercalcemia: probably through increased calcium absorption due to the lack of glucocorticoid effect on the gut
- Hypoglycemia: Glucocorticoids have permissive effects on gluconeogenesis.
- Renin levels are elevated when a mineralocorticoid deficiency is present.

 ## Emergency Care

ACUTE ADRENAL CRISIS

An intercurrent illness or surgical procedure may provoke an episode of hypotension and tachycardia, possibly leading to shock. Electrolytes reveal a decreased serum sodium, increased potassium, acidosis, and a decreased or normal glucose. Serum should be drawn and saved, but treatment should not be delayed for a diagnostic Cortrosyn stimulation test.

Treatment

- D_5NS for volume repletion
- Stress dosage of hydrocortisone: 100 mg/m² followed by 100 mg/m²/24 h of hydrocortisone divided q4h. Taper steroids over the next 1 to 2 days to a physiologic replacement dosage.
- Mineralocorticoid replacement: Florinef 0.1 mg daily when able to take PO.

 ## Therapy

CHRONIC ADRENAL INSUFFICIENCY

Treatment

- Hydrocortisone 10 to 12 mg/m²/day PO divided as t.i.d. triple dose for stress of fever, illness, vomiting. For major stress (surgery, significant illness), give hydrocortisone 50 to 100 mg/m² followed by 50 to 100 mg/M²/24 h IV divided q4h. Injectable hydrocortisone is recommended for emergency home use.
- Florinef 0.1 mg PO per day
- Patient education

—Stress dosing
—Seek medical attention for significant illness, persistent vomiting, or the inability to take fluids by mouth.
—Medic-Alert bracelet

 ## Follow-Up

An acute adrenal crisis usually improves rapidly with the administration of fluids and glucocorticoids. Steroids can usually be tapered in 12 days.

LONG-TERM MONITORING

- Clinical: reduction in hyperpigmentation
- Electrolytes, ACTH, renin
- Screen for polyautoimmune disorders.
- Growth
- Very long chain fatty acid levels and neurologic function in adrenoleukodystrophy
- Pubertal development

PITFALLS

- The symptoms of primary adrenal insufficiency are nonspecific and are similar to those found in many disease processes. The electrolyte picture of adrenal insufficiency can be seen in renal disorders, obstructive uropathy, and isolated aldosterone deficiency.
- Cosyntropin testing should definitively separate out those with true adrenal insufficiency.

 ## Common Questions and Answers

Q: What are the indications for stress dosing and how rapidly can the stress hydrocortisone dose be tapered?
A: Patients will require stress dosing of hydrocortisone for surgical procedures, fever (>100°F), vomiting, diarrhea, and particularly vigorous exercise. The stress dose is typically given for 24 hours, after which the usual dose is resumed. Should it be necessary to administer the stress dosage for a more prolonged period, the dosage can usually be tapered to a physiologic dosage over 12 days, once the patient's clinical condition has improved.

ICD-9-CM 255.4

BIBLIOGRAPHY

Baker JR. Autoimmune endocrine disease. *JAMA* 1997;278(22):1931–1937.

Grinspoon SK, Biller BMK. Clinical review: laboratory assessment of adrenal insufficiency. *J Clin Endocrinol Metab* 1994;79(4):923–931.

Guo W, Mason JS, Stone CG Jr, et al. Diagnosis of X-linked adrenal hypoplasia congenita by mutation analysis of the DAX1 gene. *JAMA* 1995;274(4):324–330.

Listenberg MJL, Kemp S, Sarde CO. Spectrum of mutations in the gene encoding the adrenoleukodystrophy protein. *Am J Hum Genet* 1995;56:44–50.

Moser HW, Loes DJ, Melhem ER, et al. X-Linked adrenoleukodystrophy: overview and prognosis as a function of age and brain magnetic resonance imaging abnormality. A study involving 372 patients. *Neuropediatrics* 2000;31(5):227–239.

Moser HW, Moser AE, Singh I, et al. Adrenoleukodystrophy: survey of 303 cases: biochemistry, diagnosis, and therapy. *Ann Neurol* 1984;16:628–641.

Peter M, Viemann M, Partsch CJ, et al. Congenital adrenal hypoplasia: clinical spectrum, experience with hormonal diagnosis, and report on new point mutations of the DAX-1 gene. *J Clin Endocrinol Metab* 1998;83(8):2666–2674.

Tsigos C. Isolated glucocorticoid deficiency and ACTH receptor mutations. *Arch Med Res* 1999;30(6):475–480.

Tsigos C, Arai K, Hung W, et al. Hereditary glucocorticoid deficiency is associated with abnormalities of the adrenocorticotropin gene. *J Clin Invest* 1993;92:2458–2461.

Vaidya B, Pearce S, Kendall-Taylor P. Recent advances in the molecular genetics of congenital and acquired primary adrenocortical failure. *Clin endocrinol* 2000;53(4):403–418.

Author: Lorraine Katz

Prion Diseases (Transmissible Spongiform Encephalopathies, TSE)

 Database

DEFINITION

- The transmissible spongiform encephalopathies (TSEs) or prion diseases are a family of slowly progressive neurodegenerative diseases of humans and animals that are uniformly fatal, causing irreversible cumulative brain damage.
- The human TSEs include Creutzfeldt-Jakob disease (CJD), the recently identified new variant CJD (vCJD), kuru, Gerstmann-Sträussler-Scheinker syndrome, and fatal familial insomnia syndrome.
- Six TSEs in animals have been described: bovine spongiform encephalopathy (BSE, also known as mad cow disease) scrapie in sheep and goats, feline spongiform encephalopathy, transmissible mink encephalopathy, exotic ungulate encephalopathy, and chronic wasting disease of mule deer and elk.

CAUSES

Prions are infectious proteins lacking nucleic acids that are believed to cause TSE. Infection arises when normal protease-sensitive host proteins, involved in neuronal function, undergo spontaneous misfolding to yield the abnormal protease-resistant form associated with infectivity. Prions reproduce by recruiting neighboring normal cellular prion protein and stimulating its conversion to the infectious form. Not all scientists believe the prion hypothesis and some have argued that the causative agent is virus-like and possesses nucleic acids.

PATHOLOGY/PATHOPHYSIOLOGY

- Progressive accumulation of abnormal prion protein in the central nervous system disrupts function leading to vacuolization and cell death. There is no host immune response or inflammation involved in the pathologic process.
- Neuropathologic findings include neuronal loss, atrophy, vacuolization or spongiform change, reactive astrogliosis, and cell death.

ASSOCIATED DISEASES AND EPIDEMIOLOGY

CJD

- CJD is the most prevalent form of TSE in humans and occurs as both a sporadic and familial disease.
- Approximately 90% of cases are sporadic because there is no family history, and no known source of transmission, and occurs throughout the world at a rate 1/1,000,000 people.
- Familial cases are associated with a gene mutation in the gene encoding normal prion protein and account for approximately 10% of cases.

- Less than 5% of CJD cases are iatrogenic resulting from accidental transmission of the causative agent via contaminated surgical equipment, as a result of cornea or dura mater transplants, or administration of human-derived pituitary growth hormones.
- There is no evidence of person-to-person transmission among family members via direct contact, by droplet or by airborne spread.
- Disease is characterized by progressive dementia, myoclonus, visual or cerebellar disturbance, pyramidal/extrapyramidal dysfunction, and/or akinetic mutism.
- Classic sporadic CJD most often occurs between the ages of 50 and 70 and affects both sexes equally.
- Death usually occurs within 1 year of onset of symptoms.

Variant CJD (vCJD)

- vCJD is a new form of CJD, first reported in 1994, which has unique clinical features.
- vCJD, in contrast to CJD, affects younger patients including adolescents (average age, 29 years) and has a longer duration of illness with median of 14 months as opposed to 4.5 months with CJD.
- There is strong epidemiologic evidence that links vCJD to BSE. BSE is a TSE affecting cattle and was first reported in the United Kingdom. The most likely route of exposure is through bovine-based foods derived from BSE-infected cattle. The highest incidence of vCJD is seen in the U.K., the country with the largest potential exposure to BSE. There are no confirmed cases of vCJD in North America.
- Clinical features, early in the illness, include prominent psychiatric symptoms such as depression and schizophrenia-like psychosis, and ataxia. Other neurologic signs such paresthesia/dysesthesia, chorea, dystonia, myoclonus, and akinetic mutism develop as the disease progresses.

Fatal-Familial Insomnia

- An autosomal-dominant disorder, caused by genetic mutation in normal prion protein gene.
- Clinical features include insomnia, dysautonomia, ataxia, myoclonus, and late dementia.
- Pathology reveals minimal vacuolization and no plaques.

Gerstmann-Sträussler-Scheinker Syndrome

- A disorder with autosomal-dominant inheritance
- Clinical features include ataxia and dementia
- Pathology reveals amyloid plaques.

 Differential Diagnosis

- Neurodegenerative disorders—mostly seen in older adults with the exception of Alpers disease

—Alzheimer disease
—Parkinson disease
—Frontotemporal dementia
—Pick disease
—Alpers disease (progressive cerebral hemiatrophy)
—Amyotrophic lateral sclerosis
—Huntington disease
—Spinocerebellar ataxia

- Psychiatric disorders—especially when considering vCJD as a diagnosis

—Depression
—Schizophrenia
—Drug-induced psychosis

- Encephalitis—infectious
- Sydenham chorea
- Subacute sclerosing panencephalitis
- Progressive multifocal leukoencephalopathy
- Toxic encephalopathy
- Inborn errors of metabolism
- Hashimoto thyroiditis
- CNS vasculitis
- CNS tumors

 Data Gathering

HISTORY

- Evidence of a familial form of TSE
- Potential iatrogenic exposures such as administration of human-derived pituitary growth hormones, implantation of dura mater or corneal grafts from humans, epilepsy surgery or other CNS surgery involving stereotactic electrodes.
- Duration of symptoms greater than 6 months.
- Afebrile illness
- In vCJD, progressive neuropsychiatric symptoms including:

—Depression, anxiety, apathy, withdrawal, or delusions
—Painful sensory symptoms including pain and/or dysesthesia.
—Ataxia
—Myoclonus, chorea, or dystonia
—Dementia

Prion Diseases (Transmissible Spongiform Encephalopathies, TSE)

 Physical Examination

- Afebrile
- Abnormal mental status examination with defects in memory, personality, and other higher cortical functions, or psychosis
- Neurologic signs include unsteady gait and the presence of involuntary movements.
- Late findings include mutism and complete immobility.

 Laboratory Aids

The diagnosis of TSE in humans can only be confirmed following pathologic examination of the brain. Microscopic examination of patients with all types of human TSEs reveals spongiform change accompanied by neuronal loss and gliosis. Amyloid plaques or immunohistochemical demonstration of abnormal prion protein in the brain may also be seen. "Florid" plaques (amyloid plaques encircled by holes or vacuoles resulting in a daisy-like appearance) are consistently present in patients with vCJD. Tonsil biopsy may be helpful in suspected cases of vCJD; the biopsy may reveal accumulation of abnormal prion protein.

LABORATORY TESTS

Most laboratory tests are of little value in the diagnosis of TSE. Examination of the CSF may reveal a mild elevation of protein, but otherwise the CSF is normal.

ELECTROENCEPHALOGRAM (EEG)

- In CJD, generalized slowing is seen early in the disease with progression to periodic burst of biphasic or triphasic sharp-wave complexes.
- In vCJD, the EEG does not show the wave forms characteristic of sporadic CJD. Although EEG abnormalities are seen in the majority of patients, these findings are not specific.

IMAGING

- In patients with vCJD, MRI reveals abnormal bilateral pulvinar high signal.
- In CJD, MRI often demonstrates hyperintense signals in the basal ganglia.
- In later stages of CJD and vCJD, imaging studies such as MRI or CT scan reveal generalized atrophy with large ventricles.

 Therapy

No treatment is effective in slowing or stopping the progression of disease. Appropriate supportive care should be provided. The prognosis for human TSEs is uniformly poor.

INFECTION CONTROL

Standard universal precautions are indicated for infection control. Strict isolation is not necessary. Caution should be used in obtaining CSF and handling tissues obtained at autopsy. Equipment contaminated by high-risk tissue should be soaked in ≥ 1 N sodium hydroxide solution for at least 1 hour and then autoclaved at 134°C for at least 1 hour.

 Common Questions and Answers

Q: Is transmission of TSEs from human blood possible?
A: There are no known cases of TSEs attributed to transfusion of blood products or reuse of devices contaminated with blood products.

Q: Is our food supply safe?
A: No cases of vCJD or BSE have been recognized in North America. The incidence in the U.K. has been low and is not increasing rapidly. Measures have been taken by the World Health Organization and the FDA to reduce the risk of TSE, including a ban on the use of ruminant tissues in animal feed, and surveillance systems to detect TSE in animals and to prevent any part or product of an animal with suspected TSE to enter the human or animal food chain. The FDA has banned biologic agents of bovine origin produced in countries at risk of BSE.

ICD-9-CM

Creutzfeldt-Jakob 046.1
Kuru 046.0
Sträussler-Scheinker syndrome 784.69

BIBLIOGRAPHY

American Academy of Pediatrics. Prion diseases. In: Pickering LK, ed. *2000 red book: report of the Committee on Infectious Diseases*, 25th ed. Elk Grove Village IL: American Academy of Pediatrics, 2000:471–473.

MacKnight C. Clinical implications of bovine spongiform encephalopathy. *Clin Infect Dis* 2000;32:1726–1731.

Prusiner SB. Shattuck Lecture— neurodegenerative diseases and prions. *N Engl J Med* 2001;344:1516–1526.

Whitley RJ, MacDonald N, et al. Technical report: transmissible spongiform encephalopathies: a review for pediatricians. *Pediatrics* 2000;106:1160–1165.

Author: Theoklis Zaoutis

Prolonged QT Interval Syndrome

 ## Database

DEFINITION

Prolonged QT interval syndrome, also known as congenital long QT syndrome (LQTS), is characterized by prolongation of the surface ECG QT interval, syncope, and sudden death as a result of malignant ventricular tachyarrhythmias. This electrical instability is due to an abnormality in ventricular repolarization.

PATHOPHYSIOLOGY

There are two hypotheses to explain the pathogenesis of congenital LQTS:

- An abnormality or imbalance in the sympathetic innervation to the heart, which would explain the sinus bradycardia, abnormal repolarization, adrenergic dependence of arrhythmias, and response to antiadrenergic medications associated with the syndrome
- An intrinsic abnormality in the mechanisms responsible for cardiac repolarization. Because some of the identified gene mutations resulting in congenital LQTS occur at loci that also encode a cardiac ion protein, ion channels have been proposed as the intrinsic abnormality that is responsible for abnormal repolarization.

GENETICS

- Autosomal dominant (Romano-Ward syndrome)
- Autosomal recessive [associated congenital nerve deafness (Jervell and Lange-Nielsen syndrome)]
- Genetic linkage analysis studies have attributed the autosomal-dominant LQTS to at least four known gene loci (chromosomes 11, 3, 7, and 4).

	LQT1	LQT2	LQT3	LQT4	LQT5	LQT6
Chromosome	11	7	3	4	21	21
Gene	KVLQT1	HERG	SCN5A			

EPIDEMIOLOGY

- Exact prevalence of LQTS is not known, but it may be a common cause of syncope and sudden unexplained death in children and young adults.
- Extrapolation from sudden death data suggests that the frequency may be as high as 1 in 5,000.

COMPLICATIONS

- Complications, especially in untreated patients, include:

—Ventricular tachyarrhythmias, specifically torsades de pointes
—Syncope
—Sudden death

- In patients with the inherited form of the condition, as opposed to those with a new mutation, asymptomatic family members may be affected.

PROGNOSIS

- Children have a higher incidence of sudden death than do adults, which may reflect a bias that adult patients have already survived childhood.
- Pediatric patients with greatest risk for sudden death are believed to be those with QT$_c$ greater than 600 msec. Beta-blocker therapy has been shown to reduce the incidence of sudden death.

 ## Differential Diagnosis

Congenital LQTS is most commonly misdiagnosed as vasovagal syncope or a seizure disorder. All patients who have a syncopal event or who are diagnosed with epilepsy should have a baseline screening ECG. Sudden infant death syndrome (SIDS) may be related to congenital LQTS (controversial). QT interval prolongation may be subtle, such that up to 10% of affected individuals may have a normal screening ECG and up to 40% may have borderline prolongation of the QT interval.

- Electrolyte abnormalities: hypokalemia, hypocalcemia, hypomagnesemia, and metabolic acidosis
- Toxins: organophosphates
- CNS trauma
- Malnutrition: anorexia
- Primary myocardial disease: myocarditis, ischemia
- Medications

—Cardiac medications: quinidine, procainamide, disopyramide, sotalol, amiodarone
—Antibiotics/antifungals: erythromycin, trimethoprim/sulfa, pentamidine, ketoconazole, fluconazole
—Psychotropic medications: tricyclics, phenothiazines, haloperidol
—Antihistamines: Seldane, Hismanal, Benadryl
—Gastrointestinal: cisapride.

 ## Data Gathering

HISTORY

- The history may be notable for:

—Palpitations
—Symptoms of presyncope
—Syncope

- These symptoms may be related to provocative stimuli, especially emotional or physical stress. The use of medications known to prolong the QT$_c$ interval should be established.
- Most importantly, a thorough family history for arrhythmia, syncope, epilepsy, or sudden unexplained death should be obtained.

 ## Physical Examination

Usually normal, may have bradycardia

 ## Laboratory Aids

Bazett's formula: QT$_c$ = QT/(square root of RR interval). Generally, a QT$_c$ greater than 500 msec is considered abnormal, although some clinicians allow a slightly longer QT$_c$ for infants younger than 6 months of age. In addition, some clinicians argue that the QT$_c$ should not be corrected at heart rates less than 60 bpm. The measurement should be taken in lead II without significant sinus arrhythmia. Children frequently have a prominent U wave, and it should generally be included in the measurement of the QT$_c$ if it is greater than half the amplitude of the T wave. A single measured prolonged QT$_c$ interval does not make the diagnosis of LQTS, and there is currently no single diagnostic test to confirm the diagnosis. Scoring systems may help stratify patients into high, moderate, and low probability of having the syndrome. See the table Diagnostic Criteria for Long QT Syndrome.

Diagnostic Criteria for Long QT Syndrome

Family history	
Family members with definite LQTS	1
Unexplained sudden cardiac death before age 30 among immediate family members	0.5
Symptoms	
Syncope[a]	
With stress	2
Without stress	1
Congenital deafness	0.5
Electrocardiographic findings	
QT_c	
>480 msec	3
460–470 msec	2
450 msec (in males)	1
Torsades de pointes	2
T-wave alternans	1
Notched T wave in 3 leads	1
Low heart rate for age	0.5
Prominent U waves	1
Miscellaneous	1

[a] Mutually exclusive

Total score: 0–2 = unaffected; 2.5–4.0 = intermediate; ≥4.5 = affected

Atrioventricular block can be seen in infants with relatively rapid heart rates and P waves that occur during the prolonged repolarization period and ventricular refractoriness. Other tests that may help confirm the diagnosis include 24-hour ambulatory Holter monitoring. This recording may disclose asymptomatic ventricular ectopy or arrhythmias, T-wave alternans, or variability in the QT_c interval during different periods of the day. Exercise stress testing may also be helpful in identifying ventricular arrhythmias or prolongation of the QT_c interval, particularly during the early recovery phase. The echocardiogram should demonstrate normal cardiac structure and function.

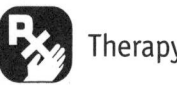

Therapy

Many clinicians support medically treating asymptomatic children because of a high incidence of sudden death occurring as the first symptom.

• Patients are usually treated based on symptoms and the clinical severity of their disease. The primary mode of therapy is β-blockade, most commonly with propranolol, atenolol, or nadolol. The class Ib antiarrhythmic medications, such as mexiletine, are also used in patients with congenital LQTS. Medications do not generally help treat patients with acquired LQTS.

• Occasionally, implantation of a permanent pacemaker is indicated based on the theory that long pauses may help to promote the induction of tachyarrhythmias, such as torsades de pointes.

• Left stellate ganglionectomy is a controversial therapy performed to eliminate the hyperactive left sympathetic ganglion output.

• Automatic implantable cardioverter-defibrillators (AICDs) are usually reserved for older children and adolescents who have significant symptoms and documented ventricular arrhythmias. Recent identification of disease genes in congenital LQTS may lead to the development of therapy specific to the ion channel defect.

Follow-Up

Follow-up outpatient appointments should include the review of new or recurrent symptoms, including palpitations, near-syncope or syncope, and the efficacy and adverse effects of medical therapy. The ECG may demonstrate a normal or prolonged QT_c. Follow-up 24-hour ambulatory Holter monitor recordings and exercise stress tests may help in the assessment of adequate beta-blocker therapy and the identification of ventricular arrhythmias.

PREVENTION

Preventive measures should focus on the avoidance of exposure to medications or situations that may provoke prolongation of the QT_c interval or the induction of torsades de pointes, such as certain antihistamines and antibiotics, sympathomimetics, caffeine, electrolyte abnormalities, and highly stressful environments.

PITFALLS

As reviewed in the Differential Diagnosis section, the primary pitfall is missed recognition of the syndrome. This may occur when an affected patient has a normal screening ECG (up to 10% of patients) or when a wrong diagnosis is made (epilepsy, for example). Once a diagnosis is made, family members should be thoroughly screened.

Common Questions and Answers

Q: Should activity be restricted in patients with congenital LQTS?
A: Because sudden rises in serum catecholamine levels may precipitate symptoms, it is appropriate to restrict competitive and vigorous athletics. Symptomatic patients may require greater restrictions. Documentation of appropriate β-blockade, by a lower maximal heart rate at peak exercise, on follow-up exercise stress test may be helpful.

Q: If someone is identified as having LQTS, should family members be evaluated?
A: Yes, with a high degree of suspicion. Most cases of congenital LQTS are inherited in an autosomal-dominant pattern, so that each child of an affected parent has a 50% chance of having the gene. This does not predict the severity of symptoms, but parents, all siblings, and children of patients should have ECGs. Holter monitoring and exercise stress testing may be helpful in provoking an abnormal QT_c interval in suspected family members.

ICD-9-CM 426.8

BIBLIOGRAPHY

Ackerman MJ. The long QT syndrome. *Pediatr Rev* 1998;19(7):232–238.

Garson A Jr, Dick M II, Fournier A, et al. The long QT syndrome in children: an international study of 287 patients. *Circulation* 1993;87:1866–1872.

Hoffman JI. The prolonged QT syndrome. *Adv Pediatr* 2001;48:115–156.

Roden DM, Lazzara R, Rosen M, et al. Multiple mechanisms in the long QT syndrome: current knowledge, gaps, and future directions. *Circulation* 1996;94:1996–2012.

Schwartz PJ, Moss AJ, Vincent GM, et al. Diagnostic criteria for the long QT syndrome: an update. *Circulation* 1993;88:782.

Zupancic JA, Triedman JK, Alexander M, et al. Cost-effectiveness and implications of newborn screening for prolongation of QT interval for the prevention of sudden infant death syndrome. *J Pediatr* 2000;136(4): 481–489.

Author: Ronn E. Tanel

Prune-Belly Syndrome

 Database

DEFINITION

The prune-belly syndrome is a rare congenital disorder characterized by the triad of:

- Deficiency of the abdominal musculature
- Bilateral cryptorchidism
- Dilated, anomalous development of the bladder and upper urinary tract

It presents in a broad spectrum of severity, from severe renal dysplasia and pulmonary hypoplasia to mild uropathy with stable renal function.

CAUSES

The etiology of the prune-belly syndrome remains unclear. Two theories have been proposed:

- The triad of congenital defects may be the result of a primary mesodermal defect in development with congenital deficiency of smooth muscle in the bladders, ureters, and renal pelvis.
- Outflow obstruction of the bladder *in utero* may result in dilation of the bladder and upper urinary tract with subsequent renal injury. The expanded bladder may block the route of the descending testicles and may cause abdominal distention and abdominal wall muscle atrophy.

PATHOPHYSIOLOGY

- Prune-belly bladder is large, irregular in shape, and thick walled. Many patients have poor urinary flow and high residual volumes.
- Ureters are usually markedly dilated, tortuous, and elongated. Peristalsis is ineffective and the distal ureters are most severely affected.
- Renal involvement is variable; the most severe dysplasia occurs in patients with worse dilation of the urinary tract. The dysplastic changes are usually symmetric.
- Usually, the bladder neck is wide and the prosthetic urethra is dilated and triangular. Most patients do not have anatomic obstruction at this point.

GENETICS

- The genetic basis of prune-belly syndrome remains unclear.
- A majority of patients have normal karyotypes.
- A majority of cases are sporadic, although rare cases in siblings have been reported.

EPIDEMIOLOGY

- Most patients are detected during the neonatal period or prenatally during maternal ultrasound.
- Prune-belly syndrome is much more common in males.

COMPLICATIONS

Many patients have other associated anomalies:

- *Gastrointestinal anomalies* include imperforate anus and increased risk of volvulus.
- *Lower extremity musculoskeletal anomalies* include talipes equinovarus and congenital hip dislocation.

Complications of the syndrome include:

- Pulmonary hypoplasia
- Vulnerability to recurrent pulmonary infections and postoperative atelectasis secondary to chest wall instability and ineffective cough because of abdominal wall deficiency
- Frequent urinary tract infections (UTIs) secondary to upper urinary stasis, vesicoureteral reflux, and bacteriuria
- Sequelae of progressive renal insufficiency

PROGNOSIS

- Patients with the most severe renal dysplasia die in the neonatal period.
- Those with a mild form do not require surgical treatment of the urinary tract; renal function is usually stable and the prognosis is excellent.
- For patients with moderate involvement, the degree of renal dysplasia and insufficiency determines outcome. In addition, upper urinary tract stasis, poor bladder emptying, vesicoureteral reflux, and bacteriuria are factors that may combine to result in a worse long-term prognosis.

 Differential Diagnosis

- The distinctly abnormal physical examination of the affected infant results in an early, accurate diagnosis in most cases.
- Pseudo–prune-belly syndrome (prune-belly syndrome uropathy, normal abdominal wall examination, and incomplete or absent cryptorchidism)

 Data Gathering

HISTORY

In patients with mild involvement of the abdominal wall that are not detected in the neonatal period, evaluation of UTIs may reveal the dilated urinary tract.

 Physical Examination

- In most cases, the abdominal wall is characterized by multiple wrinkles and redundant skin.
- A large, distended bladder creates a suprapubic mass.
- Ureters and kidneys are readily palpable.
- Intestinal loops and peristalsis may be observed.
- Testes are undescended.
- Myopathy results in difficulty in sitting up from a supine position.

Laboratory Aids

TESTS

- The initial evaluation should include assessment of renal function.
- May see elevated serum levels of creatinine and BUN
- Renal failure may result in anemia and elevated levels of potassium, phosphorus, hydrogen ion, and uric acid, and decreased concentrations of sodium, calcium, and bicarbonate.

IMAGING

- An ultrasound will demonstrate the dilatation and redundancy of the upper urinary tract.
- When considering a voiding cystourethrogram, consider the risk of introducing infection into the dilated, poorly draining urinary tract.
- Renal function and drainage of the dilated tract can be assessed by radioisotope renal scan or an excretory urogram.

 Therapy

SUPPORTIVE

- The basic principles of supportive care and management of renal failure apply.
- Antibiotics in the neonatal period and antibiotic prophylactic of indefinite duration are indicated to prevent infection.

SPECIFIC

- The dilated, tortuous urinary tract is managed by urologists. The optimal approach to patients with severe uropathy who survive the newborn period is very controversial.
- Some advocate minimal surgical intervention, based on the observation that there is no functional obstruction and the dilated system has a low pressure owing to the deficient smooth musculature. If renal function deteriorates, the urinary tract dilation progresses or the patient develops a urinary tract infection despite antibiotic prophylaxis; cutaneous vesicostomy is recommended to facilitate drainage.
- Others advocate extensive surgical remodeling. Possible procedures include, as indicated:

—Internal urethrotomy, reduction cystoplasty
—Excision of the redundant ureter with reimplantation of the remaining segment
—Cutaneous ureterostomy
—Pyelostomy

- Reconstruction of the abdominal wall has yielded good cosmetic results with questionable improvements in function.
- Bilateral orchiopexy is indicated.

 Follow-Up

Regardless of how patients might be managed, they require long-term follow-up, with meticulous attention to renal function, pulmonary function, and urine bacteriology.

 Common Questions and Answers

Q: Are patients with prune-belly syndrome candidates for renal transplantation?
A: Yes. However, special pretransplant consideration should be given to the dilated urinary tract in order to optimize function.

Q: How does the urinary tract function in older children?
A: A tendency for bladder tone and ureteral peristalsis to improve with age has been noted.

Q: Are these patients infertile?
A: Normal sexual activity has been described. However, there are no reports of fertility, and the patients usually have azoospermia.

Q: What is the usual cause of morbidity in the newborn period?
A: Respiratory failure.

ICD-9-CM 756.7

BIBLIOGRAPHY

Coplen DE, Snow BW, Duckett JW. Prune-belly syndrome. In: Gilwater JY, Grayhack JT, Howards SS, et al., eds. *Adult and pediatric urology*, 3rd ed. St. Louis: Mosby, 1996: 2297–2310.

Greskovich FJ III, Nyberg LM Jr. The prune belly syndrome: a review of its etiology, defects treatment and prognosis. *J Urol* 1988;140:707–712.

Jennings RW. Prune belly syndrome. *Semin Pediatr Surg* 2000;9(3):115–120.

Loder RT, Guiboux JP, Bloom DA, et al. Musculoskeletal aspects of prune-belly syndrome. *Am J Dis Child* 1992;146: 1224–1229.

Noh PH, Cooper CS, Winkler AC, et al. Prognostic factors for long-term renal function in boys with the prune-belly syndrome. *J Urol* 1999;162(4):1399–1401.

Pagon RA, Smith DW, Shepard TH. Urethral obstruction malformation complex: a cause of abdominal deficiency and the "prune-belly." *J Pediatr* 1979;94:900.

Sutherland RS, Mevorach RA, Kogan BA. The prune-belly syndrome: current insights. *Pediatr Nephrol* 1995;9(6):770–778.

Wheatley JM, Stephens FD, Hutson JM. Prune-belly syndrome: ongoing controversies regarding pathogenesis and management. *Semin Pediatr Surg* 1996;5(2):95–106.

Woodard JR. Current management of the dilated urinary tract in prune-belly syndrome. *J Urol* 1988;159(5):1680.

Woodard JR, Zucker I. Lessons learned in 3 decades of managing the prune-belly syndrome. *Urol Clin North Am* 1990;17:407.

Author: Mary B. Leonard

Pseudotumor Cerebri

 Database

DEFINITION

Diagnostic criteria of pseudotumor cerebri include:

- Signs and symptoms of increased intracranial pressure, such as headache, vomiting, visual changes and papilledema
- Elevated CSF pressure with otherwise normal CSF
- Normal neurologic examination except for papilledema (and occasional abducens nerve palsy)
- Normal neuroimaging study

CAUSES

- Pathogenesis may involve decreased CSF absorption secondary to arachnoid villi dysfunction or elevated intracranial venous pressure. For example, obesity may lead to increased intraabdominal, intrathoracic, and cardiac filling pressure, eventually leading to elevated intracranial venous pressure.
- Numerous precipitants of pseudotumor have been reported. In adolescents, it is clearly associated with obesity and weight gain, but is not clearly linked to obesity in children below age 11 years. Many weaker associations may be due to chance. Pseudotumor is often linked to tetracycline, sulfonamides, withdrawal from corticosteroids, isotretinoin, and thyroid replacements; it is also linked to vitamin A deficiency or intoxication, chronic anemia, and hypothyroidism.

GENETICS

Sporadic, no clear genetic predisposition, unless related to an underlying hormonal, toxic, or inflammatory condition.

EPIDEMIOLOGY

- Incidence in children is unknown.
- Males and females are affected equally in childhood, but not in adulthood.
- Pseudotumor has been reported as early as 4 months of age, with a median age of 9 years.

ASSOCIATED CONDITIONS

- Visual loss due to optic nerve pressure
- Endocrinopathies, exogenous steroids, craniosynostosis, lead exposure, growth hormone treatment, and tetracycline may be associated with pseudotumor.

 Differential Diagnosis

The following may all be confused with pseudotumor, but the clinical picture, neuroimaging, and CSF analysis usually permit their distinction.

- Chronic meningitis (such as CNS Lyme disease), encephalitis, or cerebral edema (may show minimal changes on neuroimaging with elevated CSF protein and little pleocytosis)
- Cerebral venous sinus thrombosis (as in otitic hydrocephalus), most easily seen on MRI/MR venogram (MRV).

 Data Gathering

HISTORY

- Headache is the most common presenting complaint.
- Blurred vision, diplopia, transient visual obscurations, and dizziness may be present.
- Infants and young children may present with irritability, somnolence, stiff neck, or ataxia.
- Directed history for signs of associated endocrinopathy, antibiotic or steroid exposure, sleep disturbance, sinus infection, connective tissue, tendency for thrombosis

 Physical Examination

- Papilledema is almost always present in older children.
- Most infants have some degree of papilledema, even with open fontanelles and split sutures.
- Sixth cranial nerve palsies are common in children with pseudotumor; they were found in 29 of 68 patients in one series.
- Other cranial nerve deficits are rarely seen.
- Recording baseline visual acuity and visual fields in older children is essential.

 Laboratory Aids

TESTS

- Cranial CT or MRI should be normal. MRI is preferred because of superior imaging of brainstem, posterior fossa, and sinuses. MRA/MRV is useful in evaluating dural venous sinus thrombosis.
- Lumbar puncture manometry with the patient in a relaxed position should show an opening pressure of greater than 250 mm H_2O, but otherwise normal CSF composition.
- Goldmann perimeter visual field testing or computerized visual fields are useful in children over 5 years of age to document field deficits and monitor response to therapy.
- CBC and thyroid function tests (TFTs) should be obtained because anemia, hypothyroidism, and hyperthyroidism have rarely been associated with pseudotumor.

The following may be useful in selected cases:

- ANA
- ESR
- Urine cortisol
- Serum lead level
- Serologic testing for Lyme disease (though false positives can be misleading)

 Emergency Care

The urgency of diagnosis and treatment depends on the severity of visual loss. Most patients present with mild-to-moderate visual loss, rather than severe or progressive visual loss.

Therapy

- Treatment depends on the degree of visual loss.
- For patients with no visual loss, removal of possible causative agents may be the only intervention needed, along with treatment of associated conditions (obesity, anemia, thyroid disease). Headache can be treated symptomatically if needed.
- For patients with mild-to-moderate visual loss, acetazolamide (Diamox), a carbonic anhydrase inhibitor that decreases CSF production, is the drug of choice.

—The pediatric dosage is 60 mg/kg/d divided q.i.d. for the standard form and b.i.d. for the long-acting form (Diamox sequels).
—The initial adult dose is 250 mg q.i.d. or 500 mg b.i.d., increased to 750 mg q.i.d. or 1,500 mg b.i.d. if tolerated.

- Furosemide can be used if acetazolamide is ineffective or has intolerable side effects.
- Serial lumbar punctures are not recommended as standard therapy, although the initial LP can be useful to relieve symptoms acutely.
- Surgical therapy (optic nerve sheath fenestration or lumboperitoneal shunt) is indicated for progressive visual loss despite medical therapy or for severe visual loss at presentation. Optic nerve sheath fenestration may be the preferred surgical treatment, because of the high-failure rates of lumboperitoneal shunting. Retrospective studies support use of corticosteroids, and acetazolamide is indicated while awaiting surgical therapy.

 Follow-Up

- Patients should have visual acuity, visual fields, and fundi evaluated weekly or biweekly initially.
- If vision is stable, then monthly visits may be adequate for 3 to 6 months.
- More frequent follow-up is required for any signs of progressive visual loss.
- Follow-up and tapering of acetazolamide should be done in conjunction with a neurologist or neuro-ophthalmologist.
- If visual loss resolves, acetazolamide can be tapered after 2 months of therapy.

PITFALLS

- Children are *not* exempt from permanent visual loss as a sequela of pseudotumor.
- Headache may transform to "chronic daily headache" after objective signs have resolved.
- Pseudotumor may be diagnosed erroneously if:

—Pseudopapilledema is mistaken for papilledema
—CSF abnormalities (i.e., isolated increase in protein) are overlooked
—Noncontrast CT fails to identify a cerebral venous sinus thrombosis (contrast CT or MRI should be done)

 Common Questions and Answers

Q: What are the side effects of acetazolamide?
A: Side effects of acetazolamide include GI upset, paresthesias, loss of appetite, drowsiness, metabolic acidosis, and renal stones. An alternative is furosemide.

Q: If pseudotumor occurs on tetracycline, can the child take penicillin?
A: Penicillins/cephalosporins have not been reported as a significant cause of pseudotumor.

Q: Are there any limitations on physical activity?
A: Activity can be graded entirely according to the child's symptoms.

ICD-9-CM 348.2

BIBLIOGRAPHY

Jones JS, Nevai J, Freeman MP, et al. Emergency department presentation of idiopathic intracranial hypertension. *Am J Emerg Med* 1999;17:517–521.

Liu GT, Volpe NJ, Galetta SL. *Neuro-ophthalmology: diagnosis and management.* Philadelphia: WB Saunders, 2001:204–14.

Phillips PH, Repka MX, Lambert SR. Pseudotumor cerebri in children. *J AAPOS Am Assoc Pediatr Ophthalmol Strabismus* 1998;2:33–38.

Scott IU, Siatkowski RM, Eneyni M, et al. Idiopathic intracranial hypertension in children and adolescents. *Am J Ophthalmol* 1997;124:253–255.

Soler D, Cox T, Bullock P, et al. Diagnosis and management of benign intracranial hypertension. *Arch Dis Child* 1998;78:89–94.

Soler D, Lessell S. Pediatric pseudotumor cerebri (idiopathic intracranial hypertension). *Surv Ophthalmol* 1992;37:155.

Author: Dennis J. Dlugos

Psittacosis

Database

DEFINITION

Psittacosis is an acute febrile disease characterized by pneumonitis and other systemic symptoms. The name is derived from the Greek word for parrot, *psittakos*.

CAUSE

Chlamydia psittaci (an obligate intracellular parasitic bacterium)

PATHOPHYSIOLOGY

- Inhalation of aerosolized organisms into the respiratory tract
- Incubation period of 5 to 21 days
- Spreads via bloodstream to lungs, liver, and spleen
- Lymphocytic inflammatory alveolar response

EPIDEMIOLOGY

- Birds are the major reservoir (pigeons, parrots, parakeets, turkeys, chickens, ducks).
- Infecting agent present in bird nasal secretions, urine, feces, feathers, viscera, carcasses
- While inhalation is the most common route of infection, bird bites and mouth-to-beak contact also spread infection.
- Birds may be healthy or sick.
- Most reported cases (70%) are the result of exposure to pet caged birds (especially parrots, parakeets).
- Most common mammalian source of infection is sheep.
- Occupational hazard of workers in poultry plants, pet shops, zoos, farms.
- Rarely transmitted person to person.
- Only 100 to 200 total cases reported in United States each year.
- Very rare disease in young children.

COMPLICATIONS

- Hepatitis, anemia
- Thrombophlebitis, pulmonary embolus
- Arthritis, keratoconjunctivitis
- Endocarditis, myocarditis, pericarditis
- Encephalitis: agitation, delirium, confusion, stupor

PROGNOSIS

Complete recovery is expected in all but a few rare cases (even without antibiotic use).

ASSOCIATED ILLNESS

Pneumonitis, along with severe headache, is the most common presentation.

Differential Diagnosis

- Psittacosis should be considered in all fevers of unknown origin or atypical pneumonitis.
- *Mycoplasma* and *Chlamydia pneumoniae*, *Legionella* spp., *Coxiella burnetii* (Q fever), tuberculosis, viral and fungal pneumonitis, as well as pneumococcal pneumonia

Data Gathering

HISTORY

- Abrupt onset of symptoms is usual.
- Fever, headache, cough, weakness, chills, muscle aches, and joint pain are common.
- A nonproductive cough is usual.
- Vomiting, confusion, and photophobia are less common.

PITFALLS

Failure to question parents as to the exposure of the patient to any type of bird—wild or domestic

Physical Examination

- Ill appearance, tachypnea, rales, and splenomegaly are common.
- A relative bradycardia is a unique finding in some cases.
- Rash, meningismus, pharyngeal injection, cervical adenopathy, hepatomegaly, and mental status changes less common.

Laboratory Aids

TESTS

- Chest x-ray demonstrates diffuse interstitial infiltrates.
- Routine laboratory studies are not helpful.
- Complement fixation titers (see Common Questions and Answers, below)
- Isolation of the organism is diagnostic.

PITFALLS

Note that the complement fixation titers do not distinguish between the various chlamydial infections (*C. psittaci, C. pneumoniae,* and *C. trachomatis*)

Therapy

- Tetracycline (40 mg/kg/d) or doxycycline (100 mg b.i.d.) for at least 10 to 14 days in children older than 8 years
- Erythromycin (40 mg/kg/d) in children 8 years and younger
- Azithromycin, clarithromycin, and chloramphenicol are additional options.
- Oxygen and other supportive care (especially respiratory) as needed

Follow-Up

- Resolution of fever and most other systemic symptoms can be expected within 48 hours of antibiotic therapy.
- Untreated patients may have severe pulmonary symptoms for 1 to 3 weeks.

PREVENTION

- Epidemiologic investigation is indicated in all possible cases.
- Birds suspected to be infected should be sacrificed, transported, and analyzed by appropriate experts.
- Potentially contaminated bird areas should be disinfected and aired.

Common Questions and Answers

Q: In children with pneumonia who have a pet bird, how is the diagnosis confirmed?
A: A fourfold rise in antibody titers by complement fixation or microimmuno-fluorescence (acute and convalescent specimens; 2–3 weeks apart); a single titer of 1:32 or higher (highly suggestive); culture (done through the CDC).

Q: Does the source bird usually exhibit signs of infection or illness?
A: No. While the bird may show signs like anorexia, ruffled feathers, depression, or watery green droppings, often the bird is totally asymptomatic.

ICD-9-CM 073.9

BIBLIOGRAPHY

American Academy of Pediatrics. *Chlamydia psittaci.* In: Pickering LK, ed. *2000 red book: report of the Committee on Infectious Diseases,* 25th ed. Elk Grove Village, IL: American Academy of Pediatrics, 2000:206–207.

Butler JC, Whitney CG. Compendium of measures to control *Chlamydia psittaci* infection among humans (psittacosis) and pet birds (avian chlamydiosis), 1998. *MMWR* 1998;47(RR-10):1–14.

Cotton MM, Partridge MR. Infection with feline *Chlamydia psittaci. Thorax* 1998;53:75–76.

Gregory DW, Schaffner W. Psittacosis. *Semin Respir Infect* 1997;12(1):7–11.

Hammerschlag MR. Atypical pneumonias in children. *Adv Pediatr Infect Dis* 1995;10:1–39.

Kirchner JT. Is Contact with birds causing your patient's pneumonia? *Postgrad Med* 1997;102(2):181–182,187–188,193–194.

Schlossberg D, Delgado J, Moore MM, et al. An epidemic of avian and human psittacosis. *Arch Intern Med* 1993;153:2594.

Scully RE, ed. Weekly clinicopathological exercises: psittacosis causing acute respiratory distress syndrome. *N Engl J Med* 1998;338(21):1527–1535.

Author: Nicholas Tsarouhas

Psoriasis

 Database

DEFINITION

Psoriasis is a skin disease characterized by a chronic relapsing nature and, most commonly, clinical features of scaly, erythematous papules and plaques with thick white scale usually involving elbows, knees, and scalp (psoriasis vulgaris). Other variants include guttate, erythrodermic, and pustular psoriasis (see Physical Examination, below, for details).

CAUSES

The pathogenesis is unknown. Trigger factors are well defined and include:

- Trauma to normal skin, producing psoriasis in the area (Koebner phenomenon)
- Infections (upper respiratory infections, *Streptococcus pyogenes,* human immunodeficiency virus)
- Stress
- Winter
- Certain drugs (systemic corticosteroids, lithium, (β-adrenergic blockers, nonsteroidal antiinflammatory drugs, and antimalarials)

PATHOPHYSIOLOGY

- Plaque-type psoriasis is characterized by a thickened, parakeratotic epidermis with an absent granular layer above dermal papillae containing dilated tortuous capillaries.
- Collections of polymorphonuclear leukocytes extend from the dermal papillae into the epidermis (Munro microabscesses).
- A mixed perivascular infiltrate is confined to the papillary dermis.

GENETICS

- Psoriasis has a strong genetic influence.
- The mode of genetic transmission is not defined. It is likely multifactorial with more than one gene involved and modified by environmental influence.

—One third of patients with psoriasis report a relative with the disease.
—8.1% of offspring develop psoriasis in family studies, when one parent is affected.
—When both parents have psoriasis, the percentage increases to 41%.
—In twin studies, 65% of monozygotic twins are concordant for the disease, while only 30% of dizygotic twins are concordant.

EPIDEMIOLOGY

- Psoriasis is universal in occurrence, but the prevalence varies in different populations. The average prevalence in the United States is estimated at 1% to 3%.
- Males and females are equally affected.
- Onset of psoriasis is bimodal, commonly presenting in the third decade with a smaller second peak of onset in the sixth decade; however, it can present at any age, with a mean age of onset in children of 8.1 years.
- Earlier onset is associated with more severe disease.

PROGNOSIS

- Once psoriasis appears, it generally persists throughout life.
- Spontaneous remissions of variable length and frequency occur but are unpredictable.

 Differential Diagnosis

Classic plaque psoriasis is easily diagnosed. Variants of psoriasis, including guttate, erythrodermic, and pustular disease, are more difficult to recognize. The differential varies with the type of psoriasis and includes:

- Nummular eczema
- Cutaneous T-cell lymphoma
- Tinea corporis
- Pityriasis rosea
- Pityriasis lichenoides et varioliformis acuta
- Secondary syphilis
- Atopic dermatitis
- Drug eruption
- Candidiasis
- Seborrheic dermatitis

 Data Gathering

HISTORY

- When the eruption first appeared
- Area involved
- Recent illness, particularly sore throat
- Recent medications, particularly systemic steroids
- Any appearance of lesions with trauma to skin
- Joint pain
- Previous treatments and response
- Improvement with sun exposure
- Family history of psoriasis

 Physical Examination

- A complete cutaneous examination is necessary.
- In psoriasis vulgaris, sharply demarcated erythematous plaques with white scale are located most commonly on the elbows, knees, scalp, lumbar area, and umbilicus, but they can cover any surface and large areas of the body. Intertriginous regions are often involved, but scale is absent.
- Guttate psoriasis presents often in children and young adults as small papules (0.5–1.5 cm), with limited scale over the trunk and proximal extremities, and is frequently associated with streptococcal infection.
- Erythema with variable scale involving the majority of the body accompanied by chills is characteristic of erythrodermic psoriasis.
- Generalized pustular psoriasis is the most serious variant, with 23-mm sterile pustules arising on erythematous skin over large areas of the body and accompanied by high fevers.
- A chronic and localized variant of pustular disease involves only the palms and soles.

PHYSICAL EXAMINATION TRICKS

Classic plaque psoriasis is easily diagnosed, but variants and mild cases require careful examination for physical clues.

- Nails are frequently involved, with pinpoint pits, hyperkeratosis, and oil spots.
- Areas of hidden disease are the retroauricular portion of the scalp and the perianal region.
- Removal of scale on plaques results in bleeding points, a feature known as the Auspitz sign.
- The Koebner phenomenon may produce linear or geometric lesions corresponding to areas of trauma.
- Swollen or deformed joints suggest associated psoriatic arthritis.

 Laboratory Aids

TESTS

- An elevated uric acid level is a common finding.
- *Streptococcus pyogenes* infection is frequent in guttate disease, and throat culture is appropriate.
- Other laboratory values are generally within normal limits. However, in more severe variants, anemia, elevated erythrocyte sedimentation rate, and decreased albumin levels can be seen.
- In pustular psoriasis, leukocytosis and hypocalcemia are associated.

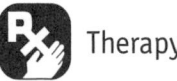

Therapy

- Therapy is delivered by topical medications, phototherapy, or systemic medications.
- Localized disease is treated with topical therapy and more diffuse disease with phototherapy.
- Systemic medications are reserved for resistant cases.
- Except in the most severe cases, therapy for children should be limited to topical medication and ultraviolet B (UVB) phototherapy.
- General skin care should include gentle washing, soaking to remove scale, and application of emollients, preferably ointments and creams.

DRUGS

Topical

- Topical corticosteroids

—Mid- to high-potency topical corticosteroid ointments are applied twice daily.
—Midpotency preparations (0.025% fluocinolone ointment, 0.1% triamcinolone acetonide) are preferred in children.
—Low-potency corticosteroids (1.0% and 2.5% hydrocortisone) are used on the face and intertriginous regions to prevent atrophy.
—Can also be found in shampoo preparations (Dermasmoothe FS and Capex)

- Anthralin

—Anthralin is applied to plaques for a 30-minute application, and is washed off carefully.
—Lower concentrations are used initially (0.1%, 0.25%) and are increased gradually as tolerated (0.5%, 1.0%).
—Irritation and staining are common, and the face and intertriginous regions cannot be treated with this approach.

- Calcipotriene

—Calcipotriene ointment is a vitamin D_3 derivative often used for treatment of adults.
—It is applied twice daily, with avoidance of the face and intertriginous regions.
—Maximum use in adults is 100 g/wk.
—Rare cases of hypercalcemia have been reported.
—Although effective in children, safety guidelines have not been established.

Tazarotene Gel

- A topical retinoid (0.05% and 0.1%)
- Can be mildly to moderately irritating when used as monotherapy.
- Often combined with topical steroids as adjunctive therapy applied once or twice daily.
- Coal tar

—A weak therapeutic agent when employed as monotherapy

—More effective when combined with UVB phototherapy
—Used in multiple shampoo preparations

PHOTOTHERAPY

UVB

- Administered between three and seven times weekly in a booth with bulbs that emit the appropriate wavelength of ultraviolet radiation
- Very effective for guttate and plaque psoriasis
- Average treatment time: 3 months and gradually increasing the time. Sunscreen should be used on the face.
- Narrowband UVB represents a form of monochromatic UVB using wavelengths of 311 nm and appears to be a somewhat more effective form of delivering UVB phototherapy.
- PUVA (psoralen and UVB)

—PUVA and oral medications (methotrexate and etretinate) should be reserved for severe cases and carefully monitored by a dermatologist.

Possible Conflicts with Other Drugs

Photosensitizing medication (tetracyclines, sulfa derivatives, phenothiazines, and others) should be avoided with phototherapy.

DURATION

- Topical therapy is administered chronically with breaks to minimize side effects.
- Remissions occur in summer with sun exposure, and medications may often be discontinued.
- The average treatment course with UVB therapy is 3 months; if the patient clears, treatment may be followed by an average remission period of 5 months.

Follow-Up

WHEN TO EXPECT IMPROVEMENT

- Response will depend on the potency of medication and frequency of treatment.
- Improvement with topical medication is obvious at 2 weeks and usually maximum at 2 months.
- One month of UVB therapy produces a decrease in disease.

SIGNS TO WATCH FOR

Pustules, a significant increase in degree or extent of erythema, or fever suggest progression of the disease to more serious variants and may require hospitalization and systemic therapy.

PITFALLS

- If therapy is too aggressive, disease may become irritated and worsen.
- Scrubbing by the patient to remove scale also irritates the disease.
- Psychological aspects of the disease, particularly in children, should be addressed.

Common Questions and Answers

Q: Will my disease get worse?
A: It is impossible to predict the course of an individual's disease, since it is influenced by both heredity and everyday factors in the environment. While there is no cure, with treatment the disease can be kept under control. Remissions do occur and maybe for prolonged periods of time.

Q: When my disease is in remission, what can I do to prevent it from returning?
A: Avoidance of trauma and frequent moisturization of the skin is important. In the summer, controlled sun exposure is helpful. You may have to continue other treatments at less frequent intervals. Any sore throats should be cultured and treated if streptococcal disease is present. However, frequently it is impossible to prevent recurrence of the disease.

Q: Will my other children get psoriasis?
A: If neither parent has psoriasis, the chances are <10% that another child will develop the disease; if one parent is affected, the chances increase to 15%; if both parents are affected, the chances are 50%. Therefore, unless both parents are affected, it is more likely that other children will not have psoriasis.

Q: Does stress make psoriasis worse?
A: Some studies have suggested that flare-ups of psoriasis are associated with increased stress. It is difficult to evaluate whether stress is the cause or the result of the disease. Do all you can to reasonably relieve stress, but do not focus on this as the cause of your psoriasis.

ICD-9-CM 696.1

BIBLIOGRAPHY

Christophers E, Sterry W. Psoriasis. In: Fitzpatrick TB, Eisen AZ, Wolff K, et al., eds. *Dermatology in general medicine*, 4th ed. New York: McGraw-Hill, 1993:489.

de Jong EM. The course of psoriasis. *Clin Dermatol* 1997;15(5):687–692.

Farber EM. Early intervention can reduce risks for problems later. *Postgrad Med* 1998;103(4): 89–92,95–96,99–100 passim.

Stern RS. Epidemiology of psoriasis. *Dermatol Clin* 1995;13(4):717–722.

Author: Albert C. Yan
Cynthia Guzzo, 2nd edition

Pubertal Delay

Database

DEFINITION

Pubertal delay is delay in age of onset of puberty. It is also delay in the rate of progression of pubertal development [greater than two standard deviations from the mean (2.5% of the population)].

Constitutional or Physiologic Delay of Puberty

• Late onset of puberty as a normal variant
• Patients grow slowly through childhood, enter puberty late and then progress through it at a normal rate.

Male pubertal development is considered delayed if:

• Genital stage 1 persists beyond 13.7 years.
• Pubic hair stage 1 persists beyond 15.1 years.
• More than 5 years pass before completion of genital growth.
• Pubertal development begins but progression stalls, such that the duration of a given sexual maturity rating is longer than expected:

—Genital 2: 2.2 years
—Genital 3: 1.6 years
—Genital 4: 1.9 years
—Pubic hair 2: 1.0 year
—Pubic hair 3: 0.5 year
—Pubic hair 4: 1.5 years

Female pubertal development is considered delayed if:

• Breast stage 1 persists beyond 13.4 years.
• Pubic hair stage 1 persists beyond 14.1 years.
• No menarche beyond age 16 years
• More than 5 years pass between initiation of breast stage 2 and menarche
• Pubertal development begins but progression stalls, such that the duration of a given sexual maturity rating is longer than expected:

—Breast 2: 1.0 year
—Breast 3: 2.2 years
—Breast 4: 6.8 years
—Pubic hair 2: 1.3 years
—Pubic hair 3: 0.9 year
—Pubic hair 4: 2.4 years

PATHOPHYSIOLOGY

• Constitutional delay is a normal variant that is believed to result from persistence of the prepubertal (childhood) hypogonadotropic state.
• Delayed puberty and short stature associated with chronic disease is not well explained.

GENETICS

• Patients with constitutional delay will often have a family history of late pubertal onset with subsequent normal stature and development.
• The genetic transmission of delayed puberty otherwise depends on the underlying disorder.

EPIDEMIOLOGY

• Constitutional delay of puberty explains 90% to 95% of pubertal delay.
• Constitutional delay occurs in 2.5% of adolescents of both sexes.
• More than 60% of patients with constitutional delay of puberty have a positive family history.

Differential Diagnosis

• Infection

—Viral or tuberculosis infection resulting in acquired panhypopituitarism

• Tumors (may result in panhypopituitarism)

—Craniopharyngioma
—Hypothalamic glioma
—Astrocytoma
—Pituitary adenoma

• Trauma

—Panhypopituitarism resulting from severe head trauma

• Congenital

—Congenital panhypopituitarism
—Mixed gonadal dysgenesis
—Turner syndrome, Noonan syndrome
—Prader-Willi syndrome

• Immunologic

—Juvenile rheumatoid arthritis
—Systemic lupus erythematosus

• Psychosocial

—Anorexia nervosa

• Environmental

—Postradiation
—Chemotherapy

• Miscellaneous

—Constitutional delay of puberty (majority of cases)
—Glucocorticoid excess
—Chronic disease

Data Gathering

HISTORY

• Obtain long-term growth record. Patients with gonadotropin or gonadal disorders usually have had normal growth during childhood but no increase in growth during the expected pubertal spurt (i.e., where growth retardation is a new event). Most children with constitutional delay have slow growth throughout childhood.
• Obtain history of progression of secondary sex characteristics. Adolescents with complete gonadal or gonadotropin deficiencies will not enter puberty, unless initiated by exogenous or adrenal hormones, whereas those with constitutional delay will progress at a normal rate after initiation of puberty. Adolescents with partial deficiencies may reach pubarche at a normal time, but will fail to progress.
• Obtain family history of pubertal development.
• Assess nutrition and socioeconomic history to rule out chronic malnutrition or eating disorder.
• Elicit history of drug use (e.g., glucocorticoids or cytotoxins).

Physical Examination

Examine all patients with pubertal delay thoroughly, with particular attention to:

• Thyroid examination
• Neurologic and funduscopic examinations to check for intracranial pathology
• Genital and gynecologic examination: external examination for all patients; internal gynecologic examination for females with amenorrhea may be indicated; breast, pubic hair, and genital examination to assess sexual maturity ratings
• The first sign of puberty in males is when testicular size is greater than 2.5 cm. Find which one of your finger segments approximates 2.5 cm, and use it as a gross measure. As a means of screening size, using a finger is more subtle than using an orchidometer. However, when a clinician needs to follow pubertal progression closely, an orchidometer is necessary to accurately establish testicular size.

Pubertal Delay

Laboratory Aids

TESTS

Routine Screening

Routine screening tests for chronic or systemic disease:

- Complete blood count
- Urinalysis
- Sedimentation rate
- Chemistry profile

Special Tests

Special tests to order based on history or physical examination findings:

- Thyroid function tests
- Gonadotropin levels (low levels suggest prepuberty or hypothalamic-pituitary failure; high levels suggest gonadal failure or absence)
- Karyotype
- Growth hormone levels

—Somatomedin C (IGF-I) level as baseline
—For true growth hormone levels, growth hormone (GH) stimulation tests are necessary. Consultation with a specialist or experienced laboratory personnel is recommended before obtaining stimulation tests.

- Dynamic tests of hypothalamic-pituitary-gonadal function are usually performed by a specialist.

Imaging

- Bone age: plain film of the epiphyseal growth centers in the hand. Epiphyses change in response to growth hormone, thyroxine, and steroids of adrenal or gonadal origin. Comparison to chronologic age can help to differentiate constitutional delay from organic disorders. A bone age is almost always indicated in the initial workup of delayed puberty.
- Pelvic ultrasound: can be useful in localization of intraabdominal testicular structures, or in determination of the presence or absence of müllerian structures. Pelvic ultrasound is indicated when testes cannot be detected in patients with a male phenotype or when müllerian structures cannot be confirmed on physical examination in patients with a female phenotype.
- CT or MRI of the head: useful in assessing pituitary or hypothalamic structures, mass lesions, pathologic calcifications, or increased intracranial pressure if a central cause of delayed puberty is suspected.

Therapy

PSYCHOSOCIAL INTERVENTIONS

Most patients with pubertal delay do not require drugs, but all need psychological and social support.

DRUGS

- In cases of presumed constitutional delay, hormones can be used to affect hypothalamic maturation, thereby initiating endogenous puberty.
- Referral to an endocrinologist or adolescent specialist is usually recommended prior to the initiation of hormonal therapy to aid in diagnosis and in monitoring response.

Follow-Up

In cases of permanent hypogonadism, because of gonadal absence, failure, or gonadotropin deficiency, long-term hormonal therapy is necessary.

PREVENTION

- Undue stress and unneeded tests can be avoided by discussing pubertal changes with patients and their families at the outset, in late childhood.
- Even though they will not ask health care providers, teens with chronic disease may be actively worrying about slow growth and pubertal development. Open discussion with a caring provider can help allay fears and stress.

PITFALLS

- No test can make a definitive diagnosis of constitutional delay.
- Levels of sex steroids and gonadotropins vary significantly in a single patient because of pulsatile or rhythmic secretions. Consult an endocrinologist to interpret these tests.
- Sex steroid therapy in a patient with hypopituitarism can affect adult height if given before growth hormone therapy is optimized.
- Consultation with a specialist or experienced laboratory personnel is recommended before obtaining stimulation tests, as they may require special conditions.

Common Questions and Answers

Q: Since approximately 95% of pubertal delay is constitutional or physiologic in nature, when can I avoid an expensive workup and just observe the patient?

A: Unfortunately, only the spontaneous onset of puberty confirms the diagnosis of constitutional delay. Anxiety from delayed puberty may preclude waiting. To make a presumptive diagnosis of constitutional delay, pathology must be ruled out. Physical examination, including genital anatomy and smell sense, must be normal. There should be no signs or symptoms consistent with chronic disease. The history, including nutritional history and review of systems, must be negative. The screening blood work must be negative. Growth must progress at least 3.7 cm per year, and bone age must be delayed no more than 4.0 years compared with chronologic age. Although not always indicated, the next level of tests can be ordered. Normal prepubertal levels of LH and FSH must be present. Presumptive diagnosis is strongly supported, but not proven, by a positive family history and a height between the 3rd and 25th percentiles.

Q: When should patients with pubertal delay be seen by an endocrinologist or adolescent specialist?
A: Often, the initial workup of pubertal delay can be completed by the primary care provider. For complex stimulation tests, or if help is needed in interpreting test results, referral to an experienced specialist is warranted. If a specific chronic disease is suspected as the underlying etiology, then referral should be made to the appropriate subspecialist.

Q: Do racial differences exist concerning pubertal onset and development?
A: Several recent studies indicate that the mean ages for onset of breast development and menarche are younger for African-American females than for Caucasian females. One such study reported the mean age of onset for breast development as 8.87 years for African-American girls and 9.96 years for Caucasian girls. Mean age at menarche was found to be 12.16 and 12.88 years for African-American and Caucasian girls, respectively.

ICD-9-CM 255.0

BIBLIOGRAPHY

Argente J. Diagnosis of late puberty. *Horm Res* 1999;51(suppl 3):95–100.

Brook CG. Treatment of late puberty. *Horm Res* 1999;51(suppl 3):101–103.

Gordon C, Mansbach J. Demystifying delayed puberty. *Contemp Pediatr* 2001;4:43.

Lee PA, O'Dea LS. Tests and variants of male sexual development. In: Hung W, ed. *Clinical pediatric endocrinology*. Philadelphia: Mosby-Yearbook, 1992:268–312.

Styne DM. New aspects in the diagnosis and treatment of pubertal disorders. *Pediatr Clin North Am* 1997;44(2):505–529.

Authors: Jonathan R. Pletcher and Kenneth R. Ginsburg

Pulmonary Embolism

 Database

DEFINITION
Pulmonary embolism (PE) is the occlusion of a pulmonary vessel by a thrombus.

PATHOPHYSIOLOGY
• Thromboemboli may develop anywhere in the systemic venous system.
• PE is characterized by the triad of hypoxemia, pulmonary hypertension, and right ventricular failure.
• Diminished pulmonary perfusion causes ventilation/perfusion (V/Q) mismatch, resulting in hypoxemia.
• Hyperventilation occurs secondary to stimulation of proprioceptors in the lung.
• Hypercapnia is seen with severe occlusion of the pulmonary artery (not often seen with smaller emboli).
• Pulmonary infarction is uncommon owing to the presence of collateral pulmonary and bronchial arteries along with the airways providing additional sources of oxygen to the tissues.

EPIDEMIOLOGY
• PEs are seen more frequently in adults.
• They are underdiagnosed in children; the incidence in children is 3.7%.
• Increasing incidence is secondary to increased central catheter utilization.
• Approximately 10% of adults who present with acute pulmonary embolus die within 1 hour of onset.
• The mortality rate can be as high as 30% if delays in diagnosis are made.
• Death occurs with 85% obstruction of the pulmonary artery.
• Risk factors vary according to age groups and sex.
• In children, risk factors include:
—Presence of a central venous catheter
—Lack of mobility
—Congenital heart disease
—Ventriculoatrial shunt
—Trauma
—Solid tumors or leukemia
—Postsurgical procedures (especially scoliosis repair)
—Hypercoagulable states
• In adults, the most common risk factor is the presence of a deep vein thrombosis, usually in the legs or pelvis.

PROGNOSIS
• If treated promptly, prognosis is good.
• If treatment is delayed (especially if the patient is hemodynamically compromised prior to the event), prognosis is poor.

 Differential Diagnosis

• Cardiac
—Cardiac tamponade
—Constrictive pericarditis
—Restrictive cardiomyopathy
• Pulmonary
—Chronic cough
—Status asthmaticus
—Pneumonia with empyema
—Pneumothorax

 Data Gathering

HISTORY
• Are there any chest symptoms?
• PE should be suspected in children who present with:
—Pleuritic chest pain
—Shortness of breath
—Hemoptysis
—Cough
—Acute respiratory distress
—Apprehension or anxiety
—Syncope
—Cardiovascular shock
• Symptoms may be nonspecific and indicative of other disorders.
• The clinician must have a high index of suspicion and recognize risk factors in order to establish the correct diagnosis.

 Physical Examination

Findings in physical examination are nonspecific.
• General
—Fever
—Diaphoresis
—Nervousness or apprehension (altered mental status is uncommon)
• Cardiovascular
—Increased intensity of the pulmonic component of S_2
—Tachycardia
—Gallop rhythm
—New murmur
• Pulmonary
—Tachypnea
—Rales
—Cyanosis (present with 65% obstruction of the pulmonary artery)
—Pleuritic chest pain
—Dyspnea
—Cough
—Hemoptysis
—Wheezing (uncommon)
• Extremities
—Deep venous thrombosis is frequently found in the adult population.
—Phlebitis
—Edema

PITFALLS
Failure to make the diagnosis is the most common mistake. PE must be suspected in the critically ill children who have a central venous catheter who develop sudden respiratory failure. Since the symptoms for severe lung disease and PE are similar, the diagnosis might be missed if the index of suspicion is low.

 Laboratory Aids

TESTS
Blood Tests
• In general, blood tests are nonspecific and of no significant value in the diagnosis of a pulmonary embolus.
• Arterial blood gas:
—Decreased P_{O_2} and P_{CO_2}
—Increased alveolar arterial (A-a) gradient

Cardiac Studies
ECG
• Useful in ruling out other conditions
• May show sinus tachycardia or nonspecific ST-T wave changes

Echocardiogram
• Useful for identifying:
—Abnormalities of cardiac anatomy
—Thrombi on catheter tips
• If there are emboli seen on echocardiogram, there is a 40% to 50% mortality rate. Also if signs of right ventricular dysfunction are noted such as right ventricular dilatation, dilated right pulmonary artery, abnormal right ventricular movement, and increased tricuspid regurgitation jet velocity, then there is associated poor outcome.

Pulmonary Function Testing
Results are nonspecific.

Evaluation of the Lower Extremities
• Finding deep vein thrombosis via:
—Impedance plethysmography
—Doppler technology
—Venography

Imaging
Spiral CT
• Fairly new modality in diagnosis of PE
• Greater sensitivity in the diagnosis of PE than V/Q scan due to ability to image abnormal pulmonary pathology.

Chest Radiograph
• May be abnormal in 70% of patients with pulmonary embolus
• Most frequent findings:
—Parenchymal infiltrates
—Atelectasis
—Pleural effusions: seen in 33% of cases, most unilateral
—Hampton hump (pyramid-shaped wedge pointing toward the hilum)

Ventilation/Perfusion (V/Q) Scan

- A V/Q scan performed to rule out a pulmonary embolus is reported in one of five categories, ranging from high probability to normal.
- An abnormal V/Q scan with normal ventilation and decreased perfusion in the appropriate clinical setting is 90% specific for a pulmonary embolus.
- A normal V/Q scan does not completely rule out pulmonary embolus, although if the patient is at low risk, a pulmonary embolus is highly unlikely.

Pulmonary Angiography

- Most sensitive and specific test
- Not done as frequently in children as in adults because of complications of the procedure
- With the introduction of newer, improved catheters and safer contrast solutions, this test is now safe to be performed in the pediatric population.
- Indicated for cases:
—Intermediate-probability V/Q scans
—High-probability scans in patients who are:
—Poor candidates for anticoagulation
—Hemodynamically unstable or require an embolectomy

 Therapy

DRUGS

- Stabilize the patient before anticoagulation or thrombolytic therapy is begun:
—Improve oxygenation
—Correct acidosis
—Stabilize blood pressure
—Analgesia for severe pleuritic chest pain. Avoid use of opiates if patient is in cardiovascular collapse.
- The goal of therapy is anticoagulation and/or thrombolysis
- In patients with intermediate or high suspicion of PE begin anticoagulation prior to investigations

ANTICOAGULATION THERAPY

To prevent further thrombus formation

Heparin

- Bolus dose: 100–200 U/kg
- Maintenance dose: 10 to 25 U/kg/h
- Keep PTT 55 to 60 seconds
- Should be given for 7 to 10 days

Coumadin

- Coumadin should be started 24 to 48 hours after heparin therapy is begun.
- Maintenance dose: 2.5 to 10.0 mg/d
- Keep PT twice normal and maintain INR between 2.0 and 3.0
- Should be continued for 3 to 6 months

Thrombolytic Therapy

Agents Available

- Streptokinase: No difference in outcome has been found using streptokinase over urokinase.
- Urokinase
- rtPA (tissue plasminogen activator): Same efficacy as streptokinase and lower chance of allergic reactions

Indications

- Hemodynamically unstable
- Large embolus
- Low-molecular-weight heparins have been used as prophylaxis or as treatment for preexisting conditions in both adults and children.
- A synthetic, nonthrombocytopenic heparin pentasaccharide with a purely antifactor Xa activity is currently being tested.
- Ticlopidine and clopidogrel have been used successfully for the prevention of thrombotic strokes and arterial thrombotic syndromes.

Contraindications to Anticoagulant Therapy

- Active internal bleeding
- Recent cerebrovascular accident
- Major surgery
- Recent gastrointestinal bleed

EMBOLECTOMY

- Indicated when hemodynamic instability persists; is reserved for patients who have failed thrombolytic therapy or dose where medical treatment is contraindicated.
- Late results are excellent if the patient has not suffered from a perioperative cardiac arrest, which is associated with early mortality.

Percutaneous Caval Filtration

- Indicated if commencement or continuation of anticoagulation is strongly contraindicated or if full anticoagulation has failed to prevent recurrent embolism.
- This should be considered in patients undergoing venous thrombolysis since up to 20% may have embolism during treatment.

 Follow-Up

Patients on Coumadin therapy should have the usual follow-up for those on anticoagulant.

 Common Questions and Answers

Q: Is it safe for children on Coumadin to play contact sports?
A: The general recommendation is that no contact sports should be allowed while children are on Coumadin therapy because of the increased risk of bleeding.

ICD-9-CM 415.1

BIBLIOGRAPHY

Arcasoy SM, Kreit JW. Thrombolytic therapy of pulmonary embolism: a comprehensive review of current evidence. *Chest* 1999;115(6): 1695–1707.

Buck JR, Connors RH, Coon WW, et al. Pulmonary embolism in children. *J Pediatr Surg* 1981;16:385.

Burki N. The dead space to tidal volume ratio in the diagnosis of pulmonary embolism. *Am Rev Respir Dis* 1986;133:679.

Cvitanic O, Marino PL. Improved use of arterial blood gas analysis in suspected pulmonary embolism. *Chest* 1989;95:48.

Derish MT, Smith DW, Frankel LR. Venous catheter thrombus formation and pulmonary embolism in children. *Pediatr Pulmonol* 1995;20(6):349–354.

Dobkin J, Reichel J. Pulmonary embolism. Diagnosis and treatment. *Cardiol Clin* 1987;5:577.

Evans DA, Wilmott RW. Pulmonary embolism in children. *Pediatr Clin North Am* 1994;41:569.

Fulkerson WJ, Coleman RE, Ravin CE, et al. Diagnosis of pulmonary embolism. *Arch Intern Med* 1986;146:961.

Iwasaki YN, Nakanishi MN, Harada HK. Spiral CT findings in septic pulmonary emboli. *Eur J Radiol* 2001;37(3):179–183.

Kutty K. Pulmonary embolism: how to nail down the diagnosis. *Postgrad Med* 1990;88:72.

Massicotte P, Adams M, Brooker LA, et al. Low-molecular-weight heparin in pediatric patients with thrombotic disease: a dose finding study. *J Pediatr* 1996;128(3):313–318.

McCoy KS, Grossman NJ. *Pediatric respiratory diseases: diagnosis and treatment.* Philadelphia: WB Saunders, 1993:509.

Tai NRM, Atwai AS, Hamilton G. Modern management of pulmonary embolism [review]. *Br J Surg* 1999;86(7):853–868.

Velmahos GC, Vassiliu P, Wilcox A. Spiral computed tomography for the diagnosis of pulmonary embolism in critically ill surgical patients: a comparison with pulmonary angiography. *Arch Surg* 2001;136(5):505–511.

Walenga JM, Fareed J. Current status on new anticoagulant and antithrombotic drugs and devices. *Curr Opin Pulmon Med* 1997;3(4): 291–302.

Author: Akinyemi O. Ajayi
Hector L. Flores-Arroyo, 2nd edition

Pulmonary Hypertension

 Database

DEFINITION

Pulmonary hypertension is increased pulmonary vascular resistance.

CAUSES

- Hypoxemia-induced pulmonary hypertension:
  - Chronic lung disease

  —Cystic fibrosis
  —Bronchopulmonary dysplasia
  —Interstitial lung disease

  - Upper airway obstruction

  —Tonsillar and/or adenoid hypertrophy
  —Obesity

  - Hypoventilation

  —Neurologically mediated process
  —Secondary to muscle weakness

- High pulmonary blood flow secondary to left-to-right shunting (seen in congenital heart disease):

—Patent ductus arteriosus
—Atrial septal defect
—Ventricular septal defect

- Left-sided cardiac disorders that increase pulmonary venous pressure:

—Left ventricular failure
—Mitral valve stenosis
—Obstructed anomalous pulmonary veins

- Occlusion of pulmonary vessels:

—Sickle cell disease
—Veno-occlusive disease
—Thromboembolism

- Pulmonary vasculitis

—Systemic lupus erythematosus
—Rheumatoid arthritis
—Scleroderma

- Persistent pulmonary hypertension of the newborn
- Idiopathic cases (primary pulmonary hypertension)

PATHOPHYSIOLOGY

Structural alternations in pulmonary vessel architecture (remodeling):

- Smooth muscle hypertrophy
- Extension of blood vessel's smooth muscle into smaller vessels

EPIDEMIOLOGY

Incidence in children is unknown.

COMPLICATIONS

- Chronic hypoxia
- Exercise intolerance
- Right-sided heart failure (cor pulmonale)
- Death

PROGNOSIS

- Dependent on the underlying disease
- In cases of primary pulmonary hypertension, improvement of pulmonary hypertension with administration of vasodilators during initial catheterization is associated with a better survival rate than if there is no response.
- 10–40% mortality in treated patients
- Near 100% mortality if patient is untreated

 Differential Diagnosis

- Pulmonary

—Asthma
—Cystic fibrosis
—Chronic obstructive pulmonary disease (COPD)
—Emphysema

- Miscellaneous

—Congestive heart failure
—Noncardiogenic pulmonary edema
—Fatigue

 Data Gathering

HISTORY

- Dyspnea (earliest complaint usually reported)
- Fatigue:

—Early on with exercise or exertion
—At rest in later stages or if severe

- Exercise intolerance
- Feeding intolerance
- Failure to thrive
- Excessive sleeping
- Diaphoresis
- Chest pain
- Syncope
- Palpitations (late finding)

 Physical Examination

Typically governed by the signs of the underlying lung or heart disease

COMMON FINDINGS

- Tachypnea
- Arrhythmias
- Narrowed splitting of S_2 heart sound
- Increased P_2 heart sound
- Presence of S_3 and/or S_4 heart sounds
- Murmur of pulmonary or tricuspid insufficiency (pulmonary insufficiency more common)
- Jugular venous distention
- Peripheral edema
- Hepatomegaly

SPECIAL QUESTIONS

Consider obstructive sleep apnea as cause of pulmonary hypertension. Ask about snoring if suspecting pulmonary hypertension in the absence of overt cardiac or pulmonary disease.

 Laboratory Aids

TESTS

- Arterial blood gas

—Measurement of P_{O_2} assesses degree of hypoxia
—Evaluation of P_{CO_2} determines presence or absence of hypoventilation

- Electrocardiogram (ECG)

—Can be normal if cor pulmonale has not yet developed
—If cor pulmonale present, ECG can demonstrate:
  —Right QRS axis deviation
  —Right ventricular hypertrophy
  —Right atrial hypertrophy

IMAGING

- Chest radiograph

—Will vary according to the underlying disorder and extent of pulmonary hypertension
—Pulmonary hypertension correlates poorly with chest radiograph findings
—In primary pulmonary hypertension:
   —Cardiomegaly
   —Enlarged pulmonary artery
   —Peripheral lung appears underperfused ("pruning" of pulmonary vessels)

- Echocardiogram with Doppler flow

—Increased pulmonary artery pressure
—Right ventricular hypertrophy
—Paradoxical movement of the intraventricular septum
—Pulmonic and tricuspid valve regurgitation
—Right-to-left shunting via an open foramen ovale

- Cardiac catheterization

—The most accurate measurement of pulmonary artery pressure is done by right heart catheterization.
—Criteria for pulmonary hypertension in children:
   —Mean pulmonary arterial pressure >20 mm Hg
   —Pulmonary artery systolic pressure >30 mm Hg
   —Pulmonary vascular resistance >3 U/m^2
—Pressures should be measured before and after vasodilator to assess reversibility of pulmonary hypertension

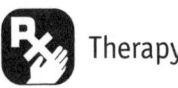 Therapy

- Therapy is directed toward:

—Treating the underlying disease
—Vasodilators to decrease the pulmonary hypertension and improve right heart function

DRUGS

- Oxygen

—Keep Sao$_2$ ≥95%

- Anticoagulation therapy (Coumadin)

—Prevents clot formation in the narrowed pulmonary vessels
—Helpful even in the absence of thromboembolic disease

- Vasodilators

—Calcium-channel blockers (e.g., nifedipine)
—Prostacyclin (IV)
—Nitric oxide (inhaled)

MECHANICAL VENTILATION

Useful for correcting hypoxia and hypercarbia secondary to hypoventilation

SURGERY

- Tonsillectomy and/or adenoidectomy if obstructive sleep apnea is present
- Transplantation (lung or heart-lung transplantation): reserved for patients with refractory, severe pulmonary hypertension

DURATION

Treatment can be lifelong unless the primary cause of the pulmonary hypertension can be corrected.

 Follow-Up

WHEN TO EXPECT IMPROVEMENT

- In acute pulmonary hypertension, response to most treatment modalities will be almost immediate.
- Oxygen has been shown to reverse hypoxia-related remodeling of the airways after a month of therapy.

PITFALLS

- Signs and symptoms of pulmonary hypertension are not specific and can easily be missed.
- In patients with severe disease, catheterization is associated with increased risk of complications.
- Supplemental oxygen can sometimes cause hypercapnia by blunting the hypoxia-driven respiratory drive.
- Vasodilators should be used under close supervision because of their effect on systemic blood pressure (systemic hypotension can be a significant problem).

 Common Questions and Answers

Q: How many hours per day should supplemental oxygen be used?
A: Studies have shown decreased mortality in patients using oxygen 24 hours per day compared with patients using supplemental oxygen for only part of the day.

Q: Should the dosage of oxygen be adjusted during the day as per the patient's activity?
A: Increasing the supplemental oxygen should be considered for activities that require increased oxygen consumption (e.g., exercise, eating, sleeping).

ICD-9-CM 416.0

BIBLIOGRAPHY

Barst RJ. Recent advances in the treatment of pediatric pulmonary hypertension. *Pediatr Clin North Am* 1999;46:331–345.

Butt AY, Higenbottam T. New therapies for primary pulmonary hypertension. *Chest* 1994;105:21S.

Redding GJ. *Respiratory disease in children: diagnosis and management*. Baltimore: Williams & Wilkins, 1994:639.

Rich S, Kaufmann E, Levy PS. The effect of high doses of calcium-channel blockers on survival in primary pulmonary hypertension. *N Engl J Med* 1992;327:76.

Rich S. The medical treatment of primary pulmonary hypertension: proven and promising strategies. *Chest* 1994;105:17S.

Soifer SJ. Pulmonary hypertension: physiologic or pathologic disease? *Crit Care Med* 1993;21:S370.

Wanstall JC, Jeffery TK. Recognition and management of pulmonary hypertension. *Drugs* 1998;56:989–1007.

Author: Richard M. Kravitz

Purpura Fulminans

 Database

DEFINITION

Purpura fulminans is a congenital, acquired, or idiopathic condition of rapidly progressive microvascular hemorrhage into the skin. It is associated with an underlying acquired or congenital disorder of coagulation, and may lead to skin necrosis.

PATHOPHYSIOLOGY

• Common features of purpura fulminans

—Inflammation: Endothelial injury from bacterial endotoxin or other trigger may initiate secretion of inflammatory cytokines or activation of coagulation and complement proteins.
—Purpura: extravasation of formed elements of the blood from injured capillaries into the skin
—Dermal vascular thrombosis: formation of microthromboses in blood vessels of the skin, leading to hemorrhage in the skin (purpura), necrosis of skin, and gangrene

• Infection-associated purpura fulminans

—Overwhelming sepsis, usually bacterial; *Neisseria meningitidis* most common
—May be a complication of varicella infection.
—Disseminated intravascular coagulation (DIC): state of sustained activation of coagulation cascade and fibrinolytic mechanisms, leading to consumption of platelets, fibrinogen, and often formation of microthromboses

• Inherited defect of coagulation presenting as neonatal purpura fulminans

—Deficiency of protein C: leads to a loss of important inhibitory regulation of coagulation and uncontrolled clotting
—Protein C slows ("brakes") the coagulation cascade at two steps: by degrading activated coagulation factor Va in the common part of the coagulation pathway, and by degrading factor VIIIa in the intrinsic pathway.
—Protein S is a cofactor for protein C.

• Idiopathic

—Postinfectious complication—formation of antibodies to protein S causing protein S deficiency has been described as a postinfectious autoimmune phenomenon.
—Complication of Coumadin therapy
—Other unknown mechanisms

GENETICS

• Deficiencies of protein C and protein S are autosomally inherited with variable penetrance.
• Many different genetic mutations, leading to both qualitative and quantitative defects of the proteins, have been described.

• Heterozygous protein C and S deficiency states usually cause a hypercoagulable condition, with increased risk of venous or arterial thrombosis throughout life.
• Homozygous protein C or S deficiency states lead to severe deficiency (less than 5% of normal factor activity) and neonatal purpura fulminans and are usually fatal.
• Factor V Leiden, a known risk factor for thrombosis, may also predispose to infection-associated purpura fulminans. May also predispose to purpura fulminans in patients who are heterozygotes for protein C or S deficiency.

EPIDEMIOLOGY

Depends on underlying cause:

• Neonatal purpura fulminans related to homozygous protein C deficiency: 1 in 250,000 to 1 in 500,000 births. Homozygous protein S deficiency is rarer.
• Purpura frequently seen in bacterial sepsis with meningococcus and other pathogens

COMPLICATIONS

• Skin necrosis and gangrene
• Scarring
• Acral amputations, from tips of digits to whole limbs
• Thrombosis in internal organs
• Death

PROGNOSIS

• Related to underlying cause of purpura fulminans
• Overall, poor for homozygous deficiencies of proteins C and S

 Differential Diagnosis

• Infection

—*N. meningitidis,* most common infectious cause of purpura fulminans
—Streptococci
—*Haemophilus* species
—Staphylococci
—Gram-negative bacteremia: *Escherichia coli, Klebsiella, Proteus, Enterobacter*
—Rickettsia: Rocky Mountain spotted fever
—Varicella

• Environmental

—Coumadin-induced skin necrosis: 1 in 500 to 1 in 1,000 individuals starting Coumadin therapy develop necrosis in subcutaneous fat, thought to be due to relative depletion of anticoagulant protein C (a vitamin K—dependent factor) during the initial phase of Coumadin effect.

• Tumor

—Myeloid leukemia

• Congenital

—Inherited deficiencies of protein C and protein S. Only severe, homozygous (less than 5% activity) deficiencies of proteins C and S are associated with purpura fulminans. Milder, heterozygous deficiencies of protein C and protein S, as well as deficiency of antithrombin III, dysfibrinogenemias, the carrier state for factor V Leiden, and other prothrombotic defects all give rise to hypercoagulable states, but not neonatal purpura fulminans. Patients with one or more risk factors for thrombosis may be more likely to develop purpura fulminans with an environmental stimulus.

• Immune
• Heparin-induced thrombocytopenia: Antibody to heparin-platelet complex causes platelet activation, thrombocytopenia, and microthrombosis, including dermal vessels.
• Antiphospholipid antibody syndrome: Predisposition to thrombosis can include skin necrosis.
• Miscellaneous

—Thrombotic thrombocytopenic purpura
—Paroxysmal nocturnal hemoglobinuria
—Henoch-Schönlein purpura

 Data Gathering

HISTORY

• Current bacterial sepsis: fever, weakness, dizziness, nausea, vomiting, onset of petechial rash
• Family history suggestive of hypercoagulable state: blood clots or thromboses at an early age, such as stroke, deep vein thrombosis, pulmonary embolism; family members taking Coumadin or heparin
• Previous affected child with purpura fulminans or hypercoagulable state
• Prior exposure to heparin, therapeutically or via intravenous "heplock"
• Medications, including anticoagulation

 Physical Examination

• Signs of sepsis: fever, hypotension, tachycardia, poor perfusion, cool extremities, decreased pulses, shock
• Nonblanching purpura
• Acral purpura and necrosis: Check fingers, nose, toes, and penis for black areas.
• An erythematous border may surround purpuric areas.
• Bullae may form over purpuric skin.
• Oozing at sites of venipuncture
• Pain, ischemia, and edema of extremities, or internal organ dysfunction may result from deep vein thrombosis or arterial thrombosis, depending on location and severity.

PHYSICAL EXAMINATION TRICKS

Depress the purpuric area with a glass slide to determine whether it blanches.

 ## Laboratory Aids

TESTS

Screening

- CBC: Platelet count may be low; hemoglobin may be low.
- Prothrombin time (PT): prolonged as in DIC
- Partial thromboplastin time (PTT): prolonged as in DIC
- Fibrinogen: decreased with consumption and fibrinolysis
- Fibrin split products: increased fibrinolysis as in DIC

Etiologic

- Protein C activity in patient and parents
- Protein S antigen (total and free) in patient and parents
- Test for antiphospholipid antibodies: usually lupus anticoagulant or anticardiolipin antibody
- Factor V Leiden mutation assay

Imaging

To document presence and extent of suspected large vessel thrombosis:

- Ultrasound with Doppler flow study
- CT
- MRI: better for visualization of vessels
- Angiography: Most invasive, requires vascular injury for access

Imaging is potentially useful to:

- Distinguish thrombosis from other pathology
- Judge age of thrombus (based on collateralization)
- Assess clot size prior to anticoagulant or thrombolytic therapy
- Distinguish baseline old clot from new thrombosis

The most useful imaging strategy depends on location and clinical situation.

False Positives

- Protein C and S levels may decrease during a thrombotic episode that is not related to an underlying deficiency. Low measurements often need to be repeated at baseline after recovery.
- Protein C and S levels may be below adult normal ranges for the first 3 to 6 months of life in healthy infants.

PITFALLS

- Proteins C and S are vitamin K-dependent. Level may be affected if vitamin K is not administered at birth.

- Protein C determination is affected by Coumadin therapy. It is difficult to confirm a deficiency state, especially mild deficiency, by repeat testing if Coumadin is started empirically.

 ## Therapy

DRUGS

- Antiinfective agents depending on underlying cause
- Fresh frozen plasma (FFP) every 12 hours to replace proteins C and S in acute DIC of purpura fulminans
- Periodic FFP infusions for chronic replacement
- Prothrombin complex concentrates
- Protein C concentrate
- Oral Coumadin

DURATION

- Protein C has half-life of 10 hours in circulation.
- Protein C replacement by periodic infusion of protein C concentrate
- Oral Coumadin therapy indefinitely usually recommended for documented protein C or S deficiency

DIET

Patients on Coumadin therapy may need to avoid foods with high vitamin K content, especially if there is variation in the dose of Coumadin required to maintain adequate anticoagulation.

POSSIBLE CONFLICTS

- Many drugs can affect Coumadin metabolism.
- Chronic infusion therapy for neonates may run into access problems.

 ## Follow-Up

WHEN TO EXPECT IMPROVEMENT

Related to underlying cause of purpura fulminans

SIGNS TO WATCH FOR

Spread of purpura, hypotension, gangrene

PITFALLS

- Individuals with protein C and protein S deficiency may have increased risk of Coumadin-induced skin necrosis when starting Coumadin. Patients should be heparinized for several days prior to the start of oral anticoagulation.

- Management of an infant on oral anticoagulation is difficult because of the practical problem of obtaining reliable measurements of PT, the increased risk associated with deep venipunctures for blood samples, and difficulty in establishing a stable Coumadin dose.

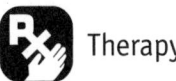 ## Common Questions and Answers

Q: What is the risk of a second affected child with protein C or S deficiency?
A: If the diagnosis is confirmed by family studies that show both parents to be carriers of the deficiency and the affected child to be homozygous, then there is a 25% chance that each subsequent infant would have purpura fulminans, and 50% chance that each child would be a carrier. However, other hypercoagulable states have been described that may be risk factors for purpura fulminans.

Q: Should a child with purpura fulminans be followed by a specialist?
A: Generally yes, with a pediatric hematologist, to assist in acute management of purpura, establishment of diagnosis, and management of oral anticoagulation.

ICD-9-CM 286.6

BIBLIOGRAPHY

Adcock DM, Brozna J, Marlar RA. Proposed classification and pathologic mechanisms of purpura fluminans and skin necrosis. *Semin Thromb Hemost* 1990;16:333.

Francis RB. Acquired purpura fulminans. *Semin Thromb Hemost* 1990;16:310.

Gerson WT, Dickerman JD, Boville G, et al. Severe acquired protein C deficiency in purpura fulminans associated with disseminated intravascular coagulation: treatment with protein C concentrate. *Pediatrics* 1993;91:418.

Leclerc F, Leteurtre S, Cremer R, et al. Do new strategies in meningococcemia produce better outcomes? *Crit Care Med* 2000;28:S60.

Marlar RA, Neumann A. Neonatal purpura fulminans due to homozygous protein C or protein S deficiencies. *Semin Thromb Hemost* 1990;16:299.

Rivard GE, David M, Farrell C, Schwarz HP Treatment of purpura fulminans in meningococcemia with protein C concentrate. *J Pediatr* 1995;126:646.

Smith OP, White B. Infectious purpura fulminans: diagnosis and treatment. *Br J Haematol* 1999;104:202.

Author: David F. Friedman

Pyelonephritis

 Database

DEFINITION

Acute pyelonephritis (upper urinary tract infection) is defined clinically by fever and flank pain, and histologically by acute renal parenchymal (interstitial) inflammation secondary to bacterial invasion.

PATHOPHYSIOLOGY

Specific factors relating to the development of pyelonephritis:

• Host related

—Anatomic abnormalities (e.g., obstruction, fistula)
—Functional abnormalities (e.g., dysfunctional voiding)

• Pathogen related

—Adherence factors (P-fimbriae)
—Virulence factors (lipopolysaccharide, capsular antigen)

CAUSES

• Enterobacteriaceae: [*Escherichia coli*, most frequent cause (80%); *Proteus*; *Klebsiella*; *Enterobacter*]
• Gram-positive organisms (cause 10–15%): *Staphylococcus aureus, epidermidis, saprophyticus,* enterococci
• Other organisms: *Pseudomonas, Haemophilus influenzae, Streptococcus* group B

PATHOLOGY

• Patchy infiltration of the medullary parenchyma by polymorphonuclear leukocytes and lymphocytes, tubular disruption and interstitial edema occurs
• Parenchymal scarring may result as a consequence of the infection.

EPIDEMIOLOGY

• 5% of girls develop urinary tract infection (UTI) during childhood.
• Urinary infections are more likely to involve the upper renal tracts in children younger than 3 years of age.
• UTIs are more common in females, except in uncircumcised males under 6 months of age.

COMPLICATIONS

• Acute: reduced concentrating ability, hyperkalemic RTA, bacteremia
• Chronic: focal renal scarring, hypertension, proteinuria, azotemia, xanthogranulomatous pyelonephritis

 Differential Diagnosis

• Cystitis
• Sterile pyuria

—Vulva-vaginitis
—Balanitis
—Systemic viral illness
—Postvaccination
—Pregnancy
—Appendicitis
—Cystic renal disease
—Tuberculosis

• Lower lobe pneumonia
• Acute appendicitis

HISTORY

• A fever of 38.5°C may represent the only complaint.
• In the neonate inquire about vomiting, lethargy, irritability, fever, hypothermia, and jaundice.
• Older children will be able to tell the examiner about flank pain, dysuria, frequency, urgency, and incontinence.

The following are important factors that predispose to the development of UTIs and should be specifically inquired after:

• Constipation
• Bubble baths
• Incorrect toilet training
• Perineal skin irritation
• Antibiotic exposure
• Uncircumcised males

 Physical Examination

• Findings may be nonspecific.
• Fever, irritability, rigors, lethargy
• Flank tenderness

—May be related to the underlying renal tract abnormality such as flank mass due to obstruction with hydronephrosis or cystic kidney disease, spina bifida apparent or occult as evidenced by a dimple, pilonidal sinus, or hemangioma.

SPECIAL QUESTIONS

• Previous UTIs
• Investigations already performed
• A family history of UTIs or reflux nephropathy
• Symptoms suggestive of dysfunctional voiding such as the bladder always feels full, infrequent use of the bathroom, and urgency incontinence
• Previous surgery or trauma to the lower back, lower motor milestones, and gait to assess the lower limb neuromuscular status and stool continence.

PHYSICAL EXAMINATION TRICKS

• Gentle posterior punch test will reveal tenderness at the costovertebral angle.
• Bimanual palpation of the kidneys for tenderness and size
• Careful neuromuscular exam of the lower limbs and of the back to evaluate for a neurogenic bladder
• Assess the rectal tone

Laboratory Aids

TESTS

• Collect urine via one of the sterile methods (midstream, catheter, or suprapubic).
• Urine dip for WBC and nitrites as a rapid screen for infection
• As a screening test, an unspun clean-catch urine specimen with bacteria on stained microscopic examination correlates (80–90%) with culture results of greater than 100,000 colonies per milliliter of urine.
• Urine for culture and sensitivity: A positive culture is defined by the growth of a single pathogenic organism of clean-catch 100,000 colonies/mL, catheter 1,000 colonies/mL, and by any growth from a suprapubic specimen.

IMAGING

• *Renal ultrasound* to rule out obstruction and to assess the renal size and parenchyma
• *Voiding cystourethrogram* (VCUG) to rule out anatomic anomalies including obstruction (e.g., posterior urethral valves) and vesicoureteric reflux
• *^{99m}Tc-dimercaptosuccinic acid* (DMSA) can be done to confirm the presence of acute pyelonephritis and to look for renal scarring. This is a sensitive and specific test that some clinicians believe to be the imaging study of choice for diagnosing acute pyelonephritis and renal scarring.

FALSE POSITIVES

May be owing to nonsterile collection techniques, allowing the urine to stand unrefrigerated, or owing to prior antibiotic exposure.

FALSE NEGATIVES

The rapid test for nitrites requires the urine to stay in the bladder for several hours and is therefore not good for infants who do not store urine in the bladder.

PITFALLS

• Imaging evaluation of the urinary tract following a UTI should be individualized based on the child's clinical presentation and on clinical judgment.
• All children 5 years or younger should have an ultrasound and VCUG; over 5 years of age an ultrasound is recommended.
• Once the urine is sterile, a VCUG can be performed; there is no need to wait 4 weeks.
• Administer antibiotic prophylaxis prior to the VCUG.

REQUIREMENTS FOR TESTING

Educate the caregivers in the use and interpretation of the dipstick, and about the symptoms and signs of urinary tract infection.

 ## Therapy

DRUGS

• Antibiotics such as co-trimoxazole, Augmentin, and the second-generation cephalosporins
• Familiarity with local antibiotic patterns of resistance is particularly important in treating hospital-acquired infections.
• Antipyretics such as acetaminophen

DURATION

• Give intravenous antibiotics until afebrile for at least 24 hours, then change to an oral formulation.
• In total, 10 to 14 days of antibiotic therapy are required.
• Patients with first-time urinary infections should receive low-dose antibiotic prophylaxis until their workup is completed.
• Children with frequent symptomatic recurrences of UTI and those with vesico-ureteric reflux (VUR) require long-term antibiotic prophylaxis.

DIET

Ensure adequate hydration.

 ## Follow-Up

• The fever usually defervesces in 3 to 5 days.
• Ongoing fever or persistent flank pain requires further evaluation to exclude a resistant organism and or an unrecognized urinary tract obstruction.
• The diagnosis and treatment of any underlying voiding dysfunction and constipation is required for the successful management of UTIs in children.
• The outcome of acute pyelonephritis (APN) is usually good, but may result in parenchymal scarring.
• Risk factors for renal damage include obstruction, reflux with dilation, young age, delay in treatment, number of episodes of pyelonephritis, and bacterial virulence factors.

 ## Common Questions and Answers

Q: Should a DMSA scan be used to help diagnose APN?
A: Routine use of the DMSA scan to diagnose APN is controversial as there is disagreement about the therapeutic implications of a positive test and routine testing will be costly. Children with hypertension and previous UTIs require a DMSA scan to look for renal cortical scarring.

Q: Does renal parenchymal scarring occur in the absence of reflux?
A: Yes. The causal relationship between reflux, acute pyelonephritis, and renal parenchymal scarring is complex.

ICD-9-CM 590.10

BIBLIOGRAPHY

Agarwal S. Vesicoureteral reflux and urinary tract infections. *Curr Opin Urol.* 2000;10(6): 587–592.

Hellerstein S. Urinary tract infections in children: why they occur and how to prevent them. *Am Fam Physician* 1998;57(10): 2440–2446,2452–2454.

Jodal U, Hansson S. Urinary tract infection. In: Holliday M, Barratt TM, Avner ED, eds. *Pediatric nephrology*, 3rd ed. Baltimore: Williams & Wilkins, 1994:950.

Kawashima A, Sandler CM, Goldman SM. Current roles and controversies in the imaging evaluation of acute renal failure. *World J Urol* 1998;16(1):9–17.

Martinell J, Hansson S, Claesson I, et al. Detection of urographic scars in girls with pyelonephritis followed for 13–38 years. *Pediatr Nephrol* 2000;14(10–11):1006–1010.

Rushton HG. Urinary tract infections in children. Epidemiology, evaluation and management. *Pediatr Clin North Am* 1997;44(5):1133–1169.

Author: Kevin E. C. Meyers

Pyloric Stenosis

 Database

DEFINITION

Pyloric stenosis is hypertrophy of the muscular layers of the pylorus with elongation and thickening, leading to obstruction of the gastric outlet.

ETIOLOGY

- Unknown
- No specific pattern of inheritance established
- Multifactorial inheritance likely
- Neonatal hypergastrinemia and gastric hyperacidity have a role.
- An association between infantile hypertrophic pyloric stenosis and the administration of oral erythromycin given for postexposure prophylaxis for pertussis has been described.

PATHOPHYSIOLOGY

- There is diffuse hypertrophy and hyperplasia of the pylorus, leading to narrowing of the gastric antrum.
- The antrum becomes thickened, elongated, and firm in consistency.
- Hypergastrinemia associated with hyperactivity, elevations of prostaglandins and deficiency of nitric oxide as a smooth muscle neurotransmitter have been suggested as etiologic factors.

INCIDENCE AND EPIDEMIOLOGY

- Exceedingly rare in newborns as well as in patients older than 6 months of age
- Occurs in approximately 1 in 950 live births; increased incidence in males
- More frequent among Caucasians

COMPLICATIONS

- Dehydration
- Electrolyte abnormalities, primarily hypochloremic metabolic alkalosis from loss of hydrochloric acid caused by persistent vomiting

PROGNOSIS

Morbidity and mortality are very low, and surgery is curative.

ASSOCIATED ANOMALIES

Increased occurrence of esophageal atresia and malrotation was noted in 5% of infants with pyloric stenosis.

 Differential Diagnosis

- Gastroesophageal reflux
- Gastroenteritis
- Pyloric atresia
- Antral web

 Data Gathering

HISTORY

- Nonbilious vomiting, classically projectile in an otherwise well and hungry child between 2 and 8 weeks of age. The infant is typically a "hungry vomiter," refeeding immediately, only to vomit again.
- Possible weight loss, varying degrees of dehydration and lethargy

 Physical Examination

- Visible peristalsis may be appreciated just after the infant feeds; this is seen as a waveform proceeding from the left upper quadrant toward the pylorus in the right upper quadrant.
- A palpable, hard, mobile, and nontender mass in the epigastrium to the right of the midline, referred to as an olive
- Best palpated after the infant has vomited

 Laboratory Aids

TESTS

- Hypochloremia and alkalosis
- Hyponatremia
- Hypokalemia
- 1–2% of infants have indirect hyperbilirubinemia associated with jaundice.

RADIOLOGIC FEATURES

Gastrointestinal Studies

- An upper gastrointestinal study can differentiate between antral webs and pylorospasm.
- In pyloric stenosis, it reveals vigorous gastric peristalsis with little or no gastric emptying.
- An elongated narrow pyloric anal canal can be seen as a single or sometimes a double tract of barium, commonly known as the "string sign."
- A pyloric bulge into the distal antrum, producing an umbrella appearance, also may be seen.

Ultrasound

- Ultrasonography identifies the hypertrophic pyloric musculature as a broad ring with low-echo density and an inner layer of high-echo density corresponding to the mucosa.
- To confirm the diagnosis, the muscle thickness should be greater than 4 mm or the pyloric length greater than 16 mm.

Emergency Care

Early identification of electrolyte abnormalities and correction with appropriate IV fluids.

 ## Therapy

- Correction of the metabolic abnormalities by replacing sodium, chloride, and potassium
- Pyloromyotomy (Ramstedt procedure): longitudinal incision of the antropyloric muscle. Laparoscopic pyloromyotomy is a minimally invasive version of the Ramstedt procedure.
- Pyloric stenosis is a medical emergency, not a surgical emergency.
- Postoperative vomiting is well recognized and is most likely caused by persistent local edema.
- Initiate feedings very slowly; most patients can be advanced to maintenance oral feedings 48 hours after surgery.

 ## Follow-Up

Vomiting may persist for several days after surgery.

PITFALLS

- Failure to appreciate that chloride loss is the most significant electrolyte disorder when replacing fluids and electrolytes
- Failure to appreciate that this disorder does occur in girls as well as boys

 ## Common Questions and Answers

Q: Can ultrasound help make the diagnosis?
A: Yes. Many will order this test first to avoid the possible aspiration of contrast material.

Q: Why is there so much chloride loss?
A: The chloride loss occurs with the loss of gastric acid, which contains HCl.

Q: What plan should I follow when replacing electrolytes?
A: Correct the deficiency of fluids with twice maintenance fluid volumes. Correct the chloride loss with normal saline, and correct the potassium loss with KCl.

ICD-9-CM 537.0

BIBLIOGRAPHY

Bissounette B, Sullivan PJ. Pyloric stenosis. *Can J Anesth* 1991;38(5):668.

Deluca SA. Hypertrophic pyloric stenosis. *Am Fam Physician* 1993;47(8):1771.

Hypertrophic pyloric stenosis in infancy following pertussis prophylaxis with erythromycin—Knoxville, Tennessee, 1999. *MMWR* 1999;48:1117.

Klein BA. Pyloric stenosis, infantile hypertrophic. In: Barkin RM, ed. *Pediatric emergency medicine: concepts and clinical practice*. St Louis: Mosby Year Book, 1997:856.

Mitchell LE, Risch N. The genetics of infantile hypertrophic pyloric stenosis: a reanalysis. *Am J Dis Child* 1993;147(11):1203.

Rogers, IM. The enigma of pyloric stenosis. Some thoughts on the etiology. *Acta Paediatr* 1997;86:6.

Zenn MR, Redo SF. Hypertrophic pyloric stenosis in the newborn. *J Pediatr Surg* 1993;28(12):1577–1578.

Author: Helen Anita John-Kelly

Rabies

Database

DEFINITION

Rabies is a viral infection of the central nervous system (CNS) that is transmitted from animals to people.

CAUSES

Transmission of the virus, a rhabdovirus containing single-stranded RNA, occurs through animal bites and, rarely, via corneal transplants (from donors with unexplained encephalitis) or inhalation among laboratory workers.

PATHOPHYSIOLOGY

Except for rare cases, the rabies virus enters the body through a bite that causes a break in the skin and introduces infected saliva. From there, the virus gains access to muscle, where it is sequestered. The virus then enters the peripheral nerves, where it moves centripetally to the CNS at a rate of approximately 3 mm/h. Once in the CNS, infection spreads rapidly to involve nearly all neurons. This, if untreated, leads to cardiopulmonary arrest and death shortly thereafter by poorly understood mechanisms.

EPIDEMIOLOGY

• While the current U.S. annual incidence of reported human rabies is about one to two cases per year, incidence rates elsewhere in the world are much higher. In addition, thousands of infected animals are identified each year in the United States.
• Endemic regions of the United States include the mid-Atlantic, southeast, south central, and north central areas, and California.
• Common vectors: Seven species of animals account for 98% of all reported U.S. animal rabies cases: skunks (38–43%), raccoons (28–31%), bats (14%), cats (4%), foxes (4%), cattle (4%), dogs (3%), and other (2%).
• Uncommon vectors: As noted, transmission rarely occurs via corneal transplants or inhalation among laboratory workers.

CLINICAL MANIFESTATIONS

• The *incubation period* can range between 10 days and 2 years! Most cases, however, present within 20 to 90 days postexposure.
• *Prodrome:* 2 to 10 days with vague and insidious symptoms such as sore throat, malaise, anxiety, depression, and, at times, fever or nausea. A fairly specific prodromal symptom is itching, pain, or tingling at the site of the bite.
• *Acute neurologic phase:* furious (80%) versus paralytic (20%) rabies

—*Furious rabies:* agitation, hyperactivity, bizarre behavior—nuchal rigidity, sore throat, and hoarseness. The pathognomonic sign is hydrophobia and, at times, aerophobia.
—*Paralytic rabies:* starts with flaccid paralysis in the limb that was bitten; subsequently spreads to other limbs. Cranial nerve involvement can give an expressionless face.
—*Coma:* follows the acute neurologic phase; May persist up to 2 weeks and is followed by death almost universally.

PROGNOSIS

• Once the patient is infected with the rabies virus, the prognosis is grim.
• Without postexposure rabies immunization, the disease is uniformly fatal.
• There are three documented cases of rabies in humans in which the patient survived after receiving postexposure immunization and intensive medical management.

Differential Diagnosis

• Other causes of encephalitis (e.g., HSV, enterovirus) can mimic rabies.
• Paralytic rabies can present much like Guillain-Barré syndrome or poliomyelitis.
• Pseudorabies is hysteria in an individual who thinks he or she has rabies, but does not. Here, though, normal blood gases and lack of variation in bizarre behavior are distinguishing.

Data Gathering

HISTORY

• Rabid animals: While signs of rabies in animals vary greatly, atypical behavior for the animal is the norm (e.g., passive animals become aggressive, nocturnal animals roam in daylight). Foaming at the mouth and lack of coordination may be present.
• A small minority of humans with rabies have no identifiable preceding animal exposure.

Physical Examination

• Although the neurologic findings can vary, cranial nerve paralysis (palate, vocal cords) is common. Therefore, hoarseness and stridor can be seen.
• Meningismus is also fairly common, along with involuntary movements. Beyond this, findings depend on type of presentation (furious versus paralytic) (see Clinical Manifestations, above).

SPECIAL QUESTIONS

• Type of animal inflicting the bite (domestic versus wild)?
• Location of the animal and availability for observation?
• History of previous rabies vaccination of the animal and patient?

Laboratory Aids

- There are no known methods for identification of rabies virus infection prior to the onset of clinical signs. However, once signs appear, laboratory diagnosis is now possible before death by several techniques:

—*Fluorescent antibodies (FA) stain* of corneal epithelial cell smears or a section of skin from the neck at the hairline
—*Serologic diagnosis* is possible if the patient survives beyond the acute period. A rise in virus-neutralizing antibody will be seen.
—*Viral isolation* from saliva, CSF, urine sedimentation, and brain is, at times, possible between days 4 and 24.

- Postmortem diagnosis is made by the presence of pathognomonic cytoplasmic inclusions (Negri bodies) in brain tissue (sensitivity, 80%).

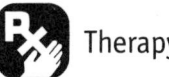 Therapy

LOCAL WOUND CARE

- The first step in preventing infection is washing out the virus mechanically or inactivating it before it has a chance to attach to and enter a neuron.
- The wound should be flushed with copious amounts of soap and water or saline.
- For puncture wounds, insertion of a catheter (i.e., angiocatheter) and irrigation with fluid by means of an attached syringe should be performed. If irrigation is too painful, infiltration of the area with local anesthesia can help.

IMMUNIZATION

Passive

- Human rabies immune globulin (HRIG) should be given to those who are bitten by any variety of wild animal known to be at high risk for rabies infection (skunk, raccoon, fox, coyote, bat) and any domestic dog or cat not in good health and in the custody of someone able to observe the animal for a 10-day period.
- The present recommendation for HRIG vaccination is 20 IU/kg, half injected locally into the tissue at the site of the bite and half administered IM. In cases of multiple wounds, to ensure that all wounds receive an injection of HRIG, dilution in saline (twofold to threefold) is acceptable.

Active

- Human diploid cell rabies vaccine (HDCV) is an inactivated rabies vaccine. This should be administered by the same criteria given above for passive immunization.
- Dosing: 1 mL IM in the deltoid region on days 0, 3, 7, 14, and 28 postexposure. Discontinue the vaccine series if fluorescent antibody testing of the animal is conducted and is negative.

PREVENTION

Immunoprophylaxis: Preexposure vaccines are offered to persons at high risk, such as veterinarians and animal handlers. Because wild animals are the largest source of rabies in the United States today, avoiding unnecessary contact is helpful. More importantly, attempts are being made to orally vaccinate wild animals by using vaccine-laden food in several areas of the United States. Last, it is essential that pet owners vaccinate their pets.

 Common Questions and Answers

Q: Does a wild squirrel or rabbit bite necessitate rabies prophylaxis?
A: In general, rodents (squirrels, rats, mice, hamsters, gerbils), lagomorphs (rabbits and hares), and opossums are not known to serve as natural rabies reservoirs. They should not be considered rabid unless they exhibit unusual behavior.

Q: Is there any evidence of human-to-human spread?
A: No.

Q: Are there any countries that require routine rabies vaccination?
A: Yes, Nepal.

Q: What if a severe allergic reaction occurs during postexposure rabies prophylaxis?
A: The reaction should be treated at the time, as you would any systemic anaphylactic reaction. Subsequently, the rabies vaccine adsorbed (RVA), produced in rhesus diploid cells, can be given on the same schedule as HDCV.

Q: If a bat is found in the house, should the family members receive immunoprophylaxis?
A: If a bat is found in the room of a sleeping person, previously unattended child, or mentally disabled person, prophylaxis should be considered. The injury inflicted by a bat bite or scratch may not be noticed in the above situations.

ICD-9-CM 071

BIBLIOGRAPHY

American Academy of Pediatrics. Rabies. In: Pickering LK, ed. *2000 red book: report of the Committee on Infectious Diseases*, 25th ed. Elk Grove Village, IL: American Academy of Pediatrics, 2000.

Centers for Disease Control. Rabies surveillance, United States, 1987. *MMWR* 1988;37:1.

Gomez-Alonso J. Rabies: a possible explanation for the vampire legend. *Neurology* 1998;51(3):856–859.

NASPHV Compendium Committee. Compendium of animal rabies control. *MMWR* 1987;35:815.

Nicholson KG. Modern vaccines. *Lancet* 1990;335:1201.

Plotkin SA. Rabies. *Clin Infect Dis* 2000;30(1):4–12.

Author: Louis M. Bell
Susan Dibbs, 2nd edition

Rectal Prolapse

 Database

DEFINITION

There are three types of rectal prolapse:

- *Complete:* The full thickness of the rectum prolapses through the anus (two layers of rectum with an intervening peritoneal sac, which may contain small bowel).
- *Incomplete:* The prolapse is limited to the two layers of mucosa only.
- *Concealed:* an internal intussusception of the upper rectum into the lower rectum, which does not emerge through the anus

CAUSES

The exact etiology is uncertain, but is related to the following:

- Constipation
- Excessive straining with bowel movements
- Diarrhea; may be more of a cause in tropical countries
- Cystic fibrosis (CF)
- Malnutrition; can cause loss of the ischiorectal fat pad
- Complete prolapse more rare in children, but when occurs may be related to poor fixation of rectum to sacrum and weak pelvic and anal musculature
- Complication of past surgery, such as imperforate anus repair
- Infections: hookworms

GENETICS

- No known inheritance pattern aside from the association with CF
- An autosomally recessive inherited disease

EPIDEMIOLOGY

- Occurs in more than 19% of children with CF
- It usually presents between 1 and $2\frac{1}{2}$ years of age in patients with CF. Presentation in these children after age 5 is rare.
- In older children and adults, it is six times more common in women than in men.
- It is seen more in underdeveloped countries, perhaps secondary to poor nutrition.

COMPLICATIONS

- In certain older patients who may also have an overactive external sphincter, the need to generate high rectal pressures in order to defecate, together with the rectal prolapse, may cause venous congestion; it may lead to the solitary rectal ulcer syndrome.
- The repetitive trauma to the mucosa can lead to a proctitis.

PROGNOSIS

With proper medical management, excellent prognosis; surgery not usually required

 Differential Diagnosis

- Tumors
- Prolapsing rectal tumor: very rare
- Trauma
- Sexual abuse (e.g., anal penetration)
- Metabolic
- CF: Of significance is the fact that many (anywhere from 10–50%) of the patients who are diagnosed with CF after age 4 have experienced rectal prolapse (either at the time of the diagnosis or as a past event).
- Anatomic

—Solitary rectal ulcer syndrome: an uncommon benign condition usually affecting older children (teenagers). Rectal bleeding on defecation common. Some studies report an association between this entity and rectal prolapse.
—Prolapsing polyp
—Large hemorrhoids
—Surgical
—Colonic intussusception

 Data Gathering

HISTORY

- It is usually first noted by a parent after the child has defecated, and may be associated with painless rectal bleeding.
- It often reduces spontaneously. If not, it is usually easily reduced manually by the parent.
- Rectal prolapse may cause some discomfort during bowel movements.
- Trauma to the recurrently prolapsed mucosa may lead to ulceration and mucus discharge.

 Physical Examination

- Usually, prolapse is not seen on examination while the patient is at rest, unless it is irreducible.
- May see poor anal tone and/or large anal orifice, especially within hours after the prolapse
- In complete rectal prolapse, concentric mucosal rings can be seen, whereas incomplete prolapse reveals radial folds. If one sees more than 5 cm of rectum emerging, it is most likely a complete prolapse.

SPECIAL QUESTIONS

- Has the patient had history of wheezing, pneumonia, or failure to thrive?
- Does this patient have CF?

PHYSICAL EXAMINATION TRICKS

- Asking the patient to strain may allow the mucosa to prolapse. However, this is obviously not very helpful in the very young patient.
- A polyp is differentiated in that it is plum-colored and does not involve the entire anal circumference.
- In an intussusception, it is possible to insert the finger around the prolapsing apex of the intussusception, between it and the lining of the anal canal.

Laboratory Aids

TESTS

- Sweat test: All children with prolapse should have a sweat test to rule out CF. This is a simple, noninvasive, inexpensive test with good specificity and sensitivity.
- Stool cultures: for bacterial and parasitic infestations, if diarrhea is present as a possible causative factor

IMAGING

Evacuation proctography: A barium enema is given, and the movement of barium is observed under fluoroscopy during defecation. This may reveal an internal prolapse not easily recognizable on examination alone. This is not commonly used in children, as good cooperation is necessary.

PITFALLS

Although the history of rectal prolapse may be evident, it is often difficult to elicit on examination, and by the time the patient is seen after a prolapse at home, it may already be spontaneously reduced. Thus, the assumption of the diagnosis may have to rest primarily on the parental history for some time.

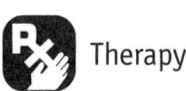 ## Therapy

- Rectal prolapse has a tendency to spontaneously resolve over time.
- The prolapse will more successfully and quickly resolve if the patient is treated for constipation. This should include both dietary manipulations (increased fiber, water) and improved toilet regime. It also will usually necessitate the use of supplemental aids such as mineral oil and, occasionally, laxatives. A small child should try to defecate on a regular toilet and not a potty. In this way, the feet are off the floor, relieving pressure on the abdomen.
- In the rare case of stool infection with diarrhea as the underlying etiology, the appropriate therapy for that infection should be instituted.

DRUGS

In a patient with CF, the addition of pancreatic enzyme supplementation, if not already a part of the regime, has been shown to cause dramatic improvement in rectal prolapse.

DURATION

The treatment of constipation should continue indefinitely, or until the child has demonstrated regular bowel habits on a high-fiber diet on his or her own without evidence of prolapse for at least several months.

SURGICAL

Numerous approaches have been attempted and advocated with varying degrees of enthusiasm, suggesting that none is perfect. These include:

- *Perianal sutures:* has poor results and high complication rate
- *Delorme procedure:* The rectal mucosa is excised and underlying rectal muscle is plicated with sutures.
- *Abdominal rectopexy:* The rectum is mobilized and attached to the sacrum by prosthetic material. Although this procedure provides good results, it has a high complication rate of constipation (greater than 50%).
- *Anterior resection rectopexy:* includes resection of the sigmoid loop and upper rectum; good results, but again, high complication rate because of the anastomosis
- *Perineal resection:* perineal rectosigmoidectomy with a coloanal anastomosis; good results

 ## Follow-Up

WHEN TO EXPECT IMPROVEMENT

Over a period of months to years on a good dietary and behavioral regime

SIGNS TO WATCH FOR

The child is beginning to strain in order to defecate.

PITFALLS

- Although usually a benign event, rectal prolapse is a very distressing condition to both the parents and the child.
- Although surgery seems to be a quicker and more definite solution, in most cases it is more prudent to allow time and medical management to solve the problem. The results from surgical procedures are not foolproof and may lead to further complications.

 ## Common Questions and Answers

Q: What should I do if my child has a rectal prolapse but I cannot reduce it?
A: You should wrap the prolapse in moist towels and bring your child to the emergency room. There, the physicians will try to reduce it. Rarely, if a prolapse is irreducible and left for a period of time, it can cause bowel ischemia and may require surgery.

Q: My child has rectal prolapse and now he is supposed to have a sweat test to determine whether or not he has cystic fibrosis. Is this very likely?
A: No. Although it is important to rule out this disease, the majority of patients with rectal prolapse do not have CF. On the other hand, many children with CF suffer from rectal prolapse.

Q: My child, who has rectal prolapse, is in day care. How will I know if he is having the prolapse?
A: You should inform someone in the school (a teacher or guardian) of his condition and he or she should check the child for prolapse after a movement. Although, if present, it usually spontaneously resolves, the teacher should inform you so you can do a manual reduction, if necessary.

ICD-9-CM 569.1

BIBLIOGRAPHY

Andrews NJ, Jones DJ. Rectal prolapse and associated conditions. *BMJ* 1992;305:242.

Bartolo DC, Kamm MA, et al. Working party report: defecation disorders. *Am J Gastroenterol* 1994;89(8):S154.

Du Boulay DF, Fairbrother J, et al. Mucosal prolapse syndrome: a unifying concept for solitary ulcer syndrome and related disorders. *J Clin Pathol* 1983;36:1264.

Kuijpers HC. Treatment of complete rectal prolapse: to narrow, to wrap, to suspend, to fix, to encircle, to plicate, or to resect? *World J Surg* 1992;16:S26.

Author: Andrew E. Mulberg

Refractive Error

 Database

DEFINITION
For the eye to be able to see, incoming light must be focused on the retina. Refractive errors are aberrations in the optical components of the eye that cause it to be out of focus. Uncorrected refractive error result in blurred vision in one or both eyes, and in children may cause strabismus and amblyopia.

PATHOPHYSIOLOGY
The most important optical components of the eye are the cornea and the lens, which refract light coming into the pupil to focus an image on the retina, and the length of the eye (distance from cornea to retina). A sharply focused image on the retina is necessary for perception of a sharp image; refractive errors cause blurring. Refractive errors can be classified in three groups based on the optical effects:
• Myopia, also called "near-sightedness," correctable with concave lenses with negative diopteric power. Myopic eyes may be in focus for closer targets, but blurred for more distant targets.
• Hyperopia, correctable with convex lenses with positive diopteric power. Although hyperopia is sometimes called "far-sightedness," this is a misnomer in children. Small hyperopic refractive errors are easily overcome by focusing the eye, or accommodation, and many hyperopic children have no difficulty seeing near or distant targets. Larger amounts of hyperopia may blur both near and distant targets, or cause eye strain or esotropia because of the focusing effort required for focusing (see Strabismus).
• Astigmatism, correctable with toric lenses, is caused by aspheric aberration. Uncorrected astigmatism creates images that are not focusable for near or distant targets. Astigmatism may occur with myopia and hyperopia.

Other terms referring to refractive error are:
• Emmetropia—neutral refraction (no refractive error)
• Anisometropia—unequal refractive error between the two eyes
• Accommodation—the ability to change the focus the eyes for near targets, and to overcome hyperopia

In children under 8 years of age, because of visual development and plasticity, refractive errors may have a significant effect on life-long vision. Amblyopia, which may cause permanent, uncorrectable vision loss, and strabismus are among the risks of untreated refractive errors in young children (see Amblyopia and Strabismus).

PATHOLOGY
The refractive components of the eye (cornea, lens, eye length) normally develop simultaneously to allow focused images during early childhood. Factors determining the relative growth and development of these ocular features are not completely understood, and abnormal growth of any component may result in refractive error. Normally, infants and young children are mildly hyperopic (+1.5 to +3.00 diopters), and growth of the eye (primarily increase in eye length) causes a progressive loss of hyperopia, becoming emmetropic during late childhood. Because of this refractive growth, hyperopic refractive errors are much more common in early childhood, and myopic errors in older children and adults. Except for patients with other ocular and systemic abnormalities, the retina, sclera, cornea, and lens are normal in patients with moderate refractive errors. High myopia may lead to retinal thinning, retinal holes, and retinal detachment.

GENETICS
Both genetic and environmental factors are important determinants of refractive status. It has been estimated that 60% of myopia can be predicted by parental refraction, although inheritance seems to be polygenic in most cases.
Some genetic syndromes associated with refractive errors include:
• Myopia
—Stickler syndrome
—Albinism
—Marfan syndrome
—Down syndrome
—Ehlers-Danlos syndrome
• Hyperopia
—Senior-Loken syndrome
—WAGR syndrome
• Astigmatism
—Down syndrome
—Cruzon syndrome
—Albinism

EPIDEMIOLOGY
Because of the age-related growth of the optical components of the eye, the prevalence of refractive errors varies during childhood. At birth the median refractive error is low hyperopia, approximately +2.00 diopters. In adults, the median is emmetropia. The distribution of refractive errors in large populations is a bell-curve around these averages, skewed toward myopia.
In school-aged children in the U.S., 7% to 25% have refractive error significant enough to affect visual acuity. About 25% of the U.S. adult population has myopia, with about 5% with hyperopia.
Certain populations have increased prevalence of myopia, including individuals of Native-American, Chinese, and Japanese descent. Refractive errors are frequently associated with other ocular conditions. These include:

• Myopia
—Retinitis pigmentosa
—Coloboma
—Microphthalmia
—Retinopathy of prematurity
—Congenital cataract
—Glaucoma
—Achromatopsia
• Hyperopia
—Esotropia
—Leber congenital amaurosis
—Surgically treated cataracts (aphakia)
• Astigmatism
—Congenital ptosis
—Coloboma
—Forceps birth injury
—Glaucoma
—Retinopathy of prematurity

COMPLICATIONS
In children, the most significant complications of uncorrected refractive errors are strabismus and amblyopia.
• Accommodative esotropia: uncorrected hyperopia in young children can be overcome by focusing, or accommodation. This involuntary change in the lens of the eye to focus (increase the positive diopteric power of the lens) is controlled reflexively, and is integrated with convergence (crossing the eyes inward). Usually, accommodation is used to focus on near targets, and convergence keeps both eyes pointed at the near target. If there is excessive hyperopia, or if there is an abnormal ratio of accommodative convergence to accommodation (AC/A ratio), the eyes may cross with accommodation. This is accommodative esotropia (see Strabismus).
• Amblyopia: amblyopia—poor visual development—results from a poorly focused image. Anisometropia (unequal refractive error), which blurs vision in one eye, is the most frequent cause of unilateral amblyopia, and occurs in about 3% to 5% of children. Less frequently, bilateral high refractive errors (>4 diopters of hyperopia, >6 diopters of myopia, or >2 diopters of astigmatism) may cause bilateral amblyopia (see Amblyopia).

 Differential Diagnosis

Any cause of monocular or binocular vision loss can simulate refractive error. Since refraction is not easily measured without eye drops and special equipment, the possibility of refractive error must be considered in all children with reduced visual acuity, and should also be considered in children with strabismus and normal vision. Cycloplegic refraction (measuring refraction after the use of eye drops to relax accommodation), and in younger children, a trial of correction with glasses is necessary to eliminate the possibility of residual amblyopia or other causes of poor vision.

Data Gathering

HISTORY
- Age of onset of vision loss
- Associated ocular abnormalities, trauma, injury or surgery
- History of strabismus, amblyopia
- History of prematurity, genetic disorders, collagen disorders (Ehlers-Danlos, Marfan syndromes)
- History of headaches, squinting, or subjective vision problems
- Family history of glasses or refractive error, amblyopia, strabismus

Physical Examination

Visual acuity is the most effective diagnostic tool for detecting refractive errors. Vision must be tested with each eye separately, using a patch, opaque card, or plastic occluder. Testing charts are available with letters as well as pictures and illiterate figures (E's). In children who are too young to test with charts, the Bruchner simultaneous red reflex examination can detect high refractive errors and anisometropia, which appear as asymmetric or distorted red pupillary reflex using the direct ophthalmoscope. Strabismus is frequently a secondary sign of refractive error in children, and can be detected by cover test, Hirschberg corneal light reflex test, or Bruchner test. Photoscreening, which uses the principle of red reflex testing, is also effective in detecting high or asymmetrical refractive errors.

Laboratory Aids

TESTS
There are no effective laboratory tests for refractive errors.

Therapy

Refractive errors are treated by corrective lenses. In young children, this is usually glasses, although contact lenses are frequently used in teenagers.
Unlike adults, children with neglected refractive error are at great risk for significant long-term complications, including amblyopia and strabismus. Hyperopia and anisometropic hyperopia pose the greatest risk for amblyopia. Therefore, smaller amounts of hyperopia and anisometropia are generally corrected with glasses. Glasses are prescribed to improve vision and treat or prevent amblyopia in children for:
- Myopia, −3.00 diopters or more in infants and young children, −1.00 diopter or more in school-age children, or −3.00 diopters or more anisometropia

- Hyperopia, +4.00 diopters or more in infants, +3.00 diopters or more in school-age children, or +1.50 diopters or more anisometropia.
- Any hyperopia in accommodative esotropia. Bifocals may also be prescribed to treat residual esotropia for near targets (high AC/A ratio).
- Astigmatism of >3.00 diopters in infants and young children, or >1.50 diopters in school-age children

In general, children accept full correction of all refractive error, although undercorrection of hyperopia by 0.50–1.00 diopter may enhance the acceptance of new glasses. Occasionally, if hyperopic correction is not well accepted, a brief period of cycloplegia with topical atropine can reinforce use of the glasses. When there is suspicion of amblyopia, vision should be retested after glasses have been worn for several weeks to measure visual improvement. Children wearing glasses must be remeasured regularly, usually at least annually, until they have reached visual maturity and the risk of amblyopia has passed (8–10 years old). Hyperopic patients may develop accommodative esotropia when their glasses are off, after wearing the glasses for some time. Full correction of hyperopia and continuous correction is the best approach to this unusual complication.

Follow-Up

Refractive errors will change over time due to growth of the eye and its optical components. In general, the younger children will need re-refraction and new glasses more frequently. All children wearing glasses should have acuity tested and be re-refracted at least annually.

PITFALLS
- Early detection and correction of refractive errors is important to prevent amblyopia and strabismus. Recognition visual acuity testing using charts should start by age 4 years.
- Children with significant refractive errors will not necessarily be symptomatic. All children should be screened for visual acuity in each eye.
- Glasses may not reverse amblyopia, even if the refractive error is appropriately corrected. Patients with suspected amblyopia (anisometropia, unilateral poor vision, and strabismus) should be followed closely even after wearing the glasses.

Common Questions and Answers

Q: Will my child always need glasses?
A: Not necessarily. Many children who wear glasses are able to see well without correction as adults. Contact lenses and refractive surgery are also possible if correction remains necessary.

Q: Will wearing glasses weaken my child's eyes?
A: No, wearing correction for refractive errors will not weaken the eyes or vision, and is important to prevent amblyopia and permanent vision loss. Occasionally, children with hyperopia will develop accommodative esotropia when the glasses are off, after wearing correction for some time. This is rarely a problem as long as the glasses are worn continuously.

Q: Is my child too young for glasses?
A: Glasses can be worn in children as young as a few months old, with appropriate frames. Usually, children get used to glasses quickly and accept correction easily.

Q: My child can see well. Why does he need glasses?
A: Some children with hyperopia can see charts well, but the accommodation (focusing) necessary to overcome the refractive error may cause eye strain, fatigue, and esotropia. Others may need glasses for unilateral refractive error, and seem to see well with both eyes open. In these children, wearing correction may treat or prevent problems even though they may seem to see well without correction.

Q: Everyone in my family has needed glasses for myopia in childhood. Is there anything we can do for my child that will prevent the development of myopia?
A: Unfortunately, very few environmental factors have been clearly identified to affect the development of myopia. Reading, particularly at an early age; excessively close visual targets (holding books or toys too close to the face); and light exposure during nighttime have been suggested as factors in myopia development. Avoiding long periods of reading, avoiding intensive near work, using a reasonable reading distance (16–18 inches), and avoiding night lights may reduce some of the environmental stimuli.

ICD-9-CM 367.9

BIBLIOGRAPHY
Drack AV. Inheritance of refractive errors. In: Traboulsi EI, ed. *Genetic diseases of the eye.* New York: Oxford University Press, 1998.

Lattimore MR Jr, Schrimsher RH. Refractive error distribution and incidence among U.S. Army aviators. *Milit Med* 1993;158:553–556.

Miller RE 2nd, Woessner WM, Dennis RJ, et al. Survey of spectacle wear and refractive error prevalence in USAF pilots and navigators. *Optom Vis Sci* 1990;67(11):833–839.

Mills, MD. The eye in childhood. *Am Fam Physician* 1999;60:907–918.

Rubin ML. *Optics for clinicians*, 2nd ed. Gainesville, FL: Triad, 1974.

Thorn F. Development of refraction and strabismus. *Curr Opin Ophthalmol* 2000;11(5):301–305.

Author: Monte Mills

Renal Artery Stenosis

 Database

DEFINITION

Renal artery stenosis is narrowing of one or both renal arteries or their more distal branches, resulting in decreased perfusion, increased renin release, increased vascular resistance, and systemic hypertension.

PATHOPHYSIOLOGY

- The most common cause is fibromuscular dysplasia (FMD).
- Other causes include hypoplasia of the renal artery, partial obstruction from a thromboembolism, severe dehydration, extrinsic compression of the artery, vasculitis, neurofibromatosis (NF), and following renal artery surgery (e.g., renal transplantation).
- Arterial narrowing by atheroma is very common in adults but rarely is seen in childhood.

PATHOLOGY

- FMD is a segmental sclerotic process involving smooth muscle hyperplasia. In 75% of patients it is unilateral. Stenosis is usually distal in the renal artery and sometimes involves intrarenal branches. FMD frequently gives a beaded appearance on angiography.
- In NF, the arterial narrowing is proximal, often at the vessel ostium.

GENETICS

- FMD is sporadic.
- NF is autosomal dominant.

EPIDEMIOLOGY

The majority of children with elevated blood pressure have primary or idiopathic hypertension. Of those with secondary hypertension, the majority have intrinsic renal disease (e.g., glomerulonephritis or renal scarring). Only 5% to 10% have renal artery stenosis. Its importance, therefore, is not its frequency but rather the fact that it is potentially curable.

COMPLICATIONS

- Renal artery stenosis often causes severe blood pressure elevation and may be associated with encephalopathy, seizures, or stroke.
- Chronic hypertension may cause damage to end-organs, including the heart and kidney.

PROGNOSIS

- Long-term outcome of percutaneous transluminal angioplasty (PTA) in FMD is excellent, and most children require no medications.
- Restenosis of the vessel is very infrequent.

ASSOCIATED ILLNESSES

- FMD is not associated with other conditions.
- Renal artery stenosis may occur in many other conditions, including NF, vasculitis including polyarteritis nodosa and Takayasu arteritis, moyamoya syndrome, William syndrome, Marfan syndrome, tuberous sclerosis, congenital rubella, and following trauma.
- In neonates, renal artery stenosis is usually the result of a thromboembolus, which is a complication of an umbilical artery catheter.

 Differential Diagnosis

- Renal artery stenosis should be suspected and investigated in children with sudden, severe, progressive, and/or difficult-to-manage hypertension.
- The differential diagnosis consists of other causes of significant hypertension, including coarctation of the aorta, rapidly progressive glomerulonephritis, and renal failure and pheochromocytoma.

 Data Gathering

HISTORY

- Symptoms in infants may include irritability, vomiting, and poor feeding.
- In children, symptoms may include headaches, vomiting, dizziness, and seizures.
- Many children are asymptomatic.

Special Question

Has the child ingested any medication that can increase blood pressure, such as sympathomimetic drugs, steroids, amphetamines, oral contraceptives, and so on?

 Physical Examination

- Accurate determination of blood pressure with appropriate-size cuff; done in the upper and lower extremities
- Blood pressure should be repeated until the patient is judged to be relaxed.
- Pulses should be checked in all four extremities.
- The skin must be examined for signs of neurofibromatosis (e.g., café-au-lait spots and neurofibromas) and vasculitis.
- The optic fundi must be checked for hypertensive vascular changes. Often, an ophthalmologist's examination is necessary.
- Auscultation of the lower back and abdomen should be checked for the presence of bruits.
- In infancy, signs of congestive heart failure may be present.

PHYSICAL EXAMINATION TRICKS

- The resting, relaxed blood pressure is likely to be obtained when the pulse rate has reached a basal resting level.
- Listen for an abdominal bruit just to the left of and superior to the umbilicus.
- Listen over the flanks with a bell stethoscope for a bruit.

Renal Artery Stenosis

 Laboratory Aids

TESTS

- *BUN* and *creatinine* to exclude intrinsic renal disease
- *Electrolytes:* A hyper-renin state leads to hyperaldosteronism and may produce hypokalemia and mild metabolic alkalosis.
- *Selective renal vein renin determinations* are suggestive of unilateral stenosis if one side is less than one and a half times the contra-lateral (normal). Random venous renin concentrations have little value and may be misleading.
- *Electrocardiogram* and/or *echocardiogram* to investigate the presence of ventricular strain or hypertrophy

IMAGING

- Although a variety of imaging studies are available that may suggest renal artery stenosis, the only definitive tests are *selective* renal arteriography, and, if indicated, transluminal angioplasty.
- Renal ultrasonography may demonstrate a smaller kidney on the suspected side, but this study cannot make or exclude the diagnosis. Special applications of *Doppler ultrasonography* and color-coded duplex sonography have shown promise, especially in the postoperative transplant period when immediate information regarding the renal artery is essential.
- Other *more invasive studies,* such as captopril-enhanced nuclear medicine scans, digital subtraction angiography, CT scans, and MRI, have not proved to be confirmatory for all patients, but they may be useful when used in selective children with a high likelihood of renal artery stenosis.

 Therapy

DRUGS

- Hypertension that accompanies renal artery stenosis is often difficult to control with antihypertensive medications. In small infants, however, long-term medical therapy may be necessary until the child is large enough for definitive correction.
- Because renal artery stenosis results in a high renin state, the angiotensin-converting enzyme (ACE) inhibitors, captopril and enalopril, are most effective. When used in conjunction with renal scintigraphy or selective renin measurements, ACE inhibitors may improve diagnosis of renal artery stenosis.
- ACE inhibitors may significantly decrease renal perfusion and function and should not be used in cases of known or suspected bilateral renal artery stenosis.
- Thrombolytic therapy with urokinase should be considered in instances of bilateral renal artery thrombosis.

DEFINITIVE CORRECTION

- PTA dilatation of the stenosis, using an intravascular balloon catheter during arteriography, is the treatment of choice. This therapy is very effective in FMD but less effective in the proximal stenosis associated with NF. Stent implantation is occasionally used as an adjunct to angioplasty.
- Surgery is indicated in cases in which PTA is not possible or successful. Autotransplantation may be effective, especially in children with bilateral renal artery and aortic narrowing.

DURATION

- Effective medical therapy should be monitored closely and continued until the renal artery stenosis can be corrected.
- Medication is generally discontinued prior to the angioplasty and used postprocedure only if the blood pressure remains elevated.

 Follow-Up

- If effective, response to antihypertensive therapy with ACE inhibitors should occur within 12 days.
- Response to dilation of the renal artery stenosis is often immediate, although transient vessel spasm may occur postprocedure and temporarily be associated with hypertension significant enough to require treatment.

PITFALLS

- Excessive investigation for renal artery stenosis or other secondary causes of hypertension in the majority of children identified with elevated blood pressure
- Failure to proceed rapidly to an arteriogram in a child appropriately suspected of having renal artery stenosis

ICD-9-CM 440.1

BIBLIOGRAPHY

Airoldi F, Palatresi S, Marana I, et al. Angioplasty of atherosclerotic and fibro-muscular renal artery stenosis: time course and predicting factors of the effects on renal function. *Am J Hypertens* 2000;13(11): 1210–1217.

Deal JE, Shell MF, Barratt TM, et al. Renovascular disease in childhood. *J Pediatr* 1992;121:378.

Ellis D, Shapiro R, Scantlebury VP, et al. Evaluation and management of bilateral renal artery stenosis in children: a case series and review. *Pediatr Nephrol* 1995;9:259.

Guzzetta PC, Davis CF, Ruley EJ. Experience with bilateral renal artery stenosis as a cause of hypertension in childhood. *J Pediatr Surg* 1991;26:532.

Lillehei CW, Shamberger RC. Staged reconstruction for middle aortic syndrome. *J Pediatr Surg* 2001;36(8):1252–1254.

Author: Thomas L. Kennedy III

Renal Failure—Acute

 Database

DEFINITION

Acute renal failure is a rapidly progressive, and potentially reversible, cessation of renal function that results in the inability of the kidney to control body homeostasis. It manifests in retention of nitrogenous waste products and fluid and electrolyte imbalances.

- Oliguria: urine output less than 0.5 mL/kg/h in infants or less than 500 mL/1.73 m² per day in older children
- Anuria: total cessation of urinary output

PATHOPHYSIOLOGY

Acute renal failure has many causes, which can be categorized into three subgroups:

- Prerenal

—Decreased perfusion of the kidney secondary either to decreased extracellular volume or diminished cardiac output
—It is the most common form of acute renal failure in children.

- Postrenal

—An obstructive process (either structural or functional)
—The obstruction can reside in the lower tract or bilaterally in the upper tracts unless the patient has a single kidney.
—This form of renal failure is more common in newborns.

- Intrinsic
- Disorders that directly affect the kidney. This form can be subcategorized:

—*Acute tubular necrosis* is the most common form of intrinsic renal failure and usually follows hypoxic or nephrotoxic injury.
—*Glomerular disorders* include the various forms of acute glomerulonephritis (AGN) such as postinfectious AGN and rapidly progressive (crescentic) AGN.
—*Vascular lesions* compromise glomerular blood flow. Hemolytic-uremic syndrome is the most common disease that causes intrinsic acute renal failure in children.
—*Interstitial nephritis* can be idiopathic or caused by reactions to drugs or infections.

- Acute renal failure is commonly precipitated by an ischemic or nephrotoxic event. Initial vasodilatation is followed by intense vasoconstriction, with blood redistributed from the cortex to the juxtamedullary nephrons. The delivery of oxygen to the kidney is impaired, leading to acute tubular necrosis. Intratubular debris and cast formation develop. Tubular fluid leaks backward across the injured tubular membrane, which, in addition to tubular obstruction, causes further hemodynamic changes.

EPIDEMIOLOGY

Acute renal failure secondary to acute tubular necrosis is commonly seen in the hospitalized patient. The combination of ischemia plus nephrotoxic agents such as aminoglycosides, amphotericin B, contrast, or chemotherapeutic agents place these individuals at increased risk.

COMPLICATIONS

- Fluid overload, resulting in congestive heart failure and hypertension
- Hyperkalemia, affecting cardiac function by causing arrhythmias
- Uremia, manifest by mental status changes, increased risk of bleeding, and infection
- Metabolic acidosis
- Hypocalcemia, causing tetany

PROGNOSIS

- Generally, patients with nonoliguric renal failure have a lower mortality rate than patients with oliguria or anuria.
- The mortality rate increases in patients with multisystem organ failure, despite good supportive care.

 Differential Diagnosis

- Chronic renal failure: insidious, associated with poor growth, polyuria, and anemia
- Azotemia: caused by corticosteroid therapy, upper gastrointestinal bleeding, hyper-catabolic state
- Elevated creatinine: caused by rhabdomyolysis, drugs (trimethoprim-sulfa, cimetidine)

 Data Gathering

Key: POST, obstruction; PRE, prerenal; ATN, acute tubular necrosis; AIN, acute interstitial nephritis; AGN, acute glomerulonephritis; HUS, hemolytic-uremic syndrome

HISTORY

- Symptoms: fever, rash (AIN, AGN), bloody diarrhea, pallor (HUS), severe vomiting or diarrhea (PRE), abdominal pain (POST), hemorrhage, shock (ATN), anuria (AGN, POST), polyuria (ATN, AIN)
- Medical history: previous infection (AGN), neurogenic bladder, single kidney (POST)
- Medications: exposure to various medications such as nonsteroidal antiinflammatory agents, β-lactam antibiotics, acyclovir (AIN), nephrotoxic drugs such as aminoglycosides, amphotericin B, cisplatinum (ATN)
- Toxins: exposure to heavy metals, organic solvents (ATN)
- Family: history of HUS
- Trauma: crush injury (ATN)
- Review of symptoms: various systemic symptoms (AGN)

 Physical Examination

- General: dehydration, shock (PRE, ATN), edema (AGN), jaundice (HUS, ATN)
- Eyes: uveitis (AIN)
- Lungs: rales (AGN)
- Heart: gallop (AGN)
- Abdomen/pelvis: mass (POST)
- Skin: rash (AIN, AGN), petechia (HUS)
- Joints: arthritis (AGN)

Laboratory Aids

TESTS

• Urinalysis: normal sediment or eumorphic RBCs, crystalluria (POST), eosinophiluria, pyuria (AIN), granular casts (PRE, ATN), pigmenturia (ATN), RBC casts, proteinuria (HUS, AGN), U_{osm} less than 350 mOsm (POST, AIN, ATN), U_{osm} greater than 500 mOsm (PRE, AGN, HUS)
• Serum chemistries: hyponatremia, hyperchloremic acidosis (POST), hyperkalemia (POST, AGN, HUS), BUN:Cr greater than 20 (PRE)
• CBC: microangiopathic hemolytic anemia, thrombocytopenia (HUS), eosinophilia (AIN)
• Serologies: hypocomplementemia (AGN), antineutrophil cytoplasmic antibodies (AGN), antinuclear antibodies (AGN)
• Renal ultrasound: hydronephrosis, trabeculated bladder (POST), increased echogenicity (ATN, AIN, AGN, HUS)
• Renal biopsy: indicated in patients with prolonged, unexplained acute renal failure

SPECIAL LABORATORY TRICKS

The *fractional excretion of sodium* (FE_{Na}) is a useful urinary index that determines tubular function.

$$FE_{Na} = [(U_{Na}/P_{Na})/(U_{creat}/P_{creat})] \times 100$$

The FE_{Na} should not be obtained after diuretics are administered.
FE_{Na} greater than 2 (AIN, ATN), FE_{Na} less than 1 (HUS, AGN, PRE)

 ## Emergency Care

• If severe hyperkalemia is present, consider:
—Calcium gluconate (0.5–1.0 mL/kg IV) over 5 to 10 minutes if severe
—Glucose (0.5 g/kg) and insulin (0.1 U/kg) IV over 30 minutes
—Sodium bicarbonate (1–2 mEq/kg) IV over 10 to 30 minutes if acidotic
—Kayexalate (1 g/kg) PO or PR in sorbitol
—Furosemide (1–2 mg/kg) if renal function is adequate
—Hemodialysis or peritoneal dialysis

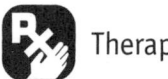 ## Therapy

Therapy is preventive, supportive, or specific.

PREVENTIVE

The use of mannitol or furosemide to prevent acute renal failure is controversial. They may be used prophylactically (amphotericin B, cisplatinum, contrast) or in cases of hemoglobinuria or myoglobinuria to augment urine flow. Some feel this may convert oliguric renal failure to nonoliguric renal failure.

SUPPORTIVE

• Establish an effective circulatory volume. If the patient is in shock, administer fluids (normal saline, lactated Ringer's) liberally, even if there is no urine output.
• Maintain a normal intravascular volume. Carefully monitor urine output and provide appropriate fluids accordingly. Consider fluid restriction and diuretics if the patient is volume overloaded.
• Monitor serum potassium levels frequently. Avoid potassium-containing drugs, fluids, or foods in patients with oligo/anuria.
• Hyponatremia is usually secondary to free water excess and should be managed with fluid restriction. Hypertonic saline should be used if only CNS symptoms are present.
• Hypocalcemia, if mild, may be treated by phosphate restriction. Severe hypocalcemia requires treatment with calcium gluconate (100 mg/kg) given slowly.
• Severe acidosis (pH <7.2) requires supplementation with bicarbonate. However, this may cause hypernatremia, fluid overload, and symptomatic hypocalcemia.
• The effect of aggressive nutritional support is controversial, with the exception of use for a significantly malnourished or hypercatabolic child.
• Hypertension should be treated aggressively if encephalopathy is present.
• Dialysis is indicated for refractory acidosis, severe hyperkalemia, volume overload, and uremic symptoms (pericarditis, lethargy), or for the removal of toxins (uric acid, salicylate).

SPECIFIC

Each cause of renal failure may have a specific treatment, such as fluid resuscitation (PRE), urologic intervention (POST), and corticosteroids (AIN, some forms of AGN).

 ## Follow-Up

Patients usually remain hospitalized until their renal function improves. Long-term follow-up to monitor sequelae is indicated in patients with prolonged anuria.

PITFALLS

The excretion of many medications is influenced by acute renal failure. Careful attention to drug dosing and levels can minimize toxicity.
A significant postobstructive diuresis can be seen after treatment for obstructive acute renal failure.

 ## Common Questions and Answers

Q: What is the expected recovery time in patients with acute renal failure who present with anuria?
A: Recovery time depends on the etiology of the acute renal failure. Children with HUS may recover in days to weeks. Others with ATN recover days after treatment of the inciting cause. Finally, children with an obstructive etiology usually recover as soon as the obstruction is relieved.

Q: When should renal function return to normal values?
A: Renal function may not return to normal in patients with prolonged periods of anuria. In other cases, once recovery starts, a normal serum creatinine is seen within weeks.

Q: What indices should be followed after a patient recovers from acute renal failure?
A: Patients recovering from acute renal failure should have blood pressures and urinalysis for proteinuria monitored regularly. Serum creatinine should be checked if the course of acute renal failure was prolonged.

ICD-9-CM 584.0

BIBLIOGRAPHY

Flynn JT. Causes, management approaches, and outcome of acute renal failure in children. *Curr Opin Pediatr* 1998;10:184–189.

Sehic A, Chesney RW. Acute renal failure: diagnosis. *Pediatr Rev* 1995;16:101–106.

Sehic A, Chesney RW. Acute renal therapy: therapy. *Pediatr Rev* 1995;16:137–141.

Thadhani R, Pascual M, Bonventre JV. Acute renal failure. *N Engl J Med* 1996;334: 1448–1460.

Author: Seth L. Schulman

Renal Failure—Chronic

Database

DEFINITION

- Chronic renal failure is a reduction in the glomerular filtration rate to <25% of normal for at least 3 months' duration.
- Chronic renal insufficiency describes a reduction in the glomerular filtration rate between 25% and 50%.

PATHOPHYSIOLOGY

- Infants younger than 2 years of age develop chronic renal failure secondary to either obstructive uropathy or renal hypodysplasia.
- Children 2 to 5 years of age develop chronic renal failure secondary to neonatal vascular accidents and hemolytic uremic syndrome, obstructive uropathy, or renal hypodysplasia.
- More common etiologies of chronic renal failure in older children and adolescents include glomerulonephritis (focal segmental glomerulosclerosis, crescentic glomerulonephritis, lupus nephritis), reflux nephropathy, or hereditary causes such as Alport syndrome.

GENETICS

Several hereditary diseases can cause chronic renal failure, including:

- Alport disease (partially X-linked dominant)
- Polycystic kidney disease (autosomal recessive or dominant)
- Familial juvenile nephronophthisis (autosomal recessive)
- Cystinosis (autosomal recessive)
- Hyperoxaluria (autosomal recessive)
- Congenital nephrotic syndrome (autosomal recessive)
- Nail patella syndrome (autosomal dominant)
- Sickle cell disease (autosomal recessive)

EPIDEMIOLOGY

- The incidence of chronic renal failure is not known.
- Approximately three to eight new cases of end-stage renal failure are reported per 1 million children per year
- Prevalence of chronic renal failure has been reported to be 32.4 per 1 million children in Western Europe, with 6% younger than 3 years of age, 30% between 3 and 9 years of age, and 64% between 9 and 15 years of age.
- Among children in the United States with chronic renal insufficiency entered into the North American Pediatric Renal Transplant Cooperative Study, 65.9% are male and 63.9% are white.

COMPLICATIONS

- Growth retardation is particularly severe when chronic renal failure develops in the first year of life. The etiology of growth failure may be secondary to poor nutrition, bone disease, acidosis, or a direct effect on the growth hormone-IGF-1 axis.
- Renal osteodystrophy may be seen early in chronic renal insufficiency and manifest as growth failure, bowing of the lower extremities, and slipped epiphysis. Vitamin D deficiency and secondary hyperparathyroidism are the major factors leading to bone disease.
- Anemia develops secondary to decreased erythropoietin secretion and decreased red cell survival. The anemia is normocytic, associated with a low reticulocyte count.
- Neurodevelopmental delay is increased in children with chronic renal failure. This is probably secondary to uremic effects on the developing brain.
- Hypertension may be seen in some patients with chronic renal failure secondary either to hyperreninemia or hypervolemia.
- Platelet abnormalities, protein-calorie malnutrition, and immunologic disturbances are also seen in uremic patients.

PROGNOSIS

Depends on underlying cause, child's age, degree of renal insufficiency, and need for dialysis or transplantation

Differential Diagnosis

- Differentiate acute from chronic renal failure.
- Usually chronic renal failure is insidious and associated with poor growth, polyuria, and anemia. The kidneys may be small on renal ultrasound. A renal biopsy may be indicated to determine the cause of renal failure if genetic causes are suspected (for counseling) or if treatment is being considered.

Data Gathering

HISTORY

Question: Symptoms?
Significance:

- Malaise
- Poor appetite
- Vomiting
- Bone pain
- Headache (if hypertensive)
- Polyuria

Question: Past history?
Significance:

- Perinatal complications
- Oligohydramnios
- Recurrent urinary tract infections
- Enuresis

Question: Familial history?
Significance:

- Renal disease
- Hearing impairment

Physical Examination

Finding: General
Significance:

- Short stature
- Poor weight gain
- Pale
- Fetid breath

Finding: HEENT
Significance:

- Retinal changes
- Preauricular pits
- Hearing deficit

Finding: Chest
Significance: Rales

Finding: Heart
Significance:

- Flow Murmur
- Gallop
- Rub

Finding: Abdomen
Significance:

- Palpable kidneys
- Suprapubic mass

Finding: Extremities
Significance:

- Rachitic changes
- Edema
- Absent patella

Finding: Neurologic
Significance:

- Developmental delay
- Altered mental status
- Hypotonia
- Irritability

Laboratory Aids

Test: Serum chemistries
Significance: Azotemia, hyperkalemia (if advanced), acidemia, hypocalcemia, hyperphosphatemia, elevated alkaline phosphatase

Test: CBC
Significance: Normocytic anemia with low reticulocyte count

Test: Urinalysis
Significance: Isosthenuria, mild proteinuria

Test: Intact parathyroid hormone
Significance: Elevated

Test: Chest x-ray
Significance: Pulmonary edema, cardiomegaly

Test: Bone films
Significance: Delayed bone age, rickets, osteitis fibrosa

Test: Renal ultrasound
Significance: Small echogenic kidneys, cystic kidneys, hydronephrosis

Test: ECG (if hyperkalemic)
Significance: Peaked T waves

SPECIAL LABORATORY TRICKS

Test: 24-hour urine collection
(= 1440 minutes)
Significance: The glomerular filtration rate can be estimated with concomitant blood sampling by calculating the creatinine clearance:

$$\frac{U_{creat} \times (volume\ voided/1440)}{P_{creat}} \times \frac{1.73}{BSA}$$

where BSA is the body surface area. The resultant value is expressed as mL/min/1.73 m^2. Normal range is 80 to 120 mL/min/1.73 m^2.
A simpler calculation that is already corrected for surface area and does not require a urine collection:

$$\frac{Height(cm) \times 0.55}{P_{creat}}$$

The correction factor (0.55) is applicable to most children 1 year of age. A lower factor (0.45) is suggested for infants <1 year of age and a higher one (0.7) for adolescent males. Plotting the reciprocal of the serum creatinine versus time can approximate the rate of decline of renal function.
This may be useful in determining when renal replacement therapy will be necessary.

 ## Therapy

MEDICATIONS

- Phosphate binders (calcium carbonate, calcium acetate, sevelamer; avoid aluminum if possible)
- 1,25-dihydroxy vitamin D
- Alkali therapy (sodium bicarbonate/citrate)
- Diuretic therapy
- Recombinant erythropoietin
- Recombinant human growth hormone

DIETARY RESTRICTIONS

- Protein
- Phosphate
- Potassium
- Sodium (indicated if edematous)
- Fluid (indicated in oliguric conditions)

RENAL REPLACEMENT THERAPY

- Dialysis: Indications similar to those for acute renal failure or when glomerular filtration rate <10 mL/min/1.73 m^2 and patient is experiencing fatigue, poor school performance, or weight loss secondary to severe dietary restrictions.
- Transplantation: In some cases a preemptive transplant may be offered in lieu of dialysis.

 ## Follow-Up

General pediatricians should follow patients with chronic renal failure with assistance from a pediatric nephrologist.

PITFALLS

During episodes of gastroenteritis infants with chronic renal failure may be prone to dehydration because they have obligatory polyuria secondary to a concentrating defect. Do not use urine output or specific gravity as indices for hydration.

 ## Common Questions and Answers

Q: What over-the-counter medications should be avoided in children with chronic renal failure?
A: Nonsteroidal antiinflammatory drugs, pseudoephedrine (if hypertensive), and magnesium or aluminum-containing antacids should not be taken.

Q: Can children with chronic renal failure receive immunizations?
A: Children with chronic renal failure should receive all necessary immunizations especially since after transplantation some vaccines are contraindicated. In some cases booster immunizations are necessary because of an inadequate response to the initial series (e.g., hepatitis B, MMR).

Q: When is recombinant human erythropoietin indicated?
A: Generally this medication should be considered when the hematocrit is <33%.

ICD-9-CM 585.0

BIBLIOGRAPHY

Benfield MR, McDonald R, Sullivan EK, et al. *The 1997 annual renal transplantation in children.* Report of the North American Pediatric Renal Transplant Cooperative Study. *Pediatr Transplant* 1999;3:152–167.

Dabbagh S. Renal osteodystrophy. *Curr Opin Pediatr* 1998;10:190–196.

Friedman AL. Etiology, pathophysiology, diagnosis, and management of chronic renal failure in children. *Curr Opin Pediatr* 1996;8:148–151.

Seidman A, Freidman A, Boineau F. Nutritional management of the child with mild to moderate chronic renal failure. *J Pediatr* 1996;129:13–18.

Author: Seth L. Schulman

Renal Tubular Acidosis

 Database

DEFINITION

• Renal tubular acidosis (RTA) is a clinical syndrome of disordered renal acidification in which the kidney fails to maintain a normal plasma concentration of bicarbonate in the setting of a normal rate of acid production from diet and metabolism.
• This syndrome is characterized by a hyperchloremic metabolic acidosis, bicarbonaturia, decreased production of titratable acids and ammonium, with, usually, an elevated urinary pH.

TYPES

• Distal (type I)

—Distal RTA is a primary renal acidification defect secondary to either an inability to secrete hydrogen ions or a back-leak in the collecting tubule. In some cases there may be bicarbonate wasting as well.
—These infants and children present with failure to thrive, hypokalemia, nephrolithiasis, nephrocalcinosis, or rickets. The nephrolithiasis is secondary to the persistent alkaline urine, hypercalciuria, and hypocitraturia.
—Patients with complete distal RTA can never acidify their urine and, therefore, always have a urine pH higher than 6.0.

• Proximal (type II)

—This form of RTA is caused by a defect in the sodium-hydrogen ion exchange mechanism. These infants and children spill bicarbonate into their urine because the renal threshold for reabsorption is reduced. Because the distal mechanism is intact, acidification of the urine is possible once the serum bicarbonate falls below the threshold.
—Isolated proximal RTA is rare; most children present with this abnormality as part of the Fanconi syndrome (bicarbonaturia, amino aciduria, glycosuria, and phosphaturia).
—Hypokalemia is usually present but hypercalciuria and hypocitraturia are not. Therefore, nephrocalcinosis, nephrolithiasis, and rickets are not the presenting features of this form of RTA.

• Distal hyperkalemic (type IV)

—Type IV RTA is the most common form of RTA in adults and children.
—Hyperkalemia distinguishes this form from types I and II.
—There are five subtypes of type IV RTA but the predominant feature is aldosterone deficiency or unresponsiveness.
—One form in children occurs with obstructive uropathy and renal insufficiency. This causes a defect in the juxtaglomerular apparatus leading to hyporeninemia with secondary hypoaldosteronism. Children with this form of RTA may present with failure to thrive.

GENETICS

• In infants and children type I RTA is usually inherited as an autosomal-dominant trait. It may occur in association with other diseases such as elliptocytosis, sickle cell disease, and the Ehlers-Danlos syndrome.
• Type II RTA with Fanconi syndrome occurs with several disorders that are autosomal recessive, including cystinosis, Lowe syndrome, Wilson disease, tyrosinemia, hereditary fructose intolerance, and galactosemia.
• Certain subtypes of type IV RTA have been reported to be familial.

EPIDEMIOLOGY

Renal tubular acidosis is an extremely rare condition.

COMPLICATIONS

• Children with RTA may develop severe growth failure, rickets, nephrocalcinosis, and nephrolithiasis.

—During episodes of vomiting or diarrhea they may be at risk of developing profound acidosis and hypokalemia.

PROGNOSIS

• Prognosis depends on the underlying etiology.
• Growth velocity increases following treatment with alkali for isolated type I and II RTA and normal stature can be achieved.
• Isolated type I RTA is a chronic condition that requires constant monitoring to avoid nephrocalcinosis.

 Differential Diagnosis

• Renal tubular acidosis is associated with a normal anion gap ($Na^+ - [Cl^- + HCO_3^-] = 8$ to 16 mEq/L).
• Other causes of metabolic acidosis with a normal anion gap include diarrhea, acetazolamide, ileal conduits, and fistulas draining the small bowel, pancreas, or biliary tree.

 Data Gathering

HISTORY

Question: Symptoms?
Significance: Failure to thrive, renal colic, bone pain, photophobia (cystinosis)

Question: Past medical history?
Significance: Prior admissions for dehydration and acidosis not associated with significant diarrhea

Question: Medications/drugs?
Significance: Amphotericin B, lithium, tetracycline (outdated), toluene

Question: Familial history?
Significance: See Genetics, above.

Question: Review of symptoms?
Significance: Other systemic diseases

Physical Examination

Finding: General
Significance: Failure to thrive

Finding: Head
Significance: Frontal bossing

Finding: Eyes
Significance:

- Cystine deposition
- Kayser-Fleischer ring
- Cataracts

Finding: Chest
Significance: Rachitic rosary

Finding: Abdomen
Significance:

- Hepatosplenomegaly
- Enlarged kidneys

Finding: Extremities
Significance:

- Bowing
- Widening of the epiphysis of wrists

Laboratory Aids

Test: Serum electrolytes
Significance: Identify the presence of a normal anion gap metabolic acidosis, hyper/hypokalemia.

Test: Urinalysis
Significance: Exclude features of Fanconi syndrome.

Test: Urine pH
Significance: Can exclude type I RTA if <6.0; best if performed in the face of acidosis. Best if determined with a pH probe as quickly as possible after collection

Test: Serum creatinine
Significance: To exclude renal insufficiency

Test: Urine anion gap
Significance:

- Negative ($Cl^- > Na^+ + K^+$) seen in gastrointestinal losses, proximal RTA
- Positive ($Cl^- < Na^+ + K^+$) seen in distal RTA

Test: Urine
Significance: Should be measured by pH meter from a fresh specimen. If this is not possible, oil should be added to cover urine and protect dissipation of CO_2.

IMAGING

Test: Abdominal flat plate
Significance: Nephrocalcinosis, nephrolithiasis

Test: Bone films
Significance: Rachitic changes, delayed bone age

Therapy

- Alkali administration is the primary therapy for children with RTA.
- Sodium/potassium citrate (Polycitra 2 mEq HCO_3^-/mL) is preferable for children with types I or II RTA.
- Sodium citrate (Bicitra 1 mEq HCO_3^-/mL) is used in infants with type IV RTA.
- Older children can take sodium bicarbonate tablets (7.7 mEq HCO_3^-)
- Patients with type I RTA require 1 to 4 mEq/kg of alkali therapy per day in three to four divided doses. This usually decreases the chances of complications such as nephrolithiasis, nephrocalcinosis, and rickets.
- Patients with type II RTA require considerably more alkali therapy (5 to 20 mEq/kg/d in four to six divided doses).
- The dosage of alkali in children with type IV RTA ranges from 1 to 5 mEq/kg/d, which is usually sufficient to correct the hyperkalemia.

Follow-Up

- Patients with RTA should be closely monitored with frequent serum potassium and plasma bicarbonate levels until a steady state is reached.
- Normal growth may be attained once the metabolic acidosis is corrected.

PITFALLS AND PREVENTION

- Avoid hemolyzed specimens that may artificially increase the serum potassium and reduce the plasma bicarbonate levels.
- Administer alkali over several divided doses.
- Closely monitor patients during episodes of gastroenteritis to avoid dehydration and severe metabolic acidosis.

Common Questions and Answers

Q: Do children outgrow renal tubular acidosis?
A: Types I and II RTA are chronic disorders that require lifelong treatment. Some children outgrow certain subtypes of type IV RTA.

Q: Can children with renal tubular acidosis develop renal failure?
A: Untreated type I RTA can lead to renal failure by causing progressive nephrocalcinosis. Children with inherited disorders associated with Fanconi syndrome such as cystinosis can also develop renal insufficiency.

ICD-9-CM 588.8

BIBLIOGRAPHY

Battle DC, Hizon M, Cohen E, et al. The use of the urinary anion gap in the diagnosis of hyperchloremic metabolic acidosis. *N Engl J Med* 1988;318:594.

Gregory MJ, Schwartz GJ. Diagnosis and treatment of renal tubular disorders. *Semin Nephrol* 1998;18:317–329.

McSherry E. Renal tubular acidosis in children (nephrology forum). *Kidney Int* 1981;20:799.

Rodriguez-Soriano J. New insights into the pathogenesis of renal tubular acidosis—from functional to molecular studies. *Pediatr Nephrol* 2000;14:1121–1136.

Zelikovic I. Renal tubular acidosis. *Pediatr Ann* 1995;24:48–54.

Author: Seth L. Schulman

Renal Venous Thrombosis

 Database

DEFINITION

• Renal venous thrombosis (RVT) is the thrombotic process that begins in the intrarenal venous radicals and usually progresses forward toward the main renal vein.
• Rarely, the thrombosis progresses in the opposite direction.

PATHOPHYSIOLOGY

• RVT in newborns and infants is commonly associated with asphyxia, dehydration (as with diarrhea), shock, sepsis, hypertonicity, and hemoconcentration.
• Additional predisposing factors in the newborn include congenital renal anomalies and maternal diabetes.
• In older children it is associated with the nephrotic syndrome, cyanotic heart disease, and hyperosmolar states such as with the use of angiography contrast agents.
• In many children, no underlying cause is apparent.
• The slow double circulation of the kidney is especially vulnerable to thrombosis.
• Thrombus formation may be initiated by vascular endothelial cell injury in conjunction with diminished vascular flow.
• RVT usually starts in the small venous radicals with progression through the arcuate and interlobular veins toward the main renal vein.
• RVT causes renal congestion and occasionally infarction.

GENETICS

• Familial occurrence is rare.
• No hereditary factors have been described.

EPIDEMIOLOGY

• RVT is predominantly a disease of the newborn.
• The incidence and prevalence are poorly defined.
• There is a small male preponderance.
• The disease is more frequently unilateral than bilateral.

COMPLICATIONS

• Bilateral RVT may lead to chronic renal failure.
• Scarring may result in hypertension.

 Differential Diagnosis

• The differential diagnosis includes other causes of renal enlargement such as hydronephrosis, cystic renal disease, renal tumors, abscess, and hematoma.
• Hemolytic uremic syndrome should also be considered because RVT may also result in fragmented red blood cells and thrombocytopenia.

PROGNOSIS

• The degree of irreversible renal damage depends on the degree of involvement and associated conditions.
• Recovery of function in affected kidneys may occur.
• Hypertension is seen in 20%.
• The majority have residual renal structural abnormalities, such as atrophy and coarse renal scarring.

 Data Gathering

HISTORY

• The majority present in the newborn period.
• Most of the symptoms are due to an underlying disorder.
• RVT is usually heralded by the sudden onset of hematuria and unilateral or bilateral flank masses.

 Physical Examination

• 60% will have a palpably enlarged kidney.
• Associated signs and symptoms include pallor, tachypnea, abdominal distention, shock, flank pain, fever, oliguria, or anuria.
• If in the thrombosis, the lower limbs may become edematous, cyanotic, and hypothermic; the inferior vena cava (IVC) is involved.

 Laboratory Aids

• Proteinuria is common.
• The majority have macroscopic hematuria.
• 90% have progressive thrombocytopenia, and the majority also have microangiopathic hemolytic anemia.
• Fibrin split products may be elevated with low-plasma fibrinogen levels.
• Azotemia and other biochemical evidence of acute renal failure may be present.
• Variations in plasma electrolytes depend on the presence of diarrhea or renal failure.

IMAGING

Test: Intravenous urograms
Significance: Almost always contraindicated because of the osmolar load of intravenous contrast material.

Test: Ultrasonography
Significance: The most useful study; it will differentiate between renal enlargement and extrarenal masses. It will also identify obstruction, cystic changes, and many congenital anomalies, and show renal enlargement, increased echogenicity, and loss of corticomedullary differentiation.

Test: Doppler evaluation
Significance: Of renal arterial and renal venous flow, and radioisotopic reperfusion and excretion studies may be helpful.

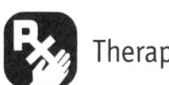 Therapy

GENERAL

- Treatment is supportive and includes correction of fluid and electrolyte disturbances and treatment of infection.
- Correction of underlying pathophysiologic abnormalities should be attempted.
- Management of the complications of azotemia and uremia, including metabolic acidosis, hyperphosphatemia, fluid overload, and hyperosmolality, may require dialysis, particularly in infants.

ANTICOAGULANT

- The effect of anticoagulant therapy has not been documented in controlled studies and remains controversial.
- Heparin should be considered if there is laboratory evidence of continuing disseminated intravascular coagulation.
- Because the lesions are often asynchronous and asymmetrical, prophylactic heparin has been proposed for cases of RVT that are identified early and do not appear to have bilateral involvement.

SURGERY

- A surgical approach in the acute phase is rarely indicated. Surgery, complicated by disturbed fluid balance and acid-base status and altered coagulation, is risky.
- Because the thrombosis begins deep within the kidney and spreads to the larger veins, thrombectomy should be considered only in the event of bilateral involvement with IVC involvement.
- Ultimately, if the kidney has negligible function and contributes to hypertension or recurrent infections, nephrectomy may be indicated.

 Follow-Up

PROGNOSIS

- Depends on the degree of involvement and associated conditions
- Mortality in infants is approximately 30%.
- Recovery of function in affected kidneys may occur. Varying degrees of renal impairment is seen in 30%.
- Hypertension is seen in 20%.
- The majority have residual renal structural abnormalities, such as atrophy and coarse renal scarring.

SIGNS TO WATCH FOR

All patients should be followed closely for evidence of hypertension.

PREVENTION

Infants at increased risk should be recognized. The infant of a diabetic mother should be followed for evidence of RVT. Patients with nephrotic syndrome are at increased risk of thrombosis in general when treated with diuretics. If cyanotic congenital heart disease is present, contrast agents should be used judiciously. Parents and caregivers should be educated about the importance of adequate intake and good hydration in the newborn and infant. Finally, there should be an increased index of suspicion among medical staff when faced with an infant with diarrhea or a hyperosmolar state.

 Common Questions and Answers

Q: Can RVT occur in the absence of gross hematuria?
A: Most patients have hematuria that may be gross. However, the hematuria is often microscopic or absent.

Q: Do patients with RVT usually have hypertension during the acute phase?
A: Hypertension is uncommon at presentation.

ICD-9-CM 453.3

BIBLIOGRAPHY

Adelman RD. Long-term follow-up of neonatal renovascular hypertension. *Pediatr Nephrol* 1987;1:35.

Arneil GC, MacDonald AM, Murphy AV, et al. Renal venous thrombosis. *Clin Nephrol* 1973;1:119.

Duncan RE, Evans TA, Martin LW. Natural history and treatment of renal vein thrombosis in children. *J Pediatr Surg* 1977;12:639.

Jobin J, O'Regan S, Demay G, et al. Neonatal renal vein thrombosis—long-term follow-up after conservative management. *Clin Nephrol* 1982;17:36.

Kaplan BS, Chesney RW, Drummond KN. The nephrotic syndrome and renal vein thrombosis. *Am J Dis Child* 1978;132:367.

Markowitz GS, Brignol F, Burns ER, et al. Renal vein thrombosis treated with thrombolytic therapy: case report and brief review. *Am J Kidney Dis* 1995;25:801–806.

Mocan H, Beattie TJ, Murphy AV. Renal venous thrombosis in infancy: long term follow-up. *Pediatr Nephrol* 1991;5:45.

Oliver WJ, Kelsch RC. Renal venous thrombosis in infancy. *Pediatr Rev* 1982;4:61.

Schmidt B, Andrew M. Neonatal thrombosis: report of a prospective Canadian and international registry. *Pediatrics* 1995;96:939–943.

Author: Mary B. Leonard

Respiratory Syncytial Virus (RSV)

 Database

DEFINITION

• RSV is a pleomorphic enveloped RNA virus of the family Paramyxoviridae. There are two major groups, A and B, that differ in the largest surface glycoprotein, the G protein. The fusion protein, F protein, is approximately 95% homologous between the two subgroups.
• It is the most common cause of bronchiolitis, a viral lower respiratory disease of infants and young children.

PATHOPHYSIOLOGY

• The F protein is responsible for fusing infected cells to adjacent cells, generating a syncytium.
• Infection is initiated in the upper respiratory tract with inoculation of the nose or eyes and may spread to the lower respiratory tract in the younger age child and in those with a primary infection.
• Obstruction of smaller airways occurs secondary to edema, necrotic tissue, and inflammatory cells.
• Virus-induced epithelial damage may expose certain receptors for environmental irritants. Receptor-irritant complexes may contribute to the signs and symptoms of reactive airway disease.

EPIDEMIOLOGY

• Incubation period for RSV is 2 to 4 days.
• Virus is detected in secretions 4 days prior to clinical symptoms and 7 days after the resolution of symptoms (viral shedding demonstrated for as long as 20 days).
• Most effective mode of transmission is via person-to-person spread: by droplet or hand-to-nose contact.
• Nosocomial spread occurs from infected hospital personnel–to-patient spread.
• Peak incidence is the first 2 years of life.
• 50% of children are infected by their first birthday with similar attack rate for the uninfected child during the second year of life.
• 40% to 70% of preschool children and 20% of school-age children are reinfected with exposure.
• There is a worldwide distribution. Temperate climates experience an annual, midwinter epidemic, while epidemics are less predictable in the tropics.
• United States epidemics may begin in November (or as late as May) and last as long as 12 weeks in urban areas.
• One antigenic strain predominates during any given epidemic.

COMPLICATIONS

• Apneic episodes in very young and premature patients.
• Pneumonia, rarely bacterial
• Pneumonitis
• Croup
• Respiratory failure
• Hypoxemia
• Hypercarbia
• Acute otitis media
• Dehydration

Those at greatest risk for severe infection include:

• Age less than 1 year, especially those between the ages of 6 weeks and 6 months
• Children with compromised cardiorespiratory status (e.g., bronchopulmonary dysplasia, congenital heart disease)
• Prematurity
• Immune deficits

PROGNOSIS

• The majority of patients have a mild-to-moderate disease course with symptomatic support.
• Some infected children proceed to more serious illness, necessitating hospitalization. An average hospital stay for previously healthy children is 5 to 7 days; full recovery is 2 weeks.
• Infants with underlying cardiac or pulmonary disease are at increased risk for more severe and longer duration of disease; mortality as high as 30%.
• Reinfections occur throughout life.

 Differential Diagnosis

INFECTION

• Influenza virus
• Parainfluenza virus type 3
• Adenovirus
• Chlamydia

ENVIRONMENTAL

• Foreign body in airway

TUMORS

• Mass compressing upper airway

CONGENITAL

• Tracheomalacia

 Data Gathering

HISTORY

Question: Initial symptoms?
Significance: Nasal discharge, cough, and fever

Question: Cough?
Significance: Typically progresses over 1 to 2 days, with tachypnea developing

Question: Duration of symptoms?
Significance: This will help in the assessment of the typical clinical progression of illness and the anticipated time course for the child.

Other significant points within the history:

• Lethargy, apnea, and possible cyanotic episodes
• Dehydration is secondary to decreased oral intake as well as increased insensible losses. Assess oral intake and urine output to rule out dehydration.
• Increasing respiratory distress?
• Did the child stop breathing/have apnea?

 Physical Examination

• Nasal discharge
• Otitis media
• Pharyngeal injection
• Conjunctivitis
• Respiratory distress with nasal flaring and retractions, grunting, rales, rhonchi, and expiratory wheezing noted on auscultation.
• Risk for hypoxemia increases as the respiratory rate approaches and surpasses 60 breaths per minute.
• Chest may become barrel-shaped in appearance as respiratory distress increases.
• Hyperinflation of the lungs will push liver and spleen into palpable positions within the abdomen.

 Laboratory Aids

• Rapid tests
• Immunofluorescent techniques or ELISA for antigen detection.
• Nasopharyngeal washing with inoculation into culture media.
• Growth should be detected by the appearance of the syncytial cytopathic effect in 3 to 14 days.
• Pulse oximetry to rule out hypoxemia

RADIOGRAPHIC STUDIES

Test: Chest radiograph
Significance: Reveals hyperexpansion, increased bronchial markings, and areas of atelectasis/infiltrate. Note: the pulmonary densities, referred to as "RSV pneumonia," are frequently areas of atelectasis but may represent bacterial infection, especially in the seriously ill patient.

 Emergency Care

Life-threatening apnea may require emergent ventilatory support with mechanical ventilation.

 Therapy

• Supportive care: hydration therapy and supplemental oxygen as needed
• Cardiorespiratory monitoring and pulse oximetry are necessary for infants at risk for apnea and hypoxemia.
• Mechanical ventilation as clinically indicated

DRUGS

• Ribavirin: an antiviral agent, has *in vitro* antiviral activity against RSV but ribavirin aerosol treatment for RSV infections is controversial. The controversy centers around the teratogenicity of ribavirin in humans, its high cost, as well as efficacy trials with conflicting results.
• Corticosteroids have not been shown to be effective.
• β_2-adrenergic agents have not been proven to be effective, but some studies have shown that 25% to 50% of patients with bronchiolitis respond to this therapy. A trial of a bronchodilator is frequently recommended.
• Mist use is considered controversial because it may irritate the airways.
• Antibiotics are rarely indicated since bacterial disease (lung or blood) are uncommon in hospitalized infants with RSV bronchiolitis.

 Follow-Up

• Bronchiolitis will peak in severity over 48 to 72 hours; therefore, reassess the patient if seen early in the disease course.
• Symptoms usually last 7 days but may last up to 2 to 3 weeks with the evidence of reactive airway disease persisting for months to years.
• Periodic breathing may occur 48 to 72 hours postextubation, but recurrent apneic episodes are rare, and home monitoring is usually not indicated.

• Fever commonly resolves over 48 hours.
• Respiratory symptoms commonly improve between days 2 and 5 of illness.
• Evidence of airway hyperactivity may continue for months to years in patients who have had bronchiolitis.

SIGNS TO WATCH FOR

• Respiratory rates greater than 60 per minute and other signs of respiratory failure
• Lethargy, altered mental status
• Prolonged high fever

PREVENTION

• Nosocomial and household spread can be minimized by strict hand washing and avoidance of contact with infected individuals.
• Routine use of gowns and gloves has been shown to decrease RSV nosocomial spread.
• Patients with RSV infection should be isolated in private or RSV-cohorted rooms.
• Nursing care should be cohorted so that nurses are not caring for both RSV infected and noninfected patients.
• Two products are available for the prevention of RSV infection: Respiratory Syncytial Virus Immune Globulin Intravenous (RSV-IGIV), made from RSV antibody positive donor serum and Palivizumab, a humanized monoclonal antibody produced by recombinant DNA technology. Both products are approved for the prevention of RSV disease in select children younger than 2 years of age with bronchopulmonary dysplasia or with a history of prematurity (birth at less than 35 weeks' gestation). Specific recommendations are available from the American Academy of Pediatrics Committee on Infectious Diseases and Committee on Fetus and Newborn for the use of Palivizumab and RSV-IGIV and these criteria should guide the use of these products. RSV-IGIV is given 1 month prior to and monthly throughout RSV season while Palivizumab is given intramuscularly monthly throughout RSV season.

PITFALLS

• RSV is labile at room temperature. Samples should be placed in viral transport media at the bedside and transported to the lab for immediate inoculation to cell culture.
• Instillation and aspiration of 5 mL of isotonic saline is the preferred method of viral collection as opposed to nasal swabs.

 Common Questions and Answers

Q: How did my child get this illness?
A: RSV bronchiolitis is caused by a virus, respiratory syncytial virus, and is passed from one person to another by contact with nasal secretions and through airborne transmission.

Q: For how long is my child contagious?
A: Viral shedding occurs for 24 hours prior to the onset of clinical symptoms and for up to 21 days from the onset of symptoms.

Q: Will my child develop asthma because of the wheezing that is occurring now?
A: Evidence of airway hyperactivity following RSV bronchiolitis may continue for months or even years in some children. It is impossible to predict future episodes of reactive airway disease, but the child should be monitored clinically over time.

Q: If a patient has severe chronic lung disease with a supplemental oxygen requirement and is less than 2 years of age at the onset of the RSV season, should RSV-IGIV or Palivizumab be recommended for this patient?
A: The risks and benefits of each therapy must be evaluated on a patient-by-patient basis. RSV-IGIV provides additional protection against other respiratory viral illnesses and may be considered for some selected high-risk infants. However, palivizumab is preferred for most high-risk children secondary to its ease of administration, safety and effectiveness.

ICD-9-CM 466.1

BIBLIOGRAPHY

AAP Committee on Infectious Diseases and Committee on Fetus and Newborn. Prevention of respiratory syncytial virus infections: indications for the use of Palivizumab and update on the use of RSV-IGIV. *Pediatrics* 1998;102(5):1211–1215.

American Academy of Pediatrics. Respiratory syncytial virus. In: Pickering LK, ed. *Red book 2000: report of the Committee on Infectious Diseases*, 25th ed. Elk Grove Village, IL: American Academy of Pediatrics, 2000: 483–487.

Barton LL, Grant KL, Lemen RJ. Respiratory syncytial virus immune globulin: decisions and costs. *Pediatr Pulmon* 2001;32:20–28.

Darville T, Yamauchi T. Respiratory syncytial virus. *Pediatr Rev* 1998;19(2):55–61.

DeVincenzo JP, Malley R, Ramilo O, et al. Viral concentration in upper and lower respiratory secretions from respiratory syncytial virus (RSV) infected children treated with RSV monoclonal antibody (MEDI-493). *Pediatr Res* 1998;43:144A(abstract 830).

Midulla F, Villani A, Panuska Jr, et al. Respiratory syncytial virus lung infection in infants: immunoregulatory role of infected alveolar macrophages. *J Infect Dis* 1993;168(6):1515–1519.

Author: Kathy Wholey Zsolway

Retinoblastoma

 Database

DEFINITION
- The most common primary intraocular tumor of childhood
- Malignant tumor of the embryonic neural retina

PATHOPHYSIOLOGY
- Originates in retinal cell precursor (retinoblast)
- Histology: small round blue cells with large hyperchromatic nuclei and scant cytoplasm
- Growth of tumor may be endophytic (from inner surface of retina to vitreous) or exophytic (from outer layer of retina into subretinal space); may cause retinal detachment.
- Spread is via optic nerve (common) with potential to invade CNS, direct extension beyond the eye, and lymphatic or hematogenous spread (uncommon).
- Tumor cells may break off from primary mass and grow independently within the eye (called vitreous seeding); single tumor with seeding may be confused with multifocal disease.

GENETICS
- Tumor development depends on loss of function of both copies of the *RB1* gene (located on chromosome 13) in a retinoblast.
- Hereditary and nonhereditary (sporadic) forms exist.

HEREDITARY RB
- 45% of all retinoblastoma.
- One *RB1* gene is dysfunctional in all cells (germline mutation); mutation in remaining *RB1* gene in any retinal cell will lead to development of a tumor.
- 90% probability of second mutation occurring in at least one (but usually more) retinal cells leading to tumor development (high penetrance)
- Therefore, multiple tumors are common (bilateral and/or multifocal).
- Mean age at diagnosis: 12 months
- Only 8% have positive familial history; remainder are new germline mutations.
- Approximately 40% to 45% of offspring will develop RB (autosomal-dominant transmission, 90% penetrance).
- *RB1* gene mutation in all cells predisposes to second (nonretinoblastoma) malignancies as well.

NONHEREDITARY RB
- 55% of all retinoblastoma
- No germline *RB1* mutation; two acquired (somatic) *RB1* mutations must occur in a single retinal cell (a rare event).
- Always unilateral
- Rarely diagnosed before 6 months (mean, 24 months)
- No increased risk of RB in offspring
- No increased risk of second malignancy

EPIDEMIOLOGY
- 1:16,000 to 1:25,000 live births
- The most common primary intraocular tumor of childhood (ocular leukemia most common overall)
- Represents 3% of all pediatric malignancies
- No sex, race, geographic, or socioeconomic predilection
- 90% diagnosed before age 4 years
- Median age at diagnosis for unilateral disease is 24 months and 12 months for bilateral disease (see Genetics, above)

COMPLICATIONS
- Metastatic spread: local spread within orbit, through the optic nerve to brain, or to distant sites (uncommon)
- Loss of eye: surgical enucleation in advanced cases
- Blindness: in advanced, bilateral disease; bilateral enucleation rarely required
- Cosmetic deformity: from enucleation, ocular prosthesis lacks normal eye movements; potential orbital bone hypoplasia secondary to external beam radiation therapy
- Second malignancy: patients with hereditary RB have a predisposition to cancer; this risk is greatly increased by exposure to radiotherapy.

PROGNOSIS
- Mortality from retinoblastoma is 8% (U.S.)
- Survival depends on extent (stage) of disease
- Metastatic disease is uncommon in the U.S. but can occur up to 5 years after diagnosis and has a poor outcome (same for hereditary and nonhereditary).
- Prognosis for vision depends on size and location of tumor(s)
- Second malignancy is most common cause of death in hereditary RB
—These include osteosarcoma (most frequent), pineal blastoma, melanoma, fibrosarcoma, and others.
—Rates of second malignancy in hereditary RB are 10% at 10 years and as high as 40% at 30 years in patients who received XRT (70% of second tumors occur in the field of radiation, 30% elsewhere).

 Differential Diagnosis

- Coats disease: acquired anomaly, males, retinal telangiectasias
- Persistent hyperplastic primary vitreous (PHPV)
- Inflammatory conditions: hypopyon, uveitis, iritis, endophthalmitis
- Toxoplasmosis, *Toxocara canis,* other ocular infections
- Retinopathy of prematurity (ROP)

 Data Gathering

HISTORY
Question: Familial history of retinoblastoma or any eye tumors?
Significance: Hereditary retinoblastoma; siblings may require eye exam

Question: Leukocoria (white pupil, "cat's eye reflex")?
Significance: Often noted in photographs of children with advanced intraocular RB (60%)

Question: Strabismus, either eso- or exotropic (20%)?
Significance: Esotropia is more common in the general population, so exotropia is more suspicious.

Question: Eye complaints?
Significance: RB is rarely painful (unless secondary glaucoma or inflammation is present); vision problems are rare complaints because tumor is usually unilateral.

Question: Inflammation, heterochromia, and glaucoma?
Significance: Rare presentations (<10%)

Question: Neurologic signs, orbital/periorbital masses, bone pain, anorexia, signs of cytopenias?
Significance: May represent metastatic disease

Question: Associated conditions?
Significance: 13q deletion syndrome has RB, dysmorphism, mental retardation, and GU or other anomalies.

 Physical Examination

- Only 3% diagnosed with routine funduscopic examination. Leukocoria more common as presenting sign.

Finding: Proptosis and orbital/periorbital masses
Significance: Late sequelae of mass effect

Finding: Check for red reflex in darkened room.
Significance: Screen for RB in office.
- Evaluate for anisocoria.
- Cover test to assess for strabismus (20%)
- Test vision of each eye independently to identify unilateral RB.

 Laboratory Aids

Test: Ophthalmologic examination
Significance: Confirmation of diagnosis based on ophthalmologic examination by a specialist in pediatric ocular tumors via direct and indirect ophthalmoscopy (and examination under anesthesia, EUA) and by imaging modalities (MRI or CT). Parents and siblings should also undergo ophthalmologic screening in many cases.

Test: Biopsy
Significance: Biopsy confirmation is rarely necessary.

Test: CBC
Significance: Assess for bone marrow involvement

Test: CSF cytology
Significance: Evaluate for leptomeningeal spread (only necessary if tumor has spread beyond the globe).

Test: Chromosome analysis
Significance: Should be performed, but even in hereditary cases only 5% have mutations detectable by this means.

IMAGING
Test: CT or MRI
Significance: Evaluate primary tumor (80% have calcification) and optic nerve extension, leptomeningeal spread, pineal blastoma (in 4% of patients with hereditary RB = "trilateral RB").

STAGING
• Intraocular and extraocular staging systems exist.
• Most RB in the United States is intraocular without metastatic disease.
• Patients with tumor extension outside the globe should have an LP and bone marrow evaluation for complete staging.

 ## Therapy

• Primary goals
—Eradicate tumor.
—Prevent metastasis.
• Secondary goals
—Salvage the eye and retain useful vision.
—Cosmetic considerations

Treatment must be individualized, depending on bilateral or unilateral disease, potential for salvageable vision, and evidence of local extension or metastatic disease. Referral to a center with oncologic and ophthalmologic specialists is essential.
• Minimal (nonbulky) intraocular disease
—Plaque radiotherapy (sewn to episcleral surface above RB lesion): local XRT to tumor in selected solitary RBs, up to 16 mm in diameter with or without vitreous seeds
—Photocoagulation (laser): for selected small RBs, usually less than 3 mm
—Cryotherapy (topical freeze technique): for selected RBs less than 3 to 4 mm in diameter without vitreous seeding, which are located anteriorly in the eye
• Bulky intraocular disease
—Current trend is toward eye salvage therapy: initial chemotherapy for tumor reduction followed by local definitive therapy (as for nonbulky disease).

—Tumor resection without enucleation is not possible because of risk of tumor spillage; enucleation of involved eye (with long segment of optic nerve removal to ensure tumor-free margins) may be required for large tumors refractory to chemoreduction or when vision is not salvageable.
—External beam radiation therapy (EBRT): RB is extremely radiosensitive; however, increases risk of second malignancy (especially in hereditary RB). Other effects: dry eye, cataract, retinopathy, and cosmetic deformity from bone maldevelopment. EBRT is still an important modality but is avoided whenever effective alternative therapies are available.
• Metastatic disease
—Multiagent chemotherapy with or without autologous bone marrow transplantation; poor results to date
—Effective treatment requires multidisciplinary collaboration between ophthalmologists, oncologists, and radiation oncologists.

 ## Follow-Up

• Frequent ophthalmologic examinations (including EUA) are mandatory to evaluate response to therapy and to screen for disease progression, particularly in hereditary RB.
• Therapy must include genetic counseling regarding the risk of second malignancies (with or without adjuvant XRT), risk to siblings, as well as the risk to future children of affected patients with hereditary RB.
• Primary care physicians must be aware of the risks of second malignancies (see Prognosis, above) and maintain an appropriately high index of suspicion for their development.
• Primary care physicians should be aware of the genetics of RB and screen siblings appropriately.

PREVENTION
Siblings and children of patients with RB should undergo ophthalmologic examinations under anesthesia to detect the presence of RB early.

PITFALLS
• Missed or delayed diagnosis: ophthalmologic examination by a specialist in pediatric ocular tumors required to establish diagnosis and follow regression or recurrence in treated eyes, follow for development of new tumors in hereditary cases
• Failure to recognize the possibility that a child with RB has a genetic predisposition, especially in the frequent setting where there is no familial history of RB
• Failure to refer for appropriate genetic counseling

 ## Common Questions and Answers

Q: What is the risk that a child with RB will become blind?
A: Vision is salvageable in 100% of eyes with low-stage involvement, and in 81% overall. In less than 10% of patients are both eyes affected severely enough to threaten vision (bilateral disease only occurs in hereditary RB).

Q: What is the chance that a child with RB in one eye will get it in the other?
A: Bilateral disease is seen with hereditary RB. A child with unilateral disease has a 15% chance of having hereditary RB, which would put the contralateral eye at risk; this risk is much higher if the child has multifocal involvement or is less than 1 year of age.

Q: What happens to the eye socket after an enucleation?
A: Prostheses can be made to fit the socket of the enucleated eye to give excellent cosmetic results.

Q: Is there a test to identify hereditary cases?
A: Routine chromosome analysis does not reveal the defective RB gene in the majority (95%) of hereditary cases. Specialized molecular tests may be used in research labs, but since there are many possible mutations, this is costly and time-consuming. In general, hereditary cases are determined clinically because of young presentation, family history, and/or bilateral or multifocal unilateral disease.

ICD-9-CM 190.5

BIBLIOGRAPHY
Abramson DH, Frank CM, Susman M, et al. Presenting signs of retinoblastoma. *J Pediatr* 1998;132(3 pt 1):505–508.

Donaldson SS, Eghert PR, Newsham I, et al. Retinoblastoma. In: Pizzo PA, Poplack DG, eds. *Principles and practice of pediatric oncology*, 3rd ed. Philadelphia/New York: Lippincott-Raven, 1997:699–715.

Gallie BL, Dunn JM, Chan HS, et al. The genetics of retinoblastoma: relevance to the patient. *Pediatr Clin North Am* 1991;38:299–315.

Magramm I. Amblyopia: etiology, detection, and treatment. *Pediatr Rev* 1992;13(1):7–14.

Nahum MP, Gdal-On M, Kuten A, et al. Long-term follow-up of children with retinoblastoma. *Pediatr Hematol Oncol* 2001;18(3):173–179.

Shields JA, Shields CL. Clinicopathologic factors related to metastasis in retinoblastoma. *Mayo Clinic Proc* 1994;69:50–56.

Author: Michael D. Hogarty

Retropharyngeal Abscess

 Database

DEFINITION

A relatively rare but potentially life-threatening infection occurring in the potential space bounded by the layers of cervical fascia posterior to the esophagus and anterior to the deep cervical fascia.

CAUSES

• Infectious: Cultures usually reveal multiple organisms, predominantly.
• *Streptococcus* (group A and others)
• *Staphylococcus aureus*
• Various anaerobic species (*Bacteroides, Peptostreptococcus,* and *Fusobacterium*)
• One pediatric study cultured *Haemophilus influenzae* type b in 20% of cases; however, the study took place before the routine use of *H. influenzae* type b conjugate vaccines.
• Many of the isolates are β-lactamase producers.

PATHOPHYSIOLOGY

The majority of infections follow a pharyngitis or supraglottitis and occur secondary to suppuration of the retropharyngeal lymph nodes, which lie in two paramedial chains and drain various nasopharyngeal structures. Other sources of infection in this space include penetrating trauma, such as from foreign object aspiration, dental procedures, or attempts at intubation. Extension of infection into this space can arise from vertebral body osteomyelitis or petrositis.

EPIDEMIOLOGY

Most large children's hospital centers report one to three cases per year. Children younger than 6 years of age are most at risk, with half of the cases occurring in infants younger than 36 months of age.

COMPLICATIONS

• Spontaneous rupture with aspiration of infected material, with subsequent asphyxia or overwhelming pulmonary infection
• Hemorrhage from extension into local arteries, and/or venous thrombosis from involvement of major neck vessels
• Extension of the infection inferiorly can occur, leading to a subdiaphragmatic or psoas abscess.

PROGNOSIS

Excellent with appropriate antibiotics, expectant care, and surgery, if needed, at optimal time

 Differential Diagnosis

• Pharyngitis
• Peritonsillar or lateral wall abscess
• Epiglottitis/supraglottitis

 Data Gathering

HISTORY

• Symptoms may be present from hours to days before correct diagnosis. Many patients will have been on oral antibiotics for presumed pharyngitis/sinusitis.
• Most frequent symptoms include sore throat, decreased oral intake, muffled voice, drooling, stiff or painful neck, fever, dysphagia, and stridor.
• Preceding neck trauma? Especially penetrating injuries, recent surgery (especially dental), and history consistent with aspiration of a foreign object.

Physical Examination

Most frequent signs are:

- Fever
- Stridor (seen in up to 50% of children)
- Drooling
- A tender cervical neck region with restricted range of motion
- Classic diagnostic finding of a bulging posterior pharyngeal wall. May be absent or difficult to appreciate in an ill, apprehensive child.

 ## Laboratory Aids

Test: CBC
Significance: Frequently reveals an elevated total WBC, with a significant left shift

Test: Lateral neck x-ray
Significance: Reveals widening of retropharyngeal space and at times an air fluid level

Test: CT scan or MRI of the neck
Significance: The most definitive test, which can usually differentiate abscess from local cellulitis/adenitis

 ## Therapy

- Emergent therapy requires maintaining patent airway; be wary of sudden spontaneous drainage of the abscess, with catastrophic aspiration.
- Careful in-hospital monitoring of airway and fluid intake.
- Start broad-spectrum parental antibiotics, active against *Streptococcus pneumoniae, S. aureus,* and oral anaerobic organisms. If patient does not improve, broaden coverage to include drugs active against β-lactamase producing organisms and anaerobic organisms. Clindamycin or ampicillin/sulbactam are good initial choices.
- Immediate consultation with otolaryngology surgical team. Schedule of incision/aspiration of abscess at optimal time, with team experienced in airway management of small children. CT-guided aspiration of the abscess has aided the surgical approach at many sites.
- In selected mild, early cases (especially if the CT scan is consistent with cellulitis rather than true abscess), parenteral antibiotics may be sufficient for therapy. Recent data suggest that up to 50% of patients can be successfully managed without surgical intervention. Patients treated with antibiotics alone must be followed closely for signs of worsening clinical status.

PITFALLS

- Physicians must maintain a high index of suspicion. The presentation of a retropharyngeal abscess can be subtle, with the most frequent initial diagnostic impression usually epiglottitis or severe pharyngitis.
- Both plain films and CT scan have false positives and false negatives.
- Once diagnosis is made, urgent consultation with experienced surgical staff is mandatory.

ICD-9-CM 478.24

BIBLIOGRAPHY

Brook I. Microbiology of retropharyngeal abscess in children. *Am J Dis Child* 1987;141:202–204.

Gaglani MJ, Edwards MS. Clinical indicators of childhood retropharyngeal abscess. *Am J Emerg Med* 1995;13:333–336.

Hammerschlag PE, Hammerschlag MR. Retropharyngeal abscess. In: Feigin R, Cherry JD, eds. *Textbook of pediatric infectious diseases*, 3rd ed. Philadelphia: WB Saunders, 1992:168–171.

Lee SS, Schwartz RH, Babadori RS. Retropharyngeal abscess: epiglottitis of the new millennium. *J Pediatr* 2001;178:435–437.

Lee SS, Schwartz RH, Bahadori RS. Retropharyngeal abscess: epiglottitis of the new millennium. *J Pediatr* 2001;138(3):435–437.

Morrison JE Jr, Pashley RT. Retropharyngeal abscess in children: a ten year review. *Pediatr Emerg Care* 1988;4:9–11.

Nagy M, Pizzuto M, Backstrom J, et al. Deep neck infections in children: a new approach to diagnosis and treatment. *Laryngoscope* 1997;107:1627–1634.

Toback SA, Carcillo J. Index of suspicion. Case #3. Discussion: retropharyngeal abscess. *Pediatr Rev* 2000;21(11):389–392.

Author: Richard M. Rutstein

Reye Syndrome

 Database

DEFINITION

Acute encephalopathy and fatty degeneration of the liver

PATHOPHYSIOLOGY

- Mitochondrial injury of unknown etiology results in reduction of hepatic intramitochondrial enzymes.
- Salicylates exacerbate condition when ingested after mitochondrial injury

EPIDEMIOLOGY

- Peak incidence age 6
- Most children range from 4 to 12 years
- More common among whites in rural and suburban communities
- Association with ingestion of aspirin-containing medicines by children with varicella or influenza B

COMPLICATIONS

- Elevated intracranial pressure secondary to cerebral edema
- Mortality greater than 40%

 Differential Diagnosis

- CNS infections (e.g., meningitis, encephalitis)
- Toxins
- Drug ingestion (e.g., salicylates, valproate)
- Metabolic diseases: In a report by Hou and colleagues, Reye-like syndrome was secondary to hereditary organic acidemias ($n = 13$), urea cycle defects ($n = 4$), mitochondrial disorders ($n = 3$), fulminant hepatitis ($n = 2$), tyrosinemia ($n = 1$), and valproate-associated hepatotoxicity ($n = 1$).

 Data Gathering

HISTORY

Question: Prodromal illness?
Significance: URI—influenza A (90%), hepatitis A, and varicella

Question: Abrupt onset of vomiting?
Significance: Onset within 4 to 7 days of initial illness.

Question: What is the natural history?
Significance: Followed by neurologic deterioration in which delirium may progress to seizures, coma, or death

 Physical Examination

- Slight liver enlargement without jaundice
- Absence of focal neurologic signs

Neurologic examination varies with stage of disease:

- Stage I: vomiting with obtundation, subtle cognitive and behavioral disturbances
- Stage II: agitated delirium and coma, may see decorticate posturing
- Stage III: hyperventilation, tachycardia, decerebrate posturing, sluggishness
- Stage IV: respiratory failure with signs of elevated intracranial pressure
- Stage V: respiratory arrest, loss of deep tendon reflexes, fixed dilated pupils

Laboratory Aids

Test: Ammonia
Significance: May be normal at the onset of vomiting

Test: Liver and muscle function testing
Significance: Elevated transaminases, creatinine kinase, lactate dehydrogenase, ammonia, and prothrombin time (PT)

Test: CSF
Significance: Normal except for elevated intracranial pressure (ICP)

Test: EEG
Significance: Characteristic of metabolic encephalopathy with generalized slow wave abnormalities

PATHOLOGY (POSTMORTEM)

Test: Liver
Significance: Grossly yellowish white in appearance secondary to increased triglycerides; foamy cytoplasm with increased microvesicular fat, decreased glycogen.

Test: Brain
Significance: Marked edema with increased intracellular fluid, and abnormal neuronal mitochondria

 Therapy

- Should be tailored based on severity of presentation
- IV glucose to counteract effects of glycogen depletion
- Fluid restriction in patients with cerebral edema (1,500 mL/m^2/d), along with mannitol to increase serum osmolality and induce cerebral dehydration.
- Vitamin K, fresh frozen plasma, and platelets as needed for treatment of secondary coagulopathy

 Follow-Up

- Cerebral function at presentation is the best predictor of outcome.
- Majority have mild illness without progression
- Patients with mild disease (stage I) recover completely.
- Patients with stage II disease may show complete recovery or subtle neurologic sequelae.
- Patients with stage III to IV disease often do not survive.

PITFALLS

Failure to recognize early and central or prevent cerebral edema—the immediate cause of death

 Common Questions and Answers

Q: Is Reye syndrome fatal?
A: More than 40% of children will die secondary to cerebral edema. Mortality rates are best predicted by neurologic state at the onset of presentation.

Q: How can the neurologic findings of Reye syndrome be differentiated from meningitis?
A: Aside from an elevated ICP, the lumbar taps of patients with Reye syndrome are at best remarkable. Elevated white count is not seen in these cases.

ICD-9-CM 331.81

BIBLIOGRAPHY

DeVivo DC. Acute encephalopathies of childhood. In: Rudolph AM, ed. *Rudolph's pediatrics*, 19th ed. Norwalk, CT: Appleton & Lange, 1991:1713–1720.

Duerksen DR, Jewell LD, Mason AL, et al. Co-existence of hepatitis A and adult Reye's syndrome. *Gut* 1997;41(1):121–124

Green CL, Blitzer MG, Shapiro E. Inborn errors of metabolism and Reye's syndrome: differential diagnosis. *J Pediatr* 1988;113:156.

Hou JW, Chou SP, Wang TR. Metabolic function and liver histopathology in Reye-like illnesses. *Acta Paediatr* 1996;85(9):1053–1057.

Lichtenstein PK, Heubi JE, Dougherty CC, et al. Grade I Reye's syndrome: a frequent cause of vomiting and liver dysfunction after varicella and upper respiratory tract infection. *N Engl J Med* 1983;309:133.

Reye RDK, Morgan G, Baral J. Encephalopathy and fatty degeneration of the viscera: a disease entity in childhood. *Lancet* 1963;2:749.

Author: Andrew E. Mulberg

Rhabdomyolysis

 Database

DEFINITION

- Muscle injury resulting from trauma, infection, or inadequate delivery, production, or consumption of energy or oxygen relative to demands. The release of intracellular contents may cause severe electrolyte disturbances including life-threatening hyperkalemia, myoglobinuria, and acute renal failure.
- Rhabdomyolysis is uncommon in childhood.

PATHOPHYSIOLOGY

- The most common causes include muscle trauma from crush injury, burns, or electric shock. Others include viral illnesses such as influenza and Epstein-Barr virus infection, heat stroke, severe exertion, status epilepticus, and vasculitis with myositis.
- Rare causes in childhood include many congenital muscle enzyme and energy substrate deficiencies, acute dystonic reactions complicating hereditary torsion dystonia, other infections, exposure to certain medications (e.g., inhalation anesthetics, propofol, and chemotherapeutic agents), toxins (e.g., snake venom, hydrocarbons), and illicit drugs, and severe electrolyte abnormalities including hypophosphatemia, hypokalemia, and hypernatremia. Copper-induced rhabdomyolysis has been reported in patients with Wilson disease.
- Rhabdomyolysis is more likely to occur following exertion in the dystrophinopathies, which include all forms of muscular dystrophy.
- The insult may lead to muscle cell destruction or failure of membrane function with release of intracellular contents including proteins and electrolytes.
- Although not approved for use in pediatric patients, the lipid lowering "statin" drugs, for example, Mevacor, may cause rhabdomyolysis.

GENETICS

Many of the rare causes of rhabdomyolysis, including muscle enzyme deficiencies, muscular dystrophy, and disorders of mitochondrial metabolism, are heritable disorders, and a familial history should be sought.

EPIDEMIOLOGY

Rhabdomyolysis is more common in adults, where it is seen most frequently in comatose patients resulting from heroin or cocaine abuse.

COMPLICATIONS

- Electrolyte release from muscle can lead to hyperkalemia, hyperphosphatemia, and secondarily to hypocalcemia.
- Acute renal failure may occur secondary to myoglobinuria.

ASSOCIATED ILLNESSES

In addition to the previously mentioned causes, rhabdomyolysis has also been reported associated with diverse conditions, including asthma, hemolytic uremic syndrome, and diabetes mellitus.

PROGNOSIS

The prognosis depends on the amount of permanent renal disease, delay in treatment, and the response to treatment. Many cases recover completely.

 Differential Diagnosis

- Includes any condition associated with muscle pain, tenderness, and/or weakness
- Examples include many viral illnesses, Lyme disease, suppurative myositis, Guillain-Barré syndrome, and collagen vascular diseases.

 Data Gathering

HISTORY

Question: Has there been increased exertion, viral illness, muscle injury, or electrical shock?
Significance: These conditions are associated with muscle breakdown and rhabdomyolysis.

Question: Is there familial history of muscle disease or reaction to anesthesia?
Significance: Rhabdomyolysis is associated with muscular dystrophy and reaction to drugs such as anesthetics.

SPECIAL QUESTIONS

- Antecedent history of illness or insult associated with rhabdomyolysis? Rhabdomyolysis may follow certain illnesses (e.g., influenza) and insults (e.g., crush injury) and thus a history of these should be sought.
- Muscle pain or weakness? These may result from rhabdomyolysis and may help suggest the diagnosis if present.
- Brownish discoloration of the urine?

Physical Examination

- Palpation of muscle for tenderness
- Testing for motor strength
- Eliciting reflexes to exclude neuropathy
- Examination of skin and mucous membranes for signs of vasculitis

 ## Laboratory Aids

- Serum electrolytes (high K_1, normal or low NA_1), calcium, and phosphorus
- BUN and creatinine: creatinine is elevated out of proportion to BUN.
- Creatine phosphokinase will be elevated greater than 100 times normal in rhabdomyolysis.
- Urinalysis
- CBC

Finding: Definitive tests for myoglobinuria
Significance: Immunoelectrophoresis and radioimmunoassay, are not generally available in clinical laboratories. Ammonium sulfate solubility testing is a reasonable test to differentiate myoglobin from hemoglobin.

Finding: Muscle biopsy
Significance: To demonstrate immunohisto-chemical features and immunoblotting to show abnormalities of the dystrophin gene may be required to evaluate the dystrophinopathies.

Finding: False positives
Significance: The dipstick for blood is positive, but examination of a freshly voided urinary sediment reveals few or no erythrocytes. In this instance, the possibilities are myoglobinuria or hemoglobinuria.

Finding: Very rapid rise in serum creatinine
Significance: May occur as a result of release from muscle

 ## Therapy

GENERAL

- Treatment is supportive. If an underlying cause is identified, it should be corrected or removed.
- Adequate hydration (e.g., 2–3 times maintenance fluids) should be sufficient to provide brisk urine flow (e.g., greater than 4 mL/kg/h). Myoglobinuric nephrotoxicity is the only entity where acute renal failure can be averted by maintaining good urine flow. Alkalinization of the urine is probably beneficial. Furosemide and/or mannitol may be helpful to maintain urine output.
- Dialysis is indicated if oliguric acute renal failure occurs and/or if severe electrolyte disturbances are present.

DRUGS

- With myoglobinuria, bicarbonate therapy should be given intravenously to maintain the urine pH above 7.
- If urine output falls in the face of adequate hydration, furosemide (1–4 mg/kg/dose IV) should be given to attempt to prevent oliguric renal failure.
- If severe hyperkalemia occurs, measures should be taken to prevent cardiac dysrhythmias (calcium, bicarbonate, glucose, and insulin) and to maximize elimination of potassium by the kidneys (furosemide) and/or gastrointestinal tract (Kayexalate).
- With hypocalcemia, give calcium only if symptoms are present.

POSSIBLE CONFLICTS

- Furosemide may interfere with alkalinization of the urine.
- Use of bicarbonate may precipitate symptomatic hypocalcemia.
- Calcium therapy for severe hyperkalemia is necessary, but its use with hyperphos-phatemia increases risk of metastatic calcification.
- Risk factors for acute renal failure include preexisting renal disease, concurrent use of nephrotoxic agents, volume depletion, and either hypotension or hypertension.
- Failure to discontinue intravenous fluids if oligoanuric renal failure develops could result in iatrogenic fluid overload.

 ## Follow-Up

WHEN TO EXPECT IMPROVEMENT

- Prompt cessation of rhabdomyolysis may be expected when the inciting cause is corrected or resolves.
- With resolution of the myoglobinuria, return to normal renal function is the rule.

PITFALLS

Failure to check for muscle breakdown in cases of child abuse

ICD-9-CM 728.89

BIBLIOGRAPHY

Brumback RA, Feeback DL, Leech RW. Rhabdomyolysis in childhood. *Pediatr Clin North Am* 1992;39:821–858.

Chamberlain MC. Rhabdomyolysis in children: a 3-year retrospective study. *Pediatr Neurol* 1991;7:226–228.

DiGiacomo JC, Frankel H, Haskell RM, et al. Unsuspected child abuse revealed by delayed presentation of periportal tracking and myoglobinuria. *J Trauma* 2000;49(2): 348–350.

Singh U, Scheld, WM. Infectious etiologies of rhabdomyolysis: three case reports and review. *Clin Infect Dis* 1996;22:642–649.

Sungur M, Guven M. Rhabdomyolysis caused by electric injury. *J Emerg Med* 2001;20(2): 195–196.

Author: Thomas L. Kennedy III

Rhabdomyosarcoma

 Database

DEFINITION
Malignant tumor of mesenchymal cells committed to skeletal muscle lineage. Etiology is unknown.

PATHOLOGY
• One of the "small round blue" cell tumors of childhood.
• Two major subtypes:
—Alveolar (19% of cases): small round cells with dense appearance, line up along spaces resembling pulmonary alveoli, associated with translocation between chromosomes 2 and 13, or less commonly 1 and 13.
—Embryonal (60% of cases): spindle-shaped cells, less densely cellular with stroma-rich appearance, associated with a chromosomal abnormality on the short arm of chromosome 11 (chromosome 11p15).
• Undifferentiated and pleomorphic types comprise the remaining cases.

GENETICS
• Majority of cases occur sporadically
• Several predisposing factors include:
—Li-Fraumeni syndrome (family cancer syndrome associated with germline mutations of the p53 gene on chromosome 17 and an autosomal-dominant inheritance) includes rhabdomyosarcoma and other soft tissue sarcomas, leukemia, brain tumors, adrenocortical carcinoma, and early-onset breast carcinoma in female relatives.
—Patients with Beckwith-Wiedemann syndrome (fetal overgrowth syndrome characterized by an abnormality at chromosome 11p15) have an increased incidence of primarily Wilms tumor, but also hepatoblastoma, rhabdomyosarcoma, and other tumors of embryonal origin.
—Neurofibromatosis type I (autosomal-dominant genetic disorder characterized by mutation of the NF1 gene on chromosome 17q11.2) is associated with an increased risk of rhabdomyosarcoma, other soft tissue sarcomas (malignant nerve sheath tumors, neurofibrosarcomas), leukemia, Wilms tumor, and brain tumors.
—Previous radiation exposure, especially in patients with Li-Fraumeni, neurofibromatosis type I or hereditary retinoblastoma (RB1 germline mutation)
—Congenital anomalies of the genitourinary system and central nervous system are more frequent than expected in children with rhabdomyosarcoma.

EPIDEMIOLOGY
• Slightly more than 200 new cases are diagnosed each year in the United States.
• Third most common extracranial solid tumor of childhood after neuroblastoma and Wilms' tumor
• 50% of cases are diagnosed in children younger than 6 years of age with smaller incidence peak in mid-adolescence.

• 1.3 times more common in males than females.
• Associations: fetal alcohol syndrome, central nervous system and genitourinary anomalies, tobacco smoking in fathers, and marijuana and cocaine use in mothers and fathers in the year prior to the child's birth

COMPLICATIONS
• Rhabdomyosarcoma can compromise function of surrounding organs.
• Metastatic spread may occur to lymph nodes, lung, bone, bone marrow, liver, or brain.

PROGNOSIS
• Overall, 70% of patients can be cured.
• Prognosis by primary site (5-year survival):

Orbit	95%
Other head and neck	78%
Parameningeal	74%
Paratesticular/vagina	89%
Bladder/prostate	81%
Extremities	74%
Other sites	67%

• Although 50% of patients with distant metastatic disease can be placed into remission, only 20% can be cured.
• Tumors with alveolar histology (typically extremity lesions) tend to metastasize early.
• Recurrence can occur many years after completion of therapy but is rare after 3 years.

 Differential Diagnosis

• Malignant
—Ewing sarcoma
—Neuroblastoma
—Non-Hodgkin lymphoma
—Leukemic chloroma
—Germ cell tumor
—Rare soft tissue sarcomas
• Nonmalignant
—Trauma
—Benign tumors: lipoma, rhabdomyoma, neurofibroma
—Langerhans cell histiocytosis
—Abscess

 Data Gathering

HISTORY
• A painless, firm swelling or mass is the most common presentation.
• Other symptoms depend on site of origin:
—Head/neck: nasal congestion or discharge, otorrhea, cranial nerve palsies, proptosis, headache, vomiting or systemic hypertension (with intracranial growth of tumor)
—Genitourinary/pelvic: urinary frequency or retention, hematuria, constipation, vaginal discharge or bleeding
—Extremity: painful or painless lumps or erythema
—Trunk: usually few symptoms until tumor widespread

 Physical Examination

• Can occur in any location, even in sites in which skeletal muscle is not normally found
• Distribution of primary tumor sites include the following:
—Head and neck (38%): parameningeal (middle ear, nasal cavity, paranasal sinuses, nasopharynx, infratemporal fossa, pterygopalatine fossa, parapharyngeal area); orbit (orbit, eyelid); nonparameningeal (scalp, parotid, oral cavity, larynx, oropharynx, cheek, hypopharynx, thyroid, parathyroid, neck)
—Genitourinary tract (21%): bladder and prostate; uterus, vagina, vulva, and paratesticular region
—Extremity (18%)
—Trunk (7%)
—Retroperitoneum (7%)
• Special attention should be given to physical examination of lymphatic structures and surrounding tissues as this may identify local invasion and/or lymphatogenous spread.

 Laboratory Aids

TESTS
Laboratory Tests
• CBC
• Electrolytes, liver and renal function tests, serum calcium, phosphorus in anticipation of starting chemotherapy

Imaging and Other Tests
To evaluate primary site and confirm diagnosis:
• CT scan or, preferably, MRI scan
• Biopsy: In addition to routine morphologic and immunohistochemical stain assessments, analysis of tumor chromosomes by traditional cytogenetics, fluorescent in situ hybridization or reverse-transcriptase PCR is helpful in making the diagnosis and may provide information regarding prognosis. Because of the importance of these studies, consultation with a pediatric oncologist before the biopsy is strongly encouraged.

To evaluate for evidence of distant metastases (present in 20% of patients at diagnosis):
• Chest radiograph and CT scan
• ^{99m}Tc-diphosphonate bone scan
• Bilateral aspiration and biopsy of iliac bone marrow
• Lumbar puncture for CSF cytology (parameningeal tumors only; to determine if CNS invasion has occurred)

Therapy

- Therapy is a multimodal approach based on location and extent of disease.
—Surgery
—Chemotherapy: common agents used include vincristine, dactinomycin, cyclophosphamide, doxorubicin, etoposide, and ifosfamide.
—Radiation therapy.
- Duration of therapy depends on location and extent of disease.
- Surgical trend is toward less radical surgery with organ preservation.
- Most children are treated according to large cooperative group protocols at pediatric oncology centers.
- Treatment is characterized by significant side effects including increased susceptibility to infection, severe mucositis, and poor nutritional status.
- Most patients require placement of an indwelling central venous catheter for the duration of their therapy.
- Experimental therapies such as high-dose chemotherapy with stem cell rescue and immunotherapy (vaccination with fusion-gene peptide products, immunomodulators such as interleukin-2 and granulocyte-macrophage colony-stimulating factor) are being investigated in clinical trials for patients with high-risk or relapsed disease.

Follow-Up

WHEN TO EXPECT IMPROVEMENT
All patients with rhabdomyosarcoma require 1 to 2 years of chemotherapy to prevent recurrence in the original site of tumor or distant spread. However, some improvement in signs and symptoms is usually seen within the first several weeks of therapy.

ACUTE EFFECTS OF THERAPY
Therapy for rhabdomyosarcoma is intensive. Patients can expect many of the following side effects:
- Frequent admissions to the hospital for chemotherapy or complications of the therapy.
- Complications from bone marrow suppressive effects of chemotherapy or radiotherapy:
—Anemia: blood transfusions are usually necessary; erythropoietin (a stimulator of erythropoiesis) is given to many patients to reduce the number of transfusions required.
—Thrombocytopenia: platelet transfusions are often necessary to reduce the risk of serious bleeding.
—Neutropenia: increased risk of bacterial and fungal infections; G-CSF (granulocyte-colony stimulating factor) is usually administered daily following chemotherapy to shorten the duration of neutropenia.

- Complications from the gastrointestinal side effects of chemotherapy or radiotherapy:
—Nausea and vomiting; relieved with ondansetron and other antiemetic agents.
—Malnutrition secondary to reduced appetite and mucosal ulcerations; nutritional supplements (oral, nasogastric, gastrostomy tube or parenteral) may be necessary.
- Complication from radiotherapy:
—Skin erythema or breakdown.

LATE EFFECTS OF THERAPY
Therapy for rhabdomyosarcoma is intensive, and is associated with significant long-term adverse effects. Regular follow-up with a pediatric oncologist is strongly recommended.
- Cardiomyopathy
—Anthracyclines (doxorubicin) weaken cardiac muscle leading to reduced left ventricular function many years after therapy.
—Approximately 5% of patients receiving cumulative doses of doxorubicin greater than 500 mg/m^2 will develop congestive heart failure.
—Radiation to the heart can lower the cumulative dose threshold to 300 mg/m^2.
—Any patient who has received an anthracycline should be cautioned against initiating strenuous physical activity without adequate preparation.
—Pregnant women who have received anthracyclines in the past should inform their obstetrician so that appropriate cardiac assessment can be completed prior to vaginal delivery.
- Kidney and bladder damage
—Urinalysis should be performed to detect hemorrhagic cystitis or tubular damage.
—Blood pressure should be monitored in patients who received irradiation to the kidneys; vascular damage and hypertension may develop many years after therapy.
- Infertility and delayed puberty
—Reduced or absent gonadal function is related to high doses of alkylating agents (cyclophosphamide, ifosfamide): males are at high risk of azoospermia; females may be fertile, but are at risk for premature menopause.
—Low-dose estrogen therapy with oral contraceptive medications may be necessary for amenorrheic women.
—Retrograde ejaculation may be seen following surgery for paratesticular tumors.
- Second malignant neoplasms
—Sarcomas may occur within the radiation field.
—Myelodysplastic syndromes and acute myeloid leukemia may occur secondary to radiation or chemotherapy (cyclophosphamide, etoposide)
- Bowel obstruction and enteritis (abdominal-pelvic tumors)
—Adhesions as a consequence of surgery or radiation
—A history of failure to gain weight or symptoms of malabsorption suggests a need for additional evaluation.

- Growth abnormalities/functional defects at the primary site
—Radiation doses greater than 20 Gy will cause growth retardation in growing children.
—Scoliosis can occur if the vertebrae are involved in the radiation field.
—Cataracts can occur after irradiation involving the head.

Common Questions and Answers

Q: Can a child with rhabdomyosarcoma receive immunizations during therapy?
A: Immunizations are not recommended during treatment because they are not likely to be effective since chemotherapy is immunosuppressive. The oral polio vaccine should not be administered to other household members, but they can receive the inactivated polio vaccine and all other immunizations.

Q: Can a child with rhabdomyosarcoma attend school?
A: As the chemotherapy for rhabdomyosarcoma is intensive, most children are unable to continue with school during this time, but will benefit from home-bound instruction.

Q: Is the treatment associated with infertility?
A: The present chemotherapy regimens include high cumulative doses of alkylating agents, placing males, in particular, at high risk for infertility. Sperm banking, therefore, is recommended in adolescent males, prior to the initiation of chemotherapy.

ICD-9-CM 171.9

BIBLIOGRAPHY
McCarville MB, Spunt SL, Pappo AS. Rhabdomyosarcoma in pediatric patients: the good, the bad, and the unusual. *AJR* 2001;176(6):1563–1569.

Pappo AS, Shapiro DN, Crist WM. Rhabdomyosarcoma: biology and treatment. *Pediatr Clin North Am* 1997;44(4):953–972.

Ruymann FB, Grovas AC. Progress in the diagnosis and treatment of rhabdomyosarcoma and related soft tissue sarcomas. *Cancer Invest* 2000;3:223–224.

Wexler LH, Helman LJ. Pediatric soft tissue sarcomas. *CA Cancer J Clin* 1994;44:211–247.

Womer RB. Soft tissue sarcomas. *Eur J Cancer* 1997;33(13):2230–2234.

Author: Kara M. Kelly

Rheumatic Fever (RF)

 Database

DEFINITION
Postinfectious immune response to group A streptococcus that results in a diffuse inflammatory disease involving multiple organ systems

PATHOPHYSIOLOGY
• Immune-mediated inflammatory reaction to specific rheumatogenic strains of group A β-hemolytic streptococci (GABHS) that affects connective tissue, namely the heart, joints, brain, blood vessels, and subcutaneous tissue. Streptococcal pharyngitis precedes the onset of acute rheumatic fever (ARF) by approximately 3 weeks.
• "Antigenic mimicry" occurs in which antigen similarities between epitopes of specific rheumatogenic streptococci and host tissue cause an autoimmune cross-reaction where produced antibodies damage the host.
• Aschoff nodules are proliferative lesions noted in the myocardium that may persist for months to years after the initiation of disease.

GENETICS
Increased familial incidence reported, therefore suggesting a genetic predisposition

EPIDEMIOLOGY
• Estimated 3% of patients with untreated or inadequately treated streptococcal pharyngitis develop ARF.
• Initial episode primarily seen between 5 to 15 years of age.
• Incidence (United States) is 0.5 to 3.1/100,000 with a resurgence in the mid-1980s.
• No longer a disease mainly found in socially and economically disadvantaged groups in the United States, yet the incidence is higher in underdeveloped countries.
• Rheumatogenic strains of group A streptococci with specific M proteins have been associated with outbreaks of ARF.

COMPLICATIONS
Cardiac
• Pancarditis (always a component of valvulitis)
—Pericarditis (including pericardial effusion) and/or myocarditis (these entities are almost always associated with valvulitis)
—Transient arrhythmias occur infrequently.
—Carditis accounts for the greatest mortality in the acute phase and significant morbidity/mortality chronically.
• Valvulitis
—Mitral valve is most commonly affected followed by aortic (usually associated with mitral involvement). Tricuspid and pulmonary valvar involvement is rare.
—Valve inflammation leads to insufficiency.
—Prolonged immune response causes fibrosis, calcification, and valve stenosis.

Arthritis
• Two or more large joints (knees, ankles, wrists, and elbows)
• Involvement is asymmetric and migratory.
• Limitation of motion may occur.
• Unusual for the symptoms to persist beyond the acute illness.
• Symptoms improve rapidly with aspirin.

Sydenham Chorea (St. Vitus Dance)
• Involuntary, purposeless, and uncoordinated movements associated with muscle weakness and/or abnormal behavior
• Due to inflammation of the basal ganglia/cerebellum
• Symptoms can occur late, up to 6 months after the onset of ARF, and usually resolve within weeks but may last months to years.

PROGNOSIS
• Patients with a previous episode of ARF are at high risk for a recurrence following streptococcal pharyngitis unless secondary prophylaxis is instituted.
• Carditis can abate spontaneously or progress. The severity of the initial carditis is a major determinant to progression to rheumatic heart disease.
• Rheumatic carditis resolves in approximately 70% to 80% of patients who adhere to prophylaxis guidelines.

 Differential Diagnosis

• Carditis: viral, bacterial, rickettsial, parasitic, or mycoplasma myocarditis; Kawasaki disease
• Arthritis: poststreptococcal arthritis, serum sickness, septic arthritis (i.e., gonococcal), Lyme disease
• Collagen vascular disease: juvenile rheumatoid arthritis (small joints, not migratory, and not relieved promptly with aspirin), systemic lupus erythematosus, bacterial endocarditis
• Chorea: congenital choreoathetosis, brain tumors, Huntington chorea, Wilson disease
• Hematologic disorders with joint involvement: sickle cell anemia, leukemia
• Congenital heart defects: previously undiagnosed valvar heart disease, mitral valve prolapse with regurgitation

 Data Gathering

HISTORY
Question: How do you use the Jones criteria to make the diagnosis of ARF?
Significance: Jones criteria for diagnosis (two major versus one major and two minor criteria with evidence of a recent streptococcal infection)

Exceptions to the Jones criteria include:
• Sydenham chorea alone or indolent carditis alone (each of which may appear late and, therefore, may not be associated with supporting evidence of a recent streptococcal pharyngitis).
• Patients with a previous diagnosis of ARF who have a recurrence may not fulfill the Jones criteria due to the subtle presentation.
• Major criteria
—Carditis: 50% of patients with ARF and always associated with a murmur of valvulitis
—Polyarthritis: 70% of patients and manifested by a migratory arthritis of major joints
—Sydenham chorea: 15% of patients and manifested by abnormal behavior and/or involuntary, purposeless movements
—Erythema marginatum: 10% of patients and is an evanescent, pink rash with serpiginous borders
—Subcutaneous nodules: 2% to 10% of patients and manifested by painless nodules over extensor surfaces of large joints, the occiput, and/or vertebral processes
• Minor criteria
—Arthralgia: can only be considered in the absence of arthritis
—Fever
—Elevated acute phase reactants (ESR, C-reactive protein)
—Prolongation of the PR interval on ECG

 Physical Examination

CARDIAC
Finding: Murmur of valvulitis
Significance: Holosystolic mitral regurgitant murmur, Carey-Coombs apical mid-diastolic murmur, or a basal diastolic murmur of aortic insufficiency

Finding: Murmur could be associated with a pericardial friction rub.
Significance: Pericardial effusion

MUSCULOSKELETAL
Finding: Pain, limited motion, erythema, warmth of two or more large joints
Significance: Arthritis criterion

NEUROLOGIC
Finding: Chorea must be differentiated from tics, athetosis, and hyperkinesis.
Significance: Sydenham's chorea criterion

SKIN
Finding: Evanescent, pink rash with pale centers and serpiginous borders on the trunk and proximal extremities.
Significance: Erythema marginatum criterion

Finding: Firm, painless nodules over the extensor surface of large joints, occiput and/or spinous processes
Significance: Subcutaneous nodules

Rheumatic Fever (RF)

Laboratory Aids

SPECIFIC TESTS
Test: No diagnostic test is available.

NONSPECIFIC TESTS
Test: Throat culture
Significance: May be negative in two thirds of patients or the patient may be a chronic carrier

Test: Rapid streptococcal antigen test
Significance: Evidence for infection with GABHS

Test: Elevated or rising streptococcal antibody titers [antistreptolysin O (ASO), anti-DNase B, antihyaluronidase]
Significance: Evidence for recent infection with GABHS

Test: Additional hematologic evaluation
Significance: Leukocytosis on complete blood count (may be normal)

Test: ESR and C-reactive protein
Significance: Minor criteria if elevated

Test: ECG
Significance: Prolonged PR interval, junctional rhythm, transient arrhythmias, ST-T wave changes

Test: CXR
Significance: Cardiomegaly may indicate carditis or pericardial effusion.

Test: Echocardiogram
Significance: Assess valve involvement, ventricular dilatation, function, and pericardial effusions

Therapy

• Primary prevention
—Full treatment of streptococcal pharyngitis infection
—Penicillin V 250 mg PO t.i.d. for 10 days; or
—Benzathine penicillin G IM (600,000 U/IM ≤27 kg or 1,200,000 U/IM >27 kg); or
—Erythromycin estolate
• Secondary prevention
—Benzathine penicillin G (1,200,000 U/IM every 3 weeks); or
—Penicillin V 250 mg PO b.i.d.; or
—Sulfadiazine PO daily; or
—Erythromycin 250 mg PO daily
—Duration depends on clinical presentation and cardiac impact of ARF.
—Patients without rheumatic carditis require prophylaxis for 5 years or until age 21, whichever comes later.

—Patients with a history of rheumatic carditis but with no residual cardiac disease (clinical or echo) require prophylaxis for at least 10 years and well into adulthood, whichever is longer.
—Patients with rheumatic heart disease should have prophylaxis for at least 10 years and at least until 40 years of age.
• Treatment of inflammation
—Aspirin: 100 mg/kg/d for 6 to 8 weeks
—Prednisone: 2 mg/kg/d for 3 to 4 weeks (usually recommended for patients with severe carditis)
—Treatment length is controversial, but often antiinflammatories are used until the sedimentation rate or C-reactive protein normalizes
• Cardiac support
—Digoxin or other inotropic agents
—Afterload reducing agents such as captopril, intravenous nitroprusside, or milrinone
—Bed rest indicated during episode of acute carditis
—Surgical valvuloplasty or valve replacement if indicated
• Treatment of chorea
—Usually supportive
—Phenobarbital, haloperidol, chlorpromazine, diazepam, valproic acid

Follow-Up

• Patients without carditis
—Close follow-up is needed for 2 to 3 weeks to assess for development of acute carditis.
—Long-term pediatric follow-up is needed to diagnose patients with indolent carditis.
—Patients with new murmurs or clinical evidence of heart failure should be referred to a cardiologist.
—Long-term follow-up is needed to evaluate those who develop chorea.
—Prophylaxis should be stressed even in individuals without carditis.
• Patients with carditis
—Cardiology follow-up is needed to assess the development or evolution of rheumatic heart disease.
—Symptoms of worsening heart failure suggest progression of valvar or myocardial disease, recurrent ARF, or endocarditis.
—Secondary prophylaxis and bacterial endocarditis prophylaxis should be stressed.

PITFALLS
No definitive diagnostic test exists and certain clinical criteria must be present and excluded from other disease states to assure the proper diagnosis.

Common Questions and Answers

Q: Does a negative throat culture rule out ARF?
A: No. Throat cultures may be negative in two thirds of patients.

Q: Is there a vaccine available to prevent ARF?
A: Not presently; however, research efforts have been promising. Antigenic strains of group A streptococcus have been identified. Additionally, progress has been made in determining factors that cause a genetic predisposition to ARF. In the future, a vaccine may be available to those patients known to be at an increased genetic risk.

Q: Can echocardiographic evidence of carditis alone be used to diagnose rheumatic fever?
A: No. At the present time, carditis can only be diagnosed with a murmur consistent with valvulitis. An echocardiographic finding of valvar insufficiency without the appropriate auscultation findings cannot be used to fulfill the Jones criterion of carditis.

Q: Can intravenous gamma globulin be used as a treatment for ARF?
A: Recent study revealed that IVIG did not alter the natural history of ARF with no detectable difference in the cardiac outcome, laboratory findings, or echocardiographic parameters when compared to placebo.

ICD-9-CM 398.99

BIBLIOGRAPHY
Aron AM, Freeman JM, Caters S. The natural history of Sydenham's chorea. *Am J Med* 1965;38:83–95.

Ayoub E. Acute rheumatic fever. In: Emmanouilides GC, ed. *Moss and Adams heart disease in infants, children, and adolescents including the fetus and young adult*, 5th ed. Baltimore: Williams & Wilkins, 1995:1400–1416.

Dajani A, Taubert K, Ferrieri P, et al. Treatment of acute streptococcal pharyngitis and prevention of rheumatic fever. *Pediatrics* 1995;96(4):758–764.

Jones TD. Diagnosis of rheumatic fever. *JAMA* 1944;126:481–484.

Special Writing Group of the Committee on Rheumatic Fever, Endocarditis, and Kawasaki's Disease of the Council on Cardiovascular Disease in the Young of the American Heart Association. Guidelines for the diagnosis of rheumatic fever, Jones criteria update. *JAMA* 1992;268(15):2069–2073.

Stollerman GH. Rheumatic fever. *Lancet* 1997;349:935–942.

Voss LM, Wilson NJ, Neutze JM, et al. Intravenous immunoglobulin in acute rheumatic fever: a randomized controlled trial. *Circulation* 2001;103(3):401–406.

Author: Timothy M. Hoffman

Rhinitis—Allergic

Database

DEFINITION
- Inflammation of the nasal and sinus mucosae, associated with sneezing, swelling, increased mucus production, and nasal obstruction
- May be seasonal (periodic symptoms, involving the same season for at least 2 consecutive years; most often due to pollens), perennial (year-long, may be due to multiple seasonal allergies or continual exposure to allergens, such as dust mites), or perennial with seasonal exacerbations

CAUSES
- Indoor allergens: house dust mite, cockroaches, animal dander, cigarette smoke, hair spray, paint, molds
- Pollens: tree pollens in early spring, grass in late spring and early summer, ragweed in late summer and autumn
- Multiple environmental factors
- Changes in air temperature

ASSOCIATED PROBLEMS
- Asthma
- Allergic conjunctivitis
- Atopic dermatitis (eczema)
- Urticaria
- Otitis media
- Sleep, taste, and/or smell disturbance
- Nasal polyps
- Mouth breathing
- Snoring
- Adenoidal hypertrophy and sleep apnea
- Decreased appetite

PATHOPHYSIOLOGY
Early-Phase Allergic Responses to Antigen Exposure (Within First Several Hours)
- Mediators, including histamine, leukotrienes, and prostaglandins, are released (mast cell degranulation) into the extracellular environment.
- Smooth muscle contraction, vasodilatation, edema, and secretions result, leading to narrowing and obstruction of the sinus ostia.
- Itching of the nose and sneezing occur after physical and chemical stimulation of nerve endings in the nose.
- Hypersecretion occurs as a result of parasympathetic pathways and reflex mechanisms.

Late-Phase Allergic Response (Several to 8 Hours After Allergen Exposure)
- Chemotactic factors lead to eosinophil, basophil, and neutrophil infiltration, and increased numbers of lymphocytes.
- Cytotoxic proteins released by activated eosinophils may cause damage to epithelial cells.
- Characterized by erythema, induration, nasal blockage, and/or wheezing

EPIDEMIOLOGY
- Most common allergic disease, affecting more than 20 million Americans; affects 8% to 20% of children and 15% to 30% of adolescents
- Estimated that up to 75% of children with asthma also have allergic rhinitis
- Most commonly begins during childhood and young adulthood, with the peak incidence being in mid-adolescence
- Perennial allergic rhinitis can occur at any age; seasonal allergic rhinitis is rare before age 3 years.

GENETICS
- Increased incidence in families with atopic disease
- If one parent has allergies, each child has a 30% chance of having an allergy; if both parents have allergies, each child has a 70% chance of having an allergy.

COMPLICATIONS
- Chronic sinusitis
- Recurrent otitis media
- Hoarseness
- Loss of smell
- Loss of hearing
- High-arched palate and dental malocclusion from chronic mouth breathing

Differential Diagnosis

INFECTION
- Viral upper respiratory tract infection
- Bacterial sinusitis

ENVIRONMENTAL
- Foreign body

TUMORS
- Nasal polyps
- Dermoid cyst
- Nasal glioma

CONGENITAL
- Cystic fibrosis
- Choanal atresia
- Immotile cilia syndrome
- Septal deviation
- Primary atrophic rhinitis

IMMUNOLOGIC
- Sarcoidosis
- Wegener granulomatosis

MISCELLANEOUS
- Idiopathic (vasomotor) rhinitis
- Nonallergic perennial rhinitis
- Rhinitis medicamentosa
- Rhinitis associated with pregnancy/other hormonal rhinitis
- Hypothyroidism
- Idiopathic neonatal rhinitis
- Drug-induced rhinitis
- Food-induced rhinitis

Data Gathering

HISTORY
Question: What are typical symptoms?
Significance: Patient often reports stuffy nose, sneezing, itching, runny nose, noisy breathing, snoring, cough, halitosis, and repeated throat clearing. Sensation of plugged ears and wheezing may occur.
Question: Are eyes red and itchy?
Significance: Suggestive of allergic conjunctivitis
Question: Are symptoms seasonal, perennial, or episodic?
Significance: May help to identify potential allergens
Question: Any exacerbating factors including pollen, animals, cigarette smoke, dust, molds?
Significance: Useful information to prevent symptoms from occurring
Question: Is there a family history of atopic disease, such as asthma or atopic dermatitis?
Significance: Supports the diagnosis
Question: Any related illnesses?
Significance: Asthma, urticaria, eczema, ear infections, and delayed speech are common associated conditions.

Physical Examination

- Allergic shiners: dark discoloration beneath the eyes due to obstruction of lymphatic and venous drainage, chronic nasal obstruction, and suborbital edema
- Dennie-Morgan lines: creases in the lower eyelid radiating outward from the inner canthus; caused by spasm in the muscles of Müller around the eye due to chronic congestion and stasis of blood
- Allergic salute: a gesture characterized by rubbing the nose with the palm of the hand upward to decrease itching and temporarily open the nasal passages
- Allergic crease: transverse crease near the tip of the nose, secondary to rubbing
- Nasal mucosa may appear pale and/or edematous; mucoid or watery material may be seen in the nasal cavity; check for nasal polyps, septal deviation.

Laboratory Aids

- Nasal cytology: specimen of nasal discharge to check for the presence of eosinophils. Have the patient blow his/her nose into a piece of nonporous paper or collect discharge with a cotton swab and transfer the discharge to a glass slide. Greater than 10% eosinophils is considered positive for nasal eosinophilia. Note: use of intranasal steroids may reduce the number of eosinophils found in nasal discharge.
- Sweat test if cystic fibrosis suspected or if nasal polyps are present.

- Audiometry and tympanometry when indicated.
- RAST (radioallergosorbent tests): *in vitro* test to measure allergen-specific IgE; very expensive; useful in patients who have diffuse atopic dermatitis.
- Enzyme-linked immunosorbent assay to measure allergen-specific IgE
- Total IgE: elevated in allergic rhinitis; not routinely indicated
- CBC: may show eosinophilia; not routinely indicated

SKIN TESTING
- *Prick test:* percutaneous, qualitative test in which antigen concentrate is placed on the skin of the volar surface of the arm or upper back, and a needle is inserted; the skin reaction is subjectively graded from 0 to 4.
- *Intradermal test:* qualitative test in which antigen is introduced intradermally (0.02 mL with a 26- to 30-gauge needle); more sensitive than the prick test and often used if prick test is negative or equivocal; the degree of swelling and erythema is graded from 0 to 4.

PROCEDURES
Rhinoscopy to assess the nasal turbinates and to look for nasal polyps

Therapy

AVOIDANCE THERAPY
Identify and eliminate known/suspected allergens.

DRUGS
- Mucolytics: act to thin the mucus and thereby improve mucociliary flow; include steam inhalation, normal saline drops, bicarbonate spray, N-acetylcysteine orally or inhaled, and oral guaifenesin
- Antihistamines: competitively blocking H1 receptors; suppress itching, ocular symptoms, sneezing, and rhinorrhea; not very effective against nasal congestion
—Second-generation: minimally or do not cross the blood–brain barrier and therefore do not have CNS side effects such as drowsiness. Loratadine (Claritin, Schering): FDA-approved for children as young as 2 years. Dose: ages 2 to 5 years—5 mg PO daily; ages 6 years or older—10 mg PO daily. Cetirizine HCl (Zyrtec, Pfizer): FDA-approved for children as young as 2 years. Dose: age 2 to 5 years: 2.5 mg = 1/2 tsp (1 mg/mL banana-grape flavored syrup) PO daily with max. dose of 5 mg/day. Fexofenadine (Allegra, Aventis): ≥12 years, 60 mg tab b.i.d.
—First-generation [e.g., diphenhydramine (Benadryl) 5 mg/kg/day divided q.i.d.]: side effects include drowsiness, performance impairment, paradoxical excitement; anticholinergic side effects (e.g., dry mouth, tachycardia, urinary retention, and constipation) may occur.
- Intranasal steroids: Blunt early phase reactions and block late phase reactions; may not be fully effective until several days to 2 weeks after initiation of therapy; must be used regularly; best when administered lying down with the head back. Agents include beclomethasone (Vancenase, Beconase); flunisolide (Nasalide); fluticasone propionate (Flonase 0.05%) in patients as young as 4 years; budesonide (Rhinocort); triamcinolone acetonide (Nasacort); mometasone furoate monohydrate (Nasonex).
- Topical cromolyn (Nasalcrom): mast-cell stabilizer; minimal side effects; does not provide immediate relief (may take 2 to 4 weeks to see clinical effect).
- Oral decongestants: α_1- and α_2-adrenergic agonists, which act to cause vasoconstriction, decreased blood supply to the nasal mucosa, and decreased mucosal edema. Cardiovascular and central nervous system side effects including tremors, agitation, hypertension, insomnia, and headaches. Agents include ephedrine, pseudoephedrine, and phenylephrine.
- Topical decongestants: Sympathomimetics; may be useful for a few days to open nasal passages to allow for delivery of topical steroids; side effects include drying of the mucosa and burning. Use for more than a few (3–5) days results in rebound vasodilation and congestion (rhinitis medicamentosa). Agents include phenylephrine (Neo-Synephrine), which is short acting; and oxymetazoline (Afrin), which is long acting.
- Combined oral decongestants and antihistamines: numerous preparations on the market.

IMMUNOTHERAPY
- Also, referred to as hyposensitization, desensitization. Consists of a series of injections with specific allergens, with increasing concentrations of allergens, once or twice weekly
- Recommended for patients who have not responded to pharmacologic therapy
- Extremely effective and long-lasting. After several months to years of treatment, total serum IgE levels decrease, and the intensity of the early-phase response is reduced.
- Side effects include urticaria, bronchospasm, hypotension, anaphylaxis

SURGERY
- Removal of allergic polyps
- Inferior turbinate surgery to reduce the size of the turbinate and relieve obstruction
- Endoscopic sinus surgery to relieve obstruction

PREVENTION
- Minimize exposure to dust mites: consider removing carpets, upholstered furniture, and curtains; washing bedding in hot water frequently, at least every 1 to 2 weeks; using pillow and mattress covers
- Minimize exposure to animal danders: minimize exposure to all animals, consider using solutions containing tannic acid, which will denature animal allergens; shampoo pets frequently if pets cannot be removed from the household; use air vent filters.
- Minimize exposure to pollens: keep windows closed, use air conditioning, avoid leaf-raking or lawn-mowing.
- Minimize exposure to molds: keep houseplants out of the bedroom, avoid spending time in the basement, keep humidity at 35% to 50%.

Follow-Up

Two to 4 weeks after initial evaluation; then every 3 to 6 months

SIGNS TO WATCH FOR
Fever, prolonged or severe headache, dizziness, pain, or purulent discharge should suggest a diagnosis other than allergic rhinitis alone.

PROGNOSIS
Generally good. Complete recovery occurs in 5% to 10% of patients.

PITFALLS
- Skin tests may be difficult to interpret in patients with diffuse eczema and dermatographism.
- Cardiac arrhythmias have been seen with patients taking terfenadine and astemizole.

Common Questions and Answers

Q: How does one minimize exposure to dust mites?
A: Keep household temperature low; maintain humidity at approximately 40% to 50%; wash linens at hot temperatures, weekly; use a microfilter when vacuum cleaning; place mattress and box spring in tightly woven casing; use air conditioning; use high-efficiency particulate air filter units.
Q: How often are nasal polyps associated with cystic fibrosis?
A: In up to 40% of children, nasal polyps are associated with cystic fibrosis. Less than 0.5% of children with asthma and rhinitis have nasal polyps.
Q: When used on a daily basis, are intranasal steroids safe?
A: Yes. It is generally accepted that inhaled steroids are safe. However, there is increasing evidence that inhaled and intranasal steroids are associated with a decrease in linear growth velocity.

ICD-9-CM 477.9

BIBLIOGRAPHY
Dykewicz MS, Fineman S. Executive summary of Joint Task Force practice parameters on diagnosis and management of rhinitis. *Ann Allergy Asthma Immunol* 1998;81:463–468.

Lasley MV, Shapiro GG. Testing for allergy. *Pediatr Rev* 2000;21:39–43.

Meltzer EO. Treatment options for the child with allergic rhinitis. *Clin Pediatr* 1998;37:1–10.

Nash DR. Allergic rhinitis. *Pediatr Ann* 1998;27(12):799–808.

Author: Esther K. Chung

Rickets

 Database

DEFINITION

Undermineralization of growing bone.

CAUSES

• See table Causes and Management of Rickets.
• Children at high risk for rickets:

—Small premature infants
—Urban breast-fed infants who do not receive supplemental vitamin D
—Children with chronic renal insufficiency
—Children with biliary atresia or chronic liver disease
—Children with inflammatory bowel diseases

 Data Gathering

HISTORY

• Symptoms of hepatic, renal, or gastrointestinal disease?
• Calcium intake? Dairy products, legumes, green vegetables.
• Factors influencing calcium absorption? Calciferol supply, steatorrhea, antacids, anticonvulsants
• Vitamin D fortified milk?
• Exposure to sunlight?: Vitamin D metabolism

Question: Factors influencing calcium excretion?
Significance: Diuretics, polyuria, or glycosuria suggestive of renal tubular dysfunction.

• Bone pain? Fractures.
• Delayed standing, walking?
• Anorexia?
• Seizures?
• Pathologic fractures?
• Tetany?
• Calcium: Familial history of rickets?

Physical Examination

• Calcification: slowed growth (short stature)
• Bossing deformity of the head
• Craniotabes: soft sutures
• Premature fusion of the sutures
• Dental caries: calcium in teeth
• Hepatic or renal enlargement: may be etiology
• Alterations in the long bones: calcification
• Keep mass of uncalcified bone matrix
• Muscle weakness: serum calcium
• Rachitic rosary: enlarged costochondral junctions
• Awkward gait: fractures and bowed leg

Causes and Management of Rickets

CAUSE	MANAGEMENT
Calcium deficiency	
Low intake	Include at least 500 mg/d of Ca
Extreme prematurity (birth weight <1,500 g)	Adjust intake to 200 mg/kg/d
Steatorrhea	25-OH-D$_3$ (5–7 μg/kg/d) if serum levels are low; supplement dietary Ca
Anticonvulsants (phenobarbital or phenytoin)	Vitamin D, 1,000–2,000 IU/d
Renal tubular acidosis	Base supplement: 3–10 mM/kg/d as NaHCO$_3$ or citrate
Vitamin D deficiency	
Insufficient UV light	400 IU/d of vitamin D
No vitamin D supplement	400 IU/d of vitamin D
Liver disease	25-OH-D, 5–7 mg/kg/d
Renal disorders that may reduce calcitriol formation	Calcitriol, 0.25–1.0 mg/d
Hypoplasia or parenchymal damage	CaCO$_3$ to restrict P absorption and supplement dietary Ca
Specific hydroxylase deficiency	Calcitriol, 0.5–1.0 mg/d
Phosphorus deficiency	
Diet (limited to premature infants)	Adjust formula or parenteral source to give 10 mg/kg/d
Antacid excess	Alternative gastric HCl control
Excessive phosphaturia from tubular dysfunction	Supplemental P and calcitriol if low

Laboratory Aids

See table Classification of Rickets and Vitamin D Metabolite Levels.

- Circulating vitamin D metabolites (25-hydroxyvitamin D, 1,25-dihydroxyvitamin D)
- Circulating levels of parathyroid hormone (PTH)
- Serum Ca, P, Mg, alkaline phosphatase, and total CO_2
- Urinary Ca, P, Mg, pH, creatinine, and amino acids, exclude Fanconi syndrome and proximal renal tubular acidosis.
- Alkaline phosphatase

IMAGING

- Order one view because rickets is symmetrical.
- Knee and wrist films
- Radiographic findings: irregular cortices and bony margins, widened metaphyses, widened growth plates, osteopenia
- DEXA (dual energy x-ray absorptiometry) is the "gold standard."

 Therapy

See table Causes and Management of Rickets.

 Follow-Up

- To avoid side effects of hypercalciuria and hypercalcemia, frequent monitoring (every 2–3 months) of blood and urinary calcium levels (calcium/creatinine ratio) should be done when vitamin D therapy is used.
- Should see radiographic improvement within 6 weeks.

 Common Questions and Answers

Q: Why are premature infants prone to rickets?
A: Premature infants have higher calcium and phosphorus requirements than full-term infants. They also tend to be sicker at birth, sometimes having feeding difficulties or malabsorption.

Q: What is the best way to diagnose rickets?
A: The most precise way to diagnose rickets is with a DEXA scan, which gives accurate measures of bone density. A routine x-ray may not show osteopenia until the disease is at a moderately severe stage.

Q: What are the sequelae of rickets?
A: The most common medical sequelae of rickets include pathologic bone fractures, slowed growth (short stature), and muscle weakness.

Q: Can rickets be treated effectively?
A: Yes, rickets can be treated effectively with the right amount and combination of calcium, phosphorus, or vitamin D supplementation. Radiographic improvement can usually be seen within 6 weeks.

ICD-9-CM 268

Renal rickets 588.0

BIBLIOGRAPHY

Behrman RM, ed. Metabolic bone disease. In: *Nelson textbook of pediatrics*, 14th ed. Philadelphia: W.B. Saunders. 1997; 1748–1752.

Bergsrom WH. Twenty ways to get rickets in the 1990s. *Contemp Pediatr* 1991;8:88.

Chesney RW. Nutrition in bone disease. In: Grand RJ, Sutphen JL, Dietz WH, eds. *Pediatric nutrition: theory and practice*. Boston: Butterworth, 1987:727–742.

Authors: Timothy A. S. Sentongo and Andrew E. Mulberg

Classification of Rickets and Vitamin D Metabolite Levels

	CALCIUM	PHOSPHORUS	ALKALINE PHOSPHATE	25 (0)
Deficient synthesis and supply	N or ↓	↓	↑	↓
No sunlight				
Poor diet				
Immaturity				
Malabsorption	N or ↓	↓	↑	↓
Liver disease	N or ↓	↓	↑	↓
Chronic renal failure	N or ↓	↑	↑	N
Vitamin D–dependent rickets (recessively inherited)	↓	↓	↑	N
Vitamin D–resistant rickets (sex-linked dominant)	N	↓	↑	N
Renal tubular disorders (defect of phosphate reabsorption)	N	↓	↑	N

N, normal; ↓, decreased; ↑, increased.

Rickettsial Disease

 Database

DEFINITION
- The rickettsial diseases are a group of illnesses caused by the Rickettsiaceae family of organisms. Despite some minor differences in epidemiologic, clinical, and laboratory characteristics, the illnesses caused by these organisms have similar manifestations and treatment.
- The rickettsial diseases can be divided into subgroups based on clinical presentation: the spotted fever group, the typhus group, Q fever, and ehrlichiosis.
- Because these illnesses are organized primarily by clinical similarities, the spotted fever group includes the tick-borne typhus classification.

CAUSES
- The rickettsial illnesses are transmitted to humans via insect vectors such as ticks, fleas, lice, or mites.
- Rickettsial diseases occur in patients of all ages. Rocky Mountain spotted fever (RMSF) has a predilection for children.
- The rickettsial diseases that occur in the United States are RMSF (see Rocky Mountain Spotted Fever), murine typhus, rickettsialpox, epidemic typhus, Q fever, and ehrlichiosis.

PATHOLOGY/PATHOPHYSIOLOGY
- For the spotted fever, typhus, and ehrlichiosis groups: vasculitis caused by proliferation of organisms in the endothelial lining of small blood vessels
- Q fever: pneumonitis

COMPLICATIONS
- Venous thrombosis
- Pneumonitis
- Pericarditis, myocarditis, heart failure
- Severe disease occurs more commonly in patients with G6PD deficiency, cardiac insufficiency, or immunocompromise.

 Differential Diagnosis

INFECTION
- Before the appearance of the rash, the constitutional symptoms associated with the spotted fevers result in a very wide differential diagnosis. After the appearance of the rash, the diagnoses are more limited: measles, meningococcemia, secondary syphilis, viral infections, coxsackievirus (hand-foot-and-mouth disease), infectious mononucleosis, enteroviral infection.
- Environmental (poisons): drug hypersensitivity reaction (toxicodermatosis)
- Tumors: leukemia with thrombocytopenia
- Immunologic: idiopathic thrombocytopenia purpura (ITP)
- Miscellaneous: leukocytoclastic angiitis, erythema multiforme/Stevens-Johnson syndrome

 Data Gathering

Differentiating the illnesses listed depends on the travel history, history of exposure to certain mammals or insects, and the initial clinical presentation of the patient. This clinical presentation is categorized by the grouping: spotted fever group, typhus group, Q fever, and ehrlichiosis.

HISTORY
Question: Fever, headache, and rash?
Significance: In general, rickettsial disease should be considered in a patient with these complaints. The progression of the rash can be particularly helpful in considering the diagnosis.

 Physical Examination

Differentiating clinical findings of each group are described subsequently, and the rashes associated with each illness are described in the table Characteristics of the Generalized Rashes of the Rickettsial Diseases.
- Constitutional symptoms
- Hepatosplenomegaly
- "Tache noir" (black spot): the earliest finding in the spotted fever group originates at the site of the infecting bite; becomes necrotic, forming eschar; regional lymphadenopathy related to eschar; lesion usually found on the head in children and on the legs in adults; is present in between 30% and 90% of cases. *Significance:* These symptoms suggest illness caused by the spotted fever group. Tache noir is present in 30% to 90% of cases.
- Impaired level of consciousness
- Myocardial and renal involvement
- Brill-Zinsser disease (BZD) is actually a recrudescence of a previous infection with epidemic (louse-borne) typhus caused by *R. prowazekii;* BZD can occur years after the initial infection and is usually less severe than the initial episode of louse-borne typhus. *Significance:* These symptoms suggest illness caused by the typhus group.
- A self-limited febrile illness characterized by headache, myalgias, and chest pain
- Pulmonary symptoms occur in some form in over 50% of cases: mild pneumonitis/cough usually an incidental finding; radiographically confirmed pneumonia in moderately ill patients; rapidly progressive pneumonia
- Endocarditis may occur.
- Hepatitis may range in severity.

Characteristics of the Generalized Rashes of the Rickettsial Diseases

	APPEARANCE	DISTRIBUTION	ASSOCIATED FINDINGS
Spotted fever group			Tache noir in 30–90% of patients
Tick typhus	Macular → papular	Extremities → palms/ soles → trunk	
Rickettsialpox	Macular → papular → Vesicles	Extremities → palms/ soles → trunk	
Scrub typhus	Macular	Limited to trunk	Rash of shorter duration lymphadenopathy is a prominent symptom
Typhus group			No tache noir
Epidemic (louse-borne) typhus	Macules → maculopapules → petechiae → hemorrhage	Trunk → extremities	
Murine typhus		Trunk → extremities	Less extensive rash of shorter duration
Miscellaneous			
Q fever	Macular or maculopapular or petechial	Trunk and extremities	No rash
Ehrlichiosis			Rash common in children; rare in adults

- Nervous system findings range from headache to meningitis and encephalitis. *Significance:* These symptoms suggest illness caused by *Coxiella burnetii,* the organism responsible for Q fever.
- Acute febrile illness characterized by headache, anorexia, and vomiting
- A relative bradycardia is often noted.
- Hyponatremia, leukopenia, and thrombocytopenia
Significance: These symptoms and signs suggest illness caused by *Ehrlichia chaffeensis*, the organism primarily responsible for human ehrlichiosis.

PHYSICAL EXAM TRICKS
Rashes that involve the palms and soles present a limited differential diagnosis. This list includes rickettsial diseases, certain viral infections such as coxsackievirus (hand-foot-and-mouth), syphilis, erythema multiforme, and urticarial rash.

 ## Laboratory Aids

Test: Polymerase chain reaction (PCR) from blood or tissue
Significance:
- Allows the identification of rickettsial-specific DNA sequences
- *R. rickettsii, R. typhi,* and *R. prowazekii*
Test: Immunofluorescent (IgM) tests
Significance:
- Sensitive, specific, and simple
- Can differentiate acute from past infection
- This technique is only useful early in the course of *R. tsutsugamushi* (scrub typhus) infection.
- Biopsy of the tache noir may reveal rickettsial organisms of the spotted fever group by direct immunofluorescent staining. Similar testing of the generalized rash is not useful for rickettsial illnesses other than RMSF.
Test: Serologic tests
- Complement fixation tests
- Enzyme-linked immunosorbent assay (ELISA)
- Latex agglutination test
- The Weil-Felix reaction assays the patients' serologic response to rickettsiae; the highest titers occur during the second and third weeks of illness; this test will be negative in patients with rickettsialpox and Q fever.
- PCR tests in blood and tissue are available for many rickettsial diseases.

FALSE-POSITIVES
The Weil-Felix reaction may be falsely positive in testing for any of the above organisms.

PITFALLS
The headache associated with rickettsial infections can be severe. However, radiographic imaging is not necessary if there are no signs or symptoms of increased intracranial pressure.

 ## Therapy

EMERGENCY
- Fluid resuscitation for patients who appear moderately to severely ill.
- Antimicrobial therapy should be instituted as soon as the diagnosis is suspected.
- Therapy is most effective if instituted within the first week of illness. There is little benefit in waiting for confirmatory diagnostic tests.

DRUGS
- All of the rickettsial diseases respond rapidly to treatment with tetracycline; the dose is 30 to 40 mg/kg/d orally or 20 mg/kg/d IV in four divided doses (maximum dose of 2 g/d); alternatively, doxycycline may be given at dosage of 100 to 200 mg/d.
- For moderate to severely ill children under the age of 8 years, doxycycline, 3 to 4 mg/kg/day in two divided doses, is still considered the drug of choice.
- Erythromycin and trimethoprim-sulfamethoxazole have been used with variable success against rickettsial infections.

DURATION
The optimum duration of treatment for rickettsial infections has not been determined. In general, the more severe infections warrant 7 to 10 days of antimicrobial therapy.

POSSIBLE CONFLICTS
Prevention
- Except for *R. tsutsugamushi* (scrub typhus) and *Ehrlichia*, all of the rickettsial diseases produce long-term immunity to the etiologic organisms within the same group.
- Fleas, ticks, and mites should be controlled in endemic areas with the appropriate insecticides.
- Clothing to cover the entire body should be worn in tick-infested areas.
- In areas where louse-borne typhus is epidemic, periodic delousing and dusting of insecticide into clothes is recommended.
- No vaccines are currently available in the United States.

 ## Follow-Up

WHEN TO EXPECT IMPROVEMENT
Improvement in the patient's clinical status usually takes place within 1 to 2 days of initiation of therapy. This improvement is delayed in severe cases, particularly if there is endocardial involvement (Q fever) or treatment is begun after the first week of illness.

PITFALLS
- Paradoxical effect of rodenticides: fleas, mites will seek alternate hosts such as humans when mice or rats are "unavailable." Therefore, rodenticides should not be the only prevention measure taken in endemic areas.
- In children younger than 8, failure to treat rickettsial infections with doxycycline can result in the development of severe disease. The benefits of a single, short course of doxycycline outweighs the very small risk of dental staining in these children.

 ## Common Questions and Answers

Q: What do I do if I or my child receives a tick bite in an endemic area to rickettsial disease?
A: There is no role for prophylaxis against rickettsial diseases for patients who have suffered tick bites.
Q: Are there differences between typhoid and typhus?
A: Typhoid, or typhoid fever, is a separate entity from typhus. Typhoid is an enteric infection caused by *Salmonella typhi* and is unrelated to the rickettsial diseases.
Q: If I contract a rickettsial illness, can I get that illness or a similar illness again?
A: With the exception of scrub typhus and *Ehrlichia*, infection with a rickettsial organism confers immunity to other rickettsia within the same group.

ICD-9-CM 083.9

BIBLIOGRAPHY
American Academy of Pediatrics. *2000 red book: report of the committee on infectious diseases*, 25th edition. Elk Grove Village, IL: American Academy of Pediatrics, 2000.

Boyd AS. Rickettsialpox. *Dermatol Clin* 1997;15:313–318.

Dumler JS, Dey C, Meier F. Human monocytic ehrlichiosis: a potentially severe disease in children. *Arch Pediatr Adolesc Med* 2000;154:847–849.

Feigin RD, Snider RL, Edwards MS. Rickettsial diseases. In: Feigin RD, Cherry JD, eds. *Textbook of pediatric infectious diseases*, 3rd ed. Philadelphia: WB Saunders, 1992.

Purvis JJ, Edward MS. Doxycycline use for rickettsial disease in pediatric patients. *Pediatr Infect Dis J* 2000;19:871–874.

Author: Joel A. Fein

Rocky Mountain Spotted Fever (RMSF)

 Database

DEFINITION

Systemic illness (small vessel vasculitis) caused by infection with obligate intracellular gram-negative bacterium, *Rickettsia rickettsii*, carried by tick vectors: wood tick (*Dermacentor andersoni*) in West; dog tick (*Dermacentor variabilis*) in East; Lone star tick (*Amblyomma americanum*) in Southwest

PATHOPHYSIOLOGY

• Transmission usually from tick (reservoir) bite; can be by transfusion and aerosol route
—Usually takes more than 6 to 10 hours (often 24 hours) to be transmitted with tick bite
• Incubation period 2 to 14 days, average approximately 7 days
• After exposure, *Rickettsia* multiply in small-vessel endothelium and disseminate via bloodstream, with focal areas of endothelial proliferation, thrombus, blood, and protein leakage
• Local vascular lesions account for signs and symptoms

EPIDEMIOLOGY

• Most prevalent rickettsial disease in United States (600–1,200 cases/year, most by *D. variabilis* ticks)
• Seasonal (April to September most common) and geographic (0–20% prevalence in tick population reported)
—Endemic to south Atlantic and west south central regions
—Less often seen in Rocky Mountain states
—Also in Mexico, Central, and South America
—Has been reported in family and local clusters
• Two thirds of patients younger than 15 years of age (usually 5 to 9 years of age)

COMPLICATIONS

• Complications uncommon with early and appropriate treatment
• Neurologic sequelae
—More common in children with severely impaired states of consciousness
—Behavioral disturbances and learning disabilities common
—Emotional lability, hyperactivity, memory loss, seizures
• Skin
—Gangrene of extremities, end-organs, skin necrosis
—Skin rash usually heals without sequelae
• Hematologic
—Can progress to DIC
• Gastrointestinal
—Hepatic dysfunction
—Hypoalbuminemia from protein loss, hepatic dysfunction, protein leak from damaged vessels
• Cardiac
—Can have persistent cardiac findings, congestive heart failure, cardiovascular collapse
• Metabolic
—Hyponatremia from water shift to intracellular spaces, sodium loss in urine

• Renal
—Acute tubular necrosis

PROGNOSIS

• No known asymptomatic infection
—May be mild if treated early
• Recovery the rule if treated in 5 to 7 days
• Case fatality approximately 3% to 7% if treated, 25% if untreated (23% before antibiotics in 1939–1945)
—Higher with older age (adult >30–40 years of age), nonwhite, male, glucose-6 phosphate diesterase deficiency (G6PD), CNS involvement, renal failure, cardiovascular collapse, late rash, hepatomegaly, jaundice, thrombocytopenia, DIC, absence of headache, GI symptoms, inappropriate or delayed antibiotics (none by 5th day) or diagnosis, no history of tick exposure
—Death usually between 9th and 12th day (fulminant cases with death in 5–6 days)

 Differential Diagnosis

• Infection
—Sepsis, meningitis, encephalitis, rubeola, atypical measles, meningococcemia, typhoid fever, leptospirosis, toxic shock, rubella, scarlet fever, disseminated gonococcal disease, *Haemophilus influenzae,* secondary syphilis, rheumatic fever, bacterial pneumonitis, poliomyelitis, pharyngitis, mumps, hepatitis, mononucleosis, enterovirus and other virus infections, fever of unknown origin, ehrlichiosis (has been reported to occur concurrently), other rickettsial disease, Kawasaki disease, gastroenteritis, meningitis, URI, pneumonitis
• Other
—Immune thrombocytopenic purpura (ITP), thrombotic thrombocytopenic purpura (TTP), immune complex vasculitis, drug reaction, ischemic heart disease, rheumatoid arthritis, erythema multiforme, intraabdominal process, acute surgical abdomen

 Data Gathering

HISTORY

Question: Abrupt or gradual onset of fever
Significance: Often unresponsive to antipyretics or antibiotics, headache (retrobulbar, frontal), rash, confusion, myalgia, nausea, vomiting, abdominal pain

• Classic triad of fever, headache, and rash only in approximately 50%
• Headache: characteristic; intense, persistent night and day, intractable; young child may not complain of headache
• Fever to more than 40°C (104°F) with oscillations of approximately 2°C [two thirds with fever >38.9°C (>102°F) in first 3 days]
• Onset usually 2 to 8 days post—tick bite
• Tick bite history obtained in only 50% to 70% of cases

 Physical Examination

Finding: Rash
Significance: Usually appears by second or third day of illness; may be delayed until sixth day or later; small percentage (10–15%) never develop rash; absence of rash should not delay presumptive diagnosis or appropriate therapy if disease suspected.
• Usually small, irregular, erythematous macules that blanch, become maculopapular and petechial (mixed rash), and confluently hemorrhagic
• Appears first (usually) on wrists and ankles, spreads centrally within hours to extremities to trunk, neck, and face; regularly occurs on palms and soles (may be spared) and scrotum; may initially appear on trunk or diffusely in some patients; can progress to necrosis of toes, ears, nose, scrotum, fingers
• May be more difficult to detect in African Americans
Finding: CNS
Significance: Meningismus, restless, irritable, apprehensive, confusion, delirium, lethargy, stupor, coma, ataxia, opisthotonos, aphasia, papilledema, seizures, cortical blindness, central deafness, ataxia, spastic paralysis, cranial nerve palsy
Finding: Cardiac
Significance: CHF, myocarditis, arrhythmias, vascular collapse (often volume related)
Finding: Pulmonary
Significance: Pneumonitis, cough, dyspnea, pulmonary edema, hypoxemia, pleural effusions, alveolar infiltrates
Finding: Gastrointestinal
Significance: Nausea, vomiting, abdominal pain, diarrhea, hepatomegaly, splenomegaly, anorexia, jaundice, mild pancreatitis
Finding: Myalgias
Significance: Especially calf or thigh
Finding: Ocular involvement
Significance: Conjunctivitis, venous engorgement, papilledema, cotton wool spots, retinal hemorrhages, retinal artery occlusion, uveitis
Finding: Other
Significance: Edema of extremities or face; parotitis, orchitis, pharyngitis

 Laboratory Aids

Make presumptive diagnosis on signs, symptoms, and epidemiologic considerations rather than on laboratory aids.
• No quick or early specific laboratory test; serologic data reliable by days 10 to 12; negative test does not exclude diagnosis.
• Culture impractical and potentially dangerous

SPECIFIC TESTS

Test: Serology
Significance: Not usually useful in acute management due to time required for serology

to become positive (6–10 days after clinical onset of disease)

Test: Probable confirmation

Significance: Fourfold increase in antibody titer by complement fixation (CF), indirect hemagglutination (IHA), indirect fluorescent antibody (IFA), latex agglutination (LA), microagglutination (MA), or single titer of at least 1:320 by *Proteus* OX-19 or OX-2 (Weil-Felix); 1:128 by LA, IHA, MA, 1:64 by IFA, or at least 1:16 by CF

Test: Enzyme-linked immunosorbent assay (ELISA)

Significance: Sensitive and accurate, but not useful until seroconversion at approximately day 6

Test: Direct immunofluorescence

Significance: Most sensitive and specific, but observer bias; can see immunofluorescent *Rickettsia* from skin rash biopsy between days 4 and 8

Test: IFA

Significance: Sensitivity 94% to 100%; specificity 100%

Test: IHA

Significance: Sensitivity 91% to 100%; specificity 99%

Test: LA

Significance: Sensitivity 71% to 94%; specificity 96% to 99%; false positive noted during pregnancy

Test: DNA polymerase chain reaction (PCR)

Significance: Takes 48 hours but can detect the organism from lesion or blood (depends on organism load; therefore, lesion usually better than blood), specific, low sensitivity.

Test: Weil-Felix

Significance: Nonspecific and insensitive, but readily available and rapid (3 to 5 minutes); sensitivity 47% to 70%, specificity 78% to 96%; positive early in course; titer greater than 1:160 suspicious. False positive with *Proteus* infections (UTI), leptospirosis, brucellosis, typhoid fever, liver disease, pregnancy. Not recommended for RMSF evaluation.

Test: CF

Significance: Sensitivity 0% to 63%, specificity 100%

Test: MA

Significance: Specific, not sensitive

NONSPECIFIC TESTS

Test: CBC, electrolytes, BUN, CR, LFT, DIC screen, CXR, ABG, ECG, echocardiogram

Significance: Nonspecific, not especially helpful in diagnosis. WBC normal or low for first 4 to 5 days; after that, leukocytosis (11,000–30,000/mm³) associated with secondary bacterial disease; elevated band count; anemia (30%); thrombocytopenia (consumptive coagulopathy); hyponatremia; hypoalbuminemia, prolonged prothrombin time, decreased fibrinogen (consumption), increased transaminases, and creatine kinase.

Test: CSF

Significance: Usually clear (WBC <10), but may see pleocytosis in one third and increased protein one half of patients.

 Therapy

- Supportive care very important
- —Volume, electrolyte support as indicated
- Platelets as indicated for thrombocytopenia
- Vitamin K (IM) for prolonged clotting time
- Hyponatremia management with fluid restriction as able (avoid sodium supplements)
- Albumin if indicated

MEDICATIONS

- All rickettsiostatic, not rickettsicidal
- —Hinder replication so host can eradicate disease
- —Duration: 5 to 10 days of therapy or until afebrile 2 to 5 days
- Doxycycline (usual medication of choice in all patients, except those who are pregnant)
- —Dosage: child: 2.2 mg/kg PO b.i.d. for 1 day, then 2.2 mg/kg/d PO in single dose; adult: 100 mg PO b.i.d.
- —Also treats ehrlichiosis if diagnosis uncertain
- —Side effects: less likely to stain teeth than tetracycline, contraindicated during pregnancy
- Chloramphenicol
- —Dosage: child: 75 to 100 mg/kg/d IV (initially) (modify if age <1 month), follow by 50 mg/kg/d divided q.i.d.; adult: 500 to 1000 mg q.i.d.
- —Side effects: peripheral neuropathy, aplastic anemia, "gray baby syndrome" with high levels, possible association with leukemia, hemolytic anemia with G6PD
- Tetracycline
- —Dosage: child: 25 to 50 mg/kg/d PO divided q.i.d. or 20 to 30 mg/kg/d IV; adult: 500 mg q.i.d. PO or IV
- —Side effects: tooth discoloration if child younger than 8 years of age (dose and duration related); pseudotumor cerebri, photosensitivity reaction, contraindicated during pregnancy
- Corticosteroids
- —May be helpful in severe cases, though no controlled studies
- —Not recommended for mild or moderately ill patients

 Follow-Up

- Expect improvement in 24 to 36 hours and defervescence in 2 to 3 days.
- Majority improve if treated early (<1 week)

CONTROL MEASURES

- Avoidance of tick-infested areas and tick contact; wear long clothing, pants tucked in socks or boots, limit skin access to ticks, frequent inspection (buddy checks)
- Tick repellants
- Early removal; ticks must attach and feed for 4 to 6 hours or longer to transmit disease; avoid direct contact with tick during removal; remove tick with tweezers (or gloved fingers

if tweezers not available) at point of attachment (as close to skin as possible), apply steady upward traction until tick's grip released and clean wound. Don't crush tick as this may increase disease transmission. Matches, petroleum jelly, fingernail polish, and rubbing alcohol do not appear to be effective for removal.

- Vaccine not available in United States; may not prevent disease but does prevent deaths
- Immunity conferred after disease

PITFALLS

- Not considering diagnosis until rash present; fatal disease often without rash at initial presentation
- Not treating empirically if strong suspicion of diagnosis
- Do not exclude diagnosis even if without history or evidence of tick bite and/or negative serologic test(s).
- Disease may occur outside endemic areas and the usual summer months.
- Classic descriptions of RMSF occur in second week. Initial presentations often are not classic.

 Common Questions and Answers

Q: For whom should RMSF as a differential diagnosis be entertained?

A: Anyone with a fever during the spring and summer who has been in an RMSF endemic area, regardless of presence of rash or history of known tick bite. Nonspecific symptoms or signs (GI, respiratory, rashes) may lead to misdiagnosis and delay in therapy.

Q: Should a child with a tick bite receive antibiotic prophylaxis when a tick is discovered?

A: To contract disease, one must be bitten by a tick that actually carries the disease (low risk), the tick must transmit the *Rickettsia* before it is removed (low risk), and the *Rickettsia* must be pathogenic if inoculated (low risk). There is no evidence that prophylaxis is necessary or efficacious in preventing disease. If considered, one must weigh risks and benefits of the therapy to be used.

ICD-9-CM 082.0

BIBLIOGRAPHY

Bleck TP. Central nervous system involvement in rickettsial diseases. *Neurol Clin* 1999;17(4)801–812.

Shapiro ED. Tick-borne diseases. *Adv Pediatr Infect Dis* 1997;13:187–218.

Thorner AR, Walker DH, Petri Jr. WA. Rocky Mountain spotted fever. State-of-the-art clinical article. *Clin Infect Dis* 1998;27: 1353–1360.

Author: George Anthony Woodward

Roseola—Herpes 6,7,8

 Database

DEFINITION

Roseola infantum is a common illness in preschool-aged children characterized by fever lasting 3 to 7 days followed by rapid defervescence and the appearance of a blanching maculopapular rash (usually on the 4th day of illness) lasting only 1 to 2 days.

CAUSES

- Roseola-like illnesses have been associated with a number of different viruses including enteroviruses (Coxsackie virus A and B, echoviruses); adenoviruses (types 1, 2, 3); parainfluenza virus; measles vaccine virus.
- A major cause of roseola appears to be human herpesvirus 6 (HHV-6). HHV-6 is a herpes virus similar to Epstein-Barr virus and cytomegalovirus.
- HHV-6 was first associated with roseola infantum by Yamanishi et al. in 1988.

PATHOPHYSIOLOGY

- Unknown
- The typical pattern of rash appearing as the fever disappears may represent virus neutralization in the skin.

EPIDEMIOLOGY

- Roseola can occur throughout the year; outbreaks have occurred in all seasons of the year.
- Roseola affects children from 3 months to 4 years. The peak age is 7 to 13 months.
- 90% of cases occur in the first 2 years of life.
- Cases occur in males and females equally.
- Incubation period is 5 to 15 days.

COMPLICATIONS

- Seizures are the most common complication of roseola. Between 5% and 10% of children will have a generalized tonic-clonic seizure associated with fever.
- Aseptic meningitis with less than 200 cells with primarily mononuclear cells have been reported.
- Encephalitis
- Thrombocytopenic purpura

PROGNOSIS

The vast majority of children with roseola infantum recover without sequelae.

 Differential Diagnosis

- Roseola has a distinctive presentation but resembles other viral exanthems.
- Antibiotic-associated rash in a child taking oral antibiotics when rash develops after defervescence.
- Rubella and enteroviral infections.

 Data Gathering

HISTORY

Question: Febrile?
Significance: Period of 3 to 5 days; commonly in the 38.9°C to 40.6°C range (102–105°F)

Question: Rash?
Significance: Appears as the fever disappears and lasts for 1 to 2 days

Question: Mild cough and coryza?
Significance: Common symptoms

Question: Appearance?
Significance: Usually children remain alert and are not ill appearing.

Question: Lymphadenopathy?
Significance: Common in the suboccipital, posterior cervical, and postauricular regions

Question: Eyelid edema and a bulging fontanelle?
Significance: Has also been noted

Laboratory Aids

Laboratory tests are not helpful in diagnosis. Commercial assays for antibody and/or antigen detection for HHV-6 are being developed.

Test: CBC
Significance: Occasionally, leukopenia with lymphocytosis is noted.

 Therapy

Supportive care

PREVENTION

• The virus associated with roseola infantum is usually transmitted via respiratory secretions or the fecal/oral spread.
• Outbreaks in hospitals have been reported, and infection control measures, such as bedside secretion precaution, should be instituted.

PITFALLS

Calling viral exanthems in preschool-aged children roseola even when fever is concomitant with rash

 Common Questions and Answers

Q: When can the child with roseola return to day care?
A: As soon as the child is afebrile; then there is no infectious risk of spread. The child may return to day care even with the rash visible.

Q: Will there be long-term sequelae in the child who has a seizure associated with roseola?
A: In general, these seizures are typical febrile seizures that hold no risk for long-term neurologic sequelae, e.g., epilepsy.

ICD-9-CM 056.9

BIBLIOGRAPHY

American Academy of Pediatrics. Human herpes virus 6. In: Peter G, ed. *1994 red book: report of the committee on infectious diseases*, 23rd ed. Elk Grove Village, IL: American Academy of Pediatrics, 1994:272–273.

Cherry JD. Roseola infantum. In: Feigin RD, Cherry JD, eds. *Textbook of pediatric infectious diseases*, 3rd ed. Philadelphia: WB Saunders, 1992:1789–1791.

Leach CT. Human herpes virus 6 and 7 infections in children: agents of roseola and other syndromes.

Leach CT, Sumaya CV, Brown NA. Human herpes virus-6: clinical implication of a recently discovered, ubiquitous agent. *J Pediatr* 1991;121:173–181.

Stoeckle MY. The spectrum of human herpes virus 6 infection: from roseola infantum to adult disease. *Annu Rev Med* 2000;51:423–430.

Author: Louis M. Bell

Salmonella Infections

 Database

DEFINITION

Salmonella is responsible for a broad spectrum of pathologic states ranging from asymptomatic infection to acute gastroenteritis to enteric fever.

EPIDEMIOLOGY

• Three species are responsible for most human salmonellosis: *S. enteritidis* (over 2,000 serotypes exist), *S. choleraesuis,* and *S. typhi.*
• Reservoirs
—*Salmonella* species other than *S. typhi:* animals and animal products (mammals, birds, reptiles, and insects); contaminated food and water; infected humans (fecal excretion may persist several months).
—Humans are the only natural reservoir for *S. typhi:* most commonly transmitted via fecally contaminated food and water; may be transmitted congenitally; chronic carriers may excrete *S. typhi* in stool for years.
• Incubation period
—Salmonella species other than *S. typhi:* 6 to 72 hours; symptoms typically begin within 24 hours.
• Incubation period of invasive *Salmonella* strains and *S. typhi* is 1 to 3 weeks.
• Age distribution: children under 5 and the elderly most commonly infected with nontyphoidal *Salmonella; S. typhi* most common in 5- to 25-year-olds.

COMPLICATIONS

• Dehydration and/or electrolyte imbalance is the most common complication arising from acute gastroenteritis.
• Invasive *Salmonella* may lead to complications of bacteremia:
—Sepsis: most common in neonates and immunosuppressed individuals
—Meningitis: vast majority of cases occur in first month of life
—Osteomyelitis: most common in patients with sickle cell anemia
—Other local infections: pneumonia, pericarditis
• Complications of enteric fever include intestinal or splenic rupture (at areas of lymphoid hypertrophy), hepatitis, pancreatitis, parotitis, orchitis, arthritis, myocarditis.
• A postinfectious form of hemolytic uremic syndrome may occur following *Salmonella* infection.

PROGNOSIS

• Most normal hosts with *Salmonella* gastroenteritis will recover spontaneously.
• Some individuals will develop a chronic carrier state, persistently shedding bacteria in the stool.
• The relapse rate of enteric fever may approach 15% of patients.

ASSOCIATED ILLNESSES

• Acute asymptomatic infection
—No clinical signs or symptoms become apparent.
—Probably most common *Salmonella* syndrome
—Patients can be identified only by recovery of organisms in stool.
• Acute gastroenteritis
—*Salmonella* is the most common type of infectious "food poisoning" in the United States.
—Symptoms begin 6 to 48 hours after *Salmonella* ingestion.
—Predominant manifestations are nausea, vomiting, crampy (often severe) abdominal pain, diarrhea (rarely, gross blood can be found).
—Other common features are malaise, myalgia, headache, and fever.
—Symptoms usually resolve spontaneously in 2 to 7 days.
• Bacteremia
—*Salmonella* organisms may produce acute or intermittent bacteremia.
—Symptoms: fever/chills, diaphoresis, myalgia, anorexia
—Bacteremia may occur before clinical gastroenteritis or, in infants, present as a persistent bacteremic state with failure to thrive.
—Up to 1 in 20 patients with *Salmonella* gastroenteritis may develop bacteremia (perhaps as high as 1 in 4 in infants).
• Enteric fever (typhoid fever, paratyphoid fever)
—Caused by *S. typhi* and several other *Salmonella* serotypes
—Incubation period 1 to 3 weeks
—Insidious onset of symptoms over 2 to 7 days: fever as high as 41°C, malaise, anorexia, abdominal pain, constipation.
—Additional symptoms and signs: lethargy, myalgia, headache, cough, either diarrhea or constipation, rigors, delirium, lymphadenopathy, organomegaly, "rose spots"
—Progression of illness: when untreated, illness with high fevers may last weeks; severe morbidity or death can result from especially virulent *Salmonella* strains.
• Asymptomatic chronic carriage
—Approximately 1% of patients infected with *Salmonella* gastroenteritis or enteric fever will continue to shed *Salmonella* in the stool for more than 1 year.

 Differential Diagnosis

The following illnesses may mimic *Salmonella* gastroenteritis and/or enterocolitis:
• *Shigellosis:* severe abdominal pains often are present, associated with high fevers, ulcers of the gastrointestinal lining are common, stools are often grossly bloody with "sheets" of fecal leukocytes.
• *Staphylococcal* food poisoning
• Other bacterial infections of the gastrointestinal tract

• Viral enteritis: rotavirus, Norwalk virus, and other viruses
• Parasitic infections
• Toxic ingestion
• Noninfectious systemic illnesses marked by inflammatory colitis

Enteric fever from *Salmonella* infection may be confused with:
• Invasive bacterial disease
• Spirochetal infection

 Data Gathering

HISTORY

• Exposure?
• Common historical features of *Salmonella* gastroenteritis:
—Nausea and vomiting begin 6 to 48 hours after ingestion.
—Diarrhea and abdominal pain with tenesmus follow; pain is typically periumbilical and in the right lower quadrant.
—Diarrhea lasts 2 to 4 days.
—Fever seldom exceeds 39°C; occurs in half of affected patients.
• Common historical features of enteric fever
—Symptoms begin 3 to 60 days after exposure.
—Commonly acquired during foreign travel
—Diarrhea uncommon early in course
—Fever ensues, which gradually increases in magnitude.
—Malaise, anorexia, myalgia, headache, abdominal pain, and vomiting may occur.

 Physical Examination

Salmonella gastrointestinal disease may display certain features:
• Dehydration may be evident.
• Abdominal pain may closely mimic appendicitis and/or cholecystitis.
• Stools may be bloody, watery, or mucousy.

Finding: Important signs of enteric fever
Significance:
• Enlarged liver and spleen
• Relative bradycardia for height of fever is a frequently distinguishing finding.
• Rose spots: 2 to 4 mm in diameter; blanching pink papules; most commonly found on anterior thorax; 5 to 20 are generally apparent at a time; fade in 3 to 4 days after appearance; characteristic of enteric fever, but not specific.

Laboratory Aids

There are several nonspecific laboratory aids to diagnosis:

Test: Stool examination
Significance: May have Hemoccult-positive stools; stool may be positive for fecal leukocytes in enterocolitis

Test: Complete blood cell count with differential
Significance: Normal in simple gastroenteritis; neutropenia, thrombocytopenia, and mild anemia are common in enteric fever.

Test: Serum chemistries
Significance: Metabolic acidosis and electrolyte abnormalities may occur with severe enteritis; a mild hepatitis is frequently found in enteric fever.

Test: Stool and blood culture and identification of *Salmonella* organisms
Significance: The "gold-standard" method for laboratory confirmation of infection

Test: Bone marrow aspirate
Significance: The most sensitive source for isolation of *Salmonella* in patients with enteric fever; early in the course of invasive illness bone marrow culture may be positive even when stool samples fail to grow the bacteria; may provide positive cultures even after initial antibiotic pretreatment.

Test: Urine culture
Significance: May be a source of *Salmonella* organisms in the young or elderly and in those with enteric fever

Test: Biopsy
Significance: Needle aspiration of purulent material may yield positive cultures; punch biopsy and culture of rose spots may confirm diagnosis of *S. typhi*.

FALSE POSITIVES
Leukocytes in the stool are suggestive of colitis but are more typical of *Campylobacter*, *Shigella*, or milk allergy.

PITFALLS
Enteric fever may precede enteritis symptoms and fecal shedding of bacteria.

Therapy

• Acute asymptomatic infection
—Should not be treated with antibiotics: antibiotics do not have impact on duration of diarrhea and may lengthen duration of carrier state.
• Acute gastroenteritis (see Common Questions and Answers, below)
—Supportive care: maintain intravascular volume; correct electrolyte abnormalities
—Do *not* administer antidiarrheal agents; they prolong gastrointestinal transit time.

—Consider antibiotics in individuals at high risk of subsequent systemic invasive illness: children younger than 3 months of age; immunocompromised hosts; patients with hemoglobinopathies; patients with chronic gastrointestinal tract disease.
• Bacteremia, enteric fever, and/or chronic carrier state:
—Supportive care
—Antibiotics are indicated; initial therapy usually to be administered intravenously
—Surgical drainage of local suppuration is indicated as in most other infections.
—Corticosteroids (3 mg/kg load, 1 mg/kg every 6 hours) may be beneficial to critically ill patients with enteric fever exhibiting neurologic complications.
—Antipyretics are controversial in enteric fever syndromes because they may cause precipitous declines in temperature and shock.
• Various antibiotics may be used to treat *Salmonella* infection:
• *Salmonella* gastroenteritis at high risk of invasive disease: increasing resistance to amoxicillin, ampicillin, and trimethoprim-sulfa; parenteral third-generation cephalosporins or fluoroquinolones preferred.
• Invasive *Salmonella* disease: intravenous ampicillin for 2 weeks has been first-line therapy; chloramphenicol, a third-generation cephalosporin, or a quinolone may be used for resistant organisms; cefotaxime for treatment of meningitis; meningitis or osteomyelitis may require 4 to 6 weeks of parenteral antibiotic therapy.
• Some authorities treat chronic carriers of *Salmonella* who shed more than 1 year: high-dose parenteral ampicillin; high-dose oral amoxicillin (with or without probenecid), ciprofloxacin; consider cholecystectomy for recalcitrant cases.

PREVENTION
Personal hygiene and sanitation measures are the primary means by which to prevent *Salmonella* infections:
• Carriers of *Salmonella* are a public health concern:
—Hospitalized patients: enteric precautions for length of illness
—Outpatients: should be restricted from food preparation for others

Follow-Up

• Acute gastrointestinal illness
—Symptoms usually resolve spontaneously within 7 days.
—Supportive care to prevent or treat dehydration may be required.
—Young children and those with underlying disease processes may be at higher risk of complications.
• Enteric fever
—Untreated, this illness will have a prolonged course over weeks.

—Life-threatening complications are most common during the second or third week of illness, often after a period of apparent clinical improvement.
—Even with appropriate treatment up to 15% of patients may suffer relapse.
• Chronic carriage
—1% to 3% of patients with *Salmonella* infection will shed bacteria in the stool for longer than 1 year.
—Chronic carriers should be identified because they represent a public health threat.

PITFALLS
• More people with *Salmonella* infestation are asymptomatic than are symptomatic.
• Antibiotic resistance is a growing problem.
• Even with appropriate therapy, patients may shed bacteria on a persistent basis or may suffer relapse.

Common Questions and Answers

Q: Should all infants with *Salmonella* gastroenteritis be treated with antibiotics?
A: Clinicians caring for children younger than 1 year of life with proven, or suspected, *Salmonella* infection face many treatment dilemmas. Any toxic-appearing infant and any infant with proven *Salmonella* bacteremia should be admitted to the hospital for parenteral antibiotics. High-risk infants (those under 3 months of age) with positive stool cultures should be treated with antibiotics after obtaining blood cultures. Well-appearing infants above the age of 3 months with *Salmonella* enterocolitis and fever can be observed off antibiotics once surveillance blood cultures are obtained.

ICD-9-CM 003.9

BIBLIOGRAPHY
Fierer J, Swancutt M. Non-typhoid salmonella: a review. *Curr Clin Top Infect Dis* 2000;20: 134–157.

Goldberg MB, Rubin RH. The spectrum of Salmonella infection. *Infect Dis Clin North Am* 1988;2:571–598.

Nataro JP. Treatment of bacterial enteritis. *Pediatr Infect Dis J* 1998;17:420–421.

St. Geme JW, Hodes HL, Marcy M, et al. Consensus: management of salmonella infection in the first year of life. *Pediatr Infect Dis J* 1988;7:615–621.

Author: Kevin C. Osterhoudt

Sarcoidosis

 Database

DEFINITION

A multisystem chronic granulomatous disease that has two distinct variations often differentiated by age of onset

CAUSES

Unknown

PATHOLOGY

• A T-cell–mediated disease, resulting in noncaseating granulomas in affected organs

EPIDEMIOLOGY

• Disease occurs before age 4 as arthritis, uveitis, fever, and rash, and in adolescence as Lofgren syndrome of erythema nodosum, polyarteritis, and hilar adenopathy. Adult-type disease with marked pulmonary involvement may also occur in older adolescents.

GENETICS

Blacks are more commonly affected than whites; specific genetic tendencies not identified.

COMPLICATIONS

In children, usually related to uveitis, or from hypercalciuria resulting in renal injury; in older adolescents, pulmonary problems such as restrictive lung disease can occur, as well as severe growth delay.

 Differential Diagnosis

• Infection: tuberculosis, bacterial sepsis, mumps, HIV, gonorrhea, Lyme disease, pulmonary mycoses
• Tumors: leukemia, neuroblastoma, lymphoma
• Immunologic: pauciarticular JRA (for early-onset type), systemic JRA, SLE, dermatomyositis, Behçet syndrome
• Genetic: Blau syndrome

 Data Gathering

HISTORY

Question: Malaise, fever, rash, evanescent painful arthritis, swollen lymph nodes, cough, and hematuria?
Significance: May be initial complaints.

 Physical Examination

• Peripheral lymphadenopathy is most common manifestation
• Eyes may be injected.
• Bilateral parotid gland enlargement and hepatosplenomegaly can be present.
• The arthritis, usually in the ankles, is extremely tender.
• Rash is diffuse, erythematous, and macular, or plaque-like.

SPECIAL QUESTIONS

Finding: History of papule?
Significance: Forming after needlestick (pathergy)

 Laboratory Aids

• CBC
• ESR
• Synovial effusions are typically noninflammatory.
• Biopsy of peripheral lymph gland, skin, conjunctivae, or minor salivary gland demonstrating noncaseating granuloma is helpful.

Test: Angiotensin-converting enzyme (ACE) level
Significance: Produced in most granulomatous diseases, but is useful where index of suspicion is high

Test: Lysozyme level
Significance: May be more sensitive than ACE level for detecting sarcoidosis

Test: Serum calcium and creatinine levels
Significance: Are important for baseline

Test: Urine for blood
Significance: Seen in patients with hypercalciuria

IMAGING

Test: CXR
Significance: May demonstrate hilar adenopathy

Test: Gallium scan
Significance: Will demonstrate uptake diffusely in lungs (extremely sensitive test)

FALSE POSITIVES

Test: ACE level
Significance: May be elevated in patients with miliary TB and biliary cirrhosis. Not a good single-screening test; however, can follow levels in response to treatment

PITFALLS

Uveitis may be occult; ophthalmology evaluation is important.

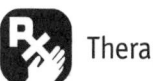 Therapy

DRUGS

Nonsteroidal antiinflammatory drugs, analgesics, and steroids all have a role. In cases of chronic disease, immunosuppressive drugs, such as corticosteroids and methotrexate, may have roles to play. In cases of hypercalciuria/hypercalcemia, hydration and Lasix should be considered.

DURATION

During times of disease activity causing clinical symptoms

DIET

Hydration is important in patients with hypercalcemia.

 Follow-Up

WHEN TO EXPECT IMPROVEMENT

Early childhood sarcoid and Lofgren syndrome may resolve over several months. Rarely, older children with pulmonary manifestations may develop chronic interstitial lung disease or bony infiltrates over years of disease.

SIGNS TO WATCH FOR

Climbing creatinine, shortness of breath, or persistent uveal tract inflammation

PROGNOSIS

Generally good for most children. Lofgren disease resolves. Over 40% of older children with adult-type disease have persistent pulmonary changes, but only a few will have pulmonary symptoms.

PITFALLS

Overtreatment of asymptomatic lymphadenopathy and not detecting hypercalciuria

 Common Questions and Answers

Q: Why is the outcome better in childhood sarcoid compared with adults with sarcoid?
A: These may be two distinct granulomatous diseases. The two clearly have different patterns of organ involvement.

ICD-9-CM 135.0

BIBLIOGRAPHY

Cron RQ, Wallace CA, Sherry DD. Childhood sarcoidosis—does age of onset predict clinical manifestations? *J Rheumatol* 1997;24: 1654–1656.

Fink CW, Cimaz R. Early onset sarcoidosis: not a benign disease. *J Rheumatol* 1997;24: 174–177.

Gedalia A, Molina JF, Ellis GS Jr, et al. Low-dose methotrexate therapy for childhood sarcoidosis. *J Pediatr* 1997;130:3–4.

Hafner R, Vogel P. Sarcoidosis of early onset. A challenge for the pediatric rheumatologist. *Clin Exp Rheumatol* 1993;11:685–691.

Lindsley CB, Petty RE. Overview and report on international registry of sarcoid arthritis in childhood. *Curr Rheumatol Rep* 2000;2: 343–348.

Pattishall EN, Kendig EL Jr. Sarcoidosis in children. *Pediatr Pulmonol* 1996;22(3): 195–203.

Shetty AK, Gedalia A. Sarcoidosis: a pediatric perspective. *Clin Pediatr* 1998;37:707–717.

Tomita H, Sato S, Matsuda R, et al. Serum lysozyme levels and clinical features of sarcoidosis. *Lung* 1999;177:161–167.

Author: Randy Q. Cron

Scabies

 Database

DEFINITION

• Scabies results from the infestation of the stratum corneum by the human mite, *Sarcoptes scabiei* (subspecies hominis, phylum Arthropoda, class Arachnida, and order Acarina). Etiologic agent is the gravid female mite, 0.2 to 0.4 mm in size.
• Animal scabies, sarcoptic mange, occurs from contact with an infested canine and produces only a transient rash in humans.
• Norwegian scabies, a variant of human scabies, occurs in institutional settings and is highly contagious, requiring isolation measures and diligent use of antiscabetics for elimination.
• Postscabetic syndrome consists of persistent pruritus, caused by hypersensitivity to the mite antigen and may persist for several days after the live mite has been eliminated.

PATHOPHYSIOLOGY

• The female mite burrows into the stratum corneum, rarely penetrating through the epidermis, for 15 to 30 days traveling 2 to 4 mm per day and laying 1 to 3 eggs per day.
• Egg laying is completed in 4 to 5 weeks when the female dies within the burrow. Eggs, hatching within the burrow, will undergo several molts and emerge on the skin surface as nymphs. After a 2- to 3-week maturation period, mating will occur; the male will die, and the gravid female will restart the cycle with burrowing.
• Ten to 30 days after scabies infestation, perhaps the time lag necessary for the body to develop humoral or cellular hypersensitivity to the mite and/or its by-products or the time necessary for an adequate mass of mites to exist, signs and symptoms will develop.

EPIDEMIOLOGY

• Affects all age groups
• Epidemics are reported to occur in 15-year cycles.
• Sole reservoir of *S. scabiei* is the human.
• Close personal contact with an infested human (with or without clinical symptoms) is required for transmission
• Mites can live isolated from a human body for 2 to 3 days; however the extent of fomite transmission is unclear.

COMPLICATIONS

• Secondary infections, including impetigo and folliculitis, may occur.
• Pruritus is often intense.

PROGNOSIS

Excellent outcome with therapy. Resistant cases, necessitating referral to a dermatologist and consideration for oral therapy, have been reported.

 Differential Diagnosis

INFECTION

• Impetigo
• Papular viral exanthem

ENVIRONMENTAL

• Contact dermatitis

IMMUNOLOGIC

• Atopic dermatitis
• Papular urticaria

MISCELLANEOUS

• Drug eruptions
• Psoriasis
• Infantile acropustulosis

 Data Gathering

HISTORY

Question: Pruritus?
Significance: Intensity worse at night when mite activity increases secondary to a rise in body temperature

Question: Evolution of the rash?
Significance: Characteristically changes over time both in appearance and distribution

Question: Symptoms in other family members or close contacts?
Significance: Close contact is required for transmission.

 Physical Examination

• Examine the entire body surface area with particular attention to the web spaces in the hands.
• Distribution of the rash is usually from the neck down in infants while in children the neck and face also may be involved.
• Lesions are typically more numerous on the hands, especially the web spaces, as well as the thenar and hypothenar eminences in older children and adults. The palms and proximal half of the foot and heel are sites of numerous lesions in infants.
• Lesions are also seen on the wrists, in the axillae, around the waistline, on the gluteal cleft, and surrounding the nipples and genitalia.
• A burrow, the characteristic lesion of scabies, is present in 90% to 95% of all symptomatic patients, and forms a "lazy S" shape with a broad base and a punctate brown-black dot at the leading edge of the mite's path. If burrows are not easily identified, washable felt tip marker can be rubbed across the web space, and after the superficial ink is removed with alcohol or water, the ink will have penetrated through the stratum corneum outlining the burrow.
• Secondary lesions are more numerous and obvious than the burrows and consist of crusted papules, small vesicles, pustules, excoriated broad areas of dermatitis, and areas of secondary infection from impetigo and folliculitis.

 Laboratory Aids

Skin scrapings may be done to secure a definitive diagnosis. The burrows most commonly found on the hands and feet should be moistened with alcohol or mineral oil. A no. 15 round-bellied blade attached to a scalpel handle should be briskly scraped across the burrows. Scraped material is placed on a slide with a drop of KOH or mineral oil with a coverslip. Under a scanning microscope, the gravid female, eggs, larvae, or feces are diagnostic.

Therapy

DRUGS

• 5% permethrin cream (Elimite) is used for infants older than 2 months and children. Apply to the entire body surface and leave on for 8 to 14 hours, then wash off. One application is usually effective, though some recommend a second application 10 to 14 days later.
• 1% lindane is effective for older children and nonpregnant adults; should remain on the body for 8 to 12 hours. Lindane use in young children is considered to be potentially toxic and hence lindane use in young children is generally not recommended.
• 10% crotamiton cream may be used for infants older than 6 months and is applied for 2 days followed by a cleansing bath 48 hours after the last application. There have been reported frequent treatment failures with crotamiton.
• 6% sulfur in a petrolatum base may be used; it is applied for 3 consecutive days in older children and adults.
• Mild-to-moderate topical steroids (e.g., 1% hydrocortisone, 0.025–0.1% triamcinolone) may be beneficial in the postscabetic syndrome.
• Oral agents, such as ivermectin, are sometimes used in adult patients for resistant scabies. Ivermectin, in a solution of propylene glycol, has been used as a topical agent in some trials. Referral to a dermatologist is recommended prior to the consideration of oral therapy or topical use of ivermectin to verify the diagnosis and to assess treatment alternatives.

Follow-Up

• Pruritus may take up to 4 weeks to resolve after effective treatment. Use of a mild-to-moderate topical steroid may improve these symptoms.
• Continued appearance of new burrows may indicate ineffective treatment (most commonly misapplication) and warrants repeat physician evaluation.

PREVENTION

• Bedding, clothing, and items of close contact should be washed and dried in hot temperatures at the time of treatment.
• All family members and close contacts should be treated concurrently regardless of clinical symptoms. Contacts may be infested without symptoms.

PITFALLS

There is a need to treat close contacts, symptomatic and asymptomatic, to eliminate the mite and prevent immediate reinfestation.

Common Questions and Answers

Q: How did my child get scabies?
A: From close contact with an infected person

Q: How long will my child continue to itch?
A: Pruritus may continue for weeks; the use of topical hydrocortisone may be helpful.

Q: Do I need to wash my child's bedding in a special detergent?
A: Simply wash all bedding in hot soapy water after your child has been treated.

ICD-9-CM 133.0

BIBLIOGRAPHY

American Academy of Pediatrics. Scabies. In: Pickering LE, ed. *2000 red book: report of the Committee on Infectious Diseases*, 25th ed. Elk Grove Village, IL: American Academy of Pediatrics, 2000:506–508.

Cestari SC, Petri V, Rotta O, et al. Oral treatment of crusted scabies with ivermectin: report of two cases. *Pediatr Dermatol* 2000;17(5):410–414.

Dourmishev AL, Serafimova DK, Dourmishev LA, et al. Crusted scabies of the scalp in dermatomyositis patients: three cases treated with oral ivermectin. *Int J Dermatol* 1998;37(3):231–234.

Rasmussen JE. Scabies. *Pediatr Rev* 1994;15(3):110–114.

Victoria J, Trujillo R. Topical ivermectin: a new successful treatment for scabies. *Pediatr Dermatol* 2001;18(1):63–65.

Author: Kathy Wholey Zsolway

Scarlet Fever

 Database

DEFINITION

- A clinical syndrome consisting of fever, pharyngitis, cervical lymphadenitis, and the characteristic "sandpaper rash," which results from infection with a strain of *Streptococcus pyogenes* (group A β-hemolytic *Streptococcus*) that elaborates streptococcal pyrogenic toxin.
- Toxins include A, B, or C. Toxin A is associated with more virulent disease.
- Similar syndrome may also be seen after infection with certain toxin-producing (enterotoxin G, I) strains of *Staphylococcus aureus*, dubbed "staphylococcal scarlet fever"
- Some investigators feel that both streptococcal and staphylococcal forms of scarlet fever and toxic shock syndrome (TSS) are on a continuum of disease. Bacteria may produce multiple toxins and the severity of disease is determined by the relative amounts of pyrogenic and TSS-producing toxins produced by the offending strain.

PATHOPHYSIOLOGY

- Susceptible individuals thought to lack toxin-specific immunity. Supported by results of "Dick test" in which a small amount of toxin introduced intradermally produces local erythema in susceptible individuals, but no reaction in those with toxin-specific immunity.
- Rash and other toxic manifestations of scarlet fever have been attributed to the development of hypersensitivity to the toxin, which therefore would require prior exposure to the toxin.
- Toxin production is dependent on lysogeny of the infecting streptococcus by a temperate bacteriophage.
- Pharyngitis characterized by mucosal erythema and frequently by small crypt abscesses with punctate exudate in enlarged tonsils.
- Edematous papillae protrude from coated mucosa to produce "strawberry tongue."
- Histologic examination of affected skin shows dilated blood and lymphatic vessels and engorged capillaries, most prominently around hair follicles.
- Acute, edematous polymorphonuclear inflammatory reaction is seen microscopically within affected tissues.
- Epidermal inflammatory reaction is usually followed by hyperkeratosis, which accounts for scaling during defervescence.

EPIDEMIOLOGY

- Peak incidence during the first few school years
- Occurs uncommonly before the age of 3 years or after the age of 15 years, possibly related to the requirement for prior sensitization and toxin-specific immunity.
- By age 10, 80% of children have developed toxin-specific antibodies.
- No sex predilection
- All forms of streptococcal pharyngitis (i.e., with or without pyrogenic toxin) are more common in temperate and cold climates, and winter and spring months, with some areas reporting an increased incidence in the fall.
- Incubation period is usually 24 to 48 hours.

COMPLICATIONS

- Acute otitis media
- Sinusitis
- Suppurative cervical lymphadenitis
- Pneumonia with or without effusion/empyema
- Peritonsillar cellulitis/abscess
- Retropharyngeal abscess
- Meningitis
- Brain abscess
- Thrombosis of intracranial venous sinuses
- Osteomyelitis
- Hepatitis
- Arthritis
- Acute rheumatic fever (ARF)
- Acute postinfectious glomerulonephritis (APGN)
- Erythema nodosum, possibly

PROGNOSIS

- Overall prognosis is excellent.
- Few patients suffer suppurative complications.
- Risk of developing ARF in untreated streptococcal infections is about 3% under epidemic conditions (0.3% in endemic situations).
- Risk of developing APGN depends on nephritogenicity of infecting strain. Attack rate is 10% to 15% with nephritogenic strains.

 Differential Diagnosis

- Nonscarlatinal streptococcal pharyngitis/tonsillitis
- Viral exanthems (measles, rubella, erythema infectiosum)
- Drug eruptions
- Staphylococcal scalded skin syndrome (SSSS)
- Toxic epidermal necrolysis (TEN)
- Toxic shock syndrome (streptococcal or staphylococcal)
- Kawasaki disease

UNCOMMON ENTITIES

- Infection with *Corynebacterium hemolyticum*
- Mercury poisoning (acrodynia)
- Atropine intoxication
- Boric acid poisoning
- Rifampin overdose

 Data Gathering

HISTORY

Question: Was there sudden onset of fever up to 40.5°C, sore throat, headache, nausea, vomiting, and toxicity?
Significance: Classic for group A streptococcal disease.

Question: Does the rash feel like sandpaper?
Significance: Texture is more important than appearance.

Question: When did the rash start?
Significance: Characteristic rash typically occurs 12 to 48 hours after onset of fever.

Question: Any abdominal pain or muscle aches prior to rash?
Significance: May complain of abdominal pain before onset of rash, as well as aching in extremities or back

Question: Any close contacts with streptococcal infection?
Significance: Helps in identification

 Physical Examination

Finding: Fine maculopapular (sandpaper texture) rash on erythematous background
Significance: Usually begins on the trunk and spreads to involve almost the entire body within hours to days

Finding: Circumoral pallor present
Significance: Classic finding

Finding: Rash blanches with pressure and ultimately desquamates.
Significance: Desquamation occurs within 7 to 21 days from onset of illness.

Finding: Characteristic toxin-induced scarlet fever exanthem
Significance: Can rarely be seen without pharyngitis in the setting of pyoderma or an infected wound (known as "surgical scarlet fever")

Finding: May see scattered petechiae
Significance: Common finding

Finding: Systemic toxicity
Significance: May indicate incorrect diagnosis

Finding: Deep red nonblanching lesions
Significance: "Pastia lines" develop in the skin folds of joints.

Finding: Dorsum of tongue
Significance: Has white coat early in illness with edematous red papillae. White covering desquamates and reveals swollen, red and mottled "strawberry tongue."

Other Findings

- Pharynx and tonsils are beefy red and may contain exudate.
- Hemorrhagic spots on interior pillar of tonsils and soft palate
- Large, tender anterior cervical nodes

Laboratory Aids

Test: Rapid streptococcal antigen tests
Significance: Effective as screening tests; 50% to 80% sensitivity and greater than 95% specificity. Positive rapid tests do not require culture confirmation.

Test: Throat culture
Significance: The "gold standard" with best sensitivity (>90%) for group A β-hemolytic streptococci. A culture should be performed when rapid test is negative.

Test: White blood cell count
Significance: Usually elevated, though may be elevated in viral pharyngitis as well. Low count would be rare with streptococcal infection.

Test: Eosinophilia (up to 30%)
Significance: is common in the recovery phase.

Test: Dick test
Significance: Of historic interest, no longer used clinically

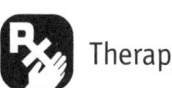

Therapy

- Identical to therapy for streptococcal pharyngitis
- Therapy started as late as 9 days after illness onset should be effective in preventing ARF.
- May withhold treatment until throat culture result is available
- Immediate therapy probably shortens symptomatic period.

DRUGS

- Oral penicillin V: drug of choice except in penicillin-allergic individuals. Resistant strains have not been documented in the U.S. Dose: 25,000–50,000 units/kg (1,600 units = 1 mg) divided into three to four doses for 10 days; 400,000 units (250 mg) twice daily for 10 days has also been shown to have comparable efficacy and is endorsed by the American Academy of Pediatrics.
- Intramuscular benzathine penicillin G: equally effective as oral penicillin. Dose: 600,000 units for children less than 60 pounds; 1,200,000 units in larger children and adults. Assures compliance. Bringing to room temperature reduces discomfort. Benzathine/procaine penicillin combinations are less painful.

- Oral erythromycin is indicated in penicillin-allergic individuals. Dose: erythromycin ethyl succinate (40 to 50 mg/kg/d in two to four divided doses). Resistance is rare in the U.S.
- Clarithromycin (10-day regimen) and azithromycin (5-day regimen) have also shown excellent clinical and bacteriologic cure rates in recent clinical trials.
- There are reports of acute rheumatic fever after the 3-day course of azithromycin.
- Amoxicillin, clindamycin, and first-generation oral cephalosporins (up to 15% of penicillin-allergic persons are also allergic to cephalosporins) are reasonable alternatives to penicillin.
- Tetracyclines and sulfonamides should *not* be used due to resistance.
- Recent trials comparing 10-day course of penicillin with shorter duration of therapy with newer oral cephalosporins have shown similar bacteriologic and clinical cure rates, but efficacy in prevention of nonsuppurative sequelae is unknown.
- Positive posttreatment cultures in asymptomatic patients: re-treatment not recommended.

Follow-Up

- Fever and symptoms usually resolve within 24 to 48 hours of antibiotic treatment.
- Nonsuppurative complications occur after unrecognized disease and when treatment is delayed for more than 9 days. ARF occurs an average of 18 days after untreated infection. APGN occurs an average of 10 days after untreated infection.

PREVENTION

- Prompt treatment leads to fewer secondary cases of streptococcal disease.
- Chemoprophylaxis with penicillin recommended by some experts in children with repeated documented episodes occurring at short intervals.

PITFALLS

- A positive throat culture may only be evidence of carriage in some cases of pharyngitis that are truly viral (e.g., Epstein-Barr virus).
- Milder disease is becoming more common, and is easier to miss. Rash may involve only the bridge of the nose, face, shoulders, and upper chest. Circumoral pallor and severe exudative pharyngitis are being seen less frequently.

Common Questions and Answers

Q: Should household contacts have throat cultures performed?
A: Only obtain cultures from symptomatic household contacts. Cultures should not routinely be obtained in asymptomatic contacts.

Q: Should posttreatment throat cultures be performed?
A: Only in symptomatic individuals and patients at risk for ARF and APGN

Q: Can scarlet fever recur?
A: Yes, there have been documented reports of recurrent scarlet fever.

Q: Have there been documented day-care outbreaks of scarlet fever?
A: Yes, outbreaks have been traced back to a single strain.

Q: How soon can children return to school or day care?
A: When they are afebrile after at least 24 hours of therapy.

ICD-9-CM 034.1

BIBLIOGRAPHY

Altemeier WA. A pediatrician's view. A brief history of group A beta hemolytic strep. *Pediatr Ann* 1998;27:264–267.

American Academy of Pediatrics. Group A streptococcal infections. In: Pickering LK, ed. *2000 red book: report of the Committee on Infectious Diseases,* 25th ed. Elk Grove Village, IL: American Academy of Pediatrics, 2000:526–536.

Barnett BO, Frieden IJ. Streptococcal skin diseases in children. *Semin Dermatol* 1992;11:3–10.

Breese BB. Streptococcal pharyngitis and scarlet fever. *Am J Dis Child* 1978;132: 612–616.

Efstratiou A. Group A streptococci in the 1990s. *J Antimicrob Chemother* 2000; 45(suppl):3–12.

Jarraud S, Cozon G, Vandenesch F, et al. Involvement of enterotoxins G and I in staphylococcal toxic shock syndrome and staphylococcal scarlet fever. *J Clin Microbiol* 1999;37:2446–2449.

Shiseki M, Miwa K, Nemoto Y, et al. Comparison of pathogenic factors expressed by group A streptococci isolated from patients with streptococcal toxic shock syndrome and scarlet fever. *Microb Pathogen* 1999;27:243–252.

Shulman ST. Evaluation of penicillins, cephalosporins, and macrolides for therapy of streptococcal pharyngitis. *Pediatrics* 1996;97:955–959.

Author: Mark L. Bagarazzi

Scleroderma

Database

DEFINITION

Scleroderma means hard skin.

• Systemic sclerosis (SSc) or progressive systemic sclerosis (PSS)

—Diagnostic criteria: one major or two minor
—Major: sclerodermatous changes (tightness, thickening, induration) proximal to the MCP or MTP
—Minor: sclerodactyly-sclerodermatous changes limited to the digits; digital pitting; bibasilar pulmonary fibrosis not due to primary lung disease
—CREST (a variant form of SSc)
  —Calcinosis
  —Raynaud phenomenon
  —Esophageal dysmotility
  —Sclerodactyly
  —Telangiectases
  —Affects approximately one half of patients with SSc
  —Females more than males
  —Earlier age of onset than SSc
  —Same characteristics as SSc, but calcinosis is more severe
  —Distal symptoms are more severe
  —Associated with anticentromere antibody

• Localized: fibrosis limited to the skin, subcutaneous tissue, and muscle

—Systemic features
—Rare: visceral involvement later in the disease
—Occasional: evolution into another connective tissue disease such as MCTD or SLE
—Very rarely: Raynaud
—Forms
  —Morphea: one or more oval or round indurations that become hard and whitish early on, have active inflammatory border with violaceous color; forms: plaque or guttate; limited number of lesions; generalized: extensive; nodular: subcutaneous
  —Linear: one or more linear areas affecting subcutaneous tissue, muscle, and bone
  —Coup de sabre: involving face or scalp may be associated with seizures
  —Parry-Romberg syndrome: form of linear scleroderma; congenital dysplasia of the subcutaneous tissue, neurologic changes such as TIAs.

PATHOPHYSIOLOGY

The following theories have been proposed:

• Alteration of normal glycosylation and hydroxylation of collagen
• Serum factors: endothelin
• Vasculopathy: based on high association with Raynaud
• Immune dysfunction: autoimmunity directed against connective tissue antigen such as laminin or type IV collagen

• May represent distinct early and late processes:
—Early: increase of hydrophilic glycosaminoglycan; increased T cells, macrophages, and plasma cells; mast cell hyperplasia
—Late: increase collagen content; collagen is embryonic with narrow fibrils and immature cross banding; atrophy of rete pegs

EPIDEMIOLOGY

• Systemic

—Incidence: annually 4.5 to 12 per million
—Age of onset: 30 to 50 years; very rare in children
—Sex ratio: younger than 7 years no difference; older than 7 years, F/M 3:1; 15 to 44 years, F/M 15:1
—Genetics: unknown

• Localized

—More common than SSc
—Exact incidence is unclear

COMPLICATIONS

• Systemic

—see Physical Examination, below

• Localized

—Skin thickening
—Joint contractures
—Leg length discrepancies

PROGNOSIS

• Natural course includes several phases: initial: inflammation; late: sclerotic, occasional regression over 3 to 5 years
• Ultimate prognosis depends on severity of skin tightness, joint contracture, and visceral involvement
• Mortality: males more than females and nonwhites more than whites
• Most common cause of death in children is secondary to cardiac, renal, and pulmonary complications

Differential Diagnosis

• Graft-versus-host disease
• Phenylketonuria
• *Borrelia* infection: acrodermatitis chronica atrophicans
• Porphyria cutanea tarda
• Scleredema

Data Gathering

HISTORY

• Thickening of skin
• Tightness of joints
• Discoloration of skin
• Often insidious onset
• Morning stiffness
• Heartburn, dysphagia, reflux, cough with swallowing

Physical Examination

Finding: Skin
Significance:

• Stage 1: Edema: tense, nonpitting, perhaps warm or tender, but often asymptomatic
• Stage 2: Sclerosis: waxy hard texture, bound to subcutaneous structures, back of digits, face (loss of forehead wrinkles, reduced mouth orifice)
• Stage 3: Atrophy: shiny appearance, hypo- or hyperpigmented, calcium deposits in subcutaneous tissue. Telangiectases: macular dilatations that fill slowly, unlike spider telangiectasias.

Finding: Raynaud phenomenon associated with underlying disease
Significance:

• Subtypes:

—Phenomenon: associated with underlying disease
—Disease
—Triple phase: blanching, cyanosis, erythema
—Present in approximately 90% of patients with systemic sclerosis
—Usually fingers, also toes, nose, ears, and tongue, often spares the thumb
—Pathophysiology: arterial vasoconstriction, venous stasis to cyanosis, reflex vasodilatation to erythema

• Calcinosis, especially over extensor joint surfaces
• Musculoskeletal
• "Creaking" of thickened tendons
• Contractures, especially PIP and elbows
• No intraarticular inflammation
• Muscle inflammation in approximately 30% of cases
• Gastrointestinal
• Mucosal telangiectasias of mouth
• Decreased incisor distance secondary to skin thickening
• Sicca syndrome with parotitis
• Loosening of teeth secondary to periodontal membrane disease
• Esophageal disease: esophagitis, occasional ulceration or stricture
• Large bowel disease less common
• Cardiac
• Primary cause of morbidity

- Possibly due to Raynaud of coronary arteries
- Pulmonary forms
- Interstitial fibrosis with gradual obliteration of vascular bed and resulting cor pulmonale
- Parenchymal disease is almost universal, frequently asymmetric, may have hacking cough, dyspnea on exertion, pleural rub
- Combined pulmonary vascular and pulmonary parenchymal
- Primary pulmonary vascular disease with right ventricular failure
- Renal, due to decreased renal plasma flow, ominous, proteinuria, hypertension
- CNS: cranial nerve involvement, especially sensory branch of trigeminal nerve
- Sicca syndrome
- Xerostomia (dry mouth)
- Keratoconjunctivitis sicca (dry eyes)
- Diagnosis: lip biopsy; rose bengal staining of cornea

PROCEDURES

- Schirmer test for dry eyes
- Periungual nailfold changes: capillary dropout and dilated loops; occasional redundant cuticular growth and digital pitting

 Laboratory Aids

There are no specific diagnostic tests.

NONSPECIFIC TESTS

Systemic Form

- ANA often positive

Test: Hb
Significance: 25% have anemia due to chronic disease or vitamin B_{12} and folate deficiencies due to chronic malabsorption in sclerodermatous gut.

Test: Eosinophilia
Significance: 15%

Test: Sclero-70 (Scl-70 or Topoisomerase 1)
Significance: 26% of adults; more common with diffuse disease than peripheral vascular disease

Test: Anticentromere antibody
Significance: 22%; almost exclusively with CREST

Histologic Findings

Test: Muscle
Significance: Increased collagen and fat; negative immunofluorescence

Test: Esophageal
Significance: Atrophic muscle replaced by fibrous tissue more commonly affects smooth muscle of lower two thirds of esophagus

ECG Findings

- ECG: first-degree block
- Right and left bundle-branch block (BBB)
- PACs and PVCs: Nonspecific T-wave changes, ventricular hypertrophy

PFTs

Test: Restrictive lung disease
Significance: 34% of SSc

Test: Decreased DLCO
Significance: 18% SSc

Test: Acro-osteolysis
Significance: Resorption of tufts of distal phalanges, especially with severe Raynaud

- Earliest changes are decreased FVC and small airway disease
- Bone x-ray
- Periarticular or subcutaneous calcification (15–25% patients)
- Bony erosions

CXR

- Bibasilar pulmonary fibrosis
- Rib notching
- Calcifications (in CREST)

High-Resolution Chest CT

- Ground glass attenuation
- Honeycombing

Esophageal Studies

Test: Manometry and pH probe
Significance: Decreased or absent peristalsis of distal esophagus: distal dilatation, hiatus hernia, stricture

- Dilatation of second and third part of duodenum and proximal jejunum

LOCALIZED FORMS

- 25% to 50% eosinophilia during active disease
- 37% to 67% have positive ANA

 Therapy

- Disease modification: Many agents have been tried; however, there are few controlled trials and no proven treatment. Medications include D-penicillamine: breaks down collagen cross-linkages; colchicine: inhibits fibroproliferative process; immunosuppressives: steroids, chlorambucil, MTX, cyclosporine, cyclophosphamide
- Supportive care: avoid cold, trauma, and excessive cold.
- Management of Raynaud: avoid cold, beta-blockers, biofeedback.

 Follow-Up

- Localized forms

—Physical examination for joint mobility, muscle bulk, and growth

- Systemic forms

—Physical examination for joint mobility, muscle bulk, and growth
—Yearly PFTs
—Yearly barium swallow

PITFALLS

- Difficulty following slow disease progression, thus recommend photography of lesions every 3 to 6 months
- Failure to appreciate limited mouth opening
- Insufficient physical therapy resulting in permanent joint contractures
- Excessive use of immunosuppressive therapy late in disease when inflammatory component has resolved.

 Common Questions and Answers

Q: Is a biopsy necessary?
A: Biopsy is often useful to confirm diagnosis and assess degree of inflammation.

Q: Is the sclero-70 antibody useful?
A: Not for diagnosis; it is only positive in a subset of individuals with the systemic form and, therefore, useful for predicting more severe disease.

ICD-9-CM 710.1

BIBLIOGRAPHY

Cron RQ, Swetter SM. Scleroderma revisited. A poststreptococcal complication. *Clin Pediatr* 1994;33:606–610.

Emery H. Pediatric scleroderma. *Semin Cutan Med Surg* 1998;17:41–47.

Foeldvari I. Diffuse and limited cutaneous systemic scleroderma. *Curr Opin Rheumatol* 2000;12:435–438.

Lehman TJ. Systemic and localized scleroderma in children. *Curr Opin Rheumatol* 1996;8:576–579.

Seely JM, Jones LT, Wallace C, et al. Systemic sclerosis: using high-resolution CT to detect lung disease in children. *AJR* 1998;170: 691–697.

Uziel Y, Feldman BM, Krafchik BR, et al. Methotexate and corticosteroid therapy for pediatric localized scleroderma. *J Pediatr* 2000;136:91–95.

Authors: Randy Q. Cron
Emily von Scheven, 2nd edition

Scoliosis/Kyphosis

 Database

DEFINITION

Lateral curvature of the spine exceeding 10 degrees (with rotation of the spine); considered idiopathic only after other causes have been excluded

POSSIBLE CAUSES

- By definition, unknown; listed are some theories, none proven in isolation
- Genetic

—Positive familial history for scoliosis in 30% (not predictive for severity)

- Connective tissue disorder

—Associated with several connective tissue disorders

- Neurologic (equilibrium system)

—Most widely supported theory
—Abnormalities noted in vestibular, ocular, proprioceptive, and vibratory functions

- Hormonal

—Lower levels of melatonin secreted from pineal body in those with adolescent idiopathic scoliosis
—Growth stimulating hormone: more of an influential factor than etiologic factor studies

PATHOLOGY

Lateral curvature of the spine with rotation

EPIDEMIOLOGY

- Prevalence

—Generally considered 1% for curves exceeding 10 degrees
—0.3% for curves exceeding 20 degrees

- Female/male ratios

—1.4:1 for curves 11 degrees to 20 degrees
—5:1 for curves more than 20 degrees

GENETICS

Positive familial history for idiopathic scoliosis in 30% (not predictive for severity)

COMPLICATIONS (NATURAL HISTORY)

- Reduced pulmonary function for patients with thoracic curves over 60 degrees
- Progression of lumbar curves over 50 degrees in adult life with degenerative disc disease and pain in some
- Cosmetic and emotional factors

PROGNOSIS

- Risk of curve progression is related to patient's maturity (Risser sign, menarcheal status) and to the size of the curve.
- Curves less than 20 to 25 degrees have a low risk of progression, even if patient is immature.
- Curves 25 to 45 degrees have higher risk of progression, particularly in the immature.
- Curves >45 to 50 degrees have much higher risk of progression, regardless of maturity.

 Differential Diagnosis

- Adolescent idiopathic scoliosis: onset after 10 years of age
- Juvenile idiopathic scoliosis: onset between 3 and 10 years of age
- Infantile idiopathic scoliosis: onset younger than 3 years of age
- Congenital scoliosis
- Scoliosis associated with neurofibromatosis
- Scoliosis associated with tumors (osteoid osteoma, other)
- Neuromuscular scoliosis
- Postural scoliosis (from leg length discrepancy for example)

—No rib hump or rotation
—Disappears with forward bending
—Long curve
—No progression

 Data Gathering

HISTORY

Question: Onset?
Significance: Consider when first noted, by whom, rate of worsening, previous treatment, associated signs or symptoms, familial history, etc.

Question: Pain?
Significance: Patients with idiopathic scoliosis should not have pain.

Question: Night pain?
Significance: If night pain, consider tumor such as osteoid osteoma or other tumor.

Question: Other signs or symptoms?
Significance: Review of systems (especially neurologic)

 Physical Examination

Finding: General inspection to look for skin changes such as:

- Café-au-lait spots, pigmentation, or other signs of neurofibromatosis; also dysraphic signs (hairy patches, etc.)
- Assess for maturity, hyperelasticity, contracture, congenital anomalies
- Assess for deformity; symmetry of spine, shoulders, and trunk, including decompensation; abnormalities of thoracic kyphosis, or cervical or lumbar lordosis
- The Adam's forward bending test is used to look for rib or paraspinous elevations.
- Assess for leg length discrepancy, congenital anomalies, and neurologic abnormalities (including abnormal abdominal reflex).

SPECIAL QUESTIONS

Finding: Crankshaft phenomenon
Significance: Progression of curve size and rotation following posterior spinal fusion in a young child, due to continued anterior spinal growth

Finding: Patient is Risser 0, open triradiate cartilages, younger than 10 years old, and is prior to the occurrence of peak height velocity (the time of maximum spinal growth).
Significance: Consider anterior fusion in addition to posterior fusion.

PHYSICAL EXAMINATION TRICKS

Finding: Scoliometer
Significance: To measure rib rotation

Finding: Abnormal abdominal reflex
Significance: May suggest intraspinal pathology including syrinx

Laboratory Aids

- Usually not helpful unless to rule out associated metabolic conditions
- Pulmonary function testing is useful preoperatively.

IMAGING STAGES

- Plain standing PA and lateral scoliosis films on a long 3-foot x-ray cassette
- Risser classification of iliac apophysis ossification is an indicator of maturity.
- MRI is not routinely necessary.
- 7% prevalence of intraspinal abnormalities found in left thoracic curves
- Curve patterns are classified according to the King classification.
- Renal ultrasound or IVP is used for evaluation of patient with congenital scoliosis.

Therapy

- Treatment

—Concepts for treatment are based on the severity of the deformity and on the likelihood of progression.

- Observation

—Curves less than 25 degrees
  —Immature patients (Risser 0, 1, 2) should be reevaluated in 4 to 6 months.
  —Skeletally mature patients (Risser 4 or 5) usually do not require follow up unless there are special circumstances.

—Curves 25 to 45 degrees
  —Risser 4 or 5 patients usually reevaluated in 1 year

BRACE TREATMENT

- Curves 25 to 45 degrees (Risser 0, 1): brace on initial evaluation; 30 to 45 degrees (Risser 2 or 3): brace on initial evaluation.
- Curves 25 degrees or greater (in Risser 0–3 patient) that have demonstrated more than 10-degree progression during the period of observation
- Continue brace treatment until maturity (2 years postmenarchal and Risser 4 in females, Risser 5 in males).

OPERATIVE MANAGEMENT

- Recommended when curves exceed 45 to 50 degrees

—Exception: Balanced thoracic and lumbar curves less than 55 degrees may be observed for progression.

- Thoracic curves and double major curves

—Posterior segmental fixation instrumentation remains current state-of-the-art
—Anterior spinal instrumentation for selected curves
—Thoracoscopic technique being developed

- Thoracolumbar and lumbar curves

—Anterior spinal fusion using solid rod segmental constructs

GENERAL TREATMENT MODALITIES

- Brace types

—Thoracolumbosacral orthosis (TLSO): success reported with use more than 16 hours daily; significantly improved outcome when compared to natural history.
—Milwaukee: seldom needed except higher thoracic or cervical curves

DRUGS

Postoperative continuous epidural infusion helpful for pain control

SIGNS TO WATCH FOR

- Back pain associated with idiopathic scoliosis (may indicate other diagnosis)

—Present in 23% at time of initial evaluation (additional 9% during follow-up)
—Of those with back pain, only 9% found to have identifiable cause such as spondylolysis, Scheuermann, syrinx, disc herniation, tumor, tether cord

PROGNOSIS

Overall, good prognosis for the majority of patients

Common Questions and Answers

Q: How long do you observe a patient with spinal asymmetry before ordering an x-ray?
A: It depends on the presence or absence of abnormalities on the physical examination. If any of the signs mentioned here are seen in conjunction with significant back pain, an x-ray or referral is indicated. The scoliometer is also a useful tool in screening patients.

Q: If a child presents with scoliosis and back pain, which occurs especially at night and is relieved with aspirin, what diagnosis is suggested?
A: Scoliosis associated with osteoid osteoma

ICD-9-CM

Scoliosis idiopathic 737.30
Scoliosis infantile progressive 737.32

BIBLIOGRAPHY

Lonstein JE. Scoliosis. In: Morrissy RT, Weinstein SL, eds. *Lovell and Winter's pediatric orthopaedics*, 4th ed. Philadelphia: Lippincott-Raven, 1996:625–685.

Lonstein JE, Carlson JM. The prediction of curve progression in untreated idiopathic scoliosis during growth. *J Bone Joint Surg* 1984;66A:1061–1071.

Author: John P. Dormans

Seborrheic Dermatitis

 Database

DEFINITION

• Seborrheic dermatitis is a yellow to erythematous, scaly, greasy lesion located in areas of high concentrations of sebaceous glands (the scalp, face, postauricular, and intertriginous areas).
• The pattern of seborrheic dermatitis varies with different age groups. In infants, it is commonly referred to as "cradle cap" and located on the vertex of the scalp.
• The term *seborrhea* refers to excessively oily skin.

PATHOPHYSIOLOGY

• Specific etiology is controversial; both genetic and environmental factors seem to influence the course of the illness.
• Infections: does not appear to be bacterial, although some suggest that the yeast *Pityrosporum ovale* is a causative factor. Seborrheic dermatitis is one of the most common cutaneous manifestations of AIDS in adults and may present before other symptoms.
• May be hormonally driven since it first appears in infancy and disappears until puberty.
• Histopathologic findings are nonspecific and include evidence of low-grade inflammation, parakeratosis, acanthosis, elongation of the rete ridges, and slight intracellular edema and spongiosis.

GENETICS

Controversial whether there is a constitutional predisposition. There is evidence that it is more common in families, but not spouses of affected patients.

EPIDEMIOLOGY

This skin disorder is first seen in infancy, and usually spontaneously resolves by the end of the first year of life. It is not usually seen again until adolescence.

COMPLICATIONS

Usually none

PROGNOSIS

The infantile form will self-resolve by the end of the first year of life. The adolescent forms may persist through middle age as a chronic skin dermatitis.

 Differential Diagnosis

• Infection: Fungal infections such as *Trichophyton tonsurans* and *Candida* may complicate these lesions, and are commonly confused with seborrhea. Tinea capitis results in a diffuse or patchy, fine, white, adherent scale on the scalp with tiny, perifollicular pustules and/or hair stubs that have broken off at the level of the scalp. Less commonly, there is patchy or diffuse hair loss. Adenopathy is often present. These can be differentiated by microscopic examination of hairs using a potassium hydroxide wet mount preparation and by fungal culture.
• Tumors: Letterer-Siwe (or Langerhans cell histiocytosis) is an uncommon disease that may present with a rash that begins with a scaly erythematous eruption on the scalp, behind the ears, in the intertriginous regions; differentiated by the presence of small reddish-brown papules or vesicles, purpuric lesions, hepatosplenomegaly, and adenopathy.
• Immunologic: Atopic dermatitis (usually affects infants at a later onset, is very pruritic, and often accompanied by a familial history of atopy). Recurrence after treatment is more indicative of atopic dermatitis. Psoriasis lacks the reddish color of seborrhea and is characterized by a micaceous scale and a tendency to locate on the flexural aspects of the extremities; it is less likely to be confined to the scalp.
• Miscellaneous: Leiner disease results in a severe generalized erythematous, exfoliative seborrheic dermatitis, and is accompanied by severe diarrhea, recurrent infections, and failure to thrive. It is the phenotypic appearance of a number of nutritional and immunologic disorders, such as acrodermatitis enteropathica, and complement deficiencies.

 Data Gathering

HISTORY

These infants usually lack a personal or familial history of atopy. The lesions are typically not pruritic and may begin early in the first few months of life. As with other dermatologic disorders, it is important to learn what treatments (especially topical steroids) have previously been tried.

 Physical Examination

• Characteristic lesions are yellow to erythematous, scaly, and greasy.
• In infants, the disorder may be confined to the scalp or may spread downward to the face and back of head.
• Thickened lesions of the scalp in infants are commonly referred to as cradle cap.
• Blepharitis is red eyelid margins with fine white scales.
• After adolescence, this disorder frequently manifests as dandruff, an increase over the normal desquamation of the scalp.
• Axillary involvement, the absence of pruritus, oozing, and weeping help distinguish seborrhea from atopic dermatitis.

Laboratory Aids

SPECIFIC TESTS

There are no specific tests for seborrhea.
Test: Microscopic examination of hairs and fungal culture
Significance: Fungal infections can be differentiated by using a potassium hydroxide wet mount preparation, and by fungal culture. Culture is often necessary to make the diagnosis because only 29% of affected patients have a positive potassium hydroxide examination.

NONSPECIFIC TESTS

Test: Skin biopsy
Significance: May help in situations that are confusing; however, findings are not necessarily diagnostic for seborrhea.

 ## Therapy

- Infantile seborrhea commonly affects the scalp and may respond to a mild shampoo. A sulfur or salicylic acid shampoo (leave on 5 minutes before rinsing off, use two to three times in the first week, then weekly afterward) may be used if no improvement. If particularly thick, the scales can be loosened first with warm mineral oil or petrolatum, and then gently scrubbed.
- Lesions resistant to treatment may respond to a short course of topical steroid lotion rubbed into the scalp with the fingertips.
- Adolescents should use shampoos with zinc pyrithione (e.g., Head and Shoulders), selenium sulfide (e.g., Selsun), or tar. Those with erythema and severe pruritus can consider treatment with topical corticosteroid lotions. Dense, diffuse scalp involvement can be treated overnight with Derma-Smoothe FS lotion (peanut oil, mineral oil, fluocinolone acetonide 0.01%) under a shower cap, and then shampoo off in the morning. This should be done nightly for no longer than 1 to 3 weeks.
- Ketoconazole cream applied once a day may be tried with resistant and widespread cases.
- Blepharitis should be treated with warm compresses, cleansing with a baby shampoo, and, if necessary, sodium sulfacetamide ophthalmic ointment. Topical steroids can suppress this lesion, but the side effects of its use around the eye (such as glaucoma) make this a poor choice for chronic therapy.

 ## Follow-Up

Some improvement should be seen with therapy by 10 to 14 days. Although this dermatitis is usually self-limited in infancy, it often takes months to resolve completely. Seborrhea may rarely be complicated by secondary bacterial or candidal infections, with erythema, tenderness, and ulceration. Long-term therapy may be required in the adolescent. Seborrhea may be caused or complicated by associated underlying disorders, such as immune defects such as acquired immunodeficiency syndrome. This should be considered with seborrhea resistant to treatment.

PREVENTION

Frequent washing with selenium lotions (such as Exsel or Selsun) can suppress activity and maintain a remission. There are no other preventative measures.

PITFALLS

Treatments to infant scalp should be left on long enough to allow the scales to loosen, and then can be scrubbed off. Parents may need to be reassured that for stubborn and persistent seborrhea, scrubbing the scalp is safe (even over the fontanelles) and may be necessary to keep the lesions under control.

 ## Common Questions and Answers

Q: Does therapy speed resolution of the disorder?
A: Treatment does not appear to influence the underlying cause of this disorder (presumably hormonal influence on the sebaceous glands), although some suggest use of an antifungal therapy to presumptively treat *Pityrosporum ovale* may resolve the lesion.

Q: Does seborrheic dermatitis cause permanent hair loss?
A: Patients can be reassured that it does not cause permanent hair loss.

ICM-9-CM 690

BIBLIOGRAPHY

Habif T. *Clinical dermatology*, 3rd ed. St Louis: CV Mosby, 1996.

Hay RJ, Graham-Brown RAC. Dandruff and seborrhoeic dermatitis. *Clin Exp Dermatol* 1997;22:3–6.

Hurwitz S. *Clinical pediatric dermatology*, 2nd ed. Philadelphia: WB Saunders, 1993.

Janniger C, Schwartz R. Seborrheic dermatitis. *Am Fam Physician* 1995;52(1):149–155.

Mimouni K, Mukamel M, Zeharia A, et al. Prognosis of infantile seborrheic dermatitis. *J Pediatr* 1995;127(5):744–746.

Author: Robert Kamei

Seizures—Febrile

Database

DEFINITION

Single, brief (less than 15 minutes), generalized seizures occurring during rise of fever in developmentally and neurologically normal children between the ages of 6 months and 5 years without intracranial infection or other underlying cause. Febrile seizures are called complex if they last longer than 15 minutes, are focal, or recur within 1 day.

GENETICS

Inheritance is thought to be multifactorial in the majority of cases. In a small subgroup of patients it is a dominantly inherited trait with about a 60% penetrance rate. To date, at least five different genetic loci have been identified.

EPIDEMIOLOGY

Two percent to 5% of children experience a febrile seizure. It is strongly age dependent: 4% occur before 6 months, 90% in the first 3 years, and 6% after age 3.

ASSOCIATED CONDITIONS

Associated with rapid rise in fever; familial history of febrile seizures

Differential Diagnosis

Consideration of nonepileptic causes of seizures. Fever may be the precipitant of seizure due to any other cause of an epileptic spell. History, physical exam, and (especially if patient is under 18 months) lumbar puncture are usually sufficient to exclude:

- CNS infection
- Anoxia
- Trauma
- Stroke/hemorrhage
- Intoxication
- Metabolic encephalopathy
- Neurodegenerative disorder
- Brain tumor
- Neurocutaneous syndromes (tuberous sclerosis, Sturge-Weber, neurofibromatosis)
- Previous brain injury (history of stroke, intracranial hemorrhage, birth asphyxia, cerebral palsy, head trauma, meningitis)

Data Gathering

HISTORY

Question: Previous history of seizures, febrile or afebrile, or neurologic abnormality?
Significance: One third of children with one simple febrile seizure will have another. Neurologic abnormality or prior afebrile seizure increases risk of subsequent epilepsy.

Question: Precipitating factors including height and duration of fever, length and symptoms of preceding illness, recent history of head trauma, possibility of ingestion?
Significance: Low fever, prolonged length of illness before seizure, ingestion, or head trauma suggest cause other than fever alone.

Question: Past medical history including gestation, birth, general health, growth and development, and current medications?
Significance: Birth complications and developmental delay may increase risk of epilepsy.

Question: Familial history?
Significance: Both febrile and afebrile seizures can be hereditary.

Question: Any recent onset of headaches, vomiting, lethargy, weakness, sensory deficits, or change in vision, behavior, balance, or gait?
Significance: Suggests underlying brain pathology and need for neuroimaging.

Physical Examination

Check vital signs for:

- Degree of fever
- Tachycardia or hypotension, suggesting possible sepsis
- Tachypnea, suggesting respiratory infection
- Head circumference

Finding: Retinal hemorrhages and evidence of intracranial hypertension such as bulging fontanelle should be noted on HEENT exam.
Significance: Signs of head trauma or possible child abuse.

Finding: Kernig and Brudzinski signs.
Significance: Possible meningitis.

Finding: Careful neurologic examination. Specific attention to mental status and any focal abnormalities of motor strength, tone, or sensation should be performed.
Significance: Suggest possible meningitis or structural brain pathology.

Laboratory Aids

Test: No routine blood testing necessary
Significance: Routine blood testing after a simple febrile seizure if the child appears well. Otherwise consider electrolytes, calcium, glucose, toxin screen.

Test: Lumbar puncture
Significance: Should be performed in any child who is thought to have a possible infection of the nervous system. This generally includes any child under 18 months of age with new presentation of probable febrile seizure but in whom clinical signs of meningitis may be difficult to accurately assess; also, any older child who appears toxic or has clinical signs suggesting CNS infection should undergo a spinal tap.

Test: EEG
Significance: Not routinely indicated after a simple febrile seizure. EEG should be performed on children who are neurologically abnormal or experience a complex seizure.

Test: MRI
Significance: Generally reserved for children with complex (focal or prolonged) febrile seizures; focal neurologic deficits, even transitory, after a seizure; and children with focal abnormality on EEG.

Therapy

- Because only one third of children with an initial febrile seizure have a second seizure, treatment of a single febrile seizure is not indicated.
- Anticonvulsant prophylaxis may be considered in children with an underlying neurologic abnormality and in children who have had two prolonged or more than three brief febrile seizures.
- When the initial febrile seizure is multiple, prolonged, or focal but the child recovers rapidly and completely, further investigations including EEG and possibly MRI are indicated. Decisions regarding anticonvulsant prophylaxis in these children must be individualized.

DRUGS

- Oral administration of diazepam, 0.3 mg/kg every 8 hours, during all febrile illnesses reduces the risk of recurrent febrile seizures.
- Alternatively, rectal diazepam, 0.3 to 0.5 mg/kg, can be administered at the time of a febrile seizure if it persists for greater than 5 minutes.
- The oral route is generally simpler but has the disadvantage of significant associated sedation during every febrile illness and may not be able to be initiated early enough to be effective in children whose seizures occur immediately at the onset of fever.
- Phenobarbital prophylaxis (3–6 mg/kg daily) is often avoided because of possible behavioral and cognitive side effects.
- Daily valproate and primidone are considered as effective as phenobarbital but also have limiting side effects.
- Phenytoin and carbamazepine are ineffective as prophylaxis.

 ## Follow-Up

PROGNOSIS

- One third of children who have a first simple febrile seizure will have a second at the time of subsequent febrile illnesses, and half of these will have a third febrile seizure.
- One half of the recurrences occur within 6 months of the first febrile seizure, three fourths within a year, and 90% within 2 years.
- Less than 9% of children with febrile seizures have more than three.
- The risk of recurrence is increased if the child has a familial history of febrile seizures, first febrile seizure occurs before 12 months of age, or at a body temperature less than 40°C. Only 2% of children whose first seizure is associated with fever have nonfebrile seizures by age 7. Prolonged or focal seizures, a prior neurologic deficit, or a family history of epilepsy is associated with an increased probability of subsequent epilepsy.
- There is no evidence that occasional febrile seizures or even febrile status epilepticus causes neurologic damage, mental retardation, a decrease in IQ, cerebral palsy, or learning problems.

PITFALLS

- Diagnosis of febrile seizure in a child less than 18 months old usually entails spinal fluid examination with normal cell count, chemistry, Gram stain, and culture.
- Continued seizures with fever beyond age 6 are not compatible with diagnosis of febrile seizure.
- Infants with febrile seizures may have serious bacterial infections, bacteremia, causing fever of primary clinical significance.

 ## Common Questions and Answers

Q: What should be done if the child has another febrile seizure?
A: Emergency measures include placement of the child recumbent or supine with head turned to avoid aspiration; place nothing in the mouth. Antipyretic medication that can be administered PR should be kept in the home. For children who have had prolonged seizures, arrangements and instructions to administer rectal diazepam can be considered.

Q: What restrictions should be placed on general activity of a child with recurrent febrile seizures?
A: No specific activity restrictions are recommended. Children at risk for recurrent seizures should not be left unattended when bathing or swimming.

ICD-9-CM 780.3

BIBLIOGRAPHY

Baumann RJ, Duffner PK. Treatment of children with simple febrile seizures: the AAP practice parameter. American Academy of Pediatrics. *Pediatr Neurol* 2000;23(1):11–17.

Berkovic SF, Scheffer IE. Febrile seizures: genetics and relationship to other epilepsy syndromes. *Curr Opin Neurol* 1998;11(2): 129–134.

Knudsen FU. Febrile seizures: treatment and prognosis. *Epilepsia* 2000;41(1):2–9.

Verity CM, Greenwood R, Golding J. Long-term intellectual and behavioral outcomes of children with febrile convulsions. *N Engl J Med* 1998;338(24):1723–1728.

Vining EP. Gaining a perspective on childhood seizures. *N Engl J Med* 1998;338(26): 1916–1918.

Author: Amy R. Brooks-Kayal

Seizures—Partial and Generalized

 Database

DEFINITION

A transient involuntary alteration of consciousness, behavior, motor activity, sensation, or autonomic function due to an excessive rate and hypersynchrony of neuronal discharges. Seizures are classified based on the location of their onset as partial (beginning in a localized area of cerebral cortex) or primary generalized (beginning simultaneously in both hemispheres). Partial seizures are additionally divided into simple partial (consciousness not impaired), complex partial (consciousness impaired), and partial seizures evolving to generalized tonic-clonic convulsions. Primary generalized seizure types include absence, atypical absence, myoclonic, clonic, tonic, atonic, and tonic-clonic seizures.

GENETICS

Idiopathic seizures may have a multifactorial genetic pattern. Several epilepsy syndromes have recently been associated with defined genetic loci (e.g., generalized epilepsy with febrile seizures plus; autosomal-dominant nocturnal frontal lobe epilepsy; benign familial neonatal convulsions). Other common epilepsy syndromes, including benign rolandic, childhood and juvenile absence, and juvenile myoclonic epilepsy, appear to be genetically heterogeneous and have an autosomal-dominant inheritance pattern with variable penetrance.

EPIDEMIOLOGY

Four to 6% of children will have at least one seizure in the first 16 years of life; the highest incidence is in childhood, with 30% of first seizures occurring before age 4 years and nearly 80% occurring before age 20 years.

RISK FACTORS

- History of previous seizure (afebrile or febrile)
- Recent withdrawal of anticonvulsant medication
- Brain tumor
- Neurodegenerative disorder
- History of remote neurologic insult (stroke, intracranial hemorrhage, cerebral palsy, head trauma, meningitis)
- Familial history of seizures

 Differential Diagnosis

- Idiopathic
- Remote symptomatic (previous history of stroke, intracranial hemorrhage, birth asphyxia, cerebral palsy, head trauma, meningitis)
- Febrile

- Acute symptomatic: CNS infection, anoxia, trauma, stroke/hemorrhage, intoxication, metabolic encephalopathy, anticonvulsant withdrawal
- Neurodegenerative disorder
- Brain tumor
- Neurocutaneous syndromes (tuberous sclerosis, Sturge-Weber, neurofibromatosis)

CAUSES OF NONEPILEPTIC SEIZURES

- Syncope
- Hyperventilation
- Narcolepsy-cataplexy
- Night terrors
- Startle disease
- Breath-holding spells
- Migraine
- Shuddering spells, paroxysmal dyskinesias, tics
- Drug-induced dystonia, psychogenic seizure, movements related to GE reflux
- Segmental myoclonus

 Data Gathering

HISTORY

Question: Previous history of seizures or neurologic abnormality?
Significance: Suggests child at risk of epilepsy

Question: Precipitating factors?

- Fever
- Preceding illness
- Recent history of head trauma
- Possibility of ingestion or recent change in antiepileptic medication
- Risk factors (see Database, above)
- Gestation, birth, general health, growth and development, and current medications, recent onset of headaches, weakness, sensory deficits, change in vision, behavior, balance, or gait

Significance: May provide clue to underlying cause of seizures

 Physical Examination

Finding: Vital signs
Significance: Indications of fever, adequacy of air exchange and perfusion, abnormal respiratory pattern, bradycardia, or hypertension, suggesting intracranial hypertension

Finding: Head circumference, signs of head trauma including retinal hemorrhages and evidence of intracranial hypertension, such as bulging fontanelle
Significance: Microcephaly suggests underlying neurologic abnormality. Signs of head trauma can indicate child abuse. Bulging fontanelle can be a sign of meningitis, trauma, or tumor.

Finding: Signs of systemic infection
Significance: Meningismus, suggesting CNS infection

Finding: Café-au-lait or ash leaf spots, facial hemangioma
Significance: Suggest neurocutaneous disorders

Finding: Convulsions
Significance: If the patient is actively convulsing, neurologic examination is often limited and should be directed toward determining possibility of intracranial hypertension and any focal abnormalities (see Status Epilepticus).

Finding: Pupillary asymmetries, altered mental status, fixed eye deviations, and focal motor weakness (Todd paresis)
Significance: May be secondary to seizure activity or indicate underlying structural lesions

 Laboratory Aids

Test: Initial
Significance: Glucose, electrolytes, BUN, antiepileptic drug levels, complete blood count, liver function tests, toxicology screen, urinalysis. Oximetry or arterial blood gas may be indicated if child is actively seizing.

Test: Lumbar puncture (LP)
Significance: Indicated in nearly all children under 2 years of age and any older child in whom CNS infection is suspected, unless a contraindication such as intracranial hypertension, cerebral mass lesion, or obstructive hydrocephalus is present. LP should be deferred until after head CT if focal abnormalities or signs of intracranial hypertension are present on examination.

Test: EEG
Significance: Indicated immediately if convulsions continue, or the patient fails to awaken within hours after convulsions cease (though children with neurologic deficits may have longer recovery). EEG also indicated in all children with first afebrile, children with complicated febrile seizure, and children with established epilepsy who have had a significant change in clinical status.

Test: Brain imaging with CT or MRI
Significance: Indicated in the initial evaluation of children with partial-onset seizures, focally abnormal EEG, focal neurologic signs, history of head trauma, or difficult-to-control seizures. Repeat brain imaging may be indicated in children with established epilepsy who have had a significant change in clinical status. MRI is preferred because it provides more detailed images; however, CT can be obtained more rapidly and is appropriate if urgent imaging is needed or patient is medically unstable.

Seizures—Partial and Generalized

 Emergency Care

See Status Epilepticus.

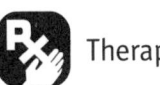 Therapy

PREVENTION

Need for long-term antiepileptic drug (AED) therapy after a first seizure depends on the etiology, patient's age, and circumstances in which seizure occurred. Chronic AED therapy generally not indicated after a seizure resulting from a transient metabolic disturbance (hyponatremia, intoxication) or after a single unprovoked seizure in a child with normal neurologic examination and EEG. Chronic AED therapy usually indicated after first seizure symptomatic of a structural brain lesion; after two or more unprovoked seizures; and in patients with known epilepsy with recurrent seizures.

MEDICATIONS

- The choice of AED for long-term management depends on the specific seizure type. Therapy should be started with a single drug, because approximately 75% of children with epilepsy will be fully controlled with monotherapy, and polytherapy increases the risk of toxicity and decreases compliance.
- For treatment of partial-onset seizures (with or without secondary generalization), carbamazepine is frequently chosen as initial therapy and is begun at 5 to 10 mg/kg/d and slowly advanced to 20 to 30 mg/kg/d divided b.i.d. (sustained release preparations only) or t.i.d. Therapeutic blood concentrations range from 8 to 12 mg/mL. LFTs and CBC must be monitored because of potential risk of thrombocytopenia, aplastic anemia, and hepatotoxicity.
- Valproate (10–15 mg/kg/d increased to 20–60 mg/kg/d for blood levels of 50 to 100 mg/dL), topiramate (4–10 mg/kg/d), lamotrigine (5–15 mg/kg/d in patients *not* taking valproate; 1–5 mg/kg/day in patients on VPA), gabapentin (20–30 mg/kg/d), and oxcarbazepine (20–30 mg/kg/d) also all have pediatric labeling and formulations and provide alternatives in children with partial seizures for whom carbamazepine is ineffective or poorly tolerated.
- Phenytoin (5–7 mg/kg/d) and pheno-barbital (3–7 mg/kg/d) are older AEDs that are frequently used acutely to rapidly control seizures but tend to be used less for chronic maintenance therapy because of concerns regarding cognitive, behavioral, and cosmetic side effects. In young infants (less than 1 year), phenobarbital continues to be used as a first-line agent.

- Ethosuximide is the initial AED of choice for childhood absence seizures. Initial dose is 20 mg/kg/d in two to three divided doses, increased as needed for blood levels of 40 to 100 mg/mL. For primary generalized epilepsies including myoclonic, tonic, or clonic seizures or for refractory absence, valproate, lamotrigine, and topiramate can be used. Adverse effects of valproate include thrombocytopenia, pancreatitis, hyper-ammonemia, and fatal hepatotoxicity. CBC and LFTs should be routinely monitored. Be aware that children under 5 years have an increased risk of hepatotoxicity from valproate, and children under 10 years have an increased risk of serious rash from lamotrigine. Zonisamide is a new AED effective for both partial and generalized seizures, but it does not yet have pediatric formulations or labeling.
- For prolonged seizures (greater than 5 minutes) or acute repetitive seizures, rectal diazepam (0.3–0.5 mg/kg/dose) can be administered. This is typically very effective at stopping the seizure and carries a minimal risk of respiratory suppression, but none-theless families should be trained in CPR prior to its usage.
- For patients with seizures that are refractory to medical therapy, other therapeutic options include the ketogenic diet, vagal nerve stimulator, and surgical resection.

 Follow-Up

PROGNOSIS

- The reported risk of recurrence after a single unprovoked seizure in children varies from 27% to 40%.
- The risk is lowest in children with normal neurologic examinations and normal EEGs and is increased in children with abnormal examinations, focally abnormal EEGs, positive familial history of seizures, partial seizure, or postictal (Todd) paralysis.

COMPLICATIONS

No convincing evidence exists that an isolated brief seizure causes brain damage. Serious injury from a brief seizure is rare and usually related to loss of consciousness and resultant falls. Few restrictions need to be placed on patients with epilepsy, with the exceptions of driving or operating heavy machinery in adolescents or particularly dangerous sports, such as scuba diving, parachuting, and rock climbing. Very frequent seizures, even if brief, may impair learning. Prolonged seizures (>30 minutes) can be associated with secondary brain injury related to exhaustion of cellular energy stores and hypoxia due to respiratory compromise (see Status Epilepticus).

PITFALLS

- Hyponatremic seizures occur in infants with gastroenteritis usually with serum sodium below 120 mEq/dL. Judicious correction of hyponatremia may prevent neurologic effects of rapid shifts in osmolarity: many clinicians administer normal saline to bring the sodium up to 120 mEq/dL, with slower correction thereafter.
- Apnea and hypoventilation may result from excessive administration of benzodiazepines or phenobarbital to children with repetitive or prolonged seizures. In general, patients treated with these drugs IV should have their ventilation and oxygenation closely monitored, and excessively large or rapidly administered doses should be avoided when possible.
- Febrile seizure is a diagnosis of exclusion in a child with first seizure associated with fever. History may suggest other possibilities; those under 18 months should undergo lumbar puncture (see Seizures—Febrile).

 Common Questions and Answers

Q: How do you know my child has epilepsy?
A: The term *epilepsy* is applied to children with recurrent seizures (more than one) not due to fever or other transient toxic/metabolic disturbance, since in general these children have a high (greater than 60%) probability of additional recurrences.

Q: Will my child always be an epileptic?
A: Depending on the circumstances, children may grow out of their seizure disorder. In many cases, anticonvulsants can be discontinued if the child has been seizure-free for 2 years.

Q: Why take an anticonvulsant(s)?
A: The purpose of anticonvulsant medication is to prevent status epilepticus and to prevent accidents and interference with normal behavior associated with brief seizures.

ICD-9-CM 345.1

BIBLIOGRAPHY

Bourgeois BF. New antiepileptic drugs in children: which ones for which seizures? *Clin Neuropharmacol* 2000;23(3):119–132.

Glauser TA. Expanding first-line therapy options for children with partial seizures. *Neurology* 2000;55(11 suppl 3):S30–37.

Morton LD, Pellock JM. Overview of childhood epilepsy and epileptic syndromes and advances in therapy. *Curr Pharmacol Des* 2000;6(8):879–900.

Pellock JM. Managing pediatric epilepsy syndromes with new antiepileptic drugs. *Pediatrics* 1999;104(5):1106–1116.

Author: Amy R. Brooks-Kayal

Sepsis

Database

DEFINITION

The terms *sepsis, bacteremia, sepsis syndrome*, and *septic shock* have been used inter-changeably in the medical literature, leading to confusion regarding the correct definition of each:
- Sepsis: the presence of pathogenic organisms or their toxins in the blood or tissues, and the systemic response to them.
- Bacteremia: the presence of viable bacteria in the bloodstream.
- Sepsis syndrome: sepsis accompanied by evidence of altered end-organ perfusion (e.g., changes in mental status, oliguria, elevated plasma lactate levels). This term has recently been used interchangeably with the systemic inflammatory response syndrome, which can be related to infection, trauma, burns, and other etiologies.
- Septic shock: sepsis syndrome with hypotension (systolic blood pressure <5% for age).

CAUSES

The etiology of sepsis varies with age in otherwise healthy children.
- Most common pathogens in the first 4 weeks of life: group B *Streptococcus*, gram-negative enterics (particularly *Escherichia coli*); *Listeria monocytogenes*.
- When there is a history of hospitalization, instrumentation, or mechanical ventilation: *Staphylococcus aureus, Staphylococcus epidermidis, Pseudomonas aeruginosa*.
- In older infants and children: *Streptococcus pneumoniae, Neisseria meningitidis,* group A *Streptococcus, Salmonella* spp.

EPIDEMIOLOGY

- Sepsis is among the most common (10–25%) medical diagnoses on admission to pediatric intensive care units.
- Mortality rates from sepsis vary with age from 5.6 deaths per 100,000 in infants less than 1 year to 0.5 per 100,000 age 1 to 4, and 0.1 per 100,000 age 5 to 14 years.
- Although sepsis may occur in previously healthy children, it is a particular concern for children with a number of chronic underlying conditions that may render them either immunosuppressed or vulnerable to invasive infections.
- Hyposplenism, either surgical or functional (e.g., sickle cell anemia), highly prone to sepsis from encapsulated organisms—*S. pneumoniae* and *H. influenzae* type b
- Neutropenia (<1,000 neutrophils/mm³ of blood), whether resulting from disease (e.g., leukemia) or from chemotherapy
- Congenital or acquired syndromes of immunodeficiency (AIDS, SCID)
- Organ transplant recipients
- Chronic use of high doses of steroids
- Patients with indwelling central venous catheters

COMPLICATIONS

The most common complications of sepsis are those resulting primarily from either acute hypoperfusion of vital organs, or to organ injury incurred by the uncontrolled systemic inflammatory response:
- Acute lung injury
- Acute renal failure
- Disseminated intravascular coagulation (DIC)
- Hypoglycemia
- Adult respiratory distress syndrome (ARDS)
- Refractory shock
- Multiple organ dysfunction syndrome (MODS)

PROGNOSIS

- Case fatality rates range from 10% to 50%.
- Mortality higher if shock exists on initial presentation
- Development of ARDS or MODS associated with increased mortality
- Survival improved in patients receiving greater than 40 mL/kg of volume resuscitation in the first hour of management
- Presence of coagulopathy (elevated PT and PTT) associated with elevated mortality from meningococcal sepsis

ASSOCIATED ILLNESSES

See Epidemiology, above, for identification of subgroups of children at high risk of sepsis.

Differential Diagnosis

The differential diagnosis of the "septic-appearing" child varies somewhat with age:
- For children, <2 months:
—Viral infections (e.g., enterovirus, respiratory syncytial virus)
—Congenital heart disease [e.g., congestive heart failure due to hypoplastic left heart syndrome, coarctation of the aorta, ventricular septal defect (VSD), valvular insufficiency]
—Myocarditis, pericarditis
—Cardiac arrhythmia (e.g., supraventricular tachycardia)
—Myocardial infarction secondary to anomalous coronary artery insertion
—Congenital adrenal hyperplasia
—Inborn errors of metabolism (e.g., maple syrup urine disease, methylmalonic or propionic acidemia, urea cycle disorders)
—Hypoglycemia
—Severe anemia
—Methemoglobinemia
—Gastroenteritis with dehydration
—Pyloric stenosis
—Volvulus
—Infant botulism
—Occult trauma: child abuse
- For older infants and children:
—Viral infections
—Myocarditis, pericarditis
—Cardiac arrhythmia (e.g., supraventricular tachycardia, ventricular tachycardia)
—Intussusception

—Toxic ingestion/poisoning (e.g., iron, salicylates, tricyclic antidepressants, oral hypoglycemic agents, ethanol, calcium channel blockers, beta-blockers, clonidine, opioids)
—(Occult) trauma
—Infant botulism
—Diabetic ketoacidosis

Data Gathering

HISTORY

Identify children at risk of sepsis (see Epidemiology, above).

Question: Duration of illness before presentation?
Significance: Abrupt onset of symptoms more typical of invasive bacterial infection
Question: Presence of chronic underlying illness?
Significance: Identifies children at higher risk of sepsis
Question: Change in behavior?
Significance: May be initial sign of systemic infection

Physical Examination

All patients with suspected sepsis should have a full set of vital signs (e.g., temperature, pulse, respiratory rate, blood pressure).

Finding: Temperature
Significance: Fever is the hallmark of an infection; however, infants in particular may demonstrate hypothermia.
Finding: Stertor, stridor
Significance: Assess for signs of airway obstruction.
Finding: Auscultation of the chest
Significance: Assess adequacy of breathing (tachypnea, rales)
Finding: Tachycardia, hypotension, poor skin perfusion, delayed capillary refill, presence of mottling
Significance: Evidence of inadequate circulatory function
Finding: Altered mental status (somnolence, confusion, disorientation, agitation)
Significance: Evidence of severe systemic disease, possible poor cerebral perfusion
Finding: Presence of petechiae and purpura
Significance: Meningococcemia or DIC
Finding: Thorough physical examination
Significance: Looking for focus of infection

Laboratory Aids

All patients with suspected sepsis should have a thorough laboratory evaluation including:

Test: CBC with WBC differential, platelet count
Significance: Elevated WBC count with increased band count suggestive of invasive infection

Test: Electrolytes, glucose
Significance: Metabolic acidosis, hypoglycemia
Test: Blood culture
Significance: Identification of causative organism
Test: Arterial blood gas
Significance: Monitoring acid-base status
Test: Urinalysis and urine culture
Significance: Potential source of infection
Test: Lumbar puncture (when hemodynamically stable)
Significance: Required for diagnosis of meningitis
Test: Chest x-ray
Significance: Potential source of infection
Test: Prothrombin time, partial thromboplastin time
Significance: Monitor development of DIC
Test: Fibrinogen, fibrin degradation products
Significance: Monitor development of DIC
Test: Gram stain and culture of petechiae or abscess contents
Significance: May yield causative organism

Therapy

- Ensure a patent airway (consider endotracheal intubation).
- Provide supplemental oxygen.
- Assist ventilation (e.g., bag-valve-mask device) as needed.
- Obtain intravenous access (consider placement of a femoral venous line or intraosseous line if difficulty securing peripheral IV).
- Volume resuscitation: bolus 20 mL/kg of normal saline solution, repeat as needed; consider colloid solutions (5% albumin, plasma) after initial 60–80 mL/kg of crystalloid)
- Correct hypoglycemia (0.5–1 g/kg of dextrose)
- Antibiotics (depends on age, presence of meningitis, central venous catheter, immune function of patient); generally given IV for at least 10 days
—Neonates, <6 weeks, no meningitis: ampicillin and gentamicin; meningitis: vancomycin and cefotaxime
—Infants and children, ≥6 weeks: cefotaxime or ceftriaxone
—Suspected meningitis with penicillin-resistant *S. pneumoniae*: vancomycin and cefotaxime or ceftriaxone
—Suspected *Salmonella* sepsis: third-generation cephalosporin or trimethoprim-sulfamethoxazole
—Nosocomially acquired infections or patients with immunosuppression and/or central venous catheters: antistaphylococcal penicillin or vancomycin, plus aminoglycoside, and third-generation cephalosporin
—Patients with an intraabdominal focus of infection: ampicillin/sulbactam or ampicillin, gentamicin, and clindamycin
- Drainage and/or eradication of focus of infection

- Inotropic agents: dopamine (begin at 5 mg/kg/min, titrate up to 20 mg/kg/min as needed), dobutamine (begin at 5 mg/kg/min), epinephrine (begin at 1–2 mg/kg/min); to be used for persistent hemodynamic instability after adequate volume resuscitation

PREVENTION
- Routine vaccination for *Haemophilus influenzae* type b and *S. pneumoniae,* particularly in high-risk patients (e.g., sickle cell anemia, asplenia)
- Rifampin prophylaxis for household or day-care exposure to *H. influenzae* type b or *N. meningitidis*
- Prompt evaluation for fever in immunosuppressed patients

Follow-Up

- Admit all patients with suspected sepsis to the hospital; consider intensive care unit admission.
- Continuous blood pressure monitoring for the development of refractory shock
- Serial vital signs and physical examinations to monitor response to therapy
- Monitor for complications of sepsis and the development of MODS.
- Chest x-ray and serial arterial blood gases for evidence of acute lung injury/ARDS
- Urine output, BUN, creatinine for acute renal failure
- Serial coagulation studies (PT/PTT) for development of DIC
- Serial blood glucose levels for hypoglycemia
- Serial liver function tests (glucose, albumin, ALT, AST, GGT, bilirubin) for evidence of hepatic dysfunction
- Serial neurologic examinations for evidence of central nervous system dysfunction

PITFALLS
- Recognize the patient at risk for sepsis (see Epidemiology, above).
- Initial priorities in management are the proper assessment of airway, breathing, and circulation.
- Provide adequate initial volume resuscitation; improved outcome is associated with giving greater than 40 mL/kg isotonic saline in the first hour of resuscitation.
- Eradicate the focus of infection (abscess) if present.
- Continuous monitoring and reassessment of the patient is essential.

Common Questions and Answers

Q: What are the earliest signs and symptoms of compensated shock?
A: Unexplained tachycardia and widened pulse pressure are among the earliest signs of septic shock and warrant additional observation and laboratory investigation.

Q: Are colloid solutions (e.g., 5% albumin, fresh frozen plasma) better than isotonic crystalloid (e.g., Ringer's lactate, normal saline) for volume resuscitation?
A: Both are effective for intravascular volume expansion, though less (approximately 25%) of the crystalloid volume initially given ultimately remains in the intravascular compartment. Generally, because of their ready availability and lower cost, crystalloid solutions are given for the first 60 to 80 mL/kg of resuscitation, and consideration is then given to the addition of colloid solutions for additional volume resuscitation.

ICD-9-CM 638.9

BIBLIOGRAPHY
Anderson MR, Blumer JL. Advances in therapy for sepsis in children. *Pediatr Clin North Am* 1997;44(1):179–205.

Angus DC, Wax RS. Epidemiology of sepsis: an update. *Crit Care Med* 2001;29(7):S109–116.

Beal AL, Cerra FB. Multiple organ failure syndrome in the 1990s. *JAMA* 1994;271:226–233.

Bone RC. A critical evaluation of new agents for the treatment of sepsis. *JAMA* 1991;266:1686–1691.

Bone RC. Let's agree on terminology: definitions of sepsis. *Crit Care Med* 1991;19:973–976.

Carcillo JA, Davis AL, Zaritsky A. A role of early fluid resuscitation in pediatric septic shock. *JAMA* 1991;266:1242–1245.

Marshall JC. Inflammation, coagulopathy, and the pathogenesis of multiple organ dysfunction syndrome. *Crit Care Med* 2001;29(7):S99–S106.

Martinot A, Leclerc F, Cremer R, et al. Sepsis in neonates and children: definitions, epidemiology, and outcome. *Pediatr Emerg Care* 1997;13(4):277–281.

Saez-Llorens X, McCracken GH. Sepsis syndrome and septic shock in pediatrics: current concepts of terminology, pathophysiology and management. *J Pediatr* 1993;123:497–508.

Selbst SM. Septic-appearing infant. In: Fleisher GR, Ludwig S, eds. *Textbook of pediatric emergency medicine*, 3rd ed. Baltimore: Williams & Wilkins, 1993:456–463.

Ziegler EJ, Fisher CJ, Sprung CL, et al. Treatment of gram-negative bacteremia and septic shock HA-1A human monoclonal antibody against endotoxin. *N Engl J Med* 1991;324:429–436.

Author: Dennis R. Durbin

Septic Arthritis

 ## Database

DEFINITION
Septic arthritis is an inflammatory response to the presence of infectious organisms within the joint space. See table Types of Organisms.

CAUSES
Bacterial
- *Staphylococcus aureus*
- Streptococci
- *Haemophilus influenzae*
- *Salmonella*
- *Neisseria gonorrhoeae*
- *Neisseria meningitidis*

Aseptic Arthritis
- Rubella
- Parvovirus
- Hepatitis B or C
- Mumps
- Herpesviruses (EBV, CMV, HSV, VZV)
- Epstein-Barr virus
- Varicella
- *Candida albicans* (neonatal)

PATHOLOGY/PATHOPHYSIOLOGY
- Entry of bacteria into joint space
- —Hematogenous spread
- —Direct inoculation (penetrating trauma) or extension from bone infection
- —Influx of inflammatory cells within the joint capsule
- —Destruction of cartilaginous structures within the joint by bacterial and lysosomal enzymes
- —If left untreated, can progress to necrosis of the intraarticular epiphysis

EPIDEMIOLOGY
- Predominant age: 2 to 6 years, adolescent (*N. gonorrhea*)
- Sex predominance: male/female 2:1
- Predominantly affected joints: knee, hip, elbow, ankle

COMPLICATIONS
- Permanent limitation of range of motion due to tissue destruction and scarring
- Growth disturbance if the epiphysis is involved

PROGNOSIS
Depends on duration of illness prior to institution of appropriate therapy

ASSOCIATED ILLNESSES
- *Neonatal septic arthritis* can be associated with *S. aureus*, group B streptococcus, *Escherichia coli*, and *Candida*.
- *Sickle cell disease* is associated with *Salmonella* infection, although *S. aureus* is still the most common.
- *Immunocompromise* associated with *Mycoplasma, Ureaplasma, Aspergillus* infection

 ## Differential Diagnosis

INFECTION
- Osteomyelitis with contiguous spread of infection
- Lyme arthritis
- Tuberculous arthritis
- Psoas abscess or retroperitoneal abscess with associated hip pain
- Cellulitis causing decreased range of motion of joint secondary to pain
- Tumors
- —Osteogenic sarcoma (long-bone pain spreading to joint space)
- —Leukemia/lymphoma
- Trauma
- —Occult fracture in proximity to growth plate
- —Ligamentous injury (sprain)
- —Foreign-body synovitis
- —Traumatic knee effusion/hemarthrosis
- Immunologic
- —Toxic synovitis
- —Postinfectious
- —Acute rheumatic fever
- —Reactive arthritis
- —*Campylobacter, Shigella*
- —Reiter syndrome (after gastrointestinal or chlamydial infection) arthritis, uveitis, urethritis
- —Collagen vascular
  - —Systemic lupus erythematosus
  - —Juvenile rheumatoid arthritis
- —Henoch-Schönlein purpura
- —Behçet syndrome (iridocyclitis, genital and oral ulcerations)
- —Inflammatory bowel disease (Crohn disease, ulcerative colitis)
- —Serum sickness
- —Erythema multiforme/Stevens-Johnson syndrome
- Miscellaneous
- —Knee
- —Apophysitis (e.g., Osgood-Schlatter disease)
- —Patellofemoral pain syndrome (chondromalacia patella)
- —Osteochondritis desiccans
- —Hip
- —Slipped capital femoral epiphysis

 ## Data Gathering

HISTORY
Question: Was there trauma?
Significance: History of recent trauma does not rule out septic arthritis.
Question: Can you describe the pain?
Significance: Pain of bacterial arthritis worsens over 1 to 3 days and does not wax and wane.
Question: How many joints are involved?
Significance: Septic arthritis is rarely polyarticular.

 ## Physical Examination

- Fever occurs within the first few days of illness in 75% of patients, but less commonly in infants. Only 50% of children with gonococcal arthritis will have fever.
- Children with septic arthritis usually appear ill.
- The joint appears warm and swollen.
- Pseudoparalysis: decreased range of motion
- Hip effusion causes the leg to be held flexed and externally rotated.
- The child with septic arthritis will usually have pain through *any* range of motion. In contrast, most traumatic injuries will allow some painless range of motion of that joint.
- There are usually no external findings when the hip or shoulder joints are infected.
- Consider hip involvement when the patient complains of knee or thigh pain.
- In the frightened or uncooperative child, it is possible to have the parent perform an examination for tenderness and range of motion while the physician observes from a distance.

 ## Laboratory Aids

TESTS
Joint Fluid in Septic Arthritis
- The WBC is often greater than 100,000/mm^3, but can be as low as 50,000/mm^3 in early infections.
- The glucose level in the synovial fluid is less than 50% that of the serum.
- Culture of the joint reveals an organism in 70% to 80% of cases (except for gonorrhea).
- A Gram stain of synovial fluid reveals pathogens in 50% of cases.

Other Supportive Tests
- The ESR is elevated (>30 mm/h) in 95% of cases. Retain suspicion if >20 mm/h.
- The C-reactive protein is increased.
- Blood cultures are positive in 30% to 40% of cases.
- A high peripheral WBC count is neither sensitive nor specific for septic arthritis.

IMAGING
- Radiography is rarely helpful in diagnosis, can show widening of joint space and/or displacement of the normal fat pads in the knee or elbow, and is less often positive in the shoulder or hip.
- A technetium-99 bone scan reveals increased uptake in the perimeter of the joint during the "blood pool" phase of the study.
- Ultrasound of the affected joint usually delineates the amount of fluid within the joint capsule. However, this test cannot differentiate between an infectious and a purely inflammatory disease.

Septic Arthritis

FALSE POSITIVES

• Bone scan cannot easily differentiate septic arthritis from epiphyseal osteomyelitis.
• Evaluation of synovial fluid from patients with rheumatologic disease can mimic that of infectious arthritis; however, the clinical picture should allow differentiation of these entities.

Emergency Care

• Drainage of infection: should occur *as soon as possible* if bacterial cause is suspected
• Indications for open surgical drainage/irrigation:
—Hip involvement
—Shoulder involvement (controversial)
—Thick, purulent, or fibrinous exudate unable to pass through 18-gauge needle
—All other joints not undergoing open drainage should undergo needle aspiration.
• Antibiotic administration as soon as possible after joint aspiration is performed
• Immobilization of extremity
• Pain management

DRUGS

Choice of antibiotics depends on age of child as outlined in the tables below.

DURATION OF THERAPY (IV AND PO) FOR VARIOUS ORGANISMS

• Treat for at least 2 weeks after resolution of fever and joint effusion.
• ≥28 days: *S. aureus*, gram-negative organisms, group B streptococcus
• ≥14 days: *H. influenzae*, *N. meningitidis*, streptococci
• ≥7 days: *N. gonorrhoeae*

Therapy

See table Empiric Therapy Prior to Identification of Organism.

Follow-Up

• Involve orthopedic surgery and physical therapy services in follow-up.
• Once the patient is receiving oral therapy, serum bactericidal titers (SBTs) must be monitored on a weekly basis if possible. Oral antibiotic titers should be kept at eight times the SBT.

WHEN TO EXPECT IMPROVEMENT

With appropriate antibacterial therapy, one should see improvement of symptoms with 2 days of initial administration.

SIGNS TO WATCH FOR

• Continued pain, fever, or lack of improvement of range of motion after 3 to 4 days of appropriate antibiotic treatment.
• Rising ESR or CRP in the face of antibiotic treatment.

PITFALLS

• Clinical examination in conjunction with the history of acute onset should raise the suspicion of septic arthritis even in the face of "negative" laboratory screening tests. The most accurate determinations can be inferred from analysis of the synovial fluid.
• Realize that some children, especially neonates and young infants, will not manifest signs of systemic disease early in the course of the illness.
• Observe failure or success of therapy, especially when the extremity is immobilized.

Common Questions and Answers

Q: How can one differentiate toxic synovitis from septic arthritis on the initial visit?
A: Although this is sometimes a difficult diagnosis to make with certainty, patients with toxic synovitis usually exhibit certain characteristics that patients with septic arthritis do not:
• Almost always involves the hip joint
• History of previous viral infection
• Some painless range of motion of the involved joint is possible.
• The ESR is lower than 20 mm/h.
• Fever is low grade.

BIBLIOGRAPHY

Adebajo AO. Rheumatic manifestations of infectious diseases in children. *Curr Opin Rheumatol* 1998;10:79–85.

Dagan RZ. Management of acute hematogenous osteomyelitis and septic arthritis in the pediatric patient. *Pediatr Infect Dis J* 1993;12:88–93.

Del Beccaro MA, Champoux AN, Bockers T, et al. Septic arthritis versus transient synovitis of the hip: the value of screening laboratory tests. *Ann Emerg Med* 1992;21:1418–1422.

Do TT. Transient synovitis as a cause of painful limps in children. *Curr Opin Pediatr* 2000;12:48–51.

Pioro MH, Mandell BF. Septic arthritis. *Rheum Dis Clin North Am* 1997;23:239–258.

Rose CD, Eppes SC. Infection-related arthritis. *Rheum Dis Clin North Am* 1997;23:677–695.

Wall EJ. Childhood osteomyelitis and septic arthritis. *Curr Opin Pediatr* 1998;10:73–76.

Author: Joel A. Fein

Types of Organisms

AGE	MOST COMMON ORGANISM	OTHER ORGANISMS
Newborn	Staphylococcus aureus	Candida albicans
		Group B streptococcus
		Gram-negative organisms
	(Klebsiella, Salmonella)	
Infants and children ≤5 years	S. aureus	Haemophilus influenzae[a]
		Streptococcus pneumoniae
Children >5 years	S. aureus	S. pneumoniae
		Neisseria meningitidis
Adolescents	Neisseria gonorrhoeae	S. aureus
		S. pneumoniae
		N. meningitidis

[a] Less likely in fully immunized children.

Empiric Therapy Prior to Identification of Organism

AGE	FIRST CHOICE	SECOND CHOICE	DURATION
Neonatal	Cefotaxime	O/N/M	IV for ≥14 days
	O/N/M	Ampicillin	PO for ≥14 days
		Gentamicin	
≤5 years	Cefuroxime	O/N/M	IV + PO = 28 days
		Chloramphenicol	
>5 years	O/N/M	Cefazolin	IV + PO = 28 days
		Clindamycin	
Adolescent			
Gonococcal	Ceftriaxone	Penicillin	IV + PO = 7–10 days
Nongonococcal	O/N/M	Cefazolin	IV + PO = 28 days

O/N/M = oxacillin or nafcillin or methicillin.

Serum Sickness

 Database

DEFINITION

- Serum sickness: type III hypersensitivity reaction that occurs 7 to 21 days after injection of foreign protein or serum (usually in the form of antiserums). The clinical syndrome consists of skin rash, itching, fever, malaise, proteinuria, vasculitis, and joint pain.
- Serum sickness–like reactions are characterized by fever, rash, lymphadenopathy, and arthralgia which occurs 1 to 3 weeks after drug exposure. Immune complexes, vasculitis, and hypocomplementemia are absent. This is the type of reaction associated with cefaclor. They are commonly referred to as serum sickness.
- Serum sickness–like reactions are more common than true serum sickness since equine serum antitoxins have been replaced with human antitoxin sera. Clinically, they present identically and are treated the same.
- Common causative agents: horse antithymocyte globulins, human diploid-cell rabies vaccine, streptokinase, hymenoptera venom, penicillins, cephalosporins, sulfonamides, hydralazine, thiouracils, metronidazole, naproxen, and dextrans.

PATHOPHYSIOLOGY

- Type III immune complex antigen-antibody complement reaction.
- Antibodies are formed 6 to 10 days after the introduction of foreign material. Antibodies interact with antigens forming immune complexes that diffuse into vascular walls. They become fixated in tissue and activate the complement cascade. C3a and C5a are produced, resulting in increased vascular permeability and activated inflammatory cells. Polymorphonuclear cells and monocytes cause diffuse vasculitis.

GENETICS

People with a genetic predisposition to produce IgE are more susceptible.

EPIDEMIOLOGY

- Limited information is available regarding the incidence of adverse drug reactions in children; generally believed to occur less frequently in children than in adults.
- More than 90% of serum sickness cases are drug induced.
- Less than 5% of serum sickness cases are fatal.

COMPLICATIONS

- Shock
- Digital necrosis
- Guillain-Barré syndrome (rare)
- Generalized vasculitis (rare)
- Peripheral neuropathy (rare)
- Glomerulonephritis (rare)
- Increased risk of anaphylaxis with repeat exposure to substance
- Fatality (rare, usually due to continued administration of antigen)

PROGNOSIS

- Excellent. Most cases are mild and transient with no sequela.
- Symptoms resolve in a few days to a few weeks.

 Differential Diagnosis

- Erythema multiforme
- Mononucleosis
- Systemic lupus erythematosus
- Rocky mountain spotted fever
- Henoch Schönlein purpura
- Hypersensitivity syndrome reaction
- Drug-induced pseudoporphyria
- Acute generalized exanthematous pustulosis
- Wegener granulomatosis

 Data Gathering

HISTORY

- Suspect in any patient with an unexplained vasculitic rash who has been taking any new drug during the last 2 months.
- Ask about presentation and evolution of rash. Typically, the rash first appears on the sides of the fingers, hands, and feet before becoming widespread.
- Is there associated pruritus? Often present.
- Fever? Often present, usually mild.
- Ask about the presence of arthritis or arthralgia. Present over half the time; usually involves the metacarpophalangeal and knee joints.
- Is there associated abdominal pain? Some cases may have visceral involvement.
- Is there a history of hematuria? There can be modest renal involvement usually presenting as proteinuria and microscopic hematuria.
- Does the patient report any neurologic symptoms? Peripheral neuropathy, brachial plexus involvement and Guillain-Barré syndrome have been reported associations.
- Is there a previous history of a similar rash? Was it associated with any medications in the past? The rash and symptoms of serum sickness will occur sooner on repeat exposure. Try to differentiate from simple drug rash, timing of rash after exposure is important in differentiating the two.
- Have you had any drug or antitoxin exposure in the last month, especially to penicillins, cephalosporins, sulfonamides, hydralazine, thiouracils, streptokinase, metronidazole, naproxen, dextrans, bupropion?

 Physical Examination

- Erythematous purpuric rash starts at the sides of the feet, toes, hands, and fingers and then becomes more widespread.
- Erythema multiforme, maculopapular, purpuric, or urticarial type rash.
- Mild to severe fever.
- Generalized lymphadenopathy; may be localized to lymph nodes that drain the injection site.
- Splenomegaly, occasionally.
- Edema of the face and neck
- Joint pain.

Laboratory Aids

Not extremely helpful in establishing diagnosis since no abnormality is universally present. Diagnosis usually apparent by classic findings and history of foreign protein or drug exposure.

- Urinalysis: may show proteinuria and/or hematuria.
- Complements levels variably reduced before returning to normal.
- Leukocytosis or leukopenia with or without eosinophilia.
- Erythrocyte sedimentation rate may be slightly elevated.
- Direct immunofluorescent staining of rash biopsy (not routinely recommended as part of workup) shows deposits of IgM and C3 complement in capillary walls.

 ## Therapy

- Stop suspected medication/antigen immediately and avoid its future use.
- Topical steroids to relieve itching.
- Antihistamines to inhibit the action of vasoactive mediators.
- NSAIDs to relieve joint pain.
- Oral corticosteroids for severe cases. Recommended to administer and taper over 10- to 14-day period. Shorter course may result in relapse and recurrent symptoms are more difficult to alleviate.
- Admit if symptoms are severe or diagnosis is unclear.

 ## Follow-Up

WHEN TO EXPECT IMPROVEMENT

- Usually self-limited illness that resolves in a few days to weeks.
- If symptoms persist for more than 1 month, reconsider the diagnosis.

PREVENTION

- No known way to prevent first occurrence.
- Take careful history of previous allergic reactions.
- Skin testing prior to antiserum administration will prevent anaphylaxis but not serum sickness.
- When the need for antiserum arises, consider prophylactic antihistamines.

PITFALLS

- A history of fever, rash, and arthralgias is commonly seen with many childhood illnesses. One must always consider differential diagnoses.
- Symptoms may be so minimal that patient does not seek medical attention.
- Often misdiagnosed as simple drug allergy

 ## Common Questions and Answers

Q: What is the difference between serum sickness and drug allergies?
A: Drug allergies are type I IgE-mediated hypersensitivity reactions that occur very soon after drug exposure in a previously sensitized individual. Serum sickness is a type III antibody-antigen immune complex and complement amplified hypersensitivity reaction that occurs 1 to 3 weeks after an initial exposure.

Q: If my child has had serum sickness, is she at risk for getting it again?
A: Yes, if she receives the same medication or related medications again. The symptoms will occur more quickly, usually in 2 to 4 days and may be more severe.

Q: Will my child have long-term effects from this illness?
A: No, this is a self-limited disease and as long as the offending agent is stopped your child will completely recover.

Q: Is there any way to prevent my child from getting serum sickness?
A: Unfortunately, there is no way to predict if your child will have a serum sickness–like reaction to a particular medication. It is extremely important to be aware of your child's exact allergies to medications and to inform all health care providers caring for your child.

Q: My child has had serum sickness while taking an antibiotic. Can he take other antibiotics?
A: Yes, but your child should never receive that particular antibiotic or any closely related antibiotic again. Repeat exposure will likely result in serum sickness occurring more quickly than after the first exposure. Your child can safely take antibiotics from other drug families.

Q: If one of my children has had serum sickness from an antibiotic, are my other children at risk?
A: No, there is no known genetic predisposition for serum sickness. Your other children do not need to avoid the medication that caused serum sickness.

Q: How is the Arthus reaction different from serum sickness?
A: The Arthus reaction is also a type III hypersensitivity reaction but only causes a local reaction. It is a local vasculitis caused by formation of antigen-antibody complexes in local vessel walls, which then activate the inflammation process. The reaction occurs within hours after an individual is injected intradermally with an antigen against which he/she has been actively immunized.

ICD-9-CM 999.5

BIBLIOGRAPHY

Erffmeyer JE. Serum sickness. *Ann Allergy* 1986;56:105–109.

Evans R, Kim K, Mahr TA. Current concepts in allergy: drug reactions. *Curr Probl Pediatr* 1991;21:185–192.

Heckbert SR, Stryker WS, et al. Serum sickness in children after antibiotic exposure: estimates of occurrence and morbidity in a health maintenance organization population. *Am J Epidemiol* 1990;132:336–342.

Knowles S, Shapiro L, Shear NH. Serious dermatologic reactions in children. *Curr Opin Pediatr* 1997;9:388–395.

Lawley TJ, Frank MM. Immune complexes and allergic disease. In: Middleton E, ed. *Allergy principles and practice*, 5th ed. St. Louis: Mosby Yearbook, 702–712.

McCollum R, Elbe DH, Ritchie AA. Bupropion indirect serum sickness like reaction. *Ann Pharmacother* 2000;34(4):471–473.

Roujeau J, Stern RS. Severe adverse cutaneous reactions to drugs. *N Engl J Med* 1994;331:1272–1285.

Author: Denise Salerno

Severe Combined Immunodeficiency

 Database

DEFINITION

Severe combined immunodeficiency (SCID) is primary immunodeficiency characterized by onset of severe, life-threatening infections in infancy due to defective or absent T- and/or B-lymphocyte–mediated immunity.

CAUSES

• A variety of defects lead to a similar clinical presentation.
• The X-linked subset is caused by defective transcription of the gamma chain of the IL-2 receptor.
• The autosomal-recessive (AR) subset is due to various defects. The most common:

—Adenosine deaminase deficiency
—Purine nucleoside phosphorylase deficiency
—JAK3 deficiency
—Absent expression of MHC class I or II molecules

GENETICS

X-linked and autosomal-recessive inheritance (see table Disorders and Diagnostic Tests)

EPIDEMIOLOGY

• Incidence: estimated to be 1 in 66,000 to 100,000 live births
• Most patients present by 6 months of age.
• The X-linked form accounts for 50% to 60% of SCID cases.
• ADA deficiency accounts for 20% to 25% of SCID cases.
• JAK3 deficiency accounts for 8% of SCID cases.
• PNP deficiency accounts for 2% to 4% of SCID cases.

COMPLICATIONS

• Untreated, most patients succumb to overwhelming infection.
• Graft-versus-host disease (GVHD) may result from transfusion of nonirradiated blood products.
• Clinical disease can be caused by live vaccines in previous undiagnosed SCID patients.
• Increased incidence of malignancy:

—Overall risk of malignancy is approximately 5%
—Thirty-fold increased incidence of lymphoma

 Differential Diagnosis

• Specific diagnosis of ADA deficiency as the cause of SCID is important, because enzyme replacement therapy is available.
• Reticular dysgenesis
• Letterer-Siwe syndrome (histiocytosis)
• Omenn syndrome
• HIV infection
• Failure to thrive is the most common presenting problem.
• Recurrent and or life-threatening infections in infancy with a variety of pathogens (both common and atypical organisms)
• Chronic diarrhea
• Persistent thrush
• Skin rashes are commonly in unusual patterns or locations. They may be the presenting symptom of GVHD.

 Data Gathering

HISTORY

• Description of infections, severity, duration, response to treatment
• Family history of unexplained deaths or unusual infections

Disorders and Diagnostic Tests

DISORDER (YEAR OF DEFINITION OF MOLECULAR BASIS)	CHROMOSOMAL LOCATION	GENE	DIAGNOSTIC TESTS OTHER THAN DIRECT MUTATION ANALYSIS
X-linked severe combined immunodeficiency (1993)	Xq13	Common γ chain (γ_c)	γ_c expression by FACS analysis
Adenosine deaminase (ADA) deficiency (1983)	20q12–13	Adenosine deaminase	Red cell ADA levels and metabolites
Purine nucleoside phosphorylase (PNP) deficiency (1987)	14q11	Purine nucleoside phosphorylase	Red cell PNP levels and metabolites
Recombinase activating gene (RAG 1&2) deficiency (1996), Omenn's syndrome (1998)	11p13	RAG 1 and RAG 2	
T-cell receptor deficiency (1987)	11q23	$CD3\gamma$/$CD3\epsilon$	
Zap 70 deficiency (1994)	2q12	ZAP 70	ZAP 70 expression
JAK3 deficiency (1995)	19p13	JAK3	JAK3 expression/signaling
IL-7 receptor deficiency (1998)	5p13	IL-7 receptor α	IL-7 receptor α expression
MHC class II deficiency			
(1993)	16p13	CIITA	HLA-DR expression
(1998)	19p12	RFX-B	
(1995)	1q21	RFX5	
(1997)	13q13	RFXAP	

From Gaspar HB, Gilmour KC, Jones AM. *Arch Dis Child* 2001;84(2):169–173.

Physical Examination

- Evaluation should focus on the presence of infection.
- Often an emaciated-appearing infant
- Marked absence of lymphoid and tonsillar tissue
- Dermatologic evaluation may reveal atypical rashes.

 ## Laboratory Aids

TESTS

- CBC with differential to assess for degree of lymphopenia
- T- and B-lymphocyte enumeration:

—T lymphocytes are markedly decreased or absent.
—B lymphocytes are variable but can be normal.

- Mitogen and antigen stimulation tests are markedly decreased or absent.
- Immunoglobulin levels are usually low or absent.

—Patients can have normal IgG levels in the first few months of life due to trans-placentally derived maternal IgG.

- Appropriate cultures to identify pathogens

 ## Therapy

- Bone marrow transplant (BMT) is the definitive treatment in most cases. Because of the impairment of recipient immune function, conditioning for BMT may be less rigorous than in other situations requiring BMT.
- Aggressive and early specific antibiotic/antifungal/antiviral therapy for infections
- *Pneumocystis carinii* prophylaxis
- If required, patients should receive only irradiated blood products. There is a risk of GVHD due to viable donor leukocytes that may survive in nonirradiated products.
- Intravenous immunoglobulin replacement: This may be required even after BMT because of variable B-lymphocyte reconstitution.
- Enzyme replacement therapy has been used in ADA-deficient patients.

 ## Follow-Up

- Close monitoring of clinical status should be done before BMT. This may be every 2 to 4 weeks, depending on the patient's status.
- The posttransplant course is variable.

—The overall success rate for matched BMT in SCID is approximately 65%. Success is also being seen in partially matched BMT.
—Patients should still be followed closely for signs of infection, graft failure, and GVHD.

 ## Common Questions and Answers

Q: How should children with SCID be managed before BMT?
A: Children suspected to have SCID should be isolated from potential sources of infection. They should not attend public places such as school because of the risk of obtaining an infection. They should be kept away from ill siblings or relatives. This is especially true if there has been an exposure to chickenpox or other viral illnesses.

Q: Should patients with SCID receive live viral vaccines?
A: Live viral vaccines are *contraindicated* in SCID. Patients suspected of severe immuno-deficiency should not receive live viral vaccines until their immunodeficiency is defined. If the patient is receiving IVIG therapy, vaccinations are not required. In addition, siblings of patients with SCID who live in the same household should not receive live viral vaccines. This is due to the risk of viral shedding in the siblings.

Q: What is the chance of another child being affected with SCID?
A: The risk of another child being born with SCID in a family with a previously affected child will depend on the type of SCID. X-linked: 50% chance of an affected male or carrier female. Autosomal-recessive causes: 25% chance of an affected child. Genetic counseling should be offered to female carriers of X-linked SCID.

Q: Can SCID be diagnosed prenatally?
A: Prenatal testing is available. Amnio-centesis can be performed, and fetal cells can be tested for the presence of ADA and PNP enzymes. Fetal cord blood sampling can be done to determine the presence or absence of fetal T and/or B cells.

ICD-9-CM 279.2

BIBLIOGRAPHY

Gaspar HB, Gilmour KC, Jones AM. Severe combined immunodeficiency-molecular pathogenesis and diagnosis. *Arch Dis Child* 2001;84(2):169–173.

Gelfand EW, Dosch HM. Diagnosis and classi-fication of severe combined immuno-deficiency. *Birth Defects* 1983;19:65–72.

Stephan JL, Vlekova V, Le Deist F. Severe combined immunodeficiency: a retrospective single center study of clinical presentation and outcome in 177 patients. *J Pediatr* 1990;123:564–572.

Stites DP, Terr AI, eds. *Basic and clinical immunology*, 7th ed. Norwalk, CT: Appleton & Lange, 1991:341–344.

Winkelstein JA, et al., eds. *Immune Deficiency Foundation. Patient and family handbook: for the primary immune deficiency diseases*, 3rd ed. Towson, MD: Immune deficiency foundation, 1999-2000.

Author: Timothy Andrews
Alex G. Yip, 2nd edition

Sexual Abuse

 ## Database

DEFINITION
Sexual abuse is the involvement of children in sexual activities that they cannot understand, for which they are not developmentally prepared, to which they cannot give informed consent, and that violate societal norms. It is due to a complex interaction of societal, familial, and individual factors. Associated problems are:
- Physical abuse
- Domestic violence
- Neglect
- Emotional abuse

EPIDEMIOLOGY
- Approximately 150,000 substantiated cases are identified each year in the United States. This is likely to be a significant under-estimation of the actual numbers.
- Girls are victimized more than boys; boys represent approximately 20% of cases reported to child protection agencies each year.
- Sexual abuse of boys is believed to be underreported.
- Children of all ages are victimized, with a peak age of vulnerability being 7 to 13 years.
- Race and socioeconomic status are not believed to play a role in the epidemiology of sexual abuse.

COMPLICATIONS
- Sexually transmitted infections, such as gonorrhea, genital warts, *Chlamydia trachomatis*, syphilis, and herpes simplex virus, are identified in only a small percentage of sexually abused children.
- Emotional problems such as posttraumatic stress disorder (PTSD), feelings of helpless-ness, impaired trust, low self-esteem, depression, adolescent substance abuse, and suicide attempts.
- Aggressive, hypersexual, withdrawn behaviors may be consequences of having been abused.

PROGNOSIS
- Varies greatly depending on specifics of abuse sustained, available support systems
- More extensive injuries (e.g., deep lacerations, tears) may take weeks to months to heal.
- The emotional impact of abuse is very slow to resolve, and may take years to resolve.

 ## Differential Diagnosis

- Infection
—With genital discharge: sexually transmitted infections (*Neisseria gonorrhoeae, C. trachomatis, Trichomonas vaginalis*), group A streptococcus, *Haemophilus influenzae, Staphylococcus aureus, Corynebacterium diphtheriae, Mycoplasma hominis, Gardnerella vaginalis, Shigella* (discharge may be bloody)
—With genital bleeding: urinary tract infection, vulvovaginitis
—With genital inflammation/pruritus: sexually transmitted infections, pinworms, scabies, *Candida albicans*, group A streptococcal perianal cellulitis
—With genital bruising that may be complicated by purpura fulminans, disseminated intravascular coagulation
- Tumors
—Sarcoma botryoid: a highly malignant sarcoma, typically of the urogenital tract
- Trauma
—Accidental trauma, including straddle and impaling injuries
—Mechanical friction from tight clothing or obesity
—Accidental tourniquet of genitals by hair
- Congenital
—Variations in hymenal configuration (septated, cribriform, microperforate, imperforate hymens)
—Urethral caruncles; vestibular bands
—Ectopic ureterocele; hemangiomas
—Syndromes associated with anogenital anomalies
- Psychosocial
—Normal behaviors (masturbation, playing doctor)
—Inappropriate viewing of sexual activity (e.g., in which the child witnesses others or sees adult videos/movies)
—False allegations of sexual abuse
- Dermatologic
—Contact dermatitis
—Seborrhea
—Diaper dermatitis
—Lichen sclerosis et atrophica
—Balanitis xerotica
—Nevi
- Endocrine
—Neonatal withdrawal bleeding
—Leukorrhea
- Miscellaneous
—Nonspecific vulvovaginitis
—Rectovaginal fistula
—Labial adhesion (agglutination)
—Urethral prolapse
—Phimosis, paraphimosis
—Foreign body

 ## Data Gathering

HISTORY
- The physician interview should be detailed if the physician is the first professional to interview the child. Prior to the examination, however, the child may have been interviewed by the police, social service workers, or a forensic interviewer. In this case, the history does not need to include all of the following details, but should include information needed to perform an appropriate medical assessment of the child.
- The interview should be conducted with the child alone in the room; diagnosis often depends on the history obtained from the child.
- Ask nonleading questions.
- Use developmentally appropriate language.

Special Questions
Ask about:
- Identity of alleged perpetrator/relationship to child
- Time of last possible contact
- Method of disclosure
- Frequency of abuse (one time versus chronic)
- Specific types of sexual contact included in the abuse
- Whether the perpetrator ejaculated, if a male
- Threats made to child by alleged perpetrator
- Previous official reports of the abuse

 ## Physical Examination

- Varies depending on age of child
- Adolescent girls require a full pelvic examination.
- Prepubertal children require careful genital inspection only.
- A few physical findings are diagnostic of abuse. These include the finding of semen or sperm, acute genital/anal injuries without an adequate accidental explanation, gonorrhea, or syphilis (excluding perinatal infection).
- Look for acute genital injuries in the absence of an appropriate history, and marked disruptions in hymenal tissue.
- Many genital findings are unlikely to be related to abuse. These include small labial adhesions in girls who are not yet toilet trained, *Candida albicans* dermatitis, erythema of the vestibule, and small mounds or projections on an otherwise normal hymen.

PROCEDURE
- The labial traction technique (gently grabbing labia majora and pulling laterally, down and toward the examiner) allows for the best visualization of the hymenal edges.
- A Wood's lamp is useful for identification of possible semen. Note: Materials other than semen may fluoresce with a Wood's lamp.

Laboratory Aids

TESTS
- Universal STD screening is not necessary.
- Vaginal cultures are obtained from within the vaginal canal. Allow 10 to 15 seconds for swabs to absorb secretions.
- Cultures for *N. gonorrhoeae* from rectum, vagina (prepubertal), cervix (adolescent), penile urethra, throat. Misidentification of *N. gonorrhoeae* can be a problem if confirmatory tests (e.g., sugar fermentation, latex agglutination) are not properly done. Be familiar with the laboratory's methods of identification and confirmation. Cultures are the gold standard and are the only acceptable method for diagnosing STDs in prepubertal children.
- *Chlamydia* cultures from rectum, vagina, cervix, penile urethra. Obtain cells for *Chlamydia* culture by gently scraping the vaginal wall with a swab (in young children). Because of the low prevalence of *Chlamydia* in the prepubertal population and normal flora that can produce false-positive results, culture remains the gold standard for *Chlamydia* testing. Rapid tests are *not* recommended for young children. PCR and LCR diagnostic techniques have not been approved for young children.
- General genital culture
- Rapid plasma reagin (RPR), hepatitis serology, HIV if indicated
- Forensic evidence collection (for an acute assault)

Therapy

- Ensure the safety of the child.
- Report *suspected* abuse to the local child welfare agency.
- Report *suspected* sexual abuse to law enforcement.
- Consult a social worker.
- Inform the parents of the report.

DRUGS
- Prophylactic antibiotics that are effective against common STDs, such as gonorrhea, *Chlamydia*, and syphilis, are generally not used for prepubertal children, because these infections are uncommon. Prophylaxis against STDs may be considered for stranger assaults.
- Identified STDs should be treated with the appropriate regimen.
- Consider pregnancy prevention (e.g., hormonal contraceptive) for adolescents.
- Tetanus booster for patients with acute, serious genital or other injuries.
- Sitz baths for comfort

Follow-Up

- Cases will be investigated by child welfare and/or the police.
- Need for foster care placement and/or ongoing supervision is decided by investigators.
- Most children are referred for short- or long-term counseling.
- Persistent physical/genital complaints, which may indicate ongoing abuse, an STD, or psychological problems
- Patient victimizing younger child: young perpetrators are often victims of previous abuse.
- It is important to get help for the child perpetrator so that the pattern of abuse does not continue.

PREVENTION
The efficacy of sexual abuse prevention programs is difficult to measure. Although children who are taught about personal safety learn from the experience, it is unknown whether their behavior is changed by such education.

PITFALLS
- Failing to consider sexual abuse in the differential diagnosis of nonspecific behavioral and physical complaints
- If cultures are not properly performed, the results may be uninterpretable or misleading.

Common Questions and Answers

Q: What does an "intact hymen" mean?
A: "Intact hymen" is not a medical term and should be avoided in describing the medical examination of the genitals. The hymen is a membranous structure at the entrance to the vaginal canal. It should have an opening that varies in size depending on the child, the child's age, the position in which the child was examined, and so on. The hymen should be inspected for signs of trauma. There is a wide variation of normal hymenal appearances, and caution should be used in interpreting findings.

Q: Can there be penetration without physical findings?
A: Yes. Although full penetration of an erect penis into the prepubertal vaginal canal (through the hymen) will leave injury, the healing properties of the hymenal tissue are great, so that past injuries are sometimes difficult or impossible to identify. Furthermore, penetration may be partial (as in vulvar coitus) and may not leave any injuries to the tissue. For these reasons, physical injuries may not be identified despite a history of penetration.

Q: Are STDs always transmitted sexually?
A: No. All STDs may be transmitted vertically (from mother to infant). The incubation periods of different infections vary, so they are expressed at different ages accordingly. Casual transmission of STDs is postulated for some organisms, but not for others. Gonorrhea and syphilis are considered diagnostic of sexual abuse outside of congenital infection. *Chlamydia*, herpes simplex virus 2, and trichomonas are probably due to sexual abuse and should be reported for evaluation. *Condyloma acuminata* is quite controversial at this time, is probably related to sexual abuse in school-aged and older children, and should be referred for evaluation. Herpes simplex virus 1 and bacterial vaginosis are nonspecific infections that are not usually related to sexual abuse. *Candida* is unlikely to be related to sexual abuse.

Q: How often do sexually abused children have physical evidence of the abuse?
A: In the majority of cases, there are no specific physical indicators of abuse. Only a small minority of patients have physical evidence considered diagnostic of abuse. Many children have nonspecific abnormalities of the physical examination, and many have normal examinations.

ICD-9-CM 995.5

BIBLIOGRAPHY
Adams JA, Harper K, Knudson S, et al. Examination findings in legally confirmed child sexual abuse: it's normal to be normal. *Pediatrics* 1994;94:310–317.

American Academy of Pediatrics. Guidelines for the evaluation of sexual abuse of children. *Pediatrics* 1999;103:186–191.

Bays J, Chadwick D. Medical diagnosis of the sexually abused child. *Child Abuse Negl* 1993;17:91–110.

Bays J, Jenny C. Genital and anal conditions confused with child sexual abuse trauma. *Am J Dis Child* 1990;144:1319–1322.

Berenson AB, Chacko MR, Wiemann CM, et al. A case-contol study of anatomic changes resulting from sexual abuse. *Am J Obstet Gynecol* 2000;182:820–834.

Christian CW, Lavelle JM, De Jong AR, et al. Forensic evidence findings in prepubertal victims of sexual assault. *Pediatrics* 2000;106:100–104.

Kellogg ND, Parra JM, Menard S, et al. Children with anogenital symptoms and signs referred for sexual abuse evaluations. *Arch Pediatr Adolesc Med* 1998;153:634–641.

Author: Cindy W. Christian

Sexual Ambiguity

 Database

DEFINITION

Genitalia can be defined as ambiguous when it is not possible to categorize the gender of the child based on outward appearances.

PATHOPHYSIOLOGY

Gonadal Dysgenesis

• Partial dysgenesis of the gonads following differentiation into testes will result in a spectrum of abnormalities ranging from phenotypically female external genitalia with the absence of müllerian structures to micropenis or cryptorchidism.
• Mixed gonadal dysgenesis: Individuals with the mosaic genotypes XO/XY and XX/XY have gonads containing both ovarian and testicular elements and external genitalia ranging from normal female, intersex, to normal male.
• Hermaphroditism: True hermaphrodites have gonads possessing both ovarian and testicular elements. This condition includes the patients with mixed gonadal dysgenesis discussed above, in addition to those with the karyotype 46XX, and less commonly 46XY.

Disorders of Sexual Phenotype

• *Female pseudohermaphroditism:* Masculinization of the female fetus is usually caused by androgens produced by the fetus or transferred across the placenta from the mother. The most common cause is CAH.
• *Male pseudohermaphroditism:* Incomplete masculinization of the male fetus can be caused by enzyme disorders of testosterone synthesis (e.g., CAH, 5α-reductase deficiency) or unresponsiveness to testosterone action (androgen resistance syndromes).

GENETICS

• Gonadal dysgenesis is associated with chromosomal aberrations.
• The mutations causing congenital adrenal hyperplasia are autosomal recessive and display HLA linkage.
• 5α-Reductase deficiency is an autosomal-recessive disorder that manifests only in genetic males.
• Androgen resistance syndromes follow an X-linked recessive pattern.

EPIDEMIOLOGY

Incidence

Inherited adrenal enzymatic defects of adrenal biosynthesis are the most common cause of virilization of the newborn female. Ninety percent of these females have 21-hydroxylase deficiency.

Age

Disorders causing sexual ambiguity occur congenitally, and the time of presentation is the newborn period. Children with 5α-reductase deficiency demonstrate virilization with puberty.

COMPLICATIONS

• 21-hydroxylase, 3β-hydroxysteroid dehydrogenase, and cholesterol desmolase deficiencies are associated with life-threatening salt-losing adrenal crises presenting in the first 2 weeks of life.
• Dysgenetic testes and ovotestes have an increased risk of malignant degeneration and should be removed.
• An incorrect or hastily made sexual assignment can cause family members undue emotional stress.

PROGNOSIS

The cosmetic outcome from surgery is usually good. The potential for gender-appropriate sexual function is usually good with therapy. The potential for reproductive function depends on the diagnosis. Long-term studies of psychological adjustment are underway.

 Differential Diagnosis

• Gonadal dysgenesis

—Partial dysgenesis of the gonads
—Mixed gonadal dysgenesis
—Hermaphroditism

• Female pseudohermaphroditism

—Congenital adrenal hyperplasia: Inherited adrenal enzymatic defects, including 21-hydroxylase, 11-hydroxylase, and 3β-hydroxysteroid dehydrogenase (3β-HSD) deficiencies, are associated with cortisol deficiency and the production of excessive amounts of adrenal androgens, which can cause virilization. Mineralocorticoid deficiency is seen with 21-hydroxylase and 3β-HSD deficiencies, as well.
—Maternal androgen exposure
—Exogenous androgens or endogenous production (e.g., maternal virilizing tumor)
—Multiple congenital anomalies
—Ambiguous genitalia can be a part of a spectrum of congenital anomalies, especially those of the urologic system and rectum.
—Idiopathic

• Male pseudohermaphroditism

—Congenital adrenal hyperplasia (CAH): Deficiencies in 3β-HSD, 17α-hydroxylase, and cholesterol desmolase result in insufficient androgen synthesis.
—5α-Reductase deficiency prevents the conversion of testosterone to dihydro-testosterone (DHT), which is necessary for the development of the male external genitalia.
—Syndromes of androgen resistance are due to abnormalities in androgen receptor or postreceptor defects. Patients with incomplete forms of androgen resistance may present with sexual ambiguity.
—Multiple congenital anomalies
—Idiopathic

 Data Gathering

Ambiguous genitalia in the neonate should be treated as an emergency, and the diagnostic evaluation undertaken as soon as possible.

HISTORY

Obtain a careful pregnancy and family history addressing:

• Drug ingestion
• Exposure to teratogens
• Infections during the pregnancy
• Androgenic changes in the mother
• Family history suggestive of CAH

Physical Examination

Notable features include:

- Palpable gonads: imply the presence of Y-chromosome material
- Fusion of the labia
- Existence of a vagina
- Position of the urethra
- Length and diameter of the penis
- Development of the scrotum
- Other dysmorphic features
- Hypertension is seen with 17α-hydroxylase and 11-hydroxylase deficiencies.

See table Features of the Classic Disorders of Adrenal Steroidogenesis.

Laboratory Aids

TESTS

Specific Tests

- Karyotype
- Steroid levels

—17-Hydroxyprogesterone
—17-Hydroxypregnenolone
—DHEA
—Testosterone
—Dihydrotestosterone
—11-Deoxycortisol
—Androstenedione

Imaging

- Pelvic ultrasound
- Urethrogram

Nonspecific Tests

Electrolytes: Hyponatremia, hyperkalemia, and acidosis are associated with several adrenal enzyme deficiencies.

Emergency Care

- Gender assignment

—The results of the diagnostic evaluation should be available within 48 to 72 hours, and gender assignment made by this time. A team approach with consultations from endocrinology, urology, and psychiatry is useful.

- Treatment of CAH

—Acute salt-wasting adrenal crisis
—Volume resuscitation with D5NS
—Stress hydrocortisone 25 to 50 mg IV immediately after the serum studies are drawn. This should be followed by 100 mg/m^2/24 h of hydrocortisone IV divided q4h.
—Hydrocortisone is gradually tapered over the next few days.
—Fludrocortisone 0.05 to 0.3 mg/d when able to take PO

Therapy

- Surgery

—Surgery may be necessary so that the sexual phenotype and gonads are consistent with the gender assignment. Dysgenetic testes and ovotestes should be removed.

- Treatment of CAH

—Acute salt-wasting adrenal crisis
—Volume resuscitation with D5NS
—Stress hydrocortisone 25 to 50 mg IV immediately after the serum studies are drawn. This should be followed by 100 mg/m^2/24 h of hydrocortisone IV divided q4h.
—Hydrocortisone is gradually tapered over the next few days.
—Fludrocortisone 0.05 to 0.3 mg/d when able to take PO
—Chronic management of CAH consists of cortisol replacement 12 to 25 mg/m^2/24 h divided as q8h and fludrocortisone 0.05 to 0.3 mg/d.

- Counseling of families

Follow-Up

- Hormone replacement therapy at puberty may be necessary.
- Long-term follow-up may involve monitoring hormone levels, linear growth, and sexual development.

PREVENTION

- Avoid the use of androgenic steroids during pregnancy.
- Prenatal diagnosis of CAH/maternal steroid treatment is available.

PITFALLS

Girls with CAH may appear quite virilized at birth and be mistaken for boys. Nevertheless, they have good female reproductive potential with adequate control of their disease, and should be assigned a female sex.

Common Questions and Answers

Q: Should a child's sex assignment be consistent with the karyotype?
A: Karyotype should not be the major factor in gender determination because gonadal and future sexual function are more important.

Q: What clues can the physical examination give to the timing of *in utero* events causing sexual ambiguity?
A: In the virilized female, labioscrotal fusion results from androgen exposure prior to 12 weeks' gestation. Thereafter, androgen exposure can only cause clitoromegaly.

ICD-9-CM 752.7

BIBLIOGRAPHY

Anhalt H, Neely EK, Hintz RK. Ambiguous genitalia. *Pediatr Rev* 1996;(6):213–220.

Carlson AD, Obeid JS, Kanellopoulou N, et al. Congenital adrenal hyperplasia: update on prenatal diagnosis and treatment. *J Steroid Biochem Mol Biol* 1999;69(1–6):19–29.

Mercado AB, Wilson RC, Cheng WK, et al. Prenatal treatment and diagnosis of congenital adrenal hyperplasia owing to steroid 21-hydroxylase deficiency. *J Clin Endocrinol Metab* 1995;80:2014–2020.

Moshang T, Thornton PS. Endocrine disorders. In: Avery GS, ed. *Neonatology: pathophysiology and management*. Philadelphia: JB Lippincott, 1993.

Styne DM. The testes. In: Kaplan S, ed. *Clinical pediatric endocrinology*. Philadelphia. WB Saunders, 1990:367–425.

White PC, Curnow KM, Pascoe L. Disorders of steroid 11 beta-hydroxylase isoenzymes. *Endocr Rev* 1994;15:421–438.

White PC, Speiser PW. Congenital adrenal hyperplasia due to 21-hydroxylase deficiency. *Endocr Rev* 2000;21:245–291.

Yong EL, Lim J, Qi W, et al. Molecular basis of androgen receptor diseases. *Ann Med* 2000;32(1):15–22.

Author: Lorraine Katz

Features of the Classic Disorders of Adrenal Steroidogenesis

ENZYME	CLINICAL MANIFESTATIONS	SEXUAL AMBIGUITY		PREDOMINANT STEROIDS
		FEMALE	MALE	
Desmolase	Salt losing	No	Yes	Low levels (all steroids)
3β-HSD	Salt losing	Yes	Yes	17-OH pregnenolone, DHEA
21-Hydroxylase	Salt losing	Yes	No	17-OH progesterone Androstenedione
11-Hydroxylase	Hypertension	Yes	No	11-Deoxycortisol
17-Hydroxylase	Hypertension	No	Yes	DOC, corticosterone

Sexual Precocity

Database

DEFINITION

Sexual precocity has traditionally been maintained as physical signs of sexual development before age 8 years in girls and age 9 years in boys. Recently, new guidelines were proposed for lowering the age considered to be normal for sexual development in girls. Signs of puberty as young as age 7 years in white girls and age 6 in African-American girls may be normal. These new guidelines have not been adopted the entire clinical picture, including rate of progression and the presence of neurologic symptoms, must be taken into account.

CAUSES

• Central precocious puberty (GnRH-dependent): associated with gonadotropin (LH and/or FSH) levels that are elevated beyond the normal prepubertal range
• Peripheral precocious puberty (GnRH-independent): gonadotropin-independent elevation of sex steroids arising from gonads/adrenals

PATHOPHYSIOLOGY

• Central precocious puberty is associated with CNS disorders.
• Peripheral precocious puberty is associated with gonadal and adrenal disorders.
• Peripheral precocious puberty can progress to central precocious puberty, due to maturation of the hypothalamic-pituitary axis by sex steroids.

GENETICS

• Familial male precocious puberty (testitoxicosis): sex-limited, autosomal-dominant inheritance of activating mutation in the LH receptor
• McCune-Albright syndrome: sporadic, postzygotic, somatic mutation in the stimulatory subunit of G-protein receptor; more common in females

EPIDEMIOLOGY

• Precocious puberty is more common in girls.
• Precocious puberty in boys is more likely to be associated with underlying pathology.

COMPLICATIONS

• Short stature
• Psychosocial stresses of early puberty

PROGNOSIS

• With treatment, improvement in predicted height is achieved, but most do not reach target height predicted by midparental height measurements. Early treatment improves final height.
• Effect of GnRH agonists on fertility has not been fully elucidated.

Differential Diagnosis

• Tumors

—CNS tumors
—Hypothalamic hamartoma: The CNS mass most commonly causing precocious puberty, it is a nonprogressive (benign), congenital malformation of neurons that secrete GnRH.
—Hypothalamic-chiasmatic glioma: often associated with neurofibromatosis
—Astrocytoma
—Ependymoma
—hCG-secreting tumors: may arise from pineal gland or liver
—Gonadal tumors
—Adrenal tumors

• Post-CNS trauma or damage

—Surgery
—Radiation: may occur after 18-Gy exposure

• Hydrocephalus
• Infection: brain abscess, meningitis, encephalitis, granuloma. These CNS lesions may result in abnormal stimulation or lack of inhibition of the GnRH-secreting area of the hypothalamus, resulting in early activation of the pituitary gland.
• Environmental: exogenous estrogen exposure (such as creams and oral contraceptives) and/or exogenous androgen exposure (such as anabolic steroid injections)
• Congenital adrenal hyperplasia (CAH): Poorly controlled CAH can activate the hypothalamic-pituitary-gonadal axis in either gender.
• Severe acquired hypothyroidism: High levels of TSH may cross-stimulate gonadal FSH and/or LH receptors.
• McCune-Albright syndrome: triad of precocious puberty, café-au-lait spots, and polyostotic fibrous dysplasia
• Familial male precocious puberty (familial testitoxicosis)
• Refeeding after severe undernutrition during early development (such as adopted children who had kwashiorkor)
• Premature thelarche
• Premature adrenarche
• Obesity

Data Gathering

HISTORY

• Careful chronology of physical changes, growth spurt, onset of menses
• Presence of neurologic, visual, or behavioral changes may suggest a CNS lesion.
• Family history of early puberty

SPECIAL QUESTIONS

• Family history suggestive of familial male precocious puberty

Physical Examination

• Plot accurate height (using wall-mounted stadiometer), weight, and growth velocity.
• Carefully stage breasts, color of vaginal mucosa, and pubic hair in girls.
• Carefully stage testicular volume, penile size, and pubic hair in boys.
• Carefully evaluate for abdominal masses.
• Examine skin for acne (comedones) and café-au-lait spots.
• Perform comprehensive neurologic evaluation to assess for possible CNS pathology.

PROCEDURE

Use standard beads (Prader gonadometer) to assess testicular volumes accurately.

Laboratory Aids

TESTS

Nonspecific Tests

Bone age: If advanced, further studies are warranted, guided by history and physical examination. If not advanced, or if the patient has only mild breast or pubic hair development (but not both), premature thelarche or premature adrenarche, respectively, is the most likely diagnosis.

Specific Tests

- Bone age
- Sex steroids: estradiol, testosterone
- Adrenal steroids: dehydroepiandrosterone sulfate (DHEA-S)
- Gonadotropins: FSH, LH (ultrasensitive or ICMA-LH if possible)
- Prolactin: often elevated with CNS tumors
- TSH and T_4
- In males, hCG levels
- Provocative tests should be done in cases in which the aforementioned tests are abnormal or equivocal:

—GnRH test for central precocious puberty; prepubertal GnRH response is predominately FSH, whereas pubertal response is predominately LH.
—ACTH stimulation test for adrenal abnormalities. Exogenous corticosteroid therapy will interfere with ACTH test but does not interfere with GnRH test of pituitary-gonadal axis.

IMAGING

- MRI of head: as indicated by history, physical examination, and laboratory tests; almost always done in males because boys are much less likely than are girls to have idiopathic sexual precocity.
- Ultrasound of gonads/adrenals: as indicated by examination and studies

 ## Therapy

As indicated by cause of the precocious puberty, for example, removal of CNS lesions or cessation of exogenous sex steroids

DRUGS

- Central precocious puberty: GnRH agonists such as Lupron are the treatment of choice. Adjunctive therapy with recombinant human growth hormone may improve final adult height; calcium supplementation may preserve bone mass accretion in girls during GnRH agonist therapy.
- Peripheral precocious puberty: aromatase inhibitors (testolactone) and antiandrogens (spironolactone or ketoconazole). Glucocorticoids for CAH.

DURATION

Until endocrinologist and family agree that pubertal progression is appropriate, guided by bone age and predicted final adult height

DIET

No restrictions

 ## Follow-Up

WHEN TO EXPECT IMPROVEMENT

- Depends on cause. For example, sexual changes of McCune-Albright syndrome are due to autonomously functioning ovarian cysts, which regress variably over time.
- Treatment of central precocious puberty with a GnRH agonist usually results in cessation of menses within 2 months, slowing or nonprogression of pubertal changes over 4 to 6 months, and decreased acceleration of bone age within 12 months.

SIGNS TO WATCH FOR

Typically, GnRH agonists are given in a depot form every 28 days, but some children require shortening of this time interval. Such dosing is often prompted by parental reports of moodiness, development of acne near the time of injection, or breakthrough menses (failure to suppress).

PITFALLS

- Obese children often have advanced bone age.
- Palpation of breast tissue (buds) can be difficult due to adiposity.

 ## Common Questions and Answers

Q: If my child is treated with GnRH agonists, will he/she go through puberty when we stop the medication?
A: Yes, children on GnRH agonist treatment do proceed through normal puberty when the medication is stopped. Effects upon fertility have not been fully elucidated.

Q: If a child already has some pubertal changes, can they be reversed?
A: If GnRH agonists are used, menses will cease, and breast tissue and pubic hair often regress.

ICD-9-CM 259.1

BIBLIOGRAPHY

Antoniazzi F, Bertoldo F, Lauriola S, et al. Prevention of bone demineralization by calcium supplementation in precocious puberty during gonadotropin-releasing hormone agonist treatment. J Clin Endocrinol Metab 1999;84(6):1992–1996.

Egli CA, Rosenthal SM, Grumbach MM, et al. Pituitary gonadotropin-independent male limited autosomal dominant sexual precocity in nine generations: familial testitoxicosis. J Pediatr 1985;106:33–40.

Herman-Giddens ME, Slora EJ, Wasserman RC, et al. Secondary sexual characteristics and menses in young girls seen in office practice: a study from the pediatric research office in settings network. Pediatrics 1997;99:505–512.

Kaplowitz P, Oberfield SE, and the Drug and Therapeutics and Executive Committees of the Lawson Wilkins Pediatric Endocrine Society. Reexamination of the age limit for defining when puberty is precocious in girls in the United States: implications for evaluation and treatment. Pediatrics 1999;104:936–941.

Oostdijk W, Rikken B, Schreuder S, et al. Final height in central precocious puberty after long term treatment with a slow release GnRH agonist. Arch Dis Child 1996;75(4):292–297.

Pasquino AM, Pucarelli I, Segni M, et al. Adult height in girls with central precocious puberty treated with gonadrotropin-releasing hormone analogues and growth hormone. J Clin Endocrinol Metab 1999;84(2):449–452.

Shankar RR, Pescovitz OH. Precocious puberty. Adv Endocrinol Metab 1995;6:55–89.

Styne DM. New aspects in diagnosis and treatment of pubertal disorders. Pediatr Clin North Am 1997;44(2):505–529.

Authors: Andrea Kelly and Robert J. Ferry, Jr.

Short-Bowel Syndrome

 Database

DEFINITION

Short-bowel syndrome is defined by malnutrition, malabsorption, fluid, and electrolyte loss after extensive small-bowel resection.

PATHOPHYSIOLOGY

- Markedly decreased mucosal surface area due to resection
- Abnormal transit
- Malabsorption of protein, fat, carbohydrate, vitamins, electrolytes, and trace elements, depending on site of resected intestine (see table Site of Absorption of Various Nutrients in the Intestine). The patient can lose as much as half of the intestine if the duodenum, distal ileum, and ileocecal valve (ICV) are present. If the ICV is gone, patients may not be able to tolerate even a 25% loss of intestine without the help of total parenteral nutrition (TPN).
- Normal bowel length: at 26 weeks' gestation: 150 to 200 cm; at birth in full-term infant: 200 to 300 cm; adult: 600 to 800 cm
- Infants have no intestinal reserve and do not tolerate small-bowel resection as well as adults. However, the long-term prognosis may be better because of hypertrophy and hyperplasia of the intestine.
- Gastric acid hypersecretion occurs soon after intestinal resection, but is transient.
- Complications include:

—Bacterial overgrowth and D-lactic acidosis due to stasis
—Renal stones due to fat malabsorption and increased oxalate absorption
—Gallstones due to disturbed enterohepatic circulation of bile salts and lithogenic bile formation

- Bowel adaptation can occur over time. Increased surface area due to bowel dilatation and villus hypertrophy and bowel lengthening can occur. Need stimulation of luminal contents for bowel growth, and factors such as glutamine, short-chain fatty acids, tropic hormones, and growth factors may be important for bowel growth.

COMPLICATIONS

- Fluid and electrolyte loss, resulting in diarrhea and dehydration and metabolic acidosis
- Calcium and magnesium deficiency, resulting in bone disease and osteoporosis
- Carbohydrate malabsorption
- Fat malabsorption
- Vitamin A deficiency: increased susceptibility to infections
- Vitamin D deficiency: bone disease (e.g., rickets)

Site of Absorption of Various Nutrients in the Intestine

SITE	NUTRIENT
Stomach	Fat
Duodenum	Calcium
	Magnesium
	Iron
	Zinc
Jejunum	Monosaccharides
	Disaccharides
	Fat-soluble vitamins A and D
	Water-soluble vitamins: thiamin, riboflavin, pyridoxine, folic acid, ascorbic acid
	Protein
Ileum	Fat
	Vitamin B_{12}
	Bile salts
Colon	Fluid
	Electrolytes
	Short-chain fatty acids

- Vitamin E deficiency: peripheral neuropathy, hemolysis
- Vitamin K deficiency: prolonged clotting time, bruising
- Vitamin B_{12}: macrocytic anemia and thrombosis
- Folic acid: macrocytic anemia
- Gallstones
- Renal stones
- Failure to thrive
- TPN-dependent liver disease: cholestasis, end stage is cirrhosis and portal hypertension
- Zinc deficiency: poor growth, infections
- Carnitine deficiency: contributes to development of steatosis

PROGNOSIS

- Depends on site and amount of bowel resected
- The more of the bowel resected, the worse is the prognosis.
- Loss of ICV, worse prognosis
- Loss of jejunum and ileum worse than loss of colon
- The longer it takes to tolerate full enteral feeds in a patient, the worse is the prognosis. Most progress is made in the first year after bowel resection.
- Development of severe TPN liver disease: poor prognosis

 Differential Diagnosis

- Infants: necrotizing enterocolitis, volvulus, atresia (jejunal and ileal), gastroschisis, meconium peritonitis, congenital short-bowel syndrome

- Older children: midgut volvulus (due to malrotation), Crohn disease, adhesions causing intestinal obstruction, strictures, trauma, aganglionosis of the intestine

 Data Gathering

HISTORY

- Stooling pattern: number, size, nature (watery, bulky, foul smelling), presence of blood and mucus
- Weight loss or gain; gaining length/height
- Abdominal distention and flatulence
- Bad perianal rashes related to stool acidity and malabsorption of carbohydrates
- Appetite
- Abdominal pain and characteristics
- Vomiting and characteristics
- Diet history: oral intake, tube feeds, parenteral nutrition
- Medication history
- Surgical history

 Physical Examination

- Weight, length, and head circumference measurements (if applicable); try to get previous growth chart if available
- Look for signs of vitamin deficiencies in examination of mouth, lips, and skin.
- Abdominal examination: surgical scars, ostomies, distention, hepatosplenomegaly, bowel sounds
- Rectal examination: consistency of stool, heme positivity, perianal rash

 Laboratory Aids

TESTS

Blood Tests

- CBC: Check for anemia and MCV.
- Electrolytes: sodium, potassium, chloride and bicarbonate; check for losses and adequacy of replacement.
- Minerals: calcium, phosphorus magnesium, iron; check for losses and adequacy of replacement therapy.
- Albumin and prealbumin: Check for protein stores and nutritional status.
- PT/PTT: Assess vitamin K status.
- Liver function tests: ALT, GGT, bilirubin if on parenteral nutrition (PN) to check for PN-associated liver disease
- Vitamin levels: vitamin A, 25-hydroxy vitamin D, vitamin E, folic acid, B_{12}; check for adequacy
- Zinc level: Check status and adequacy of supplementation.

- Carnitine: Check status if on long-term parenteral nutrition and have liver disease.
- Breath tests: lactose and lactulose breath test to check for lactase deficiency and bacterial overgrowth, respectively

Stool Tests

- Stool for pH and reducing substances: Check for carbohydrate malabsorption.
- Stool smear for fat (Sudan stain-qualitative): Check for excessive fat loss.
- Stool for blood: Check for mucosal damage.

Tests of Absorption

- Xylose absorption test and lactose breath test to check for carbohydrate malabsorption
- Seventy-two-hour quantitative fecal fat collection along with concomitant diet record
- Carotene levels to check for fat absorption
- Twenty-four-hour stool collection for α_1-antitrypsin clearance to check for protein absorption

IMAGING

Upper GI series with small-bowel follow-through and barium enema to evaluate length, caliber, and location of remaining bowel

ENDOSCOPY

- Upper endoscopy: Look for presence of inflammation that may be contributing to malabsorption; get cultures for bacterial overgrowth.
- Lower endoscopy: Look for presence of colitis, especially eosinophilic colitis, as well as caliber of anastomotic site if in colon.

 ## Therapy

DRUGS

- Supplementation of vitamin (E, D, K, B_{12}, folic acid) deficiency, calcium, magnesium, iron, and zinc
- H_2-receptor antagonists decrease gastric acid hypersecretion and reduce gastric secretory volume.
- Antidiarrheal drugs: codeine, diphenoxylate, and anticholinergic drugs (e.g., loperamide) to decrease motility
- Ion-exchange resins: Cholestyramine binds intraluminal dihydroxy bile acids to prevent bile acid—induced diarrhea.
- Octreotide: decreases gastric, pancreatic, and intestinal secretions; slows gastrointestinal motility and splanchnic blood flow
- Bacterial overgrowth: Commonly used oral antibiotics are metronidazole, trimethoprim-sulfamethoxazole, vancomycin, and gentamicin.
- Prokinetic agents: Reglan to treat delayed gastric emptying
- Miscellaneous: sucralfate to treat bile reflux

DURATION

Depends on amount and site of bowel resected and degree of intestinal adaptation that occurs. The more the resection, the longer is the therapy. Successful enteral feeds decrease the duration of parenteral nutrition. Macronutrient losses decrease with intestinal adaptation. Micronutrient supplementation may be lifelong (e.g., vitamin B_{12}).

SURGICAL/TRANSPLANT

Surgery is useful in patients who develop strictures and partial obstruction, or in those who have very short intestine length. Intestinal interpositions (isoperistaltic or antiperistaltic) can be used to delay gastric emptying, slow intestinal transit, and increase absorption. Intestinal lengthening and tapering procedures increase absorptive surface area. In patients with extremely short intestines and PN dependency, small-bowel transplantation is considered.

DIET

- Oral diet: In those patients who are able to avoid PN or tube feeds, a low-lactose diet may be well tolerated. Low-oxalate diets are helpful in preventing oxalate stones.
- Fluid and electrolyte therapy: extremely important in the acute phase immediately after bowel resection. In the chronic phase, it is important to keep up with ongoing losses, especially when enteral feeds are started.
- Enteral feeds: more successful in the patient with less extensive resection, intact ICV, and colon in continuity; no advantage of elemental formulas over intact formulas, with respect to tolerance, unless small-bowel damage is present.
- Parenteral nutrition: important in the acute phase postoperatively when nutrition must be maintained in the face of paralytic ileus; indispensable in the chronic phase when full enteral feeds cannot be instituted and nutrition needs to be maintained. Balanced solutions of protein, glucose, and fat should be administered. Prophylactic measures to prevent parenteral nutrition-induced liver damage should be instituted (e.g., prevention of overfeeding, early introduction of enteral feeds, cycling of parenteral nutrition when patient is stable). Need permanent central access to deliver concentrated PN solutions.

 ## Follow-Up

WHEN TO EXPECT IMPROVEMENT

Depends on site and extent of bowel resection

SIGNS TO WATCH FOR

Vomiting, diarrhea, weight loss, severe fluid and electrolyte abnormalities, sepsis, bowel dilatation, intestinal obstruction

 ## Common Questions and Answers

Q: What are the favorable prognostic factors in short-bowel syndrome?
A: Poor prognosis is related to the greater length of the bowel resected, loss of the ICV, loss of jejunum and ileum, longer time to tolerate full enteral feeds, and development of severe TPN-liver disease. Neonates have greater chances of bowel adaptation than do adults.

Q: Are elemental formulas better than intact formulas in the management of patients with short-bowel syndrome?
A: Recent studies have shown similar rates of absorption, stomal output, and electrolyte losses between elemental and intact formulas. The disadvantages of elemental formulas include high osmolality and cost.

ICD-9-CM 579.3

BIBLIOGRAPHY

Jona JZ. Advances in neonatal surgery. *Pediatr Clin North Am* 1998;45(3):605–617.

Kocoshes SA. Small bowel transplantation in infants and children. *Gastroenterol Clin North Am* 1994;23:727–742.

Purdum PP, Kirky DF. Short bowel syndrome: a review of the role of nutrition support. *J Parenter Enter Nutr* 1991;15:93–101.

Scolapio JS, Fleming CR. Short bowel syndrome. *Gastroenterol Clin North Am* 1998;27(2):467–479.

Sigalet DL. Short bowel syndrome in infants and children: an overview. *Semin Pediatr Surg* 2001;10(2):49–55.

Thompson JS, Rikkers LF. Surgical alternatives for the short bowel syndrome. *Am J Gastroenterol* 1987;82:97–106.

Treem WR. Short bowel syndrome In: Wyllie R, Hyams JS, eds. *Pediatric gastrointestinal disease: pathophysiology, diagnosis and management*, 2nd ed. Philadelphia: WB Saunders, 1999:315–333.

Vanderhoof JA. Invited review: short bowel syndrome. *J Pediatr Gastroenterol Nutr* 1992;14:359–370.

Warner BW, Zeigler MM. Management of the short bowel syndrome in the pediatric population. *Pediatr Clin North Am* 1993;40:1335–1350.

Author: Maria R. Mascarenhas

Sickle Cell Disease

 Database

DEFINITION

Sickle cell disease (SCD) is a group of hemoglobin disorders in which sickle hemoglobin (HbS) predominates. SCD is characterized by hemolysis, vascular occlusion, and an increased risk of bacterial infection. Common genotypes include SCD-SS, SCD-SC, SCD-Sβ^+ thalassemia, and SCD-Sβ^0 thalassemia.

GENETICS

SCD has an autosomal-recessive pattern of inheritance.

PATHOPHYSIOLOGY

- The production of HbS is caused by a genetic mutation leading to a valine for glutamic acid substitution at the sixth position of the β-globin chain.
- HbS polymerizes within red cells, particularly under deoxygenated conditions, which leads to (1) changes in red blood cell shape, (2) vascular occlusion, and (3) subsequent ischemic tissue/organ injury.

EPIDEMIOLOGY

- One in 375 African American newborns has SCD.
- One in 12 African Americans has sickle cell trait.
- The frequencies of SCD genotypes from highest to lowest are SCD-SS (60%), SCD-SC (25–30%), SCD-Sβ^+ thalassemia, SCD-Sβ^0 thalassemia, and other relatively infrequent variants.
- Although population data indicate that patients with SCD-SS and SCD-Sβ^0 thalassemia experience more complications than patients with other variants, disease severity varies widely among all individuals with SCD regardless of disease genotypes.

COMPLICATIONS

Acute

- Painful episodes: sudden, unpredictable pain that develops anywhere in the body
- Dactylitis: painful swelling of hands and feet
- Bacterial infection: Younger children are at greatest risk for sepsis/meningitis due to *Streptococcus pneumoniae,* whereas older children and adults are at greatest risk for sepsis with gram-negative organisms. *Salmonella* infections are problematic for patients of all ages.
- Acute chest syndrome: a pneumonia-like illness defined as a new infiltrate on chest x-ray
- Neurologic: including stroke (infarctive and hemorrhagic) and transient ischemic attack (TIA)
- Acute splenic sequestration: acute enlargement of the spleen, with a decreased hemoglobin and increased reticulocyte count
- Aplastic episode: transient decrease in RBC production characterized by a decrease in hemoglobin and reticulocyte count; parvovirus B19 is most common cause

- Cholecystitis: risk is greatest after age 10 years
- Priapism: a prolonged penile erection, which can be seen in males of all ages

Chronic

- Delayed linear growth and puberty
- Cholelithiasis
- Retinopathy: particularly in children with SCD-SC
- Neurologic: neurologic sequelae of stroke, silent infarction, cerebral vasculopathy and/or abnormal cerebral blood flow velocity [flow rates ≥ 200 cm/sec by transcranial Doppler (TCD) ultrasonography], arterial-venous malformations, moyamoya, neuropsychological abnormalities
- Hypersplenism: particularly in young children or patients with SCD-SC or SCD-Sβ^+ thalassemia
- Avascular necrosis: particularly of the hips
- Renal: nephrotic syndrome, acute glomerulonephritis
- Pulmonary function abnormalities
- Primary nocturnal enuresis

PROGNOSIS

Population estimates of life expectancy from 1978–1988 data range from 42 to 48 years for SCD-SS and 60 to 68 years for SCD-SC. However, many believe that early SCD diagnosis (newborn screening), penicillin prophylaxis, comprehensive medical care, and hydroxyurea therapy may increase life expectancy. Children ages 2 to 16 years with SCD-SS or SCD-Sβ^0 thalassemia are at increased risk for developing stroke if they have repeatedly abnormal TCDs. This risk is reduced with chronic transfusion therapy (see Measures for Specific Complications).

 Data Gathering

HISTORY

- SCD-phenotype
- Baseline hemoglobin and reticulocyte count
- Baseline pulse oximetry values (Spo$_2$)
- History of SCD complications
- Prior blood transfusions and complications

 Physical Examination

- Fever
- Pallor (may be accentuated at time of splenic sequestration or transient aplastic episode)
- Scleral icterus
- Signs of respiratory distress (due to acute chest syndrome)
- A flow murmur may be present (due to anemia).
- Splenomegaly
- Warmth, tenderness, decreased range of motion at site of pain
- Abnormal neurologic findings suggestive of CNS infarction or hemorrhage

 Laboratory Aids

TESTS

Diagnostic

- Hemoglobin electrophoresis: definitive test along with DNA analysis
- Screening test: "Sickledex" or "shake" tests are not recommended to establish a diagnosis or carrier status; do not use for screening in children less than 12 months of age due to false-negative results.
- CBCs: Hemoglobin values vary depending on age and SCD genotype; peripheral blood smear-sickled forms, targets, nucleated RBCs, and increased polychromasia are common RBC findings (sickle forms may be absent in transfused patients or in patients with phenotypes other than SCD-SS).
- Reticulocyte count: increased
- Quantitative hemoglobin electrophoresis
- Chemistry panel: elevated LDH, unconjugated bilirubin, AST
- Prior to the first transfusion in any sickle cell patient, draw blood for a red-cell antigen profile for future reference. (This is because of the high risk of alloimmunization in repeatedly transfused patients.)
- Neuropsychological testing: strongly recommended for children with a history of stroke, silent infarction, abnormal TCD, or learning difficulties

Imaging

- Bone scan and bone marrow scan (to help differentiate osteomyelitis from bony infarction)
- Chest x-ray study (at the time of pulmonary complications): cardiomegaly
- Abdominal ultrasound (if considering cholecystitis)
- TCD examinations at least yearly in children with SCD-SS or SCD-Sβ^0 thalassemia ages 2 to 16 years; these studies should be performed by trained examiners, experienced with the procedural modifications used for children with SCD
- CT/MRI/MR angiography (MRA) (if considering stroke)

 Therapy

GENERAL MEASURES (GENERAL WELL-PATIENT CARE)

- Children should be seen by a pediatric hematologist at least twice a year for: (1) an interim history, physical examination, and laboratory tests; (2) other ancillary studies, including TCD when appropriate; (3) patient and parent education; (4) psychosocial evaluation; and (5) referrals to other specialists, such as ophthalmology, urology, and general surgery when needed.
- Infection prophylaxis with penicillin starting by 2 months of age

- Pneumococcal vaccines (7-valent as per AAP recommendations and 23-valent at 2 and 5 years)
- Routine immunizations, including hepatitis B series; consider yearly influenza vaccine
- Consider folic acid supplementation.
- Parental monitoring for fever, splenomegaly, pain (including dactylitis), increased jaundice
- Encourage good oral hydration and supply family with medications to treat uncomplicated painful episodes at home.
- Transfusion therapy can prevent the development of SCD complications and decrease associated morbidity or recurrence of complications when used appropriately. When children with SCD-SS receive erythrocyte transfusions, avoid posttransfusion hemoglobin levels above 12 g/dL. Erythrocyte antigen matching for ABO as well as C, D, E, and Kell is recommended. Monitor children carefully for erythrocyte antibodies and/or delayed transfusion reactions.

MEASURES FOR SPECIFIC COMPLICATIONS

- Fever (rule out sepsis)
—History, physical examination, CBC, reticulocyte count, blood culture (urine, CSF culture, throat culture as indicated by examination)
—Parenteral antibiotics to provide 24- to 48-hour coverage until blood cultures are negative
—Close monitoring for other SCD complications
- Pain (vaso-occlusive episode)
—History, physical examination; consider CBC, reticulocyte count
—Hydration
—Analgesics: Therapy should be directed toward the level of pain the child is experiencing, the medications that have been used prior to presentation, and the past experience of the child with certain interventions. Patients and their families can often tell physicians what therapies have been helpful in the past. In general, for mild pain, start with mild nonnarcotic medications (acetaminophen, ibuprofen) and mild oral narcotic analgesics (codeine, oxycodone). Consider stronger agents such as oral ketorolac, hydromorphone, and morphine for initial management of moderate pain. For severe pain, use parenteral medications such as morphine, hydromorphone, and ketorolac.
—Comfort measures (massage, heating pad, warm soaks)
—Frequent reassessment for pain control and side effects of medications is mandatory.
- Acute chest syndrome
—History, physical examination, CBC, reticulocyte count, chest x-ray film (blood culture as indicated)
—Initial findings: chest pain, cough, hypoxia, fever, infiltrate on chest radiograph
—Management
—Parenteral antibiotics
—Pain management
—Supplemental oxygen for hypoxia
—Incentive spirometry or chest physiotherapy
—Red blood cell transfusion for severe disease

- Splenic sequestration
—History, physical examination, CBC, reticulocyte count (blood culture as indicated), type, and crossmatch
—Initial findings: increased spleen size, acute pallor, shock (if episode severe), anemia, and thrombocytopenia
—A sequestration episode may have a more insidious onset or be chronic in nature.
—Management
—Fever management (if indicated)
—Close, frequent observation of hemoglobin level, reticulocyte count, spleen size, and cardiovascular (CV) status
—Fluid bolus and maintenance hydration
—Red blood cell transfusion: Avoid transfusing to hemoglobin values above 10 g/dL as hemoglobin may increase as the episode resolves and red cells are released from the spleen.
—Repeated sequestration episodes may be an indication for splenectomy.
- Transient aplastic episode
—History, physical examination, CBC, reticulocyte count (blood culture as indicated), type and crossmatch, human parvovirus B19 serology
—Initial findings: pallor, tachycardia, *no* jaundice or splenomegaly, anemia, absent reticulocytes
—Management
—Fever management (if indicated)
—Close observation of hemoglobin level, reticulocyte count, and CV status
—Respiratory isolation (95% of cases are due to infection with parvovirus B19)
—Red-cell transfusion for evidence of CV compromise
- Stroke: *acute care*
—History, physical examination, CBC, reticulocyte count (blood culture as indicated), type, and crossmatch
—Initial findings: Syncope, weakness, numbness, limp, hemiparesis, seizure, slurred speech, aphasia, somnolence, coma
—Imaging: head CT, MRI, MRA; consider arteriogram
—Management
—Intravenous fluid bolus and maintenance hydration
—Red blood cell transfusion (given as simple or exchange transfusion)
—Supportive (anticonvulsives, etc.)
- Stroke (primary and secondary stroke prevention): *chronic care*
—Monthly red-cell transfusions to keep HbS level below 30%

 ## Common Questions and Answers

Q: How long will my baby with SCD live?
A: No one can predict how long a child with SCD will live. When studies were done on a large number of individuals with SCD almost two decades ago, these individuals were living, on average, into their 40s if they had the SS type of SCD and into their 60s with the SC type of SCD. Most likely, new treatments

such as daily penicillin, comprehensive medical care, and hydroxyurea therapy have prolonged the life expectancy of children with SCD.

Q: Is there any "cure" for sickle cell disease?
A: Bone marrow transplantation (BMT) is the only known cure for sickle cell disease in children. BMT requires destroying all the bone marrow of the child with SCD with strong drugs and/or radiation and replacing it with the bone marrow of a person without SCD. This marrow donor should be a relative, preferably a full sibling, whose bone marrow matches that of the child with SCD. Only those children with SCD who have experienced severe illness complications should be exposed to the morbidity and mortality risks of BMT at this time.

Q: What is hydroxyurea therapy?
A: Hydroxyurea is a medication that has been shown to reduce the number of painful episodes and acute chest syndrome events in adults with sickle cell disease. Individuals who receive this medication must be monitored closely for serious side effects, such as a decreased white blood count, hemoglobin, or platelets. Once these problems are detected and the drug is stopped, these problems usually resolve. The results of studies evaluating the safety of hydroxyurea therapy in children have not been published.

Q: What triggers or starts off a pain episode?
A: Some children say that changes in the weather (e.g., hot to cold or vice versa) will bring on painful episodes. Others say that jumping into a cold swimming pool will bring on pain. Trauma (e.g., being tackled in football), fatigue, stress, infection, and menses can also exacerbate painful episodes. However, in the majority of painful episodes, the triggers are unknown.

ICD-9-CM 282.6

BIBLIOGRAPHY

Adams RJ. Lessons from the stroke prevention trial in sickle cell anemia (STOP) study. *J Child Neurol* 2000;15:344–349.

Nathan DG, Orkin SH, eds. *Nathan and Oski's hematology of infancy and childhood*, 5th ed. Philadelphia: WB Saunders, 1993.

Reid CD, Charache S, Lubin B, eds. Management and therapy of sickle cell disease. National Institutes of Health, National Heart, Lung and Blood Institute. NIH publication No. 96-2117, 1995.

Vinchinsky E, Lubin BH. Suggested guidelines for the treatment of children with sickle cell disease. *Hematol Oncol Clin North Am* 1987;1:483–501.

White DA. DeBaun M. Cognitive and behavioral function in children with sickle cell disease: a review and discussion of methodological issues. *J Pediatr Hematol Oncol* 1998;20(5):458–462.

Author: Kim Smith-Whitley

Sinusitis

Database

DEFINITION
Sinusitis is inflammation of the mucous membranes lining the paranasal sinuses, but most commonly is used to describe bacterial rhinosinusitis, which is a clinical diagnosis made by the presence of upper respiratory tract symptoms that have not improved in 10 days or have worsened after 5 to 7 days.

May be classified by duration of symptoms:
• Acute: persistent nasal and sinus symptoms for 10 to 30 days
• Subacute: clinical symptoms 4 to 12 weeks
• Chronic: symptoms lasting at least 12 weeks
• Recurrent: acute sinusitis with complete resolution between episodes; three episodes in 6 months or four or more episodes in 1 year

May be classified by severity of illness:
• Mild: otherwise healthy, but with 10 days of persistent anterior and posterior rhinorrhea and fatigue
• Moderate: 10 days of nasal congestion with the development of low-grade fever and increasing unilateral maxillary or frontal tenderness that worsens with bending over

CAUSES
• Bacterial pathogens: *Streptococcus pneumoniae* (30–40%) with an increasing prevalence of penicillin-resistance; *Haemophilus influenzae,* non-typeable (approximately 20–28%) with an increasing prevalence of β-lactamase producing organisms; *Moraxella catarrhalis* (approximately 20–28%) with an increasing prevalence of (β-lactamase–producing organisms; group A streptococci; group C streptococci; peptostreptococci; other *Moraxella* species; *S. viridans; Eikenella corrodens; Staphylococcus aureus; Pseudomonas aeruginosa* (in patients with cystic fibrosis); anaerobic organisms
• Viral pathogens (e.g., rhinovirus, parainfluenza virus) have been recovered in respiratory isolates, but their significance is unknown.
• Fungal pathogen: *Aspergillus*
• The majority of cases begin as viral infections. Local/systemic immunity, virulence of virus, bacterial colonization of the nasopharynx, and other environmental factors may lead to conditions that allow for bacterial entry into the sinuses and growth.

COMPLICATIONS
• Orbital subperiosteal abscess
• Intracranial abscess
• Periorbital cellulitis
• Orbital cellulitis
• Orbital abscess
• Optic neuritis
• Meningitis
• Cavernous or sagittal sinus thrombosis
• Epidural, subdural, and brain abscesses
• Osteomyelitis of the maxilla
• Osteomyelitis of the frontal bone (Pott puffy tumor)

PROGNOSIS
• Spontaneous resolution in 40% to 50% of patients
• Should see improvement within 72 hours of initiation of antibiotics
• Excellent for those who are otherwise healthy

Differential Diagnosis

INFECTION
Viral URI with or without mucopurulent rhinitis

Environmental
Allergic rhinitis

Drug-Induced
Rhinitis medicamentosa

Tumors
• Nasal polyps
• Hypertrophied adenoids
• Neoplasms

Trauma
Foreign body (e.g., bead, cotton, tissue)

Congenital
• Septal deviation
• Unilateral choanal atresia
• Immotile cilia

OTHER
• Vasomotor rhinitis

Data Gathering

HISTORY
Some or all of the following may be present:
• Nasal discharge: consistency, color. In older patients, nasal discharge may *not* be the primary complaint, but concurrent rhinitis is a common feature.
• Postnasal drainage
• Nasal congestion
• Fever
• Recent history of a URI.
• Sore throat from mouth-breathing due to nasal obstruction
• Cough present during the day and may be worse at night.
• Malodorous breath
• Hyposmia/anosmia
• Maxillary dental pain
• Ear pressure or fullness
• Headache
• Fatigue
• Irritability
• Snoring
• Hyponasal speech

Physical Examination

• Fever may be present.
• Nasal-sounding voice may be present.
• Malodorous breath may be noted.
• Purulent drainage in the nose and/or oropharynx may be appreciated.
• Nasal mucosa may be erythematous, pale, boggy.
• Frontal, maxillary, and ethmoid areas may be tender to palpation/percussion.
• Headache and/or facial pain may change with position, increasing in intensity as the patient leans forward.
• Failure to transilluminate the sinuses of older children is suggestive.
• Proptosis, eye swelling, and impaired extraocular movements suggest orbital infection.

Laboratory Aids

Keep in mind that the overall clinical impression is thought to be more accurate than any single test.
• Maxillary sinus aspiration: if unresponsive to multiple antibiotics, severe facial pain, and orbital or intracranial complications; should be performed by a trained otolaryngologist

For chronic or recurrent sinusitis, consider:
• Sweat chloride test to rule out cystic fibrosis
• Immunoglobulin levels, IgG subclass levels, complement levels, and testing for human immunodeficiency virus
• Mucosal biopsy to assess ciliary function

RADIOGRAPHIC STUDIES
Imaging is *not* recommended in uncomplicated cases of sinusitis
• Sinus radiographs [including anteroposterior (Caldwell), lateral, and occipitomental (Waters) views]: several studies show that they do not always correlate with CT scans in chronic sinusitis; they are not felt to be reliable screens for chronic sinusitis. In acute sinusitis, however, they may be useful if air-fluid levels are seen. Abnormal findings consistent with sinusitis include opacification, air-fluid levels, and mucosal thickening of at least 4 mm.
• CT scans of the paranasal sinuses: useful in complicated, recurrent and chronic sinusitis; poor response to medical therapy; and/or history of polyposis
• CT scan of the head with contrast: indicated when sinusitis is accompanied by signs of increased intracranial pressure, meningeal irritation, proptosis, toxic appearance, limited extraocular movements or focal neurologic deficits; or in patients being considered for sinus-related surgery
• MRI of the sinuses: reserve for complicated cases; will show mucosal thickening and fluid

PITFALLS
• Sinus radiographs may be abnormal in asymptomatic children.
• Studies have shown a relatively high incidence of sinus abnormalities on CT scan in asymptomatic children, especially in infants

less than 12 months. The significance of opacified sinuses in asymptomatic children is not well understood.

• Up to one third of patients with symptoms of chronic sinusitis may have normal CT scans.

Therapy

If orbital or central nervous system infection is suspected by history and examination, antibiotics should be started immediately, and emergent CT studies should be performed.

DRUGS

• Mild disease in patients without a history of antibiotics in the previous 4 to 6 weeks:
—Amoxicillin (45–90 mg/kg/d divided in two to three doses): first-line agent for uncomplicated cases of acute sinusitis. Side effects include hypersensitivity, diarrhea. If dramatic improvement of symptoms within 3 to 4 days of antibiotic therapy, a minimum of 10 days of therapy is adequate. Treat for 10 to 14 days or until symptom-free and then for an additional 7 days.
—Macrolides (including azithromycin, clarithromycin, and erythromycin) or trimethoprim/sulfamethoxazole: if patient allergic to penicillin.

• Moderate disease without a history of antibiotics in the previous 4 to 6 weeks; mild disease treated with antibiotics in the previous 4 to 6 weeks; patients not responsive to first-line agents; consider for patients less than 2 years of age, patients living where there is well-described antibiotic resistance or living with smokers, patients attending day care:
—Amoxicillin, high-dose (80–90 mg/kg/d divided in two to three doses)
—Amoxicillin/clavulanic acid (45 mg/kg/d divided in two doses alone or in combination with amoxicillin (45 mg/kg/d divided in two doses): expensive; side effects include vomiting and diarrhea
• Cefpodoxime proxetil (10 mg/kg/d divided in two doses): second-generation cephalosporin; side effects include nausea, vomiting, diarrhea
• Cefuroxime axetil (30 mg/kg/d divided in two doses): second-generation cephalosporin

• Moderate disease with a history of antibiotics in the previous 4 to 6 weeks and patients not responsive to second-line agents:
—Amoxicillin/clavulanic acid (45 mg/kg/d divided in two doses alone or in combination with amoxicillin (45 mg/kg/d divided in two doses): second-line therapy
—Amoxicillin or clindamycin plus a third-generation cephalosporin (e.g., cefixime)

• Complicated sinusitis—with central nervous system or orbital involvement
—Intravenous antibiotics and hospitalization

Chronic sinusitis, use a broad-spectrum antibiotic for 4 weeks:

—Amoxicillin/clavulanic acid (45 mg/kg/d divided in two doses)
—Erythromycin/sulfisoxazole (50 mg/kg/d of the erythromycin component divided in four doses), cefuroxime axetil (250–500 mg in two divided doses), or trimethoprim-sulfamethoxazole (8 mg/kg/d of the trimethoprim component divided in two doses) may also be. Erythromycin may increase levels of theophylline.

• Normal saline: squirt into each nostril daily or twice per day; removes sensitizing agents, increases humidity, and enhances mucociliary transport; vasoconstricts and improves drainage and ventilation.
• Decongestants: these decrease nasal airway resistance and increase ostia patency in some studies, but the overall effect on acute sinusitis is unknown. Topical decongestants should be used only for short-term therapy (5 to 7 days) because rebound mucosal congestion may occur. Systemic decongestants (e.g., pseudoephedrine) have side effects that include tachycardia, hypertension, jitteriness, and insomnia.
• Mucolytics, such as guaifenesin: may improve mucous clearance
• Topical nasal steroids: reduce and prevent mucosal swelling, which can lead to osteal occlusion; particularly useful for patients with allergic rhinitis; used empirically by some experts, though there are no controlled studies for nasal steroids and sinusitis.

OTHER

• Humidifier: improves mucociliary clearance.
• Surgery: performed as a last resort after medical therapy attempted and in patients with orbital or CNS complications.

Follow-Up

• Radiographic soft tissue changes may last for up to 8 weeks; therefore, reimaging is of limited value.
• Referral to an ear, nose, and throat (ENT) specialist when the sinusitis is chronic and not responsive to medical therapy; recurrent; complicated; or when there is polyposis

PITFALLS

• Diagnosis of sinusitis is being made with increasing frequency and may result in overtreatment, given that up to 45% will have spontaneous resolution.
• With widespread antibiotic use, there are increasing numbers of resistant organisms.

PREVENTION

• Use prophylactic amoxicillin or sulfisoxazole for refractory sinusitis.
• Avoid allergen exposure and treat allergies if present.
• Practice daily nasal hygiene through the use of normal saline drops/spray.
• Improve mucociliary clearance by increasing ambient humidity with a humidifier.

Common Questions and Answers

Q: Are all of the sinuses present at birth?
A: No, the maxillary and ethmoid sinuses form during the third and fourth gestational month, and are present at birth. They continue to enlarge until the preteen years. The sphenoid sinuses develop between 3 and 7 years; isolated sphenoid sinusitis is rare. The frontal sinuses are present at age 5 to 6 years and are not completely developed until late adolescence.
Q: Does the nasal discharge seen with sinusitis have to be purulent and thick?
A: No. Though the nasal discharge is often described as purulent and thick, it may also be clear or mucoid, or thick or thin. Multiple studies have shown that a change in color or consistency is not a specific sign of a bacterial infection.
Q: Are radiographs useful in the diagnosis of sinusitis?
A: There is evidence to suggest that x-rays have limited value in the diagnosis of sinusitis, and are not recommended in cases of uncomplicated sinusitis. Mucosal thickening may be seen with viral upper respiratory tract infections and allergic rhinitis. Studies have shown that x-rays do not correlate well with CT scans in the diagnosis of chronic sinusitis.
Q: Can one make the diagnosis of sinusitis based on CT scan results alone?
A: No. Up to 50% of patients who had CTs performed for other reasons had soft tissue changes in their sinuses. Mucosal thickening and opacification on CT imaging have been seen in large numbers of asymptomatic patients. These findings seem to occur more frequently in infants younger than 12 months. Given the poor specificity of CT imaging of the paranasal sinuses, results must be used in the context of the patient's clinical presentation.

ICD-9-CM
Chronic 473.9
Frontal 461.1
Maxillary 461.0
Ethmoid 461.2

BIBLIOGRAPHY
Aitken M, Taylor JA. Prevalence of clinical sinusitis in young children followed up by primary care pediatricians. *Arch Pediatr Adolesc Med* 1998;152:244–248.

Brooks I, Gooch WM, Jenkins SG, et al. Medical management of acute bacterial sinusitis. *Ann Otol Rhinol Laryngol Suppl* 2000;182(9):2–20.

Sinus and Allergy Health Partnership. Antimicrobial treatment guidelines for acute bacterial rhinosinusitis. *Otolaryngol Head Neck Surg* 2000;123(1 pt 2):S1–S32.

Author: Esther K. Chung

Sleep Apnea—Obstructive Sleep Apnea Syndrome

 Database

DEFINITION

Obstructive sleep apnea syndrome (OSAS) refers to the clinical spectrum of disorders associated with upper airway obstruction during sleep. In children, the incidence is estimated to be between 1% and 2%. Obstructive apnea is defined as the cessation of airflow at the nose and mouth despite respiratory effort. OSAS is usually associated with some degree of gas exchange abnormality and sleep fragmentation. This form of apnea is distinct from central apnea, which implies cessation of airflow that is not accompanied by respiratory effort and may indicate immaturity of mechanisms that control breathing during sleep or central nervous system (CNS) dysfunction.

- Many children with OSAS exhibit partial airway obstruction. This is known as obstructive hypoventilation or hypopnea.
- OSAS may be subdivided into mild, moderate, and severe forms according to the degree of severity.
- Upper airway resistance is a respiratory disorder characterized by partial airway obstruction and arousals leading to sleep fragmentation and not associated with gas-exchange abnormalities.
- Primary snoring or habitual snoring implies snoring that does not lead to abnormalities in gas-exchange or sleep fragmentation.
- Central apneas up to 20 seconds may be a normal finding in premature or newborn infants during the first months of life.
- Periodic breathing is a breathing pattern associated with three or more central apneas of at least 3 seconds' duration each and separated by less than 20 seconds. Periodic breathing may be found in the newborn; however, it should not exceed more than 4% of sleep time and not be associated with bradycardia or hypoxemia.

PATHOPHYSIOLOGY

- The peak incidence of OSAS in children is between 2 and 6 years of age and most commonly is associated with adenotonsillar hypertrophy.
- In infants, OSAS is uncommon; however, it may exist with craniofacial anomalies, neurologic disorders associated with low muscle tone, laryngeal or tracheal malacia, and gastroesophageal reflux.
- In older children OSAS may be associated with obesity. This form may resemble the adult type of OSAS.

GENETICS

- In prepubertal children, OSAS occurs equally in boys and girls. However, in adults, OSAS is more common in men.

- Several genetic disorders with associated craniofacial anomalies, hypotonia, and obesity may lead to OSAS. These include:

—Pierre Robin syndrome
—Treacher Collins syndrome
—Down syndrome
—Prader-Willi syndrome
—Hereditary neuromuscular disorders

COMPLICATIONS

Complications are due to chronic hypoxemia, hypercarbia, acidosis, as well as sleep fragmentation and include:

- Pulmonary hypertension and later cor pulmonale
- Systemic hypertension, which has been reported in adults
- Congestive heart failure; arrhythmias are common in adults with an underlying coronary heart disease
- Neurodevelopmental complications: daytime somnolence, poor school performance, hyperactivity, and social withdrawal
- Poor growth and failure to thrive
- Respiratory failure and death have also been reported in children with OSAS postanesthesia.

ASSOCIATED CONDITIONS

- Adenotonsillar hypertrophy
- Craniofacial anomalies including midfacial hypoplasia and mandibular hypoplasia and affecting airway patency during sleep
- Neurologic and neuromuscular disorders causing hypotonia and upper airway and poor ventilation during sleep
- Gastroesophageal reflux
- Obesity
- Allergic rhinitis, nasal septal deviation, nasal polyps
- Some sedative as well as anesthesia may worsen OSAS symptoms

 Differential Diagnosis

- Primary snoring or habitual snoring: This condition is not associated with sleep-disordered breathing.
- Upper airway resistance: This condition is associated primarily with sleep fragmentation and daytime sleepiness but no gas exchange during sleep.
- Obesity-hypoventilation syndrome
- Central apnea and periodic breathing

Other causes of excessive daytime sleepiness include:

- Narcolepsy: onset rare before adolescence; associated cataplexy, sleep paralysis
- Epilepsy: absence spells of unresponsiveness; EEG changes
- Drug intoxication: antihistamines, anticonvulsants, narcotics

- Causes of obstructive apnea include any cause of lymphoidal hypertrophy in the upper airway; allergies; acute upper airway; infections (viral/bacterial tonsillitis, epiglottitis, retropharyngeal abscess); chronic phenytoin exposure; excessive storage material in upper airway submucosa
- Causes of abnormal laxity of upper airway soft tissues: Down syndrome, chronic neuromuscular disease, Prader-Willi syndrome, myasthenia gravis
- Causes of abnormal control/coordination of upper airway musculature: Almost any cause of diffuse CNS dysfunction may cause obstructive apnea, most commonly cerebral palsy and acquired lesions of the CNS such as stroke and head trauma
- Causes of central apnea: beyond infancy, most commonly due to drugs suppressing ventilatory drive; in premature infants may be due to nonspecific immaturity of neural ventilatory control mechanism, sepsis, and, rarely, seizures, brainstem compression, brain tumors, Arnold Chiari type 2
- Reflux may potentiate central apnea and should be investigated (see below).
- Androgen steroid replacement has been shown to cause central apnea in adults

 Data Gathering

HISTORY

- Children with OSAS frequently have a history of specific night and day symptoms. Night symptoms include difficulty breathing when asleep, snoring, apneas, and restless sleep with frequent arousals. Day symptoms include frequent upper respiratory infections and recurrent ear infections, conductive hearing loss, mouth breathing, poor appetite, and a hyponasal voice.
- Other concerns that may ultimately be attributed to or linked with sleep apnea include attention-deficit hyperactivity, poor school performance, and headaches (especially morning time and on awakening)

—Obstructive sleep apnea syndrome rarely produces these symptoms acutely, but tends to occur over weeks to months. However, parents may notice that at times of upper respiratory infections the symptoms worsen.

 Physical Examination

- Complete physical examination may disclose signs suggestive for OSAS and its complications.
- Assessment of the child's growth should be made. In severe cases of OSAS, failure to thrive has been reported.
- Obesity remains a risk factor especially in older children.

- Assessment of tonsils size
- Presence of mouth breathing, adenoidal facies, midfacial hypoplasia, retrognathia, micrognathia, or other craniofacial anomalies may be present at times and may suggest the diagnosis.
- Observation for nasal obstruction due to polyps, nasal septal deviation, turbinate hypertrophy, or congestion
- Tongue size as its relative size in comparison to the pharynx
- Mobility and size of the soft palate; hard palate integrity
- In extreme cases cardiac involvement may lead to cor pulmonale and heart failure. Examination may suggest signs of pulmonary hypertension or congestive heart failure.
- A neurologic examination should be performed to evaluate general muscle strength and tone and developmental status, especially in infants and in children who do not improve after adenotonsillectomy.
- Children evaluated for attention-deficit hyperactivity should be evaluated for sleep-disordered breathing or a primary sleep disorder.

 ## Laboratory Aids

TESTS

Polysomnography

The definitive method to establish diagnosis of OSAS and to assess the degree of severity and differentiate the type of sleep apnea is an overnight polysomnography. This is a dynamic, 8- to 10-hour long multichannel study that can assess simultaneously for any respiratory or sleep abnormality. Important indices such as oxygenation, ventilation, apnea density (apnea index), and hypopnea density are determined along with sleep parameters such as sleep efficiency, sleep stages, number of arousals, and movements throughout the night. During polysomnography the patient is monitored by electro-encephalogram, electro-oculogram, electro-myogram, arterial oxygen saturation, end tidal CO_2 tension, airflow, respiratory effort, and electrocardiogram. Normative respiratory and sleep variables have recently been published.

Other Studies

- Lateral neck x-ray is easy to perform to assess adenoid and tonsillar size as well as patency of the nasopharyngeal airway.
- Validated questionnaires are helpful to screen for OSAS even in the office.
- Upper airway endoscopy as well as bronchoscopy may be performed to evaluate for an anatomic or dynamic cause for airway obstruction (pharyngeal hypotonia, pharyngeal stenosis, laryngotracheomalacia, vocal cord polyps, papilloma).

- Head or neck CT or MRI should be considered when complex craniofacial anomalies are present and surgical considerations are needed.
- In severe cases of OSAS, a cardiac evaluation, including ECG, chest x-ray, and Doppler echocardiogram, may be indicated.
- Routine blood work is generally non-contributory. However, in severe forms of OSAS, polycythemia, hypercarbia, and elevated levels of bicarbonate may be noted.
- Evaluation for gastroesophageal reflux may include pH monitoring during sleep, barium swallow, or radionuclide studies (milk scan).

 ## Therapy

- In most cases upper airway obstruction in children is caused by adenotonsillar hypertrophy, and therefore adenoton-sillectomy is the first choice of therapy. However, some patients continue to have significant OSAS after surgery; in these cases further evaluation for the reason for OSAS is indicated.
- Use of noninvasive ventilatory support such as continuous positive airway pressure (CPAP) or BiPAP may be helpful.
- In complicated cases when craniofacial malformations are involved, surgical procedures such as tongue reduction, uvulopalatopharyngoplasty, and mandibular or maxillary advancement may be indicated.
- When there is evidence of gastroesophageal reflux, treatment with antacids, prokinetic agents, and chalasia precautions is indicated.
- Weight loss may be useful in children who are obese.
- Dental appliances were shown to be useful in adults with mild OSAS; however, there is no such experience in children.
- In extreme cases, a tracheostomy may be indicated.

 ## Follow-Up

In most children between 2 and 6 years of age with mild to moderate OSAS, clinical improvement is expected soon after adenotonsillectomy. However, in young children <1 year of age, in severe forms of OSAS, or if there is an underlying craniofacial anomaly or a neurologic disorder, a repeat overnight polysomnogram is indicated 6 to 8 weeks after surgery to ensure relief from OSAS.

- Regrowth of adenoid tissue may occur several months to years after adenoidectomy. Therefore, if clinical symptoms such as snoring, difficulty breathing while asleep, or decline in school performance recur, a reevaluation is indicated.
- Follow-up sleep studies may help to monitor therapy.

PITFALLS

- Habitual snoring may be confused with snoring related to upper airway obstruction. These could be easily differentiated by polysomnography.
- Normal-size tonsils does not exclude OSAS.
- Treatment of reflux in infants with obstructive apnea may be helpful even in the absence of obvious symptoms of reflux.

 ## Common Questions and Answers

Q: Can my child have OSAS after he underwent adenotonsillectomy?
A: Yes, at times the adenoid tissue can grow back again. In addition, some cases of OSAS are related to a small upper airway that is restricted by anatomic or neurologic conditions; in these cases adenotonsillectomy will not always resolve OSAS.

Q: Does OSAS cause neurologic problems?
A: Few studies suggest neurocognitive deficits in children with OSAS. The most common findings include reduced school performance and attention deficit and hyperactivity. However, more studies are indicated to establish this association.

ICD-9-CM 780.53

BIBLIOGRAPHY

Brouillette R, Hanson D, David R, et al. A diagnostic approach to suspected obstructive sleep apnea in children. *J Pediatr* 1984;105:10–14.

Cunningham S, Harris M. Are sleep studies worth doing? *Arch Dis Child* 2001;84(1):92.

Gozal D. Sleep-disordered breathing and school performance in children. *Pediatrics* 1998;102:616–620.

Groswasser J, Simon T, Scaillet S, et al. Reduced arousals following obstructive apneas in infants sleeping prone. *Pediatr Res* 2001;49(3):402–406.

Marcus CL, Omlin KJ, Basinski DJ, et al. Normal polysomnogram values for children and adolescents. *Am Rev Respir Dis* 1992;146:1235–1239.

Redline S, Tishler PV, Schluchter M, et al. Risk factors for sleep-disordered breathing in children. Associations with obesity, race, and respiratory problems. *Am J Respir Crit Care Med* 1999;159:1527–1532.

Authors: Raanan Arens and Peter M. Bingham

Slipped Capital Femoral Epiphysis

 Database

DEFINITION

Slipped capital femoral epiphysis is displacement of the epiphysis of the head of the femur.

PATHOPHYSIOLOGY

• Unclear: abnormal stress on normal physeal plate versus a process that weakens the plate
• The femoral head slips posteriorly and inferiorly, exposing the anterior and superior aspects of the metaphysis of the femoral neck.
• Associations: endocrine dysfunction, primary hypothyroidism, pituitary dysfunction, hypogonadism, cryptorchidism, chemotherapy, pelvic radiotherapy, renal rickets

GENETICS

Five percent of cases are associated with parental disease.

EPIDEMIOLOGY

• Incidence: 1 to 3 per 10,000
• Race: blacks more than whites
• Sex: males more than females (3:2)
• Age of onset: boys, 14 to 16 years; girls, 11 to 13 years (essentially never postmenarche)
• Associated with obesity, increased height, genital underdevelopment, pituitary tumors

COMPLICATIONS

• Ischemic necrosis of epiphysis: usually due to manipulative reduction of the slippage; more common in males; x-ray reveals increased density, irregularity, and ultimately collapse of epiphysis.
• Chondrolysis (acute cartilage necrosis): 1% to 40%, more common in females and blacks; etiology unclear; x-ray reveals narrowed joint space, sclerosis of acetabular rim, and osteoporosis of femoral head.

 Differential Diagnosis

• Severe sepsis
• Ischemic necrosis
• Tuberculosis of the hip; however, pain is associated with movement in all directions, and there should be other evidence of disease.
• Renal rickets
• Achondroplasia
• Schwachman syndrome: metaphyseal chondrodysplasia with pancreatic insufficiency

 Data Gathering

HISTORY

• Pain in hip or knee
• Occasional history of trauma; however, usually not sufficient to explain the findings
• Three patterns:

—Chronic: most common, onset of symptoms greater than 3 weeks, lack of full internal rotation of hip
—Acute: sudden onset with inability to walk or severe pain and difficulty walking
—Acute-on-chronic: sudden exacerbation of symptoms that have been present for a while

 Physical Examination

• Limp if unilateral, or waddling gait if bilateral
• Tenderness and occasional palpable thickening over hip
• Thigh atrophy
• Lack of full internal rotation of hip and decreased motion in all planes secondary to synovitis

PROCEDURE

When the hip is flexed, the thigh is forced into lateral rotation.

Laboratory Aids

TESTS

Radiographs

- Lateral view: frog leg or Lowenstein
- Measure degree of displacement:

—Minimal: alteration in plane of epiphysis relative to femoral neck; significant if angle less than 82%
—Mild: displacement less than 1 cm
—Moderate: displacement greater than 1 cm, less than two-thirds diameter of femoral neck

- Epiphyseal plate widened and irregular
- Decreased height of physis
- "Blanch sign" dense area in femoral neck
- A "Klein line" drawn along the superior femoral neck transects less of the physis than on the normal side.
- Hormonal evaluation if suspected

Pathology

Histologic findings include widening of the epiphyseal plate, large clefts, and necrotic debris in the cartilage and synovitis.

 ## Therapy

- Designed to prevent complications and further slipping
- Conservative: bed rest with traction; probably does not reduce slipping; temporizing until surgery can be scheduled
- Manipulative reduction: risk of damage to epiphyseal vessels or breakdown of callus; probably only to be considered if within 24 hours of acute slip
- Epiphyseal fixation: risk of damage to articular surface or growth plate
- Intertrochanteric osteotomy
- Salvage: hip fusion

PITFALLS

- Diagnosis is most often missed when slipped capital femoral epiphysis is not considered.
- Hip pain may be absent; there may be no pain, or only thigh or knee pain due to referred pain.

 ## Follow-Up

Chondrolysis and avascular necrosis are uncommon side effects of slipped capital femoral epiphysis.

 ## Common Questions and Answers

Q: What type of x-ray should be obtained?
A: Lateral or frog lateral of hips.

Q: Is there a role for CT or MRI?
A: CT can be useful to demonstrate degree of slip. MRI may demonstrate early changes not detectable by radiograph and CT.

ICD-9-CM 732.9

BIBLIOGRAPHY

Loder RT. Slipped capital femoral epiphysis. *Am Fam Physician* 1998;57:2135–2142.

Lubicky JP. Chondrolysis and avascular necrosis: complications of slipped capital femoral epiphysis. *J Pediatr Orthop B* 1996;5:162–167.

Rattey T, Piehl F, Wright JG. Acute slipped capital femoral epiphysis. Review of outcomes and rates of avascular necrosis. *J Bone Joint Surg* 1996;78A:398–402.

Reynolds RA. Diagnosis and treatment of slipped capital femoral epiphysis. *Curr Opin Pediatr* 1999;11:80–83.

Umans H, Liebling MS, Moy L, et al. Slipped capital femoral epiphysis: a physeal lesion diagnosed by MRI, with radiographic and CT correlation. *Skeletal Radiol* 1998;27:139–144.

Weiner D. Pathogenesis of slipped capital femoral epiphysis: current concepts. *J Pediatr Orthop B* 1996;5:67–73.

Author: Randy Q. Cron
Emily von Scheven, 2nd edition

Smallpox (Variola Virus)

 Database

DEFINITION

Smallpox is an acute eruptive contagious disease caused by the poxvirus family. The disease has the characteristics of fever, chill, backache, and headache. These symptoms progress to a papular rash, to a vesicular rash, and then to a pustular rash. The vesicles in time fall off, leaving scars that are known as pockmarks.

The two most fatal forms of smallpox are the hemorrhagic and the malignant.

• The hemorrhagic form is uniformly fatal to patients of all ages and both sexes, but especially to pregnant women. There is a shorter incubation time with the hemorrhagic form that causes the skin to become dusky and to bleed; the mucous membranes also bleed. Death occurs 5 days after the onset of the rash.

• Malignant smallpox has an abrupt onset of the prodromal phase, with lesions present but never progressing to pustules. The skin lesions remain flat and appear red and fine-grained. If the patient survives, there is minimal scarring, but in severe cases there can be large losses of the epidermis.

There has not been a smallpox case in the United States since the late 1940s, and the last documented case was in Somalia in 1977.

CAUSES

Smallpox are particles that contain double-stranded DNA, a disk-shaped core, and a lipoprotein envelope. It is a member of the poxvirus family Orthopoxvirus.

TRANSMISSION

• Transmitted via respiratory aerosol or by direct contact with the virus via the skin lesions
• After entering the bloodstream, which is the primary viremia, the virus infects the upper respiratory tract and local lymph nodes.
• The internal organs are infected as the virus enters the bloodstream for a second time, which is the secondary viremia (this occurs around day 8 of the disease).
• After the secondary viremia, the virus spreads to the skin. These events occur during the incubation period when the infected individual is well.
• Humans are the only vector that transmits the disease.
• Infected clothes or bedding can spread smallpox virus.

COMPLICATIONS

The risk of secondary infection is common when the pustules are present. The risk of mortality is estimated at 30%.

 Differential Diagnosis

• Varicella
• Viral exanthem
• Meningococcemia (in the hemorrhagic form of smallpox)

HISTORY

• The incubation period usually lasts 7 to 14 days.
• There is an abrupt onset of the fever and malaise.
• A rash follows, which usually starts in the face and spreads over the body to the extremities.
• The rash starts with macules and then progresses to papules, to vesicles, to pustules, and then to crusting lesions, which occur at around 2 to 3 weeks.
• The patient is infectious during the entire illness until the scabs fall off. The patient is most infectious during days 7 to 10 of the rash.

Smallpox (Variola Virus)

Laboratory Aids

- In the past the diagnosis was made by growing virus in cell culture or by detecting viral antigens in the vesicular fluid by immunofluorescence.
- Electron microscopy of pustular fluid can assist in the diagnosis. Active skin lesions under the microscope have the appearance of altered epithelial cells that contain Guarnieri bodies, which are eosinophilic intracytoplasmic bodies.

TREATMENT

- There is no proven treatment for smallpox, but research to evaluate new antiviral agents is ongoing.
- Patients with smallpox can benefit from supportive therapy (e.g., intravenous fluids, medicine to control fever or pain) and antibiotics for any secondary bacterial infections that may occur.

PREVENTION

Prior to 1972, all children in the United States were vaccinated at age 1. The smallpox vaccine is also known as vaccinia. The vaccine immunity lasts 10 years. There is lifelong immunity after the smallpox illness. Vaccinia is effective because:

- There is only one serotype of the virus.
- Humans are the sole reservoir of the virus.
- There is no subclinical or carrier state.
- There is a rapid antibody response that helps protect people exposed to smallpox.
- The illness is easily recognized to help vaccinate persons exposed to the disease.

Vaccination is inoculated intradermally on the arm or hip. The formation of a vesicle is an indication of successful vaccination. Patients cannot get smallpox from the vaccination. Smallpox vaccine does not contain smallpox virus but rather another live virus called vaccinia virus. Since this virus is related to the smallpox virus, vaccination with vaccinia provides immunity against infection from smallpox virus.
With possible threats of bioterrorism after the September 11, 2001, terrorist attacks, the U.S. Government has plans to increase the production of vaccine. Currently, there is no recommendation to restart routine vaccination.
In the event of an outbreak of smallpox, rapid inoculation of vaccine would be given to those people exposed to the smallpox within 4 days. The vaccination can help prevent or ameliorate the illness. It would be imperative to immunize all health care officials, police, firefighters, morticians, transit workers, and emergency management workers.

Complications of Vaccination

- Encephalitis, generalized vaccinia, and vaccinia gangrenosa.
- Incidence of complications of vaccination has been estimated to be 1 in 4,000.
- With the presence of human immunodeficiency virus (HIV), immunosuppression due to organ/bone marrow transplants and other types of immunocompromised illness, the incidence of vaccine side effects could be much higher in these groups of people.
- Vaccinia immune globulin could be administered with the vaccine to help reduce complications in those who are at higher risk of side effect from the vaccine.

—The availability of vaccinia immune globulin is limited.

Infection Control

- Home care for those infected with smallpox should be tried initially, because there is a medical antiviral treatment for smallpox.
- Home care would also prevent infecting other patients in the hospital who do not have smallpox. Supportive care is most helpful in maintaining fever and pain control and fluid management.
- Any patient admitted to the hospital suspected of having smallpox should be placed in a negative pressure isolation room with high-efficiency particulate air filtration.
- Gowns and mask should be worn.
- Used gowns and laundry should be placed in biohazard bags and be autoclaved prior to laundering or incinerated.
- Persons who die of smallpox should be cremated, if possible.
- Any suspected case should be reported immediately to local/state health departments.

PITFALLS

- In those case of hemorrhagic or malignant smallpox, diagnosis can be delayed because of absence of classic symptoms.
- Laboratory tests can assist in making the diagnosis.
- The major obstacle is that most physicians and health care workers have not seen this disease in a patient, only in textbooks. The lack of familiarity with the disease's initial symptoms could delay the diagnosis and delay vaccination of close contact individuals.

Common Questions and Answers

Q: Can I go to my doctor and request the smallpox vaccine?
A: The last case of smallpox was in 1977. The vaccine has not been recommended since 1972; therefore, no vaccine is available. The CDC has an emergency supply of vaccine for small outbreaks. The United States government has ordered a larger supply of vaccine.

Q: Is smallpox fatal?
A: Death may occur in up to 30% of cases, but the majority of people survive.

Q: How many people have not had the vaccination?
A: About half of the population has not been vaccinated. Those people immunized are not protected from smallpox because the vaccine immune efficacy wanes after 10 years.

ICD-9-CM 050.9

BIBLIOGRAPHY

Henderson DA, et al. Small pox as a biological weapon. Medial and Public Health Management. *JAMA* 1999;281(22):2127–2137

Levinson WE, Jawetz E. *Medical microbiology and immunology.* East Norwalk: Appleton & Lange, 1992:174–175

Internet Web site at Centers for Disease Control (CDC) for small pox. *http://www.bt.cdc.gov/Agent/Smallpox/Smallpox.asp*

Author: Charles I. Schwartz

Snake and Insect Bites

 Database

DEFINITION

Injury to the human skin and/or subcutaneous tissues caused by bite, envenomation, or sting, causing usually local, but in some cases systemic effects
- Snake bites
—Crotalinae (pit vipers: cotton mouths, copperheads and rattlesnakes)
—Elapidae (coral snakes)
- Spider bites
—Black widow (*Lactrodectus mactans*)
—Brown recluse (*Loxosceles reclusa*)
- Insect stings
—Hymenoptera: fire ants (*Solenopsis*), yellow jackets, wasps, bees

PATHOPHYSIOLOGY

- Snake bites
—While there are about 120 snake species in the U.S., only 15% envenomate substances capable of causing fatal reactions.
—Snake venom consists of numerous enzymes and polypeptides that are neurotoxic, cytotoxic, and hemotoxic.
—Pit viper venom produces significant local inflammation, injury to the vascular endothelium, and may lead to coagulopathy, thrombocytopenia, and shock.
—The venom of coral snake is primarily neurotoxic and may produce neuromuscular paralysis and respiratory depression.
- Spider bites
—Although there are about 20,000 species of predominantly venomous spiders in the U.S., most lack fangs capable of penetrating human skin or toxin strong enough to produce more than a mild reaction. The black widow and brown recluse spiders can cause significant harm, however.
—The black widow venom, α-atrotoxin, is a neurotoxin that stimulates myoneural junctions and nerve terminals by increasing synaptic release of acetylcholine and by initiating a massive influx of calcium. Its toxicity is mostly systemic causing severe skeletal muscle pain and cramping, and autonomic disturbances such as hypertension and sweating.
—The brown recluse venom, mainly sphingomyelinase D, acts on red blood cell membranes, platelets, endothelial cells, and other cells, resulting in tissue infarction and necrosis. It causes the destruction of tissues at the site of the envenomation and triggers coagulopathy. Systemic symptoms are more likely to occur in children, presumably due to a smaller ratio of body weight to venom volume. Hemolysis, hemoglobinuria, disseminated intravascular coagulation, shock, seizures, and death rarely may occur.
- Insect stings
—The fire ant bites with its jaws, and then swings its head around to inflict multiple stings. The venom has a direct toxic effect on mast cell membranes causing an immediate wheal-and-flare reaction at the bite site.

—The venom of the bee, hornet, yellow jacket, and wasp contain antigens that trigger an immunoglobulin E (IgE) antibody response, resulting in allergic reactions. The allergic reaction can vary in severity from mild local effects to profound anaphylactic reactions.

EPIDEMIOLOGY

- Snake bites
—Only 15% of all snake bites are from poisonous snakes, and only about two thirds of those involve true envenomation. Coral snake bites constitute less than 1% of all snake bites.
—About 8,000 people sustain a poisonous snake bite annually in the U.S., and 12 to 15 fatalities occur.
- Spider bites
—The incidences of black widow and brown recluse spider bites are unknown mainly due to the inability to identify the species of spider involved in the majority of cases.
—The black widow is found in most areas of North America but especially in southern New England. The brown recluse is found mainly in southern and midwestern states.
- Insect bites
—One percent to 4% of American population is at risk for anaphylaxis from Hymenoptera stings; 50 to 150 people die each year from sting anaphylaxis.

PROGNOSIS

- Snake bites
—Since the majority of snake bites are from nonvenomous snakes, and about one third of bites from venomous snakes do not involve envenomation, the majority of bites cause only local injury.
—Significant envenomation can result in considerable tissue destruction, and severe envenomation can cause death.
—Aggressive supportive care and early consideration of antivenom may improve outcome.
- Spider bites
—Most bites do not produce serious effects; some bites can cause severe local and systemic reactions, including death.
—The most severe reactions and the rare fatalities occur with greater frequency in children.
- Insect bites
—Most bites and stings cause minimal local effects, although some cause series systemic reactions and, rarely, death.

 Differential Diagnosis

- Black widow spider bites: acute abdomen, renal colic, opioid withdrawal, and tetanus
- Poisonous snake bites: nonpoisonous snake bite (leaves scratches, not punctures), rodent bites, thorn wounds
- Brown recluse spider bite: other spider bites, insect bites and stings (including Lyme), cellulitis, poison ivy/oak, Stevens-Johnson syndrome, toxic epidermal necrolysis, erythema nodosum, chronic herpes simplex, purpura fulminans, diabetic ulcer, gonococcal hemorrhagic lesion

HISTORY

- Snake bites
—A description of the snake can be used to differentiate poisonous from nonpoisonous snakes. Poisonous snakes have triangular-shaped heads, a pit (heat sensor in front of each eye), fangs, slit-like pupils, a single row of subcaudal plates, and may have a rattle. Nonpoisonous snakes have oval heads, no pits, rows of small teeth, round pupils, a double row of subcaudal plates, and no rattles. The corals have oval heads, yet are still poisonous.
—In the Elapidae family, the coral snake can be differentiated from the benign king snake by the pattern of the colored bands: "Red on yellow, kill a fellow; red on black, venom lack."
—If the snake is brought in for identification, use caution! The head of the dead snake can deliver a venomous bite for up to 1 hour after death/decapitation.
—Onset of symptoms in relation to time of bite
- Spider bites
—Identification of spider (rare). The black widow is about the size of a quarter, glossy black, gray or brown, with a red, orange, or yellow hourglass-shaped marking on the ventral surface. The brown recluse is small (1–1.5 cm), gray or reddish/brown, with a brown fiddle-shaped mark on the dorsum of the cephalothorax.
—Onset of symptoms in relation to time of bite (history of bite is uncommon)
- Insect bites
—Type of insect
—Previous history of insect bite allergy

 Physical Examination

- Crotalinae (pit viper) bites
—Intense local pain and burning occur in first few minutes, followed by edema and perioral numbness that may extend to the scalp and periphery. Paresthesias may be accompanied by a metallic taste in the mouth.
—Local ecchymosis and vesicles appear within the first few hours, and by 24 hours hemorrhagic blebs are present. Lymphadenitis may result.
—Necrosis extending throughout the bitten extremity generally ensues without treatment.
—Nausea, vomiting, weakness, chills, and sweating can also occur with systemic absorption of venom.
—Within several hours neuromuscular involvement can develop (diplopia, dysphagia, lethargy, etc.).
—Sign of hypovolemic shock, hemorrhagic diathesis, and neuromuscular dysfunction may occur in life-threatening envenomations.
- Elapidae (coral snake) bites
—Mild, often unimpressive local signs and symptoms (pain, swelling), but significant neurologic effects that include extremity paresthesias, weakness, fasciculations, and bulbar dysfunction that can progress to flaccid paralysis.

—Inspect bite wound for fang punctures.
—Carefully assess neurovascular integrity, consider compartment pressures if severe edema
- Black widow spider bites
—No local symptoms associated with bite
—1 to 8 hours after bite, generalized pain and muscle rigidity, cramping abdominal pain
—Children often have nausea and vomiting.
—Respiratory difficulty may occur.
—Hypertension, tachycardia, and cholinergic effects (diaphoresis, salivation, lacrimation, and bronchorrhea)
- Brown recluse spider bites
—Spectrum from minor local reaction to severe necrosis
—Local reaction: pain, erythema, swelling, and pruritus
—Ischemia and skin necrosis: A bright red papule appears within a few hours of the bite and can evolve within 48 to 72 hours into a hemorrhagic vesicle surrounded by purple discoloration (necrosis) or blanching (vasospasm). Shortly after, a firm, purple necrotic lesion appears, and within 7 to 14 days black eschar is visible. Ulcer healing can take weeks to months.
- Insect bites
—Small local reactions: painful, pruritic, urticarial lesion at the sting site
—Large local reaction: swelling and erythema, may become several centimeters in diameter.
—Anaphylaxis is rare with fire ants but occurs more frequently with bee stings.

DIAGNOSTIC AIDS
- Snake bites
—CBC, platelet count, PT/PTT, fibrinogen, fibrin split products, serum electrolytes, CPK, creatinine, urinalysis
- Spider bites
—CBC, serum electrolytes, creatinine, CPK, urinalysis
- Insect bites
—No tests routinely done

Therapy

- Crotalinae (pit vipers) bites:
—Prehospital: Remove constrictive items (jewelry or clothing) and immobilize extremity at or below level of heart. Cryotherapy, arterial tourniquets, excision and incision are not recommended. Oral suctioning is never recommended!
—Rapid transport to medical facility
—Address airway, breathing, and circulation
—The use of a constrictive band to decrease systemic absorption of venom is controversial. Its main indication is for cases of prolonged transport time to a medical facility or rapid progression of systemic symptoms. A flat band is placed 5 to 10 cm proximal to the bite, with enough pressure to impede lymphatic and superficial venous flow but not arterial flow. One to two fingers should fit easily between the band and the patient's extremity.
—Wound care: irrigation and dressing.

—Determine if envenomation has occurred via serial examinations (every 30 minutes) and laboratory studies (every 4 hours).
—Antivenom is the mainstay of therapy. Administration of antivenom should be made in consultation with a toxicologist and/or herpetologist. General indications include progressive local swelling, pain or ecchymosis, and any systemic signs or symptoms.
—Two Crotalinae antivenoms are available: Antivenin [Crotalidae Polyvalent (ACP) (Wyeth Laboratories)] and Crotalidae Polyvalent Immune Fab (Ovine) (Altana, Inc.) approved by the FDA in October 2000. Some hospitals (in endemic areas) and many zoos may stock antivenoms. In addition, the regional poison control center may have access to *The Antivenom Index* and will be able to help locate the nearest supply.
—Administration of ACP antivenom commonly is associated with the development of serum sickness and may be complicated by anaphylaxis. Skin testing prior to administration is recommended.
—Early data suggest that the use of Fab preparations is associated with fewer immediate and delayed hypersensitivity reactions.
—Supportive care: volume replacement, packed red blood cells, platelets, fresh-frozen plasma, cryoprecipitate as indicated for hypovolemia and bleeding diathesis. Observe closely for respiratory and renal failures.
—Fasciotomy only for elevated compartment pressures
—Empiric antibiotics are controversial but may be indicated in cases of extensive tissue involvement.
—Analgesia and tetanus prophylaxis
- Elapidae (coral snakes)
—Constriction bands, suction, and drainage do not prevent coral snake venom absorption.
—Crotalinae antivenom is ineffective in treating Elapidae envenomation. Antivenom is available from Wyeth Laboratories to treat envenomation by *Micrurus* (Eastern and Texas coral snakes) but no antivenom is available for the Arizona coral snake (*Micruroides*)
—Local wound care, supportive care, analgesia, and tetanus vaccination as above.
- Black widow spider bites
—To alleviate muscle pain and cramping, parenteral opioids and benzodiazepines can be administered.
—10% calcium gluconate has been used anecdotally, but is not of proven benefit.
—Lactrodectus-specific antivenom is available for more severe envenomations. Specific indications include young age, pregnancy, life-threatening hypertension and tachycardia, or severe symptoms refractory to other treatment measures. Administration of an equine serum preparation has been associated with hypersensitivity reactions and occasionally death. One vial is generally all that is needed.

- Brown recluse spider bites
—Most bites can be treated on an outpatient basis with local wound care and symptomatic treatment for pain and pruritus.
—Patients with systemic symptoms, serious infection, or extensive necrosis warrant hospitalization for aggressive supportive care.
—Large, necrotic areas may require surgical excision and skin grafting. Early surgical excision is contraindicated as it may lead to further necrosis. The area of necrosis may not be fully demarcated until 4 to 8 weeks after the bite.
—There have been several anecdotal reports of treatment of some severe brown recluse spider bites with dapsone and others with hyperbaric oxygen therapy. Neither of these treatment modalities has proved efficacy. The administration of dapsone to children has been associated with the development of methemoglobinemia.
- Insect bites or stings
—Rarely require more than local wound care and symptomatic treatment (antihistamine) for pruritus.
—If stinger remains in skin, remove by pinching or scraping. Emphasis should be on quick removal (to decrease exposure to venom) rather than method of removal.
—Life-threatening anaphylaxis should be treated with subcutaneous epinephrine (0.01 mL/kg 1:1,000 max of 0.5 mL), methylprednisolone (2 mg/kg), diphenhydramine (1.25 mg/kg).
—Bacterial superinfection is rare, but if present can usually be treated with oral and/or topical antibiotics with activity against common skin flora.

ICD-9-CM
Chigger 133.8
Snake and Spider 989.5

BIBLIOGRAPHY
Abstracts and Commentary from the Recent Clinical Toxicology Literature. Black widow spider bite: Who should get the antivenom? *AACT Clin Toxicol Update* 1994;7(3):1.

Bunzli WF, Wright DH, Hoang AD, et al. Current management of human bites. *Pharmacotherapy* 1998;18:227–234.

Clark RF, Wethern-Kestner S, Vance MV, et al. Clinical presentation and treatment of black widow spider envenomation: a review of 163 cases. *Ann Emerg Med* 1992;21:782–787.

Dart RC, McNally J. Efficacy, safety, and use of snake antivenoms in the United States. *Ann Emerg Med* 2001;37:181–188.

Walter FG, Bilden EF, Gibly RL. Envenomations. *Crit Care Clin* 1999;15:353–386.

Author: Jill C. Posner

Spinal Muscular Atrophy

 Database

DEFINITION

Spinal muscular atrophy (SMA) is a disorder of motor neurons that causes progressive weakness. The milder form (type III, Kugelberg-Welander) usually begins after age 2, while the severe, early infantile form (type I, Werdnig-Hoffman) usually starts before age 6 months. Although in type I death due to respiratory failure is common, some individuals survive for years or decades.

PATHOPHYSIOLOGY

The gene product for the most common type of SMA (type I) is involved in the regulation of RNA transcription. For some reason motor neurons are peculiarly susceptible to downstream effects that may include programmed cell death, excitotoxic amino acid, insufficiency of a trophic factor, or mitochondrial injury/free radical accumulation.

GENETICS

• Most commonly autosomal recessive: a clinical DNA test is available for the most common type; rare forms of SMA are X-linked (adult-onset, male-restricted spinal and bulbar muscular atrophy).
• Juvenile amyotrophic lateral sclerosis (ALS) (see Differential Diagnosis, below), which also involves upper motor neurons, may be autosomal dominant.

EPIDEMIOLOGY

Worldwide incidence is approximately 1 per 4,000 live births (though areas with higher incidence have been identified), making SMA one of the most common lethal hereditary disorders in humans. No known ethnic predilection for the most common genetic forms.

COMPLICATIONS

• Respiratory complications from hypoventilation (infection, aspiration, hypercapnia-induced stupor, hypoxia) are most prominent.
• Associated swallowing difficulty may necessitate a feeding tube.
• Contractures may occur.
• Though sphincteric function is normal, immobility may cause bowel stasis

ASSOCIATED CONDITIONS

• Rare forms are associated with cardio-myopathy or congenital heart disease.
• Arthrogryposis with degeneration of brainstem neurons (infantile neuronal degeneration)

 Differential Diagnosis

Other disorders that may resemble SMA include:

• Prader-Willi or Down syndrome (because of hypotonia)
• Metabolic disorders, especially those effecting muscle, e.g., Pompe disease (glycogen excess on muscle biopsy), mitochondrial disease
• Hexosaminidase-A deficiency, organic aciduria

Other neurologic disorders in the differential diagnosis of SMA include:

• Riley Day/familial dysautonomia (features prominent gut/autonomic dysfunction)
• Hypomyelinating neuropathy
• Congenital myopathy/congenital muscular dystrophy
• Myotonic dystrophy (DNA test, dominant inheritance)
• Myasthenia gravis (prominent ptosis, preserved reflexes)
• Juvenile ALS (upper motor neuron signs)
• Cervical spinal cord injury (history of birth trauma, breech)
• Polio
• Fazio-Londe disease: disproportionate bulbar dysfunction affecting swallowing
• Guillain-Barré syndrome (slowed nerve conduction velocity, increased CSF protein)
• Infant botulism (rapid onset, pupillary involvement)
• Spinal cord tumor

 Data Gathering

HISTORY

• In some cases, onset in mid-infancy with hypotonia, poor head control, and generalized weakness may come to light during a well checkup.
• In other cases, newborns present with acute respiratory insufficiency shortly after birth and require mechanical ventilation.
• Delay or loss of motor milestones in the setting of hypotonia should always raise the possibility of SMA.
• Family history of prior floppy infants, even in the extended family, may be present.
• Rarely there is variation in age of onset within families—neonatal to juvenile or adolescent onset

 Physical Examination

Evidence supporting diagnosis of SMA includes:

• Abducted, externally rotated limbs, paucity of movement
• Tongue fasciculations (80%)
• Proximal pattern symmetric weakness
• Sparing of extraocular muscles and diaphragm (hence paradoxical abdominal excursions)
• Moro and grasp reflexes are useful in assessing neuromuscular weakness in newborns.
• Note posture on ventral suspension and degree of head control while prone, sitting, and pulling to sit.
• The presence of deep tendon reflexes weighs against the diagnosis of SMA.

Laboratory Aids

TESTS

• DNA test for "SMN" mutation is the starting point of diagnosis and can obviate further testing if abnormal; if this test is normal, electromyography and muscle biopsy are done to exclude alternate diagnoses.
• Laboratory testing for alternative diagnoses is noted in the differential diagnosis.
• Prenatal diagnosis is available when the proband is known to have a DNA abnormality.

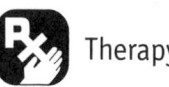 ## Therapy

• There is no effective therapy for motor neuron disease; experimental agents for related conditions in adults (e.g., amyotrophic lateral sclerosis) may prove useful in pediatric motor neuron disease.
• Supportive/anticipatory care directed toward respiratory complications, postural support, and genetic counseling
• Careful monitoring of nutritional status: catabolic state may accelerate the condition, and should be avoided.

 ## Follow-Up

• Anticipatory/preventive medical issues: respiratory condition, physical therapy to prevent contractures, and so on.
• Ongoing planning and counseling regarding prognosis and appropriate medical intervention
• Follow-up genetic counseling

PITFALLS

• A seemingly minor respiratory infection in an infant or child with quadriparesis calls for close monitoring and follow-up, because it may rapidly become serious.
• Phenocopies of SMA: neonatal myasthenia, Guillain-Barré syndrome, sometimes mitochondrial disease; make laboratory confirmation of SMA important, because prognosis or genetic implications of these conditions may be very different from those of SMA.
• Because SMA is hereditary, genetic counseling should not be neglected once the diagnosis is established.
• Survival to the end of the first decade or later can occur in type I SMA!

 ## Common Questions and Answers

Q: What are prospects for specific therapy for SMA?
A: Gene therapy or use of neurotrophic factors may come to clinical trials in the next 5 years. Cell biology studies on the role of the gene product in ribosomes hold promise. The Muscular Dystrophy Association and several national parents' groups have up-to-date information on therapy trials.

Q: Can routine vaccinations be given to infants with SMA?
A: Yes. In addition to routine vaccinations, yearly influenza vaccinations are recommended for older children with quadriparesis, because they are at high risk from common respiratory pathogens.

ICD-9-CM 335.10

BIBLIOGRAPHY

Crawford TO. From enigmatic to problematic; the new molecular genetics of childhood spinal muscular atrophy. *Neurology* 1996;46(2):335–340.

Cole N, Siddique T. Genetic disorders of motor neurons. *Semin Neurol* 1999;19:407–418.

Matthijs G, Devriendt K, Fryns JP. The prenatal diagnosis of spinal muscular atrophy. *Prenat Diagn* 1998;18(6):607–610.

Pearn JH, Gardner-Medwin D, Wilson J. A clinical study of chronic childhood spinal muscular atrophy: a review of 141 cases. *J Neurol Sci* 37:227–248.

Russman BS, Melchreit R, Drennan JC. Spinal muscular atrophy: the natural course of disease. *Muscle Nerve* 1983;6:179.

Author: Peter M. Bingham

Staphylococcal Scalded Skin Syndrome (SSSS)

 Database

DEFINITION

• A spectrum of generalized exfoliative skin eruptions, which resemble scalding injuries but are caused by an epidermolytic toxin produced by certain strains of *Staphylococcus aureus*
• Known as Ritter disease or pemphigus neonatorum in neonates

Spectrum of disease ranges from:

• Bullous impetigo: characterized by discrete, flaccid bullae containing clear or cloudy yellow fluid
• Staphylococcal scarlet fever: a mild generalized scarlatiniform eruption with exfoliation, but without the strawberry tongue and palatal enanthem of streptococcal scarlet fever.
• Evidence based on toxin production now suggests that staphylococcal scarlet fever often represents an abortive form of toxic shock syndrome (TSS).
• Classic SSSS: characterized by abrupt onset of fever, irritability and diffuse, blanchable erythema in association with marked skin tenderness

PATHOPHYSIOLOGY

• A soluble exotoxin, referred to as exfoliative (epidermolytic) toxin A or B (ETA or ETB), produced by certain strains of *S. aureus* and usually belonging to phage group II in the U.S.
• Generalized desquamation with early intraepidermal bullae demonstrating a cleavage plane just beneath the granular cell layer.
• Nikolsky sign develops within 12 hours to 3 days accompanied by flaccid thin-walled bullae. Bullae spontaneously rupture within hours, separating the superficial epidermis into large sheets revealing moist red surfaces resembling burns. One to 3 days later the denuded areas dry and the entire body surface undergoes a secondary flaky desquamation. Entire skin heals within a total of 10 to 14 days.

EPIDEMIOLOGY

• Most cases are caused by type 71 (75% of cases) or type 70, with occasional cases due to types 3A, 3B, 3C, and 55.
• The vast majority of cases occur in neonates or even intrauterine (as Ritter disease) and young children <5 years of age.
• Large screening experiments reveal toxin-producing strains in 5% to 6% of individuals.
• Antibodies to ETA have been found in 88% of cord blood samples and are absent in acute sera of patients with SSSS.
• Rarely occurs in adults due to increased circulating antibodies and adult kidney excretion of the toxin.
• Most frequently occurs in association with immunosuppression or renal impairment in adults.
• No differences in incidence based on gender or socioeconomic status.

COMPLICATIONS

• Occasional shedding of hair and nails
• Fungal or bacterial superinfection following desquamation
• Serious fluid and electrolyte disturbances in cases involving large surface areas that may lead to poor temperature control, hypovolemia, sepsis syndrome, and death; neonates are particularly susceptible.

PROGNOSIS

• Exfoliated areas eventually dry with a flaky desquamation in 3 to 5 days of initiating appropriate antibiotic therapy.
• Usually complete recovery within 10 to 14 days without scarring.
• More guarded in infants and those with underlying illness.
• Mortality reported as 1% to 10% in neonates and 3% in children.

 Differential Diagnosis

• Toxic epidermal necrolysis (TEN)
• Kawasaki disease
• Erythema multiforme bullosum
• Erythema multiforme major (Stevens-Johnson syndrome)
• Streptococcal or staphylococcal TSS
• Bullous varicella
• Burns
• Primary bullous disorders
• Chronic bullous disease of childhood
• Pemphigus vulgaris or foliaceus
• Epidermolysis bullosa

 Data Gathering

HISTORY

Question: Was there a nonspecific virus-like prodrome with irritability?
Significance: This is the typical presentation.

Question: Where did the rash begin?
Significance: It typically begins periorally and then extends to the trunk and extremities and finally desquamates.

Question: Was there any recent, seemingly trivial, localized extracutaneous infection?
Significance: Infections involving the nasopharynx, middle ear, conjunctiva, pharynx, tonsils, umbilicus, or urinary tract are frequently recalled.

Question: Was there any recent medication use?
Significance: A history of recent drug use suggests TEN.

 Physical Examination

Finding: Erythroderma
Significance: Usually extremely painful

Finding: Fever
Significance: Usually abrupt onset after prodrome

Finding: Large flaccid bullae that leave behind denuded skin resembling a burn after bursting
Significance: Often appear in areas of trauma, or in areas that are rubbed or even touched, including intertriginous zones

Finding: Distribution of lesions
Significance: Usually involve perineal, periumbilical, and intertriginous areas of the neonate, while the extremities are usually involved in older children

Finding: Crusting seen in a radial pattern (sunburst) around the mouth, nose, and eyes
Significance: Occurs without mucous membrane involvement

Finding: Sandpaper texture of rash and increased erythema or petechiae in skin creases
Significance: Pastia lines are seen in the scarlatiniform variant.

Finding: Nikolsky sign
Significance: Gentle friction applied obliquely to apparently healthy skin will cause wrinkling then sloughing.

 Laboratory Aids

TESTS

Test: Skin biopsy
Significance: Used to differentiate SSSS from TEN, as the cornified skin layer is recovered in SSSS whereas the entire necrotic epidermis should be recognized in TEN.

Test: Excision of some exfoliated skin for frozen or permanent histologic section
Significance: Easier to obtain than a biopsy and is often useful in arriving at the diagnosis.

Staphylococcal Scalded Skin Syndrome (SSSS)

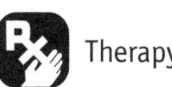 Therapy

- Apply principles of good burn care in severe cases including:

—Fluid and electrolyte management should include daily maintenance requirements as well as replacement of "third-space" fluid loss based on the percentage of affected body surface area (BSA). Fluid should be replaced as an isotonic solution calculated at 3 mL/kg of affected BSA. Most experts recommend replacement of one half of losses over the first 8 hours and the other half over the next 16 hours.
—Children should be allowed to rest unclothed upon sterilized linens, and handling of the child should be kept to a minimum. Wound care should focus on relief of pressure on peripheral circulation by the developing eschars. This is usually followed by débridement, and affected areas are eventually dressed with silver sulfadiazine or similar agent.

DRUGS

- Antistaphylococcal agents: parenteral antibiotic therapy (e.g., nafcillin, oxacillin, cephalosporins, clindamycin) should be employed for extensive skin involvement or serious systemic disease. Oral therapy (e.g., dicloxacillin, cloxacillin, amoxicillin/clavulanate, cephalexin, clindamycin) is generally sufficient for bullous impetigo. Duration of therapy is typically 7 to 10 days. Topical preparations are of no benefit.
- Corticosteroids have been shown to be detrimental in both experimental animal models and clinical trials.

 Follow-Up

Patients may be followed via telephone as long as lesions are healing well and parents do not report significant complications.

PREVENTION

- Eradication of staphylococci to prevent recurrences after first attack
- Preventing skin from becoming overly moist or macerated

ISOLATION OF HOSPITALIZED PATIENT

- Suspected or documented cases should be placed in contact isolation.

PITFALLS

- Confusion with TEN may lead to possible use of corticosteroids or simple discontinuation of antibiotics, resulting in enhanced infection from prolonged toxin production.
- Differentiation from streptococcal disease with need for penicillinase-resistant antibiotic therapy (e.g., nafcillin).
- A methicillin-resistant strain of *S. aureus* has been reported to cause SSSS.

 Common Questions and Answers

Q: Can SSSS recur?
A: Yes.

Q: Is SSSS contagious?
A: Yes, the staphylococci are primarily spread from person to person, even maternal-fetal, most efficiently by someone with lesions, but asymptomatic carriers may also spread infection. Spread of organisms does not necessarily lead to signs of toxin production in those acquiring infection.

Q: How can one distinguish TEN from SSSS?
A: TEN is frequently confused with SSSS and may be differentiated by skin biopsy showing cleavage plane at the dermal-epidermal junction. TEN or Lyell disease is more common in adults and is usually secondary to drug hypersensitivity (e.g., sulfonamides, barbiturates, pyrazolone derivatives).

Q: Can staphylococcus be isolated from the bullae?
A: SSSS bullae are sterile, although organisms may be found in a distant focus, such as the nares or conjunctivae. In bullous impetigo, staphylococci may be isolated from the bullae.

ICD-9-CM 695.1

BIBLIOGRAPHY

Eichenfield LF, Honig PJ. Blistering disorders in childhood. *Pediatr Clin North Am* 1991;38:959–976.

Farrell AM. Staphylococcal scalded skin syndrome. *Lancet* 1999;354:880–881.

Gemmell CG. Staphylococcal scalded skin syndrome. *J Med Microbiol* 1995;43:318–327.

Ladhani S, Evans RW. Staphylococcal scalded skin syndrome. *Arch Dis Child* 1998;78:85–88.

Lina G, Gillet Y, Vandenesch F, et al. Toxin involvement in staphylococcal scalded skin syndrome. *Clin Infect Dis* 1997;25:1369–1373.

Pollack S. Staphylococcal scalded skin syndrome. *Pediatr Rev* 1996;17:18.

Resnick SD. Staphylococcal toxin-mediated syndromes in childhood. *Semin Dermatol* 1992;11:11–18.

Schenfeld LA. Images in clinical medicine. Staphylococcal scalded skin syndrome. *N Engl J Med* 2000;342:1178.

Yokota S, Imagaura T, Katakura S, et al. Staphylococcal scalded skin syndrome caused by exfoliative toxin-B-producing methicillin-resistant *Staphylococcal aureus*. *Eur J Pediatr* 1996;155:722.

Authors: Mark L. Bagarazzi and Daniel H. Conway

Status Epilepticus

 ## Database

DEFINITION

Status epilepticus (SE) is defined as more than 30 minutes of continuous seizure activity or two or more sequential seizures in 30 minutes without full recovery of consciousness between seizures. SE presents in several forms:

- Repeated generalized convulsive seizures with persistent postictal depression of neurologic function between seizures
- Nonconvulsive seizures that produce a continuous or fluctuating alteration in consciousness
- Repeated partial seizures manifested as focal motor convulsions or sensory symptoms not associated with altered consciousness (epilepsia partialis continua)

Generalized convulsive SE is characterized by loss of consciousness and convulsive movements that may be symmetric or asymmetric. Nonconvulsive SE may be manifested only by alteration in consciousness. In epilepsia partialis continua (EPC), recurrent focal clonic activity or sensory symptoms occur without alteration of consciousness.

GENETICS

Some inherited conditions increase risk of SE, including neurocutaneous syndromes (tuberous sclerosis, Sturge-Weber) and familial epilepsy syndromes.

EPIDEMIOLOGY

There are 50,000 to 60,000 cases per year, and there is increased risk in young children and the elderly.

PATHOLOGY

SE is most commonly due to metabolic derangements, intoxications, trauma, neoplasm, circulatory brain injury, and acute infection. Idiopathic cases may be due to abnormality of brain development (beyond MRI resolution).

RISK FACTORS

History of seizure disorder, recent withdrawal of anticonvulsant medication, brain tumor, neurodegenerative disorder, history of remote neurologic insult (stroke, cerebral palsy, head trauma, meningitis)

PROGNOSIS

The morbidity and mortality of SE are primarily a function of etiology and are lower in children than in adults. Recent mortality estimates in children range from 1% to 3%, with risk of new neurologic sequelae estimated at 9%.

 ## Differential Diagnosis

- Idiopathic
- Remote symptomatic (previous history of stroke, intracranial hemorrhage, birth asphyxia, cerebral palsy, head trauma, meningitis)
- Febrile
- Acute symptomatic (CNS infection, anoxia, trauma, stroke/hemorrhage, intoxication, metabolic encephalopathy, anticonvulsant withdrawal)
- Neurodegenerative disorder
- Brain tumor
- Neurocutaneous syndromes (tuberous sclerosis, Sturge-Weber)
- Nonepileptic seizures (including psychogenic seizures or pseudoseizures) may mimic status epilepticus.

 ## Data Gathering

HISTORY

- A history of seizures or neurologic abnormality can be clue to etiology.
- Ask specifically about precipitating factors, including:

—Fever, preceding illness
—History of head trauma
—Change in antiepileptic medication
—Family history of seizures

 ## Physical Examination

- Vital signs for indications of fever, adequacy of air exchange and perfusion, or abnormal respiratory pattern, bradycardia, or hypertension suggesting intracranial hypertension
- Signs of head trauma, including retinal hemorrhages and evidence of intracranial hypertension such as bulging fontanelle
- Look for signs of systemic infection, especially meningismus suggesting CNS infection.
- A careful skin examination, including Wood lamp examination, should be performed for evidence of neurocutaneous disorders.
- If the patient is actively convulsing, a neurologic examination is limited to observation, or asymmetry of movement.
- Epileptic activity can produce transient neurologic abnormalities such as pupillary asymmetries, eye deviation, and focal motor weakness (Todd paresis), which may *not* correlate with the underlying structural lesion. Once seizure activity is controlled, conduct a neurologic examination with specific attention to mental status, abnormalities of motor strength, tone, or sensation.

 ## Laboratory Aids

TESTS

Initial

- Glucose
- Electrolytes, calcium, magnesium
- BUN
- Arterial blood gas
- Antiepileptic drug levels
- CBC
- Liver function tests
- Toxicology screen
- Urinalysis

Other Tests

- A lumbar puncture is indicated to rule out CNS infection unless a contraindication, such as intracranial hypertension, cerebral mass lesion, or obstructive hydrocephalus, is suspected; it may be deferred until after the head CT if suspicion of CNS infection is low.
- Brain imaging with CT or MRI is indicated in children with SE, including partial-onset seizures (including aura), focally abnormal EEG, focal neurologic signs, or history of head trauma. MRI provides more detailed images; however, CT can be obtained more rapidly and is appropriate if urgent imaging is needed or the patient is medically unstable.
- An EEG is indicated if convulsions continue and interventions such as pentobarbital-induced coma are considered, or if the patient remains comatose for 2 hours or longer after convulsions cease. An EEG also is indicated in children with first seizure and children with established epilepsy who have had a significant change in clinical status.

Status Epilepticus

 Therapy

- Initial management includes stabilization of airway, supporting respiration, maintaining blood pressure, and gaining intravascular access. Body temperature, blood pressure, ECG, and respiratory function should be monitored.
- Airway control may be maintained by head positioning, and oral airway placement and oxygen supplementation provided via nasal cannula, mask, or bag-valve-mask ventilation. If the need for respiratory assistance persists, endotracheal intubation may be required.
- Blood glucose level should be determined promptly, and if hypoglycemia is documented, 2 to 4 mL/kg of D25 (25% dextrose) administered.
- Body temperature should be closely monitored and if elevated, rectal acetaminophen and a cooling blanket used.
- Antiepileptic drug administration should be initiated whenever seizure activity persists for longer than 10 to 15 minutes. Benzodiazepines are generally used in initial management of patients with active convulsions. The benzodiazepines most commonly used in SE are lorazepam (0.05–0.1 mg/kg/dose at 2 mg/min maximum, up to a total dose of 0.3–0.5 mg/kg) and diazepam (0.1–0.2 mg/kg/dose at 5 mg/min, up to a total dose of 1.0 mg/kg, not to exceed a total dose of 10 mg). Be aware that hypotension and respiratory depression can occur after benzodiazepine administration.
- If SE persists, administer a loading dose of 20 mg (phenytoin-equivalents)/kg fosphenytoin IV. Additional doses of 5 mg/kg may be given if needed to stop convulsion (to maximum total dose of 30 mg/kg). Especially for phenytoin infusion, BP and ECG should be monitored and the rate of infusion reduced if hypotension or cardiac arrhythmias occur.
- Intravenous phenobarbital at a loading dose of 20 mg/kg (maximum rate, 100 mg/min) is generally a third-line drug for older children and adults but is usually given before phenytoin in infants younger than 1 year of age. Additional 5- to 10-mg/kg increments (to total maximum dose of 30–40 mg/kg) may be given as necessary to stop convulsions. Sedation, respiratory depression, and hypotension are potential side effects.
- If intravenous access is difficult to obtain, diazepam (0.5 mg/kg to a maximum of 20 mg), paraldehyde (0.3–0.5 mL/kg diluted 1:1 in vegetable oil), and valproic acid (20 mg/kg of liquid formulation diluted 1:1 in water) can be administered.

 Follow-Up

PREVENTION

Need for long-term antiepileptic drug (AED) therapy after SE depends on the etiology, patient's age, and circumstances in which SE occurred. Chronic AED therapy is indicated when SE is caused by structural brain lesions or in patients with known epilepsy. Chronic AED therapy may not be needed in children who have SE solely as a result of transient metabolic disturbances such as hyponatremia, intoxication, or fever, or in neurologically normal children who experience SE as their first seizure and no cause is found.

PITFALLS

- *Anticonvulsant intoxication* may occasionally cause SE (phenytoin, carbamazepine); check levels on any patient known to take anticonvulsants.
- *Neuromuscular blockers* used in intubation may obscure ongoing electrical seizures. EEG monitoring is mandatory for all patients who have had pharmacologic paralysis for airway control during SE.
- *Psychogenic status* may be characterized by asynchronous limb movements, pelvic thrusting, and purposeful resistance to passive movement. Induction of a seizure by suggestion further supports this diagnosis.

 Common Questions and Answers

Q: Does SE cause brain injury?
A: Two principal determinants of outcome are hypoxic brain injury due to hypoventilation during a seizure and brain injury because of an identifiable underlying cause of SE, such as encephalitis. Outcome in children with idiopathic SE without hypoxia is usually very good.

Q: What is the value of PET or other functional imaging in refractory epilepsy?
A: Functional imaging studies may help localize "hot spots" for staging of surgical therapy of refractory epilepsy.

Q: How safe is administration of rectal diazepam by parents for children with cluster seizures?
A: Studies suggest that when dosing guidelines are closely followed, this agent is safe and effective in terminating clusters of seizures, obviating a trip to the emergency room.

ICD-9-CM 345.3

BIBLIOGRAPHY

Mitchell WG, Conry JA, Crumrine PK, et al. An open-label study of repeated use of diazepam rectal gel (Diastat) for episodes of acute breakthrough seizures and clusters: safety, efficacy, and tolerance. North American Diastat Group. *Epilepsia* 1999;40:1610–1617.

Parker AP, Ferrie CD, Keevil S, et al. Neuroimaging and spectroscopy in children with epileptic encephalopathies. *Arch Dis Child* 1998;79:39–43.

Perry HE, Shannon MW. Diagnosis and management of opioid- and benzodiazepine-induced comatose overdose in children. *Curr Opin Pediatr* 1996;8(3):243–247.

Author: Keith Nagle
Amy R. Brooks-Kayal, 2nd edition

Stevens-Johnson Syndrome

 Database

DEFINITION

Stevens-Johnson syndrome (SJS) is a distinctive acute hypersensitivity syndrome marked by widespread bullous rash with mucocutaneous involvement, pronounced constitutional symptoms, and fever.

ETIOLOGY

- Hypersensitivity to viral (especially herpes simplex), bacterial, fungal, or *Mycoplasma pneumoniae* infections
- Food or drugs (especially sulfonamides, penicillins, and anticonvulsants)
- Less commonly, immunologic disorders, malignancies, and biologic products, such as vaccines and immunoglobulin

PATHOPHYSIOLOGY

Acute hypersensitivity reaction, causing epidermal and dermal inflammation and destruction by invading lymphocytes and deposition of immune complexes, resulting in the following findings:

- Erythema multiforme rash and bullae diffusely involving skin
- Extensive bullae with crusting and superficial ulceration of the mucous membranes of the lips, eyes, nares, genitalia, and rectum
- Severe conjunctivitis with corneal involvement, including ulceration, keratitis, and uveitis
- Extension of oral lesions into the respiratory mucosa
- Hematuria and nephritis

EPIDEMIOLOGY

- Occurs at any age
- Highest incidence in spring and fall

COMPLICATIONS

- Severe dehydration and secondary infection (similar to burn patients)
- Sepsis
- Corneal ulceration and blindness
- Pneumonitis, pneumonia, and respiratory failure
- Nephritis and renal failure
- Stress ulcers and gastric perforation

PROGNOSIS

- Recovery can take several weeks or longer if there are complications.
- SJS can resolve completely over time with little or no scarring.
- May have corneal scars, which may impair vision

 Differential Diagnosis

INFECTION

- Varicella
- Staphylococcal or streptococcal scalded skin syndrome
- Disseminated herpes simplex virus
- Measles

TRAUMA

- Burns (chemical or heat)

METABOLIC

- Drug reaction

CONGENITAL

- Epidermolysis bullosa

IMMUNOLOGIC

- Primary immunobullous dermatoses (pemphigus, pemphigoid, linear IgA dermatosis)
- Henoch-Schönlein purpura
- Lupus erythematosus

MISCELLANEOUS

- Erythema multiforme minor

 Data Gathering

HISTORY

Question: Were there any exposures to drugs within the last several weeks, especially sulfa drugs, penicillins, and anticonvulsants?
Significance: These drugs are common causes of SJS.

Question: Does the patient have another medical condition?
Significance: It is important to identify the underlying cause (infectious or toxic) and investigate underlying medical problems. Ask about recent or current medications, vaccinations, and toxic exposures.

 Physical Examination

- Determine the surface area of skin involved.
- Examine all orifices (including anus and urethral meatus) for mucocutaneous involvement.
- Determine hydration, respiratory, gastrointestinal, and urologic status.
- Assess presence of infection or sepsis.

 Laboratory Aids

TESTS

Specific Tests

- CBC (infection); electrolytes (dehydration); BUN/creatinine (renal function); erythrocyte sedimentation rate; Tzanck smear of skin/mucosal lesions (HSV)
- Consider serologic tests, looking for specific viral etiologies and mycoplasma titers.
- Pulse oximetry

Radiographic Tests

- Chest radiograph (pneumonia)

 Emergency Care

- Address life-threatening complications: sepsis, shock, hypovolemia, hypoxia, gastrointestinal bleeding.
- Admit to the intensive care unit or burn unit if indicated.

Stevens-Johnson Syndrome

 Therapy

- Eliminate the cause if identified.
- Intravenous access is critical to provide fluid resuscitation and maintenance of large fluid requirements.
- Débridement and meticulous skin care are critical.
- Nutritional support is critical and often achieved with high-calorie nasogastric feeds or intravenous hyperalimentation.
- Ophthalmology consult
- Monitor closely for secondary infection.
- Monitor closely for airway complications.
- Skin grafts may be indicated.

DRUGS

- Cover open lesions with bacitracin ointment and gauze or Xeroform-impregnated gauze.
- Do *not* use Silvadene skin dressing because the sulfadiazine component may aggravate the condition.
- Reserve antibiotics for identified infections only. Do not use prophylactic antibiotics.
- Acyclovir is indicated if active herpes simplex infection is suspected.
- Prevent and treat stress ulcers with antacids and H_2 blockers.
- Steroids are currently *not* indicated.
- Intravenous immune globulin has been associated with decreased duration of fever and length of hospital stay.

 Follow-Up

- Skin care until all areas healed
- Ophthalmology consult if corneal involvement
- Follow renal function if impaired
- Education to avoid the causative agent

PREVENTION

None known

PITFALLS

- Discontinuation of the causative agent (e.g., anticonvulsants or antibiotics) may leave another problem untreated.
- Delay in recognition of complications

 Common Questions and Answers

Q: Why should steroids not be used?
A: Steroids are currently not indicated for SJS. A possible association with herpes simplex infection makes their use risky. Efficacy has not been shown.

Q: How do you differentiate between SJS and erythema multiforme (EM)?
A: Mucous membrane involvement is present in SJS but not in EM. SJS is more extensive and associated with more systemic symptoms.

Q: Who should be admitted to the intensive care unit?
A: Any patient with pulmonary involvement and serious infection, or if close monitoring of fluids and electrolytes, or extensive skin care is not available in the regular inpatient unit.

ICD-9-CM 695.1

BIBLIOGRAPHY

Cohen B. The many faces of erythema multiforme. *Contemp Pediatr* 1994;11:19–39.

Hurwitz S. Pediatric dermatology. *Pediatr Clin North Am* 1991;38(4):972–974.

Leaute-Labreze C, Lamireau T, et al. Diagnosis, classification, and management of erythema multiforme and Stevens-Johnson syndrome. *Arch Dis Child* 2000;83:347–352.

Leaute-Labreze C, Lamireau T, Chawki D, et al. Diagnosis, classification, and management of erythema multiforme and Stevens-Johnson syndrome. *Arch Dis Child* 2000;83(4):347–352.

Morici MV, Galen WK, Shetty AK, et al. Intravenous immunoglobulin therapy for children with Stevens-Johnson syndrome. *J Rheumatol* 2000;27(10):2494–2497.

Stewart MG, Duncan NO III, Franklin DJ, et al. Head and neck manifestations of erythema multiforme in children. *Otolaryngol Head Neck Surg* 1994;111(3,1):236–242.

Author: Deborah L. Silver

Stomatitis

 Database

DEFINITION

- Stomatitis is inflammation of the mucous membranes of the mouth. There are multiple etiologies, with viral infections (e.g., herpes simplex virus, HSV, type 1) and recurrent aphthous stomatitis being the most common in children.
- Stomatitis may occur as part of a more generalized disease as in hand-foot-and-mouth disease, often due to coxsackievirus A16 and enterovirus 71.
- Recurrent aphthous stomatitis, known more commonly as canker sores, does not have an identified infectious agent. These lesions are believed to be mediated by immunologic response to a variety of insults, including trauma, stress, hormonal fluctuations, infections, vitamin deficiencies, food allergies, or nutritional deficiencies.
- Herpangina is a disease caused by coxsackievirus group A and marked by stomatitis consisting of 1- to 2-mm oral vesicles and ulcers, and systemic symptoms, most notably fever.

PATHOPHYSIOLOGY

- Infection, inflammation, or trauma leads to interruption of the integrity of the mucosal epithelium.
- Ongoing inflammation leads to further denudation of the epithelium.
- Inflammatory cells and mediators can produce exudates and erythema of the ulceration. The most common causes of this process are enteroviruses (such as coxsackievirus), HSV (particularly type 1), and recurrent aphthous ulcers (usually caused by microtrauma, stress, vitamin deficiencies and food allergies).

EPIDEMIOLOGY

- HSV type 1: up to 90% of the adult population has serologic evidence of previous infection.
- Enteroviral infections occur commonly in summer and fall months.

COMPLICATIONS

Infectious

- Cellulitis
- Lymphadenitis

Miscellaneous

- Dehydration
- Pain

PROGNOSIS

- Most cases of stomatitis are mild and resolve within 1 to 2 weeks.
- HSV stomatitis is most severe during the initial infection; however, it tends to recur in response to stress or trauma as the virus has a long latent period within the nerves of the face, particularly the trigeminal nerve.
- Recurrent aphthous stomatitis also recurs in response to stress or trauma.

 Differential Diagnosis

- Coxsackie viruses
- HSV
- Varicella
- Trauma
- Medications (e.g., chemotherapeutic agents)
- Stevens-Johnson syndrome
- Candidal infections
- Lichen planus
- Reiter syndrome (reactive arthritis, rash, conjunctivitis, urethritis, diarrhea, and stomatitis with painless erosive ulcers)
- Behçet syndrome (associated with ulcerations of the oral and genital mucous membranes)
- Crohn disease
- HIV-associated aphthous ulcers
- Cyclic neutropenia
- PFAPA syndrome: periodic fever, aphthous stomatitis, pharyngitis, and adenitis

 Data Gathering

HISTORY

Question: How old is the child?
Significance: Herpangina and herpetic gingivostomatitis occur in infants, toddlers, and preschool-aged children. Coxsackievirus (hand-foot-and-mouth disease) occurs most frequently in toddlers and young school-aged children. Aphthous stomatitis occurs in older children and adults.

Question: Are there any associated symptoms?
Significance: Fever, malaise, diarrhea, or other constitutional symptoms occur with coxsackievirus, herpangina, and primary herpetic gingivostomatitis.

Question: Does the child have chronic medical problems?
Significance: Immunodeficiency states (e.g., HIV and neutropenia), poor nutritional status, and inflammatory bowel disease are associated with development of mucosal ulceration.

Question: Does the child take any medications?
Significance: Medications, particularly penicillins, sulfa-containing drugs, and antiepileptics, have been associated with Stevens-Johnson syndrome, which has oral mucositis as part of its constellation of symptoms.

Question: Does the child have other lesions on the body?
Significance: Varicella consists of lesions mainly on the trunk and extremities. Coxsackievirus when part of hand-foot-and-mouth disease consists of lesions in the mouth as well as the palms and soles. HSV can cause lesions on the lips.

Physical Examination

- Enteroviral infections are associated with small shallow ulcerations with smooth borders on the posterior oral cavity structures such as the tonsils, soft palate, and pharynx. Also vesicular lesions may be present on the palms and soles.
- Herpes simplex infections are shallow ulcers with irregular, erythematous borders that coalesce; they are found on the lips, tongue, and gingiva.
- Varicella infections are shallow ulcers with erythematous borders that usually do not coalesce. In addition, diffuse vesicles in varying stages of healing can be found on the skin, particularly the trunk and extremities.
- Stevens-Johnson syndrome presents with large irregular ulcers, which may occasionally be deep. There is occasionally a hemorrhagic component to these ulcers. Ulcers are also sometimes present on other mucosal surfaces. Target lesions, bullae, and urticarial lesions may also be present.
- Behçet syndrome and Reiter syndrome may have painless ulceration of the oral mucous membranes.
- Gingivitis in association with stomatitis is usually present in drug-induced causes of stomatitis, as well as with HSV.
- Herpetic whitlow is the transmission of herpes virus and development of lesions on the extremities, notably the fingers due to direct contact with lesions in the mouth.
- Herpangina consists of oral vesicles and ulcers typically around the fauces, near the tonsillar pillars.

 ## Laboratory Aids

- Usually there is no need for laboratory testing for simple stomatitis. If there are other systemic signs of illness (e.g., diarrhea or arthritis), a more thorough workup for more severe illnesses such as Crohn disease, Reiter syndrome, or cyclic neutropenia should be done.
- HSV can be diagnosed with direct fluorescent antibody staining, rapid enzyme immunoassay, or viral culture of the lesion. Usually there is no need for diagnostic testing of the oral lesions unless cases are severe, the patient is immunocompromised, or there is concern there may be another etiology (e.g., Stevens-Johnson, cyclic neutropenia).
- Enteroviruses can be cultured from stool, nasopharyngeal, throat, CSF, and blood specimens. PCR of CSF fluid also can diagnose an enteroviral infection. Usually there is no need for diagnostic testing of the oral lesions unless cases are severe, the patient is immunocompromised, or there is concern that there may be another etiology (e.g., Stevens-Johnson, cyclic neutropenia).

 ## Therapy

RINSES

- Salt water rinses (normal saline or 1 tsp of table salt mixed with 16 oz of tepid water or 1 tsp of baking soda with 32 oz of water) every 1 to 2 hours while ulcers are present may aid in reducing pain and shortening the duration of the ulceration.
- Magic mouthwash equal parts of diphenhydramine and Maalox or Kaopectate. In severe cases, 2% viscous lidocaine can be added in an equal amount, but care must be taken to limit the application of lidocaine on ulcerated mucosa, as it may be absorbed, leading to arrhythmias. Also, when applied to the posterior pharynx lidocaine can decrease the gag reflex, leading to an increased risk of aspiration.

ANALGESICS

- Viscous lidocaine 2% (see caution above)
- Acetaminophen or ibuprofen
- Acetaminophen with codeine may be used in severe cases, when intake of fluids is greatly affected by pain. Codeine should be used cautiously as it may cause constipation and central nervous system depression.
- Acyclovir can be given orally for herpes simplex infections to decrease the length of the infection, but usually needs to be given within the first 48 hours of development of oral lesions. Acyclovir usually is more beneficial when used for household contacts who begin to exhibit symptoms, and when treatment can be initiated early.

 ## Follow-Up

In young children, the greatest risk is their inability to take in liquids adequately, leading to dehydration. They should be followed closely. If dehydration occurs due to poor oral intake, intravenous rehydration should be considered.

PREVENTION

- Hand washing can prevent spread of viral infections.
- Due to the long life of enteroviruses on surfaces, toys and other objects used by affected children should be sterilized before being used by other children.
- Contact isolation should be observed for children with viral stomatitis in the hospital setting.

 ## Common Questions and Answers

Q: Is stomatitis contagious?
A: Yes, this is a contagious infection. To avoid spreading the illness, careful hand washing should be done. In cases of suspected enteroviral infections, careful sterilization of toys and surfaces with which the affected child has contact should be done before use by unaffected children.

Q: How can I get my child to take food and liquids if stomatitis is painful?
A: The inability to stay hydrated is one of the complications of stomatitis. Children will not have their regular intake of solids due to mechanical effects of these on painful ulcers. Using regular analgesics, such as acetaminophen or ibuprofen, can help decrease pain. Topical administration of magic mouthwash (see above) before offering fluids may be helpful. Offering small amounts of cool liquids frequently may be better tolerated than large amounts given all at once. If your child has decreased urine output or altered mental status, seek medical attention.

Q: When can my child return to school/day care?
A: Young children with herpes or enteroviral stomatitis can transmit these from oral secretions. In cases of young children who drool frequently, or place toys in their mouths, this is a high risk for transmitting the illness. Children become less contagious when the lesions heal. In the case of varicella, children are contagious until *all* vesicles are crusted over.

ICD-9-CM 528.0

BIBLIOGRAPHY

American Academy of Pediatrics. Summaries of infectious diseases. In: Peter G, ed. *2000 red book: report of the Committee on Infectious Diseases*, 25th ed. Elk Grove Village, IL: American Academy of Pediatrics, 2000:236–238, 309–318, 624–638.

Feder HM. Periodic fever, aphthous stomatitis, pharyngitis, adenitis: a clinical review of a new syndrome. *Clin Opin Pediatr* 2000;12: 233–236.

Pichichero ME, McLinn S, Rotbart HA, et al. Clinical and economic impact of enterovirus illness in private pediatric practice. *Pediatrics* 1998;102(5)1126–1134.

Scott DA, Coulter WA, Lamey P-J. Oral shedding of herpes simplex virus type 1: a review. *J Oral Pathol Med* 1997;26:441–447.

Siegel MA. Strategies for management of commonly encountered oral mucosal disorders. *J Calif Dent Assoc* 1999;27(3):210–227.

Woo S-B, Sonis ST. Recurrent aphthous ulcers: a review of diagnosis and treatment. *J Am Dent Assoc* 1996;127:1202–1213.

Author: Lee R. Atkinson

Strabismus

Database

DEFINITION

From the Greek *strabismos* (condition of squinting), strabismus is an abnormal misalignment of the eyes. The misalignment can be constant or intermittent, and the eyes can be misaligned in any direction.

• When the deviation between the eyes is constant in all gaze positions, the deviation is *comitant*. Most childhood strabismus is comitant.
• *Incomitant* strabismus, with a variable angle depending on the direction of gaze, is seen with palsy of cranial nerves III, IV, or VI, and in some strabismus syndromes such as Duane and Brown syndromes and Graves ophthalmopathy.
• The strabismus is identified by the relative direction of the eyes. *Esotropia* is an inward deviation or crossing; *exotropia* is an outward deviation; *hypertropia* and *hypotropia* are deviations up and down.

PATHOPHYSIOLOGY

• The pathophysiology of the most common forms of childhood strabismus is poorly understood. Infants with strabismus demonstrate subtle abnormalities in both motor function (asymmetrical smooth pursuit movements) and binocular sensory function (suppression, anomalous retinal correspondence). No neuroanatomic abnormalities have been consistently demonstrated in infants with idiopathic strabismus.
• Accommodative esotropia, a common strabismus syndrome, is caused by abnormalities in the reflexive convergence that is necessary for looking at near objects. If the ratio of accommodation (focusing for near) to convergence (rotating eyes inward to keep each eye on the target) is abnormally high, focusing on near targets leads to excessive convergence and esotropia.
• Less often, strabismus syndromes are caused by anatomic restriction to extraocular rotation (Graves disease, Brown syndrome), congenital or acquired paresis or palsy of extraocular muscles (III, IV, or VI palsy, Duane syndrome, Möbius syndrome) or abnormalities of vision (sensory strabismus).

PATHOLOGY

No specific pathologic abnormality of the motor nerves, extraocular muscles, or orbits is seen in most patients with idiopathic, comitant strabismus. Patients with paretic strabismus demonstrate atrophy of cranial nerves and extraocular muscles. Graves disease, myasthenia, and other neuromotor diseases causing strabismus have specific pathologic features in the extraocular muscles.

GENETICS

Genetic factors are clearly important in the development of many strabismus patterns, with about 30% of strabismus patients having affected family members. The inheritance appears to be multigenic. No specific genes have been associated with idiopathic childhood strabismus syndromes, but genetic causes have been identified for some rarer strabismus syndromes including congenital fibrosis syndromes (chromosome 12p) and Kearns-Sayre syndrome (mitochondrial deletion).

EPIDEMIOLOGY

• Strabismus of all types has an overall prevalence of 4% to 5%.
• Frequent coincident ophthalmic diagnoses are amblyopia (30–60%), nystagmus (8–10%), and refractive error (30–50%).
• Premature birth, cerebral palsy, seizure disorders, and developmental delays are frequently associated with strabismus, but most patients with idiopathic comitant strabismus are otherwise developmentally and neurologically normal.

COMPLICATIONS

• Amblyopia occurs in 30% to 60% of children with strabismus, and may require additional treatment. Amblyopia must be recognized and treated early in childhood, during the sensitive period of visual development, to restore normal vision.
• Loss of binocularity (ability to use both eyes together, for example depth perception) frequently occurs with strabismus in early childhood. Restoration of normal alignment is necessary for binocularity, and the best binocularity is associated with treatment of strabismus in early childhood (before 2 years of age). In older children and adults, diplopia (double vision) may occur.
• The disfigurement of strabismus, with secondary psychological and social effects, may be a significant problem for children and adults with strabismus.

Differential Diagnosis

• The most common reason for mistaken referral of infants for esotropia is "pseudoesotropia," caused by wide epicanthal folds giving the false appearance of esotropia. This can be easily recognized by the normal corneal light reflex (Hirschberg test) and the normal cover test.
• Sensory strabismus, due to reduced vision in one or both eyes, can be comitant or incomitant and can be caused by any ocular, optic nerve, or central cause of vision loss. Sensory deviations are most frequently exotropic, but may be in any direction.
• The differential diagnosis of abnormal eye movement in childhood includes palsy of cranial nerves III, IV, or VI, orbital fracture or

craniofacial anomaly, systemic or localized motor abnormalities like myasthenia gravis, orbital fibrosis syndrome, infantile botulism, and idiopathic orbital pseudotumor.
• Special strabismus syndromes include Duane syndrome (congenital aberrant innervation of cranial nerve III), Möbius syndrome (congenital absence of cranial nerve VI and VII), Brown syndrome (congenital or acquired monocular elevation defect due to abnormality of the trochlea-superior oblique tendon complex), and thyroid ophthalmopathy (Graves disease).

Data Gathering

HISTORY

• Age of onset of deviation
• Frequency, duration, and direction of deviation
• Subjective vision problems or complaints
• History of eye or head trauma, premature birth, seizure disorder, neurologic abnormality, or other motor problems
• Previous use of glasses, patching, or other therapy
• Family history of strabismus, amblyopia, refractive error, or childhood vision problems

Physical Examination

• Vision: patients capable of recognition are tested with charts (letters, pictures, E's), and younger patients are tested by the ability to fixate and hold visual fixation on targets (toys, lights) in each eye. It is very important to test each eye separately, to detect possible amblyopia and other causes of monocular vision loss. Patients capable of reading charts should have complete ophthalmic examination if they cannot recognize at least the 20/40-size target with each eye, or if there is a difference of two lines between eyes.
• Ocular alignment:

—Hirschberg test: With patient looking at a flashlight, observe the location of the reflection of the light on the corneal surface. Normally, the reflection should be centered in the pupil and symmetric. In strabismus, the reflection will be displaced laterally (esotropia) or medially (exotropia) in one eye.
—Bruchner test: With a direct ophthalmoscope using the largest light, and the patient looking directly at the light, the light is shone into the patient's eyes. Normally, the pupils should be orange or red and the pupils should symmetrically fill with light. Asymmetrical brightness or color between the two eyes or shadows in the pupil of either eye are abnormal, and may indicate strabismus or other eye problems.

—Cover test (alternate cover test): With the patient holding visual attention on a single target, the eyes are alternately occluded to force the patient to switch fixation between eyes. Normally, switching fixation should not cause the eyes to move. Movement of the eyes with alternate occlusion signifies strabismus, and merits complete evaluation.

• Ocular rotations: Comitant strabismus will demonstrate a consistent angle of deviation in all gaze directions. Incomitant strabismus, including cranial nerve palsies, thyroid ophthalmopathy, and Duane and Brown syndromes, will be greater in one direction and smaller or absent in others. Ductions (movements of each eye) may be restricted in certain directions with incomitant strabismus.
• Complete ophthalmic examination, including evaluation of vision, alignment, ocular anatomy, and cycloplegic refraction, is indicated whenever there is suggestion or suspicion of strabismus or abnormal vision based on history, screening tests, or examination.

 ## Laboratory Aids

TESTS

The diagnosis of strabismus is based on clinical examination, and no laboratory or radiologic tests are routinely necessary. Depending on the clinical situation, imaging studies of the orbits and brain may be helpful in evaluating cranial nerve palsies, suspected traumatic strabismus, and strabismus associated with neurologic disease. Serologic testing for antiacetylcholine receptor antibodies is a specific test for myasthenia gravis, but may be negative in some cases.

 ## Emergency Care

Acute-onset strabismus, especially if incomitant and associated with diplopia, can be a neurologic emergency and require urgent or emergent evaluation. The significance of acute incomitant strabismus is the possibility of acquired cranial nerve palsy, which may be caused by intracranial aneurysm or other lesions that might need immediate attention.

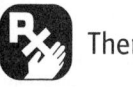 ## Therapy

• Prompt diagnosis and treatment are important for successful outcome from childhood strabismus. Depending on the diagnosis, treatment may include glasses, patching, orthoptic exercises, surgery, or a combination of these therapies.
• Glasses are useful, and may be curative, in certain forms of strabismus, especially *accommodative esotropia*. With accommodative esotropia, glasses reduce or eliminate esotropia by reducing the need to focus the eyes to overcome hyperopia.
• Occlusive therapeutic patching is used to treat amblyopia. In addition to the improved prognosis for long-term stability of surgical correction after amblyopia is treated, patching may sometimes improve alignment even without surgery. However, patching and other amblyopia treatments are usually only an adjunct to strabismus treatment.
• Surgery is frequently necessary to realign the eyes to treat strabismus. The ocular insertions of the extraocular muscles are shifted, either weakening or strengthening the muscle's effectiveness relative to the other muscles. In most patients, strabismus surgery can be performed in an ambulatory setting with minimal operative risk and postoperative morbidity. In large case series, approximately 20% of patients require more than one surgery for satisfactory alignment.

 ## Follow-Up

Recurrences of strabismus and amblyopia are common. Close monitoring of treatment, and frequent follow-up until visual maturity is achieved at 8 to 10 years of age is important due to the frequently unstable outcome of strabismus and amblyopia treatment. Most patients will benefit from reassessment every 6 to 12 months after treatment is complete, until age 10 years.

PITFALLS

• Strabismus is frequently recognized by parents and primary care practitioners, but amblyopia may be asymptomatic. Visual acuity testing with each eye separately, and long-term follow-up until patients reach the age of visual maturity (about 10 years) is important even after successful treatment.
• Patients rarely "grow out of" strabismus. Infants as young as 3 months can have careful eye movement and alignment examinations. Delayed diagnosis may worsen prognosis.
• Patients with intermittent strabismus may benefit from treatment, even if the deviation is not present constantly.
• Strabismus can be a sign of more significant ocular or neurologic abnormality. Retinoblastoma, retinal detachment, brain tumor, and other treatable conditions may initially present with ocular misalignment.

 ## Common Questions and Answers

Q: Does strabismus interfere with learning?
A: No. Patients with normal vision and childhood strabismus should not necessarily have difficulty learning. Learning problems should not be blamed solely on strabismus.

Q: Is "vision training therapy" an effective treatment for strabismus?
A: Eye exercises are rarely helpful in treating childhood strabismus. There is very little practical or scientific evidence that vision training therapy as commonly practiced has value in patients with comitant childhood strabismus.

Q: Does early surgical correction of strabismus improve the long-term outcome?
A: Correction of esotropia prior to 2 years of age has been demonstrated to improve the chance of developing normal binocularity. However, many patients do not develop binocularity even after early treatment. Many other factors influence the visual outcome in strabismus patients.

Q: Is correction of strabismus in older children and adults just cosmetic?
A: No. Older children and adults may have measurable visual improvement after treatment of strabismus, including expansion of visual fields and restoration of binocularity. In addition, the psychological and social effects of disfiguring strabismus may justify corrective surgery even if no visual improvement is expected.

Q: In patients with accommodative esotropia treated with glasses, will the glasses be necessary for the rest of the patient's life?
A: Many patients wearing glasses for accommodative esotropia are able to stop wearing glasses later in childhood (12–14 years) without recurrence of esotropia.

ICD-9-CM 378.9

BIBLIOGRAPHY

Engle EC. The genetics of strabismus: Duane, Moebius, and fibrosis syndromes. In: Traboulsi EI, ed. *Genetic diseases of the eye*. New York: Oxford University Press, 1998.

Mills MD. The eye in childhood. *Am Fam Physician* 1999;60:907–918.

Mills MD. Fundamental principles of strabismus surgery. In: Albert DM, ed. *Ophthalmic surgery: principles and techniques*. Malden, MA: Blackwell Science, 1999.

Robb RM. Strabismus in childhood. In: Albert DM, Jakobiec FA, eds. *Principles and practice of ophthalmology*, 2nd ed. Philadelphia: WB Saunders, 2000.

Von Noorden GK. *Binocular vision and ocular motility: theory and management of strabismus*, 5th ed. St. Louis: Mosby–Year Book, 1996.

Wright KW, ed. *Pediatric ophthalmology and strabismus*. St. Louis: Mosby–Year Book, 1995.

Author: Monte D. Mills

Strep Infection—Invasive Group A β-Hemolytic Streptococcus

 Database

DEFINITION

Infection associated with isolation of group A β-hemolytic streptococci (GABHS) from a normally sterile body site.

Syndromes

• Deep and systemic infections (e.g., bacteremia, meningitis, pneumonia, osteomyelitis, septic arthritis, surgical wound infection)
• Necrotizing fasciitis (NF)
• Streptococcal toxic shock syndrome (STSS)

Case Definition for STSS

• I. Isolation of GABHS

—A. From a normally sterile site (e.g., blood, CSF, tissue, peritoneal fluid)
—B. From a nonsterile site (e.g., throat, vagina, sputum)

• II. Clinical signs of severity

—A. Hypotension
—B. ≥2 of the following signs:
—Renal impairment
—Coagulopathy
—Hepatic involvement
—Adult respiratory distress syndrome
—A generalized erythematous macular rash that may desquamate
—Soft tissue necrosis, including NF or myositis, or gangrene

• Definite case: an illness fulfilling criteria IA and II (A and B)
• Probable case: an illness fulfilling criteria IB and II (A and B) and no other identifiable cause

CAUSES

Streptococcus pyogenes is the only species within this group of β-hemolytic streptococci. The M1 and M3 strains predominate in cases of severe GABHS infections.

PATHOPHYSIOLOGY

• The pathogenic mechanism has not been fully elucidated; however, an association with streptococcal pyrogenic exotoxin (SPE) has been suggested. These toxins, especially SPE A and C, as well as mitogens and superantigens stimulate large numbers of T cells to release a variety of cytokines.
• Portal of entry may be inapparent or unimpressive.
• Shock and multiorgan system failure may ensue.
• In NF, an area of cellulitis develops initially followed by bullous skin changes and the rapid progression of subcutaneous tissue necrosis involving fat and fascia. Skeletal muscle is rarely involved.

EPIDEMIOLOGY

• In children, the most common antecedent is varicella.
• Since the mid-1980s there has been a notable increase in the incidence, morbidity, and mortality.
• The CDC has estimated that the annual incidence in the U.S. is 4 to 5 cases per 100,000 persons, approximately 10,000 cases per year.
• Several reports have suggested a relationship between the use of nonsteroidal antiinflammatory drugs and invasive GABHS infection.
• Other high-risk groups include patients with diabetes mellitus, chronic cardiac or pulmonary disease, HIV infection or AIDS, and intravenous drug use.
• The rate of STSS and fatal cases of invasive GABHS appears to be lower in children as compared with adults.

COMPLICATIONS

From Deep and Systemic Infections

• Sepsis syndrome
• Hematologic seeding and development of focal infection
• Complications associated with specific site of involvement (e.g., meningitis—neurologic impairment, septic arthritis—joint destruction, etc.)

From NF

• Severe tissue necrosis usually requires extensive surgical débridement and often results in amputation of involved extremities.
• Compartment syndrome
• Functional disabilities
• Cosmetic sequelae

From STSS

• Multiorgan system failure from systemic hypotension and direct effects of inflammatory mediators:
• Adult respiratory distress syndrome
• Disseminated intravascular coagulopathy (DIC)
• Acute tubular necrosis resulting in renal failure
• Hepatic failure
• Cardiac insufficiency
• Cerebral ischemia and edema
• Metabolic derangements

PROGNOSIS

• Fulminant course with rapid deterioration is characteristic of invasive GABHS infections.
• Improved prognosis with early recognition and aggressive management.
• Case-fatality rate in pediatric series approximately 5% to 10%.

 Differential Diagnosis

INFECTION

• Bacterial sepsis
• Staphylococcal toxic shock syndrome
• Other soft tissue infections: cellulitis, erysipelas, clostridial or mixed anaerobic and aerobic fasciitis/gangrene

 Data Gathering

HISTORY

Historical features vary depending on the GABHS syndrome

• Consider GABHS infection in any child with varicella who has any of the following:

—Return of fever after defervescence
—A temperature of ≥39°C beyond the third day of illness
—A fever persisting beyond the fourth day of illness

• In children without varicella, presentation can be nonspecific with fever, chills, myalgias, malaise, pain, macular erythematous rash.
• Severe pain and hyperesthesia out of proportion to the clinical findings
• Portal of entry is unknown in 25% to 50% of cases.
• A preceding clinical pharyngitis is not common.

 Physical Examination

• Vital signs: elevated temperature, tachycardia early, hypotension is a later sign
• Toxic appearance is common but not the rule, especially early in the disease course.
• Skin exam varies. In many instances there are no cutaneous findings or, in cases of varicella, the lesions may not appear superinfected. Alternatively, there may be an initial erythematous cellulitic area that rapidly progresses to a violaceous color with bullous formation.
• A generalized macular erythematous rash is sometimes observed with STSS.
• Deep infections will have physical examination findings consistent with the specific focus (e.g., joint pain and limitation of mobility in septic arthritis, respiratory symptoms in GABHS pneumonia, etc.)

Strep Infection—Invasive Group A β-Hemolytic Streptococcus

 Laboratory Aids

TESTS

- CBC, electrolytes, BUN, CR, glucose, LFTs, DIC screen
- WBC not elevated in all pediatric case series
- Blood culture positive for *S. pyogenes* in >50%
- Culture of wound and tissue aspirates
- Throat culture positive in 50%

IMAGING

MRI to define the extent of involvement in NF

 Therapy

SUPPORTIVE CARE

- Volume resuscitation
- Replete electrolytes as indicated
- Blood products as indicated for anemia or thrombocytopenia
- Airway support for severe depression of level of consciousness or respiratory insufficiency

DRUGS

- Intravenous antibiotic therapy covering for both GABHS and *Staphylococcus aureus* should be instituted promptly. Oxacillin (150 mg/kg/day divided q6) or nafcillin (200 mg/kg/day divided q4–6h, max 12 g daily) *plus* clindamycin (25–40 mg/kg/day divided q6 or q8). In penicillin allergic patients, consider vancomycin (40 mg/kg/day divided q6) plus clindamycin.
- Following the identification of GABHS from blood, body fluid, or tissue specimens, the drugs of choice are high-dose penicillin G (200,000 to 400,000 U/kg/day in four to six divided doses) plus clindamycin.
- There have been no penicillin G–resistant isolates of GABHS reported. There are strains resistant to clindamycin, so this drug should not be used alone until it is shown to be sensitive.
- Large numbers of GABHS organisms can overcome the efficacy of penicillin. The synergistic use of clindamycin should be considered in cases of NF and STTS.
- Inotropes should be administered as indicated.
- There are a few case reports suggesting that the use of intravenous immunoglobulin may be beneficial in patients with STSS. Various regimens have been used: 150 to 400 mg/kg per day for 5 days; 1 to 2 g/kg as single dose
At this time, the optimal regimen is unknown

SURGICAL TREATMENT IN NF

- Consider surgical consult early in management of NF

- Fasciotomy to relieve compartment syndrome
- Extensive débridement of necrotic tissue is often indicated.

PREVENTION

Routine immunization against varicella

ISOLATION OF HOSPITALIZED PATIENTS

In addition to standard precautions, droplet precautions are recommended for children with pneumonia, and contact precautions should be used for children with extensive or draining cutaneous infections for at least 24 hours after the start of antimicrobial therapy.

PITFALLS

- Not considering the diagnosis until hemodynamic instability is apparent
- Do not exclude diagnosis even in the absence of rash, cellulitis, or superinfected varicella lesions. Rash is only one of six clinical signs of severity in the criteria for STSS.
- Recognize that the involvement of subcutaneous structures in NF may be much more extensive than what might be suggested on physical examination.
- Failing to search for a localized infection as a source of toxin in STTS

 Common Questions and Answers

Q: For whom should the diagnosis of invasive GABHS be entertained?
A: Consider GABHS in any child with varicella who experiences recrudescence of fever, fever ≥39°C beyond the third day of illness, or any fever beyond the fourth day of illness. A high index of suspicion should be maintained in patients with septicemia, and in febrile patients with pain and hyperesthesia out of proportion to the clinical findings.

Q: Should the use of nonsteroidal antiinflammatory drugs (NSAIDs) be restricted in patients with varicella?
A: There have been several reports suggesting an association between the use of NSAIDs and the development of NF or STTS, however, there has been no study to establish a causal relationship. It has been demonstrated that NSAIDs inhibit immune-mediated defense mechanisms, enhance the production of cytokines, and suppress the pain and fever that might encourage a patient with invasive GABHS infection to seek medical attention sooner. No formal recommendations for restricting the use of NSAIDs are being made at this time.

Q: Should close contacts of patients with invasive GABHS infections receive chemoprophylaxis?
A: No formal recommendations for chemoprophylaxis for household contacts are being made at this time. There are no data available to demonstrate the magnitude of the increased risk of developing disease or the effectiveness of chemoprophylaxis.

ICD-9-CM

Streptococcal infection 034.0
Necrotising fasciitis 728.86

BIBLIOGRAPHY

American Academy of Pediatrics. Group A streptococcal infections. In: *Red book: report of the Committee on Infectious Diseases*, 25th ed. Washington, DC: American Academy of Pediatrics, 2000.

American Academy of Pediatrics, Committee on Infectious Diseases. Severe invasive group A streptococcal infections: a subject review. *Pediatrics* 1998;101:136–140.

Barry W, Hudgins L, et al. Intravenous immunoglobulin therapy for toxic shock syndrome. *JAMA* 1992;267:3315–3316.

Doctor A, Harper MB, Fleisher GR. Group A β-hemolytic streptococcal bacteremia: historical overview, changing incidence, and recent association with varicella. *Pediatrics* 1995;96:428–433.

Kaul R, McGeer A, Norrby-Teglund A, et al. Intravenous immunoglobulin therapy for streptococcal toxic shock syndrome—a comparative observational study. The Canadian Streptococcal Study Group. *Clin Infect Dis* 1999;28(4):800–807.

Lamothe F, D'Amico P, et al. Clinical usefulness of intravenous human immunoglobulins in invasive Group A streptococcal infections: case report and review. *Clin Infect Dis* 1995;21:1469–1470.

Laupland KB, Davies HD, Low DE, et al. Invasive group A streptococcal disease in children and association with varicella-zoster virus infection. *Pediatrics* 2000;105(5):E60.

Shulman ST, Ranz RR. Streptococcus pyogenes (Group A streptococcus). In: Long, SS, ed. *Principles and practice of pediatric infectious diseases*. New York: Churchill Livingstone, 1997.

Stevens DL. Could nonsteroidal antiinflammatory drugs (NSAIDs) enhance the progression of bacterial infections to toxic shock syndrome? *Clin Infect Dis* 1995;21:977–980.

The Working Group on Severe Streptococcal Infections. Defining the group A streptococcal toxic shock syndrome. *JAMA* 1993;269:390–391.

Wheeler MC, Row MH, et al. Outbreak of group A streptococcus septicemia in children. *JAMA* 1991;266:533–537.

Wilson GJ, Talkington DF, et al. Group A streptococcal necrotizing fasciitis following varicella in children: case reports and review. *Clin Infect Dis* 1995;20:1333–1338.

Author: Jill C. Posner

Stroke

Database

DEFINITION

Stroke is a neurologic deficit progressing over minutes to hours due to insufficient perfusion of the brain or spinal cord.

PATHOPHYSIOLOGY

Abnormalities of the blood, vasculature, or the heart (dysrhythmia or anatomic) lead to embolism or intravascular thrombosis.

PATHOLOGY

Edema, neuronal swelling, cellular infiltrate, and cavitation starting from 8 hours until months after an ischemic brain injury

GENETICS

Various hereditary and metabolic disorders, especially coagulation disorders, hereditary AVM, and hyperhomocystinemia.

EPIDEMIOLOGY

Overall incidence is approximately 2.5 per 100,000, but certain groups are at higher risk (heart disease, sickle cell disease, hereditary thrombophilias).

COMPLICATIONS

- Seizures
- Respiratory insufficiency
- Intracranial hypertension
- Motor, visual, and cognitive deficits
- Autonomic disturbances
- Infection susceptibility

Differential Diagnosis

- Several disorders may mimic the presentation of stroke:

—Migraine
—Demyelinating disease
—Focal encephalitis
—Postepileptic paralysis (Todd paresis)
—Conversion disorder
—Rarely intracranial neoplasm, abscess, subdural empyema, or mitochondrial disease may present as stroke.

- Underlying causes of stroke include hematologic, circulatory, and cardiac disorders:

—*Hematologic:* factor V deficiency, lupus anticoagulant, anticardiolipin syndrome, sickle cell, hyperhomocystinemia, dyslipidemia, proteins S or C, antithrombin III deficiency, asparaginase treatment, hyperviscosity syndromes (including leukemia), thrombocythemia, extreme dehydration, hemorrhagic stroke.
—*Vascular:* carotid or vertebral dissection, intracranial AVM, carotid trauma, moyamoya, cavernous angioma ("occult cerebrovascular malformations"), vasculitis (especially due to bacterial meningitis); rarely, aneurysm, Takayasu arteritis, chronic meningitides (tuberculosis, Lyme, or sarcoidosis)
—*Cardiac:* especially rheumatic heart disease, cyanotic congenital heart disease, or heart failure due to acquired or cardiomyopathy, or perioperatively; weak association with mitral prolapse, atrial septal defects; rarely, atrial myxoma, aortic dilatation (Marfan), pulmonary AVM

Data Gathering

HISTORY

- Occurrence of stroke in specific settings may point to the diagnosis; previous migraines may point to complicated migraine (rare); details of the timing and circumstances of symptom onset may be critical in establishing diagnosis.
- Recent trauma, infection, excessive bleeding or spontaneous clotting, or history of heart disease should be established.
- Family history of premature thrombosis, hemoglobinopathy, or vascular malformations (e.g., cavernous hemangioma or hereditary hemorrhagic telangiectasia).
- Perinatal stroke may be related to a pre-, peri-, or postpartum cerebrovascular event and frequently presents with neonatal seizures.
- Complications of labor or fetal exposure to vasoactive compounds may sometimes be associated.

Physical Examination

- Vital signs, color, and respiratory pattern may disclose existing or impending respiratory failure due to loss of protective airway reflexes.
- General examination should include peripheral pulses and perfusion; palpation and auscultation of the precordium and cervical area may reveal evidence of dysrhythmia or anatomic lesions.
- Neurologic findings important to note include level of alertness, speech fluency and comprehension, confrontation visual fields, funduscopy (especially for papilledema), eye movements, facial symmetry, pattern of most severely affected limbs, and extensor response of great toe to plantar stimulation (Babinski sign).
- In the absence of sensory complaints, detailed sensory exam is often fruitless.

Laboratory Aids

TESTS

Laboratory Tests

- Blood chemistry, particularly glucose, should be tested; mild hyperglycemia may reflect stress response; marked elevation (e.g., in diabetics) should be treated, since hyperglycemia may aggravate ischemic brain injury.
- Complete blood count and PT/PTT may prompt important therapeutic decisions.

IMAGING

- Individuals with stable vital signs and suspected stroke should undergo a brain imaging study promptly. Noncontrasted images are important to look for possible hemorrhage and may be followed by contrasted images for possible focal encephalitis, or to identify underlying vascular lesions.
- Many diagnostic questions can be resolved equally well by CT or MRI, though CT may be preferable in suspected subarachnoid hemorrhage; MRI is much more sensitive in the first 24 hours after symptom onset, and may identify venous or sinus thrombosis, or smaller bilateral lesions pointing to systemic embolization.

OTHER TESTS

More extensive testing in undiagnosed cases may include:

- Tests for specific coagulopathies (see Differential Diagnosis, above)
- Varicella serology (may be a common cause of stroke in children)
- Amino acid screening (for homocysteine)
- Hemoglobin electrophoresis (sickle hemoglobin)
- Lipid profile (hypercholesterolemia)
- Echocardiography (ASD, luminal lesion)
- Carotid Doppler (stenosis/dissection)
- Specialized neuroradiologic studies (MR angiogram, standard angiography)

 Emergency Care

- Airway compromise due to impaired protective reflexes
- Stroke may present as new onset seizures—follow protocol for emergent treatment of seizures
- Urgent neurosurgical evaluation indicated in cases of intracranial hemorrhage or posterior fossa ischemic stroke (see below)
- Empiric antibiotics indicated in the setting of stroke and fever (abscess, septic emboli, empyema)

 Therapy

- *Hospitalization:* Patients with radiologically documented or clinically suspected stroke who have stable airway, breathing, and circulation are most often hospitalized for observation and supportive therapy. Those with a diminished or fluctuating level of alertness or with radiographically extensive area(s) of infarction are often monitored in an intensive care unit for changes in respiratory status or signs of increased intracranial pressure.
- Strokes involving the posterior fossa or cerebellum are of particular concern because of the risk of tentorial herniation; a neurosurgical consult should be obtained for these cases and for those with intracranial hemorrhage above or below the tentorium.
- *Consultation* with neurology, neurosurgery, cardiology, hematology, or other pediatric subspecialists is often helpful.
- *Drugs:* In most cases, there is no contraindication to pharmacotherapy appropriate to any identified underlying condition; the decision to use antiplatelet therapy or anticoagulation is complex and depends on risk of hemorrhage or other potential side effects.
- *Rehabilitation and physical therapy* may improve outcome and should be instituted as soon as the patient's condition permits.
- *Investigational therapies* include hypervolemic hemodilution, thrombolytic agents, calcium channel antagonists, and antagonists of glutamate receptors.

 Follow-Up

- The usual course in stroke of any cause is for gradual improvement after the acute onset of symptoms. Significant recovery of neurologic function may continue as long as months after the ictus, especially in infants and toddlers.
- Involvement of child developmentalists and/or ophthalmologists in follow-up depends on the etiology and residual deficits of the stroke.
- *Remote sequelae* that may not be evident for months or years after stroke include epilepsy, hydrocephalus, learning difficulties, short attention span, posture disturbances (especially cerebral palsy), sphincter disturbances, pressure sores, and susceptibility to infection if airway protective reflexes are impaired.

PITFALLS

- AVMs may not be seen on angiography immediately after a primary intracerebral hemorrhage. Some clinicians repeat angiography several weeks or months later.
- CT may be normal in the first 24 hours after nonhemorrhagic stroke. A follow-up study may be necessary.
- Diagnosis of transient ischemic attack (TIA) may depend on history; a vigorous diagnostic evaluation should be pursued.

 Common Questions and Answers

Q: Will my child have another stroke?
A: Anecdotal evidence suggests that children with no identifiable underlying basis for stroke do not have recurrence. Otherwise, the chance of recurrence depends on remediation of the underlying cause.

Q: Aren't there any medicines for acute stroke?
A: Tissue plasminogen activator (TPA) appears to be useful in some cases of adult nonhemorrhagic stroke, but its usefulness in childhood stroke has not been studied.

ICD-9-CM 436

BIBLIOGRAPHY

Gunther G, Junker R, Strater R, et al. Symptomatic ischemic stroke in full-term neonates: role of acquired and genetic prothrombotic risk factors. *Stroke* 2000;31:2437–2441.

Isaels SJ, Seshia SS. Childhood stroke associated with protein C or S deficiency. *J Pediatr* 1987;3:562–564.

Kittner SJ, Adams RJ. Stroke in children and young adults. *Curr Opin Neurol* 1996;9(1):53–56.

Natowicz M, Kelley RI. Mendelian etiologies of stroke. *Ann Neurol* 1987;22:175–192.

Rivkin MJ, Volpe JJ. Strokes in children. *Pediatr Rev* 1996;17(8):265–278.

Yamamoto LG, Yim GK, Bart RD Jr. Emergency department presentations of cerebrovascular disease in children. *Am J Emerg Med* 1999;17:163–171.

Author: Peter M. Bingham

Stuttering

 Database

DEFINITION

Stuttering is a common, involuntary speech dysfluency, which results in disruption of speech flow. Children who stutter experience blocks in their speech from syllable repetitions, truncated sentences or words, or alteration of sentence structure.
Stuttering typically begins between the ages of 2 and 5 years, with the majority of individuals experiencing onset by the age of 10 years. The most common form of stuttering is developmental stuttering (DS), which is characterized by gradual onset in childhood. Persistent developmental stuttering (PDS) is DS that does not resolve. While many toddlers and preschoolers experience occasional disrupted fluency, which is normal, it is important not to overlook true stuttering. The diagnosis of stuttering needs to be made in a timely matter so that necessary interventions can be made.

PATHOPHYSIOLOGY

- The cause of stuttering is unknown.
- Neuroimaging research data indicate a hyperdopaminergic origin of stuttering. These findings are corroborated with effective clinical experience using dopamine receptor antagonists (see Treatment, below).
- The type of word seems to play a role in stuttering. For example, children younger than 9 years old tend to stutter more often on function words, such as pronouns, prepositions, and articles. In contrast, older children who stutter have difficulty with content words, such as nouns, main verbs, adverbs, and adjectives.
- Environmental variables do not cause stuttering, but communicative stress has been shown to affect fluency. People who stutter experience fewer symptoms in the low-stress situation of speaking with children, and experience worse dysfluency in high-stress settings, such as when speaking to a large group of people.

GENETICS

- Twin studies and familial aggregation patterns strongly indicate a relationship between stuttering and genetics. At this time no specific "stuttering gene" has been identified and there is no genetic test for stuttering available.
- Individuals who recover from stuttering do not appear to have a different genetically independent disorder than those who continue to stutter as adults.

EPIDEMIOLOGY

- Overall prevalence in children is 5%.
- 80% have resolution of their stuttering, while 20% continue to stutter as adults.
- Males are more frequently and more severely affected than females.
- Male/female ratio of early childhood stuttering is 2:1.
- In adults who persistently stutter, the male/female ratio is 4–5:1.

COMPLICATIONS

- Underestimation of the intellectual capacity of the child who stutters is common since they may appear slow in communication. This can undermine the academic potential and eventual achievement of the child that stutters.
- The emotional complications of stuttering include tension, anxiety, social isolation, and difficulty with forming relationships.

PROGNOSIS

- 75% to 80% of children who stutter have resolution.
- Stuttering does not disappear overnight. In the individuals for whom stuttering resolves, it is important to note that the path is one of gradually decreasing severity and frequency.
- The longer stuttering exists, the more difficult it is to change and the more likely that secondary complications develop.

 Differential Diagnosis

OTHER SPEECH PROBLEMS

- Disrupted fluency—seen between the ages of 2 to 5 years, with spontaneous remission
- Cluttering—disturbance in the rhythm, stress, intonation, and rate of speech
- Spasmodic dysphonia—spastic movements of muscles of the larynx causing speech disruption

NEUROLOGIC

- Degenerative disorder
- Focal brain lesions
- Cerebral blood flow alterations
- Segmental or focal action dystonia
- Gilles de la Tourette syndrome—defined by multiple tics, shouting, and grunting

 Data Gathering

HISTORY

- At what age did the stuttering start?
- Does the child seem to get frustrated or upset with the stuttering?
- Is the stuttering exacerbated with competition for attention?
- Are there any neurologic symptoms present? Any tics?
- Any history of CNS trauma?
- Birth history?
- Are there any relatives who stutter?
- Medication history?

Physical Examination

- Observe the child for any evidence of tics or movement disorder.
- Assess the child's development; patients who stutter should have otherwise normal development.
- Observe the child's speech, bearing in mind that in the office setting the speech patterns may or may not reflect the patient's baseline. Factors to look for:

—Pattern of speech—fast vs. slow, pressured, monotone
—Types of words that cause stuttering and word avoidance
—Evidence of frustration with stuttering

- Perform a complete neurologic examination

Laboratory Aids

- There are no known laboratory tests for stuttering.
- Neuroimaging should be considered if the neurologic examination is not normal and/or if the stuttering is associated with neurologic symptoms.

Therapy

The old adage, "Ignore it and it will go away," does not apply to stuttering. Once speech therapy is in place, the primary care provider can help the family to reduce focus on the issue in hopes of reducing tension and frustration.

SPEECH AND LANGUAGE PATHOLOGIST REFERRAL

- May improve the speech of children who stutter
- The threshold for referral to a speech-language pathologist should be low.
- Speech-language pathologists may employ breath-control and rhythm-of-speech exercises.

PHARMACOLOGIC THERAPY

- Pharmacologic therapies are emerging.
- Risperidone, a serotonin-dopamine antagonist, decreases stuttering severity when compared to placebo; it does not have impact on the amount of time spent stuttering or the social alienation that accompanies stuttering.
- Haloperidol, a dopamine antagonist, has been shown to be effective in controlling stuttering symptoms.
- Three case reports with olanzapine, a serotonin-dopamine antagonist, indicate that it may be a future treatment option.

Follow-Up

The speech-language pathologist will determine the follow-up, which will depend on the patient's age and degree of dysfluency.

PITFALLS

- Delayed diagnosis
- Delayed referrals to specialists
- Inappropriate response to child's stuttering by parents

Common Questions and Answers

Q: If my child stutters, does that mean (s)he will have decreased language abilities?
A: No. This is a common misconception. Children at all ages who stutter have language abilities near or above normative age expected levels.

Q: How will I know if speech therapy will cure my child's stuttering?
A: There is good evidence that speech-language pathologists can improve the speech of children who stutter. However, it is impossible to predict which children will go on to stutter as adults.

Q: Is there a particular length of speech therapy that is recommended?
A: No. The duration of therapy varies with each individual.

ICD-9-CM 307.0

BIBLIOGRAPHY

Au-Yeung J. Phonological words and stuttering on function words. *J Speech Lang Hear Res* 1998;41(5):1019–1030.

Conture EG. Treatment efficacy: stuttering. *J Speech Hear Res* 1996;39(5):S18–S26.

Costa D. Stuttering: an update for physicians. *Can Med Assoc J* 2000;162(13):1849–1855.

Dalton R. Habit disorders. In: *Nelson textbook of pediatrics*, 16th ed. Philadelphia: WB Saunders, 2000.

Lavid N. Management of child and adolescent stuttering with olanzapine: three case reports. *Ann Clin Psychiatry* 1999;11(4):233–236.

Maguire GA. Stuttering: neuropsychiatric features measured by content analysis of speech and the effect of risperidone on stuttering severity. *Compr Psychiatry* 1999;40(4)308–314.

Watkins RV. Early childhood stuttering III: initial status of expressive language abilities. *J Speech Lang Hear Res* 1999;42(5): 1125–1135.

Yairi E. Early childhood stuttering I: persistency and recovery rates. *J Speech Lang Hear Res* 1999;42(5):1097–1112.

Yairi E. Genetics of stuttering: a critical review. *J Speech Hear Res* 1996;39(4): 771–784.

Author: Lisa Chamberlain

Subdural Hematoma

 ## Database

DEFINITION

A subdural hematoma (SDH) is a collection of blood between outer pial and inner dural meningeal layers. The bleeding is usually venous in origin, although either cortical arteries or bridging veins may be torn.

PATHOPHYSIOLOGY

- SDHs may be acute or chronic. Arterial SDHs present quickly, whereas venous SDHs may accumulate slowly, not detected for weeks or months. Acute SDHs contain blood, whereas chronic SDHs contain proteinaceous exudate and blood-breakdown products. Rebleeding may be the underlying cause of many chronic SDHs.
- Significant force is usually required for SDH unless there are predisposing circumstances; SDH is only rarely due to trivial or minor trauma. However, SDH can occur with relatively minor trauma in individuals with bleeding disorders, children on chronic dialysis, and those with enlarged extracerebral spaces (cortical atrophy).
- Some metabolic disorders, such as glutaric aciduria type I, can be associated with both acute and chronic SDHs.
- SDHs in nonaccidental trauma may be due to the striking of the infant's head against a surface (like a mattress). The sudden deceleration associated with the impact may tear bridging veins traveling in the subdural space. The term *shaking-impact syndrome* may be more accurate than *shaken-baby syndrome*.
- SDHs can also occur after ventricular shunting.

GENETICS

There is no clear genetic predisposition, except when hereditary coagulopathy or metabolic disease is implicated.

EPIDEMIOLOGY

- SDHs occur in all age groups. Neonatal SDHs occur with spontaneous deliveries, but may be more frequent following deliveries with forceps or vacuum extraction. SDHs related to birth usually resolve.
- SDHs in infants and young children are frequently the result of nonaccidental trauma. Risk factors for nonaccidental trauma include disability or prematurity of the child, unstable family situations, parents of young age, and low socioeconomic status. One study found that fathers were the most frequent perpetrators, followed by boyfriends, female baby-sitters, and mothers, in descending order of frequency.
- SDHs in older children are often the result of motor vehicle accidents, and may be associated with other intracranial injuries, such as diffuse axonal injury.

COMPLICATIONS

- Traumatic SDHs are often associated with cerebral contusions. Other associated injuries include skull fractures, diffuse axonal injury, and penetrating injuries.
- SDHs may result in mass effect, focal neurologic signs, and coma.
- Increased intracranial pressure (ICP) and seizures are other serious complications.

PROGNOSIS

In general, long-term outcome is related to the condition of the child at time of presentation. Prolonged ICP or significant cerebral edema before treatment is worrisome.

 ## Differential Diagnosis

- SDHs are almost always traumatic, but separating accidental from nonaccidental trauma may be difficult. Falls in infants may cause linear skull fractures, rarely SDHs.
- Macrocephaly or other signs/symptoms since birth may help to date the origin of the SDH to the perinatal or neonatal period.
- Epidural hematomas, subarachnoid hemorrhages, and acute SDHs cannot be distinguished clinically. The lucid interval sometimes seen with epidural hematomas in adults is not a reliable sign. A head CT should differentiate.

Approach to the Patient

A careful history and detailed physical exam are essential in order to explore possible causes of the SDH, assess the child's neurologic status, and look for evidence of other injuries. Prompt neuroimaging is critical.

 ## Data Gathering

HISTORY

- Newborn: SDHs due to birth trauma may present with lethargy, pallor, poor feeding, apnea, and seizures.
- Infants and young children: SDHs may also present with a nonspecific history of lethargy, irritability, vomiting, poor feeding, apnea, and seizures.
- Older children present with a history of trauma and alteration of consciousness.
- Chronic SDHs present with nonspecific signs, such as vomiting, irritability, failure to thrive, anemia, and seizures.

 ## Physical Examination

- Newborns may present with decreased responsiveness, a bulging fontanelle, hypotonia, or hypertonia. Retinal hemorrhages are not specific at this age, because they are seen in up to 40% of newborns following a vaginal delivery.
- Infants and young children may also present with nonspecific physical signs, but focal neurologic signs may be present. Retinal hemorrhages are most often associated with nonaccidental trauma, but they have been reported after accidental trauma leading to SDH. Bilateral retinal hemorrhages with retinal folds or detachments are particularly associated with nonaccidental trauma.
- Other signs of child abuse include burns, lacerations, and bruises in various stages of healing, and belt marks, choke marks, and multiple fractures of different ages.
- Older children present with signs of external head trauma, decreased responsiveness, and focal neurologic signs.

 ## Laboratory Aids

TESTS

Imaging

- CT scan is the imaging study of choice in acute head trauma with neurologic signs. SDH appears as an extraaxial area of increased density, crescentic in shape, and often associated with cerebral contusion or mass effect. CT also may show evidence of cerebral edema, with loss of gray matter/white matter differentiation and small ventricles.
- Subacute SDHs may be difficult to distinguish from adjacent gray matter on CT scan; loss of gray/white matter differentiation is helpful. Chronic SDHs appear as areas of low density on CT scan, often bilateral.
- MRI is helpful to clarify subacute and chronic SDHs and to identify small SDHs missed by CT.
- Ultrasound is less helpful since it may be difficult to distinguish the subdural space from the subarachnoid space.
- If child abuse is suspected, a skeletal survey or bone scan is useful to look for fractures of different ages.
- Incidental SDH is frequently found on neuroimaging studies in newborns; frequently no intervention is required other than close follow-up.

Emergency Care

Children with SDHs may be critically ill on presentation. The aggressiveness of acute therapy depends on the child's clinical condition. Neuroimaging studies and, if necessary, prompt neurosurgical consultation should not be delayed.

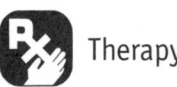 ## Therapy

- The treatment of choice for large, acute SDHs is surgical evacuation. Smaller SDHs may be managed conservatively, with careful monitoring for signs of neurologic deterioration.
- While awaiting surgery, attention to airway, breathing, and circulation (ABCs) is critical. Tracheal intubation should be performed if the child's Glasgow Coma Scale score is less than 8 or if airway protective reflexes are impaired.
- Isotonic fluids should be given, because hypotonic fluids may worsen cerebral edema.
- Measures to control ICP include elevating the head of the bed 30% to promote venous drainage, hyperventilation to a Pco_2 of 25 to 30 torr, and osmotic therapy with mannitol or furosemide. The efficacy of these measures in improving long-term outcome following large SDHs has not been established.
- Seizures should be treated promptly. Phenytoin is the drug of choice, with phenobarbital as a second option. Prophylactic phenytoin given for a few weeks is effective in reducing early posttraumatic seizures but does not affect long-term risk of epilepsy.
- Treatment of chronic SDHs is more controversial. If there are no signs of ICP, conservative treatment is reasonable, and most collections will resolve. Subdural taps are indicated if ICP rises. If taps are not successful, a subdural-peritoneal shunt may be placed.
- Treatment of SDHs that develop after ventricular shunting is particularly challenging.

 ## Follow-Up

- Neurologic sequelae of SDHs are more severe than epidural hematomas because of associated cerebral contusions.
- In general, long-term outcome is related to the condition of the child at the time of surgical evacuation of the hematoma. Prolonged ICP or significant cerebral edema before surgery indicates a poor prognosis.
- Children generally have a better outcome from head injury than do adults, but children younger than 7 years old often do worse than older children, especially if the SDH is the result of nonaccidental trauma.
- Long-term problems include headache, seizures, hydrocephalus, vertigo, difficulty concentrating, poor school performance, fixed neurologic deficits, and neurobehavioral problems.
- Epilepsy eventually develops in approximately 10% to 15% of patients after severe head injury. This risk generally does not warrant the use of long-term prophylactic anticonvulsants.
- Children with neurologic sequelae from head injury may benefit from admission to a rehabilitation hospital.
- Social work services should be consulted in cases of known or suspected child abuse.

PREVENTION

- Parents should be counseled about appropriate methods to channel frustration and anger with infants and children. Shaking an infant is never appropriate.
- Bicycle helmets, car seats, and seat belts are all valuable in preventing head injuries in children.

PITFALLS

- Be suspicious if the stated history does not fit with the pattern or severity of the injury. Physicians and other health care professionals with experience in child abuse should be consulted early if abuse is suspected.
- Chronic SDHs must be differentiated from benign external hydrocephalus, a self-limited condition characterized by increasing head size and low-density extraaxial fluid collections. MRI can differentiate benign external hydrocephalus.

 ## Common Questions and Answers

Q: When did the bleed occur?
A: With chronic SDHs, the time and type of injury may be difficult to establish, since no trauma may be reported and the trauma may have occurred weeks or months before. Neuroimaging can give some indication of the injury's timing.

Q: What limitations should be imposed after an acute SDH?
A: Because SDH may recur with minor trauma, it is prudent to avoid any activities that have significant risk of fall or a blow to the head.

Q: Why are anticonvulsants not used to prevent seizures following SDHs?
A: Seizure medications may be given for a few weeks to present early seizures following a SDH. After a few weeks, the risks and side effects of the medications outweigh the risk of developing seizures. If seizures begin at a time remote to the injury, then seizure medications can be restarted.

Q: My baby twisted out of my arms, fell head-first onto a tile floor, and suffered a head injury. Will I be reported for child abuse?
A: Not if the injuries fit with the stated history. In this case, the most likely injury would be a linear skull fracture. If more serious intracranial injuries do occur, they will probably not be associated with retinal hemorrhages or other injuries, such as older fractures in multiple stages of healing.

ICD-9-CM 852.2

BIBLIOGRAPHY

Duhaime AC, Christian CW, Rorke LB, et al. Nonaccidental head injury in infants—the "shaken-baby syndrome." *N Engl J Med* 1998;338:1822–1829.

Goldstein B, Powers KS. Head trauma in children. *Pediatr Rev* 1994;15:213–219.

Hartley LM, Khwaja OS, Verity CM. Glutaric aciduria type I and nonaccidental head injury. *Pediatrics* 2001;107:174–175.

Haviland J, Russell RI. Outcome after severe non-accidental head injury. *Arch Dis Child* 1997;77:504–507.

Perrin RG, Rutka JT, Drake JM, et al. Management and outcomes of posterior fossa subdural hematomas in neonates. *Neurosurgery* 1997;40:1190–1199.

Swift DM, McBride L. Chronic subdural hematoma in children. *Neurosurg Clin North Am* 2000;11:439–446.

Author: Dennis J. Dlugos

Sudden Infant Death Syndrome

 Database

DEFINITION

Sudden infant death syndrome (SIDS) is sudden and unexpected death of an infant (<1 year old) that remains unexplained after a complete postmortem investigation, including autopsy, death scene evaluation, and review of the case history. Associated problems:

- Acute life-threatening event (ALTE)
- Poverty
- Low birth weight; small for gestational age (SGA)
- Prematurity
- Maternal smoking
- Maternal substance abuse
- Soft bedding, covered airway, overheating

PATHOPHYSIOLOGY

- Unknown
- There are multiple theories, including central apnea associated with brain abnormalities, upper airway obstruction, and cardiac arrhythmias; metabolic diseases such as glycogen storage disease and medium-chain acyl-CoA dehydrogenase deficiency; and environmental factors such as hyperthermia, unsafe bedding, and prone sleeping position. Each attempts to explain SIDS, although none can adequately explain all SIDS deaths.
- "Negative" autopsy
- May see punctate petechial hemorrhages

EPIDEMIOLOGY

- Five thousand deaths per year in the United States
- 1.4 cases per 1,000 live births
- Ninety percent of cases occur before 6 months of age.
- Peak incidence: age 2 to 4 months
- Incidence of SIDS has decreased by >40% with the decrease in prone sleeping since the early 1990s.
- African Americans infants have SIDS rates more than 2 times the national average.

 Differential Diagnosis

- Infection

—Sepsis (bacterial, viral)
—Pneumonia
—Bronchiolitis
—Myocarditis

- Environmental

—Accidental asphyxiation
—Hyperthermia
—Hypothermia
—Toxins
—Poisonings

- Trauma

—Child abuse, including nonaccidental suffocation
—Drowning

- Metabolic

—Medium-chain acyl-CoA dehydrogenase (MCAD) deficiency
—Long-chain acyl-CoA dehydrogenase deficiency
—Pyruvate carboxylase deficiency
—Phosphoenolpyruvate carboxykinase deficiency
—Defects in glycogenolysis
—Defects in pyruvate oxidation
—Defects in oxidative phosphorylation
—Biotinidase deficiency
—3-hydroxy-3-methylglutaric aciduria
—Urea cycle defects
—Lactic acidemias
—Aminoacidopathies
—Glycogen storage disease

- Congenital

—Congenital heart disease

- Miscellaneous

—Adrenal insufficiency
—Arrhythmias

 Data Gathering

HISTORY

- Previously healthy infant, with or without recent upper respiratory tract infection
- Found dead after a nap or in the morning
- No struggle or crying heard

Special Questions

- Have there been previous infant or child deaths in the family? It is unusual to have more than one SIDS death in a family. When multiple SIDS deaths occur in a family, the possibility of sequential homicide needs to be considered.
- When was the last time the baby was seen alive?
- Where was the baby found?
- In what position was the baby found?
- What was the child wearing?
- Were there blankets, stuffed toys, or bumpers at the baby's head?
- Were there any recent illnesses?
- What is the prenatal history?
- Is there a history of previous maternal miscarriages?
- What is the date of the last immunizations?
- Have there been prior medical problems?
- Is there a history of apnea?

 Physical Examination

- Postmortem lividity
- Pink, frothy discharge at nose and mouth
- Look for signs of injury.
- Check for dysmorphic features.

Laboratory Aids

A full autopsy must be done on all infants who die suddenly and unexpectedly.

IMAGING

A postmortem skeletal survey is indicated if there is suspicion of abuse.

 ## Therapy

Resuscitation is almost always initiated before receiving the baby at the hospital. If rigor mortis or lividity is present, resuscitation efforts should not be initiated.

 ## Follow-Up

- The medical examiner or coroner's office should be notified of all SIDS deaths. Remember, it's not officially SIDS until the autopsy has been completed.
- Provide support to the family.
- Refer to a SIDS center.

PITFALLS

- Not completing full postmortem examination, including autopsy, death scene review, and careful review of case and family history

PREVENTION

- Avoid a prone sleeping position for young, healthy infants.
- Provide a safe sleeping environment. Avoid soft materials in the infant's sleeping environment.
- Avoid overheating.
- Use apnea monitors for infants with ALTE. These monitors, although widely used, have not been shown to decrease mortality related to SIDS.

 ## Common Questions and Answers

Q: Do all infants who die suddenly and unexpectedly require an autopsy?
A: Yes. It is estimated that autopsy reveals a cause of death in approximately 15% of SIDS deaths. The diagnosis of SIDS cannot be made without an autopsy!

Q: Does SIDS run in families?
A: Recurrence rates in families in which a sibling has died of SIDS vary greatly among studies, but large, controlled studies indicate no increased risk of SIDS in subsequent siblings. In families with recurrent SIDS death, especially after the third infant death, the possibility of serial homicide needs to be investigated.

Q: How can you tell the difference between SIDS and intentional suffocation?
A: Because the physical findings of an autopsy cannot distinguish between SIDS and intentional suffocation, other factors related to the death must be considered when attempting to distinguish the two. In comparing the features of suffocated children with the clinical features associated with SIDS, Meadow makes the following comparisons:

- The percent of suffocated children with previous apnea is approximately 90%, compared with less than 10% of SIDS infants.
- Forty-four percent of the suffocated children had a previously unexplained medical problem, whereas greater than 95% of SIDS infants were previously healthy.
- Fifty-five percent of suffocated children were older than 6 months at the time of diagnosis.
- Forty-eight percent of suffocated children had a sibling who had died, compared with 2% of SIDS deaths.

—Although these important differences may identify some children who are intentionally suffocated, differentiating fatal abuse by suffocation from SIDS is difficult.

ICD-9-CM 789.0

BIBLIOGRAPHY

American Academy of Pediatrics Task Force on Infant Sleep Position and Sudden Infant Death Syndrome. Changing concepts of sudden infant death syndrome: implications for infant sleeping environment and sleep position. *Pediatrics* 2000;105:650–656.

American Academy of Pediatrics. Distinguishing sudden infant death syndrome from child abuse fatalities. Committee on Child Abuse and Neglect. *Pediatrics* 2001;107(2):437–441.

Carolan PL, Moore JR, Luxenberg MG. Infant sleep position and the sudden infant death syndrome. A survey of pediatric recommendations. *Clin Pediatr* 1995;34(8):402–409.

Keens TG, Davidson Ward SL. Apnea spells, sudden death and the role of the apnea monitor. *Pediatr Clin North Am* 1993;40:897–911.

Kohlendorfer U, Kiechl S, Sperl W. Sudden infant death syndrome: risk factor profiles for distinct subgroups. *Am J Epidemiol* 1998;147(10):960–968.

Meadow R. Suffocation, recurrent apnea, and sudden infant death. *J Pediatr* 1990;117(3):351–357.

Peterson DR, Sabotta EE, Daling JR. Infant mortality among subsequent siblings of infants who died of sudden infant death syndrome. *J Pediatr* 1986;108:911–914.

Reece RM. Fatal child abuse and sudden infant death syndrome: a critical diagnostic decision. *Pediatrics* 1994;91:423–429.

Southall DP, Plunkett MC, Banks MW, et al. Covert video recordings of life-threatening child abuse: lessons for child protection. *Pediatrics* 1997;100:735–760.

Author: Cindy W. Christian

Suicide

Database

DEFINITION
- Suicide is an intentional self-harming act that ends life.
- Attempted suicide occurs when the act does not succeed in its goal (also, failed or near suicide).
- Suicidal behavior is any voluntary act that can potentially end one's life.
- Suicidal ideation is defined as thoughts or plans to end one's own life.

ETIOLOGY
Suicidal behavior in adolescents results from the interaction of long-standing individual and family conditions, social environment, and acute stressors:
- Psychiatric disorders: Suicidal behavior is included in the diagnostic criteria for major depressive episode and borderline personality disorder (DSM-IV). Additionally, psychotic disorders, conduct disturbance, adjustment disorder, and panic disorders have all been found to be associated with suicidal behavior.
- Intense emotional state, in particular shame or humiliation, can be "trigger events" for a suicidal act.
- Personality and social factors can also contribute, such as antisocial behavior, aggressive or impulsive proclivities, and social isolation.
- Suicidal behavior runs in families. There is evidence of a genetic component and of learned behavior or suicidal behavior as a communicative or expressive act.
- While there are significant demographic differences between adolescents who complete and those who attempt suicide, completed suicide victims have previous attempt rates of 30% to 50%, while teens who attempt suicide have a nearly 50-fold increased risk of completing suicide in the future.

PATHOPHYSIOLOGY
- Decreased central serotonergic activity may result in aggressive or impulsive behaviors, which may be aimed at oneself.
- An underlying psychiatric or personality disorder acutely worsened by a stressful life event can trigger a suicidal act.
- Feelings of isolation and lack of external support (particularly from caregivers) can result in hopelessness and despair.
- Suicide may be an impulsive act designed to punish loved ones or express frustration or rage. Because there is no reliable way to tell which individual attempting suicide will terminate his/her life, all suicidal behavior must be carefully evaluated and taken seriously.

EPIDEMIOLOGY
- Suicide is a leading cause of mortality and morbidity for 15- to 24-year-olds.
- Adolescent mortality from suicide has significantly increased since 1970, leveling off somewhat since 1994.

- Peak mortality occurs in the 15- to 19-year-old age group, with the highest rate of suicidal ideation and behavior occurring in tenth graders.
- Overall, suicide accounted for 8.9 deaths per 100,000 persons aged 15 to 19 years in 1998.
- Suicide rates for 10 to 14 year olds were 1.6 per 100,000 persons in 1998, and have remained stable since 1985.
- There are an estimated 50 to 200 attempts for every completed suicide.
- As many as 19% of youth in grades 9 through 12 reported seriously considering suicide at some point in 1999, with 8% reporting a prior suicide attempt.
- Females *attempt* suicide at a rate three to four times that of males. Females are most likely to attempt suicide through ingestion.
- Males *complete* suicide at a rate three to four times that of females. Males are most likely to use the more lethal methods of firearm use (rural) or hanging (urban) in attempting suicide.
- White teens have a higher rate of completing suicide than African-American teens, with African-American teenaged females having the lowest rate of suicide completion.

COMPLICATIONS
- Long-term organ damage or physical disability, depending on the method used
- Long-lasting emotional scars in families of victims, resulting from frustration, anger, and guilt
- Repeat suicide attempt or completion

PROGNOSIS
- Twenty percent to 50% of those attempting suicide will make a repeat attempt.
- Psychiatric hospitalization has not been shown to decrease risk of attempted suicide in patients with a history of mood disorder and substance abuse.
- Multiple reports show that adolescents who attempt suicide routinely terminate treatment after just a few visits.

Differential Diagnosis

- Central nervous system
—Any insult to cerebral cortex can result in disinhibitory behaviors.
- Psychiatric disorders, with particular attention to depression, personality disorder, and substance abuse
- Psychosocial trauma or maladjustment
—Emotional or physical abuse, with the suicide attempt being a way to gain attention, obtain help, or serve as a means of escape
—Feelings of isolation or abandonment, such as following the revelation of pregnancy or homosexuality

Data Gathering

HISTORY
- Communication should be nonjudgmental and supportive.
- The provider should sensitively ascertain if the patient has a weapon or other method of self-harm.
A comprehensive history should always be obtained or reviewed by a trained mental health worker. Components of a comprehensive history include:
- Method and timing (particularly if method is ingestion)
- Lethality of attempt (e.g., number of pills, seriousness of physical injury)
- Circumstances of attempt (e.g., remote site, public display)
- History of prior attempts
- Level of planning of attempt
- Current affect and psychological status (e.g., feelings and/or level of depression, hopelessness, impulsivity, self-esteem, etc.)
- Family consistency and dynamics
- Pharmaceuticals available at home; what is missing
- History of interpersonal conflict or personal loss
- Family history of suicide
- History of substance use
- History of psychological disorder or disease state
- History of abuse, neglect, or incest
- Social supports and coping strategies
- Feelings of regret or continued desire for self-harm
The following historical information increases the risk for a future, potentially lethal suicide attempt:
- History of potentially lethal attempt
- Family history of suicide or attempted suicide
- Unstable family structure
- Poor social support system, lack of feeling connected

Physical Examination

- Physical signs or sequelae of prior attempts
- Adolescents do not have to have the classic findings of depressed adults.
- Even without a history of ingestion, closely observe vital signs, skin, mucous membranes, and pupils for evidence of toxidrome.
- Examine the skin for signs of physical abuse or self-mutilation.
- If indicated or suspected, examine the genitalia for signs of sexual abuse.
- A complete neurologic examination is essential for the evaluation of intracranial processes, acute mental status changes, and ingestions.

Laboratory Aids

TESTS
- Serum and urine toxicology screens
- Urine pregnancy test to assess pregnancy as a potential precipitating factor and to recognize potential danger to the fetus

- Acetaminophen level, as it is highly hepatotoxic and used frequently by teenagers
- Other laboratory tests will depend on the history of method of attempt (e.g., trauma labs, metabolic screens, etc.).
- Electrocardiograms are indicated for many pharmacologic ingestions, including antidepressants and benzodiazepines.

IMAGING
- Abdominal plain film, if history of iron or vitamin ingestion, or severe trauma
- Other imaging studies may be indicated, depending on method of attempt.

 Emergency Care

- Trauma response as indicated
- Monitoring of behavior and vital signs if history of ingestion
- Decontamination of GI tract and circulation as indicated.
- When available, the Poison Control Center can be very helpful with evaluation and treatment of most drug ingestions.
- Ongoing safety is of primary concern: immediate physical protection (remove all weapons) and enforce around-the-clock observation
- After medical evaluation and stabilization, the need for psychiatric hospitalization or outpatient follow-up can be assessed. Psychiatric disposition should be determined by, or in conjunction with, a mental health professional. Considerations for admission include:
- Historical factors indicating high risk for repeat attempt
- Ongoing suicidal ideation
- Family stability and support
- Current mental status
- Availability of alternative interventions (e.g., intensive psychiatric follow-up, day treatment program)

When discharge to a caregiver is being considered, the following minimal criteria should be in place at the time of discharge:
- The patient expresses regret and denies ongoing suicidal thoughts.
- The patient is medically stable.
- The patient's family is involved and reports understanding of the seriousness of the attempt.
- The patient and parents agree to contact a health professional or go to the emergency department if suicidal intent recurs. The patient and family must have 24-hour access to mental health or physical health professionals.
- The patient must not have impaired mental status (e.g., severely depressed, psychoses, delirium, intoxication, etc.).
- Lethal methods of self-harm are not immediately available to the patient (e.g., guns, dangerous pharmaceuticals).
- Follow-up and treatment of underlying psychological disorders have been arranged. This ideally involves more than just providing a phone number to psychiatric services.
- Acute precipitants and crises have been addressed.

- There is nothing to indicate to the provider that the patient and family will be noncompliant.
- Caregivers and patients are in agreement with the discharge plan.
- Barriers to obtaining follow-up treatment, in particular insurance and fear of stigma, have been addressed and will not preclude ongoing treatment.

 Therapy

DRUGS
- Medications that reverse toxidromes may be indicated (flumazenil, naloxone).
- Charcoal for recent ingestions
- *N*-acetylcysteine (Mucomyst) therapy should be initiated as soon as an ingestion of acetaminophen is reported.
- Tricyclic antidepressants (TCAs) do not exhibit the same efficacy in children and adolescents that they do in adults. Additionally, they may take a week or longer to work.
- Selective serotonin reuptake inhibitors have been shown to be effective in treating mild depressive disorders in adolescence and are much less toxic than TCAs.
- Other psychotropic medicines may be used in the acute setting for sedation or psychoses.

 Follow-Up

Long-term therapy is often needed for adolescents who attempt suicide. Therefore, improvement may be slow and punctuated by frequent setbacks.

SIGNS TO WATCH FOR
- Acute life stressors
- Failure to comply with therapy or follow-up
- A sudden sense of calm or resolution may occur when a patient has decided to end life.

PREVENTION
Screening of all adolescents for suicidal thoughts and behaviors and associated risk factors should occur at routine office visits as well as during evaluation of emotional distress or physical symptoms (e.g., chronic headache, abdominal pain). Screening should include:
- Change in level of functioning in school, work, or home
- Changes in mood or affect
- Direct inquiry about suicidal ideation and plans
- Exploration and discussion of coping strategies
- Discussion of social support

If suicidal ideation is reported, the risk of attempt should be assessed. Components of risk assessment include:
- Frequency and timing of suicidal thoughts
- Method of self-injury considered
- Plan to follow through
- History of past suicide attempt
- Consultation with a psychiatrist if there is any question of risk for suicide attempt

- Confidentiality does not extend to potentially suicidal adolescents. Parents, or the appropriate authority, should be made aware of the risk, as well as a plan, for self-harm on the part of the adolescent.

PITFALLS
- Adolescents often present to medical personnel before attempting suicide. The practitioner should be particularly aware of constitutional or vague complaints.
- Management must always occur in conjunction with a mental health professional.
- Parents and professionals should avoid minimizing attempts as "not serious" or as "just seeking attention." Different laboratories offer different spectra and sensitivities in their toxicology screens. Providers must be familiar with their laboratories and should determine whether additional studies are indicated.

 Common Questions and Answers

Q: Do I keep suicide attempts or plans confidential?
A: No. The limits of confidentiality should be clearly outlined to patients and families at the first visit or early in the patient's adolescence. These limits include anything that will directly place the patient's life in danger, such as suicidal plans, abuse, or homicidal intentions.

Q: If I directly question my patients about suicide, won't that put the idea in their head?
A: No. In most cases, patients will be relieved by having a professional who wants to talk about it. There is only risk in asking if nothing is done with the answer. Appropriate referral to mental health services or counseling can save patients' lives.

ICD-9-CM 300.9

BIBLIOGRAPHY
Greenhill LL, Waslick B. Management of suicidal behavior in children and adolescents. *Psychiatr Clin North Am* 1997;20:641–665.

Press BR, Khan SA. Management of the suicidal child or adolescent in the emergency department. *Curr Opin Pediatr* 1997;9:237–241.

U.S. Department of Health and Human Services, Office of the Assistant Secretary for Planning and Evaluation. *Trends in the well-being of America's children and youth, 2000*. Washington, DC: US Government Printing Office, 2000:106–107, 134–137.

Authors: Jonathan R. Pletcher and Kenneth R. Ginsburg

Superior Mesenteric Artery Syndrome

 Database

DEFINITION

Superior mesenteric artery (SMA) syndrome is obstruction of the distal duodenum by the superior mesenteric artery or its branches.

CAUSES

- The mesenteric artery forms an acute downward aorto-mesenteric angle as it leaves the aorta. The duodenum lies within this angle and in some individuals can be compressed by the SMA anteriorly and the vertebra posteriorly, leading to symptoms of obstruction.
- Some of the conditions that predispose to narrowing of this angle are:

—Increase in lordosis of the back, such as immobilization by body cast, scoliosis surgery, prolonged bed rest in a supine position
—Rapid growth in children
—Weight loss resulting in loss of mesenteric fat
—Variations of the ligament of Treitz. A short ligament lifts the third or fourth part of the duodenum into the narrower segment in the aorto-mesenteric angle.

PROGNOSIS

Most patients improve without need for surgery and are asymptomatic on follow-up.

 Differential Diagnosis

- Anorexia nervosa/bulimia/hysterical
- Luminal obstruction: foreign body
- Intramural obstruction: duplication cyst, web, tumor, and stricture
- Extramural obstruction: tumor, annular pancreas, bands, adhesions, volvulus, and intussusception
- Dysmotility disorder, which can be due to an intrinsic neuronal disorder, muscular weakness (holovisceral myopathy), or fibrosis (scleroderma, retroperitoneal fibrosis)

 Data Gathering

HISTORY

- Vomiting (bilious and nonbilious), nausea, postprandial nausea and vomiting, weight loss, early satiety, dehydration, bloating, abdominal pain, and failure to thrive
- The symptoms are chronic and acute, and most patients have vague abdominal pain from 18 months to 10 years in duration.
- None of the symptoms or signs for SMA syndrome are pathognomonic, but a history of weight loss, immobilization, or back surgery followed by symptoms of early satiety, bloating, and vomiting after meals would suggest the diagnosis.

 Physical Examination

- Abdominal pain
- Increased bowel gas
- Dehydration in some cases

Laboratory Aids

IMAGING

• A plain abdominal radiograph could show gas predominantly in a distended stomach with a dilated proximal duodenum with a sharp cutoff at the level where the SMA crosses the duodenum.
• An upper contrast radiography would demonstrate passage of contrast when the patient is maneuvered into a prone position, which increases the aorto-mesenteric angle by gravity.
• A determination of the aorto-mesenteric angle in severe cases may help in decision making when surgery is contemplated. In normal patients, this angle has a range of 45 to 60 degrees, whereas in patients with SMA syndrome, it is reported to be between 10 and 22 degrees.

 Therapy

• Refeeding to gain weight. Feeding in a prone position may help, but if this fails, a jejunal tube bypassing the obstruction or a period of parenteral feeding can be used.
• Frequent repositioning of patients in body cast
• A decrease in viscosity in feeds has a theoretical advantage.
• Reversal of back surgery may be necessary in some patients.
• Bypass surgery is unnecessary in most cases. Refractory cases in which duodenojejunostomy or derotation surgery has been tried are associated with very good results. The latter surgery consists of dividing the ligament of Treitz, and the whole small intestine is passed beneath the SMA and lies in the right abdomen; the colon is separated from the retroperitoneal attachments and placed in the left abdomen.

 Common Questions and Answers

Q: When the diagnosis of SMA syndrome is suspected, what sequence do you follow?
A: The logical sequence is to see if the patient improves with refeeding and mobilization first, followed by an imaging study, such as an upper GI contrast study. CT does not improve diagnosis, and an aorto-mesenteric angle study is almost never required.

Q: The following treatment modalities are known to be useful in treatment of SMA syndrome: do nothing, or feed with a jejunal tube, a liquid diet, prone feeding, or TPN. Which program works?
A: All of the above have been used in SMA syndrome. There is a probability that some patients have a functional disorder and do not require any of these feeding modalities. Weight gain has also been accomplished with total parenteral nutrition.

Q: Does radiographic testing or a feeding clinical trial help in confirming the diagnosis?
A: Yes, it may be helpful to confirm the diagnosis if the classical to-and-fro motion of barium is seen on radiographic studies during fluoroscopy. In addition, a clinical trial of feeding and weight gain often becomes the criteria for confirmation of the diagnosis.

ICD-9-CM 557.1

BIBLIOGRAPHY

Atkin JT, Skandalakis JE, Gray S. The anatomic basis of vascular compression of the duodenum. *Surg Clin North Am* 1974;54: 1361–1370.

Gustafsson L. Diagnosis and treatment of superior mesenteric syndrome. *Br J Surg* 1984;71:499–501.

Marchant EA, Alvear DT, Fagelman KM. True clinical entity of vascular compression of the duodenum in adolescence. *Surg Gynecol Obstet* 1989;168:381–386.

Author: Andrew E. Mulberg

Supraventricular Tachycardia

 ## Database

DEFINITION

Supraventricular tachycardia (SVT) is a rapid and regular narrow complex tachycardia originating at or above the atrioventricular (AV) node. The heart rates in infants range from 220 to 320 beats/min and in older children may be slower (150 to 250 beats/min).

- Fifty percent of cases are idiopathic and occur in young infants and children.
- Twenty percent of cases have associated conditions such as postcardiac surgery, infection, fever, or drug exposure (e.g., cold medications).
- Ten percent to 20% of cases have Wolff-Parkinson-White (WPW) syndrome, which may be associated with congenital heart disease (Ebstein anomaly, L-looped transposition of the great arteries, or hypertrophic cardiomyopathy).

PATHOPHYSIOLOGY

There are three different mechanisms for SVT:

- Reentry tachycardia: This is the most common mechanism for SVT. It involves a circuit rhythm within the atria (atrial flutter or fibrillation), AV node (AV nodal reentry tachycardia), or accessory pathway (atrioventricular reentrant tachycardia).
- Ectopic (automatic) atrial tachycardia: This is a rare mechanism for SVT and includes automatic atrial tachycardia, ectopic atrial tachycardia, and multifocal atrial tachycardia. A single focus in the atrium is responsible for rapid firing, and the heart rate may vary substantially throughout the day.
- Nodal tachycardia: This originates from the AV node and may resemble atrial tachycardia. The heart rates are relatively slower (120–200 beats/min).

GENETICS

SVT has been noted in several families, but no specific genetic inheritance has been described.

EPIDEMIOLOGY

- SVT is the most common arrhythmia in childhood.
- Forty percent of patients present between birth and 6 months, 30% present between 4 and 9 years.

COMPLICATIONS

Complications from SVT can arise from one of three causes:

- Persistent tachycardia can lead to congestive heart failure and cardiovascular collapse. This is especially true in the infant who may go unrecognized for 24 to 48 hours.
- A few patients with WPW syndrome (<5%) can have rapid conduction down the accessory pathway. If this occurs during atrial flutter/fibrillation, it can lead to a rapid ventricular response and ventricular fibrillation. Patients with WPW syndrome receiving digoxin and/or verapamil are at increased risk.
- Side effects of pharmacologic agents used to treat SVT include bradycardia, other ventricular arrhythmias due to the proarrhythmic effects of antiarrhythmic agents (digoxin, procainamide, amiodarone, flecainide), or noncardiac side effects (gastrointestinal, liver, pulmonary, and thyroid dysfunction).

 ## Differential Diagnosis

- Narrow complex SVT needs to be distinguished from normal sinus rhythm, sinus and junctional tachycardia, ventricular tachycardia, and sick-sinus syndrome with tachyarrhythmia. Structural heart disease should be excluded in all cases of newly diagnosed SVT.
- Wide complex tachycardia from either aberrantly conducted SVT or SVT with antegrade conduction down an accessory pathway can be seen in a small percentage of patients and may be confused with ventricular tachycardia. As a general rule, unless there are preexisting data that the patient has SVT, *wide complex tachycardia should always be interpreted as ventricular tachycardia until proven otherwise.*

 ## Data Gathering

HISTORY

- Signs and symptoms include those suggestive of low cardiac output if the tachycardia has gone unnoticed, especially in infants: tachypnea, retractions, irritability, decreased feedings, excessive sweating, hypotension, poor perfusion, and decreased urine output.
- The toddler and older child may experience palpitations, shortness of breath, chest pain, and dizziness or syncope. It is important to know what the child was doing at the time the arrhythmia started and whether the rhythm had an abrupt onset and termination.

 ## Physical Examination

The following need to be assessed in all patients presenting with SVT:

- Heart rate
- Respiratory rate
- Blood pressure
- Hydration status
- Peripheral perfusion
- Liver size
- Mental status
- Presence of gallop rhythm on auscultation
- Older children often report being able to terminate episodes of tachycardia by performing the Valsalva maneuver (e.g., gagging or standing on their head).

 ## Laboratory Aids

TESTS

- Diagnosis can be made by a 12-lead ECG, 24-hour Holter recording, transtelephonic monitor (TTM), or a transesophageal recording.
- Patients with WPW syndrome have diagnostic ventricular preexcitation (short PR and a delta wave) on the surface ECG.
- An exercise stress test and/or electrophysiologic testing may be indicated in older patients with WPW syndrome to help prognosticate this condition.
- Nonpharmacologic maneuvers (ice, vagal) and pharmacologic maneuvers (e.g., IV adenosine, 50–300 μg/kg/dose) may distinguish tachycardias that involve the AV node from other types of SVT.

IMAGING

A chest x-ray may reveal cardiomegaly, suggesting congestive heart failure or underlying structural heart disease.

Therapy

- Always assess the child's ABCs (airway, breathing, and circulation).
- Initial management of SVT depends on the child's hemodynamic condition.
- Presentation in cardiovascular collapse due to SVT warrants treatment with synchronized DC cardioversion (0.5–2.0 joules/kg).
- In a stable child, adenosine (IV bolus 50–350 μg/kg) may be used to block the AV node and achieve pharmacologic cardioversion. The half-life of the drug is less than 1 minute. Verapamil should be avoided as acute treatment of SVT in children less than 12 months of age because of its vasodilating and negative inotropic effect. Nonpharmacologic vagal maneuvers, including ice to the face, Valsalva, gag, and headstand, may be tried in older children. Pacing via an esophageal catheter may also be used.
- Oral digoxin is the agent of choice in hemodynamically stable SVT needing chronic therapy. Digoxin, however, is contraindicated in patients with WPW because it may potentiate faster conduction down the accessory pathway and lead to ventricular fibrillation in some patients.
- Beta-blockers (propranolol or nadolol) are the treatment of choice in individuals with WPW. Procainamide and amiodarone may be used in more resistant cases. Beta-blockers are usually given to patients with exercise-induced SVT.
- Radiofrequency catheter ablation is an alternative to long-term drug therapy and may be employed for the following reasons: (1) SVT refractory to medical therapy, (2) side effects from the medical regimen, (3) patient choice, (4) life-threatening arrhythmias, (5) rapid conduction properties of an accessory pathway (e.g., WPW), or (6) concomitant congenital or acquired heart disease.

Other forms of SVT, including automatic tachycardias (ectopic atrial and multifocal atrial tachycardia) and atrial flutter and fibrillation, may be responsive to antiarrhythmics such as procainamide, flecainide (should generally be avoided if the patient has structural heart disease), amiodarone or beta-blockers either alone or in different combinations.

 Follow-Up

- As SVT may recur, neonates and infants generally should receive maintenance therapy for the first year of life and then be observed off medications, assuming that they are not having frequent breakthrough episodes of SVT.
- Individuals with recurrences in the first year of life or those requiring multiple medications should be treated for 1- to 2-year periods during which they are episode-free, and then closely followed off medications.
- In children presenting beyond infancy, the likelihood for spontaneous resolution of the tachycardia is less likely, and treatment may need to be continued into adulthood. These patients may be considered for a radiofrequency ablation.
- Over-the-counter sympathomimetic cold medications and caffeine products should be avoided, as they may increase the likelihood of SVT.

 Common Questions and Answers

Q: How should infants on chronic therapy be monitored?
A: Parents with infants on chronic therapy for SVT should be educated about counting the heart rate by palpation or auscultation at least one or two times daily. This method of surveillance is just as effective as HR monitors. Alarm monitors can increase anxiety level by frequent false alarms and are generally not recommended.

Q: What is the concern with verapamil?
A: Verapamil is an L-type calcium channel blocker that blocks conduction in the AV node and is very effective in treating SVT in adults. Since myocardial contractility in infants depends mostly on the transsarcolemmal L-type calcium channels, hypotension and cardiovascular collapse have been reported with its use in children younger than 1 year of age.

Q: What are the indications and success rate of electrophysiology testing and radio-frequency catheter ablation?
A: Refractory arrhythmias, need for multiple medications, undesirable side effects from the medications, life-threatening events (syncope, cardiac arrest), wide complex tachycardia (cannot determine whether SVT or VT), and elective ablation after 6 to 8 years of age are some of the indications. The success rate of RFA varies from 80% to 90%, depending on the location of the bypass tract or ectopic foci.

ICD-9-CM 427.89

BIBLIOGRAPHY

Brinder LS, Boeche R, Atkinson D. Evaluation and management of supraventricular tachycardia. *Ann Emerg Med* 1992;21:1499.

Fleisher G, Ludwig S. *Textbook of pediatric emergency medicine*. Baltimore: Williams & Wilkins, 1993:549–554.

Kirk CR, Gibbs JL, Thomas R, et al. Cardiovascular collapse after verapamil in supraventricular tachycardia. *Arch Dis Child* 1987;62:1265–1282.

Levin DL, Morriss FC. *Essentials of pediatric intensive care*, vol 1. New York: Churchill Livingstone, 1997:225–227.

Moss AJ, Adams FH. *Heart disease in infants, children, and adolescents*, vol 2, 5th ed. Baltimore: Williams & Wilkins, 1995: 1555–1586.

Author: Pamela S. Ro

Syncope

 ## Database

DEFINITION

Syncope is loss of consciousness, typically lasting no longer than 1 to 2 minutes, due to a transient drop in cerebral perfusion pressure.

PATHOPHYSIOLOGY

The most common mechanism of syncope is vasovagal or neurocardiogenic, in which a variety of external stimuli—pain, emotional upset, carotid pressure—trigger increased vagal tone, leading to slowed heart rate and peripheral vasodilation and decreased cerebral perfusion pressure. Rarer causes include cardiac arrhythmia (heart block or tachy-arrhythmia) and intracranial hypertension.

ASSOCIATED CONDITIONS

Over one third of syncopal spells in children are accompanied by a convulsion that may last several minutes (EEG is normal).

 ## Differential Diagnosis

Alternative causes of loss of consciousness not due to syncope include:

- Head trauma
- Epilepsy ("temporal lobe syncope")
- Psychogenic
- Stroke, hypoglycemia (rare except in certain metabolic disorders)

Underlying causes of syncope in any age group may include congenital heart malformations, arteriovenous malformation; pulmonary hypertension; intracranial hypertension due to hydrocephalus, mass, or pseudotumor; and tachyarrhythmia or heart block (Stokes-Adams).
Other causes of syncope by age group include the following:

- Toddlers

—Pallid or cyanotic breath-holding spells; these occur in response to pain, excitement, or frustration, begin with a deep inspiration or exhalation, though the precipitating "gasp" may not be apparent. (Anemia may be associated.)
—Mastocytosis—syncope preceded by dyspnea

- Older children:

—Prolonged QT syndrome or arrhythmogenic right ventricular dysplasia; may be familial; may occur as unprovoked syncope or as exercise-induced syncope that may resemble an epileptic convulsion
—Adrenal insufficiency
—Dysautonomia—orthostatic hypotension

 ## Data Gathering

HISTORY

- Detailed history of the spell are the most important information used to distinguish syncope from seizure or head trauma.
- Questions addressing a possible family history of spells or syncope is essential.
- The child or observers may recall "presyncopal" signs—such as diaphoresis, light-headedness, palpitations, visual changes—all lasting only a few seconds before loss of consciousness.
- Increasing duration of unconsciousness suggests increasing probability that the event is epileptic, rather than syncopal.
- Several generalized tonic-clonic movements may occur with syncope—presyncopal signs point to the nonepileptic nature of the event.
- Details of body position, eye movements, and respiratory pattern

Physical Examination

It is rare for children with syncope to have physical findings that could indicate the cause of syncope. Key findings to document include:

- Vital signs, peripheral/central pulses
- Orthostatic pulse and blood pressure changes
- Right and left arm blood pressures
- Funduscopy—papilledema?
- Cranial bruits
- Heart sounds (gallop, clicks, murmurs?)

 ## Laboratory Aids

Some children may have a clear history of vasovagal syncope and no laboratory testing will be required. If the event is suspected to be symptomatic of a heart condition, ECG and chest x-ray studies may be useful screening tests.

- Children with unexplained syncope may undergo more extensive testing to rule out arrhythmia: treadmill ECG, Holter monitoring, EEG (looking for evidence of epilepsy)
- Other laboratory testing (CBC, blood gases, echocardiogram, brain imaging, spinal tap) may be appropriate based on clinical suspicion of underlying causes (see Differential Diagnosis, above).
- Clinical intervention is primarily aimed at training the patient in prevention/anticipation:

—Avoiding circumstances predisposing to the most common form of syncope (vasovagal)
—Sitting or lying down when warning signs occur
—Maintaining adequate hydration especially during illness/exertion

- Therapy is otherwise addressed to underlying causes, in the unusual circumstance that one is found.

PITFALLS

- Syncope with exercise always warrants an electrocardiogram and echocardiography.
- Recurrent syncope due to prolonged QT interval may be missed on routine ECG; QT interval may be prolonged only on treadmill testing.
- Carbon monoxide poisoning may cause syncopal-like spells; ask about potential exposure.
- Epilepsy may rarely mimic a syncopal episode or recurrent presyncopal symptoms; "temporal lobe syncope" seems to occur principally in adults or adolescents.
- A family history of sudden death, syncope, or seizures should trigger further laboratory studies.
- Syncope may trigger a convulsion in an epileptic patient.

 ## Follow-Up

- A record should be kept once a child has had two or more syncopal spells within 6 months.
- Many children seem to outgrow a developmental stage when, for unknown reasons, they have frequent vasovagal episodes; they may retain a tendency to syncopal spells through adulthood.
- Persistent and frequent spells may prompt more extensive laboratory testing, as described above.

Common Questions and Answers

Q: Do breath-holding spells cause brain damage?
A: Pallid breath-holding spells appear to be uniformly benign; in rare cases, older children with cyanotic breath-holding spells have had neurologic sequelae of recurrent hypoxemia.

Q: What limitations in activity are appropriate for children with recurrent syncope?
A: Precautions should be taken similar to those for children of similar age who have epilepsy—closely monitored water recreation, and restrictions on climbing; however, most children with recurrent syncope do not experience spells in the midst of vigorous activity.

ICD-9-CM 780.2

BIBLIOGRAPHY

Freed MD. Advances in the diagnosis and therapy of syncope and palpitations in children. *Curr Opin Pediatr* 1994;6(4): 368–372.

Kapoor WN. Syncope. *N Engl J Med* 2000;343:1856–1862.

Lerman-Sagie T, Lerman P, Mukamel M, et al. A prospective evaluation of pediatric patients with syncope. *Clin Pediatr* 1994;33(2):67–70.

Author: Nancy Drucker

Synovitis—Transient

 Database

DEFINITION

A transient inflammatory process resulting in arthralgia and arthritis (especially affecting the hip) and occasionally rash precipitated by an exposure to an infectious agent or drug

CAUSES

Usually viral (especially enteroviruses), postvaccine, or drug-mediated (especially antibiotics)

PATHOLOGY

A type III hypersensitivity reaction mediated by immune complex deposition within the skin and joint spaces

EPIDEMIOLOGY

Any age at risk, common in ages 3 to 10, with males affected 1.5 times more commonly

GENETICS

No specific associations

COMPLICATIONS

In affected hips, rarely avascular necrosis of femoral head and coxa magna

 Differential Diagnosis

- Infection: Lyme, septic, gonorrhea
- Environment: trauma (fracture, or soft tissue injury), slipped capital femoral epiphysis, avascular necrosis
- Tumors: osteoid osteoma
- Immunologic: juvenile rheumatoid arthritis, SEA syndrome
- Psychological: psychogenic limp
- Miscellaneous: hypothyroidism

 Data Gathering

HISTORY

- Exposure to individuals with viral syndromes
- Day care
- Recent use of antibiotics
- Recent vaccination, especially MMR
- Relatively rapid onset of symptoms, with refusal to bear weight, in a nontoxic appearing child
- Recent nonspecific upper respiratory infection

 Physical Examination

Finding: General examination usually benign with occasional low-grade fever.
Significance: Child refuses to bear weight but may tolerate slight ranging of joint. Effusions in peripheral joints are usually small and evanescent.

PROCEDURE

Extreme pain on passive ranging raises suspicion for septic joint.

 Laboratory Aids

Test: CBC
Significance: Usually mild leukocytosis

Test: ESR
Significance: Usually midrange elevation (35–60)

IMAGING

Test: X-ray
Significance: Usually normal or demonstrates small effusion; no evidence of periosteal changes

Test: Ultrasound
Significance: Affected hip joints may have demonstrable effusions

Test: MRI
Significance: Normal signal intensity may help differentiate transient synovitis from septic hip.

Test: Joint aspirate culture
Significance: Be wary of contaminated joint aspiration cultures

Test: Culture
Significance: Be wary of contaminated joint aspiration cultures.

PITFALLS

Distinctions between the septic joints may be difficult.

Therapy

DRUGS

- Usually very responsive to NSAIDs such as ibuprofen (up to 10 mg/kg/dose four times a day).
- Rarely, a short course of oral steroids is necessary.

DURATION

Usually 1 to 3 weeks of a tapering course of NSAIDs is effective.

POSSIBLE CONFLICTS

- Avoid initiation of therapy until septic joint is not a major concern, because early use of NSAIDs can mask disease progression in septic joints

 Follow-Up

WHEN TO EXPECT IMPROVEMENT

Usually significant improvement in 24 to 48 hours

SIGNS TO WATCH FOR

Ongoing synovitis despite therapeutic levels of NSAIDs or any bony changes indicates need to change diagnosis.

PROGNOSIS

Excellent, though on occasion patients will experience recurrence of symptoms with subsequent viral syndrome or reexposure to a previously associated drug.

PITFALLS

Overinvestigation/therapy of child with features by history, physical examination, and laboratory supportive of diagnosis of serum sickness

 Common Questions and Answers

Q: Are there any chronic sequelae from transient synovitis?
A: Not usually. This is generally a benign disease; injury to the femoral head in affected hips is extremely rare but long-term sequelae include Legg-Calvé-Perthes disease.

Q: Is there an association with chronic arthritis?
A: No, there is no known increased risk for chronic arthritis in affected children.

ICD-9-CM 726.90

BIBLIOGRAPHY

Cassidy JT, Petty RE. *Textbook of pediatric rheumatology*, 4th ed. Philadelphia: WB Saunders, 2001.

Del Baccaro MA, Champoux AN, Bockers T, et al. Septic arthritis verus transient synovitis of the hip: the value of screening laboratory tests. *Ann Emerg Med* 1992;21:1418–1422.

Do TT. Transient synovitis as a cause of painful limps in children. *Curr Opin Pediatr* 2000;12:48–51.

Authors: Randy Q. Cron
Gregory F. Keenan, 2nd edition

Syphilis

Database

DEFINITION
Systemic infection caused by the spirochete *Treponema pallidum*.

Congenital Syphilis
• Transmitted from an infected mother to her unborn or newborn baby. Early congenital syphilis refers to the symptoms appearing in the first 2 years of life, and late congenital syphilis refers to those occurring later in childhood. Clinical manifestations range from asymptomatic to death or stillbirth.
• Manifestations include periostitis, osteochondritis, persistent rhinorrhea, maculopapular or vesiculobullous rash, hepatitis, pneumonia.
• Late manifestations may cause central nervous system (CNS), dental, and skeletal disease.

Acquired Syphilis
• Sexually transmitted from an infected individual to an uninfected individual. Sexual abuse must be considered when syphilis is diagnosed in children.
• Primary stage: painless chancre(s) (indurated ulcers) at the site of inoculation; typically lasts 1 to 6 weeks.
• Secondary stage: generalized rash, which is often maculopapular and involves the palms and soles; condyloma lata, hypertrophic papular lesions; fever, malaise, lymphadenopathy; follows the primary stage by 2 to 10 weeks and lasts up to 2 to 10 weeks.
• Relapse: symptoms of secondary syphilis may recur one or more times before the latent period.
• Latent period: variable, occurs after the secondary stage; first 4 years of latent period are referred to as "early latent," and subsequent years as "late latent" or "syphilis of unknown duration;" lasts 1 to 40 years or more; patients in this period are seroreactive but there is no other evidence of disease.
• Tertiary stage: many years after the primary infection; may see manifestations of gummatous changes of the skin, bone, and/or viscera, or cardiovascular syphilis.
• Neurosyphilis: evidence of CNS infection with *T. pallidum*; may occur at any stage.

PATHOPHYSIOLOGY
• Congenital: transplacental (hematogenous) infection of the fetus at any stage of pregnancy; rarely from contact with infectious lesions during passage through the birth canal
• Acquired: exposure to an infected genital or nongenital skin lesion
• In late congenital syphilis, a late hypersensitivity reaction is believed to cause the findings of interstitial keratitis, deafness, and Clutton joints.

COMPLICATIONS
• Stillbirth, spontaneous abortion, perinatal death: 40% of pregnancies in mothers with untreated early syphilis

• Hydrops fetalis
• Prematurity
• Nephrosis
• Failure to thrive
• Disseminated intravascular coagulation
• Pseudoparalysis of Parrot: paralysis of one of the limbs of an infant affected by congenital syphilis; usually unilateral
• Acute syphilitic leptomeningitis
• Cranial nerve palsies
• Hearing loss (e.g., eighth nerve deafness; 10–40 years after birth)
• Interstitial keratitis (5–20 years after birth)
• Cerebral infarction
• Seizure disorder
• Mental retardation
• Rhagades: cluster of scars radiating around the mouth
• Mulberry molars: maldevelopment of the cusps in the first molars
• Clutton joints: painless arthritis of the knees and, rarely, other joints
• Hutchinson triad: Hutchinson teeth (notched upper central incisors), interstitial keratitis, eighth nerve deafness
• Saber shins: anterior bowing of the midportion of the tibia

PROGNOSIS
• The prognosis is better the earlier syphilis is detected and treated. Following appropriate therapy, the disease is usually totally arrested. With late findings of syphilis, involving the nervous system and/or cardiovascular system, there may not be clinical improvement.
• Untreated infection in the neonate progresses to neurosyphilis within 1 year.

Differential Diagnosis

• Neonate: herpes simplex virus, toxoplasmosis, cytomegalovirus, rubella, sepsis, neonatal hepatitis, osteomyelitis
• Primary syphilis: chancroid, granuloma inguinale, lymphogranuloma venereum, scabies, mycotic infections, herpes progenitalis
• Secondary syphilis: infectious mononucleosis, scabies, viral exanthem, e.g., enteroviruses may cause a maculopapular rash involving the palms and soles

Data Gathering

HISTORY
Newborn/Infants
• Always obtain a detailed prenatal history; inquire about all syphilis testing done on the mother; if mother has a history of syphilis, ensure documented treatment; the local department of health should have records on all cases of syphilis.
• Newborns should be evaluated for congenital syphilis if:
—Mother not adequately treated for syphilis
—Mother treated with nonpenicillin regimen, such as erythromycin

—Mother treated adequately but without a fourfold decrease in antibody titers in early or high-titer syphilis
—Maternal syphilis treated less than 1 month (30 days) before delivery
—Maternal syphilis treated prior to pregnancy with insufficient follow-up to assess serologic response to treatment
—Maternal titer has increased fourfold or if the infant titer is fourfold greater than the mother's titer or if the infant is symptomatic

Older Children/Adolescents
• Ask about possible sexual abuse in children and sexual activity in adolescents.
• Ask about a history of other sexually transmitted diseases/lesions.
• Ask about risk factors for HIV exposure.

Physical Examination

Early congenital syphilis, may see:
• Low birth weight
• Irritability, bulging fontanel, if neurosyphilis is present
• Loss of hair, eyebrows
• Fissures in the lips, nares, anus; mucocutaneous lesions
• Rhinitis ("snuffles") may occur at one to several weeks of age and may be blood-tinged and purulent
• Lymphadenopathy
• Pneumonia: check for tachypnea, respiratory distress
• Myocarditis
• Hepatosplenomegaly with or without jaundice
• Pseudoparalysis of an extremity
• Rash: bullous ("syphilitic pemphigus") and/or maculopapular; symmetrically distributed on palms, soles, and other parts of the body
• Condyloma lata (flat, wart-like, moist) around the anus/vagina, chancres
Late congenital syphilis, may see:
• Bony deformities, such as short maxilla, high arched palate, saddle nose, mulberry molars, Higouménaki sign (enlargement of the sternoclavicular portion of the clavicle), protuberance of the mandible, saber shins, scaphoid scapulae
• Rhagades, neurologic involvement
Acquired syphilis:
• Primary syphilis: chancre: painless ulcer, single, most commonly located on the genitalia; painless, inguinal adenopathy
• Secondary syphilis: may see a flu-like illness: fever, headache, sore throat, nasal discharge, generalized arthralgias and myalgias, malaise, generalized adenopathy (painless and mobile nodes); hepatosplenomegaly; maculopapular rash involving the palms and soles and may involve the mucous membranes; condyloma lata (moist, papular lesions); alopecia; also, look for signs of meningitis, hepatitis, nephropathy, ocular involvement.

Laboratory Aids

—VDRL slide test: congenital infection if infant's titer is at least fourfold greater than the maternal titer; VDRL should be done on CSF, when syphilis is suspected to rule out neurosyphilis.

—RPR (rapid plasma reagin): a simplified variation of the VDRL test; more sensitive than VDRL

—False-positive nontreponemal test results may occur with lab error, autoimmune disease, tuberculosis, lymphoma, viral infections (incl. infectious mononucleosis, hepatitis, varicella, and measles), endocarditis, malaria, contamination with Wharton jelly on cord specimens and intravenous drug abuse. In newborns, nontreponemal testing of the cord blood may result in false-positive (e.g., from contamination with Wharton jelly) and false-negative results. Therefore, serum from the infant is preferable.

—Usually becomes nonreactive after therapy within 1 year in low-titer (≤1:8) primary syphilis, and within 2 years in secondary and congenital syphilis. In late latent and tertiary syphilis, the nontreponemal test may remain positive in spite of therapy.

• *Treponemal antibody tests:* nonquantitative; used to confirm the diagnosis of syphilis; do *not* correlate with disease activity; positive for life once infected; more difficult and expensive than the nontreponemal tests

—FTA-ABS (fluorescent treponemal antibody) and MHA-TP (microhemagglutination assay for antibodies to *T. pallidum*) are available.

—Positive treponemal tests may be seen in other spirochetal diseases (e.g., Lyme disease, leptospirosis), and rarely in autoimmune disease and viral infections.

• *Complete blood count (CBC):* if anemia or thrombocytopenia suspected

• *Liver function tests:* if liver disease suspected

• *Pathologic evaluation of the placenta and umbilical cord:* using specific fluorescent antitreponemal antibody staining is recommended

• *CSF analysis:* in syphilis, findings include mononuclear pleocytosis, moderately elevated protein, normal glucose; should be performed in all patients with acquired syphilis of greater than 1 year's duration.

In infants, perform when congenital syphilis suspected, if the physical examination is consistent with syphilis, if infant titer fourfold greater than that of mother, darkfield or fluorescent antibody test positive on body fluids, and all children being treated with antibiotics for syphilis.

• *Microscopy:* treponemes may be seen on darkfield microscopy of fresh exudate from skin lesions, regional lymph node, placenta, umbilical cord; or by direct fluorescent antibody staining of acetone-fixed exudate.

RADIOGRAPHIC STUDIES

• Long bones: to rule out metaphyseal osteochondritis and/or diaphyseal periostitis

• Chest radiograph: if pneumonia is suspected (fluffy diffuse infiltrates are seen with pneumonia alba); if cardiac symptoms are present

Therapy

In congenital syphilis, treat if physical, laboratory, and/or x-ray evidence of disease, positive test confirming syphilis, CSF VDRL reactive, nontreponemal titer at least fourfold greater than that of mother.

DRUGS

• In high-risk and symptomatic patients, treatment should be started while awaiting confirmatory treponemal test results.

• *Congenital syphilis:*

—IV aqueous crystalline penicillin G (100,000–150,000 U/kg/d divided b.i.d. or t.i.d.; administered as 50,000 U/kg per dose IV q12h during first 7 days of life and q8h thereafter for total of 10 days) or IM procaine penicillin G (50,000 U/kg/d) for 7 to 10 days is the recommended therapy for neonates. After 4 weeks of age, use aqueous penicillin G, 200,000 to 300,000 U/kg/d divided q.i.d. times 10 days. Data supporting the use of ampicillin are not available.

• *Acquired syphilis, less than 1 year duration:* IM benzathine penicillin G 50,000 U/kg (maximum 2.4 million units) in a single dose; if penicillin-allergic, tetracycline (in patients older than 8 years) 500 mg PO q.i.d. or doxycycline, 100 mg PO b.i.d. for 2 weeks for patients older than 9 years; erythromycin 500 mg PO q.i.d. or ceftriaxone is an alternative that should be used in consultation with an infectious disease specialist.

• *Acquired syphilis, greater than 1 year duration:* IM benzathine penicillin G, 50,000 U/kg, weekly for 3 consecutive weeks; if penicillin-allergic, tetracycline, 500 mg PO q.i.d. or doxycycline 100 mg PO b.i.d. for 4 weeks.

• *Neurosyphilis:* Penicillin: aqueous penicillin G 200,000 to 300,000 U/kg/d (not to exceed 24 million U/d) divided q4–6h for 10 to 14 days. There is some variability in treatment, following this regimen. Consultation with an infectious disease specialist is therefore recommended.

Follow-Up

• For all infants born to positive mothers, follow-up at 1, 2, 3, 6, and 12 months of age. Serologic tests should be performed 3, 6, and 12 months after therapy until they become nonreactive. If titers have not shown a decline by 3 months, re-treatment should be considered.

• For patients with neurosyphilis, clinical, serologic, and CSF evaluation should occur every 6 months until the CSF is normal. A reactive CSF VDRL at 6 months is an indication for re-treatment.

• Osteochondritis and periostitis in the newborn are usually self-limited and heal in the first 6 months of life.

• Hemolytic anemia seen in congenital syphilis may persist for weeks.

PREVENTION

• All cases should be reported to the local department of health.

• All sexual contacts of persons with acquired syphilis should be evaluated for other STDs as well as syphilis.

• Prenatal screening early in pregnancy is recommended in all states. In high-risk patients and in areas of high prevalence, screening should be repeated at 28 weeks' gestation.

• Mothers of infants with congenital syphilis should also be tested for gonorrhea, chlamydia, HIV, and hepatitis B infection.

Common Questions and Answers

Q: Does pregnancy cause a false-positive VDRL result?

A: There are conflicting studies regarding this issue. A positive VDRL in an otherwise healthy pregnant woman should never be considered a false-positive test. A treponemal-specific test should be performed to confirm the diagnosis of syphilis, and the patient should be treated appropriately.

Q: Can an infant have congenital syphilis if the mother had a negative VDRL during pregnancy?

A: A mother with a negative VDRL during pregnancy may have acquired syphilis late in pregnancy and transmitted it to her fetus. If the mother was not tested at delivery, then the diagnosis may have been missed. Some recommend that VDRLs be performed at the time of delivery for mothers who are at high risk for syphilis.

Q: What is the prozone phenomenon?

A: When a nontreponemal test is falsely negative due to high concentrations of antibody to *T. pallidum*, diluting the serum will result in positive test results.

ICD-9-CM 079.9

BIBLIOGRAPHY

Centers for Disease Control and Prevention. Primary and secondary syphilis—United States, 1999. *MMWR* 2001;50:113–117.

Sanchez PJ. Laboratory tests for congenital syphilis. *Pediatr Infect Dis J* 1998;17:70–71.

St. Louis ME, Wasserheit JN. Elimination of syphilis in the United States. *Science* 1998;281:353–354.

Author: Esther K. Chung

Tapeworm

Database

CAUSES
- *Taenia saginata* (beef tapeworm)
- *Taenia solium* (pork tapeworm)
- *Diphyllobothrium latum* (fish tapeworm)
- *Dipylidium caninum* (dog tapeworm)
- *Echinococcus granulosus*

PATHOLOGY
- Tapeworms cause two major types of zoonotic disease syndromes depending on whether humans are the definitive or intermediate host.
- When humans serve as definitive hosts, adult tapeworms infect the GI tract and interfere with nutrition. These infections are often asymptomatic and seldom life threatening.
- When humans serve as intermediate hosts for the larval cestode, serious pathology can result.

PATHOPHYSIOLOGY
- Beef tapeworm: Cattle (intermediate host) ingest the eggs of *T. saginata* in contaminated feeds. The eggs hatch, releasing embryos. The embryos penetrate the intestinal mucosa, enter the bloodstream, and settle in various tissues where they develop into larvae. Larvae in undercooked meat are consumed by humans and mature into adult tapeworms within the human (definitive host) GI tract. They can grow up to 25 m in length.
- Pork tapeworm: Humans are the only definitive host for the adult pork tapeworm, whereas both humans and pigs are intermediate hosts for its embryonic form, cysticercus.
—Eggs of *T. solium* are ingested by the pig (intermediate host). In the intestine, the eggs release embryos that penetrate the mucosa, enter the bloodstream, and settle in various tissues to differentiate into cysticerci (infective larvae). Cysticerci are ingested by humans consuming undercooked pork. Cysticerci mature into adult worms in the small intestine of humans (definitive host). These adult worms can reach a length of 2 to 7 m.
—Humans, as intermediate hosts, ingest food contaminated with human feces containing *T. solium* eggs. The eggs hatch, liberating embryos (oncospheres). Penetration through the intestinal mucosa leads to blood-borne distribution to the brain, subcutaneous tissues, muscle, and eye, where they develop into a cysticerci.
- Fish tapeworm: When sewage containing *D. latum* eggs contaminates freshwater lakes and streams, larvae hatch into the water. These larvae are eaten by crustaceans and fish. Humans are infected when they consume these undercooked fish. The larvae mature into adult tapeworms in the intestines of humans.
- Dog tapeworm: Larvae develop in fleas (intermediate host) after ingestion of the eggs; humans infected through accidental ingestion of infected fleas.
- Echinococcosis (hydatid disease): Humans ingest eggs of *E. granulosus* through contaminated dog feces. After ingestion, the eggs hatch and release embryos (oncospheres) in the small intestine. Penetration through the mucosa leads to blood-borne distribution to the liver, lungs, and other sites, where development of cysts begins. Within the cysts, new larvae (scolices) develop, accumulate fluid, and enlarge to encroach on surrounding structures.

EPIDEMIOLOGY
- Beef tapeworm: Widespread in cattle-breeding areas of the world, with a prevalence of >10% in areas of Africa, such as Ethiopia and Kenya, and the former Soviet Union. Slightly lower rates of infection exist in Europe, Southeast Asia, and South America.
- Pork tapeworm: Cysticercosis has a high prevalence in developing areas of Central and South America. In the U.S., immigrants account for >90% of patients with cysticercosis.
- Fish tapeworm: Infection is most prevalent in populations whose culinary habits result in consumption of undercooked fish. In the U.S., infected salmon have been implicated in the majority of cases on the West Coast.
- Dog tapeworm: This infection is found in dogs and cats worldwide, but is uncommon in the U.S.
- Echinococcosis: It is associated with the practice of feeding sheep viscera to dogs. It is hyperendemic in sheep-raising areas of South America, Australia, and areas of Africa, such as Kenya and Uganda. Also seen in China, central Asia, and parts of the western U.S.

COMPLICATIONS
- Echinococcosis: Cysts grow slowly, causing symptoms only when they are relatively large. They frequently develop in the liver (50–70%) and lung (20–30%); 5% to 10% of cysts involve other organs, including the eye, brain, spleen, heart, bone, and kidneys. Pulmonary lesions cause cough and hemoptysis. Bone involvement leads to pathologic fractures. Renal involvement can lead to pain and hematuria. Spontaneous rupture of cysts can cause anaphylaxis.

Differential Diagnosis

- Tapeworm infections should be considered in all cases of diarrhea and abdominal pain. Larval infection should be considered in individuals with cystic end-organ disease.
- Abdominal pain, anemia, and vitamin B_{12} deficiency can be seen with fish tapeworm infections, Crohn disease, and intestinal bacterial overgrowth.
- Echinococcal cysts must be differentiated from benign cysts, cavitary tuberculosis, abscesses, and neoplasms.

Data Gathering

HISTORY
Question: Recent travel or immigration?
Significance: Tapeworm infections are more prevalent in other countries.
Question: GI tract complaints?
Significance: Symptoms related to the GI tract include nausea, weight loss, diarrhea, abdominal pain, and intestinal obstruction.
Question: Respiratory tract symptoms?
Significance: Cough, dyspnea, and hemoptysis are associated with rupture of pulmonary hydatid cyst due to *E. granulosus*. Anaphylaxis may result from rupture of a hydatid cyst in any organ.
Question: Alteration in mental status or development of partial or generalized seizures?
Significance: Onset of new CNS pathology is seen with neurocysticercosis and some species of *Echinococcus*. CNS symptoms in neurocysticercosis typically appear 5 to 7 years after initial infection (latencies as short as 6 months and as long as 30 years have occurred).
Question: Symptoms of anemia?
Significance: Anemia due to vitamin B_{12} deficiency is seen with 2% of fish tapeworm infections.

Physical Examination

Finding: Pallor
Significance: Signs of anemia secondary to vitamin B_{12} deficiency can be seen with fish tapeworm infections. Other signs of pernicious anemia include glossitis, peripheral neuropathy, decreased vibration sense, and ataxia.
Finding: Jaundice
Significance: Hepatic cysts from echinococcosis may be palpable in the RUQ; biliary tree extension can lead to obstructive jaundice and cholangitis.
Finding: Cough, wheeze, or signs of respiratory distress
Significance: Rupture hydatid cysts in echinococcosis can cause an immediate hypersensitivity syndrome or anaphylaxis. Rupture of pulmonary cysts also cause cough and hemoptysis.
Finding: Abdominal tenderness
Significance: Can be seen with any tapeworm infection. Beef tapeworm and dog tapeworm infections are usually asymptomatic.
Finding: Abdominal distention
Significance: Fish tapeworm and, rarely, dog tapeworm infections can be complicated by intestinal obstruction.

Finding: Alteration in mental status or signs of elevated intracranial pressure or meningitis
Significance: The initial sign of neurocysticercosis in children is most often a generalized seizure. Elevated intracranial pressure, meningitis, and encephalitis are other complications. Both neurocysticercosis and vitamin B_{12} deficiency due to fish tapeworm can simulate a psychotic illness with delirium or hallucinations.
Finding: Proglottids in stool
Significance: In dog tapeworm infections, proglottids, resembling rice or seeds, are noted in the stool.

 ## Laboratory Aids

Test: Beef tapeworm
Significance: Identification of scolex in stool; Ziehl-Neelsen stain of stool or perianal adhesive tape preparations identifies eggs; collection of proglottids in saline with microscopic examination; ELISA test can detect antigens from the genus *Taenia* in stools.
Test: Pork tapeworm
Significance: ELISA test and immunoblot in combination for parenchymal cysticercosis; stool samples for intestinal worms as for beef tapeworm. Contrast-enhanced CT or MRI of the brain may reveal cysticerci with surrounding edema, granuloma, or calcification.
Test: Fish tapeworm
Significance: Stool samples for eggs and proglottids are diagnostic. Mild eosinophilia (5–15%) may be present. Fifty percent of patients have low vitamin B_{12} levels, 2% have megaloblastic anemia.
Test: Dog tapeworm
Significance: Characteristic egg packets (loose membrane containing up to 20 eggs) may be identified in stool or perianal adhesive tape preparations.
Test: Echinococcosis
Significance: The diagnosis is usually suspected on the basis of clinical or radiologic findings plus a history of residence in an endemic area.
—IgE levels are elevated. Eosinophilia is present in <25% of infected persons. Mild elevation of hepatic enzymes may be present with hepatic hydatid cysts.
—On radiograph, pulmonary cysts demonstrate a sharply demarcated, smooth-bordered cyst; there is a crescent-shaped air level after cyst rupture. Lesions in the liver and spleen may calcify but only over many years.
—The Casoni skin test (injection of hydatid fluid into the dermis) yields an erythematous papule in <60 minutes in 50% to 80% of infected patients. There is a false-positive result in 30% of uninfected patients.
—Serologic testing is falsely negative in 10% to 50% of cases. False-negative results are more likely in patients with pulmonary hydatid

cysts and in children. No current serologic test excludes the diagnosis of hydatid cysts.
—In seronegative persons, a presumptive diagnosis can be confirmed by demonstrating protoscolices or hydatid membranes in the liquid obtained from percutaneous aspiration of the cyst under ultrasound guidance. This procedure is controversial due to the risk of anaphylaxis if rupture occurs during aspiration.
—Demonstration of internal septa or daughter cysts (after cyst rupture) by CT, MRI, or ultrasound indicates hydatid cysts. Such findings are present in approximately 50% of patients with unilocular liver cysts.

 ## Therapy

• Beef tapeworm:
—Praziquantel: 5 to 10 mg/kg as a single dose; no safety profile exists for children under the age of 4.
—Alternative: Niclosamide: children 11 to 34 kg, 1 g as a single dose; children >34 kg, 1.5 g as a single dose (not available in U.S.).
• Pork tapeworm:
—Intestinal disease: praziquantel: 5 to 10 mg/kg as a single dose
—Neurocysticercosis: albendazole: 15 mg/kg/d (max. 800 mg/d) in two divided doses for 28 days
Alternative or if albendazole results in only partial response: praziquantel: 50 mg/kg/d in three divided doses for 14 days. Dexamethasone to reduce cerebral edema should be given 2 days before cysticidal therapy and continued during and shortly after drug therapy. Anticonvulsant therapy may be required.
• Fish tapeworm: Same as in beef tapeworm. In addition, supplement with vitamin B_{12}.
• Dog tapeworm: Same as in beef tapeworm.
• Echinococcosis:
—Surgical resection of intact hydatid cysts, especially if >10 cm or secondarily infected.
—Albendazole 15 mg/kg/d (max. 800 mg/d) in two divided doses for 28 days, may require up to three courses of therapy with drug-free intervals of 14 days between courses.
Note: The benzimidazoles, including albendazole, are contraindicated in patients with blood dyscrasias, leukopenia, and liver disease. Prolonged courses require monitoring of liver function and hematopoiesis.
Note: Dexamethasone lowers plasma levels of praziquantel by as much as 50% but raises the level of albendazole by 50%.

PREVENTION

• Adult tapeworms: In general, avoiding contamination of food and drink with human feces, as well as proper cooking of meat and fish prevents transmission of beef, pork, and fish tapeworms.
• Beef tapeworm: Proper disposal of human feces would disrupt the life cycle of this parasite because humans are the only known definitive host for *T. saginata*.
• Pork tapeworm: The refrigeration of pork infested with cysticerci at temperatures above

0°C does not affect parasite survival. However, storage of pork for 4 days at −5°C or 1 day at −24°C kills most cysticerci.
• Fish tapeworm: Human eating habits must be altered since regulations for proper disposal of human feces won't prevent contamination of water supplies with eggs from animal sources. Brief cooking (≥56°C for 5 minutes) or freezing (−18°C for 24 hours) renders the fish safe for consumption.
• Dog tapeworm: Regular veterinary care of pets with periodic deworming prevents most infections.
• Echinococcosis: Control measures can interrupt the life cycle of *E. granulosus* as the cestode moves between sheep and carnivore hosts. Measures include careful disposal of sheep viscera and mass chemotherapy of dogs.

 ## Follow-Up

• Beef tapeworm: Stool should be checked for eggs and proglottids 1 month after completion of therapy.
• Pork tapeworm: CNS imaging studies should be repeated at 2-month intervals (with continued therapy) until successful elimination of parenchymal brain cysticerci.
• Fish tapeworm: Stool examinations to evaluate for cure should be performed 6 weeks or longer after therapy.
• Dog tapeworm: No follow-up stool examination is indicated, but the appearance of proglottids 1 week or longer after therapy is indication of treatment failure.
• Echinococcosis: Prolonged follow-up with ultrasound or other imaging procedures, depending on the extent and location of the cysts, is required.

 ## Common Questions and Answers

Q: How may one prevent tapeworm infections when traveling to other countries?
A: Proper food preparation is essential to prevent infections. Avoid uncooked or undercooked food products. In addition, avoid drinking potentially contaminated water by using bottled water.
Q: Is treatment for cerebral cysticercosis always indicated?
A: No, for an isolated cystic lesion in the brain parenchyma treatment is not needed. In many children, the lesion disappears spontaneously within 2 or 3 months.

ICD-9-CM 123.9

BIBLIOGRAPHY
Anonymous. Drugs for parasitic infections. *Med Lett Drugs Ther* 1998;40:1–12.

Bruckner DA. Helminthic food-borne infections. *Clin Lab Med* 1999;19:639–660.

Schantz PM. Tapeworms (cestodiasis). *Gastroenterol Clin* 1996;25:637–653.

Author: Samir S. Shah

Tendonitis

 ## Database

DEFINITION

Inflammation of a tendon at its insertion or along its tendon sheath

CAUSES

Frequently associated with repetitive motion/overuse type activities

PATHOLOGY

Inflammation, microtearing, and microfracture may be present.

EPIDEMIOLOGY

Increases with age and at time of puberty. There may be a slight increase in incidence in girls.

GENETICS

Hypermobile individuals may be prone to these injuries.

COMPLICATIONS

Ongoing pain and predisposition for recurrence

 ## Differential Diagnosis

- Infection: septic arthritis, osteomyelitis
- Environmental: fracture
- Metabolic: homocystinuria
- Congenital: generalized hypermobility, Marfan syndrome, Ehlers-Danlos
- Immunologic: ankylosing spondylitis and the reactive spondyloarthropathies (Crohn disease, Reiter syndrome), inflammatory arthritides
- Psychological: "Touch me not" psychogenic pain

 ## Data Gathering

HISTORY

Question: Trauma or overuse?
Significance: Verify acute nature of injury.

 ## Physical Examination

Question: Any evidence of hematoma?
Significance: Palpate around and about affected areas, detecting point tenderness especially at tendon insertions as well as over bony prominences.

SPECIAL QUESTIONS

Question: Was a pop or snap felt at the time of the event?
Significance: Sometimes this is felt when tendons and ligaments are torn.

 ## Laboratory Aids

Test: ESR
Significance: Occasionally, an ESR will be helpful to rule out inflammatory conditions if history and/or physical examination are suggestive.

IMAGING

Test: X-ray
Significance: Affected area may be indicated to rule out a fracture or identify a bone spur.

FALSE POSITIVES

Patients may have torn ligaments, fractures, or arthritis, not just tendonitis on examination.

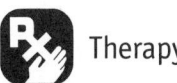 Therapy

Rest/reduced use of the affected tendon/muscle group is essential, occasionally requiring splinting

PT/OT

Either self-directed or formal help with resumption of desired activity, through gentle range of motion exercises against low resistance and advanced as tolerated

DRUGS

Nonsteroidal antiinflammatory drugs; rarely do soft tissue steroid injections have a role in children.

DURATION

1 to 4 weeks

 Follow-Up

WHEN TO EXPECT IMPROVEMENT

Improvement often takes 2 to 6 weeks.

SIGNS TO WATCH FOR

If the provocative activity is resumed too soon, the irritation will recur.

PROGNOSIS

Usually good for children; however, many will suffer recurrences if proper exercises before desired activity are not continued.

PITFALLS

Overdiagnosis in young children, in whom overuse is rare and other diagnoses should be considered; underdiagnosis in older children in whom repetitive activities are likely to occur

 Common Questions and Answers

Q: Which activities can result in overuse syndromes and tendonitis?
A: Virtually any repetitive activity in which children engage can cause tendonitis. For example, pain in the tendons of the thumb has occurred in children overusing video games.

ICD-9-CM 726.90

BIBLIOGRAPHY

Athreya BH, Cheh ML, Kingsland LC 3rd. Computer assisted diagnosis of pediatric rheumatic disease. *Pediatrics* 1998;102(4): E48.

Marsh JS, Daigneault JP. Ankle injuries in the pediatric population. *Curr Opin Pediatr* 2000;12(1):52–60.

Micheli LJ, Fehlandt AF. Overuse injuries to tendons and apophyses in children and adolescents. *Clin Sports Med* 1992;11: 713–726.

Authors: Randy Q. Cron
Gregory F. Keenan, 2nd edition

Teratoma

 Database

DEFINITION

An embryonal neoplasm that contains tissue derived from all three germ layers (endoderm, mesoderm, and ectoderm). Teratomas are mature or immature and may occur with or without malignant elements. They are a subset of the broader class of germ cell tumors.

PATHOPHYSIOLOGY

- Abnormal migration of germ cells at about the 6th week of embryonal development, causing germ cells to come to rest outside the gonads.
- Mature teratoma: contains well-differentiated, nonmitotic tissues from all three germ layers, such as squamous epithelium, neuronal tissue, muscle, teeth, cartilage, bone, gastrointestinal, and respiratory tract linings.
- Immature teratoma: contains only immature embryonic components of the three germinal layers. Divided histologically into four grades, 0 to 3, dependent on immature elements and mitotic activity.
- Teratoma with malignant germ cell elements: foci of malignant tissue that resemble other germ cell tumors such as embryonal carcinoma, endodermal sinus tumor, and choriocarcinoma, in addition to mature or immature tissues.

EPIDEMIOLOGY

- Germ cell tumors account for approximately 3% of childhood malignancies (<15 years) and 15% of malignancies of ages 15 to 19 years.
- Incidence of germ cell tumors as a whole is approximately 2.5 per million in Caucasian children and 3.0 per million in African-American children under 15 years of age.
- Males and females are equally affected.
- One suggestive epidemiologic association is with high maternal hormone levels during pregnancy.
- More controversial associations include younger gestational age; viral infections including HSV, VZV, CMV, mumps; other congenital anomalies; maternal UTI or tuberculosis; paternal occupation in chemical industries.
- Sacrococcygeal tumors: Most prevalent in infants; females more frequently affected
- Testicular and ovarian tumors: most prevalent in infants and adolescents
- Vaginal tumors: most prevalent in girls under age 3 years
- Mediastinal tumors: average age of the pediatric patient is 3 years, but also found in adolescents; most common extragonadal germ cell tumor in adults

GENETICS

- Most consistent (80% of germ cell tumors) structural chromosomal abnormality is an isochromosome 12p [i(12p)]
- No pattern of inheritance is known.

 Differential Diagnosis

- Sacrococcygeal: pilonidal cyst, meningocele, lipomeningocele, hemangioma, abscess, bone tumor, epidermal cyst, chondroma, lymphoma, ependymoma, neuroblastoma, glioma
- Abdominal: Wilms tumor, neuroblastoma, lymphoma, rhabdomyosarcoma, hepatoblastoma, retained twin fetus
- Vaginal: rhabdomyosarcoma (sarcoma botryoides), clear cell carcinoma
- Ovarian: cyst, appendicitis, pregnancy, pelvic infection, hematocolpos, sarcoma, lymphoma, other ovarian tumors
- Testicular: epididymitis, testicular torsion, infarct, orchitis, hernia, hydrocele, hematocele, rhabdomyosarcoma, lymphoma, leukemia, other testicular tumors
- Mediastinal: Hodgkin and non-Hodgkin lymphoma, leukemia, thymoma

 Data Gathering

HISTORY

Question: External mass, constipation, urinary abnormalities, lower extremity weakness?
Significance: Sacrococcygeal mass may impinge on nerve structures. Anterior sacrococcygeal mass may have no external component.

Question: Cough, wheeze, dyspnea, hemoptysis, SVC syndrome?
Significance: Suggests anterior mediastinal mass

Question: Blood-tinged vaginal discharge?
Significance: Vaginal teratoma

Question: Abdominal pain, nausea, vomiting, constipation, urinary tract symptoms?
Significance: Ovarian tumors present late with a large mass.

Question: Painless scrotal swelling or painful testicular torsion?
Significance: Testicular mass may be teratoma

Question: Cryptorchidism?
Significance: Associated with germ cell tumors in boys

 Physical Examination

Finding: Palpable mass either externally or internally, signs of spinal cord compression?
Significance: Sacrococcygeal tumor

Finding: Vaginoscopy reveals a polyploid lesion arising from the vaginal wall?
Significance: Examination under anesthesia usually necessary

Finding: Palpable abdominal mass, peritoneal symptoms?
Significance: Ovarian mass may be large

Finding: Palpable mass in scrotum?
Significance: Testicular origin

Finding: Decreased breath sounds, consolidation, wheezing, SVC syndrome?
Significance: Mediastinal mass may be an emergency

Laboratory Aids

Test: Serum α-fetoprotein (AFP) and β-human chorionic gonadotropin (β-hCG)
Significance: Pure teratomas are not associated with elevated tumor markers. The elevation of either of these markers indicates the presence of more malignant germ cell elements and requires review of the histologic material.

Test: CBC and chemistry profile, with electrolytes, blood urea nitrogen, creatinine, liver function tests, uric acid, and lactate dehydrogenase
Significance: Workup to rule out other malignancies or associated organ dysfunction

IMAGING

Test: Plain x-ray
Significance: May reveal mature calcified tissues, such as bone or teeth, within the tumor

Test: Chest x-ray
Significance: Shows mediastinal mass

Test: CT scan
Significance: Necessary to evaluate the primary site and regional disease

Test: Chest CT and bone scan
Significance: If malignancy is suspected or proven, these are indicated for evaluation of metastasis.

Test: Ultrasound, if CT is not readily available
Significance: May be helpful, but it will rarely suffice as the sole imaging study of the primary site. May be first evidence of anterior sacrococcygeal mass or to differentiate testicular mass from hydrocele.

 ## Therapy

• Mature teratoma: full surgical excision, irrespective of the site, is curative.
• Immature teratoma: complete surgical resection is the therapy of choice. In cases of elevated α-fetoprotein, many suggest a short course of postoperative adjuvant chemotherapy.
• Teratoma with malignant components: surgery plus chemotherapy with etoposide, cisplatin or carboplatin, and bleomycin. Patients with residual disease should have additional surgery and additional chemotherapy if total resection not possible. Radiation is reserved for salvage therapy in recurrent disease.

 ## Follow-Up

• Serial physical exams and imaging studies of primary site
• Tumor markers (AFP or β-hCG), if elevated at diagnosis
• If chemotherapy or radiation therapy utilized, need to monitor for secondary malignancies, long term. Short term, need to monitor blood counts, chemistries, renal function, and audiology.

PREVENTION

There is no known prevention for the development of teratomas and other germ cell tumors.

PITFALLS

All that appears to be a teratoma is not. Be prepared for other malignant and nonmalignant histologies on biopsy.

 ## Common Questions and Answers

Q: What is the chance of cure for malignant teratomas?
A: With current chemotherapy as outlined above, disease-free survival is 85%.

Q: Can a benign tumor recur? If so, can it then be malignant?
A: Yes. If there is residual tissue left behind, the tumor can recur. If there were unrecognized areas of malignancy, the recurrence can be a malignant teratoma. The greatest risk for the latter is with the immature teratomas.

ICD-9-CM

Benign 186.9
Sacral 653.7

BIBLIOGRAPHY

Gobel U, Calaminus G, Engert J, et al. Teratomas in infancy and childhood. *Med Pediatr Oncol* 1998;31:8–15.

Lazar EL, Stolar CJ. Evaluation and management of pediatric solid ovarian tumors. *Semin Pediatr Surg* 1998;7:29–34.

Wagner RB. The history of mediastinal teratoma. *Chest Surg Clin North Am* 2000;10:213–222.

Walsh C, Rushton HG. Diagnosis and management of teratomas and epidermoid cysts. *Urol Clin North Am* 2000;27:509–518.

Weidner N. Germ-cell tumors of the mediastinum. *Semin Diagn Pathol* 1999;16:42–50.

Author: Jane E. Minturn
Debra L. Friedman, 2nd edition

Tetanus

Database

DEFINITION
Tetanus is a disease characterized by tonic spasms of the skeletal muscles and occasionally the glottis and larynx due to intoxication with an exotoxin tetanospasmin produced by *Clostridium tetani*.

CAUSE
• Tetanus is caused by an anaerobic, spore-forming bacterium, *C. tetani*. In anaerobic conditions, present in wounds with significant tissue damage, inoculated spores become vegetative and produce the disease-causing toxin.
• *C. tetani* is a gram-positive rod found in superficial layers of soil, especially in agricultural areas. Spores may survive in soil for months to years if not exposed to sunlight.
• *C. tetani* spores are found as part of the normal intestinal flora in many domesticated animals, rats, and humans.

PATHOPHYSIOLOGY
• Spores are inoculated into a variety of wounds when they are contaminated by soil or dust from houses or buildings. Under appropriate anaerobic conditions the spores become the vegetative bacillus and produce toxin. Anaerobic conditions in wounds are promoted by larger amounts of necrosis, the presence of foreign bodies, or other ongoing infections with suppuration.
• *C. tetani* produces two exotoxins, but only tetanospasmin is clinically important.
• Tetanospasmin is one of the most powerful exotoxins known, second in lethality only to botulinum toxin. It seems to travel from the wound site to the central nervous system (CNS) through the neurons. There may be some distribution of the toxin via the hematogenous route as well.
• The toxin may be absorbed directly into skeletal muscle adjacent to the injury and affects the motor end plates, producing sustained contractions in that area, a condition known as local tetanus.
• Once absorbed into peripheral nerves, the toxin is carried to the CNS by an as yet unclear mechanism.
• The toxin has four major effects on the nervous system. At motor end plates in skeletal muscle release of acetylcholine from neurons is inhibited. Toxin also seems to interfere with contraction and relaxation mechanisms directly. In the spinal cord action on interneurons leads to inhibition of antagonist mechanisms and uncontrolled muscle spasms result. In the brain there is also an inhibition of antagonist mechanisms leading to uncontrolled spasms. The toxin also binds to receptors in the medullary center and can lead to direct respiratory depression. Finally, the sympathetic nervous system seems to be affected, leading to profuse sweating, vasoconstriction, labile hypertension, tachycardia, and dysrhythmias, and later hypotension.
• Tetanospasmin does not seem to affect cognitive processes directly. "Tetanic seizures" are actually uncontrolled, generalized tetanic muscle spasms.
• The toxin binds irreversibly to neurons and resolution occurs slowly over 2 to 4 weeks.
• Secondary complications may be associated with findings including pneumonia (often secondary to aspiration), pulmonary hemorrhage, CNS hemorrhage, and fractures, including vertebral body compressions related to the severe tetanic spasms.

EPIDEMIOLOGY
• Tetanus, especially neonatal tetanus, remains a major problem in developing countries but is rare in the developed world because of widespread immunization. In the United States, there are 50 to 200 cases reported annually including occasional cases of neonatal tetanus. Most cases are among the elderly but unimmunized children are also at risk. Rare cases have been reported in patients with seemingly protective levels of antitetanus antibodies.
• About two thirds of cases in the United States occur between May and November. People from rural areas and who are involved in agriculture are more likely to have contact with the organisms, although many cases are reported among intravenous drug abusers. In the United States, there have been cases reported in patients after body piercing.

COMPLICATIONS
• Most complications are related to the severe tetanic muscle contractions experienced by these patients.
• Severe spasm of the paraspinal muscles has led to compression fractures of vertebral bodies. Other bones may be broken as well, and muscle hemorrhages are not uncommon. Spasm of the chest wall as well as laryngospasm may precipitate respiratory failure and arrest. Spasms cause severe pain for patients.
• Spasms also cause dysphagia, hydrophobia, neck stiffness, and urinary retention.
• Repeated or continuous spasms may lead to elevations in body temperature.
• Cerebrovascular hemorrhages may be seen in rare cases, especially in neonatal tetanus.
• Pneumonia, including aspiration, may be a complication.

PROGNOSIS
• With advances in the ability to provide respiratory support in an intensive care setting, the prognosis has improved significantly. Overall mortality rates have decreased from approximately 66% in the 1950s in the United States to 30% in the 1980s.
• Children and young adults have a much better prognosis than older individuals.
• In developing nations, mortality rates remain very high, reflecting an inability to provide technologically advanced tertiary care.
• A more rapid onset of disease and a more rapid progression from trismus to generalized spasms is associated with a more severe course.
• In the absence of complications, recovery is usually complete in survivors without long-term sequelae.
• Signs and symptoms usually progress for about 1 week after presentation before reaching their worst. The patient's condition then plateaus for about 1 week and then gradually improves over 2 to 6 weeks.

Differential Diagnosis

• Infections: retropharyngeal and peritonsillar abscesses, poliomyelitis, viral encephalitis, and meningoencephalitis may present with trismus or cranial nerve findings that would suggest a diagnosis of tetanus.
• Toxin: dystonic reactions to phenothiazine medications may resemble tetanus in presentation. Diphenhydramine will effectively treat these reactions.
• Metabolic: hypocalcemia due to rickets or other disorders is usually not as severe as the tetanic contractions seen with tetanus.

Data Gathering

HISTORY
Question: Incubation period?
Significance: Usually between 3 and 21 days. Cases have been reported with shorter periods, and at times it may be as long as several months. Sites of inoculation farther from the CNS are associated with longer incubation periods.
Question: Pain?
Significance: Local tetanus is associated with painful muscle contractions and stiffness limited to the area near the wound. This may persist for several weeks and resolve, or it may progress to generalized tetanus.
Question: Trismus?
Significance: The classic initial complaint of trismus is seen in about half of cases. Other early complaints include dysphagia, neck pain and stiffness, stiffness and pain in other muscle groups, urinary retention, restlessness, irritability, and headache.
Question: Progression of symptoms?
Significance: Usually occur over the first week but may progress more rapidly.
Question: Neonatal tetanus?
Significance: Usually complicates deliveries where aseptic conditions were not maintained, and the mother is either unimmunized or not up to date in her immunization status.

Physical Examination

Finding: Initial presenting sign is usually trismus.
Significance: Persistent trismus gives rise to the classic sardonic smile (wrinkling of the forehead and distortion of the eyebrows and the corners of the mouth).
Finding: Fever?
Significance: Initially, patients are usually afebrile.
Finding: As the disease progresses, other muscle groups develop tetanic contractions.
Significance: Tonic contractions of the paraspinal muscles lead to a significant opisthotonic posture. Severe spasmodic contractions, "tetanic seizures," also occur. These are extremely painful and can be associated with laryngospasm and tetany of the respiratory musculature with fatal results.
Finding: Tetanus spasms
Significance: Precipitated by a variety of stimuli including a cold draft, noise, pain, anxiety, and light touch. Because tetanus toxin does not affect the sensorium, the severe anxiety and pain associated with these spasms may precipitate additional spasms.
Finding: Tachycardia, flushing, severe and labile episodes of hypertension and tachycardia
Significance: Autonomic nervous system involvement. Hypotension may be a late feature of the disease.
Finding: Fever
Significance: With sustained contractions, fever may develop, although it may also be a result of complications including pneumonia, infected in-dwelling catheters, or infected decubiti.
Finding: Cephalic tetanus
Significance: Involves only the cranial nerves and occurs after wounds of the face, scalp, or neck. It may also complicate chronic infections of the head and neck including chronic otitis media. Loss of airway control is a frequent and often fatal complication. Cephalic tetanus may progress to generalized tetanus.

Laboratory Aids

Test: Laboratory investigations
Significance: Yield little useful information in cases of tetanus. Anaerobic wound cultures may rarely yield *C. tetani.* The WBC is usually normal or mildly elevated. CSF studies are unremarkable. EEG and EMG are nonspecific. The diagnosis is made clinically.

Emergency Care

• It is important to recognize the presentation of tetanus so that emergency care may be begun promptly.
• In the emergency department, supportive care including aggressive airway management (including tracheostomy when indicated),

ventilatory support, and pharmacologic interventions to promote sedation and muscle relaxation (e.g., diazepam) are the most important therapies.
• Treatment with tetanus immune globulin should be initiated.

Therapy

SPECIFIC

• Specific therapy is aimed at eradication of the vegetative organism and thereby the source of ongoing toxin production and neutralization of any toxin that has not already been irreversibly bound to neurons.
• Human tetanus immune globulin (TIG) should be administered in a dose of 500 to 3,000 units in three divided doses at three separate sites. Repeat doses do not seem to be indicated. Infants with neonatal tetanus should be given a dose of 250 units.
• If TIG is not available, tetanus antitoxin (TAT) may be administered if a skin test for sensitization to this equine-derived product is negative. If the skin test is positive, desensitization must be accomplished before TAT can be administered. The dose of TAT is 50,000 to 100,000 units with half given intramuscularly and half intravenously.
• Penicillin G, 200,000 U/kg/d should be given intravenously in four divided doses for 10 days. Oral tetracycline or intravenous vancomycin may be used in penicillin-sensitive individuals. Cephalosporins are not effective.
• Aggressive surgical débridement and removal of foreign bodies from the infected wound must be undertaken. If a wound is gangrenous, amputation may be considered.
• After resolution of the illness complete, active immunization is required in individuals who have tetanus.

SUPPORTIVE CARE

• Patients suspected of having tetanus should be rapidly transferred to a tertiary care center capable of providing sophisticated ventilatory and cardiovascular support in an intensive care setting. Transfer should occur early in the disease before these sophisticated techniques are necessary.
• Patients should be kept in a quiet, darkened room with minimum stimulus. Cardiac and respiratory status should be monitored closely.
• Tracheostomy may prevent fatal laryngospasm. It is preferable that this be done on a semi-emergent rather than emergent basis.
• Parenteral nutrition is usually required to maintain adequate nutrition and hydration.

DRUGS

• Diazepam should be given to promote sedation and muscle relaxation. A dose of 0.1 to 0.2 mg/kg IV every 4 to 6 hours is an appropriate initial dose. Phenothiazines, especially chlorpromazine, may be helpful if additional sedation is needed. Sedation must be titrated to desired effect and in an attempt to avoid respiratory depression. If spasms cannot be adequately controlled or if

laryngospasm or spasm of the respiratory musculature compromises ventilation, then neuromuscular blockade and mechanical ventilation should be instituted.
• Nondepolarizing neuromuscular blocking agents are usually used. Vecuronium in an initial dose of 0.1 to 0.2 mg/kg IV followed by a continuous infusion or hourly dosing intervals seems to have less cardiovascular effects than other agents.
• Beta-blockers are used as needed to manage hypertension, with propranolol in a dose of 0.01 to 0.1 mg/kg every 6 to 8 hours being a popular choice.

PREVENTION

• The mainstays of prevention are good hygiene and aggressive active immunization of all individuals. All wounds should be cleaned thoroughly with soap and water, and foreign bodies should be sought aggressively and removed.
• Tetanus prophylaxis should be initiated at the time of injury in the following manner:
—If the patient has had at least three prior doses of tetanus toxoid, no TIG should be given. A dose of tetanus toxoid should be given if it has been longer than 7 years since the last dose or if it has been longer than 5 years and the wound is considered to be dirty or tetanus-prone.
—If the patient has had fewer than three doses of tetanus toxoid, TIG should be given if the wound is considered tetanus-prone. The dose is 250 to 500 U IM. All of these patients should receive tetanus toxoid regardless of the nature of the wound.

Common Questions and Answers

Q: What is a tetanus-prone wound?
A: Deep puncture wounds, wounds causing a large amount of tissue necrosis including crushing wounds, large ragged lacerations, and wounds clearly contaminated with soil or feces are generally considered tetanus-prone. All wounds, including minor wounds such as corneal abrasions, insect bites, small lacerations, and burns, may be inoculated with spores and lead to the development of tetanus.

ICD-9-CM 037.0

BIBLIOGRAPHY
Abrahamian FM, Pollack CV Jr, LoVecchio F, et al. Fatal tetanus in a drug abuser with protective antitetanus antibodies. *J Emerg Med* 2000;18(2):189–193.

Dyce O, Bruno JR, Hong D, et al. Tongue piercing: the new "rusty nail"? *Head Neck* 2000;22(7):728–732.

Loscalzo IL, Ryan J, Loscalzo J, et al. Tetanus: a clinical diagnosis. *Am J Emerg Med* 1995;13:488–490.

Thayaparan B, Nicoll A. Prevention and control of tetanus in childhood. *Curr Opin Pediatr* 1998;10(1):4–8.

Author: James M. Callahan

Tetralogy of Fallot (TOF)

 Database

DEFINITION

• Anatomic hallmark is anterior malalignment of infundibular septum:

—A large and unrestrictive ventricular septal defect (VSD)
—Various degrees of right ventricular outflow tract obstruction (RVOTO)
—Overriding aorta
—(Resultant) right ventricular hypertrophy (RVH)

PATHOPHYSIOLOGY

Severity of clinical signs and symptoms are dependent on the degree of RVOTO and related right-to-left shunt.

GENETICS

• Some TOFs are associated with a chromosome 22q11 microdeletion.
• May be associated with other syndromes including Down, fetal alcohol, and a variety of limb abnormality syndromes. TOF may also be associated with midline abdominal defects (e.g., omphalocele).

EPIDEMIOLOGY

3.5% to 8% of all CHD

COMPLICATIONS

• Paroxysmal hypoxic spells (hypercyanotic spells a.k.a. "tet spell")
• Bacterial endocarditis
• Cerebrovascular accident (CVA) secondary to cyanosis, polycythemia, and microcytic anemia
• Right ventricular dysfunction and ventricular arrhythmia
• Postoperative sudden death (ventricular arrhythmias and/or complete heart block)

PROGNOSIS

• Generally good if treated surgically in a timely manner
• More than 85% of patients with TOF are expected to survive to adulthood.

 Differential Diagnosis

TOF should be considered in all infants with heart murmur and/or various degrees of cyanosis and otherwise acyanotic infants or children with history of hypercyanotic spells.

 Data Gathering

HISTORY

• Heart murmur in the newborn period
• Various degrees of progressive cyanosis
• History of paroxysmal cyanosis especially when crying or with exercise

 Physical Examination

• Various degrees of cyanosis may be present at birth or may appear later during infancy or childhood as a result of progression of the pulmonary stenosis.
• Normal S_1 and single loud S_2 secondary to a more anteriorly located aorta
• Systolic ejection murmur at left upper sternal border secondary to RVOTO

 Laboratory Aids

Test: ECG
Significance: Right axis deviation (+90 to 180 degrees), RVH

IMAGING

Test: CXR
Significance: Right aortic arch (30%), decreased pulmonary vascular markings, boot-shaped heart ("coeur en sabot") with concave main pulmonary artery segment

Test: Echocardiogram
Significance: Anterior malalignment type VSD, presence of other VSDs, degree of infundibular stenosis, presence of valvar pulmonary stenosis and/or branch pulmonary artery stenosis, overriding aorta, arch sidedness, coronary artery anatomy

Test: Cardiac catheterization
Significance: Presence of multiple VSDs (other than single malalignment type VSD), degree and levels of stenosis in the RVOT and pulmonary arteries, arch sidedness, coronary artery anatomy

Therapy

MEDICAL

- Hypercyanotic spells:

—Knee-chest position
—Oxygen
—Morphine sulfate (0.1 mg/kg IV or IM)
—Intravenous fluid bolus and/or NaHCO$_3$
—Beta-blocker
—Phenylephrine (0.02 mg/kg IV)
—Polycythemia: oral Fe supplement
—SBE prophylaxis

SURGICAL

- Palliative surgery: Blalock-Taussig shunt
- Corrective surgery: VSD patch closure and RVOT reconstruction

 Follow-Up

PROGNOSIS

- Surgical mortality is quite low in most centers
- Residual hemodynamic abnormalities are quite common:

—Pulmonary insufficiency (with transannular patch repair)
—Residual RVOTO right ventricular outlet track obstruction
—RV dysfunction
—Left pulmonary artery stenosis
—Residual VSD

- Conduction abnormalities (complete heart block)
- Supraventricular and ventricular arrhythmias

 Common Questions and Answers

Q: What is the etiology of the "tet spell"?
A: There is an increase in obstruction/vasospasm of the RVOT and/or pulmonary vascular bed that leads to a dramatic decrease in pulmonary blood flow and increased right-to-left shunt at the level of the VSD. Therefore, treatment should be aimed at increasing pulmonary blood flow either by decreasing pulmonary vascular resistance (O$_2$, morphine) or increasing systemic vascular resistance (knee-chest position, phenylephrine).

Q: When is an optimal time for elective surgical repair of TOF?
A: Still controversial. At Children's Hospital of Philadelphia, we recommend elective repair of TOF in early infancy (3–6 months).

ICD-9-CM 745.2

BIBLIOGRAPHY

Neches WH, Park SC, Ettedgui JA. Pediatric cardiology. In: *Tetralogy of Fallot and tetralogy of Fallot with pulmonary atresia.* Philadelphia: Lea & Febiger, 1990:1073–1100.

Rosenthal A. Adults with tetralogy of Fallot: repaired, yes; cured, no. *N Engl J Med* 1993;329:355–356.

Walsh EP, Rockenmacher S, Keane JF, et al. Late results in patients with tetralogy of Fallot repaired during infancy. *Circulation* 1988;77:1062–1067.

Zuberbuhler JR. *Moss and Adams: Heart diseases in infants, children and adolescents,* 5th ed. Baltimore: Williams & Wilkins, 1995:998–1017.

Author: Pamela S. Ro

Thalassemia

Database

DEFINITION

- Thalassemia syndromes are hereditary microcytic anemias occurring as a result of mutations that quantitatively reduce globin synthesis.
- Normal hemoglobin is a tetramer of two α and two β chains.

—α-Thalassemia: decrease or lack of α globin synthesis
—β-Thalassemia: decrease or lack of β globin synthesis

PATHOPHYSIOLOGY

- Decrease in either α- or β-globin synthesis leads to fewer completed $\alpha_2\beta_2$ tetramers produced per red cell, which results in a decrease in intracellular hemoglobin and microcytosis.
- Unpaired globin chains lead to ineffective erythropoiesis.
- The red cell life span is shortened as a result of hemolysis and splenic sequestration.
- Varying degrees of anemia depending on gene defect.

GENETICS

- α-Thalassemia

—Each diploid cell normally has four α-globin genes, two on each chromosome 16.
—Some mutations completely abolish the expression of an α-globin gene (α^0).
—Other mutations decrease the expression of α-globin gene (α^+).
—The four α-thalassemia syndromes reflect the inheritance of molecular defects affecting the output of one, two, three, or four α genes. See table Alpha Thalassemia Syndromes.

- β-Thalassemia

—Each diploid cell normally has two β-globin genes, one on each chromosome 11.
—Many mutations abolish the expression completely (β^0), while others cause variable decrease in quantitative expression (β^+).
—Heterozygous state for β-globin mutation produces β-thalassemia trait.
—Homozygous state produces β-thalassemia major (β^0) or thalassemia intermedia (β^+).

CLINICAL CLASSIFICATION

EPIDEMIOLOGY

- α-Thalassemia

—Predominantly in Chinese subcontinent, Malaysia, Indochina, and Africa, and African-American population.

- β-Thalassemia

—Mediterranean countries, Africa, India, Pakistan, Mideast, and China.

COMPLICATIONS

Most complications occur in patients with homozygous β-thalassemia. They include:

- Skeletal abnormalities secondary to hyperplastic marrow
- Growth retardation
- Congestive heart failure due to severe anemia
- Postsplenectomy sepsis
- Gallstones
- Well-transfused patients will develop iron overload if not chelated which can lead to:

—Endocrine disturbances: delayed puberty, growth retardation, diabetes mellitus, hypothyroidism, hypoparathyroidism
—Cardiac abnormalities: pericarditis, arrhythmias, congestive heart failure (young adults)
—Hepatic abnormalities: cirrhosis and liver failure (onset after second decade usually)

PROGNOSIS

- Life expectancy has improved over the years with regular transfusions and chelation therapy
- Bone marrow transplant from a histocompatible sibling donor may be curative.

Differential Diagnosis

- Differential includes other microcytic anemias

—Iron deficiency anemia—can be determined with Fe studies
—Anemia of chronic disease

Data Gathering

HISTORY

Question: Age of onset?
Significance: Severe α- or β-thalassemia is symptomatic within first year of life.

Question: Mediterranean, African, or Asian descent?
Significance: Common ethnic background in thalassemia

Question: Familial history of anemia or chronic transfusions?
Significance: Siblings and/or parents may be affected.

Physical Examination

Finding: Pallor
Significance: Indicates anemia

Finding: Heart murmur
Significance: Flow murmurs are often heard in significant anemia. Patients with severe anemia may present with congestive heart failure.

Finding: Variable degrees of icterus
Significance: Hemolysis is part of thalassemia.

Finding: Abnormal facies (frontal bossing)
Significance: Facial bone expansion by hypertrophic marrow in poorly transfused patients with β-thalassemia

Finding: Failure to thrive
Significance: Related to anemia and energy expended in ineffective erythropoiesis

Finding: Variable degrees of hepatosplenomegaly
Significance: Extramedullary hematopoiesis

Alpha Thalassemia Syndromes

SYNDROME	CLINICAL FEATURES	α-GLOBIN GENES AFFECTED
Silent carrier	No anemia, normal CBC	1
α-Thalassemia trait	Mild microcytic anemia, usually asymptomatic	2
HbH disease	Moderate microcytic anemia, splenomegaly	3
Hydrops fetalis	Death *in utero* due to severe anemia	4

Laboratory Aids

- CBC with RBC indices

—MCV, MCH, and MCHC are decreased in both α- and β-thalassemia

- RDW is usually normal
- Peripheral smear may reveal microcytosis, hypochromia, anisocytosis, poikilocytosis, target cells, nucleated red cells, polychromasia
- Hb 9 to 12 g/dL in α- or β-thalassemia trait
- Hb usually 6 to 10 g/dL in HbH disease
- Hb usually 7 to 10 g/dL in thalassemia intermedia
- Hb less than 5 g/dL in thalassemia major
- Reticulocyte count

—Usually elevated in HbH and β-thalassemia intermedia and major

- Indirect bilirubin

—May be elevated in severe thalassemia where there is significant red cell destruction

- Hemoglobin electrophoresis

—α-Thalassemia trait (two defective genes) will have 5% to 10% Hb Bart's (a tetramer of four γ chains) at birth, which should be detected on the newborn screen. This disappears in 1 to 2 months, after which the electrophoresis will be normal in α-thalassemia trait.
—β-thalassemia trait: HbF 1% to 5%, HbA₂ 3.5% to 8%, remainder HbA. The elevated HbA2 will distinguish α- from β-thalassemia trait.
—HbH disease (three defective α genes): 5% to 30% HbH (β four), remainder HbA.
—Hydrops fetalis (four defective α genes): mainly Hb Bart's.
—Thalassemia major (two defective β genes): HbF 20% to 100%, HbA₂ 2% to 7%, HbA 0% to 80%. In most cases no HbA is detected.

- Iron studies, serum ferritin

—Useful to help distinguish thalassemia from iron deficiency

 ## Therapy

- Silent carriers α- and β-thalassemia trait: genetic counseling only
- HbH disease

—Folic acid daily
—Transfusions whenever necessary
—Splenectomy if evidence of hypersplenism
—Cholecystectomy if necessary

- Homozygous β-thalassemia

—Regular transfusions of red cells every 3 to 4 weeks to maintain Hb at 9 to 10 g/dL
—Chelation therapy with desferrioxamine to avoid iron overload
—Splenectomy if transfusion requirement more than 200 mL/kg/y
—Folic acid daily
—Penicillin prophylaxis (125–250 mg b.i.d.) for all splenectomized patients
—Pneumococcal and *Haemophilus influenzae* vaccine prior to splenectomy
—Cholecystectomy if indicated
—No iron supplements
—Genetic counseling
—Bone marrow transplantation using histocompatible sibling donor can cure the disease and is being increasingly utilized.

 ## Follow-Up

Transfusion-dependent patients need to be transfused every 3 to 4 weeks. In these patients serum ferritin and liver function tests should be done every 3 months. Liver biopsy may be needed to assess the status of iron overload.

PREVENTION

Thalassemia can be prevented by identifying and counseling potential parents who can have children with thalassemia. Diagnosis can be made in early pregnancy by chorionic villus sampling.

PITFALLS

Thalassemia trait is often treated presumptively as iron deficiency anemia. Iron studies should be done to confirm the diagnosis if there is no improvement in hemoglobin level after a few weeks of iron therapy.

 ## Common Questions and Answers

Q: Is prenatal testing available?
A: Yes.

Q: In a transfused patient, when does iron overload become a problem and when is chelation started?
A: Usually after the age of 5 years

ICD-9-CM 282.4

BIBLIOGRAPHY

Giardina PJ, Hilgartner MW. Update on thalassemia. *Pediatr Rev* 1992;13(2):55–62.

Giardini C. Treatment of beta-thalassemia. *Curr Opin Hematol* 1997;4(2):79–87.

Piomelli S. Management of thalassemia major (Cooley's anemia). *Semin Hematol* 1995;32(2):262–268.

Piomelli S, Loew T. The management of patients with Cooley's anemia: transfusions and splenectomy. *Hematol Oncol Clin North Am* 1991;5(3):557–569.

Weatherall DJ. The hereditary anaemias. *BMJ* 1997;314:492–496.

Author: Leslie Raffini
Sadhna M. Shankar, 2nd edition.

Tick Fever

Database

DEFINITION

• Relapsing fever in its endemic form is a vector-borne infection with characteristic recurrent fevers caused by several species of spirochetes of the genus *Borrelia*. In the United States the vector for endemic relapsing fever are ticks of the genus *Ornithodoros*. Epidemic relapsing fever is transmitted by the body louse and is no longer found in the United States.
• Colorado tick fever (CTF) is a febrile, usually benign, systemic illness caused by an arbovirus in the family Reoviridae and transmitted by ticks in the genus *Dermatocentor*.

CAUSES

• Relapsing fever is caused by several spirochetes in the genus *Borrelia* including *B. hermsii, B. parkerii,* and *B. turicatae.* Epidemic relapsing fever (louse-borne) is caused by *B. recurrentis.*
• Colorado tick fever is caused by an arbovirus in the family Reoviridae.

PATHOPHYSIOLOGY

• Endemic relapsing fever is characterized by repeated episodes of spirochetemia.
• *Borreliae* are able to undergo plasmid-mediated, antigenic variation. An antibody response against a particular strain leads to immobilization, opsonization, agglutination, and phagocytosis, and symptoms abate. The infecting organism can then again undergo antigenic variation and a recurrent episode of spirochetemia and symptoms occurs. Tick-borne disease may relapse 10 to 12 times before final resolution.
• Transmission of the infecting organism occurs when ticks of the genus *Ornithodoros* take blood meals and then detach themselves. These bites are usually painless, and the tick may remain attached for up to 15 minutes. Ticks are maintained by intermediate hosts including rodents and other small mammals.
• When a tick feeds on an infected individual, spirochetes invade all tissues including the female genital tract. Once infected, ticks remain capable of transmitting disease for many years. In addition, transovarial infection of offspring leads to increased transmission of spirochetes and increased survival.

• In the human host, organisms persist in the central nervous system (CNS), bone marrow, liver, and spleen during remissions. Pathologic findings in humans include petechial hemorrhages on visceral surfaces, hepatosplenomegaly, and a histiocytic myocarditis.
• Pneumonia, CNS hemorrhages, meningitis, disseminated intravascular coagulation (DIC), splenic rupture, hepatic coma, and dysrhythmias may result. Spirochetes may cross the placenta and lead to spontaneous abortion or severe infection in neonates.
• CTF is acquired when infected, adult ticks of the genus *Dermatocentor* (including *D. andersonii,* the wood tick) attach and ingest a blood meal from a human host instead of porcupines, elk, marmot, or deer (usual hosts).
• Ticks are infected while larvae as they feed on viremic, intermediate hosts such as chipmunks and ground squirrels.
• Aseptic meningitis, encephalitis, myocarditis, atypical pneumonia, epididymo-orchitis, and hepatitis have been reported. Generalized hemorrhage and death have been rarely reported in children. Granulocytopenia and thrombocytopenia are often seen.

EPIDEMIOLOGY

• Endemic relapsing fever occurs in the United States among people who are exposed to the habitat of the ticks that serve as vectors. In the U.S., most cases are found in the West among people who have spent time in old summer cabins in forested mountain areas. In several series, cabins that were found to be the source of cases contained large rodent nests with infected ticks in them.
• Colorado tick fever is also found among humans who travel to a location where the vector (ticks of the genus *Dermacentor*) is found. The wood tick is found in the Rocky Mountains and western Black Hills at elevations of 4,000 to 10,000 feet. Cases usually occur between April and July when adult ticks are most active. Cases have been reported as early as March and as late as November. Most cases are reported in males, and two thirds of cases are reported in individuals between the ages of 10 and 49 years.

COMPLICATIONS

• Relapsing fever may be associated with hepatosplenomegaly with necrotic foci. Diffuse histiocytic interstitial myocarditis may be associated with dysrhythmias. Pneumonia, CNS hemorrhages, splenic rupture, meningitis, DIC, hepatitis, and hepatic coma may result. *In utero* infection may result in fetal loss or severe neonatal infection.
• Treatment may be associated with a marked Jarisch-Herxheimer reaction, which may require intravenous fluids and other supportive measures.
• CTF may lead to aseptic meningitis, encephalitis, myocarditis, atypical pneumonia, hepatitis, and epididymo-orchitis. A prolonged convalescence with persistent lassitude, fatigability, headache, musculo-skeletal pain, and fevers may persist for weeks to months in patients who experience persistent viremia.

PROGNOSIS

• Relapsing fever generally responds rapidly to appropriate antibiotic therapy and leaves no significant sequelae. Even when untreated, the vast majority of cases are benign and self-limited. Louse-borne, epidemic relapsing fever in developing countries has been associated with mortality rates of up to 40%.
• CTF resolves without sequelae in most patients. Symptoms may persist for at least 3 weeks in a majority of patients. Patients older than 30 years are at a much greater risk of developing prolonged symptoms. Infection usually leads to permanent immunity.

Differential Diagnosis

• Relapsing fever and CTF resemble each other clinically, but leukopenia is more often seen with CTF. Exposure to ticks or a history of travel to an area where appropriate vectors are found is a helpful clue in diagnosing either disease.
• Relapsing fever and CTF may be misdiagnosed as influenza or enteroviral infections.
• Spirochetes may be seen on peripheral blood smears in cases of relapsing fever.

Data Gathering

HISTORY

Question: Fever?
Significance: Endemic relapsing fever has a sudden onset of high fever after an incubation period of 5 to 11 days. Patients complain of chills, headache, and myalgias. Symptoms resolve after 3 to 6 days but then recur within several days. Repeated recurrences continue with decreasing severity and lengthening periods of lack of symptoms. CTF has a usual incubation period of 4 days (range, 1–14 days). There is a history of tick exposure in 90% of patients. Patients complain of abrupt onset of fever, chills, fatigue, headache, myalgias, photophobia, and stiff neck.

Question: Headache?
Significance: Patients may complain of headache, photophobia, stiff neck, and rash, which usually begins on the trunk. There may be epistaxis.

Question: Other symptoms of CTF?
Significance: Gastrointestinal symptoms, pharyngitis, and rash may be noted by some patients.

Question: How long do symptoms of CTF last?
Significance: In about half of patients symptoms resolve after 2 to 4 days and then recur after 1 to 3 days. Symptoms then last for another 2 to 3 days. Some patients will have a third symptomatic period, whereas others will only have the initial symptomatic period.

 ## Physical Examination

Finding: High fever
Significance: Relapsing patients have high fevers (39°–41°C).

Finding: Tender hepatosplenomegaly
Significance: Characteristic of relapsing fever

Finding: A macular rash
Significance: May be seen on the trunk in approximately 10% of cases, but it may fade quickly or become generalized or petechial.

Finding: Meningismus and signs of iridocyclitis
Significance: May be seen

Finding: CTF
Significance: Patients with CTF have mostly nonspecific findings. There are often signs of CNS involvement or meningismus. Myalgias and muscle tenderness are usually seen.

 ## Laboratory Aids

Test: Peripheral blood smear
Significance: In relapsing fever the diagnosis is often made when spirochetes are noted on a peripheral blood smear. Increased sensitivity can be obtained by examining dehemoglobinized thick smears or buffy coat preparations.

Test: Weil-Felix agglutination tests
Significance: May be positive but are nonspecific. Indirect fluorescent antibody tests are more sensitive but may be falsely positive in cases of Lyme disease.

Test: Specific test for relapsing fever
Significance: Intraperitoneal inoculation of immature laboratory mice with infected blood leads to spirochetemia in the mice and is a specific and sensitive diagnostic tool.

Test: Nonspecific laboratory findings
Significance: Include thrombocytopenia, hyperbilirubinemia, and elevated hepatic transaminases

Test: Electrocardiograms and chest roentgenogram
Significance: Should be performed to exclude the possibility of myocarditis

Test: Diagnostic test for CTF
Significance: May be confirmed by serologic testing, immunofluorescence testing for viral antigens on the surface of red blood cells, or by viral culture

Test: Associated laboratory findings in CTF
Significance: Include leukopenia and thrombocytopenia. Initially, both granulocytopenia and lymphopenia occur. Lymphopenia resolves first, and an atypical lymphocytosis may occur.

Test: CSF studies in CTF
Significance: Pleocytosis may be found, especially in children.

 ## Therapy

DRUGS

• Endemic relapsing fever may be treated with oral tetracycline (in patients older than 8 years of age) or erythromycin at doses of 40 mg/kg/d in four divided doses for 10 days.
• Patients who are symptomatic at the time treatment is begun are at significant risk of developing the Jarisch-Herxheimer reaction (severe fevers, rigors, sweating, hypotension, and prostration) related to rapid clearing of the spirochetemia. In symptomatic patients it is suggested that treatment is initiated with a single dose of oral phenoxymethyl penicillin (7.5 mg/kg) or intravenous penicillin G (10,000 U/kg given over 30 minutes). These therapies should lead to a slower clearing of the organisms and a less severe reaction.
• Close observation, intravenous fluids, and good supportive care are important in treating possible reactions.
• When the patient is afebrile, a course of tetracycline or erythromycin should be completed to prevent relapse, which has been associated with the use of penicillin alone.
• There is no specific therapy for patients with CTF. Good supportive care is usually all that is required.

PREVENTION

• Both of these diseases can be prevented by avoidance or elimination of the vector.
• Dwellings should be made of rodent-proof construction. Rodent-nesting materials should be removed from buildings where this is not possible.
• Light-colored, long-sleeved shirts, and long trousers with legs tucked inside of one's socks should be worn when infested areas cannot be avoided. Persons should inspect themselves and each other frequently for adherent ticks.
• Confirmed cases should be reported to health authorities so control measures can be instituted.

ICD-9-CM 066.1

BIBLIOGRAPHY

Boyer KM. Borrelia: relapsing fever. In: Feigin RD, Cherry JD, eds. *Textbook of pediatric infectious disease*, 3rd ed. Philadelphia: WB Saunders, 1992:1058–1062.

Doan-Wiggins L. Tick-borne diseases. *Emerg Med Clin North Am* 1991;9:303–325.

Tsai TF. Arboviral infections in the United States. *Infect Dis Clin North Am* 1991;5:73–102.

Author: James M. Callahan

Tics

Database

DEFINITION

Tics are rapid, irregular stereotyped movement (motor tics) or vocalizations (vocal tics) that are under partial voluntary control. The movements usually involve the muscles of the face, neck, and shoulder. Tics are often (but not always) brought on by stress and excitement. They typically occur in clusters, and they can be simple or complex. Simple motor tics are blinking; grimacing; neck, arm, or leg jerking; shoulder shrugging; etc. Simple vocal tics include coughing, grunting, barking, yelping, etc. Complex motor tics include jumping, smelling objects, shaking wrists, copropraxia, and echopraxia. Complex vocal tics include coprolalia, echolalia, and neologism.

• Gilles de la Tourette syndrome (GTS) is defined as a condition of chronic vocal and motor tics of more than 1 year's duration.
• Typical onset in childhood with motor tics followed by vocalizations (grunts, snorts, barks); later in adolescence 50% to 60% develop coprolalia and echolalia. Obsessive-compulsive behavior, attention deficits, learning disabilities, and sleep disorders are also frequently seen.
• The natural history of GTS is exacerbation of tics in adolescence, but 80% of children improve as they reach adulthood. The lifetime prevalence in GTS has been estimated to be between 0.1 and 1.0 in 1,000.

PATHOPHYSIOLOGY

• The pathophysiology of tics or GTS is not known.
• Most theories regarding GTS have implicated abnormalities in central dopaminergic transmission, but other neurotransmitters such as serotonin and norepinephrine as well as sex hormones have been implicated.

GENETICS

No single gene has been associated with tics or GTS. However, tics are frequently seen in families and GTS may be transmitted as an autosomal-dominant trait.

EPIDEMIOLOGY

• Tics can occur in any age group from 2 years up.
• Simple motor tics are considered a part of normal development and occur in 10% to 20% of all school-aged children.
• There is no gender or race preference.
• The average age of onset is 7 years.

COMPLICATIONS

• Tics are usually harmless. However, patients with complex motor tics that persist for years may develop repetitive motion injuries with arthritic changes of the neck and spine, resulting in increased risk of radiculopathy, disc herniation, and myelopathy.
• Children with tics and particularly GTS are often teased by their peers and have difficulty with social adjustments, isolation, and depression. Comorbid learning difficulties may also contribute to these problems.

PROGNOSIS

Most children outgrow their tics within a year. If the tics last longer than 1 year they may remain as a simple tic disorder or develop into GTS.

Differential Diagnosis

• Movements resembling tics include:

—Hemifacial spasm: a spastic contraction of one-half the muscles of the face. Frequency varies from occasional to constant, but the spasm usually lasts longer than a tic. Spasm results from:
  —Abnormal activity in the facial nerve
  —Aberrant regeneration after a Bell palsy
  —Arteriovenous malformation
  —Aneurysms
  —Brainstem or posterior fossa tumors
  —Idiopathic

—Myoclonus: may be difficult to differentiate as this movement can be very fast
—Myokymia: fine repetitive, arrhythmic twitching of muscle bundles around eyes and lips; benign and common, although severe myokymia can be seen in posterior fossa tumors, Guillain-Barré syndrome, and severe multiple sclerosis (MS).
—Paroxysmal dyskinesia: often familial, movement is more sustained and complex, may be triggered by movement
—Partial epilepsy: may look like a tic disorder, but there is no voluntary control; EEG may show corresponding abnormalities
—Tremors: simple tics can resemble tremor; tics are more variable and lack the oscillatory appearance of tremor.
—Sleep myoclonus: tics do not occur during sleep; erratic movements during sleep are most commonly benign sleep myoclonus.

Data Gathering

HISTORY

Good record-keeping helps to adjust medication appropriately.

• When did the first tic occur?
• What exacerbates and alleviates the tics?
• History of vocal tics (including throat-clearing, coughing, grunting, sniffing)?
• Is there some degree of voluntary control?
• Have the tics changed in character?
• Is there any other associated behavior in the child, e.g., attention deficit/hyperactivity disorder, obsessive-compulsive disorder, sleep disorders?
• Does anyone else in the family have tics?

Physical Examination

• General and neurologic examinations are unrevealing. Spontaneous movements or vocalizations may be absent during the visit.
• Often the child can reproduce the tic at will.

Laboratory Aids

Because tics are generally not a symptom of an underlying brain disorder, laboratory testing is usually not indicated.

Test: MRI of the brain
Significance: Not necessarily indicated, but should be normal

Test: EEG
Significance: May be helpful if there is a concern of partial seizures

Test: Psychological testing
Significance: May be the most useful ancillary assessment (if any testing is to be done) because of high incidence of associated learning disabilities, attention deficit/hyperactivity disorder, obsessive-compulsive disorder

Tics

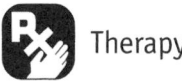 Therapy

Decision to treat is based on the severity of tics/vocalizations as reported by the child and parent. Medications are not needed in the majority of children with simple tics. Learning and attention difficulties associated with GTS may be the primary focus of attention.

- Haloperidol: started at 0.5 mg qhs and increased each week to effect. A usual maintenance dose is 1 to 3 mg/d divided b.i.d. Side effects include sedation, irritability, decreased appetite, rare neuroleptic malignant syndrome, tardive dyskinesia. Risperdal has similar pharmacodynamic properties to haloperidol and is useful in treatment of GTS but appears to have significantly fewer side effects.
- Pimozide: started at 2 mg/d divided b.i.d., increased 2 mg q week to effect. Maintenance dose is 0.2 mg/kg/d or 10 mg (whichever is less); side effects similar to haloperidol.
- Clonidine: started at 0.05 mg/d, increased 0.05 q week. Maintenance is 0.1 to 0.6 mg/d. Sedation is the main side effect; rebound hypertension is a concern if withdrawn rapidly.
- Alternatives include fluphenazine, clonazepam (primarily used as an anticonvulsant; may cause sedation), and desipramine (primarily used as an antidepressant; potential for arrhythmia).
- Clomipramine may improve associated obsessive-compulsive behavior.
- SSRIs, including fluoxetine, may be useful for tics, GTS, particularly when comorbid obsessive-compulsive symptoms are a problem.
- CNS stimulants used for attention deficits, such as Ritalin, may exacerbate tics, or be associated with onset of tics, though they do not appear to cause tic disorder per se, and are not strictly contraindicated for patients with GTS.
- Biofeedback and behavioral modification have been recommended.

 Follow-Up

The tics in GTS often become refractory to medication after prolonged use. May help to switch to another drug or to alternate between two drugs.

PREVENTION

Tics cannot be prevented. However, social isolation, adjustment difficulties, and depression can be prevented or minimized by informing teachers, sports coaches, and other caregivers of the child's condition.

PITFALLS

Avoid exclusive focus on the tics in a child: Is he or she adjusting in school? Is there a learning disability? Does he or she have friends? Are there other stressors in the family? GTS is frequently misdiagnosed—there is an approximate 10-year interval between onset of symptoms and treatment.

 Common Questions and Answers

Q: My child just started school and now she blinks excessively. When I tell her to stop it just gets worse. What can I do?
A: Tics are considered part of normal development. They can last anywhere from a few weeks to a year, and they usually disappear if you ignore them. If they last longer than a year, they are probably not a simple tic and you should contact your doctor. If there is any concern of eye irritation or a visual disturbance, an ophthalmologic checkup is appropriate.

Q: Our son has been diagnosed with GTS. His tics are increasing in frequency, and now he has developed vocalizations with obscenities. He has already lost his friends in school and was suspended twice last week because of his foul mouth. I tell him to stop but he does not listen. What should I do?
A: Children with GTS cannot control their vocalizations. Swearing is not intentional. Telling a child to control his vocalizations will only increase the level of anxiety and increase the tics. Once a child has been diagnosed with GTS (particularly if vocalizations are present), it may help to inform teachers, school personnel, and peers about the disease so that misunderstandings can be minimized and the child can feel comfortable at school. A review of medication with the child's physician (child psychiatrist or neurologist) is appropriate.

ICD-9-CM 307.20

BIBLIOGRAPHY

Anouti A, Koller WC. Diagnostic testing in movement disorders. *Neurol Clin* 1996;14(1):169–182.

Coats DK, Paysse EA, Kim DS. Excessive blinking in childhood: a prospective evaluation of 99 children. *Ophthalmology* 2001;108(9):1556–1561.

Kurlan R. Tourette syndrome. Treatment of tics. *Neurol Clin* 1997;1592:403–409.

Lumar R, Lang AE. Tourette syndrome. Secondary tic disorders. *Neurol Clin* 1997;15(2):309–331.

Moll GH, Heinrich H, Trott GE, et al. Children with comorbid attention-deficit-hyperactivity disorder and tic disorder: evidence for additive inhibitory deficits within the motor system *Ann Neurol* 2001;49(3):393–396.

Scahill L, Tanner C, Dure L. The epidemiology of tics and Tourette syndrome in children and adolescents. *Adv Neurol* 2001;85:261–271.

Author: A. G. Christina Bergqvist

Toddler's Diarrhea

Database

DEFINITION

Chronic diarrhea lasting at least 3 to 4 weeks in a child between 1 and 5 years of age, in a child who is normally active and growing well. Abdominal pain may be present; straining and eating and sleeping problems are not part of the syndrome. The condition is also known as chronic nonspecific diarrhea and may follow a gastroenteritis.

CAUSES

- Excess fruit juice intake usually leading to carbohydrate intolerance due to excess fructose and sorbitol.
- Motility disorder, i.e., variant of irritable bowel syndrome of infancy.
- Diet that is high in fluid but low in fat and fiber.

PATHOPHYSIOLOGY

- Chronic nonspecific diarrhea is often preceded by acute gastroenteritis or other viral infection that results in dietary restrictions. Increased oral fluids, including juices are used to stay ahead of stool losses and prevent dehydration.
- Carbohydrate malabsorption

—Capacity of small intestine to absorb fructose is limited. Foods that contain equivalent amounts of fructose and glucose are more readily absorbed because of the additive effect of a glucose-dependent fructose cotransport mechanism. An excess of fructose over glucose will result in fructose malabsorption by the small intestine.
—Sorbitol is nonabsorbable and inhibits fructose absorption and may cause gastrointestinal symptoms.
—Excessive intake of juices high in sorbitol and those with a high fructose to glucose ratio will result in fructose malabsorption and gastrointestinal symptoms.

- Motility disorder:

—Persistence of immature bowel motility pattern. There is failure of initiation of normal postprandial delayed gastric emptying and rapid transit due to persistence of small-bowel fasting motility pattern.
—Meals with high dietary fat delay gastric emptying. High-fluid, low-fat meals lack this benefit.

- Low-fiber diet

—Dietary fiber (pectin) important for purpose of binding water to help form solid stools

GENETICS

Family members often report nonspecific gastrointestinal complaints or functional bowel disorders.

EPIDEMIOLOGY

It is the most common cause of prolonged diarrhea without failure to thrive (FTT) in children.

PROGNOSIS

Good

Differential Diagnosis

All causes of diarrhea without malnutrition should be considered.

- Infection: giardiasis, cryptosporidiosis, bacterial gastroenteritis, and bacterial overgrowth
- Congenital: cystic fibrosis, sucrase-isomaltase deficiency
- Immunologic: celiac disease, cow's milk-sensitive enteropathy, food allergy (multiple)
- Miscellaneous: postinfectious enteropathy, constipation, and hormone secreting tumors like vasoactive intestinal peptide (VIP)-oma, neuroblastoma, laxatives, Munchausen-by-proxy.

Data Gathering

HISTORY

Question: Detailed history?
Significance: Essential with special attention to the "four F's": fiber, fluid, fat, and fruit juices

Question: Chronic diarrhea?
Significance: Usually chronic diarrhea is preceded by a gastroenteritis.

Question: Stool characteristics?
Significance: Typically first stool of the day is large and has better consistency than those occurring later on in the day.

Question: Timing of diarrhea?
Significance: Usually no stools passed at night

Question: Stools foul smelling and contain undigested food particles?
Significance: Usually present due to very rapid transit

Question: Physical appearance?
Significance: Children are healthy appearing, eat well, and are growing normally, although weight might be influenced by the dietary measures.

Question: Are other children affected?
Significance: Presence of other affected family members or day-care mates makes infectious etiology more likely.

Physical Examination

Finding: Normal
Significance: Although weight might be influenced by the dietary practices and measures

Laboratory Aids

Test: Stool culture
Significance: Usually normal

Test: Infectious workup
Significance: Negative

Test: Stool test
Significance: Negative for WBC and blood

Test: CBC normal
Significance: No anemia

Test: Serum electrolytes normal
Significance: No dehydration

Therapy

DIET

• The child's feeding pattern should be normalized according to the "four F's":

—Overconsumption of fruit juices should be discouraged, especially those that contain sorbitol and a high fructose-to-glucose ratio.
—Fiber intake should be normalized by introduction of whole meal bread and fruits.
—Increase dietary fat to at least 35% to 40% of total energy intake. Substitution of low-fat milk with whole milk may be sufficient.
—Restrict fluid intake to less than 150 cc/kg/d.

• Improvement occurs within a few days to a couple of weeks after initiating the above therapy. Parental reassurance is confirmed by good response to dietary therapy.

MEDICATIONS

Not routinely recommended and should be left to specialist's discretion. Loperamide and aspirin have been successfully used to normalize bowel patterns in cases refractory to dietary therapy but should be discouraged.

REFERRAL

• Failure of response to the above therapy
• Weight loss despite adequate intake
• Presence of other symptoms like anorexia, irritability, fever, and vomiting
• Blood and mucus in diarrhea

TESTS TO PREPARE FOR CONSULTATION

Sweat chloride, celiac disease panel (antigliadin and antiendomysial antibodies), serum albumin, sedimentation rate, stool Sudan III stain for fecal fat

SPECIAL INSIGHTS

• It is important to take a good history because all the illnesses in the DDx are associated with morbidity, if diagnosis is delayed.
• Consider constipation, if diarrhea alternates with normal or hard stools. KUB will show colonic fecal retention.
• Need to make follow-up phone call to parents within a few days of instituting diet. If no improvement within a week despite good compliance with dietary recommendations, then rethink diagnosis and consider referral to a specialist.
• Improvement with dietary changes confirms the diagnosis and also reassures the parents.
• Excessive fruit juice consumption has been linked to decreased weight and height, and also obesity in children. It is prudent to limit its consumption to less than 12-fl oz/d.

Common Questions and Answers

Q: Is growth normal in a patient with toddler's diarrhea?
A: Growth is usually normal; weight may be mildly influenced by the prior dietary practices and measures, and failure to thrive has also been reported recently.

Q: What are the components of a successful treatment plan?
A: Attention to the "four F's": decreased fruit juice intake, increased fat intake, decreased fluid, and increased fiber intake

Q: When should care by a pediatric gastroenterologist be sought?
A: If no response after 2 weeks of compliance with dietary therapy, growth delay or other gastrointestinal or systemic complaints

ICD-9-CM 787.91

564.5 (functional diarrhea)

BIBLIOGRAPHY

Dennison BA. Fruit juice consumption by infants and children: a review. *J Am Coll Nutr* 1996;15(5 suppl):4S–11S.

Hamdi I, Dodge JA. Toddler diarrhea: observations on the effects of aspirin and loperamide. *J Pediatr Gastroenterol Nutr* 1985;4:362–365.

Hoekstra JH. Toddler diarrhea: more a nutritional disorder than a disease. *Arch Dis Child* 1998;79(1):2–5.

Hoekstra JH, Van den Aker JHL, Kneepkens CMF, et al. Evaluation of $^{13}CO_2$ breath tests for the detection of fructose malabsorption. *J Lab Clin Med* 1996;127(3):303–309.

Huffman S. Toddler's diarrhea. *J Pediatr Health Care* 1999;13(1):32–33.

Kneepkens CMF, Hoekstra JH. Chronic nonspecific diarrhea of childhood. *Pediatr Clin North Am* 1996;43:375–390.

Lifshitz F, Ament ME, Kleinman RE, et al. Role of juice carbohydrate malabsorption in chronic nonspecific diarrhea in children. *J Pediatr* 1992;120:825–829.

Author: Timothy A. S. Sentongo

Toxic Shock Syndrome (TSS)

Database

DEFINITION
- TSS is caused by group A β-hemolytic streptococci (GABHS or *Streptococcus pyogenes*) or TSS toxin-1 (TSST-1) producing strains of *Staphylococcus aureus*.
- Acute febrile illness characterized by myalgia, vomiting, diarrhea, pharyngitis, diffuse desquamating macular erythroderma, mucous membrane and conjunctival erythema, multiorgan system involvement by direct inflammatory damage or ischemia, disseminated intravascular coagulopathy, and frequently hypotension.
- CDC criteria for diagnosis of staphylococcal TSS:
—Fever 38.9°C or higher
—Diffuse macular erythroderma
—Desquamation 1 to 2 weeks after onset, particularly of palms and soles
—Hypotension below fifth percentile for children, or orthostatic changes greater than 15 mm Hg or orthostatic syncope or dizziness
—Involvement of three or more organ systems: gastrointestinal, muscular, mucous membrane, renal, hepatic, hematologic, or neurologic
All five of the above with negative blood cultures, except for *S. aureus* and negative serology for Rocky Mountain spotted fever (RMSF), leptospirosis, and measles. Four of five criteria termed "probable." Four criteria plus death prior to desquamation yields complete syndrome.
- CDC criteria for diagnosis of streptococcal TSS:
—Hypotension or shock.
—Any two of the following: renal impairment, disseminated intravascular coagulopathy, thrombocytopenia, hepatic impairment, adult respiratory distress syndrome, erythematous macular rash that may desquamate, soft tissue necrosis.
—Isolation of GABHS from a normally sterile site constitutes a definite case. Isolation of GABHS from a nonsterile site constitutes a probable case.
Associated risk factors:
- Superabsorbent tampon use
—Local staphylococcal or streptococcal infection
—Surgical wounds
—Diaphragm or contraceptive sponge use
—Childbirth and abortion

PATHOPHYSIOLOGY
- TSST-1 causes extensive interstitial edema of all tissues and minimal perivascular mononuclear cellular infiltrate either directly or through cytokine (e.g., interleukin-1 and tumor necrosis factor) induction.
- Streptococcal toxins probably act similarly.
- Cytokines, as well as the TSST-1 toxin itself, act to decrease peripheral vascular resistance with its resultant interstitial edema. Intravas-

cular volume becomes increasingly depleted and hypotension develops.
- An early sign of decreased intravascular volume is tachycardia out of proportion to the patient's fever, This is an attempt to increase tissue perfusion by increasing cardiac output.
- Direct toxin effects and resultant inflammatory infiltration of the myocardium may produce decreased contractility resulting in cardiogenic shock.
- Additionally, activation of coagulation and thrombolytic enzyme systems promote a consumptive coagulopathy.

EPIDEMIOLOGY
- Early 1980s: over 90% of cases occurred in menstruating females; associated with "super-absorbent" tampon use. The frequency of cases occurring in menstruating females dropped in the mid-1980s because of changes to less absorbent or different composition tampons.
- Currently, ~60% of cases occur in females.
- Mean age: 22 years
- Current incidence of menses-related disease: 1 to 5 per 100,000 women of menstrual age per year
- Incubation period for postoperative *S. aureus*–mediated TSS can be less than 12 hours.
- Streptococcal TSS incidence highest among children
- Preceding varicella infection dramatically increases the risk for acquiring invasive disease due to GABHS including TSS.

COMPLICATIONS
Multisystem organ failure secondary to distributive shock/hypotension including:
- Pulmonary edema
- Disseminated intravascular coagulopathy (DIC)
- Acute renal failure (oliguric and nonoliguric)
- Hepatic failure
- Myocardial edema and decreased contractility with or without arrhythmias
- "Stunned" myocardium demonstrating severe ventricular contractile dysfunction
- Cerebral edema with toxic or ischemic encephalopathy
- Metabolic disturbances
- Telogen effluvium; temporary hair and nail loss
- Neuropsychologic disturbances including memory loss; abnormal EEG rare

PROGNOSIS
- Recurrences are associated with inadequate treatment (parenteral antibiotics).
- Mortality approximately 7% for staphylococcal disease. Myocardial failure and pulmonary failure are the most common causes of death.
- Mortality higher in nonmenstrual TSS due to delayed recognition.
- Death usually occurs within the first few days; may occur as late as 2 weeks following onset.
- Permanent renal damage is extremely rare.

Differential Diagnosis

- Septic shock due to *Neisseria meningitidis*
- Streptococcal and staphylococcal scarlatiniform eruptions
- Leptospirosis
- RMSF without characteristic rash
- Fulminant viral infection (e.g., adenovirus)
- Kawasaki disease, although TSS may present simultaneously with Kawasaki disease. Coronary artery dilatation has been reported in cases presenting as TSS.
- Toxic epidermal necrolysis (TEN)

Data Gathering

HISTORY
Question: Any recent use of tampons, contraceptive sponge, and/or diaphragm? Any surgical or nonsurgical wounds, burns, childbirth, abortion, or puerperal infections?
Significance: These are all known risk factors.
Question: Any other active streptococcal or staphylococcal infections?
Question: Was there an abrupt onset of high fever, chills, malaise, headache, pharyngitis, myalgias, fatigue, vomiting, diarrhea, abdominal pain, and dizziness or syncope?
Significance: Findings seen in TSS.
Question: Was there diffuse erythroderma, severe watery diarrhea (often with fecal incontinence), decreased urine output, and altered mental status 24 to 48 hours following the influenza-like prodrome?
Significance: Seen in 20% of cases.
Question: What is written on the tampon package?
Significance: polyacrylate, polyester foam, and cross-linked carboxymethylcellulose, and claims of "super-absorbency" are associated with TSS.

Physical Examination

Finding: Any sign of soft tissue infection such as cellulitis, necrotizing fasciitis, myositis, soft tissue abscesses, sinusitis.
Significance: Often seen prior to TSS
Finding: Overall appearance
Significance: Moderately to severely ill
Finding: Vital signs
Significance: Fever, tachycardia, tachypnea, orthostasis, or frank hypotension. Tachycardia is the prelude to hypotension.
Finding: Skin, mucous membranes, and soft tissues
Significance: Erythroderma, peripheral cyanosis and edema, bulbar conjunctival hyperemia, subconjunctival hemorrhages, beefy red mucous membranes, muscle tenderness
Finding: Mental status
Significance: Altered, including somnolence, agitation, disorientation, obtundation within 24 to 72 hours

Toxic Shock Syndrome (TSS)

Finding: Intensity of erythroderma
Significance: May be most intense surrounding the infected focus (e.g., perineum)
Finding: Desquamation
Significance: Begins on trunk and extremities 5 to 7 days after onset. Full thickness desquamation of fingers, toes, palms, and soles begins 10 to 12 days after onset.
Finding: Vesicle or bullae formation, or presence of violaceous hue
Significance: These are ominous findings.

 Laboratory Aids

Test: Antibodies to TSST-1
Significance: Will be positive several weeks after acute presentation
Test: Antibodies to antistreptolysin O (ASO), antideoxyribonuclease B, or other streptococcal extracellular products
Significance: May increase 4 to 6 weeks after infection in streptococcal-mediated disease
Test: CBC
Significance: Usually reveals thrombocytopenia early in the course of disease, thrombocytosis during the recovery phase, anemia early in disease, normal or slightly elevated leukocyte count with left shift and absolute lymphopenia. Neutropenia is more ominous than lymphopenia.
Test: Blood cultures
Significance: Positive in 60% of streptococcal TSS, rarely positive in staphylococcal TSS
Test: Local cultures
Significance: S. aureus may be isolated from vagina or cervix in menstrual TSS, from other infectious focus in nonmenstrual cases. Isolation of group A streptococci from a sterile site is a definite case, while isolation from a nonsterile site constitutes a probable case.
Test: Coagulation studies
Significance: May reveal prolonged prothrombin and partial thromboplastin times (PT/PTT) with or without evidence of DIC; low fibrinogen, elevated fibrin degradation products
Test: Urinalysis
Significance: May reveal sterile pyuria
Test: Lumbar puncture
Significance: May reveal CSF pleocytosis
Test: Chemistry panel
Significance: May show elevated BUN/creatinine, abnormal liver enzymes and elevated bilirubin, hypoproteinemia, hypocalcemia, and/or hypophosphatemia
Test: Creatinine phosphokinase
Significance: May be elevated, reflecting skeletal muscle involvement.

 Emergency Care

- Aggressive fluid resuscitation and often vasopressors in severe cases.
- Correction of coagulopathy and anemia with plasma and blood products

 Therapy

- Removal of all foreign bodies
- Surgical débridement with myositis and necrotizing fasciitis; abscess drainage
- Antibiotics: parenteral administration with antistreptococcal and staphylococcal therapy. Eradicates source of the toxin, but does not affect the course of the acute illness.
- Use both a bacterial cell wall inhibitor such as semisynthetic antistaphylococcal penicillins (e.g., nafcillin, oxacillin, dicloxacillin, and cefuroxime or ampicillin/ sulbactam) as well as a protein synthesis inhibitor such as clindamycin to end toxin, enzyme, and cytokine production.
- Continue therapy for 10 to 15 days or until causative bacteria are eradicated on follow-up cultures.
- Clindamycin, erythromycin if penicillin allergic
- Intravenous immunoglobulin:
—Anecdotal reports of efficacy for streptococcal TSS.
—May be considered for infections refractory to aggressive therapy.
—Optimal regimen is not known, although single doses of 1 to 2 g/kg, as well as several days of 150 to 450 mg/kg/d have been studied.
- Corticosteroids: have not been systematically studied.

 Follow-Up

- Poor prognosis is often heralded by development of pulmonary edema, falling cardiac index, and rising pulmonary capillary wedge pressure.
- Renal failure and cerebral edema (complication of fluid resuscitation) are other indications of complicated course.
- Temperature usually returns to normal within 2 days.
- Toxin-mediated cardiomyopathy should resolve if fatal arrhythmia does not occur during decompensated stage.
- Gastrointestinal, hepatic, and musculoskeletal changes resolve rapidly with rare permanent sequelae except for muscle weakness.
- Hair and nail loss may occur 4 to 16 weeks after onset; resolve within 5 to 6 months.
- Encephalopathy is common, rarely causes seizures; both resolve within 4 to 5 days.

PREVENTION
- Avoidance of tampon use after first episode of TSS.
- Scrupulous wound care.
- Limitation of intravaginal foreign body use (e.g., tampon, sponge, etc.) and strict adherence to manufacturer directions.

PITFALLS
- S. aureus isolated from nares or vagina may represent a false-positive finding because 10% to 30% of individuals are healthy carriers.
- The production of TSST-1 by isolate is only presumptive evidence unless case meets diagnostic criteria.
- Failure to meet CDC diagnostic criteria
- Failure to identify soft tissue or muscular site of local infection
- Failure to identify or remove foreign body
- Erythroderma may not be appreciated if already hypotensive

 Common Questions and Answers

Q: Can TSS recur?
A: Yes. Inadequate eradication of the nidus of infection, such as sinusitis or a foreign body, may promote TSS recurrence. Also, individuals with some immune system defects may develop recurrent TSS.
Q: Is there a test that proves TSS?
A: No, even if TSST-1 antibodies are present, they do not prove TSS unless criteria for the case definition are met.
Q: Can TSS be diagnosed in persons who have no risk factors?
A: Yes, there have been reports meeting the case definition where none of the known associated factors were present.

ICD-9-CM 040.89

BIBLIOGRAPHY
American Academy of Pediatrics. Toxic shock syndrome. In: Pickering LK, ed. 2000 red book: report of the Committee on Infectious Diseases, 25th ed. Elk Grove Village, IL: American Academy of Pediatrics, 2000:567–583.

Alejandro MM, Lansang MA, Dans LF, et al. Intravenous immunoglobulin for treating sepsis and septic shock. Cochrane Database Syst Rev 2000;CD001090.

Ayoub EM, Ahmed S. Update on the complication of group A streptococcal infections. Curr Probl Pediatr 1997;27:90–101.

Bisno AL, Stevens DC. Streptococcal infection of skin and soft-tissues. N Engl J Med 1996;334:240–245.

Crew JR, Harrison K, Corey RG, et al. Stunned myocardium in the toxic shock syndrome. Ann Intern Med 1992;117:912–913.

Manders SM. Toxin-mediated streptococcal and staphylococcal disease. J Am Acad Dermatol 1998;39:383–398.

Authors: Mark L. Bagarazzi and Daniel H. Conway

Toxoplasmosis

 Database

DEFINITION

Toxoplasma gondii is an intracellular protozoan parasite with a complex life cycle, whose definitive host is the cat. In addition to causing asymptomatic infection and clinical disease in humans, the organism is capable of causing asymptomatic and symptomatic infections in a wide range of mammals and birds.

PATHOPHYSIOLOGY

- Toxoplasmosis is acquired by the ingestion of oocysts or intact viable tissue cysts in inadequately cooked meat.
- After ingestion, the oocysts and cysts are disrupted by the digestive process, and viable infective organisms cross the gastrointestinal lining. Hematologic spread leads to infection of multiple organs, most notably the heart, skeletal muscle, and the brain. There, slowly growing or dormant cysts remain for the patient's lifetime.
- Congenital toxoplasmosis generally occurs during a primary maternal infection. An exception may be when the pregnant woman is severely immunocompromised; congenital infection has occurred in offspring of HIV-infected women with latent toxoplasmosis infection.
- Primary infection in the first trimester is associated with a higher incidence of symptomatic congenital disease, though the majority of congenital infections occur late in pregnancy, and the neonates have subclinical infection at birth. Overall, 30% to 40% of infants born to mothers with primary infection during pregnancy will be congenitally infected.

EPIDEMIOLOGY

- The rate of acquired infection, usually asymptomatic, varies widely through the world and increases with age.
- Seroprevalence rates among pregnant women vary from 4% to 80% worldwide; in the United States a recent serologic survey found 15% of women of childbearing age were seropositive. Worldwide, the incidence of congenital infection ranges from 1 to 7/1,000 live births; in the United States incidence is estimated at 0.1 to 1/1,000 live births. It is believed that 400 to 4,000 infants are born in the U.S. with congenital toxoplasmosis.
- 70% to 90% of children with congenital toxoplasmosis are asymptomatic at birth. Late sequelae (chorioretinitis, mental retardation, seizures, sensorineural hearing loss) occur in greater than 50% of untreated infants considered asymptomatic at birth.

COMPLICATIONS

- Congenital infection: retardation, retinitis, hydrocephalus, seizures, microcephaly, sensorineural hearing loss
- Acquired infection (all rare): adenopathy, mononucleosis-like syndrome, myocarditis, pneumonia, meningitis/encephalitis

PROGNOSIS

- Majority of acquired infections are asymptomatic or associated with mild short-lived symptoms.
- Majority of congenital infections are asymptomatic, though late sequelae occur in greater than 50% of untreated infants.
- Symptomatic newborns are at significant risk for sequelae, most frequently neurologic (hydrocephalus, retardation) or ophthalmic (retinitis, blindness).
- Prenatal treatment appears to decrease risk to newborn; therapy of all infected infants appears to improve outcome.

 Differential Diagnosis

- Primary infection: acute disease symptoms of adenopathy, fever, rash: primary EBV, CMV, HIV infection
- For the newborn with micro/macrocephaly, hepatosplenomegaly, eye disease; other congenital infections: CMV, syphilis, rubella

 Data Gathering

HISTORY

- For acquired infection, history of contact with cats, eating raw or undercooked meat (especially pork)
- For congenital infection, history of maternal exposure or positive titers (IgG and/or IgM)

 Physical Examination

- Acquired infection: adenopathy, rash, fever, malaise, hepatosplenomegaly
- Congenital infection: micro- or macrocephaly, hydrocephalus, chorioretinitis, hepatosplenomegaly, petechiae, sensorineural hearing loss, intracerebral calcifications

Laboratory Aids

- Screen all pregnant women or their infants in high-incidence areas by use of toxoplasmosis-specific IgM or rise in IgG titer over time.
- Prenatal diagnosis by PCR on amniotic fluid appears promising, with high degree of sensitivity/specificity
- For the at-risk neonate, diagnosis is made by demonstration of specific IgM, IgA, or IgE titers, or rise in IgG titers, and/or clinical symptoms in infant of mother with recent primary infection.
- Head CT or MRI demonstrating calcifications
- Thrombocytopenia
- Early and frequent audiologic and ophthalmic evaluations are a necessity. Many affected infants will have normal neonatal examinations.
- Elevated liver function tests

 ## Therapy

Pyrimethamine and sulfadiazine for the first year of life for all congenitally infected infants, symptomatic or not. Folic acid is given during the course of therapy to minimize hematologic side effects.

PREVENTION

- Avoidance of undercooked meats
- Seronegative women need to exercise caution in caring for cats.
- Maternal/neonatal antibody screening is important in areas with a significant incidence of toxoplasmosis.
- Treatment of pregnant women with documented seroconversion may prevent congenital infection in many cases.
- If fetal infection is established, aggressive treatment during pregnancy with spiramycin, pyrimethamine, and sulfonamide may ameliorate the severity of the disease in the infant.

 ## Follow-Up

- Continued attention to neurologic development and frequent audiologic and ophthalmic evaluations throughout the first few years of life.
- For children with early symptomatic disease, careful attention to neurologic condition and early intervention services to optimize outcome.

PITFALLS

- Failure to consider diagnosis in at-risk or symptomatic infant.
- Failure to consider the significant risk of late sequelae in asymptomatic exposed/infected neonate and therefore failure to offer therapy to asymptomatic infected neonate.

 ## Common Questions and Answers

Q: What is the risk of congenital infection in a mother with stable toxoplasmosis?
A: The risk of congenital infection in the offspring of a mother with long-standing toxoplasmosis infection is considered very low; the exception would be for mothers with a significant degree of immunosuppression or deficiency.

Q: What is the risk of congenital infection in offspring of a mother with documented primary infection during pregnancy?
A: Approximately 30% to 40% of infants born to mothers with primary infection during pregnancy will be infected themselves. This rate may be lower if the mother receives therapy (spiramycin or pyrimethamine/sulfadiazine) prenatally. Of the infected infants, the majority (70–90%) are normal at birth; with treatment for 12 months, it appears most will have a favorable outcome.

ICD-9-CM 130.9

BIBLIOGRAPHY

Hohlfeld P, Daffos F, Costa JM, et al. Prenatal diagnosis of congenital toxoplasmosis with a polymerase-chain-reaction test on amniotic fluid. *N Engl J Med* 1994;331:695–699.

Jones JL, Lopez A, Wilson M, et al. Congenital toxoplasmosis: a review. *Obstet Gynecol Surv* 2001;56:296–305.

Koppe JG, Loewer-Sieger DH, de Roever-Bonnet H. Results of 20-year follow-up of congenital toxoplasmosis. *Lancet* 1986;1:254–256.

Lappalainen M, Koskiniemi M, Hiilesmaa V, et al. Outcome of children after maternal primary toxoplasma infection during pregnancy with emphasis on avidity of specific IgG. *Pediatr Infect Dis J* 1995;14:354–361.

Lynfield R, Guerina NG. Toxoplasmosis. *Pediatr Rev* 1997;18:75–83.

Roizen N, Swisher CN, Stein MA, et al. Neurological and developmental outcome in treated congenital toxoplasmosis. *Pediatrics* 1995;95:11–20.

Author: Richard M. Rutstein

Tracheitis

 Database

DEFINITION

• Acute tracheitis: potentially life-threatening bacterial infection of the trachea, which presents acutely in the otherwise normal child.
• Subacute tracheitis: infectious complication of long-term intubation or tracheostomy, predominately in children with an underlying respiratory, neurologic, or other chronic disorder.

CAUSES

• Acute

—*Staphylococcus aureus* predominately
—*Moraxella catarrhalis, Haemophilus influenza* including type b (Hib) and nontypeable, group A β-hemolytic streptococcus (GABHS), and oral anaerobes less commonly
—*Mycobacterium tuberculosis;* uncommon but known pathogen
—Herpes simplex virus (after burn injury and intubation)
—Influenza A virus often recovered from cultures, but is felt to be a predisposing factor rather than an etiology of tracheitis
—Measles virus uncommon, but should be considered in known measles case

• Subacute

—Organisms as above
—Organisms associated with nosocomial infections in a particular institution (e.g., *Pseudomonas aeruginosa,* other gram-negative enteric bacteria, *Moraxella catarrhalis,* etc.)
—Fungus (e.g., *Candida* spp.) with underlying immunodeficiency or chronic steroid use

PATHOPHYSIOLOGY

• Not clearly known; postulated disruption of the mucociliary elevator, leading to decreased clearance of bacterial pathogens
• In children with artificial airways, natural airway protective mechanisms are bypassed and pathogens are inoculated directly into the trachea with suctioning.
• Viral infection may precede bacterial tracheitis.
• Infection causes destruction of the tracheal wall, sloughing of mucosa, and mucus and pus production, leading to airway obstruction.

EPIDEMIOLOGY

• Infancy through early adolescence, mean age in early school age (5.7 years)
• Younger patients more likely to require intubation
• Increased incidence during viral respiratory season
• No gender predisposition

COMPLICATIONS

• Pneumonia
• Prolonged mechanical ventilation with associated complications (including pneumothorax, pneumonia, tracheal stenosis)
• Staphylococcal toxin syndromes (e.g., toxic shock syndrome)
• Adult respiratory distress syndrome (ARDS)
• Death

PROGNOSIS

• Acute tracheitis: outcome ranges from recovery without sequelae to tracheal stenosis (even without intubation); most patients recover fully
• Subacute tracheitis: frequent recurrences not unusual (because of altered airway mechanics and/or underlying disease)

 Differential Diagnosis

INFECTIOUS

• Epiglottitis
• Pharyngitis
• Laryngitis
• Bronchitis
• Pneumonia, including *Pneumocystis carinii* pneumonia (PCP)

ENVIRONMENTAL

Chemical or inhalation burns to airway

TUMORS

Laryngeal tumors (rare)

TRAUMA

Blunt trauma to neck

CONGENITAL

Underlying airway stenosis compromised by acute viral infection, tracheal papillomatosis (human papillomavirus aspirated at birth)

 Data Gathering

HISTORY

• Immunization history, especially Hib vaccine
• Upper respiratory infection prodrome?

Tracheitis Subgroups

• Acute: symptoms progress over 8- to 10-hour period; fever, lethargy, cough, dyspnea, hoarseness, stridor, noisy respirations.
• Subacute: Same as for acute with more indolent progression, increased supplemental oxygen requirement, change in pattern of breathing, stridor, noisy respirations.

 Physical Examination

Finding: Acute
Significance: Toxic appearance, anxiety, and "air hunger," lethargy, fever, shortness of breath, cyanosis, labored respiration with retractions, cough, may have concomitant signs of pneumonia.

Finding: Subacute
Significance: Same as for acute with changes in secretions suctioned from trachea (thickening, change in color).

Laboratory Aids

Test: Tracheal culture
Significance: Obtain specimen directly from the trachea in controlled setting (for emergent airway management), throat swab not adequate, endotracheal tube cultures not adequate.

Test: Gram stain tracheal material
Significance: For predominant organism and white blood cells (especially polymorpho-nuclear leukocytes)

Test: Blood culture
Significance: Should be obtained, but bacteremia not common.

Test: CBC
Significance: Increased white count with a left shift.

Test: Erythrocyte sedimentation rate, C reactive protein
Significance: Usually elevated.

Test: Laryngoscopy or bronchoscopy
Significance: Diagnostic and therapeutic; visualize airway and suction material that obstructs airway (must be performed in setting with preparation to intubate or place tracheotomy if necessary).

RADIOGRAPHIC STUDIES

• Radiographs must be performed in controlled setting with trained personnel available to intubate if necessary.
• Lateral neck and anteroposterior (AP) neck radiographs: distention of the hypopharynx, subglottic narrowing, cloudiness of the tracheal air column, irregularity of the tracheal wall, sloughing of mucosa (may mimic foreign body), radiographs have a good correlation with findings on bronchoscopy.

Therapy

• Control of airway essential; not all patients require intubation, but preparation must be made to perform emergent intubation or tracheotomy at any time (decline may occur gradually or suddenly if debris in airway obstructs).
• Children with preexisting artificial airway may require increase in ventilatory support.

DRUGS

• Acute (community acquired)

—If up-to-date Hib immunization: antistaphylococcal coverage with a semisynthetic penicillin (e.g., oxacillin, nafcillin); if penicillin allergy, clindamycin
—Inadequate Hib immunization: ampicillin/sulbactam

• Subacute (hospital-acquired, preexisting artificial airway)

—Guide therapy by known prior colonization and pathogens common in particular institution
—Mildly ill patient: empiric therapy with amoxicillin/clavulanate for 10 to 14 days
—Severely ill patient: empiric therapy with ticarcillin/clavulanate or ampicillin/sulbactam, then guide therapy by cultures (unless a predominant organism is cultured, results may reflect colonizing organisms and/or mouth flora, rather than the etiologic organism)

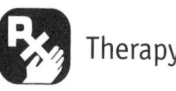

Follow-Up

• Acute tracheitis: because of the possibility of tracheal stenosis, which may be mild and asymptomatic until the child experiences the next respiratory tract infection, the parents must be counseled to bring the child for care any time there is noisy breathing, especially stridor.
• Chronic tracheitis: no follow-up cultures should be taken; the child should be monitored the same way all children with abnormal/artificial airways would be.

SIGNS TO WATCH FOR

• Obstruction of endotracheal tube with secretions is not unusual and would be indicated by a sudden deterioration.
• Persistent fever may indicate nosocomial infection (e.g., pneumonia, urinary tract infection, etc.).
• Sudden worsening while on ventilator may indicate pneumothorax.

PREVENTION

• Routine immunization, especially for Hib in all children; immunization for influenza in children with artificial airways
• Avoid overaggressive suctioning of children with artificial airways.

PITFALLS

Patients may have rapid progression of symptoms; initial radiographic studies may be negative, close clinical observation is critical.

Common Questions and Answers

Q: Are routine surveillance cultures of patients with artificial airways helpful in prevention of tracheitis?
A: No. Children who have been hospitalized and have artificial airways rapidly become colonized with the organisms that are common within the institution. These organisms will persist for months, are difficult to eradicate, and even if eradicated will be replaced with other, possibly more resistant flora. Routine culture is expensive and will only identify colonization.

Q: How can you differentiate a child with severe pharyngitis from tracheitis?
A: In many ways, the clinical presentation of tracheitis is similar to that of severe pharyngitis, but in tracheitis there will be signs of respiratory compromise (e.g., stridor) and toxic appearance. The two illnesses may look very similar early in the disease course.

Q: How can you differentiate a child with tracheitis and one with tracheitis who also has systemic toxin-mediated complications?
A: Children with a toxic shock syndrome presentation will usually have a diffuse erythroderma, nonpurulent conjunctivitis, and inflamed oral mucosa (strawberry tongue). The hypotension and tachycardia will be out of proportion to the degree of illness and may be refractory to fluid resuscitation.

ICD-9-CM 616.0

BIBLIOGRAPHY

Bernstein T, Brilli R, Jacobs B. Is bacterial tracheitis changing? A 14-month experience in a pediatric intensive care unit. *Clin Infect Dis* 1998;27(3):458–462.

Britto J, Habibi P, Walters S, et al. Systemic complications associated with bacterial tracheitis. *Arch Dis Child* 1996;72:249–250.

Horowitz IN. Staphylococcal tracheitis, pneumonia, and adult respiratory distress syndrome. *Pediatr Emerg Care* 1996;12(4):288–289.

Jones R, Santos J, Overall J. Bacterial tracheitis. *JAMA* 1979;242:721–726.

Author: Jill A. Foster

Tracheoesophageal Fistula (TEF) and Esophageal Atresia

 Database

DEFINITION

- Abnormal communication between the trachea and esophagus.
- Major types:

—Esophageal atresia (EA) with distal tracheoesophageal fistula (TEF) (85%)
—Pure esophageal atresia (8%)
—"H-type" TEF (5%)
—Esophageal atresia with proximal TEF with or without distal TEF (<1%)

PATHOPHYSIOLOGY

- Poorly understood and likely different for the variants of EA and TEF.
- For TEF, incomplete separation of the esophagus and trachea that normally occurs before the sixth week of gestation.

EPIDEMIOLOGY

- Incidence: 1:3,000 to 1:4,500 live births
- Minimal male preponderance
- Possible association with maternal vitamin A and riboflavin deficiency, and maternal use of thalidomide and progesterone

GENETICS

- Unlikely that inherited factors play a dominant role.
- Nonrandom association with the other abnormalities in the VACTERL syndrome—vertebral, anorectal, cardiac, renal, and limb—suggests some insults to the fetus that result in disordered embryogenesis.
- Associated chromosomal abnormalities (trisomies 18 and 21) seen.

COMPLICATIONS

- Tracheomalacia
- Gastroesophageal reflux (50%) and esophageal dysmotility
- Anastomotic strictures (30%)
- Anastomotic leaks (15%)
- Respiratory distress/failure
- Aspiration pneumonia
- Chronic "barking" cough
- Dysphagia (50%)/obstructing esophageal foreign bodies
- Recurrent TEF (5%)

PROGNOSIS

- Previous classification systems were used to identify relative risks of primary repair. These were based on the patient's weight, the presence of other congenital anomalies, and the degree of pneumonitis. Advances in ventilatory support and neonatal care have lessened the validity and usefulness of these systems. The complications dictate the resultant morbidity of this anomaly.

 Differential Diagnosis

- Traumatic or spontaneous pharyngeal or esophageal perforation
- Pharyngeal diverticulum
- Laryngotracheoesophageal cleft
- Esophageal webs and duplication cysts
- Gastroesophageal reflux
- Paraesophageal hernia

 Data Gathering

HISTORY

Question: Was there any maternal polyhydramnios?
Significance: This is highly suggestive of a proximal intestinal bowel obstruction—esophageal, gastric (rare), and duodenal atresias.

Question: Is there severe drooling and coughing with or without feeding?
Significance: This is suggestive of an esophageal atresia with or without a TEF.

Question: Is there severe choking with feedings in the neonate?
Significance: This is suggestive of an esophageal atresia with or without a TEF.

Question: Are there any associated anomalies (e.g., anomalies seen with VACTERL)?
Significance: Significant association of specific anomalies with EA/TEF.

 Physical Examination

- Cyanotic with feeding
- Excessive secretions
- Excessive drooling
- Inability to pass the orogastric (OG) tube—usually passes less than 10 cm, unless an 8-French (F) tube or smaller is used, which may coil in the proximal pouch
- Scaphoid abdomen with pure EA; and distended, tympanitic abdomen with EA/TEF
- Associated anomalies (VACTERL)

 Laboratory Aids

TESTS

Preoperative laboratory tests should include

- CBC
- Blood type and cross
- Electrolytes and serum calcium

Karyotyping may be done at this time; however, the results are usually unavailable at the time of surgery.

RADIOGRAPHIC STUDIES

- Chest and abdominal x-rays with a 10-F OG tube in the proximal esophageal pouch: only air should be injected into the OG tube as it is pushed into the pouch while the x-ray is taken. This will help to delineate the length of the pouch. Liquid contrast agents are to be avoided due to the increased risk of aspiration. Pulmonary infiltrates are common, particularly in the right upper lobe. The chest x-ray will also provide information regarding the side of the aortic arch and the heart shape.
- Plain x-rays are useful to evaluate for vertebral or other bony abnormalities.
- Renal ultrasounds: to evaluate for any renal abnormalities.
- Ultrasound of the spine: to evaluate for a tethered spinal cord.
- Preoperative echocardiogram: identifies structural cardiac anomalies. This will help to determine the surgical approach.
- Contrast esophagram—patient prone and contrast injected as catheter is withdrawn from the stomach. This study is done *only* if an OG tube passes and an "H-type" TEF is suspected.

 Therapy

SURGERY

Preoperative

- OG tube—10 F or larger; for continuous or intermittent aspiration of proximal esophageal pouch.
- Head elevated at a 30- to 45-degree angle with patient prone or supine to minimize the risk of aspiration.
- NPO and adequate intravenous fluids. Umbilical catheters may be useful, especially if a transanastomotic feeding tube or gastrostomy are not placed at the time of surgery.
- Timely pediatric surgery consultation. Rapid deterioration in the patient's clinical status may occur, especially in the premature, high-risk patient.

- Avoid CPAP and other positive pressure ventilation to limit gastric distention, aspiration, and respiratory compromise. If respiratory distress worsens, an endotracheal tube should be placed with the tip above the carina but below the fistula.
- H_2-blockers may reduce the risk of gastric contents resulting in aspiration pneumonitis prior to surgical repair.

Intraoperative

- Bronchoscopy—locates the fistula in TEF and identifies possible other fistulae or anomalies; done selectively or routinely.
- Primary repair: division of TEF and esophageal anastomosis via thoracotomy— side opposite the aortic arch—done within the first several days of life; usually possible if distance between esophageal segments is less than that of three vertebral bodies.
- Delayed repair: division of TEF and gastrostomy tube placement with delayed esophageal repair. This procedure is indicated for pure esophageal atresia, long-gap EA/TEF (which is a gap that is more than three vertebral bodies long), and very high risk infants with severe respiratory failure.
- Staged repair: initial gastrostomy with esophageal repair up to 2 years later. Usually reserved for pure atresia with a very long gap.
- Cervical esophagostomy (spit fistula): used for very long gap atresias (usually pure EA), and chronic aspiration prior to definitive repair, which is either an esophageal substitute or a delayed primary repair.
- Esophageal replacement performed using gastric transposition, reversed gastric tube, colon, or jejunum.

Postoperative

- Frequent, gentle suctioning of the mouth and pharynx. It is helpful intraoperatively to measure the distance from the teeth to the level of the esophageal anastomosis and tracheal repair to avoid trauma to the repaired area.
- Avoid aggressive suctioning and hyperextension of the neck.
- CPAP and positive pressure ventilation is to be avoided. If patient needs endotracheal intubation, it should be performed by the most skilled person available.
- Prophylactic paralysis and endotracheal intubation for 5 to 7 days may help prevent anastomotic disruption and strictures in long-gap atresias with significant anastomotic tension.
- Fluids given as maintenance IV fluids, TPN via PICC or central venous lines, or enteral feedings via a gastrostomy or transanastomotic feeding tube placed at the time of surgery. This tube is not to be replaced or repositioned if it becomes dislodged.

- Pleural/retropleural tube left in place until esophagram 5 to 7 days postoperatively demonstrates no leak or oral feedings are advanced without clinical evidence of a leak. Placement of a pleural/retropleural tube and postoperative esophagram are not always indicated, especially in very short gap anastomoses and low-risk patients.

DRUGS

- Prophylactic antibiotics to cover skin and oral anaerobic flora—duration is variable. Antibiotics may be discontinued before pleural tube is removed. Antibiotics should be continued for 7 to 10 days for aspiration pneumonia.
- H_2-blockers may reduce the risk of postoperative stricture formation.

 Follow-Up

SIGNS TO WATCH FOR

- Postoperative anastomotic leak: most close spontaneously over 1 to 3 weeks; complete disruptions require repair. Suspect a leak when there is a postoperative pleural effusion, pneumothorax, or pneumomediastinum, or if there is significant saliva-like chest tube output.
- Anastomotic stricture: more common after anastomotic leak and long-gap repair with significant anastomotic tension. Frequently requires one or more dilatations; esophageal replacement rarely required.
- Gastroesophageal reflux: major source of postoperative strictures and long-term pulmonary problems—aspiration pneumonias and reactive airway disease. Fundoplication may be necessary but should be avoided due to inherently increased risk of postoperative dysphagia and esophageal dysmotility.
- Recurrent TEF: presentation similar to GERD; need to evaluate for recurrent TEF prior to therapy/surgery for GERD.
- Tracheomalacia: commonly seen with barky cough and intermittent stridor (especially when suffering from URI); most outgrow the problems as the diameter of the trachea increases.
- Dysphagia: usually improves with time; frequent prolonged difficulty with certain solid foods—carrots, meats, celery.

PITFALLS

- Aggressive airway management involving endotracheal intubation and mechanical ventilation is reported to result in gastric perforation or the need for emergent gastrostomy placement.
- Failure to place an enteric tube large enough for suction in the esophageal pouch, resulting in aspiration.

- Failure to maintain the infant with an elevated head of the bed, even during transport of the infant, which may result in aspiration.
- Premature removal of the retropleural drainage tube may result in mediastinitis.

 Common Questions and Answers

Q: When will my baby be able to begin to feed?
A: The usual time to initiate feedings in a primary repair of an EA-TEF is after 1 week, when the anastomosis is healed. In delayed repairs, feedings can begin via the gastrostomy tube shortly after surgery.

Q: Will my baby have any problems when he/she goes home?
A: Any baby with EA-TEF may have complications that include GER, feeding difficulties, tracheomalacia, and dysphagias.

Q: Is there anything specific that caused this to happen to my baby? Could anything have been done during the pregnancy to prevent or treat this problem?
A: EA with TEF develops *in utero* without specific known causes. There is currently no known fetal treatment or therapy for this problem.

ICD-9-CM 750.3

BIBLIOGRAPHY

Clark DC. Esophageal atresia and tracheoesophageal fistula. *Am Fam Physician* 1999;59:910–920.

Foker JE, Linden BC, Boyle EM, et al. Development of a true primary repair for the full spectrum of esophageal atresia. *Ann Surg* 1997;226:533–543.

Kay S, Shaw K. Revisiting the role of routine retropleural drainage after repair of esophageal atresia with distal esophageal fistula. *J Pediatr Surg* 1999;34:1082–1085.

Marshall AL. Survivors of neonatal congenital lung disease. *Pediatr Pulmonol Suppl* 1997;16:252–253.

Stoll C, Alembik Y, Dott B, et al. Evaluation of prenatal diagnosis of congenital gastrointestinal atresias. *Eur J Epidemiol* 1996;12:611–616.

Teich S, Barton DP, Ginn-Pease ME, et al. Prognostic classification for esophageal atresia and tracheoesophageal fistula: Waterston versus Montreal. *J Pediatr Surg* 1997;32:1075–1080.

Authors: Douglas Katz and Daniel H. Conway

Tracheomalacia/Laryngomalacia

 Database

DEFINITION

- Laryngomalacia (LM)

—Narrowing and collapse of the supraglottic structures of the larynx
—Most common congenital anomaly of the larynx
—Most common noninfectious cause of stridor in children

- Tracheomalacia (TM)

—Narrowing and collapse of the extrathoracic or intrathoracic trachea
—Common cause of chronic wheezing in children
—Classified as primary and secondary:
  —Primary—congenital; results from immature development of the tracheal structures; may occur with other congenital anomalies such as tracheoesophageal fistula, laryngomalacia, and facial anomalies
  —Secondary—acquired in a normally developed trachea after some insult such as prolonged positive-pressure ventilation, recurrent infection or aspiration, or external compression

PATHOPHYSIOLOGY

- Laryngomalacia

—Multiple factors likely involved
—Inward collapse of aryepiglottic folds (cuneiform cartilages) during inspiration
—Elongated, flaccid omega-shaped epiglottis prolapses posteriorly into the pharynx during inspiration
—Immaturity of the laryngeal cartilage results in weakness and collapse during inspiration
—Immaturity of neuromuscular control results in hypotonia of pharyngeal muscles

- Tracheomalacia

—Weakness of the tracheal wall secondary to softening of the anterior cartilaginous rings and to decreased tone of the posterior membranous wall
—With increasing age, the length, area, thickness, and amount of cartilage increases in the anterior rings, as well as the size and contractility of the membranous wall
—During exhalation, increased collapsing pressure across a compliant airway wall causes invagination of the posterior membrane

 Differential Diagnosis

- Laryngomalacia—differential diagnosis of chronic stridor

—Abnormalities of the vocal cords: vocal cord paralysis
—Laryngeal abnormalities: laryngeal cleft, laryngeal web, subglottic hemangioma, papilloma
—Subglottic stenosis
—External compression from mediastinal mass, vascular ring

- Tracheomalacia—differential diagnosis of chronic homophonous wheeze
- Structural abnormalities: vascular compression/ring, tracheal stenosis/web, cystic lesion, mass/tumor
- Nonstructural abnormalities: gastroesophageal reflux disease, retained foreign body, chronic bacterial bronchitis

 Data Gathering

HISTORY

Laryngomalacia?

- Symptoms may be present at birth or delayed until 1 to 2 months of age.
- Inspiratory stridor
- May be asymptomatic during sleep or quiet breathing
- Worsens with crying, agitation, feeding, and upper respiratory infections, supine positioning

Tracheomalacia

- Primary: symptoms may be delayed until 2 to 3 months of age
- Secondary: symptoms delayed until after causative insult occurs
- Expiratory wheeze or inspiratory stridor
- Harsh barking cough
- May be asymptomatic during sleep or quiet breathing
- Worsens with crying, agitation, feeding, and upper respiratory infections

 Physical Examination

Laryngomalacia

- Vibratory, low-pitched inspiratory stridor
- Suprasternal retractions
- Positional changes noted: usually worsens with flexion of neck, supine position
- Stridor transmitted throughout the chest on auscultation

Tracheomalacia

- Homophonous expiratory wheeze (intrathoracic)
- High-pitched inspiratory stridor (extrathoracic)
- Intercostal retractions, worse during acute respiratory infections.

Laboratory Aids

Test: Flexible fiberoptic laryngo/bronchoscopy
Significance:

- Performed during spontaneous breathing
- Most efficient method to evaluate stridor or chronic wheezing
- Visualize the degree and extent of laryngomalacia and/or tracheomalacia
- Evaluate for other airway lesions in the differential diagnosis

Test: Barium swallow
Significance:

- Best noninvasive test to evaluate stridor or chronic wheeze
- Especially of value in evaluation of patients with concomitant swallowing abnormalities
- May see external compression of esophagus from vascular malformation

Test: Chest radiograph
Significance:

- Usually normal in both laryngomalacia and tracheomalacia
- Important to rule out other abnormalities that may cause external airway compression

Test: Airway fluoroscopy
Significance:

- Lateral views are the most useful to visualize the defect
- May be normal; does not rule out diagnosis
- Inspiratory collapsing larynx may be seen in laryngomalacia
- Expiratory narrowing or collapse of the trachea may be seen in tracheomalacia.

Test: MRI
Significance

- Evaluates for thoracic/vascular anomalies that may cause external compression of the airway
- May provide more precise measurements of airway size
- May be performed dynamically to show changes in airway caliber during respiratory cycle

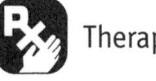

Therapy

- Laryngomalacia

—Usually resolves spontaneously by 18 months of age
—Observation and reassurance
—Treatment of exacerbating factors, such as asthma or gastroesophageal reflux disease
—Tracheostomy may be needed in severe cases to bypass airway obstruction.

—In rare situations, laryngeal surgery is necessary—epiglottoplasty, resection of arytenoids

- Tracheomalacia

—Usually resolves spontaneously by 18 to 24 months of age
—Observation and reassurance
—Treatment of exacerbating factors, such as asthma or gastroesophageal reflux disease
—Bronchoconstrictor therapy to increase tone of airway wall—bethanecol chloride, ipratropium bromide
—Continuous positive airway pressure (CPAP) may be needed in more severe cases.
—Tracheostomy may be needed in severe cases to bypass lesion or to provide CPAP.
—Humidification of secretions may help some patients, especially during respiratory infections.
—Aortopexy may be needed in severe cases to suspend the anterior trachea and widen the airway.

Follow-Up

Monitor for recurrent respiratory symptoms, poor growth, other exacerbating conditions (asthma, gastroesophageal reflux disease).

PROGNOSIS

- In cases of isolated laryngomalacia and/or tracheomalacia, prognosis is usually excellent.
- In patients with history of tracheoesophageal fistula or other airway anomalies, tracheal dysfunction may persist after corrective surgery.

PITFALLS

- Missing other causes for presenting symptoms (see Differential Diagnosis, above)
- Not investigating lower airway in more severe cases of laryngomalacia for other airway anomalies
- Not treating diseases that may exacerbate symptoms and delay spontaneous resolution
- The use of bronchodilators (β_2-agonist) *may* increase the tracheal wall collapsibility by decreasing muscular tone, thereby making the symptoms worse.
- Bronchoscopy should ideally be done under conscious sedation during spontaneous breathing, to avoid altering vocal cord movement and airway dynamics.
- The use of rigid bronchoscopy may stent open the trachea, making tracheomalacia more difficult to identify.

Common Questions and Answers

Q: When will the symptoms improve?
A: As anatomic structures mature with age, laryngomalacia symptoms may improve by 6 months of age with usual resolution by 18 months of age. Tracheomalacia may last longer, but in both entities symptoms usually resolve completely by age 2.

Q: Should all patients have an endoscopic evaluation?
A: No. Diagnosis is usually made based on the appropriate history and physical examination. Infants with mild to moderate typical presentation need only careful monitoring for recurrence or worsening of symptoms and for poor growth. However, airway evaluation should be performed in all cases where a different pathology is considered or when symptoms worsen or persist past the expected age of resolution.

Q: What should I do when symptoms worsen?
A: Calm the patient, provide humidification of secretions and treatment of intercurrent infection. In cases where associated bronchospasm is suspected, a trial of steroids or bronchodilators may be considered.

ICD-9-CM 748.3

BIBLIOGRAPHY

Altman K, et al. Congenital airway abnormalities in patients requiring hospitalization. *Arch Otolaryngol Head Neck Surg* 1999;125(5):525–528.

Baxter J, Dunbar J. Tracheomalacia. *Ann Otol Rhinol Laryngol* 1963;72:1013–1023.

Deoras K, et al. Developmental changes in tracheal structure. *Pediatr Res* 1991;30(2):170–175.

Jacobs I, et al. Tracheobronchomalacia in children. *Arch Otolaryngol Head Neck Surg* 1994;120(2):154–158.

Schidlow D, Smith D. *A practical guide to pediatric respiratory diseases*. St. Louis: Mosby, 1994.

Author: Laura T. Mulreany

Transfusion Reaction

 Database

DEFINITION

Any acute or subacute adverse reaction that develops as a consequence of the administration of blood components. Types include:

- Acute reactions: hemolytic, febrile, allergic, hypervolemia, bacterial sepsis
- Delayed reactions: hemolytic
- Late complications of transfusion: infection, alloimmunization, iron overload, graft-versus-host disease (GVHD)

EPIDEMIOLOGY

10% of blood product recipients develop some type of transfusion reaction.

ACUTE HEMOLYTIC

Cause

Incompatibility of donor RBC antigens and recipient RBC antibodies; usually ABO blood group incompatibility

Pathophysiology

Antigen-antibody interaction leads to complement activation on the surface of the transfused red cells, resulting in acute intravascular hemolysis and vasomotor instability.

History and Physical Examination

Fever, chills, abdominal or flank pain, pink or tea-colored urine, tachycardia, hypotension, oliguria

Laboratory Aids

- Direct Coombs test: positive
- CBC: anemia
- UA: hemoglobinuria
- PT/PTT/fibrinogen/FSP: disseminated intravascular coagulation (DIC)

Therapy

- As needed to maintain circulation and urine output

—Stop transfusion immediately.
—Hydration
—Pressors
—Diuretics

- Treat DIC with plasma

Prevention

Proper labelling of blood specimens and products and correct identification of product and recipient will eliminate most acute hemolytic transfusion reactions.

FEBRILE

Cause

Reaction between recipient antibodies to donor leukocyte or plasma protein antigens

Pathophysiology

Prior exposure to blood products may result in the formation of antibodies to leukocytes or plasma protein antigens; upon reexposure the antigen-antibody interaction causes the release of pyrogens; these reactions develop more frequently in individuals with a history of prior transfusion or pregnancy; alternatively, cytokines in the product can cause fever in the recipient.

History and Physical Examination

Fever, chills

Laboratory Aids

- Direct Coombs test
- Blood culture of the patient and product
- Stat Gram stain of the product; all should be negative
- This is a diagnosis of exclusion.

Therapy

Stop transfusion; antipyretics (acetaminophen); may resume transfusion if patient is stable and acute hemolytic transfusion reaction is ruled out.

Prevention

Pretransfusion antipyretic or administration of leukodepleted products; the latter is recommended for chronically transfused patients who have a high incidence of febrile transfusion reactions.

ALLERGIC

Cause

Reaction between recipient antibodies and donor plasma proteins; the incidence is sporadic and donor dependent.

Pathophysiology

Unknown

History and Physical Examination

Urticaria; sometimes bronchospasm; rarely anaphylaxis

Laboratory Aids

None

Therapy

Stop transfusion; antihistamine (diphenhydramine); steroids or epinephrine in severe reactions

Prevention

Pretransfusion antihistamine or administration of washed RBC products (in patients with repeated or severe allergic reactions)

HYPERVOLEMIA

Cause

Administration of an excessive volume of a blood product or infusion at an excessive rate

Pathophysiology

Circulatory overload leading to heart failure

History and Physical Examination

Hypertension, dyspnea, rales, cardiac arrhythmia

Laboratory Aids

CXR: increased pulmonary vascular markings

Therapy

Diuretics (furosemide)

Prevention

Administer appropriate volumes (typically 10 mL/kg) at appropriate rate; most RBC transfusions are administered over 3 to 4 hours unless the patient is acutely hypovolemic or actively hemorrhaging; individuals with chronic anemia are frequently euvolemic and should be transfused gradually (smaller volumes over longer time period).

BACTERIAL SEPSIS

Cause

Contaminated blood product; most common in platelet products near the end of their shelf life

Pathophysiology

Intravascular infusion of viable bacteria and endotoxins leads to acute septic shock.

History and Physical Examination

Fever, chills, hypotension

Laboratory Aids

Stat Gram stain and blood culture of the transfused product; positive for bacteria

Therapy

Stop transfusion, fluids if hypotensive, and antibiotics to cover *Staphylococcus* and *Yersinia* species

Prevention

Sterile technique in blood collection, storage and administration; careful inspection of product prior to transfusion

DELAYED HEMOLYTIC

Cause

Incompatibility of donor RBC antigens and recipient RBC antibodies; usually minor blood group antigens

Pathophysiology

Previously transfused individuals who have been sensitized to a minor blood group antigen develop an anamnestic response upon reexposure; at the time of the current transfusion, antibody titers are below detectable levels; after the transfusion is complete, titers rise (usually within 3 to 10 days) and extravascular hemolysis occurs.

History and Physical Examination

Fever, malaise, dark urine, jaundice; rarely shock, renal failure

Laboratory Aids

CBC: anemia; bilirubin: elevated; indirect Coombs test (antibody screen): positive; direct Coombs test: positive (mixed field) if done early

Therapy

Depends on degree of hemolysis; if profound, may need management as described under Acute Hemolytic above

Prevention

Appropriately performed antibody screen at time of transfusion; check blood bank records for previously identified antibodies.

LATE COMPLICATIONS

Infection

- Posttransfusion hepatitis: caused by hepatitis B or C
- Acquired immunodeficiency syndrome (AIDS): caused by human immunodeficiency virus (HIV)
- Cytomegalovirus (CMV): problematic in individuals with inherited or acquired immunodeficiency states; these individuals should receive CMV-negative products
- Other infection: Epstein-Barr virus, syphilis, malaria, toxoplasmosis, HTLV-I, Chagas disease, babesiosis, filariasis

Alloimmunization

Formation of antibodies to RBC, platelet, and human leukocyte antigens (HLA) can develop in an individual who has been multiply transfused; this can cause cross-matching problems, febrile transfusion reactions, delayed hemolytic transfusion reactions, and platelet transfusion refractoriness.

Iron Overload

Chronically transfused individuals will accumulate iron as a byproduct of RBC breakdown; an iron-chelating drug (desferrioxamine) will enhance its excretion.

Graft-Versus-Host Disease (GVHD)

Individuals with inherited or acquired T-cell immunodeficiency states can develop GVHD from transfused immunocompetent T cells; can also occur if donor and recipient are related and share HLA types; these individuals should receive irradiated blood products.

 ## Common Questions and Answers

Q: What is the risk of acquiring certain infections?
A: Hepatitis B—1:63,000 units
Hepatitis C—1:103,000 units
HIV—1:676,000 units

Q: Is directed donor blood safer?
A: No, there is no evidence that the infection risk is lower, and some studies suggest that the infection risk actually may be higher.

Q: Is it safe to give a transfusion to a patient with fever?
A: Yes. However, if the temperature rises during the transfusion or if symptoms such as chills or hypotension develop, the transfusion should be stopped and the patient evaluated for a transfusion reaction.

ICD-9-CM 999.8

BIBLIOGRAPHY

Busch MP. Transfusion and HIV. *Curr Opin Hematol* 1994;1:438.

Capon SM, Goldfinger D. Acute hemolytic transfusion reaction, a paradigm of the systemic inflammatory response: new insights into pathophysiology and treatment. *Transfusion* 1995;35(6):513–520.

Jones DS, Byers RH, et al. Epidemiology of transfusion-associated acquired immuno-deficiency syndrome in children in the United States. *Pediatrics* 1992;89:123.

Manno CS. What's new in transfusion medicine. *Pediatr Clin North Am* 1996;43: 793–808.

Petz LD, Swisher SN, Kleinman S, et al., eds. *Clinical practice of transfusion medicine*, 3rd ed. New York: Churchill Livingstone, 1996.

Schreiber, et al. The risk of transfusion transmitted infection. *N Engl J Med* 1996;96:1685–1690.

Author: Cynthia F. Norris

Transient Erythroblastopenia of Childhood

 Database

DEFINITION

An acquired, self-limited suppression of red cell production in an otherwise healthy child.

PATHOPHYSIOLOGY

Unknown. Possible viral etiology is parvovirus B19, but this remains hypothetical. A serum inhibitor, such as an IgG directed at the committed erythroid stem cell progenitor, has also been proposed but not yet proven.

GENETICS

There is no simple genetic pattern; familial TEC has been reported (rarely), suggesting a combination of environmental factors and genetic propensity.

EPIDEMIOLOGY

- Mean age at diagnosis is 26 months; less than 10% are older than 3 years of age at diagnosis.
- Slight male predominance (male/female 5.1:3.1)
- There is no seasonal predominance.

COMPLICATIONS

- Cardiovascular compromise secondary to severe anemia is often less than expected given the level of anemia. High-output congestive heart failure is unusual.
- Neurologic symptoms including confusion and transient hemiparesis have been reported but are rare.
- A significant number of patients also have neutropenia (ANC <1500/μL) during either the acute or recovery phases of the illness.

PROGNOSIS

- All children recover usually within 1 to 2 months from diagnosis (up to 8 months to recovery).
- Prognosis is excellent.
- Recurrence is rare.

 Differential Diagnosis

- Environmental: iron-deficiency anemia
- Metabolic: hypothyroidism
- Congenital: Diamond-Blackfan anemia (this diagnosis usually made within first year of life)
- Neoplasm: leukemia, myelodysplastic syndromes
- Miscellaneous: renal disease, anemia of chronic disease

 Data Gathering

HISTORY

Question: Pallor?
Significance: Typically slow in onset and, therefore, often missed by parents. Often noted by an adult who sees the child less frequently.

Question: Activity level?
Significance: Often preserved because of slow onset of anemia. An extremely anemic child may be irritable, sleepy, and/or lethargic.

SPECIAL QUESTIONS

Question: History of fever, easy bruisability, or frequent/severe infections (especially bacterial)?
Significance: Should alert the clinician to consider other diagnoses such as leukemia and bone marrow failure syndromes.

 Physical Examination

- Child is generally well appearing and not chronically ill.
- Pallor
- Tachycardia secondary to anemia
- Usually no organomegaly, ecchymosis, petechiae, or jaundice

 Laboratory Aids

Test: CBC
Significance: Low Hgb, normal MCV, normal RBC morphology. Total WBC count/morphology and platelet count should be normal; if not, consider leukemias. ANC may be decreased (rarely below 500/μL) but morphology must be normal. RDW may be elevated during recovery.

Test: Reticulocyte count
Significance: Low to zero during anemic phase, should be high during recovery

Test: Chemistry/blood bank
Significance: Bilirubin, LDH, ferritin, iron levels, and Coombs testing should be normal to rule out iron-deficiency anemia and immune hemolysis.

Test: Hemoglobin electrophoresis with quantitative HbF
Significance: Should be normal in TEC, elevated in Diamond-Blackfan anemia

Test: Chest x-ray
Significance: To determine degree of cardiomegaly

Test: Bone marrow aspiration
Significance: May be necessary to rule in TEC and rule out other diagnoses such as Diamond-Blackfan and the leukemias. Presence or absence of early RBC precursors may help predict time to recovery. Maturation of megakaryocytes and the myeloid cell line must be normal, especially if neutropenia is present.

Transient Erythroblastopenia of Childhood

 Therapy

- Initial inpatient observation for complications of severe anemia. Daily CBC at least initially to gauge rate of fall of hemoglobin/rise of reticulocyte count and to estimate time to recovery.
- PRBC transfusion only if there is evidence of cardiovascular compromise. If a transfusion is needed, transfuse slowly to prevent fluid overload. A good rule of thumb is to transfuse the same number of mL/kg as the patient's hemoglobin, over 3 to 4 hours. A second transfusion is rarely required.
- Normal activity and diet for age, as tolerated
- Instruct family on signs and symptoms of severe anemia.

DRUGS

No role for prednisone, iron supplements, anabolic steroids, or other immunosuppressive agents. Short-term folic acid may be indicated during reticulocytosis.

 Follow-Up

WHEN TO EXPECT IMPROVEMENT

- Clinic visits weekly to monitor hemoglobin and reticulocytes. (These visits may need to be more frequent in the beginning of the illness and less frequent as recovery becomes evident.)
- Elevation of reticulocyte count is the first sign of recovery.

PREVENTION

There is no known way to prevent TEC.

ISOLATION

Because of possible teratogenicity of parvovirus 19 and contagion within hospital

PITFALLS

- TEC must be an isolated normocytic, normochromic anemia. If the other cell lines are affected or if the anemia is macrocytic, consider bone marrow failure syndromes.
- Iron therapy has no place in the treatment of TEC. Be sure to check RBC indices and reticulocyte count prior to instituting iron therapy for anemia.

 Common Questions and Answers

Q: Can other children in a family get this illness?
A: The cause(s) of this illness in otherwise normal children is unknown. It is very rare for other family members to be affected. It is appropriate to reassure parents with regard to this issue.

Q: Are transfusions always necessary?
A: No. Only in cases of heart failure is a transfusion necessary. Most often, children can be managed with watchful waiting.

Q: How can TEC be distinguished from Diamond-Blackfan syndrome?
A: Children with Diamond-Blackfan syndrome are usually less than 1 year old and can have elevated hemoglobin F levels. If a bone marrow aspirate is obtained during the recovery phase of TEC, then the diagnosis will be clear. Often, however, only time will tell. Children with TEC always recover; those with Diamond-Blackfan syndrome do not.

ICD-9-CM 284.8

BIBLIOGRAPHY

Bhambhani K, Inoue S, Sarnaik SA. Seasonal clustering of transient erythroblastopenia of childhood. *Am J Child Dis* 1988;142:175–177.

Cherrick I, Karayalcin G, Lanzkowsky P. Transient erythroblastopenia of childhood: prospective study of fifty patients. *Am J Pediatr Hematol Oncol* 1994;16(4):320–324.

Nathan DG, Oski FA, eds. *Hematology of infancy and childhood*, 4th ed. Philadelphia: WB Saunders, 1993.

Author: Julie W. Stern
Therese B. West, 1st edition

Transient Tachypnea of the Newborn (TTN)

 Database

DEFINITION

Early onset of tachypnea (respiratory rate >60 breaths per minute) following uneventful normal preterm or term, vaginal or cesarean delivery; sometimes with retractions, expiratory grunting, or cyanosis relieved by minimal oxygenation (<40%).

PATHOPHYSIOLOGY

• Slow or decreased absorption of fetal lung fluid, including fluid accumulation in the interstitial space, resulting in decreased pulmonary compliance, decreased tidal volume, and increased dead space
• Mild immaturity of the surfactant system may contribute to decreased pulmonary compliance and result in increased respiratory rate. In some infants with TTN, a decreased amount of phosphatidyl glycerol has been found in their amniotic fluid.

EPIDEMIOLOGY

11 per 1,000 live births

COMPLICATIONS

• Hypoxia
• Respiratory failure requiring CPAP or mechanical ventilation (rare)

PROGNOSIS

Generally considered a self-limited condition with no recurrence and no residual pulmonary dysfunction. Some studies, however, have demonstrated associations with persistent fetal circulation in the neonatal period and asthma during childhood.

 Differential Diagnosis

RESPIRATORY

• Meconium aspiration
• Respiratory distress syndrome
• Pneumothorax
• Pneumomediastinum

INFECTION

• Pneumonia
• Sepsis

NEUROLOGIC

• Cerebral hypoventilation
• Birth asphyxia

CARDIAC

• Congenital cyanotic heart disease

METABOLIC

• Conditions manifesting as metabolic acidosis

MISCELLANEOUS

• CCAM (congenital cystic adenomatoid malformation)

 Data Gathering

HISTORY

Question: When was the onset of tachypnea?
Significance: In general, TTN usually presents as early onset of tachypnea (within first few hours of life)

Question: Are there maternal risk factors?
Significance: Recent research has demonstrated that TTN was twice as likely for infants of mothers with asthma compared to infants of mothers without asthma.

Question: Are there birth-related risk factors?
Significance: Birth risk factors include maternal sedation, maternal fluid administration, maternal exposure to β-mimetic agents, prolonged labor, cesarean section, preterm birth, fetal asphyxia, and infant male sex. The mechanisms are unknown. The presence of risk factors for other conditions (e.g., maternal fever) may make a TTN diagnosis less likely and other diagnoses more likely (e.g., pneumonia or sepsis).

 Physical Examination

• Respiratory rate >60 per minute
• Cyanosis, grunting, flaring, intercostal retractions
• Lungs clear on auscultation, without rales or rhonchi
• Absence of signs and symptoms more specific for infection, and neurologic and cardiac conditions (e.g., fever, cyanosis without respiratory distress)

 Laboratory Aids

TESTS

Test: Pulse oxymetry
Significance: Oxygen saturation should be maintained above 96%.

Test: Arterial blood gas
Significance: Metabolic acidosis with base deficit suggestive of asphyxia

Test: CBC
Significance: Decreased or increased white cell count and increased immature forms (e.g., bands) suggests infection.

Test: Blood culture
Significance: Positive results indicate infection.

RADIOGRAPHIC STUDIES

Test: Chest x-ray
Significance: TTN indicated by prominent central pulmonary vascular markings (central perihilar streaking), fluid lines in the fissures, hyperaeration, flat diaphragms and, occasionally, pleural fluid.

Emergency Care

• NPO (initially, nothing by mouth until respiratory status stabilized and diagnosis clarified)
• Oxygen (may help reduce respiratory distress if patient hypoxic)
• CPAP or mechanical ventilation if indicated
• Antibiotics if pneumonia or sepsis suspected
• Furosemide (diuretic) has not been shown to improve TTN

SUPPORTIVE CARE

• IV fluids if NPO
• Monitoring of respiratory status (e.g., pulse oximetry)

Transient Tachypnea of the Newborn (TTN)

 Therapy

 Follow-Up

WHEN TO EXPECT IMPROVEMENT

- Rapid respirations slow gradually.
- 12 to 72 hours

SIGNS TO WATCH FOR

- Fever, lethargy, poor feeding, early jaundice
- Persistent or increased need for oxygen

PITFALLS

Since TTN is a diagnosis of exclusion, it is important to consider and exclude other diagnoses by carefully relying on history, examination, and appropriate laboratory aids.

 Common Questions and Answers

Q: Will my baby have breathing problems afterward?
A: No.

Q: Is my baby at risk for breathing problems such as asthma?
A: No. Although there is a relationship between maternal asthma and TTN, there is no consistent evidence thus far of a relationship between TTN and the development of asthma.

Q: When can my baby go home?
A: When his/her breathing rate is low enough so that s/he does not need oxygen and can feed well.

ICD-9-CM 770.6

BIBLIOGRAPHY

Dani C, Reali MF, Bertini G, et al. Risk factors for the development of respiratory distress syndrome and transient tachypnea in newborn infants. *Eur Respir J* 1999;14:155–159.

Demissie K, Marcella SW, Breckenbridge MB, et al. Maternal asthma and transient tachypnea of the newborn. *Pediatrics* 1998;102:84–90.

Hansen T, Corbet A. Disorders of transition. In: Taeusch HW, Ballard R, eds. *Avery's diseases of the newborn*, 7th ed. Philadelphia: WB Saunders, 1998:613–615.

Hook B, Kiwi R, Amini SB, et al. Neonatal morbidity after elective repeat cesarean section and trial of labor. *Pediatrics* 1997;100:348–353.

Martin RJ, Sosenko I, Bancalari E. Respiratory problems. In: Klaus MH, Fanaroff AA, eds. *Care of the high-risk neonate*, 5th ed. Philadelphia: WB Saunders, 2001:262–263.

Miller MJ, Fanaroff AA, Martin RJ. Respiratory disorders in preterm and term infants. In: Fanaroff AA, Martin RJ, eds. *Neonatal-perinatal medicine: diseases of the fetus and infants*, 7th ed. St. Louis: Mosby Year Books, 2001:1030–1031.

Schaubel D, Johansen H, Dutta M, et al. Neonatal characteristics as risk factors for preschool asthma. *J Asthma* 1996;33: 255–264.

Whitsett JA, Pryhuber GS, Rice WR, et al., eds. *Neonatology, pathophysiology and management of the newborn*, 5th ed. Philadelphia: Lippincott Williams & Wilkins, 1999:505–506.

Author: John I. Takayama

Transposition of the Great Arteries

 Database

DEFINITION

Abnormal anatomic relationship between the great arteries and the ventricles in which the aorta arises from the anatomic right ventricle and the pulmonary artery arises from the anatomic left ventricle.

PATHOLOGY

• In transposition of the great arteries (TGA) the aorta originates anteriorly from the right ventricle carrying desaturated blood to the body, and the pulmonary artery originates posteriorly from the left ventricle carrying oxygenated blood to the lungs. There is fibrous continuity between the pulmonary and mitral valves and subaortic conus (infundibulum) is present. In the normal heart the aorta arises posteriorly from the left ventricle, there is fibrous continuity between the aortic and mitral valves, and subpulmonary conus is present.
• The most common type of TGA, known as D-transposition or D-TGA is TGA (S,D,D): situs solitus of the atria and viscera (S), dextroventricular segment situs (D), aortic valve annulus to the right of the pulmonary artery (D).
• Other variations include TGA (S,D,L), in which the aortic valve annulus is to the left of the pulmonary artery (L), and TGA (S,L,L) or "corrected transposition," in which there is situs solitus of the atria and the viscera (S), levoventricular segment situs (L), and the aortic valve annulus is to the left of the pulmonary artery (L).
• Associated abnormalities: PDA and PFO with intact ventricular septum (50%), dynamic obstruction of the left ventricular outflow tract (subpulmonary obstruction)(20%), ventricular septal defect (VSD) (40%), VSD and left ventricular outflow tract obstruction (10%), subaortic stenosis, aortic stenosis, coarctation of the aorta or interruption of the aortic arch (10%), subpulmonic stenosis, pulmonary stenosis, pulmonary atresia, coronary branching abnormalities (33%), straddling or overriding atrioventricular valve, leftward juxtaposition of the atrial appendages (5%).

PATHOPHYSIOLOGY

• Systemic and pulmonary circulation are separated and function in parallel.
• Desaturated systemic venous blood passes through the right heart to the aorta, while the oxygenated pulmonary venous blood passes through the left heart and returns to the lungs.
• Survival depends on defects that permit mixing between the two circulations [PDA, PFO/atrial septal defect (ASD), VSD].

EPIDEMIOLOGY

• TGA represents 5% to 7% of all congenital heart disease.
• Incidence is 20 to 30 per 100,000 live births, with a 60% to 70% male preponderance.

 Differential Diagnosis

The differential diagnosis for the neonate with transposition of the great arteries is that of the cyanotic neonate.

• Cardiac

—Lesions with ductal dependent pulmonary blood flow:
  —Tricuspid atresia with normally related great arteries
  —Tetralogy of Fallot
  —Tetralogy of Fallot with pulmonic atresia
  —Critical pulmonic stenosis
  —Pulmonary atresia with intact ventricular septum
  —Ebstein anomaly
  —Heterotaxy (most forms)

—Ductal independent mixing lesions:
  —Total anomalous pulmonary venous connection without obstruction
  —Truncus arteriosus

—Lesions with ductal dependent systemic blood flow:
  —Hypoplastic left heart syndrome
  —Interrupted aortic arch
  —Critical coarctation of the aorta
  —Critical aortic stenosis

• Pulmonary

—Primary lung disease
—Airway obstruction
—Extrinsic compression of the lungs

• Neurologic

—CNS dysfunction
—Respiratory neuromuscular dysfunction

• Hematologic

—Methemoglobinemia
—Polycythemia

 Data Gathering

HISTORY

• Infants of normal birth weight or sometimes larger than normal.
• Cyanosis within the first few hours (intact atrial septum) or first few days of life.
• Tachypnea often without retractions
• Poor feeding

 Physical Examination

• General: moderate to severe cyanosis in a large male newborn with "comfortable" tachypnea
• Cardiovascular: single loud S_2, no heart murmur is heard in infants with intact ventricular septum, soft systolic murmur in those infants with a VSD, and a systolic ejection murmur of valvar or subvalvar aortic or pulmonic stenosis may be heard.
• Respiratory: generally there is dyspnea and tachypnea without retractions in the neonate without a VSD; in cases of a large VSD with congestive heart failure, retractions will be present.
• Abdomen: hepatomegaly occurs when there is a large VSD and congestive heart failure.

 Laboratory Aids

TESTS OR STUDIES

• *Arterial blood gas*: hypoxemia (Po_2 often in low 30s) unchanged in 100% Fio_2. Infants with marginal mixing have Po_2 <20 with metabolic acidosis.
• *Chest radiograph*: mild cardiomegaly with an egg-shaped heart with narrow superior mediastinum and increased pulmonary vascular markings (egg on a string)
• *Electrocardiogram*: initially normal, progressing to right ventricular hypertrophy and right axis deviation
• *Echocardiogram*: two-dimensional echocardiography and color-flow Doppler studies usually provide all the anatomic and functional information required for management of infants with D-TGA. The study should focus on the alignment of the great arteries, and other associated anomalies, specifically defects that promote intercirculatory mixing, the presence of left or right ventricular outflow tract obstruction, and the coronary anatomy.

 Therapy

DRUGS

• Correction of metabolic acidosis, hypoglycemia, and hypocalcemia improves myocardial function.
• PGE_1 is used for severe cyanosis to promote mixing at the ductus arteriosus. Instituting PGE_1 may increase pulmonary venous congestion if there is an inadequate interatrial communication by increasing the pulmonary blood flow). Side effects of PGE_1 include apnea, fever, and hypotension.

INTERVENTIONAL CATHETERIZATION

• Balloon atrial septostomy (Rashkind procedure) is used in the severely hypoxemic infant with an intact or restrictive atrial septum to promote intercirculatory mixing at the atrial level to stabilize the neonate prior to definitive or palliative surgery.

SURGERY

• Definitive surgery for D-TGA includes procedures that redirect the right- and left-sided pulmonary and systemic venous returns at the atrial, ventricular, and great artery level, and include:

—Atrial inversion: Atrial inversion procedures involve baffling the pulmonary venous blood flow to the tricuspid valve (systemic circulation), and the systemic venous blood flow to the mitral valve (pulmonary circulation). The two atrial inversion operations include the *Mustard* procedure, in which prosthetic or pericardial baffles are used to redirect the blood, and the *Senning* procedure, in which the baffles are made of an atrial septal flap and the RA free wall. The Senning procedure, a modification of the Mustard procedure, is used in the following infants:
  —Infants with D-TGA with intact ventricular septum, who have not been repaired within the first month of life
  —Neonates with D-TGA with intact ventricular septum and moderate to severe pulmonic stenosis
  —Neonates with D-TGA with "unswitchable coronaries" (<1% of cases)

—Ventricular inversion:
  —D-TGA/VSD with severe pulmonic stenosis: The *Rastelli* operation may be used to redirect the blood at the ventricular level. In the operation the left ventricular blood flow is baffled to the aorta by creating an intraventricular tunnel between the VSD and the aortic valve. A conduit is placed from the right ventricle to the pulmonary artery to redirect the right ventricular blood flow.
  —D-TGA/VSD with severe aortic stenosis: The Damus-Kaye-Stansel operation in conjunction with the Rastelli operation may be used to redirect ventricular blood flow.

—Arterial switch: Surgical switching of the great arteries with coronary reimplantation.

PROGNOSIS

• Without treatment, 30% mortality in first week of life, 50% within first month, 70% within first 6 months, and 90% within first year.
• In most centers, the mortality rate after arterial switch operation for D-TGA with intact ventricular septum or D-TGA/VSD is less than 3%. Factors that have been shown to increase the mortality risk include an intramural course of the left coronary artery, retropulmonary course of the left coronary artery, complex arch abnormalities, right ventricular hypoplasia, multiple VSDs, and straddling atrioventricular valves.

 Follow-Up

COMPLICATIONS

• Complications of the *intraatrial surgeries* include obstruction of the pulmonary venous return (<2% of the cases), obstruction of the systemic venous return (<5% of cases), residual intraatrial baffle shunt (<20% of all cases), tricuspid regurgitation (5–10%), absence of sinus rhythm (>50% of cases), frequent supraventricular arrhythmias (50%), and moderate to severely depressed RV function (10%). Follow-up is recommended every 6 to 12 months to detect arrhythmias, TR, or depressed right ventricular function, which generally occurs years after surgery. Arrhythmias include sick-sinus syndrome, marked sinus bradycardia, ectopic atrial rhythm, slow junctional rhythm, and supraventricular tachycardia, especially aflutter and ectopic atrial tachycardia.
• Complications after the *Rastelli* operation include conduit obstruction and complete heart block (rare). Follow-up is recommended every 12 months to monitor for conduit obstruction, left ventricular outflow tract obstruction, and various forms of heart block.
• Complications after the *arterial switch operation* are much rarer relative to the atrial and ventricular inversion operations, and include supravalvar pulmonary stenosis at the anastomotic site (<5% of cases), supravalvar aortic stenosis at the anastomotic site (<5% of cases), neo-aortic regurgitation is a late finding in 25% of patients, and coronary artery obstruction, which may lead to ischemia and infarction. *These complications are generally rare and hemodynamically insignificant.* Mortality results from the following:

—*Early mortality* is usually related to kinking or obstruction of the coronary arteries during transfer to the neoaorta, an "unprepared" left ventricle, or hemorrhage from the multiple suture lines.
—*Late mortality* (1–2%) usually occurs from myocardial ischemia, pulmonary vascular obstructive disease, or during reoperation for supravalvular stenosis.

• Follow-up is recommended every 6 to 12 months to monitor for supravalvar aortic or pulmonic stenosis, neo-aortic valve insufficiency and coronary ischemia.

ICD-9-CM 745.10

BIBLIOGRAPHY

Blume ED, Wernovsky G. Long-term results of the arterial switch operation for transposition of the great vessels. *Semin Thorac Cardiovasc Surg* 1998;1:129–137.

Dunbar-Masterson C, Wypij D, Bellinger DC, et al. General health status of children with D-transposition of the great arteries after the arterial switch operation. *Circulation* 2001;104(12 suppl 1):I138–142.

Paul MH, Wernovsky G. Transposition of the great arteries. In: Emmanouilides GC, Riemenschneider TA, Allen HD, et al., eds. *Moss and Adams' heart disease in infants, children and adolescents including the fetus and young adult*, 5th ed. Baltimore: Williams & Wilkins, 1995:1154–1225.

Wernovsky G, Hougen TJ, Walsh EP, et al. Midterm results after the arterial switch operation for transposition of the great arteries with intact ventricular septum: clinical, hemodynamic, echocardiographic and electrophysiologic data. *Circulation* 1988;77:1333–1344.

Wernovsky G, Mayer JE Jr, Jonas RA, et al. Factors influencing early and late outcome of the arterial switch operation for transposition of the great arteries. *J Thorac Cardiovasc Surg* 1995;109:289–302.

Author: Bradley S. Marino

Transverse Myelitis

 Database

DEFINITION

Demyelination in the spinal cord causing acute/subacute loss of motor sensory and autonomic function, often preceded by midback pain; may be postviral, postvaccinal, or associated with multiple sclerosis. Pathophysiology suspected: autoimmune versus direct viral invasion versus vasculitis.

ASSOCIATED CONDITIONS

• Rarely, primary inflammatory disorders (e.g., lupus erythematosus, Sjögren disease) present with transverse myelitis
• Rare metabolic causes of myelopathy include vitamin B_{12} deficiency, adrenomyeloneuropathy/leukodystrophy

EPIDEMIOLOGY

4.6/million per year

 Differential Diagnosis

Presentation of transverse myelitis in a toddler may resemble osteomyelitis, arthritis, toxic synovitis, or even an acute abdominal process: extreme irritability, unwillingness to bear weight. In many cases extremity weakness seen in transverse myelitis may resemble an acute neuromuscular disorder such as Guillain-Barré syndrome (GBS) or polymyositis. Definitive myelopathic signs (spastic tone, hyperreflexia, up-going toes, sensory level) require exclusion of alternative causes of myelopathy that are treated differently:

• Compressive myelopathies:

—Vertebral osteomyelitis/discitis
—Intrinsic or extrinsic tumor
—Spine trauma
—Epidural abscess

• Infectious causes of myelopathy:

—Polio: raises concern of underlying immunodeficiency
—Lyme disease: in children with possible exposure; serology is nonspecific but is sensitive unless antibiotics given early in the course (ablating immune response)
—Syphilis: usually chronic, tertiary form (tabes dorsalis), though meningovascular lues may cause acute myelopathy

• Inflammatory diseases: especially lupus erythematosus
• Vascular: cord ischemia (postcardiac surgery), cord AVM
• Metabolic: leukodystrophy usually chronic myelopathy:
• Pelizaeus-Merzbacher, adrenoleukodystrophy (both X-linked)
• Transverse myelitis may be part of a more generalized demyelinative disorder.
• If multiple lesions occur at different times, diagnosis of multiple sclerosis is made.
• Transverse myelitis in association with demyelination of optic nerves (optic neuritis) is referred to as Devic disease.
• Multiple coincident demyelinating lesions: best seen on MRI; indicate acute disseminated encephalomyelitis (ADEM)

 Data Gathering

HISTORY

The most prominent symptom is often unwillingness or inability to bear weight, possibly with decreased spontaneous use of hands. History of neoplastic illness or immunodeficiency may suggest alternate causes of acute myelopathy. Details of the temporal course of the symptoms are important, since sudden onset of weakness, although not inconsistent with transverse myelitis, raises the possibility of acute structural or vascular causes of myelopathy. After 2 to 3 days, the patient's signs usually plateau and evolve toward spasticity/hyperreflexia.

• Transverse myelitis may be suggested by history of back pain or urinary or fecal incontinence/retention.
• Episodes are often preceded by respiratory illness, trauma, or surgery.

 Physical Examination

• Children often appear extremely irritable, and extent of weakness is assessed by how vigorously the child resists examination.
• Fever, hypertension, tachycardia, meningeal signs can appear; point tenderness over the spine may point to an alternative diagnosis.
• Neurologic exam directed to visual acuity and color vision, funduscopic examination for optic nerve head pallor (optic neuritis)
• Motor signs of abnormal tone: weakness is usually symmetric, legs more than arms
• Reflexes are normal or brisk.
• Sensory ataxia, a sensory level that can spare joint position and vibration, can be present.
• Sphincter dysfunction can lead to emergent complication of *urinary retention* or incontinence; check for loss of anal wink, bladder dilatation, postvoid residual.

Laboratory Aids

- Urgent imaging of the spine must be done in acute myelopathy to rule out a surgically remediable lesion.
- MRI of spine (at lowest level that could explain level of weakness or sensory) excludes structural causes of myelopathy and can be diagnostic of transverse myelitis: cord swelling with abnormal signal within the cord.
- CSF, usually done after imaging, often shows normal or slightly increased protein, mild pleocytosis with lymphocyte predominance.
- Investigation for underlying inflammatory disorder including ESR and ANA, is appropriate.
- Investigation for granulomatous disease or spirochetal infection includes PPD/anergy panel, serum ACE (angiotensin-converting enzyme, elevated in sarcoidosis), RPR, Lyme titer.
- Viruses associated with TM include the herpesviruses (EBV, VZV, HSV), mumps, rubella, influenza, HIV.
- Investigation for underlying metabolic disorder can include very-long-chain fatty acid (VLCFA) (looking for adrenoleuko-dystrophy) and B_{12} (looking for subacute combined degeneration).

 ## Therapy

- Intravenous glucocorticoids may be most useful in acute demyelinative disease if used within 48 hours of symptom onset.
- patients with transverse myelitis whose symptoms are progressing require close monitoring, in some cases in an intensive care setting, to anticipate respiratory embarrassment or autonomic instability; mechanical ventilation or use of antihypertensive agents may be necessary.
- Autonomic deficits may require bowel/bladder regimen, catheterization, prophylactic antibiotics, stool softeners.
- Neurosurgical consultation if imaging reveals a surgically remediable cause of myelopathy (e.g., epidural abscess, neuroblastoma)
- Cyclophosphamide reported useful in myelitis associated with inflammatory diseases (lupus).
- Treatments indicated for other causes of myelopathy that may be found (e.g., emergent radiation/steroid therapy for neoplastic cord compression)

 ## Follow-Up

- 60% of individuals with transverse myelitis resolve (gradually); neurologic complications include fixed weakness, sensory, or autonomic deficits.
- In cases of suspected MS, check brainstem auditory evoked potentials (BAERs), visual evoked responses (VERs) for evidence of other foci of demyelination.
- Physical and occupational therapy may help promote functional recovery and prevent contractures.

PITFALLS

- A high index of suspicion of abnormal autonomic reflexes may prevent perforated bladder.
- GBS is frequently confused with transverse myelitis, particularly when the latter presents with hyporeflexia; also, the "cytoalbuminemic dissociation" (high-protein, low-grade pleocytosis) in CSF from patients with GBS helps distinguish the two conditions.

 ## Common Questions and Answers

Q: What makes you think this could be MS instead?
A: History of other similar episodes that have now resolved completely, association with internuclear ophthalmoplegia, association with optic neuritis, multiple lesions in space of different ages on MRI of brain/spine.

Q: What is the usual clinical course?
A: Symptoms usually worsen for 2 to 3 days, then plateau and change to upper motor neuron (UMN) before 60% resolve gradually to baseline.

Q: What causes the pain and irritability commonly seen in children with TM?
A: Pain in TM may be due to (1) neuropathic pain from nerve root inflammation, (2) nociceptive pain from passive dural inflammation, (3) muscle spasm from motor dyscontrol, (4) bladder distention from dysautonomia, (5) psychological distress from loss of motor control, or (6) dysesthesia from demyelination of spinothalamic tract.

ICD-9-CM 323.9

BIBLIOGRAPHY

Knebusch M, Strassburg HM. Acute transverse myelitis in childhood: nine cases and review of the literature. *Dev Med Child Neurol* 1998;40:631–639.

Sebire G, Hollenberg H, Meyer L, et al. High dose methyl prednisolone in severe acute transverse myelopathy. *Arch Dis Child* 1997;76:167–168.

Wilmshurst J, Walker MC. Rapid onset transverse myelitis in adolescence: implications for pathogenesis and prognosis. *Arch Dis Child* 1999;80:137–142.

Author: D. Elizabeth McNeil

Trichinosis

Database

DEFINITION

Disease caused by ingestion of inadequately cooked meat containing the nematode (roundworm) *Trichinella* larvae cysts (parasitic food poisoning).

- Other names: trichinosis, trichinelliasis, trichinellosis

PATHOPHYSIOLOGY

- *Trichinella* larvae (eggs, cysts, obligate intracellular parasites) in poorly cooked meat (primarily pork) eaten by patient
- Symptoms related to absolute number of ingested larvae
- Organisms released after cyst wall digestion by gastric enzymes, pass to small intestine, invade mucosa with edema, hyperemia, and ulcerations, and then develop into adult worms. Fertilized females release larvae (500–5,000) over approximately 2 to 6 weeks. Adult worms then expelled in feces (do not multiply in human host).
- Larvae travel via lymphatic and venules to the bloodstream and into skeletal muscle fibers to grow (10×), coil, and encyst. Muscle fibers enlarge, become edematous; may have granulomatous reactions in nonskeletal muscle, but larvae are only found in skeletal muscle.
- Symptoms occur approximately 7 to 14 days after ingestion, maybe sooner.
- Cysts (hyaline capsules) may calcify over several months to years.

EPIDEMIOLOGY

- Worldwide distribution; virulence varies with location and strain.
- Five species and three additional phenotypes: most infections from *Trichinella spiralis*
- Infections occur sporadically and in epidemics (families, small communities).
- CDC reported 138 outbreaks from 1973 to 1992 (1,038 cases).
- Approximately 4% of cadavers in 1970 study with evidence of previous infection (16% in 1941 study)
- Certain nationalities may be more likely to contract disease due to dietary habits.
- Should be considered in patients with recent foreign travel (especially Mexico, Southeast Asia, Africa)
- Most infections involve ingestion of poorly cooked pork, wild game (bear, cougar, hyena, lion, fox), horse, or walrus meat
- Decreasing number of cases per year in United States due to increased public awareness leading to better-cooked meat, home and commercial freezing, and laws preventing feeding of garbage to swine

COMPLICATIONS

- Myocarditis (most frequent serious complication), meningoencephalitis, CNS granulomas, pneumonitis, pericardial effusion, pleural effusion, pulmonary embolism or infarction, fatty changes of the liver, glomerulonephritis, severe enteritis, prolonged muscle aches, ocular disturbances, cardiac complaints and headaches
- Can be fatal (4–8 weeks postinfection)
- Rarely permanent damage

PROGNOSIS

- Usually resolves spontaneously over several months
- Muscle swelling and weakness may persist.
- Poorer prognosis (can be fulminant and fatal) if cardiac, CNS, or pulmonary involvement
- Children may be more symptomatic, but fewer complications and quicker recovery than adults

Differential Diagnosis

- Infection: viral syndromes, parasitic, spirochetal, gastroenteritis, influenza, sinusitis, typhoid fever, measles, scarlet fever, meningitis, rheumatic fever, encephalitis, encephalomyelitis, poliomyelitis
- Miscellaneous: Fever of unknown origin, dermatomyositis, myocarditis, inflammatory bowel disease, angioneurotic edema, glomerulonephritis, polyneuritis, eosinophilic leukemia, polyarteritis nodosa, nonabsorption syndromes

Data Gathering

HISTORY

Question: Most ingestions asymptomatic (subclinical)?
Significance: Nonspecific signs and symptoms may mimic other nonspecific illnesses. Lack of specificity of presentation may make diagnosis less obvious in some instances.

Question: Ingestion of poorly cooked or raw meat?
Significance: Infection is transmitted by ingestion of inadequately prepared meat. History of this diet should raise suspicion of potential trichinosis infection.

Question: Ingestion of game animal?
Significance: Game animals have been associated with transmission of trichinosis. This diet may also be associated with less than ideal storage or cooking issues.

Question: Others with same diet and similar symptoms?
Significance: Because this is a dietary acquired disease, others with similar diet may be at risk of developing trichinosis. Epidemics have been reported in families and communities.

Physical Examination

- Classic presentation includes myositis, fever, periorbital edema, and eosinophilia
- Symptomatic orderly progression (includes three stages):

—GI stage (first days to week postingestion)
—Nausea, vomiting, diarrhea (may be prolonged), abdominal pain, cramps, constipation, fever (rare), malaise
—Dissemination ("muscular phase," muscle invasion) stage (weeks 2–6)
—Fever, periorbital edema, myalgias most common symptoms
—Malaise, fatigue, facial edema and pain, tenderness, swelling, aching, weakness, or fasciculations of muscles (includes extraocular, face, tongue, larynx, neck, shoulder, chest, back, upper extremity muscles, and diaphragm), sweating, cough, rash
—Convalescent (encystment) stage (weeks 3–6)
—May have continued, prolonged (months) weakness, myalgias, paralysis, neurologic, circulatory or metabolic issues

Finding: Other reported signs and symptoms include cough, shortness of breath, hoarseness, headache, dysphagia, conjunctivitis, chemosis, maculopapular, urticarial or petechial rash, trunk or limb edema, conjunctival or splinter (subungual) hemorrhages, facial flushing, photophobia, blurred vision, diplopia, neck mass, cranial nerve abnormalities, meningoencephalitis, seizures, intracranial vessel thrombosis, focal neurologic findings, pericardial effusion

Laboratory Aids

SPECIFIC TESTS

- Pitfalls

—Serology takes time (3 weeks)
—No stool, body fluid (other than serology), or radiographic aid for routine specific diagnosis

- Trichinella serology (through CDC or state labs): requires several weeks to become positive; use two tests to increase sensitivity: bentonite flocculation (1:5 or fourfold increase), latex flocculation test, ELISA, immunofluorescence

- Skeletal muscle biopsy

—Most direct diagnostic tool, though usually not needed
—Best source swollen muscle, at least 2 weeks postinfection
—Encysted larvae in necrotic muscle fibers surrounded by inflammatory cells
—Granulomatous reaction in nonskeletal muscle, but not encysted larvae

- Skin test: becomes positive in 2nd to 3rd week; does not distinguish between acute or old infection as test remains positive for years after infection

NONSPECIFIC TESTS

- CBC and differential: eosinophilia (to 70%), peaks 10 to 21 days postinfection
- Serum CPK, LDH, SGOT, SGPT often elevated; ESR may be normal or elevated
- ECG: abnormal with myocarditis
- Imaging studies: small CNS lesions, some with ring calcifications; intravenous enhancement on CT scan
- Electromyography: results resemble polymyositis and inflammatory myopathies

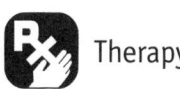 ## Therapy

- No ideal or totally satisfactory therapy
- Symptomatic: bed rest, salicylates
- Most recover without specific therapy

MEDICATIONS

- Intestinal phase
- Mebendazole (Vermox)

—Variable dosing recommendations (~10 days)
—200 to 400 mg t.i.d. ×3 days, followed by 400 to 500 mg t.i.d. ×10 days
—May be helpful during the disseminated (muscular) phase
—Successful in animal treatments
—Less toxic than thiabendazole

- Thiabendazole (Mintezol):

—Best if used within 24 hours of ingestion
—25 mg/kg PO for 7 days
—Kills some but not all established larvae
—Does not appear to alter established infection
—Better absorbed than mebendazole
—Has antiinflammatory, antipyretic, and analgesic effects

- Albendazole (Albenza)

—Best if used within 24 hours of ingestion
—400 mg PO b.i.d. × 8 to 14 days

- Pyrantel pamoate (Antiminth):

—11 mg/kg/d for 4 days
—Effective against GI worms, not encysted worms

- Muscular phase
- Systemic corticosteroids (high and low dose):

—Alleviate inflammatory reaction and help if CNS or cardiac involvement
—May be useful, but unproven
—Should not be used alone as may prolong symptomatic disease state

 ## Follow-Up

- Expect improvement over several weeks.
- Cardiac, neurologic, or pulmonary involvement indicates more severe problems.
- Prognosis usually good

PREVENTION

Isolation

Standard precautions

Control Measures

- Eat only fully cooked meat, especially pork and ground beef that may have been mixed with pork and game.

—Cook until no trace of pink
—Thermal death at 55°C (usually cook to 77°C [170°F])
—Freeze for 3 weeks at −15°C (5°F).

- Smoking, salting, and drying meat are not reliable sterilization methods.
- Avoid feeding swine uncooked meat scraps.
- Active rat control
- Avoid breast-feeding by infected mother.

PITFALLS

- Assuming only pork can transmit disease
- Not considering trichinosis in differential diagnosis

 ## Common Questions and Answers

Q: How can I prevent infection?
A: Be sure meat is fully cooked [55–77°C (101–170°F)] (not pink) or has been stored in a freezer at less than −15°C (5°F) for greater than 3 weeks (or −23°C (−10°F) for 10 days). *Trichinella* larvae in game may be relatively resistant to freezing.

Q: Is trichinosis contagious from person to person?
A: No, except through infected breast-milk.

Q: Do special precautions need to be taken when treating a patient with presumed trichinosis?
A: Only good hand washing. No isolation required.

Q: What should we recommend for a patient who has eaten contaminated meat?
A: Treatment with mebendazole or thiabendazole should be considered.

Q: What are the classic hallmarks of trichinosis?
A: Periorbital edema, myositis, fever, eosinophilia, especially with history of poorly cooked meat products.

ICD-9-CM 124

BIBLIOGRAPHY

American Academy of Pediatrics. Trichinosis (Trichinella spiralis). In: Pickering LK, ed. *2000 red book: report of the Committee of Infectious Diseases* , 25th ed. Elk Grove Village, IL: American Academy of Pediatrics, 2000:587–588, 715, 767–770.

Bia FJ, Barry M. Parasitic infections of the central nervous system. *Neurol Clin* 1986;4: 171–206.

Clausen MR, Meyer CN, Krantz T, et al. Trichinella infection and clinical disease. *QJM* 1996;89(8):631–636.

Grove DI. Tissue nematodes (trichinosis, dracunculiasis, filariasis). In: Mandell GL, Bennett JE, Dolin R, eds. *Principles and practice of infectious diseases*, 5th ed. Philadelphia: Churchill-Livingstone, 2000:526–528, 1151, 2943–2945.

Kreel L, Poon WS, Nainby-Luxmoore JC. Trichinosis diagnosis by computed tomography. *Postgrad Med J* 1988;64: 626–630.

MacLean JD, Viallet J, Law C, et al. Trichinosis in the Canadian Arctic: report of five outbreaks and a new clinical syndrome. *J Infect Dis* 1989;160:513–520.

McAuley JB, Michelson MK, Schantz PM. Trichinosis infection in travelers. *J Infect Dis* 1991;164:1013–1016.

McAuley JB, Michelson MK, Schantz PM. Trichinosis surveillance, United States, 1987–1990. *MMWR CDC Surveill Summ* 1991;40:35–42.

Moore TA, Nutman TB. Travel medicine: eosinophilia in the returning traveler. *Infect Dis Clin North Am* 1998;12(2)503–521.

Morse JW, Ridenour R, Unterseher P. Trichinosis: infrequent diagnosis or frequent misdiagnosis? *Ann Emerg Med* 1994;24: 969–971.

Author: George Anthony Woodward

Tuberculosis

 Database

DEFINITION

Pediatric tuberculosis (TB) is the disease state caused by *Mycobacterium tuberculosis*, an acid-fast bacillus (AFB). Pediatric TB should be regarded as a spectrum of exposure, from infection to disease, because progression from an infected individual (exposure) to infection and subsequently disease can occur much faster in children under 2 years of age (occurring within the incubation of the disease stated below). Progression through this spectrum is age-dependent, being 40% to 50% for 0- up to 2-year-old, approximately 20% for 2- to 4-year-olds, and 10% to 15% for those 5 years old and over, the 5- to 10-year-olds being the most protected age group.

EPIDEMIOLOGY

- The most common route of infection is via the respiratory tract. TB is spread from a person with disease by droplet nuclei that are inhaled by other individuals. A child becomes infected with TB after close and prolonged contact with an adult or adolescent who has active, untreated infectious disease, usually pulmonary TB, in a poorly ventilated space. The sole risk factor is breathing air containing droplet nuclei that contain the tubercle bacillus. Thus there are individuals who develop TB without knowledge of an infectious contact.
- Congenital infection occurs, rarely, in the setting of an untreated mother in the last trimester of pregnancy.
- Infection with the tubercle bacillus needs to be differentiated from disease (i.e., tuberculosis).
- Approximately 8% (19 million) Americans have been infected with TB; 45% are African Americans and 25% are whites over 70 years of age.
- The number with active contagious disease is approximately 25,000.
- The interval between onset of infection and disease is 10 to 12 weeks to many years.
- Of adults, only 10% of those infected will develop disease, and this is reduced by 60% to 90% if preventative INH is taken within the first 2 years of infection. This is the most likely time when infection replicates sufficiently to progress to a disease state. In most, untreated infection becomes dormant and does not progress.
- The greatest chance of disease occurring is within the first 2 years after infection [of developing a positive purified protein derivative (PPD) reaction]. However, for infants and children younger than 5 years old, progression through the spectrum of pediatric TB (exposure-infection-disease) is age-dependent (see Definition, above).
- Postpubertal adolescents and immunosuppressed individuals, including persons with diabetes, with chronic renal failure, malnourished individuals, and persons on steroids for whatever reasons (including pulse doses), have higher risks of progression of infection to disease.
- Nationwide, the past 4 years have documented an increase in TB in children under 2 years of age in the states where TB is common.

PATHOPHYSIOLOGY

- Pathology of disease includes the formation of a primary focus of infection, usually in the lung (Ghon focus), with recruitment of cell-mediated immune responses, which lead to formation of adenopathy of the hilar, cervical, mediastinal, and/or other nodes, depending on the dissemination of infection.
- Development of a PPD reaction is dependent on an adequate cell-mediated immune response, which often is not fully developed in infants younger than 2 years of age and in those infected with overwhelming disease, such as miliary TB or meningitis or large pleural effusions.

COMPLICATIONS

- Missed diagnosis: failure to consider TB in a child who is failing to thrive and whose PPD is negative
- TB meningitis: Outcome is dependent on the stage at which anti-TB medication is begun.
—If Rx is started at stage I, complete recovery occurs in 94%, with neurologic sequelae in 6%.
—If delayed until stage II, complete recovery occurs in 51%, with neurologic sequelae in 40% and death in 7%.
—If delayed until stage III, complete recovery occurs in 18%, with neurologic sequelae in 61% and death in 20%.
- Miliary TB
- Bony TB: Most commonly spinal
- Renal TB: Presents as a fever of undetermined origin (FUO), with or without urinary symptoms
- Congenital TB manifests with hepatosplenomegaly; may have CSF abnormalities and CXR abnormalities
- Evolution of multidrug-resistant TB (MDRTB): The cost of medication alone to treat an individual with a sensitive organism is $10,000 per year; the cost of drug treatment with a resistant organism is $250,000 per year, not including any hospitalization costs.
- Drug toxicity: Pediatric patients are much more tolerant of anti-TB medications than are adults; thus regular monitoring of liver function tests is not routinely required.
- Hepatitis with INH, rifampin, and pyrazinamide (PZA); neurologic complications with INH; skin rashes with rifampin; ototoxicity with streptomycin; but ocular toxicity with EMB in the pediatric age group has not been documented, and therefore is a safe drug to use.

PROGNOSIS

- The death rate for untreated TB is 40% over 4 years.
- For miliary TB and meningeal TB, prognosis is dependent on the stage of presentation (as above).
- For outbreaks of MDRTB, death rates have ranged from 70% to 90%.

ASSOCIATED DISEASES

- The following diseases are associated with progression of infection to disease:
—HIV infection: factor in the increase in TB, since 1 in 240 Americans is infected with HIV, and the bacillus grows better, evades detection (chest x-rays may appear normal), and is more contagious
—Lymphoma
—Diabetes
—Chronic renal failure
—Malnutrition
—Immunosuppression, including daily potential steroid use

 Differential Diagnosis

TB can do anything malignancy can do.
- Pulmonary infiltrate: other chronic organisms such as *Nocardia* and histoplasmosis. Infiltrates due to bacterial or viral pathogens resolve faster than TB; thus, reevaluation of a suspect in 8 to 12 weeks clarifies this differential.
- Hilar adenopathy: In TB it is usually unilateral, but EBV, adenovirus, pertussis, and malignancy are possible mimickers.
- Miliary disease: pulmonary, hepatosplenomegaly with or without CNS involvement
- Gastrointestinal disease: The most common differential is Crohn disease.
- Meningitis: fungal meningitis, partially treated bacterial meningitis (rarely)

 Data Gathering

HISTORY

Inquire about the factors that are associated with tuberculosis infection:
- Exposure
- Migrant farmers
- Immigration from a high-TB area such as Haiti, Southeast Asia, Africa (any part), South American, or Russia
- Higher incidence in Native Americans
- Contact with adults who have active TB
- HIV-positive persons
- Immunosuppressed state
- Incarcerated adolescents and relatives
- Homeless persons
- Poor city dwellers
- Exposure to milk from untested herds
- Malnutrition
- Chronic steroid usage

 Physical Examination

- May reflect underlying disease such as HIV, malnutrition, chronic steroid use
- Pulmonary rales
- Presence of sputum
- May be normal especially in 5- to 10-year-olds

Laboratory Aids

TESTS
Skin Testing
- The Mantoux test is 5 tuberculin units of PPD administered intradermally.
- The CDC does not recommend routine skin testing in low-risk groups in communities with low prevalence of TB except for one-time testing during childhood.
- Children at high risk should be tested. The Philadelphia Department of Public Health TB Control recommends periodic testing for high-risk patients at 1 to 2 years old, 4 to 5 years old, or 11 to 12 years old.
  —High-risk children include those in contact with adults from regions of the world with high prevalence; adults with TB, HIV, and immunosuppressed states; those with Hodgkin disease, lymphoma, diabetes, chronic renal failure, and malnutrition; incarcerated adolescents; and those with exposure to high-risk adults.
- Skin tests become positive 3 to 6 weeks after exposure but may not turn positive for 3 months.

Other Tests
- Culture of sputum, gastric washings, pleural fluid, CSF, urine
- In children, the best source is early-morning gastric washings.
- Culture may take 2 to 3 weeks by the radiometric method.
- Positive cultures are found in fewer than 50% of children.

IMAGING
Chest radiographs may show hilar adenopathy with or without atelectasis.

 ## Therapy

HOSPITALIZATION
- Treatment initiated as an outpatient may not be complied with; thus hospitalization reinforces the issue of disease and allows time for education and linkage to TB control programs, which can then supervise direct observed therapy (DOT); however, in the era of managed care, direct linkage of the patient to the local TB control program through the health department and provision of DOT can avert the need to hospitalize for starting therapy, especially since the positivity rate of gastric aspirates for TB is 10% in the best hands.
- In cases of extensive disease, such as miliary or meningitis, and when an adult source case is not known, aggressive attempts should be made to obtain an organism from gastric aspirates, bronchoalveolar lavage, CSF, pleural or joint aspirate, bone aspirate, liver or tissue biopsy, and, in some cases, blood cultures.

ISOLATION POLICIES
- In the past, children under 8 years of age did not require isolation for pulmonary disease, because the disease is usually a primary infection; that is, there is less organism load and more lymphatic enlargement. However, unless one knows that the parent and/or any adult visitors are *not* contagious, many infection control units require isolation of the child because the family members' state of contagion is unknown at the time of admission.
- Nonpulmonary, such as GI TB, meningitis, bone, joint, also do not require isolation
- Children older than 8 years of age and adolescents should be isolated until they have completed 10 days of four-drug therapy (listed below).

DRUGS
- Initial treatment in areas with MDRTB of more than 4%: Until sensitivities are known, a four-drug regimen should be started: INH, 10 mg/kg/d; rifampin, 10 mg/kg/d; PZA, 30 mg/kg/d; and either streptomycin, 20 mg/kg/d (depending on whether it is meningitis or miliary TB, for which a cidal antibacterial agent is desired) or ethambutol, 25 mg/kg/d.
- If the organism is sensitive, treatment with the initial four primary drugs should continue for the first 2 months, followed by 4 months of INH and rifampin. When this regimen is adhered to, prognosis and a complete cure is achieved in 97% to 98% of patients.

PREVENTION
- Prevention of disease by using INH, 10 mg/kg/d for 6 months orally, or if compliance is an issue, two times a week as DOT at 20 mg/kg, with a maximum dose of 900 mg, *without breaks in treatment,* is 60% to 90% effective against the development of active TB for 20 years in *nonimmunosuppressed* children. This recommendation prevents disease in the treated individual and, as a public health measure, interrupts transmission to contacts of the infected person with an efficacy of 60% to 90%.
- However, use of other regimens in cases of a contact of MDRTB is still being evaluated in children; therefore, this situation should be discussed with a specialist who has experience, usually one who is associated with the CDC or local TB control programs. Children with HIV or other immunodeficiency states require 12 months of prophylaxis. Any child (usually older children and adolescents) whose x-ray is consistent with past infection (granuloma or fibrosis) and who has not received INH prophylaxis previously requires 12 months of INH.
- BCG (bacille of Calmette and Guérin) vaccine is recommended only for infants and children who are PPD-negative, who are continually and intimately exposed to contagious adults or to adults with TB that is resistant to both INH and rifampin, and who cannot take long-term preventative medication or be removed from the contagious adult. These recommendations are currently under review.
- Follow-up and contact tracing are key to making TB a preventable disease.

 ## Common Questions and Answers

Q: If the child has completed a course of INH and is reexposed, what are the risks of infection?
A: One course of preventive therapy is believed to confer immunity to subsequent exposure, even to MDRTB (data are preliminary).
Q: Should all children in close proximity to inner-city areas with a prevalence of TB be screened annually with PPD?
A: No. One needs to consider the risk/benefit. Children under 5 years of age progress to disease more rapidly and are harder to diagnose when ill with TB; therefore, children who are under 5 years of age and live in high-risk parts of a city should be screened; otherwise, screening, according to the American Academy of Pediatrics, at ages 1, 5, and 11 is sufficient.
Q: Because parents return for the PPD reading only 26% to 50% of the time, depending on which clinic they use, are there other ways to ensure that parents receive the PPD reading?
A: This is a tough question. An improved public health surveillance system, use of child care providers, or school programs requiring examination and utility are all shown to be more effective than patient education by the provider.

ICD-9-CM 011.9

BIBLIOGRAPHY
Control of tuberculosis in the United States. *Am Rev Respir Dis* 1992;142:1623–1633.

Diagnostic Standards and Classification of Tuberculosis in Adults and Children. This official statement of the American Thoracic Society and the Centers for Disease Control and Prevention was adopted by the ATS Board of Directors, July 1999. This statement was endorsed by the Council of the Infectious Disease Society of America, September 1999. *Am J Respir Crit Care Med* 2000;161 (4 pt 1):1376–1395.

Heymann SJ, Brewer TF, Wilson ME, et al. Pediatric tuberculosis: what needs to be done to decrease morbidity and mortality. *Pediatrics* 2000;106(1).

Inselman LS. Tuberculosis in children: an update. *Pediatr Pulmonol* 1996;21(2): 101–120.

New directions in diagnostics. *Pediatr Infect Dis J* 1997;16(suppl 3):S43–S48.

Author: Barbara Watson

Tuberous Sclerosis

 ## Database

DEFINITION

Tuberous sclerosis (TSC) is a neurocutaneous syndrome characterized by hamartomatous growths involving multiple regions of the body, such as the brain, retina, heart, kidney, and skin. First described by Bourneville in 1880, the classic diagnostic triad of adenoma sebaceum, mental retardation, and seizures has been revised to include other manifestations, because many patients with TSC do not exhibit this triad.

CAUSES

TSC either is inherited in an autosomal-dominant pattern or results from a spontaneous, sporadic mutation.

PATHOLOGY

Findings reflect the primary tissue in which lesions are identified (*denotes lesions that confirm the diagnosis of TSC).

• Brain

—Three characteristic lesions include *cortical tubers, *subependymal nodules, and giant-cell astrocytomas.
—In tubers, cerebral cortical architecture is disrupted, and these regions may undergo calcification, which can be visible on skull radiographs or brain CT.
—Subependymal nodules consist of large abnormal astrocytes emanating from the lateral ventricular surface.
—Giant-cell astrocytomas are low-grade benign astrocytic neoplasms.

• Skin

—Facial angiofibromas are highly suggestive of TSC and consists of pinkish-yellow plaques on the malar regions and nasolabial folds.
—Ash leaf spots are hypopigmented, hypomelanotic macules occurring anywhere on the body.

• Ungual fibromas are fleshy growths along the lateral borders of the nailbed. Shagreen patches are areas of shaggy, leathery skin typically in the lumbosacral area.

• Retina

—Whitish-yellow angiolipomas or *astrocytic hamartomas occur near the optic nerve head or the retinal periphery, which may calcify.

• Heart
• Rhabdomyomas in the ventricular wall occur in infancy and contain abundant nodules of large eosinophilic cells; this is the most common cardiac tumor of infancy and early childhood.
• Kidney

—Renal cysts, polycystic kidneys, *angiomyolipomas, and, rarely, renal carcinomas

• Other organ systems

—Less commonly affected are the lungs, gastrointestinal tract, spleen, vascular bed, and lymphatics.

GENETICS

Two clearly identified loci for familial and sporadic cases based on linkage analyses are 9q34 and 16p13, corresponding to *TSC1* and *TSC2* genes, respectively. *TSC1* encodes the protein hamartin. The *TSC2* gene encodes a protein named tuberin. It is hypothesized that hamartin and tuberin may function as a tumor suppressor. There is a loss of allelic *TSC2* heterozygosity in TSC hamartomas, suggesting that an inactivating mutation of the *TSC2* occurring in somatic or germ-cell lines reflects a second-hit mutation.

EPIDEMIOLOGY

Current estimates suggest an incidence of 1 in 5,000 to 1 in 15,000 births. Approximately 60% to 70% of cases reflect sporadic mutation; 30% to 40% of cases are familial; it affects males and females equally.

PROGNOSIS

Mental retardation unfortunately will not improve unless cognitive impairment results from uncontrolled seizures. Seizure control is often difficult, and many children require epilepsy surgery to remove cortical tubers or subependymal nodules. Cardiac tumors may require surgical intervention. Renal angiomyolipomas can be embolized angiographically or surgically corrected. Subependymal giant cell astrocytomas that cause hydrocephalus may require resection.

 ## Differential Diagnosis

Neurocutaneous syndromes in which skin lesions, mental retardation, and seizures are characteristic features should be considered:

• Neurofibromatosis
• Sturge-Weber syndrome
• von Hippel–Lindau disease
• Neurocutaneous melanosis
• Albright syndrome
• Incontinentia pigmenti
• Linear sebaceous nevus

 ## Data Gathering

HISTORY

• Primary symptoms include seizures, mental defect, and skin lesions.
• Seizures may begin at any time. In infancy, infantile spasms are a common presenting seizure.
• Mental retardation may manifest as developmental delay, but some patients are without cognitive defect.
• Skin lesions may appear in infancy or during early childhood.
• It is important to take a full family history, including consanguinity.
• Inquire about history of TSC, seizures, mental retardation, skin lesions, and cardiac or renal disease/cancers.

Physical Examination

- Need to maintain high level of suspicion for TSC in any patient evaluated with:

—Infantile spasms
—Seizures
—Mental retardation/developmental delay
—Peculiar skin lesions.

- Ash leaf and café-au-lait spots are small (often less than 5 mm) but may be found anywhere on skin and are often present at birth.
- Facial angiofibromas are typically on the face around the nose and cheeks and appears similar to acne, appearing in the later childhood to adolescent years. It does not itch or suppurate.
- Ungual fibromas appear around the nailbed.
- Shagreen patches are brownish, leathery skin patches near the sacrum.
- Funduscopic examination may reveal whitish-yellow areas in epi- and peripapillary regions around the optic nerve head. They rarely cause visual impairment.
- Clinical signs of congestive heart failure in infants may be seen with cardiac TSC.
- Flank pain, nausea and vomiting, and hematuria may reflect renal involvement.

PROCEDURE

- In any suspected neurocutaneous syndrome, skin examination with a Wood's lamp may be especially helpful in identifying hypopigmented lesions such as ash leaf spots. Dilated funduscopic examination may also aid in full visualization of optic nerve head.
- One rare sign of TSC is the presence of small dental enamel pits.

 ## Laboratory Aids

TESTS

- Routine blood and CSF lab tests are typically normal unless renal function is significantly compromised by renal cysts or renal angiomyolipomas.
- In patients with mental retardation or seizures, EEG is essential to evaluate cerebral activity.
- In infants, an EEG may also help diagnose infantile spasms, which are associated electrographically with a highly disorganized pattern of large-amplitude, asynchronous, sharp waves called hypsarrhythmia.
- Later in childhood, children with TSC may develop the Lennox-Gastaut syndrome, which consists of mental retardation, seizures, and a characteristic EEG pattern of slow (2.5-Hz) spike-wave complexes.

IMAGING

- MRI of the brain with gadolinium administration performed serially every 1 to 2 years will identify tubers, subependymal nodules, and giant-cell tumors. These appear hyperintense on T-weighted images and may enhance with gadolinium. Rarely, a giant-cell astrocytoma may obstruct the foramen of Monro, resulting in hydrocephalus, which can also be detected with MRI.
- Echocardiography can detect cardiac rhabdomyomas in infants with TSC.
- Renal ultrasound (every 1–2 years) or CT will demonstrate renal lesions.

 ## Therapy

DRUGS

Anticonvulsant therapy as needed and ACTH for infantile spasms; medical management of congestive heart failure or cardiac dysrhythmias in TSC patients with cardiac rhabdomyomas

 ## Follow-Up

SIGNS TO WATCH FOR

- A persistent change in mental status may reflect status epilepticus, an expanding mass lesion with obstructive hydrocephalus, or a new CNS neoplasm.
- Worsening renal function may reflect progressive renal involvement.

 ## Common Questions and Answers

Q: Can TSC be transmitted in subsequent pregnancies?
A: An affected individual with the TSC gene mutation has a 50% chance of transmitting the mutation to his or her offspring.

Q: Is genetic testing available?
A: A commercial diagnostic test is under development for TSC1 and TSC2 gene mutations.

Q: Will my child need brain surgery?
A: In the event of refractory seizures, removal of cortical tubers may help seizure control. If a brain tumor is detected by MRI, neurosurgical evaluation is indicated.

ICD-9-CM 759.5

BIBLIOGRAPHY

Crino P, Henske C. New developments in the neurobiology of the tuberous sclerosis complex. *Neurology* 1999;53:1384–1391.

Gomez MR. *Tuberous sclerosis*, 2nd ed. New York: Raven Press, 1988.

Jozwiak S, Schwartz RA, Janniger CK, et al. Usefulness of diagnostic criteria of tuberous sclerosis complex in pediatric patients. *J Child Neurol* 2000;15(10):652–659.

Sarnat H. *Cerebral dysgenesis*. New York: Oxford University Press, 1991.

Webb DW, Osborne JP. Tuberous sclerosis. *Arch Dis Child* 1995;72(6):471–474.

Author: Peter B. Crino

Tularemia

 Database

DEFINITION

Tularemia is an infection with *Francisella tularensis,* a small, nonmotile, gram-negative coccobacillus that requires cysteine for growth. Two types have been described:

• Type A (Neartica): found in arthropods; highly virulent to rabbits and humans
• Type B (Palaeartica): found in water and aquatic animals; less virulent

Tularemia is characterized by six clinical forms, depending on the site of entry:

• Ulceroglandular tularemia constitutes 75% of all cases. A papule, which ruptures and ulcerates, occurs at the site of entry. Lymphadenopathy and hepatosplenomegaly accompany systemic symptoms of fever, chills, and headache.
• Glandular tularemia is identical to the ulceroglandular form, but without a skin lesion.
• Oculoglandular tularemia occurs when the organism gains access via the conjunctival sac, usually from rubbing the eyes with contaminated fingers. The eyelids are inflamed and the conjunctiva is infected. Yellow nodules and ulcers may appear on the palpebral conjunctiva.
• Typhoidal tularemia presents as fever of unknown origin, without localizing lymphadenopathy or skin findings. Shock, pleuropulmonary findings, odynophagia, diarrhea, and bowel necrosis are often associated.
• Oropharyngeal tularemia occurs after the ingestion of infected, improperly cooked meat. An exudative or membranous tonsillitis is seen. Lower gastrointestinal tract involvement with vomiting, diarrhea, and abdominal pain may be associated.
• Pneumonic tularemia occurs after inhalation of the organism. This presentation is seen in laboratory workers and is the most fulminant and lethal form. Tularemia in this form has been produced as a biologic weapon.

PATHOPHYSIOLOGY

• Infection follows contact with rabbits or rodents.
• Ticks or deerflies are the most common vector.
• Entry into the human is via skin or mucous membranes.
• A papule or ulcer may be seen at the inoculation site.
• Bacteremia occurs after a 3- to 5-day incubation period, accompanied by fever and lymphadenopathy.
• The organism produces localized disease in reticuloendothelial organs, with areas of focal necrosis that may form granulomas.

EPIDEMIOLOGY

• *F. tularensis* is found in the northern hemisphere between 30° and 71° latitude.
• Wild mammals (rabbits, hares, squirrels, beavers, and deer) may be infected, as well as invertebrates (ticks, deerflies, and mosquitoes).
• Humans acquire tularemia after a bite by an infected arthropod or contact with tissues or body fluids of an infected animal.
• Most frequently affected are hunters, trappers, and farmers.

COMPLICATIONS

• Lymph node suppuration occurs in 40% of pediatric patients, regardless of treatment.
• Infection with *F. tularensis* may be complicated by necrotic and granulomatous lesions in the liver and spleen, as well as parenchymal degeneration.
• A sepsis syndrome with shock, fever, myalgias, and severe headache can be seen.
• Pneumonia and pleural involvement are frequently encountered in adults with typhoidal tularemia.

PROGNOSIS

When recognized and treated with appropriate antibiotics, the course is generally less than 1 month. Mortality is low, except in fulminant disease.

 Differential Diagnosis

Tularemia should be considered in the following differentials:

• Fever of unknown origin
• Fever with purulent conjunctivitis
• Fever with hepatosplenomegaly
• Fever with skin ulcer

Data Gathering

HISTORY

• A history of any of the following contacts with affected animals should be sought: ingestion of wild animal meat, hunting or cleaning wild animals, and playing with dead wild animals.
• History of a recent tick bite is common among affected patients.
• A history of a papule that became ulcerated is classic for the ulceroglandular form.
• Fever greater than 101°F for 2 to 3 weeks is common, with associated weight loss.

Physical Examination

• Skin lesions should be sought.
• Hepatosplenomegaly, purulent conjunctivitis, adenopathy, and exudative tonsillitis are other localized findings.

Laboratory Aids

TESTS

• Serum agglutination titers to *F. tularensis* are positive if 1:160 or greater.
• A fourfold rise in titers after the second week of illness is characteristic and diagnostic.
• Cultures of blood, skin, ulcers, lymph nodes, gastric washings, and respiratory secretions require special media.
• Laboratory personnel should be made aware of the infection risk from specimens.

Therapy

• If respiratory compromise is present, oxygen supplementation and/or assisted ventilation must be rapidly addressed.
• Recognition and prompt, aggressive treatment of shock should be a major priority.
• Intravenous antibiotic therapy should be administered. Streptomycin has been used traditionally, but gentamicin has recently been found to be equally effective.

Follow-Up

PREVENTION

Isolation of the Hospitalized Patient

Infection control measures should include protection against secretions and respiratory isolation of the pneumonic form.

Control Measures

• Protective clothing and insect repellent should be used to minimize insect bites.
• Inspection for ticks (and immediate removal) should be routine after outdoor activity in endemic areas.
• Rubber gloves should be worn while cooking or handling wild rabbit meat.
• Laboratory workers should wear rubber gloves and masks when working with potentially infectious specimens.

ICD-9-CM 021.9

BIBLIOGRAPHY

Boyce JM. Francisella tularensis. In: Mandell GL, Douglas GR, Bennett JE, eds. *Principles and practice of infectious diseases*, 3rd ed. New York: Churchill-Livingstone, 1990:1742–1746.

Cross JT, Schutze GE, Jacobs RF. Treatment of tularemia with gentamicin in pediatric patients. *Pediatr Infect Dis J* 1995;14(2): 151–152.

Dennis DT, Inglesby TV, Henderson DA, et al. Tularemia as a biological weapon: medical and public health management. *JAMA* 2001; 285(21):2763–2773.

Kaye D. Tularemia. In: Braunwald E, ed. *Harrison's principles of internal medicine*, 14th ed. New York: McGraw-Hill, 1987: 613–615.

Yow MD. Tularemia. In: Oski FA, ed. *Principles and practice of pediatrics*. Philadelphia: JB Lippincott, 1990:1132–1133.

Author: Louis M. Bell
Janet H. Friday, 2nd edition

Ulcerative Colitis

Database

DEFINITION

Ulcerative colitis (UC) is a disease characterized by remitting and relapsing inflammation of the large intestine. UC and Crohn disease (CD) are the disorders that represent the idiopathic inflammatory bowel diseases (IBDs). The hallmark symptoms of UC are abdominal cramping, diarrhea, and bloody stools.
There are multiple patterns of presentation in children. UC always affects the rectum, with contiguous involvement extending proximally, including up to the entire large intestine.

CAUSES

UC is thought to be a multifactorial disease. It likely results from a combination of individual genetic susceptibility and several environmental risk factors that may include:
- Hygiene/exposure to bacteria/parasites/viruses/allergens
- Breast versus bottle feeding
- Specific bacteria that colonize the colon
- Dietary influences
- Smoking

PATHOLOGY

- Inflammation and ulceration of colonic mucosa with acute inflammatory cells infiltrating the villi, lamina propria, and crypts, giving rise to crypt abscesses
- Inflammation is mucosal, but can infiltrate all layers of the bowel.
- Site of colon affected:
—Rectum (100%)
—Left side (50%–60%)
—Pancolitis (10%)
- Small intestine should not be involved, but occasionally the terminal ileum can show some inflammation on radiologic or histologic examination. This is thought to be from refluxed colonic contents (backwash ileitis).
- Skip lesions are not seen in ulcerative colitis.

GENETICS

- HLA association: Bw52, DR2 (Japan); A2, Bw35, Bw40 (Ashkenazi Jews); A7, A11 (Netherlands)
- Higher concordance in monozygotic than in dizygotic twins

EPIDEMIOLOGY

- Yearly incidence is 2/100,000 in 10- to 19-year-olds
- 20% of patients with UC present before the age of 20
- Incidence peaks between 15 and 30 years of age
- Total prevalence is 50 to 75 per 100,000

COMPLICATIONS

- Bleeding
- Anemia
- Toxic megacolon
- Extraintestinal manifestations hepatobiliary disease (3% to 5%), uveitis (up to 4%), arthritis affecting large joints (10%), spondylitis (6%), erythema nodosum (<5%), pyoderma gangrenosum (<1%), renal calculi (5%)
- Malignancy risk is 0.51% per year after a decade of onset of disease. The risk for adenocarcinoma of the colon in children who developed disease before 14 years of age is 40% by 40 years of age.
- Colonic stricture

Differential Diagnosis

- Crohn disease
- Infectious colitis: *Salmonella, Shigella, Campylobacter, Yersinia, Escherichia coli* (enterohemorrhagic), *Aeromonas,* Amebiasis, *Clostridium difficile,* cytomegalovirus
- Sexually transmitted disease (herpes simplex, lymphogranuloma inguinale, *Chlamydia*)
- Trauma due to anal sex or sexual abuse
- Congenital Hirschsprung enterocolitis
- Bleeding juvenile polyps
- Milk protein allergy
- Eosinophilic colitis
- Autoimmune enteropathy
- Irritable bowel syndrome (IBS)
- Appendicitis
- Hemolytic-uremic syndrome
- Henoch-Schönlein purpura

Data Gathering

HISTORY

A detailed history is important in making the diagnosis:
- Rectal bleeding (90%)
- Abdominal pain (90%)
- Diarrhea (50%)
- Weight loss (10%)
- Growth failure
- Recent travel (enteric infections)
- Antibiotic use (*C. difficile*)
- Family history of IBD
- Appendectomy

Physical Examination

- Fever
- Evidence of weight loss or poor growth
- Signs of anemia
- Uveitis
- Mouth sores
- Arthritis
- Abdominal tenderness
- Abdominal distention
- Perianal/rectal examination (UC should not be associated with perianal disease)
- Evidence of hepatobiliary disease

Laboratory Aids

TESTS

- CBC (anemia, iron deficiency)
- Iron studies (iron deficiency)
- ESR (disease activity)
- Electrolytes (hydration)
- Hepatic function panel (hepatobiliary disease)
- pANCA (positive in 80% of UC patients, 20% of CD patients)
- Stool for blood, white cells (colitis)
- Stool cultures, *C. difficile* toxin A and B (infection)

IMAGING

- Plain abdominal radiograph: This is important in diagnosing perforation, ileus, obstruction, and toxic megacolon. In toxic megacolon, the colon is dilated, and there are multiple air-fluid levels indicative of ileus. Serial x-rays are mandatory.
- Barium enema demonstrates strictures and mucosal disease.
- An upper GI and small-bowel follow-through (UGI/SBFT) can demonstrate the entire gastrointestinal tract to exclude small intestinal disease.
- MRI is gaining efficacy for differentiation between transmural and mucosal inflammation.
- Ultrasound may be useful for evaluating associated hepatobiliary disease.
- Radionuclide imaging can differentiate between CD (small and large bowel involvement) and UC (only large bowel involvement).

PROCEDURES

- Colonoscopy (with biopsies) is necessary to confirm the diagnosis of ulcerative colitis.
- Endoscopic retrograde cholangiopancreatography (ERCP) is useful in diagnosing primary sclerosing cholangitis (3% of UC patients).

PITFALLS

- The combination of positive pANCA and negative ASCA (anti–*Saccharomyces cerevisiae* antibody) has a reported sensitivity of 60% to 70% and a specificity of 95% to 97% for ulcerative colitis in adults. The sensitivity and specificity is poorer in pediatric patients.

Ulcerative Colitis

- Inflammation of the small intestine demonstrated by colonoscopy, UGI/SBFT, or radionuclide imaging is indicative of CD, not UC.
- Perianal disease (perianal skin tags, perianal fistulae, perianal abscess) is indicative of CD, not UC.
- Infectious colitis (especially *C. difficile*) can mimic the findings of UC. *C. difficile* infection must be evaluated with assays for both toxin A and toxin B, or up to 40% of infections can be missed.
- Toxic megacolon is a surgical emergency. The patient has a dilated colon with breakdown of its barrier to toxins entering the systemic circulation. Signs and symptoms include peritonitis, mental status changes, and fluid and electrolyte imbalance. Plain abdominal radiograph shows a segment or total colonic dilatation. Risk factors include first attack, pancolitis, concurrent use of opiates or anticholinergics, and recent barium enema or colonoscopy.

HOME TESTING
Home testing of stool for occult blood can alert patients and physicians to active disease.

Emergency Care

Emergency care is indicated for fulminant disease. Initial evaluation should include abdominal examination, laboratory evaluation (CBC, ESR, electrolytes), and abdominal obstruction series (supine and upright abdominal films). Surgical consultation should be obtained in cases of suspected toxic megacolon.

Therapy

- Mild disease can be treated with oral mesalamine, topical corticosteroid enema or foam, or mesalamine enema/suppositories.
- Moderate disease: mesalamine, a short course of oral corticosteroid, low-residue diet
- Fulminant disease: hospitalization, complete bowel rest with total parenteral nutrition, broad-spectrum antibiotics (intravenous ampicillin, gentamicin, and metronidazole), intravenous corticosteroids, serial abdominal radiographs, frequent examinations, stool chart (frequency, amount of blood, and volume of stool output), early surgical consult.
- If treatment of severe disease fails after 2 weeks, intravenous cyclosporine is started. Those who respond to cyclosporine are started on oral cyclosporine, which is discontinued after 6 to 8 months. The risk of relapse after discontinuation of cyclosporine is high, and it is useful to start 6-mercaptopurine (6-MP) or azathioprine as a maintenance therapy.
- Those who fail therapy with cyclosporine or demonstrate chronic unresponsive disease for 6 months should be referred for colectomy.
- Infliximab has recently been demonstrated to have efficacy in UC and may represent an alternative to cyclosporine for unresponsive disease.

- Therapy of toxic megacolon is aimed at preventing perforation with decompression of the bowel. Management includes complete bowel rest, discontinuation of anticholinergics and narcotics, not performing endoscopy or barium enema, and broad-spectrum antibiotics; frequent examinations are required. Close communication with surgical colleagues is crucial. In the absence of improvement after 24 to 72 hours, the patient requires urgent surgery.
- Maintenance of remission: The corticosteroid dose is tapered and discontinued over weeks to months after initial presentation. Mesalamine is started before discharge.

SURGERY
- Urgently required for perforation, significant and persistent bleeding, toxic megacolon, and failure of medical treatment for fulminant colitis
- Can be electively performed for chronic incapacitating disease, growth failure, disease greater than 10 years' duration
- Ileoanal anastomosis and pouch construction is surgery of choice for most pediatric patients

DRUGS
- Methylprednisolone (intravenous): 1 to 2 mg/kg/d (equivalent to prednisone 60 mg maximum)
- Prednisone (oral): 1 to 2 mg/kg/d oral (up to maximum 60 mg/d)
- Mesalamine (oral): 40 to 60 mg/kg/day (maximum 4.8 g/day)
- Mesalamine (enema): 4 g at bedtime
- Mesalamine (suppository): 500 mg b.i.d.
- Hydrocortisone enema: 100 mg qd–b.i.d.
- Hydrocortisone foam: 80 mg qd–b.i.d.
- Cyclosporine (intravenous): 4 mg/kg/d for 2 weeks (therapeutic levels vary depending on the technique used in the laboratory)
- Cyclosporine (oral): 6 to 8 mg/kg/d for 6 to 8 months
- 6-MP (oral): 1.0 to 1.5 mg/kg to start (keep ANC greater than 500)
- Azathioprine (oral): 2.0 mg/kg (keep ANC greater than 500)
- Infliximab (intravenous): 5 mg/kg 2 weeks apart, then every 6–12 weeks as needed.

Follow-Up

Outpatient follow-up with a pediatric gastroenterologist should be arranged. Important parameters to follow as an outpatient include abdominal symptoms, stool frequency/consistency, height/weight, hemoglobin, WBC (for patients on immunosuppressives), ESR, albumin, bilirubin and liver enzymes, fecal occult blood testing, colonoscopic cancer screening (patients with long-standing disease).

Common Questions and Answers

Q: Will my child have this disease forever?
A: Some people will have only the initial attack and then be symptom-free, but usually an individual will have episodes of recurrences and remissions. Surgical removal of the colon represents a curative procedure, although some patients may develop inflammation in the pouch created out of the remaining bowel (pouchitis).
Q: What is the cause of ulcerative colitis?
A: Both genetic and environmental factors are important in the development of ulcerative colitis.
Q: Where can I learn more about Crohn disease?
A: The Crohn and Colitis Foundation of America (*www.CCFA.org*) is a nonprofit organization dedicated to the care and education of people with Crohn disease and ulcerative colitis.
Q: What new therapies will be used in the near future?
A: Biologic agents, a type of therapy that uses our recently improved knowledge of the immune system, represent a new type of therapy.

ICD-9-CM 556

BIBLIOGRAPHY
Baldassano RN, Piccoli DA. Inflammatory bowel disease in pediatric and adolescent patients. *Gastroenterol Clin North Am* 1999;28(2):445–458.

Becker JM. Surgical therapy for ulcerative colitis and Crohn's disease. *Gastroenterol Clin North Am* 1999;28(2):371–90, viii–ix.

Lewis JD, Deren JJ, Lichtenstein GR. Cancer risk in patients with inflammatory bowel disease. *Gastroenterol Clin North Am* 1999;28(2):459–477.

Michetti P, Peppercorn MA. Medical therapy of specific clinical presentations. *Gastroenterol Clin North Am* 1999;28(2):353–70, viii.

Papadakis KA, Targan SR. Current theories on the causes of inflammatory bowel disease. *Gastroenterol Clin North Am* 1999;28(2):283–296.

Stein RB, Hanauer SB. Medical therapy for inflammatory bowel disease. *Gastroenterol Clin North Am* 1999;28(2):297–321.

Authors: Jonathan E. Markowitz and Robert N. Baldassano

Ureteropelvic Junction Obstruction

 ## Database

DEFINITION

Ureteropelvic junction (UPJ) obstruction is a partial blockage of the kidney at the point where the renal pelvis transitions into the proximal ureter.

ETIOLOGIES

• Intrinsic: a congenital narrowing of the UPJ, which is most commonly due to abnormal musculature and fibrosis of this area, resulting in an adynamic segment.
• Extrinsic: kinking at the UPJ, which is most commonly due to the renal pelvis draping over a lower pole crossing vessel. This type of obstruction can be intermittent.

PATHOPHYSIOLOGY

The obstruction can cause varying degrees of hydronephrosis.

• Mild forms of UPJ obstruction result in dilation of the renal pelvis without loss of function.
• More severe forms result in dilation of the renal pelvis and calyces with loss of renal parenchyma and decreased function.
• In the most severe cases the kidney may have cystic dysplasia and very poor function. Congenital hydronephrosis due to an intrinsic narrowing is often asymptomatic.
• When the obstruction is intermittent due to a crossing vessel, the renal pelvis becomes distended (most likely due to transient increase in urine output), which drapes it over the vessel and kinks the ureter, resulting in an acute obstruction. The acute distention of the renal pelvis results in pain (renal colic).

EPIDEMIOLOGY

• 75% of all cases of prenatal hydronephrosis are due to UPJ obstruction
• Occurs more commonly in males (M/F 2:1)
• Left-sided lesion more common (66%)
• Bilateral in 10% to 40%
• 50% of patients have an additional genitourinary malformation (most common are vesicoureteral reflux, contralateral UPJ obstruction, multicystic dysplastic kidney, and renal agenesis)
• Of patients with VATER association, 21% have UPJ obstruction and thus should be screened with renal ultrasound

 ## Differential Diagnosis

• Vesicoureteral reflux: Higher grades of reflux will result in dilation of the upper urinary tract.
• Distal ureteral obstruction: obstruction at the level of the bladder due to ureterovesical junction obstruction, ureterocele, or an ectopic ureter
• Bladder outlet obstruction: dilation of the upper urinary tract secondary to obstruction of the lower urinary tract due to posterior urethral valves, urethral atresia, or stricture
• Megacalycosis: congenital dilation and increased numbers of calyces without significant renal pelvis dilation or obstruction
• Multicystic-dysplastic kidney: can be difficult to differentiate severe hydronephrosis from cysts by ultrasound. Renal scan will demonstrate no function in multicystic-dysplastic kidneys.
• Triad syndrome: a triad of hypoplastic abdominal wall musculature, bilateral undescended testes, and dilation of the urinary tract (also known as prune-belly syndrome or Eagle-Barrett syndrome).

 ## Data Gathering

HISTORY

• Antenatal: if unilateral, timing and severity of hydronephrosis, if detected during prenatal ultrasonography, and status of contralateral kidney. When bilateral or affecting a solitary kidney, renal insufficiency is a concern. The presence of oligohydramnios, increased renal echogenicity, and cystic changes point to poor renal function postnatally.
• Postnatal: feeding intolerance (very rarely due to massive UPJ obstruction)
• Older children: history of episodic abdominal (may not lateralize well), flank or back pain. Length of episodes (usually 30 min to several hours). Associated nausea and vomiting. Relation of episodes to fluid intake. History of urinary tract infections or gross hematuria.

 ## Physical Examination

• Newborn: Palpate kidneys. Affected kidney may feel enlarged but should not be tense. A tense mass can indicate a severe obstruction and should be imaged promptly.
• Older child: careful abdominal exam for enlarged kidney and tenderness. Costal-vertebral angle tenderness.

 ## Laboratory Aids

TESTS

• Newborn: if bilateral or a solitary kidney need serial assessments of renal function (serum electrolytes and creatinine) starting at 24 to 48 hours of age. With a normal contralateral kidney no immediate laboratory testing is necessary.
• Older children: urinalysis to detect hematuria or pyuria. Culture if infection suspected.

IMAGING

Antenatally detected hydronephrosis: Infants with antenatally detected hydronephrosis typically are evaluated with three imaging studies: a renal/bladder ultrasound, voiding cystourethrogram, and renal scan.

• Renal/bladder ultrasound: In most cases immediate imaging is not necessary. Because of a period of relative oliguria of a newborn in the first 24 to 48 hours of life, an ultrasound may underestimate the degree of hydronephrosis. This should not preclude evaluating an infant during this time as long any normal study is followed up with a repeat study in 4 to 6 weeks. Evaluation should reveal the severity of dilation of the renal pelvis and calyces, changes in the amount and echogenicity of the parenchyma, and presence of cortical cysts. The evaluation of the full bladder is important for excluding dilated distal ureters, thickening of the bladder wall due to outlet obstruction, and ureteroceles. In cases of bilateral hydronephrosis, a solitary hydronephrotic kidney, or a tense kidney on physical exam, imaging should be promptly performed.
• Voiding cystourethrogram: This study will detect the presence of vesicoureteral reflux as well as exclude the presence of posterior urethral valves and other abnormalities of the bladder. The test can be delayed until after discharge from the nursery unless there is concern about posterior urethral valves, in which case it should be performed early.

Ureteropelvic Junction Obstruction

• Renal scan: This study can quantitate the differential renal function or the amount each kidney contributes to overall renal function. The two most commonly used radionuclides are 3-mercaptoacetyl triglycine (MAG-3) and diethylenetriamine pentaacetic acid (DTPA). MAG-3 is a better choice for the immature kidneys in infants. In addition to the ability to detect diminished function, if there is poor drainage of the affected kidney, furosemide is given when the radiotracer reaches its maximum level of accumulation to attempt to wash out the radiotracer. The time for washing out half of the accumulated radiotracer ($T_{1/2}$) is often given in the report. A prompt (less than 10 minutes) washout time (expressed as the time to wash out half of the radiotracer) is indicative of a nonobstructed kidney. A slower washout time may be indicative of obstruction when it is greater than 20 minutes. An intermediate time (10–20 minutes) is indeterminate.

• Intravenous pyelogram (IVP): This study is most useful for evaluating the anatomy of the kidney and the ureters. It is also quite useful for evaluating an older child with intermittent symptoms if it can be done during a symptomatic episode. A normal study during a symptomatic episode excludes an intermittent UPJO as the cause of the child's pain. On the other hand, if a normal study is obtained while the child is asymptomatic, an intermittent UPJ obstruction remains a possible cause.

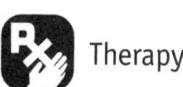

Therapy

The decision to observe or surgically correct a UPJ obstruction depends on several factors. One must consider the age and overall health of the neonate, the amount of functional impairment of the kidney, whether it is a unilateral or bilateral process, the drainage pattern on renal scan, and whether or not it is symptomatic. There is no strict rule for who should be observed and who should undergo surgery. This decision should be made on an individual basis.

• Antibiotic prophylaxis: Newborns should be started on a once-a-day dose of amoxicillin or cephalexin at 1/4 to 1/2 the therapeutic dose. The theory is to suppress the growth of bacteria in the bladder but not give a dose high enough to develop resistant organisms in the intestine. The antibiotic can be switched to trimethoprim/sulfamethoxazole or nitrofurantoin at 3 months of age. The duration that infants should be left on antibiotics is controversial among practicing pediatric urologists. Almost all agree that infants should be started on prophylactic antibiotics at birth. They should be continued at least until the infant undergoes a VCUG to exclude reflux. Several factors including age, sex, and degree of hydronephrosis are taken into account when deciding whether or not to stop the prophylaxis.

• Observation: Infants with hydronephrosis thought to be due to a narrowing at the UPJ are typically observed when there is preserved function (greater than 40%) in the affected kidney and the contralateral kidney is normal. The pattern of drainage is taken into account, and if there is prompt drainage and normal (50% ± 5%) these patients are followed with less frequent follow-up studies than those with less function and poor drainage. Most patients have follow-up imaging studies done at 3- to 6-month intervals during their first year of life, and they are gradually spaced out as time goes by if the hydronephrosis remains stable or improves.

• Older children with hydronephrosis due to a UPJ obstruction are often detected during a symptomatic episode. If the UPJ obstruction is asymptomatic and the function of the kidney is preserved, the child may be observed as well.

• Surgery: The gold standard for the repair of the UPJ obstruction has been a pyeloplasty. During the procedure the narrowed UPJ is most commonly excised and the ureter is reanastomosed to the renal pelvis. This procedure is successful 95% of the time. There are less invasive approaches such as endoscopically incising the narrowing (endopyelotomy) or balloon dilation. These approaches have been used in adults with rates of success in the 50% to 70% range but are considerably less invasive. Endoscopic procedures have not been routinely offered as first-line therapy for the treatment of UPJ obstructions because of their limited experience in children and the lower rates of success. Laparoscopic pyeloplasty is being performed in older children and adolescents and be more common in the next several years. It offers a similar rate of success to a traditional pyeloplasty with decreased perioperative morbidity because of the small incisions for the laparoscopic instruments.

Common Questions and Answers

Q: My unborn baby has hydronephrosis. My obstetrician told me that it is most likely a UPJ obstruction. Is my baby going to need surgery to correct this?
A: Not necessarily, only about one third of babies with significant hydronephrosis ultimately require surgical correction.

Q: Will my child's kidney look normal after the surgery to fix it?
A: Often the kidney has less dilation and looks better but not completely normal. Of greater importance is that there is no longer obstruction and the function is preserved or improved.

ICD-9-CM 593.4

BIBLIOGRAPHY

Bauer SB. Anomalies of the kidney and ureteropelvic junction. In: Walsh PC, Retik AB, Vaughan ED, et al., eds. *Cambell's urology*. 1998:1708–1755.

Mandell J, Peters CA, Retik AB. Perinatal urology. In: Walsh PC, Retik AB, Vaughan ED, et al., eds. *Cambell's urology*. Philadelphia: Saunders. 1601–1618.

Authors: J. Christopher Austin and Michael C. Carr

Urethral Prolapse

 Database

DEFINITION

Circular eversion of the distal urethral mucosa through the external urethral meatus.

GENETICS

Predominance in African-American females indicates a hereditary pattern.

ETIOLOGY

• Etiology unclear, proposed theories include:

—Poor adherence between smooth muscle layers of the urethra
—Estrogen deficiency

EPIDEMIOLOGY

• Prepubertal girls younger than 10 years of age
• Preponderance among African-American females (90–100% of patients in reported series)
• Patients above average for height and weight

 Differential Diagnosis

• Prolapsing ureterocele (or ectopic ureter, urethral polyp, bladder)
• Sarcoma botryoides
• Condyloma
• Hydrometrocolpos
• Periurethral abscess
• Trauma

 Data Gathering

HISTORY

• Ninety-five percent present with bleeding/bloody spotting in underwear.
• Twenty-one percent have dysuria, frequency.
• Occasionally a patient presents with urinary retention.
• Some are asymptomatic and detected only incidentally.

 Physical Examination

• Circular (doughnut-shaped) protrusion of urethral meatus with a reddish-purple mass filling the introitus with the urethral meatus at the center.
• Tissue appears inflamed and friable.

IMAGING

• If the appearance is atypical for urethral prolapse, ultrasound may be used to rule out bladder tumor (sarcoma botryoides) or prolapsed ureterocele.
• Urethral prolapse with typical presentation requires no imaging.

Therapy

- Do not try to manually reduce the prolapsed tissue.
- Conservative—Sitz baths followed by topical estrogen cream b.i.d.
- Surgical—Most typical surgical approach is excision of prolapsed segment over a urethral Foley catheter, suturing the proximal urethral margin to the adjacent vestibule.

Follow-Up

Outpatient visit to assess success of estrogen cream or surgical repair

Common Questions and Answers

Q: What is the most common presenting complaint?
A: Bleeding

Q: What is the "first aid" for this problem?
A: Avoid infection and respect the tissue. Keep tissue moist. You may use antibiotic cream. Do not push the tissue back into the urethra.

ICD-9-CM 599.5

BIBLIOGRAPHY

Baldwin D, Landa H. Common problems in pediatric gynecology. *Urol Clin North Am* 1995;22:173.

Kelalis P, King K, Belman A, eds. *Clinical pediatric urology*. Philadelphia: WB Saunders, 1992:653–654.

Valerie E, Gilchrists B, Frischer J, et al. Diagnosis and treatment of urethral prolapse in children. *Urology* 1999;54(6):1082.

Authors: Michele Clement and Stephen A. Zderic

Urinary Tract Infection

Database

DEFINITION

Urinary tract infection (UTI) is growth of bacterial urinary tract pathogen(s) at:

- $\geq 10^2$ colony-forming units (CFU)/mL for suprapubic aspirate
- $\geq 10^4$ CFU/mL for urine obtained by catheterization
- $\geq 10^5$ CFU/mL for urine obtained by clean-catch technique

PATHOLOGY

- Urinary tract pathogens include:

—Common: *Escherichia coli, Klebsiella* spp., *Enterococcus, Proteus mirabilis*
—Less common: *Enterobacter cloacae,* group B hemolytic streptococci, *Citrobacter, Staphylococcus aureus,* and *Staphylococcus saprophyticus* (teenage girls)

- A specimen must be obtained sterilely, not by applying a bag to the perineum.
- Ninety percent of patients will also have pyuria [5 WBC/high-power field (HPF) or urine dipstick for leukocyte esterase (LE)] and bacteriuria on examination of the urine.
- Upper tract infection or pyelonephritis: infection of the renal parenchyma; vast majority of febrile babies with a positive culture have upper tract infection.
- Lower tract infection: infection limited to bladder, not involving the kidneys; occurs more in older children and adolescents; no fever.

EPIDEMIOLOGY

- Ascending infection from bladder instrumentation, perineal irritation, bacterial soilage, sexual activity
- Dysfunctional voiding
- Urinary tract abnormalities: vesicoureteral reflux (VUR), neurogenic bladder, urethral obstruction

RISK FACTORS

- Sex/age: boys most at risk for UTI during first year of life; girls until school age and again in adolescence
- Circumcision status: Uncircumcised males have ten times the incidence of UTI compared with circumcised males.
- Race: Caucasians have a higher incidence of UTI; Caucasian females have the highest rate.
- Abnormal urinary tract: Children with VUR and obstruction are at higher risk for UTI.
- Voiding dysfunction

COMPLICATIONS

- Repeated febrile UTIs in young children may lead to renal scarring.
- Renal scarring in childhood carries a risk of hypertension, preeclampsia, and end-stage renal disease as an adult.

PROGNOSIS

Prompt treatment of febrile UTIs reduces the risk for scarring and its sequelae.

ASSOCIATED ILLNESSES

Approximately 10% of babies with febrile UTIs (pyelonephritis) are bacteremic.

Differential Diagnosis

- Lower tract infections

—Urethral irritation for irritants such as bubble baths
—Diabetes
—Excessive drinking
—Masses adjacent to the bladder
—Normal potty training
—Dyes from ingested fluids
—Dehydration with concentrated urine

- Upper tract infections

—Gastroenteritis
—Pelvic inflammatory disease or tubo-ovarian abscess (TOA)
—Appendicitis
—Ovarian torsion

Data Gathering

HISTORY

- Babies: Symptoms are nonspecific, such as vomiting, irritability, poor feeding, and fever.
- Older children: Classic symptoms of the lower tract include urgency, frequency, dysuria, hesitancy, suprapubic discomfort, hematuria, and malodorous urine. Classic symptoms of the upper tract include chills, nausea, flank pain, and fever.

Physical Examination

BABIES

- Fever is the most common finding.
- Abdominal pain or distention
- Poor growth or weight gain
- Malodorous urine

OLDER CHILDREN

- Lower tract: suprapubic tenderness
- Upper tract: fever, costovertebral angle tenderness to percussion

SPECIAL QUESTION

Has the young child had a history of UTI, unexplained fevers, or urinary tract anomaly?

PROCEDURE

Suspect UTI in any febrile baby less than 1 year of age or in a preschool girl, even in the absence of signs and symptoms, especially if there is not a definite source of fever, fever has been present ≥ 2 days, or temperature is $\geq 39°C$.

Laboratory Aids

TESTS

• Urinalysis: 5 WBC/HPF or bacteria on Gram stain microscopy per HPF.
• Urine dipstick is equivalent to conventional microscopy: trace color changes on the LE test strip indicate 5 WBC/HPF; nitrite indicates the presence of nitrate-splitting bacteria.
• Rapid filter testing for bacteriuria is equivalent to microscopic examination for bacteria; it is not as sensitive as the dipstick for detecting UTI.

—Enhanced urinalysis: 10 WBC/cm³ or higher, or bacteria on Gram stain, may be most sensitive for detecting UTI in the neonate

• Urine culture collected sterilely is the gold standard for diagnosis.

FALSE POSITIVES

Contaminated urine by perineum or stool organisms

PITFALLS

• Ten percent of babies will have a negative urinalysis despite culture or nuclear scan-documented UTI.
• Failure to culture by sterile means: unable to interpret a contaminated urine culture result

HOME TESTING

Urine dipstick for LE or nitrite with first morning void can be used to screen children at risk for repeated infections.

REQUIREMENTS

• Obtain urine sterilely to avoid false-positive results.
• The nitrite test requires urine to be in the bladder for 4 hours; therefore, the first morning specimen is best.

 ## Therapy

UPPER TRACT INFECTION

• Drugs: ampicillin and gentamicin intravenously until afebrile (48 hours); sterile urine, and sensitivity of the organisms to antibiotics known for neonates or infants who may have urinary tract abnormalities.
• Length of treatment: Complete a 10- to 14-day course orally.
• Outpatient oral treatment may be satisfactory in babies older than 6 months who look well, can take oral fluids, have normal urinary tract anatomy, and have good follow-up.

LOWER TRACT INFECTION

• Drugs: amoxicillin, trimethoprim-sulfamethoxazole, cefprozil, nitrofurantoin orally
• Length of treatment: 7 to 10 days

PREVENTION

• Teaching correct wiping—front to back—to young children.
• Prophylactic antibiotics for selected children with recurrent infection, VUR, pyelonephritis
• Attention to good voiding habits

 ## Follow-Up

• Repeat urine culture if persistent fever >2 days, not improving.
• Radiologic evaluation
• Renal cortical scan: all febrile children
• Ultrasound: boys, girls less than 12 years
• Voiding cystourethrogram (VCUG): all boys, all infants younger than 1 year, history of voiding dysfunction, upper tract infection, or abnormal RCS or ultrasound

PITFALLS

• Not obtaining urine by a sterile method for culturing; unable to interpret contaminated results; not knowing if the child should have a radiographic workup
• Not culturing febrile babies without a documented source of fever; increased risk of long-term sequelae, untreated pyelonephritis

 ## Common Questions and Answers

Q: Which children require radiologic evaluation after their first UTI?
A: All boys, any girl with an upper tract infection, and all girls younger than 3 years of age.

Q: Does a urine culture need to be done if the dipstick or urinalysis is negative?
A: Approximately 10% of febrile infants with pyelonephritis will have a false-negative screening test (dipstick, urinalysis). A sterile urine culture should be done.

ICD-9-CM 599.0

BIBLIOGRAPHY

Al-Orifi F, McGillivray D, Tange S, et al. Urine culture from bag specimens in young children: are the risks too high? *J Pediatr* 2000;137: 221–226.

American Academy of Pediatrics, Committee on Quality Improvement, Subcommittee on Urinary Tract Infection. Practice parameter: the diagnosis, treatment, and evaluation of the initial urinary tract infection in febrile infants and young children. *Pediatrics* 1999;103:843:852.

Friedman AL. Urinary tract infection. *Curr Opin Pediatr* 1998;10(2):197–200.

Gorelick MH, Shaw KN. Clinical decision rule to identify young febrile children at risk for UTI. *Arch Pediatr Adol Med* 2000,154:386–390.

Gorelick MH, Shaw KN. Screening tests for UTI in children: a meta-analysis. *Pediatrics* 1999;104(5):e1.

Heldrich FJ. UTI diagnosis: getting it right the first time. *Contemp Pediatr* 1995;12:110–133.

Hoberman A, Chao HP, Keller DM, et al. Prevalence of urinary tract infection in febrile infants. *J Pediatr* 1993;23(1):17–23.

Hoberman A, Wald ER, Hickey RW, et al. Oral versus initial intravenous therapy for urinary tract infections in young febrile children. *Pediatrics* 1999;104:79–86.

Shaw KN, Gorelick M, McGowan KL, et al. Prevalence of UTI in febrile young children in the emergency department. *Pediatrics* 1998;102(2):1–5, *http://www.pediatrics.org/cgi/content/full/102/2/e16.*

Winberg J. Commentary: progressive renal damage from infection with or without reflux. *J Urol* 1992;148:1733–1734.

Author: Kathy N. Shaw

Urticaria

 Database

DEFINITION

Acute urticaria is a common, allergic skin disorder characterized by well-circumscribed, localized, or generalized erythematous, raised skin lesions (wheals or welts) of various sizes; it is usually intensely pruritic. Chronic urticaria is a type that recurs frequently or lasts longer than 6 weeks.

ETIOLOGY

- Ingestions (usually foods: seafood, nuts, eggs, food additives; antibiotics, especially penicillin and sulfa drugs)
- Direct contact (plants)
- Injected agents (antibiotics, blood products, insect stings and bites)
- Inhalants (pollens, danders)
- Infectious agents [viral, especially hepatitis and Epstein-Barr virus (EBV), bacterial, parasitic]
- Physical factors (cold, pressure, sun exposure, water exposure)
- Systemic diseases (collagen-vascular, serum sickness, malignancy, hyperthyroidism, mastocytosis)
- Associated illnesses include angioedema and anaphylaxis.

PATHOPHYSIOLOGY

IgE or non–IgE-mediated hypersensitivity reaction causing extravasation of fluid from small blood vessels mediated by various chemicals, including histamine, kinins, prostaglandins, and serotonin

GENETICS

Rarely hereditary (cold urticaria)

EPIDEMIOLOGY

Nonspecific

COMPLICATIONS

- Swelling of the oropharynx or airways can be life threatening.
- Progression to anaphylaxis with wheezing and hypotension may also be life threatening.

PROGNOSIS

- Good
- Usually self-limited and benign
- Chronic urticaria: may persist intermittently for weeks to years

 Differential Diagnosis

Appearance is very distinctive and diagnosis usually straightforward.

INFECTION

Varicella

TRAUMA

Insect bites (fleas, mosquitoes, spiders)

IMMUNOLOGIC

Erythema multiforme

 Data Gathering

HISTORY

- History of urticaria
- Known exposures and ingestions
- Evanescent lesions
- Family history
- Underlying medical problems
- History of atopy
- For chronic urticaria: symptom diary including activity, diet, illnesses, sun exposure, and medications

Special Questions

- Cold/heat exposure?
- Exertion or emotional stress (cholinergic urticaria)?
- Water exposure (aquagenic urticaria)?
- Sun exposure (solar urticaria)?

 Physical Examination

- Blanching "wheal and flare" lesions
- Migratory lesions
- Examine mucous membranes and airway.
- Evaluate for wheezing (may be part of anaphylaxis).
- Check blood pressure (hypotension may be part of anaphylaxis).
- Apply an ice cube, rewarm the area, and examine for a wheal: cold urticaria.

Laboratory Aids

TESTS

Testing is useful if a specific cause is suspected (must be individualized):

• Suspected underlying infectious agent: throat culture, titers for hepatitis or EBV, etc.
• Suspected underlying systemic disease: ANA, RF, ESR, CBC, thyroid studies, as indicated
• Suspected IgE-mediated urticaria: skin testing to confirm causal relationship (RAST is alternative to skin testing)

 Emergency Care

Acute situations: epinephrine 1:1,000, 0.1 to 0.3 mL; rapid relief of itching; antihistamines relieve itching less quickly. See the Anaphylaxis topic for further management of acute reactions.

 Therapy

DRUGS

• Antihistamines: diphenhydramine (Benadryl) 1.25 mg/kg/dose, or hydroxyzine (Atarax) 0.5 mg/kg/dose q4–6h, cetirizine (Zyrtec) 5 mg for 2 to 6 years, once daily, or 5 to 10 mg/d for 6 to 12 years or loratadine (Claritin) 5 to 10 mg/d for 6 to 12 years; cyproheptadine (Periactin) 2 to 4 mg q8–12h for cold urticaria
• Combination H1 (Benadryl, Atarax) and H2-receptor antagonists (ranitidine, cimetidine) for chronic urticaria
• Corticosteroids may work in chronic urticaria; high doses are often necessary, with predictable side effects.

 Follow-Up

SIGNS TO WATCH FOR

• Airway compromise
• Wheezing
• Hoarse voice
• Difficulty breathing or swallowing

PREVENTION

• Sunscreens, protective clothing, or sun avoidance for solar urticaria
• Avoid causative agents (foods, contacts, inhalants, medications, etc.)

PITFALLS

Discontinuation of a medication needed to treat another condition may result in problems.

 Common Questions and Answers

Q: What duration of observation in acute urticaria is necessary to avoid missing serious sequelae?
A: In uncomplicated cases that respond rapidly to antihistamines, observation can be brief—minutes to hours. If the allergic reaction is complicated by angioedema or airway problems, or if epinephrine is administered, observation should be prolonged (several hours or overnight) to observe for worsening symptoms or anaphylaxis.

Q: Should patients with chronic urticaria be referred to a specialist?
A: If urticaria persists for more than 6 weeks and no underlying etiology is identified, the patient should be referred to an allergist or immunologist for evaluation and treatment, because it may be a sign of underlying systemic disease.

ICD-9-CM 708.9

BIBLIOGRAPHY

Dalal I, Levine A, et al. Chronic urticaria in children: expanding the "autoimmune kaleidoscope." *Pediatrics* 2000;106(5): 1139–1141.

Dalal I, Levine A, Somekh E, et al. Chronic urticaria in children: expanding the "autoimmune kaleidoscope." *Pediatrics* 2000;106(5):1139–1141.

Greaves MW. Chronic urticaria. *N Engl J Med* 1995;332(26):1767–1771.

Hurwitz S. *Clinical pediatric dermatology: a textbook of skin disorders of childhood and adolescence*, 2nd ed. Philadelphia: WB Saunders, 1993:516–519.

Kwong KY, Maalouf N, Jones CA. Urticaria and angioedema: pathophysiology, diagnosis and treatment. *Pediatr Ann* 1998;27(11):719–724.

Mortureux P, Leaute-Labreze C, Lamireau T, et al. Acute urticaria in infancy and early childhood. *Arch Dermatol* 1998;134:319–323.

Volonakis M, Katsarov-Katsari A, Stratigos J. Etiologic factors in childhood chronic urticaria. *Ann Allergy* 1992;69:61–65.

Author: Deborah L. Silver

Vaginitis

 Database

DEFINITION

Vaginitis: disruption of the normal vaginal flora, which involves an inflammatory response
Vaginosis: disruption of the normal vaginal flora that does not involve an inflammatory response; may represent colonization; not thought to be sexually transmitted
Vaginal discharge: secretions found in the vagina and often noted by patients on their undergarments or when wiping. Normal vaginal discharge appears clear or white, varies from odorless to a mild odor, and in postmenarchal girls often varies in amount and consistency throughout the menstrual cycle
Vulvovaginal pruritus: vulvar itching often associated with changes in vaginal discharge and/or vulvar dermatitis

COMPLICATIONS

• **Labial adhesions:** following trauma and certain dermatoses
• **Toxic shock syndrome:** associated with retained foreign body, especially tampon
• **Pelvic inflammatory disease:** from untreated cervicitis and possibly bacterial vaginosis (BV). May result in subsequent fertility problems and/or ectopic pregnancies.
• **Vulvar dysesthesia syndrome:** pain syndrome from chronic vulvar/vaginal infections
• **Preterm labor, preterm rupture of membranes, and chorioamnionitis:** all associated with concurrent BV

PROGNOSIS

Depends on etiology, but generally excellent with appropriate treatment. Infections may recur.

 Differential Diagnosis

PREMENARCHAL GIRLS

• The majority of vulvovaginitis in premenarchal girls is diagnosed as "nonspecific vulvovaginitis."
—Vaginal discharge is usually a brown or green color, malodorous, and has a pH of 4.7 to 6.5.
—Long-standing symptoms are more likely to be caused by a mixed bacterial infection or irritant dermatitis, whereas acute onset of symptoms is more likely to be associated with a specific bacterial cause.
• Bloody or blood-tinged discharge should prompt consideration of excoriations, onset of menarche/precocious puberty, streptococcal vaginitis, trauma, trichomoniasis, foreign body, or tumor.
• Common etiologies of pediatric vulvovaginitis:
—Overgrowth of coliform bacteria from poor perineal hygiene
—Hemolytic streptococci and coagulase-positive staphylococci transmitted manually from the nasopharynx
—Irritant dermatitis from chemicals, soaps, detergents, bubble bath, undergarment materials, particularly nylon and/or tight fitting ones
• Less common etiologies:
—Vulvovaginal candidiasis
—Foreign body, most commonly toilet paper
—STIs from sexual abuse (gonorrhea, chlamydia, trichomonal vaginitis)
—Trauma (acute, sexual abuse, masturbation behaviors)
—Systemic diseases (giardiasis, shigellosis, Stevens-Johnson syndrome)
—Congenital anomalies (fistulas, ectopic ureter, urethral prolapse)
—Precocious puberty

• Additional causes of isolated vulvar itching:
—Infestations: pinworm, scabies, lice
—Molluscum contagiosum (umbilicated vulvar papules with white core of curd-like or seed-like material caused by pox virus)
—Dermatologic disorders: lichen sclerosis, psoriasis, seborrhea

PARA- AND POSTMENARCHAL GIRLS

In para- (6–12 months before menarche) and postmenarchal girls, the amount and consistency of the discharge tends to vary throughout the month, with the most discharge in menarchal girls usually seen midcycle.
• Common etiologies: vulvovaginal candidiasis (the overgrowth of yeast forms), BV (the overgrowth of *Gardnerella vaginalis* and *M. hominis* and other anaerobes), allergic/irritant reactions (soaps, latex, spermicides, etc.), trichomonal vaginitis (sexually transmitted parasite), cervicitis (gonorrhea and chlamydia)
• Less common causes: nonspecific cervicitis, foreign body (most commonly tampons), sloughed debris from condyloma (caused by some types of sexually transmitted human papilloma virus).
• Additional causes of isolated vulvar itching: contact/allergic dermatitis, vulvar dermatoses (lichen simplex chronicus, lichen sclerosis, lichen planus), vulvar dysplasia (HPV), molluscum contagiosum

 Data Gathering

HISTORY

• Ask about breast development and onset of menarche.
• Ask about risk factors for vulvovaginal candidiasis: underlying medical conditions such as diabetes, immunosuppression, current/recent use of antibiotics or steroids; predisposition to perineal moisture, such as diaper use and enuresis.

DDx of Vaginal Infections in Para- and Postmenarchal Girls

DIAGNOSTIC CRITERIA	NORMAL	VULVOVAGINAL CANDIDIASIS	BACTERIAL VAGINOSIS	TRICHOMONAL VAGINITIS
Symptoms	None or increased d/c	Itching, burning, d/c	Irritation, foul odor, d/c	Frothy d/c, odor, itching, dysuria
Inspection	Normal	Vulvar erythema ± satellite lesions	± Vulvar erythema	± Cervical erythema
Discharge	Clear, white	Little or none, or white, curdy, adherent	Homogeneous, white-gray to yellow, green thin	Gray to green, frothy
Vaginal pH	3.8–4.2	<4.5 usually	>4.5	>4.5
Amine odor	No	No	Yes, fishy	Sometimes fishy
Microscopic	Lactobacilli; few or no WBCs	Budding yeast, pseudo-hyphae in KOH, few or no WBCs	Clue cells; absent or few lactobacilli, few or no WBCs	Swimming trichomonads and usually WBC >10/HPF

Amsel's clinical criteria for BV (any three of the following): clue cells, pH >4.5, + whiff test, homogeneous gray or white discharge. Gram-stain criteria may also be used. Note: culture is unreliable for BV. d/c, discharge.

- Use of possible irritants, including bubble baths, soaps, detergents, douches, nylon underwear
- Likelihood of foreign body (e.g., toilet paper, toy, tampon)
- Duration, color, consistency, odor of abnormal discharge
- Presence of itching, burning, and/or vulvar irritation; dysuria
- Attempted therapies
- Prior history of vaginal discharge or itching, diagnosis and treatment
- Family history of atopy

Physical Examination

- Perform a thorough abdominal exam.
- Assess Tanner staging.
- Examine discharge on undergarments/pads.
- Examine external genitalia for erythema, evidence of trauma, excoriations suggestive of scratching, labial adhesions, hypo/hyperpigmentations, warts, other irregular lesions.

Laboratory Aids

If suspect possible infectious etiology, obtain discharge for pH testing (Nitrazine paper), wet mount slide with saline and another with KOH, and perform whiff test. If patient had possible sexual exposure or many WBCs on wet mount with negative trichomonads, do test for gonorrhea and chlamydia.

TESTS
- **pH test:** Nitrazine paper runs green-blue when >4.5, and yellow <4.5.
- **Wet mount:** Mix discharge with one to two drops saline on slide, and place coverslip, look for *Lactobacilli* (small rods), assess for WBCs suggestive of inflammation, BV ≥20% of clue cells (epithelial cells coated with bacteria, best seen along the edges of the cells, like a fried egg with lots of pepper on it); trichomonads—usually see swimming parasite slightly larger than WBCs.
- **KOH prep:** Mix sample of discharge with one to two drops 10% KOH, look for hyphae ± buds (moderately sensitive).
- **Whiff test:** KOH drop on speculum, positive if fishy amine odor
- **Gram stain:** Smear discharge evenly over slide and let dry, usually send to lab.
- **Vaginal culture:** Used more with premenarchal girls, usually not necessary in postmenarchal girls, but may be helpful if negative microscopic exam with KOH prep but clinically suspect yeast, especially atypical species
- **Gonorrhea and chlamydia assays:** If suspect sexual exposure, and/or if discharge has >10 WBC/HPF
- **Pap test:** Clue cells and "shift in vaginal flora" found incidentally on Pap test are 97% specific for BV. May also incidentally diagnose *Trichomonas vaginalis*.

Tips for Collecting and Examining Vaginal Discharge
- Use a Peterson (thin) or pediatric speculum.
- Use a cotton-tip swab to collect the vaginal discharge (either cotton-tip side to smear onto dry slide or wooden side to mix into solution previously put on slide). The vaginal fornices usually have the highest volume of discharge for collection, but also try to get a sample of any discharge clinging to the vaginal side walls.
- If not doing a speculum exam, collect discharge with a cotton swab by placing patient in the frog-leg position, separating her labia with your or her fingers, and gently placing the swab into vagina to the anticipated level of the top of the vagina and withdraw moving in a small circular motion to get discharge from the side walls, too. If you encounter resistance, change your angle a little, but never force the swab in. If the patient is particularly sensitive, you can moisten the cotton tip with nonbacteriostatic saline, but you might collect less discharge that way.
—Another option, particularly for younger girls, is to do a nonbacteriostatic saline wash (2–3 mL) of vagina with small catheter attached to syringe (butterfly catheter with needle portion cut off, or small red rubber catheter cut off to create a 5- to 6-cm distal portion).

Therapy

- In premenarchal girls, unless suspect sexual abuse or foreign body, prior to doing a vaginal examination, can usually start with education regarding hygiene and eliminating possible irritants. If discharge persistent, it is often necessary to search for infectious etiologies or other pathologies.
- Sitz baths and then application of barrier ointment/cream such as petroleum jelly or SBR-lipocream may help relieve irritation and discomfort.
- **Streptococcal vaginitis:** penicillin VK
- **Staphylococcal vaginitis:** cephalexin
- **Yeast vaginitis:** topical clotrimazole, miconazole, butoconazole, terconazole, or single-dose oral fluconazole in adolescent or adults
- **Bacterial vaginosis:** metronidazole PO or metronidazole gel or clindamycin cream per vagina
- **Trichomonal vaginitis:** metronidazole PO. Treat sexual partners and/or consider need for evaluation for child abuse.
- **Cervicitis**
- **Gonorrhea:** cefixime PO single dose, ceftriaxone IM single dose, ciprofloxacin PO single dose (older girls).
Because of legal implications, only conventional cultures should be used for children.
- **Chlamydia:** doxycycline (7-day course), azithromycin (1-g single dose for adolescent/adult), erythromycin. Treat sexual

partners and/or consider need for evaluation for child abuse.
- **Foreign body:** removal, sometimes requires anesthesia
- **Vulvar dermatoses:** topical corticosteroids
- **Infestations:** specific therapies

Follow-Up

- To ensure resolution of symptoms, especially when treating for nonspecific vaginitis
- Culture for test of cure after treating for chlamydia or gonorrhea.

PREVENTION
- Teach young girls to wipe front to back and to avoid bubble baths and harsh soaps, nylon undergarments, and tight fitting clothes.
- For recurrent yeast vaginitis or during antibiotic treatments, it may be helpful to eat yogurt with live cultures or to take a "probiotic" supplement such as *Acidophilus* or *Lactobacillus*.

CONTROL MEASURES
- Standard universal precautions
- Gonorrhea and chlamydia are reportable infections.

PITFALLS
- An itchy vagina/vulva isn't always a yeast infection.
- *Gardnerella* is a common colonizer of the vaginal tract; therefore, positive culture alone is unreliable in diagnosing BV.

Common Questions and Answers

Q: How sensitive for yeast vaginitis is microscopy using KOH prepared slide?
A: Less than 50%; therefore, if other causes of discharge and itching have been ruled out, consider culture for yeast or a trial of empiric therapy.
Q: Are bacterial vaginosis and vulvovaginal candidiasis sexually transmitted infections?
A: Probably not. They are found in girls and women who have never had sexual contact.
Q: Is douching a good method to prevent bacterial infections?
A: No. Douching tends to disrupt the normal protective vaginal flora and actually increase the likelihood of developing a vaginal infection and may lead to upper genital tract infections.

ICD-9-CM 616.10

BIBLIOGRAPHY
Centers for Disease Control and Prevention. 1998 Guidelines for treatment of sexually transmitted diseases. *MMWR* 1998;47(RR-1).

Nyirjesy P. Vaginitis in the adolescent patient. *Pediatr Clin North Am* 1999;46(4):733–745.

Authors: Lisa Bernard-Pearl and Deirdre Bernard-Pearl

Vein of Galen Malformations

 Database

DEFINITION

Vein of Galen malformations are congenital arteriovenous malformations (AVMs). The vein of Galen connects the deep cerebral venous system with the intracranial venous sinuses. After draining the internal cerebral veins and basal veins, the vein of Galen flows into the straight sinus.

PATHOPHYSIOLOGY

Vein of Galen malformations may consist of a simple arteriovenous (AV) fistula or a more complicated AVM. Clinical symptoms develop because of high-output congestive heart failure (CHF), cerebral ischemia or hemorrhage, or hydrocephalus. Cerebral ischemia may result from the shunting of blood from the brain parenchyma to the malformation.

GENETICS

No known genetic predisposition

EPIDEMIOLOGY

- Forty to sixty percent of cases present as neonates, almost always with CHF. Occasional infants will present with hydrocephalus, subarachnoid hemorrhage, or intraventricular hemorrhage.
- Older infants and children present with hydrocephalus, focal neurologic signs, headache, and subarachnoid hemorrhage.
- The incidence is unknown, but clinical experience suggests that this is a very rare condition.

COMPLICATIONS

- High-output CHF, cerebral ischemia or hemorrhage, and hydrocephalus may result from this congenital vascular anomaly.
- In severe cases, 80% of cardiac output may be delivered to the head because of the low vascular resistance within the malformation. Cardiac ischemic may occur because of decreased coronary artery blood flow.
- In a recent series, three of 34 children had hemorrhagic complications: two children presented with acute intracranial hemorrhage, and a third developed acute intracranial hemorrhage following endovascular treatment of the malformation.
- Longer-term complications include mental retardation, seizures, and cerebral palsy.

PROGNOSIS

Prognosis depends on the size of the malformation, the severity of the CHF, and the extent of cerebral injury prior to therapy. Historically, the prognosis has been poor for patients presenting as neonates with CHF. Recent advances in endovascular embolization techniques may improve prognosis.

 Differential Diagnosis

- The diagnosis must be considered in any newborn with unexplained CHF (especially high-output failure), hydrocephalus, or intracranial hemorrhage.
- Other causes of high-output CHF in the newborn include anemia, hyperthyroidism, and other AVMs.
- In older infants and children, presenting symptoms may be nonspecific and raise suspicion of hydrocephalus or a mass lesion.
- Tumors that may obstruct the sylvian aqueduct include common posterior fossa tumors in children, pinealoma, hemangioblastoma, ependymoma, and hamartomas (e.g., in tuberous sclerosis).

Approach to the Patient

First priority is the hemodynamic stability of the patient, since life-threatening CHF may be the presenting symptom. After a history and physical exam, neuroimaging studies must be promptly obtained, so treatment plans can be formulated.

 Data Gathering

HISTORY

- Ninety-five percent of newborns with vein of Galen malformations present in CHF. The history discloses weight gain, edematous appearance, feeding difficulty, and irritability consistent with heart failure. Changes in head circumference over time should be documented in older patients presenting with macrocephaly and loss or stasis of developmental milestones.
- Infants and older children usually present with hydrocephalus, headache, exercise-induced syncope, or subarachnoid hemorrhage. Irritability, stupor, or limitation of neck mobility may occur in patients with these complications or with intraventricular hemorrhage.

 Physical Examination

- In newborns, tachycardia, respiratory distress, hepatomegaly, a continuous cranial bruit heard over the posterior skull, and bounding carotid pulses and peripheral pulses may be present. The resting pulse may increase over time as the volume of blood shunted to the malformation increases.
- As CHF worsens, the peripheral pulses may lose their bounding character, but the prominent carotid pulses persist.
- Older infants and children also may present with CHF but more often demonstrate increased head circumference, focal neurologic signs, and failure to thrive. Less common presenting signs include visual loss, proptosis, syncope, seizures, acute or progressive hemiparesis, developmental regression, epistaxis, and vertigo.
- The "sunset eyes" sign, indicative of dorsal midbrain dysfunction, usually occurs in the setting of hydrocephalus with impaired consciousness.

 Laboratory Aids

TESTS

As with other AVMs, CBC and blood gases are often normal. Chest x-ray and ECG may reveal typical changes of high-output CHF, even in patients with resting tachycardia but no overt circulatory symptoms.

IMAGING

- Neuroimaging studies are definitive.
- Prenatal diagnosis is now possible with fetal ultrasound. This allows planning for the appropriate location of delivery and postnatal management.
- In newborns, cranial ultrasound shows a large, hypoechoic structure in the region of the vein of Galen. CT shows a high-density mass that enhances with contrast. MRI shows an area of decreased signal intensity or signal void because of high flow within the malformation. CT and MRI may also show areas of cerebral ischemia or hemorrhage.
- Magnetic resonance angiography can detail the arterial supply and venous drainage of the malformation, but most surgeons require standard angiography before intervention.

Emergency Care

The need for emergency intervention depends on the clinical presentation of the patient. Treatment usually depends on the severity of the CHF. Decompensated hydrocephalus causing coma and status epilepticus represent other possible emergent complications of this condition.

Therapy

• Treatment of choice in all ages is endovascular embolization. This treatment depends on the availability of an interventional radiologist. A venous or arterial approach may be used, depending on the anatomy of the lesion. Direct surgical intervention has unacceptable risks and is no longer recommended.
• Refractory CHF prompts intervention (i.e., embolization of the malformation).
• The initial goal is not total obliteration of the lesion, but a reduction in blood flow to the lesion to improve cardiac function. Embolization can be completed in stages over a few months once CHF is controlled.
• Treatment in older infants and children is indicated to prevent cerebral ischemia from arterial steal or from venous infarction, and to prevent hydrocephalus and its sequelae.
• Therapy for associated conditions may include positive inotropes, diuretics, anticonvulsants, and CNS ventricular shunting.
• Radiosurgery (gamma surgery) is a newer treatment option for older children who are clinically stable.

 ## Follow-Up

• Both the circulatory and neurologic complications of this condition can be progressive, and either may recur following surgery.
• Survival depends largely on the severity of the CHF and the age of the patient. In the past, mortality in newborns approached 100%. Today, approximately 50% of newborns with severe CHF will survive. Critically ill infants requiring embolization in the first week of life continue to have the poorest prognosis.
• In one series of 28 children, 45% of those younger than 1 year of age had good outcomes, 61% of those ages 1 to 2 years had good outcomes, and 100% of those older than 2 years had good outcomes.
• Resting tachycardia may be an early sign of recurrent CHF in patients previously embolized.
• Patients who survive with neurologic deficits are at risk for the sequelae of stroke.
• Ophthalmologic complications of hydrocephalus require close follow-up of visual function.
• A follow-up CT or MRI is indicated in evaluating patients with new neurologic signs or symptoms.

PREVENTION

There is no known prevention for these congenital malformations.

PITFALLS

• Advent of seizures may not necessarily signal recurrence or progression of the original lesion—repeat scan and comparison to prior studies are usually indicated.
• Overly rapid reduction in blood flow to the malformation can result in overperfusion of normal brain, systemic hypertension, cerebral edema, or hemorrhage.
• *Hydrocephalus* may occur in patients who have had hemorrhage from the malformation.
• *Shunt failure* may cause acute hydrocephalus, even if the malformation has not changed.

 ## Common Questions and Answers

Q: Can the malformation recur?
A: AVMs have a propensity to recur. Imaging studies give a good indication of the likelihood of recurrence.

Q: How does the malformation cause seizures?
A: Seizures are most often due to ischemia, acute hydrocephalus, infection, or metabolic disturbances.

ICD-9-CM 747.40

BIBLIOGRAPHY

Borthne A, et al. Vein of Galen malformations in infants: clinical, radiological and therapeutic aspects. *Eur Radiol* 1997;7:1252–1258.

Brunelle F. Arteriovenous malformations of the vein of Galen in children. *Pediatr Radiol* 1997;27:501–513.

Meyers PM, Halbach VV, Phatouros CP, et al. Hemorrhagic complications in vein of Galen malformations. *Ann Neurol* 2000;47:748–755.

Payne BR, Prasad D, Steiner M, et al. Gamma surgery for vein of Galen malformations. *J Neurosurg* 2000;93:229–236.

Rodesch G, et al. Prognosis of antenatally diagnosed vein of Galen malformations. *Childs Nerv Syst* 1994;10:79–83.

Volpe JJ. *Neurology of the newborn*, 4th ed. Philadelphia: WB Saunders, 2001:849–854.

Author: Dennis J. Dlugos

Ventricular Septal Defect

 Database

DEFINITION

A ventricular septal defect (VSD) is an opening in the ventricular septum. The ventricular septum can be divided into several portions:

- The canal (a.k.a. inlet) septum
- The membranous septum
- The conal (a.k.a. infundibular) septum
- The muscular septum

There are several corresponding types of VSDs, which have different natural histories and associated problems:

- Inlet VSD: part of an AV canal defect (see Atrial Septal Defect); 5% to 7% of all VSDs.
- Conoventricular (a.k.a. perimembranous) VSDs; 80% of all VSDs.
- Conal septal malalignment VSD: abnormal alignment of this portion of the septum usually results in obstruction of the right ventricular outflow tract (anterior malalignment, e.g., tetralogy of Fallot) or left ventricular outflow tract (posterior malalignment). Always large and unrestrictive.
- Conal septal hypoplasia VSD
- Muscular VSD: can be single or multiple and of variable size in any given patient; 5% to 20% of all VSDs.

There also may be multiple VSDs of different types in a single patient.

PATHOPHYSIOLOGY

Direction of shunting (left to right or right to left) depends on the relative pulmonary (PVR) and systemic vascular resistances (SVR). Determinants of the amount of shunting depend on the size of the defect.

- Small VSD: defect imposes high resistance to flow. There is a large left ventricular (LV) to right ventricular (RV) pressure gradient and a small left to right shunt, directly related to the size of the defect. The work load of the ventricles is normal.
- Moderate sized VSD: defect imposes some resistance to flow, but the amount of shunting can still be large and is affected by the relative PVR and SVR. The RV pressure is normal or only mildly increased.
- Large (unrestrictive) VSD: generally the same size as or larger than the aortic orifice. The RV and LV pressures are equal and the amount of shunting is purely determined by the PVR and SVR. The lower the PVR, the greater the degree of left-to-right shunting.

A large left-to-right shunt leads to increased pulmonary blood flow, left atrial and left ventricular dilation, tachypnea, and congestive heart failure (CHF). Typical onset of CHF is at 2 to 8 weeks of age with postnatal fall of PVR.

When a large VSD is left untreated, pulmonary vascular disease (irreversible increase in PVR) may develop, leading to reversal of the shunt, cyanosis, and right ventricular failure (Eisenmenger syndrome).

GENETICS

Three percent of children with VSDs have a parent with a VSD. VSD is the most common lesion in trisomy 21, 13, and 18, but >95% of children with VSDs have normal chromosomes. Conal septal malalignment VSDs are associated with 22q11 deletions.

EPIDEMIOLOGY

VSD is the most common form of congenital heart disease, occurring in approximately 1.5 to 5.7 per 1,000 live births and 4.5 to 7.0 per 1,000 preterm births; isolated VSD accounts for 20–50% of all congenital heart disease; 56% of patients are female.

COMPLICATIONS

- All VSDs

—endocarditis: overall rate of 15 cases per 10,000 person-years of follow-up

- Moderate to large VSDs

—Left ventricular volume overload, left atrial hypertension, CHF, poor growth, Eisenmenger syndrome

- Specific types

—Conoventricular VSDs: development of aortic insufficiency (AI), subaortic membrane, or double-chambered RV
—Conal septal hypoplasia VSDs: development of aortic insufficiency.

PROGNOSIS

- Spontaneous closure: 80% of small muscular VSDs and 8% to 35% of small conoventricular VSDs, usually by age 2 years
- Prognosis with surgical closure is excellent; see Therapy, below.
- The risk of Eisenmenger syndrome can be eliminated by surgical closure of large VSDs by age 2 years.

 Data Gathering

HISTORY

- Small VSD: The child is usually asymptomatic, with normal growth and development. Most commonly, a murmur is detected at 1 to 6 weeks of age.
- Moderate VSD: There is poor weight gain, with sparing of longitudinal growth. There may be an increased incidence of respiratory infections. Sweating and fatigue with feeding may be present.
- Large VSD: The symptoms are the same as above but may be more severe.
- Children with Eisenmenger syndrome may have cyanosis, fatigue and symptoms of right heart failure.

 Physical Examination

- Small VSD: The child appears healthy. A systolic thrill along the left sternal border may be palpable. Heart sounds are normal. A harsh, high-pitched, holosystolic or less than holosystolic murmur is best heard at the left lower sternal border.
- Moderate to large defect: Tachycardia and tachypnea are present. The precordial impulse is increased. The S_2 is wide, with slight respiratory variation. The P_2 component of S_2 may be normal or accentuated. A harsh, low-pitched holosystolic murmur is heard at the left lower sternal border. A diastolic rumble at the apex due to increased flow across the mitral valve is present if the shunt is $\geq$2:1. Hepatomegaly may be present.
- In children with elevated PVR, the S_2 is narrowly split or single and the P_2 component is loud. The murmur may decrease in duration and intensity or disappear.
- If AI develops, a high-pitched, early diastolic murmur may be heard along the left sternal border.
- In Eisenmenger syndrome, there is cyanosis, an increased RV impulse, a single or narrowly split S_2 with a loud P_2 component and a minimal or absent VSD murmur. There may be a harsh systolic murmur of TR, a high-pitched early diastolic murmur of pulmonary insufficiency, or an S_3. Jugular venous distention and hepatomegaly indicate high right-sided filling pressures.

Laboratory Aids

TESTS

Electrocardiogram

- Small defect: normal
- Moderate defect: LVH
- Large defect: biventricular hypertrophy and left atrial enlargement
- Eisenmenger syndrome: RVH

Chest X-Ray

- Small defect: normal
- Moderate-large defect: hyperinflation, cardiomegaly, increased pulmonary vascular markings
- Eisenmenger syndrome: normal heart size with prominent central pulmonary arteries and decreased peripheral vascular markings

Echocardiography

- All children with a VSD-type murmur should undergo echocardiographic evaluation to define the location, size, and number of VSDs and any associated defects. Color Doppler enables visualizing the shunt direction.

Cardiac Catheterization

- Generally reserved for children with poorly defined anatomy, associated lesions, or pulmonary hypertension with unknown reactivity.

 ## Therapy

- Small defect: no intervention; observation and SBE prophylaxis for indicated procedures.
- Moderate-to-large defects: If signs of congestive heart failure develop, digoxin, diuretics, increased caloric intake, and close follow-up are indicated.
- Perimembranous and muscular defects may become smaller or close spontaneously. An early surgical repair should be undertaken during infancy if there is evidence of intractable heart failure, FTT, or pulmonary hypertension. Otherwise, the patient can be followed conservatively.
- Conoseptal hypoplasia and malalignment defects do not close spontaneously; surgical closure is indicated in infancy.
- After 1 year of life, a significant left-to-right shunt (Qp/Qs $\geq$2:1) is an indication for surgery.
- Children with controlled congestive heart failure but who have elevated pulmonary artery pressures (at least half-systemic) should undergo repair before the age of 2 years.
- Development of complications including AI, subaortic membrane, and double-chambered RV are indications for surgical repair.
- Surgical correction may be contraindicated if the PVR is greater than 8 Wood's units/m^2.
- The mortality of surgical repair is less than 5%.
- Complete heart block occurs in less than 2% of patients.

 ## Follow-Up

A significant residual VSD may need early reoperation.

 ## Common Questions and Answers

Q: Should children with a VSD-type murmur undergo echocardiographic evaluation to define the location, size, and number of VSDs?
A: Yes.

Q: Should children with VSD have SBE prophylaxis?
A: Yes.

Q: Should asymptomatic children with VSD have restricted activity?
A: No, if there are no other problems.

ICD-9-CM 745.4

BIBLIOGRAPHY

Gumbiner CH, Takao A. Ventricular septal defect. In: Garson A, et al., eds. *The science and practice of pediatric cardiology*, 2nd ed. Baltimore, Williams & Wilkins, 1998:1119–1140.

Kidd L, et al. Second natural history study of congenital heart defects: results of treatment of patients with ventricular septal defects. *Circulation* 1993;87(2 suppl I):I38–I51.

McDaniel NL, Gutgesell HP. Ventricular septal defects. In: Allen HD, et al., eds. *Moss and Adams' heart disease in infants, children and adolescents*, 6th ed. Philadelphia: Lippincott Williams & Wilkins, 2001:636–651.

Weinberg PM. Anatomy and classification of congenital heart disease. In: Kaiser LR, et al., eds. *Mastery of cardiothoracic surgery*. Philadelphia: Lippincott-Raven, 1998:589–602.

Author: Amy B. Hirshfeld
Song-Gui Yang, 2nd edition

Ventricular Tachycardia

 Database

DEFINITION

Ventricular tachycardia (VT) is a series of three or more repetitive beats originating from the ventricle at a rate faster than 120 bpm. It usually has a wide complex rhythm but can be narrow in infants. VT may, but not always, have atrioventricular dissociation.

- *Sustained ventricular tachycardia:* lasts longer than 30 seconds or causes hemodynamic compromise
- *Nonsustained ventricular tachycardia:* lasts from 3 beats to 30 seconds but without hemodynamic compromise
- May be monomorphic or polymorphic
- *Torsades de pointes:* associated with congenital long QT syndrome, acquired long QT, Brugada syndrome; the QRS complexes gradually change shape throughout the tachycardia.

ETIOLOGY

- Idiopathic
- Myocarditis
- Dilated cardiomyopathy
- Long QT syndrome (LQT)
- RV dysplasia
- Brugada syndrome
- Congenital heart disease (CHD) (e.g., tetralogy of Fallot, transposition of the great arteries, aortic stenosis, hypertrophic cardiomyopathy, mitral valve prolapse, Ebstein anomaly, and pulmonary vascular occlusive disease)
- Ventricular tumors
- Metabolic disturbances (hypoxia, acidosis, hypo/hyperkalemia)
- Drug ingestion (e.g., digitalis toxicity, antiarrhythmic agents)
- Myocardial ischemia (e.g., Kawasaki disease, congenital coronary problems)
- Trauma

PATHOPHYSIOLOGY

VT may result from a reentrant mechanism, triggered mechanism, or abnormal automaticity.

GENETICS

Long QT syndrome may be inherited as an autosomal-recessive or -dominant pattern. It is related to a variety of potential ion channel defects, and may be associated with hearing loss and/or a family history of sudden death. Brugada syndrome is related to a defect in the sodium channel and appears to be inherited as an autosomal-dominant pattern.

EPIDEMIOLOGY

VT may present at any age. Premature ventricular contractions (PVCs) have been reported in 0.8% to 2.2% of otherwise healthy children.

COMPLICATIONS

- Cardiovascular compromise (sudden death)
- Acquired cardiomyopathy (from long-standing VT and lack of AV synchrony)

PROGNOSIS

- Generally very good in patients with idiopathic VT and a structurally normal heart
- Suppression of ventricular ectopy with exercise has a favorable prognosis.
- In patients with heart disease (congenital or acquired) or the LQT syndrome, VT may increase the risk of presyncope, syncope, and possibly sudden death.

 Differential Diagnosis

- Supraventricular tachycardia with aberrancy
- Antidromic tachycardia (antegrade conduction down an accessory pathway, e.g., WPW)
- Atrial flutter or fibrillation with rapid conduction over an accessory pathway

 Data Gathering

HISTORY

- Mostly asymptomatic
- Palpitations
- Presyncope or syncope
- Exercise intolerance
- Dizziness
- Cardiac arrest

 Physical Examination

- Typically normal, occasional irregularity secondary to frequent PVCs
- Signs of underlying heart disease, if any are present

Laboratory Aids

TESTS

- ECG: three or more consecutive ventricular complexes faster than 120 bpm. The bundle branch morphology (right or left) may point to the origin of the VT. Similar morphology to isolated PVCs. May have AV dissociation. Typically, repolarization (T-wave) abnormalities are present. Always measure the QTc in lead II in sinus rhythm.
- ECHO: Rule out congenital heart disease, tumors, and assess ventricular function.
- Holter monitor: Quantitative assessment of ventricular ectopy, frequency of VT, and measurement of QTc interval.
- Exercise stress test (5 years and up): The characteristic response is that benign PVCs are suppressed with exercise and return in the immediate recovery period. Exacerbation or worsening of ventricular arrhythmias is very concerning.
- Cardiac catheterization: assessment of hemodynamics and possible coronary artery imaging
- Electrophysiologic study—Possible indications: (1) diagnosis of a wide complex rhythm; (2) suspected VT in the setting of an abnormal heart, syncope, or cardiac arrest; (3) nonsustained VT in patients with CHD; (4) determination of appropriate medical treatment in a patient with inducible VT; (5) syncope in the setting of palpitations (SVT versus VT); and (6) characterization of the VT and consideration for radiofrequency ablation. *Note:* Electrophysiologic studies are generally not helpful in individuals with LQT syndrome.

 ## Therapy

ACUTE

- If the patient is hemodynamically compromised, prompt synchronized direct-current (1–2 joules/kg; adult, 100–400 joules) is indicated.
- CPR as necessary
- Lidocaine (1 mg/kg bolus over 1 minute, followed by an infusion at 20–50 μg/kg/min, assuming normal kidney function)
- If *torsades de pointes*, $MgSO_4$ may be given.
- Overdrive ventricular pacing may terminate the tachycardia. However, pacing may accelerate the VT or induce ventricular fibrillation.
- Intravenous amiodarone (side effect: hypotension, responds to volume)

CHRONIC

- Medications

—Class IB (mexiletine and phenytoin): beta-blockers (propranolol, atenolol, nadolol) are used in LQT syndrome; may be effective in exercise-induced VT and postoperative congenital heart defects
—Class III (amiodarone and sotalol): avoid in patients with the LQT syndrome
—Class IC (flecainide): proarrhythmia and sudden death have been reported in patients with structural heart disease while on class IC agents.

- Atrial pacing at rates slightly faster than VT rates may suppress tachycardia
- Radiofrequency ablation
- Automatic implantable cardioverter defibrillators

 ## Follow-Up

- Depends on the underlying etiology
- ECG, ECHO, Holter, and exercise stress test

PITFALLS

Misdiagnosis of VT for SVT with aberrancy. Wide-complex tachycardia should always be considered to be ventricular tachycardia until proven otherwise.

 ## Common Questions and Answers

Q: Do frequent single PVCs require treatment?
A: In an otherwise healthy child with a structurally normal heart, normal QT interval, and suppressed PVCs with exercise, no treatment is indicated.

Q: Should siblings of patients with the LQT syndrome be evaluated?
A: Yes, siblings and parents (even if asymptomatic) should have an electrocardiogram, Holter monitor, and exercise stress test for definitive evaluation of the QT interval.

ICD-9-CM 427.1

BIBLIOGRAPHY

Carboni MP, Garson A Jr. Ventricular arrhythmias. In: Garson A Jr, Bricker JT, Fisher DJ, et al., eds. *The science and practice of pediatric cardiology*, 2nd ed. Philadelphia: Williams & Wilkins, 1998:2121–2168.

Garson A Jr, Smith RT, Moak JP, et al. Ventricular arrhythmias and sudden death in children. *J Am Coll Cardiol* 1985;5(6): 134B–137B.

Pfammatter JP, Paul T, et al. Idiopathic ventricular tachycardia in infancy and childhood. *J Am Coll Cardiol* 1999;33: 2067–2072.

Yabek SM. Ventricular arrhythmias in children with an apparently normal heart. *J Pediatr* 1991;119:1–11.

Author: Mitchell I. Cohen

Vesicoureteral Reflux

 Database

DEFINITION

Vesicoureteral reflux (VUR) occurs when urine passes backward from the bladder to the ureters or kidneys.

CAUSES

• A combination of abnormal anatomy and abnormal voiding pressure

—Primary VUR results from either a short ureteral tunnel through the bladder wall, or transient high pressure voiding, which occurs normally in the first 18 months of life.
—Patients with primary VUR can expect improvement and even resolution of the VUR with time as the ureteral tunnel grows or when bladder pressures decrease.

• Secondary VUR occurs when there is an associated lesion responsible for the abnormal anatomy or increased intravesical (bladder) pressure.

—Patients with secondary reflux require treatment of their primary problem, and still may require surgery to treat their secondary reflux. Causes of secondary reflux are dysfunctional voiding, neuropathic bladder due to spina bifida, ureteroceles, posterior ureteral valves, and prune belly syndrome.
—Although it may seem arbitrary, the distinction between primary and secondary reflux is important because the large prospective trials have been conducted on patients with primary reflux, and it is not appropriate to extend those findings to patients with secondary reflux.
—Another important distinction is whether the diagnosis of VUR was made as a result of a prenatal diagnosis of hydronephrosis, or whether the child presented with urinary tract infection.

PATHOLOGY

VUR in combination with urinary tract infection can lead to pyelonephritis, renal scarring, and possibly end-stage renal disease. Primary VUR is classified into five grades based on the voiding cystourethrogram (VCUG).

• Grade I: reflux into ureter
• Grade II: reflux into renal pelvis without dilation of calyces
• Grade III: blunting of calyces, mild dilation of ureter
• Grade IV: grossly dilated ureter, moderate calyceal dilation with maintained papillary impressions
• Grade V: grossly dilated ureter with loss of papillary impressions

The grading scale is important because spontaneous resolution rates are significantly different between grades I to III and grades IV to V.

GENETICS

30% of siblings will have low-grade reflux, but the great majority will have been asymptomatic, and renal scarring is rare. Parents with VUR have a 60% chance of having children with reflux. Whether or not to screen siblings is controversial. We elect to screen the patients with a history of recurrent febrile illnesses and girls who have not yet toilet trained.

EPIDEMIOLOGY

VUR occurs in about 1% of children. There are now clearly two different groups of patients:

—Those who were detected prenatally without any history of urinary tract infection (UTI).

• Approximately 30–50% of patients with prenatal hydronephrosis have VUR.
• The ratio of males to females in this group is 3:1. This is believed to be caused by a period of high-pressure voiding in boys, which resolves by 18 months.

—Those who were detected after an acute UTI.

• About 30–50% of children with UTI will have reflux, and they tend to be 2- to 3-year-old girls.
• Since most children achieve urinary continence by this point, the cause of the UTI tends to be infrequent voiding caused by overlearning the ability to tighten the pelvic floor.

PROGNOSIS

• In primary VUR, 80% of grades I and II reflux, 70% of grade III, 40% of grade IV, and 25% of grade V resolve over a 5-year period.
• The annual rate of spontaneous resolution is between 15% and 20% for grades I to III.
• Ultimately the goal is prevention of renal scarring, rather than resolution of the reflux, since low-pressure sterile reflux does not lead to renal scarring.
• Therefore, the patient's propensity toward UTI must be considered as well as whether the reflux is resolving.

 Differential Diagnosis

In the prenatally detected group, hydronephrosis can also be due to ureteropelvic junction obstruction. The important task is to differentiate primary from secondary VUR so that the parents can be appropriately counseled.

 Data Gathering

HISTORY

• Prenatal diagnosis or UTI
• Family or sibling history of VUR
• Family history of renal failure
• Voiding history: age at potty training
• Daytime or nighttime incontinence
• Frequency of urination
• Sensation of emptying the bladder completely
• Signs of dysfunctional voiding:

—Urgency
—Frequency
—Damp underwear
—Associated constipation

• Evidence of delaying urination:

—Squattino, crossing legs
—Compressing urethra

 Physical Examination

• Abdominal palpation (mainly to check for hard stool)
• Check for labial adhesions in girls
• Phimosis in boys
• Palpation of spine
• Blood pressure

Laboratory Aids

A serum creatinine may be obtained if the renal ultrasound suggests significant renal scarring.

IMAGING

• Renal/bladder ultrasound: This is usually obtained at the time of UTI, or if the patient had a prenatal diagnosis of hydronephrosis, at 1 week of life. The ultrasound is not as sensitive as DMSA scan for renal scarring. The lack of hydronephrosis does not mean that the patient does not have VUR. However, it is a useful tool for following renal growth.
• VCUG: A contrast study is necessary for the first VCUG, to delineate the urethral anatomy in boys, and to accurately grade the reflux in both sexes. Follow-up VCUGs can be performed using radionuclide to decrease the radiation dose to the child.
• DMSA renal scan: The most accurate way to diagnose pyelonephritis and renal scarring. Unfortunately, it is not possible to predict which patients will develop scarring after an acute episode. If the diagnosis of upper tract infection vs. cystitis is important, then the DMSA scan during an acute episode is useful.

Therapy

• Four prospective randomized controlled trials have concluded that medical management (prophylactic antibiotics) and surgery have essentially equal outcomes in regard to hypertension, growth, and renal scarring. Surgery was more effective at preventing pyelonephritis.
• The rate of renal scarring was equal in the medical and surgical arms of the International Reflux Study. However, the timing of renal scarring was different: in the medically treated arm, new renal scars continued to form during 5 years of follow-up, whereas in the surgical arm, the renal scars stopped within 10 months of surgery. Surgery was 95% successful in correcting reflux with a 4% complication rate. Surgery involves creation of a longer muscular backing for the ureter to create a flap-valve mechanism.
• Patients with low-grade reflux should be maintained on prophylactic antibiotics, since grades I to III have a significant rate of spontaneous resolution. Patients with high-grade reflux should be initially maintained on prophylactic antibiotics, but earlier consideration for surgical correction should be given due to the lower rate of spontaneous resolution. Likewise, patients with reflux and renal scarring should be considered for earlier surgery since they have already shown a propensity toward UTI and renal damage.

• Antibiotic prophylaxis does not mean treatment dose antibiotics. The antibiotics chosen are highly concentrated in the urine, and the use of high doses only selects out resistant organisms and leads to complications such as yeast infections. Amoxicillin at 12.5 mg/kg qd is used for the first 2 months of life, then trimethoprim/sulfamethoxazole (40 mg/200 mg per 5 mL) at 2.5 mL/kg qd (equivalent to 2–3 mg/kg qd of trimethoprim) or nitrofurantoin at 2 mg/kg qd.
• Patients being managed on antibiotic prophylaxis undergo annual follow-up VCUG to document improvement or resolution of VUR. A renal ultrasound is also obtained to follow renal growth and check for gross renal scars.
• Indications for crossing over to surgery are:

—Patient or parent wishes
—Noncompliance with medical therapy
—Breakthrough infections while on medical therapy. (This is more of a relative indication. A careful review of voiding habits should be carried out to ensure that dysfunctional voiding is not responsible for the UTI.)
—New renal scarring
—Persistence of reflux after an appropriate period of antibiotic prophylaxis

• The use of injectable bulking agents such as Teflon is popular in Europe. Due to concerns about particle migration, Teflon is not approved for this use in the United States. Many alternative substances have been tried, with at best 80% success rates 1 year after multiple treatments. The minimally invasive nature of these treatments is balanced with a lower success rate, and no clear favorite has yet emerged.
• The management of patients who continue to have VUR after several years of prophylactic antibiotics is controversial. While most feel comfortable taking boys with VUR off antibiotics after age 6 because the risk of renal scarring is decreased and boys are at low risk for UTI, the adolescent girl is at increased risk for complications during pregnancy if she has UTI. The few studies on this subject seem to indicate that the patients with VUR and recurrent UTI are at risk for pregnancy-related complications whether or not the VUR has been surgically corrected, suggesting that the propensity toward UTI plays a more important factor.

Follow-Up

Patients with renal scarring should have annual blood pressure checks and urinalysis for proteinuria.
More detailed recommendations can be found in the article by Elder et al. (see Bibliography).

Common Questions and Answers

Q: What is the significance of reflux seen after a UTI?
A: UTI in the presence of reflux can cause pyelonephritis and renal scarring.

Q: Why not operate to repair the reflux when it is diagnosed.
A: Depending on the grade of reflux, many cases will resolve in time. See Therapy, above.

ICD-9-CM 593.7

BIBLIOGRAPHY

Atala A, Keating MA. Vesicoureteral reflux and megaureter. In: Walsh PC, Retik AB, Vaughn ED, et al., eds. *Campbell's urology*, 7th ed. Philadelphia: WB Saunders, 1998.

Elder JS, Peters CA, Arant BS, et al. Pediatric vesicoureteral reflux guidelines panel summary report on the management of primary vesicoureteral reflux in children. *J Urol* 1997;157:1846–1851.

Shortliffe LMD. Urinary tract infections in infants and children. In: Walsh PC, Retik AB, Vaughn ED, et al., eds. *Campbell's urology*, 7th ed. Philadelphia: WB Saunders, 1998.

Walker RD. Vesicoureteral reflux and urinary tract infection in children. In: Gillenwater JY, Grayhack JT, Howards SS, et al., eds. *Adult and pediatric urology*, 3rd ed. St. Louis: Mosby, 1996.

Yeung CK, Godley ML, Dhillon HK, et al. The characteristics of primary vesico-ureteric reflux in male and female infants with pre-natal hydronephrosis. *Br J Urol* 1997; 80:319–327.

Authors: Hsi-Yang Wu and Howard M. Snyder

Viral Hepatitis

 Database

DEFINITION

Viral hepatitis is inflammation of the liver caused by hepatotropic viruses, which include hepatitis A to E, as well as other hepatotropic viruses, such as EBV, CMV, HSV, VZV, enterovirus, rubella, Coxsackie B, adenovirus, parvovirus, and many others. In the United States, hepatitis B accounts for 40% of viral hepatitis cases, hepatitis A for 30%, and hepatitis C for 20%.

TYPES OF HEPATITIS

Hepatitis A
- Transmitted by the oral-fecal route
- Characterized by enteric symptoms associated with right upper quadrant pain, jaundice, diarrhea, pale stools, anorexia, nausea, hepatomegaly, and splenomegaly
- Incubation period is about 15 to 40 days, and transaminases rise about 1 week after onset of symptoms; recovery is seen in over 95% of patients within 1 to 2 weeks.
- Jaundice is seen in 88% of adults, but is present in only 65% of children with hepatitis A.

Hepatitis B
- Transmitted by body fluids
- Incubation period of 50 to 180 days and has three phases: prodrome, icteric, and convalescence. The prodrome precedes jaundice by 2 to 3 weeks, with vague symptoms of rash and arthralgia resembling serum sickness.
- Jaundice is seen less frequently in children compared with adults, and it may be accompanied by symptoms of fever, fatigue, myalgia, abdominal pain, and pruritus.
- Circulating immune complexes occasionally result in extrahepatic manifestations, which include vasculitis, nephropathy, and acrodermatitis.
- Icteric phase lasts about 4 to 6 weeks, and this is followed by clearance of circulating antigens during the convalescence phase.
- The younger the age of the child with the infection, the higher the likelihood of developing chronic infection. Ninety-five percent of infected neonates, 20% of children, and 10% of adults become carriers after an acute infection.
- Only 5% to 10% lose their carrier status spontaneously.

Hepatitis C
- Causes hepatitis and accounts for a significant number of what was previously called non-A, non-B hepatitis
- Transmitted by blood and sexual contact
- Clinical disease is insidious, with a long latency period before levels of ALT start to rise.
- Only about 25% of infected patients have an acute illness that is indistinguishable from other forms of hepatitis.

- May take up to 12 months after exposure for serology to become positive. Detection is by serology or by detection of viral RNA by RT-PCR. Rarely causes fulminant liver failure.
- After an infection, about 80% will develop viral persistence.
- After chronic hepatitis C virus (HCV) infection, liver functions may remain relatively normal for as long as 50 years. At present, one cannot predict which patients will develop end-stage liver failure after infection.
- The virus undergoes frequent mutations, which may account for the viral persistence.

Hepatitis D
- A viral parasite of the hepatitis B virus. It consists of an HDV antigen and HDV ribonucleic acid surrounded by the hepatitis B viral coat.
- Transmitted by blood or sexual activity
- Causes two types of acute hepatitis:
—Co-infection: Acute hepatitis B and D virus infection occurs simultaneously.
—Co-infection has a mortality rate of 1% to 10%.
—Chronicity in co-infection is less than 5%.
—Superinfection: Acute hepatitis D occurs in a chronic carrier of hepatitis B.
—Superinfection has a mortality rate of 5% to 20%. Fulminant liver failure occurs more frequently in superinfection.
—Chronicity is 75% in superinfection. Chronic HDV causes cirrhosis in 70% to 80% of patients and is a rapidly progressive disease compared with chronic hepatitis B alone.

Hepatitis E
- Causes epidemic hepatitis in areas where water sanitation is poor
- Transmitted via the oral-fecal route
- Resembles hepatitis A clinically
- Incubation period of 6 weeks and affects young adults mainly
- Higher mortality of 20%, which is higher than hepatitis A, and causes fulminant liver failure in pregnant women. It does not cause chronic hepatitis.

PATHOLOGY

Acute viral hepatitis tends to affect the liver parenchyma, while chronic viral hepatitis affects portal and periportal areas. Acuteness is defined by an injury period of less than 6 months in duration. In acute hepatitis, there is spotty necrosis, panlobular disarray, increased cellularity, pleomorphism of hepatocytes, and focal parenchymal necrosis. There are multinucleated hepatocytes, indicating liver regeneration, and this leads to hepatocytes of variable sizes, staining, and shapes. Inflammatory cells line the sinusoids. Chronic viral hepatitis is continuing inflammation of the liver for more than 6 months. Chronic inflammation affects the portal tracts predominantly but also extends into the parenchyma. Early on, there is periportal expansion and fibrosis initially bounded by the limiting plate. Later, it extends beyond the limiting plate into the

parenchyma (piecemeal necrosis). Portal bridging is the finding of extensive fibrosis that occurs between two portal tracts. When the injury is chronic and severe, attempts by the liver to regenerate lead to nodular changes and, finally, to cirrhosis.

 Differential Diagnosis

There are many disorders that give rise to elevated transaminases, and there are clues to a viral origin based on the history, serology, and histologic findings. One often invokes the diagnosis of non-A, non-B, non-C hepatitis when the cause is almost certainly viral but no virus is isolated.

 Data Gathering

HISTORY
- In hepatitis transmitted by blood or sexual means, the following risk factors apply:
—Positive family history of hepatitis (hepatitis B, C)
—Immigrants or travelers from endemic areas (E)
—Institution residents such as day care (hepatitis A), prisons (B, C)
—IV drug abusers (B, C, D)
—People with multiple sexual partners (B, C, D)
—Health care workers (B, C)
—Patients requiring multiple blood transfusions or hemodialysis (B, C)
—Dietary intake in some countries (e.g., shellfish) (A)
- Many are thought to have hepatitis A because they often present with symptoms of gastroenteritis.
- Persistence of elevated transaminases and symptoms that resemble chronic fatigue syndrome lead to repeat labs with serologic testing for viral hepatitis.
- There may be hepatomegaly and splenomegaly with or without jaundice.
- Cholestasis is sometimes seen with tea-colored urine and pale stools.
- Other common symptoms are myalgia, abdominal pain, anorexia, fever, and pale stools.

 Laboratory Aids

TESTS
- Routine liver function tests
- Prothrombin time
- Albumin
- Anti-HAV IgM: recent infection
- Anti-HAV IgG: past exposure
- HBsAg: current infection, either acute or chronic
- HBsAb IgM/IgG: resolution of disease
- HBeAg: significant infectivity, viral replication

- HBeAb: end of severe infectivity (except in precore mutants when HBV DNA is positive)
- HBcore IgM: early phase of acute infection, not present in chronic hepatitis B
- HBcore Ag: only found in liver, not serum
- HBV DNA: quantification useful to assess viral load
- HBV DNA: qualitative is to screen for presence or absence of viral DNA
- HDV Ag: active infection
- HDV Ab: exposure to hepatitis D
- HDV RNA: active replication
- HCV Ab: exposure
- HCV RNA: active replication
- Liver biopsy is useful in assessing the degree of liver damage and also to assess response to therapy. It is not indicated for diagnosis of acute viral hepatitis, although it is sometimes done inadvertently.

Hepatitis B and D

- Acute infection: HBsAg+, HBcore IgM+, HBV DNA+, HBe Ag+
- Chronic infection high risk: HBsAg+, HBe Ag+, HBsAb−, HBV DNA+
- Chronic infection low risk: HBsAg+, HBeAg−, HBeAb+, HBV DNA−
- Chronic active hepatitis: positive serology plus elevated transaminases plus hepatitis on liver biopsy (after 6 months of presenting with symptoms)
- HDV coinfection: HBcIgM+, HDV Ag+, HDV IgM−/−, HDV IgA−
- HDV superinfection: HBcIgM− HDV Ag+, HDV IgM+, HDV IgA+
- Chronic HDV: HBcIgM−, HDV Ag−, HDV IgM+, HDV IgA+

Therapy

HEPATITIS A

- No specific therapy is available; patients should avoid going back to the nursery or day-care center for 2 weeks after illness.
- Postexposure prophylaxis with pooled human serum globulin at dose of 0.02 mL/kg for household contacts, intimate exposure contacts, and children and staff in nursery or day-care centers with outbreaks. Preexposure (short-term, 0.02 mL/kg; long-term, 0.06 mL/kg every 4–6 months) to travelers to endemic areas.
- Havrix Junior (GSK) vaccine is given by IM injection. Ages 1 to 15 years: two doses of 0.5 mL; the second is given 2 to 4 weeks after the first dose; booster dose 0.5 mL, 6 to 12 months following the initial dose.
- It is sensible for children with liver disease to be vaccinated to prevent its exacerbation.

HEPATITIS B

Postexposure prophylaxis with HBIG is indicated for neonates born to mothers who are hepatitis B carriers, after sexual contact with carriers, and after accidental exposure to infected blood products.

DRUGS

Interferon-α

- The current recommendation to eradicate hepatitis B is by interferon. Predictive factors for response are high serum ALT prior to therapy, low serum HBV DNA, nonvertically acquired hepatitis B, active hepatitis on liver biopsy, female sex, HIV−, and HDV−. The success rate based on adult studies is 33% for the loss of HBeAg. In patients with cirrhosis, the use of interferon is more risky because it can cause the liver disease to become decompensated, and should only be done in centers with good access to liver transplantation.
- Interferon treatment for hepatitis C in children is not established. It is licensed for use, in adults, however, with response—in the region of 41% improvement in ALT; 70% of patients show improved histology, but with a 50% to 70% relapse rate. Interferon with ribavirin (Rebetron) is approved for use in adults but not in children.
- Interferon-α (dose from published pediatric trials)
—Chronic HBV: 5 to 10 MU/m^2 given three times a week for 6 to 12 months
—Chronic HCV: 3 MU/m^2 given three times a week for 6 to 12 months
—Interferon is not licensed for use in children, and it has hematologic, infectious, autoimmune, neuropsychiatric, and systemic side effects, with myelosuppression the most common dose-dependent side effect.

Other Drugs

- Lamivudine
—There may be a role for lamivudine in the treatment of chronic hepatitis B. This is an oral nucleoside analogue that inhibits viral DNA replication. It has been shown to markedly reduce HBV DNA levels in 98% of patients during therapy, but, in general, the patients return to pretreatment status after the drug is discontinued. Lamivudine dosage (trial basis) is 25 to 100 mg/d for 1 year in an adult.
- Famciclovir, adefovir, and thymosin are currently undergoing studies for efficacy and safety in the treatment of HBV.

CURIOSITIES

Hepatitis G was discovered a few years ago, and although so named, has not been found or proven to cause hepatitis.

Common Questions and Answers

Q: Why do patients infected at birth with HBV have a higher incidence of chronicity?
A: This is probably a dose effect, with the infecting dose being higher in vertical transmission than in other forms of transmission. In addition, early infection increases the time for the virus to integrate into the host genome.

Q: What is the current definition of non-A, non-B (NANB) hepatitis?
A: NANB hepatitis should now be termed non-A to non-E, with all the testing available in modern hospitals. In the past, this probably included patients who are now known to have HCV.

Q: What is the best way of eradicating hepatitis B?
A: Universal vaccination in childhood has been recommended by the U.S. Public Health Service for eradication of HBV. Vaccination is actively pursued in some Asian countries, where the disease affects about a third of the population. However, some babies born to HBsAg+ mothers develop escape mutants of hepatitis B virus.

Q: Should mothers with HCV positivity breast-feed?
A: Based on the fact that viral RNA levels are very low in breast milk, it is felt that transmission of HCV via breast milk is very unlikely.

ICD-9-CM
Hepatitis A 070.1
B 070.30
C 070.51
D 070.52
E 070.53

BIBLIOGRAPHY
Balistreri W. Acute and chronic viral hepatitis. In: Suchy FJ, ed. *Liver disease in children*. St. Louis: Mosby 1994:460–509.

Chien RN, Leung NW, et al. One year trial of lamivudine for chronic hepatitis B. *N Engl J Med* 1998;339:61–68.

Desmet MA, Gerber M, Hoofnagle JH, et al. Classification of chronic hepatitis: diagnosis, grading and staging. *Hepatology* 1994;19: 1513–1520.

Koff RS. Hepatitis vaccines. *Infect Dis Clin North Am* 2001;15(1):83–95.

Niederau CN, Heingest T, Lange S, et al. Long term follow up of HBeAg-positive patients treated with interferon alpha for chronic hepatitis B. *N Engl J Med* 1996;334: 1422–1427.

O'Connor JA. Acute and chronic viral hepatitis. *Adolesc Med* 2000;11(2):279–292.

Popper H, Schaffner F. The vocabulary of chronic hepatitis. *N Engl J Med* 1997;284:1154–1156.

Author: John Tung

Volvulus

 ## Database

DEFINITION

Volvulus is torsion of the gut upon itself or upon a narrow mesenteric pedicle. It may be acute and complete or chronic and intermittent.

CAUSES

Malrotation results in a narrow mesenteric stalk for the midgut loop and obstructing bands (Ladd bands) across the duodenum, predisposing to volvulus.

EPIDEMIOLOGY

- Malrotation with midgut volvulus is most common in neonates.
- Fifty percent to 80% of patients with abnormal rotation will be symptomatic in infancy.

COMPLICATIONS

- Intermittent or acute obstruction
- Strangulation resulting in ischemia and loss of midgut
- Protein-losing enteropathy can also result from strangulation.

 ## Differential Diagnosis

- Perforated viscus
- Necrotizing enterocolitis
- Meconium ileus
- Hirschsprung enterocolitis
- Appendicitis
- Intussusception
- Pyelonephritis

 ## Data Gathering

HISTORY

- Symptoms of acute or recurrent obstruction at birth or in the first year of life
- Recurrent bilious emesis with acute abdomen
- Feeding intolerance
- Chylous ascites and/or protein-losing enteropathy due to lymphatic congestion
- In older children, recurrent abdominal pain and emesis

 ## Physical Examination

- Abdominal tenderness and distention
- Irritability, lethargy
- Brawny edema of abdominal wall
- Bloody stools
- Drawing up of legs
- Tachypnea and tachycardia

 ## Laboratory Aids

TESTS

- May see metabolic acidosis, thrombocytopenia

IMAGING

- Abdominal x-ray may show dilated stomach and duodenum.
- Upper gastrointestinal tract radiography may show abnormal position of the ligament of Treitz and a "corkscrew" appearance of the midgut.
- The radiographic appearance, though, may be confusing because there are at least seven patterns of duodenal malrotation reported.
- In the absence of a corkscrew or Z-shaped duodenum, patterns that usually indicate volvulus or obstructing Ladd bands, colon position had greater prognostic implication, especially when the cecum is positioned in the RUQ or LUQ.
- In report by Long et al. (1996), these latter patterns were associated with the highest prevalence of volvulus.
- Barium enema shows an abnormal position of the cecum.

Therapy

- Close monitoring of fluids and electrolytes to prevent shock
- Laparotomy with resection of ischemic portions of the intestine
- Ladd procedure: volvulus is untwisted, transduodenal bands are divided, mesenteric base is broadened, and appendix is removed.
- If the entire midgut is ischemic, the volvulus may be untwisted, with reexploration in 12 to 24 hours.

 ## Follow-Up

- Prognosis depends on extent of involvement and degree of ischemia.
- Monitor closely for feeding intolerance postoperatively.

PITFALLS

- May take hours to days to become symptomatic
- Symptoms may be mistaken for colic in infants or cyclic emesis in older children.
- Delayed diagnosis may result in strangulation and infarction, leading to short-gut syndrome.

 ## Common Questions and Answers

Q: In what age group is volvulus most common?
A: Midgut volvulus is most common in the neonatal period.

Q: How can the signs and symptoms of volvulus be distinguished from gastroesophageal reflux?
A: Although both intermittent volvulus and gastroesophageal reflux (GER) may present with vomiting, the emesis in GER is not bilious. Bilious emesis, abdominal pain, and lethargy are signs of an abdominal obstruction, requiring further examination.

Q: Should one think of intermittent volvulus in the differential diagnosis of children with presentation of protein-losing enteropathy?
A: In children with unusual presentations of protein-losing enteropathy, especially with emesis as a contributing feature, exclude intermittent volvulus.

ICD-9-CM 560.9

BIBLIOGRAPHY

Gebara S, Firor HU. Congenital anomalies of the midgut. In: Wyllie R, Hyams JS, eds. *Pediatric gastrointestinal disease.* Philadelphia: WB Saunders, 1993:495–596.

Hatch EI, Sawin R. The acute abdomen. In: Wyllie R, Hyams JS, eds. *Pediatric gastrointestinal disease.* Philadelphia: WB Saunders, 1993:210–212.

Ismail A. Recurrent colonic volvulus in children. *J Pediatr Surg* 1997;32(12): 1739–1742.

Jabra AA, Eng J, Zaleski CG, et al. CT of small-bowel obstruction in children: sensitivity and specificity. *AJR* 2001; 177(2):431–436.

Kealey WD, McCallion WA, Brown S, et al. Midgut volvulus in children. *Br J Surg* 1996;83(1):105–106.

Long FR, Kramer SS, Markowitz RI, et al. Radiographic patterns of intestinal malrotation in children. *Radiographics* 1996;16(3):547–556.

Stewart DR, Colodneg AL, Daggert WC. Malrotation of the bowel infants and children: a 15 year review. *Surgery* 1976;79:716–720.

Author: Andrew E. Mulberg

Von Willebrand Disease

Database

DEFINITION

Von Willebrand disease (vWD) is a bleeding disorder in which there is a deficiency or abnormality of von Willebrand factor (vWF), which facilitates the adherence of platelets to sites of endothelial injury.

PATHOPHYSIOLOGY

- vWF is a large multimeric protein that binds to collagen at sites of endothelial injury, recruiting platelets by binding to a specific receptor on the platelet membrane (GPIb), thus initiating primary hemostasis.
- vWF also serves to stabilize coagulation factor VIII in circulation.
- When this protein is either deficient or defective, platelet "plugging" is compromised, resulting in a bleeding diathesis characterized by easy bruising, frequent epistaxis, menorrhagia, and prolonged bleeding following lacerations or abrasions.
- Type 1 vWD is due to decreased production of vWF and results in a mild bleeding diathesis.
- Type 2 vWD is the result of abnormal production of vWF.
- Type 3 vWD is due to virtually no production of vWF and therefore is associated with a severe bleeding diathesis.
- vWD is an inherited bleeding disorder; however, acquired forms of vWD have been described in association with hypothyroidism, Wilms tumor, congenital heart disease, EBV infection, and valproate therapy.

GENETICS

- The gene for vWF is found on chromosome 12.
- Type 1 follows an autosomal-dominant inheritance pattern.
- Type 2 varies, but in general follows an autosomal-dominant inheritance pattern. Compound heterozygous patients have been described.
- Type 3 follows an autosomal-recessive inheritance pattern.

EPIDEMIOLOGY

The prevalence of vWD in the general pediatric population is estimated to be about 1%. Children of all races can be affected.

COMPLICATIONS

- Significant perioperative bleeding can occur, especially with tonsillectomy, but the most common complications are recurrent epistaxis, prolonged bleeding with cuts and abrasions, and menorrhagia.
- Patients with type 3 vWD have a more severe bleeding disorder and can have bleeding complications similar to those seen in hemophilia such as hemarthroses and intracranial hemorrhage.

PROGNOSIS

- Except for rare cases of acquired vWF deficiency, vWD is inherited and therefore is lifelong.
- Most patients with vWD have a normal life expectancy and, with proper education and treatment, minimal risk for permanent disability.
- Type 3 vWD is a severe bleeding disorder; as a result life-threatening hemorrhage can occur. Types 1 and 2 tend to be mild and can even go undetected.

Differential Diagnosis

- Primary hemostatic disorders

—Platelet function abnormalities, congenital thrombocytopenia
—Mild coagulation factor deficiencies
—Hemophilia (type 3 vWD and type 2N are similar to mild and moderate factor VIII deficiency)

- Acquired and secondary hemostatic disorders

—Mild coagulopathies, resulting in bleeding or a prolongation of the PTT or bleeding time
—Uremia
—Acquired thrombocytopenia
—Drugs that affect platelet function

- Connective tissue disorders

—Ehlers-Danlos syndrome
—Osteogenesis imperfecta
—Scurvy

Data Gathering

HISTORY

- A family history of vWD or bleeding tendency is an important part of the evaluation for vWD. However, be aware that variation in frequency and severity of bleeding symptoms can occur from person to person, even within an affected family.
- Mucosal bleeding is especially common in vWD.
- Gum bleeding is common, usually the result of minor trauma associated with routine dental care.
- Bruising is common with increased number, and quite frequently, increased size (>5 cm), and often palpable rather than flat.
- Recurrent and/or prolonged epistaxis
- Menorrhagia occurs in 50% to 75% of women with vWD.
- Excessive posttraumatic or postsurgical bleeding
- In some patients with vWD, there may be no significant history of bleeding problems.

Physical Examination

- Bruises: increased number, size, and/or unusual location
- May be entirely normal

Laboratory Aids

TESTS

- PTT is elevated in 25% of patients.
- Bleeding time is prolonged in 50% of patients.
- Factor VIII activity is the least sensitive of the usual screening coagulation tests.
- Ristocetin cofactor activity is the most helpful single test for vWD.
- An ELISA-based functional vWF assay can be used in place of the ristocetin cofactor assay.
- Factor VIII antigen (vWF)
- vWF multimeric analysis helps determine specific type:

—Type 1 (65–80%): all multimers of vWF present but decreased; most common and mildest form of the disease
—Type 2A (10–12%): absence of high-molecular-weight multimers (not uncommon for ristocetin cofactor activity to be proportionally lower than vWF antigen)
—Type 2B (3–5%): decrease of the highest, high-molecular-weight multimers with increased low-dose, ristocetin-induced platelet aggregation
—Type 2N (1–2%): normal multimeric analysis, factor VIII activity low due to decreased binding to vWF
—Type 2M (1–2%): usually has normal multimeric analysis; the factor is dysfunctional due to a point mutation (not uncommon for ristocetin cofactor activity to be proportionally lower than vWF antigen).
—Type 3 (1–3%): undetectable multimers of vWF; most severe form
—Platelet type (0–1%): like type 2B

- CBC to rule out thrombocytopenia and anemia. Iron deficiency is common, and platelets can be slightly low in type 2B.
- PT to look for other coagulation abnormalities (PT is normal in vWD)

PITFALLS

- Unfortunately, false-negative laboratory evaluations for vWD do occur. Thus, a normal laboratory evaluation does not necessarily indicate the absence of disease. The laboratory tests may need to be repeated several times before declaring a patient does not have vWD. vWF is an acute-phase reactant, and tests for vWD should be done when the patient is well.

- Normal ranges for vWF are blood type specific, with levels being lower in those with blood type O.
- Steroids, oral contraceptives, and other estrogens can increase vWF levels.
- Other conditions that alter vWF levels:

—Increased levels can be associated with the newborn period, collagen vascular disorders, postsurgical states, liver disease, hyperthyroidism, high-stress states, pregnancy, and inflammatory or infectious disease.
—Decreased levels: hypothyroidism, valproate therapy
—Change in the multimeric pattern of vWF: DIC, TTP, HUS, and VSDs

REQUIREMENTS

- No aspirin within at least 7 days of the bleeding time
- Avoidance of any of the many agents (antihistamines, Ca^{2+} channel blockers, furosemide, NSAIDs) that affect platelet function 24 hours prior to the bleeding time
- Avoid cigarette smoking and heavy exercise prior to testing for vWD.

 Therapy

IMMEDIATE

- Supportive measures are often enough to stop the bleeding (e.g., compression, etc.)
- Severe bleeding in a postsurgical or posttraumatic condition may require infusion with a factor concentrate containing vWF, such as Humate-P. Severity of bleeding will be a function of the type of vWD present.

DRUGS

Knowledge of the type of vWD is required for the proper treatment of the disease.

- DDAVP (desmopressin acetate)

—Most patients with type 1 vWD will respond to DDAVP; however, a few may not; therefore, a trial of DDAVP is recommended after the age of 1 year for most patients.
—May be administered by intravenous, subcutaneous, or intranasal routes
—The dose is 0.3 to 0.4 μg/kg SC or IV (diluted in normal saline and given over 20 to 30 minutes).
—May be ineffective in type 2A and type 3 disease
—May worsen thrombocytopenia in type 2B and platelet-type vWD
—Tachyphylaxis (failure to respond after repeated doses) can occur.

- Blood products

—Cryoprecipitate: The development of a solvent detergent-treated cryoprecipitate may reduce the risk of virus transmission. May be an appropriate product for families that wish

to have a directed donor (vWF levels in the donor can be increased by administering DDAVP prior to collection).
—Humate-P and Alphanate: plasma derived, intermediate purity factor VIII concentrate products with adequate levels (especially large multimers) of vWF
—The dose of Humate-P is 40 to 60 U/kg IV every 12 to 24 hours.

- Aminocaproic acid (Amicar): helpful for mucosal bleeding and following tooth extraction to prevent bleeding. May also be helpful with menorrhagia. The dose is 100 mg/kg given PO every 6 hours.

PREVENTION

- Avoid heavy-contact sports (football, etc.); otherwise, assume normal activity for age. Type 3 patients and some type 2 patients need to be more cautious about level of activity.
- For patients with recurrent epistaxis, measures should be taken to avoid drying of the mucosa by applying petroleum jelly and to reduce trauma to the nasal mucosa by keeping the fingernails short and discouraging nose picking.
- It may be advisable for patients to wear an emergency ID bracelet indicating that they have vWD in the event they are involved in an accident that renders them unconscious.

 Follow-Up

WHEN TO EXPECT IMPROVEMENT

Except for rare cases of acquired vWD, there is a lifelong risk of bleeding.

SIGNS TO WATCH FOR

- Pattern of bleeding
- Hepatitis, if exposed to blood products
- Some patients will become iron-deficient from chronic blood loss.
- Inhibitors are extremely rare in vWD, with type 3 patients at highest risk.

 Common Questions and Answers

Q: How can a child have a bleeding disorder if he or she went through surgery without a problem?
A: In vWD, the vWF level can change as a function of stresses in the body. Many conditions will cause the vWF level to rise to a normal level. These conditions include infectious illnesses and pregnancy, as well as emotional stress. In surgery, the reason for the surgery itself (e.g., appendicitis, etc.) may cause enough stress to raise the factor levels to normal and prevent bleeding.

Q: Should the other family members be tested?
A: Yes, even if there is no history of bleeding in family members. Other affected family members may be unaware that they have the disease because vWD can be so mild.

Q: What sports activities can a person with vWD participate in safely?
A: People with type 1 vWD can participate in most activities, although it is usually advised to avoid situations in which significant trauma takes place, such as football, boxing, sky diving, and so forth. Patients with type 3 should try to avoid activities with even moderate trauma. For type 2 patients, the risk of bleeding varies.

Q: Is life expectancy lower in people with vWD?
A: For the majority of patients with vWD, their life expectancy and quality of life will be normal.

ICD-9-CM 286.4

BIBLIOGRAPHY

Blomback M, Eneroth P, Andersson OM, et al. On laboratory problems in diagnosing mild von Willebrand's disease. *Am J Hematol* 1992;40:117–120.

Lethagen S, Harris AS, Nilsson IM. Intranasal desmopressin (DDAVP) by spray in mild hemophilia Q and von Willebrand's disease type I. *Blut* 1990;60:187–191.

Mannucci PM. Desmopressin (ddavp) in the treatment of bleeding disorders: the first 20 years. *Blood* 1997;90:2515–2521.

Montgomery RR, Gill JC, Scott JP. Hemophilia and von Willebrand disease. In: Nathan DG, Orkin SH, eds. *Hematology of infancy and childhood*, 5th ed. Philadelphia: WB Saunders, 1993:1644–1659.

Sadler JE. A revised classification of von Willebrand disease. *Thromb Haemost* 1994; 71:520–525.

Werner EJ. von Willebrand disease in children and adolescents. *Pediatr Clin North Am* 1996;43(3):683–707.

Werner EJ, Abshire TC Giroux DS, et al. Relative value of diagnostic studies for von Willebrand's disease. *J Pediatr* 1992;121: 34–38.

Author: J. Nathan Hagstrom

Warts

Database

DEFINITION
Warts (verrucae) are benign, proliferative, intraepithelial tumors caused by the human papillomavirus (HPV), a small double-stranded DNA virus belonging to the family Papovaviridae. To date, there have been more than 100 types of HPV isolated *in vitro*. The major types of warts include:
- Common warts (verruca vulgaris)
- Flat warts (verruca plana)
- Plantar warts (verruca plantaris)
- Anogenital warts (venereal warts, condyloma acuminata)
- Laryngeal warts (laryngeal papillomatosis)

PATHOPHYSIOLOGY
- Warts can potentially infect any cutaneous or mucosal membrane surface. The most likely sites include areas prone to trauma, explaining the predominance of warts on the hands and feet. Most HPV types have preferred sites of infectivity. There is a great deal of overlap, and one should not use typing to infer modes of transmission.
- Histology shows marked hyperplasia of the epidermis with thin dermal papillae that contain abundant blood vessels, some of which may be thrombosed. These vessels correlate clinically with the "black dots" and pinpoint bleeding seen after paring of the wart.

EPIDEMIOLOGY
- Humans are thought to be the only reservoir of HPV.
- Incubation periods range from 1 to 6 months, but latency periods of 3 years or longer are suspected.
- Primary mode of transmission is thought to be by direct physical contact. Fomite spread has been postulated, and recently HPV has been spread to nasal mucosa from laser plumes.
- Once infected, individuals can spread virus to themselves (i.e., autoinoculation), primarily by manipulating warts or shaving.
- Vertical transmission, or transmission by passage through an infected birth canal, can lead to anogenital and laryngeal warts.
- Approximately 10% of children between 5 and 10 years of age have warts.
- Peak incidence of nongenital warts is between the ages of 12 and 16.
- Caucasians are affected more than are African Americans, for unknown reasons.
- Incidence of anogenital warts has increased dramatically in adults, but less so in children.
- Immunocompromised individuals (primarily those with impaired cell-mediated immunity), as well as individuals with preexisting skin conditions that impair skin barrier function, are at increased risk for infection.

COMPLICATIONS
Anogenital Warts
- Certain HPV types play a prominent role in the development of squamous-cell carcinoma, particularly in the anogenital skin of men and women. Most types seen in children have low oncogenic potential.
- Bowenoid papulosis is considered a premalignant variant of anogenital warts. Clinically indistinguishable from anogenital warts, these lesions show features of dysplasia on biopsy. Despite this histology, they generally behave in a benign manner.

Laryngeal Warts
- Stridor
- Dyspnea
- Dysphonia
- Airway obstruction

Epidermodysplasia Verruciformis
- A rare autosomal-recessive genodermatosis, where patients have impaired natural killer cell–mediated immunity. Consequently, they progressively develop widespread, refractory warts, particularly over bony prominences. The lesions in sun-exposed areas are at increased risk of cutaneous malignancy, namely invasive squamous cell carcinomas, strongly suggesting the contribution of ultraviolet radiation to carcinogenesis.

PROGNOSIS
Spontaneous regression is seen in up to two thirds of *untreated* common warts within 2 years. No conclusive data on anogenital warts exist.

Differential Diagnosis

- Common warts
- —Typically distinguishable on clinical grounds
- Flat warts
- —Dermal nevi
- —Epidermal nevi
- —Molluscum contagiosum
- —Milia
- —Folliculitis
- —Lichen planus
- —Lichen nitidus
- —Acrokeratosis verruciformis
- Plantar warts
- —Corns
- —Calluses
- —Foreign bodies
- Anogenital warts
- —Condyloma lata
- —Molluscum contagiosum
- —Skin tags
- —Hemorrhoids
- —Pyramidal perineal papules
- —Squamous cell carcinoma

Data Gathering

HISTORY
- Determine the duration of the warts, as well as the tempo of proliferation. If present for less than 6 months to 1 year, do not treat with aggressive modalities.
- Anogenital warts should always prompt a careful history for sexual abuse. However, the majority of children younger than 3 years of age are exposed through nonsexual contact with infected parents, siblings, and caregivers. A maternal or paternal history of anogenital warts, and history of warts in individuals in close contact with the patient, should be determined.

Physical Examination

- When assessing anogenital warts, one should examine the entire patient for a potential source of infection. Presence of other warts may suggest autoinoculation. Parents and primary caregivers should likewise be checked to rule out heteroinoculation. The practitioner must check for signs of possible physical or sexual abuse. Suspicious cases should be cultured for gonorrhea and chlamydia, with serologic tests for syphilis and HIV. In cases of suspected abuse, the appropriate authorities must be notified.
- Application of 3% to 5% acetic acid to genital warts may enhance their detection.
- Paring of warts may help differentiate diagnostic possibilities by showing evidence of "black dots" or pinpoint hemorrhage at the base.
- Because of their infectious nature, warts are more likely in areas of trauma. Due to inoculation, they may be seen in a linear array.

Laboratory Aids

TESTS
- Biopsy is rarely needed.
- Southern blot hybridization for identification of HPV type: rarely useful in the clinical setting
- Polymerase chain reaction for identification of HPV type: rarely useful in the clinical setting

Therapy

- With the likelihood for spontaneous resolution, one should never underestimate the value of benign neglect in the treatment of warts.
- The decision to treat must be based on the age and personality of the patient, and the number, size, and location of the warts.
- All therapeutic modalities work by destruction of HPV-infected epithelial cells.
- Treatment should include the clinically visible margins as well as immediately adjacent normal skin, as this has been shown to harbor viral DNA.
- Most modalities require multiple treatments and work by progressive debulking of virally infected cells.
- Painful procedures may benefit from topical anesthesia (EMLA or ELA-max) prior to treatment.
- While not all-inclusive, the following are the most accepted modes of therapy.

READILY AVAILABLE IN MOST PEDIATRIC PRACTICES

• Surgical tape occlusion
—A benign, easy, inexpensive option with variable efficacy. Anecdotal responses have been reported, but untested. The procedure requires 24-hour occlusion, and response is slow.

• Hyperthermia
—Likewise, a benign option with anecdotal success, but untested. Treatment is time consuming, as it requires immersion in 45°C water for 30 minutes daily. Response is slow.

• Salicylic acid
—Minimally invasive, inexpensive therapy that is well tolerated and can be performed at home. Many different products are available over the counter (e.g., Duofilm, Occlusol HP, Trans-Ver-Sal, Compound W) for treatment of common warts. Plantar warts often require 40% salicylic acid in an adhesive plaster. Success rates have been reported to be as high as 84%. This procedure requires dedicated application, and response can be slow.

• Cantharidin
—Minimally invasive and usually well tolerated. Vesiculation can be unpredictable, and therefore it is not recommended for facial lesions. It may cause significant pigmentary changes.

• Tretinoin (Retin-A 0.1% cream)
—Primary indication is for flat warts; not effective for common warts
—Well tolerated, with the exception of mild local irritation; not for use in intertriginous sites

• Podophyllin or podophyllotoxin
—Not FDA approved for pediatric use, but has been used in children safely. Its primary indication is for anogenital warts. It should not be used in large areas due to systemic absorption. Oral ingestion can be fatal. Podophyllin requires in-office application, but podophyllotoxin (Condylox solution or gel) can be used at home.

• Immunotherapy (Imiquimod)
—Although not FDA approved for children, it appears to be safe. It is indicated for treatment of anogenital warts. No conclusive studies with common warts exist.

• Cimetidine
—Recently, multiple anecdotal reports of success with a dosage of 30 to 50 mg/kg/d in three divided doses (maximum, 3.5-g daily dose). It is speculated to work by stimulating T-lymphocyte activity. Double-blind, placebo-controlled studies show that efficacy is no better than placebo.

TYPICALLY RESERVED FOR DERMATOLOGY PRACTICES

• Trichloroacetic/bichloracetic acid/other keratolytics
—Work similarly to salicylic acids but are more potent medications, which can hasten response; requires in-office application

• Contact sensitization (squaric acid dibutyl ester, dinitrochlorobenzene)
—Works by inducing a local allergic contact dermatitis over warts. Requires biweekly in-office application. It can be difficult to titrate

and can cause severe erythema and blistering. It is recommended that its application be done only by experienced personnel.

• Cryotherapy
—Often very effective, and relatively rapid in comparison with topical therapies. Cryotherapy is performed with two freeze-thaw cycles of 5- to 10-second duration. Disadvantages of this procedure include pain, risk of pigmentary changes, and a low risk of scarring.

• Laser ablation (CO_2, erbium:YAG, and flashlamp pulsed dye laser)
—An expensive but often effective option. Disadvantages of this procedure include pain, pigmentary changes, and a low risk of scarring. Laryngeal warts typically need aggressive therapy with laser ablation to prevent respiratory compromise.

• Surgery
—Should be reserved for refractory cases. Disadvantages include pain and the requirement for local anesthesia. Surgery will leave a scar and the recurrence risk is high.

• Electrosurgery/curettage
—Should be reserved for refractory cases. Disadvantages include pain and the requirement for local anesthesia. These procedures will leave a scar, and the recurrence risk is high.

• Bleomycin
—Should be reserved for refractory cases. Requires multiple injections, so it is typically painful. A Raynaud-like phenomenon has been seen in a small subset of individuals when bleomycin was used in the lateral distal fingers.

• Cidofovir
—Should be reserved for refractory cases. Must be compounded before use and is very expensive.

Follow-Up

• All treated warts require close follow-up, typically at 3- to 4-week intervals, to evaluate response to therapy and for possible re-treatment. Prolonged intervals between treatments can delay resolution by allowing for regrowth of the wart.

• Extensive, treatment-refractory HPV infection in the absence of obvious cause should prompt the practitioner to check for underlying immunodeficiency.

PREVENTION

Manipulation of warts, especially during treatment, by biting or picking should be discouraged to prevent spread.

PITFALLS

Warts that do not respond to conventional therapy, particularly in the anogenital skin, should be further studied to rule out other diagnostic possibilities. It must be emphasized that HPV typing gives no insight into the actual mode of transmission of anogenital warts.

Common Questions and Answers

Q: How likely are warts to spread?
A: Unfortunately, because we don't fully understand the mechanisms of transmission, we don't have good studies to predict infectivity. Those individuals with impaired skin integrity or immunodeficiency are at greater risk for infection with HPV. However, in the presence of normal, intact skin, infection is relatively uncommon. Good skin care (e.g., removing hangnails) can prevent potential spread to adjacent skin. Reduction of manipulation of lesions also will prevent spread. Infected children should not be prevented from going to day care or school.

Q: What can you give me to remove these warts once and for all?
A: Unfortunately, no definitive therapy exists. All treatments are locally destructive, and often need to be repeated. Despite clinical clearing, subclinical infection may persist, which can cause recurrence. Latent infections also occur.

Q: How did my child get venereal warts? Was she or he sexually abused?
A: Although there are conflicting studies, it is generally accepted that the most common mode of transmission of anogenital warts in children under 3 years of age is through nonsexual contact [e.g., vertical transmission, passage through the birth canal, autoinoculation, heteroinoculation (see previous discussion)]. This does not negate the obligation of the physician to investigate for physical and/or sexual abuse. Should the practitioner feel uncomfortable with this type of investigation, the patient should be referred to a specialist. Development of anogenital warts in children older than 3 years of age must be investigated thoroughly for evidence of abuse.

ICD-9-CM
Verruca vulgaris 078.10
Verruca plana 078.19
Verruca plantaris 078.19
Anogenital warts 078.11

BIBLIOGRAPHY
Handley J, Hanks E, Armstrong K, et al. Common association of HPV2 with anogenital warts in prepubertal children. *Pediatr Dermatol* 1997;14(5):339–343.

Siegfried EC. Warts on children: an approach to therapy. *Pediatr Ann* 1996;25(2):79–90.

Silverberg NB, Lim JC, Paller AS, et al. Squaric acid immunotherapy for warts in children. *J Am Acad Dermatol* 2000;42:803–808.

Author: Ho Jin Kim

West Nile Virus (and Other Arbovirus Encephalitis)

 Database

DEFINITION

- West Nile virus (WNV) is an arbovirus (arthropod-borne virus) first recognized in the United States in 1999 during an outbreak of encephalitis in New York City.
- Infection can be asymptomatic; clinical disease is characterized by a simple febrile illness, often associated with myalgias, arthralgias, headaches, conjunctivitis, lymphadenopathy, and a roseolar rash.
- Occasionally (<15% of cases), central nervous system (CNS) manifestations such as encephalitis, aseptic meningitis, or myelitis can be seen.
- Other arboviruses can produce similar syndromes or acute hemorrhagic fevers.

CAUSES

- Arboviruses can be divided into two groups based on the predominant clinical syndrome.
- In the United States, five arboviruses are important causes of encephalitis: WNV, California encephalitis virus (LaCrosse strain), Eastern equine encephalitis (EEE), Western equine encephalitis (WEE), and St. Louis encephalitis.
- Arboviruses such as yellow fever, dengue fever, and Colorado tick fever typically cause acute febrile diseases and hemorrhagic fevers and are not characterized by encephalitis.

PATHOPHYSIOLOGY

- The incubation period for WNV and other arboviral encephalitis agents is 5 to 21 days, usually 1 week.
- The incubation period reflects the time necessary for viral replication, viremia, and subsequent invasion of the CNS.
- Virus replication begins locally at the site of the insect bite, transient viremia leads to spread of virus to liver, spleen, and lymph nodes. With continued viral replication and viremia, seeding of other organs including the CNS occurs.
- Virus can rarely be recovered from blood within the first week of onset of illness but not after neurologic symptoms have developed.

EPIDEMIOLOGY

- Arboviruses are spread by mosquitoes, ticks, and sand flies. The major vector for WNV in the U.S. is the *Culex* mosquito.
- Arboviruses are maintained in nature through cycles of transmission among birds, horses, and small animals. Humans and domestic animals are infected incidentally as "dead-end" hosts.
- Disease among birds has been a hallmark of WNV in the U.S., and has served as a sensitive surveillance indicator of WNV activity.

- Each North American arbovirus has specific geographic distributions and is associated with a different ratio of asymptomatic-to-clinical infections. These agents cause disease of variable severity and have distinct age-dependent effects. WNV has been predominately identified in the northeastern U.S.
- The peak incidence of arboviral encephalitis usually occurs during the late summer and early fall. In the South, EEE can be seen throughout the year. Seasonality depends on the breeding and feeding seasons of the arthropod host.
- LaCrosse encephalitis is the most common arboviral cause of encephalitis in children in the U.S. causing approximately 70 cases per year; 90% of clinical disease occurs in children younger than 15 years of age. WNV currently ranks second (21 human cases in the year 2000) but encephalitis is most commonly seen in older adults, generally aged >50 years. Cases of WNV in children are unusual.
- A median of 3 to 5 cases of WEE and EEE are reported nationally each year. EEE tends to produce a more fulminant illness than LaCrosse or WEE.

COMPLICATIONS

- Optic neuritis
- Seizures
- Coma
- Death
- Guillain-Barré syndrome
- Severe neurologic sequelae
- Myocarditis
- Pancreatitis
- Hepatitis

 Differential Diagnosis

INFECTIOUS

Viral

- Herpes simplex virus (HSV)
- Enteroviruses
- HIV
- HHV-6
- Epstein-Barr virus
- CMV
- Lymphocytic choriomeningitis virus
- Rabies
- Mumps
- Influenza
- Adenovirus

Nonviral

- Cat scratch disease (*Bartonella henselae*)
- *Mycoplasma pneumoniae*
- Postinfectious encephalomyelitis—generally follows a vague viral syndrome, usually upper respiratory tract, by days to weeks.
- Abscess/subdural empyema
- Meningitis

—Tuberculous
—Cryptococcal or other fungal (histoplasmosis, coccidioidomycoses, blastomycoses)
—Bacterial
—Listeria

- Toxoplasmosis
- *Plasmodium falciparum* infection (malaria)
- Parasites (cysticercosis, echinococcus, amebiasis, trypanosomiasis)

NONINFECTIOUS

- Tumor
- Carcinomatous meningitis
- Systemic lupus erythematosus
- Sarcoidosis
- Vasculitis
- Hemorrhage
- Toxic encephalopathy
- Metabolic disorders

 Data Gathering

HISTORY

The diagnosis of arboviral infections of the CNS is difficult. Characteristic epidemiology that suggests a specific etiology is an important part of the history. The season of disease, prevalent diseases within the community, and animal exposures may provide clues to the diagnosis. Enteroviral infections are seen in the warmer months (summer and early fall) in temperate climates. Mosquito propagation in damp climates during the summer months may increase the likelihood of arthropod-borne viruses. History of an animal bite or bat exposure may suggest the possibility of rabies.

Physical Examination

- Encephalitis caused by arboviruses is characterized by acute onset of fever and headache in almost all patients. Associated symptoms include seizures, altered consciousness, disorientation, and behavioral disturbances. Neurologic signs are more commonly diffuse but may be focal. These clinical findings can help to distinguish patients with meningitis, which is characterized by nuchal rigidity and fever usually without an altered sensorium.
- Other symptoms reported with WNV include arthralgias, myalgias, pharyngitis, conjunctivitis, nausea, vomiting, diarrhea, abdominal pain, and rash. The rash is seen in about 50% of patients and is described as nonpruritic, roseolar, or maculopapular on the chest, back, and arms, which lasts 1 week. Diffuse lymphadenopathy is also common.
- Neurologic examination can reveal motor weakness, increased deep tendon reflexes and extensor plantar responses, tremor or abnormal movement of extremities.

Laboratory Aids

The diagnosis of arboviral encephalitis depends on the recognition of epidemiologic risk factors and typical signs and symptoms with the aid of laboratory and radiographic studies.

ROUTINE LABORATORY TESTS

- CBC typically reveals a mild leukocytosis.
- Mild increase in erythrocyte sedimentation rate.
- Mild to moderate CSF pleocytosis predominately mononuclear cells.
- Elevated CSF protein
- Normal CSF glucose

SEROLOGY

- IgM and IgG enzyme-linked immunosorbent assays (ELISAs) for WNV and other arboviruses are performed at state public health laboratories and the CDC.
- The diagnosis of arbovirus encephalitis is made by one of the following:

—A fourfold rise in serum antibody titers. Acute-phase titers should be collected 0 to 8 days after onset of symptoms. Convalescent phase titers should be collected 14 to 21 days after acute specimen. A single negative acute-phase specimen is inadequate for diagnosis, but a positive test can provide evidence of recent infection.
—Isolation of the virus from tissue, blood, or CSF
—PCR to detect viral RNA
—Capture of virus-specific IgM antibodies in the CSF by ELISA.

RADIOGRAPHIC STUDIES

Imaging studies such as MRI or CT can assist in ruling out other potential causes of encephalopathy or encephalitis. MRI has proved useful in differentiating postinfectious encephalomyelitis from acute viral encephalitis. The former is characterized by enhancement of multifocal white matter lesions.

EEG

Diffuse generalized slowing of brain waves. Periodic high-voltage spike waves originating in the temporal lobe region and slow-wave complexes at 2- to 3-second intervals are suggestive of herpes simplex virus infection.

Therapy

SPECIFIC

- No specific antiviral therapy is available.
- Supportive therapy including cardio-respiratory function, fluid and electrolyte balance, seizure control, and reduction of intracranial pressure is important.
- Recovery can often be seen after prolonged periods of coma.

PREVENTION

- Public health department efforts focus on surveillance of viral activity to predict and prevent outbreaks.
- Active bird surveillance to detect the presence of WNV activity
- Active mosquito surveillance to detect viral activity in mosquito populations
- Passive surveillance by veterinarians and human health care professionals to detect neurologic illnesses consistent with encephalitis.
- Personal precautions to avoid mosquito bites including use of repellents, protective clothing, screens, and installation of air conditioners
- Vaccines for prevention of most arbovirus infections are not available. A vaccine is available for Japanese encephalitis for travelers to endemic areas who are planning prolonged stays.

INFECTION CONTROL MEASURES

- Standard precautions are recommended for the hospitalized patient.
- Respiratory precautions are recommended when vector mosquitos are present.

Follow-Up

- Prognosis for recovery depends on the specific infecting agent and host factors such as age and underlying illness.
- Neurobehavioral follow-up should be considered in children with severe or complicated disease.

Common Questions and Answers

Q: Should testing for arboviruses, including WNV, be performed on all patients with encephalitis?
A: Diagnostic testing for arboviruses is not recommended for all patients with encephalitis. The prevalence of these diseases is low and the diagnosis of more common causes of childhood encephalitis (e.g., HSV) should be pursued initially. Patients with no other identifiable cause of encephalitis who have epidemiologic risk factors such as geographic location, season, and exposure history suggestive of arbovirus encephalitis should be evaluated. Testing of patients with aseptic meningitis or Guillain-Barré syndrome is low-yield.

ICD-9-CM

Encephalitis
ARBo 064
Eastern equine 062.2
Western equine 062.1
Viral 049.8
La Crosse 062.5

BIBLIOGRAPHY

American Academy of Pediatrics. Arboviruses. In: Pickering LK, ed. *2000 red book: report of the Committee on Infectious Diseases* , 25th ed. Elk Grove Village, ILL: American Academy of Pediatrics, 2000:170–175.

Asnis DS, Conetta R, Teixeira AA, et al. The West Nile Virus outbreak of 1999 in New York: the Flushing Hospital experience. *Clin Infect Dis* 2000;30:413–418.

CDC Guidelines for Surveillance, Prevention and Control of West Nile Virus Infection— United States. *MMWR* 2000;49(2):25–28.

Johnson RT. Acute encephalitis. *Clin Infect Dis* 1996;23:219–26.

Whitley RJ, Kimberlin DW. Viral encephalitis. *Pediatr Rev* 1999;20(6):192–198.

Author: Theoklis Zaoutis

Wilms Tumor

 Database

DEFINITION

Wilms tumor is a malignant tumor of the kidney occurring in the pediatric age group. It is also called *nephroblastoma*.

CAUSES

• 20% of Wilms tumors have a mutation in the *WT1* tumor suppressor gene.
• Causes in the remaining 80% of patients is unknown.

PATHOLOGY

• Gross: often cystic with hemorrhages and necrosis; usually no calcification (useful in differentiating from neuroblastoma, which is calcified on plain x-ray); may extend into the inferior vena cava (IVC).
• Histology: triphasic pattern blastemal, epithelial, and stromal cell. Blastemal cells aggregate into nodules like primitive glomeruli; the presence of anaplasia indicates a poor prognosis.

GENETICS

• Fifteen percent to 20% are hereditary in origin.
• Familial cases are more often bilateral and occur at an earlier age.
• A tumor-suppressor gene related to Wilms tumor (*WT1*) has been localized to chromosome 11p13.
• Mutations of this gene occurs in approximately 20% of Wilms tumors.
• Heterozygous deletions on 11p13 associated with congenital Wilms tumor/aniridia/genital anomaly/mental retardation syndrome
• Another candidate tumor suppressor gene *WT2* has been localized to 11p15.

EPIDEMIOLOGY

• Most common primary malignant renal tumor of childhood
• Five percent to 6% of all childhood cancer
• Incidence: 1 in 10,000 live births
• Higher incidence in blacks
• More common in girls than boys
• Peak age: 2 to 3 years
• May be associated with aniridia, hemihypertrophy, and cryptorchidism
• Increased incidence in children with neurofibromatosis
• Associated syndromes: WAGR (Wilms tumor, aniridia, GU abnormalities, mental retardation), Beckwith-Wiedeman syndrome (macroglossia, omphalocele, visceromegaly, hemihypertrophy), and Denys-Drash syndrome (ambiguous genitalia, progressive renal failure, and increased risk of Wilms tumor).

COMPLICATIONS

• Extension into IVC
• Metastasis to lungs and liver
• Cardiac toxicity secondary to Adriamycin
• Liver dysfunction secondary to actinomycin D and radiation therapy (XRT)

PROGNOSIS

• Stages I and II: more than 90% cured
• Stage III: 85% cured
• Stage IV: 70% cured

 Differential Diagnosis

• Polycystic kidney
• Renal hematoma
• Renal abscess
• Neuroblastoma
• Other neoplasms of kidney: clear-cell carcinoma, rhabdoid tumor

 Data Gathering

HISTORY

• Abdominal distention
• Abdominal pain (20–30% of cases)
• Hematuria (20–30% of cases)
• Fever, anorexia, vomiting
• Family history of Wilms tumor
• Rapid increase in abdominal size (suggestive of hemorrhage in the tumor)

 Physical Examination

• Asymptomatic abdominal mass extending from flank toward midline (most common presentation)
• Anemia (secondary to hemorrhage in the tumor)
• Fever
• Hypertension (due to increased renin production in 25% of cases)
• Varicocele (indicates obstruction to spermatic vein due to tumor thrombus in renal vein or IVC)
• Aniridia, hemihypertrophy, cryptorchidism, hypospadias
• Signs of Beckwith-Wiedemann and neurofibromatosis

 Laboratory Aids

TESTS

• CBC
• Electrolytes
• Urine analysis: for microscopic hematuria
• Liver and kidney function tests

IMAGING

• Ultrasound of abdomen

—Diagnostic of mass of renal origin
—Evaluate for extension of tumor into IVC

• CT scan of abdomen: useful if diagnosis doubtful
• IVP: no longer routinely used
• Chest x-ray: to evaluate for metastatic disease
• Bone scan: only if clear-cell variety on pathology
• CT of head: only for rhabdoid tumors

CLINICOPATHOLOGIC STAGING

- **Stage I:** Tumor is restricted to one kidney and completely resected. The renal capsule is intact.
- **Stage II:** Tumor extends beyond the kidney but is completely excised.
- **Stage III:** Residual nonhematogenous tumor is confined to the abdomen.
- **Stage IV:** There is hematogenous spread to lungs, liver, bone, or brain.
- **Stage V:** bilateral disease

FAVORABLE PROGNOSTIC FACTORS

- Tumor weight less than 250 g
- Age at presentation less than 24 months
- Stage I disease
- Favorable histology

POOR PROGNOSTIC FACTORS

- Anaplastic pathology
- Lymph node involvement
- Distant metastasis

 ## Therapy

SURGERY

- Nephrectomy

—Preoperative chemotherapy in case of very large tumors with IVC extension
—For bilateral disease nephrectomy of more affected side and partial nephrectomy of the other side, followed by chemotherapy and radiation

RADIATION THERAPY

- Not required for stage I and II patients
- Local XRT with 1,000 cGy for stages III and IV
- Whole-lung radiation (1,200 cGy) for pulmonary metastasis

CHEMOTHERAPY

- For stages I and II favorable histology: vincristine (VCR) and actinomycin D (AMD) every 3 weeks for 6 months
- For stages III and IV favorable histology: VCR, AMD, and doxorubicin for 6 to 15 months
- Add cyclophosphamide for higher stage anaplastic tumors

SIDE EFFECTS OF THERAPY

Temporary loss of hair, peripheral neuropathy, impaired function of the remaining kidney over years following radiation, cardiac toxicity with Adriamycin, second malignant neoplasms in few cases

 ## Follow-Up

- Every 3 months for 18 months, every 6 months for 1 year, and then yearly
- Chest x-ray, urinalysis, and abdominal ultrasound at regular intervals

PITFALLS

Rarely, Wilms tumor may present with polycythemia. It can present as fever of unknown origin without any other signs or symptoms.

 ## Common Questions and Answers

Q: What should be done to protect the remaining kidney during sports?
A: Children should wear a kidney guard to protect the unaffected kidney during contact sports.

Q: Can a child grow and live normally with one kidney?
A: Yes.

ICD-9-CM 189.0

BIBLIOGRAPHY

Blakely ML, Ritchey ML. Controversies in the management of Wilms' tumor. *Semin Pediatr Surg* 2001;10(3):127–131.

Coppes MJ, Haber DA, Grundy PE. Genetic events in development of Wilms tumor. *N Engl J Med* 1994;331(9):586–590.

Green DM, et al. Wilms' tumor. In: Pizzo PA, Poplack DG, eds. *Principles and practice of pediatric oncology*, 3rd ed. Philadelphia: Lippincott-Raven, 1997.

Mrowka C, Schedl A. Wilms' tumor suppressor gene WT1: from structure to renal pathophysiologic features. *J Am Soc Nephrol* 2000;11:S106–S115.

Neville HL, Ritchey ML. Wilms' tumor. Overview of National Wilms' Tumor Study Group results. *Urol Clin North Am* 2000;27(3):435–442.

Petruzzi MJ, Green DM. Wilms tumor. *Pediatr Clin North Am* 1997;44(4):939–952.

Ritchey ML, Haase GM, Shochat SJ. Current management of Wilms' tumor. *Semin Surg Oncol* 1993;9(6):502–509.

Shochat SJ. Wilms' tumor: diagnosis and treatment in the 1990's. *Semin Pediatr Surg* 1993;2(1):59–68.

Author: Tammy I. Kang
Sadhna Shankar, 2nd edition

Wilson Disease

 Database

DEFINITION

Wilson disease (WD) is a treatable, recessive disorder of copper metabolism affecting brain, liver, eyes, and blood.

PATHOPHYSIOLOGY

Primarily degenerative changes in brain, liver, and cornea, due to decreased copper excretion, and subsequent accumulation in other tissues. Copper ion is thought to inhibit pyruvate oxidase in brain and adenosine triphosphate (ATP) in body membranes.

GENETICS

Autosomal-recessive inheritance, defect on chromosome 13. Mutations have been detected in a gene involved in copper transport.

EPIDEMIOLOGY

Incidence of 1 in 100,000 to 500,000

ASSOCIATED CONDITIONS

• Corneal: Kayser-Fleischer rings (granular copper deposits on limbus)
• Fanconi syndrome
• Psychiatric: paranoia, delusions, schizoid-type behavior
• Pancreatitis, hepatitis
• Cardiomyopathy
• Bone disease: asymptomatic osteoporosis, osteomalacia
• Endocrinologic: gynecomastia, delayed puberty; amenorrhea due to liver disease

 Differential Diagnosis

• Liver disease resembling hepatic involvement from WD includes any cause of fulminant hepatic failure or chronic active hepatitis.
• Unexplained hemolytic anemia or thrombocytopenia may occur.
• Neurologic conditions presenting similarly to WD include Huntington disease (prominent dystonia in children), essential tremor, Sydenham chorea, hereditary dystonia, and other neurodegenerative diseases.
• Psychiatric disorders, particularly psychoses (schizophrenia, mania), may be the initial presentation of WD

 Data Gathering

HISTORY

• Children usually present with hepatic abnormalities, including fulminant hepatic failure (around 8–16 years). They can present with manifestations of subacute hepatitis followed by fulminant hepatic failure (with low ALT/AST, and low Alk Phos)
• Characteristic neurologic complications are usually not seen until puberty:

—Tremor
—Dysarthria and dystonia
—Decreased ability to perform voluntary movements
—The most prominent symptom is the new-onset difficulty with performance of voluntary motor movements.
—A family history of liver disease with or without associated psychiatric symptoms is helpful in the differential, though rarely present.

 Physical Examination

• Vital signs are generally normal unless anemia is present.
• Heart examination may reveal evidence of cardiomyopathy.
• GU examination may reveal delayed sexual development gynecomastia.
• Corneal abnormalities are uniformly present when there are CNS manifestations: ophthalmologic examination to evaluate for Kayser-Fleischer rings (though they can be seen on direct ophthalmologic examination in some cases).
• Examination may reveal hepatomegaly with or without splenomegaly.
• Edema and ascites can also be noted; abdominal palpation for ascites, hepatosplenomegaly
• Neurologic examination should focus on mental status, psychiatric review of systems, and motor examination: tremor, dystonia, and incoordination.

Laboratory Aids

TESTS

- Screening labs: CBC, PT/PTT, U/A
- Abdominal ultrasound for evaluation of liver size
- Liver biopsy is the definitive procedure for tissue diagnosis.
- Serum ceruloplasmin (usually low; 15% of patients have normal values)
- Elevated serum copper and urine copper
- 3× ceruloplasmin (mg/L) 5% serum Cu (mg/L) (usually 90–95%)

 ## Therapy

- Penicillamine or trientine (triethyl tetramine) and low-copper diet for life

—Therapy takes weeks to months to be effective.
—The amount of recovery is proportional to the amount of preexisting damage.

- Patients who present in hemolytic crisis require liver transplantation.

 ## Follow-Up

- Patients require treatment for life.
- Sudden discontinuation of therapy may precipitate fulminant hepatic failure.
- In some patients (10–20%) with neurologic symptoms, there may be temporary exacerbation before improvement.
- Patients on penicillamine require follow-up examinations, 24-hour urine copper, serum copper, CBC, and U/A before treatment: weekly during the first month, monthly for the first year, and then yearly.
- One of the side effects of penicillamine therapy is a reversible myasthenia.
- Screen family members older than age 3 years with physical examination, LFTs, serum ceruloplasmin, and ophthalmologic examination.

PITFALLS

- Identification of Kayser-Fleischer rings may require slit-lamp examination.
- Wilson disease should be considered in patients with chronic liver disease or psychosis of unspecified etiology.
- Neurologic abnormalities in WD may be markedly asymmetrical.

 ## Common Questions and Answers

Q: Why is screening not performed in children under 3 years?
A: Normal neonatal copper excretion is similar to that of patients with WD. By the age of 3 years, the excretion rate is similar to that of adults.

Q: Can my patients with Wilson disease have children?
A: Women of reproductive age who are treated can have normal pregnancies. Both penicillamine and trientine appear safe during pregnancy in patients with WD, though the number of patients who have taken the medicine during pregnancy is low.

ICD-9-CM 275.1

BIBLIOGRAPHY

Scriver CR, Beaudet AL, Sly WS, et al. *Metabolic basis for inherited disease.* New York: McGraw-Hill, 1997:1416–1423.

Sternlieb I. Wilson's disease. *Clin Liver Dis* 2000;4(1):229–239, viii–ix.

Yarze JC, Martin P, Munoz SJ, et al. Wilson's disease: current status. *Am J Med* 1992;92:643–654.

Author: D. Elizabeth McNeil

Wiskott-Aldrich Syndrome

 Database

DEFINITION

Wiskott-Aldrich syndrome (WAS) is an X-linked primary immunodeficiency with the classic clinical triad of thrombocytopenia with small platelets, eczema, and recurrent infections. It is also associated with IgA nephropathy, autoimmune disorders, and an increased incidence of hematopoietic malignancies.

CAUSES

- Mutation in a recently described novel gene, Wiskott-Aldrich syndrome protein (*WASP*), on the X chromosome, may lead to this syndrome.
- *WASP* may be important for signal transduction and the regulation of the cytoskeletal reorganization.
- Abnormalities of a cell-surface glycoprotein, sialophorin, on T lymphocytes may relate to the abnormal cell-surface cytoarchitecture seen in this syndrome.

GENETICS

- X-linked recessive disease
- Linkage analyses have localized the defective *WASP* gene to X p11.22p–11.23.
- Approximately 60% of cases will have a positive family history for WAS.
- X-linked thrombocytopenia (XLT) without the other findings is caused by mutations of the same gene.

EPIDEMIOLOGY

- Incidence is rare.
- Presents in infancy with serious bleeding episodes secondary to thrombocytopenia
- Recurrent infections usually start after 6 months of age. (Bacterial: otitis media, sinusitis, meningitis, sepsis and pneumonia. Viral infections: HSV, varicella with systemic complications)
- Milder phenotypes may lack history of recurrent infections.
- Eczema is usually present by 1 year of age. (May be resistant to therapy, sometimes requiring systemic antibiotics)

COMPLICATIONS

- Progressive decline in immunologic function with an increase in infections. Both humoral and cellular immune systems are affected.
- There is an increased frequency of autoimmune phenomena such as arthritis and vasculitis. The most common is hemolytic anemia. Vasculitis, Henoch-Schönlein purpura, inflammatory polyarthritis, and inflammatory bowel disease are also observed.
- Approximately 100-fold increased risk of malignancy compared with the general pediatric population. Malignancy is more common in adolescents.
- Bleeding episodes can be life threatening.

 Differential Diagnosis

- Other causes of thrombocytopenia such as ITP
- Severe atopic disease with dermatitis and secondary skin infections
- HIV infection
- Hyper-IgE syndrome
- Diagnosis should be considered in any boy who has congenital or early-onset thrombocytopenia with small platelets.
- Definitive diagnosis: male patient, congenital thrombocytopenia ($<$70,000/mm^3), small platelets [mean platelet volume (MPV) $<$0.5 fL], a mutation in the *WASP* gene or absent *WASP* mRNA.

 Data Gathering

HISTORY

- Persistent or severe bleeding in infancy due to thrombocytopenia
- Recurrent infections, especially by bacteria with capsular polysaccharides (e.g., *Pneumococcus*)
- Eczema can be of variable severity.
- Older patients may report recurrent viral infections.
- Maternal family history of WAS or XLT

 Physical Examination

- Evaluation should focus on presence of infection.
- Dermatologic examination is significant for the extent of eczema and the presence of petechiae or ecchymoses.
- Splenomegaly

 Laboratory Aids

TESTS

- CBC with differential
- Platelet count with mean platelet volume and platelet size by Coulter counter; hallmark of WAS is small platelets.
- Immunoglobulin levels typically reveal normal IgG, decreased IgM, and increased IgA and IgE.
- Functional antibody titers and isohemagglutinins; hallmark of WAS is reduced or absent responses to polysaccharide antigens and isohemagglutinins to ABO antigens.
- T- and B-lymphocyte enumeration and mitogen stimulation studies. These may progressively deteriorate with increasing age.

PROCEDURES

- Lymph node biopsy in suspected malignancy
- Bone marrow aspirate to evaluate thrombocytopenia

Wiskott-Aldrich Syndrome

 Therapy

- Antibiotics for acute infections and prophylactically in postsplenectomy patients
- Splenectomy may be helpful for persistent severe thrombocytopenia in select patients. However, this may greatly increase the risk of overwhelming infections with encapsulated organisms.
- Thrombocytopenia precautions: no aspirin and avoidance of situations in which trauma (especially head trauma) is likely to occur, such as contact sports.
- Platelet transfusions may be necessary for severe bleeding. Use irradiated blood products to avoid graft-versus-host disease, and CMV-negative products in case of bone marrow transplantation (BMT).
- IVIG replacement therapy is helpful in managing recurrent infections in some patients.
- BMT should be considered in these patients. If a full match is available, this is the treatment of choice. The overall success rate of HLA-identical BMT is 85%. The use of haploidentical BMT is controversial because of a lower success rate. Cord blood as a source of stem cells is also a curative therapy.
- Consider food allergy as exacerbating factor for eczema.

 Follow-Up

- Signs and symptoms of malignancy should be evaluated expeditiously.
- As patients age, a progressive increase in infectious and autoimmune complications may occur.

 Common Questions and Answers

Q: What is the life expectancy for WAS patients?
A: Before currently available therapies, most affected patients died in childhood. Currently, many patients live into their third and fourth decades, even without BMT. Major causes of mortality are infections (44%), bleeding (23%), and malignancies (26%). Incidence of malignancy increases in third decade of life. Successfully transplanted patients have a prolonged life expectancy.

Q: Should patients with WAS receive live viral vaccines?
A: These vaccines should be avoided because of the variable cellular immune defects associated with WAS. Any patients receiving IVIG do not require vaccinations.

Q: What is the chance of a sibling having WAS?
A: As with any X-linked disease, there is a 50% chance of another affected male child or asymptomatic carrier female. Genetic counseling should be offered to carrier females.

Q: Can WAS be diagnosed prenatally?
A: In families with affected males, fetal blood sampling can be performed in male fetuses to assess the size of the platelets. Small platelet size and family history of WAS suggests an affected infant.

ICD-9-CM 279.12

BIBLIOGRAPHY

Derry JMD, Ochs HD, Francke U. Isolation of novel gene mutated in Wiskott Aldrich syndrome. *Cell* 1994;78:635–644.

Litzman J, Jones A, Hann I, et al. Intravenous immunoglobulin, splenectomy, and antibiotic prophylaxis in Wiskott-Aldrich syndrome. *Arch Dis Child* 1996;75(5):43–69.

Nonoyama S, Ochs HD. Wiskott-Aldrich syndrome. *Curr Allergy Asthma Rep* 2001;1:430–437.

Ochs HD. The Wiskott-Aldrich syndrome. *Clin Rev Allergy Immunol* 2001;20(1):61–86.

Ochs HD, Skichter SJ, Harker LA, et al. The Wiskott Aldrich syndrome: studies of lymphocytes, granulocytes and platelets. *Blood* 1980;55:243–252.

Stites DP, Terr AI. *Basic and clinical immunology*, 7th ed. Norwalk, CT: Appleton-Lange, 1991:346–347.

Sullivan KS, Mullen CA, Blaise RM, et al. A multi-institutional survey of Wiskott Aldrich syndrome. *J Pediatr* 1994;125:876–885.

Winkelstein JA, et al., eds. *Patient and family handbook: for the primary immune deficiency diseases*, 2nd ed. Immune Deficiency Foundation, 1993.

Author: Elena Perez
Alexander Yip, 2nd edition

Yersinia enterocolitica

 Database

DEFINITION

Yersinia enterocolitica is a facultative, nonlactose-fermenting, urease-positive, gram-negative coccobacillus; 34 serotypes have been recognized with serotypes 0:3, 8, and 9 the most common.

PATHOPHYSIOLOGY

- *Y. enterocolitica* adheres to epithelial cells and mucus, and heat-stable enterotoxins are produced, which play a role in the development of watery diarrhea.
- Another cytotoxin then directly injures the distal small bowel and large bowel, producing the characteristic bloody or mucous diarrhea.
- An enterocolitis develops and usually persists 5 to 14 days and is seen most commonly in the younger age groups.
- A pseudoappendicular syndrome due to mesenteric adenitis and/or terminal ileitis is seen more commonly in the older child or young adult.
- Extraintestinal manifestations include pharyngitis, suppurative lymphadenitis, pyomyositis, osteomyelitis, abscess, urinary tract infection, pneumonia, endocarditis, meningitis, peritonitis, panophthalmitis, conjunctivitis, and septic arthritis.
- If septicemia is present, mortality can be as high as 50%.

EPIDEMIOLOGY

- Most infected individuals are young children.
- *Y. enterocolitica* has been isolated from contaminated water, soil, wild and domestic animals, and unpasteurized milk products.
- Epidemics have been noted in the African-American population during the winter holidays due to exposure to raw chitterlings (pork intestines) prepared for holiday meals.
- Cases due to contaminated blood transfusions from asymptomatic carriers of *Y. enterocolitica* 0:3 have been reported.
- Fecal–oral and person-to-person transmission are also possible.
- The incubation period is approximately 1 to 11 days, with symptoms persisting for 5 to 14 days. Symptoms for up to several months have been reported.
- The duration of organism excretion is approximately 6 weeks after diagnosis is made.
- A clinical state of iron overload and deferoxamine therapy are risk factors for developing systemic illness.

COMPLICATIONS

- Postinfectious sequelae of erythema nodosum and reactive arthritis involving weight-bearing joints (occurring 1–2 weeks after gastrointestinal symptoms) can occur, although these complications are seen most often in adults.
- Reiter syndrome, myocarditis, glomerulonephritis, erysipelas, chronic diarrhea persisting for months, and hemolytic anemia have also been reported.
- Intestinal perforation and ileocolic intussusception are possible.
- Septicemia is observed in patients with underlying medical conditions.
- Patients with iron overload disorders, e.g., β-thalassemia, hemochromatosis, have an increased susceptibility to *Yersinia* bacteremia.
- Following septicemia, focal abscesses of the liver, kidney, spleen, and lungs have been reported.
- The FDA has reported that contamination of the U.S. blood supply by bacterial infections, although rare, is most frequently due to *Y. enterocolitica*.

PROGNOSIS

The prognosis is usually quite good, because most infections are gastrointestinal. Systemic disease (septicemia and subsequent secondary spread) has higher morbidity and mortality.

 Differential Diagnosis

Y. enterocolitica should be considered in all patients with a diarrheal illness with bloody or mucous stools with fever and abdominal pain, as well as in patients with the extraintestinal manifestations described above.

 Data Gathering

HISTORY

- Enterocolitis is the most common manifestation in young children.
- The history taking should include exposure to unpasteurized milk products and raw pork or poultry, especially the preparation of pork chitterlings.
- A history of acute onset of abdominal pain, diarrhea with blood or mucus, and mild fever suggest the diagnosis.
- Abdominal pain can be diffuse or localized to the right lower quadrant, suggestive of pseudoappendicitis due to mesenteric adenitis or terminal ileitis.
- Duration of illness is usually 2 to 3 weeks, but may be longer, and 25% of patients will have hematochezia.

Physical Examination

Because of the wide range of clinical extraintestinal manifestations, the physical examination is nonspecific for this organism.

 ## Laboratory Aids

TESTS

• Blood, sputum, CSF, urine, and bile cultures do not require selective culture media techniques; stool samples should be plated on selective media such as cefsulodin-triclosan-novobiocin agar. If routine enteric media (MacConkey) are used, a cold enrichment technique will increase recovery of the organism.
• Serologic methods (tube agglutination assay, ELISA) are available with a rise in titers noted 1 week after onset of symptoms and peak titers observed by the second week of illness. These tests identify IgM, IgG, and IgA antibodies against *Y. enterocolitica*.
• Cross-reactivity between *Y. enterocolitica* and *Brucella abortus*, *Rickettsia* species, *Moraxella morganii*, *Salmonella* species, and thyroid tissue antigen make serodiagnosis of limited usefulness.

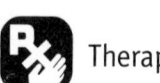 ## Therapy

• Antimicrobial therapy has been shown to benefit patients with systemic infections, focal extraintestinal infections, and enterocolitis in an immunocompromised host.
• The benefit of treatment of uncomplicated enterocolitis, mesenteric adenitis, or pseudoappendicitis has not been established.
• For most isolates, trimethoprim-sulfamethoxazole, chloramphenicol, aminoglycosides, tetracycline, quinolones, and third-generation cephalosporins are effective treatment options.
• *Y. enterocolitica* is usually resistant to most penicillins and first-generation cephalosporins.

 ## Follow-Up

• Symptoms of enterocolitis usually abate within 2 weeks of the onset of symptoms, although shedding of the organism in the stool can last at least 6 weeks after diagnosis.
• For extraintestinal manifestations, the expected course is dependent on the specific organ system involved.

PREVENTION

• Infection control: Enteric precautions are indicated for patients with enterocolitis until symptoms resolve.
• General measures: Attempts to eliminate reservoirs and reduce frequency of ingesting contaminated foods and beverages are necessary; uncooked meats, especially pork and unpasteurized milk, as well as preparation of meats near or during preparation of infant bottles for feeding, are common sources of infection.

PITFALLS

• Not all bacterial colitis presents with bloody or mucus-appearing diarrhea. Therefore, suspicion should exist if the diarrhea is prolonged or environmental exposures pose a risk for developing infection.
• The possibility of *Y. enterocolitica* bacteremia should be considered in blood transfusion–related illnesses, thalassemia, or prior history of liver disease.

 ## Common Questions and Answers

Q: How long is a child considered infectious with *Y. enterocolitica*?
A: Although the typical course of enterocolitis is approximately 14 days, shedding of the organism in the stool can last at least 6 weeks. Enteric precautions should be discussed with the child's parent or caregiver to ensure infection control.

Q: If there is no history of evidence of bloody or mucous stools, can you exclude *Y. enterocolitica* as the likely infectious agent in a child with diarrhea?
A: No. In fact, early in the course of illness, the diarrhea is more likely to be watery due to the enterotoxins produced (see Pathophysiology, above).

Q: How is the diagnosis of *Y. enterocolitica* determined if you are unable to isolate the organism from a clinical specimen?
A: When a diagnosis cannot be made during acute infection or in the clinical setting of postinfectious complications, a serologic titer of greater than 1:128 is suggestive of previous infection of *Y. enterocolitica*. Keep in mind the possibility of cross-reactivity with *Brucella, Rickettsia, Morganella,* and *Salmonella* species as well as thyroid antigens.

ICD-9-CM 027.8

(Sepsis) 020.9

BIBLIOGRAPHY

Bottone EJ. *Yersinia enterocolitica*: the charisma continues. *Clin Microbiol Rev* 1997;10:257–276.

Cover TL, Aber RC. *Yersinia enterocolitica*. *N Engl J Med* 1989;321:16–24.

Kane DR, Reuman PD. *Yersinia enterocolitica* causing pneumonia and empyema in a child and a review of the literature. *Pediatr Infect Dis J* 1992;11:59–1593.

Krishnan LAG, Brecher ME. Transfusion-transmitted bacterial infection. *Hematol Oncol Clin North Am* 1995;9:167–185.

Lee LA, Taylor J, Carter GP, et al. *Yersinia enterocolitica* 0:3: an emerging cause of pediatric gastroenteritis in the United States. *J Infect Dis* 1991;163:660–663.

Natkin J, Beavis KG. *Yersinia enterocolitica* and *Yersinia pseudotuberculosis*. *Clin Lab Med* 1999;19:523–536.

Peter G, Halsey NA, Marcuse EK, et al. *Yersinia enterocolitica*. In: *2000 red book: report of the Committee on Infectious Diseases*, 25th ed. Elk Grove Village, IL: American Academy of Pediatrics, 2000:642–643.

Author: Philip V. Scribano

SECTION III
Syndromes Glossary

4p syndrome—characterized by a round face, prominent nasal tip, polydactyly, and scoliosis.

5p syndrome—characterized by macrocephaly; small mandible; long, thin fingers; short, big toes; and anorectal and renal anomalies.

13q syndrome—typically involves malformations of the brain, heart, kidneys, and digits; usually lethal.

Aagene syndrome—hereditary (autosomal-recessive transmission); characterized by recurrent intrahepatic cholestasis, with lymphedema.

Aarskog syndrome—an x-linked recessive disorder characterized by short stature, and musculoskeletal and genital anomalies unknown etiology. Physical features include short stature (90%), hypertelorism, small nose with anteverted nares, broad philtrum and nasal bridge, abnormal auricles and widow's peak, brachyclinodactyly (80%), broad feet with bulbous toes (75%), simian crease (70%), ptosis (50%), syndactyly (60%), "shawl" scrotum (80%), cryptorchidism (75%), inguinal hernia (60%), hyperopic astigmatism, large corneas, ophthalmoplegia, strabismus, delayed puberty, mild pectus excavatum, prominent umbilicus. Radiographs show delayed bone age.

abetalipoproteinemia—recessive transmission; characterized by progressive cerebellar ataxia and pigmentary degeneration of the retina (starts with malabsorption of fat and progresses to ataxia); absent or reduced lipoproteins and low carotene, vitamin A, and cholesterol levels; and acanthocytosis [spiny projections on red blood cells (RBCs)].

acanthosis nigricans (Lawrence-Seip syndrome)—characterized by hyperpigmented lichenoid plaques in the neck and axilla; may be associated with insulin resistance.

acrodermatitis enteropathica—autosomal-recessive transmission; characterized by zinc deficiency, vesicobullous and eczematous skin lesions in the perioral and perineal areas, cheeks, knees, and elbows; photophobia, conjunctivitis and corneal dystrophy; chronic diarrhea; glossitis; nail dystrophy; growth retardation; and superinfections and *Candida* infections.

Adie syndrome—characterized by a large pupil with little or no reaction to light; pupil may react to accommodation; patients have hyperreflexia.

agenesis of corpus callosum—cause unknown (rarely, X-linked recessive); absence of the major tracts connecting the right and left hemispheres is usually associated with hydrocephalus, seizures, developmental delay, abnormal head size, and hypertelorism.

Alagille syndrome (arteriohepatic dysplasia)—characterized by paucity or absence of intrahepatic bile ducts with progressive destruction of bile ducts; patients have a broad forehead, deep-set eyes that are widely spaced and underdeveloped, a small, pointed mandible, cardiac lesions, vertebral arch defects, and changes in the renal tubules and interstitium.

Albers-Schönberg disease (osteopetrosis tarda, marble bone disease)—most cases are autosomal dominant, a few are autosomal recessive; patients are prone to fractures and have mild anemia and craniofacial disproportion; radiologic changes include increased cortical bone density, longitudinal and transverse dense striations at the ends of the long bones, lucent and dense bands in the vertebrae, and thickening at the base of the skull.

Albright syndrome—see **McCune-Albright syndrome.**

Alexander disease—unknown pathogenesis; characterized by megaloencephaly in infants, dementia, spasticity and ataxia; may cause seizures in younger children; patients become mute, immobile, and dependent; hyaline eosinophilic inclusions occur in the footplates of astrocytes in subpial and subependymal regions.

Alport syndrome—several forms are hereditary male-to-male autosomal dominant, and an X-linked form also exists; characterized by neurosensory deafness and progressive renal failure.

Anderson disease (glycogen storage disease, type IV)—caused by a defect in the glycogen branching enzyme 1, 4-α-glucan branching enzyme; characterized by hepatomegaly and failure to thrive in the first few months, progressing to liver cirrhosis and splenomegaly.

Apert syndrome (acrocephalosyndactyly)—autosomal dominant; characterized by high and flat frontal bones, underdevelopment of the middle third of the face, hypertelorism and proptosis; a narrow, high, arched palate; a short, beaked nose; and syndactyly of the toes and digits.

arthrogryposis multiplex congenita—characterized by fixed contractures of the middle joints; present at birth.

Asperger syndrome—a developmental disorder on the higher-functioning end of the autism spectrum. These patients, often viewed as brilliant, eccentric, and physically awkward, fail to develop relationships with peers, have repetitive and stereotyped behaviors, usually with hand movements. See *www.aspergersyndrome.org.*

Bart syndrome—autosomal dominant; congenital aplasia of the skin; characterized by nail defects and recurrent blistering of the skin and mucous membranes.

Bartter syndrome—hypertrophy of the juxtaglomerular apparatus; characterized by hypokalemic alkalosis, hypochloremia, and hyperaldosteronism; patients have normal blood pressure but the renin level is elevated; may lead to mental retardation and small stature.

Beckwith-Wiedemann syndrome—characterized by hypoglycemia, macrosomia, and visceromegaly; patients have umbilical anomalies and renal medullary dysplasia.

Behçet syndrome—unknown cause; involves relapsing iridocyclitis and recurrent oral and genital ulcerations; 50% of patients have arthritis.

blind loop syndrome—stasis of small intestine, usually secondary to incomplete bowel obstruction or a problem of intestinal motility.

Bloch-Sulzberger syndrome (incontinentia pigmenti)—characterized by mental retardation; one third of patients have seizures and ocular malformations.

Bloom syndrome—autosomal recessive; characterized by erythema and telangiectasia in a butterfly distribution, photosensitivity, and dwarfism.

Blount disease (tibia vara)—characterized by irregularity of the medial aspect of the tibial metaphysis adjacent to the epiphysis; bowing starts as angulation at the metaphysis.

blue diaper syndrome—defective tryptophan absorption; characterized by bluish stains on the diapers, digestive disturbances, fever, and visual difficulties.

Brill disease (Brill-Zinsser disease)—repeat episode of typhus; caused by a *Rickettsia* infection.

bronchiolitis obliterans—begins with necrotizing pneumonia secondary to viral infection (e.g., adenovirus, influenza, measles); tuberculosis (TB); or inhalation of fumes, talcum powder, or zinc; and involves the obstruction of small bronchi and bronchioles by fibrous tissue.

Byler disease—autosomal-recessive familial cholestasis; characterized by hepatomegaly, pruritus, splenomegaly, elevated bile acids, and gallstones.

Caroli disease—autosomal recessive; cystic dilatation of the intrahepatic bile ducts; characterized by recurrent bouts of cholangitis and biliary abscesses secondary to bile stasis and gallstones.

cat's eye syndrome—autosomal dominant; characterized by ocular coloboma, down-slanting eyes, congenital heart disease, and anal atresia.

Charcot-Marie-Tooth disease (peroneal muscular atrophy)—most common cause of chronic peripheral neuropathy; characterized by foot drop, high-arch foot; patients may have stocking-glove sensory loss.

Chèdiak-Higashi syndrome—autosomal-recessive disorder; involves partial oculocutaneous albinism, increased susceptibility to infection, lack of natural killer cells, and large, lysosome-like granules in many tissues; patients have splenomegaly, hypersplenism, hepatomegaly, lymphadenopathy, nystagmus photophobia, and peripheral neuropathy.

Coat disease—telangiectasia of retinal vessels, with subretinal exudate.

Cobb syndrome—intraspinous vascular anomaly and port-wine stains.

Cockayne syndrome—autosomal recessive; characterized by dwarfism, mental retardation, bird-like facies, premature senility, and photosensitivity.

Cornelia de Lange syndrome—prenatal growth retardation; characterized by microcephaly, hirsutism, anteverted nares, down-turned mouth, mental retardation, and congenital heart defects.

cri du chat syndrome—characterized by growth retardation, mental deficiency, hypotonia, microcephaly, round "moon face," hypertelorism, epicanthal folds, and down-slanting palpebral fissures.

Crigler-Najjar syndrome (congenital nonhemolytic unconjugated hyperbilirubinemia)—type 1 is recessive; a deficiency of uridine diphosphate (UDP) glucuronyl transferase causes a rapid increase in the unconjugated bilirubin level on the first day of life; no hemolysis occurs and patients have no conjugation activity; type 2 is autosomal dominant and is characterized by variable penetrance and partial activity of UDP glucuronyl transferase.

Cronkhite-Canada syndrome—diffuse intestinal polyps involving large and small intestine; characterized by alopecia, brown skin lesions, and onychatrophia; patients have diarrhea and protein-losing enteropathy (PLE).

Crouzon syndrome (craniofacial dysostosis)—autosomal dominant with a range of expressivity; characterized by exophthalmos, hypertelorism, and hypoplasia of maxilla; patients have oral cavity anomalies and premature closure of the external auditory meatus.

cyclic neutropenia—syndrome involving lack of granulocyte macrophage colony-stimulating factor (GM-CSF); characterized by fever, mouth lesions, cervical adenitis, and gastroenteritis occurring every 3 to 6 weeks; neutrophil count may be zero.

de Toni-Fanconi-Debré acute syndrome—fatal; infantile myopathy with renal dysfunction; involves abnormal mitochondria and lipid and glycogen accumulation; patient has weak cry, poor muscle tone, poor suck, and lactic acidosis.

De Sanctis-Cacchione syndrome—autosomal recessive; characterized by xeroderma pigmentosum with mental retardation, dwarfism, and hypogonadism; skin is unable to repair itself after exposure to ultraviolet light; patients may have erythema, scaling bullae, crusting telangiectasia keratoses, photophobia, corneal opacities, and tumors of the eyelids.

Diamond-Blackfan syndrome (congenital hypoplastic anemia)—failure of erythropoiesis; characterized by macrocytic anemia; patients have anemia, pallor, and weakness, no hepatomegaly, elevated fetal hemoglobin, and defect in abduction with retraction of the eye on adduction.

DiGeorge syndrome—thymic hypoplasia with hypocalcemia; patients have tetany, abnormal facies, congenital heart disease, and increased incidence of infection.

Dubin-Johnson syndrome—autosomal recessive; characterized by elevated conjugated bilirubin, large amounts of coproporphyrin I in urine, and deposits of melanin-like pigment in hepatocellular lysosomes.

Dubowitz syndrome—Children with this syndrome nearly always have a history of intrauterine growth retardation involving both low birth weight and reduced length. Primary microcephaly. Facial characteristics include triangular face; small, receding chin; and broad and sometimes flat nasal bridge. As the child matures, the nasal bridge appears less wide and often becomes prominent, producing a continuous line with the forehead when viewed in profile. Tip of nose is frequently wide, rounded, or prominent, hypertelorism, shortened palpebral fissure that may be slanted, ptosis, sloping and high forehead, scanty hair and eyebrows, ear abnormalities.

Eagle-Barrett syndrome (prune-belly syndrome)—characterized by deficiency of the abdominal musculature, dilatation and dysplasia of the urinary tract, cryptorchidism, dilatation of the posterior urethra, and a hypoplastic or absent prostate.

ectodermal dysplasia—characterized by the poor development, or absence, of teeth, nails, hair, and sweat glands; patients have hyperextensible skin, hypermobile joints, and easy bruisability.

Eisenmenger syndrome—characterized by ventricular septal defect (VSD) with pulmonary hypertension.

Fabry disease—X-linked, lipid storage disease; involves a defect of the ceramide trihexoside α-galactosidase; characterized by tingling and burning in the hands and feet; small, red maculopapular lesions on the buttocks, inguinal area, fingernails, and lips; and an inability to perspire; patients have proteinuria, progressing to renal failure.

Farber syndrome—autosomal recessive; involves a deficiency of acid ceramidase; characterized by hoarseness; painful, swollen joints; and palpable nodules over affected joints and pressure points.

fetal alcohol syndrome—characterized by a small body, head, and maxillary bone; abnormal palpebral fissures; epicanthal folds; cardiac septal defect; delayed development; and mental deficiency.

fetal hydantoin syndrome—characterized by hypoplasia of the midface, low nasal bridge, ocular hypertelorism, cupid bow upper lip; patients experience slow growth, may have mental retardation, cleft lip, and cardiac malformation.

Friedreich ataxia—mostly autosomal recessive; appears in late childhood or in adolescence; involves progressive cerebellar and spinal cord dysfunction; patients have high-arched foot, hammer toes, and cardiac failure.

fructose intolerance, hereditary—autosomal recessive; involves deficiency of fructose-1-phosphate aldolase or fructose 1,6-diphosphatase; characterized by vomiting, diarrhea, hypoglycemic seizures, and jaundice.

Gardner syndrome—characterized by multiple gastrointestinal polyps with malignant transformation, skin cysts, and multiple osteoma.

Gaucher disease—abnormal storage of glucosylceramide in the reticuloendothelial system; three types: (1) adult, or chronic, (2) acute neuropathic, or infantile, (3) subacute neuropathic, or juvenile; characterized by splenomegaly, hepatomegaly, delayed development, strabismus, swallowing difficulties, laryngeal spasm, opisthotonos, and bone pain.

Gianotti-Crosti syndrome—papular acrodermatitis and hepatitis B virus (HBV) infection; usually benign and self-limited.

Gilles de la Tourette syndrome—dominant trait with partial penetrance; characterized by multiple tics (e.g., blinking, twitching, grimacing) and involvement of muscles of swallowing and respiration; patient may exhibit swearing behavior and may have learning disabilities.

Glanzmann disease—autosomal recessive; involves defective primary platelet aggregation (size and survival of platelets is normal).

Goldenhar syndrome—characterized by oculoauriculovertebral dysplasia and mandibular hypoplasia; patients have a hypoplastic zygomatic arch; malformed, displaced pinnae, and hearing loss.

Goltz syndrome—focal dermal hypoplasia; herniations of fat through thinned dermis produce tan papillomas associated with other skin defects and skeletal anomalies (e.g., syndactyly, polydactyly, spinal defects); patients also have colobomas, strabismus, and nystagmus.

Gradenigo syndrome—acquired palsy of the abducens nerve and pain in the trigeminal nerve distribution, usually occurs after otitis media; produces diplopia, ocular and facial pain, photophobia, and lacrimation.

Hand-Schüller-Christian disease—see **histiocytosis X.**

Hartnup disease—autosomal recessive defect in transport of monoamine monocarboxylic amino acids by intestinal mucosa and renal tubules; characterized by photosensitivity and a pellagra-like skin rash; patients may have cerebellar ataxia.

histiocytosis X— (reticuloendotheliosis) formerly called eosinophilic granuloma, Hand-Schüller-Christian disease, or Letterer-Siwe disease; patients may have a few solitary bone lesions or seborrheic dermatitis of scalp, lymphadenopathy, hepatosplenomegaly, tooth loss, exophthalmos, or pulmonary infiltrates.

Hunter syndrome (mucopolysaccharidosis II)—X-linked recessive; characterized by an accumulation of heparan sulfate and dermatan sulfate and enzyme deficiency of L-iduronate sulfatase.

Hurler syndrome (mucopolysaccharidosis IH)—autosomal recessive; characterized by an accumulation of heparan sulfate and dermatan sulfate, and enzyme deficiency of α-L-iduronidase.

hyper-IgE—characterized by recurrent deep tissue and skin staphylococcal infections; patients have eosinophilia and IgE levels that are 10 times greater than normal.

incontinentia pigmenti—see **Bloch-Sulzberger syndrome.**

Jeune thoracic dystrophy—characterized by respiratory distress, short limbs, and polydactyly; may progress to renal insufficiency.

Job syndrome—characterized by severe staphylococcal infections, chronic skin disease, and cold abscesses; patients may have elevated IgE.

Kallmann syndrome—familial; characterized by isolated gonadotropin deficiency and anosmia.

Kartagener syndrome—characterized by sinusitis, bronchiectasis, and immotile cilia.

Kasabach-Merritt syndrome—characterized by hemangioma and consumption coagulopathy, platelet trapping, and microangiopathic hemolytic anemia.

Kleine-Levin syndrome—characterized by unusual hunger, somnolence, and motor restlessness.

Klinefelter syndrome—XXY karyotype; characterized by seminiferous tubule dysgenesis, testicular atrophy, eunuchoid habitus, and gynecomastia.

Klippel-Feil syndrome—characterized by a short neck, limited neck motion, and low occipital hairline.

Krabbe leukodystrophy—autosomal recessive; characterized by cerebroside lipidosis and lack of myelin in white matter; usually presents by age 1 year; patients have hyperreflexia, rigidity, swallowing difficulties, lack of development.

Larsen syndrome—usually autosomal dominant; characterized by hyperlaxity, multiple dislocations, and skin hyperplexity.

Laurence-Moon-Biedl syndrome—characterized by retinitis pigmentosa, polydactyly, obesity, and hypogonadism.

Lennox-Gastaut syndrome (childhood epileptic encephalopathy)—characterized by severe seizures, mental retardation, and characteristic electroencephalography (EEG) pattern (i.e., generalized bilaterally synchronous sharp wave and slow wave complexes); patients have seizures starting in infancy; condition is difficult to treat; mental retardation is common.

Lesch-Nyhan syndrome—X-linked recessive disorder; characterized by a defect in purine metabolism; patients have hyperuricemia as a result of diminished or absent hypoxanthine guanine phosphoribosyl transferase (HGPRT) activity, choreoathetosis, compulsive self-mutilation, mental retardation, and growth failure.

Letterer-Siwe disease—component of histiocytosis X; characterized by acute disseminated histiocytosis; patients have seborrheic-looking skin lesions, bone lesions, gingival lesions, and liver and lung infiltrates.

Lowe syndrome (oculocerebral dystrophy)—X-linked recessive; patients have congenital cataracts, glaucoma, hypotonia, hyperreflexia, severe mental retardation, rickets, osteopenia, pathologic fractures, aminoaciduria, and organic aciduria.

Maffucci syndrome—multiple enchondromata and hemangioma of the bone and overlying skin; patients have short stature, skeletal deformities, scoliosis, and limb disproportion.

Marfan syndrome—connective tissue disorder characterized by ectopia lentis; dilatation of the aorta; long, thin extremities; pectus excavatum or carinatum; scoliosis; and pneumothorax.

McCune-Albright syndrome—polyostotic fibrous dysplasia; found more commonly in girls and in patients living on the coast of Maine; characterized by prominent skin discoloration with ragged edges; patients may have precocious puberty, hyperthyroidism, gigantism headaches, epilepsy, and mental deficiency.

MELAS syndrome—*m*itochondrial *e*ncephalopathy, *l*actic *a*cidosis, and *s*troke-like episodes; causes seizures, alternating hemiparesis, hemianopsia, or cortical blindness; patients have lactic acidosis, spongy degeneration of the brain, sensorineural hearing loss, and short stature.

Menkes syndrome—X-linked recessive; patients have short scalp hair, hypopigmentation, hypothermia, growth failure, skeletal defects, arterial aneurysms, seizures, and progressive central nervous system (CNS) failure.

Möbius syndrome—characterized by cranial nerve defects and a hypoplastic tongue or digits.

Morquio syndrome (mucopolysaccharidosis)—characterized by severe skeletal deformities, pectus carinatum, kyphoscoliosis, short neck, hypoplasia of the odontoid processes, C1 and C2 dislocation, neurosensory deafness, and aortic insufficiency.

multiple cartilaginous exostosis—characterized by bony projections near the ends of the tubular bones and ribs, scapula, vertebral bodies, and iliac crest; the exostoses become calcified and cause skeletal deformities; appears after the age of 3 years.

nail-patella syndrome—autosomal dominant; characterized by dystrophic and hypoplastic nails, hypoplastic patellae and iliac horns, and malformed radial heads; may lead to nephrotic syndrome and renal failure.

Niemann-Pick disease—four types; storage of sphingomyelin and cholesterol causes hepatomegaly; patients are normal at birth but experience delayed development; 50% have a macular cherry red spot.

Noonan syndrome—normal karyotype; syndrome is characterized by cardiac lesions [atrial septal defect (ASD) or pulmonic stenosis]; facial changes (palpebral slant, broad flat nose); webbed neck; short stature; a high, arched palate; and malformed ears.

Osler-Weber-Rendu syndrome—hereditary hemorrhagic telangiectasia; patients have telangiectasia in the skin, respiratory tract mucosa, lips, nails, conjunctiva, and nasal and oral mucosae.

Parinaud syndrome—characterized by weakness of upward gaze, poor convergence and accommodation, refractive nystagmus with upward gaze, and pupillary changes.

Patau syndrome—see **trisomy 13.**

Pelizaeus-Merzbacher disease—characterized by dancing eye movements, delayed motor development and spasticity, small head, poor head control, and possible optic atrophy and seizures.

Peutz-Jeghers syndrome—autosomal dominant; patients have bluish-black macules around the mouth and intestinal polyposis in the small bowel.

Pickwickian syndrome—characterized by obesity and hypoventilation syndrome; patients may have respiratory arrest, restless sleep.

Pierre Robin syndrome—characterized by severe micrognathia, glossoptosis, and cleft palate.

Poland syndrome—characterized by a unilateral hypoplastic pectoral muscle with ipsilateral upper limb deficiency, syndactyly, and a defect of the subclavian artery.

Prader-Willi syndrome—characterized by hypotonia, hypomentia, hypogonadism, obesity, narrow bifrontal diameter, and hypotonia; patients may have a deletion in chromosome 15.

progeria—characterized by premature aging, severe growth failure, atherosclerosis, alopecia, and dystrophic nails.

prune-belly syndrome—see **Eagle-Barrett syndrome**.

Rieger syndrome—sporadic autosomal dominant; characterized by microcornea with opacity, iris hypoplasia, anterior synechiae, hypodontia, and maxillary hypoplasia.

Riley-Day syndrome—familial dysautonomia; affects sensory and autonomic functions; patients have poor feeding, aspiration, no tears, high threshold to pain, markedly decreased reflexes, smooth tongue and impaired taste, and erratic blood pressure and temperature.

Rotor syndrome—autosomal recessive; characterized by elevated conjugated bilirubin, elevated coproporphyrin I and coproporphyrin in urine, and normal liver biopsies.

Rubinstein-Taybi syndrome—characterized by broad thumbs and toes, short stature, mental retardation, beaked nose, hypoplastic mandible, and congenital heart defect.

Russell-Silver dwarf syndrome—characterized by intrauterine growth retardation (IUGR), subnormal growth velocity, triangular facies, clinodactyly, simian creases, and genitourinary malformations.

Sandhoff GM$_2$-gangliosidosis type II—characterized by deficient hexosaminidase activity leading to cherry red spot in macula, failure to develop motor skills, blindness, weakness, and seizures.

Sanfilippo type A syndrome (mucopolysaccharidosis IIIA)—autosomal recessive; characterized by accumulation of heparan sulfate, dermatan sulfate, and sulfatidase.

Sanfilippo type B syndrome (mucopolysaccharidosis IIIA)—autosomal recessive; characterized by accumulation of heparan sulfate, dermatan sulfate, and α-N-acetylglucosaminidase.

Scheie syndrome (mucopolysaccharidosis IS)—autosomal recessive; characterized by accumulation of heparan sulfate and dermatan sulfate, and an enzyme defect affecting α-L-iduronidase.

scimitar syndrome—characterized by hypoplasia of the right lung with systemic arterial supply, anomalous right pulmonary vein, and dextroposition of heart.

Seckel syndrome—characterized by intrauterine growth retardation (IUGR), microcephaly, sharp facial features with underdeveloped chin, and mental retardation.

Shwachman syndrome—characterized by pancreatic dysfunction, short stature, bone marrow dysfunction, and skeletal abnormalities.

silo filler disease—acute pneumonitis caused by inhalation of nitrogen dioxide; patients have chills, fever, cough, dyspnea, and cyanosis; associated with a high mortality rate.

Smith-Lemli-Opitz syndrome—characterized by short stature, microcephaly, ptosis, anteverted nares, micrognathia, syndactyly, cryptorchidism, and mental retardation.

Sotos syndrome—characterized by cerebral gigantism, large head and ears, prominent mandible, mental retardation, and poor coordination.

Stickler syndrome—autosomal dominant; characterized by high myopia, cataract formation, and retinal detachment.

Sturge-Weber syndrome—characterized by a port-wine stain on the face at the first branch of the trigeminal nerve; patients have seizures and mental retardation.

Swyer-James syndrome—characterized by unilateral hyperlucent lung following bronchiolitis obliterans.

Tourette syndrome—see **Gilles de la Tourette syndrome**.

Treacher Collins syndrome—autosomal dominant with incomplete penetration; characterized by mandibulofacial dysostosis; patients have hypoplastic mandible; hypoplastic zygomatic arches; antimongoloid slant to eyes; deformities of the pinna; and a high, arched palate with or without cleft palate.

trisomy 9—characterized by deep-set eyes, bulbous nasal tip, an anxious facial expression, and cleft lip.

trisomy 13 (Patau syndrome)—characterized by cleft lip, microphthalmia, postaxial polydactyly, and cardiovascular anomalies.

trisomy 18—characterized by a small face, high nasal bridge, short palpebral fissures, micrognathia, small mouth, overriding fingers, and hypoplastic nails; patients have mental

retardation and intrauterine growth retardation (IUGR).

tuberous sclerosis—characterized by epiloia; patients have seizures, mental deficiency, adenoma sebaceum foci of intracranial calcification, hypopigmented macules, ash leaf spots, connective tissue nevi (shagreen spots), adenoma sebaceum, and angiofibroma.

Turcot syndrome—characterized by adenomatous colonic polyposis associated with malignant brain tumors, especially glioblastomas.

Turner syndrome—characterized by gonadal dysplasia (streak gonads stem from XO karyotype), short stature, sexual infantilism, atypical facies, low hairline, webbed neck, congenital lymphedema of the extremities, coarctation of the aorta, and increased carrying angle.

Usher syndrome—autosomal recessive; characterized by retinitis pigmentosa, cataracts, and sensorineural deafness.

vanishing testes syndrome—characterized by bilateral gonadal failure with normal external male genitalia, normal 46,XY karyotype, absent testes, and no male puberty.

VATER syndrome—syndrome involving *v*ertebral defects, *a*nal atresia, *t*racheoesophageal atresia, radial dysplasia, *r*enal dysplasia, and congenital heart defect.

Vogt-Koyanagi-Harada syndrome—characterized by vitiligo, uveitis, dysacousia, and aseptic meningitis.

von Gierke disease (type 1 glycogenosis)—glucose-6-phosphate dehydrogenase (G6PD) is absent in the liver, kidney, and intestinal mucosa; characterized by hypoglycemia under stress (e.g., fasting), hepatomegaly, and seizures.

von Hippel–Landau disease—autosomal dominant (linked to chromosome 3); characterized by hemangioblastoma of the cerebellum and retina; patients have cystic cerebellar neoplasm with increased intracranial pressure (ICP).

Waardenburg syndrome—autosomal dominant; characterized by white forelock, heterochromic irides, displacement of the inner canthi, broad nasal root, and confluent eyebrows.

Wegener granulomatosis—necrotizing granulomatous vasculitis of the arteries and veins; involves airways, lungs, and kidneys with resultant rhinorrhea, nasal ulceration, hemoptysis, and cough; patients have hematuria caused by necrotizing vasculitis.

Werner syndrome—autosomal recessive; characterized by short stature, juvenile cataracts, hypogonadism, gray hair in second decade.

Williams syndrome—characterized by mental retardation, hypoplastic nails, periorbital

Wilson-Mikity syndrome

fullness, supravalvular aortic stenosis, growth delay, and stellate iris.

Wilson-Mikity syndrome—characterized by pulmonary immaturity; occurs in premature infants; patients have slow onset of respiratory distress, retractions, and apnea; may clear in several weeks.

Wiskott-Aldrich syndrome—characterized by thrombocytopenia, severe eczema, and recurrent skin infections.

Wolff-Parkinson-White syndrome—characterized by a short PR interval and slow upstroke of the QRS-delta wave; usually occurs in patients with a normal heart but also may occur in patients with Ebstein anomaly and cardiomyopathy.

Wolman disease—fatal condition characterized by primary xanthomatosis, adrenal insufficiency, vomiting, failure to thrive, steatorrhea, hepatomegaly, and adrenal calcification.

Zellweger syndrome—cerebrohepatorenal syndrome; characterized by hepatic fibrosis and cirrhosis; patients have seizures, mental retardation, hypotonia, glaucoma, congenital stippled epiphyses, and cysts of the renal cortex.

Zollinger-Ellison syndrome—characterized by islet cell tumors that produce duodenal and jejunal ulcers; patients have high gastrin levels and excessive acid secretion.

Cardiology Laboratory

Timothy M. Hoffman

Cardiology Laboratory

BLOOD PRESSURE MEASUREMENT

Accurate measurement of the blood pressure depends on selection of an appropriate cuff size. The recommended width of the cuff is 40% to 50% of the circumference of the measured extremity. If the cuff size is too small, then the blood pressure will be overestimated, whereas if it is too large, the blood pressure will be underestimated. Auscultation of the diastolic component of the blood pressure exhibits two endpoints: Korotkoff phases IV and V, respectively. In children, phase IV (i.e., the point of diminution or muffling of the Korotkoff sound) is generally considered a more accurate representation

of the diastolic pressure. Phase V (i.e., the disappearance of the Korotkoff sounds) should be considered the diastolic endpoint if it falls within 6 mm Hg of phase IV. Standard blood pressure measurements for children from birth to 18 years of age are shown in the figure Standard Blood Pressure Measurements in Accordance with Age and Gender.

Pulsus Paradoxus

Pulsus paradoxus, a decrease of more than 10 mm Hg in the systolic blood pressure during inspiration, may be associated with cardiac tamponade (e.g., as a result of pericardial effusion), constructive

pericarditis, or severe respiratory compromise (e.g., asthma exacerbation).

Hint: Pulsus paradoxus must not be confused with pulsus alternans (i.e., a decrease in the systolic pressure on alternate contractions that indicates left ventricular failure).

Using a sphygmomanometer, the clinician inflates the cuff until the pressure is 20 mm Hg above the systolic pressure. She then slowly deflates the bladder until the first Korotkoff sound is heard independent of the respiratory cycle—this is the first data point. She continues to slowly deflate the bladder until the Korotkoff phase I sound is noted in all respiratory cycles (in inspiration and

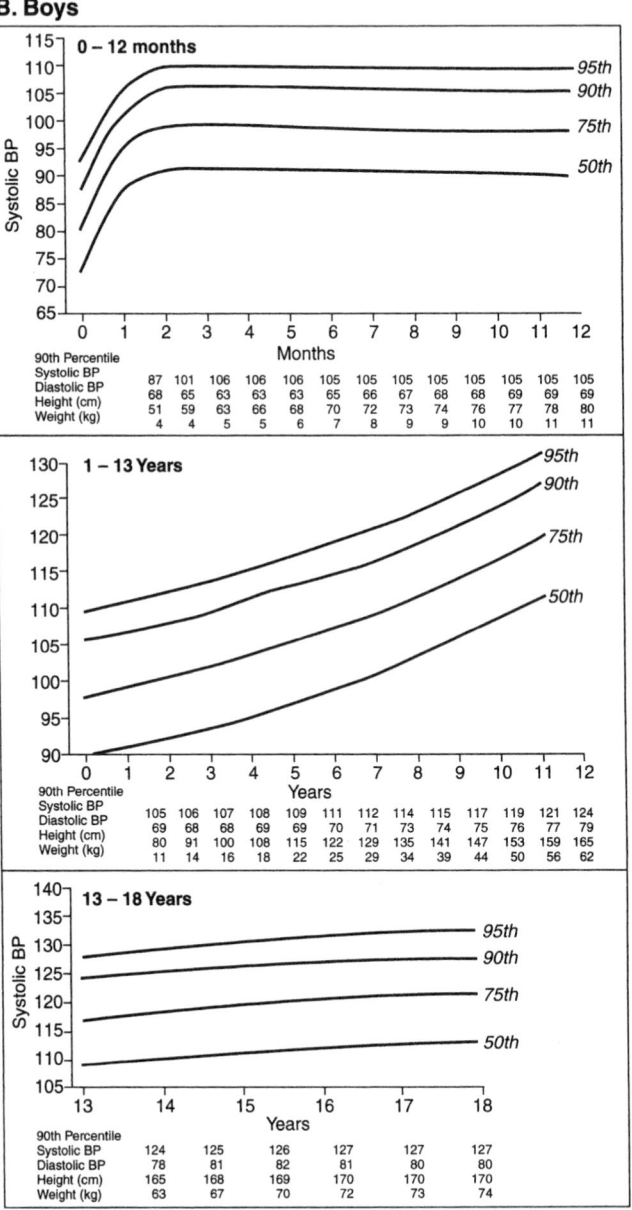

Standard blood pressure measurements in accordance with age and gender. **A:** Girls. **B:** Boys. BP, blood pressure. (From Horan MJ. Report of the Second Task Force on Blood Pressure Control in Children—1987. *Pediatrics* 1987;79:1–25, with permission.)

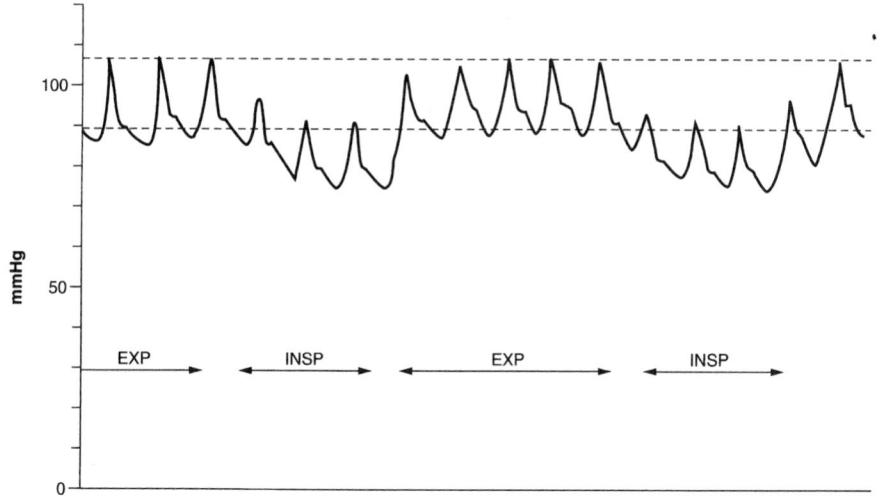

Pulsus paradoxus. EXP, expiration; INSP, inspiration. (Modified from Park MK. *Pediatric cardiology for practitioners*, 3rd ed. St. Louis: Mosby-Year Book 1996:15, with permission.)

A normal electrocardiogram showing waveforms and intervals. The standard paper speed is 25 mm per second; therefore, a single 1-mm box equals 0.04 second, and a large (5-mm) box equals 0.20 second.

expiration)—the second data point. The difference between the points is considered the reduction in systolic pressure during inspiration and is abnormal if it is greater than 10 mm Hg. See the figure Pulsus Paradoxus for a schematic depiction.

HYPEROXITEST

The hyperoxitest can be useful for differentiating cardiac and pulmonary causes of cyanosis, and is one of the first evaluations performed when confronted with a cyanotic newborn. Cyanosis usually becomes apparent at a mean capillary concentration of 3 to 4 g/dL of reduced hemoglobin, a concentration that corresponds to an oxygen saturation of 70% to 80%.

In infants with cyanosis and hypoxemia, the arterial oxygen tension (Pao_2) can range from 10 to 60 mm Hg. In an infant with a pulmonary cause for the cyanosis, administration of 100% oxygen increases the Pao_2 to a level significantly greater than 150 mm Hg. In an infant with cardiac cyanosis, the Pao_2 does not increase beyond 150 mm Hg in response to the administration of 100% oxygen. In patients with congenital heart disease, this phenomenon is attributable to right-to-left shunting (i.e., the mixing of unoxygenated blood and oxygenated blood within the circulatory system). Right-to-left shunting may be either intracardiac or extracardiac in nature.

ELECTROCARDIOGRAPHY

The electrocardiogram (ECG) provides data concerning the following:

- Rhythm
- Rate
- Intervals
- Axis
- Hypertrophy
- Wave changes (Q waves and ST/T waves)

Rhythm

Rhythm diagnosis is beyond the scope of this discussion.

Rate

The heart rate is determined accurately by dividing 60 by the RR interval (measured in seconds). For example, if the RR interval is 0.4 second (10 small boxes), the heart rate is 60 divided by 0.4, or 150 beats/min.

Intervals

See the figure A Normal Electrocardiogram Showing Waveforms and Intervals. Interval standards include the PR, QRS, and QT intervals. The normal heart rate, PR interval, and QRS duration vary with age (see the table Heart Rate, PR Intervals, and QRS Duration)

PR Interval

First-degree atrioventricular block is characterized by a PR interval that is greater

Cardiology Laboratory

Heart Rate, PR Intervals, and QRS Duration

AGE	HEART RATE (BEATS/MIN)		PR INTERVALS IN LEAD II (SECONDS)		ORS DURATION (SECONDS)	
	MEAN	RANGE	MEAN	RANGE	MEAN	RANGE
<1 day	126	95–155	0.106	0.082–0.138	0.05	0.025–0.069
1–7 days	135	100–180	0.107	0.079–0.130	0.05	0.025–0.068
8–30 days	160	120–190	0.100	0.075–0.128	0.053	0.026–0.075
<1–3 months	147	95–200	0.098	0.075–0.126	0.052	0.027–0.069
3–6 months	139	114–170	0.105	0.078–0.137	0.053	0.028–0.075
6–12 months	130	95–170	0.105	0.077–0.138	0.055	0.03 –0.070
1–3 years	121	95–150	0.113	0.090–0.140	0.056	0.032–0.070
3–5 years	98	70–130	0.119	0.092–0.150	0.058	0.03 –0.069
5–8 years	86	65–120	0.124	0.094–0.155	0.059	0.035–0.075
8–12 years	86	65–120	0.129	0.093–0.165	0.062	0.038–0.079
12–16 years	86	65–120	0.135	0.098–0.169	0.065	0.040–0.081

Adapted with permission from Liebman J, Plonsey R, Gillette PC: *Pediatric Electrocardiography*. Baltimore, Williams & Wilkins, 1982, pp 96–97 and Cassels DE, Ziegler RF: *Electrocardiography in Infants and Children*, Philadelphia, WB Saunders, 1966, p 100.

than the standard range for age. A short PR interval associated with a delta wave is indicative of Wolff-Parkinson-White syndrome.

QRS Interval

The QRS duration represents the intraventricular conduction time and is normally less than 0.09 second (in children younger than 4 years) or 0.1 second (in children older than 4 years). A QRS duration greater than normal is identified as a bundle branch block:

• *Left bundle branch block* is diagnosed when there is a monophasic R wave in lead I and no Q wave in lead V_6.
• *Right bundle branch block* is diagnosed when there is a wide S wave in leads I and V_6, right axis deviation, and an M-shaped (RSR′ pattern) QRS complex in lead V_1.

• *Left anterior hemiblock* can be diagnosed in the setting of left axis deviation associated with right bundle branch block.

QT Interval

The QT measurement is corrected for heart rate using the following formula:

$$QTc = \text{measured QT (seconds)}/\text{radRR interval (seconds)}$$

The QTc interval is less than 0.45 second for infants younger than 6 months, and less than 0.44 second for children.

Axis

The frontal axis should be determined for the P, QRS, and T waves from the limb leads (I, II, III, aVR, aVL, aVF). The hexaxial reference system (see the figure Hexaxial Reference System) is usually used. The normal axis falls between 0 and 90 degrees.
The axis is equal to the direction of the largest positive force on depolarization. A cursory way to determine the frontal axis is to note the complex that is isoelectric and locate the two planes perpendicular to it. The perpendicular plane with the greatest positive deflection is indicative of the axis.

P-Wave Axis

The location of the P-wave axis determines the origin of an atrial-derived rhythm:

• 0 to 90 degrees = a high right atrial rhythm (normal sinus rhythm)
• 90 to 180 degrees = a high left atrial rhythm
• 180 to 270 degrees = a low left atrial rhythm
• 270 to 0 degrees = a low right atrial rhythm

Hint: Classic "mirror image" dextrocardia is associated with a P-wave axis of 90 to 180 degrees in conjunction with high-amplitude forces in the right chest leads and low voltage in the left chest leads (i.e., lead V_4R has a greater amplitude than lead V_4).

QRS Axis

The QRS axis value is age-specific (see the table Age-Specific QRS Axis Values), but may correlate with congenital heart disease in certain clinical settings. For example, a northwest axis or left axis deviation (−30 to −120 degrees) may correlate with an endocardial cushion defect or tricuspid atresia. Left axis deviation is always abnormal in a newborn.

T-Wave Axis

The T-wave axis helps determine strain associated with ventricular hypertrophy. A T-wave axis that is 90 degrees different from the QRS axis suggests strain.

Age-Specific QRS Axis Values

AGE	MEAN (DEGREES)	RANGE (DEGREES)
<1 day	135	60–180
1–7 days	125	60–180
8–30 days	110	0–180
1–3 months	80	20–120
3–6 months	65	20–100
6–12 months	65	0–120
1–3 years	55	0–100
3–5 years	60	0–80
5–8 years	65	340–100
8–12 years	65	0–120
12–16 years	65	340–100

Adapted from Liebman J, Plonsey R, Gillette PC. *Pediatric electrocardiography*. Baltimore: Williams & Wilkins, 1982: 90, with permission.

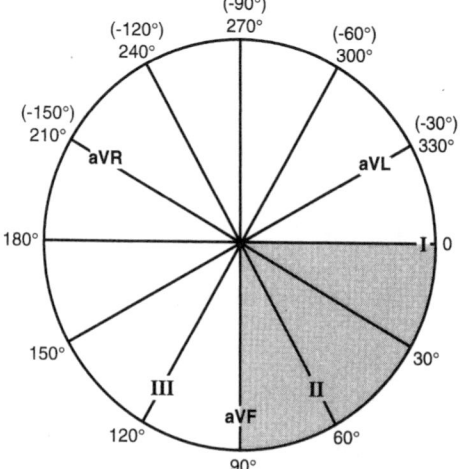

Hexaxial reference system (frontal axis). The *shaded area* represents the normal axis.

Normal Range of Values (5th–95th Percentile) for R and S Waves in Leads, V_1 and V_6

	LEAD V_6		LEAD V_1	
AGE	R WAVE (MM)	S WAVE (MM)	R WAVE (MM)	S WAVE (MM)
<1 day	7.0–20.0	2.5–27.0	2.3–7.0	1.6–10.3
1–7 days	9.0–27.4	4.6–18.8	2.2–13.1	0.8–9.9
8–30 days	4.2–19.8	2.5–12.8	1.7–20.5	0.6–9.0
1–3 months	3.6–17.9	2.0–17.4	3.6–12.9	0.8–5.8
3–6 months	6.1–16.7	2.1–11.8	5.0–15.8	0.6–4.9
6–12 months	4.0–16.0	1.9–14.4	5.5–17.6	0.7–3.3
1–3 years	3.6–15.0	2.2–20.5	5.0–17.5	0.6–3.4
3–5 years	2.6–15.6	5.0–24.8	5.4–20.6	0.6–2.4
5–8 years	2.6–13.5	5.3–21.0	7.9–20.5	0.6–2.9
8–12 years	3.6–11.3	4.8–22.3	8.4–19.2	0.6–2.8
12–16 years	2.1–11.1	5.5–22.3	7.9–17.4	0.7–3.1

Adapted from Liebman J, Plonsey R, Gillette PC. *Pediatric electrocardiography*. Baltimore: Williams & Wilkins, 1982: 84–95, with permission.

Hypertrophy

Right Atrial Hypertrophy

Diagnostic findings on ECG include a peaked P wave that exceeds 2.5 mm in any lead (often best seen in lead II).

Left Atrial Hypertrophy

A P wave with a notched contour and a duration of more than 0.08 second in lead II is diagnostic. Alternatively, a biphasic P wave in lead V_1 or V_3R with a terminal inverted portion that measures 1×1 mm will suffice to make the diagnosis.

Right Ventricular Hypertrophy

The table Normal Range of Values for R and S Waves in Leads V_1 and V_6 summarizes the normal measurements of R and S waves in leads V_1 and V_6 by age. Right ventricular hypertrophy can be diagnosed if any one of the following is seen:

- An R wave in lead V_1 that is greater than the 98th percentile for age
- An S wave in lead V_6 that is greater than the 98th percentile for age
- An upright T wave in lead V_1 in a patient older than 4 days
- Pure qR in leads V_3R or V_1
- A RSR' pattern in leads V_3R or V_1, in which the R' portion is 15 mm greater than the R wave (in a child younger than 1 year) or 10 mm greater than the R wave (in a child older than 1 year)

Left Ventricular Hypertrophy

Left ventricular hypertrophy can be diagnosed if any one of the following is seen:

- An R wave in lead V_6 that is greater than the 98th percentile for age
- A Q wave in lead V_5 or V_6 that is greater than 4 mm

- An R wave in lead V_1 that is below the 5th percentile for age
- An S wave in lead V_1 that is greater than the 98th percentile for age

Wave Changes

- ST segment elevation of greater than 2 mm in the precordial leads may indicate pericarditis, myocardial injury, ischemia, infarction, or digitalis effect.
- Tall, peaked T waves may be seen in patients with hyperkalemia.
- Flat T waves can occur in children with myocarditis, hypokalemia, or hypothyroidism.

CHEST ROENTGENOGRAPHY

When examining a chest radiograph, one must comment on the cardiac size, organ situs, and the pulmonary vascular markings (normal, increased, or decreased).

Cardiac Size

Cardiac size is determined by estimating the cardiothoracic ratio. The ratio is calculated by dividing the largest diameter of the heart by the largest internal diameter of the thorax. If the result is greater than 0.5, cardiomegaly is present.

Organ Situs

The normal cardiac silhouette in the anterior-posterior and lateral views is depicted in the figure Normal Cardiac Silhouette.

Pulmonary Vascular Markings

Pulmonary vascular markings reflect the appearance of the pulmonary arteries and veins on a chest radiograph over the lung fields. These markings can be increased in states of excessive pulmonary arterial flow [e.g., ventricular septal defect (VSD), atrial septal defect (ASD), patent ductus arteriosus

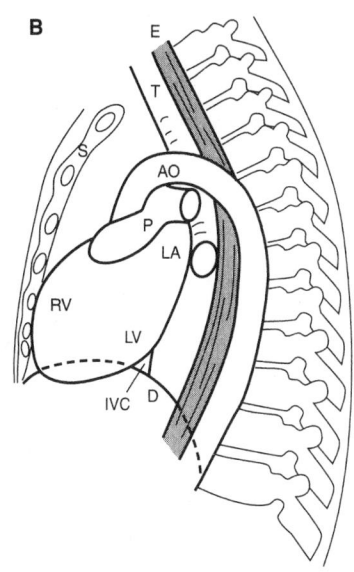

Normal cardiac silhouette. **A:** Anterior-posterior view. **B:** Lateral view. AO, aorta; C, clavicle; D, diaphragm; E, esophagus; IVC, inferior vena cava; LA, left atrium; LV, left ventricle; P, pulmonary outflow tract; RA, right atrium; RCV, right ventricle; S, sternum; T, trachea; SVC, superior vena cava. (Modified from Sapire DW. *Understanding and diagnosing pediatric heart disease.* East Norwalk, CT: Appleton & Lange, 1991:64, with permission.)

(PDA)], as well as in states characterized by excessive pulmonary venous flow (e.g., congestive heart failure, conditions characterized by pulmonary edema or pulmonary venous obstruction). On the radiograph, increased pulmonary vasculature is noted when cephalization occurs and the vascular shadows extend more than two-thirds across the lung field.

Decreased pulmonary vasculature markings are manifested radiographically as hyperlucency of the lung field and a paucity of pulmonary vasculature, as seen in patients with tetralogy of Fallot.

Cardiology Laboratory

Echocardiographic series. The numbers represent different planes along a sweep of the echocardiographic beam. **A:** Subcostal views. **B:** Apical views. **C:** Parasternal views. **D:** Suprasternal views. AO, aorta; AV, aortic valve; IA, innominate artery; LA, left atrium; LCA, left coronary artery; LPA, left pulmonary artery; LSA, left subclavian artery; MPA, middle pulmonary artery; MV, mitral valve; PA, pulmonary artery; PM, papillary muscle; PV, pulmonary valve; RA, right atrium; RCA, right coronary artery; RPA, right pulmonary artery; RV, right ventricle; RVOT, right ventricular outflow tract; SVC, superior vena cava. (Modified from Park MK. *Pediatric cardiology for practitioners*, 3rd ed. St. Louis: Mosby-Year Book, 1996:70–73, with permission.)

Hint: The following signs, seen on the anterior-posterior projection, offer clues to the diagnosis:

A "boot-shaped" heart is often seen in newborns with tetralogy of Fallot.

An "egg on a string" is noted in newborns with a narrow mediastinum owing to absence of a large thymus, and is associated with transposition of the great arteries.

A "snowman sign" is associated with supracardiac total anomalous pulmonary venous return. The left vertical vein, innominate vein, and the superior vena cava form the superior aspect of the snowman.

ECHOCARDIOGRAPHY

In pediatric patients, echocardiography is performed in a stepwise fashion to obtain subcostal views, apical four-chamber views, parasternal views, and suprasternal views (see the figure Echocardiographic Series).

M-Mode Echocardiography

A parasternal short-axis view using M-mode echocardiography reveals a cross section of the left ventricle and, therefore, can be used to estimate cardiac dimensions. Most commonly, it is used to obtain a shortening fraction (SF), calculated in the following

manner:

$$SF = 100 \times ((LV \text{ end-diastolic dimension} - LV \text{ end-systolic dimension}) \div LV \text{ end-diastolic dimension})$$

The normal value for the SF is generally considered to be 28% to 38%, independent of age.

Doppler Echocardiography

Doppler echocardiography detects a frequency shift that reflects the direction and velocity of blood flow. Doppler echocardiography is used

Normal pressure (systolic over diastolic, in mm HG), mean pressures, and oxygen saturations for children. The data are based on information compiled from healthy patients between the ages of 2 months and 20 years. AO, aorta; IVC, inferior vena cava; LA, left atrium; LV, left ventricle; PA, pulmonary artery; PV, pulmonary vein; RA, right atrium; RV, right ventricle; SVC, superior vena cava.

to detect valvular insufficiency or stenosis and abnormal vasculature flow patterns

CARDIAC CATHETERIZATION

Cardiac catheterization allows sampling of oximetric and hemodynamic data. The normal pressures and oxygen saturations for children are depicted in the figure Normal Pressures, Mean Pressures, and Oxygen Saturations for Children. Cardiac catheterization, an invasive procedure, is often used in conjunction with angiography to confirm the diagnosis and physiology of certain acquired and congenital heart diseases. The technique also has therapeutic applications, such as patent ductus arteriosus coil embolization, coil embolization of aortopulmonary collaterals, pulmonary artery angioplasty and stent placement, and balloon valvuloplasty of semilunar valvular stenosis.

Shunts

Data obtained from cardiac catheterization can be used to calculate the degree and direction of an intracardiac or extracardiac shunt. The calculation is based on the Fick principle, using oxygen as the indicator.

The oxygen content equals the dissolved oxygen (which is usually negligible) plus the oxygen capacity [hemoglobin (g/dL) $\times$ 1.36 mL O_2/dL $\times$ 10] multiplied by the oxygen saturation (as a percentage).

Flow (Q) is the oxygen consumption divided by the arteriovenous oxygen content difference:

$$Qp = \frac{VO_2}{PV - PA}$$

$$Qs = \frac{VO_2}{AO - MV}$$

where

Qp = pulmonary flow
Qs = systemic flow
VO_2 = oxygen consumption per unit time
PV = pulmonary venous oxygen content
PA = pulmonary arterial oxygen content
MV = mixed venous oxygen content
AO = aortic oxygen content

To calculate the amount of a shunt, one needs to calculate the effective pulmonary blood flow (Qp eff):

$$Qp\ eff = \frac{VO_2}{PV - MV}$$

A left-to-right shunt is the pulmonary flow less the effective pulmonary flow (Qp $-$ Qp eff), and a right-to-left shunt is the systemic flow less the effective pulmonary flow (Qs $-$ Qp eff).

Resistance

Systemic and pulmonary vascular resistance can also be calculated using the catheterization data. This calculation is based on the Ohm law (essentially, the pressure change across the vascular bed divided by flow equals resistance):

$$Rs = \frac{AO - RA}{Qs}$$

$$Rp = \frac{PA - LA}{Qp}$$

where

Rs = systemic resistance
Rp = pulmonary resistance
AO = mean aortic pressure
RA = mean right atrial pressure
PA = mean pulmonary artery pressure
LA = mean left atrial pressure

A pulmonary resistance (Rp) of 2.5 Wood units or less is considered within the normal range; however, no vascular bed is rigid, and variations in flow can affect the result obtained.

SECTION V
Surgical Glossary
Aaron E. Carroll and
Nahush A. Mokadam

aortopexy

aortopexy—a procedure in which the aorta is approximated to the anterior thoracic wall; for the treatment of tracheomalacia.

Bishop-Koop procedure—resection of a dilated loop of bowel proximal to meconium obstruction, with end-to-side anastomosis between the proximal bowel and obstructed loop, combined with end ileostomy; for the treatment of meconium ileus.

bladder augmentation—a procedure in which a portion of the intraabdominal gastrointestinal tract is used to increase the volume of the bladder.

Blalock-Taussig shunt—a procedure in which the subclavian artery is anastomosed to the pulmonary artery; for the temporary treatment of tetralogy of Fallot.

Boix-Ochoa procedure—restoration of the intraabdominal esophageal length, repair of the esophageal hiatus, fixation of the esophagus to the hiatus, and restoration of the angle of His; for the treatment of incompetent lower esophageal sphincter.

chordee correction—a procedure in which the corpus spongiosum is moved ventrally and the corpus cavernosa are approximated dorsally; for the treatment of chordee (abnormal penile curvature associated with epispadias or hypospadias).

Clatworthy mesocaval shunt—division of the common iliac veins and side-to-end anastomosis of the inferior mesenteric vein to the left renal vein; for the treatment of portal hypertension.

Cohen procedure—trigonal reimplantation of the ureter; for the treatment of vesicoureteral reflux.

colonic conduit diversion—a procedure involving two stages: (1) a loop diversion using a colonic segment, and (2) an end-to-side anastomosis of the colonic segment to the gastrointestinal tract.

colonic interposition—replacement of the esophagus with a colonic segment; for treatment of esophageal atresia or stricture when gastric mobilization is not feasible.

diaphragmatic plication—surgical shortening of the diaphragm (abdominal, transthoracic, or bilateral); for the treatment of diaphragmatic eventration.

distal splenorenal shunt—see **Warren shunt**.

Drapanas mesocaval shunt—prosthetic graft implantation from the inferior mesenteric vein to the inferior vena cava; for the treatment of portal hypertension.

Duckett transverse preputial island flap—technique in which a flap of foreskin is used to elongate the urethra; for the treatment of hypospadias.

Duhamel procedure—resection of the aganglionic colon above the dentate line with stable anastomosis to the rectal stump, normally performed in children 6 to 12 months of age for the treatment of Hirschsprung disease (see **Martin modification**).

end-to-side portocaval shunt—procedure in which the portal vein is divided and anastomosed to the inferior vena cava; for the treatment of portal hypertension.

esophagectomy—resection of the esophagus, with gastric pull-up and anastomosis with the cervical esophagus; for the treatment of esophageal atresia or stricture.

Fontan procedure—a procedure in which a graft is created to connect the pulmonary artery to the right atrium; for the treatment of hyperplastic right heart syndrome.

Glenn shunt—a shunt from the superior vena cava to the pulmonary artery; for the treatment of tricuspid atresia or stenosis.

gridiron incision—see **McBurney incision**.

Hegman procedure—surgical release of the tarsal, metatarsal, and intertarsal ligaments; for the treatment of metatarsus adductus.

Heller myotomy—myotomy of the anterior lower esophagus (always accompanied by a Thal fundoplication); for the treatment of achalasia.

ileal loop diversion—resection and implantation of ureters into an isolated ileal segment, with an ileal stoma and primary anastomosis of ileum to cecum.

ileal ureter—ileal interposition between the renal pelvis and bladder when the ureteral length is insufficient for anastomosis; for the treatment of urinary obstruction.

ileocecal conduit diversion—bilateral ureteral diversion and anastomosis to an isolated ileocecal segment and cecostomy with primary anastomosis of ileum to the right colon.

J-pouch—creation of an ileal reservoir in the distal ileum using a J-shaped configuration; used following colectomy.

Jateene procedure—arterial retransposition; for the treatment of transposition of the great vessels.

Kasai procedure—resection of atretic extrahepatic bile ducts and gallbladder with Roux-en-Y anastomosis of the jejunum to the remaining common hepatic duct; for the treatment of biliary atresia or other extrahepatic obstruction.

Kimura procedure (parasitized cecal patch)—a multistep operation in which (1) a side-to-side anastomosis is made with a portion of the distal ileum and the right colon, and (2) an ileoanal pull-through is performed; for the treatment of Hirschsprung disease.

King operation—resection of the knee with placement of a Küntscher rod to fix the femur to the tibia, followed by a Syme amputation for the treatment of proximal focal femoral deficiency (PFFD).

Koch pouch diversion—a procedure involving bilateral ureteral diversion with anastomosis to a neobladder formed from an isolated ileal segment, combined with an ileal stoma and primary anastomosis of ileum to ileum.

Ladd operation—restoration of intestinal anatomy from a malrotated state; for the treatment of intestinal malrotation.

Lanz incision—an abdominal incision made in the left iliac fossa; for colostomy formation.

left hepatectomy—resection of the left hepatic lobe (medial and lateral segments).

Magpi procedure—distal advancement of the urethral meatus and granuloplasty; for the treatment of hypospadias.

Mainz pouch diversion—a procedure involving bilateral ureteral division with anastomosis to a neobladder formed from isolated cecum and terminal ileum; combined with an ileal stoma and primary anastomosis of the ileum to the right colon.

Martin modification (of Duhamel procedure)—right and transverse colectomy with ileoanal pull-through and side-to-side anastomosis of the remaining left colon to the ileum; procedure preserves some absorptive capacity of the large bowel; for the treatment of total colonic Hirschsprung disease.

McBurney (gridiron) incision—abdominal incision from the anterior superior iliac spine to the umbilicus; used for appendectomy.

Mikulicz procedure—a diverting enterostomy performed proximal to the meconium obstruction without resection; for the treatment of meconium ileus.

mini-Pena procedure—anterior sagittal anorectoplasty; for the treatment of anterior rectoperianal fistula (boys) or rectal-fourchette fistula (girls).

Mitrofanoff technique—a modification of neobladder diversion procedures, in which vascularized appendix is used to create the stoma.

Mustard technique—redirection of blood through an atrial septal defect (ASD) using a pericardial pathway; for the treatment of transposition of the great vessels; because of associated increased turbulence, this technique is not widely used today.

Mustarde procedure—correction, using simple mattress sutures, of a prominent ear with normal or absent antihelical folds.

Nissen fundoplication—a technique involving a 360-degree wrap of the gastric fundus around the gastroesophageal junction; for the treatment of incompetent lower esophageal sphincter; patient is rendered unable to vomit or belch.

Norwood procedure—a three-stage palliative procedure including (1) atrial septectomy, transection, and ligation of the pulmonary artery, "neoaorta" formation using the proximal pulmonary artery, and creation of a synthetic porto-aortal shunt; (2) creation of a Glenn shunt; and (3) performance of a modified Fontan procedure; for the treatment of hypoplastic left heart syndrome.

onlay island flap—a technique in which a flap of foreskin is used to elongate the urethra; for the treatment of hypospadias.

orchidopexy—testicular pull-down and attachment; for the treatment of undescended testis.

orthoplasty—surgical correction of excessive penile curvature.

parasitized cecal patch—see **Kimura procedure**.

Pena procedure—posterior sagittal anorectoplasty performed in children 1 to 6 months of age; for the treatment of imperforate anus.

Pfannenstiel incision—an abdominal incision used to gain access to the lower abdomen and bring pelvic organs within reach without dividing muscular tissue.

pharyngoplasty—elevation of the posterior pharyngeal wall following a primary cleft palate repair (to narrow the pharyngeal space); for the treatment of velopharyngeal incompetence.

Potts shunt—anastomosis of the descending aorta to the pulmonary artery for the permanent treatment of tetralogy of Fallot.

proximal splenorenal shunt—end-to-side anastomosis of the splenic vein to the left renal vein with splenectomy; for the treatment of portal hypertension.

pyeloplasty—resection of an atretic ureter with primary anastomosis to the renal pelvis; for the treatment of ureteropelvic junction obstruction.

Ramstedt operation—relaxation of the pyloric sphincter; for the treatment of pyloric stenosis.

Rashkind procedure—balloon atrial septostomy; for the treatment of palliation of the great vessels.

Rastelli repair—a technique involving the closure of a ventricular septal defect (VSD) with a patch and the creation of a conduit from the distal pulmonary artery to the right ventricle; for the treatment of transposition of the great vessels.

Ravitch procedure—a procedure involving (1) creation of osteotomies between the manubrium and costal cartilages, (2) a greenstick fracture of the manubrium, and (3) the temporary insertion (for 6 to 12 months) of a stabilizing bar; for the treatment of pectus excavatum or pectus carinatum.

right colon pouch—a procedure involving bilateral ureteral division with anastomosis to a neobladder (formed from an isolated segment of the right colon), combined with an ileal stoma and primary anastomosis of the ileum to the transverse colon.

right hepatectomy—resection of the right hepatic lobes (anterior and posterior segments).

rooftop (bilateral subcostal) incision—an abdominal incision used to access the liver and portal structures.

Roux-en-Y anastomosis—division of the jejunum distal to the ligament of Treitz with end-to-side anastomosis of the duodenum to the distal jejunum and anastomosis of the proximal jejunum (typically) to the bile duct.

S-pouch—the creation of an ileal reservoir in the distal ileum using an S-shaped configuration following colectomy.

Santulli-Blanc enterostomy—a modification of the Bishop-Koop procedure that involves the resection of a distal dilated bowel segment with side-to-end anastomosis to the proximal enterostomy; for the treatment of meconium ileus.

Senning procedure (venous switch)—technique involving intraatrial redirection of venous return so that systemic caval return is shunted through the mitral valve to the left ventricle, and pulmonary return is brought through the tricuspid valve to the right ventricle; for the treatment of transposition of the great vessels.

side-to-side portocaval shunt—a procedure in which the portal vein is anastomosed to the inferior vena cava; for the treatment of portal hypertension.

side-to-side splenorenal shunt—side-to-side anastomosis of the splenic vein to the left renal vein; for the treatment of portal hypertension.

Sistrunk operation—complete excision of a thyroglossal duct cyst.

Soave procedure—a technique involving endorectal pull-through; for the correction of rectal resection.

Stamm gastrostomy—placement of an open gastrostomy tube; the opening is designed to close spontaneously on removal of the tube.

Sting procedure—subureteric Teflon injection; for the endoscopic correction of vesicoureteral reflux.

Sugiura procedure—a technique that involves lower esophageal transection and primary anastomosis, devascularization of the lower esophagus and stomach, and splenectomy; for the treatment of esophageal varices.

Swenson procedure—resection of the posterior rectal wall to the dentate line

(aganglionic region); for the treatment of Hirschsprung disease; technically difficult and rarely performed.

Syme amputation—amputation of the foot, calculated to bring the end of the stump above the opposite knee at maturity; for the treatment of proximal focal femoral deficiency (PFFD).

Thal procedure—a procedure involving a 180-degree anterior wrap of the gastric fundus around the gastroesophageal junction, preserving the patient's ability to vomit and belch; for the treatment of incompetent lower esophageal sphincter.

Thiersch operation—a procedure in which a distal rectal segment that has prolapsed is approximated to the external sphincter muscle; for the treatment of rectal prolapse.

trisegmentectomy—resection of the right hepatic lobe and the quadrate lobe of the liver (right posterior segment, right anterior segment, and medial segment).

ureteropyelostomy—partial resection and side-to-side anastomosis of a partially duplicated ureter.

uretocalycostomy—a technique for the treatment of urinary obstruction involving division of the ureter (distal to the obstruction) and intrarenal anastomosis to the most dependent renal calyx; when the renal pelvis is insufficient for anastomosis, the lower pole of the kidney is resected.

vaginal switch operation—a procedure in which the vagina is separated from the urinary tract; for treatment of duplicated vagina.

Van Ness procedure—rotational 180-degree osteotomy of the femur in which the foot and ankle are brought to the level of the opposite knee; for prosthetic attachment for the treatment of femoral deficiency.

venous switch—see **Senning procedure**.

ventricular shunt procedure—a procedure in which a Silastic catheter is positioned in a lateral ventricle and tunneled subcutaneously to drain into the central venous system or peritoneal cavity; for the treatment of hydrocephalus

Warren (distal splenorenal) shunt—a procedure in which the splenic vein is anastomosed to the left renal vein; for the treatment of portal hypertension.

Waterston aortopulmonary anastomosis—a procedure involving anastomosis of the ascending aorta and the right pulmonary artery; for the temporary treatment of tetralogy of Fallot.

Whipple procedure—resection of the pancreatic head, duodenum, and gallbladder with gastrojejunostomy, hepatojejunostomy, and pancreaticojejunostomy.

SECTION VI

Laboratory Values

Henry R. Drott

Laboratory Values

NORMAL LABORATORY VALUES

% Saturation	20%–40%
Absolute B_1 count	76–462/μL
Absolute lymphocyte count (ALC)	1266–3022/μL
Absolute T3	919–2419/μL
Absolute T4	614–1447/μL
Absolute T8	267–1133/μL
Absolute T11	1025–2587/μL
Acetaminophen	10–20 μg/mL
Acid phosphatase total	2–10 U/L
Alanine aminotransferase (ALT)	5–45 U/L
Albumin	3.7–5.6 g/dL
Aldolase	<6 U/L
Alkaline phosphatase (AP)	130–560 U/L
Alpha$_1$-antitrypsin	210–500 mg/dL
Alpha-fetoprotein (AFP)	0.6–5.6 ng/mL
Amikacin	
Peak	20–30 μg/mL
Trough	0–10 μg/mL
Ammonia	9–33 μmol/L
Amylase	30–100 U/L
Anion gap	7–20 mmol/L
Antithrombin III	91%–128%
Apolipoprotein A-I	102–215 mg/dL
Apolipoprotein B	45–125 mg/dL
Aspartate aminotransferase	
Newborn	35–140 U/L
Child	10–60 U/L
B_1 (Total B cells)	4%–21%
Bands	0%–4%
Bicarbonate	20–26 mEq/L
Bilirubin	
δ	0.3–0.6 mg/dL
Neonatal	2.0–12.0 mg/dL
Total	0.6–1.4 mg/dL
Unconjugated	0.2–1.0 mg/dL
Blasts	0%
Caffeine	5–20 μg/mL
Calcium	8.9–10.7 mg/dL
Ionized	1.12–1.30 mmol/L
Stool	0–640 mg/24 h
Carbon dioxide	20–26 mmol/L
Carboxyhemoglobin	0%–2%
CD3+ and CD8+	17.4%–34.2%
CD14+	0%–10%
CD45+ and CD14−	90%–100%
Ceruloplasmin	23–48 mg/dL
CH$_{50}$	104–356 U/mL
Chloramphenicol	5–20 μg/mL
Chloride	96–106 mmol/L
Sweat	0–40 mmol/L
Cholesterol	111–220 mg/dL
High-density lipoprotein (HDL)	35–82 mg/dL
Low-density lipoprotein (LDL)	59–137 mg/dL
Complement	
C3	
Newborn	67–161 mg/dL
Child	90–187 mg/dL
C4	16–45 mg/dL
Copper	67–147 μg/dL

NORMAL LABORATORY VALUES

Cortisol	
AM	10–25 μg/dL
PM	2–10 μg/dL
C-reactive protein (CRP), quantitative	0–1.2 mg/dL
Creatine kinase	
<age 1 year	60–305 U/L
>age 1 year	60–365 U/L
Creatinine	0.6–1.2 mg/dL
Cryoglobulin	
C3	0.0–0.028 mg/dL
IgA	0.0–0.026 mg/dL
IgG	0.0–0.157 mg/dL
IgM	0.0–0.224 mg/dL
Cyclosporin A	150–400 μg/L
Digoxin	0.5–2.0 ng/mL
DNA binding	0–149 IU/mL
D-Xylose, posttest	36–63 mg/dL (25-g dose)
Erythrocyte sedimentation rate (ESR)	0–20 mm/h
Ethosuximide	25–100 μg/mL
Factor II assay	27%–108%
Factor V assay	50%–200%
Factor VII assay	50%–200%
Factor VIII assay	50%–200%
Factor IX assay	
Newborn	14.5%–58.0%
Child	50%–200%
Factor X assay	50%–200%
Factor XI assay	50%–200%
Ferritin	23–70 ng/mL
Fibrin split products	0–10 μg/mL
Fibrinogen	180–431 mg/dL
G-6-PD assay, quantitative	4.6–13.5 U/g Hb
γ-Glutamyltransferase (GGT)	14–26 U/L
Gentamicin	
Peak	4–10 μg/mL
Trough	0–2 μg/mL
Glucose	75–110 mg/dL
CSF	32–82 mg/dL
Whole blood	60–115 mg/dL
Ham test	
Acidified	0%–1%
Unacidified	0%–1%
Haptoglobin	13–163 mg/dL
Hematocrit	36%–46%
Spun	36%–41%
Hemoglobin	13.5–17.0 g/dL
A$_1$C	3.8%–5.9%
Total	
Newborn	10–18 g/dL
Child	12–16.0 g/dL
HbA$_2$, quantitative	1.8%–3.6%
HbF, quantitative	0%–1.9%
Immunoglobulin A	
Newborn	0–5 mg/dL
Infant	27–169 mg/dL
Child	70–486 mg/dL

Continued

Laboratory Values   (continued)

Immunoglobulin E	
Newborn	0–15 IU/mL
Child	0–200 IU/mL
Immunoglobulin G	
CSF	0.5–6 mg/dL
Child	635–1775 mg/dL
Immunoglobulin M	
Child	71–237 mg/dL
Iron	50–180 μg/dL
Urine	0–2.0 mg/24 h
Iron-binding capacity	250–420 μg/dL
Lactate	
CSF	0–3.3 mmol/L
Plasma	0.6–2.0 mmol/L
Lactate dehydrogenase (LDH)	340–670 U/L
Latex IgE	0–20 U
Lead, blood	0–10.0 μg/dL
Lipase	25–110 U/L
Lyme antibodies (IgG/IgM)	0.00–0.79
Magnesium	1.5–2.5 mg/dL
Mean corpuscular hemoglobin (MCH)	26.0–34.0 pg
Mean corpuscular volume (MCV)	80.0–100.0 μm^3
Mean platelet volume	7.4–10.4 fl
Methemoglobin	0.0%–1.9%
Netilmicin	
Peak	5–10 μg/mL
Trough	0–2 μg/mL
Osmolality	
Urine	
Newborn	50–645 mOsm/kg
Child	50–1500 mOsm/kg
Whole blood	275–296 mOsm/kg
Partial thromboplastin time	25.0–38.0 seconds
Peroxide hemolysis	0%–20%
Phenobarbital	15–40 μg/mL
Phenytoin	10–20 μg/mL
Phosphorus	2.7–4.7 mg/dL
Platelet aggregation, 10 μm	>60.1%
Platelet count	150–400 10^3/μL
Potassium	3.8–5.4 mmol/L
Prealbumin	22.0–45.0 mg/dL
Primidone	5–12 μg/mL
Procainamide	4–10 μg/mL
Prolactin	2.7–15.2 ng/mL
Protein, 24-hour total	0–150 mg/24 h
Protein C	
Immunologic	50%–122%
Functional	59%–116%
Protein S, free	40%–111%

Laboratory Values   (continued)

Protein, total	6.3–8.6 g/dL
Prothrombin time	10–12 seconds
Protoporphyrin, free RBC	30–80 μmol/mol Hb
Pyruvate kinase assay	1.8–2.3 IU/mL RBC
RBC distribution width	11.5%–14.5%
Reptilase	18–22 seconds
Reticulocyte count	0.5%–1.5%
Ristocetin cofactor	48%–220%
Salicylate	<35 mg/dL
Sodium	136–145 mmol/L
Sucrose hemolysis	0%–5%
T3 (total T cells)	69%–86%
T4 (helper T cells)	39%–57%
T4–T8 ratio	0.7–2.5
T8 (suppressor T cells)	18%–45%
T11 (SRBC receptor)	75%–93%
Theophylline	10–20 μg/mL
Thrombin time	11.3–16.3 seconds
Thyroid-stimulating hormone (thyrotropin)	0.5–5.0 μIU/mL
Thyroxine	
Newborn	3.0–14.4 μg/dL
Infant	4.6–13.4 μg/dL
Child	4.5–10.3 μg/dL
Thyroxine-binding globulin	1.8–4.2 mg/dL
Tobramycin	
Peak	4–10 μg/mL
Trough	0–2 μg/mL
Total cell count	100
Total eosinophil count	100–300 mm^3
Total protein	
CSF	
Newborn	40–120 mg/dL
Child	15–40 mg/dL
Urine	0–20 mg/dL
Triglycerides	34–165 mg/dL
Triiodothyronine	0.9–2.25 ng/mL
Trypsin, stool	80–740 μg/g
Urea nitrogen	2–19 mg/dL
Uric acid	2.1–5.0 mg/dL
Urine pH	4.8–7.8
Urine specific gravity; TS meter	1.003–1.1035
Valproic acid	50–100 μg/mL
Vancomycin	
Peak	20–30 μg/mL
Trough	0–12 μg/mL
White blood cell count	
Newborn	9–30 10^3/μL
Child	4.5–11.0 10^3/μL
Zinc	68–94 μg/dL

SECTION VII
Tables

DEVELOPMENT

Table 1   Scoring System: Draw-a-Person Test

ONE POINT ASSIGNED PER FEATURE:

Head present	Fingers present
Neck present	Correct number of fingers shown
Neck, two dimensions	Opposition of thumb shown
Eyes present	(must include fingers)
Eye detail: brows or lashes	Hands present
Nose present	Arms present
Nose, two dimensions	Arms at side or engaged in activity
(not round ball)	Feet: any indication
Mouth present	Attachment of arms to legs I
Lips, two dimensions	(to trunk or anywhere)
Both nose and lips in two	Attachment of arms and legs II
dimensions	(at correct point on trunk)
Both chin and forehead shown	Trunk present
Bridge of nose (straight to eyes;	Trunk in proportion, two dimensions
narrower than base)	(if greater than breadth)
Hair I (any scribble)	Clothing I (anything)
Hair II (more detail)	Clothing II (two articles of clothing)
Ears present	

MENTAL AGE (YR)	POINTS SCORED BY BOYS	POINTS SCORED BY GIRLS
3	4	5
4	7	7
5	11	11
6	13	14
7	16	17
8	18	20

Table 1—*Continued*.   Receptive Language Development

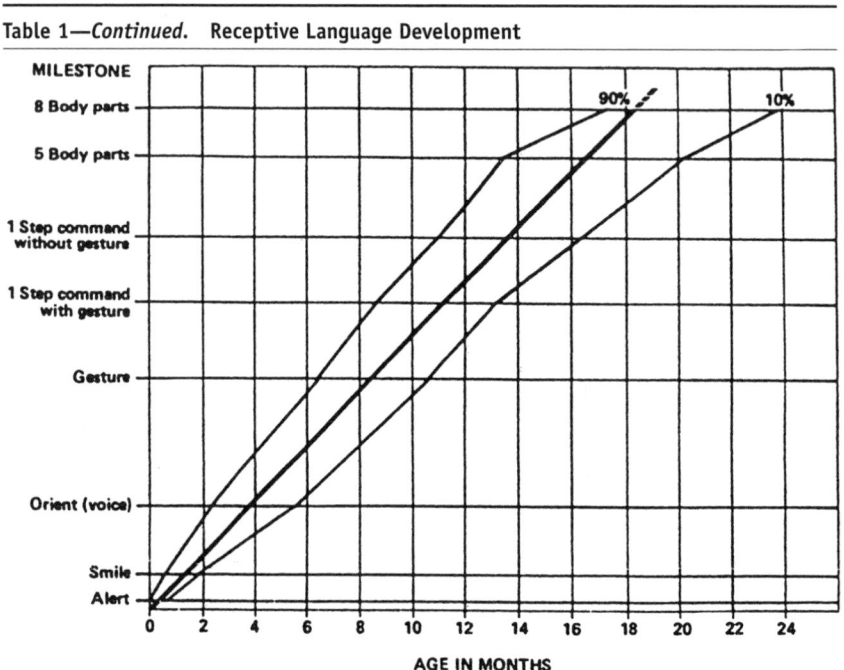

Table 1—*Continued.*   Expressive Language Development

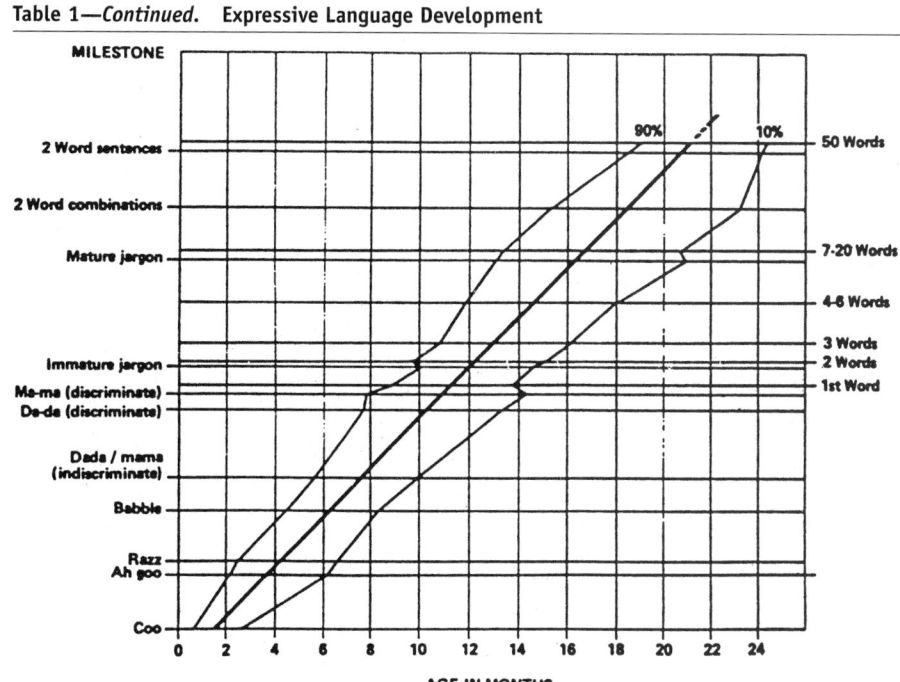

Table 2   Developmental Milestones from Birth to 5 Years

AGE (MONTHS)	ADAPTIVE/FINE MOTOR	LANGUAGE	GROSS MOTOR	PERSONAL–SOCIAL
1	Grasp reflex (hands fisted)	Facial response to sounds	Lifts head in prone position	Stares at face
2	Follows object with eyes past midline	Coos (vowel sounds)	Lifts head in prone position to 45°	Smiles in response to others
4	Hands open Brings objects to mouth	Laughs and squeals Turns toward voice	Sits: head steady Rolls to supine	Smiles spontaneously
6	Palmar grasp of objects	Babbles (consonant sounds)	Sits independently Stands, hands held	Reaches for toys Recognizes strangers
9	Pincer grasp	Says "mama," "dada" nonspecifically, comprehends "no"	Pulls to stand	Feeds self Waves bye-bye
12	Helps turn pages of book	2–4 words Follows command with gesture	Stands independently Walks, one hand held	Points to indicate wants
15	Scribbles	4–6 words Follows command no gesture	Walks independently	Drinks from cup Imitates activities
18	Turns pages of book	10–20 words Points to 4 body parts	Walks up steps	Feeds self with spoon
24	Solves single-piece puzzles	Combines 2–3 words Uses "I" and "you"	Jumps Kicks ball	Removes coat Verbalizes wants
30	Imitates horizontal and vertical lines	Names all body parts	Rides tricycle using pedals	Pulls up pants Washes, dries hands
36	Copies circle Draws person with 3 parts	Gives full name, age, and sex Names 2 colors	Throws ball overhand Walks up stairs (alternating feet)	Toilet trained Puts on shirt, knows front from back
42	Copies cross	Understands "cold," "tired," "hungry"	Stands on one foot for 2–3 sec	Engages in associative play
48	Counts 4 objects Identifies some numbers and letters	Understands prepositions (under, on, behind, in front of) Asks "how" and "why"	Hops on one foot	Dresses with little assistance Shoes on correct feet
54	Copies square Draws person with 6 parts	Understands opposites	Broad-jumps 24 inches	Bosses and criticizes Shows off
60	Prints first name Counts 10 objects	Asks meaning of words	Skips (alternating feet)	Ties shoes

Table 2A   Causes of Failure to Thrive

AGE AT ONSET	DIAGNOSTIC CONSIDERATIONS
Before birth (IUGR, prematurity)	Especially in "symmetric" IUGR, consider prenatal infections, congenital syndromes, teratogenic exposures (anticonvulsants, alcohol, etc.)
Neonatal	Incorrect formula preparation; failed breast-feeding; neglect; poor feeding interactions; metabolic, chromosomal, or anatomic abnormality (less common)
3–6 months	Underfeeding (possibly associated with poverty); improper formula preparation; milk protein intolerance; oral-motor dysfunction; celiac disease; HIV infection; cystic fibrosis; congenital heart disease; GE reflux
7–12 months	Autonomy struggles; overly fastidious parent; oral-motor dysfunction; delayed introduction of solids; intolerance of new foods
After 12 months	Coercive feeding; highly distractable child; distracting environment; acquired illness; new psychosocial stressor (divorce, job loss, new sibling, death in the family, etc.)

Reproduced from Frank DA, et al., with permission from the authors.

Table 3   Primitive Reflexes

PRIMITIVE REFLEX	AGE AT DISAPPEARANCE (MONTHS)	DESCRIPTION
Palmar grasp	3–4	Pressing against the palmar surface of the infant's hand results in flexion of all fingers.
Rooting	3–4	Stroking the perioral skin at the corners of the mouth causes the mouth to open and turn to stimulated side.
Galant	2–3	Stroking along the paravertebral area causes lateral flexion of the trunk with the concavity toward the stimulated side.
Moro	4–6	Sudden movement of the head causes symmetric abduction and extension of the arms followed by gradual adduction and flexion of the arms over the body.
Asymmetric tonic neck	4–6	Turning the head to one side leads to extension of extremities on that side and flexion on the contralateral side. This puts the infant in the fencing position.
Tonic labyrinthine	2–3	In supine neck extension leads to shoulder retraction and trunk and lower extremity extension. This is reduced by neck flexion.
Positive support	2–3	Stimulation of the ball of the foot leads to co-contraction of opposing muscle groups, allowing weight to be borne.
Placing/stepping	Variable	When the dorsal surface of one foot touches the underside of a table, the infant places the foot on the table top.

Table 4 Penile and Clitoral Length in the Newborn Infant

GESTATIONAL AGE	LENGTH (MEAN ± SD) (CM)

Male Measure from pubic ramus to the tip of the glans with gentle traction applied.[a]

30 wk	2.5 ± 0.4
34 wk	3.0 ± 0.4
Term	3.5 ± 0.4

Female Measure with labia majora separated and the prepuce skin retracted.[b]

Term Infants	4.0 ± 1.24

Preterm infants—The clitoris achieves full size by 24 wk gestation and may appear more prominent relative to the labia in premature infants.

[a]Feldman KW, Smith DW. Fetal phallic growth and penile standards for newborn male infants. *J Pediatr* 1975;86:395.

[b]Oberfield S, Mondok A, Shanrivar F, et al. Clitoral size in full-term infants. *Am J Perinatol* 1989; 6(4):453.

Table 5 Tanner Stages in the Female

STAGE	BREAST	PUBIC HAIR
1	Prepubertal, elevation of papilla only	Prepubertal
2	Enlargement of areola, elevation of breast and papilla ("breast bud")	Sparse, long, straight, slightly pigmented hair along labia
3	Further enlargement of breast and areola with no separation of contour	Hair is darker, curlier, and coarser with increased distribution on pubes
4	Areola and papilla form a second mount above the breast	Adult-type hair limited to pubes with no extension to medial thigh
5	Mature breast	Mature distribution of inverse triangle with spread to medial thighs

Table 6 Tanner Stages in the Male

STAGE	GENITAL DEVELOPMENT	PUBIC HAIR
1	Prepubertal	Prepubertal
2	Enlargement of testes (>4 mL volume) and scrotum with reddening of scrotal skin	Sparse, long, straight, slightly pigmented hair at base of penis
3	Growth of penis, primarily length, with further increase in size of testes and scrotum	Hair is darker and curlier with increased distribution on pubes
4	Further increase in length and breadth of penis with development of glans, increase in testes and scrotum	Adult-type hair limited to pubes with no extension to medial thigh
5	Adult size and shape	Mature distribution with spread to medial thighs and lower abdomen

Table 7 Normal Growth Rates

AGE	EXPECTED GROWTH RATE
First year	25 cm (10 inches)/y
Second year	12.5 cm (5 inches)/y
Childhood	6.25 cm (2.5 inches)/y
Adolescence, boys	15–38 cm (6–15 inches)
Adolescence, girls	15–25 cm (6–12 inches)

Table 8 Head Growth Velocity

FULL-TERM		PRETERM	
2 cm/mo	0–3 months	1 cm/wk	0–2 months
1 cm/mo	3–6 months	0.5 cm/wk	2–4 months
0.5 cm/mo	7–12 months	See full-term	>4 months

Table 9 Illustrations of the Primary and Permanent Dentition. *A* and *B,* The numbers represent the average age of eruption for the teeth, indicated in months for the primary teeth and years for the permanent dentition. *C* and *D,* The names of specific teeth in the primary and permanent dentition are shown.

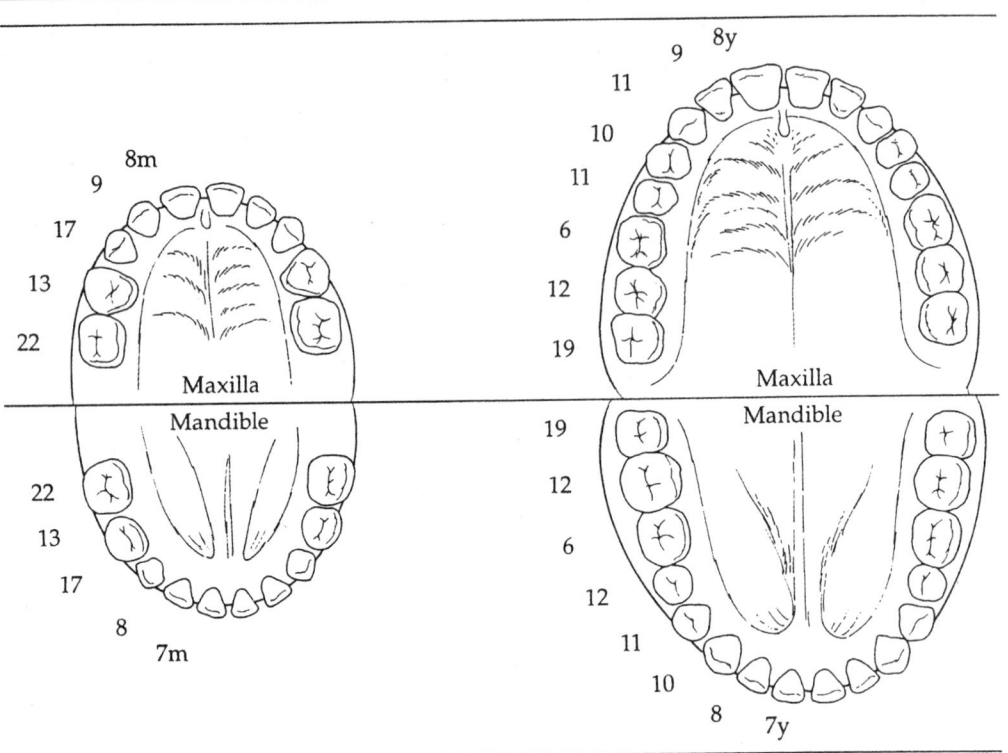

A. Primary Dentition   B. Permanent Dentition

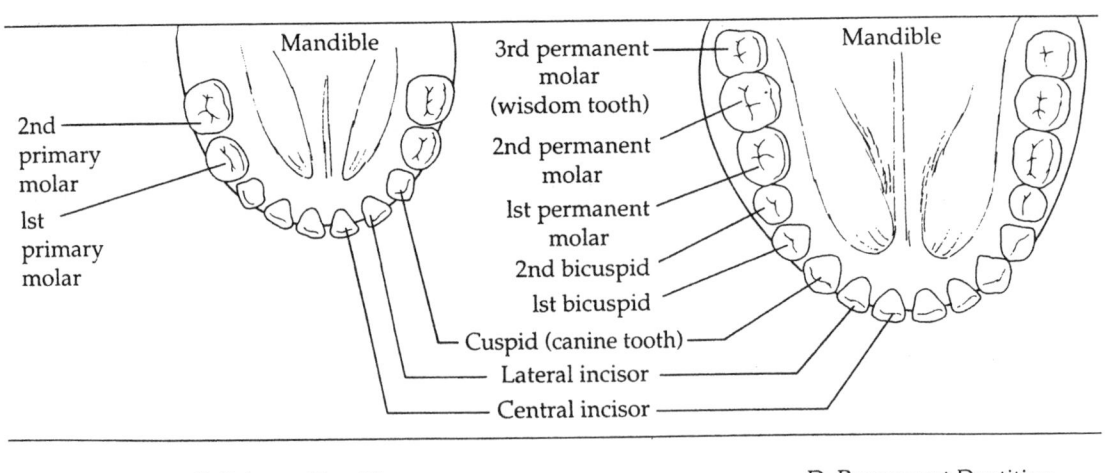

C. Primary Dentition   D. Permanent Dentition

Reproduced with permission from Nazif MM, Davis HW, McKibben DH, Roody MA. Arts of Pediatric Physical Diagnosis-3.

IMMUNIZATION

Table 10

DOWN SYNDROME GIRLS PHYSICAL GROWTH: 1 TO 36 MONTHS

NAME _____ RECORD # _____

From Cronck C, Crocker AC, Pueschel SM, et al. Growth charts for children with Down syndrome: 1 month to 18 years of age. Pediatrics. 1988;81:102–110, with permission.

Table 10A

GIRLS WITH DOWN SYNDROME
PHYSICAL GROWTH:
2 TO 18 YEARS

From Cronck C, Crocker AC, Pueschel SM, et al. Growth charts for children with Down syndrome: 1 month to 18 years of age. Pediatrics. 1988;81:102–110, with permission.

Table 11

DOWN SYNDROME BOYS
PHYSICAL GROWTH:
1 TO 36 MONTHS

From Cronck C, Crocker AC, Pueschel SM, et al. Growth charts for children with Down syndrome: 1 month to 18 years of age. Pediatrics. 1988;81:102–110, with permission.

Table 11A

From Cronck C, Crocker AC, Pueschel SM, et al. Growth charts for children with Down syndrome:
1 month to 18 years of age. Pediatrics. 1988;81:102–110, with permission.

Table 12

Recommended Childhood Immunization Schedule
United States, 2002

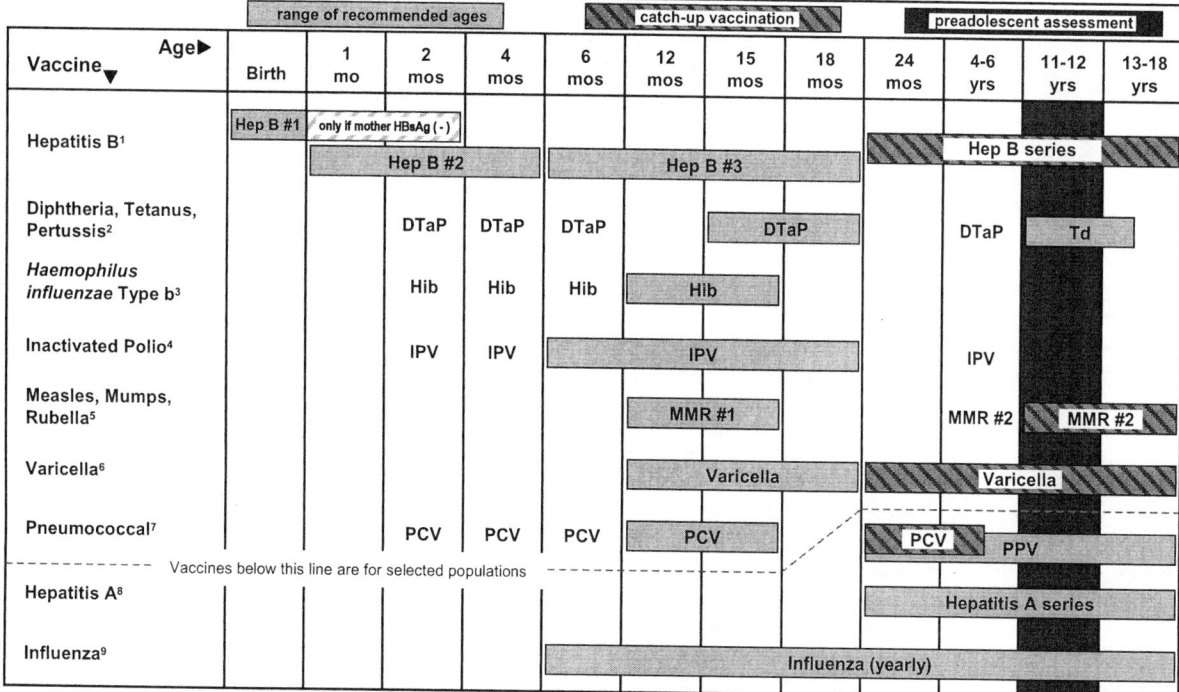

Vaccine ▼ / Age ▶	Birth	1 mo	2 mos	4 mos	6 mos	12 mos	15 mos	18 mos	24 mos	4-6 yrs	11-12 yrs	13-18 yrs
Hepatitis B[1]	Hep B #1	only if mother HBsAg (-)	Hep B #2			Hep B #3				Hep B series		
Diphtheria, Tetanus, Pertussis[2]			DTaP	DTaP	DTaP		DTaP			DTaP	Td	
Haemophilus influenzae Type b[3]			Hib	Hib	Hib	Hib						
Inactivated Polio[4]			IPV	IPV		IPV				IPV		
Measles, Mumps, Rubella[5]						MMR #1				MMR #2	MMR #2	
Varicella[6]						Varicella				Varicella		
Pneumococcal[7]			PCV	PCV	PCV	PCV			PCV	PPV		
Hepatitis A[8]										Hepatitis A series		
Influenza[9]						Influenza (yearly)						

range of recommended ages — catch-up vaccination — preadolescent assessment

Vaccines below this line are for selected populations

This schedule indicates the recommended ages for routine administration of currently licensed childhood vaccines, as of December 1, 2001, for children through age 18 years. Any dose not given at the recommended age should be given at any subsequent visit when indicated and feasible. ▨ Indicates age groups that warrant special effort to administer those vaccines not previously given. Additional vaccines may be licensed and recommended during the year. Licensed combination vaccines may be used whenever any components of the combination are indicated and the vaccine's other components are not contraindicated. Providers should consult the manufacturers' package inserts for detailed recommendations.

1. Hepatitis B vaccine (Hep B). All infants should receive the first dose of hepatitis B vaccine soon after birth and before hospital discharge; the first dose may also be given by age 2 months if the infant's mother is HBsAg-negative. Only monovalent hepatitis B vaccine can be used for the birth dose. Monovalent or combination vaccine containing Hep B may be used to complete the series; four doses of vaccine may be administered if combination vaccine is used. The second dose should be given at least 4 weeks after the first dose, except for Hib-containing vaccine which cannot be administered before age 6 weeks. The third dose should be given at least 16 weeks after the first dose and at least 8 weeks after the second dose. The last dose in the vaccination series (third or fourth dose) should not be administered before age 6 months.

Infants born to HBsAg-positive mothers should receive hepatitis B vaccine and 0.5 mL hepatitis B immune globulin (HBIG) within 12 hours of birth at separate sites. The second dose is recommended at age 1-2 months and the vaccination series should be completed (third or fourth dose) at age 6 months.

Infants born to mothers whose HBsAg status is unknown should receive the first dose of the hepatitis B vaccine series within 12 hours of birth. Maternal blood should be drawn at the time of delivery to determine the mother's HBsAg status; if the HBsAg test is positive, the infant should receive HBIG as soon as possible (no later than age 1 week).

2. Diphtheria and tetanus toxoids and acellular pertussis vaccine (DTaP). The fourth dose of DTaP may be administered as early as age 12 months, provided 6 months have elapsed since the third dose and the child is unlikely to return at age 15-18 months. **Tetanus and diphtheria toxoids (Td)** is recommended at age 11-12 years if at least 5 years have elapsed since the last dose of tetanus and diphtheria toxoid-containing vaccine. Subsequent routine Td boosters are recommended every 10 years.

3. Haemophilus influenzae type b (Hib) conjugate vaccine. Three Hib conjugate vaccines are licensed for infant use. If PRP-OMP (PedvaxHIB® or ComVax® [Merck]) is administered at ages 2 and 4 months, a dose at age 6 months is not required. DTaP/Hib combination products should not be used for primary immunization in infants at age 2, 4 or 6 months, but can be used as boosters following any Hib vaccine.

4. Inactivated poliovirus vaccine (IPV). An all-IPV schedule is recommended for routine childhood poliovirus vaccination in the United States. All children should receive four doses of IPV at age 2 months, 4 months, 6-18 months, and 4-6 years.

5. Measles, mumps, and rubella vaccine (MMR). The second dose of MMR is recommended routinely at age 4-6 years but may be administered during any visit, provided at least 4 weeks have elapsed since the first dose and that both doses are administered beginning at or after age 12 months. Those who have not previously received the second dose should complete the schedule by the visit at 11-12 years.

6. Varicella vaccine. Varicella vaccine is recommended at any visit at or after age 12 months for susceptible children (i.e. those who lack a reliable history of chickenpox). Susceptible persons aged ≥13 years should receive two doses, given at least 4 weeks apart.

7. Pneumococcal vaccine. The heptavalent **pneumococcal conjugate vaccine (PCV)** is recommended for all children aged 2-23 months and for certain children aged 24-59 months. **Pneumococcal polysaccharide vaccine (PPV)** is recommended in addition to PCV for certain high-risk groups. See *MMWR* 2000;49(RR-9);1-37.

8. Hepatitis A vaccine. Hepatitis A vaccine is recommended for use in selected states and regions, and for certain high-risk groups; consult your local public health authority. See *MMWR* 1999;48(RR-12);1-37.

9. Influenza vaccine. Influenza vaccine is recommended annually for children age ≥ 6 months with certain risk factors (including but not limited to asthma, cardiac disease, sickle cell disease, HIV, and diabetes; see *MMWR* 2001;50(RR-4);1-44), and can be administered to all others wishing to obtain immunity. Children aged ≤12 years should receive vaccine in a dosage appropriate for their age (0.25 mL if age 6-35 months or 0.5 mL if aged ≥ 3 years). Children aged ≤ 8 years who are receiving influenza vaccine for the first time should receive two doses separated by at least 4 weeks.

For additional information about vaccines, vaccine supply, and contraindications for immunization, please visit the National Immunization Program Website at www.cdc.gov/nip or call the National Immunization Hotline at 800-232-2522 (English) or 800-232-0233 (Spanish).

Approved by the Advisory Committee on Immunization Practices (www.cdc.gov/nip/acip), the American Academy of Pediatrics (www.aap.org), and the American Academy of Family Physicians (www.aafp.org).

Table 13 Recommendations for Routine Immunization of HIV-Infected Children in the United States

VACCINE	KNOWN ASYMPTOMATIC HIV INFECTION	SYMPTOMATIC HIV INFECTION
Hepatitis B	Yes	Yes
DTaP (or DTP)	Yes	Yes
IPV[a]	Yes	Yes
MMR	Yes	Yes[b]
Hib	Yes	Yes
Pneumococcal[c]	Yes	Yes
Influenza[d]	Yes	Yes
Varicella[e]	No	No

Adapted from the American Academy of Pediatrics. In Peter G, ed. *1997 red book: report of the Committee on Infectious Diseases*, 24th ed. Elk Grove Village, IL: American Academy of Pediatrics, 1997.

DTP, diphtheria and tetanus toxoids and pertussis vaccine; DTaP, diphtheria and tetanus toxoids acellular pertussis vaccine; IPV, inactivated poliovirus vaccine; MMR, live-virus measles, mumps, and rubella; Hib, *Haemophilus influenzae* type b conjugate.

[a] Only inactivated polio vaccine (IPV) should be used for HIV-infected children, HIV-exposed infants whose status is indeterminate, and household contacts of HIV-infected patients.

[b] Severely immunocompromised HIV-infected children should not receive MMR vaccine.

[c] Pneumococcal vaccine should be administered at 2 years of age to all HIV-infected children. Children who are older than 2 years of age should receive pneumococcal vaccine at the time of diagnosis. Revaccination after 3 to 5 years is recommended in either circumstance.

[d] Influenza vaccine should be provided each fall and repeated annually for HIV-exposed infants 6 months of age and older, HIV-infected children and adolescents, and for household contacts of HIV-infected patients.

[e] Varicella vaccine is not currently indicated for HIV-exposed or HIV-infected patients, but studies are in progress to determine safety and possible indication.

Table 14 Guide to Tetanus Prophylaxis in Routine Wound Management

HISTORY OF ABSORBED TETANUS TOXOID (DOSES)	CLEAN, MINOR WOUNDS		ALL OTHER WOUNDS[A]	
	TD[B]	TIG[C]	TD[B]	TIG[C]
Unknown or <3	Yes	No	Yes	Yes
≥3[d]	No[e]	No	No[f]	No

Adapted from the American Academy of Pediatrics. In Peter G, ed. *1997 red book: report of the Committee on Infectious Diseases*, 24th ed. Elk Grove Village, IL: American Academy of Pediatrics, 1997.

Td, adult-use tetanus and diphtheria toxoids; TIG, tetanus immune globulin (human).

[a] Such as, but not limited to, wounds contaminated with dirt, feces, soil, or saliva; puncture wounds; avulsions; and wounds resulting from missiles, crushing, burns, or frostbite.

[b] For children <7 years, diphtheria and tetanus toxoids and acellular pertussis (DTaP) or diphtheria-tetanus-pertussis (DTP) is recommended; if pertussis vaccine is contraindicated, diphtheria-tetanus toxoid (DT) is given. For persons ≥7 years of age, Td is recommended.

[c] Equine tetanus antitoxin should be used when TIG is not available.

[d] If only 3 doses of fluid toxoid have been received, a fourth dose of toxoid, preferably an adsorbed toxoid, should be given.

[e] Yes, if more than 10 years since the last dose.

[f] Yes, if more than 5 years since the last dose. (More frequent boosters are not needed and can accentuate side effects.)

Table 15   Suggested Intervals Between Immunoglobulin Administration and Measles Vaccination (MMR or Monovalent Measles Vaccine)

INDICATION FOR IMMUNOGLOBULIN	PREPARATION	ROUTE	DOSE		INTERVAL (MONTHS)[a]
			U OR ML	MG IgG/KG	
Tetanus	TIG	IM	250 U	10	3
Hepatitis A prophylaxis	IG				
Contact prophylaxis		IM	0.02 mL/kg	3.3	3
International travel		IM	0.06 mL/kg	10	3
Hepatitis B prophylaxis	HBIG	IM	0.06 mL/kg	10	3
Rabies prophylaxis	RIG	IM	20 lU/kg	22	4
Measles prophylaxis	IG				
Standard		IM	0.25 mL/kg	40	5
Immunocompromised host		IM	0.50 mL/kg	80	6
Varicella prophylaxis	VZIG	IM	125 U/10 kg (maximum, 625 U)	20–39	5
Blood transfusion					
Washed RBCs		IV	10 mL/kg	Negligible	0
RBCs, adenine-saline added		IV	10 mL/kg	10	3
Packed RBCs		IV	10 mL/kg	20–60	5
Whole blood		IV	10 mL/kg	80–100	6
Plasma or platelet products		IV	10 mL/kg	160	7
Replacement (or therapy) of immune deficiencies	IGIV	IV	...	300–400	8
ITP	IGIV	IV	...	400	8
RSV	IGIV	IV	...	750	9
ITP		IV	...	1000	10
ITP or Kawasaki disease		IV	...	1600–2000	11

Adapted from the American Academy of Pediatrics. In: Peter G, ed. *1997 Red Book: Report of the Committee on Infectious Diseases.* 24th ed. Elk Grove Village, IL: American Academy of Pediatrics, 1997.

IG, immune globulin; IGIV, intravenous immune globulin; IM, intramuscular; ITP, immune (idiopathic) thrombocytopenic purpura; IV, intravenous; HBIG, hepatitis B immune globulin; MMR, measles-mumps-rubella vaccine; RBCs, red blood cells; RIG, rabies immune globulin; RSV-IGIV, respiratory syncytial virus intravenous immune globulin; TIG, tetanus immune globulin; VZIG, varicella-zoster immune globulin.

[a]These intervals should provide sufficient time for decreases in passive antibodies in all children to allow for an adequate response to the measles vaccine. Physicians should not assume that children are fully protected against measles during these intervals. Additional doses of IG or measles vaccine may be indicated after exposure to measles.

FEEDING & NUTRITION

Table 16　Maternal Drug Use During Lactation

AVOID DURING LACTATION		*NO EFFECTS ON INFANT*
Alcohol	Meperidine	Ampicillin
Chloramphenicol	Oral contraceptives	Caffeine
Cimetidine	Paregoric	Cephalosporins
Clindamycin	Phenobarbital	Erythromycin
Codeine	Propoxyphene	Furosemide
Diazepam	Radionuclide material	Haloperidol
Ergot	Sulfonamides	Hydralazine
Iodine	Tetracycline	
Isoniazid		
LSD		
Marijuana		

Adapted from Roberts RJ. *Drug therapy in infants*. Philadelphia: WB Saunders, 1984.

Table 17　Commercially Available Oral Rehydration Fluids (in mEq/L)

	Na+	*K+*	*Cl−*	*BASE*	*GLUCOSE*
Pedialyte	45	20	35	30	2.5
Lytren	50	25	45	30	2.0
Rehydralyte	75	20	65	30	2.5
WHO formula	90	20	80	30	2.0

Table 18　Composition of Infant Formulas (per 100 mL)

NAME (MANUFACTURER)	*Kcal/oz*	CHO *(% of cal/type)*	Fat *(% of cal/type)*	PRO *(% of cal/type)*	*FE (mg)*	VIT D *(IU)*	*mg Ca/mg PO₄*
Cow's milk–based standard formulas							
Enfamil (Mead Johnson) with/without iron	20[a]	44%[a] Lactose	48% Palm olein, coconut oil, soy oil, sunflower oil	8% Cow's milk	1.22/0.34	41	52/36
Similac (Ross); with/without iron	20[a]	43% Lactose	48% Soy oil, coconut oil	9% Cow's milk	1.2/0.15	40	49/38
PM 60/75 (Ross)[b]	20	41% Lactose	50% Coconut oil, corn oil	9% Lactalbumin, casein	0.15	40	75/20
Gerber; with/without iron (Gerber)	20[c]	43% Lactose	49% Corn oil, coconut oil	9% Cow's milk	1.21/0.11	40	50/39
Good Start (Carnation)[b]	20[c]	44% Lactose, soy maltodextrin	46% Palm oil, safflower oil, coconut oil	10% Whey and whey protein	1.01	41	43/24
Soy-based standard formulas							
Isomil (Ross)	20	41% Corn syrup, sucrose	49% Coconut oil, soy oil	10% Soy protein isolate	1.2	40	70/50
Prosobee (Mead Johnson)	20	40% Corn syrup solids	48% Coconut oil, soy oil, palm oil	12% Soy protein isolate	1.3	42	63/49

Continued

Table 18   Composition of Infant Formulas (per 50 mL)   (continued)

NAME (MANUFACTURER)	Kcal/oz	CHO (% of cal/type)	Fat (% of cal/type)	PRO (% of cal/type)	FE (mg)	VIT D (IU)	mg Ca/mg PO₄
Preterm formulas							
Similac Special Care (Ross)	24[d]	42% Lactose (50%), polycose glucose polymers (50%)	47% MCT oil (50%), soy oil (30%), coconut oil (20%)	11% Nonfat milk whey (60%), casein (75%)	1.5/0.3	122	146/81
Enfamil Premature (Mead Johnson); with/without iron	24[d]	44% Lactose (50%), corn syrup solids	44% MCT oil (75%), soy oil (75%), coconut oil (20%)	12% Lactalbumin (60%), casein (75%)	1.5/0.2	219	134/75
Similac Neocare (Ross)[e]	22	41% Lactose (50%), glucose polymers (50%)	49% MCT oil (25%), LCT oil (75%)	10% Whey (50%), casein (50%)	1.3	59	78/46
Special formulas[f]							
Nutramigen (Mead Johnson)	20	54% Modified corn starch, corn syrup solids	35% Corn oil, soy oil	11% Casein hydrolysate and amino acids	1.25	42	63/42
Pregestimil (Mead Johnson)	20	41% Corn syrup solids, modified corn-starch, dextrose	48% MCT oil (60%), corn oil, soy oil, safflower oil	11% Casein hydrolysate, amino acids	1.25	50	63/42
Portagen (Mead Johnson)	20	46% Corn syrup solids, sucrose	75% MCT oil (85%), corn oil, Lecithin	14% Sodium caseinate	1.25	52	63/47
Alimentum (Ross)[e]	20	41% Sucrose, modified tapioca starch	48% MCT oil (50%), safflower oil (75%), soy oil (10%)	11% Casein hydrolysate, amino acids	1.2	30	70/50
Lactofree (Mead Johnson)	20	42% Corn syrup solids	49% Palm olein, soy oil, coconut oil, sunflower oil	9% Cow's milk protein isolate	1.2	75	55/37
Neocate (Scientific Hospital Supplies, Inc.)	20	47% Corn syrup solids, dextrose, maltose, maltriose, oligosaccharides	41% Hybrid safflower oil, coconut oil, soy oil	12% Synthetic free amino acids	1.2	58	83/62

CHO, carbohydrate; CF, cystic fibrosis; FE, iron; LCT, long-chain triglyceride; MCT, medium-chain triglyceride; PRO, protein.

[a] Also available as 24 kcal/oz and 27 kcal/oz.

[b] Formula with a low renal solute load.

[c] Also available as 24 kcal/oz.

[d] Also available as 20 kcal/oz.

[e] Available only as ready-to-feed.

[f] Indications for Special Formulas

NAME	INDICATIONS
Nutramigen	Cow's milk allergy, severe or multiple food allergies, severe or persistent diarrhea, galactosemia
Pregestimil	Malabsorption, intestinal resection, severe or persistent diarrhea, food allergies
Portagen	Steatorrhea secondary to CF, intestinal resections, pancreatic insufficiency, biliary atresia, lymphatic anomalies, celiac disease
Alimentum	Problems with digestion or absorption, severe or prolonged diarrhea, CF, steatorrhea, food allergies, intestinal resection
Lactofree	Lactose intolerance *without* cow's milk protein intolerance
Neocate	Cow's milk allergy, soy and protein hydrolysate intolerance, multiple food protein intolerance

Table 19   Uncommon Disorders Associated with Obesity

Alström-Hallgren syndrome
Autosomal-recessive trait, obesity, retinal degeneration with blindness in childhood, sensory nerve deafness, diabetes mellitis, small testes in males, and progressive nephropathy in adults.

Carpenter syndrome
Obesity; brachycephaly with craniosynostosis; peculiar facies with lateral displacement of inner canthi and apparent exophthalmos, flat nasal bridge, low-set ears, retrognathism, and high-arched palate; brachydactyly of hands with clinodactyly and partial syndactyly; preaxial polydactyly of feet with partial syndactyly; and mental retardation.

Cohen syndrome
Mild—childhood onset, truncal obesity, persistent hypotonia and muscle weakness, mild mental retardation, characteristic craniofacies with high nasal bridge, maxillary hypoplasia with mild downslant to palpebral fissures, high arched palate, short philtrum, small jaw, open mouth and prominent maxillary central incisors, mottled retina, myopia, strabismus, narrow hands and feet with shortening of metacarpals and metatarsals, simian crease, hyperextensible joints, lumbar lordosis, and mild scoliosis.

Cushing syndrome
Truncal obesity, hypertension, glucose intolerance, hirsutism, oligomenorrhea or amenorrhea, plethora, moon facies, buffalo hump, striae, ecchymoses, increased fatigability and weakness, and personality changes.

Growth hormone deficiency
Short stature, mild-to-moderate obesity.

Hyperinsulinemia (from an insulin-secreting pancreatic tumor, hypersecretion by pancreatic beta cells or a hypothalamic lesion)
Progressive obesity with hyperphagia, normal or excessive growth in stature, and signs and symptoms of hypoglycemia.

Hypothalamic dysfunction (due to tumor, trauma, or inflammation)
Hyperinsulinemia and hyperphagia may be accompanied by headache, papilledema, impaired vision, amenorrhea or impotence, diabetes insipidus, hypothyroidism, adrenal insufficiency, somnolence, temperature dysregulation, seizures, and coma.

Hypothyroidism
Short stature; delayed sexual maturation; delayed union of epiphyses; lethargy; cold intolerance; hoarse voice; menorrhagia; decreased appetite; dry skin; aching muscles and delayed relaxation phase of deep tendon reflexes; progression to dull expressionless face; sparse hair; periorbital puffiness; large tongue; pale, cool, rough-feeling skin; and presence or absence of goiter.

Laurence-Moon-Biedl (Bardet-Biedl) syndrome
Autosomal-recessive trait, truncal obesity, retinal dystrophy/retinitis pigmentosa with progressively decreasing acuity, mental retardation, hypogenitalism, digital anomalies (polydactyly, syndactyly, or both), and nephropathy.

Polycystic ovary (Stein-Leventhal) syndrome
Irregular or absent menses, moderate hirsutism, weight gain shortly after menarche, increased ratio of luteinizing hormone to follicle-stimulating hormone, hyperandrogenemia, and increased levels of estrone with normal levels of estradiol. May occur in association with congenital adrenal hyperplasia, Cushing syndrome, hyperprolactinemia, or insulin resistance.

Prader-Willi syndrome
Obesity, hypotonia, and feeding problems in infancy; hyperphagia in childhood and adolescence; developmental delay; mental retardation; hypogonadism; short stature; small hands and feet; and strabismus.

Pseudohypoparathyroidism (type I)
Short stature, round facies, short metatarsals and metacarpals, subcutaneous calcifications, moderate mental retardation, cataracts, coarse and dry skin, brittle hair and nails, hypocalcemia, and hyperphosphatemia.

Turner syndrome
Short stature, tendency to obesity, ovarian dysgenesis, broad chest with widely spaced nipples, prominent ears, narrow maxilla and small mandible, low posterior hairline, webbed posterior neck, elbow and knee anomalies, nail and skin anomalies, renal anomalies, and hearing impairment.

From Online Mendelian Inheritance in Man.

Table 20 1989 Recommended Daily Dietary Allowance[a]

AGE (YEARS) & SEX GROUP	WEIGHT[b] (KG)	(LB)	HEIGHT[b] (CM)	(IN)	FAT-SOLUBLE VITAMINS VITA-MIN A (µg RE)[c]	VITA-MIN D (µg)[d]	VITA-MIN E (mg TE)[e]	VITA-MIN K (µg)	WATER-SOLUBLE VITAMINS VITA-MIN C (mg)	THIA-MIN (mg)	RIBO-FLAVIN (mg)	NIACIN (mg NE)[f]	VITA-MIN B6 (mg)	FO-LATE (µg)	VITA-MIN B12 (µg)
Infants															
0.0–0.5	6	13	60	24	375	7.5	3	5	30	0.3	0.4	5	0.3	25	0.3
0.5–1.0	9	20	71	28	375	10	4	10	35	0.4	0.5	6	0.6	35	0.5
Children															
1–3	13	29	90	35	400	10	6	15	40	0.7	0.8	9	1.0	50	0.7
4–6	20	44	112	44	500	10	7	20	45	0.9	1.1	12	1.1	75	1.0
7–10	28	62	132	52	700	10	7	30	45	1.0	1.2	13	1.4	100	1.4
Males															
11–14	45	99	157	62	1000	10	10	45	50	1.3	1.5	17	1.7	150	2.0
15–18	66	145	176	69	1000	10	10	65	60	1.5	1.8	20	2.0	200	2.0
Females															
11–14	46	101	157	62	800	10	8	45	50	1.1	1.3	15	1.4	150	2.0
15–18	55	120	163	64	800	10	8	55	60	1.1	1.3	15	1.5	180	2.0

Adapted from the National Academy of Sciences-National Research Council.

[a] The allowances, expressed as average daily intakes over time, are intended to provide for individual variations among most normal persons as they live in the United States under usual environmental stresses. Diets should be based on a variety of common foods to provide other nutrients for which human requirements have been less well defined.

[b] The median weights and heights of those younger than 19 years were taken from Hammill PVV, et al. Physical growth: National Center for Health Statistics percentiles. *Am J Clin Nutr.* 1979;32:607–629. The use of these figures does not imply that the height-to-weight ratios are ideal.

[c] RE, retinol equivalent. 1 RE = 1 µg retinol or 6 µg beta-carotene.

[d] As cholecalciferol. 10 µg cholecalciferol = 400 IU of vitamin D.

[e] TE, alpha-tocopherol equivalents. 1 TE = 1 mg d-alpha-tocopherol.

[f] NE, niacin equivalent. 1 NE = 1 mg of niacin or 60 mg of dietary tryptophan.

INFECTIOUS DISEASES

Table 21 Risk Factors for Group B Streptococcal Infection

Maternal risk factors
Prolonged rupture of membranes (>18 hours)*
Premature rupture of membranes (<37 weeks' gestation)*
Preterm labor (<37 weeks' gestation)*
Fever >37.9°C (100.2°F)*
History of previous infant with GBS sepsis*
Clinical evidence of chorioamnionitis
GBS bacteriuria*
Multiple gestation
Diabetes
Fetal/neonatal risk factors
Prematurity
Meconium passed *in utero*
Low 5-minute Apgar score (<6)
Male gender (sepsis four times more common in boys than in girls)

GBS, group B streptococci.

*Risk necessitating intrapartum antibiotic administration per 1996 Centers for Disease Control (CDC) guidelines.

Table 22 Signs and Symptoms of Sepsis in the Newborn

Respiratory distress	Tachypnea (respiratory rate >60/min), grunting, nasal flaring, retractions; sometimes present even without an oxygen requirement or abnormal chest x-ray
Temperature instability	Fever >37.9°C or hypothermia
Poor feeding	Lack of interest, abdominal distention, vomiting, diarrhea
Altered neurologic status	Lethargy, irritability, hypotonia, seizures (especially if meningitis is present)
Apnea	Especially in preterm infants
Poor perfusion	Mottled, grayish, capillary refill >3 s
Tachycardia	Often a late sign
Bulging fontanelle	Meningitis

Table 23 Neutrophil Indices

NEUTROPHIL INDICES	NORMAL VALUES
Absolute neutrophil count (ANC)[a]	>1800/mm³
Absolute band count (ABC)[b]	<2000/mm³
I:T ratio[c]	<0.2

[a] ANC = % total neutrophils × WBC count

[b] ABC = % bands × WBC count

[c] I:T = % immature (bands, metamyelocytes, myelocytes): % total (immature + segmented) neutrophils

Table 24 Clinical Features Associated with Congenital Infection

Intrauterine growth retardation
Hydrops
Hepatosplenomegaly
Microcephaly, intracranial calcifications, hydrocephalus
Anemia, thrombocytopenia, petechiae
Jaundice (especially conjugated hyperbilirubinemia)
Pneumonitis
Cardiac malformations, myocarditis
Eye abnormalities (chorioretinitis, cataracts)
Bone abnormalities (osteochondritis, periostitis)

Table 25 Clinical Findings in Congenitally Infected Infants that Suggest a Specific Diagnosis

INFECTION	SUGGESTIVE FINDINGS
Rubella	Cataracts, cloudy cornea, pigmented retina
	"Blueberry muffin" syndrome
	Vertical striation
	Malformation (PDA, pulmonary artery stenosis)
CMV	Microcephaly with periventricular calcifications
	Inguinal hernias in boys
	Petechiae with thrombocytopenia
Toxoplasmosis	Hydrocephalus with generalized calcifications
	Chorioretinitis
Syphilis	Osteochondritis and periostitis
	Eczematoid skin rash
	Mucocutaneous lesions (snuffles)
Herpes	Skin vesicles
	Keratoconjunctivitis
	Acute CNS findings

Modified with permission from Stagno S, Pass RF, Alford CA. Perinatal infections and maldevelopment. In: Bloom AD, James LS, eds. *The fetus and the newborn*, vol 17, Series 1. New York: Wiley-Liss, 1981.

CMV, cytomegalovirus; CNS, central nervous system; PDA, patent ductus arteriosus.

Table 26 Interpretation of Epstein-Barr Virus (EBV) Serology[a]

	IgG-VCA	IgM-VCA	EBV NUCLEAR ANTIGENS	EBV EARLY ANTIGENS
No evidence of infection	<10	<10	<2	<10
Acute infection	>10	≥10	<2	≥20
Convalescent infection	>10	Variable	>2	Variable
Remote past infection	≥10	<10	>2	≤20

[a] Values are expressed in reciprocal titers as measured by standard immunofluorescence methods.

GASTROINTESTINAL

Table 27   Classic Clinical Findings in Disorders Characterized by Abdominal Pain

DISORDER	TYPICAL CLINICAL PICTURE	DEFINITIVE DIAGNOSTIC TEST
Peptic ulcer disease	Burning or sharp midepigastric pain that occurs 1–3 hours after meals and is exacerbated by spicy food and relieved by antacids; family history of peptic ulcer disease	Endoscopy
Pancreatitis	Episodic left upper quadrant pain that occurs 5–10 minutes after meals, radiates to the back, and is exacerbated by fatty foods	Pancreatic ultrasound or CT scan Serum amylase level ($\uparrow$)
Urinary tract infection	Suprapubic pain, burning on urination, urinary frequency, urinary urgency	Urine culture Urinalysis
Renal calculi	Severe periodic cramping pain that occurs in the flank and occasionally radiates to the groin; costovertebral angle tenderness; family history of renal calculi	Urinalysis Renal ultrasound
Periappendiceal abscess	Right lower quadrant pain; rebound and direct tenderness; anorexia and vomiting; fever	Barium enema Laparoscopy WBC count ($\uparrow$)
Gallbladder disease	Right upper quadrant pain that occurs 5–10 minutes after meals and is exacerbated by fatty foods; family history of gallstones	Gallbladder ultrasound
Menstrual pain	Cramping suprapubic pain that occurs during the menses	Trial with NSAIDs
Pelvic inflammatory disease (PID)	Suprapubic pain	Cervical culture
Functional abdominal pain (irritable bowel syndrome)	Cramping periumbilical pain that is exacerbated by eating and relieved by defecation	Trial with Metamucil
Lactose intolerance	Cramping periumbilical pain that increases following ingestion of dairy products and is accompanied by flatulence and bloating	Trial with a milk-free diet Breath hydrogen study for lactose deficiency
Inflammatory bowel disease	Right lower quadrant cramping and tenderness; anemia; guaiac-positive stool	Colonoscopy Barium enema Upper gastrointestinal series ESR ($\uparrow$), platelet count ($\uparrow$), WBC count ($\uparrow$)
Esophagitis	Epigastric and substernal pain that is relieved by antacids and exacerbated by lying down; history of iron deficiency; anemia; guaiac-positive stool	Endoscopy
Lead poisoning	Abdominal pain; history of pica; microcytic anemia; basophilic stippling	Serum lead level
Pancreatic pseudocyst	Left upper quadrant pain; recurrent vomiting; history of abdominal pain	Abdominal ultrasound
Sickle cell disease (SCD)	Periumbilical pain that responds to rest and rehydration	Sickle cell preparation Hemoglobin Electrophoresis
Abdominal epilepsy	Periodic severe abdominal pain that is often associated with seizures	Trial with anticonvulsants
Abdominal migraine	Severe abdominal pain; family history of migraine; recurrent headache, fever, and vomiting; unilateral or occipital headache; somatic complaints	Trial with antimigraine medications
Depression	Social withdrawal; decreased activity; irritability; poor attention span; difficulty sleeping	Trial with antidepressant medications
School avoidance	Nonspecific abdominal pain; severe anxiety reaction; pain that is more severe on weekdays and improves on weekends	

Modified with permission from Olson AD. Abdominal pain. In: Stockman JA, ed. *Difficult diagnosis in pediatrics*. Philadelphia: WB Saunders, 1990; p.253.

ESR, erythrocyte sedimentation rate; NSAIDs, nonsteroidal antiinflammatory drugs; WBC, white blood cell; $\uparrow$, increased.

Table 28 Abdominal Masses Commonly Associated with Calcification

Neuroblastoma
Teratoma
   Ovarian
   Sacrococcygeal
Adrenal hematoma
Hepatic hemangioma
Meconium peritonitis

Table 29 Comparison of Functional Constipation and Hirschsprung Disease

	FUNCTIONAL CONSTIPATION	*HIRSCHSPRUNG DISEASE*
Symptoms as a newborn	Rare	Almost always
Late onset (after 3 years)	Common	Rare
Difficult bowel training	Common	Rare
Stool size	Large	Small, ribbonlike
Urge to defecate	Rare	Common
Obstructive symptoms	Rare	Common
Enterocolitis	Rare	Sometimes
Failure to thrive	Rare	Common
Abdominal distention	Rare	Common
Stool in rectal ampulla	Common	None
Barium enema	Copious stool / No transition zone	Delayed evacuation / Transition zone
Rectal biopsy	Normal	No ganglion cells / Increased anticholinesterase staining
Anorectal manometry	Distention of rectum causes relaxation of the internal sphincter	No sphincter relaxation

Table 30 Commonly Used Pediatric Medications that May Cause Cholestasis and Hepatotoxicity

Anticonvulsants
   Phenobarbital
   Diphenylhydantoin
   Carbamazepine
   Valproic acid
Antimicrobials
   Tetracycline
   Erythromycin (estolate preparations)
   Sulfonamides
   Ketoconazole
   Isoniazid
   Rifampin
   Griseofulvin

Immunosuppressants
   Cyclosporine
   Azathioprine
   Methotrexate
Steroids
   Corticosteroids
   Androgens
   Oral contraceptives
Miscellaneous drugs
   Acetaminophen
   Salicylates
   Chlorpromazine
   Cimetidine
   Iron preparations (with overdosage)

A large number of less commonly encountered agents, including antineoplastic agents, antidepressants, antipsychotics, and tranquilizers can also cause cholestasis and hepatotoxicity.

Table 31 Defects in Hepatic Bilirubin Conjugation

DISEASE	*DEFECT*	*GENETICS*
Gilbert disease	Underactivity of the transferase, defective uptake of albumin-bound bilirubin from the plasma	Autosomal recessive
Crigler-Najjar syndrome		
Type I	Complete absence of the transferase enzyme	Autosomal recessive
Type II	Partial absence of the transferase enzyme (less severe than type I)	Autosomal dominant

Table 32 Foods and Drugs Mimicking Blood in the Stool

FALSE HEMATOCHEZIA	*FALSE MELENA*	*FALSE HEME-POSITIVE STOOLS*
Foods that contain red dye	Spinach	Red meat
Juice	Blueberries	Cherries
Candy	Licorice	Tomato skin
Kool-Aid	Purple grapes	Iron supplements
Jello	Chocolate	
Tomatoes	Grape juice	
Beets	Bismuth subsalicylate	
Cranberries	Iron supplements	

Table 33   Clinical Signs of Dehydration in Children

PARAMETER	MILD	MODERATE	SEVERE
Activity	Normal	Lethargic	Lethargic to comatose
Color	Pale	Gray	Mottled
Urine output	Decreased (<2–3 mL/kg/hr)	Oliguric (<1 mL/kg/hr)	Anuric
Fontanelle	Flat	Depressed	Sunken
Mucous membranes	Dry	Very dry	Cracked
Skin turgor	Slightly decreased	Markedly decreased	Tenting
Pulse	Normal to increased	Increased	Grossly tachycardic
Blood pressure	Normal	Normal	Decreased
Weight Loss	5%	10%	15%

Hypernatremic dehydration may be accompanied by moderate clinical signs. Reprinted with permission from Rogers MC: Shock. In: Rogers MC, Helfaer MA, eds. *Handbook of pediatric intensive care,* 2nd ed. Baltimore: Williams & Wilkins, 1994:140.

Table 34   Therapy for Hyperlipidemia

TYPE	MECHANISM	REDUCTION IN CHOLESTEROL (%)	EFFECT ON VLDL	EFFECT ON HDL	SIDE EFFECT	DOSE
Nonpharmacological therapy American Heart Association diet	Limits exogenous cholesterol	10–15	Decrease	Decrease		N/A
Exercise	Improves insulin resistance	Some decrease	Decrease	Increase		N/A
Weight Loss	Improves insulin resistance	Some decrease	Decrease	Mild increase		N/A
Pharmacological therapy Bile acid resins	Accelerate LDL disposal	20–30	Mild decrease	Mild increase	Epigastric distress, constipation, bloating, interferes with some drug absorption	Up to 24 g/day cholestyramine in divided doses
Nicotinic acid or niacin	Reduces VLDL and LDL synthesis increases HDL	25	50% decrease	30%–40% increase	Flushing, headache, tachycardia, gastrointestinal distress, activation of peptic ulcer disease and inflammatory bowel disease, hepatic dysfunction	Titrate up to 1 g 3 times/day
Probucol	Increases LDL disposal; reduces HDL/LDL	5–15		Decrease	Nausea, diarrhea, flatulence, eosinophelia, hepatic dysfunction, prolongation of QT interval	0.5 g 2 times/day
Gemfibrozil	Enhances VLDL breakdown; decreases VLDL production	Decrease	40%–50% decrease	20%–30% increase	Rarely myositis; should not be used in patients with renal disease, cholelithiasis, or liver dysfunction	600 mg 2 times/day
HMG CoA reductase inhibitor (lovastatin)	Inhibits cholesterol synthesis; increases LDL disposal	30–40			Elevated liver enzymes, myositis, cataracts in animals	20–40 mg 2 times/day

HDL, high-density lipoprotein; HMG CoA, 3-hydroxy-3-methylglutaryl coenzyme A; LDL, low-density lipoprotein; VLDL, very-low-density lipoprotein.

HEPATIC

Table 34A   Expected Liver Span of Infants and Children

	BOYS		GIRLS	
AGE (YR)	MEAN ESTIMATED LIVER SPAN	STANDARD ERROR OF MEAN	MEAN ESTIMATED LIVER SPAN	STANDARD ERROR OF MEAN
6 mo	2.4	2.5	2.8	2.6
1	2.8	2.0	3.1	2.1
2	3.5	1.6	3.6	1.7
3	4.0	1.6	4.0	1.7
4	4.4	1.6	4.3	1.6
5	4.8	1.5	4.5	1.6
6	5.1	1.5	4.8	1.6
8	5.6	1.5	5.1	1.6
10	6.1	1.6	5.4	1.7
12	6.5	1.8	5.6	1.8
14	6.8	2.0	5.8	2.1
16	7.1	2.2	6.0	2.3
18	7.4	2.5	6.1	2.6
20	7.7	2.8	6.3	2.9

From Lawson EE, Grand RJ, Neff RK,et al. *Am J Dis Child* 1978;132:475, with permission.

Table 34B   Review of Liver Function Tests

I. LIVER FUNCTION TESTS

AP	AST	ALT	GGT	5 = NUC
Liver	Hepatocyte	Hepatocyte	Placenta	Biliary
Bone	Muscle	Muscle	Pancreas	
Intestine			Kidney	
Placenta			Bile	
Tumors			Ducts	
			Choroid	

II. "TRUE" LIVER FUNCTION TESTS
Prothrombin time
Albumin
Bile acids and salts
Factor II, V, VII, IX, X
    Vitamin k-dependent factors: II, VII, IX, X

III. LIVER FUNCTION TESTS
Clinical pearls for daily use:

	ALKALINE PHOSPHATASE	γ-GGT
Low	Zinc deficiency	Bile acid deficiency
	Wilson disease	
	Cystic fibrosis	
High	See other List	Cholestasis, ICP

IV. LIVER FUNCTION TESTS
Clinical pearls for daily use: Elevated transaminases and normal bilirubin,
    GGT, and alkaline phosphatase

Table 34C   Clinical Disease States and Age of Presentation of Hepatomegaly

AGE	CLINICAL DISEASE STATES
Newborn (Birth–2 mo)	Intrauterine and intrapartum acquired infection (TORCH, syphilis, other)
	Erythroblastosis fetalis
	Neonatal hepatitis, α_1-antitrypsin, Alagille syndrome
	Bitiary atresia
	Congestive heart failure
	Congenital paroxysmal atrial tachycardia
	Sepsis
Infant (2–12 mo)	Cystic fibrosis
	Metabolic disease: glycogen storage, α_1-antitrypsin deficiency, galactosemia, tyrosinemia, hereditary fructose intolerance, other
	Neonatal hepatitis, hepatitis B
	HIV infection (AIDS)
	Histiocytosis
	Malnutrition
	Tumors (intrinsic, metastatic)
	Cholelithiasis
	Choledochal cyst
Young child (1–6 yrs)	Viral hepatitis
	Drug-toxic hepatitis
	Parasitic
	Tumor
	Leukemia, lymphoma
Older child, adolescent (7–20 yrs)	Viral hepatitis
	Drug-toxic hepatitis
	Wilson disease
	Chronic active hepatitis
	Congenital hepatic fibrosis
	Focal nodular hyperplasia, adenoma
	α_1-Antitrypsin deficiency
	Reye syndrome
	Sickle cell anemia
	Cholelithiasis
	Juvenile rheumatoid arthritis, lupus erythematosus, sarcoidosis
	Leukemia, lymphoma
	Gonococcal perihepatitis
	Cystic fibrosis
	Diabetes

Adapted from Walker, WA, Mathia RK. *Pediatr Clin North Am* 1975;22:929.

ELECTROLYTES

Table 35   Assessment of Hypernatremia

UNDERLYING CAUSE	ECF VOLUME	URINE OUTPUT	URINE SODIUM	SPECIFIC GRAVITY
Sodium excess	Increased	Normal or increased	Increased	High
Water loss (DI)	Decreased	Increased	Decreased	High
Sodium and water loss (water > sodium)	Normal or decreased	Decreased	Increased	Low

DI, diabetes insipidus; ECF, extracellular fluid.

Table 36 Assessment of Hyponatremia

IF URINE OUTPUT DECREASED AND UNₐ <20 mEq/L	IF URINE OUTPUT DECREASED AND UNₐ >20 mEq/L	IF URINE OUTPUT NORMAL OR INCREASED AND UNₐ >20 mEq/L	IF URINE OUTPUT NORMAL OR INCREASED AND UNₐ >20 mEq/L
Effective intravascular volume, consider: CHF, nephrotic syndrome, dehydration, liver disease, third spacing conditions	Renal failure or increased ADH	Water intoxication	Renal NaCL wasting Nonoliguric renal failure, adrenal insufficiency Osmotic diuretic use or osmotic diuresis

The column headers use UN_a notation.

Table 37 Conditions Associated with Increased ADH/ADH-Like Effect and Hyponatremia

Pain

Vomiting

CNS disorders: including injuries, infection, tumors

Intrathoracic disorders: including infections, mechanical ventilation

Drugs: narcotics, barbiturates, carbamazepine, NSAIDs, cyclophosphamide, vincristine, others not commonly used in pediatrics

Table 38 Determination of Serum Osmolality

Reliable estimate under most circumstances:

$$Serum\ Osm = 2(Na\ mEq/L) + 10$$

Estimate when there is hyperglycemia or azotemia

$$Serum\ Osm = 2(Na) + glucose/18 + BUN/2.8$$

Table 39 Drugs Associated with Hyperkalemia

Potassium-sparing diuretics (e.g., spironolactone, triamterene, amiloride)

Potassium supplements (e.g., potassium chloride)

Potassium-containing penicillins

Stored blood

Cyclosporine

Nonsteroidal antiinflammatory drugs (NSAIDs)

Heparin

Angiotensin-converting enzyme (ACE) inhibitors

β-adrenergic blockers

Chemotherapeutic agents

Table 40 Treatment of Hyperkalemia

AGENT	INDICATION	MECHANISM OF ACTION	DOSE	SIDE EFFECTS/POTENTIAL PROBLEMS
10% Calcium gluconate	ECG changes	Stabilizes membranes	1 mg/kg IV over 5–10 minutes	Hypercalcemia
Sodium bicarbonate	ECG changes or very high K^+ level	Shifts K^+ to intracellular compartment	1 mg/kg IV over 5–10 minutes	Sodium load
Glucose plus insulin	ECG changes or very high K^+ level	Shifts K^+ to intracellular compartment	0.25–0.5 gm/kg glucose plus 0.3 U insulin/gm glucose over 30–60 minutes	Hyper- or hypoglycemia
Kayexalate resin	To remove K^+ from body	K^+ binds to resin in gut	1 gm/kg PO or PR in 50%–70% sorbitol	Constipation
Furosemide	Symptomatic hyperkalemia	Enhances urinary K^+ excretion	1–2 mg/kg IV	May not be enough renal function to be effective
Hemo- or peritoneal dialysis	No renal function	Removes K^+ in dialysate	...	Risks associated with dialysis
Exchange transfusion	ECG changes or very high K^+ level	Donor blood has had most K^+ removed	Double volume	Risks associated with exchange transfusion

ECG, electrocardiogram; IV, intravenous; K^+, potassium; PO, orally; PR, parenterally.

Table 41   Drugs Associated with Hypokalemia

Drugs associated with increased renal loss
  Aminoglycoside toxicity
  Amphotericin B
  Cisplatin
  Penicillins in high doses
  Corticosteroids
  Diuretics (except for potassium-sparing ones)
Drugs associated with increased cellular uptake of potassium
  Terbutaline
  Epinephrine
  β-adrenergic agents (e.g., albuterol)
  Theophylline toxicity
  Barium toxicity
  Insulin

Table 42   Oral Potassium Supplements

PREPARATION	FORMULATION	POTASSIUM SUPPLIED
Potassium phosphate	Tablet	1.1, 2.3, or 3.7 mEq
Potassium chloride	Extentabs	10 mEq
	Powder packet	20 mEq
	Effervescent tablets	20 mEq
	Liquid	20 mEq
Potassium citrate	Tablets, crystals, or syrup	1 mEq/mL (Polycitra) or 2 mEq/mL (Polycitra-K)
Potassium gluconate	Liquid	20 mEq/15 mL

Table 43   Commonly Used Calcium Preparations

PREPARATION	ELEMENTAL CALCIUM CONTENT	ROUTE
Calcium gluconate (10%)	1 mL = 9 mg = 0.45 mEq	IV
Calcium chloride (10%)	1 mL = 27 mg = 1.36 mEq	IV
Calcium glubionate (Neocalglucon)	1 mL = 23 mg = 1.12 mEq	PO

Table 44   Calcium Needs

Maintenance calcium (not precisely known)	20–50 mg/kg/d (elemental calcium)
Emergency calcium (for severe symptoms)	10–20 mg/kg (elemental calcium) slow IV with cardiac monitor

RENAL

Table 45   Characteristics of Renal Tubular Acidosis

	TYPE 1	TYPE 2	TYPE 3
Renal function?	Normal	Normal	Normal or decreased
Failure to thrive?	Yes	Yes	Yes
Polyuria or polydipsia?	Yes	Yes	No
Potassium level?	Normal or low	Normal or low	Elevated
Bicarbonate leak?	Usually	Significant	Small
Urine maximally acid?	No (pH > 6)	Yes	Yes
Nephrocalcinosis or nephrolithiasis?	Yes	No	No
Fanconi syndrome?	No	Often	No
Osteomalacia or rickets?	Rarely	If Fanconi syndrome is present	No

Table 46   Toxins Removed by Hemodialysis

TOXIN	MEASURED LEVEL SUGGESTIVE OF NEED FOR HEMODIALYSIS[a]
Acetaminophen	>100 μg/mL in conjunction with antidote
Arsenic	Only with coexistent renal failure
Bromide	>150 mg/dL and severe symptoms
Chloral hydrate	250 mg/dL
Ethanol	600 mg/dL
Ethylene glycol	50 mg/dL
Isopropanol	400 mg/dL
Lithium	4 mEq/L in acute overdose
	As needed for severe symptoms in chronic overdose
Methanol	50 mq/dL
Salicylates	100–120 mg/dL in acute overdose
	60–800 mg/dL in chronic overdose

[a] The decision to perform hemodialysis should be based on physical findings as well as drug levels. A repeat measure should be obtained when the drug level is elevated to ensure that a laboratory error has not occurred. In addition, units of measure should be checked before instituting hemodialysis.

Table 47   Toxins Removed by Charcoal Hemoperfusion[a]

TOXIN	MEASURED LEVEL SUGGESTIVE OF NEED FOR CHARCOAL HEMOPERFUSION
Amitriptyline	Based on signs and symptoms
Chloral hydrate	250 mg/dL
Digitoxin	50 ng/mL with antidotal therapy
Digoxin	15 ng/mL with antidotal therapy
Ethchlorvinyl	150 μg/mL
Glutethimide	40 mg/L
Methaqualone	40 μg/mL
Notriptyline	Based on signs and symptoms
Pentobarbital	50 mg/L
Phenobarbital	100 mg/L
Theophylline	100 μg/mL in acute overdose
	60 μg/mL in chronic overdose

[a] The decision to perform hemoperfusion should be based on physical findings as well as drug levels. A repeat measure should be obtained when the drug level is elevated to ensure that a laboratory error has not occurred. In addition, units of measure should be checked before instituting hemodialysis.

Table 48   Normal Values for Fractional Excretion of Sodium (Fe$_{Na}$)

	PRERENAL ARF	INTRINSIC ARF
Adult or child	<1.0	>2.0
Infant (neonate)	<2.5	>2.5

ARF, acute renal failure.

Table 49   Causes of False-Positive Dipstick Reactions for Urinary Protein

Overlong immersion
Placing reagent strip directly in the urine stream
Alkaline urinary pH (pH >7.0)
Quaternary ammonium compounds and detergents
Pyuria
Bacteriuria
Mucoprotein

Table 50   Drugs that May Cause Hemolytic Anemia in Patients Who Have G6PD Deficiency

Acetanilid	Nitrofurantoin
Doxorubicin	Primaquine
Methylene blue	Pamaquine
Naphthalene	Sulfa drugs

PULMONARY

Table 51 Characteristics of the Three Stages of Parapneumonic Pleural Effusions

	EXUDATIVE STAGE	*FIBRINOLYTIC STAGE*	*ORGANIZING STAGE (EMPYEMA)*
Appearance	Nonpurulent, not turbid	Nonpurulent, not turbid	Purulent, turbid
Fluid consistency	Free flowing	Loculated	Organized
Gram stain and culture results	Negative	Transitional	Positive (before antibiotic treatment)
Glucose	>100 mg/dL	<50 mg/dL	<50 mg/dL
Protein	<3 g/dL	>3 g/dL	>3 g/dL
pH	>7.30	<7.30	<7.30
WBCs	Few	PMNs	PMNs

PMNs, polymorphonuclear neutrophils; WBCs, white blood cells.

Table 52 Pleural Fluid Diagnostic Studies

STUDY	*TRANSUDATE*	*EXUDATE*
Biochemical		
Pleural LDH	<200 IU	$\geq$200 IU
Pleural fluid/serum LDH ratio[a]	<0.6	$\geq$0.6
Pleural fluid/serum protein ratio[a]	<0.5	$\geq$0.5
Specific gravity	<1.016	$\geq$1.016
Protein level	<3.0 g/dL	$\geq$3.0 g/dL
Other studies		
Glucose	*Usually* >40 mg/dL	*Typically* <40 mg/dL
Amylase	May be elevated in some neoplasms, GI trauma, or surgery	
Rheumatoid factor, LE prep, ANA	Are occasionally helpful if collagen vascular disorders are within the differential	
Hematologic		
WBC count	Although high counts (>100/mm^3) are suggestive of an exudate, the results are quite variable	
WBC differential	May actually provide more useful information	
Lymphocyte count	May be elevated in neoplasms, tuberculosis, and some fungal infections	
Segmented neutrophils	May be elevated in bacterial infections, connective tissue disease, pancreatitis, or pulmonary infarction	
Eosinophil count	May be elevated in bacterial infections, neoplasms, and connective tissue diseases	
RBC count	If >100,000/mm^3, is suggestive of trauma, neoplasms, or pulmonary infarction	
Cytology and chromosomal studies	May show evidence of malignant cells or chromosomal abnormalities	
Microbiology		
Gram stain		
Fluid culture for aerobes and anaerobes		
Acid-fast stain (if tuberculosis is in the differential)		
Fungal culture		
Viral culture		
Counterimmune electrophoresis may aid in the detection of a bacterial infection)		

[a]These tests are more reliable in differentiating transudate from exudate than specific gravity or protein level.

Table 53 Normal Blood Gas Values from the Children's Hospital of Philadelphia Blood Gas Laboratory

PARAMETER	AGE OF PATIENT	NORMAL VALUE
pH	1 day	7.29–7.45
	3–24 months	7.34–7.46
	>7 years	7.37–7.41
Pco_2	1 day	27–40 mm Hg
	3–24 months	26–42 mm Hg
	>7 years	34–40 mm Hg
Po_2	1 day	37–97 mm Hg
	3–24 months	88–103 mm Hg
	>7 years	88–103 mm Hg
Base excess	1 day	>8-(−2)
	3–24 months	−7–0
	>7 years	−4-(+2)
HCO_3	1 day	19 mmol/L
	3–24 months	16/24 mmol/L
	>7 years	22–27 mmol/L
O_2 saturation	...	94%–99%
Venous pH	...	7.32–7.42
Venous CO_2		25–47 mm Hg
Venous O_2		25–47 mm Hg

CO_2, carbon dioxide; HCO_3, bicarbonate; O_2 = oxygen; Pco_2, carbon dioxide tension; Po_2, oxygen tension.

Table 54 Signs of Inhalation Injury

PULMONARY	CNS	SKIN
Tachypnea	Confusion	Facial burns
Stridor	Dizziness	Singed nasal hairs
Hoarseness	Headache	Cyanosis
Rales	Hallucinations	Cherry red color
Wheezing	Restlessness	
Cough	Coma	
Retractions	Seizures	
Nasal flaring		
Carbonaceous sputum		

CARDIOVASCULAR

Table 56 Common Causes of Abnormally Wide Splitting of the Second Heart Sound (S_2)

Atrial septal defect (ASD)
Mild pulmonic stenosis
Complete right bundle branch block
Left ventricular paced beats
Massive pulmonary embolus

Table 55 Pulmonary Function Test

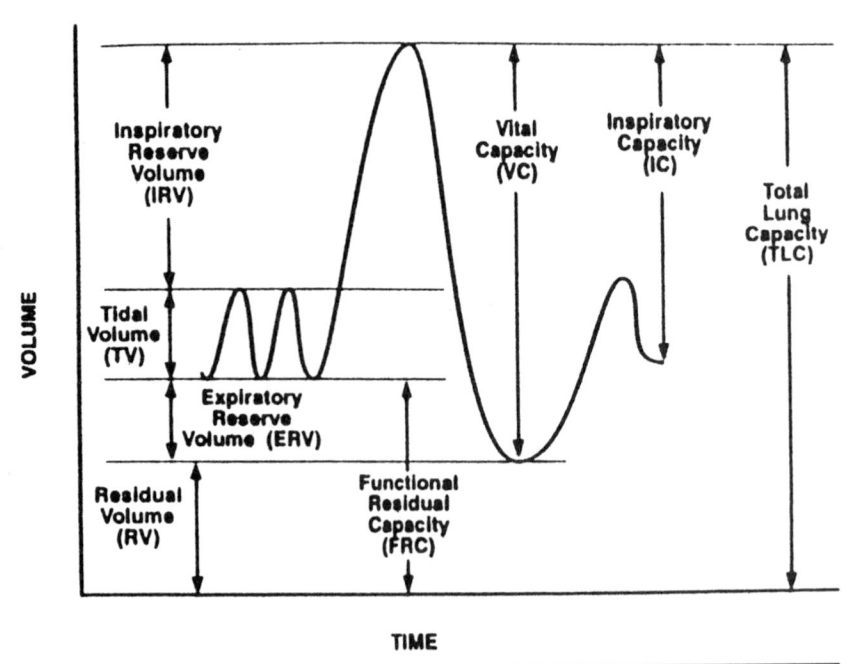

Table 57   Conditions Causing a Prominent Third Heart Sound (S₃)

Physiologic (infants and children)
Congestive heart failure (CHF)
Ventricular septal defect, with large pulmonary to systemic
   flow ratio
Mitral insufficiency
Tricuspid insufficiency
Hyperdynamic ventricle with high output (e.g., anemia, thyrotoxicosis,
   arteriovenous fistula)

Table 58   Conditions Causing a Prominent Fourth Heart Sound (S₄)

Left ventricular outflow tract obstruction (e.g., aortic stenosis)
Right ventricular outflow tract obstruction (e.g., pulmonic stenosis)
Hypertrophic cardiomyopathy
Heart block (atrium contracting against a closed valve)

Table 59   Drugs Associated with Rapid Heart Rates

Prescription drugs
   β-adrenergic agonists (e.g., albuterol)
   Methylxanthines (e.g., theophylline)
   Tricyclic antidepressants (e.g., imipramine)
   Nonsedating histamines (e.g., terfenadine)
Over-the-counter drugs
   Decongestants (e.g., pseudoephedrine)
   Diet aids (phenylpropanolamine)
   Inhaled bronchodilators (e.g., albuterol)
   Caffeine-containing products
Drugs of abuse
   Nicotine
   Cocaine
   Amphetamines
   Alcohol
   Marijuana
   LSD
   Phencyclidine
   Amyl nitrate

Table 60   Causes of Prolonged QT Interval

Congenital
   Hereditary
      Jervell and Lange-Nielsen syndrome: long QT interval, stress-induced
         syncope, congenital nerve deafness, autosomal-recessive
         inheritance
      Romano-Ward syndrome: long QT interval, stress-induced syncope,
         autosomal-dominant inheritance (usually incomplete
         penetrance)
   Sporadic
Acquired
   Electrolyte abnormalities
      Hypocalcemia
      Hypomagnesemia
   Metabolic disturbances
      Malnutrition
      Liquid protein diets
   Drugs
      Phenothiazines (e.g., haloperidol)
      Tricyclic antidepressants (e.g., imipramine)
      Nonsedating antihistamines (e.g., terfenadine)
      Class Ia antiarrhythmic agents (e.g., quinidine)
      Class III antiarrhythmic agents (e.g., amiodarone)
   CNS trauma
   Cardiac abnormalities
      Ischemia
      Mitral valve prolapse
      Myocarditis
   Intraventricular conduction abnormalities
      Bundle branch blocks

Table 61   Structural Heart Disease Associated with Tachycardia

DEFECT	_TYPE OF TACHYCARDIA_
Congenital heart disease	
Mitral valve prolapse	SVT, VT
Aortic valve stenosis or regurgitation	VT
Ebstein anomaly of the tricuspid valve	SVT (WPW) commonly, VT less commonly
Tetralogy of Fallot	VT
Mustard/Senning repair of D-TGA	SVT (particularly atrial flutter)
Fontan repair of single ventricle	SVT (particularly atrial flutter)
Cardiomyopathy	
Hypertrophic cardiomyopathy	SVT, VT
Dilated cardiomyopathy	SVT, VT
Arrhythmogenic right ventricular dysplasia	VT (monomorphic, left bundle branch block)
Miscellaneous causes	
Cardiac tumor (atrial myxoma, rhabdomyosarcoma)	VT
Eisenmenger complex (pulmonary vascular disease and pulmonary hypertension)	SVT, VT (depending on tumor site)

D-TGA, D-transposition of the great arteries; SVT, supraventricular tachycardia; VT, ventricular tachycardia; WPW, Wolff-Parkinson-White syndrome.

Table 62   Poisons Causing Tachycardia

Tachycardia and hypertension
  Amphetamines
  Antihistamines
  Cocaine
  LSD/PCP
Tachycardia and hypotension
  β_2-adrenergic agonists
    Albuterol
    Terbutaline
  Carbon monoxide
  Cyclic antidepressants
  Hydralazine
  Iron
  Phenothiazines
  Theophylline
  Any agent causing vomiting, diarrhea, or hemorrhage

LSD, lysergic acid diethylamide; PCP, phencyclidine hydrochloride.

Table 63   Poisons Causing Bradycardia

Bradycardia and hypertension
  α-Adrenergic agonists
    Phenylpropanolamine
    Ephedrine
  Clonidine
  Ergotamine
Bradycardia and hypotension
  α_1-Adrenergic antagonists
    Phentolamine
    Prazosin
  α_1-Adrenergic agonists
    Clonidine
    Tetrahydrozoline
  β-adrenergic antagonists
    Propranolol
    Atenolol
    Metoprolol
  Calcium channel blockers
  Digitalis-containing drugs and plants
  Narcotics
  Organophosphate pesticides
  Sedative/hypnotics

Table 64   Poisons Causing Cardiac Arrhythmias

Atrioventricular block
  Astemizole
  β-Adrenergic antagonists
  Calcium channel blockers
  Clonidine
  Cyclic antidepressants
  Digitalis-containing drugs and plants
Ventricular tachycardia
  Amphetamines
  Carbamazepine
  Chloral hydrate
  Chlorinated hydrocarbons
  Cocaine
  Cyclic antidepressants
  Digitalis-containing drugs or plants
  Phenothiazines (especially thioridazine)
  Theophylline
  Type Ia antiarrhythmic agents
    Quinidine
    Procainamide
  Type Ic antiarrhythmic agents
    Flecainide
    Encainide
Torsades de pointes (multifocal ventricular tachycardia)
  Amantadine
  Cyclic antidepressants
  Lithium
  Nonsedating antihistamines
    Astemizole
    Terfenadine
  Quinidine
  Phenothiazines
  Sotalol

Table 65   Revised Jones Criteria for Diagnosis of Acute Rheumatic Fever

MAJOR CRITERIA	MINOR CRITERIA
Carditis	Fever
Arthritis	Arthralgia
Rash (erythema marginatum)	Elevated ESR, CRP
Chorea (Sydenham)	Prolonged PR interval on ECG
Subcutaneous nodules	History of prior attack of rheumatic fever or rheumatic heart disease

Diagnosis is likely with the presence of two major and one minor criteria, or one major and two minor criteria. Supporting evidence of a preceding streptococcal infection includes a history of recent scarlet fever, a positive throat culture for group A *Streptococcus*, and an increased antistreptolysin O (ASO) titer (or titers for other streptococcal antibodies).

Adapted from the Report of the Ad Hoc Committee of the American Heart Association Council on Rheumatic Fever and Congenital Heart Disease. *Circulation* 1984; 69:204A–208A.

CRP, C-reactive protein; ECG, electrocardiogram; ESR, erythrocyte sedimentation rate.

MUSCULOSKELETAL

Table 66   Range of Motion of Major Joints

	FLEXION	EXTENSION	ABDUCTION	ADDUCTION	INTERNAL ROTATION	EXTERNAL ROTATION
Hip	120°	30°	50°	30°	35°	45°
Knee	135°	5°	0°	0°	10°	10°
Ankle	50°	20°	10°	20°	5° (eversion)	5° (inversion)
Shoulder	90°	45°	180°	45°	55°	45°
Elbow	135°	5°	0°	0°	90° (supination)	90° (pronation)
Wrist	80°	70°	20° (radial)	30° (lunar)	0°	0°

Table 67   Characteristics of Synovial Fluid

	APPEARANCE	WBC/MM²	% NEUTROPHILS	% GLUCOSE SYNOVIAL BLOOD
Normal	Clear	<2000	<40	>50
Infectious	Turbid	>75,000	>75	<50
Inflammatory (JRA, SLE)	Clear/turbid	5,000–75,000	50	≥ 50
Traumatic	Bloody/Clear	<5,000	<50	>50

Table 68   Relationship Between Short Stature, Bone Age, and Growth Velocity[a]

Bone age delayed—normal growth velocity	Constitutional short stature
Bone age normal—normal growth velocity	Genetic short stature
Bone age delayed—delayed growth velocity	Organic diseases

[a] Velocity = the rate of growth during a year.

ENDOCRINOLOGY

Table 69   Clinical and Biochemical Features of Congenital Adrenal Hyperplasia (CAH)

ENZYME DEFECT	SEXUAL AMBIGUITY		ADDITIONAL CLINICAL MANIFESTATIONS	PREDOMINANT STEROIDS
	FEMALE	MALE		
Desmolase	−	+	Salt wasting	. . .
3β-Hydroxysteroid dehydrogenase	+	+	Salt wasting	17-OH-pregnenolone, DHEA
21-Hydroxylase	+	−	Salt wasting	17-OH-progestone, androstenedione
11-Hydroxylase	+	−	Hypertension	11-Deoxycortisol
17-Hydroxylase	−	+	Hypertension	DOC, corticosterone

DHEA, dehydroepiandrosterone; DOE, deoxycorticosterone.

Table 70   Normal Serum Adrenal Steroid Levels in Newborn Infants

STEROID	PRETERM SICK		PRETERM WELL	FULL TERM
	24–28 WEEKS	31–35 WEEKS	31–35 WEEKS	
Cortisol (μg/dL)	7.5 ± 4	6 ± 2.7	6.9 ± 3.8	6.2 ± 3.9
17-OH-Preg (ng/dL)	1794 ± 1818	1395 ± 694	942 ± 739	245 ± 291
17-OH-Pro (ng/dL)	651 ± 661	373 ± 317	169 ± 95	36 ± 13[a]
11-deoxycortisol (ng/dL)	662 ± 548	294 ± 239	111 ± 62	87 ± 42
DHEA (ng/dL)	1872 ± 4038	675 ± 502	920 ± 1227	286 ± 238
DHEAS (μg/dL)	467 ± 312	459 ± 209	341 ± 93	162 ± 88
Androstenedione (ng/dL)	479 ± 1032	206 ± 86	215 ± 134	149 ± 67

Data based on information in Lee MM, Rajabopalan L, Berg G, et al. Serum adrenal steroid concentrations in premature infants. *J Clin Endocrinol Metab* 1989;69:1133–1136, and in Wiener D, Smith J, Dahlem S, et al. Serum adrenal steroid levels in healthy term 3-day-old infants. *J Pediatr* 1987;110(1):122–124.

17-OH-Preg, 17-OH-pregnenolone; 17-OH-Pro, 17-OH-progesterone; DHEA, dehydroepiandrosterone; DHEAS, dehydroepiandrosterone sulfate.

[a] 17-OH-Pro values in full-term sick newborns may be double or triple the baseline values. No data are available for other steroid hormones in sick full-term infants.

Table 71   Pharmacokinetics of Common Insulin Preparations

INSULIN PREPARATION	ONSET (HOURS)	PEAK (HOURS)	DURATION OF ACTION (HOURS)
Ultra-rapid-acting (Lispro)	0.25–0.50	1–2	2–3
Short-acting (Regular, Semilente)	0.5–1.0	2–4	4–6
Long-acting (NPH, Lente)	2–4	6–12	18–24
Very long-acting (Ultralente)	6–10	18–24	24–36

NPH, neutral protein Hagedorn insulin.

Table 72   Normal Thyroid Hormone Levels

T_4	Total	7.0–15.0 μg/dL
	Free	0.8–2.3 ng/dL
T_3		100–250 ng/dL
TSH		0.5–5.0 μg/dL

Table 73　Normal Ranges for Gonadotropin and Sex Steroid Levels: Females

	LH (mLU/mL)	FSH (mLU/mL)	ESTRADIOL (ng/dL)	TESTOSTERONE (ng/dL)
0–1 year	0.02–7.0	0.24–14.2	0.5–5.0	<10
Prepubertal	0.02–0.3	1.0–4.2	<1.5	<3–10
Tanner 2	0.02–4.7	1.0–10.8	1.0–2.4	7.0–28
Tanner 3	0.10–12.0	1.5–12.8	0.7–6.0	15–35
Tanner 4	0.4–11.7	1.5–11.7	2.1–8.5	13–32
Tanner 5	0.4–11.7	1.0–9.2	3.4–17.0	20–38
Adult	...	...	...	10–55
Follicular phase	2.0–9.0	1.8–11.2	3.0–10.0	...
Midcycle	18.0–49	6.0–35.0	...	...
Luteal phase	2.0–11.0	1.8–11.2	7.0–30.0	...

FSH, follicle-stimulating hormone; LH, luteinizing hormone.

Table 74　Normal Ranges for Gonadotropin and Sex Steroid Levels: Males

	LH (mLU/mL)	FSH (mLU/mL)	ESTRADIOL (ng/dL)	TESTOSTERONE (ng/dL)
0–1 year	0.02–7.0	0.16–4.1	1.0–3.2	<10
Prepubertal	0.02–0.3	0.26–3.0	<1.5	<3–10
Tanner 2	0.2–4.9	1.8–3.2	0.5–1.6	18–150
Tanner 3	0.2–5.0	1.2–5.8	0.5–2.5	100–320
Tanner 4	0.4–7.0	2.0–9.2	1.0–3.6	200–620
Tanner 5	0.4–7.0	2.6–11.0	1.0–3.6	350–970
Adult	1.5–9.0	2.0–9.2	0.8–3.5	350–1030

FSH, follicle-stimulating hormone; LH, leuteinizing hormone.

Table 75　Classification of Total and LDL Cholesterol Levels in Children and Adolescents from Families with Hypercholesterolemia or Premature Cardiovascular Disease

CATEGORY	TOTAL CHOLESTEROL, mg/dL	LDL CHOLESTEROL, mg/dL
Acceptable	<170	<110
Borderline	170–199	110–129
High	≥200	≥130

NEUROLOGIC

Table 76　Causes of Ataxia

FORM OF ATAXIA	MAJOR CAUSES	OTHER CAUSES
Acute ataxia	Ingestion	Migraine
	Postinfectious cerebellitis	Neuroblastoma
Acute recurrent ataxia	Migraine	...
	Metabolic disease	
Chronic ataxia	Congenital disorders with mental deficiency	...
Chronic progressive ataxia	Brain tumors	Ataxia-telangiectasia
	Neuroectodermal tumors	Friedreich ataxia

Table 77   Glasgow Coma Scale

Eyes open		Best motor response	
Spontaneously	4	Obey commands	6
To speech	3	Localize pain	5
To pain	2	Withdrawal	4
None	1	Flexion to pain	3
Best verbal response		Extension to pain	2
Oriented	5	None	1
Confused	4		
Inappropriate	3		
Incomprehensible	2		
None	1		

Adapted from Fleisher G, Ludwig S, eds. *Textbook of pediatric emergency medicine*, 3rd ed. Baltimore: Williams & Wilkins, 1993:272.

Table 78   Glasgow Coma Scale (GCS) for Adults and Children and Modified Score for Infants

	GLASGOW COMA SCORE (ADULTS/OLDER CHILDREN)		MODIFIED GLASGOW COMA SCORE (INFANTS)
Eye opening	Spontaneous	4	Spontaneous
	To verbal stimuli	3	To speech
	To pain	2	To pain
	None	1	None
Best verbal response	Oriented	5	Coos and babbles
	Confused speech	4	Irritable, cries
	Inappropriate words	3	Cries to pain
	Nonspecific sounds	2	Moans to pain
	None	1	None
Best motor response	Follows commands	6	Normal spontaneous movements
	Localizes pain	5	Withdraws to touch
	Withdraws to pain	4	Withdraws to pain
	Flexes to pain	3	Abnormal flexion
	Extends to pain	2	Abnormal extension
	None	1	None

Table 79   Drugs that Can Cause Delirium or Coma

DRUG	PHYSICAL FINDINGS
Barbiturates	Small, reactive pupils; hypothermia; flaccidity; doll's eye reflex may be absent
Opiates	Pinpoint, reactive pupils; hypothermia; hypotension; hypoventilation; bradycardia
Psychedelics	Small, reactive pupils; hypertension; hyperventilation; dystonic posturing
Amphetamines	Dilated pupils, hyperthermia, hypertension, tachycardia, arrhythmia
Cocaine	Dilated pupils, hyperthermia, tachycardia
Atropine-scopolamine	Dilated pupils; hyperthermia; flushing; hot, dry skin; supraventricular tachycardia
Glutethimide	Midposition, irregular fixed pupils; hypothermia; flaccidity
Tricyclic antidepressants	Hyperthermia, hypotension, supraventricular tachycardia
Phenothiazines	Hypotension, arrhythmia, dystonia
Methaqualone	Same as with barbiturates; if severe tachycardia, dystonia

From Packer RJ, Berman PH. Coma. In: Fleisher GR, Ludwig S, eds. *Textbook of pediatric emergency medicine*, 3rd ed. Baltimore: Williams & Wilkins, 1993:126, with permission.

Table 80   Prognostic Indicators of Poor Neurologic Outcome in Near-Drowning Victims[a]

At the scene
   Submersion time >4–10 minutes
   Delay in beginning CPR
   Resuscitation >25 minutes
In the emergency department
   Necessity for CPR
   Fixed, dilated pupils
   pH <7.0
   GCS score <5
After initial resuscitation
   Persistent GCS score <5
   Persistent apnea

CPR, cardiopulmonary resuscitation; GCS, Glasgow Coma Scale.

[a] Applies to victims of warm water near-drownings only. Hypothermic victims of cold water near-drownings may have a better prognosis.

Table 81   Relationship of the Lesion to the Physical Findings

LESION	*FINDINGS*
Upper motor neuron involving corticospinal tract, thalamus, centrum, semiovale, motor cortex	Altered, normal or increased reflexes, bulk normal; strength normal or decreased
Cerebellum	Uncoordinated
Spinal (upper and lower motor)	Local pain, bowel and bladder dysfunction, if anterior horn cells involved, weakness and bulk, decreased absent reflexes, fasciculations
Peripheral	Loss of distal muscles, fasciculations less than spinal lesions; sensation is affected
Muscle	Weakness, muscle atrophy, decreased reflexes, pain, cramping, stiffness
Corticospinal tract	Increased tone, clasp knife character in flexion of arms and extension of legs
Extrapyramidal (basal ganglia)	Rigidity, normal reflexes, absent Babinski, voluntary movement is preserved, may have tremor, chorea, athetosis or dystonia

Table 82   Poisons Causing Coma

Coma with miosis
  Barbiturates and other sedative/hypnotics
  Bromide
  Chloral hydrate
  Clonidine
  Ethanol
  Narcotics
  Organophosphates
  PCP
  Phenothiazines
  Tetrahydrozoline
Coma with mydriasis
  Atropine/diphenoxylate
  Carbon monoxide
  Cyanide
  Cyclic antidepressants
  Glutethimide
  LSD

LSD, lysergic acid diethylamide; PCP, phencyclidine hydrochloride.

Table 83   Poisons Causing Seizures

Amoxapine
Amphetamines
Anticonvulsants
  Phenytoin
  Carbamazepine
Antihistamines and anticholinergic drugs or plants
Camphor
Carbon monoxide
Chlorinated hydrocarbons
Cocaine
Cyanide
Cyclic antidepressants
Isoniazid
Lead
Lidocaine
Meperidine
PCP
Phenothiazines
Phenylpropanolamine
Propoxyphene
Propranolol
Theophylline

PCP, phencyclidine hydrochloride.

Table 84　Differential Diagnosis of Metabolic Neurologic Dysfunction

PROMINENT SYMPTOM	DIAGNOSES TO CONSIDER	DIAGNOSTIC TEST	METABOLIC THERAPY
Myoclonic seizures	Ceroid	DNA, tissue EM	
	Lafora body disease	Muscle biopsy	
	Prion (GSS)	DNA	
	Mitochondrial	DNA, muscle biopsy	CoQ, other vitamins
	Aminoacidopathies	Blood biochemistry	Dietary
	Biotinidase deficiency	Blood biochemistry	Biotin supplement
	Organic acidurias	Blood biochemistry	Dietary, vitamins
Stroke	Homocystinuria	Blood/urine test	B vitamins, betaine
	Mitochondrial	DNA, muscle biopsy	
Coma	Organic aciduria	Blood/urine test	
	MSUD	Blood/urine test	
	Hyperammonemias	Blood test	Dietary
Spasticity	Leukodystrophy	MRI, fibroblast analysis	Dietary
Visual loss	Leukodystrophy	MRI	
	Mitochondrial	DNA, muscle biopsy	
Psychosis	Leukodystrophy	MRI, blood biochemistry, DNA, fibroblast analysis	
	Porphyria	Blood/urine	Avoid precipitants
		Biochemistry	
	Wilson disease	Copper excretion, DNA	Penicillamine
	Homocystinuria	Blood biochemistry	(See above)
	Ceroid	DNA, tissue electron microscopy	
	Huntington disease	DNA	
Microcephaly	Ceroid	DNA, tissue EM	
	Rett syndrome	(Clinical features)	
	Krabbe disease	Blood biochemistry	
Macrocephaly	Storage disorders	DNA, blood biochemistry	
	Canavan disease	Urine biochemistry, DNA	
Neuropathy	Krabbe disease	MRI and blood biochemistry	
	Metachromatic leukodystrophy		
	Porphyria	Blood/urine biochemistry	
	Mitochondrial	DNA, muscle biopsy	
	Friedreich ataxia	(Clinical features)	
	Abetalipoproteinemia		
	Disorders/deficiency of vitamin E	Blood biochemistry	Vitamin E
	Mitochondrial	Vitamin E level	Vitamin E
	Neuroaxonal dystrophy	DNA, muscle biopsy	
		MRI, nerve biopsy	
Myopathy	Fukuyama disease	MRI	
	Mitochondrial	DNA, muscle biopsy	
	Lactic acidoses	Blood biochemistry	
Ataxia	Ataxia telangiectasia	DNA	
	Leukodystrophies	MRI, blood biochemistry	
	Friedreich		
	Mitochondrial	(Clinical features)	
	Hartnup	DNA, muscle biopsy	
	Hyperammonemias	Blood biochemistry	
	Abetalipoproteinemia	Blood biochemistry	
	Sphingolipidoses	Blood biochemistry	
	Machado-Joseph, SCA-1 (hereditary ataxias)	Blood biochemistry, fibroblast analysis, DNA	

Table 85   Acquired Disorders Associated with Progressive Neurologic Dysfunction

STRUCTURAL	*HORMONAL*	*INFECTIOUS*	*ENVIRONMENTAL*	*TOXIC*	*IMMUNOLOGIC*
Hydrocephalus	Hypothyroidism	SSPE	Malnutrition/malabsorption syndromes	Lead	Demyelination/multiple sclerosis
Brain tumor	Congenital adrenal hyperplasia (visuospatial deficits)	HIV	Vitamin/trace element deficiency (niacin, thiamine, folic acid, vitamin E, B_{12}, essential fatty acids)	Organic chemicals	Opsoclonus/myoclonus or cerebellar ataxia (neuroblastoma
Vascular anomalies		Spirochetes		Carbon monoxide	Sydenham chorea
				Cocaine, hallucinogens, hypnotics	Rasmussen encephalitis
			Physical abuse/neglect	Phenytoin (cerebellar degeneration)	

Table 86   Epidural versus Acute Subdural Hematoma

	EPIDURAL HEMATOMA	*SUBDURAL HEMATOMA*
Common mechanism	Blunt direct trauma, frequently to parietal region	Acceleration-deceleration injury
Etiology	Arterial or venous	Venous (bridging veins below dura)
Incidence	Uncommon	Common
Peak age	Usually >2 years	Usually <1 year
		Peak at 6 months
Location	Unilateral	75% Bilateral
	Commonly parietal	Diffuse, over cerebral hemispheres
Skull fracture	Common	Uncommon
Associated seizures	Uncommon	Common
Retinal hemorrhages	Rare	Common
Decreased level of consciousness	Common	Almost always
Mortality	Rare	Uncommon
Morbidity in survivors	Low	High
Clinical findings	Dilated ipsilateral pupil, contralateral hemiparesis	Decreased level of consciousness
	Period of lucidity prior to acute decompensation and rapid progression to herniation	Irritability, lethargy
Onset	Acute	Acute (within 24 hours), subacute (within 1 day–2 weeks), or chronic (after 2 weeks)
Findings on CT	Convex "lens-shaped" cerebral hemisphere	Concave, diffusely surrounding cerebral hemisphere

CT, computed tomography.

GYNECOLOGICAL

Table 87 Age-Related Prevalence of Principal Laparoscopic Findings in 121 Adolescent Females 11 to 17 Years Old with Acute Pelvic Pain (The Children's Hospital, Boston, 1980–1986)

	NUMBER OF PATIENTS		
DIAGNOSIS	AGE 11–13	AGE 14–15	AGE 16–17
Ovarian cyst	12 (50%)	16 (35%)	19 (37%)
Acute pelvic inflammatory disease	4 (17%)	7 (16%)	10 (19%)
Adnexal torsion	0 (0%)	7 (16%)	2 (4%)
Endometriosis	0 (0%)	2 (4%)	4 (7%)
Ectopic pregnancy	0 (0%)	3 (7%)	1 (2%)
Appendicitis	3 (13%)	4 (9%)	6 (12%)
No pathology	5 (20%)	6 (13%)	10 (19%)
Total	24 (20%)	45 (37%)	52 (43%)

From Goldstein DP. Acute and chronic pelvic pain. *Pediatr Clin North Am* 1989;36(3):576.

Table 88 Key Characteristics of Vaginal Discharges

	PRESENTING SYMPTOMS	DISCHARGE	NONMENSTRUAL pH	AMINE/ WHIFF TEST	VAGINAL SMEAR	TREATMENT
Nonspecific vaginitis	Foul-smelling discharge Itching	Scant to copious Brown to green in color	Variable	Negative	Leukocytes Bacteria and other debris	Improved perineal hygiene
Physiologic leukorrhea	None	Variable Scant to moderate Clear to white	<4.5	Negative	Normal epithelial cells Lactobacilli predominate	None
Bacterial vaginosis	Foul-smelling discharge	Gray-white	>4.7	Positive	Epithelial cells with bacteria ("clue cells") Gram-negative rods	Metronidazole Clindamycin
Candidiasis	Severe itching Vulvar inflammation	White, "curd-like"	<4.5	Negative	Fungal hyphae and buds	Topical or intravaginal imidazoles, triazoles Oral ketoconazole
Trichomonal vaginitis	Copious discharge Itching	Profuse Yellow to green	5.0–6.0	Occasionally present	Motile flagellated organisms	Metronidazole
Foreign body	Foul-smelling discharge	Foul-smelling Purulent Dark brown	Variable (usually >4.7)	Occasionally present	Leukocytes Epithelial cells with bacteria and debris	Remove foreign body Irrigate vagina
Contact vulvovaginitis	Vulvar inflammation Itching Edema	Scant White to yellow	Variable (usually <4.5)	Negative	Leukocytes Epithelial cells	Remove irritant Topical steroids

Table 89   Emergency Contraceptive Pills

INSTRUCTIONS FOR USE

Any of the birth control pills listed below can be used as ECPs. Use only the type of pill your health care provider prescribed for you. Use only one type of pill.

IF YOU ARE TAKING	*NUMBER OF PILLS TO SWALLOW AS SOON AS POSSIBLE (1ST DOSE)*	*NUMBER OF PILLS TO SWALLOW 12 HOURS LATER (2ND DOSE)*
Ovral	2 white pills	2 white pills
Lo/Ovral	4 white pills	4 white pills
Levlen	4 light-orange pills	4 light-orange pills
Nordette	4 light-orange pills	4 light-orange pills
Tri-Levlen	4 yellow pills	4 yellow pills
Triphasil	4 yellow pills	4 yellow pills
Alesse	5 pink pills	5 pink pills

• To reduce the chance of nausea, take an antinausea medicine (like Dramamine II or Benadryl) 1 hour **before** the first ECP dose; repeat according to labeled instructions. This may make you feel tired, so don't drive or drink any alcohol.

• Take the first ECP dose as soon as convenient **WITHIN 3 DAYS (72 HOURS)** after unprotected sex. Try to time the first dose so that the timing of the second dose will be convenient.

• Take the second ECP dose **12 hours after the first dose.**

IMPORTANT: Do not take any extra ECPs. More pills will probably not make the treatment work better. More pills will increase your risk of feeling sick to your stomach.

• Use condoms, spermicides, or a diaphragm if you have sex after taking ECPs until you get your period. Talk to your health care provider about other regular birth control methods you can use in the future.

• Your next period may be a few days early or late.

IMPORTANT: Do a home pregnancy test or see your health care provider if your period has not started **within 3 weeks** after ECP treatment. You may be pregnant.

Source: Program for Applied Technologies (PATH). *Emergency contraception: Resources for providers.* Seattle, 1997. This patient handout may be reproduced without permission of the publisher.

TRAUMA

Table 90   Classification of Burns

TYPE OF BURN	*AFFECTED SKIN LAYER*	*APPEARANCE*
First degree	Epidermis	Erythema, hypersensitivity
Second degree		
Superficial	Upper (papillary) dermis	Erythema, blistering, intact hairs, exquisite pain
Deep	Deep (reticular dermis)	Skin may be white or mottled and nonblanching, or blistered and moist; pain may or may not be present; hairs easily pulled
Third degree	Entire dermis	Dry, white or charred skin; leathery appearance, painless, no hair
Fourth degree	Subcutaneous tissue	Same as third degree; may have exposed muscle and bone

Table 91 "Rule of Nines"

	PERCENT OF BSA		
BODY PART	INFANT	CHILD	ADOLESCENT/ADULT
Head	18%	13%	9%
Anterior trunk	18%	18%	18%
Posterior trunk	18%	18%	18%
Upper extremity (each)	9%	9%	9%
Lower extremity (each)	14%	16%	18%
Genitalia	1%	1%	1%

For small burns, a rough estimate of the affected BSA can be made by comparing the burn with the size of the child's palm (which represents approximately 1% of the BSA).

BSA, body surface area.

TOXICOLOGY

Table 92 Agents with Limited or Uncertain Binding to Activated Charcoal

Iron	Gasoline
Lithium	Mineral seal oil
Heavy metals	Caustics[a]
Arsenic	NaOH
Mercury	KOH
Lead	HCL
Thallium	H_2SO_4
Alcohols	Low-molecular-weight
Methanol	compounds
Ethanol	Cyanide
Isopropanol	Pesticides
Ethylene glycol	Organophosphates
Hydrocarbons	Carbamates
Kerosene	

[a] Administration of activated charcoal may also impede further management.

Table 93 Agents Causing Hypoglycemia in Overdosed Children

Ethanol
Salicylates
Oral hypoglycemic agents
Propranolol
Insulin

Table 94 Poisons Not Detected on the Comprehensive Drug Screen[a]

β-Adrenergic antagonists
Calcium channel blockers
Carbon monoxide
Clonidine
Cyanide
Iron
LSD
Many benzodiazepines (alprazolam, midazolam, lorazepam)
Most plants and mushrooms

[a] Partial listing of some of the most common poisons.

Table 95 Poisons Causing Respiratory Depression or Apnea[a]

Antipsychotic agents	Exotic snake envenomation
Carbamate pesticides	Cobras
Chlorinated hydrocarbons	Sea snakes
Trichloroethylene	Mambas
1,1,1-trichloroethane	Mojave rattlesnake envenomation
Clonidine	Narcotics
Coral snake envenomation	Nicotine
Cyclic antidepressants	Organophosphate pesticides
Ethanol (especially when combined with sedative/hypnotics)	Sedative/hypnotics

[a] Partial list of representative poisons.

Table 96 Poisons Causing an Abnormal Anion Gap[a]

Increased anion gap with metabolic acidosis	Methanol[b]
Carbon monoxide[b]	Salicylates[b]
Cyanide	Theophylline[b]
Ethanol[b]	*Decreased anion gap*
Ethylene glycol[b]	Bromide
Iron[b]	Lithium[b]
Isoniazid	Hypermagnesemia[b]
	Hypercalcemia[b]

[a] Partial list of representative poisons; anion gap = $Na^+ - (Cl^- + CO_2^-)$.

[b] Specific levels rapidly available.

Table 97   Common Poisons and Antidotes

POISON	ANTIDOTE	ADMINISTRATION
Acetaminophen	N-Acetylcysteine	Loading dose 140 mg/kg, then 17 doses at 70 mg/kg/dose. Dilute 20% solution to 5%–10% with juice or soda to improve palatability.
Anticholinergics	Physostigmine	
Benzodiazepines	Flumazenil	
β-Adrenergic antagonists	Glucagon	
Calcium channel blockers	Glucagon	
	Calcium gluconate 10%	0.3–0.6 mL/kg (8–16 mEq calcium/kg)
Carbon monoxide	Hyperbaric oxygen	
	Sodium thiosulfate 25%[a]	
Cyanide	Sodium nitrate 3%	Dose depends on hemoglobin (see cyanide antidote kit package insert). Do not exceed recommended dosage. Do not give to patients suffering from concomitant carbon monoxide exposure.
	Sodium thiosulfate 25%	Dose depends on hemoglobin (see cyanide antidote kit package insert).
Digitalis	Digitalis Fab fragments	Calculate dose based on level or dose ingested or 10 vials if acute overdose, 5 vials if chronic overdose.
Ethylene glycol	Ethanol	0.6 g/kg load over 1 hour followed by 100 mg/kg/hr infusion
	Pyridoxine	2 mg/kg and thiamine 0.5 mg/kg
Iron	Deferoxamine	5–15 mg/kg/hr IV infusion
Isoniazid	Pyridoxine	
Lead	Lead level 45–69 μg/dL	
	Dimercaptosuccinic acid	10 mg/kg PO three times daily for 5 days, then twice daily for 14 days (may be useful at lower levels)
	or	
	Calcium NaEDTA	50–75 mg/kg/day divided, every 6 hours either IM or by slow IV infusion (IV use not FDA-approved)
	Lead level $\geq$ 70 μg/dL	
	Calcium NaEDTA and	Administer as described above
	British anti-lewisite (BAL)	3–5 mg/kg IM every 4 hours for 5 days
Methanol	Folate	50–100 mg over 6 hours
	4-Methylpyrazole (investigational)	
Methemoglobinemia	Methylene blue 1%	1–2 mg/kg (0.1–0.2 mL/kg)
Narcotics	Naloxone	
Organophosphates	Atropine	0.1–0.5 mg/kg initial dose with additional doses as needed to counteract bronchorrhea
	Pralidoxime	25–50 mg/kg (up to 1 g); for severe cases, consider 10–15 mg/kg/hr infusion
Phenothiazines (dystonia)	Diphenhydramine	1–2 mg/kg IM or IV
	Benztropine	1–2 mg/kg IM or IV

IM, intramuscularly; IV, intravenously; FDA, Food and Drug Administration; NaEDTA, sodium ethylenediaminetetraacetic acid; PO, orally.

[a] Consider for possible cyanide inhalation if the patient suffers from smoke inhalation.

Table 98   Epidemiologic Aspects of Food Poisoning

ORGANISM	PATHOGENESIS	SOURCE	PREVENTION
Salmonella	Infection	Meats, poultry, eggs, dairy products	Proper cooking and food handling, pasteurization
Staphylococcus	Preformed enterotoxin	Meats, poultry, potato salad, cream-filled pastry, cheese, sausage	Careful food handling, rapid refrigeration
Clostridium prefringens	Enterotoxin	Meats, poultry	Avoid delay in serving foods, avoid cooling and rewarming foods
Clostridium botulinum	Preformed neurotoxin	Honey, home-canned foods, uncooked foods	Proper refrigeration (see text)
Vibrio parahaemolyticus	Infection enterotoxin	Sea fish, seawater, shellfish	Proper refrigeration
Bacillus cereus			
Diarrheal type	Sporulation enterotoxin	Many prepared foods	Proper refrigeration
Vomiting type	Preformed toxin	Cooked or fried rice, vegetables, meats, cereal, puddings	Proper refrigeration of cooked rice and other foods
Enterohemorrhagic E. coli 0157-H7	Cytotoxins	Milk, beef	Thorough cooking of beef, consumption of pasteurized milk products
Enterotoxigenic E. coli (traveler's diarrhea)	Enterotoxin	Food or water	Prognosis is not recommended for infants and young children

Table 99 Clinical Aspects of Food Poisoning

ORGANISM	INCUBATION	SYMPTOMS	DURATION	TREATMENT
Bacillus cereus	Vomiting toxin 1–6 hr Diarrhea toxin 6–24 hr	Vomiting ± diarrhea; fever uncommon	8–24 hr	None
Brucella	Several days to months; usually >30 days	Weakness, fever, headache chills, arthralgia, weight loss; splenomegaly		Bactrim, tetracycline
Campylobacter	2–10 days; usually 2–5 days	Diarrhea (often bloody), abdominal pain, fever		Severe infection or immunocompromised; erythromycin, Cipro, or Norfloxacin
Clostridia botulinum	2 hr–8 days; usually 12–48 hr	Poor feeding, weak cry, constipation, diplopia, blurred vision, resp weakness; symmetric descending paralysis		Supportive, trivalent equine antitoxin to prevent further paralysis
Clostridia perfringens	6–24 hr	Diarrhea, abdominal cramps, vomiting and fever uncommon	<24 hr	None
Escherichia coli	→	→		Antibiotics in systemic infections
E. coli 0157:H7	1–10 days; usually 3–4 days	Diarrhea (often bloody), abdominal cramps, little or no fever. Can cause HUS.	5–10 days	Supportive
ETEC	6–48 hr	Diarrhea, abdominal cramps, nausea, fever, and vomiting; Uncommon	5–10 days	Supportive
Listeria monocytogenes	2–6 wk	Meningitis, neonatal sepsis, fever	Variable	Ampicillin and gentamicin
Nontyphoidal Salmonella	6–48 hr	Diarrhea often with fever and abdominal cramps	<7 days	None unless <3 months or immunocompromised
Salmonella typi	3–60 days; usually 7–14 days	Fever, anorexia, malaise, headache, myalgias, ± diarrhea or constipation	3–4 wk	Chloramphenicol, ampicillin, amoxicillin, Bactrim, Cefotaxime, Ceftriaxone
Shigella	12 hr–6 days; usually 2–4 days	Diarrhea (often bloody), frequently fever, abdominal cramps	1 day–1 month	Bactrim, Cipro
Staphylococcus aureus	30 min–8 hr; usually 2–4 hr	Vomiting, diarrhea	<24 hr	None
Vibriosis	4–30 hr	Diarrhea, cramps, nausea, vomiting	Self limited	Usually none. Treatment for patients with liver disease or immunocompromised: Cefotaxime, gentamicin, Chloramphenicol, Tetracycline
Yersinia enterocolitica	1–10 days; usually 4–6 days	Diarrhea, abdominal pain (often severe), mesenteric adenitis, pseudo-appendicular syndrome	1–3 wks	Septicemia or enterocolitis in immunocompromised: cefotaxime, aminoglycosides, tetracycline, Bactrim, chloramphenicol

Table 100   Nomogram for Estimating Severity of Acute Poisoning

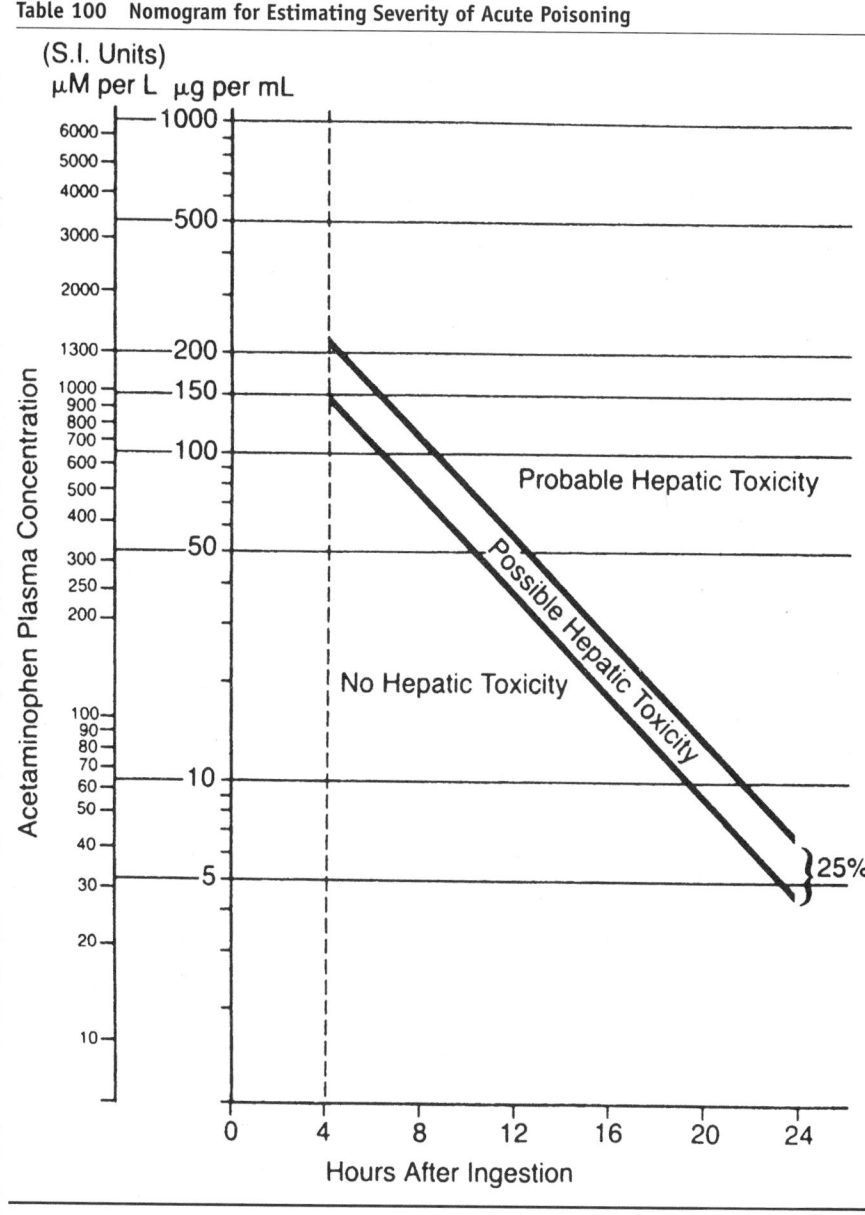

Table 101   Poisonous Plants

The following are a few common plants that are toxic:

Azalea	Laurel
Buttercup	Lily-of-the-valley
Calla lily	Mistletoe
Creeping Charlie— ground ivy	Morning glory
	Nightshade
Daffodil	Periwinkle
Delphinium	Philodendron
Elderberry	Poison ivy
Holly berries	Poison oak
Hyacinth bulbs	Rhododendron
Hydrangea	Sweet pea
Iris	Tomato vines
Ivy (Boston and English)	Tulip
	Wisteria
Jimson weed	Yew
Larkspur	

GONOCOCCAL INFECTIONS

Table 102   Regimens for the Treatment of Pelvic Inflammatory Disease (PID) in Adolescents

---

Outpatient regimens
  Regimen A
    Ofloxacin, 400 mg PO twice daily for 14 days
                    PLUS
    Metronidazole, 500 mg PO twice daily for 14 days
  Regimen B
    Ceftriaxone, 250 mg IM once
                    OR
    Cefoxitin (2 mg IM) plus probenecid (1 g PO) in a single dose
      concurrently once
                    OR
    Another parenteral third-generation cephalosporin (e.g., ceftizoxime
      or cefotaxime)
                    PLUS
    Doxycycline, 100 mg orally twice daily for 14 days
Inpatient regimens
  Parenteral regimen A
    Cefotetan, 2 g IV every 12 hours
                    OR
    Cefoxitin, 2 g IV every 6 hours
                    PLUS
    Doxycycline, 100 mg IV or PO every 12 hours
  Parenteral regimen B
    Clindamycin, 900 mg IV every 8 hours
                    PLUS
    Gentamicin loading dose IV or IM (2 mg/kg of body weight),
      followed by a maintenance dose (1.5 mg/kg) every 8 hours; single
      daily dosing may be substituted

The safety and effectiveness of fluoroquinolones (e.g., ciprofloxacin, ofloxacin, nurfloxacin, enoxacin) in patients younger than 18 years, pregnant women, and lactating women has not been established; therefore, fluoroquinolones are presently not recommended in these patients.

IM, intramuscularly; IV, intravenously; PO, orally.

Table 103   Uncomplicated Gonococcal Infection: Treatment in Children Beyond the Newborn Period and in Adolescents. Recommended Antimicrobial Regimens Include Therapy for Presumed Concomitant Infection with *Chlamydia trachomatis*[a]

DISEASE	PREPUBERTAL CHILDREN WHO WEIGH <100 LB (45 KG)	DISEASE	PATIENTS WHO WEIGH >100 LB (45 KG) AND ARE 9 YEARS OR OLDER
Uncomplicated vulvovaginitis, urethritis, proctitis, or pharyngitis	Ceftriaxone, 125 mg IM,[b] in a single dose **OR** Spectinomycin[c] (max 2 g), IM, in a single dose **PLUS** Erythromycin,[e] 40 mg/kg/d in divided doses for 7 d	Uncomplicated endocervicitis, or urethritis	Ceftriaxone, 125 mg IM,[b] in a single dose **OR** Ciprofloxacin,[d] 500 mg orally, in a single dose **OR** Cefixime, 400 mg orally, in a single dose **OR** Oftoxacin,[d] 400 mg orally, in a single dose **OR** Spectinomycin,[c] 2 g IM, in a single dose **PLUS** Doxycycline, 100 mg orally, twice daily for 7 d[f] **OR** Azithromycin, 1 g orally, in a single dose

[a] Hospitalization should be considered, especially for patients who have been treated as outpatients and have failed to respond, and for those who are unlikely to adhere to treatment regimens.

[b] Some clinicians believe the discomfort of an IM injection can be reduced by using 1% lidocaine as a diluent.

[c] Spectinomycin is not recommended for treatment of pharyngeal infections; in persons who cannot take a cephalosporin, a quinolone, or spectinomycin, a 5-d oral regimen of trimethoprim-sulfamethoxazole may be given.

[d] Quinolones are contraindicated for persons younger than 18 years, pregnant women, and nursing women.

[e] Doxycycline can be given instead of erythromycin if the child is 9 years or older.

[f] Tetracycline, 500 mg, four times daily, can be substituted for doxycycline.

From American Academy of Pediatrics. In: Peter G, ed. *1994 Red book: report of the Commitee on Infectious Diseases,* 23rd ed. Elk Grove Village, IL: American Academy of Pediatrics, 1994:199, with permission.

Table 104   Complicated Gonococcal Infection: Treatment for Children Beyond the Newborn Period and for Adolescents[a]

DISEASE	PREPUBERTAL CHILDREN WHO WEIGH <100 LB (45 KG)	DISEASE	PATIENTS WHO WEIGH >100 LB (45 KG) AND ARE 9 YEARS OR OLDER
Ophthalmia, peritonitis, bacteremia, or arthritis	Ceftriaxone, 50 mg/kg/d (max 1 g/d) IV or IM,[c] once daily for 7 d	Gonococcal pharyngitis Pelvic inflammatory disease	Ceftriaxone, 125 mg IM,[c] in a single dose See Table 86

[a] In all cases, in addition to the recommended treatment for gonococcal infection, doxycycline (100 mg orally, twice daily for 7 d), tetracycline (500 mg, 4 times daily for 7 d), or azithromycin (1 g orally, in a single dose) is recommended on the presumption that the patient has concomitant infection with *Chlamydia trachomatis,* for children younger than 9 y and pregnant women, erythromycin is recommended.

[b] Hospitalization is required; follow-up cultures are necessary to ensure that treatment has been effective.

[c] Some clinicians believe the discomfort of IM injection can be reduced by using 1% lidocaine as a diluent.

[d] Such as the arthritis-dermatitis syndrome.

[e] Spectinomycin is not recommended for treatment of pharyngeal gonococcal infection. For patients who cannot take a cephalosporin, spectinomycin, or a quinolone, a 5-d oral regimen of trimethoprim-sulfamethoxazole may be given.

[f] Alternatively, parenteral therapy can be discontinued 24–48 h after improvement begins and a 7-d course is completed with an appropriate oral antimicrobial. Some experts advise a 10- to 14-d course of therapy.

From American Academy of Pediatrics. In: Peter G, ed. *1994 Red book: report of the Committee on Infectious Diseases,* 23rd ed. Elk Grove Village, IL: American Academy of Pediatrics, 1994:200, with permission.

MISCELLANEOUS

Table 105   Late Effects of Chemotherapy and Radiation

CHEMOTHERAPY AGENT	POSSIBLE LATE EFFECTS
Cyclophosphamide	Azoospermia, amenorrhea, hemorrhagic cystitis, secondary malignancies
Doxorubicin, daunomycin	Cardiomyopathy/pericarditis, secondary leukemia
Methotrexate, actinomycin	Avascular necrosis, hepatitis or cirrhosis, learning disabilities with intrathecal use
Vincristine	Neuropathies
Steroids	Obesity, avascular necrosis, osteoporosis, cataracts
Cisplatin	Gynecomastia, nephritis, thrombotic thrombocytopenic purpura
Etoposide	Secondary leukemia
RADIATION	
Cranium/brain	Short stature or short trunk, obesity, learning disabilities, leukoencephalopathy, cranial neuropathies, alopecia, cataracts, hypothyroidism, second malignancies (brain, thyroid)
Head and neck	Nasolacrimal duct obstruction, chronic conjunctivitis, chronic otitis media, alopecia, cataracts, dental abnormalities, voice changes, facial deformities, neuropathies, esophagitis, second malignancies (thyroid, soft tissue sarcomas, bone tumors)
Mediastinum	Cardiomyopathy, hypothyroidism, second malignancies (thyroid, acute myeloid leukemia, breast cancer), pneumonitis/fibrosis, reduced cell-mediated immunity
Lungs	Pneumonitis or fibrosis
Spine	Short stature or short trunk, scoliosis, hypothyroidism, second malignancies (thyroid), delayed puberty
Bones	Atrophy or hypoplasia, avascular necrosis, osteoporosis, second malignancies (bone and soft-tissue sarcomas), osteochondromas
Total nodes	Reduced cell-mediated immunity, bone marrow dysfunction

Table 106   Red Eye: Common Causes by Location

CONJUNCTIVA	ADNEXA	GLOBE
Infectious conjunctivitis	Chalazion/hordeolum	Corneal abrasion
Neonatal conjunctivitis	Dacryocystitis	Foreign body
Allergic conjunctivitis	Orbital cellulitis	
Periorbital cellulitis		

Table 107   Helpful Specific Drug Levels

DRUG	TIME TO PEAK BLOOD LEVEL (HOURS POSTINGESTION)	POTENTIAL INTERVENTION
Acetaminophen	4	N-Acetylcysteine administration
Carbamazepine	2–4[a,b]	…
Carboxyhemoglobin	Immediate	Hyperbaric oxygen therapy
Digoxin	2–4	Fab (digoxin antibody) fragment
Ethanol	$1/2$–1[b]	…
Ethylene glycol	$1/2$–1	Ethanol infusion and hemodialysis
Iron	2–4	Deferoxamine administration
Isopropanol	$1/2$–1[b]	…
Lead	5 weeks[a]	Chelation and environmental abatement
Lithium	2–4	Hemodialysis
Methanol	$1/2$–1	Ethanol infusion and hemodialysis
Methemoglobinemia	Immediate	Methylene blue administration
Phenobarbital	2–4	Alkaline diuresis, multiple-dose activated charcoal
Phenytoin	1–2[a]	Multiple-dose activated charcoal
Salicylates	6–12[a]	Alkaline diuresis, multiple-dose activated charcoal, hemodialysis
Theophylline	1–36[a]	Multiple-dose activated charcoal, whole-bowel irrigation, charcoal hemoperfusion, hemodialysis

[a]Repeated measurement of levels is necessary because of significant variation in time to reach to peak level.

[b]The peak level is predictive of toxicity and clinical course. Adapted from Weisman RS, Howland MA, Verebey K. The toxicology laboratory. In: Goldfrank LR, Flomenbaum NE, Lewin NA, et al., eds. *Goldfrank's toxicologic emergencies,* 5th ed. East Norwalk, CT: Appleton & Lange, 1994:105.

Table 108   Human Papilloma Viruses: Preferred Sites of Infectivity

CLINICAL TYPE	HPV TYPE
Verruca vulgaris (common warts)	1, 2, 4, 7, 26, 27, 29
Verruca plana (flat warts)	3, 10, 28, 41
Verruca plantaris (plantar warts)	1, 2, 4
Anogenital warts	1–6, 10, 11, 13, 16, 18, 31, 33, 35, 39, 41, 42
Laryngeal warts	6, 11, 13, 30, 40
Anogenital carcinoma	11, 16, 18, 31, 33, 42, 47
Bowenoid papulosis	16, 18, 30
Epidermodysplasia verruciformis	5, 8–10, 12, 14, 15, 17, 19–25, 16–38, 40

Table 109   Proper Child Safety Seat Use Chart: Buckle Everyone; Children Age 12 and Under Sit in Back!

	INFANTS	TODDLER	YOUNG CHILDREN
Weight	Birth to 1 year up to 20–22 lbs	Over 1 year and >20–40 lbs	>40–80 lbs
Type of seat	Infant only or rear-facing convertible	Convertible/forward-facing	Belt positioning booster seat
Seat position	Rear-facing only	Forward facing	Forward facing
Guidelines	Children to 1 year and at least 20 lbs in rear-facing seats	Harness straps should be at or above shoulders	Belt positioning booster seats must be used with both lap and shoulder belts
	Harness straps at or below shoulder level	Most seats require top slot for forward-facing	Make sure the lap belt fits low and tight across the lap/upper thigh area and the shoulder belt fits snug crossing the chest and shoulder to avoid abdominal injuries
Warning	All children age 12 and under should ride in the back seat	All children age 12 and under should ride in the back seat	All children age 12 and under should ride in the back seat

From National Highway Traffic Safety Administration, *www.nhtsa.dot.gov.*

SECTION VIII

Medications

Monica Darby

MEDICATIONS

Table 1   Medications

DRUG	DOSE	DOSAGE FORMS
Acetaminophen (Feverall, Panadol, Tempra, Tylenol)	*Orally or rectally:* Children: 10–15 mg/kg repeated every 4–6 hours, up to 5 doses daily. Adults: 325–650 mg every 4–6 hours or 1 g t.i.d. or q.i.d. Do not exceed 4 g/day.	Drops: 100 mg/mL Suspension: 160 mg/5 mL Suppositories: 120 mg, 325 mg, 650 mg Tablets: 160 mg, 325 mg, 500 mg Tablets, chewable: 80 mg Also available in combination with codeine; see codeine monograph.
Acetazolamide (Diamox)	*Orally or IV:* Children and adults: 8–30 mg/kg/day in 4 divided doses. Do not exceed 1 g/day. *Altitude sickness (adults):* 250 mg every 8–12 hours beginning 24–48 hours before ascent and continuing for at least 48 hours after arrival.	Injection: 500 mg Tablets: 250 mg
Acetylcysteine (Mucomyst, Mucosil)	*Acetaminophen poisoning:* 140 mg/kg PO followed by 70 mg/kg for 17 doses administered every 4 hours until acetaminophen levels are nontoxic. Usually administered as a 5% solution diluted in juice or soda. *Inhalation* (administer 10% solution undiluted): Infants: 2–4 mL repeated t.i.d. or q.i.d. Children and adolescents: 6–10 mL repeated t.i.d. or q.i.d.	Solution for inhalation: 10% or 20% in 10-mL and 30-mL vials
Acyclovir (Zovirax)	*Oral doses for children and adults:* *Varicella zoster (chickenpox):* 80 mg/kg/day in 4 divided doses for 5 days. Do not exceed 800 mg/dose (3,200 mg/day). *Herpes simplex virus:* Children: 1,200 mg/m^2/day in 4–5 divided doses. Adults: 200 mg every 4 hours while awake (5 doses daily). Chronic suppressive therapy at a dose of 400 mg b.i.d. may be used for up to 1 year or longer. *IV doses for children and adults:* *Neonatal HSV encephalitis:* 30 mg/kg/day in 3 divided doses for 10–14 days. *HSV encephalitis:* 1,500 mg/m^2/day in 3 divided doses for at least 10 days and up to 21 days. *Other HSV infections:* 750 mg/m^2/day in 3 divided doses for 7 days. *Varicella zoster infections:* 1,500 mg/m^2/day in 3 divided doses for 7 days. *Topically:* apply ointment every 3 hours up to 6 times daily for 7 days. Use a disposable finger cot or glove when applying the ointment to avoid transmission of the virus. Dosage may need to be adjusted in patients with renal dysfunction.	Capsules: 200 mg Injection: 500-mg, 1-g vials Ointment: 5%, 15 g Suspension: 200 mg/5 mL
Adenosine (Adenocard)	*IV (given via rapid push followed by a saline flush):* Children: 0.1 mg/kg initially, followed by doses increasing in 0.05 mg/kg increments every 2 minutes to a maximum dose of 0.35 mg/kg or 12 mg/dose. Adults: 6 mg followed by 12 mg with a repeat dose of 12 mg, if needed.	Injection: 3 mg/mL 2-mL vial)
Albumin, human (Albuminar, Albutein, Plasbumin)	*IV (as a 5% solution for hypovolemic patients or 25% for fluid- or sodium-restricted patients):* Children: 0.5–1 g/kg infused over 2–4 hours. May repeat to a maximum of 6 g/kg/day.	Injection: 5% (50 mL, 250 mL, 500 mL); 25% (20 mL, 50 mL, 100 mL)

Continued

Table 1 **Medications** (continued)

DRUG	DOSE	DOSAGE FORMS
Albumin, human (Albuminar, Albutein, Plasbumin) (continued)	Adults: 25 g infused over 2–4 hours. Usually not to exceed 125 g/day.	
Albuterol (Proventil, Ventolin)	*Oral:* Age 2–<6: 0.3–0.6 mg/kg/day in 3 divided doses to a maximum of 12 mg/day. Age ≥6–≤12: 6–8 mg/day in 3–4 divided doses to a maximum of 24 mg/day. Over age 12: 6–16 mg/day in 3–4 divided doses to a maximum of 32 mg/day. *Inhalation:* *Metered-dose inhaler:* Under age 12: 1–2 inhalations q.i.d. Over age 12: 1–2 inhalations up to 6 times a day. *Nebulization:* 0.01–0.05 mL/kg usually repeated every 4–6 hours, but may be administered more frequently in severely ill patients under controlled conditions.	Aerosol: 90 μg/actuation Solution for inhalation: 0.5% Syrup: 10 mg/5 mL Tablets: 2 mg, 4 mg Tablets, extended release: 4 mg, 8 mg
Allopurinol (Zyloprim)	*Orally:* Under age 6: 150 mg/day in 3 divided doses. Age 6–10: 300 mg/day in 2 or 3 divided doses. Over age 10: 600–800 mg/day in 2 or 3 divided doses. Note: The metabolism of mercaptopurine and azathioprine is decreased by allopurinol. Decrease dose of mercaptopurine or azathioprine by 75%.	Tablets: 100 mg, 300 mg
Alprostadil (Prostin VR Pediatric)	A continuous infusion beginning at a dose of 0.05–0.1 μg/kg/min. Dosage may be adjusted downward or gradually upward based on the patient's response. Usual dosage range is 0.01–0.4 μg/kg/min.	Injection: 500 μg/mL (1-mL ampule)
Aluminum acetate (Domeboro, Burow's Solution)	*Topically:* as a wet dressing or soak 2–4 times daily for 30 minutes at a time. Usual concentrations are 1:10, 1:20, or 1:40. *Ear:* 4–6 drops in the ear at first every 2–3 hours, then every 4–6 hours until itching or burning subsides.	Powder (packets): 1 packet/pint of water = 1:40 dilution Solution otic, 1:10 dilution with 2% acetic acid
Aluminum and magnesium hydroxides (Maalox, Maalox Plus, Mylanta)	Children: 5–10 mL 4–6 times daily or more frequently. Adults: 15–30 mL 4–6 times daily or more frequently.	Suspension: aluminum hydroxide 225 mg and magnesium hydroxide 200 mg/5 mL Suspension with simethicone: as above with simethicone 25 mg/5 mL
Amantadine (Symmetrel)	*Orally* for prophylaxis or treatment of influenza A: Children 1–9 years of age: 5–9 mg/kg/day in 2 divided doses Children 10 years of age and adults: 200 mg daily in 1 or 2 divided doses	Solution: 50 mg/5 mL Capsules: 100 mg
Amikacin (Amikin)	*IV* (dose should be based on ideal body weight): Neonates: 0–4 weeks, <1,200 g: 7.5 mg/kg/dose every 18–24 hours. ≤7 days of age: 1,200–2,000 g: 7.5 mg/kg/dose every 12–18 hours. >2,000 g: 10 mg/kg/dose every 12 hours. Over 7 days of age: 1,200–2,000 g: 7.5 mg/kg/dose every 8–12 hours. >2,000 g: 10 mg/kg/dose every 8 hours. Infants and children: 15–22.5 mg/kg/day in 3 divided doses daily. The dose for the treatment of nontuberculous mycobacterial infections is 15–30 mg/kg/day in 2 divided doses, to a maximum of 1.5 g/day as part of a multiple-drug regimen.	Injection: 50 mg/mL, 250 mg/mL

Continued

Table 1   Medications   (continued)

DRUG	DOSE	DOSAGE FORMS
Amikacin (Amikin) (*continued*)	Adults: 15 mg/kg/day in 2–3 divided doses. Dosage adjustment is required in patients with renal dysfunction.	

Aminocaproic acid (Amicar)	*IV:*
	    Children: 100 mg/kg over the first hour followed by an infusion of 33.3 mg/kg/hr to a maximum daily dose of 30 g.
	    Older children and adults: 4–5 g over the first hour followed by an infusion of 1 g/hr for 8 hours or until control is achieved.
	Orally: doses are the same or alternatively, 100 mg/kg may be administered every 4–6 hours to a maximum of 5 g/dose.
		Injection: 250 mg/mL (20-mL vial)
		Solution: 1.25 g/5 mL (16-oz bottle)
		Tablets: 500 mg

Amiodarone (Cordarone)	*Orally:*
	    Children (use body surface area for children age 1 year or under): loading dose of 10–15 mg/kg/day or 600–800 mg/1.73 m^2/day in 1–2 divided doses for 4–14 days or until adequate control of arrhythmia is achieved or prominent adverse effects occur. Then reduce dosage to 5 mg/kg/day or 200–400 mg/1.73 m^2/day as a single dose for several weeks. A further dose reduction to 2.5 mg/kg/day should be attempted if the arrhythmia does not recur.
	    Adults: loading dose of 800–1,600 mg/day in 1–2 divided doses for 1–3 weeks, followed by dose of 600–800 mg/day in 1–2 divided doses for 1 month. Maintenance dose usually 400 mg/day, but may be lower for supraventricular arrhythmias.
	IV:
	    Children (only limited information is available): initial loading dose of 5 mg/kg over 1 hour followed by a continuous infusion of 5 μg/kg/min has been used. The continuous infusion dosage may be increased to 10 μg/kg/min and then to 15 μg/kg/min until the desired effect is achieved.
	    Adults: loading dose of 150 mg administered over 10 minutes (15 mg/min) followed by 360 mg over 6 hours at a rate of 1 mg/min, followed by the maintenance dose of 540 mg over 18 hours at a rate of 0.5 mg/min. If necessary, maintenance infusion of 0.5 mg/min may be continued past the initial 24 hours. Additional bolus doses of 150 mg may be administered over 10 minutes for breakthrough arrhythmias.
		Injection: 50 mg/mL
		Tablets: 200 mg

Amitriptyline (Elavil, Endep)	*Orally:* *Chronic pain:* 0.1 mg/kg/day at bedtime initially, advancing to 0.5–2 mg/kg/day over a 2–3 week period. *Depression:* 1 mg/kg/day to start, advancing to a maximum of 5 mg/kg or 100 mg, whichever is less. Adolescents and adults: 25–50 mg at bedtime or in divided doses, increasing daily doses by 25 mg to a maximum of 100 mg/day for adolescents and 300 mg for adults. Dosage should be decreased to the lowest effective dose after symptom control has been reached.	Tablets: 10 mg, 25 mg, 50 mg, 75 mg, 100 mg, 150 mg

Continued

Table 1 Medications (continued)

DRUG	*DOSE*	*DOSAGE FORMS*

Amoxicillin (Amoxil, Polymox, Trimox, Wymox)	*Orally:*
	  Children ≤20 kg: 20 mg/kg/day in 3 divided doses for urinary tract infections. 40 mg/kg/day in 3 divided doses for otitis media, upper respiratory infection, or skin infections. Acute otitis media due to highly resistant strains of *S. pneumoniae* may require doses of 80–90 mg/kg/day in 3 divided doses.
	  Children >20 kg and adults: 750 mg/day in 3 divided doses for urinary tract infections or 1,500 mg/day in 3 divided doses for otitis media, upper respiratory infections, or skin infections. Maximum daily dose is 3 g.
	Endocarditis prophylaxis: 50 mg/kg (up to 2 g) 1 hour before procedure
		Capsules: 250 mg, 500 mg
		Drops: 50 mg/mL
		Suspension: 125 mg/5 mL, 250 mg/5 mL
		Tablets, chewable: 125 mg, 250 mg

Amoxicillin and clavulanic acid (Augmentin)	*Orally* (based on the amoxicillin component): 20–40 mg/kg/day in 3 divided doses to a maximum of 1.5 g/day, or 25–45 mg/kg/day in 2 divided doses to a maximum of 1.75 g/day using the b.i.d. formulation of the drug. Use the higher doses for respiratory tract infections and otitis media.	Suspension: amoxicillin 125 mg and clavulanic acid 31.25 mg/5 mL; b.i.d. formulation—amoxicillin 200 mg and clavulanic acid 28.5 mg/5 mL; amoxicillin 250 mg and clavulanic acid 62.5 mg/5 mL; b.i.d. formulation—amoxicillin 400 mg and clavulanic acid 57 mg/5 mL Tablets: amoxicillin 250 mg and clavulanic acid 125 mg; amoxicillin 500 mg and clavulanic acid 125 mg; b.i.d. formulation—amoxicillin 875 mg and clavulanic acid 125 mg Tablets, chewable: amoxicillin 125 mg and clavulanic acid 31.25 mg; b.i.d. formulation—amoxicillin 200 mg and clavulanic acid 28.5 mg; amoxicillin 250 mg and clavulanic acid 62.5 mg; b.i.d. formulation—amoxicillin 400 mg and clavulanic acid 57 mg
Amphotericin B (Fungizone)	*IV* (infusion over 2–8 hours): *Test dose* (infusion over 30 minutes) <10 kg: 0.1 mg in 1 mL D_5W. ≥10 kg: 1 mg in 10 mL D_5W. *Therapeutic dose:* begin with 0.25–0.5 mg/kg immediately following test dose. Doses may be doubled on each subsequent day to a maximum of 1 mg/kg as the patient tolerates. Once therapy is established, alternate day doses at a maximum of 1.5 mg/kg/day may be used. Bladder irrigations of 15–50 mg daily in 1 L of sterile water instilled over 24 hours have been used to treat bladder infections.	Injection: 50-mg vial
Amphotericin B, cholesteryl (Amphotec)	*IV* (infusion at a rate of 1 mg/kg/hr): Children and adults: 3–4 mg/kg/day as a single infusion. Doses of 6 mg/kg/day have been used to treat invasive *Candida* or *Cryptococcus* infections. Admix with 5% dextrose injection to a final concentration of about 0.6 mg/mL for administration over 3–4 hours. In patients who tolerate the longer infusion time well, the time can be shortened to 2 hours.	Injection: 50-mg vial
Amphotericin B, liposomal complex (Abelcet)	*IV* (infusion over 2 hours): Children and adults: 5 mg/kg/day in a single infusion. Admix with 5% dextrose to a final concentration of 1 mg/mL. A final concentration of 2 mg/mL may be used for pediatric patients or patients requiring fluid restriction.	Suspension for injection: 5 mg/mL

Continued

Table 1   Medications   (continued)

DRUG	DOSE	DOSAGE FORMS

Ampicillin (Omnipen, Polycillin, Principen, Totacillin)	*IV:*
	Meningitis:
	Neonates under age 7 days:
	  <2,000 g: 100 mg/kg/day in 2 divided doses.
	  ≥2,000 g: 150 mg/kg/day in 3 divided doses.
	Neonates over age 7 days:
	  <1,200 g: 100 mg/kg/day in 2 divided doses.
	  1,200–2,000 g: 150 mg/kg/day in 3 divided doses.
	  >2,000 g: 200 mg/kg/day in 4 divided doses.
	Infants and children: 150–300 mg/kg/day in 4–6 divided doses to a maximum of 12 g/d.
	Adults: 150–200 mg/kg/day in 6–8 divided doses to a maximum total daily dose of 14 g.
	Moderate infections:
	Neonates under age 7 days:
	  <2,000 g: 50 mg/kg/day in 2 divided doses.
	  >2,000 g: 75 mg/kg/day in 3 divided doses.
	Neonates over age 7 days:
	  <1,200 g: 50 mg/kg/day in 2 divided doses.
	  1,200–2,000 g: 75 mg/kg/day in 3 divided doses.
	  >2,000 g: 100 mg/kg/day in 4 divided doses.
	Infants, children, and adults: 50–100 mg/kg/day in 4–6 divided doses to a maximum total dose of 12 g/day.
	Orally (mild to moderate infections):
	Children <20 kg: 50–75 mg/kg/day in 4 divided doses. Do not exceed adult doses for the same degree of infection.
	Children >20 kg and adults: 1–2 daily (250–500 mg/dose) in 4 divided doses.
		Capsules: 250 mg, 500 mg
		Injection: 125-mg, 250-mg, 500-mg, 1-g, 2-g vials
		Suspension: 125 mg/5 mL, 250 mg/5 mL, 500 mg/5 mL

Ampicillin and sulbactam sodium (Unasyn)	*IV:* Infants and children: 150 mg/kg/day (100 mg ampicillin + 50 mg sulbactam) in 3–4 divided doses. Adults: 1.5–3 g (1–2 g ampicillin + 0.5–1 g sulbactam) given every 6 hours.	Injection: 1.5 g (1 g ampicillin + 0.5 g sulbactam), 3 g (2 g ampicillin + 1 g sulbactam)
Amrinone (Inocor)	*IV:* a bolus dose of 0.75 mg/kg administered over 2–3 minutes is followed by a maintenance infusion of 3–5 μg/kg/min for neonates or 5–10 μg/kg/min for infants, children, or adults. The bolus doses may be repeated at 30-minute intervals to a total of 3 mg/kg. Total daily dose should not exceed 10 mg/kg.	Injection: 5 mg/mL
Aspirin (Anacin, Ascriptin, Bufferin, Easprin, Ecotrin)	*Orally or rectally:* *Analgesic, antipyretic:* Children: 10–15 mg/kg every 4–6 hours. Adults: 325–1,000 mg every 4–6 hours, up to 4 g/day. *Antiinflammatory:* Children ≤25 kg: 60–90 mg/kg/day in 3–4 divided doses initially, with a usual range of 80–100 mg/kg/day. Monitor serum levels. Children >25 kg and adults: 2.4–3.6 g/day in 4 divided doses. Maximum total daily dose usually should not exceed 5.4 g. *Kawasaki syndrome:* 100 mg/kg/day in 4 divided doses until fever resolves; then 3–8 mg/kg once daily for 6–10 weeks after onset of the disease, or longer.	Suppositories: 300 mg, 325 mg, 600 mg, 650 mg Tablets: 325 mg, 500 mg, 650 mg Tablets, chewable: 81 mg Tablets, extended release: 165 mg, 325 mg, 500 mg, 650 mg, 975 mg Also available in buffered formulation, enteric-coated tablets, and chewing gum.

Continued

Table 1   Medications   (continued)

DRUG	DOSE	DOSAGE FORMS
Atenolol (Tenormin)	*Orally:* Children: initially 0.8–1 mg/kg/day in a single dose. Dosage may be increased to 1.5 mg/kg/day or a maximum of 2 mg/kg/day if necessary. Adults: initially 25–50 mg/day, increasing to 50–100 mg/day as needed. The maximum dose for hypertension is 100 mg; for angina, 200 mg.	Tablets: 25 mg, 50 mg, 100 mg
Atropine sulfate	*Preoperative orally or IM:* 0.02 mg/kg to a maximum dose of about 1 mg. *Bradycardia:* 0.02 mg/kg with a minimum dose of 0.1 mg and a maximum dose of 0.5 mg in children, 1 mg in adolescents, and 2 mg in adults. *Ophthalmic:* 1–2 drops of 0.5–1% solution in the eye.	Injection: 0.3 mg/mL, 0.4 mg/mL, 0.5 mg/mL, 0.8 mg/mL, 1 mg/mL Ointment, ophthalmic: 0.5%, 1% Solution, ophthalmic: 0.5%, 1%, 2%
Attapulgite (Kaopectate)	*Orally* (dose after each loose bowel movement, up to 7 times a day): Age 3–5: 7.5 mL or 1 tablet. Age 6–12: 15 mL or 2 tablets. Over age 12: 30 mL or 4 tablets.	Suspension: 600 mg/15 mL Tablets, chewable: 300 mg
Azathioprine (Imuran)	*IV or orally:* Children and adults: initially 3–5 mg/kg/day as a single dose. Maintenance doses are usually 1–3 mg/kg/day. Note: Metabolism of azathioprine is decreased by allopurinol; decrease dose of azathioprine by 75%.	Injection: 100-mg vial Tablets: 50 mg
Azelastine (Astelin)	*Intranasal metered dose spray:* 12 years of age and adults: 2 sprays in each nostril twice daily	Solution, nasal: 137 μg/metered spray
Azithromycin (Zithromax)	*Orally:* *Otitis media* (6 months of age and older): 10 mg/kg (to a maximum of 500 mg) on the first day followed by 5 mg/kg/day (to a maximum of 250 mg) for 4 days. *Pharyngitis/tonsillitis:* 2 years of age and older: 12 mg/kg/day (to a maximum of 500 mg) for 5 days. Adults: 500 mg on the first day followed by 250 mg/day for 4 days. *Uncomplicated chlamydia infection:* 1 g as a single dose for patients >8 years of age weighing at least 45 kg. *Gonorrhea:* 2 g for patients weighing at least 45 kg *Chancroid:* 20 mg/kg to a maximum dose of 1 g	Capsules: 250 mg Suspension: 100 mg/5 mL, 200 mg/5 mL, 1-g packet
Aztreonam (Azactam)	*IV or IM:* Children over age 1 month: 60–100 mg/kg/day in 3–4 divided doses. Doses of up to 200 mg/kg/day have been used in severe infections. Maximum total daily dose is 8 g. Adults: 1–2 g every 6–8 hours, depending on the severity of the infection. Dose adjustment is necessary in renal impairment.	Injection: 500-mg, 1-g, 2-g vials
Bacitracin; bacitracin and polymyxin B (Polysporin); bacitracin, neomycin, and polymyxin B (Neosporin)	*Topically:* apply to affected area 1–3 times daily. *Ophthalmic:* apply to eyes every 3–4 hours.	Ointment, ophthalmic (all three): 3.5-g tube Ointment, topical (all three): 15-g, 30-g tubes

Continued

Table 1   Medications   (continued)

DRUG	_DOSE_	_DOSAGE FORMS_
Beclomethasone dipropionate (Beclovent, Beconase, Vancenase, Vanceril)	_Intranasal:_ Age 6–12: 1 inhalation in each nostril t.i.d. Over age 12 and adults 1 inhalation in each nostril b.i.d. or q.i.d. or 2 inhalations in each nostril b.i.d. _Intranasal aqueous formulation:_ Children ≥6 years of age and adults: 1–2 sprays in each nostril b.i.d. Vancenase AQ 84 μg: 1–2 sprays in each nostril daily. _Oral inhalation:_ Age 6–12: 1–2 inhalations t.i.d. or q.i.d. or 2–4 inhalations b.i.d. Do not exceed 10 inhalations/day. Over age 12 and adults: 2 inhalations t.i.d. or q.i.d. not to exceed 20 inhalations/day. Vanceril 84 μg Double Strength: use 1/2 the doses recommended above.	Intranasal aerosol spray: 42 μg/spray Intranasal nasal suspension spray pump: 42 μg/spray Intranasal nasal suspension spray pump double strength: 84 μg/spray Oral inhalation aerosol: 42 μg/spray Oral inhalation aerosol double strength: 84 μg/spray
Betamethasone (Diprolene, Diprosone, Maxivate, Uticort, Valisone)	Apply a thin film to the skin 1–3 times daily. Avoid application to the face, groin, or axillae.	Benzoate (Uticort): 0.025% cream, lotion, gel Dipropionate, augmented (Diprolene): 0.05% cream, lotion, gel, ointment Dipropionate (Diprosone): 0.05% cream, lotion, ointment, 0.1% aerosol Dipropionate with clotrimazole (antifungal) [Lotrisone] Valerate (Valisone): 0.01% cream, lotion, ointment
Bethanechol (Urecholine)	_Orally:_ _Gastroesophageal reflux:_ Children: 0.1–0.2 mg/kg given at least 30 minutes before a meal. Up to 4 doses/day may be given. Adults: 10–50 mg up to q.i.d. _Urinary retention:_ Children: 0.6 mg/kg/day in 3–4 divided doses. Adults: 10–50 mg/dose up to q.i.d.	Tablets: 25 mg
Bisacodyl (Dulcolax)	_Orally_ (higher doses for evacuation, lower for laxation): Age 3–12: 5–10 mg as a single dose. Over age 12: 5–15 mg as a single dose. Tablets are enteric coated and must not be chewed or crushed. _Rectally:_ Under age 2: 5 mg/day as a single dose. Age 2–11: 5–10 mg/day as a single dose. Age 12 or over: 10 mg/day as a single dose.	Suppositories: 5 mg, 10 mg Tablets, enteric coated: 5 mg
Brompheniramine (Dimetane)	_Orally:_ <6 years of age: 0.125 mg/kg/dose 4 times a day to a maximum of 8 mg/day. 6–12 years of age: 2–4 mg given 3–4 times a day to a maximum of 16 mg/day. Over age 12: 4–8 mg every 4–6 hours to a maximum of 24 mg/day. Extended-release tablets may be given in as 8 mg b.i.d. or t.i.d. or 12 mg b.i.d.	Elixir: 2 mg/5 mL Tablet: 4 mg, 8 mg, 12 mg Tablets, extended release: 8 mg, 12 mg
Budesonide (Rhinocort)	_Intranasal metered dose spray:_ Children ≥6 years of age and adults: 8 sprays (4 sprays in each nostril) as a single dose in the morning or as 2 divided doses. Dosage may be decreased to the lowest number of sprays that controls symptoms.	Aerosol, nasal: 50 μg/actuation

Continued

Table 1   Medications   (continued)

DRUG	DOSE	DOSAGE FORMS
Bumetanide (Bumex)	*Orally or IV:* Neonates: 0.01–0.05 mg/kg/dose every 24–48 hours. Infants and children: 0.015–0.1 mg/kg/dose every 6–24 hours to a maximum of 10 mg/day. Adults: 0.5–1 mg/dose IV or 0.5–2 mg/dose orally once or twice daily to a maximum of 10 mg/day.	Injection: 0.25 mg/mL Tablets: 0.5 mg, 1 mg, 2 mg
Caffeine	*Orally or IV:* *Loading dose:* 10 mg/kg caffeine base. If theophylline has been administered within the previous 3 days, a modified dose (50–75% of loading dose) may be given. *Maintenance:* 2.5 mg/kg caffeine base 24 hours after the loading dose. Dosage may be adjusted based on the patient's response and the results of serum level monitoring. Do not use caffeine and sodium benzoate injection in neonates.	Injection: 10 mg/mL Solution: 10 mg/mL
Calcitriol (Calcijex, Rocaltrol)	Individualize to maintain normal serum calcium levels. *Orally:* *Hypocalcemia in premature infants:* 1 μg/day for 5 days. *Renal failure:* Children 0.25–2 μg/day (hemodialysis) or 0.014–0.041 μg/kg/day (no hemodialysis). Adults: 0.25–1 μg/day. *IV:* *Hypocalcemia in premature infants:* 0.05 μg/kg/day for 4 days. *Renal failure:* Children: 0.01–0.05 μg/kg 3 times weekly (hemodialysis). Adults: 0.5–3 μg 3 times weekly (hemodialysis).	Capsules: 0.25 μg, 0.5 μg Injection: 1 μg/mL, 2 μg/mL (1-mL ampules) Solution: 1 μg/mL
Calcium salts	See dosage forms for calcium content of various salts. Dosage should be adjusted based on the desired response and serum calcium levels. *IV (gluconate or chloride salts):* *Cardiac resuscitation:* Calcium gluconate: Children: 60–100 mg/kg/dose to a maximum of 3 g. Adults: 500 mg–1 g/dose. Calcium chloride: Children: 20 mg/kg/dose to a maximum of 1 g. Adults: 2–4 mg/kg/dose to a maximum of 1 g. *Hypocalcemia* (usually the gluconate salt): Neonates: 200–800 mg/kg/day, usually as a continuous infusion. Infants and children: 200–500 mg/kg/day as a continuous infusion or in 4 divided doses. Adults: 2–15 g/day as a continuous infusion or in divided doses.	Calcium acetate = 25% Ca = 250 mg Ca per 1 g Ca acetate Calcium carbonate = 40% Ca = 400 mg Ca per 1 g Ca carbonate Calcium chloride = 27% Ca = 270 mg Ca per 1 g Ca chloride Calcium citrate = 21% Ca = 210 mg Ca per 1 g Ca citrate Calcium glubionate = 6.5% Ca = 65 mg Ca per 1 g Ca glubionate Calcium gluconate = 9% Ca = 90 mg Ca per 1 g Ca gluconate Calcium lactate = 13% Ca = 130 mg Ca per 1 g Ca lactate Injection: Chloride salt: 1 g (100 mg/mL) = 27 mg Ca/mL Gluconate salt: 1 g (100 mg/mL) = 9 mg Ca/mL Suspension: carbonate salt: 1.25 g/5 mL = 500 mg Ca/5 mL

Continued

Table 1   Medications   (continued)

DRUG	DOSE	DOSAGE FORMS

Calcium salts (*continued*)	*Orally (carbonate, glubionate, or lactate salts):*
	  Neonates: 20–80 mg calcium/kg/day in 4–6
	    divided doses.
	  Infants and children: 20–40 mg calcium/kg/day in
	    4–6 divided doses.
	  Adults: 400 mg–1.2 g calcium/day or more.
		Syrup: glubionate salt: 1.8 g/5 mL = 115 mg Ca/5 mL
		Tablets:
		  Acetate salt: 667 mg = 169 mg Ca (PhosLo)
		  Carbonate salt: 650 mg = 260 mg Ca; 1.25 g =
		    500 mg Ca; 1.5 g = 600 mg Ca
		  Citrate salt: 950 mg = 200 mg Ca (Citracal);
		    2376 mg = 500 mg Ca (Citracal Liquitab)
		  Gluconate salt: 500 mg = 45 mg Ca; 650 mg =
		    58.5 mg Ca; 975 mg = 87.75 mg Ca; 1 g =
		    90 mg Ca
		  Lactate salt: 325 mg = 42.25 mg Ca; 650 mg =
		    84.5 mg Ca

Calfactant (Infasurf)	*Intratracheally:* 3 mL/kg divided into 2–4 aliquots.
	  Patients should be ventilated and repositioned
	  between aliquots.
		Suspension, intratracheal: 8 mL

Captopril (Capoten)	*Orally:*
	  Neonates: 0.01–0.05 mg/kg up to t.i.d., initially.
	    Dose may be increased incrementally to a
	    maximum of 0.5 mg/kg administered as frequently
	    as every 6 hours (2 mg/kg/day).
	  Infants and children: 0.15–0.3 mg/kg up to t.i.d.,
	    initially. Dose may be increased incrementally to a
	    maximum of 6 mg/kg/day in divided doses.
	  Adolescents and adults: 12.5–25 mg every 8–12 hours,
	    initially. May be titrated upward to a maximum of
	    6 mg/kg/day or 450 mg.
		Tablets: 12.5 mg, 25 mg, 50 mg, 100 mg

Carbamazepine (Tegretol)	*Orally:* initially 5–10 mg/kg/day in 2–4 divided doses,
	  increasing slowly to a maximum of 30 mg/kg/day
	  (1.6–2.4 g in adults).
	Suspension formulation should be administered in
	  3–4 daily doses; tablet formulations may be
	  administered in 2–3 divided doses.
		Suspension: 100 mg/5 mL
		Tablets, chewable: 100 mg
		Tablets: 200 mg

Carbamide peroxide (Debrox, Gly-Oxide)	*Ear:* instill up to 5–10 drops in the ear and allow to
	  remain there for several minutes or longer.
	Orally: apply several drops to the affected area up to
	  q.i.d.
		Drops, oral: 10% (Cank-aid, Gly-Oxide, Orajel Brace-aid
		  Rinse)
		Drops, otic: 6.5% (Auro Ear Drops, Debrox, Murine Ear
		  Drops)

Cefaclor (Ceclor)	*Orally:* 20–40 mg/kg/24 hr in 2–3 divided doses to a maximum of 2 g/24 hr.	Capsules: 250 mg Suspension: 125 mg/5 mL, 250 mg/5 mL

Cefadroxil (Duricef, Ultracef)	*Orally:*
	  Children: 30 mg/kg/day in 2 divided doses to a
	    maximum of 2 g/day.
	  Adults: 1–2 g/day in a single or 2 divided doses.
		Capsules: 500 mg
		Suspension: 125 mg/5 mL, 250 mg/5 mL, 500 mg/5 mL
		Tablets: 1 g

Cefazolin (Ancef, Kefzol)	*IV or IM:* 50–100 mg/kg/day in 3 divided doses to a
	  maximum of 6 g/day. Usual adult doses are
	  500 mg–2 g/dose every 8 hours
	Dosing adjustment is necessary in renal impairment.
		Injection: 250-mg, 500-mg, 1-g vials

Cefdinir (Omnicef)	*Orally:*
	  Age 6 months to 12 years: 14 mg/kg/day in 1 or 2
	    divided doses.
	  >12 years or 43 kg: 600 mg daily in 1 or 2 divided
	    doses.
		Capsules: 300 mg
		Suspension: 125 mg/5 mL

Cefixime (Suprax)	*Orally:*
	  Children: 8 mg/kg/day in 1 or 2 divided doses to a
	    maximum of 400 mg.
	  Adults: 400 mg/day in 1 or 2 divided doses.
	Otitis media: use suspension formula because higher
	  serum levels are reached at the same dose when the
	  suspension is administered.
		Suspension: 100 mg/5 mL
		Tablets: 200 mg, 400 mg

Continued

Table 1   Medications   (continued)

DRUG	*DOSE*	*DOSAGE FORMS*
Cefotaxime (Claforan)	*IV:* *Sepsis:* 　Infants and children: 100–120 mg/kg/day in 3–4 divided doses. 　Adults: 1–2 g every 6–8 hours. *Meningitis:* 　Neonates under age 1 week: 50 mg/kg every 12 hours. 　Neonates age 1 week or over: 50 mg/kg every 8 hours. 　Infants over 4 weeks and children: 200 mg/kg/day in 4 divided doses. A dose of 300 mg/kg/day in 4 divided doses has been used for the treatment of pneumococcal meningitis. Maximum total daily dose is 12 g. 　Adults: 2 g every 4–6 hours. Dosing adjustment is necessary in renal impairment.	Injection: 1-g, 2-g vials
Cefoxitin (Mefoxin)	*IV:* 　Neonates: 90–100 mg/kg/day in 3 divided doses. 　Children: 80–160 mg/kg/day depending on the severity of the infection in 4 divided doses. 　Adults: 1–2 g every 6–8 hours to a maximum total daily dose of 12 g.	Injection: 1-g, 2-g vials
Cefpodoxime (Vantin)	*Orally* (with food to enhance absorption): 　Children: 10 mg/kg/day in 2 divided doses to a maximum of 400 mg/day (otitis media) or 200 mg/day (pharyngitis/tonsillitis). 　Adults: 200 mg/day in 2 divided doses for upper respiratory or uncomplicated urinary tract infection, 400 mg/day in 2 divided doses for lower respiratory tract infection (community-acquired pneumonia), 800 mg/day in 2 divided doses (skin, skin structure infection). Dosage adjustment is necessary in severe renal impairment.	Suspension: 50 mg/5 mL, 100 mg/5 mL Tablets: 100 mg, 200 mg
Cefprozil (Cefzil)	*Orally:* 　Children: 　　*Otitis media:* 30 mg/kg/day in 2 divided doses to a maximum total daily dose of 1 g. 　　*Pharyngitis, tonsillitis:* 15 mg/kg/day in 2 divided doses to a maximum total daily dose of 500 mg. 　Adults: 　　*Lower respiratory tract:* 500 mg every 12 hours. 　　*Upper respiratory tract and skin:* 500 mg every 24 hours. Dosage adjustment is necessary in renal impairment.	Suspension: 125 mg/5 mL, 250 mg/5 mL Tablets: 250 mg, 500 mg
Ceftazidime (Fortaz, Tazicef, Tazidime)	*IV:* 　Neonates: 　　<2,000 g: 60 mg/kg/day in 2 divided doses. 　　≥2,000 g: 90 mg/kg/day in 3 divided doses. 　Infants and children: 90–150 mg/kg/day in 3 divided doses to a maximum total daily dose of 6 g. 　Adults: 3–6 g/day in 3 divided doses. Dosage adjustment is necessary in renal impairment.	Injection: 500 mg, 1 g, 2 g

Continued

Table 1 Medications (continued)

DRUG	DOSE	DOSAGE FORMS
Ceftriaxone (Rocephin)	*IV or IM:* *PPNG (uncomplicated pharyngeal, urethral, endo-cervical, rectal):* <45 kg: 125 mg IM as a single dose. ≥45 kg: 250 mg IM as a single dose. *PPNG (ophthalmia):* >20 kg: 1 g IM as a single dose. *Infants born to a mother infected with PPNG:* 50 mg/kg IM to a maximum of 125 mg as a single dose. *Other serious infections (not including meningitis):* Children: 50–75 mg/kg/day in 2 divided doses. Do not exceed 2 g/day. Adults: usually 1–2 g as a single daily dose or in 2 divided doses. *Otitis media, chancroid:* 50 mg/kg as a single dose given IM. *Meningitis:* Children: 100 mg/kg/day in 1–2 divided doses to a maximum total daily dose of 4 g.	Injection: 250-mg, 500-mg, 1-g, 2-g vials
Cefuroxime (Ceftin, Kefurox, Zinacef)	*Orally* (administer with food to enhance absorption): *Otitis media* (all ages): 30 mg/kg/day in 2 divided doses to a maximum total daily dose of 1 g. *Other infections* (all ages): 20 mg/kg/day in 2 divided doses to a maximum total daily dose of 500 mg. *IV:* Children: 50–100 mg/kg/day in 3–4 divided doses. A dose of 150 mg/kg/day in 3 divided doses is recommended for bone and joint infections. Do not exceed adult doses below. Adults: 2.25–4.5 g/day in 3 divided doses. Higher dose is necessary for severe infections and bone and joint infections. Dosage adjustment is necessary in renal impairment.	Injection: 750-mg, 1.5-g vials Suspension (axetil): 125 mg/5 mL Tablets: 125 mg, 250 mg, 500 mg
Cephalexin (Keflet, Keflex)	*Orally:* Children: 50–100 mg/kg/day in 4 divided doses for otitis media and serious infections. Doses of 25–50 mg/kg/day in 2–4 divided doses may be used for less serious infections. Do not exceed adult doses. Adults: 1–4 g/day in 4 divided doses.	Capsules: 250 mg, 500 mg Drops: 100 mg/mL Suspension: 125 mg/5 mL, 250 mg/5 mL Tablets: 250 mg, 500 mg, 1 g
Cetirizine (Zyrtec)	*Orally:* Age 2–5 years: 2.5 mg/day. Dose may be increased to 5 mg/day as a single or 2 divided doses. Age 6 years–adults: 5–10 mg/day as a single dose.	Syrup: 1 mg/mL Tablets: 5 mg, 10 mg
Charcoal (Actidose-Aqua, Actidose with Sorbitol, CharcoAid, Liqui-Char)	*Orally:* usually available as premixed solutions. Solutions containing sorbitol should not be used for multiple doses because diarrhea will occur. Do not administer concomitantly with ipecac because charcoal will adsorb and inactivate the ipecac. Do not administer with milk, ice cream, or sherbet because adsorptive capacity of the charcoal will be decreased. Single dose: Children: 1–2 g/kg up to 15–30 g as soon as possible after the ingestion, preferably after emesis. Adults: 30–100 g. Dose should be 5 to 10 times the amount of the ingested poison. Multiple dose (products without sorbitol): Infants: 1 g/kg every 4–6 hours. Children and adults: 1–2 g/kg (up to 60 g) every 2–6 hours.	Liquid: 25 g/120 mL, 30 g/240 mL, 50 g/240 mL Liquid, with sorbitol: 25 g/120 mL, 50 g/240 mL

Continued

Table 1   Medications   (continued)

DRUG	DOSE	DOSAGE FORMS
Chloral hydrate (Aquachloral, Noctec)	*Orally or rectally:* *Sedation before procedures:* 60–75 mg/kg 30 minutes to 1 hour before the procedure. May repeat with a half-dose (30–37.5 mg/kg) if the first dose is ineffective. Do not exceed 120 mg/kg or 2 g total. *Sedation for anxiety:* 25 mg/kg/day in divided doses every 6–8 hours to a maximum of the usual adult dose of 750 mg/day. Continuous therapy, especially in infants, is not recommended.	Capsules: 250 mg, 500 mg Suppositories: 324 mg, 500 mg, 648 mg Syrup: 500 mg/5 mL
Chloramphenicol (Chloromycetin)	*IV or orally:* Neonates under age 7 days: 25 mg/kg/day in a single daily dose. Neonates age 7–21 days: 50 mg/kg/day in 2 divided doses daily. Infants and children: 50–75 mg/kg/day in 4 divided doses to a maximum total daily dose of 4 g. Adults: 50 mg/kg/day in 4 divided doses to a maximum total daily dose of 4 g. Serum levels must be monitored closely, especially in neonates and infants, and patients with renal or hepatic impairment.	Capsules: 250 mg Injection: 1-g vial
Chlorothiazide (Diuril)	*Orally:* Infants under age 6 months: 20–40 mg/kg/day in 2 divided doses. Children: 20 mg/kg/day in 2 divided doses. Adults: 0.5–1 g/day in 1 or 2 divided doses. *IV:* Infants under age 6 months: 20–40 mg/kg/day in 2 divided doses, but doses of 2–8 mg/kg/day may be sufficient in some patients. Children: 4–20 mg/kg/day in 2 divided doses. Adults: 0.5–1 g/day.	Injection: 500 mg Suspension: 250 mg/5 mL Tablets: 250 mg, 500 mg
Chlorpromazine (Thorazine)	*Nausea and vomiting or psychosis:* Over age 6 months: 0.3–0.5 mg/kg IV every 6–8 hours or 0.5–1 mg/kg PO every 4–6 hours or 1 mg/kg rectally every 6–8 hours as needed. Do not exceed adult doses. Adults: 25–50 mg IV every 6–8 hours or 10–25 mg PO every 4–6 hours or 50–100 mg rectally every 6–8 hours. Doses may be increased in the treatment of psychoses; some adults may require as much as 800 mg/day until control is achieved. Dose should then be decreased to the usual maintenance levels of 200 mg/day for adults.	Injection: 25 mg/mL Oral concentrate: 30 mg/mL, 100 mg/mL Suppositories: 25 mg, 100 mg Syrup: 10 mg/5 mL Tablets: 10 mg, 25 mg, 50 mg, 100 mg, 200 mg
Cholestyramine resin (Cholybar, Questran, Questran Light)	*Orally:* Children: 240 mg/kg/day of the resin administered in 3 divided doses. Adults: 3–4 g t.i.d. or q.i.d. Doses should be administered mixed in liquids (4 g in 2–6 oz) or with pulpy fruits (applesauce or pineapple). Many drugs bind with cholestyramine in the GI tract. Drugs should be administered 1 hour before or 4 hours after cholestyramine. Patients should also be cautioned to ingest plenty of fluids to avoid constipation and fecal impaction.	Bar: 4 g resin/bar (Cholybar) Powder: 4 g resin/9 g powder (Questran); 4 g resin/5 g powder (Questran Light, contains aspartame)

Continued

Table 1   Medications   (continued)

DRUG	DOSE	DOSAGE FORMS
Cimetidine (Tagamet)	*Orally, IV:* Initial dose: 　Neonates: 5–10 mg/kg/day in 2–3 divided doses daily. 　Infants: 10–20 mg/kg/day in 2–4 divided doses daily. 　Children: 20–40 mg/kg/day in 4 divided doses daily. 　Adults: 300 mg every 6 hours. Orally, doses of 800 mg at bedtime or 400 mg b.i.d. may be used. 　Doses may be adjusted upward, especially in hypersecretory states, as necessary to maintain the gastric pH of 5 or greater. A maximum total daily dose of 2.4 g should not be exceeded. 　Dosage must be adjusted in renal impairment.	Injection: 150 mg/mL Liquid: 300 mg/5 mL Tablets: 200 mg, 300 mg, 400 mg, 800 mg
Ciprofloxacin (Ciloxan, Cipro)	The drug is not approved for use in patients under age 18 due to possible adverse effects; consider risk vs. benefit if for use in patients under age 18. *Orally (on an empty stomach):* 　Children: 20–30 mg/kg/day in 2 divided doses; up to 40 mg/kg/day may be used for patients with cystic fibrosis. Do not exceed 1.5 g/day. 　Adults: 500–1,500 mg/day in 2 divided doses. *IV (administer over 1 hour at a concentration of 1–2 mg/mL):* 　Children: 15–20 mg/kg/day in 2 divided doses; up to 30 mg/kg/day may be used in patients with cystic fibrosis. Do not exceed 800 mg/day. 　Adults: 400–800 mg/day in 2 divided doses. 　Dosage must be adjusted in patients with renal dysfunction. *Ophthalmic:* administer 1–2 drops every 2 hours while awake for 2 days and then every 4 hours while awake for 5 days.	Injection: 10 mg/mL Solution, ophthalmic: 3.5% Tablets: 250 mg, 500 mg, 750 mg
Citrate and citric acid (Bicitra, Polycitra, Shohl's Solution)	*Orally (dilute in water or juice):* 　Infants and children: 2–3 mEq/kg/day in 3–4 divided doses. 　Adults: 15–30 mL given q.i.d. 　Giving doses with meals decreases the saline laxative effect.	Content per 1 mL*
Clarithromycin (Biaxin)	*Orally:* 　Children: 15 mg/kg/day in 2 divided doses, not to exceed 1 g/day. 　Adults: 500 mg–1 g/day in 2 divided doses.	Suspension: 125 mg/5 mL, 250 mg/5 mL Tablets: 250 mg, 500 mg
Clindamycin (Cleocin)	*IV:* 　Neonates under age 7 days: 　　≤2,000 g: 10 mg/kg/day in 2 divided doses. 　　>2,000 g: 15 mg/kg/day in 3 divided doses. 　Neonates over age 7 days: 　　<1,200 g: 10 mg/kg/day in 2 divided doses. 　　1,200–2,000 g: 15 mg/kg/day in 3 divided doses. 　　>2,000 g: 20 mg/kg/day in 3–4 divided doses. 　Infants and children: 25–40 mg/kg/day in 3–4 divided doses. 　Adults: 1.2–2.7 g/day in 2–4 divided doses. 　　Maximum total daily dose should not exceed 4.8 g and should be used for life-threatening infections only.	Capsules: 150 mg Injection: 150 mg/mL Solution, oral: 75 mg/5 mL Solution, topical: 1%

Continued

Table 1　Medications　(continued)

DRUG	_DOSE_	_DOSAGE FORMS_
Clindamycin (Cleocin) (*continued*)	*Orally:* Infants and children: 15–25 mg/kg/day in 3–4 divided doses for moderate to severe infections. Adults: 150–450 mg every 6–8 hours to a maximum total daily dose of 1.8 g. *Topically:* apply to the affected area b.i.d. Avoid the eyes, abraded skin, and mucous membranes.	
Clonazepam (Klonopin)	*Orally:* Under age 10 or <30 kg: initially 0.01–0.03 mg/kg/day in 2–3 divided doses. Dose may be increased gradually (every third day) until seizures are controlled or adverse effects are seen. The usual maintenance dose range is 0.1–0.2 mg/kg/day. Adults >30 kg: initially 1.5 mg/day in 3 divided doses. Dose may be increased by 0.5–1 mg every third day to a maximum total daily dose of 20 mg. Usual maintenance dose is 0.05–0.2 mg/kg/day.	Tablets: 0.5 mg, 1 mg, 2 mg
Clonidine (Catapres)	*Orally:* *Hypertension:* 5 to 10 μg/kg/day in 2 to 3 divided doses. In patients who experience sedation, the doses may be divided such that the patient receives a larger dose at bedtime and a smaller dose in the morning. Dose may be incrementally increased if necessary to 25 μg/kg/day to a maximum dose of 0.9 mg/day. *Attention deficit/hyperactivity disorder:* 5 μg/kg/day in 4 divided doses has been used in some patients who have failed conventional therapy.	Tablet: 0.1 mg, 0.2 mg, 0.3 mg
Clorazepate dipotassium (Tranxene)	*Orally:* Age 9–12: initially 3.75–7.5 mg b.i.d. Dose may be increased by 3.75 mg at weekly intervals to a maximum total daily dose of 60 mg. Over age 12 and adults: up to 7.5 mg up to t.i.d. May be increased by 7.5 mg at weekly intervals to a maximum total daily dose of 90 mg.	Capsules or tablets: 3.75 mg, 7.5 mg, 15 mg Tablets: 11.25 mg, 22.5 mg
Clotrimazole (Lotrimin, Mycelex)	*Vaginal cream:* 1 full applicator at bedtime for 7–14 days. *Vaginal suppository:* 1 suppository intravaginally at bedtime for 7 days or 2 at bedtime for 3 days or 500 mg as a single dose. *Topically:* apply to affected areas b.i.d.	Cream, topical: 1% (30-g tube) Cream, vaginal: 1% (45-g tube) Solution, topical: 1% (30-mL squeeze bottle) Suppositories, vaginal: 100 mg, 500 mg
Codeine	*Orally:* *Analgesic:* 0.5–1 mg/kg every 4–6 hours as needed, to a maximum of 60 mg. Usual adult dose is 30 mg. *Antitussive:* 0.2–0.25 mg/kg every 4–6 hours as needed, to a maximum of 30 kg. *SC:* same doses as above may be used, although the oral route is only two thirds as effective as the SC route. It should not be used IV. (For IV route, use morphine)	Injection (phosphate): 30 mg/mL, 60 mg/mL Solution, oral (phosphate): 15 mg/5 mL Tablets (sulfate): 15 mg, 30 mg, 60 mg Also available in various combinations with acetaminophen: Elixir, oral: 12 mg codeine with 120 mg acetaminophen Tablets: 7.5 mg codeine with acetaminophen 300 mg (Tylenol w/Codeine No. 1), 15 mg codeine with acetaminophen 300 mg (Tylenol w/Codeine No. 2), 300 mg codeine with acetaminophen 300 mg (Tylenol w/Codeine No. 3), 60 mg codeine with acetaminophen 300 mg (Tylenol w/Codeine No. 4)

Continued

Table 1   Medications   (continued)

DRUG	_DOSE_	_DOSAGE FORMS_
Colfosceril palmitate (Exosurf Neonatal)	_Intratracheally:_ should be used only by physicians familiar with its administration. The usual dose is 5 mL/kg divided equally between the two lungs. Second and third doses may be administered at 12-hour intervals. The infant should be suctioned before administration of colfosceril and ventilator settings should be decreased, depending on the patient's response.	Powder, lyophilized: 108 mg/10 mL
Colistin, neomycin, and hydro-cortisone (Coly-Mycin S Otic)	_Otic_ (shake bottle well before administering): Children: 3 drops in the affected ear t.i.d. or q.i.d. Adults: 4 drops in the affected ear t.i.d. or q.i.d.	Suspension, otic: 5 mL
Cortisone acetate (Cortone Acetate)	Depends on the use of the drug and patient response. _Orally:_ _Physiologic replacement:_ 0.5–0.75 mg/kg/day in 3 divided doses. _Antiinflammatory:_ 2.5–10 mg/kg/day in 3–4 divided doses. _IM:_ _Physiologic replacement:_ 0.25–0.35 mg/kg/day as a single dose. _Antiinflammatory:_ 1–5 mg/kg/day in 1 or 2 divided doses. In patients requiring physiologic replacement, dosage may need to be increased during periods of stress, including perioperatively and during illness.	Injection: 50 mg/mL Tablets: 5 mg, 10 mg, 25 mg
Cosyntropin (Cortrosyn)	_IV:_ Under age 2: 0.125 mg. Over age 2 and adults: 0.25 mg.	Injection: 0.25 mg
Co-trimoxazole (trimethoprim and sulfamethoxazole; Bactrim, Septra)	_Orally or IV (based on trimethoprim):_ Over age 2 months and adults: _Treatment doses:_ _Mild to moderate infections (urinary tract or otitis media):_ 8 mg trimethoprim/kg/day in 2 divided doses. Maximum dose is 320 mg trimethoprim/day. _Pneumocystis carinii pneumonitis:_ 20 mg trimethoprim/kg/day in 4 divided doses. _Prophylaxis doses:_ _Urinary tract infection:_ 2 mg trimethoprim/kg/day as a single dose. _Pneumocystis carinii:_ 150 mg/m^2/day in 1 or 2 divided doses daily on 3 consecutive or alternating days per week. Dosage adjustment is necessary in patients with renal impairment. IV doses must be administered over 60–90 minutes and should be well diluted (1 mL injection in 25 mL infusate).	Injection: 16 mg trimethoprim and 80 mg sulfamethoxazole per 1 mL Suspension: 8 mg trimethoprim and 40 mg sulfamethoxazole per 1 mL Tablets: 80 mg trimethoprim and 400 mg sulfamethoxazole Tablets, double strength: 160 mg trimethoprim and 800 mg sulfamethoxazole
Cromolyn sodium (Crolom, Intal, Nasalcrom, Opticrom)	Children: _Metered-dose inhaler:_ 2 inhalations q.i.d. _Spinhaler dry inhalation:_ contents of 1 capsule q.i.d. _Nebulizer solution:_ 20 mg nebulized q.i.d. _Intranasal spray:_ 1 spray in each nostril 3–6 times daily. _Ophthalmic:_ 1–2 drops in each eye 4–6 times daily.	Capsules, powder for inhalation: 20 mg Inhalation, metered dose: 800 μg/spray Solution, nasal: 5.2 mg/spray Solution, nebulizer: 20 mg/2 mL Solution, ophthalmic: 4%

Continued

Table 1   Medications   (continued)

DRUG	DOSE	DOSAGE FORMS
Crotamiton (Eurax)	*Topically:* apply a thin layer to all skin surfaces from the neck to the toes and soles of the feet. Be sure to apply to all surfaces, including skin folds. Avoid the face and mucous membranes, including the urethral meatus. A second coat is applied 24 hours later. A cleansing bath should follow 48 hours after the second application. Treatment may be repeated after 7–10 days if the mites reappear. It is safe for use in infants and young children. If signs of irritation or hypersensitivity appear, remove the product immediately by bathing. Contaminated clothing and bed linens should be washed to avoid reinfestations.	Cream: 10% Lotion: 10%
Cyclosporine (Neoral, Sandimmune)	NOTE: The two are *not* bioequivalent. Clinical condition and serum levels must be monitored carefully when a patient's therapy is changed from one to the other, especially in patients receiving large doses (>10 mg/kg/day) of Sandimmune who are changed to Neoral therapy because significant drug toxicity may result. *Orally:* *Sandimmune:* initially 10–18 mg/kg/day (dose dependent on organ being transplanted) in 2 divided doses, tapering over several weeks with frequent monitoring to a maintenance dose usually in the range of 5–10 mg/kg/day. *Neoral:* initially about 10 mg/kg/day in 2 divided doses, tapering over several weeks based on clinical condition and serum levels. *Conversion from Sandimmune to Neoral:* Consult with pharmacist *IV (Sandimmune only):* 5–6 mg/kg/day in 1 or 2 divided doses. Each dose should be administered over at least 2 hours.	Capsules (Neoral): 25 mg, 100 mg Capsules (Sandimmune): 25 mg, 50 mg, 100 mg Injection (Sandimmune): 50 mg/mL Solution, oral (Neoral and Sandimmune): 100 mg/mL
Dantrolene sodium (Dantrium)	*Orally:* *Spasticity:* Children >5 years of age: 0.5 mg/kg given b.i.d. initially, but frequency may be increased gradually to t.i.d. or q.i.d. The maximum dose is 100 mg q.i.d. Adults: 25 mg daily initially, with increases in frequency and dose to a maximum of 400 mg/day in 4 divided doses. *Malignant hyperthermia prophylaxis:* 4–8 mg/kg/day in 3–4 divided doses daily for 1–2 days prior to surgery. *Intravenously:* *Malignant hyperthermia prophylaxis:* 2.5 mg/kg administered over 1 hour about 1.25 hours before surgery. Repeat doses may be necessary. *Malignant hyperthermia crisis:* 1 mg/kg given rapidly. Repeat doses may be necessary, but it is usually not necessary to exceed 2.5 mg/kg. Maximum dose should not exceed 10 mg/kg.	Capsules: 25 mg, 50 mg, 100 mg Injection: 20 mg
Deferoxamine (Desferal)	Children: *Acute iron intoxication:* 15 mg/kg/hr IV continuous infusion; maximum 6 g/24 hr. *Chronic iron overload:* 20–25 mg/kg/day IM or 500 mg–2 g IV with each unit of blood transfused, or 20–40 mg/kg/day SC over 8–12 hours up to 1–2 g/day.	Injection: 500-mg vial

Continued

Table 1 Medications (continued)

DRUG	DOSE	DOSAGE FORMS
Desmopressin acetate (DDAVP)	*Intranasally:* *Nocturnal enuresis in patients over age 6:* 20 μg at bedtime with half of dose in each nostril. Dose may be increased or decreased depending on the patient's response. Usual range is 10–40 μg/day. *Diabetes insipidus in patients age 7 years–adults:* initially 5 μg/day as a single dose or in 2 divided doses. Dosage should be titrated to the patient's response. The usual range is 5–40 μg/day. *Orally:* *Diabetes insipidus:* Children: initially, 0.05 mg/dose with careful monitoring to prevent hyponatremia or water intoxication. Over age 12 and adults: initially, 0.05 mg b.i.d. Dosage may then be adjusted to maintain normal diurnal water turnover. The usual total daily dosage is in the range of 0.1–1.2 mg and may be administered in 2–3 divided doses. *Nocturnal enuresis in children over age 12:* 0.2–0.4 mg/day at bedtime. *IV:* *To increase factor VIII levels:* 0.3 μg/kg over 30 minutes. *Diabetes insipidus:* adult doses are 2–4 μg/day in 2 divided doses or approximately one tenth of the intranasal dose necessary to control the patient's symptoms, if that is known.	Injection: 4 μg/mL Solution, nasal: 100 μg/mL/2.4 mL bottle with calibrated intranasal tube Spray, intranasal: 10 μg/actuation metered dose Tablets: 0.1 mg, 0.2 mg
Dexamethasone (Decadron, Hexadrol, Maxidex)	*IV or orally:* *Bacteria meningitis:* 0.6 mg/kg/day in 4 divided doses for the first 4 days of antibiotic therapy. It must be started at the same time or before the first dose of antibiotic. *Cerebral edema:* 1–1.5 mg/kg/day in 4 divided doses to a maximum total daily dose of 16 mg. *Antiemetic therapy (chemotherapy-induced emesis):* 20 mg/m^2/day in 4 divided doses. *Airway edema or extubation:* 0.5–2 mg/kg/day in 4 divided doses beginning 24 hours before and continuing for at least 24 hours after extubation. Doses should be tapered when discontinuing long-term therapy. *Ophthalmic:* instill drops or apply ointment t.i.d. or q.i.d.	Elixir: 0.5 mg/5 mL Injection: 4 mg/mL, 10 mg/mL, 20 mg/mL, 24 mg/mL Ointment, ophthalmic: 0.05% Solution, ophthalmic: 0.05% Solution, oral: 1 mg/mL Tablets: 0.25 mg, 0.5 mg, 0.75 mg, 1 mg, 1.5 mg, 2 mg, 4 mg, 6 mg
Dextroamphetamine sulfate (Dexedrine)	*Orally:* Age 3–5: 2.5 mg/day given in the morning. Dosage may be increased 2.5 mg/day until a response is realized or side effects appear. Usual range is 0.1–0.5 mg/kg/day to a maximum of 40 mg. Age 6 or older: 5 mg/day in the morning or at noon. Dosage may be increased in 5-mg increments at weekly intervals. Usual range is 0.1–0.5 mg/kg/day to a maximum of 40 mg.	Capsules, sustained release: 5 mg, 10 mg, 15 mg Tablets: 5 mg, 10 mg

Continued

Table 1 Medications (continued)

DRUG	DOSE	DOSAGE FORMS
Diazepam (Diastat Rectal, Valium)	*IV:* *Status epilepticus:* 0.05–0.3 mg/kg administered over 2–3 minutes and repeated every 15–30 minutes to a total maximum dose of 0.75 mg/kg or 30 mg, whichever is less. May be repeated in 2–4 hours, if necessary. *Sedation:* 0.04–0.2 mg/kg every 2–4 hours to a maximum of 0.6 mg/kg within an 8-hour period. *Orally for sedation or muscle relaxant:* 0.12–0.8 mg/kg/day in 3–4 divided doses to an adult dose of 6–40 mg/day. *Rectally (round dose off to closest dose available from manufacturer):* Children 2–5 years of age: 0.5 mg/kg. Children 6–11 years of age: 0.3 mg/kg Children ≥12 years of age and adults: 0.2 mg/kg. Dose may be repeated every 4–12 hours as necessary.	Gel, rectal (in rectal delivery system): 2.5 mg, 5 mg, 10 mg, 15 mg, 20 mg Injection: 5 mg/mL Solution, oral: 5 mg/5 mL Solution, concentrated oral: 5 mg/mL Tablets: 2 mg, 5 mg, 10 mg
Diazoxide (Hyperstat IV, Proglycem)	*IV (hypertensive emergency):* 1–3 mg/kg to a maximum of 150 mg. Dose may be repeated in 5–15 minutes. *Orally (hypoglycemia due to hyperinsulinism):* Newborns and infants: initially 8 mg/kg/day in 2 or 3 divided doses. May be increased incrementally if response is inadequate to a maximum of 15 mg/kg/day. Children and adults: 3 mg/kg/day in 2 or 3 divided doses initially. May be increased to a maximum of 8 mg/kg/day.	Capsules: 50 mg Injection: 15 mg/mL Suspension, oral: 50 mg/mL
Dicloxacillin (Dycill, Dynapen, Pathocil)	*Orally:* Children <40 kg: 25–50 mg/kg/day in 4 divided doses. Doses of 50–100 mg/kg/day in 4 divided doses are necessary for follow-up oral therapy of osteomyelitis. Children ≥40 kg and adults: 125–500 mg/dose every 6 hours.	Capsules: 250 mg, 500 mg Suspension, oral: 62.5 mg/5 mL
Didanosine [ddI (dideoxyinisine); Videx]	*Orally:* doses must be given at 12-hour intervals on an empty stomach, but because the drug is degraded by gastric acids, each formulation contains buffers. Infants and children: 180–300 mg/m^2/day in 2 divided doses. If the tablet formulation is used, children over age 1 should receive 2 tablets per dose to assure sufficient buffering. Children under age 1 may receive doses in a single tablet. Adults: <60 kg: 125 mg (tablets) or 167 mg (buffered powder) per dose twice daily. ≥60 kg: 200 mg (tablets) or 250 mg (buffered powder) per dose twice daily.	Powder for oral solution, buffered (single-dose packets): 100 mg, 167 mg, 250 mg, 375 mg Powder for oral solution, pediatric (mixed with an antacid at the time it is dispensed by the pharmacist): 10 mg/mL tablets, buffered, chewable/dispersible: 25 mg, 50 mg, 100 mg, 150 mg
Digoxin (Lanoxicaps, Lanoxin)	Should be based on lean body weight. Dosage adjustment is required in patients with impaired renal function. Total digitalizing dose (TDD) is administered as follows: half TDD initially, then one fourth TDD 8–12 hours later, then one fourth TDD 8–12 hours after that. Maintenance doses are administered in 2 divided doses beginning 12 hours after the last digitalizing dose. Patients should be under continuous cardiographic monitoring during digitalization. IM doses are the same as oral doses, but that route of administration should be avoided.†	Capsules, liquid filled (Lanoxicaps): 0.05 mg, 0.1 mg, 0.2 mg (90–100% bioavailable) Elixir: 0.05 mg/mL (75–87% bioavailable) Injection: 0.1 mg/mL, 0.25 mg/mL (100% bioavailable IV) Tablets: 0.125 mg, 0.25 mg, 0.5 mg (60–80% bioavailable)

Continued

Table 1 Medications (continued)

DRUG	DOSE	DOSAGE FORMS
Dimercaprol [BAL (British anti-lewisite)]	*Deep IM:* *Lead toxicity:* *Severe poisoning:* 4 mg/kg 6 times a day for 3–5 days. *Arsenic, mercury, or gold toxicity:* *Mild:* Days 1 and 2: 3 mg/kg q.i.d. Day 3: 3 mg/kg b.i.d. Days 4–14: 3 mg/kg every day. *Severe:* Days 1 and 2: 3 mg/kg 6 times a day. Day 3: 3 mg/kg q.i.d. Days 4–14: 3 mg/kg b.i.d.	Injection: 100 mg/mL (3-mL ampul)
Diphenhydramine (Benadryl, Benylin, Nytol, Sleep-Eze 3, Sominex Formula 2)	*IV, orally, IM:* Children: 5 mg/kg/day in 3 or 4 divided doses to a maximum of 300 mg/day. Adults: 10–50 mg repeated as often as every 4 hours, not to exceed 400 mg/day. The drug may cause paradoxical excitement in children.	Capsules: 25 mg, 50 mg Elixir (14% alcohol): 12.5 mg/5 mL Injection: 10 mg/mL, 50 mg/mL Syrup (5% alcohol): 12.5 mg/5 mL Tablets: 25 mg, 50 mg
Dobutamine hydrochloride (Dobutrex)	*IV infusion:* 2–15 μg/kg/min to a maximum of 40 μg/kg/min. Start at the lower end of the range and titrate upward based on the patient's response.	Injection: 12.5 mg/mL
Docusate sodium (dioctyl sodium sulfosuccinate; Colace, D-S-S, Doxinate)	*Orally (in 1–4 divided doses with a glass of water):* Infants and children under age 3: 10–40 mg/day. Age 3–6: 20–60 mg/day. Age >6–12: 40–150 mg/day. Over age 12 and adults: 50–500 mg. Do not administer with mineral oil because absorption of the mineral oil may be increased.	Capsules: 50 mg, 100 mg, 240 mg, 250 mg Liquid: 150 mg/15 mL Solution: 50 mg/mL Syrup: 50 mg/15 mL, 60 mg/15 mL Also available in combination with stimulant laxatives, including senna, phenolphthalein, and casanthranol.
Dopamine hydrochloride (Dopastat, Intropin)	*Continuous IV infusion:* initially 1 μg/kg/min titrated upward based on patient's response to a maximum of 20 μg/kg/min in neonates or 50 μg/kg/min in all other patients. The hemodynamic effects of dopamine occur only at doses >15 μg/kg/min.	Injection in 5% dextrose: 0.8 mg/mL, 1.6 mg/mL, 3.2 mg/mL (premixed infusions) Injection: 40 mg/mL, 80 mg/mL, 160 mg/mL
Dornase alfa (Pulmozyme)	*Inhalation via approved compressor:* Children >5 years of age and adults: 2.5 mg/day.	Solution, inhalation: 2.5 mg/2.5 mL
Doxycycline (Doryx, Doxy-100, Vibramycin)	*Orally or IV:* Children under age 8: should not be used unless there is no alternative. $\geq$ age 8: 2–5 mg/kg/day to a maximum of 200 mg/day in 1 or 2 divided doses. Adults: 100–200 mg/day in 1 or 2 divided doses. Inpatient treatment of PID 100 mg IV b.i.d. with cefoxitin 2 g IV every 6 hours for at least 4 days or 2 days after patient improves, whichever is longer. Doxycycline should be continued orally to complete 10–14 days of therapy.	Capsules or tablets: 50 mg, 100 mg Injection: 100 mg, 200 mg
d-Xylose (wood sugar; Xylo-Pfan)	*Orally (prepared as a 5–10% aqueous solution):* 14.5 g/m^2 to a maximum dose of 25 g. Alternatively, a dose of 500 mg/kg may be used. Infants should fast for 4–5 hours before the dose and children should fast overnight. Blood xylose levels are then measured to determine extent of intestinal absorption.	Powder for preparing oral solutions: 25 g

Continued

Table 1   Medications   (continued)

DRUG	*DOSE*	*DOSAGE FORMS*

Edetate calcium disodium (Calcium Disodium Versenate, Calcium EDTA)	*Mild to moderate lead poisoning:* 25–50 mg/kg.
	 Severe lead poisoning: up to 75 mg/kg/24 hr not to exceed 1.5 g/day.
	 Usual dosage (children):
	 Asymptomatic lead toxicity:
	   Initial: up to 1 g/m^2/24 hr in a continuous IV drip if possible or in 2–4 divided doses for 5 days.
	   Subsequent courses: up to 50 mg/kg/24 hr in a continuous IV drip if possible or in 2–4 divided doses for 3–5 days.
	 Symptomatic lead toxicity or lead encephalopathy:
	   Initial: up to 1.5 g/m^2/24 hr in a continuous IV drip if possible or in 6 divided doses for 5–7 days; give with dimercaprol (BAL).
	   Subsequent courses: as for asymptomatic toxicity above.
		Injection: 200 mg/mL
		 For intravenous infusion, dilute to a maximum concentration of 5 mg/mL with D$_5$W or normal saline.
		 Infusions should be administered either continuously or over 1–2 hours if intermittent doses are used. Rapid infusion may increase intracranial pressure.

Edrophonium (Enlon, Reversol, Tensilon)	*Myasthenia gravis diagnosis:* Infants: Initially 0.1 mg; if no response, follow with an additional 0.4 mg for a maximum total dose of 0.5 mg. Children: Initial: 0.04 mg/kg followed by 0.16 mg/kg if no response; maximum total dose is 10 mg. Adults: 0.2 mg/kg up to 10 mg. Administer 2 mg initially, then titrate dose. *Titration of therapy:* 0.04 mg/kg one time; if strength improves, an increase in neostigmine or pyridostigmine dose is indicated.	Injection: 10 mg/mL May precipitate cholinergic crisis.
Enalapril, enalaprilat (Vasotec)	*Orally:* initially 0.1 mg/kg/day in 1 or 2 divided doses to the usual adult dose of 2.5–5 mg/kg/day. Dosage may be increased as required to a maximum of 0.5 mg/kg/day or 40 mg. *IV:* 5–10 μg/kg (up to 0.625–1.25 mg) may be administered every 8–24 hours as necessary for control of hypertension. Dosage must be decreased in patients with compromised renal function and also should be decreased in patients who are hyponatremic or volume depleted, in severe congestive heart failure, or in those who are receiving diuretics. The oral dosage form (enalapril) is a prodrug that is not stable in aqueous media. The injectable dosage form (enalaprilat) is the active form, but is not absorbed from the GI tract.	Injection: 1.25 mg/mL Tablets: 2.5 mg, 5 mg, 10 mg, 20 mg

Enoxaparin (Lovenox)	*SC:*
	 Prophylaxis:
	   Infants <2 months of age: 0.75 mg/kg/dose every 12 hours
	   Infants ≥2 months of age and children: 0.5 mg/kg/dose every 12 hours
	   Adults >45 kg: 30 mg every 12 hours
	 Treatment of DVT or PE:
	   Infants <2 months of age: 1.5 mg/kg/dose every 12 hours
	   Infants ≥2 months of age and children: 1 mg/kg/dose every 12 hours
	   Adults >45 kg: 1 mg/kg/dose every 12 hours.
	   Doses should be adjusted based on anti-factor Xa levels.
		Injection: 100 mg/mL

Continued

Table 1   Medications   (continued)

DRUG	*DOSE*	*DOSAGE FORMS*
Epinephrine (Adrenalin, Sus-Phrine, Vaponefrin)	*IV for asystole, or pulseless arrest:* Neonates: 0.01–0.03 mg/kg (0.1–0.3 mL/kg of a 1:10,000 solution) every 3–5 minutes as necessary. Infants to adults: 0.1 mg/kg to a maximum of 1 mg; may be repeated every 3–5 minutes as necessary. A continuous infusion may be started at a dose of 0.1–1 μg/kg/min and titrated to effect. *Nebulization:* 0.25–0.5 mL of a 2.25% racemic epinephrine solution diluted in 2.5–3 mL of normal saline for inhalation. *SC for allergic reactions:* 0.01 mg/kg to a maximum dose of 0.5 mg (of the 1:1,000 solution). For a prolonged effect, 0.005 mL/kg/dose of the 1:200 suspension in glycerin (equivalent to 0.025 mg/kg/dose) may be given every 8–12 hours.	Aerosol: 0.2–0.3 mg/spray, depending on brand (Bronkaid Mist, Primatene Mist, AsthmaHaler Mist) Injection: 1:10,000 (0.1 mg/mL), 1:1,000 (1 mg/mL) Injection pre-filled automatic syringe: 1:200 (EpiPen delivers 0.3 mg IM, EpiPen Jr. delivers 0.15 mg IM) Solution, racemic for inhalation: 2.25% (AsthmaNefrin, S-2, Vaponefrin)
Epoetin alfa (erythropoietin; Epogen, EPO, r-HuEPO)	*IV or SC:* initially 50–100 U/kg administered 1–3 times weekly until the hematocrit reaches 30–33%. Dosage should be lowered if the hematocrit exceeds that range or increases by more than 4 points in a 2-week period. It may be increased if the hematocrit does not reach the target range or fails to increase by 5–6 points in an 8-week period. The usual maintenance dose is 25 U/kg 3 times weekly. Hematocrit and serum iron levels should be monitored frequently. Blood pressure should also be monitored frequently.	Injection: 2,000 U/mL, 4000 U/mL, 10,000 U/mL
Ergocalciferol (vitamin D_2, activated ergosterol; Calciferol, Drisdol)	1 μg = 40 U. *Orally:* Healthy infants and children: 400 U/day. Infants and children with malabsorption syndromes: 1,000 U/day. Children with liver disease: 4,000–8,000 U/day. Children with vitamin D–dependent rickets: 3,000–5,000 U/day. Nutritional rickets with normal absorption: 1,000–5,000 U/day; with malabsorption: 10,000–25,000 U/day. *IM:* should be retained for patients with rickets due to severe vitamin D deficiency. The dose for vitamin D–resistant rickets ranges from 50,000–500,000 U/day, for hypoparathyroidism from 50,000–200,000 U/day, and for familial hypophosphatemia from 10,000–80,000 U/day. The range between therapeutic and toxic doses is narrow. Patients must be closely monitored.	Capsules: 50,000 U (1.25 mg) Injection (in sesame oil): 500,000 U/mL (12.5 mg/mL) Solution, oral: 8,000 U/mL (200 μg/mL)
Erythromycin (E-Mycin, Ery-Tab, Eryc, Erythrocin, E.E.S., Ilosone, Pediamycin)	*Orally* (do not exceed 2 g/day): Neonates: 20–30 mg/kg/day in 2 or 3 divided doses. Infants and children: Base or ethylsuccinate: 30–50 mg/kg/day in 3 or 4 divided doses. Estolate: 20–50 mg/kg/day in 3 or 4 divided doses. Adults: Base, estolate, or stearate: 250–500 mg every 6–12 hours. Ethylsuccinate: 400–800 mg every 6–12 hours. *Endocarditis prophylaxis* (penicillin-allergic patients): 20 mg/kg to a maximum of 1 g 2 hours before the procedure and 10 mg/kg to a maximum of 500 mg 6 hours later.	Base: Capsules, enteric-coated pellets; 250 mg Ointment, ophthalmic: 0.5% Solution, topical: 1.5%, 2% Tablets, enteric coated: 250 mg, 333 mg, 500 mg Tablets, film coated: 250 mg, 500 mg Estolate: Capsules: 250 mg Suspension: 125 mg/5 mL, 250 mg/5 mL Tablets: 500 mg Ethylsuccinate: Suspension: 200 mg/5 mL, 400 mg/5 mL Tablets, chewable: 200 mg Tablets: 400 mg Stearate: Tablets: 250 mg, 500 mg

Continued

Table 1   Medications   (continued)

DRUG	DOSE	DOSAGE FORMS
Erythromycin (E-Mycin, Ery-Tab, Eryc, Erythrocin, E.E.S., Ilosone, Pediamycin) (*continued*)	*Bowel preparation* (erythromycin base, only): 20 mg/kg to a maximum of 1 g administered at 1:00, 2:00, and 11:00 P.M. on the day before surgery, usually combined with neomycin and mechanical cleansing of the bowel. *IV:* 15–20 mg/kg/day to a maximum of 4 g/day administered in 4 divided doses. *Ophthalmic ointment* for prophylaxis of neonates: apply a 0.5–1 cm ribbon of the ointment to each conjunctival sac. *Topically for acne:* apply to the affected areas b.i.d. The skin should be washed, rinsed well, and dried before applying the erythromycin. Keep away from the eyes, nose, and mouth.	
Erythromycin and sulfisoxazole (Eryzole, Pediazole)	*Orally* (based on the erythromycin content): Up to age 2 months: 40–50 mg/kg/day in 3 or 4 divided doses to a maximum of 2 g/day. Alternatively, the following patient weights may be used: 8–15 kg: 2.5 mL every 6 hours. 16–23 kg: 5 mL every 6 hours. 24–44 kg: 7.5 mL every 6 hours. ≥45 kg: 10 mL every 6 hours.	Suspension: 200 mg erythromycin and 600 mg sulfisoxazole per 5 mL
Ethacrynic acid (Edecrin)	*Orally:* 1 mg/kg administered 1–2 times daily. Do not exceed the usual adult dose of 50–100 mg/day. *IV:* 0.4–1 mg/kg up to 50 mg administered 1 or 2 times daily. Serum electrolytes must be closely monitored during ethacrynic acid therapy.	Injection: 50 mg Tablets: 25 mg, 50 mg
Ethambutol (Myambutol)	*Orally* (patient should be old enough to cooperate with an eye exam; optic neuritis is an adverse effect): Children: 15 mg/kg/day in a single dose. Adolescents and adults: 15–25 mg/kg/day in a single dose. Do not exceed 2.5 g/day.	Tablets: 100 mg, 400 mg
Ethosuximide (Zarontin)	*Orally:* Under age 6: 15 mg/kg/day in 2 divided doses to a maximum of 250 mg/dose. ≥ age 6: 250 mg b.i.d. Dose may be increased by 250 mg/day every 4–7 days to a maximum of 1.5 g/day or 40 mg/kg/day.	Capsules: 250 mg Syrup: 250 mg/5 mL
Fentanyl citrate (Sublimaze)	*IV* (slowly over a period of 3–5 minutes to avoid chest wall rigidity and to titrate to effect): Children: 1–2 μg/kg may be repeated at 30–60-minute intervals. For continuous therapy, after a bolus dose, a dose of 1 μg/kg/hr initially may be increased or decreased as necessary to response. Older children and adults: 0.5–1 μg/kg (25–50 μg) may be repeated at 30–60-minute intervals. The doses listed are analgesic/sedation doses. Doses used for general anesthesia may be higher. *Orally (Oralet):* Children ≥2 years of age who weigh 15–40 kg: 5–15 μg/kg to a maximum of 400 μg. Children ≥40 kg and adults: 5 μg/kg to a maximum of 400 μg.	Injection: 50 μg/mL Lozenge, oral transmucosal (Oralet): 100 μg, 200 μg, 300 μg, 400 μg

Continued

Table 1   Medications   (continued)

DRUG	DOSE	DOSAGE FORMS

Ferrous sulfate (Feosol, Fer-In-Sol)	*Orally (doses are expressed as elemental iron; ferrous sulfate contains 20% iron):*
	Iron deficiency anemia:
	    Children: 3–6 mg/kg/day depending on the severity of the deficiency. Higher doses should be administered in 3 divided doses; moderate doses may be administered in 2 divided doses to avoid GI upset. For prophylaxis, 1–2 mg/kg/day in a single dose may be used.
	    Adults: 120–240 mg iron daily in 2–4 divided doses. For prophylaxis, 60 mg iron daily as a single dose.
	Administration between meals increases absorption, but may result in more GI upset. Do not administer with antacids, eggs, or milk because they may decrease absorption of the iron.
		Capsules: 50 mg Fe
		Drops: 15 mg Fe/0.6 mL
		Elixir: 44 mg Fe/5 mL
		Syrup: 18 mg Fe/5 mL
		Tablets: 60 mg Fe, 65 mg Fe

Fluconazole (Diflucan)	*Orally or IV:* *Oropharyngeal or esophageal candidiasis:* 6 mg/kg (up to 200 mg) on the first day; then 3 mg/kg/day (up to 100 mg). *Systemic candidiasis or cryptococcal meningitis:* 12 mg/kg (up to 400 mg) on the first day; then 6 mg/kg/day (up to 200 mg). *Prevention of candidiasis in bone marrow transplant:* 12 mg/kg/day (up to 400 mg) beginning several days before anticipated onset of neutropenia and continued until 7 days after neutrophil count is >1,000/mm^3. *Vaginal candidiasis:* 150 mg as a single dose. Dosage should be adjusted in patients with renal dysfunction.	Injection: 2 mg/mL (ready to administer) Suspension: 10 mg/mL, 40 mg/mL Tablets: 50 mg, 100 mg, 150 mg, 200 mg

Flucytosine (Ancobon)	*Orally:*
	    Neonates: 50–100 mg/kg/day in 1–2 divided doses.
	    Children and adults: 50–150 mg/kg/day in 4 divided doses. Dosage must be adjusted in renal impairment.
		Capsules: 250 mg, 500 mg

Fludrocortisone (Florinef)	*Orally:*
	    Infants and children: 0.05–0.1 mg/day.
	    Adults: 0.05–0.2 mg/day.
		Tablets: 0.1 mg

Flumazenil (Mazicon, Romazicon)	*IV:*
	    Children (little information is available on dosing in children) The following are guidelines only: 0.01 mg/kg (to a maximum of 0.2 mg) initially, followed by 0.005 mg/kg (to a maximum of 0.2 mg) every minute until a total cumulative dose of 1 mg has been reached.
	    Adults:
	    Reversal of sedation: 0.2 mg over 15 seconds; may repeat 0.2-mg dose every 60 seconds to a maximum of 1 mg. May repeat doses every 20 minutes to a maximum of 3 mg in 1 hour.
	    Benzodiazepine overdose: 0.2 mg over 30 seconds, then 0.3 mg over 30 seconds if desired level of consciousness is not reached. Additional 0.5-mg doses may be given every minute until a cumulative dose of 3 mg has been reached. If a partial response is noted, further 0.5-mg doses may be given until a cumulative dose of 5 mg is reached.
	    Resedation may occur in patients who received long-acting benzodiazepines.
		Injection: 0.1 mg/mL

Continued

Table 1   Medications   (continued)

DRUG	DOSE	DOSAGE FORMS
Flunisolide (AeroBid, Nasalide)	*Intranasal spray:* Age 6–14: 1 spray in each nostril t.i.d. or 2 sprays in each nostril b.i.d. initially. Maintenance dose is usually 1 spray in each nostril daily. Over age 14 and adults: 2 sprays in each nostril b.i.d. or t.i.d. initially. After symptoms are controlled, dosage should be decreased to the lowest dose that will prevent symptoms from recurring. That may be as little as 1 spray in each nostril once daily for perennial rhinitis. The maximum dose is 4 sprays to each nostril daily. *Oral inhalation:* Children 6–15 years of age: 2 inhalations twice a day. Adults: 2 inhalations twice a day initially, increasing to a maximum of 8 inhalations daily. Improvement in symptoms may take from several days to several weeks to occur, but therapy should not be continued for more than 3 weeks in the absence of efficacy. Dosage should be decreased to the lowest effective dose when symptoms abate.	Oral inhalation: 250 μg/spray Spray, intranasal: 25 μg/metered spray
Fluocinolone acetonide (Fluonid, Flurosyn, Synalar, Synemol)	*Topically:* apply a thin layer to the affected area b.i.d. to q.i.d. Use the lowest effective potency product. Absorption is greater if the product is covered by anything that is occlusive (plastic pants, tight diapers).	Cream: 0.01%, 0.025%, 0.2% Ointment: 0.025% Shampoo: 0.01% Solution: 0.01%
Fluoride (Fluoritab, Karidium, Luride, Pediaflor)	*Orally:* dosage should be based on the fluoride content of the water supply. Long-term supplementation in areas with fluoridated water may result in dental fluorosis and osseous changes.* Fluoride content of drinking water <0.3 ppm: Birth–6 months: do not supplement. >6 months–3 years: 0.25 mg/day. >3–6 years: 0.5 mg/day. >6–16 years: 1 mg/day. Fluoride content of drinking water 0.3–0.6 ppm: Birth–3 years: do not supplement. 3–6 years: 0.25 mg/day. >6–16 years: 0.5 mg/day. Fluoride content of drinking water >0.6 ppm: do not supplement. *Dental gel:* usually applied by a dentist. *Rinses:* over-the-counter rinses may be used for patients over age 6 on a daily basis and contain 0.01–0.02% fluoride.	Most multivitamin combinations are available in formulations containing appropriate amounts of fluoride (Poly-Vi-Flor drops or chewable tablets, Tri-Vi-Flo drops, Vi-Daylin/F drops and chewable tablets). Products containing only fluoride: Drops: 0.125 mg/drop, 0.25 mg/drop, 0.5 mg/mL Solution: 0.2 mg/mL (may be used orally or as a rinse) Tablets, chewable: 0.5 mg, 1 mg
Fluticasone (Flonase, Flovent)	*Intranasal metered dose spray* Children ≥4 years of age: 1 spray in each nostril daily. Dosage may be increased to 2 sprays in each nostril daily if necessary. Adults: 2 sprays in each nostril daily. *Oral aerosol inhalation:* Children ≥12 years of age and adults: 88 μg twice daily for patients not previously treated with corticosteroids to a maximum of 440 μg twice daily in patients who were previously treated with inhaled corticosteroids.	Powder, oral inhalation: 50 μg (delivers 44 μg), 100 μg (delivers 88 μg), 250 μg (delivers 220 μg) Spray oral inhalation: 44 μg/actuation, 110 μg/actuation, 220 μg/actuation Suspension, nasal: 50 μg/actuation

Continued

Table 1   Medications   (continued)

DRUG	DOSE	DOSAGE FORMS
Fluticasone (Flonase, Flovent) (continued)	*Oral powder inhalation:* 　Children 4–12 years of age: 50 μg twice daily to a maximum of 100 μg twice daily. 　Children >12 years of age and adults: 100 μg twice a day up to 500 μg twice a day based on the patient's previous corticosteroid needs. Patients who previously required oral corticosteroids may require up to 1,000 μg twice a day.	
Folic acid (Folvite)	*Orally, parenterally:* 　Infants: 50 μg/day. 　Age 1–10: 1 mg/day initially, then 0.1–0.4 mg/day. 　Age 11 and over, and adults: 1 mg/day initially, then 0.5 mg/day.	Injection: 5 mg/mL, 10 mg/mL Tablets: 0.1 mg, 0.4 mg, 0.8 mg, 1 mg
Fosphenytoin–See phenytoin		
Furosemide (Lasix)	*Orally, IV, or IM:* 　Premature neonates (oral absorption may be poor): 1–2 mg/kg every 12–24 hours. Oral doses up to 4 mg/kg may be used. 　Children: 1–2 mg/kg every 6–12 hours but not to exceed 6 mg/kg/day. 　Adults: 20–80 mg/day in divided doses to a maximum of 600 mg/day. Serum electrolyte levels should be monitored closely.	Injection: 10 mg/mL Solution: 10 mg/mL, 40 mg/5 mL Tablets: 20 mg, 40 mg, 80 mg
Gabapentin (Neurontin)	*Orally (as add-on therapy):* 　Patients 3–12 years of age: 10–15 mg/kg/day in 3 divided doses. The maintenance dose for patients 3–4 years of age is usually about 40 mg/kg/day and for patients 5 years and older is 25–35 mg/kg/day. 　Age >12yr–adults: initially, 300 mg on day 1, followed by rapid titration to 300 mg t.i.d. The usual maintenance dosage range is 900–1,800 mg/day in 3 divided doses to a maximum daily dose of 3,600 mg. It is not necessary to monitor gabapentin levels or the levels of other antiepileptic drugs the patient may be taking because there are no significant drug interactions. Withdrawal of gabapentin therapy should be accomplished over a period of at least 1 week.	Capsules: 100 mg, 300 mg, 400 mg Solution: 250 mg/5 mL
Ganciclovir (Cytovene, DHPG)	*IV (as an infusion over 1 hour):* 　*Induction:* 10 mg/kg/day in 2 divided doses for 2–3 weeks. 　*Maintenance:* 5 mg/kg/day as a single dose for 7 days a week to 6 mg/kg/day for 5 days a week. 　*Orally:* 　*Maintenance therapy only:* in adults, a dose of 1,000 mg t.i.d. with food is used. There are no guidelines for oral use in children. 　Dosage must be adjusted in patients with renal dysfunction.	Capsules: 250 mg Injection: 500-mg vial
Gentamicin (Garamycin)	*IV or IM (in obese patients it should be based on ideal, rather than actual, body weight):* 　Neonates under age 7 days: 　　<1,000 g: 2.5 mg/kg every 24 hours. 　　1,000–1,500 g: 2.5 mg/kg every 18 hours. 　　>1,500 g: 2.5 mg/kg every 12 hours. 　Neonates over age 7 days: 　　1,200–2,000 g: 2.5 mg/kg every 8–12 hours. 　　>2,000 g: 2.5 mg/kg every 8 hours.	Injection: 10 mg/mL, 40 mg/mL Ointment, ophthalmic: 0.3% Solution, ophthalmic: 0.3%

Continued

Table 1   Medications   (continued)

DRUG	DOSE	DOSAGE FORMS
Gentamicin (Garamycin) (continued)	ECMO patients: 2.5 mg/kg every 18 hours. Infants and children under age 5: 2.5 mg/kg every 8 hours. Age 5–10: 2 mg/kg every 8 hours. Over age 10 and adults: 5 mg/kg/day administered in 3 divided doses. *Ophthalmic solution:* 1–2 drops in the affected eye every 2–4 hours. More frequent application (up to every hour) may be used initially in severe infections. *Ophthalmic ointment:* apply a ribbon of ointment to the eye b.i.d. or t.i.d. *Intrathecal/intraventricular* (use only a preservative-free product): Neonates: 1 mg/day as a single dose. Children over age 3 months: 1–2 mg/day. Older children and adults: 4–8 mg/day. Dosage must be adjusted in renal dysfunction. Serum levels should be monitored during therapy in all patients.	
Glucagon	*IV, IM, or SC:* *Hypoglycemia* (dose may be repeated in 20 minutes if necessary): Neonates: 0.025 mg/kg/dose. Children: 0.025–0.1 mg/kg/dose to a maximum of 1 mg. Adults: 0.5–1 mg/dose. *Infusion for the treatment of neonatal hyperinsulinemia:* 1–5 ng/kg/min to start and titrate to response. The infusion must be delivered by a pump to maintain a steady rate. Glucose levels must be monitored hourly until they are stable in an acceptable range. Rebound hypoglycemia may occur if the infusion is suddenly discontinued. *Diagnostic aid during radiography:* 0.25–2 mg 10 minutes before the procedure.	Injection: 1 mg-vial, 10 mg-vial (1 mg = 1 U)
Glycopyrrolate (Robinul)	*IM:* *Preoperatively:* Under age 2: 4.4–8.8 μg/kg 30–60 minutes before the procedure. $\geq$ age 2–adults: 4.4 μg/kg 30–60 minutes before the procedure. *Orally:* *To control respiratory secretions* (glycopyrrolate is poorly absorbed from the GI tract): 50 μg/kg administered t.i.d. or q.i.d. *Reversal of neuromuscular blockade:* 0.2 mg for each 1 mg neostigmine or 5 mg pyridostigmine administered.	Injection: 0.2 mg/mL Tablets: 1 mg, 2 mg
Gonadorelin HCl [Factrel, LHRH (luteinizing hormone-release hormone), GnRH (gonadotropin-releasing hormone)]	*IV:* 2–5 μg/kg to a maximum of 100 μg.	Injection: 100 μg

Continued

Table 1   Medications   (continued)

DRUG	DOSE	DOSAGE FORMS

Griseofulvin (Microsize products: Fulvicin U/F, Grifulvin V, Grisactin; Ultramicrosize products: Fulvicin P/G, Grisactin Ultra, Gris-PEG)	Absorption of griseofulvin from the GI tract is somewhat dependent on the size of the particles of griseofulvin. The ultramicrosize is absorbed about 1.5 times as well as the microsize. Absorption is also increased by administering the dose with a fatty meal. Duration of therapy is dependent on the site of infection and ranges from 2–4 weeks for tinea corporis, to 4–8 weeks for tinea capitis and tinea pedis, to 3–6 months for tinea unguium.
	Children:
	  Microsize: 15–20 mg/kg/day in 1 or 2 divided doses.
	  Ultramicrosize: 10–13 mg/kg/day in 1 or 2 divided doses.
	Older children and adults:
	  Microsize: 500 mg–1 g/day in a single or 2 divided doses. Use higher dose for tinea pedis or tinea unguium.
	  Ultramicrosize: 660–750 mg/day in a single or 2 divided doses.
	During long-term therapy, renal, hepatic, and hematopoietic function should be monitored.
	Patients should also be cautioned to avoid sunlight because photosensitivity reactions have occurred.
		Microsize:
		  Capsules: 125 mg, 250 mg
		  Suspension: 125 mg/5 mL
		  Tablets: 250 mg, 500 mg
		Ultramicrosize:
		  Tablets: 125 mg, 165 mg, 250 mg, 330 mg

Haloperidol (Haldol)	*Orally:*
	Age 3–12:
	  Agitation or hyperkinesia: 0.01–0.03 mg/kg/day once daily.
	  Tourette disorder: 0.05–0.075 mg/kg/day in 2 or 3 divided doses.
	  Psychotic disorders: 0.05–0.15 mg/kg/day in 2 or 3 divided doses.
	  IM: 1–3 mg every 4–8 hours; maximum, 0.1 mg/kg/day.
	  Dose should be individually adjusted to patient. Not recommended for children under age 3. Oral dosage range is 2–100 mg/24 hr.
		Injection: 5 mg/mL
		Solution, concentrated oral: 2 mg/mL
		Tablets: 1 mg, 2 mg, 5 mg, 10 mg

Heparin sodium	*IV:*
	  Anticoagulation:
	  Children and adults:
	    Continuous infusion: 50 U/kg then 15–25 U/kg/hr. Dose may be increased by 2–4 U/kg/hr every 6–8 hours based on the results of the APTT.
	    Intermittent infusion: 50–100 U/kg every 4 hours. This method is less desirable than continuous infusion.
	  Line flushing:
	  Central catheters: may be flushed as infrequently as once daily with 2–3 mL of solution containing 10 U/mL for patients under age 1 or 100 U/mL for patients age 1 or older.
	  Peripheral catheters, locks: usually flushed every 6–8 hours with 10 U/mL concentration with a volume determined by the length of the catheter, but usually about 1 mL.
	  Lines should be flushed before and after medication or blood administration or if blood is seen in the catheter.
	  Preservative-free heparin solutions should be used for all line flushes in children under age 2 months.
		Injection: 1,000 U, 5,000 U, 10,000 U, 20,000 U, 40,000 U/mL
		Injection, preservative-free: 1,000 U, 5,000 U, 10,000 U/mL
		Solution, lock flush: 10 U/mL, 100 U/mL (available preserved and preservative-free)

Continued

Table 1   Medications   (continued)

DRUG	DOSE	DOSAGE FORMS

Hydralazine (Apresoline)	*Orally:*
	  Children: 0.75–1 mg/kg/day in 2–4 divided doses, but not to exceed 25 mg/dose initially. May be increased slowly over 3 or 4 weeks to a maximum of 7.5 mg/kg/day (or 200 mg).
	  Adults: initially 10 mg q.i.d. May be increased by 10–25 mg/dose every 2–5 days to a maximum of 300 mg/day.
	IV (ratio of oral to IV dosing is about 4:1):
	  Children: initially 0.1–0.2 mg/kg (to a maximum of 20 mg) every 4–6 hours. May be increased to a maximum of 1.7–3.5 mg/kg/day.
	  Adults: initially 10–20 mg every 4–6 hours. May be increased to 40 mg/dose. Dose must be adjusted in renal impairment.
		Injection: 20 mg/mL
		Tablets: 10 mg, 25 mg, 50 mg, 100 mg

Hydrochlorothiazide (Esidrix, HydroDIURIL, Oretic)	*Orally* (chlorothiazide, which is available as a suspension, is usually a better choice for children requiring low doses):
	  Children over age 6 months: 2 mg/kg/day in 2 divided doses.
	  Adults: 25–100 mg/day in 1 or 2 doses.
		Tablets: 25 mg, 50 mg, 100 mg

Hydrocortisone (Cortef, Cortenema, Cortifoam, Cortril, Hydrocortone, Solu-Cortef)	*Orally:*
	Congenital adrenal hyperplasia: initially 30–36 mg/m^2/day divided as one third in the morning and two thirds in the evening or one fourth in the morning, one fourth midday, and half in the evening.
	Physiologic replacement: 0.5–0.75 mg/kg/day.
	Antiinflammatory: 2.5–10 mg/kg/day in 3 or 4 divided doses.
	IV:
	Adrenal insufficiency:
	  Infants and young children: 1–2 mg/kg bolus, then 25–150 mg/day in 3 or 4 divided doses.
	  Older children: 1–2 mg/kg bolus, then 150–250 mg/day in 3 or 4 divided doses.
	  Adults: 15–240 mg/day in 1 or 2 divided doses.
	Antiinflammatory:
	  Infants and children: 1–5 mg/kg/day in 2–4 divided doses.
	  Adults: 15–240 mg every 12 hours.
	Shock (succinate salt):
	  Children: 50 mg/kg then in 4 hours or every 24 hours as needed.
	  Adults: 500 mg–2 g every 2–6 hours.
	Rectal retention enemas: 1 enema nightly for 21 days. May be continued for a longer period if effective or discontinued if no effect is seen.
	Intrarectal foam: 1 full applicator rectally nightly or b.i.d. for 2 or 3 weeks. Absorption of hydrocortisone may be greater from the foam formulation than the enema. Discontinue if not effective after 3 weeks.
	Topically (low-potency corticosteroid in most formulations): apply a thin layer to the affected area t.i.d. or q.i.d.
		Cream, topical: 0.5%, 1%, 2.5%
		Enema: 100 mg/60 mL (Cortenema)
		Foam, intrarectal: 90 mg/full applicator (Cortifoam), rectal/anal 1% (Proctofoam-HC)
		Injection (sodium phosphate): 50 mg/mL
		Injection (sodium succinate): 100-mg, 250-mg, 500-mg, 1-g vials
		Ointment, topical: 0.5%, 1%, 2.5%
		Suspension (cypionate): 10 mg/5 mL
		Tablets: 5 mg, 10 mg, 20 mg

Continued

Table 1   Medications   (continued)

DRUG	*DOSE*	*DOSAGE FORMS*

Hydromorphone (Dilaudid)	*IV:*
	  Young children: 0.015–0.03 mg/kg every 3–4 hours.
	  Older children and adults: 1–4 mg every 3–4 hours.
	Orally:
	  Young children: 0.04–0.07 mg/kg every 3–4 hours.
	  Older children and adults: 1–6 mg every 3–4 hours
	    depending on size and pain severity.
	To convert a patient from oral to IV therapy: start with
	  a ratio of 5:1. Ratios of up to 2:1 may be required in
	  some patients on long-term chronic therapy.
	To convert a patient from IV to oral therapy: in a
	  patient who is receiving a stable dose, use an IV to
	  oral ratio of 1:3.
	Equianalgesic doses:
	  Oral: 7.5 mg hydromorphone = 30 mg morphine.
	  Parenteral: 1.5 mg hydromorphone = 10 mg
	    morphine.
		Injection: 1 mg/mL, 2 mg/mL, 4 mg/mL, 10 mg/mL
		Solution, oral: 1 mg/mL
		Suppositories, rectal: 3 mg
		Tablets: 2 mg, 4 mg, 8 mg

Hydroxyzine (Atarax, Vistaril)	*Orally:*
	  Children: 2 mg/kg/day in 3 or 4 doses.
	  Adults: 100–400 mg/day in 3 or 4 doses. Use
	    lower doses for pruritus and higher doses
	    for sedation.
	Parenterally: the use of hydroxyzine parenterally
	  (IM, IV, SC) has been associated with severe adverse
	  effects at the site of the injection. The reactions are
	  characterized by local discomfort, sterile abscess,
	  erythema, and tissue necrosis. Phlebitis and
	  hemolysis have been reported after IV
	  administration. The manufacturers recommend
	  administration by deep IM injection into a
	  well-developed large muscle. SC infiltration of the
	  drug from an IM injection or extravasation of an
	  IV injection must be avoided.
		Capsule (pamoate): 25 mg, 50 mg, 100 mg
		Injection for IM use: 25 mg/mL, 50 mg/mL
		Solution, oral: 10 mg/5 mL
		Suspension, oral (pamoate): 25 mg/5 mL
		Tablets: 10 mg, 25 mg, 50 mg, 100 mg

Ibuprofen (Advil, Motrin, Nuprin)	*Orally:*
	Antipyretic:
	  Age 6 months–12 years (repeat doses up to every
	    6 hours):
	    Temperature <39°C (102.2°F): 5 mg/kg/dose.
	    Temperature ≥39°C (102.2°F): 10 mg/kg/dose.
	  Over age 12 and adults: 200–400 mg/dose to a
	    maximum of 1,200 mg/day.
	Juvenile rheumatoid arthritis: 30–70 mg/kg/day in
	  4 divided doses to a maximum of 2400 mg/day.
	Adult antiinflammatory dose: 400–800 mg every
	  6–8 hours to a maximum of 3200 mg/day.
		Suspension, oral: 100 mg/5 mL
		Tablets: 200 mg, 300 mg, 400 mg, 600 mg, 800 mg

Imipenem and cilastatin (Primaxin)	*IV infusion over 1 hour* (expressed as mg of imipenem):
	  Children: 50–100 mg/kg/day in 4 divided doses to a
	    maximum of 4 g/day.
	  Adults: 2–4 g/day in 3 or 4 divided doses.
	Dosage adjustment is required in renal impairment.
		Injection: imipenem 250 mg and cilastatin 50 mg,
		  imipenem 500 mg and cilastatin 500 mg

Imipramine (Tofranil)	*Orally:*
	Enuresis in children under age 6: initially 25 mg 1 hour
	  before bedtime nightly. Dose may be increased to
	  50 mg in children age 6–12 or 75 mg in children
	  over age 12 if the initial dose is ineffective.
		Tablets: 10 mg, 25 mg, 50 mg

Continued

Table 1   Medications   (continued)

DRUG	*DOSE*	*DOSAGE FORMS*
Imipramine (Tofranil) (*continued*)	*Depression:* Children: 1.5 mg kg/day in 1–4 divided doses initially. May be increased in increments of about 1 mg/kg/day to a maximum of 5 mg/kg/day. Adolescents: 25–50 mg/day increased gradually to a maximum of 100 mg/day in a single or divided doses. Adults: 75–100 mg/day increased gradually to a maximum of 300 mg/day in a single or divided doses. Dosage should be decreased to the minimum effective dose after symptom control has been achieved. *Doses used to treat pain:* generally lower than those used in the treatment of depression. A starting dose of 0.2–0.4 mg/kg/day administered at bedtime may be used initially. A gradual increase to 1–3 mg/kg/day may be necessary for some patients. Administration of the total daily dose at bedtime may decrease the daytime sedative effects.	
Immune globulin, intramuscular	*IM:* *Measles prophylaxis:* 0.25 mL/kg within 6 days of exposure. In immunocompromised patients, use 0.5 mL/kg (15 mL maximum). *Hepatitis A preexposure prophylaxis:* Risk of exposure within 3 months: 0.02 mL/kg. Risk of exposure greater than 3 months: 0.06 mL/kg. *Hepatitis A postexposure:* 0.02 mL/kg given within 2 weeks of exposure. *Immunodeficiency:* IV has largely replaced use of the IM form. An initial dose of 1.2 mL/kg is followed with doses of 0.6 mL/kg at 2–4-week intervals. The usual maximum volumes are 20–30 mL in infants and small children and 30–50 mL in adults.	Injection, IM: 165 ± 15 mg (of protein) per mL (2 mL and 10 mL)
Immune globulin, intravenous (Gamimune N, Gammagard S/D, Gammar-P IV, Iveegam, Polygam S/D, Sandoglobulin, Venoglobulin-I, Venoglobulin-S)	*IV as a slow infusion:* The rate of infusion varies from product to product but should always be initiated at a very slow rate and may be increased every 30 minutes to the manufacturer's maximum recommended rate or less as the patient tolerates. Infusion-related reactions usually abate if the rate of infusion is decreased. Anaphylactic hypersensitivity reactions may occur and are more likely in patients with IgA deficiency. *Immunodeficiency syndromes:* 100–400 mg/kg every 2–4 weeks. *Idiopathic thrombocytopenic purpura:* either 400 mg/kg/day for 2–5 consecutive days or 1 g/kg/day for 1 or 2 consecutive days may be used for induction. Maintenance doses are usually 400 mg/kg/dose every 4–6 weeks but may be increased to 800–1,000 mg/kg if the lower dose is insufficient and are based on platelet counts and clinical response. *Kawasaki disease:* usually 2 g/kg as a single dose. Alternatively, 400 mg/kg/day for 4 days may be used.	Gamimune N: 5% or 10% solution in vials Gammagard S/D: powder with diluent to make 5% solution Gammar-P IV: powder with diluent to make 5% solution Iveegam: powder with diluent to make 5% solution Polygam S/D: powder with diluent to make 5% solution Sandoglobulin: powder with diluent to make 3%, 6%, or 12% solution Venoglobulin-I: powder with diluent to make 5% solution Venoglobulin-S: solution 5%, 10%

Continued

Table 1   Medications   (continued)

DRUG	DOSE	DOSAGE FORMS
Indomethacin IV (Indocin IV)	*IV push:* Further dilution of the reconstituted injection may result in precipitation of insoluble indomethacin. An initial 0.2 mg/kg/dose is followed by 2 doses based on the patient's postnatal age (PNA) *at the time of the first dose:* PNA <48 hours: 0.1 mg/kg at 12–24-hour intervals. PNA 2–7 days: 0.2 mg/kg at 12–24-hour intervals. PNA >7 days: 0.25 mg/kg at 12–24-hour intervals. The patient's renal and hepatic function should be monitored. Oral use in children is generally not recommended.	Injection (sodium trihydrate): 1 mg
Insulin	*IV:* *Treatment of diabetic ketoacidosis:* loading dose of 0.1 U/kg followed by a continuous infusion of 0.1 U/kg/hr (usual range 0.05–0.2 U/kg/hr) to maintain steady, but slow, decrease of serum glucose levels of 80–100 mg/dl/hr. Only regular insulin should be used by this route. *SC:* *Maintenance:* most patients require 0.5–1 U/kg/day in 2–4 divided doses depending on how well controlled the patient's glucose levels have been. Patients should be warned not to change insulins without prior approval of their physicians. If regular insulin is to be mixed with other types of insulin, the regular insulin should always be measured first. Extemporaneously prepared doses of mixed insulins should be used as soon as possible after mixing to minimize the amount of the regular insulin that will be bound by excess protamine or zinc in the other insulin. The activity of regular insulin has a time to onset of 1/2 to 1 hour, peaks at 2–3 hours, and has a duration of 5–7 hours. The activity of isophane (NPH) insulin has a time to onset of about 1–2 hours, peaks at 4–12 hours, and has a duration of 18–24 hours.	All insulins below are 100 U/mL. Regular insulin: available in beef and pork; pork; human, recombinant DNA; and human, semisynthetic Isophane (NPH) insulin: available in beef and pork; pork, human, recombinant DNA Lispro (Humalog): human, recombinant DNA Prompt zinc (semilente) insulin: available in beef and pork; pork; and human, recombinant DNA Extended zinc (ultralente) insulin: available in beef and pork; and human, recombinant DNA Fixed combinations: regular insulin 30 U/mL with isophane insulin 70 U/mL; available as pork; human, recombinant DNA; and human, semisynthetic isophane insulin 50 U/mL available as human, recombinant DNA
Ipecac	*Orally* (followed by 10–20 mL/kg (up to 300 mL) of water. May be repeated after 20 minutes if vomiting does not occur): Age 6–12 months: 5–10 mL. Age >1–12 years: 15 mL. Over age 12 years: 30 mL. Do not administer at the same time as activated charcoal, or with milk or carbonated beverages.	Syrup
Ipratropium bromide (Atrovent)	*Oral metered dose inhalation:* Children 3–14 years of age: 1–2 inhalations t.i.d. Children >14 years of age and adults: 2 inhalations q.i.d. Maximum dose should not exceed 12 inhalations in 24 hours. *Nebulization* Children 3–14 years of age: 125–250 μg t.i.d. Children >14 years of age and adults: 500 μg 3 to 4 times daily.	Aerosol, metered dose: 18 μg/actuation Solution for nebulization: 0.02%, 2.5 mL

Continued

Table 1   Medications   (continued)

DRUG	DOSE	DOSAGE FORMS

Isoniazid (isonicotinic acid hydrazide, isonicotinyl hydrazide; INH, Nydrazid)	*Orally or IM:*
	Treatment:
	  Children: 20 mg/kg/day in 1 or 2 divided doses (up to 300 mg/day).
	  Adults: 5 mg/kg/day up to 300 mg; 10 mg/kg should be used for disseminated disease.
	Prophylaxis:
	  Children: 10 mg/kg/day in a single dose up to 300 mg/day.
	  Adults: 300 mg/day.
	Liver function should be monitored during therapy because hepatitis may occur at any time. Patients whose diets are low in milk or meat should receive pyridoxine supplements at a dose of about 10–50 mg/day.
		Injection: 100 mg/mL
		Solution, oral: 50 mg/5 mL (with sorbitol 70%)
		Tablets: 100 mg, 300 mg

Isoproterenol (Isuprel)	*IV (by continuous infusion):* 0.05–3 μg/kg/min up to 2–20 μg/min.
	Oral inhalation: 1–2 metered doses up to 6 times daily.
	Nebulization:
	  Age 2–9: 0.25 mL (1:200) in 2.5 mL normal saline solution up to every 4 hours.
	  Over age 9: 0.5 mL (1:200) in 2.5 mL normal saline solution up to every 4 hours.
		Aerosol, metered dose inhaler: 1:400 (0.25%)
		Injection: 1:5,000 (0.2 mg/mL, 1 mg/5 mL)
		Solution for inhalation: 1:200 (0.5%)

Ketoconazole (Nizoral)	*Orally* (acid must be present in the GI tract for the dissolution and absorption of ketoconazole):
	  Children: 3.3–6.6 mg/kg/day in 1 or 2 divided doses to a maximum dose of 400 mg/day.
	  Adults: 200–400 mg/day in a single dose.
	Do not administer antacids or H_2 antagonists at the same time as ketoconazole.
	Monitor liver function during therapy.
	Topically: apply to the affected area once or twice daily.
	Shampoo for dandruff: apply shampoo and lather, allow to remain on the scalp for at least 1 minute before rinsing. Reapply shampoo and lather again, allow to remain on the scalp for 3 minutes, and then rinse. Treatments should be done twice weekly with at least 3 days between treatments, for 4 weeks. The frequency of subsequent treatments should be determined individually.
		Cream: 2%
		Shampoo: 2%
		Tablets: 200 mg

Lamivudine (Epivir)	*Orally:*
	  Age 3 months–12 years: 4 mg/kg b.i.d., to a maximum of 150 mg b.i.d.
	  Adolescents and adults: 150 mg b.i.d.
	  Dosage adjustment may be necessary in patients with renal dysfunction.
		Solution: 10 mg/mL
		Tablets: 150 mg

Leuprolide acetate (Lupron, Lupron Depot)	*SC:* *Anterior pituitary gonadotropic testing:* 10 μg/kg/dose. *Precocious puberty:* 50 μg/kg/day. Dosage may be titrated upward in 10-μg/kg increments if suppression of ovarian or testicular function is incomplete.	Injection for SC use (Lupron): 5 mg/mL Injection, suspension for IM use (Lupron Depot): 3.75 mg, 7.5 mg

Continued

Table 1   Medications   (continued)

DRUG	DOSE	DOSAGE FORMS
Leuprolide acetate (Lupron, Lupron Depot) (continued)	*IM for precocious puberty* (higher doses may be necessary for younger children. Doses should be based on the patient's weight and age): Girls over age 8 and boys over age 9: 0.3 mg/kg (minimum 7.5 mg) repeated every 4 weeks using the depot product. Dosage may be increased in 3.75-mg increments every 4 weeks until an effective dose is achieved. Therapy should generally be discontinued at age 11 for girls or age 12 for boys.	
Levothyroxine sodium (Levothroid, Synthroid)	*Orally:* Age 0–6 months: 8–10 μg/kg or 25–50 μg/day. Age >6–<12 months: 6–8 μg/kg or 50–75 μg/day. Age 1–5: 5–6 μg/kg or 75–100 μg/day. Age 6–12: 4–5 μg/kg or 100–150 μg/day. Over age 12 and adults: 2–3 μg/kg or >150 μg/day. *IV:* one half to three fourths of the oral dose for children or about half the oral dose for adults. The parenteral form of the drug is very unstable and should be used immediately after reconstitution without admixing with other solutions.	Injection: 200 μg, 500 μg Tablets: 25 μg, 50 μg, 75 μg, 88 μg, 100 μg, 112 μg, 125 μg, 150 μg, 175 μg, 200 μg, 300 μg
Lidocaine hydrochloride (Xylocaine)	*IV for cardiac arrhythmias:* 1 mg/kg loading dose followed by a continuous infusion of 20–50 μg/kg/min. The loading dose may be repeated twice at 10–15-minute intervals, if necessary. *Infiltration for local anesthesia:* dose depends on procedure, degree, and duration of anesthesia required and the vascularity of the site. Maximum recommended dose is 4.5 mg/kg. Doses should not be repeated sooner than 2 hours. *Topical:* apply to affected area as needed. Maximum dose should not exceed 3 mg/kg or be repeated within 2 hours. Patients treated with oral lidocaine viscous should be cautioned about the hazards of biting the numbed areas and swallowing difficulties.	Aerosol, metered dose: 10% (for use before endotracheal intubation) Injection: 0.5%, 1%, 1.5%, 2%, 4%; 0.5% with epinephrine 1:200,000; 1% with epinephrine 1:100,000 or 1:200,000; 1.5% with epinephrine 1:200,000; 2% with epinephrine 1:100,000 or 1:200,000 Jelly: 2% Liquid, viscous: 2% Ointment: 2.5%, 5% Solution, topical: 2%, 4%
Lindane (gamma benzene hexachloride; Kwell)	*Topically:* *Pediculosis:* apply 15–30 mL of shampoo to the scalp and lather for 4–5 minutes, then rinse. The hair should be combed with a fine-toothed comb to remove nits. Treatment may be repeated after 1 week, if necessary. *Scabies:* apply a thin layer of the lotion to the skin from the neck to the toes (include the head in infants). The lotion should be removed by bathing after 6 hours for infants, 6–8 hours for children or 8–12 hours for adults. Treatment may be repeated after 1 week, if necessary. Percutaneous absorption may occur and cause toxicity. Do not apply to inflamed or raw skin.	Lotion: 1% Shampoo: 1%
Loperamide (Imodium)	*Orally:* *Acute diarrhea* (dosage is for the initial 24 hours): Age 2 up to age 6 (13–20 kg): 1 mg t.i.d. Age >6–8 (20–30 kg): 2 mg b.i.d. Age >8–12 (>30 kg): 2 mg t.i.d. Adults: 4 mg initially followed by 2 mg after each unformed stool to a maximum of 8 mg in 24 hours (16 mg/24 hr under a physician's care). For subsequent days, use a dose of 0.1 mg/kg for children after each loose stool, but do not exceed dosage guidelines for the first day.	Capsules: 2 mg Solution, oral: 1 mg/5 mL Tablets: 2 mg

Continued

Table 1   Medications   (continued)

DRUG	*DOSE*	*DOSAGE FORMS*
Loperamide (Imodium) (*continued*)	*Chronic diarrhea:* Children: 0.08–0.24 mg/kg/day in 2 or 3 doses daily to a maximum of 2 mg/dose. Adults: 4 mg followed by 2 mg after each unformed stool until symptoms are controlled, then decreased to the lowest dose that will control symptoms. Usual maintenance dose is 4–8 mg/day.	
Loracarbef (Lorabid)	*Orally* (administer doses on an empty stomach): Age 6 months–12 years: *Otitis media:* 30 mg/kg/day in 2 divided doses. Administer only the suspension for otitis because it is absorbed more quickly and results in higher blood levels. *Other infections:* 15 mg/kg/day in 2 divided doses. Older children and adults: 200–400 mg/day in 2 divided doses.	Capsules: 200 mg Suspension, oral: 100 mg/5 mL, 200 mg/5 mL
Loratadine (Claritin)	*Orally:* Age 2–12: 5 mg/day in a single dose. Adults >30 kg: 10 mg/day in a single dose.	Tablets: 10 mg
Lorazepam (Ativan)	*IV:* *Status epilepticus:* Neonates: 0.05 mg/kg over 2–5 minutes. Dose may be repeated in 10–15 minutes. Infants and children: 0.1 mg/kg over 2–5 minutes to a maximum of 4 mg/dose. A second dose of 0.05 mg/kg may be given. Adolescents: 0.07 mg/kg over 2–5 minutes to a maximum of 4 mg. Dose may be repeated in 10–15 minutes. Adults: 4 mg over 2–5 minutes. Dose may be repeated in 10–15 minutes. *Adjunct to antiemetic therapy:* 0.02–0.04 mg/kg up to every 6 hours. Do not exceed a maximum of 2 mg/dose. *Orally or IV:* *Anxiety and sedation:* Infants and children: 0.03–0.04 mg/kg/day, in 3–4 divided doses. Adults: 2–6 mg/day, usually orally, in 2 or 3 divided doses.	Injection: 2 mg/mL, 4 mg/mL Solution, oral: 2 mg/mL Tablets: 0.5 mg, 1 mg, 2 mg
Magnesium citrate (Citrate of Magnesia, Evac-Q-Mag)	*Orally* (chill for better palatability): Under age 6: 2–4 mL/kg. Age 6–12: 100–150 mL. Over age 12: 150–300 mL.	Solution: 300 mL (carbonated; contains 3.85–4.71 mEq Mg/5 mL)
Magnesium gluconate (Almora, Magonate, Magtrate)	*Orally* (expressed in terms of mEq of magnesium): Children: 0.5–0.75 mEq/kg/day in 3 or 4 divided doses. Adults: 2.2–4.4 mEq administered b.i.d. or t.i.d.	Liquid: 1,000 mg/5 mL (54 mg Mg = 4.4 mEq Mg) Tablets: 500 mg (27 mg Mg = 2.2 mEq Mg)
Magnesium hydroxide (Milk of Magnesia)	*Orally:* Under age 2: 0.5 mL/kg/dose. Age 2–5: 5–15 mL/day. Age 6–12: 15–30 mL/day. Over age 12: 30–60 mL/day.	Suspension: contains about 13.7 mEq Mg/5 mL

Continued

Table 1 Medications (continued)

DRUG	DOSE	DOSAGE FORMS
Magnesium sulfate (Epsom Salts)	*IV* [expressed in terms of magnesium sulfate (and mEq Mg)]: *Hypomagnesemia* (monitor serum magnesium levels closely): Neonates: 25–50 mg/kg (0.2–0.4 mEq/kg) every 8–12 hours for 2–3 doses. Infants and children: 25–50 mg/kg (0.2–0.4 mEq/kg) every 4–6 hours for 3 or 4 doses with a maximum single dose of 2,000 mg (16 mEq). Doses up to 100 mg/kg have been used in severe hypomagnesemia. Adults: 1 g (8 mEq) every 6 hours for 4 doses. Doses of 2–3 g (16–24 mEq) have been used for severe hypomagnesemia. *Maintenance dose:* 30–60 mg/kg/day (0.25–0.5 mEq/kg/day) in 3 or 4 divided doses. *Management of seizures or hypertension in children:* 25–100 mg/kg (0.2–0.8 mEq/kg) every 4–6 hours as needed. Administer the drug slowly (over 1–2 hours) in a concentration not greater than 10 mg/mL. Blood pressure should be monitored frequently during infusions because hypotension has been reported with too-fast administration.	Injection: 500 mg/mL (4 mEq magnesium = 49 mg Mg)
Mannitol (Osmitrol)	*IV:* initial dose of 2 g/kg followed by doses of 0.25–0.5 g/kg every 4–6 hours. A test dose of 0.2 g/kg (to a maximum of 12.5 g) over 3–5 minutes should produce a urine flow of about 1 mL/kg/hr for 2 or 3 hours. It should be used for patients with marked oliguria or inadequate renal function.	Injection: 5%, 10%, 15%, 20%, 25%
Mebendazole (Vermox)	*Orally:* Over age 2 and adults: *Enterobiasis (pinworm):* 100 mg as a single dose. May be repeated at 2 weeks. *Ascariasis (roundworm), trichuriasis (whipworm), hookworm, or mixed infections:* 200 mg/day in 2 divided doses for 3 days. A second course may be administered 3–4 weeks later.	Tablets, chewable: 100 mg
Meperidine hydrochloride (Demerol)	Oral doses are about half as effective as IV doses but are generally used for less severe pain; therefore, the doses listed are for all routes of administration, but that should be kept in mind if a patient is being switched from parenteral to oral therapy. Children: 1–1.5 mg/kg every 3–4 hours. A single dose of 3 mg/kg (to a maximum of 100 mg) may be used preoperatively. Adults: 50–150 mg every 3–4 hours. Dosage adjustment is necessary in renal impairment. Long-term or high-dose therapy may result in accumulation of normeperidine, an active metabolite that is a CNS stimulant, especially in patients with renal failure.	Injection: 25 mg/mL, 50 mg/mL, 75 mg/mL, 100 mg/mL Solution, oral: 50 mg/5 mL Tablets: 50 mg, 100 mg
Meropenem (Merrem IV)	*IV:* *Intraabdominal infections:* Age 3 months–adults: 60 mg/kg/day in 3 divided doses to a maximum total daily dose of 3 g. *Meningitis:* Age 3 months–adults: 120 mg/kg/day in 3 divided doses to a maximum total daily dose of 6 g.	Injection: 500 mg, 1 g

Continued

Table 1   Medications   (continued)

DRUG	DOSE	DOSAGE FORMS
Mesalamine (Asacol, Pentasa, Rowasa)	*Orally:* Adults: 1 g (capsules) q.i.d. or 800 mg (tablets) t.i.d. *Rectally:* 4 g enema administered at bedtime daily. The enema should be retained overnight (8 hours) for best results. The oral forms of the drug are formulated with an enteric coating to slowly release the drug.	Capsules (Pentasa): 250 mg Suspension, rectal: 4 g/60 mL Tablets (Asacol): 400 mg
Metaproterenol (Alupent, Metaprel)	*Orally:* Under age 6: 1.3–2.6 mg/kg/day in 3 or 4 divided doses. Age 6–9 (<27 kg): 10 mg/dose t.i.d. or q.i.d. Over age 9 (>27 kg) and adults: 20 mg/dose t.i.d. or q.i.d. *Oral inhalation:* Over age 12 and adults: 2–3 inhalations every 3–4 hours, up to 12 inhalations daily. *Nebulizer:* Age 6–12: 0.1 mL of a 5% solution diluted in 0.9% sodium chloride solution to 3 mL, repeated up to every 4 hours. Over age 12 and adults: 0.2–0.3 mL of 5% solution (or 2.5 mL of 0.4% or 0.6% commercially available diluted solution) administered t.i.d. or q.i.d.	Inhalation: Aerosol: 0.65 mg/inhalation spray Solution: 5%, 0.4% in normal saline solution, 0.6% in normal saline solution Solution, oral: 10 mg/5 mL Tablets: 10 mg, 20 mg
Methylene blue (Urolene Blue)	*IV for methemoglobinemia:* 1–2 mg/kg injected slowly over a period of several minutes. The dose may be repeated in 1 hour, if necessary. *Orally for adults with chronic methemoglobinemia:* 100–300 mg/day.	Injection: 10 mg/mL Tablets: 65 mg
Methylphenidate (Ritalin)	*Orally:* Over age 6: initially 0.3 mg/kg/day (2.5–5 mg/dose) before breakfast and lunch. That may be increased to the usual dosage range of 0.5–1 mg/kg/day or a maximum of 2 mg/kg/day or 60 mg. The sustained-release form may be given as a single dose at breakfast.	Tablets: 5 mg, 10 mg, 20 mg Tablets, extended release: 20 mg
Methylprednisolone (A-methaPred, Depo-Medrol, Medrol, Solu-Medrol)	*IV:* *Status asthmaticus:* 1 mg/kg every 6 hours. *Acute spinal cord injury:* 30 mg/kg over 15 minutes followed in 45 minutes by an infusion of 5.4 mg/kg/hr for 23 hours. *Shock:* 30 mg/kg and may be repeated every 4–12 hours, but not to continue for longer than 48–72 hours. *"Pulse" therapy for lupus nephritis in older children and adults:* 1 g/day for 3 days. A dose of 30 mg/kg every other day for 6 doses has been used for children. *Orally:* Children: 0.117–1.6 mg/kg/day in 4 divided doses. Adults: 2–60 mg/day in 4 divided doses. *Intraarticular, intralesional doses (acetate):* 4–40 mg or up to 80 mg for large joints every 1–5 weeks.	Injection (acetate; Depo-Medrol): 20 mg/mL, 40 mg/mL, 80 mg/mL Injection (sodium succinate): 40-mg, 125-mg, 500-mg, 1-g, 2-g vials Tablets: 2 mg, 4 mg, 8 mg, 16 mg, 24 mg, 32 mg
Metoclopramide (Maxolon, Octamide, Reglan)	*Orally or IV:* *Gastroesophageal reflux:* Children: initially 0.1–0.5 mg/kg/day in 4 divided doses before meals. Dosage may be increased to a maximum of 0.8 mg/kg/day. Adults: 10–15 mg 30 minutes before meals and at bedtime.	Injection: 5 mg/mL Solution, oral: 5 mg/5 mL, 10 mg/5 mL Tablets: 5 mg, 10 mg

Continued

Table 1   Medications   (continued)

DRUG	DOSE	DOSAGE FORMS
Metoclopramide (Maxolon, Octamide, Reglan) (continued)	*IV:* *Intubation of GI tract or radiographic exam:* Under age 6: 0.1 mg/kg. Age 6–14: 2.5–5 mg. Adults: 10 mg. *Antiemetic in chemotherapy-induced nausea:* 1–2 mg/kg administered 30 minutes before the chemotherapy and every 2–4 hours as necessary thereafter to a maximum of 3 doses. Extrapyramidal reactions are common at this dose and may be treated with diphenhydramine IV (1 mg/kg up to 50 mg) every 6 hours.	
Metolazone (Zaroxolyn)	*Orally:* Infants and children: 0.2–0.4 mg/kg/day in 1–2 divided doses. Adults: 2.5–5 mg/day for the treatment of hypertension. Edema due to cardiac or renal disease may require doses of 5–20 mg/day.	Tablets: 2.5 mg, 5 mg, 10 mg
Metronidazole (Flagyl, Protostat)	*Orally or IV:* *Anaerobic bacterial infections* (IV initially, then orally): Infants other than neonates to adults: 30 mg/kg/day in 4 divided doses, not to exceed 4 g/day. *Amebiasis* (usually orally): Infants and children: 35–50 mg/kg/day in 3 divided doses. Adults: 500–750 mg every 8 hours. *Other parasitic infections* (usually orally): Infants and children: 15–30 mg/kg/day in 3 divided doses. Adults: 250 mg every 8 hours or a single 2-g dose. *Pelvic inflammatory disease:* Adults: 500 mg every 12 hours. *Antibiotic-associated pseudomembranous colitis:* Infants and children: 20 mg/kg/day in 4 divided doses. Adults: 250–500 mg t.i.d. or q.i.d. Oral doses may be taken with food to minimize stomach upset.	Injection: available 5 mg/mL ready to infuse solution or 500-mg vial Tablets: 250 mg, 500 mg
Midazolam (Versed)	*IV* (titrate dose slowly to avoid excessive dosing): *Conscious sedation:* Children: 0.05 mg/kg just before the procedure to a maximum dose of 2 mg. Dose may be repeated every 3 or 4 minutes up to 4 times. Adults: 0.5–2 mg over 2 minutes. Titrate to effect by repeating doses every 2–3 minutes to a usual dose of 2.5–5 mg. *Infusion for sedation during mechanical ventilation:* administer a loading dose of 0.05–0.2 mg/kg followed by a continuous infusion of 1–2 μg/kg/min and titrate to effect. *Orally:* 0.5 mg/kg to a maximum dose of 15 mg. *Intranasally:* 0.2–0.3 mg/kg/dose. The oral and intranasal routes of administration are not FDA approved.	Injection: 1 mg/mL, 5 mg/mL
Mineral oil	*Orally* (do not administer concomitantly with docusate): Children: 5–20 mL/day. Adults: 15–45 mL/day.	Enema: 133 mL Liquid

Continued

1000

Table 1   Medications   (continued)

DRUG	DOSE	DOSAGE FORMS
Mineral oil (continued)	*Rectally* (as a retention enema): Children: 30–60 mL. Adults: 60–150 mL.	
Mometasone Elocon	*Topically:* Apply a thin film to the affected area once daily. The cream and ointment have been used twice daily.	Cream: 0.1% Lotion: 0.1% Ointment: 0.1%
Montelukast (Singulair)	*Orally:* Children 2–6 years of age: 4 mg once daily. Children >6–14 years of age: 5 mg once daily. Children >14 years of age and adults: 10 mg once daily.	Tablets, chewable: 4 mg, 5 mg Tablets: 10 mg
Morphine sulfate (Astramorph PF, Duramorph, MSIR, MS Contin, Roxanol)	*IV or IM:* Neonates and infants under age 6 months: these patients are particularly sensitive to the respiratory depressant effects of opiates; therefore, the doses recommended are lower: 0.03 mg/kg every 3 or 4 hours. Infusions have been used in neonatal patients at a dose of 0.01 mg/kg/hr. The dose may be increased if necessary but should not exceed 0.015–0.02 mg/kg/hr. Infants over 6 months and children: 0.025–0.1 mg/kg every 3 to 6 hours. Doses of up to 2.5 mg/kg have been used in severe pain such as sickle cell or cancer pain. The usual maximum dose is 10 mg. Adults: 2.5–10 mg every 2–6 hours. *Epidurally:* 0.5–5 mg in the lumbar region. Dose may be repeated every 24 hours. Maximum dose is 10 mg/24 hr. *Intrathecally:* one tenth of epidural dose or about 0.2–1 mg/dose. Repeat doses are not recommended. *Orally:* prompt-release preparations are administered every 3 or 4 hours; controlled-release preparations are administered every 8–12 hours. Oral doses are about one third as effective as IV doses. Infants over 6 months and children: 0.3 mg/kg every 3 or 4 hours (prompt release) or 0.3–0.6 mg/kg every 8–12 hours (extended release). Adults: 10–30 mg every 3–4 hours (prompt release) or 15–30 mg every 8–12 hours (extended release).	Injection: 0.5 mg/mL, 1 mg/mL, 2 mg/mL, 3 mg/mL, 4 mg/mL, 5 mg/mL, 8 mg/mL, 10 mg/mL, 15 mg/mL Solution: 10 mg/5 mL, 20 mg/5 mL, 20 mg/mL Suppositories: 5 mg, 10 mg, 20 mg, 30 mg Tablets: 15 mg, 30 mg Tablets, controlled release: 15 mg, 30 mg, 60 mg, 100 mg
Mumps virus vaccine (Mumpsvax)	*SC into the outer aspect of the upper arm:* 0.5 mL at age 15 months or older. Trivalent MMR vaccine is preferred for most vaccinations. Federal law requires that the date of administration, manufacturer, lot number, and expiration date of the vaccine, and the name, title, and address of the person administering the dose be entered into the patient's permanent medical record. It also requires providers to distribute information on vaccines before each vaccination.	Injection: $\geq$20,000 $TCID_{50}$/0.5 mL
Mupirocin (pseudomonic acid A; Bactroban)	*Topically:* *Impetigo:* apply ointment to affected area t.i.d. for 3–5 days. *Lacerations, minor suture infections or abrasions:* apply cream to the affected area t.i.d. for 10 days. *Intranasal Staphylococcus aureus infection:* apply 1/2 of the contents of a unit-dose tube of intranasal cream into each nostril 2–4 times daily for 5–14 days.	Cream (as mupirocin calcium): 2% mupirocin Cream, intranasal (as mupirocin calcium): 2% Ointment: 2%

Continued

Table 1 Medications (continued)

DRUG	DOSE	DOSAGE FORMS
Nafcillin (See oxacillin)	Neonates: 60 mg/kg/24 hr in 4–6 divided doses. Children: 100–200 mg/kg/24 hr in 4–6 divided doses.	Injection: 500 mg, 1 g, 2 g
Nalbuphine (Nubain)	*Parenterally:* *Reversal of morphine infusion side effects:* 0.025–0.05 mg/kg repeated every 6 hours as necessary. *Analgesia:* Children over age 10 months: 0.1–0.14 mg/kg every 3–6 hours as necessary to a maximum dose of 10 mg. Adults: 10–20 mg every 3–6 hours. Its use in narcotic-dependent patients may cause symptoms of withdrawal.	Injection: 10 mg/mL, 20 mg/mL
Naloxone (Narcan)	*IV (preferred), IM, or SC:* *Neonatal opiate depression:* 0.01 mg/kg every 2 or 3 minutes until the desired response is obtained. Additional doses may be necessary at 1–2-hour intervals. *Opiate overdosage:* 0.1 mg/kg to a dose of 2 mg administered every 2 or 3 minutes until 5 doses (up to 10 mg) have been given. If the depressive condition is not reversed, causes other than opiate ingestion should be considered. Additional doses may be necessary because the duration of effect of the opiate is generally longer than that of naloxone. The drug may also be administered via continuous infusion, especially if higher doses are necessary. *Postoperative narcotic reversal (partial reversal):* 0.005–0.01 mg/kg every 2–3 minutes until the desired degree of reversal is achieved. Care should be taken to avoid excessive dosage because that might result in a decrease in analgesia and an increase in blood pressure.	Injection (neonatal): 0.02 mg/mL Injection: 0.4 mg/mL, 1 mg/mL
Naproxen (Aleve, Naprosyn)	*Orally:* 5–10 mg/kg every 8–12 hours to a maximum daily dose of 1 g.	Suspension: 125 mg/5 mL Tablets: 250 mg, 375 mg, 500 mg
Nelfinavir (Viracept)	*Orally* (to be used in combination with nucleoside analogs): Age 2–13: 60–90 mg/kg/day in 3 divided doses with food. Adolescents and adults: 750 mg/dose t.i.d.	Powder: 50 mg/g (1 g scoop provided to measure doses) Tablets: 250 mg
Neomycin, polymyxin B, and hydrocortisone (Cortisporin)	*Ophthalmic:* Solution: 1–2 drops to the affected eye every 4–6 hours; apply finger pressure to the lacrimal sac for 1 minute after instillation. Ointment: apply about 1/2-inch ribbon of ointment to the eye t.i.d. or q.i.d. *Otic* (both a suspension and a solution formulation are available. The solution form may sting when instilled, but allows the ear canal to be examined easily): instill 3–4 drops into the affected ear t.i.d. or q.i.d.	Ointment, ophthalmic: neomycin 0.35%, bacitracin 400 U, polymyxin B 10,000 U, and hydrocortisone 1% Solution or suspension, otic: neomycin 5 mg/mL, polymyxin B 10,000 U/mL, and hydrocortisone 1% Suspension, ophthalmic: neomycin 0.35%, polymyxin B 10,000 U, and hydrocortisone 1%
Neomycin sulfate (Mycifradin)	*Orally:* *Bowel preparation:* 15 mg/kg (up to 1 g) at 1 P.M., 2 P.M., and 11 P.M. on the day before surgery (with erythromycin, cleansing enemas). *Hepatic coma:* 50–100 mg/kg/day in 3 or 4 divided doses up to 12 g/day.	Solution, oral: 125 mg/5 mL Tablets: 500 mg

Continued

Table 1   Medications   (continued)

DRUG	DOSE	DOSAGE FORMS
Neostigmine (Prostigmin)	*IM:* *Myasthenia gravis test:* 0.04 mg/kg single dose *IV:* *Reversal of nondepolarizing neuromuscular blockade after surgery in conjunction with atropine or glycopyrrolate:* Infants: 0.025–0.1 mg/kg/dose. Children: 0.025–0.08 mg/kg/dose. Adults: 0.5–2.5 mg, total dose not to exceed 5 mg.	Injection: 0.25 mg/mL, 0.5 mg/mL, 1 mg/mL
Nitrofurantoin (Furadantin, Macrodantin)	*Orally:* *Active infection:* Children: 5–7 mg/kg/day in 4 divided doses to a maximum of 400 mg/day. Adults: 200–400 mg/day in 4 divided doses. *Chronic suppression therapy:* Children: 1–2 mg/kg/day in 1 or 2 divided doses. Adults: 50–100 mg at bedtime daily. Administer with food or milk to decrease rate of absorption because high peak levels are associated with increased GI upset.	Capsules (macrocrystals): 25 mg, 50 mg, 100 mg Suspension: 25 mg/5 mL
Nitroprusside sodium (Nipride, Nitropress)	*IV as a continuous infusion:* 0.3–0.5 μg/kg/min initially, then titrate to effect. Usual dose is 3 μg/kg/min. The maximum dose is 10 μg/kg/min. Cyanide toxicity may occur during prolonged therapy or in patients with hepatic dysfunction. Administration of sodium thiosulfate may decrease blood cyanide levels. Thiocyanate may accumulate in patients with renal impairment.	Injection: 50 mg Protect solutions from light. Do not use if highly colored (blue, green, or red).
Norepinephrine (Levarterenol, Levophed, Noradrenalin)	*IV as a continuous infusion:* initially 0.05–0.1 μg/kg/min, titrated to response. Maximum dose: 1–2 μg/kg/min.	Injection: 1 mg/mL
Nystatin (Mycostatin, Nilstat)	*Orally:* Neonates: 100,000 U administered q.i.d. Infants: 200,000 U administered q.i.d. Children and adults: 400,000–1 million U administered q.i.d. *Topically:* apply ointment or cream to the affected area t.i.d. or q.i.d.	Cream: 100,000 U/g [also available with triamcinolone, a topical steroid (Mycolog)] Ointment: 100,000 U/g [also available with triamcinolone, a topical steroid (Mycolog)] Suspension: 100,000 U/mL Tablets: 500,000 U (intestinal infections only) Troches: 200,000 U
Octreotide (somatostatin analog; Sandostatin)	*IV or SC:* the subcutaneous route is generally preferred because absorption is not immediate and the activity is somewhat prolonged. The drug may also be administered as a continuous infusion. Pediatric experience is limited, but initial doses of 1–10 μg/kg with total daily doses of 2–50 μg/kg in 2–4 divided doses. Usual adult doses are 50 μg 1 or 2 times daily initially, then titrate dose to the patient's response. The long-term effects of octreotide on growth hormone release have not been determined.	Injection: 50 μg/mL, 100 μg/mL, 200 μg/mL, 500 μg/mL, 1,000 μg/mL
Ofloxacin (Floxin Otic, Ocuflox)	*Ophthalmic infections:* *Bacterial conjunctivitis:* 1–2 drops in the affected eye every 2–4 hours while awake for 2 days, then 4 times a day for up to 5 more days. *Bacterial keratitis:* 1–2 drops in the affected eye every 30 minutes while awake and 4–6 hours after retiring for 2 days, then every hour while awake for up to 4–6 more days, then 4 times a day until cure is affected.	Solution, ophthalmic: 0.3% Solution, otic: 0.3%

Continued

Table 1   Medications   (continued)

DRUG	_DOSE_	_DOSAGE FORMS_
Ofloxacin (Floxin Otic, Ocuflox) (_continued_)	_Otic infections:_ _Otitis externa:_ 　Children 1–12 years of age: 5 drops in the affected ear canal twice a day for 10 days. 　Children >12 years of age and adults: 10 drops in the affected ear canal twice a day for 10 days. _Suppurative otitis media in patients with perforated tympanic membranes:_ 10 drops in the affected ear twice a day for 14 days. The tragus of the ear should be pumped several times to make sure the solution is in the ear canal and the patient should remain in a position with the ear up for 5 minutes. _Otitis media in patients with tympanostomy tubes:_ 　5 drops in the affected ear twice a day for 10 days. The tragus of the ear should be pumped as above and the patient should remain in a position with the ear up for 5 minutes.	
Olopatadine (Patanol)	_Ophthalmic:_ 　Children ≥3 years of age to adults: 1–2 drops in each eye twice daily at 6–8 hours intervals.	Solution, ophthalmic: 0.1%
Omeprazole (Prilosec)	_Orally with food or a meal:_ 　Children: while safety and efficacy in children has not been established, a dose of 0.6–0.7 mg/kg/day as a single dose in the morning has been used. If necessary, a second dose may be given 12 hours later. The usual range of doses used is 0.3–3.3 mg/kg/day. 　Adults: 20 mg daily. Higher doses may be used for pathologic hypersecretory conditions. The usual starting dose is 60 mg daily, but doses of up to 360 mg daily have been used. Doses >80 mg/day should be given in 2–3 divided doses. 　Capsules: 10 mg, 20 mg, 40 mg. The capsules contain enteric coated spheres. If the patient is unable to swallow capsules, the spheres may be put into an acidic juice, such as apple juice, for administration. Do not crush the spheres. The spheres may be crushed for administration through a jejunostomy tube if a 650-mg tablet of sodium bicarbonate is added.	Capsules: 10 mg, 20 mg, 40 mg. The capsules contain enteric coated spheres. If the patient is unable to swallow capsules, the spheres may be put into an acidic juice, such as apple juice, for administration. Do not crush the spheres. The spheres may be crushed for administration through a tube if a 650 mg tablet of sodium bicarbonate is added to the diluent.
Oseltamivir (Tamiflu)	_Orally (within 2 days of onset of symptoms):_ 　≥13 years of age: 75 mg twice a day for 5 days.	Capsules: 75 mg
Oxacillin (Bactocill)	_IV:_ Neonates under age 7 days: 　<2,000 g: 50 mg/kg/day in 2 divided doses. 　≥2,000 g: 100 mg/kg/day in 2 divided doses. Neonates over age 7 days: 　<1,200 g: 50 mg/kg/day in 2 divided doses. 　1,200–2,000 g: 75 mg/kg/day in 3 divided doses. 　>2,000 g: 100 mg/kg/day in 4 divided doses. Infants and children (depends on severity and site of infection): 　_Mild to moderate infections:_ 50 mg/kg/day in 4 divided doses. 　_Severe infections, including osteomyelitis:_ 100–200 mg/kg/day in 4–6 divided doses. Total maximum dose is 12 g/day.	Capsules: 250 mg, 500 mg Injection: 250 mg, 500 mg, 1 g, 2 g, 4 g, 10 g Solution, oral: 250 mg/5 mL

Continued

Table 1   Medications   (continued)

DRUG	*DOSE*	*DOSAGE FORMS*

Oxacillin (Bactocill) (*continued*)	Adults:
	  Mild to moderate infections: 250–500 mg every 6 hours.
	  Severe infections: 1–2 g every 4–6 hours.
	Orally:
	  Infants and children: 50–100 mg/kg/day in 4 divided doses.
	  Adults: 500 mg–1 g every 4–6 hours.	

Oxybutynin (Ditropan)	*Orally:*
	  Children ≤age 5: 0.2 mg/kg/dose given 2–3 times daily.
	  Children over age 5: 5 mg administered b.i.d. or t.i.d.
	  Adults: 5 mg b.i.d. or t.i.d., to a maximum of q.i.d.
		Solution, oral: 5 mg/5 mL
		Tablets: 5 mg

Pancrelipase (Cotazym, Cotazym-S, Creon, Pancrease MT, Ultrase, Zymase)	*Orally:* depends on the condition being treated and the dietary content of the patient. Dosage is usually determined by the fat content of the diet. The usual starting dose is 4,000–8,000 U of lipase activity before or with each meal or snack for children age 1–7, 4,000–12,000 U for children age >7–12, or 4,000–33,000 U for adults. Further dosage adjustments may be made based on the patient's symptoms. The newer, enteric-coated products are designed to release the enzymes at pH >6 and are therefore more resistant to destruction by gastric acids.	Capsules, delayed release, containing enteric-coated spheres, microspheres, or microtablets‡
Paregoric	*Analgesic:* 0.25–0.5 mL/kg from once daily to q.i.d. *Antidiarrheal:* 0.1 mL/kg after each loose stool up to q.i.d. Contains 0.4 mg/mL morphine.	Tincture: 16-oz bottle

Penicillamine (Cuprimine, Depen)	Do not exceed a dose of 30 mg/kg/day.
	Rheumatoid arthritis:
	Children:
	  Initial: 3 mg/kg/day (≤250 mg/day) for 3 months, then 6 mg/kg/day (≤500 mg/day) in divided doses b.i.d. for 3 months. Maximum: 10 mg/kg/day in 3 or 4 divided doses.
	Wilson disease:
	  Children: 20 mg/kg/day in 4 divided doses.
		Capsules: 125 mg, 250 mg
		Tablets: 250 mg

Penicillin G, aqueous (potassium and sodium salts)	*IV:*
	Neonates under age 7 days:
	  <2,000 g: 25,000 U/kg every 12 hours. For meningitis, use 50,000 U/kg every 12 hours.
	  >2,000 g: 20,000 U/kg every 8 hours. For meningitis, 50,000 U/kg every 8 hours.
	Neonates over age 7 days:
	  <2,000 g: 25,000 U/kg every 8 hours. For meningitis, 50,000 U/kg every 8 hours.
	  >2,000 g: 25,000 U/kg every 6 hours. For meningitis, 50,000 U/kg every 6 hours.
	  Infants and children: 100,000–250,000 U/kg/day in 6 divided doses. Up to 500,000 U/kg/day may be used for severe infections to a maximum of 20 million U/day.
	  Adults: 2–20 million U/day in 6 divided doses.
	The potassium salt contains 1.7 mEq of potassium and 0.3 mEq of sodium per 1 million U.
	The sodium salt contains 2 mEq of sodium per 1 million U.
	The potassium salt must be administered slowly at high doses due to the effect of the potassium.
		Injection, potassium salt: 1 million U, 5 million U, 10 million U
		Injection, sodium salt: 5 million U

Continued

Table 1   Medications   (continued)

DRUG	DOSE	DOSAGE FORMS
Penicillin G procaine, benzathine	*Deep IM:* results in low but prolonged serum levels. May be given as a single daily dose. A dose of penicillin G benzathine will result in low serum levels for up to 4 weeks. Newborns: avoid use in these patients because sterile abscess and procaine toxicity are of greater concern. Infants: 50,000 U/kg up to 600,000 U. Children and adults: 600,000–1.2 million U/day. Maximum dose is 4.8 million U.	Injection, benzathine: 600,000 U/mL Injection, benzathine and procaine: combined equal parts of each in 300,000 U, 600,000 U, 1.2 million U, 2.4 million U; 900/300 (900,000 U benzathine, 300,000 U procaine) Injection, procaine: 600,000 U/mL
Penicillin V potassium (phenoxymethylpenicillin; Pen Vee K, V-Cillin K, Veetids)	*Orally:* Children: 25–50 mg/kg/day in 4 divided doses. Adults: 125–500 mg/dose every 6 hours. *Prophylaxis:* Under age 5: 125 mg b.i.d. Over age 5 and adults: 250 mg b.i.d.	Liquid, oral: 250 mg/5 mL Tablets: 125 mg, 250 mg, 500 mg
Pentobarbital (Nembutal)	*Orally, IM:* *Sedation before surgery:* Children: 2–6 mg/kg/day to a maximum of 100 mg. *IV:* *For sedation before procedures:* dose should be administered slowly and incrementally to avoid oversedation. Patients must be closely observed. Dosing is very patient-specific. The rate of injection should not exceed 1 mg/kg/min (50 mg/min in adults). Allow at least 1 minute to reach full effect. Children: initially 2 mg/kg to a maximum of 100 mg. Incremental doses of 1–2 mg/kg may be used to a maximum total dose of 200 mg. Adults: initially 100 mg. Incremental doses of 100–200 mg may be given to a maximum dose of 500 mg for healthy adults. *Barbiturate coma:* 10–15 mg/kg administered over 1–2 hours, followed by a maintenance infusion of 1 mg/kg/hr. Dosage may be increased to 2–3 mg/kg/hr to maintain burst suppression on EEG. Hypothermia may necessitate a decrease in dosage. *Rectally* (do not divide suppositories): 4.5–9 kg: 30 mg. >9–18 kg: 30–60 mg. 19–36 kg: 60 mg. >36–50 kg: 60–120 mg. >50 kg: 120–200 mg.	Capsules: 50 mg, 100 mg Elixir: 20 mg/5 mL Injection: 50 mg/mL Suppositories: 30 mg, 60 mg, 120 mg, 200 mg
Permethrin (Elimite Cream, Nix Cream Rinse)	*Scabies:* Children >2 months of age and adults: apply cream from head to toe. Wash cream off after 8–14 hours. May be reapplied after 1 week if live mites appear. *Head lice:* apply cream rinse to hair that has been thoroughly washed, rinsed and towel dried. Saturate hair and scalp with cream rinse. Also apply to the ears and hairline at the nape of the neck. Rinse off after 10 minutes and remove remaining nits with the comb provided. May be repeated after 1 week if necessary.	Cream, topical 5% Cream rinse: 1%

Continued

Table 1   Medications   (continued)

DRUG	DOSE	DOSAGE FORMS
Phenobarbital	*IV or orally:* *Loading doses (usually IV for status epilepticus):* Neonates: 20 mg/kg in a single or 2 divided doses. Infants, children and adults: 15–18 mg/kg a single or 2 divided doses. Allow 15–30 minutes for the drug to distribute into the CNS and for the seizures to stop. *Maintenance doses:* Neonates: 5 mg/kg/day in 2 divided doses. Infants: 5–6 mg/kg/day in 2 divided doses. Age 1–5: 6 mg/kg/day in 2 divided doses. Age >5–12: 4 mg/kg/day in 1 or 2 divided doses. Over age 12 and adults: 1–2 mg/kg/day in 1 or 2 divided doses.	Elixir: 15 mg/5 mL, 20 mg/5 mL Injection (sodium): 30 mg/mL, 60 mg/mL, 65 mg/mL, 130 mg/mL Tablets: 15 mg, 30 mg, 60 mg, 100 mg
Phentolamine mesylate Phenylephrine (Neo-Synephrine, Mydfrin ophthalmic)	*Test dose (pheochromocytoma):* 1 mg IM or IV. *Intranasally (do not use for longer than 3–5 days):* Under age 6: 0.125% solution 2–3 drops every 4 hours as needed. Age 6–12: 0.25% solution 2–3 drops or 1–2 sprays every 4 hours as needed. Over age 12 and adults: 0.5% solution 2–3 drops or 1–2 sprays every 4 hours as needed. 1% solution may be used in adults with extreme congestion. *Ophthalmic:* Infants: 1 drop of 2.5% solution 15–30 minutes before procedure. Children and adults: 1 drop of 2.5% or 10% solution; may repeat in 15–30 minutes. *IV for severe hypotension or shock:* a bolus dose of 5–20 μg/kg (2–5 mg in adults) may be repeated every 10–15 minutes. For infusion, initial doses of 0.1–0.5 μg/kg/min are titrated to effect.	Injection: 5-mg ampul Drops only: 0.125% Injection: 10 mg/mL Solution, nasal drops or spray: 0.25%, 0.5%, 1% Solution, ophthalmic: 2.5%, 10%
Phenytoin (Dilantin) and fosphenytoin (Cerebyx)	Care must be taken when changing from one dosage form of the drug to another because some contain phenytoin sodium and some contain the free acid form of the drug. The free acid form is used for the Infatabs and the suspension. Phenytoin sodium is used for the injection and capsules. Phenytoin sodium contains 92% phenytoin. Injection labeled as 50 mg/mL phenytoin sodium contains 46 mg of phenytoin and capsules labeled 100 mg contain 92 mg phenytoin. Fosphenytoin should be ordered in terms of phenytoin equivalents. The patient's serum levels should be monitored whenever the dosage form is changed. In addition, the different brands of phenytoin capsules have different dissolution characteristics. Dilantin capsules are considered extended and may be dosed in adults as a single daily dose. The serum level range usually associated with clinical effectiveness is 10–20 μg/mL; that associated with mild to moderate toxicity may be as low as 25–30 μg/mL. *Loading dose (IV or PO):* 15–20 mg/kg in a single or divided doses.	Capsule, phenytoin sodium, extended: 30 mg, 100 mg Injection, for phenytoin: 75 mg/1 mL (equivalent to 50 mg phenytoin sodium) Injection, phenytoin sodium: 50 mg/mL Suspension, phenytoin: 125 mg/5 mL Tablet, chewable, phenytoin: 50 mg

Continued

Table 1   Medications   (continued)

DRUG	DOSE	DOSAGE FORMS
Phenytoin (Dilantin) and fosphenytoin (Cerebyx) (*continued*)	*Maintenance dose (IV or PO):* 5 mg/kg/day in 2 or 3 divided doses initially and then adjusted to response and serum levels. Usual ranges based on age (divided into 2 or 3 doses daily): Neonates: 5–8 mg/kg/day. Age 6 months–3 years: 8–10 mg/kg/day. Age 4–6: 7.5–9 mg/kg/day. Age 7–9: 7–8 mg/kg/day. Age 10–16: 6–7 mg/kg/day. Adults: 5–6 mg/kg/day may be given as a single dose if extended-capsule preparation is used. Higher doses are required in infants and young children due to lower absorption of the drug from the GI tract. IV doses of phenytoin should be administered at a maximum rate of about 1 mg/kg/min (50 mg/min in adults) to avoid cardiovascular side effects. The injection is not compatible with many solutions or medications. The line must be flushed well with saline before administration to avoid precipitation of phenytoin in the line. Extravasation of the drug must also be avoided because it is very alkaline and may cause severe tissue necrosis. Thorough flushing of the vessel after phenytoin administration will also decrease the incidence of local tissue inflammation that may occur even in the absence of extravasation. Fosphenytoin injection should be diluted with either 5% dextrose or normal saline to a concentration of 1.5–25 mg of phenytoin equivalents (2.3–37.5 mg fosphenytoin) per mL of diluent and may be administered at a rate of 2–3 mg phenytoin equivalents/kg/min (100–150 mg phenytoin equivalents/min in adults).	
Phosphate (potassium and/or sodium)	Should be guided by the patient's serum phosphorus and potassium levels. Severe deficits should be replaced by the IV route because the oral route may result in diarrhea and oral absorption is unreliable. In general, the deficit should be made up by incorporating it into the patient's maintenance fluids. Intermittent infusions should follow the guidelines outlined below for potassium infusions because the IV form is potassium phosphate and each 3 mmol of phosphate will also deliver 4.4 mEq of potassium. The guidelines below are meant for use in patients with severe hypophosphatemia (<1 mg/dL in adults): Neonates: 0.5 mmol/kg up to 1–2 mmol/kg/day. Children: 0.15–0.3 mmol/kg with subsequent doses only after serum levels are checked and if the patient is symptomatic. Adults: 0.08 mmol/kg (uncomplicated hypophosphatemia) or 0.16 mmol/kg for prolonged deficits. Do not exceed 0.24 mmol/kg/day (serum phosphorus ≥0.5 mg/dL) or 0.5 mmol/kg/day (serum phosphorus <0.5 mg/dL). IV doses should be administered over a 6-hour period. *Maintenance doses:* Children: 0.5–1.5 mmol/kg/day. Adults: 15–30 mmol/day.	Injection (potassium phosphate): 3 mmol (94 mg) phosphorus and 4.4 mEq potassium per milliliter Packets or capsules (Neutra-Phos): 250 mg (8 mmol) phosphorus, 7 mEq potassium, and 7 mEq sodium Packets or capsules (Neutra-Phos K): 250 mg (8 mmol) phosphorus, 14.25 mEq potassium Tablets (K-Phos Neutral): 250 mg (8 mmol) phosphorus, 1.1 mEq potassium, and 13 mEq sodium Tablets (Uro-KP-Neutral): 250 mg (8 mmol) phosphorus, 1.27 mEq potassium, and 10.9 mEq sodium

Continued

Table 1   Medications   (continued)

DRUG	DOSE	DOSAGE FORMS
Phosphate (potassium and/or sodium) (continued)	*Orally:* should be taken with food to increase GI tolerance. Each packet or capsule should be mixed in 75 mL of water. Tablets should be taken with a full glass of water. *Maintenance doses:* Children: 2–3 mmol/kg/day in 4 divided doses. Adults: 32–64 mmol/day (4–8 packets) in 4 divided doses. Do not administer at the same time as aluminum- and/or magnesium-containing antacids, sucralfate, or calcium because they may act to bind phosphorus.	
Phytonadione (vitamin K; AquaMEPHYTON, Konakion, Mephyton)	*IM or SC:* *Hemorrhagic disease of the newborn, prophylaxis:* 0.5–1 mg within 1 hour of birth and again 6–8 hours later, if needed. *Treatment:* 1–2 mg/day. *Treatment of deficiency caused by malabsorption or decreased synthesis or due to drugs (administer IV cautiously and slowly):* Children: 1–2 mg/day. Adults: 10 mg/day *Treatment of oral anticoagulant overdose:* Infants: 1–2 mg repeated every 4–8 hours. Children and adults: 2.5–10 mg repeated in 6–8 hours. *Orally:* *Prevention of deficiency in malabsorption:* Children: 2.5–5 mg every other day or daily. Adults: 5–25 mg/day.	Injection: 2 mg/mL, 10 mg/mL Tablets: 5 mg
Piperacillin (Piperacil)	*IV:* Neonates: 150 mg/kg/day in 3 divided doses. Infants and children: 300 mg/kg/day in 4–6 divided doses. Doses of 300–500 mg/kg/day in 6 divided doses have been used in the treatment of children with cystic fibrosis. Adults: 2–4 g every 4–8 hours. Do not exceed 18 g/day.	Injection: 2-g, 3-g, 4-g, 40-g bulk package
Piroxicam (Feldene)	*Orally:* Children: 0.2–0.3 mg/kg/day in a single daily dose to a maximum of 15 mg/day. Adults: 10–20 mg/day in a single dose.	Capsules: 10 mg, 20 mg
Polyethylene glycolelectrolyte solution (Colovage, Colyte, GoLYTELY, OCL)	*Orally after a 3–4-hour fast:* Children: 25–40 mL/kg/hr. Adults: 240 mL every 10 minutes. The patient should continue to drink the solution until the rectal effluent is clear. Rapid drinking of each portion is more effective than slow consumption. The first bowel movement should occur about an hour after starting. The solution is more palatable if chilled, but must not be poured over ice. Nothing, including other flavorings, should be added to the solution. *Nasogastric tube administration:* Adults: 240 mL every 10 minutes.	Powder for oral solution to make 4 L: PEG3350 236 g, sodium sulfate 22.74 g, sodium bicarbonate 6.74 g, sodium chloride 5.86 g, and potassium chloride 2.97 g

Continued

Table 1   Medications   (continued)

DRUG	DOSE	DOSAGE FORMS
Potassium chloride	*Orally:* liquid doses must be well diluted before administration to avoid GI adverse effects. Capsules or tablets should be taken with a full glass of water. Capsules may be opened and emptied onto a soft food, but the beads should not be crushed or chewed. Total daily dose may be given in 1 or 2 divided doses if tolerated, or may be given in 3 or 4 divided doses to decrease GI upset. Dose is usually based on each patient's requirements and may depend on concurrent medications or medical conditions that result in potassium losses. The following may be used as general guidelines: *Normal daily requirement for either PO or IV replacement:* Newborn: 2–6 mEq/kg/day. Children: 2–3 mEq/kg/day. Adults: 40–80 mEq/day. *During diuretic therapy:* Children: 1–2 mEq/kg/day. Adults: 20–40 mEq/day. *For treatment of hypokalemia:* Children: 2–5 mEq/kg/day. Adults: 40–100 mEq/day. *IV:* doses should be well diluted. Usually they are incorporated into the patient's daily fluid requirement. The maximum desirable concentration is 80 mEq/L. Greater concentrations should be used cautiously and only in patients with documented hypokalemia with a serum potassium level <2.5 mEq/L. In the case of a patient in whom a shorter infusion of potassium is necessary, the following guidelines may be used: Maximum concentration of the solution must not exceed 30 mEq/100 mL (1 mEq/3 mL) and rate of infusion should not exceed 1 mEq/kg/hr in children or 40 mEq/hr in adults. The solutions should be infused using a pump to control the infusion rate. Infusion over 2–3 hours (0.3–0.5 mEq/kg/hr) is more desirable. Administration of doses greater than 0.3 mEq/kg/hr should be done only if the patient has an ECG monitor in place. Solutions should be mixed well to prevent layering of the potassium chloride, which may result in inadvertent rapid administration.	Capsules, controlled release: 8 mEq (600 mg), 10 mEq (750 mg) Injection, concentrated: 2 mEq/mL, 3 mEq/mL Liquids: 20 mEq/15 mL (10%), 30 mEq/15 mL (15%), 40 mEq/15 mL (20%) Powders, effervescent packets: 15 mEq, 20 mEq, 25 mEq Tablets, effervescent: 20 mEq, 25 mEq, 50 mEq Tablets, extended release: 6.7 mEq (500 mg), 8 mEq (600 mg), 10 mEq (750 mg) Other potassium salts are also available and may be desirable in patients who are acidotic. They include bicarbonate, citrate, acetate, and gluconate salts.
Prednisolone and prednisone	*Orally:* depends on the condition being treated and the patient's response. The lowest dose possible should be used. Withdrawal of long-term therapy must be accomplished slowly by gradually tapering the dose. The guidelines below may be used for initial dosing. Children: *Antiinflammatory or immunosuppressive:* 0.1–2 mg/kg/day in 1–4 divided doses. *Acute asthma:* 1–2 mg/kg/day in 1 or 2 divided doses for up to 5 days. *Inflammatory bowel disease:* 1–3 mg/kg/day in 1–2 divided doses. *Nephrotic syndrome:* 2 mg/kg/day in 3 or 4 divided doses. *Organ transplants:* 1 mg/kg/day in 2 divided doses, tapering gradually to 0.15 mg/kg/day or lowest effective dose.	Prednisolone: Liquid, as sodium phosphate: 5 mg/5 mL (Pediapred), 15 mg/5 mL (OraPred) Syrup (Prelone): 15 mg/5 mL Tablets: 5 mg Prednisone: Solution: 5 mg/5 mL Syrup (Liquid Pred): 5 mg/5 mL Tablets: 1 mg, 2.5 mg, 5 mg, 10 mg, 20 mg, 50 mg

Continued

1010

Table 1   Medications   (continued)

DRUG	DOSE	DOSAGE FORMS
Primidone (Mysoline)	*Orally:* Under age 8: initially 50–125 mg/day at bedtime or in 2 divided doses. Increase dose by 50–125 mg/day at weekly intervals to the normal range of 125–250 mg t.i.d. or 10–25 mg/kg/day. Over age 8 and adults: initially 125–250 mg/day at bedtime or in 2 divided doses. Increase dose by 125–250 mg/day at weekly intervals to the usual maintenance dose of 250 mg t.i.d. or q.i.d. Do not exceed 500 mg q.i.d. (2 g). Primidone is metabolized to phenobarbital and phenyl-ethylmalonamide (PEMA). Phenobarbital levels should be monitored in addition to primidone levels.	Suspension: 250 mg/5 mL Tablets: 50 mg, 250 mg
Probenecid (Benemid)	*Uricosuric:* Children under age 2: not recommended. Age 2–14: *Initial:* 25 mg/kg for 1 dose. *Maintenance:* 40 mg/kg/24 hr in 4 divided doses.	Tablets: 500 mg
Procainamide (Procanbid, Pronestyl)	*IV:* Children: loading dose of 3–6 mg/kg to a maximum of 100 mg over 5 minutes. This may be repeated every 5–10 minutes to a maximum of 15 mg/kg. Follow with a maintenance infusion at a dose of 20–80 μg/kg/min. Adults: loading dose of 50–100 mg, repeated every 5–10 minutes to a maximum of 15–18 mg/kg or 1–1.5 g. Follow with a maintenance infusion at a usual dose of 3–4 mg/min (range 1–6 mg/min). *Orally* (immediate-release products must be administered every 3 hours; controlled-release products must be administered every 6 hours or every 12 hours depending on the formulation used): Children: 15–50 mg/kg/day to a maximum dose of 4 g/day. Adults: usual range is 1–4 g/day in divided doses as above.	Capsules, immediate release: 250 mg, 375 mg, 500 mg Injection: 100 mg/mL, 500 mg/mL Tablets, immediate release: 250 mg, 375 mg, 500 mg Tablets, sustained release: 250 mg, 500 mg, 750 mg, 1,000 mg Tablets, sustained release, 12-hour duration (Procanbid): 500 mg, 1,000 mg
Prochlorperazine (Compazine)	*Orally or rectally as an antiemetic:* 0.4 mg/kg/day in 3 or 4 divided doses or alternatively by the patient's weight: 9–14 kg: 2.5 mg every 12–24 hours as needed, to a maximum of 7.5 mg/day. >14–18 kg: 2.5 mg every 8–12 hours as needed, to a maximum of 10 mg/day. >18–39 kg: 2.5 mg every 8 hours or 5 mg every 12 hours as needed, to a maximum of 15 mg/day. >40 kg: Rectally: 25 mg every 12 hours. Orally: 5–10 mg t.i.d. or q.i.d. *IM* (IV is not recommended in children): 0.13 mg/kg; may be repeated if necessary up to t.i.d. or q.i.d. Usual adult dose is 5–10 mg every 4 hours to a maximum of 40 mg/day.	Capsules, sustained release: 10 mg, 15 mg, 30 mg Injection: 5 mg/mL Suppositories: 2.5 mg, 5 mg, 25 mg Syrup: 5 mg/5 mL Tablets: 5 mg, 10 mg, 25 mg

Continued

Table 1   Medications   (continued)

DRUG	DOSE	DOSAGE FORMS
Promethazine (Phenergan)	*Antihistamine* (usually orally): Children: 0.1 mg/kg every 6 hours during the day. A dose of 0.5 mg/kg may be used at bedtime. Adults: 12.5 mg every 6 hours during the day with a 25-mg dose at bedtime. *Antiemetic* (orally, IV, IM, or rectally): Children: 0.5 mg/kg up to every 4 hours. Adults: 12.5–25 mg every 4 hours as needed. *Motion sickness* (orally): Children: 0.5 mg/kg 30 minutes to 1 hour before traveling; then every 12 hours as needed. Adults: 25 mg 30 minutes to 1 hour before traveling; then every 12 hours as needed. *Sedation* (all routes): Children: 0.5–1 mg/kg every 6 hours as needed. Adults: 25–50 mg every 6 hours as needed.	Injection: 25 mg/mL, 50 mg/mL Suppositories: 12.5 mg, 25 mg, 50 mg Syrup: 6.25 mg/5 mL, 25 mg/5 mL Tablets: 12.5 mg, 25 mg, 50 mg
Propranolol (Inderal)	*Orally:* *Arrhythmias:* Children: 0.5–1 mg/kg/day in 3 or 4 divided doses. Dosage may be titrated upward at 3–7-day intervals to the usual range of 2–4 mg/kg/day. If higher doses are necessary, up to 16 mg/kg/day (up to 640 mg) may be used. Adults: usually 10–30 mg every 6–8 hours. *Hypertension:* Children: 0.5–1 mg/kg/day in 2–4 divided doses, increasing at 3–7-day intervals to the usual range of 1–5 mg/kg/day. Adults: 40 mg b.i.d., increasing at 3–7-day intervals to a maximum dose of 640 mg/day. *Migraine prophylaxis:* Children: 0.6–1.5 mg/kg/day in 3 divided doses. Adults: 80 mg/day in 3 or 4 divided doses. Dose may be increased to a maximum of 240 mg/day in divided doses. *Tetralogy spells:* Children: 1–2 mg/kg every 6 hours. *Thyrotoxicosis:* Neonates: 2 mg/kg/day in 2–4 divided doses. Children: 1 mg/kg/day q.i.d. Adolescents and adults: 10–40 mg every 6 hours. *IV:* reserve for life-threatening arrhythmias. To be administered as an IV bolus *slowly* under ECG monitoring. The IV dose is much smaller than the oral dose. Children: 0.01–0.1 mg/kg to a maximum of 1 mg for arrhythmias. For tetralogy spells, 0.15–0.25 mg/kg, which may be repeated once after 15 minutes. Adults: 1–3 mg. A second dose may be given, if necessary, after 2 minutes.	Capsules, sustained release: 60 mg, 80 mg, 120 mg, 160 mg Injection: 1 mg/mL Solution: 4 mg/mL, 8 mg/mL Tablets: 10 mg, 20 mg, 40 mg, 60 mg, 80 mg, 90 mg
Propylthiouracil	*Orally:* Initially: Neonates: 5–10 mg/kg/day in 3 divided doses. Under age 10: 5–7 mg/kg/day in 3 divided doses. ≥ age 10: 150–300 mg/day in 3 divided doses. Adults: 300 mg/day in 3 divided doses. After control of symptoms has been achieved, the dose may be decreased to the lowest dose possible, usually one third to two thirds of the initial dose, administered in 3 doses daily.	Tablets: 50 mg

Continued

Table 1   Medications   (continued)

DRUG	DOSE	DOSAGE FORMS
Protamine sulfate	*IV:* 1 mg of protamine sulfate neutralizes 90 mg of lung-derived heparin or 115 U of intestinal mucosa-derived heparin. Because heparin disappears rapidly from the circulation, the dose of protamine decreases rapidly with time elapsed since the heparin infusion. The dose of protamine necessary after 30 minutes is half the dose above and that necessary after 2 hours is one fourth the dose above. Because protamine itself is an anticoagulant, avoid overdosing. Protamine should be administered slowly, over a 1-minute period, and the dose should not exceed 50 mg.	Injection: 10 mg/mL
Protirelin (Thyrel TRH)	*IV* (as a bolus over 15–30 seconds with the patient remaining supine for an additional 15 minutes): Children: 7 μg/kg to a maximum of 500 μg. Adults: 500 μg.	Injection: 500 μg/mL
Psyllium (Fiberall, Hydrocil, Konsyl, Metamucil, Perdiem Fiber, Serutan).	*Orally* (each dose should be accompanied by a full glass of water or other liquid): Children: half the adult dose (1/2 to 1 packet or 1.7–3.4 g of psyllium) once daily to t.i.d. Adults: 1–2 packets or 3.4–6.8 g of psyllium once daily to t.i.d.	Powder: ~3.4 g/dose Powder, effervescent
Pyrantel pamoate (Antiminth)	*Orally* (may be taken with juice or milk and without regard to the ingestion of food): 11 mg/kg to a maximum of 1 g.	Suspension: 50 mg/mL
Ranitidine (Zantac)	*Orally:* Children: 2–4 mg/kg/day in 2 divided doses initially. Dose may be higher in hypersecretory conditions. Adults: 150 mg b.i.d. or 300 mg at bedtime. Dose may be higher or more frequently administered. Up to 6 g/day has been used. *IV:* Children: 1–2 mg/kg/day in 3 or 4 divided doses. Do not exceed 6 mg/kg/day or 300 mg/day. Adults: 50 mg every 6–8 hours. Do not exceed 400 mg/day.	Injection: 25 mg/mL Syrup: 15 mg/mL Tablets: 75 mg, 150 mg, 300 mg
Ribavirin (Virazole)	Aerosol administered via the manufacturer's small particle aerosol generator (SPAG). 6 g of the drug are solubilized in sterile water and aerosolized over 12–18 hours daily for 3–7 days. Therapy must be started within the first 3 days of lower respiratory tract infection due to RSV. The manufacturer recommends against using the drug for patients who require assisted ventilation. Precipitation of the drug in respiratory equipment has occurred, as has accumulation of fluid in tubing. Either condition may compromise the patient.	Powder for reconstitution for aerosol: 6 g
Rifampin (Rifadin, Rimactane)	*Orally* (on an empty stomach): *Tuberculosis:* Children: 10–20 mg/kg/day as a single daily dose to a maximum of 600 mg. Adults: 600 mg/day. *Meningococcal carriers:* Under age 1 month: 10 mg/kg/day in 2 divided doses for 2 days. Infants and children: 20 mg/kg/day in 2 divided doses for 2 days, to a maximum dose of 1,200 mg/day. Adults: 600 mg/dose b.i.d. for 2 days.	Capsules 150 mg, 300 mg Injection: 600 mg Suspension: not commercially available, but may be made by mixing the powder from the capsules with simple syrup to form a 10 mg/mL suspension. Such suspensions are stable for 4 weeks at room temperature or refrigerated.

Continued

Table 1   Medications   (continued)

DRUG	DOSE	DOSAGE FORMS
Rifampin (Rifadin, Rimactane) (continued)	*Haemophilus influenzae type b prophylaxis:* Under age 1 month: 10 mg/kg/day as a single dose for 4 days. Over age 1 month and children: 20 mg/kg/day as a single dose for 4 days. Adults: 600 mg/day for 4 days. *IV* (over 30 minutes to 3 hours): same doses as for the oral route. Rifampin may cause a red-orange discoloration of the sweat, urine, tears, and other body fluids; soft contact lenses may be permanently stained.	
Rimantadine (Flumadine)	*Orally:* Under age 10: 5 mg/kg once daily to a maximum dose of 150 mg. Over age 10 and adults: 100 mg b.i.d. Therapy may be continued for up to 6 weeks. Rimantadine does not completely prevent an immune response to influenza vaccine; therefore, vaccination is not contraindicated. Rimantadine should be continued for 2–4 weeks after vaccination to allow for antibody production.	Syrup: 50 mg/5 mL Tablets: 100 mg
Ritonavir (Norvir)	*Orally with food to increase absorption:* Children 2–12 years of age: 250 mg/m^2/dose given twice a day initially to decrease the nausea that usually occurs. The dose is gradually increased by 50 mg/m^2/dose every 2–3 days as tolerated to a maximum of 400 mg/m^2/dose (or 600 mg/dose). Children >12 years of age and adults: 300 mg/dose twice daily initially, increasing by 100 mg/dose over 3–5 days to a maximum dose of 600 mg twice a day.	Capsule, liquid filled: 100 mg Solution, oral: 80 mg/mL
Salmeterol (Serevent, Serevent Diskus)	*Powder (Diskus) for oral inhalation:* Children ≥4 years of age to adults: 1 inhalation (50 μg) twice daily about 12 hours apart is used for chronic asthma. *Metered dose inhalation:* Children ≥12 years of age and adults: 2 inhalations (42 μg) twice daily about 12 hours apart. For exercise-induced asthma, 1 puff should be inhaled 30–60 minutes prior to exercise and may be repeated 12 hours later. Patients on regular twice a day doses should not add a third dose prior to exercise.	Inhalation, metered dose: 21 μg/actuation Inhalation, powder: 50 μg/foil blister
Scopolamine (hyoscine; Isopto Hyoscine)	*IM, SC, or IV:* Children: 0.006 mg/kg to a maximum dose of 0.3 mg. Adults: 0.3–0.65 mg. *Ophthalmic:* Children: 1 drop (up to q.i.d. for uveitis). Adults: 1–2 drops (up to q.i.d. for uveitis).	Injection: 0.3 mg/mL, 0.4 mg/mL, 0.86 mg/mL, 1 mg/mL Solution, ophthalmic: 0.25%
Sermorelin acetate (growth hormone-releasing hormone; Geref)	*IV* (in the morning after an overnight fast): 1 μg/kg IV push followed by a 3-mL saline flush.	Injection: 50-μg vials
Silver sulfadiazine (Silvadene, SSD, Thermazene)	*Topically:* applied to a thickness of 1/16-inch under sterile conditions (using a sterile glove) once or b.i.d. to a clean, debrided wound. Wound should always be covered with cream; reapply if it rubs off.	Cream: 10 mg/g

Continued

Table 1   Medications   (continued)

DRUG	*DOSE*	*DOSAGE FORMS*

Sodium bicarbonate (baking soda, $NaHCO_3$)	*IV:*
	Cardiac arrest (only after adequate ventilation has been established): 1 mEq/kg IV push initially; may repeat with a dose of 0.5 mEq/kg. Further doses should not be given until the patient's acid–base status has been determined. In infants, the concentration should not exceed 4.2% (0.5 mEq/mL).
	Metabolic acidosis (after measurement of blood gases and pH):
	  Children: mEq HCO_3 = 0.3 × weight (kg) × base deficit (mEq/L) *OR* mEq HCO_3 = 0.5 × weight (kg) × [24-serum HCO_3 (mEq/L)].
	  Adults: mEq HCO_3 = 0.2 × weight (kg) × base deficit (mEq/L) *OR* mEq HCO_3 = 0.5 × weight (kg) × [24-serum HCO_3 (mEq/L)].
	Doses should be administered slowly with frequent monitoring of acid–base balance.
	Orally:
	Urine alkalinization (titrate dose to desired pH):
	  Children: 1–10 mEq/kg/day in divided doses.
	  Adults: 48 mEq initially followed by 12–24 mEq every 4 hours. Doses up to 192 mEq/day have been used.
		Injection: 4.2% (0.5 mEq/mL), 7.5% (0.9 mEq/mL), 8.4% (1 mEq/mL)
		Tablets: 325 mg, 650 mg

Sodium polystyrene sulfonate (Kayexalate)	*Orally:*
	  Children: base the dose on the exchange rate of 1 mEq K^+/g of resin in smaller children.
	  Alternatively, a dose of 1 g/kg every 6 hours may be used.
	  Adults: 15 g administered once daily to q.i.d.
	Rectally as a retention enema:
	  Children: 1 g/kg every 2–6 hours.
	  Adults: 30–50 g every 6 hours.
	Enemas should be retained for as long as possible to increase ion exchange. Evacuation of the enema should be followed by a non–sodium-containing cleansing enema. Sorbitol is frequently used for making solutions because it helps to prevent constipation.
	Administer cautiously to patients who may be at risk of serum sodium level increases. It is not totally selective for potassium; small amounts of calcium and magnesium may also be lost.
		Powder
		Suspension: 15 g/60 mL (with sorbitol)

Sodium sulfacetamide (Ak-Sulf, Bleph-10, Cetamide, Sodium Sulamyd)	*Topically to the eye:*
	  Solutions: apply 1–2 drops in the affected eye up to every 2 or 3 hours while awake.
	  Ointment: apply to the eye once daily to q.i.d.
	  Drops will cause burning or stinging sensation.
	  Ointment will cause blurred vision.
		Ointment, ophthalmic: 10%
		Ointment, ophthalmic: 10% with prednisolone 0.2%, 0.25%, or 0.5%
		Suspension, ophthalmic: 10%, 15%, 30%
		Suspension, ophthalmic: 15% with phenylephrine 0.125% (Vasosulf)
		Suspension, ophthalmic: 10% with prednisolone 0.2%, 0.25%, or 0.5%

Spironolactone (Aldactone)	*Orally:*
	Edema (response may not be evident for up to 5 days):
	  Children: 1–3 mg/kg/day in 1 or 2 divided doses.
	  Adults: 100 mg/day with a range of 25–200 mg/day.
	Primary aldosteronism:
	  Children: 125–375 mg/m^2/day in divided doses.
	  Adults: 400 mg/day in 1 or 2 divided doses.
		Tablets: 25 mg, 50 mg, 100 mg (a stable suspension may be made by crushing tablets and suspending the powder in simple syrup or cherry syrup.)

Continued

Table 1   Medications   (continued)

DRUG	DOSE	DOSAGE FORMS
Stavudine (Zerit)	*Orally:* Age 6 months–15 years: dose has not been established, but doses of 1–2 mg/kg/day have been well tolerated. Adults: <60 kg: 30 mg b.i.d. ≥60 kg: 40 mg b.i.d. Dosage must be adjusted in patients with renal dysfunction.	Capsules: 15 mg, 20 mg, 30 mg, 40 mg
Streptomycin	*IM:* Newborn: 20–30 mg/kg/24 hr in 2 divided doses for 10 days. Children: 20–40 mg/kg/24 hr in 2 divided doses for 10 days. Adults: 1–2 g in 1 or 2 doses daily. Maximum dose 2 g/24 hr.	Injection: 400 mg/mL
Sucralfate (Carafate)	Sucralfate is not absorbed from the GI tract. It may bind with other drugs administered at the same time, lowering their effectiveness; therefore, it should be administered at least 2 hours before or after other drugs. *Orally:* Children: dosage has not been established, but 40–80 mg/kg/day in 4 divided doses has been used. Adults: 1 g q.i.d. The dose for stomatitis or mucositis is about 500 mg–1 g of suspension swished around the mouth and then spit out or swallowed, repeated q.i.d.	Suspension: 1 g/10 mL Tablets: 1 g
Sulfasalazine (Azulfidine)	*Orally:* Over age 2: initially 40–60 mg/kg/day in 3–6 divided doses (not to exceed 6 g/day) then decreasing to a maintenance dose of 20–40 mg/kg/day in 4 divided doses to a maximum dose of 2 g/day. Adults: initially 3–4 g/day in equally divided doses. Although doses as high as 12 g/day have been used, they are generally accompanied by an increased incidence of adverse effects. Maintenance doses are usually 2 g/day in 4 divided doses. The drug may cause a yellow discoloration of urine and skin.	Tablets: 500 mg Tablets, enteric coated: 500 mg
Sulfisoxazole (Gantrisin)	*Orally:* Over age 2 months: 150 mg/kg/day in 4 or 6 divided doses to a maximum daily dose of 6 g. An initial dose of 75 mg/kg may be given. Adults: 2–4 g initially followed by 4–8 g/day in 4–6 divided doses.	Solution or suspension: 500 mg/5 mL Tablets: 500 mg
Sumatriptan (Imitrex)	*SC:* Children ≥6 years of age and ≤30 kg: 0.06 mg/kg or 3 mg. Children >30 kg and adults: 6 mg. A second dose may be given at least 1 hour after the first dose if necessary. Do not exceed 2 doses in 24 hours.	Injection: 12 mg/ml

Continued

Table 1   Medications   (continued)

DRUG	*DOSE*	*DOSAGE FORMS*

Tacrolimus (FK-506, Prograf)	Patients are usually treated concurrently with an adrenal corticosteroid.
	Orally:
	    Children: 0.1–0.5 mg/kg/day in 2 divided doses.
	    Adults: 0.15–0.3 mg/kg/day in 2 divided doses.
	Doses may be decreased to a lower maintenance dose.
	IV (as a continuous infusion):
	    Children: 0.1 mg/kg/day.
	    Adults: 0.05–0.1 mg/kg/day.
	Conversion to oral therapy should take place as soon as the patient is able to tolerate oral medication.
		Capsules: 1 mg, 5 mg
		Injection: 5 mg/mL

Terbinafine (Lamisil AF)	*Topically:* ≥12 years of age: apply to affected area and surrounding skin for at least 1 week, but not more than 4 weeks.	Cream: 1%

Terbutaline (Brethine, Bricanyl)	*Orally:*
	    Under age 12: initially 0.05 mg/kg t.i.d., increased gradually as required to a maximum of 0.15 mg/kg t.i.d. or total of 5 mg/24 hr.
	    Over age 12: initially 2.5 mg t.i.d.
	Maintenance: usually 5 mg or 0.075 mg/kg t.i.d.
	Parenteral, SC:
	    Under age 12: 0.01 mg/kg to a maximum of 0.3 mg every 15–20 minutes for 3 doses.
	    Over age 12: 0.25 mg, repeated in 15–30 minutes if needed once only; a total dose of 0.5 mg should not be exceeded within a 4-hour period.
	Inhalation: 2 puffs every 4–6 hours.
		Aerosol, oral: 0.2 mg/activation
		Injection: 1 mg/mL (1-mL ampul)
		Tablets: 2.5 mg, 5 mg

Tetracycline (Achromycin V, Panmycin, Robitet, Sumycin)	*Orally* (should be given on an empty stomach):
	    Over age 8: 25–50 mg/kg/day in 4 divided doses.
	    Adults: 1–2 g/day in 2–4 divided doses.
		Capsules: 250 mg, 500 mg
		Suspension: 125 mg/5 mL
		Tablets: 250 mg, 500 mg

Theophylline	*IV or orally for apnea in infants:*
	    Premature neonates (postconceptional age under 40 weeks): 2 mg/kg/day in 2 divided doses.
	    Term neonates under age 4 weeks: 5 mg/kg loading dose followed by 2–4 mg/kg/day in 2 or 3 divided doses.
	    Term neonates over age 4 weeks: 5–7.5 mg/kg loading dose followed by 3–6 mg/kg/day in 3 divided doses.
	Acute bronchospasm (all dosing should be based on lean body weight):
	Loading dose: 1 mg/kg will increase serum theophylline concentration by 2 μg/mL. Patients who have received no theophylline in the previous 24 hours may be given 6 mg/kg. Patients who have received theophylline within the previous 24 hours may receive 3 mg/kg. Serum theophylline level should be monitored 30 minutes after the end of a bolus infusion. Loading dose should be administered IV over 30 minutes or PO using an immediate-release product. For patients requiring a continuous IV infusion of theophylline, it should be started at the completion of the bolus dose at the following rate for children:
	Age 6 months–1 year: 0.5 mg/kg/hr.
	Age >1–9: 0.9 mg/kg/hr.
	Age >9–12 and adolescent smokers: 0.8 mg/kg/hr.
	Age >12–16 (nonsmokers): 0.7 mg/kg/hr.
		Immediate release:
		  Capsules: 100 mg, 200 mg
		  Injection in D_5W: 0.4 mg/mL, 0.8 mg/mL, 1.6 mg/mL, 2 mg/mL, 3.2 mg/mL, 4 mg/mL
		  Solution: 27 mg/5 mL, 50 mg/5 mL, 90 mg/5 mL (provided by 105 mg/5 mL of aminophylline)
		  Tablets: 100 mg, 125 mg, 200 mg, 250 mg, 300 mg
		Controlled release:
		  Capsules and tablets of various strengths and release properties: Frequency of dosing must be based on the characteristics of the product chosen. Immediate-release products must be administered every 6 hours. Extended-release products may be administered every 8–12 hours or even every 24 hours in adolescents using products designed for daily administration. Serum levels should be monitored frequently during early therapy to maintain serum levels between 10–20 μg/mL. After a stable dose is achieved, monitoring should be done at least every 6–12 months.

Continued

Table 1   Medications   (continued)

DRUG	DOSE	DOSAGE FORMS
	Theophylline levels should be monitored 12–24 hours after beginning the infusion and daily while therapy continues. *Oral therapy for chronic bronchospasm:* Age 6 months–1 year: 12–18 mg/kg/day. Age >1–9: 20–24 mg/kg/day. Age >9–12 and adolescent smokers: 20 mg/kg/day. Age >12–16 (nonsmokers): 18 mg/kg/day. Over age 16 (nonsmokers): 13 mg/kg/day (not to exceed 900 mg/day).	
Ticarcillin (Ticar)	*IV (for the treatment of severe infections):* Neonates under age 1 week: <2 kg: 75 mg/kg every 12 hours. ≥2 kg: 75 mg/kg every 8 hours. Neonates from age 1–4 weeks: <2 kg: 75 mg/kg every 8 hours. ≥2 kg: 100 mg/kg every 8 hours. Infants over age 4 weeks and children: 200–300 mg/kg/day in 4–6 divided doses. Children weighing over 40 kg and adults: 200–300 mg/kg/day in 4–6 divided doses to a maximum daily dose of 24 g. Dosage must be adjusted in patients with renal or hepatic dysfunction.	Injection: 1 g, 3 g, 6 g (20-g and 30-g pharmacy bulk packages)
Ticarcillin and clavulanate potassium (Timentin)	*IV (may be expressed in terms of ticarcillin content alone or in terms of the fixed ratio (30:1) of the commercially available combination product):* Children: <60 kg: 200–300 mg/kg/day of ticarcillin (207–310 mg of ticarcillin/clavulanic acid) in 4–6 divided doses. ≥60 kg: 3 g ticarcillin + 0.1 g clavulanic acid (3.1 g of combination) every 4–6 hours to a maximum of 24 g of ticarcillin daily. Dosage must be adjusted in patients with renal or hepatic dysfunction.	Injection: 3 g ticarcillin + 0.1 g clavulanic acid labeled as a combined total potency of 3.1 g (pharmacy bulk package containing 30 g ticarcillin + 1 g clavulanic acid)
Tobramycin (Nebcin, TobraDex, Tobrex)	*IV:* Infants and children: 7.5 mg/kg/day in 3 divided doses. Older children and adults: 5 mg/kg/day in 3 divided doses. Patients with cystic fibrosis usually require higher doses (10 mg/kg/day in 3 divided doses). Dosage may be increased based on the results of serum level monitoring. Dosage must be adjusted in patients with renal dysfunction. *Ophthalmic:* Ointment: apply a 1-cm ribbon of ointment to the eye b.i.d. or t.i.d. Solution: apply 1–2 drops into the eye up to every 30–60 minutes in severe infections or every 3–4 hours for moderate infections.	Injection: 10 mg/mL, 40 mg/mL Ointment, ophthalmic: 0.3% Ointment, ophthalmic: 0.3% with dexamethasone 0.1% Solution, ophthalmic: 0.3% Solution, ophthalmic: 0.3% with dexamethasone 0.1%
Tolmetin (Tolectin)	*Orally for rheumatoid arthritis:* Over age 2: initially 20 mg/kg/day in 3 or 4 divided doses, adjusted to the patient's response. Usual maintenance dosage range is 15–30 mg/kg/day. Adults: 600 mg–1.8 g/day in 3 divided doses.	Capsules: 400 mg Tablets: 200 mg, 600 mg

Continued

Table 1   Medications   (continued)

DRUG	DOSE	DOSAGE FORMS
Topiramate (Topomax)	*Orally* Children 2–16 years of age: initially, 1–3 mg/kg/day (or 25 mg) given daily at bedtime for 1 week. Gradually increase dose by 1–3 mg/kg/day and increase frequency to twice daily to the usual maintenance dosage range of 5–9 mg/kg/day. Children >16 years of age and adults: initially, 50 mg daily in two divided doses, then increase at weekly intervals by 50 mg/day to a usual adult dose range of 200–400 mg daily in 2 divided doses.	Capsule, sprinkle: 15 mg, 25 mg Tablet: 25 mg, 100 mg, 200 mg. Tablets should not be crushed since the drug has a very bitter taste. Broken tablets should be used immediately as the drug is not stable.
Tretinoin (retinoic acid; Retin-A)	*Topically:* apply to the affected area once daily after cleaning, generally at bedtime. Avoid application to areas not being treated. Use should be discontinued if severe reddening, swelling, or peeling occurs. After healing, therapy may be restarted with the same or a different formulation administered less frequently.	Cream: 0.025%, 0.05%, 0.1% Gel: 0.01%, 0.025% Solution: 0.05%
Trifluridine (Viroptic)	*Topically to the eye:* apply 1 drop every 2 hours while awake until re-epithelialization has occurred. Maximum daily dose of 9 drops should not be exceeded. After re-epithelialization has occurred, dosage should be reduced to 1 drop every 4 hours for an additional 7 days to prevent recurrence, but the total length of therapy should not exceed 21 days.	Solution, ophthalmic: 1%

Trimethobenzamide (Tigan)	*IM* (not for infants or young children): 200 mg t.i.d. or q.i.d.
	Rectally (not for neonates or infants):
	  <13.6 kg: 100 mg t.i.d. or q.i.d.
	  13.6–45 kg: 100–200 mg t.i.d. or q.i.d.
	  >45 kg: 200 mg t.i.d. or q.i.d.
	Orally:
	  13.6–45 kg: 100–200 mg t.i.d. or q.i.d.
	  >45 kg: 250 mg t.i.d. or q.i.d.
	Alternatively, a dose of 5 mg/kg administered t.i.d. or q.i.d. rectally or orally may be used.
		Capsules: 100 mg, 250 mg
		Injection: 100 mg/mL
		Suppositories: 100 mg, 200 mg

Trimethoprim (Primsol, Proloprim, Trimpex)	*Orally:*
	UTI:
	  Infants and children <12 years of age: 4–6 mg/kg/day in 2 divided doses for 10 days.
	  Children ≥12 years of age and adults: 100 mg twice daily or 200 mg once daily for 10 days
	  Pneumocystis carinii pneumonia treatment (given with dapsone): 15–20 mg/kg/day in 4 divided doses.
		Solution: 50 mg/5 mL
		Tablet: 100 mg, 200 mg

Tropicamide (Mydriacyl, Ocu-Tropic, Tropicacyl)	*Topically to the eye:* 1 to 2 drops into the eye(s) 15–20 minutes before exam. 0.5% solution is usually sufficient for exam. If cycloplegia for refraction is necessary, 1% solution must be used and repeated in 5 minutes. Exam must take place within 30 minutes because its effect is short.	Solution, ophthalmic: 0.5%, 1%

Continued

Table 1   Medications   (continued)

DRUG	DOSE	DOSAGE FORMS
Valproic acid, valproate sodium, and divalproex sodium (Depacon, Depakene, Depakote)	*Orally* (expressed in terms of valproic acid): initially 15 mg/kg/day increasing by 5–10 mg/kg/day at weekly intervals until seizures are controlled or side effects occur. Usual maximum total daily dose is 60 mg/kg. Frequency of administration in part depends on dosage form, but dosage is usually divided. To prevent adverse GI effects, capsules (valproic acid) and solution are usually administered in 2 or 3 divided doses. Divalproex usually may be administered in 2 divided doses. The usual therapeutic serum concentration range is 50–100 μg/mL. The oral solution has been administered rectally in patients who are NPO by diluting it 1:1 with tap water and administering it as a retention enema. *IV* (over 1 hour): for patients who are not on valproic acid therapy, use the dosing and frequency of administration guidelines outlined above for oral dosing. For patients already on valproic acid therapy, use the patient's total oral daily dose and frequency of dosing for the IV route. The use of the injectable form for periods of more than 14 days has not been studied.	Capsules (divalproex sodium): 125 mg valproic acid Capsules (valproic acid): 250 mg Injection: 100 mg/mL Solution (valproate sodium): 250 mg valproic acid/5 mL Tablets (divalproex sodium): 125 mg, 250 mg, 500 mg valproic acid

Vancomycin (Lyphocin, Vancocin, Vancoled)	*IV* (over at least 1 hour):
	Neonates under age 7 days:
	  <1,000 g: 10 mg/kg every 24 hours.
	  1,000–2,000 g: 10 mg/kg every 18 hours.
	  >2,000 g: 10 mg/kg every 12 hours.
	Neonates age 7–30 days:
	  <1,000 g: 10 mg/kg every 18 hours.
	  1,000–2,000 g: 10 mg/kg every 12 hours.
	  >2,000 g: 10 mg/kg every 8 hours.
	Infants age 31–60 days: 10 mg/kg every 8 hours.
	Infants over age 2 months and children: 40 mg/kg/day in 4 divided doses to a maximum dose of 2 g/day.
	Adults: 0.5 g every 6 hours or 1 g every 12 hours. Dosage adjustment is necessary in renal impairment.
	Higher doses, up to 60 mg/kg/day, may be required in children with staphylococcal central nervous system infections.
	Intrathecal:
	Neonates: 5–10 mg/day.
	Children: 5–20 mg/day.
	Adults: 20 mg/day.
	Orally (not absorbed; do not use for systemic infections):
	Children: 40 mg/kg/day in 4 divided doses to a maximum daily dose of 2 g.
	Adults: 0.5–2 g/day in 3 or 4 divided doses.
		Capsules: 125 mg, 250 mg
		Injection: 500 mg, 1 g, (5-g, 10-g pharmacy bulk packages)
		Solution, oral: 1 g, 10 g

Continued

Table 1   Medications   (continued)

DRUG	*DOSE*	*DOSAGE FORMS*

Verapamil (Calan, Isoptin, Verelan)	*IV* (push over 2 to 3 minutes):
	  Under age 1: 0.1–0.2 mg/kg (usually 0.75–2 mg).
	  Age 1–16: 0.1–0.3 mg/kg to a maximum of 10 mg.
	    May be repeated once in 30 minutes if not
	    effective.
	  Over age 16: 0.075–0.15 mg/kg (5–10 mg) with a
	    repeat dose in 30 minutes if necessary.
	Orally (not well established in children):
	  Age 1–5: 4–8 mg/kg/day in 3 divided doses or
	    about 40–80 mg every 8 hours.
	  Over age 5: 80 mg every 6–8 hours.
	  Adults: 240–480 mg/day in 3 or 4 divided doses
	    (1–2 doses daily using extended-release products
	    for the treatment of hypertension).
		Capsules, extended release: 120 mg, 180 mg, 240 mg
		Injection: 2.5 mg/mL
		Tablets: 40 mg, 80 mg, 120 mg
		Tablets, extended release: 120 mg, 180 mg, 240 mg

Vitamin A (Aquasol A)	*Orally:*
	For malabsorption syndromes (water miscible product):
	  Under age 8: 5,000–15,000 U/day.
	  Over age 8 and adults: 10,000–50,000 U/day.
	For severe deficiency with xerophthalmia:
	  Age 1–8: 5,000 U/kg/day for 5 days or until
	    recovery.
	  Over age 8 and adults: 500,000 U/day for 3 days,
	    then 50,000 U/day for 14 days, then 10,000–
	    20,000 U/day for 2 months.
	Deficiency (without corneal change):
	  Under age 1: 10,000 U/kg/day for 5 days, then
	    7,500–15,000 U/day for 10 days.
	  Age 1–8: 5,000–10,000 U/kg/day for 5 days, then
	    17,000–35,000 U/day for 10 days.
	  Over age 8 and adults: 100,000 U/day for 3 days,
	    then 50,000 U/day for 14 days.
	Dietary supplementation:
	  Infants up to age 6 months: 1,500 U/day.
	  Age >6 months–3 years: 1,500–2,000 U/day.
	  Age 4–6: 2,500 U/day.
	  Age 7–10: 3,300–3,500 U/day.
	  Over age 10 and adults: 4,000–5,000 U/day.
		Capsules: 10,000 U, 25,000 U, 50,000 U

Vitamin E [alpha tocopherol, alpha tocopheryl acetate, tocopherol polyethylene glycol succinate (TPGS), Aquasol E]	*Orally* (water miscible or water soluble TPGS products
	  are recommended, especially for patients with
	  malabsorption):
	Deficiency:
	Infants: 25–50 U/day.
	Children with malabsorption: 15–25 U/kg/day to raise
	  and maintain plasma tocopherol levels.
	Patients with cystic fibrosis, thalassemia, or sickle-cell
	  disease may require larger daily doses (400–800
	  U/day).
	Adults: 60–75 U/day.
		Capsules: 100 U, 200 U, 400 U, 600 U, 1,000 U
		Capsules, water miscible: 100 U, 200 U, 400 U
		Solution, water miscible: 50 U/mL
		Solution (TPGS): 400 U/15 mL

Warfarin sodium (Coumadin)	*Orally:*
	  Infants and children: 0.1 mg/kg/day with a range of
	    0.05–0.34 mg/kg/day adjusted to achieve the
	    desired PT.
	  Adults: 5–15 mg/day initially for 2–5 days until
	    desired PT is reached. Usual maintenance dosage
	    range is 2–10 mg/day.
		Tablets: 1 mg, 2 mg, 2.5 mg, 4 mg, 5 mg, 7.5 mg,
		  10 mg

Zafirlukast (Accolate)	*Orally on an empty stomach:*
	  Children 7–12 years of age: 10 mg twice daily.
	  Children >12 years of age and adults: 20 mg twice
	    daily.
		Tablet: 10 mg, 20 mg

Continued

Table 1   Medications   (continued)

DRUG	_DOSE_	_DOSAGE FORMS_
Zalcitabine (ddC, Hivid)	_Orally:_ Under age 13: 0.01 mg/kg/dose given every 8 hours. Adolescents age 13–adults: 0.75 mg every 8 hours on an empty stomach. Adjust dose in patients with renal dysfunction.	Tablets: 0.375 mg, 0.75 mg
Zanamivir (Relenza)	_Oral inhalation:_ Children ≥12 years of age and adults: 2 inhalations twice a day for 5 days beginning within 2 days of the onset of symptoms.	Powder for inhalation with device: 5 mg/actuation
Zidovudine (Retrovir)	_Orally:_ Age 3 months–12 years: 180 mg/m^2 every 6 hours to a maximum of 200 mg every 6 hours. Dosage may be decreased in patients who develop anemia and/or granulocytopenia. Adults: _Asymptomatic:_ 100 mg every 4 hours while awake (500 mg/day). _Symptomatic:_ 100 mg every 4 hours (600 mg/day). _IV:_ Age 3 months–13 years: 0.5–1.8 mg/kg/hr as a continuous infusion or 100 mg/m^2 by infusion over 1 hour every 6 hours. Adults: 1–2 mg/kg every 4 hours 6 times daily. _Maternal–fetal HIV transmission prevention:_ Maternal (>14 weeks of pregnancy): 100 mg every 4 hours while awake (500 mg/day) until the onset of labor. During labor and delivery, 2 mg/kg over 1 hour followed by a continuous IV infusion of 1 mg/kg/hr until the umbilical cord is clamped. Infant: 2 mg/kg orally every 6 hours starting within 12 hours of birth and continuing for 6 weeks. For infants unable to tolerate oral drugs, 6 mg/kg/day IV in 4 evenly divided doses may be used. Dosage adjustment is necessary in severe renal impairment.	Capsules: 100 mg Injection: 10 mg/mL Solution: 50 mg/5 mL
Zinc	Response may not occur for 6–8 weeks. _Orally:_ Infants and children: 0.5–1 mg/kg/day of elemental zinc in 1–3 divided doses. Adults: 25–50 mg elemental zinc t.i.d. _Acrodermatitis enteropathica:_ 10–45 mg/day elemental zinc. Zinc sulfate 4.4 mg = 1 mg elemental zinc (220 mg = 50 mg).	Zinc sulfate (23% zinc): Capsules: 220 mg (50 mg zinc) Injection: 1 mg/mL, 5 mg/mL (zinc) Tablets: 66 mg (15 mg zinc), 110 mg (25 mg zinc), 220 mg (45 mg zinc) Zinc gluconate (14.3% zinc): Tablets: 10 mg (1.4 mg zinc), 15 mg (2 mg zinc), 50 mg (7 mg zinc), 78 mg (11 mg zinc)

*See Table 83.2 for a discussion of the content of each milliliter of these products.

†See Table 83.3 for dosage recommendations.

‡See Table 83.4 for the lipase, amylase, and protease content of each form of pancrelipase.

Table 2   Citric Acid and Citrate Dosage Forms (Content per 1 mL)

PRODUCT	SODIUM CITRATE	POTASSIUM CITRATE	CITRIC ACID	BICARBONATE EQUIVALENT
Bicitra solution	100 mg (1 mEq Na)	. . .	66.8 mg	1 mEq
Oracit solution	98 mg (1 mEq Na)	. . .	128 mg	1 mEq
Polycitra K solution	. . .	220 mg (2 mEq K)	66.8 mg	2 mEq
Polycitra-LC solution	100 mg (1 mEq Na)	110 mg (1 mEq K)	66.8 mg	2 mEq

Table 3   Digoxin Dosing

	TOTAL DIGITALIZING DOSE (μG/KG)		DAILY MAINTENANCE DOSE (μG/KG DIVIDED IN 2 DOSES)	
AGE	PO	IV	PO	IV
Preterm infant	20–30	15–25	5–7.5	4–6
Full-term infant	25–40	20–30	6–10	5–8
1 month to 2 years	35–60	30–50	10–15	7.5–12
2 years to adult	30–40	25–35	7.5–15	6–9
Maximum dose	0.75–1.5 mg	0.5–1 mg	0.125–0.5 mg	0.1–0.4 mg

IV, intravenously; PO, orally.

Table 4   Pancrelipase Dosage Forms

	LIPASE (USP UNITS)	AMYLASE (USP UNITS)	PROTEASE (USP UNITS)
Capsules (enteric-coated or delayed-release microspheres)			
Cotazym-S	5,000	20,000	20,000
Creon	8,000	30,000	13,000
Creon-10	10,000	33,200	37,500
Creon-20	20,000	66,400	75,000
Pancrease	4,500	20,000	25,000
Pancrease MT-4	4,500	12,000	12,000
Pancrease MT-10	10,000	30,000	30,000
Pancrease MT-16	16,000	48,000	48,000
Pancrease MT-20	20,000	56,000	44,000
Ultrase MT-12	12,000	39,000	39,000
Ultrase MT-20	20,000	65,000	65,000
Zymase	12,000	24,000	24,000
Capsules (filled with non–enteric coated powder)			
Cotazym, Ku-Zyme HP	8,000	30,000	30,000
Powder (not enteric-coated)			
Viokase (per 0.7 g)	16,800	70,000	70,000
Tablets (not enteric-coated)			
Ilozyme	11,000	30,000	30,000
Viokase	8,000	30,000	30,000

Index

Page numbers in boldface indicate major discussion; page numbers in italics denote figures; those followed by "t" denote tables.

Index

Index

Index

Index

Index

Index

Index

Index

Index

Index

Index

Index

Index

Index

Index

Index

Index

Index